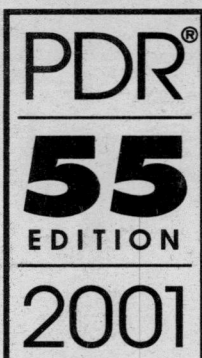

PHYSICIANS' DESK REFERENCE®

Supplement A

For important errata, turn the page.

IMPORTANT NOTICE

Supplements to PHYSICIANS' DESK REFERENCE are published twice yearly to provide readers with significant revisions of existing product listings as well as comprehensive information on new drugs and other products not included in the current annual edition. Before prescribing or administering any product described in PHYSICIANS' DESK REFERENCE, be sure to consult this supplement to determine whether revisions have occurred since the 2001 edition of PDR went to press.

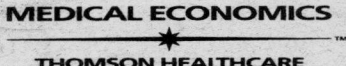

This supplement is a compilation of information submitted by the products' manufacturers. Each entry has been prepared, edited, and approved by the manufacturer's medical department, medical director, and/or medical consultant. The publisher does not warrant or guarantee any of the products described herein nor is the publisher responsible for misuse of a product due to typographical error. The publisher does not perform any independent analysis in connection with the product information contained herein.

Officers of Thomson Healthcare: *Chief Executive Officer:* Michael Tansey; *Chief Operating Officer:* Richard Noble; *Chief Financial Officer and Executive Vice President, Finance:* Paul Hilger; *Executive Vice President, Directory Services:* Paul Walsh; *Senior Vice President, Planning and Business Development:* William Gole; *Vice President, Human Resources:* Pamela M. Bilash

ERRATA

Dermik Laboratories

The contact information listed on page 1113 of the 2001 edition should read as follows:

Direct Inquiries to:
Customer Service
Somerset Corporate Center, Building 3
300 Somerset Corporate Blvd.
Bridgewater, NJ 08807-2854
(800) 207-8049

For Medical Information Contact:
Medical Information Services
Somerset Corporate Center, Building 3
300 Somerset Corporate Blvd.
Bridgewater, NJ 08807-2854
(800) 633-1610

Merck

In a recent PDR Addendum announcing the new, once-weekly dosage of **Fosamax**, as well as the drug's new indication for treatment of osteoporosis in men, the Product Identification photos failed to include the *round* 10-milligram tablet which, along with the *oval* 10-milligram tablet, remains available for once-daily dosing.

Otsuka America

The fax number for inquiries that appears on page 14 of the 2001 edition is incorrect and should read (301) 212-8577.

Purdue Pharma

In the Product Identification photos of **Chirocaine** on page 332 of the 2001 edition, the 30 mL single dose vial color-coded yellow contains 0.5% levobupivacaine injection, not the 0.25% injection indicated in the caption.

Westwood-Squibb

On page 3325 of the 2001 edition, in the entry for **Dovonex** Ointment (calcipotriene ointment, 0.005%), the name of the product is shown incorrectly as "Donovex."

Key to Controlled Substances Categories

Products listed with the symbols shown below are subject to the Controlled Substances Act of 1970. These drugs are categorized according to their potential for abuse. The greater the potential, the more severe the limitations on their prescription.

CATEGORY	INTERPRETATION
ℂII	**HIGH POTENTIAL FOR ABUSE.** Use may lead to severe physical or psychological dependence. Prescriptions must be written in ink, or typewritten and signed by the practitioner. Verbal prescriptions must be confirmed in writing within 72 hours, and may be given only in a genuine emergency. No renewals are permitted.
ℂIII	**SOME POTENTIAL FOR ABUSE.** Use may lead to low-to-moderate physical dependence or high psychological dependence. Prescriptions may be oral or written. Up to 5 renewals are permitted within 6 months.
ℂIV	**LOW POTENTIAL FOR ABUSE.** Use may lead to limited physical or psychological dependence. Prescriptions may be oral or written. Up to 5 renewals are permitted within 6 months.
ℂV	**SUBJECT TO STATE AND LOCAL REGULATION.** Abuse potential is low; a prescription may not be required.

Key to FDA Use-in-Pregnancy Ratings

The U.S. Food and Drug Administration's use-in-pregnancy rating system weighs the degree to which available information has ruled out risk to the fetus against the drug's potential benefit to the patient. The ratings, and their interpretation, are as follows:

CATEGORY	INTERPRETATION
A	**CONTROLLED STUDIES SHOW NO RISK.** Adequate, well-controlled studies in pregnant women have failed to demonstrate a risk to the fetus in any trimester of pregnancy.
B	**NO EVIDENCE OF RISK IN HUMANS.** Adequate, well-controlled studies in pregnant women have not shown increased risk of fetal abnormalities despite adverse findings in animals, or, in the absence of adequate human studies, animal studies show no fetal risk. The chance of fetal harm is remote, but remains a possibility.
C	**RISK CANNOT BE RULED OUT.** Adequate, well-controlled human studies are lacking, and animal studies have shown a risk to the fetus or are lacking as well. There is a chance of fetal harm if the drug is administered during pregnancy; but the potential benefits may outweigh the potential risk.
D	**POSITIVE EVIDENCE OF RISK.** Studies in humans, or investigational or post-marketing data, have demonstrated fetal risk. Nevertheless, potential benefits from the use of the drug may outweigh the potential risk. For example, the drug may be acceptable if needed in a life-threatening situation or serious disease for which safer drugs cannot be used or are ineffective.
X	**CONTRAINDICATED IN PREGNANCY.** Studies in animals or humans, or investigational or post-marketing reports, have demonstrated positive evidence of fetal abnormalities or risk which clearly outweighs any possible benefit to the patient.

NEW PRODUCT LISTINGS INDEX

Listed below are new *PDR* listings first appearing in 2001 *PDR* Supplement A. These listings include comprehensive descriptions of new pharmaceutical products introduced since publication of the 2001 *PDR*, new dosage forms of products already described, and existing pharmaceutical products not described in the 2001 *PDR*.

REVISED PRODUCT INFORMATION INDEX

As new research data and clinical findings become available, the product information in *PDR* is revised accordingly. Revisions submitted since the 2001 edition went to press can be found below. To remind yourself of a revision, write "See Supplement A" next to the product's heading in the book.

NEW PRODUCT LISTINGS

This section contains comprehensive descriptions of new pharmaceutical products introduced since publication of the 2001 *PDR*, new dosage forms of products already described, and existing pharmaceutical products not described in the 2001 *PDR*.

Allergan, Inc.
2525 DUPONT DRIVE
P.O. BOX 19534
IRVINE, CA 92623-9534

Direct Inquiries to:
(714) 246-4500

LUMIGAN™   ℞
(bimatoprost ophthalmic solution) 0.03%

DESCRIPTION
LUMIGAN™ (bimatoprost ophthalmic solution) 0.03% is a synthetic prostamide analog with ocular hypotensive activity. Its chemical name is (Z)-7-[(1R,2R,3R,5S)-3,5-Dihydroxy-2-[1E,3S)-3-hydroxy-5-phenyl-1-pentenyl]cyclopentyl]-5-N-ethylheptenamide, and its molecular weight is 415.58. Its molecular formula is $C_{25}H_{37}NO_4$. Its chemical structure is:

Bimatoprost is a powder, which is very soluble in ethyl alcohol and methyl alcohol and slightly soluble in water. LUMIGAN™ is a clear, isotonic, colorless, sterile ophthalmic solution with an osmolality of approximately 290 mOsmol/kg.
Each mL contains: Active: bimatoprost 0.3 mg; Preservative: Benzalkonium chloride 0.05 mg; Inactives: Sodium chloride; sodium phosphate, dibasic; citric acid; and purified water. Sodium hydroxide and/or hydrochloric acid may be added to adjust pH. The pH during its shelf life ranges from 6.8–7.8.

CLINICAL PHARMACOLOGY
Mechanism of Action
Bimatoprost is a prostamide, a synthetic structural analog of prostaglandin with ocular hypotensive activity. It selectively mimics the effects of naturally occurring substances, prostamides. Bimatoprost is believed to lower intraocular pressure (IOP) in humans by increasing outflow of aqueous humor through both the trabecular meshwork and uveoscleral routes, Elevated IOP presents a major risk factor for glaucomatous field loss. The higher the level of IOP, the greater the likelihood of optic nerve damage and visual field loss.
Pharmacokinetics
Absorption: After one drop of bimatoprost ophthalmic solution 0.03% was administered once daily to both eyes of 15 healthy subjects for two weeks, blood concentrations peaked within 10 minutes after dosing and were below the lower limit of detection (0.025 ng/mL) in most subjects within 1.5 hours after dosing. Mean C_{max} and AUC_{0-24hr} values were similar on days 7 and 14 at approximately 0.08 ng/mL and 0.09 ng•hr/mL, respectively, indicating that steady state was reached during the first week of ocular dosing. There was no significant systemic drug accumulation over time.
Distribution
Bimatoprost is moderately distributed into body tissues with a steady-state volume of distribution of 0.67 L/kg. In human blood, bimatoprost resides mainly in the plasma. Approximately 12% of bimatoprost remains unbound in human plasma.

Metabolism
Bimatoprost is the major circulating species in the blood once it reaches the systemic circulation following ocular dosing. Bimatoprost then undergoes oxidation, N-deethylation and glucuronidation to form a diverse variety of metabolites.
Elimination
Following an intravenous dose of radiolabeled bimatoprost (3.12 µg/kg) to six healthy subjects, the maximum blood concentration of unchanged drug was 12.2 ng/mL and decreased rapidly with an elimination half-life of approximately 45 minutes. The total blood clearance of bimatoprost was 1.5 L/hr/kg. Up to 67% of the administered dose was excreted in the urine while 25% of the dose was recovered in the feces.
Clinical Studies:
In clinical studies of patients with open angle glaucoma or ocular hypertension with a mean baseline IOP of 26 mm Hg, the IOP-lowering effect of LUMIGAN™ (bimatoprost ophthalmic solution) 0.03% once daily (in the evening) was 7–8 mm Hg.

INDICATIONS AND USAGE
LUMIGAN™ (bimatoprost ophthalmic solution) 0.03% is indicated for the reduction of elevated intraocular pressure in patients with open angle glaucoma or ocular hypertension who are intolerant of other intraocular pressure lowering medications or insufficiently responsive (failed to achieve target IOP determined after multiple measurements over time) to another intraocular pressure lowering medication.

CONTRAINDICATIONS
LUMIGAN™ (bimatoprost ophthalmic solution) 0.03% is contraindicated in patients with hypersensitivity to bimatoprost or any other ingredient in this product.

WARNINGS
LUMIGAN™ (bimatoprost ophthalmic solution) 0.03% has been reported to cause changes to pigmented tissues. These reports include increased pigmentation and growth of eyelashes and increased pigmentation of the iris and periorbital tissue (eyelid). These changes may be permanent.
LUMIGAN™ may gradually change eye color, increasing the amount of brown pigment in the iris by increasing the number of melanosomes (pigment granules) in melanocytes. The long-term effects on the melanocytes and the consequences of potential injury to the melanocytes and/or deposition of pigment granules to other areas of the eye are currently unknown. The change in iris color occurs slowly and may not be noticeable for several months to years. Patients should be informed of the possibility of iris color change. Eyelid skin darkening has also been reported in association with the use of LUMIGAN™.
LUMIGAN™ may gradually change eyelashes; these changes include increased length, thickness, pigmentation, and number of lashes.
Patients who are expected to receive treatment in only one eye should be informed about the potential for increased brown pigmentation of the iris, periorbital tissue, and eyelashes in the treated eye and thus, heterochromia between the eyes. They should also be advised of the potential for a disparity between the eyes in length, thickness, and/or number of eyelashes.

PRECAUTIONS
General:
There have been reports of bacterial keratitis associated with the use of multiple-dose containers of topical ophthalmic products. These containers had been inadvertently contaminated by patients who, in most cases, had a concurrent corneal disease or a disruption of the ocular epithelial surface (see Information for Patients).
Patients may slowly develop increased brown pigmentation of the iris. This change may not be noticeable for several months to years (see Warnings). Typically the brown pig-

mentation around the pupil is expected to spread concentrically towards the periphery in affected eyes, but the entire iris or parts of it may also become more brownish. Until more information about increased brown pigmentation is available, patients should be examined regularly and, depending on the clinical situation, treatment may be stopped if increased pigmentation ensues. The increase in brown iris pigment is not expected to progress further upon discontinuation of treatment, but the resultant color change may be permanent. Neither nevi nor freckles of the iris are expected to be affected by treatment.
LUMIGAN™ (bimatoprost ophthalmic solution) 0.03% should be used with caution in patients with active intraocular inflammation (e.g., uveitis).
Macular edema, including cystoid macular edema, has been reported during treatment with bimatoprost ophthalmic solution. LUMIGAN™ should be used with caution in aphakic patients, in pseudophakic patients with a torn posterior lens capsule, or in patients with known risk factors for macular edema. LUMIGAN™ has not been evaluated for the treatment of angle closure, inflammatory or neovascular glaucoma.
LUMIGAN™ should not be administered while wearing contact lenses.
LUMIGAN™ has not been studied in patients with renal or hepatic impairment and should therefore be used with caution in such patients.
Information for Patients:
Patients should be informed that LUMIGAN™ has been reported to cause increased growth and darkening of eyelashes and darkening of the skin around the eye in some patients. These changes may be permanent.
Some patients may slowly develop darkening of the iris, which may be permanent.
When only one eye is treated, patients should be informed of the potential for a cosmetic difference between the eyes in eyelash length, darkness or thickness, and/or color changes of the eyelid skin or iris.
Patients should be instructed to avoid allowing the tip of the dispensing container to contact the eye, surrounding structures, fingers, or any other surface in order to avoid contamination of the solution by common bacteria known to cause ocular infections. Serious damage to the eye and subsequent loss of vision may result from using contaminated solutions.
Patients should also be advised that if they develop an intercurrent ocular condition (e.g., trauma or infection) or have ocular surgery, they should immediately seek their physician's advice concerning the continued use of the multidose container.
Patients should be advised that if they develop any ocular reactions, particularly conjunctivitis and eyelid reactions, they should immediately seek their physician's advice.
Contact lenses should be removed prior to instillation of LUMIGAN™ and may be reinserted 15 minutes following its administration. Patients should be advised that LUMIGAN™ contains benzalkonium chloride, which may be absorbed by soft contact lenses.
If more than one topical ophthalmic drug is being used, the drugs should be administered at least five (5) minutes between applications.

Carcinogenesis, Mutagenesis, Impairment of Fertility:
Carcinogenicity studies were not performed with bimatoprost.
Bimatoprost was not mutagenic or clastogenic in the Ames test, in the mouse lymphoma test, or in the *in vivo* mouse micronucleus tests.
Bimatoprost did not impair fertility in male or female rats up to doses of 0.6 mg/kg/day (approximately 103 times the recommended human exposure based on blood AUC levels).

Pregnancy: Teratogenic Effects: **Pregnancy Category C.**
In embryo/fetal developmental studies in pregnant mice and rats, abortion was observed at oral doses of bimatoprost which achieved at least 33 or 97 times, respectively, the intended human exposure based on blood AUC levels.

Continued on next page

Lumigan—Cont.

At doses 41 times the intended human exposure based on blood AUC levels, the gestation length was reduced in the dams, the incidence of dead fetuses, late resorptions, peri- and postnatal pup mortality was increased, and pup body weights were reduced.

There are no adequate and well-controlled studies of LUMIGAN™ administration in pregnant women. Because animal reproductive studies are not always predictive of human response, LUMIGAN™ should be administered during pregnancy only if the potential benefit justifies the potential risk to the fetus.

Nursing Mothers:
It is not known whether LUMIGAN™ is excreted in human milk, although in animal studies, bimatoprost has been shown to be excreted in breast milk. Because many drugs are excreted in human milk, caution should be exercised when LUMIGAN™ is administered to a nursing woman.

Pediatric Use:
Safety and effectiveness in pediatric patients have not been established.

Geriatric Use:
No overall clinical differences in safety or effectiveness have been observed between elderly and other adult patients.

ADVERSE REACTIONS

In clinical trials, the most frequent events associated with the use of LUMIGAN™ (bimatoprost ophthalmic solution) 0.03% occurring in approximately 15% to 45% of patients, in descending order of incidence, included conjunctival hyperemia, growth of eyelashes, and ocular pruritus. Approximately 3% of patients discontinued therapy due to conjunctival hyperemia.

Ocular adverse events occurring in approximately 3 to 10% of patients, in descending order of incidence, included ocular dryness, visual disturbance, ocular burning, foreign body sensation, eye pain, pigmentation of the periocular skin, blepharitis, cataract, superficial punctate keratitis, eyelid erythema, ocular irritation, and eyelash darkening. The following ocular adverse events reported in approximately 1 to 3% of patients, in descending order of incidence, included: eye discharge, tearing, photophobia, allergic conjunctivitis, asthenopia, increases in iris pigmentation, and conjunctival edema. In less than 1% of patients, intraocular inflammation was reported as iritis.

Systemic adverse events reported in approximately 10% of patients were infections (primarily colds and upper respiratory tract infections). The following systemic adverse events reported in approximately 1 to 5% of patients, in descending order of incidence, included headaches, abnormal liver function tests, asthenia and hirsutism.

OVERDOSAGE

No information is available on overdosage in humans. If overdose with LUMIGAN™ (bimatoprost ophthalmic solution) 0.03% occurs, treatment should be symptomatic.

In oral (by gavage) mouse and rat studies, doses up to 100 mg/kg/day did not produce any toxicity. This dose expressed as mg/m^2 is at least 70 times higher than the accidental dose of one bottle of LUMIGAN™ for a 10 kg child.

DOSAGE AND ADMINISTRATION

The recommended dosage is one drop in the affected eye(s) once daily in the evening. The dosage of LUMIGAN™ (bimatoprost ophthalmic solution) 0.03% should not exceed once daily since it has been shown that more frequent administration may decrease the intraocular pressure lowering effect.

Reduction of the intraocular pressure starts approximately 4 hours after the first administration with maximum effect reached within approximately 8 to 12 hours.

LUMIGAN™ may be used concomitantly with other topical ophthalmic drug products to lower intraocular pressure. If more than one topical ophthalmic drug is being used, the drugs should be administered at least five (5) minutes apart.

HOW SUPPLIED

LUMIGAN™ (bimatoprost ophthalmic solution) 0.03% is supplied sterile in opaque white low density polyethylene ophthalmic dispenser bottles with turquoise polystyrene caps in the following sizes: 2.5 mL fill in 8 mL container — NDC 0023-9187-03, and 5 mL fill in 8 mL container — NDC 0023-9187-05.

Rx only

Storage: LUMIGAN™ should be stored in the original container at 15° to 25°C (59° to 77°F).

ALLERGAN
® and ™ Marks owned by Allergan, Inc.
This product is covered under US Pat. No. 6,688,819.
March 2001
©Allergan, Inc., Irvine, CA 92612

To keep your **PDR** up to date throughout the year, note these revisions on the corresponding pages of the annual volume. Simply write **"See Supplement A"** next to the product heading.

American Regent Laboratories, Inc.

ONE LUITPOLD DRIVE
SHIRLEY, NY 11967

Direct Inquiries to:
Ray Czaja
800-645-1706

VENOFER® ℞
(iron sucrose injection)
Rx Only

DESCRIPTION

Venofer® (iron sucrose injection) is a brown, sterile, aqueous, complex of polynuclear iron(III)-hydroxide in sucrose for intravenous use. Iron sucrose injection has a molecular weight of approximately 34,000–60,000 daltons and a proposed structural formula:

$$[Na_2Fe_5O_8(OH) \cdot 3(H_2O)]_n \cdot m(C_{12}H_{22}O_{11})$$

where: n is the degree of iron polymerization and m is the number of sucrose molecules associated with the iron(III)-hydroxide.

Venofer® is available in 5 mL single dose vials. Each 5 mL contains 100 mg (20 mg/mL) of elemental iron as iron sucrose in water for injection. The drug product contains approximately 30% sucrose w/v (300 mg/mL) and has a pH of 10.5–11.1. The product contains no preservatives. The osmolarity of the injection is 1250 mOsmol/L.

Therapeutic class: Hematinic

CLINICAL PHARMACOLOGY

Pharmacodynamics: Following intravenous administration of Venofer®, iron sucrose is dissociated by the reticuloendothelial system into iron and sucrose. In 22 hemodialysis patients on erythropoietin (recombinant human erythropoietin) therapy treated with iron sucrose containing 100 mg of iron, three times weekly for three weeks, significant increases in serum iron and serum ferritin and significant decreases in total iron binding capacity occurred four weeks from the initiation of iron sucrose treatment.

Pharmacokinetics: In healthy adults treated with intravenous doses of Venofer®, its iron component exhibits first order kinetics with an elimination half-life of 6 h, total clearance of 1.2 L/h, non-steady state apparent volume of distribution of 10.0 L and steady state apparent volume of distribution of 7.9 L. Since iron disappearance from serum depends on the need for iron in the iron stores and iron utilizing tissues of the body, serum clearance of iron is expected to be more rapid in iron deficient patients treated with Venofer® as compared to healthy individuals. The effects of age and gender on the pharmacokinetics of Venofer® have not been studied.

Distribution: In healthy adults receiving intravenous doses of Venofer®, its iron component appears to distribute mainly in blood and to some extent in extravascular fluid. A study evaluating Venofer® containing 100 mg of iron labeled with 52Fe/59Fe in patients with iron deficiency shows that a significant amount of the administered iron distributes in the liver, spleen and bone marrow and that the bone marrow is an iron trapping compartment and not a reversible volume of distribution.

Metabolism and Elimination: Following intravenous administration of Venofer®, iron sucrose is dissociated into iron and sucrose by the reticuloendothelial system. The sucrose component is eliminated mainly by urinary excretion. In a study evaluating a single intravenous dose of Venofer® containing 1510 mg of sucrose and 100 mg of iron in 12 healthy adults, 68.3% of the sucrose was eliminated in urine in 4 h and 75.4% in 24 h. Some iron also is eliminated in the urine. In this study and another study evaluating a single intravenous dose of iron sucrose containing 500–700 mg of iron in 26 anemic patients on erythropoietin therapy, approximately 5% of the iron was eliminated in urine in 24 h at each dose level.

Drug-drug Interactions: Drug-drug interactions involving Venofer® have not been studied. However, like other parenteral iron preparations, Venofer® may be expected to reduce the absorption of concomitantly administered oral iron preparations.

CLINICAL TRIALS

Venofer® is used to replenish body iron stores in patients with iron deficiency on chronic hemodialysis and receiving

---

erythropoietin. In these patients iron deficiency is caused by blood loss during dialysis procedure, increased erythropoiesis, and insufficient absorption of iron from the gastrointestinal tract. Iron is essential to the synthesis of hemoglobin to maintain oxygen transport and to the function and formation of other physiologically important heme and non-heme compounds. Most hemodialysis patients require intravenous iron to maintain sufficient iron stores to achieve and maintain a hemoglobin of 11–12 g/dL.

Three clinical trials were conducted to assess the safety and efficacy of Venofer®. Two studies were conducted in United States and one was conducted in South Africa.

Study A
Study A was a multicenter, open-label, historically-controlled study in 101 hemodialysis patients (77 patients with Venofer® treatment and 24 in the historical control group) with iron deficiency anemia. Eligibility for Venofer® treatment included patients undergoing chronic hemodialysis three times weekly, receiving erythropoietin, hemoglobin concentration greater than 8.0 and less than 11.0 g/dL for at least two consecutive weeks, transferrin saturation <20%, and serum ferritin <300 ng/mL. The erythropoietin dose was to be held constant throughout the study. The protocol did not require administration of a test dose; however, some patients received a test dose at the physician's discretion. Exclusion criteria included significant underlying disease, asthma, active inflammatory disease, or serious bacterial or viral infection. Venofer® 5 mL (one vial) containing 100 mg of elemental iron was administered through the dialysis line at each dialysis session either as a slow injection or a saline diluted slow infusion for a total of 10 dialysis sessions with a cumulative dose of 1000 mg elemental iron. A maximum of 3 vials of Venofer® was administered per week. No additional iron preparations were allowed until after the Day 57 evaluation. The mean change in hemoglobin from baseline to Day 24 (end of treatment), Day 36, and Day 57 was assessed.

The historical control population consisted of 24 patients with similar ferritin level as patients treated with Venofer®, who were off intravenous iron for at least 2 weeks and who had received erythropoietin therapy with hematocrit averaging 31–36 for at least two months prior to study entry. Patient age and serum ferritin level were similar between treatment and historical control patients. The mean baseline hemoglobin, hematocrit, were higher and erythropoietin dose was lower in the historical control population than the Venofer®-treated population.

Patients in the Venofer®-treated population showed a statistically significantly greater increase in hemoglobin and hematocrit than did patients in the historical control population. See Table 1.

[See table below]

Serum ferritin increased significantly (p=0.0001) at endpoint of study from baseline in the Venofer®-treated population (165.3±24.2 ng/mL) compared to this historical control population (−27.6±9.5 ng/mL). Transferrin saturation also increased significantly (p=0.0016) at endpoint of study from baseline in the Venofer®-treated population (8.8±1.6%) compared to the historical control population (−5.1±4.3%).

Study B
Study B was a multicenter, open label, study of Venofer® (iron sucrose injection) in 23 iron deficient hemodialysis patients who had been discontinued from iron dextran due to intolerance. Eligibility criteria and Venofer® administration were otherwise identical to Study A. The mean change from baseline to the end of treatment (Day 24) in hemoglobin, hematocrit, and serum iron parameters was assessed.

All 23 enrolled patients were evaluated for efficacy. Statistically significant increases in mean hemoglobin (1.1±0.2 g/dL), hematocrit (3.6±0.6%), serum ferritin (266.3±30.3 ng/mL) and transferrin saturation (8.7±2.0%) were observed from baseline to end of treatment.

Study C
Study C was a multicenter, open-label, two period (treatment followed by observation period) study in iron deficient hemodialysis patients. Eligibility for this study included chronic hemodialysis patients with a hemoglobin less than or equal to 10 g/dL, a serum transferrin saturation less than or equal to 20%, and a serum ferritin less than or equal to 200 ng/mL, who were undergoing maintenance hemodialysis 2 to 3 times weekly. Forty-eight percent of the patients had previously been treated with oral iron. Exclusion criteria were similar to those in studies A and B. Venofer®, was administered in doses of 100 mg during sequential dialysis sessions until a pre-determined (calculated) total dose of iron was administered.

Table 1. Changes from Baseline in Hemoglobin and Hematocrit

Efficacy parameters	End of treatment		2 week follow-up		5 week follow-up	
	Venofer® (n=69)	Historical Control (n=18)	Venofer® (n=73)	Historical Control (n=18)	Venofer® (n=71)	Historical Control (n=15)
Hemoglobin (g/dL)	1.0±0.12**	0.0±0.21	1.3±0.14**	−0.6±0.24	1.2±0.17*	−0.1±0.23
Hematocrit (%)	3.1±0.37**	−0.3±0.65	3.6±0.44**	−1.2±0.76	3.3±0.54	0.2±0.86

**p<0.01 and *p<0.05 compared to historical control from ANCOVA analysis with baseline hemoglobin, serum ferritin and erythropoietin dose as covariates.

Patients received Venofer® at each dialysis session, two to three times weekly. One hour after the start of each session, 5 mL iron sucrose (100 mg iron) in 100 mL 0.9% NaCl was administered into the hemodialysis line. A 50 mg dose (2.5 mL) was given to patients within two weeks of study entry. Patients were treated until they reached an individually calculated total iron dose based on baseline hemoglobin level and body weight. Twenty-seven patients (20%) were receiving erythropoietin treatment at study entry and they continued to receive the same erythropoietin dose for the duration of the study.

Changes from baseline to observation week 2 and observation week 4 (end of study) were analyzed.

The modified intention-to-treat population consisted of 130 patients. Significant ($p < 0.0001$) increases from baseline in mean hemoglobin (1.7 g/dL), hematocrit (5%), serum ferritin (434.6 ng/mL), and serum transferrin saturation (14%) were observed at week 2 of the observation period and these values remained significantly increased ($p < 0.0001$) at week 4 of the observation period.

CLINICAL INDICATIONS AND USAGE

Venofer® is indicated in the treatment of iron deficiency anemia in patients undergoing chronic hemodialysis who are receiving supplemental erythropoietin therapy.

CONTRAINDICATIONS

The use of Venofer® is contraindicated in patients with evidence of iron overload, in patients with known hypersensitivity to Venofer® or any of its inactive components, and in patients with anemia not caused by iron deficiency.

WARNINGS

HYPERSENSITIVITY REACTIONS:

POTENTIALLY FATAL HYPERSENSITIVITY REACTIONS CHARACTERIZED BY ANAPHYLACTIC SHOCK, LOSS OF CONSCIOUSNESS, COLLAPSE, HYPOTENSION, DYSPNEA, OR CONVULSION HAVE BEEN REPORTED RARELY IN PATIENTS RECEIVING VENOFER® (SEE ADVERSE REACTIONS). FATAL IMMEDIATE HYPERSENSITIVITY REACTIONS HAVE BEEN REPORTED IN PATIENTS RECEIVING THERAPY WITH MANY IRON CARBOHYDRATE COMPLEXES. FACILITIES FOR CARDIOPULMONARY RESUSCITATION MUST BE AVAILABLE DURING DOSING. SERIOUS ANAPHYLACTOID REACTIONS REQUIRE APPROPRIATE RESUSCITATION MEASURES. ALTHOUGH FATAL HYPERSENSITIVITY REACTIONS HAVE NOT BEEN OBSERVED IN VENOFER®, CLINICAL STUDIES, INSUFFICIENT NUMBERS OF PATIENTS MAY HAVE BEEN ENROLLED TO OBSERVE THIS EVENT. PHYSICIAN VIGILANCE WHEN ADMINISTERING ANY INTRAVENOUS IRON PRODUCT IS ADVISED (SEE PRECAUTIONS and ADVERSE REACTIONS).

HYPOTENSION:

HYPOTENSION HAS BEEN REPORTED FREQUENTLY IN PATIENTS RECEIVING INTRAVENOUS IRON. HYPOTENSION FOLLOWING ADMINISTRATION OF VENOFER® MAY BE RELATED TO RATE OF ADMINISTRATION AND TOTAL DOSE ADMINISTERED. CAUTION SHOULD BE TAKEN TO ADMINISTER VENOFER® ACCORDING TO RECOMMENDED GUIDELINES (SEE DOSAGE AND ADMINISTRATION).

PRECAUTIONS

General:

Because body iron excretion is limited and excess tissue iron can be hazardous, caution should be exercised to withhold iron administration in the presence of evidence of tissue iron overload. Patients receiving Venofer® require periodic monitoring of hematologic and hematinic parameters (hemoglobin, hematocrit, serum ferritin and transferrin saturation). Iron therapy should be withheld in patients with evidence of iron overload. Transferrin saturation values increase rapidly after IV administration of iron sucrose; thus, serum iron values may be reliably obtained 48 hours after IV dosing. (See **DOSAGE AND ADMINISTRATION** and **OVERDOSAGE**).

Drug Interactions:

Venofer® (iron sucrose injection) should not be administered concomitantly with oral iron preparations since the absorption of oral iron is reduced.

Carcinogenesis, Mutagenesis, and Impairment of Fertility:

No long-term studies in animals have been performed to evaluate the carcinogenic potential of Venofer®.

Venofer® was not genotoxic in the Ames test, the mouse lymphoma cell (L5178Y/TK+/−) forward mutation test, the human lymphocyte chromosome aberration test, or the mouse micronucleous test.

Venofer® at IV doses up to 15 mg iron/kg/day (about 1.2 times the recommended maximum human dose on a body surface area basis) was found to have no effect on fertility and reproductive performance of male and female rats.

Pregnancy Category B:

Teratology studies have been performed in rats at IV doses up to 13 mg iron/kg/day (about 0.5 times the recommended maximum human dose on a body surface area basis) and rabbits at IV doses up to 13 mg iron/kg/day (about 1 times the recommended maximum human dose on a body surface area basis) and have revealed no evidence of impaired fertility or harm to the fetus due to Venofer®. There are, however, no adequate and well controlled studies in pregnant women. Because animal reproduction studies are not always predictive of human response, this drug should be used during pregnancy only if clearly needed.

Nursing Mothers:

Venofer® is excreted in milk of rats. It is not known whether this drug is excreted in human milk. Because many drugs are excreted in human milk, caution should be exercised when Venofer® is administered to a nursing woman.

Pediatric Use:

Safety and effectiveness of Venofer® in pediatric patients have not been established.

In a country where Venofer® is available for use in children, at a single site, five premature infants (weight less than 1250 g) developed necrotizing enterocolitis and two of the five expired during or following a period when they received Venofer®, several other medications and erythropoietin. Necrotizing enterocolitis may be a complication of prematurity in very low birth weight infants. No causal relationship to Venofer® or any other drugs could be established.

Geriatric Use:

Clinical studies of Venofer® did not include sufficient numbers of subjects aged 65 and over to determine whether they respond differently from younger subjects. Other reported clinical experience has not identified differences in responses between the elderly and younger patients. In general, dose selection for an elderly patient should be cautious, usually starting at the low end of the dosing range, reflecting the greater frequency of decreased hepatic, renal, or cardiac function, and of concomitant disease or other drug therapy.

ADVERSE REACTIONS

Exposure to Venofer® has been documented in 1004 patients with chronic renal failure. Of these, 231 were dialysis patients in the above mentioned clinical trials, and 773 were patients described in the medical literature.

The safety of Venofer® has been documented in 231 chronic renal failure patients exposed to single doses of 100 mg iron IV as iron sucrose given up to three times weekly for up to ten doses in 3 clinical trials. Of these, 100 were U.S. (Studies A and B) and 131 were non-U.S. patients (Study C). Adverse events were recorded by the investigator using terminology of their own choosing.

Common Adverse Events Observed In 3 Clinical Trials:

Adverse events, whether or not related to Venofer® administration, reported by >5% of treated patients from a total of 231 patients in three studies are as follows: hypotension (36%), cramps/leg cramps (23%), nausea, headache, vomiting, and diarrhea.

Adverse Events Observed During 3 Clinical Trials:

Adverse events, whether or not related to Venofer® administration, reported by >1% of treated patients from a total of 231 patients in 3 studies are categorized below by body system either by investigator term or by COSTART terminology and ranked in order of decreasing frequency within each body system. Some of these symptoms may be seen in patients with chronic renal failure or on hemodialysis not receiving intravenous iron.

Body as a Whole: headache, fever, pain, asthenia, unwell, malaise, accidental injury.

Cardiovascular Disorders, General: hypotension, chest pain, hypertension, hypervolemia.

Gastrointestinal System Disorders: nausea, vomiting, abdominal pain, elevated liver enzymes.

Central and Peripheral Nervous System: dizziness.

Musculoskeletal System: cramps/leg cramps, musculoskeletal pain.

Respiratory System: dyspnea, pneumonia, cough.

Skin and appendages: pruritus, application site reaction.

Hypersensitivity reactions: See WARNINGS.

In three clinical trials (231 patients), several patients experienced pruritus and one patient experienced a facial rash. No patients experienced generalized rashes or urticaria. No serious or life-threatening anaphylactoid reaction was observed in three trials and non of these reactions led to treatment discontinuation. From the spontaneous reporting system, 27 patients reported anaphylactoid reactions including 8 patients who experienced serious or life-threatening reactions (anaphylactic shock, loss of consciousness, collapse, hypotension, dyspnea, or convulsion) associated with Venofer® administration in the estimated more than 450,000 patients exposed to Venofer® between 1992 and 1999.

OVERDOSAGE

Dosages of Venofer® (iron sucrose injection) in excess of iron needs may lead to accumulation of iron in storage sites leading to hemosiderosis. Periodic monitoring of iron parameters such as serum ferritin and transferritin saturation may assist in recognizing iron accumulation. Venofer® should not be administered to patients with iron overload and should be discontinued when serum ferritin levels equal or exceed established guidelines [1]. Particular caution should be exercised to avoid iron overload where anemia unresponsive to treatment has been incorrectly diagnosed as iron deficiency anemia.

Symptoms associated with overdosage or infusing Venofer® too rapidly included hypotension, headache, vomiting, nausea, dizziness, joint aches, paresthesia, abdominal and muscle pain, edema, and cardiovascular collapse. Most symptoms have been successfully treated with IV fluids, hydrocortisone, and/or antihistamines. Infusing the solution as recommended or at a slower rate may also alleviate symptoms.

Preclinical Data:

Single IV doses of Venofer® at 150 mg iron/kg in mice (about 3 times the recommended maximum human dose on a body surface area basis) and 100 mg iron/kg in rats (about 8 times the recommended maximum human dose on a body surface area basis) were lethal.

The symptoms of acute toxicity were sedation, hypoactivity, pale eyes, and bleeding in the gastrointestinal tract and lungs.

DOSAGE AND ADMINISTRATION

The dosage of Venofer® is expressed in terms of mg of elemental iron. Each 5 mL vial contains 100 mg of elemental iron (20 mg/mL).

Of the three clinical studies in hemodialysis patients, the two U.S. studies (100 patients) did not require a test dose; however, some patients received a test dose at the physician's discretion. In a non-U.S. study, 131 patients received a first dose of Venofer® [2.5 mL (50 mg elemental iron) diluted in 50 mL 0.9% NaCl] administered over 3 to 10 minutes.

The recommended dosage of Venofer® for the repletion treatment of iron deficiency in hemodialysis patients is 5 mL of Venofer® (100 mg of elemental iron) delivered intravenously during the dialysis session. Most patients will require a minimum cumulative dose of 1000 mg of elemental iron, administered over 10 sequential dialysis sessions, to achieve a favorable hemoglobin or hematocrit response. Patients may continue to require therapy with Venofer® or other intravenous iron preparations at the lowest dose necessary to maintain target levels of hemoglobin, hematocrit and laboratory parameters of iron storage within acceptable limits.

Administration: Venofer® must only be administered intravenously (directly into the dialysis line) either by slow injection or by infusion.

Slow Intravenous injection: In chronic renal failure patients, Venofer® may be administered by slow intravenous injection into the dialysis line at a rate of 1 mL (20 mg iron) undiluted solution per minute [i.e., 5 minutes per vial] not exceeding one vial Venofer® [100 mg iron] per injection. Discard any unused portion.

Infusion: Venofer® may also be administered by infusion (into the dialysis line for hemodialysis patients). This may reduce the risk of hypotensive episodes. The content of each vial must be diluted exclusively in a maximum of 100 mL of 0.9% NaCl, immediately prior to infusion. The solution should be infused at a rate of 100 mg of iron over a period of at least 15 minutes. Unused diluted solution should be discarded.

NOTE: Do not mix Venofer® with other medications or add to parental nutrition solutions for intravenous infusion. Parenteral drug products should be inspected visually for particulate matter and discoloration prior to adminstration, whenever the solution and container permit.

Recommended Dosage:

Adults: 100 mg iron administered one to three times per week to a total dose of 1000 mg in 10 doses, repeat if needed. Frequency of dosing should be no more than three times weekly.

HOW SUPPLIED

Venofer® is supplied in 5 mL single dose vials. Each 5 mL vial contains 100 mg elemental iron (20 mg/mL). Contains no preservatives. Packaged in cartons containing 10 single dose vials. Store in original carton at 25°C (77°F). Excursions permitted to 15°–30°C (59°–86°F). [See USP Controlled Room Temperature]. Do not freeze.

Sterile

NDC 0517-2340-10

CAUTION: Rx ONLY

[1] *NKF-DOQI Clinical Practice Guidelines for the Treatment of Anemia of Chronic Renal Failure,* National Kidney Foundation, 1997.

IN2340

Rev. 11/00

MG #15727

AMERICAN
REGENT
LABORATORIES, INC.
SHIRLEY, NY 11967

VENOFER® is a registered trademark of Vifor (International), Inc.

To keep your **PDR** up to date throughout the year, note these revisions on the corresponding pages of the annual volume. Simply write **"See Supplement A"** next to the product heading.

AstraZeneca LP
WILMINGTON, DE 19850-5437

For Medical Information,
Adverse Drug Experiences,
and Customer Service
Contact: (800) 236-9933

TABLETS   9329100
                                           610517-00
ATACAND HCT™ 16–12.5   ℞
(Candesartan Cilexetil Hydrochlorothiazide)
ATACAND HCT™ 32–12.5
(Candesartan Cilexetil Hydrochlorothiazide)

USE IN PREGNANCY
When used in pregnancy during the second and third trimesters, drugs that act directly on the renin-angiotensin system can cause injury and even death to the developing fetus. When pregnancy is detected, ATACAND HCT should be discontinued as soon as possible. See WARNINGS, Fetal/Neonatal Morbidity and Mortality.

DESCRIPTION
ATACAND HCT* (candesartan cilexetil-hydrochlorothiazide) combines an angiotensin II receptor (type AT_1) antagonist and a diuretic, hydrochlorothiazide.

Candesartan cilexetil, a nonpeptide, is chemically described as (±)-1-[[(cyclohexyloxy)carbonyl]oxy]ethyl 2-ethoxy-1-[[2'-(1H-tetrazol-5-yl)[1,1'-biphenyl]-4-yl]methyl]-1H-benzimidazole-7-carboxylate.

Its empirical formula is $C_{33}H_{34}N_6O_6$, and its structural formula is

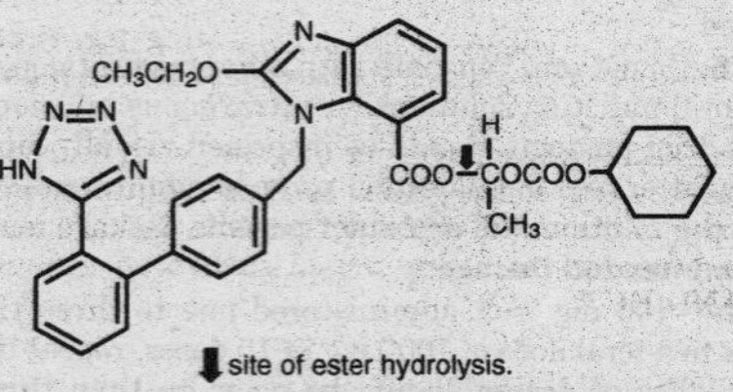

↓ site of ester hydrolysis.

Candesartan cilexetil is a white to off-white powder with a molecular weight of 610.67. It is practically insoluble in water and sparingly soluble in methanol. Candesartan cilexetil is a racemic mixture containing one chiral center at the cyclohexyloxycarbonyloxy ethyl ester group. Following oral administration, candesartan cilexetil undergoes hydrolysis at the ester link to form the active drug, candesartan, which is achiral.

Hydrochlorothiazide is 6-chloro-3,4-dihydro-2H-1,2,4-benzothiadiazine-7-sulfonamide 1,1-dioxide. Its empirical formula is $C_7H_8ClN_3O_4S_2$ and its structural formula is

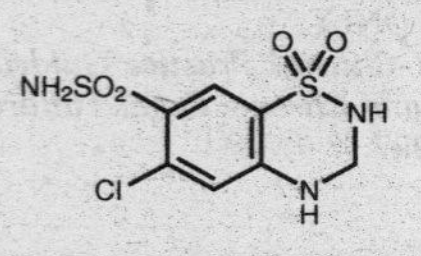

Hydrochlorothiazide is a white, or practically white, crystalline powder with a molecular weight of 297.72, which is slightly soluble in water, but freely soluble in sodium hydroxide solution.

ATACAND HCT is available for oral administration in two tablet strengths of candesartan cilexetil and hydrochlorothiazide. ATACAND HCT 16–12.5 contains 16 mg of candesartan cilexetil and 12.5 mg of hydrochlorothiazide. ATACAND HCT 32–12.5 contains 32 mg of candesartan cilexetil and 12.5 mg of hydrochlorothiazide. The inactive ingredients of the tablets are calcium carboxymethylcellulose, hydroxypropyl cellulose, lactose monohydrate, magnesium stearate, corn starch, polyethylene glycol 8000, and ferric oxide (yellow). Ferric oxide (reddish brown) is also added to the 16–12.5 mg tablet as colorant.

* Trademark of the AstraZeneca Group
© AstraZeneca 2000

CLINICAL PHARMACOLOGY
Mechanism of Action
Angiotensin II is formed from angiotensin I in a reaction catalyzed by angiotensin-converting enzyme (ACE, kininase II). Angiotensin II is the principal pressor agent of the renin-angiotensin system, with effects that include vasoconstriction, stimulation of synthesis and release of aldosterone, cardiac stimulation, and renal reabsorption of sodium. Candesartan blocks the vasoconstrictor and aldosterone-secreting effects of angiotensin II by selectively blocking the binding of angiotensin II to the AT_1 receptor in many tissues, such as vascular smooth muscle and the adrenal gland. Its action is, therefore, independent of the pathways for angiotensin II synthesis.

There is also an AT_2 receptor found in many tissues, but AT_2 is not known to be associated with cardiovascular homeostasis. Candesartan has much greater affinity (>10,000-fold) for the AT_1 receptor than for the AT_2 receptor.

Blockade of the renin-angiotensin system with ACE inhibitors, which inhibit the biosynthesis of angiotensin II from angiotensin I, is widely used in the treatment of hypertension. ACE inhibitors also inhibit the degradation of bradykinin, a reaction also catalyzed by ACE. Because candesartan does not inhibit ACE (kininase II), it does not affect the response to bradykinin. Whether this difference has clinical relevance is not yet known. Candesartan does not bind to or block other hormone receptors or ion channels known to be important in cardiovascular regulation.

Blockade of the angiotensin II receptor inhibits the negative regulatory feedback of angiotensin II on renin secretion, but the resulting increased plasma renin activity and angiotensin II circulating levels do not overcome the effect of candesartan on blood pressure.

Hydrochlorothiazide is a thiazide diuretic. Thiazides affect the renal tubular mechanisms of electrolyte reabsorption, directly increasing excretion of sodium and chloride in approximately equivalent amounts. Indirectly, the diuretic action of hydrochlorothiazide reduces plasma volume, with consequent increases in plasma renin activity, increases in aldosterone secretion, increases in urinary potassium loss, and decreases in serum potassium. The renin-aldosterone link is mediated by angiotensin II, so coadministration of an angiotensin II receptor antagonist tends to reverse the potassium loss associated with these diuretics.

The mechanism of the antihypertensive effect of thiazides is unknown.

Pharmacokinetics
General
Candesartan Cilexetil
Candesartan cilexetil is rapidly and completely bioactivated by ester hydrolysis during absorption from the gastrointestinal tract to candesartan, a selective AT_1 subtype angiotensin II receptor antagonist. Candesartan is mainly excreted unchanged in urine and feces (via bile). It undergoes minor hepatic metabolism by O-deethylation to an inactive metabolite. The elimination half-life of candesartan is approximately 9 hours. After single and repeated administration, the pharmacokinetics of candesartan are linear for oral doses up to 32 mg of candesartan cilexetil. Candesartan and its inactive metabolite do not accumulate in serum upon repeated once-daily dosing.

Following administration of candesartan cilexetil, the absolute bioavailability of candesartan was estimated to be 15%. After tablet ingestion, the peak serum concentration (C_{max}) is reached after 3 to 4 hours. Food with a high fat content does not affect the bioavailability of candesartan after candesartan cilexetil administration.

Hydrochlorothiazide
When plasma levels have been followed for at least 24 hours, the plasma half-life has been observed to vary between 5.6 and 14.8 hours.

Metabolism and Excretion
Candesartan Cilexetil
Total plasma clearance of candesartan is 0.37 mL/min/kg, with a renal clearance of 0.19 mL/min/kg. When candesartan is administered orally, about 26% of the dose is excreted unchanged in urine. Following an oral dose of ^{14}C-labeled candesartan cilexetil, approximately 33% of radioactivity is recovered in urine and approximately 67% in feces. Following an intravenous dose of ^{14}C-labeled candesartan, approximately 59% of radioactivity is recovered in urine and approximately 36% in feces. Biliary excretion contributes to the elimination of candesartan.

Hydrochlorothiazide
Hydrochlorothiazide is not metabolized but is eliminated rapidly by the kidney. At least 61% of the oral dose is eliminated unchanged within 24 hours.

Distribution
Candesartan Cilexetil
The volume of distribution of candesartan is 0.13 L/kg. Candesartan is highly bound to plasma proteins (>99%) and does not penetrate red blood cells. The protein binding is constant at candesartan plasma concentrations well above the range achieved with recommended doses. In rats, it has been demonstrated that candesartan crosses the blood-brain barrier poorly, if at all. It has also been demonstrated in rats that candesartan passes across the placental barrier and is distributed in the fetus.

Hydrochlorothiazide
Hydrochlorothiazide crosses the placental but not the blood-brain barrier and is excreted in breast milk.

Special Populations
Pediatric
The pharmacokinetics of candesartan cilexetil have not been investigated in patients <18 years of age.

Geriatric
The pharmacokinetics of candesartan have been studied in the elderly (≥65 years). The plasma concentration of candesartan was higher in the elderly (C_{max} was approximately 50% higher, and AUC was approximately 80% higher) compared to younger subjects administered the same dose. The pharmacokinetics of candesartan were linear in the elderly, and candesartan and its inactive metabolite did not accumulate in the serum of these subjects upon repeated, once-daily administration. No initial dosage adjustment is necessary. (See DOSAGE AND ADMINISTRATION.)

Gender
There is no difference in the pharmacokinetics of candesartan between male and female subjects.

Renal Insufficiency
In hypertensive patients with renal insufficiency, serum concentrations of candesartan were elevated. After repeated dosing, the AUC and C_{max} were approximately doubled in patients with severe renal impairment (creatinine clearance <30 mL/min/1.73m²) compared to patients with normal kidney function. The pharmacokinetics of candesartan in hypertensive patients undergoing hemodialysis are similar to those in hypertensive patients with severe renal impairment. Candesartan cannot be removed by hemodialysis. No initial dosage adjustment is necessary in patients with renal insufficiency.

Thiazide diuretics are eliminated by the kidney, with a terminal half-life of 5–15 hours. In a study of patients with impaired renal function (mean creatinine clearance of 19 mL/min), the half-life of hydrochlorothiazide elimination was lengthened to 21 hours. (See DOSAGE AND ADMINISTRATION.)

Hepatic Insufficiency
No differences in the pharmacokinetics of candesartan were observed in patients with mild to moderate chronic liver disease. Thiazide diuretics should be used with caution in patients with hepatic impairment. (See DOSAGE AND ADMINISTRATION.)

Pharmacodynamics
Candesartan Cilexetil
Candesartan inhibits the pressor effects of angiotensin II infusion in a dose-dependent manner. After 1 week of once-daily dosing with 8 mg of candesartan cilexetil, the pressor effect was inhibited by approximately 90% at peak with approximately 50% inhibition persisting for 24 hours.

Plasma concentrations of angiotensin I and angiotensin II, and plasma renin activity (PRA), increased in a dose-dependent manner after single and repeated administration of candesartan cilexetil to healthy subjects and hypertensive patients. ACE activity was not altered in healthy subjects after repeated candesartan cilexetil administration. The once-daily administration of up to 16 mg of candesartan cilexetil to healthy subjects did not influence plasma aldosterone concentrations, but a decrease in the plasma concentration of aldosterone was observed when 32 mg of candesartan cilexetil was administered to hypertensive patients. In spite of the effect of candesartan cilexetil on aldosterone secretion, very little effect on serum potassium was observed.

In multiple-dose studies with hypertensive patients, there were no clinically significant changes in metabolic function including serum levels of total cholesterol, triglycerides, glucose, or uric acid. In a 12-week study of 161 patients with noninsulin-dependent (type 2) diabetes mellitus and hypertension, there was no change in the level of HbA_{1c}.

Hydrochlorothiazide
After oral administration of hydrochlorothiazide, diuresis begins within 2 hours, peaks in about 4 hours and lasts about 6 to 12 hours.

Clinical Trials
Candesartan Cilexetil–Hydrochlorothiazide
Of 12 controlled clinical trials involving 4588 patients, 5 were double-blind, placebo controlled and evaluated the antihypertensive effects of single entities vs the combination. These 5 trials, of 8 to 12 weeks duration, randomized 3037 hypertensive patients. Doses ranged from 2 to 32 mg candesartan cilexetil and from 6.25 to 25 mg hydrochlorothiazide administered once daily in various combinations.

The combination of candesartan cilexetil-hydrochlorothiazide resulted in placebo-adjusted decreases in sitting systolic and diastolic blood pressures of 14-18/8-11 mm Hg at doses of 16–12.5 mg and 32–12.5 mg. The combination of candesartan cilexetil and hydrochlorothiazide 32–25 mg resulted in placebo-adjusted decreases in sitting systolic and diastolic blood pressures of 16-19/9-11 mm Hg. The placebo corrected trough to peak ratio was evaluated in a study of candesartan cilexetil-hydrochlorothiazide 32–12.5 mg and was 88%.

Most of the antihypertensive effect of the combination of candesartan cilexetil and hydrochlorothiazide was seen in 1 to 2 weeks with the full effect observed within 4 weeks. In long-term studies of up to 1 year, the blood pressure lowering effect of the combination was maintained. The antihypertensive effect was similar regardless of age or gender, and overall response to the combination was similar in black and non-black patients. No appreciable changes in heart rate were observed with combination therapy in controlled trials.

INDICATIONS AND USAGE
ATACAND HCT is indicated for the treatment of hypertension. This fixed dose combination is not indicated for initial therapy (see DOSAGE AND ADMINISTRATION).

CONTRAINDICATIONS
ATACAND HCT is contraindicated in patients who are hypersensitive to any component of this product.

Because of the hydrochlorothiazide component, this product is contraindicated in patients with anuria or hypersensitivity to other sulfonamide-derived drugs.

WARNINGS
Fetal/Neonatal Morbidity and Mortality
Drugs that act directly on the renin-angiotensin system can cause fetal and neonatal morbidity and death when administered to pregnant women. Several dozen cases have been reported in the world literature in patients who were taking

angiotensin-converting enzyme inhibitors. When pregnancy is detected, ATACAND HCT should be discontinued as soon as possible.

The use of drugs that act directly on the renin-angiotensin system during the second and third trimesters of pregnancy has been associated with fetal and neonatal injury, including hypotension, neonatal skull hypoplasia, anuria, reversible or irreversible renal failure, and death. Oligohydramnios has also been reported, presumably resulting from decreased fetal renal function; oligohydramnios in this setting has been associated with fetal limb contractures, craniofacial deformation, and hypoplastic lung development. Prematurity, intrauterine growth retardation, and patent ductus arteriosus have also been reported, although it is not clear whether these occurrences were due to exposure to the drug. These adverse effects do not appear to have resulted from intrauterine drug exposure that has been limited to the first trimester. Mothers whose embryos and fetuses are exposed to an angiotensin II receptor antagonist only during the first trimester should be so informed. Nonetheless, when patients become pregnant, physicians should have the patient discontinue the use of ATACAND HCT as soon as possible. Rarely (probably less often than once in every thousand pregnancies), no alternative to a drug acting on the renin-angiotensin system will be found. In these rare cases, the mothers should be apprised of the potential hazards to their fetuses, and serial ultrasound examinations should be performed to assess the intra-amniotic environment.

If oligohydramnios is observed, ATACAND HCT should be discontinued unless it is considered life saving for the mother. Contraction stress testing (CST), a nonstress test (NST), or biophysical profiling (BPP) may be appropriate, depending upon the week of pregnancy. Patients and physicians should be aware, however, that oligohydramnios may not appear until after the fetus has sustained irreversible injury.

Infants with histories of *in utero* exposure to an angiotensin II receptor antagonist should be closely observed for hypotension, oliguria, and hyperkalemia. If oliguria occurs, attention should be directed toward support of blood pressure and renal perfusion. Exchange transfusion or dialysis may be required as means of reversing hypotension and/or substituting for disordered renal function.

Candesartan Cilexetil–Hydrochlorothiazide
There was no evidence of teratogenicity or other adverse effects on embryo-fetal development when pregnant mice, rats or rabbits were treated orally with candesartan cilexetil alone or in combination with hydrochlorothiazide. For mice, the maximum dose of candesartan cilexetil was 1000 mg/kg/day (about 150 times the maximum recommended daily human dose [MRHD]*). For rats, the maximum dose of candesartan cilexetil was 100 mg/kg/day (about 31 times the MRHD*). For rabbits, the maximum dose of candesartan cilexetil was 1 mg/kg/day (a maternally toxic dose that is about half the MRHD*). In each of these studies, hydrochlorothiazide was tested at the same dose level (10 mg/kg/day, about 4, 8, and 15 times the MRHD* in mouse, rats, and rabbit, respectively). There was no evidence of harm to the rat or mouse fetus or embryo in studies in which hydrochlorothiazide was administered alone to the pregnant rat or mouse at doses of up to 1000 and 3000 mg/kg/day, respectively.

Thiazides cross the placental barrier and appear in cord blood. There is a risk of fetal or neonatal jaundice, thrombocytopenia, and possibly other adverse reactions that have occurred in adults.

---

*Doses compared on the basis of body surface area. MRHD considered to be 32 mg for candesartan cilexetil and 12.5 mg for hydrochlorothiazide.

Hypotension in Volume- and Salt-Depleted Patients
Based on adverse events reported from all clinical trials of ATACAND HCT, excessive reduction of blood pressure was rarely seen in patients with uncomplicated hypertension treated with candesartan cilexetil and hydrochlorothiazide (0.4%). Initiation of antihypertensive therapy may cause symptomatic hypotension in patients with intravascular volume- or sodium-depletion, eg, in patients treated vigorously with diuretics or in patients on dialysis. These conditions should be corrected prior to administration of ATACAND HCT, or the treatment should start under close medical supervision (see DOSAGE AND ADMINISTRATION).

If hypotension occurs, the patients should be placed in the supine position and, if necessary, given an intravenous infusion of normal saline. A transient hypotensive response is not a contraindication to further treatment which usually can be continued without difficulty once the blood pressure has stabilized.

Hydrochlorothiazide
Impaired Hepatic Function
Thiazide diuretics should be used with caution in patients with impaired hepatic function or progressive liver disease, since minor alterations of fluid and electrolyte balance may precipitate hepatic coma.

Hypersensitivity Reaction
Hypersensitivity reactions to hydrochlorothiazide may occur in patients with or without a history of allergy or bronchial asthma, but are more likely in patients with such a history.

Systemic Lupus Erythematosus
Thiazide diuretics have been reported to cause exacerbation or activation of systemic lupus erythematosus.

Lithium Interaction
Lithium generally should not be given with thiazides (see PRECAUTIONS, Drug Interactions, Hydrochlorothiazide, Lithium).

PRECAUTIONS
General
Candesartan Cilexetil–Hydrochlorothiazide
In clinical trials of various doses of candesartan cilexetil and hydrochlorothiazide, the incidence of hypertensive patients who developed hypokalemia (serum potassium <3.5 mEq/L) was 2.5% versus 2.1% for placebo; the incidence of hyperkalemia (serum potassium >5.7 mEq/L) was 0.4% versus 1.0% for placebo. No patient receiving ATACAND HCT 16–12.5 mg or 32–12.5 mg was discontinued due to increases or decreases in serum potassium. Overall, the combination of candesartan cilexetil and hydrochlorothiazide had no clinically significant effect on serum potassium.

Hydrochlorothiazide
Periodic determination of serum electrolytes to detect possible electrolyte imbalance should be performed at appropriate intervals.

All patients receiving thiazide therapy should be observed for clinical signs of fluid or electrolyte imbalance: namely, hyponatremia, hypochloremic alkalosis, and hypokalemia. Serum and urine electrolyte determinations are particularly important when the patient is vomiting excessively or receiving parenteral fluids. Warning signs or symptoms of fluid and electrolyte imbalance, irrespective of cause, include dryness of mouth, thirst, weakness, lethargy, drowsiness, restlessness, confusion, seizures, muscle pains or cramps, muscular fatigue, hypotension, oliguria, tachycardia, and gastrointestinal disturbances such as nausea and vomiting.

Hypokalemia may develop, especially with brisk diuresis, when severe cirrhosis is present, or after prolonged therapy. Interference with adequate oral electrolyte intake will also contribute to hypokalemia. Hypokalemia may cause cardiac arrhythmia and may also sensitize or exaggerate the response of the heart to the toxic effects of digitalis (eg, increased ventricular irritability).

Although any chloride deficit is generally mild and usually does not require specific treatment, except under extraordinary circumstances (as in liver disease or renal disease), chloride replacement may be required in the treatment of metabolic alkalosis.

Dilutional hyponatremia may occur in edematous patients in hot weather; appropriate therapy is water restriction, rather than administration of salt, except in rare instances when the hyponatremia is life-threatening. In actual salt depletion, appropriate replacement is the therapy of choice. Hyperuricemia may occur or acute gout may be precipitated in certain patients receiving thiazide therapy.

In diabetic patients dosage adjustments of insulin or oral hypoglycemic agents may be required. Hyperglycemia may occur with thiazide diuretics. Thus latent diabetes mellitus may become manifest during thiazide therapy.

The antihypertensive effects of the drug may be enhanced in the post-sympathectomy patient.

If progressive renal impairment becomes evident consider withholding or discontinuing diuretic therapy.

Thiazides have been shown to increase the urinary excretion of magnesium; this may result in hypomagnesemia.

Thiazides may decrease urinary calcium excretion. Thiazides may cause intermittent and slight elevation of serum calcium in the absence of known disorders of calcium metabolism. Marked hypercalcemia may be evidence of hidden hyperparathyroidism. Thiazides should be discontinued before carrying out tests for parathyroid function.

Increases in cholesterol and triglyceride levels may be associated with thiazide diuretic therapy.

Impaired Renal Function
Candesartan Cilexetil
As a consequence of inhibiting the renin-angiotensin-aldosterone system, changes in renal function may be anticipated in susceptible individuals treated with candesartan cilexetil. In patients whose renal function may depend upon the activity of the renin-angiotensin-aldosterone system (eg, patients with severe congestive heart failure), treatment with angiotensin-converting enzyme inhibitors and angiotensin receptor antagonists has been associated with oliguria and/or progressive azotemia and (rarely) with acute renal failure and/or death. Similar results may be anticipated in patients treated with candesartan cilexetil. (See CLINICAL PHARMACOLOGY, Special Populations.)

In studies of ACE inhibitors in patients with unilateral or bilateral renal artery stenosis, increases in serum creatinine or blood urea nitrogen (BUN) have been reported. There has been no long-term use of candesartan cilexetil in patients with unilateral or bilateral renal artery stenosis, but similar results may be expected.

Hydrochlorothiazide
Thiazides should be used with caution in severe renal disease. In patients with renal disease, thiazides may precipitate azotemia. Cumulative effects of the drug may develop in patients with impaired renal function.

Information for Patients
Pregnancy
Female patients of childbearing age should be told about the consequences of second- and third-trimester exposure to drugs that act on the renin-angiotensin system, and they should also be told that these consequences do not appear to have resulted from intrauterine drug exposure that has been limited to the first trimester. These patients should be asked to report pregnancies to their physicians as soon as possible.

Symptomatic Hypotension
A patient receiving ATACAND HCT should be cautioned that lightheadedness can occur, especially during the first days of therapy, and that it should be reported to the pre-

scribing physician. The patients should be told that if syncope occurs, ATACAND HCT should be discontinued until the physician has been consulted.

All patients should be cautioned that inadequate fluid intake, excessive perspiration, diarrhea, or vomiting can lead to an excessive fall in blood pressure, with the same consequences of lightheadedness and possible syncope.

Potassium Supplements
A patient receiving ATACAND HCT should be told not to use potassium supplements or salt substitutes containing potassium without consulting the prescribing physician.

Drug Interactions
Candesartan Cilexetil
No significant drug interactions have been reported in studies of candesartan cilexetil given with other drugs such as glyburide, nifedipine, digoxin, warfarin, hydrochlorothiazide, and oral contraceptives in healthy volunteers. Because candesartan is not significantly metabolized by the cytochrome P450 system and at therapeutic concentrations has no effects on P450 enzymes, interactions with drugs that inhibit or are metabolized by those enzymes would not be expected.

Hydrochlorothiazide
When administered concurrently the following drugs may interact with thiazide diuretics:

Alcohol, barbiturates, or narcotics—Potentiation of orthostatic hypotension may occur.

Antidiabetic drugs (oral agents and insulin)—Dosage adjustment of the antidiabetic drug may be required.

Other antihypertensive drugs—Additive effect or potentiation.

Cholestyramine and colestipol resins—Absorption of hydrochlorothiazide is impaired in the presence of anionic exchange resins. Single doses of either cholestyramine or colestipol resins bind the hydrochlorothiazide and reduce its absorption from the gastrointestinal tract by up to 85 and 43 percent, respectively.

Corticosteroids, ACTH—Intensified electrolyte depletion, particularly hypokalemia.

Pressor amines (eg, norepinephrine)—Possible decreased response to pressor amines but not sufficient to preclude their use.

Skeletal muscle relaxants, nondepolarizing (eg, tubocurarine)—Possible increased responsiveness to the muscle relaxant.

Lithium—Generally should not be given with diuretics. Diuretic agents reduce the renal clearance of lithium and add a high risk of lithium toxicity. Refer to the package insert for lithium preparations before use of such preparations with ATACAND HCT.

Non-steroidal Anti-inflammatory Drugs—In some patients, the administration of a non-steroidal anti-inflammatory agent can reduce the diuretic, natriuretic, and antihypertensive effects of loop, potassium-sparing and thiazide diuretics. Therefore, when ATACAND HCT and non-steroidal anti-inflammatory agents are used concomitantly, the patient should be observed closely to determine if the desired effect of the diuretic is obtained.

Carcinogenesis, Mutagenesis, Impairment of Fertility
Candesartan Cilexetil–Hydrochlorothiazide
No carcinogenicity studies have been conducted with the combination of candesartan cilexetil and hydrochlorothiazide. There was no evidence of carcinogenicity when candesartan cilexetil was orally administered to mice and rats for up to 104 weeks at doses up to 100 and 1000 mg/kg/day, respectively. Rats received the drug by gavage whereas mice received the drug by dietary administration. These (maximally-tolerated) doses of candesartan cilexetil provided systemic exposures to candesartan (AUCs) that were, in mice, approximately 7 times and, in rats, more than 70 times the exposure in man at the maximum recommended daily human dose (32 mg). Two-year feeding studies in mice and rats conducted under the auspices of the National Toxicology Program (NTP) uncovered no evidence of a carcinogenic potential of hydrochlorothiazide in female mice (at doses of up to approximately 600 mg/kg/day) or in male and female rats (at doses of up to approximately 100 mg/kg/day). The NTP, however, found equivocal evidence for hepatocarcinogenicity in male mice.

Candesartan cilexetil, alone or in combination with hydrochlorothiazide, tested negative for mutagenicity in bacteria (Ames test), for unscheduled DNA synthesis in rat liver, for chromosomal aberrations in rat bone marrow and for micronuclei in mouse bone marrow. In addition, candesartan (the active metabolite) was not genotoxic in the microbial mutagenesis, mammalian cell mutagenesis, and *in vitro* and *in vivo* chromosome aberration assays. In the *in vitro* Chinese hamster lung cell chromosomal aberration and mouse lymphoma assays, mutagenic effects were detected when hydrochlorothiazide was tested in the presence of candesartan. Hydrochlorothiazide was not genotoxic *in vitro* in the Ames test for point mutations and the Chinese Hamster Ovary (CHO) test for chromosomal aberrations, or *in vivo* in assays using mouse germinal cell chromosomes, Chinese hamster bone marrow chromosomes, and the *Drosophila* sex-linked recessive lethal trait gene. Positive test results were obtained for hydrochlorothiazide in the *in vitro* CHO Sister Chromatid Exchange (clastogenicity) and in the Mouse Lymphoma Cell (mutagenicity) assays and in the *Aspergillus nidulans* nondisjunction assay.

No fertility studies have been conducted with the combination of candesartan cilexetil and hydrochlorothiazide. Fertil-

Continued on next page

Atacand HCT—Cont.

ity and reproductive performance were not affected in studies with male and female rats given oral doses of up to 300 mg candesartan cilexetil/kg/day (83 times the maximum daily human dose of 32 mg on a body surface area basis). Hydrochlorothiazide had no adverse effects on the fertility of mice and rats of either sex in studies wherein these species were exposed, via their diet, to doses of up to 100 and 4 mg/kg, respectively, prior to conception and throughout gestation.

Pregnancy

Pregnancy Categories C (first trimester) *and D* (second and third trimesters). See WARNINGS, Fetal/Neonatal Morbidity and Mortality.

Nursing Mothers

It is not known whether candesartan is excreted in human milk, but candesartan has been shown to be present in rat milk. Thiazides appear in human milk. Because of the potential for adverse effects on the nursing infant, a decision should be made whether to discontinue nursing or discontinue the drug, taking into account the importance of the drug to the mother.

Pediatric Use

Safety and effectiveness in pediatric patients have not been established.

Geriatric Use

Of the total number of subjects in all clinical studies of ATACAND HCT (2831), 611 (22%) were 65 and over, while 94 (3%) were 75 and over. No overall differences in safety or effectiveness were observed between these subjects and younger subjects. Other reported clinical experience has not identified differences in responses between the elderly and younger patients, but greater sensitivity of some older individuals cannot be ruled out.

ADVERSE REACTIONS

Candesartan Cilexetil–Hydrochlorothiazide

ATACAND HCT has been evaluated for safety in more than 2800 patients treated for hypertension. More than 750 of these patients were studied for at least six months and more than 500 patients were treated for at least one year. Adverse experiences have generally been mild and transient in nature and have only infrequently required discontinuation of therapy. The overall incidence of adverse events reported with ATACAND HCT was comparable to placebo. The overall frequency of adverse experiences was not related to dose, age, gender, or race.

In placebo-controlled trials that included 1089 patients treated with various combinations of candesartan cilexetil (doses of 2–32 mg) and hydrochlorothiazide (doses of 6.25–25 mg) and 592 patients treated with placebo, adverse events, whether or not attributed to treatment, occurring in greater than 2% of patients treated with ATACAND HCT and that were more frequent for ATACAND HCT than placebo were: ***Respiratory System Disorder:*** upper respiratory tract infection (3.6% vs 3.0%); ***Body as a Whole:*** back pain (3.3% vs 2.4%); influenza-like symptoms (2.5% vs 1.9%); ***Central/Peripheral Nervous System:*** dizziness (2.9% vs 1.2%).

The frequency of headache was greater than 2% (2.9%) in patients treated with ATACAND HCT but was less frequent than the rate in patients treated with placebo (5.2%).

Other adverse events that have been reported, whether or not attributed to treatment, with an incidence of 0.5% or greater from the more than 2800 patients worldwide treated with ATACAND HCT included: ***Body as a Whole:*** inflicted injury, fatigue, pain, chest pain, peripheral edema, asthenia; ***Central and Peripheral Nervous System:*** vertigo, paresthesia, hypesthesia; ***Respiratory System Disorders:*** bronchitis, sinusitis, pharyngitis, coughing, rhinitis, dyspnea; ***Musculoskeletal System Disorders:*** arthralgia, myalgia, arthrosis, arthritis, leg cramps, sciatica; ***Gastrointestinal System Disorders:*** nausea, abdominal pain, diarrhea, dyspepsia, gastritis, gastroenteritis, vomiting; ***Metabolic and Nutritional Disorders:*** hyperuricemia, hyperglycemia, hypokalemia, increased BUN, creatine phosphokinase increased; ***Urinary System Disorders:*** urinary tract infection, hematuria, cystitis; ***Liver/Biliary System Disorders:*** hepatic function abnormal, increased transaminase levels; ***Heart Rate and Rhythm Disorders:*** tachycardia, palpitation, extrasystoles, bradycardia; ***Psychiatric Disorders:*** depression, insomnia, anxiety; ***Cardiovascular Disorders:*** ECG abnormal; ***Skin and Appendages Disorders:*** eczema, sweating increased, pruritus, dermatitis, rash; ***Platelet/Bleeding Clotting Disorders:*** epistaxis; ***Resistance Mechanism Disorders:*** infection, viral infection; ***Vision Disorders:*** conjunctivitis; ***Hearing and Vestibular Disorders:*** tinnitus.

Reported events seen less frequently than 0.5% included angina pectoris, myocardial infarction and angioedema.

Candesartan Cilexetil

Other adverse experiences that have been reported with candesartan cilexetil, without regard to causality, were: ***Body as a Whole:*** fever; ***Metabolic and Nutritional Disorders:*** hypertriglyceridemia; ***Psychiatric Disorders:*** somnolence; ***Urinary System Disorders:*** albuminuria.

Hydrochlorothiazide

Other adverse experiences that have been reported with hydrochlorothiazide, without regard to causality, are listed below:

Body As A Whole: weakness; ***Cardiovascular:*** hypotension including orthostatic hypotension (may be aggravated by alcohol, barbiturates, narcotics or antihypertensive drugs); ***Digestive:*** pancreatitis, jaundice (intrahepatic cholestatic jaundice), sialadenitis, cramping, constipation, gastric irritation, anorexia; ***Hematologic:*** aplastic anemia, agranulocytosis, leukopenia, hemolytic anemia, thrombocytopenia; ***Hypersensitivity:*** anaphylactic reactions, necrotizing angiitis (vasculitis and cutaneous vasculitis), respiratory distress including pneumonitis and pulmonary edema, photosensitivity, urticaria, purpura; ***Metabolic:*** electrolyte imbalance, glycosuria; ***Musculoskeletal:*** muscle spasm; ***Nervous System/Psychiatric:*** restlessness; ***Renal:*** renal failure, renal dysfunction, interstitial nephritis; ***Skin:*** erythema multiforme including Stevens-Johnson syndrome, exfoliative dermatitis including toxic epidermal necrolysis, alopecia; ***Special Senses:*** transient blurred vision, xanthopsia; ***Urogenital:*** impotence.

Laboratory Test Findings

In controlled clinical trials, clinically important changes in standard laboratory parameters were rarely associated with the administration of ATACAND HCT.

Creatinine, Blood Urea Nitrogen— Minor increases in blood urea nitrogen (BUN) and serum creatinine were observed infrequently. One patient was discontinued from ATACAND HCT due to increased BUN. No patient was discontinued due to an increase in serum creatinine.

Hemoglobin and Hematocrit— Small decreases in hemoglobin and hematocrit (mean decreases of approximately 0.2 g/dL and 0.4 volume percent, respectively) were observed in patients treated with ATACAND HCT, but were rarely of clinical importance.

Potassium— A small decrease (mean decrease of 0.1 mEq/L) was observed in patients treated with ATACAND HCT. In placebo-controlled trials, hypokalemia was reported in 0.4% of patients treated with ATACAND HCT as compared to 1.0% of patients treated with hydrochlorothiazide or 0.2% of patients treated with placebo.

Liver Function Tests— Occasional elevations of liver enzymes and/or serum bilirubin have occurred.

OVERDOSAGE

Candesartan Cilexetil–Hydrochlorothiazide

No lethality was observed in acute toxicity studies in mice, rats and dogs given single oral doses of up to 2000 mg/kg of candesartan cilexetil or in rats given single oral doses of up to 2000 mg/kg of candesartan cilexetil in combination with 1000 mg/kg of hydrochlorothiazide. In mice given single oral doses of the primary metabolite, candesartan, the minimum lethal dose was greater than 1000 mg/kg but less than 2000 mg/kg.

Limited data are available in regard to overdosage with candesartan cilexetil in humans. The most likely manifestations of overdosage with candesartan cilexetil would be hypotension, dizziness, and tachycardia; bradycardia could occur from parasympathetic (vagal) stimulation. If symptomatic hypotension should occur, supportive treatment should be initiated. For hydrochlorothiazide, the most common signs and symptoms observed are those caused by electrolyte depletion (hypokalemia, hypochloremia, hyponatremia) and dehydration resulting from excessive diuresis. If digitalis has also been administered, hypokalemia may accentuate cardiac arrhythmias.

Candesartan cannot be removed by hemodialysis. The degree to which hydrochlorothiazide is removed by hemodialysis has not been established.

Treatment

To obtain up-to-date information about the treatment of overdose, consult your Regional Poison Control Center. Telephone numbers of certified poison control centers are listed in the Physicians' Desk Reference (PDR). In managing overdose, consider the possibilities of multiple-drug overdoses, drug-drug interactions, and altered pharmacokinetics in your patient.

DOSAGE AND ADMINISTRATION

The usual recommended starting dose of candesartan cilexetil is 16 mg once daily when it is used as monotherapy in patients who are not volume depleted. ATACAND can be administered once or twice daily with total daily doses ranging from 8 mg to 32 mg. Patients requiring further reduction in blood pressure should be titrated to 32 mg. Doses larger than 32 mg do not appear to have a greater blood pressure lowering effect.

Hydrochlorothiazide is effective in doses of 12.5 to 50 mg once daily.

To minimize dose-independent side effects, it is usually appropriate to begin combination therapy only after a patient has failed to achieve the desired effect with monotherapy.

The side effects (see WARNINGS) of candesartan cilexetil are generally rare and apparently independent of dose; those of hydrochlorothiazide are a mixture of dose-dependent phenomena (primarily hypokalemia) and dose-independent phenomena (eg, pancreatitis), the former much more common than the latter.

Therapy with any combination of candesartan cilexetil and hydrochlorothiazide will be associated with both sets of dose-independent side effects.

Replacement Therapy: The combination may be substituted for the titrated components.

Dose Titration by Clinical Effect: A patient whose blood pressure is not controlled on 25 mg of hydrochlorothiazide once daily can expect an incremental effect from ATACAND HCT 16–12.5 mg. A patient whose blood pressure is controlled on 25 mg of hydrochlorothiazide but is experiencing decreases in serum potassium can expect the same or incremental blood pressure effects from ATACAND HCT 16–12.5 mg and serum potassium may improve.

A patient whose blood pressure is not controlled on 32 mg of ATACAND can expect incremental blood pressure effects from ATACAND HCT 32–12.5 mg and then 32–25 mg. The maximal antihypertensive effect of any dose of ATACAND HCT can be expected within 4 weeks of initiating that dose.

Patients with Renal Impairment: The usual regimens of therapy with ATACAND HCT may be followed as long as the patient's creatinine clearance is >30 mL/min. In patients with more severe renal impairment, loop diuretics are preferred to thiazides, so ATACAND HCT is not recommended.

Patients with Hepatic Impairment: Thiazide diuretics should be used with caution in patients with hepatic impairment; therefore, care should be exercised with dosing of ATACAND HCT.

ATACAND HCT may be administered with other antihypertensive agents.

ATACAND HCT may be administered with or without food.

HOW SUPPLIED

No. 3825 — Tablets ATACAND HCT 16–12.5, are peach, oval, biconvex, non-film-coated tablets, coded ACS on one side and 162 on the other. They are supplied as follows:

NDC 0186-0162-28 unit dose packages of 100.

NDC 0186-0162-54 unit of use bottles of 90.

No. 3826 — Tablets ATACAND HCT 32–12.5, are yellow, oval, biconvex, non-film-coated tablets, coded ACJ on one side and 322 on the other. They are supplied as follows:

NDC 0186-0322-28 unit dose packages of 100.

NDC 0186-0322-54 unit of use bottles of 90.

Storage

Store at 25°C (77°F); excursions permitted to 15–30°C (59–86°F) [see USP Controlled Room Temperature]. Keep container tightly closed.

ATACAND HCT is a trademark of the AstraZeneca Group

Issued September 2000

Manufactured under the license from Takeda Chemical Industries, Ltd.

by: AstraZeneca AB, S-151 85 Södertälje, Sweden

for: AstraZeneca LP, Wilmington, DE 19850

Made in Sweden

610517-00

NEXIUM™ ℞

(esomeprazole magnesium)

DELAYED-RELEASE CAPSULES

Rx only

DESCRIPTION

The active ingredient in NEXIUM™ (esomeprazole magnesium) Delayed-Release Capsules is bis(5-methoxy-2-[(S)-[(4-methoxy-3,5-dimethyl-2-pyridinyl)methyl]sulfinyl]-1*H*-benzimidazole-1-yl) magnesium trihydrate, a compound that inhibits gastric acid secretion. Esomeprazole is the S-isomer of omeprazole, which is a mixture of the S- and R-isomers. Its empirical formula is $(C_{17}H_{18}N_3O_3S)_2Mg \times 3\ H_2O$ with molecular weight of 767.2 as a trihydrate and 713.1 on an anhydrous basis. The structural formula is:

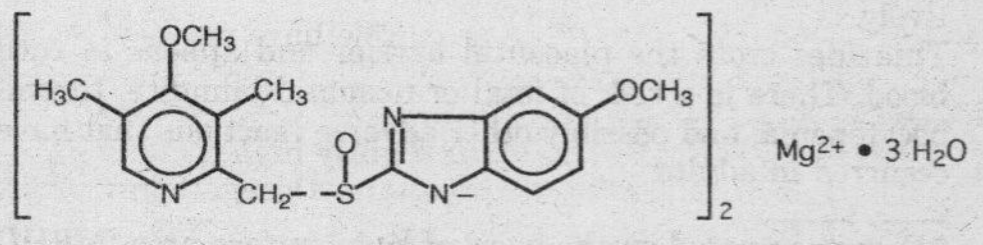

The magnesium salt is a white to slightly colored crystalline powder. It contains 3 moles of water of solvation and is slightly soluble in water.

The stability of esomeprazole magnesium is a function of pH; it rapidly degrades in acidic media, but it has acceptable stability under alkaline conditions. At pH 6.8 (buffer), the half-life of the magnesium salt is about 19 hours at 25°C and about 8 hours at 37°C.

NEXIUM is supplied as Delayed-Release Capsules for oral administration. Each delayed-release capsule contains 20 mg or 40 mg of esomeprazole (present as 22.3 mg or 44.5 mg esomeprazole magnesium trihydrate) in the form of enteric-coated pellets with the following inactive ingredients: glyceryl monostearate 40-50, hydroxypropyl cellulose, hydroxypropyl methylcellulose, magnesium stearate, methacrylic acid copolymer type C, polysorbate 80, sugar spheres, talc, and triethyl citrate. The capsule shells have the following inactive ingredients: gelatin, FD&C Blue #1, FD&C Red #40, D&C Red #28, titanium dioxide, shellac, ethyl alcohol, isopropyl alcohol, n-butyl alcohol, propylene glycol, sodium hydroxide, polyvinyl pyrrolidone, and D&C Yellow #10.

CLINICAL PHARMACOLOGY

Pharmacokinetics

Absorption

NEXIUM Delayed-Release Capsules contain an enteric-coated pellet formulation of esomeprazole magnesium. After oral administration peak plasma levels (C_{max}) occur at approximately 1.5 hours (T_{max}). The C_{max} increases proportionally when the dose is increased, and there is a three-fold increase in the area under the plasma concentration-time curve (AUC) from 20 to 40 mg. At repeated once-daily dosing with 40 mg, the systemic bioavailability is approximately 90% compared to 64% after a single dose of 40 mg. The mean exposure (AUC) to esomeprazole increases from 4.32 μmol*hr/L on day 1 to 11.2 μmol*hr/L on day 5 after 40 mg once daily dosing.

The AUC after administration of a single 40 mg dose of esomeprazole is decreased by 33–53% after food intake compared to fasting conditions. Esomeprazole should be taken at least one hour before meals.

The pharmacokinetic profile of esomeprazole was determined in 36 patients with symptomatic gastroesophageal reflux disease following repeated once daily administration of 20 mg and 40 mg capsules of NEXIUM over a period of five days. The results are shown in the following table:

Pharmacokinetic Parameters of NEXIUM Following Oral Dosing for 5 days

Parameter	NEXIUM 40 mg	NEXIUM 20 mg
AUC (µmol*h/L)	12.6	4.2
Coefficient of variation	42%	59%
C_{max} (µmol/L)	4.7	2.1
T_{max} (h)	1.6	1.6
$t_{1/2}$ (h)	1.5	1.2

Values represent the geometric mean, except the T_{max}, which is the arithmetic mean.

Distribution
Esomeprazole is 97% bound to plasma proteins. Plasma protein binding is constant over the concentration range of 2–20 µmol/L. The apparent volume of distribution at steady state in healthy volunteers is approximately 16 L.

Metabolism
Esomeprazole is extensively metabolized in the liver by the cytochrome P450 (CYP) enzyme system. The metabolites of esomeprazole lack antisecretory activity. The major part of esomeprazole's metabolism is dependent upon the CYP2C19 isoenzyme, which forms the hydroxy and desmethyl metabolites. The remaining amount is dependent on CYP3A4 which forms the sulphone metabolite. CYP2C19 isoenzyme exhibits polymorphism in the metabolism of esomeprazole, since some 3% of Caucasians and 15–20% of Asians lack CYP2C19 and are termed Poor metabolizers. At steady state, the ratio of AUC in Poor metabolizers to AUC in the rest of the population (Extensive metabolizers) is approximately 2.

Following administration of equimolar doses, the S- and R-isomers are metabolized differently by the liver, resulting in higher plasma levels of the S- than of the R-isomer.

Excretion
The plasma elimination half-life of esomeprazole is approximately 1–1.5 hours. Less than 1% of parent drug is excreted in the urine. Approximately 80% of an oral dose of esomeprazole is excreted as inactive metabolites in the urine, and the remainder is found as inactive metabolites in the feces.

Special Populations
Geriatric
The AUC and C_{max} values were slightly higher (25% and 18%, respectively) in the elderly as compared to younger subjects at steady state. Dosage adjustment based on age is not necessary.

Pediatric
The pharmacokinetics of esomeprazole have not been studied in patients < 18 years of age.

Gender
The AUC and C_{max} values were slightly higher (13%) in females than in males at steady state. Dosage adjustment based on gender is not necessary.

Hepatic Insufficiency
The steady state pharmacokinetics of esomeprazole obtained after administration of 40 mg once daily to 4 patients each with mild (Child Pugh A), moderate (Child Pugh Class B), and severe (Child Pugh Class C) liver insufficiency were compared to those obtained in 36 male and female GERD patients with normal liver function. In patients with mild and moderate hepatic insufficiency, the AUCs were within the range that could be expected in patients with normal liver function. In patients with severe hepatic insufficiency the AUCs were 2 to 3 times higher than in the patients with normal liver function. No dosage adjustment is recommended for patients with mild to moderate hepatic insufficiency (Child Pugh Classes A and B). However, in patients with severe hepatic insufficiency (Child Pugh Class C) a dose of 20 mg once daily should not be exceeded (See **DOSAGE AND ADMINISTRATION**).

Renal Insufficiency
The pharmacokinetics of esomeprazole in patients with renal impairment are not expected to be altered relative to healthy volunteers as less than 1% of esomeprazole is excreted unchanged in urine.

Pharmacokinetics: Combination Therapy with Antimicrobials
Esomeprazole magnesium 40 mg once daily was given in combination with clarithromycin 500 mg twice daily and amoxicillin 1000 mg twice daily for 7 days to 17 healthy male and female subjects. The mean steady state AUC and C_{max} of esomeprazole increased by 70% and 18%, respectively during triple combination therapy compared to treatment with esomeprazole alone. The observed increase in esomeprazole exposure during co-administration with clarithromycin and amoxicillin is not expected to produce significant safety concerns.

The pharmacokinetic parameters for clarithromycin and amoxicillin were similar during triple combination therapy and administration of each drug alone. However, the mean AUC and C_{max} for 14-hydroxyclarithromycin increased by 19% and 22%, respectively, during triple combination therapy compared to treatment with clarithromycin alone. This increase in exposure to 14-hydroxyclarithromycin is not considered to be clinically significant.

Pharmacodynamics
Mechanism of Action
Esomeprazole is a proton pump inhibitor that suppresses gastric acid secretion by specific inhibition of the H^+/K^+-ATPase in the gastric parietal cell. The S- and R-isomers are protonated and converted in the acidic compartment of the parietal cell forming the active inhibitor, the achiral sulphenamide. By acting specifically on the proton pump, esomeprazole blocks the final step in acid production, thus reducing gastric acidity. This effect is dose-related up to a daily dose of 20 to 40 mg and leads to inhibition of gastric acid secretion.

Antisecretory Activity
The effect of esomeprazole on intragastric pH was determined in patients with symptomatic gastroesophageal reflux disease in two separate studies. In the first study of 36 patients, NEXIUM 40 mg and 20 mg capsules were administered over 5 days. The results are shown in the following table:

Effect on Intragastric pH on Day 5 (N=36)

Parameter	NEXIUM 40 mg	NEXIUM 20 mg
% Time Gastric pH >4[†] (Hours)	70%* (16.8 h)	53% (12.7 h)
Coefficient of variation	26%	37%
Median 24 Hour pH	4.9*	4.1
Coefficient of variation	16%	27%

[†]Gastric pH was measured over a 24-hour period
*p< 0.01 NEXIUM 40 mg vs NEXIUM 20 mg

In a second study, the effect on intragastric pH of NEXIUM 40 mg administered once daily over a five day period was similar to the first study, (% time with pH>4 was 68% or 16.3 hours).

Serum Gastrin Effects
The effect of NEXIUM on serum gastrin concentrations was evaluated in approximately 2,700 patients in clinical trials up to 8 weeks and in over 1,300 patients for up to 6–12 months. The mean fasting gastrin level increased in a dose-related manner. This increase reached a plateau within two to three months of therapy and returned to baseline levels within four weeks after discontinuation of therapy.

Enterochromaffin-like (ECL) Cell Effects
In 24-month carcinogenicity studies of omeprazole in rats, a dose-related significant occurrence of gastric ECL cell carcinoid tumors and ECL cell hyperplasia was observed in both male and female animals (see **PRECAUTIONS**, Carcinogenesis, Mutagenesis, Impairment of Fertility). Carcinoid tumors have also been observed in rats subjected to fundectomy or long-term treatment with other proton pump inhibitors or high doses of H_2-receptor antagonists.

Human gastric biopsy specimens have been obtained from more than 3,000 patients treated with omeprazole in long-term clinical trials. The incidence of ECL cell hyperplasia in these studies increased with time; however, no case of ECL cell carcinoids, dysplasia, or neoplasia has been found in these patients.

In over 1,000 patients treated with NEXIUM (10, 20 or 40 mg/day) up to 6–12 months, the prevalence of ECL cell hyperplasia increased with time and dose. No patient developed ECL cell carcinoids, dysplasia, or neoplasia in the gastric mucosa.

Endocrine Effects
NEXIUM had no effect on thyroid function when given in oral doses of 20 or 40 mg for 4 weeks. Other effects of NEXIUM on the endocrine system were assessed using omeprazole studies. Omeprazole given in oral doses of 30 or 40 mg for 2 to 4 weeks had no effect on carbohydrate metabolism, circulating levels of parathyroid hormone, cortisol, estradiol, testosterone, prolactin, cholecystokinin or secretin.

Microbiology
Esomeprazole magnesium, amoxicillin and clarithromycin triple therapy has been shown to be active against most strains of *Helicobacter pylori (H. pylori)* in vitro and in clinical infections as described in the **Clinical Studies** and **INDICATIONS AND USAGE** sections.

Helicobacter
Helicobacter pylori
Susceptibility testing of *H. pylori* isolates was performed for amoxicillin and clarithromycin using agar dilution methodology, and minimum inhibitory concentrations (MICs) were determined.

Pretreatment Resistance
Clarithromycin pretreatment resistance rate (MIC ≥ 1 µg/mL) to *H. pylori* was 15% (66/445) at baseline in all treatment groups combined. A total of > 99% (394/395) of patients had *H. pylori* isolates which were considered to be susceptible (MIC ≤ 0.25 µg/mL) to amoxicillin at baseline. One patient had a baseline *H. pylori* isolate with an amoxicillin MIC = 0.5 µg /mL.

Clarithromycin Susceptibility Test Results and Clinical/Bacteriologic Outcomes
The baseline *H. pylori* clarithromycin susceptibility results and the *H. pylori* eradication results at the Day 38 visit are shown in the table below:

Clarithromycin Susceptibility Test Results and Clinical/Bacteriological Outcomes[a] for Triple Therapy - (Esomeprazole magnesium 40 mg once daily/amoxicillin 1000 mg twice daily/clarithromycin 500 mg twice daily for 10 days)

Clarithromycin Pretreatment Results	*H. pylori* negative (Eradicated)	*H. pylori* positive (Not Eradicated) Post-treatment susceptibility results			
		S[b]	I[b]	R[b]	No MIC
Susceptible[b] 182	162	4	0	2	14
Intermediate[b] 1	1	0	0	0	0
Resistant[b] 29	13	1	0	13	2

[a]Includes only patients with pretreatment and post-treatment clarithromycin susceptibility test results
[b]Susceptible (S) MIC ≤ 0.25 µg/mL, Intermediate (I) MIC =0.5 µg/mL, Resistant (R) MIC ≥ 1.0 µg/mL

Patients not eradicated of *H. pylori* following esomeprazole magnesium/amoxicillin/clarithromycin triple therapy will likely have clarithromycin resistant *H. pylori* isolates. Therefore, clarithromycin susceptibility testing should be done, when possible. Patients with clarithromycin resistant *H. pylori* should not be re-treated with a clarithromycin-containing regimen.

Amoxicillin Susceptibility Test Results and Clinical/Bacteriological Outcomes
In the esomeprazole magnesium/amoxicillin/clarithromycin clinical trials, 83% (176/212) of the patients in the esomeprazole magnesium/amoxicillin/clarithromycin treatment group who had pretreatment amoxicillin susceptible MICs (≤ 0.25 µg/mL) were eradicated of *H. pylori*, and 17% (36/212) were not eradicated of *H. pylori*. Of the 36 patients who were not eradicated of *H. pylori* on triple therapy, 16 had no post-treatment susceptibility test results and 20 had post-treatment *H. pylori* isolates with amoxicillin susceptible MICs. Fifteen of the patients who were not eradicated of *H. pylori* on triple therapy also had post-treatment *H. pylori* isolates with clarithromycin resistant MICs. There were no patients with *H. pylori* isolates who developed treatment emergent resistance to amoxicillin.

Susceptibility Test for Helicobacter pylori
The reference methodology for susceptibility testing of *H. pylori* is agar dilution MICs. One to three microliters of an inoculum equivalent to a No.2 McFarland standard (1×10^7 $- 1 \times 10^8$ CFU/mL for *H. pylori*) are inoculated directly onto freshly prepared antimicrobial containing Mueller-Hinton agar plates with 5% aged defibrinated sheep blood (≥ 2 weeks old). The agar dilution plates are incubated at 35°C in a microaerobic environment produced by a gas generating system suitable for *Campylobacter*. After 3 days of incubation, the MICs are recorded as the lowest concentration of antimicrobial agent required to inhibit growth of the organism. The clarithromycin and amoxicillin MIC values should be interpreted according to the following criteria:

Clarithromycin MIC (µg/mL)[a]	Interpretation	
≤ 0.25	Susceptible	(S)
0.5	Intermediate	(I)
≥ 1.0	Resistant	(R)
Amoxicillin MIC (µg/mL)[a,b]	Interpretation	
≤ 0.25	Susceptible	(S)

[a] These are breakpoints for the agar dilution methodology and they should not be used to interpret results obtained using alternative methods.
[b] There were not enough organisms with MICs > 0.25 µg/mL to determine a resistance breakpoint.

Standardized susceptibility test procedures require the use of laboratory control microorganisms to control the technical aspects of the laboratory procedures. Standard clarithromycin and amoxicillin powders should provide the following MIC values:

Microorganism	Antimicrobial Agent	MIC (µg/mL)[a]
H. pylori ATCC 43504	Clarithromycin	0.016–0.12 (µg/mL)
H. pylori ATCC 43504	Amoxicillin	0.016–0.12 (µg/mL)

[a]These are quality control ranges for the agar dilution methodology and they should not be used to control test results obtained using alternative methods.

Clinical Studies
Healing of Erosive Esophagitis
The healing rates of NEXIUM 40 mg, NEXIUM 20 mg, and omeprazole 20 mg (the approved dose for this indication) were evaluated in patients with endoscopically diagnosed erosive esophagitis in four multicenter, double-blind, randomized studies. The healing rates at weeks 4 and 8 were evaluated and are shown in the table below:

Continued on next page

Nexium—Cont.

[See table below]
In these same studies of patients with erosive esophagitis, sustained heartburn resolution and time to sustained heartburn resolution were evaluated and are shown in the table below:
[See table at bottom of next page]
In these four studies, the range of median days to the start of sustained resolution (defined as 7 consecutive days with no heartburn) was 5 days for NEXIUM 40 mg, 7–8 days for NEXIUM 20 mg and 7–9 days for omeprazole 20 mg.
There are no comparisons of 40 mg of NEXIUM with 40 mg of omeprazole in clinical trials assessing either healing or symptomatic relief of erosive esophagitis.
Long-Term Maintenance of Healing of Erosive Esophagitis
Two multicenter, randomized, double-blind placebo-controlled 4-arm trials were conducted in patients with endoscopically confirmed, healed erosive esophagitis to evaluate NEXIUM 40 mg (n=174), 20 mg (n=180), 10 mg (n=168) or placebo (n=171) once daily over six months of treatment.
No additional clinical benefit was seen with NEXIUM 40 mg over NEXIUM 20 mg.
The percentage of patients that maintained healing of erosive esophagitis at the various time points are shown in the figures below:

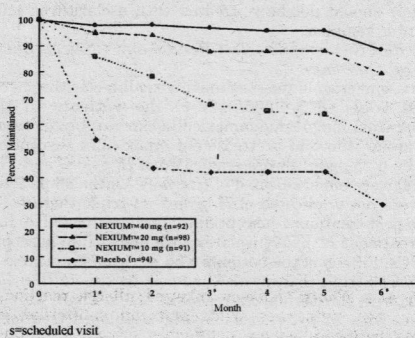

Maintenance of Healing Rates by Month (Study 177)

s=scheduled visit

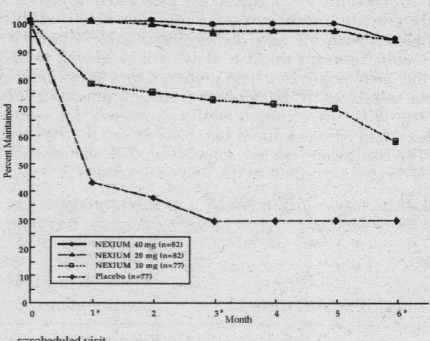

Maintenance of Healing Rates by Month (Study 178)

s=scheduled visit

Patients remained in remission significantly longer and the number of recurrences of erosive esophagitis was significantly less in patients treated with NEXIUM compared to placebo.
In both studies, the proportion of patients on NEXIUM who remained in remission and were free of heartburn and other GERD symptoms was well differentiated from placebo.
In a third multicenter open label study of 808 patients treated for 12 months with NEXIUM 40 mg, the percentage of patients that maintained healing of erosive esophagitis was 93.7% for six months and 89.4% for one year.
Symptomatic Gastroesophageal Reflux Disease (GERD)
Two multicenter, randomized, double-blind, placebo-controlled studies were conducted in a total of 717 patients

comparing four weeks of treatment with NEXIUM 20 mg or 40 mg once daily versus placebo for resolution of GERD symptoms. Patients had ≥ 6-month history of heartburn episodes, no erosive esophagitis by endoscopy, and heartburn on at least four of the seven days immediately preceding randomization.
The percentage of patients that were symptom-free of heartburn was significantly higher in the NEXIUM groups compared to placebo at all follow-up visits (Weeks 1, 2, and 4). No additional clinical benefit was seen with NEXIUM 40 mg over NEXIUM 20 mg.
The percent of patients symptom-free of heartburn by day are shown in the figures below:

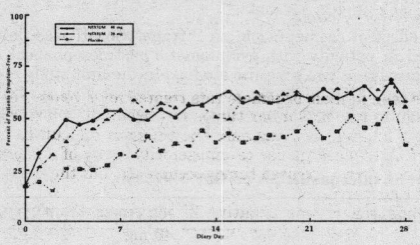

Percent of Patients Symptom-Free of Heartburn by Day
(Study 225)

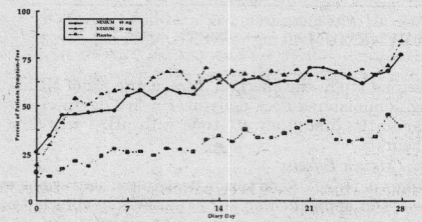

Percent of Patients Symptom-Free of Heartburn by Day
(Study 226)

In three European symptomatic GERD trials, NEXIUM 20 mg and 40 mg and omeprazole 20 mg were evaluated. No significant treatment related differences were seen.
Helicobacter pylori (H. pylori) Eradication in Patients with Duodenal Ulcer Disease
Triple Therapy (NEXIUM/amoxicillin/clarithromycin):
Two multicenter, randomized, double-blind studies were conducted using a 10 day treatment regimen. The first study (191) compared NEXIUM 40 mg once daily in combination with amoxicillin 1000 mg twice daily and clarithromycin 500 mg twice daily to NEXIUM 40 mg once daily plus clarithromycin 500 mg twice daily. The second study (193) compared NEXIUM 40 mg once daily in combination with amoxicillin 1000 mg twice daily and clarithromycin 500 mg twice daily to NEXIUM 40 mg once daily. *H. pylori* eradication rates, defined as at least two negative tests and no positive tests from CLOtest®, histology and/or culture, at 4 weeks post-therapy were significantly higher in the NEXIUM plus amoxicillin and clarithromycin group than in the NEXIUM plus clarithromycin or NEXIUM alone group. The results are shown in the following table:

**H. pylori Eradication Rates at 4 Weeks after 10 Day
Treatment Regimen
% of Patients Cured
[95% Confidence Interval]
(Number of patients)**

Study	Treatment Group	Per-Protocol[†]	Intent-to-Treat[‡]
191	NEXIUM plus amoxicillin and clarithromycin	84%* [78, 89] (n=196)	77%* [71, 82] (n=233)
	NEXIUM plus clarithromycin	55% [48, 62] (n=187)	52% [45, 59] (n=215)
193	NEXIUM plus amoxicillin and clarithromycin	85%** [74, 93] (n=67)	78%** [67, 87] (n=74)
	NEXIUM	5% [0, 23] (n=22)	4% [0, 21] (n=24)

[†]Patients were included in the analysis if they had *H. pylori* infection documented at baseline, had at least one endoscopically verified duodenal ulcer ≥ 0.5 cm in diameter at baseline or had a documented history of duodenal ulcer disease within the past 5 years, and were not protocol violators. Patients who dropped out of the study due to an adverse event related to the study drug were included in the analysis as not *H. pylori* eradicated.
[‡]Patients were included in the analysis if they had documented *H. pylori* infection at baseline, had at least one documented duodenal ulcer at baseline, or had a documented history of duodenal ulcer disease, and took at least one dose of study medication. All dropouts were included as not *H. pylori* eradicated.
*p < 0.05 compared to NEXIUM plus clarithromycin
**p < 0.05 compared to NEXIUM alone

The percentage of patients with a healed baseline duodenal ulcer by 4 weeks after the 10 day treatment regimen in the NEXIUM plus amoxicillin and clarithromycin group was 75% (n=156) and 57% (n=60) respectively, in the 191 and 193 studies (per-protocol analysis).

INDICATIONS AND USAGE
Treatment of Gastroesophageal Reflux Disease (GERD)
Healing of Erosive Esophagitis
NEXIUM is indicated for the short-term treatment (4 to 8 weeks) in the healing and symptomatic resolution of diagnostically confirmed erosive esophagitis. For those patients who have not healed after 4–8 weeks of treatment, an additional 4–8-week course of NEXIUM may be considered.
Maintenance of Healing of Erosive Esophagitis
NEXIUM is indicated to maintain symptom resolution and healing of erosive esophagitis. Controlled studies do not extend beyond 6 months.
Symptomatic Gastroesophageal Reflux Disease
NEXIUM is indicated for treatment of heartburn and other symptoms associated with GERD.
H. pylori Eradication to Reduce the Risk of Duodenal Ulcer Recurrence
Triple Therapy (NEXIUM plus amoxicillin and clarithromycin): NEXIUM, in combination with amoxicillin and clarithromycin, is indicated for the treatment of patients with *H. pylori* infection and duodenal ulcer disease (active or history of within the past 5 years) to eradicate *H. pylori*. Eradication of *H. pylori* has been shown to reduce the risk of duodenal ulcer recurrence. (See **Clinical Studies** and **DOSAGE AND ADMINISTRATION**.)
In patients who fail therapy, susceptibility testing should be done. If resistance to clarithromycin is demonstrated or susceptibility testing is not possible, alternative antimicrobial therapy should be instituted. (See **CLINICAL PHARMACOLOGY, Microbiology** and the clarithromycin package insert, **CLINICAL PHARMACOLOGY, Microbiology**.)

CONTRAINDICATIONS
NEXIUM is contraindicated in patients with known hypersensitivity to any component of the formulation or to substituted benzimidazoles.
Clarithromycin is contraindicated in patients with a known hypersensitivity to any macrolide antibiotic.
Concomitant administration of clarithromycin with pimozide is contraindicated. There have been post-marketing reports of drug interactions when clarithromycin and/or erythromycin are co-administered with pimozide resulting in cardiac arrhythmias (QT prolongation, ventricular tachycardia, ventricular fibrillation, and torsade de pointes) most likely due to inhibition of hepatic metabolism of pimozide by erythromycin and clarithromycin. Fatalities have been reported. (Please refer to full prescribing information for clarithromycin.)
Amoxicillin is contraindicated in patients with a known hypersensitivity to any penicillin. (Please refer to full prescribing information for amoxicillin.)

WARNINGS
CLARITHROMYCIN SHOULD NOT BE USED IN PREGNANT WOMEN EXCEPT IN CLINICAL CIRCUMSTANCES WHERE NO ALTERNATIVE THERAPY IS APPROPRIATE. IF PREGNANCY OCCURS WHILE TAKING CLARITHROMYCIN, THE PATIENT SHOULD BE APPRISED OF THE POTENTIAL HAZARD TO THE FETUS. (See WARNINGS in prescribing information for clarithromycin.)
Amoxicillin: Serious and occasionally fatal hypersensitivity (anaphylactic) reactions have been reported in patients on penicillin therapy. These reactions are more apt to occur in individuals with a history of penicillin hypersensitivity and/or a history of sensitivity to multiple allergens.
There have been well documented reports of individuals with a history of penicillin hypersensitivity reactions who have experienced severe hypersensitivity reactions when treated with a cephalosporin. Before initiating therapy with any penicillin, careful inquiry should be made concerning previous hypersensitivity reactions to penicillins, cephalosporins, and other allergens. If an allergic reaction occurs, amoxicillin should be discontinued and the appropriate therapy instituted.
SERIOUS ANAPHYLACTIC REACTIONS REQUIRE IMMEDIATE EMERGENCY TREATMENT WITH EPINEPH-

Erosive Esophagitis Healing Rate (Life-Table Analysis)

Study	No. of Patients	Treatment Groups	Week 4	Week 8	Significance Level*
1	588	NEXIUM 20 mg	68.7%	90.6%	N.S.
	588	Omeprazole 20 mg	69.5%	88.3%	
2	654	NEXIUM 40 mg	75.9%	94.1%	p < 0.001
	656	NEXIUM 20 mg	70.5%	89.9%	p < 0.05
	650	Omeprazole 20 mg	64.7%	86.9%	
3	576	NEXIUM 40 mg	71.5%	92.2%	N.S.
	572	Omeprazole 20 mg	68.6%	89.8%	
4	1216	NEXIUM 40 mg	81.7%	93.7%	p < 0.001
	1209	Omeprazole 20 mg	68.7%	84.2%	

*log-rank test vs omeprazole 20 mg
N.S. = not significant (p > 0.05).

RINE. OXYGEN, INTRAVENOUS STEROIDS, AND AIRWAY MANAGEMENT, INCLUDING INTUBATION, SHOULD ALSO BE ADMINISTERED AS INDICATED.

Pseudomembranous colitis has been reported with nearly all antibacterial agents, including clarithromycin and amoxicillin, and may range in severity from mild to life threatening. Therefore, it is important to consider this diagnosis in patients who present with diarrhea subsequent to the administration of antibacterial agents.

Treatment with antibacterial agents alters the normal flora of the colon and may permit overgrowth of clostridia. Studies indicate that a toxin produced by *Clostridium difficile* is a primary cause of "antibiotic-associated colitis".

After the diagnosis of pseudomembranous colitis has been established, therapeutic measures should be initiated. Mild cases of pseudomembranous colitis usually respond to discontinuation of the drug alone. In moderate to severe cases, consideration should be given to management with fluids and electrolytes, protein supplementation, and treatment with an antibacterial drug clinically effective against *Clostridium difficile colitis*.

PRECAUTIONS

General

Symptomatic response to therapy with NEXIUM does not preclude the presence of gastric malignancy.

Atrophic gastritis has been noted occasionally in gastric corpus biopsies from patients treated long-term with omeprazole, of which NEXIUM is an enantiomer.

Information for Patients

Patients should be informed of the following:

NEXIUM Delayed-Release Capsules should be taken at least one hour before meals.

For patients who have difficulty swallowing capsules, one tablespoon of applesauce can be added to an empty bowl and the NEXIUM Delayed-Release Capsule can be opened, and the pellets inside the capsule carefully emptied onto the applesauce. The pellets should be mixed with the applesauce and then swallowed immediately. The applesauce used should not be hot and should be soft enough to be swallowed without chewing. The pellets should not be chewed or crushed. The pellet/applesauce mixture should not be stored for future use.

Antacids may be used while taking NEXIUM.

Drug Interactions

Esomeprazole is extensively metabolized in the liver by CYP2C19 and CYP3A4.

In vitro and *in vivo* studies have shown that esomeprazole is not likely to inhibit CYPs 1A2, 2A6, 2C9, 2D6, 2E1 and 3A4. No clinically relevant interactions with drugs metabolized by these CYP enzymes would be expected. Drug interaction studies have shown that esomeprazole does not have any clinically significant interactions with phenytoin, warfarin, quinidine, clarithromycin or amoxicillin.

Esomeprazole may potentially interfere with CYP2C19, the major esomeprazole metabolizing enzyme. Coadministration of esomeprazole 30 mg and diazepam, a CYP2C19 substrate, resulted in a 45% decrease in clearance of diazepam. Increased plasma levels of diazepam were observed 12 hours after dosing and onwards. However, at that time, the plasma levels of diazepam were below the therapeutic interval, and thus this interaction is unlikely to be of clinical relevance.

Esomeprazole inhibits gastric acid secretion. Therefore, esomeprazole may interfere with the absorption of drugs where gastric pH is an important determinant of bioavailability (e.g., ketoconazole, iron salts and digoxin).

Coadministration of oral contraceptives, diazepam, phenytoin, or quinidine did not seem to change the pharmacokinetic profile of esomeprazole.

Combination Therapy with Clarithromycin

Co-administration of esomeprazole, clarithromycin, and amoxicillin has resulted in increases in the plasma levels of esomeprazole and 14-hydroxyclarithromycin. (See **CLINICAL PHARMACOLOGY, Pharmacokinetics: Combination Therapy with Antimicrobials.**)

Concomitant administration of clarithromycin with pimozide is contraindicated. (See clarithromycin package insert.)

Carcinogenesis, Mutagenesis, Impairment of Fertility

The carcinogenic potential of esomeprazole was assessed using omeprazole studies. In two 24-month oral carcinogenicity studies in rats, omeprazole at daily doses of 1.7, 3.4, 13.8, 44.0 and 140.8 mg/kg/day (about 0.7 to 57 times the human dose of 20 mg/day expressed on a body surface area basis) produced gastric ECL cell carcinoids in a dose-related manner in both male and female rats; the incidence of this effect was markedly higher in female rats, which had higher blood levels of omeprazole. Gastric carcinoids seldom occur in the untreated rat. In addition, ECL cell hyperplasia was present in all treated groups of both sexes. In one of these studies, female rats were treated with 13.8 mg omeprazole/kg/day (about 5.6 times the human dose on a body surface area basis) for 1 year, then followed for an additional year without the drug. No carcinoids were seen in these rats. An increased incidence of treatment-related ECL cell hyperplasia was observed at the end of 1 year (94% treated vs 10% controls). By the second year the difference between treated and control rats was much smaller (46% vs 26%) but still showed more hyperplasia in the treated group. Gastric adenocarcinoma was seen in one rat (2%). No similar tumor was seen in male or female rats treated for 2 years. For this strain of rat, no similar tumor has been noted historically, but a finding involving only one tumor is difficult to interpret. A 78-week mouse carcinogenicity study of omeprazole did not show increased tumor occurrence, but the study was not conclusive.

Esomeprazole was negative in the Ames mutation test, in the *in vivo* rat bone marrow cell chromosome aberration test, and the *in vivo* mouse micronucleus test. Esomeprazole, however, was positive in the *in vitro* human lymphocyte chromosome aberration test. Omeprazole was positive in the *in vitro* human lymphocyte chromosome aberration test, the *in vivo* mouse bone marrow cell chromosome aberration test, and the *in vivo* mouse micronucleus test.

The potential effects of esomeprazole on fertility and reproductive performance were assessed using omeprazole studies. Omeprazole at oral doses up to 138 mg/kg/day in rats (about 56 times the human dose on a body surface area basis) was found to have no effect on reproductive performance of parental animals.

Pregnancy

Teratogenic Effects. Pregnancy Category B

Teratology studies have been performed in rats at oral doses up to 280 mg/kg/day (about 57 times the human dose on a body surface area basis) and in rabbits at oral doses up to 86 mg/kg/day (about 35 times the human dose on a body surface area basis) and have revealed no evidence of impaired fertility or harm to the fetus due to esomeprazole. There are, however, no adequate and well-controlled studies in pregnant women. Because animal reproduction studies are not always predictive of human response, this drug should be used during pregnancy only if clearly needed.

Teratology studies conducted with omeprazole in rats at oral doses up to 138 mg/kg/day (about 56 times the human dose on a body surface area basis) and in rabbits at doses up to 69 mg/kg/day (about 56 times the human dose on a body surface area basis) did not disclose any evidence for a teratogenic potential of omeprazole. In rabbits, omeprazole in a dose range of 6.9 to 69.1 mg/kg/day (about 5.5 to 56 times the human dose on a body surface area basis) produced dose-related increases in embryo-lethality, fetal resorptions, and pregnancy disruptions. In rats, dose-related embryo/fetal toxicity and postnatal developmental toxicity were observed in offspring resulting from parents treated with omeprazole at 13.8 to 138.0 mg/kg/day (about 5.6 to 56 times the human doses on a body surface area basis). There are no adequate and well-controlled studies in pregnant women. Sporadic reports have been received of congenital abnormalities occurring in infants born to women who have received omeprazole during pregnancy.

Amoxicillin

Pregnancy Category B. See full prescribing information for amoxicillin before using in pregnant women.

Clarithromycin

Pregnancy Category C. See **WARNINGS** (above) and full prescribing information for clarithromycin before using in pregnant women.

Nursing Mothers

The excretion of esomeprazole in milk has not been studied. However, omeprazole concentrations have been measured in breast milk of a woman following oral administration of 20 mg. Because esomeprazole is likely to be excreted in human milk, because of the potential for serious adverse reactions in nursing infants from esomeprazole, and because of the potential for tumorigenicity shown for omeprazole in rat carcinogenicity studies, a decision should be made whether to discontinue nursing or to discontinue the drug, taking into account the importance of the drug to the mother.

Pediatric Use

Safety and effectiveness in pediatric patients have not been established.

Geriatric Use

Of the total number of patients who received NEXIUM in clinical trials, 778 were 65 to 74 years of age and 124 patients were ≥ 75 years of age.

No overall differences in safety and efficacy were observed between the elderly and younger individuals, and other reported clinical experience has not identified differences in responses between the elderly and younger patients, but greater sensitivity of some older individuals cannot be ruled out.

ADVERSE REACTIONS

The safety of NEXIUM was evaluated in over 10,000 patients (aged 18–84 years) in clinical trials worldwide including over 7,400 patients in the United States and over 2,600 patients in Europe and Canada. Over 2,900 patients were treated in long-term studies for up to 6–12 months. In general, NEXIUM was well tolerated in both short and long-term clinical trials.

The safety in the treatment of healing of erosive esophagitis was assessed in four randomized comparative clinical trials, which included 1,240 patients on NEXIUM 20 mg, 2,434 patients on NEXIUM 40 mg, and 3,008 patients on omeprazole 20 mg daily. The most frequently occurring adverse events (≥1%) in all three groups was headache (5.5, 5.0, and 3.8, respectively) and diarrhea (no difference among the three groups). Nausea, flatulence, abdominal pain, constipation, and dry mouth occurred at similar rates among patients taking NEXIUM or omeprazole.

Additional adverse events that were reported as possibly or probably related to NEXIUM with an incidence < 1% are listed below by body system:

Body as a Whole: abdomen enlarged, allergic reaction, asthenia, back pain, chest pain, chest pain substernal, facial edema, peripheral edema, hot flushes, fatigue, fever, flu-like disorder, generalized edema, leg edema, malaise, pain, rigors; ***Cardiovascular:*** flushing, hypertension, tachycardia; ***Endocrine:*** goiter; ***Gastrointestinal:*** bowel irregularity, constipation aggravated, dyspepsia, dysphagia, dysplasia GI, epigastric pain, eructation, esophageal disorder, frequent stools, gastroenteritis, GI hemorrhage, GI symptoms not otherwise specified, hiccup, melena, mouth disorder, pharynx disorder, rectal disorder, serum gastrin increased, tongue disorder, tongue edema, ulcerative stomatitis, vomiting; ***Hearing:*** earache, tinnitus; ***Hematologic:*** anemia, anemia hypochromic, cervical lymphoadenopathy, epistaxis, leukocytosis, leukopenia, thrombocytopenia; ***Hepatic:*** bilirubinemia, hepatic function abnormal, SGOT increased, SGPT increased; ***Metabolic/Nutritional:*** glycosuria, hyperuricemia, hyponatremia, increased alkaline phosphatase, thirst, vitamin B12 deficiency, weight increase, weight decrease; ***Musculoskeletal:*** arthralgia, arthritis aggravated, arthropathy, cramps, fibromyalgia syndrome, hernia, polymyalgia rheumatica; ***Nervous System/Psychiatric:*** anorexia, apathy, appetite increased, confusion, depression aggravated, dizziness, hypertonia, nervousness, hypoesthesia, impotence, insomnia, migraine, migraine aggravated, paresthesia, sleep disorder, somnolence, tremor, vertigo, visual field defect; ***Reproductive:*** dysmenorrhea, menstrual disorder, vaginitis; ***Respiratory:*** asthma aggravated, coughing, dyspnea, larynx edema, pharyngitis, rhinitis, sinusitis; ***Skin and Appendages:*** acne, angioedema, dermatitis, pruritus, pruritus ani, rash, rash erythematous, rash maculo-papular, skin inflammation, sweating increased, urticaria; ***Special Senses:*** otitis media, parosmia, taste loss, taste perversion; ***Urogenital:*** abnormal urine, albuminuria, cystitis, dysuria, fungal infection, hematuria, micturition frequency, moniliasis, genital moniliasis, polyuria; ***Visual:*** conjunctivitis, vision abnormal.

Endoscopic findings that were reported as adverse events include: duodenitis, esophagitis, esophageal stricture, esophageal ulceration, esophageal varices, gastric ulcer, gastritis, hernia, benign polyps or nodules, Barrett's esophagus, and mucosal discoloration.

The incidence of treatment-related adverse events during 6-month maintenance treatment was similar to placebo. There were no differences in types of related adverse events seen during maintenance treatment up to 12 months compared to short-term treatment.

Two placebo-controlled studies were conducted in 710 patients for the treatment of symptomatic gastroesophageal reflux disease. The most common adverse events that were reported as possibly or probably related to NEXIUM were diarrhea (4.3%), headache (3.8%), and abdominal pain (3.8%).

Other adverse events not observed with NEXIUM, but occurring with omeprazole can be found in the omeprazole package insert, **ADVERSE REACTIONS** section.

Combination Treatment with Amoxicillin and Clarithromycin

In clinical trials using combination therapy with NEXIUM plus amoxicillin and clarithromycin, no adverse events pe-

Continued on next page

Sustained Resolution‡ of Heartburn (Erosive Esophagitis Patients)

Study	No. of Patients	Treatment Groups	Cumulative Percent# with Sustained Resolution: Day 14	Day 28	Significance Level*
1	573 555	NEXIUM 20 mg Omeprazole 20 mg	64.3% 64.1%	72.7% 70.9%	N.S.
2	621 620 626	NEXIUM 40 mg NEXIUM 20 mg Omeprazole 20 mg	64.8% 62.9% 56.5%	74.2% 70.1% 66.6%	p <0.001 N.S.
3	568 551	NEXIUM 40 mg Omeprazole 20 mg	65.4% 65.5%	73.9% 73.1%	N.S.
4	1187 1188	NEXIUM 40 mg Omeprazole 20 mg	67.6% 62.5%	75.1% 70.8%	p <0.001

‡Defined as 7 consecutive days with no heartburn reported in daily patient diary.
#Defined as the cumulative proportion of patients who have reached the start of sustained resolution
*log-rank test vs omeprazole 20 mg
N.S. = not significant (p > 0.05).

Nexium—Cont.

culiar to these drug combinations were observed. Adverse events that occurred have been limited to those that had been observed with either NEXIUM, amoxicillin, or clarithromycin alone.

The most frequently reported drug-related adverse events for patients who received triple therapy for 10 days were diarrhea (9.2%), taste perversion (6.6%), and abdominal pain (3.7%). No treatment-emergent adverse events were observed at higher rates with triple therapy than were observed with NEXIUM alone.

For more information on adverse events with amoxicillin or clarithromycin, refer to their package inserts, **ADVERSE REACTIONS** section.

Laboratory Events

The following potentially clinically significant laboratory changes in clinical trials, irrespective of relationship to NEXIUM, were reported in ≤ 1% of patients: increased creatinine, uric acid, total bilirubin, alkaline phosphatase, ALT, AST, hemoglobin, white blood cell count, platelets, serum gastrin, potassium, sodium, thyroxine and thyroid stimulating hormone (see **CLINICAL PHARMACOLOGY**, *Endocrine Effects* for further information on thyroid effects). Decreases were seen in hemoglobin, white blood cell count, platelets, potassium, sodium, and thyroxine.

In clinical trials using combination therapy with NEXIUM plus amoxicillin and clarithromycin, no additional increased laboratory abnormalities particular to these drug combinations were observed.

For more information on laboratory changes with amoxicillin or clarithromycin, refer to their package inserts, **ADVERSE REACTIONS** section.

OVERDOSAGE

A single oral dose of esomeprazole at 510 mg/kg (about 103 times the human dose on a body surface area basis), was lethal to rats. The major signs of acute toxicity were reduced motor activity, changes in respiratory frequency, tremor, ataxia, and intermittent clonic convulsions.

There have been no reports of overdose with esomeprazole. Reports have been received of overdosage with omeprazole in humans. Doses ranged up to 2,400 mg (120 times the usual recommended clinical dose). Manifestations were variable, but included confusion, drowsiness, blurred vision, tachycardia, nausea, diaphoresis, flushing, headache, dry mouth, and other adverse reactions similar to those seen in normal clinical experience (see omeprazole package insert - **ADVERSE REACTIONS**). No specific antidote for esomeprazole is known. Since esomeprazole is extensively protein bound, it is not expected to be removed by dialysis. In the event of overdosage, treatment should be symptomatic and supportive.

As with the management of any overdose, the possibility of multiple drug ingestion should be considered. For current information on treatment of any drug overdose, a certified Regional Poison Control Center should be contacted. Telephone numbers are listed in the Physicians' Desk Reference (PDR) or local telephone book.

DOSAGE AND ADMINISTRATION

The recommended adult dosages are outlined in the table below. NEXIUM Delayed-Release Capsules should be swallowed whole and taken at least one hour before eating.

For patients who have difficulty swallowing capsules, one tablespoon of applesauce can be added to an empty bowl and the NEXIUM Delayed-Release Capsule can be opened, and the pellets inside the capsule carefully emptied onto the applesauce. The pellets should be mixed with the applesauce and then swallowed immediately. The applesauce used should not be hot and should be soft enough to be swallowed without chewing. The pellets should not be chewed or crushed. The pellet/applesauce mixture should not be stored for future use.

The pellets have also been shown *in vitro* to remain intact when exposed to tap water, orange juice, apple juice and yogurt.

Recommended Adult Dosage Schedule of NEXIUM

Indication	Dose	Frequency
Gastroesophageal Reflux Disease (GERD)		
Healing of Erosive Esophagitis	20 mg or 40 mg	Once Daily for 4 to 8 Weeks*
Maintenance of Healing of Erosive Esophagitis	20 mg	Once Daily**
Symptomatic Gastroesophageal Reflux Disease	20 mg	Once Daily for 4 Weeks***
***H. pylori* Eradication to Reduce the Risk of Duodenal Ulcer Recurrence**		
Triple Therapy:		
NEXIUM	40 mg	Once Daily for 10 Days
Amoxicillin	1000 mg	Twice Daily for 10 Days
Clarithromycin	500 mg	Twice Daily for 10 Days

* (see **CLINICAL STUDIES**). The majority of patients are healed within 4 to 8 weeks. For patients who do not heal

after 4–8 weeks, an additional 4–8 weeks of treatment may be considered.
** Controlled studies did not extend beyond six months.
*** If symptoms do not resolve completely after 4 weeks, an additional 4 weeks of treatment may be considered.

Please refer to amoxicillin and clarithromycin full prescribing information for **CONTRAINDICATIONS, WARNINGS** and dosing in elderly and renally-impaired patients.

Special Populations

Geriatric: No dosage adjustment is necessary. (See **CLINICAL PHARMACOLOGY, Pharmacokinetics**.)

Renal Insufficiency: No dosage adjustment is necessary. (See **CLINICAL PHARMACOLOGY, Pharmacokinetics**.)

Hepatic Insufficiency: No dosage adjustment is necessary in patients with mild to moderate liver impairment (Child Pugh Classes A and B). For patients with severe liver impairment (Child Pugh Class C), a dose of 20 mg of NEXIUM should not be exceeded (See **CLINICAL PHARMACOLOGY, Pharmacokinetics**.)

Gender: No dosage adjustment is necessary. (See **CLINICAL PHARMACOLOGY, Pharmacokinetics**.)

HOW SUPPLIED

NEXIUM Delayed-Release Capsules, 20 mg, are opaque, hard gelatin, amethyst colored capsules with two radial bars in yellow on the cap and 20 mg in yellow on the body. They are supplied as follows:
NDC 0186-5020-31 unit of use bottles of 30
NDC 0186-5022-28 unit dose packages of 100
NDC 0186-5020-54 bottles of 90
NDC 0186-5020-68 bottles of 100
NDC 0186-5020-82 bottles of 1000
NEXIUM Delayed-Release Capsules, 40 mg, are opaque, hard gelatin, amethyst colored capsules with three radial bars in yellow on the cap and 40 mg in yellow on the body. They are supplied as follows:
NDC 0186-5040-31 unit of use bottles of 30
NDC 0186-5042-28 unit dose packages of 100
NDC 0186-5040-68 bottles of 100
NDC 0186-5040-82 bottles of 1000

Storage

Store at 25°C (77°F); excursions permitted to 15–30°C (59–86°F). [See USP Controlled Room Temperature]. Keep container tightly closed. Dispense in a tight container if the product package is subdivided.

REFERENCES

1. National Committee for Clinical Laboratory Standards. Methods for Dilution Antimicrobial Susceptibility Tests for Bacteria That Grow Aerobically. Fifth Edition: Approved Standard NCCLS Document M7-A5, Vol. 20, no. 2, NCCLS, Wayne, PA, January 2000.
NEXIUM is a trademark of the AstraZeneca group
©AstraZeneca 2001
Manufactured for:
AstraZeneca LP
Wilmington, DE 19850
By: AstraZeneca AB
Sodertalje, Sweden
Product of France

Axcan Scandipharm Inc.
22 INVERNESS PARKWAY
BIRMINGHAM, AL 35242

Direct Inquiries to:
Customer Service
(800) 950-8085
Fax: (205) 991-8426
For Medical Information Contact:
John S. Cipriano, M.S., R.Ph.
(205) 991-8085
Fax: (205) 991-8047

CANASA™ ℞
(Mesalamine)
Rectal Suppositories 500 mg
NDC 58914-500-56
Rx Only

DESCRIPTION

The active ingredient in CANASA™, is mesalamine, also known as 5-aminosalicylic acid (5-ASA). Chemically, mesalamine is 5-amino-2-hydroxybenzoic acid, and is classified as an anti-inflammatory drug.
The empirical formula is $C_7H_7NO_3$, representing a molecular weight of 153.14. The structural formula is:

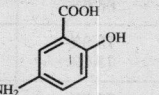

Each CANASA™ Rectal Suppository contains 500 mg of mesalamine in a base of Hard Fat NF.

CLINICAL PHARMACOLOGY

Sulfasalazine has been used in the treatment of ulcerative colitis for over 55 years. It is split by bacterial action in the colon into sulfapyridine (SP) and mesalamine (5-ASA). It is thought that the mesalamine component only is therapeutically active in ulcerative colitis.

Mechanism of Action

The mechanism of action of mesalamine (and sulfasalazine) is unknown, but appears to be topical rather than systemic. Although the pathology of inflammatory bowel disease is uncertain, both prostaglandins and leukotrienes have been implicated as mediators of mucosal injury and inflammation. Recently, however, the role of mesalamine as a free radical scavenger or inhibitor of tumor necrosis factor (TNF) has also been postulated.

Pharmacokinetics

Absorption: Mesalamine (5-ASA) administered as a rectal suppository is variably absorbed. In patients with ulcerative colitis treated with mesalamine 500 mg rectal suppositories, administered once every eight hours for six days, the mean mesalamine peak plasma concentration (C_{max}) was 353 ng/mL (CV=55%) following the initial dose and 361 ng/mL (CV=67%) at steady state. The mean minimum steady state plasma concentration (C_{min}) was 89 ng/mL (CV=89%). Absorbed mesalamine does not accumulate in the plasma.

Distribution: Mesalamine administered as rectal suppositories distributes in rectal tissue to some extent. In patients with ulcerative proctitis treated with CANASA™ 500 mg rectal suppositories, rectal tissue concentrations for 5-ASA and N-acetyl-5-ASA have not been rigorously quantified.

Metabolism: Mesalamine is extensively metabolized, mainly to N-acetyl-5-ASA. The site of metabolism has not been elucidated. In patients with ulcerative colitis treated with one 500 mg mesalamine rectal suppository every eight hours for six days, peak concentration (C_{max}) of N-acetyl-5-ASA ranged from 467 ng/mL to 1399 ng/mL following the initial dose and from 193 ng/mL to 1304 ng/mL at steady state.

Elimination: Mesalamine is eliminated from plasma mainly by urinary excretion, predominantly as N-acetyl-5-ASA. In patients with ulcerative proctitis treated with one mesalamine 500 mg rectal suppository every eight hours for six days, ≤12% of the dose was eliminated in urine as 5-ASA and 8–77% as N-acetyl-5-ASA following the initial dose. At steady state, ≤ 11% of the dose was eliminated as 5-ASA and 3–35% as N-acetyl-5-ASA. The mean elimination half-life was five hours (CV=73%) for 5-ASA and six hours (CV=63%) for N-acetyl-5-ASA following the initial dose. At steady state, the mean elimination half-life was seven hours for both 5-ASA and N-acetyl-5-ASA (CV=102% for 5-ASA and 82% for N-acetyl-5-ASA).

Drug-Drug Interactions: The potential for interactions between mesalamine, administered as 500 mg rectal suppositories, and other drugs has not been studied.

Special Populations (Patients with Renal or Hepatic Impairment): The effect of renal or hepatic impairment on elimination of mesalamine in ulcerative proctitis patients treated with mesalamine 500 mg suppositories has not been studied.

Preclinical Toxicology

Preclinical studies of mesalamine were conducted in rats, mice, rabbits and dogs and kidney was the main target organ of toxicity. In rats, adverse renal effects were observed at a single oral dose of 600 mg/kg (about 3.2 times the recommended human intra-rectal dose, based on body surface area) and at IV doses of >214 mg/kg (about 1.2 times the recommended human intra-rectal dose, based on body surface area). In a 13-week oral gavage toxicity study in rats, papillary necrosis and/or multifocal tubular injury were observed in males receiving 160 mg/kg (about 0.86 times the recommended human intra-rectal dose, based on body surface area) and in both males and females at 640 mg/kg (about 3.5 times the recommended human intra-rectal dose, based on body surface area). In a combined 52-week toxicity and 127-week carcinogenicity study in rats, degeneration of the kidneys and hyalinization of basement membranes and Bowman's capsule were observed at oral doses of 100 mg/kg/day (about 0.54 times the recommended human intra-rectal dose, based on body surface area) and above. In a 14-day rectal toxicity study of mesalamine suppositories in rabbits, intra-rectal doses up to 800 mg/kg (about 8.6 times the recommended human intra-rectal dose, based on body surface area) was not associated with any adverse effects. In a six-month oral toxicity study in dogs, doses of 80 mg/kg (about 1.4 times the recommended human intra-rectal dose, based on body surface area) and higher caused renal pathology similar to that described for the rat. In a rectal toxicity study of mesalamine suppositories in dogs, a dose of 166.6 mg/kg (about 3.0 times the recommended human intra-rectal dose, based on body surface area) produced chronic nephritis and pyelitis. In the 12-month eye toxicity study in dogs, Keratoconjunctivitis sicca (KCS) occurred at oral doses of 40 mg/kg (about 0.72 times the recommended human intra-rectal dose, based on body surface area) and above.

CLINICAL STUDIES

Two double-blind placebo-controlled multicenter studies were conducted in North America in patients with mild to moderate active ulcerative proctitis. The primary measures of efficacy were the same in all trials (clinical disease activity index, sigmoidoscopic and histologic evaluations). The main difference between the studies was dosage regimen: 500 mg three times daily (1.5 g/d) in Study 1; and 500 mg twice daily (1.0 g/d) in Study 2. A total of 173 patients were studied (Study 1, N=79; Study 2, N=94). Eighty-nine (89) patients received mesalamine suppositories and eighty-four (84) patients received placebo suppositories. Patients were evaluated clinically and sigmoidoscopically after three and six weeks of suppository treatment. In Study No. 1 patients were 17 to 73 years of age (mean = 39 yrs), 57% were female, and 97% were white. Patients had an average extent of proctitis (upper disease boundary) of 10.8 cm. Eighty-four percent (84%) of the study patients had multiple prior episodes of proctitis. In Study No. 2, patients were 21 to 72 years of age (mean = 39 yrs), 62% were female, and 96% were white. Patients had an average extent of proctitis (upper disease boundary) of 10.3 cm. Seventy-eight percent (78%) of the study patients had multiple prior episodes of proctitis.

Compared to placebo, mesalamine suppository treatment was statistically (p<0.01) superior to placebo in all trials with respect to improvement in stool frequency, rectal bleeding, mucosal appearance, disease severity, and overall disease activity after three and six weeks of treatment. Daily diary records indicated significant improvement in rectal bleeding in the first week of therapy while tenesmus and diarrhea improved significantly within two weeks. Investigators rated patients receiving mesalamine much improved compared to patients receiving placebo (p<0.001).

The effectiveness of mesalamine suppositories was statistically significant irrespective of sex, extent of proctitis, duration of current episode or duration of disease.

INDICATIONS AND USAGE

CANASA™ Suppositories are indicated for the treatment of active ulcerative proctitis.

CONTRAINDICATIONS

CANASA™ Suppositories are contraindicated for patients known to have hypersensitivity to mesalamine (5-aminosalicylic acid) or to the suppository vehicle [saturated vegetable fatty acid esters (Hard Fat, NF)].

PRECAUTIONS

Mesalamine has been implicated in the production of an acute intolerance syndrome characterized by cramping, acute abdominal pain and bloody diarrhea, sometimes fever, headache and a rash; in such cases prompt withdrawal is required. The patient's history of sulfasalazine intolerance, if any, should be re-evaluated. If a rechallenge is performed later in order to validate the hypersensitivity it should be carried out under close supervision and only if clearly needed, giving consideration to reduced dosage. In the literature, one patient previously sensitive to sulfasalazine was rechallenged with 400 mg oral mesalamine; within eight hours she experienced headache, fever, intensive abdominal colic, profuse diarrhea and was readmitted as an emergency. She responded poorly to steroid therapy and two weeks later a pancolectomy was required. The possibility of increased absorption of mesalamine and concomitant renal tubular damage as noted in the preclinical studies must be kept in mind. Patients on CANASA™, especially those on concurrent oral products which contain or release mesalamine and those with preexisting renal disease, should be carefully monitored with urinalysis, BUN and creatinine testing.

In a clinical trial most patients who were hypersensitive to sulfasalazine were able to take mesalamine enemas without evidence of any allergic reaction. Nevertheless, caution should be exercised when mesalamine is initially used in patients known to be allergic to sulfasalazine. These patients should be instructed to discontinue therapy if signs of rash or fever become apparent.

A small proportion of patients have developed pancolitis while using mesalamine. However, extension of upper disease boundary and/or flare-ups occurred less often in the mesalamine-treated group than in the placebo-treated group.

Rare instances of pericarditis have been reported with mesalamine containing products including sulfasalazine. Cases of pericarditis have also been reported as manifestations of inflammatory bowel disease. In the cases reported there have been positive rechallenges with mesalamine or mesalamine containing products. In one of these cases, however, a second rechallenge with sulfasalazine was negative throughout a 2 month follow-up. Chest pain or dyspnea in patients treated with mesalamine should be investigated with this information in mind. Discontinuation of CANASA™ may be warranted in some cases, but rechallenge with mesalamine can be performed under careful clinical observation should the continued therapeutic need for mesalamine be present.

There have been two reports in the literature of additional serious adverse events: one patient who developed leukopenia and thrombocytopenia after seven months of treatment with one 500 mg suppository nightly, and one patient with rash and fever which was a similar reaction to sulfasalazine.

Information for Patients: See patient information printed at the end of this insert.

Carcinogenesis, Mutagenesis, Impairment of Fertility
Mesalamine caused no increase in the incidence of neoplastic lesions over controls in a two-year study of Wistar rats fed up to 320 mg/kg/day of mesalamine admixed with diet (about 1.7 times the recommended human intra-rectal dose, based on body surface area).

Mesalamine was not mutagenic in the Ames test, the mouse lymphoma cell (TK$^{+/-}$) forward mutation test, or the mouse micronucleus test.

No effects on fertility or reproductive performance of the male and female rats were observed at oral mesalamine doses up to 320 mg/kg/day (about 1.7 times the recommended human intra-rectal dose, based on body surface area). The oligospermia and infertility in men associated with sulfasalazine have not been reported with mesalamine.

Pregnancy, Teratogenic Effects, Pregnancy Category B
Teratology studies have been performed in rats at oral doses up to 320 mg/kg/day (about 1.7 times the recommended human intra-rectal dose, based on body surface area) and in rabbits at oral doses up to 495 mg/kg/day (about 5.4 times the recommended human intra-rectal dose, based on body surface area) and have revealed no evidence of impaired fertility or harm to the fetus due to mesalamine. There are, however, no adequate and well controlled studies in pregnant women. Because animal reproduction studies are not always predictive of human response, this drug should be used in pregnancy only if clearly needed.

Nursing Mothers
It is not known whether mesalamine or its metabolite(s) are excreted in human milk. Because many drugs are excreted in human milk, caution should be exercised when CANASA™ is administered to a nursing woman.

Pediatric Use
Safety and effectiveness in pediatric patients have not been established.

Geriatric Use
Clinical studies of CANASA™ did not include sufficient numbers of subjects aged 65 and over to determine whether they respond differently from younger subjects. Other reported clinical experience has not identified differences in responses between the elderly and younger patients. In general, dose selection for an elderly patient should be cautious, reflecting the greater frequency of decreased hepatic, renal, or cardiac function, and of concomitant disease or other drug therapy.

Mesalamine is known to be substantially excreted by the kidney, and the risk of toxic reactions to this drug may be greater in patients with impaired renal function. Because elderly patients are more likely to have decreased renal function, it may be useful to monitor renal function.

ADVERSE REACTIONS
Clinical Adverse Experience

ADVERSE REACTIONS OCCURRING IN MORE THAN 1% OF MESALAMINE SUPPOSITORY TREATED PATIENTS (COMPARISON TO PLACEBO)

Symptom	Mesalamine (n=177)		Placebo (n=84)	
	N	%	N	%
Dizziness	5	3.0	2	2.4
Rectal Pain	3	1.8	0	0.0
Fever	2	1.2	0	0.0
Rash	2	1.2	0	0.0
Acne	2	1.2	0	0.0
Colitis	2	1.2	0	0.0

In addition, the following adverse events have been associated with mesalamine containing products: nephrotoxicity, pancreatitis, fibrosing alveolitis and elevated liver enzymes. Cases of pancreatitis and fibrosing alveolitis have been reported as manifestations of inflammatory bowel disease as well.

Hair Loss
Mild hair loss characterized by "more hair in the comb" but no withdrawal from clinical trials has been observed in seven of 815 mesalamine patients but none of the placebo-treated patients. In the literature there are at least six additional patients with mild hair loss who received either mesalamine or sulfasalazine. Retreatment is not always associated with repeated hair loss.

OVERDOSAGE

There have been no documented reports of serious toxicity in man resulting from massive overdosing with mesalamine. Under ordinary circumstances, mesalamine absorption from the colon is limited.

DOSAGE AND ADMINISTRATION

The usual dosage of CANASA™ (mesalamine) Suppositories is one 500 mg rectal suppository 2 times daily with possible increase to 3 times daily if inadequate response at two weeks. The suppository should be retained for one to three hours or longer, if possible, to achieve the maximum benefit. While the effect of CANASA™ Suppositories may be seen within three to twenty-one days, the usual course of therapy would be from three to six weeks depending on symptoms and sigmoidoscopic findings. Studies have suggested that CANASA™ Suppositories will delay relapse after the six-week short-term treatment.

Patient Instructions:
NOTE: CANASA™ Suppositories will cause staining of direct contact surfaces, including but not limited to fabrics, flooring, painted surfaces, marble, granite, vinyl, and enamel.

I. Detach one suppository from strip of suppositories.
II. Hold suppository upright and carefully remove the plastic wrapper.
III. Avoid excessive handling of suppository, which is designed to melt at body temperature.
IV. Insert suppository completely into rectum with gentle pressure, pointed end first.
V. A small amount of lubricating gel may be used on the tip of the suppository to assist insertion.

HOW SUPPLIED

CANASA™ Suppositories: CANASA™ Suppositories for rectal administration are available as bullet shaped, light tan suppositories containing 500 mg mesalamine supplied in boxes of 30 individually plastic wrapped suppositories (NDC 58914-500-56).
Boxes of 30.
Store at controlled room temperature, preferably between 20° to 25°C (68° to 77° F) [See USP Controlled Temperature]. Keep away from direct heat, light or humidity. Do not refrigerate.
Rx only
Axcan Scandipharm, Inc.
Birmingham, AL 35242
Date: January 4, 2001

Patient Information
CANASA™ Rectal Suppositories (mesalamine)

Read this information carefully before you begin treatment. Also, read the information you get whenever you get more medicine. There may be new information. This information does not take the place of talking with your doctor about your medical condition or your treatment. If you have any questions about this medicine, ask your doctor or pharmacist.

What is CANASA™?
CANASA™ (can-AH-sah) is a medicine used to treat ulcerative proctitis (ulcerative rectal colitis). CANASA™ works inside your rectum (lower intestine) to help reduce bleeding, mucous and bloody diarrhea caused by inflammation (swelling and soreness) of the rectal area. You use CANASA™ by inserting it into your rectum.

Who should not use CANASA™?
Do not use CANASA™ if you are allergic to the active ingredient mesalamine (also found in drugs such as Rowasa, Asacol, Pentasa, Azulfidine, and Dipentum), if you are allergic to the inactive ingredients, or if you have had any unusual reaction to the ingredients.
Tell your doctor if you
• Have kidney problems. Using CANASA™ may make them worse.
• Have had inflamed pancreas (pancreatitis).
• Are pregnant. You and your doctor will decide if you should use CANASA™.
• Have ever had pericarditis (inflamed sac around your heart).
• Are allergic to sulfasalazine. You may need to watch for signs of an allergic reaction to CANASA™.
• Are allergic to aspirin.
• Are allergic to other things, such as foods, preservatives, or dyes.

How should I use CANASA™?
Follow your doctor's instructions about how often to use CANASA™ and how long to use it. The usual dose of adults and teenagers is 1 suppository 2 times a day for 3–6 weeks. We do not know if CANASA™ will work for children or is safe for them.
Follow these steps to use CANASA™:
1. For best results, empty your rectum (have a bowel movement) just before using CANASA™.
2. Detach one CANASA™ suppository from the strip of suppositories.
3. Hold the suppository upright and carefully peel open the plastic at the pre-cut line to take out the suppository.
4. Insert the suppository with the pointed end first completely into your rectum, using gentle pressure.
5. For best results, keep the suppository in your rectum for 3 hours or longer, if possible.
If you have trouble inserting CANASA™, you may put a little bit of lubricating gel on the suppository.
Do not handle the suppository too much, since it may begin to melt from the heat from your hands and body.
If you miss a dose of CANASA™, use it as soon as possible, unless it is almost time for next dose. Do not use 2 suppositories at the same time to make up for a missed dose.
Keep using CANASA™ as long as your doctor tells you to use it, even if you feel better.
CANASA™ can cause stains on things it touches. Therefore keep it away from clothing and other fabrics, flooring, painted surfaces, marble, granite, plastics, and enamel. Be careful when you use CANASA™ to avoid stains.

What should I avoid while taking CANASA™?
Do not breast feed while using CANASA™. We do not know if CANASA™ can pass through the milk and harm the baby. Tell your doctor if you become pregnant while using CANASA™.

What are the possible side effects of CANASA™?
• The most common side effects of CANASA™ are: headache, gas or flatulence, and diarrhea. These events also occurred when patients were given an inactive suppository.
• Less common, but possibly serious side effects include a reaction to the medicine (acute intolerance syndrome) that includes cramps, sharp abdominal (stomach area) pain, bloody diarrhea, and sometimes fever, headache and rash. Stop use and tell your doctor right away if you get any of these symptoms.
• In rare cases, the sac around the heart may become inflamed (pericarditis). Tell your doctor right away if you develop chest pain or shortness of breath, which are signs of this problem.
• In rare cases, patients using CANASA™ develop worsening colitis (pancolitis).

Continued on next page

Canasa—Cont.

- A very few patients using CANASA™ may have mild hair loss.
- Other side effects not listed above may also occur in some patients. If you notice any other side effects, check with your doctor or pharmacist.

How should I store CANASA™?

Store CANASA™ at controlled room temperature. It is best to keep it between 68° and 77°F (20°–25°C). Keep it away from direct heat, light, or humidity. Keep it out of the reach of children. **Do not refrigerate it.**

General advice about prescription medicines

Medicines are sometimes prescribed for conditions that are not mentioned in patient information leaflets. Do not use CANASA™ for a condition for which it was not prescribed. Do not give CANASA™ to other people, even if they have the same symptoms you have.

This leaflet summarizes the most important information about CANASA™. If you would like more information, talk with your doctor. You can ask your pharmacist or doctor for information about CANASA™ that is written for health professionals.

Biovail Pharmaceuticals Inc.

808 AVIATION PARKWAY
SUITE 1400
MORRISVILLE, NC 27560

Direct Inquiries to:
Phone: 1-866-Biovail
1-866-246-8245

Product Information on Cedax®, D.A. Chewable™, Dura-vent®, D.A. 11®, Dura-Vent®/DA, Fenesin™, Fenesin™ DM, Guai-vent™/PSE, Keftab® and Rondec® please refer to the 2001 PDR under DJ Pharma Inc.

Boehringer Ingelheim Pharmaceuticals, Inc.

A subsidiary of Boehringer Ingelheim Corporation
900 RIDGEBURY ROAD
POST OFFICE BOX 368
RIDGEFIELD, CT 06877-0368

For Medical Information Contact:
1–800–542–6257
or email:
druginfo@rdg.boehringer-ingelheim.com

MICARDIS® HCT ℞

(telmisartan and hydrochlorothiazide)
Tablets 40 mg/12.5 mg
and 80 mg/12.5 mg

Prescribing Information

> **USE IN PREGNANCY**
> **When used in pregnancy during the second and third trimesters, drugs that act directly on the renin-angiotensin system can cause injury and even death to the developing fetus.** When pregnancy is detected, MICARDIS HCT tablets should be discontinued as soon as possible (see WARNINGS, Fetal/Neonatal Morbidity and Mortality).

DESCRIPTION

MICARDIS HCT is a combination of telmisartan, an orally active angiotensin II antagonist acting on the AT_1 receptor subtype, and hydrochlorothiazide, a diuretic.

Telmisartan, a nonpeptide molecule, is chemically described as 4′-[(1,4′-dimethyl-2′-propyl[2,6′-bi-1H-benzimidazol]-1′-yl)methyl]-[1,1′-biphenyl]-2-carboxylic acid. Its empirical formula is $C_{33}H_{30}N_4O_2$, its molecular weight is 514.63, and its structural formula is:

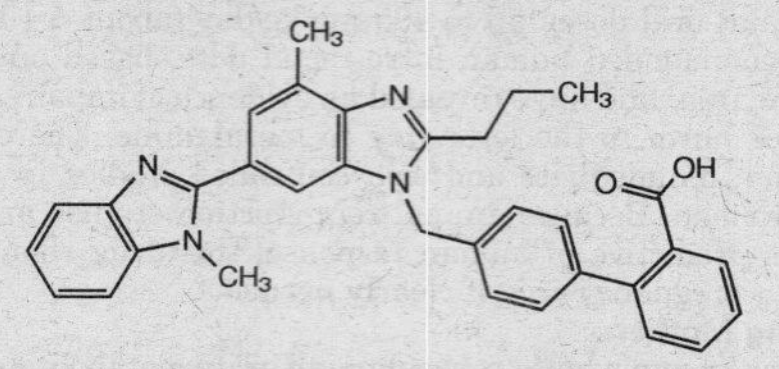

Telmisartan is a white to off-white, odorless crystalline powder. It is practically insoluble in water and in the pH range of 3 to 9, sparingly soluble in strong acid (except insoluble in hydrochloric acid), and soluble in strong base.

Hydrochlorothiazide is a white, or practically white, practically odorless, crystalline powder with a molecular weight of 297.74. It is slightly soluble in water, and freely soluble in sodium hydroxide solution. Hydrochlorothiazide is chemically described as 6-chloro-3,4-dihydro-2*H*-1,2,4-benzothiadiazine-7-sulfonamide 1,1-dioxide. Its empirical formula is $C_7H_8ClN_3O_4S_2$, and its structural formula is:

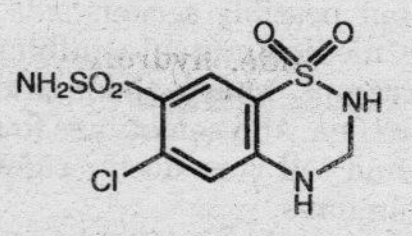

MICARDIS HCT tablets are formulated for oral administration with a combination of 40 mg or 80 mg of telmisartan and 12.5 mg hydrochlorothiazide. The tablets contain the following inactive ingredients: sodium hydroxide, meglumine, povidone, sorbitol, magnesium stearate, lactose monohydrate, microcrystalline cellulose, maize starch, iron oxide red, sodium starch glycolate. MICARDIS HCT tablets are hygroscopic and require protection from moisture.

CLINICAL PHARMACOLOGY

Mechanism of Action

Angiotensin II is formed from angiotensin I in a reaction catalyzed by angiotensin-converting enzyme (ACE, kininase II). Angiotensin II is the principal pressor agent of the renin-angiotensin system, with effects that include vasoconstriction, stimulation of synthesis and release of aldosterone, cardiac stimulation, and renal reabsorption of sodium. Telmisartan blocks the vasoconstrictor and aldosterone-secreting effects of angiotensin II by selectively blocking the binding of angiotensin II to the AT_1 receptor in many tissues, such as vascular smooth muscle and the adrenal gland. Its action is therefore independent of the pathways for angiotensin II synthesis.

There is also an AT_2 receptor found in many tissues, but AT_2 is not known to be associated with cardiovascular homeostasis. Telmisartan has much greater affinity (>3,000 fold) for the AT_1 receptor than for the AT_2 receptor.

Blockade of the renin-angiotensin system with ACE inhibitors, which inhibit the biosynthesis of angiotensin II from angiotensin I, is widely used in the treatment of hypertension. ACE inhibitors also inhibit the degradation of bradykinin, a reaction also catalyzed by ACE. Because telmisartan does not inhibit ACE (kininase II), it does not affect the response to bradykinin. Whether this difference has clinical relevance is not yet known. Telmisartan does not bind to or block other hormone receptors or ion channels known to be important in cardiovascular regulation.

Blockade of the angiotensin II receptor inhibits the negative regulatory feedback of angiotensin II on renin secretion, but the resulting increased plasma renin activity and angiotensin II circulating levels do not overcome the effect of telmisartan on blood pressure.

Hydrochlorothiazide is a thiazide diuretic. Thiazides affect the renal tubular mechanisms of electrolyte reabsorption, directly increasing excretion of sodium salt and chloride in approximately equivalent amounts. Indirectly, the diuretic action of hydrochlorothiazide reduces plasma volume, with consequent increases in plasma renin activity, increases in aldosterone secretion, increases in urinary potassium loss, and decreases in serum potassium. The renin-aldosterone link is mediated by angiotensin II, so coadministration of an angiotensin II receptor antagonist tends to reverse the potassium loss associated with these diuretics.

The mechanism of the antihypertensive effect of thiazides is not fully understood.

Pharmacokinetics

General

Telmisartan:

Following oral administration, peak concentrations (C_{max}) of telmisartan are reached in 0.5–1 hour after dosing. Food slightly reduces the bioavailability of telmisartan, with a reduction in the area under the plasma concentration-time curve (AUC) of about 6% with the 40 mg tablet and about 20% after a 160 mg dose. The absolute bioavailability of telmisartan is dose dependent. At 40 and 160 mg the bioavailability was 42% and 58%, respectively. The pharmacokinetics of orally administered telmisartan are nonlinear over the dose range 20–160 mg, with greater than proportional increases of plasma concentrations (C_{max} and AUC) with increasing doses. Telmisartan shows bi-exponential decay kinetics with a terminal elimination half-life of approximately 24 hours. Trough plasma concentrations of telmisartan with once daily dosing are about 10–25% of peak plasma concentrations. Telmisartan has an accumulation index in plasma of 1.5 to 2.0 upon repeated once daily dosing.

Hydrochlorothiazide:

When plasma levels have been followed for at least 24 hours, the plasma half-life has been observed to vary between 5.6 and 14.8 hours.

Metabolism and Elimination

Telmisartan:

Following either intravenous or oral administration of ^{14}C-labeled telmisartan, most of the administered dose (>97%) was eliminated unchanged in feces via biliary excretion; only minute amounts were found in the urine (0.91% and 0.49% of total radioactivity, respectively).

Telmisartan is metabolized by conjugation to form a pharmacologically inactive acylglucuronide; the glucuronide of the parent compound is the only metabolite that has been identified in human plasma and urine. After a single dose, the glucuronide represents approximately 11% of the measured radioactivity in plasma. The cytochrome P450 isoenzymes are not involved in the metabolism of telmisartan. Total plasma clearance of telmisartan is >800 mL/min. Terminal half-life and total clearance appear to be independent of dose.

Hydrochlorothiazide:

Hydrochlorothiazide is not metabolized but is eliminated rapidly by the kidney. At least 61% of the oral dose is eliminated as unchanged drug within 24 hours.

Distribution

Telmisartan:

Telmisartan is highly bound to plasma proteins (>99.5%), mainly albumin and α_1-acid glycoprotein. Plasma protein binding is constant over the concentration range achieved with recommended doses. The volume of distribution for telmisartan is approximately 500 liters, indicating additional tissue binding.

Hydrochlorothiazide:

Hydrochlorothiazide crosses the placental but not the blood-brain barrier and is excreted in breast milk.

Special Populations

Pediatric: Telmisartan pharmacokinetics have not been investigated in patients <18 years of age.

Geriatric: The pharmacokinetics of telmisartan do not differ between the elderly and those younger than 65 years (see DOSAGE AND ADMINISTRATION).

Gender: Plasma concentrations of telmisartan are generally 2–3 times higher in females than in males. In clinical trials, however, no significant increases in blood pressure response or in the incidence of orthostatic hypotension were found in women. No dosage adjustment is necessary.

Renal Insufficiency: Renal excretion does not contribute to the clearance of telmisartan. Based on modest experience in patients with mild-to-moderate renal impairment (creatinine clearance of 30–80 mL/min, mean clearance approximately 50 mL/min), no dosage adjustment is necessary in patients with decreased renal function. Telmisartan is not removed from blood by hemofiltration (see PRECAUTIONS, and DOSAGE AND ADMINISTRATION).

Hepatic Insufficiency: In patients with hepatic insufficiency, plasma concentrations of telmisartan are increased, and absolute bioavailability approaches 100% (see PRECAUTIONS, and DOSAGE AND ADMINISTRATION).

Drug Interactions: See PRECAUTIONS, Drug Interactions.

Pharmacodynamics

Telmisartan:

In normal volunteers, a dose of telmisartan 80 mg inhibited the pressor response to an intravenous infusion of angiotensin II by about 90% at peak plasma concentrations with approximately 40% inhibition persisting for 24 hours.

Plasma concentration of angiotensin II and plasma renin activity (PRA) increased in a dose-dependent manner after single administration of telmisartan to healthy subjects and repeated administration to hypertensive patients. The once-daily administration of up to 80 mg telmisartan to healthy subjects did not influence plasma aldosterone concentrations. In multiple dose studies with hypertensive patients, there were no clinically significant changes in electrolytes (serum potassium or sodium), or in metabolic function (including serum levels of cholesterol, triglycerides, HDL, LDL, glucose, or uric acid).

In 30 hypertensive patients with normal renal function treated for 8 weeks with telmisartan 80 mg or telmisartan 80 mg in combination with hydrochlorothiazide 12.5 mg, there were no clinically significant changes from baseline in renal blood flow, glomerular filtration rate, filtration fraction, renovascular resistance, or creatinine clearance.

Hydrochlorothiazide:

After oral administration of hydrochlorothiazide, diuresis begins within 2 hours, peaks in about 4 hours and lasts about 6 to 12 hours.

Clinical Trials

Telmisartan:

The antihypertensive effects of telmisartan have been demonstrated in six principal placebo-controlled clinical trials, studying a range of 20–160 mg; one of these examined the antihypertensive effects of telmisartan and hydrochlorothiazide in combination. The studies involved a total of 1773 patients with mild to moderate hypertension (diastolic blood pressure of 95–114 mmHg), 1031 of whom were treated with telmisartan. Following once daily administration of telmisartan, the magnitude of blood pressure reduction from baseline after placebo subtraction was approximately (SBP/DBP) 6-8/6 mmHg for 20 mg, 9-13/6-8 mmHg for 40 mg, and 12-13/7-8 mmHg for 80 mg. Larger doses (up to 160 mg) did not appear to cause a further decrease in blood pressure.

Upon initiation of antihypertensive treatment with telmisartan, blood pressure was reduced after the first dose, with a maximal reduction by about 4 weeks. With cessation of treatment with telmisartan tablets, blood pressure gradually returned to baseline values over a period of several days to one week. During long-term studies (without placebo control) the effect of telmisartan appeared to be maintained for up to at least one year. The antihypertensive effect of telmisartan is not influenced by patient age, gender, weight or body mass index. Blood pressure response in black patients (usually a low-renin population) is noticeably less than that in Caucasian patients. This has been true for most, but not all, angiotensin II antagonists and ACE inhibitors.

The onset of antihypertensive activity occurs within 3 hours after administration of a single oral dose. At doses of 20, 40, and 80 mg, the antihypertensive effect of once daily administration of telmisartan is maintained for the full 24-hour dose interval. With automated ambulatory blood pressure monitoring and conventional blood pressure measurements, the 24-hour trough-to-peak ratio for 40–80 mg doses of telmisartan was 70–100% for both systolic and diastolic blood pressure. The incidence of symptomatic orthostasis after the first dose in all controlled trials was low (0.04%).

There were no changes in the heart rate of patients treated with telmisartan in controlled trials.

Telmisartan & Hydrochlorothiazide:

In controlled clinical trials with over 2500 patients, 1017 patients were exposed to telmisartan (20 to 160 mg) and concomitant hydrochlorothiazide (6.25 to 25 mg). These trials included one factorial trial with combinations of telmisartan (20, 40, 80, 160 mg, or placebo) and hydrochlorothiazide (6.25, 12.5, 25 mg and placebo). Four other studies of at least six months duration allowed add-on of hydrochlorothiazide for patients who either were not adequately controlled on the randomized monotherapy dose or had not achieved adequate response after completing the up-titration of telmisartan.

The combination of telmisartan and hydrochlorothiazide resulted in additive placebo-adjusted decreases in systolic and diastolic blood pressure at trough of 16-21/9-11 mmHg at 40/12.5 mg and 80/12.5 mg, compared to 9-13/7-8 mmHg for telmisartan 40 mg to 80 mg and 4/4 mmHg for hydrochlorothiazide 12.5 mg alone.

In active controlled studies, the addition of 12.5 mg hydrochlorothiazide to titrated doses of telmisartan in patients who did not achieve or maintain adequate response with telmisartan monotherapy further reduced systolic and diastolic blood pressure.

The antihypertensive effect was independent of age or gender.

There was essentially no change in heart rate in patients treated with the combination of telmisartan and hydrochlorothiazide in the placebo controlled trial.

INDICATIONS AND USAGE

MICARDIS HCT is indicated for the treatment of hypertension. This fixed dose combination is not indicated for initial therapy (see DOSAGE AND ADMINISTRATION).

CONTRAINDICATIONS

MICARDIS HCT is contraindicated in patients who are hypertensive to any component of this product.

Because of the hydrochlorothiazide component, this product is contraindicated in patients with anuria or hypersensitivity to other sulfonamide-derived drugs.

WARNINGS

Fetal/Neonatal Morbidity and Mortality

Drugs that act directly on the renin-angiotensin system can cause fetal and neonatal morbidity and death when administered to pregnant women. Several dozen cases have been reported in the world literature in patients who were taking anigotensin converting enzyme inhibitors. When pregnancy is detected, MICARDIS HCT tablets should be discontinued as soon as possible.

The use of drugs that act directly on the renin-angiotensin system during the second and third trimesters of pregnancy has been associated with fetal and neonatal injury, including hypotension, neonatal skull hypoplasia, anuria, reversible or irreversible renal failure, and death. Oligohydramnios has also been reported, presumably resulting from decreased fetal renal function; oligohydramnios in this setting has been associated with fetal limb contractures, craniofacial deformation, and hypoplastic lung development. Prematurity, intrauterine growth retardation, and patent ductus arteriosus have also been reported, although it is not clear whether these occurrences were due to exposure to the drug. These adverse effects do not appear to have resulted from intrauterine drug exposure that has been limited to the first trimester. Mothers whose embryos and fetuses are exposed to an angiotensin II receptor antagonist only during the first trimester should be so informed. Nonetheless, when patients become pregnant, physicians should have the patient discontinue the use of MICARDIS HCT tablets as soon as possible.

Rarely (probably less often than once in every thousand pregnancies), no alternative to an angiotensin II receptor antagonist will be found. In these rare cases, the mothers should be apprised of the potential hazards to their fetuses, and serial ultrasound examinations should be performed to assess the intra-amniotic environment.

If oligohydramnios is observed, MICARDIS HCT tablets should be discontinued unless they are considered life-saving for the mother. Contraction stress testing (CST), a non-stress test (NST), or biophysical profiling (BPP) may be appropriate, depending upon the week of pregnancy. Patients and physicians should be aware, however, that oligohydramnios may not appear until after the fetus has sustained irreversible injury.

Infants with histories of *in utero* exposure to an angiotensin II receptor antagonist should be closely observed for hypotension, oliguria, and hyperkalemia. If oliguria occurs, attention should be directed toward support of blood pressure and renal perfusion. Exchange transfusion or dialysis may be required as a means of reversing hypotension and/or substituting for disordered renal function.

A developmental toxicity study was performed in rats with telmisartan/hydrochlorothiazide doses of 3.2/1.0, 15/4.7, 50/15.6, and 0/15.6 mg/kg/day. Although the two higher dose combinations appeared to be more toxic (significant decrease in body weight gain) to the dams than either drug alone, there did not appear to be an increase in toxicity to the developing embryos.

No teratogenic effects were observed when telmisartan was administered to pregnant rats at oral doses of up to 50 mg/kg/day and to pregnant rabbits at oral doses up to 45 mg/kg/day. In rabbits, embryolethality associated with maternal toxicity (reduced body weight gain and food consumption) was observed at 45 mg/kg/day [about 12 times the maximum recommended human dose (MRHD) of 80 mg on a mg/m^2 basis]. In rats, maternally toxic (reduction in body weight gain and food consumption) telmisartan doses of 15 mg/kg/day (about 1.9 times the MRHD on a mg/m^2 basis), administered during late gestation and lactation, were observed to produce adverse effects in neonates, including reduced viability, low birth weight, delayed maturation, and decreased weight gain. Telmisartan has been shown to be present in rat fetuses during late gestation and in rat milk. The no observed effect doses for developmental toxicity in rats and rabbits, 5 and 15 mg/kg/day, respectively, are about 0.64 and 3.7 times, on a mg/m^2 basis, the maximum recommended human dose of telmisartan (80 mg/day).

Studies in which hydrochlorothiazide was administered to pregnant mice and rats during their respective periods of major organogenesis at doses up to 3000 and 1000 mg/kg/day, respectively, provided no evidence of harm to the fetus.

Thiazides cross the placental barrier and appear in cord blood. There is a risk of fetal or neonatal jaundice, thrombocytopenia, and possibly other adverse reactions that have occurred in adults.

Hypotension in Volume-Depleted Patients

Initiation of antihypertensive therapy in patients whose renin-angiotensin system are activated such as patients who are intravascular volume- or sodium-depleted, e.g., in patients treated vigorously with diuretics, should only be approached cautiously. These conditions should be corrected prior to administration of MICARDIS HCT. Treatment should be started under close medical supervision (see DOSAGE AND ADMINISTRATION).

If hypotension occurs, the patients should be placed in the supine position and, if necessary, given an intravenous infusion of normal saline. A transient hypotensive response is not a contraindication to further treatment which usually can be continued without difficulty once the blood pressure has stabilized.

Hydrochlorothiazide

Hepatic Impairment: Thiazide diuretics should be used with caution in patients with impaired hepatic function or progressive liver disease, since minor alterations of fluid and electrolyte balance may precipitate hepatic coma.

Hypersensitivity Reaction: Hypersensitivity reactions to hydrochlorothiazide may occur in patients with or without a history of allergy or bronchial asthma, but are more likely in patients with such a history.

Systemic Lupus Erythematosus: Thiazide diuretics have been reported to cause exacerbation or activation of systemic lupus erythematosus.

Lithium Interaction: Lithium generally should not be given with thiazides (see PRECAUTIONS, Drug Interactions, Hydrochlorothiazide, *Lithium*).

PRECAUTIONS

Serum Electrolytes

Telmisartan & Hydrochlorothiazide:

In controlled trials using the telmisartan/hydrochlorothiazide combination treatment, no patient administered 40/12.5 mg or 80/12.5 mg had a decrease in potassium ≥1.4 mEq/L, and no patient experienced hyperkalemia. No discontinuations due to hypokalemia occurred during treatment with the telmisartan/hydrochlorothiazide combination. The absence of significant changes in serum potassium levels may be due to the opposing mechanisms of action of telmisartan and hydrochlorothiazide on potassium excretion on the kidney.

Hydrochlorothiazide:

Periodic determinations of serum electrolytes to detect possible electrolyte imbalance should be performed at appropriate intervals. All patients receiving thiazide therapy should be observed for clinical signs of fluid or electrolyte imbalance: hyponatremia, hypochloremic alkalosis, and hypokalemia. Serum and urine electrolyte determinations are particularly important when the patient experiences excessive vomiting or receives parenteral fluids. Warning signs or symptoms of fluid and electrolyte imbalance, irrespective of cause, include dryness of mouth, thirst, weakness, lethargy, drowsiness, restlessness, confusion, seizures, muscle pains or cramps, muscular fatigue, hypotension, oliguria, tachycardia, and gastrointestinal disturbances such as nausea and vomiting.

Hypokalemia may develop, especially with brisk diuresis, when severe cirrhosis is present, or after prolonged therapy. Interference with adequate oral electrolyte intake will also contribute to hypokalemia. Hypokalemia may cause cardiac arrhythmia and may also sensitize or exaggerate the response of the heart to the toxic effects of digitalis (e.g., increased ventricular irritability).

Although any chloride deficit is generally mild and usually does not require specific treatment except under extraordinary circumstances (as in liver disease or renal disease), chloride replacement may be required in the treatment of metabolic alkalosis.

Dilutional hyponatremia may occur in edematous patients in hot weather; appropriate therapy is water restriction, rather than administration of salt except in rare instances when the hyponatremia is life-threatening. In actual salt depletion, appropriate replacement is the therapy of choice.

Hyperuricemia may occur or frank gout may be precipitated in certain patients receiving thiazide therapy.

In diabetic patients dosage adjustments of insulin or oral hypoglycemic agents may be required.

Hyperglycemia may occur with thiazide diuretics. Thus latent diabetes mellitus may become manifest during thiazide therapy.

The antihypertensive effects of the drug may be enhanced in the post sympathectomy patient.

If progressive renal impairment becomes evident consider withholding or discontinuing diuretic therapy.

Thiazides have been shown to increase the urinary excretion of magnesium; this may result in hypomagnesemia.

Thiazides may decrease urinary calcium excretion. Thiazides may cause intermittent and slight elevation of serum calcium in the absence of known disorders of calcium metabolism. Marked hypercalcemia may be evidence of hidden hyperparathyroidism. Thiazides should be discontinued before carrying out tests for parathyroid function.

Increases in cholesterol and triglyceride levels may be associated with thiazide diuretic therapy.

Impaired Hepatic Function

Telmisartan:

As the majority of telmisartan is eliminated by biliary excretion, patients with biliary obstructive disorders or hepatic insufficiency can be expected to have reduced clearance. MICARDIS HCT tablets should therefore be used with caution in these patients.

Impaired Renal Function

Telmisartan:

As a consequence of inhibiting the renin-angiotensin-aldosterone system, changes in renal function may be anticipated in susceptible individuals. In patients whose renal function may depend on the activity of the renin-angiotensin-aldosterone system (e.g., patients with severe congestive heart failure), treatment with angiotensin-converting enzyme inhibitors and angiotensin receptor antagonists has been associated with oliguria and/or progressive azotemia and (rarely) with acute renal failure and/or death. Similar results may be anticipated in patients treated with telmisartan.

In studies of ACE inhibitors in patients with unilateral or bilateral renal artery stenosis, increases in serum creatinine or blood urea nitrogen were observed. There has been no long-term use of telmisartan in patients with unilateral or bilateral renal artery stenosis but an effect similar to that seen with ACE inhibitors should be anticipated.

Hydrochlorothiazide:

Thiazides should be used with caution in severe renal disease. In patients with renal disease, thiazides may precipitate azotemia. Cumulative effects of the drug may develop in patients with impaired renal function.

Information for Patients

Pregnancy: Female patients of childbearing age should be told about the consequences of second- and third-trimester exposure to drugs that act on the renin-angiotensin system, and they should also be told that these consequences do not appear to have resulted from intrauterine drug exposure that has been limited to the first trimester. These patients should be asked to report pregnancies to their physicians as soon as possible.

Symptomatic Hypotension: A patient receiving MICARDIS HCT should be cautioned that lightheadedness can occur, especially during the first days of therapy, and that it should be reported to the prescribing physician. The patients should be told that if syncope occurs, MICARDIS HCT should be discontinued until the physician has been consulted.

All patients should be cautioned that inadequate fluid intake, excessive perspiration, diarrhea, or vomiting can lead to an excessive fall in blood pressure, with the same consequences of lightheadedness and possible syncope.

Potassium Supplements: A patient receiving MICARDIS HCT should be told not to use potassium supplements or salt substitutes that contain potassium without consulting the prescribing physician.

Drug Interactions

Telmisartan:

Digoxin: When telmisartan was coadministered with digoxin, median increases in digoxin peak plasma concentration (49%) and in trough concentration (20%) were observed. It is, therefore, recommended that digoxin levels be monitored when initiating, adjusting, and discontinuing telmisartan to avoid possible over- or under-digitalization.

Warfarin: Telmisartan administered for 10 days slightly decreased the mean warfarin trough plasma concentration; this decrease did not result in a change in International Normalized Ratio (INR).

Other Drugs: Coadministration of telmisartan did not result in a clinically significant interaction with acetaminophen, amlodipine, glibenclamide, hydrochlorothiazide or ibuprofen. Telmisartan is not metabolized by the cytochrome P450 system and had no effects *in vitro* on cytochrome P450 enzymes, except for some inhibition of CYP2C19. Telmisartan is not expected to interact with drugs that inhibit cytochrome P450 enzymes; it is also not expected to interact with drugs metabolized by cytochrome P450 enzymes, except for possible inhibition of the metabolism of drugs metabolized by CYP2C19.

Hydrochlorothiazide:

When administered concurrently, the following drugs may interact with thiazide diuretics:

Continued on next page

Micardis HCT—Cont.

Alcohol, barbiturates, or narcotics: Potentiation of orthostatic hypotension may occur.
Antidiabetic drugs (oral agents and insulin): Dosage adjustment of the antidiabetic drug may be required.
Other antihypertensive drugs: Additive effect or potentiation.
Cholestyramine and colestipol resins: Absorption of hydrochlorothiazide is impaired in the presence of anionic exchange resins. Single doses of either cholestyramine or colestipol resins bind the hydrochlorothiazide and reduce its absorption from the gastrointestinal tract by up to 85% and 43%, respectively.
Corticosteroids, ACTH: Intensified electrolyte depletion, particularly hypokalemia.
Pressor amines (e.g., norepinephrine): Possible decreased response to pressure amines but not sufficient to preclude their use.
Skeletal muscle relaxants, nondepolarizing (e.g., tubocurarine): Possible increased responsiveness to the muscle relaxant.
Lithium: Should not generally be given with diuretics. Diuretic agents reduce the renal clearance of lithium and add a high risk of lithium toxicity. Refer to the package insert for lithium preparations before use of such preparations with MICARDIS HCT.
Non-steroidal anti-inflammatory drugs: In some patients, the administration of a non-steroidal anti-inflammatory agent can reduce the diuretic, natriuretic, and antihypertensive effects of loop, potassium-sparing and thiazide diuretics. Therefore, when MICARDIS HCT and non-steroidal anti-inflammatory agents are used concomitantly, the patient should be observed closely to determine if the desired effect of the diuretic is obtained.

Carcinogenesis, Mutagenesis, Impairment of Fertility
Telmisartan & Hydrochlorothiazide:
No carcinogenicity, mutagenicity, or fertility studies have been conducted with the combination of telmisartan and hydrochlorothiazide.
Telmisartan:
There was no evidence of carcinogenicity when telmisartan was administered in the diet to mice and rats for up to 2 years. The highest doses administered to mice (1000 mg/kg/day) and rats (100 mg/kg/day) are, on a mg/m^2 basis, about 59 and 13 times, respectively, the maximum recommended human dose (MRHD) of telmisartan. These same doses have been shown to provide average systemic exposure to telmisartan >100 times and >25 times, respectively, the systemic exposure in humans receiving the MRHD (80 mg/day).
Genotoxicity assays did not reveal any telmisartan-related effects at either the gene or chromosome level. These assays included bacterial mutagenicity tests with Salmonella and *E coli* (Ames), a gene mutation test with Chinese hamster V79 cells, a cytogenetic test with human lymphocytes, and a mouse micronucleus test.
No drug-related effects on the reproductive performance of male and female rats were noted at 100 mg/kg/day (the highest dose administered), about 13 times, on a mg/m^2 basis, the MRHD of telmisartan. This dose in the rat resulted in an average systemic exposure (telmisartan AUC as determined on day 6 of pregnancy) at least 50 times the average systemic exposure in humans at the MRHD (80 mg/day).
Hydrochlorothiazide:
Two-year feeding studies in mice and rats conducted under the auspices of the National Toxicology Program (NTP) uncovered no evidence of a carcinogenic potential of hydrochlorothiazide in female mice (at doses of up to approximately 600 mg/kg/day) or in male and female rats (at doses of up to approximately 100 mg/kg/day). The NTP, however, found equivocal evidence for hepatocarcinogenicity in male mice.
Hydrochlorothiazide was not genotoxic *in vitro* in the Ames mutagenicity assay of *Salmonella typhimurium* strains TA 98, TA 100, TA 1535, TA 1537, and TA 1538 and in the Chinese Hamster Ovary (CHO) test for chromosomal aberrations, or *in vivo* in assays using mouse germinal cell chromosomes, Chinese hamster bone marrow chromosomes, and the *Drosophila* sex-linked recessive lethal trait gene. Positive test results were obtained in the *in vitro* CHO Sister Chromatid Exchange (clastogenicity) and in the Mouse Lymphoma Cell (mutagenicity) assays, and in the *Aspergillus nidulans* non-disjunction assay.
Hydrochlorothiazide had no adverse effects on the fertility of mice and rats of either sex in studies wherein these species were exposed, via their diet, to doses of up to 100 and 4 mg/kg, respectively, prior to mating and throughout gestation.

Pregnancy
Pregnancy Categories C (first trimester) and D (second and third trimesters) (See WARNINGS, Fetal/Neonatal Morbidity and Mortality).

Nursing Mothers
It is not known whether telmisartan is excreted in human milk, but telmisartan was shown to be present in the milk of lactating rats. Thiazides appear in human milk. Because of the potential for adverse effects on the nursing infant, a decision should be made to discontinue nursing or discontinue the drug, taking into account the importance of the drug to the mother.

Pediatric Use
Safety and effectiveness in pediatric patients have not been established.

Geriatric Use
In the controlled clinical trials (n=1017), approximately 20% of patients treated with telmisartan/hydrochlorothiazide were 65 years of age or older, and 5% were 75 years of age or older. No overall differences in effectiveness and safety of telmisartan/hydrochlorothiazide were observed in these patients compared to younger patients. Other reported clinical experience has not identified differences in responses between the elderly and younger patients, but greater sensitivity of some older individuals cannot be ruled out.

ADVERSE REACTIONS
MICARDIS HCT (telmisartan/hydrochlorothiazide) has been evaluated for safety in over 1700 patients, including 716 treated for over six months and 420 for over one year. In clinical trials with MICARDIS HCT, no unexpected adverse events have been observed. Adverse experiences have been limited to those that have been previously reported with telmisartan and/or hydrochlorothiazide. The overall incidence of adverse experiences reported with the combination was comparable to placebo. Most adverse experiences were mild in intensity and transient in nature and did not require discontinuation of therapy.
Adverse events occurring at an incidence of 2% or more in patients treated with telmisartan/hydrochlorothiazide and at a greater rate than in patients treated with placebo, irrespective of their causal association, are presented in Table 1.
[See table below]
The following adverse events were reported at a rate less than 2% in patients treated with telmisartan/hydrochlorothiazide and at a greater rate than in patients treated with placebo: back pain, dyspepsia, vomiting, tachycardia, hypokalemia, bronchitis, pharyngitis, rash, hypotension postural, abdominal pain.
Finally, the following adverse events were reported at a rate of 2% or greater in patients treated with telmisartan/hydrochlorothiazide, but were as, or more common in the placebo group: pain, headache, cough, urinary tract infection.
Adverse events occurred at approximately the same rates in men and women, older and younger patients, and black and non-black patients.
In controlled trials (n=1017), 0.2% of patients treated with MICARDIS HCT 40/12.5 mg or 80/12.5 mg discontinued due to orthostatic hypotension, and the incidence of dizziness was 4% and 7%, respectively.

Telmisartan:
Other adverse experiences that have been reported with telmisartan, without regard to causality, are listed below:
Autonomic Nervous System: impotence, increased sweating, flushing; *Body as a Whole:* allergy, fever, leg pain, malaise, chest pain; *Cardiovascular:* palpitation, dependent edema, angina pectoris, leg edema, abnormal ECG, hypertension, peripheral edema; *CNS:* insomnia, somnolence, migraine, vertigo, paresthesia, involuntary muscle contractions, hypoaesthesia; *Gastrointestinal:* flatulence, constipation, gastritis, dry mouth, hemorrhoids, gastroenteritis, enteritis, gastroesophageal reflux, toothache, non-specific gastrointestinal disorders; *Metabolic:* gout, hypercholesterolemia, diabetes mellitus; *Musculoskeletal:* arthritis, arthralgia, leg cramps, myalgia; *Psychiatric:* anxiety, depression, nervousness; *Resistance Mechanism:* infection, fungal infection, abscess, otitis media; *Respiratory:* asthma, rhinitis, dyspnea, epistaxis; *Skin:* dermatitis, eczema, pruritus; *Urinary:* micturition frequency, cystitis; *Vascular:* cerebrovascular disorder; *Special Senses:* abnormal vision, conjunctivitis, tinnitus, earache. A single case of angioedema was reported (among a total of 3781 patients treated with telmisartan).

Hydrochlorothiazide:
Other adverse experiences that have been reported with hydrochlorothiazide, without regard to causality, are listed below:
Body as a whole: weakness;
Digestive: pancreatitis, jaundice (intrahepatic cholestatic jaundice), sialadenitis, cramping, gastric irritation;
Hematologic: aplastic anemia, agranulocytosis, leukopenia, hemolytic anemia, thrombocytopenia;
Hypersensitivity: purpura, photosensitivity, urticaria, necrotizing angiitis (vasculitis and cutaneous vasculitis), fever, respiratory distress including pneumonitis and pulmonary edema, anaphylactic reactions;
Metabolic: hyperglycemia, glycosuria, hyperuricemia;
Musculoskeletal: muscle spasm;
Nervous System/Psychiatric: restlessness;
Renal: renal failure, renal dysfunction, interstitial nephritis;
Skin: erythema multiforme including Stevens-Johnson syndrome, exfoliative dermatitis including toxic epidermal necrolysis;
Special Senses: transient blurred vision, xanthopsia.

Clinical Laboratory Findings
In controlled trials, clinically relevant changes in standard laboratory test parameters were rarely associated with administration of MICARDIS HCT (telmisartan/hydrochlorothiazide) tablets.
Hemoglobin and Hematocrit: Decreases in hemoglobin (≥2 g/dL) and hematocrit (≥9%) were observed in 1.2% and 0.6% of telmisartan/hydrochlorothiazide patients, respectively, in controlled trials. Changes in hemoglobin and hematocrit were not considered clinically significant and there were no discontinuations due to anemia.
Creatinine, Blood Urea Nitrogen (BUN): Increases in BUN (≥11.2 mg/dL) and serum creatinine (≥0.5 mg/dL) were observed in 2.8% and 1.4%, respectively, of patients with essential hypertension treated with MICARDIS HCT in controlled trials. No patient discontinued treatment with MICARDIS HCT due to an increase in BUN or creatinine.
Liver Function Tests: Occasional elevations of liver enzymes and/or serum bilirubin have occurred. No telmisartan/hydrochlorothiazide treated patients discontinued therapy due to abnormal hepatic function.
Serum Electrolytes: See PRECAUTIONS.

OVERDOSAGE
Telmisartan:
Limited data are available with regard to overdosage in humans. The most likely manifestations of overdosage with telmisartan would be hypotension, dizziness and tachycardia; bradycardia could occur from parasympathetic (vagal) stimulation. If symptomatic hypotension should occur, supportive treatment should be instituted. Telmisartan is not removed by hemodialysis.
Hydrochlorothiazide:
The most common signs and symptoms observed in patients are those caused by electrolyte depletion (hypokalemia, hypochloremia, hyponatremia) and dehydration resulting from excessive diuresis. If digitalis has also been administered, hypokalemia may accentuate cardiac arrhythmias. The degree to which hydrochlorothiazide is removed by hemodialysis has not been established. The oral LD_{50} of hydrochlorothiazide is greater than 10 g/kg in both mice and rats.

DOSAGE AND ADMINISTRATION
The usual starting dose of telmisartan is 40 mg once a day; blood pressure response is dose related over the range of 20–80 mg. Patients with depletion of intravascular volume should have the condition corrected or telmisartan tablets should be initiated under close medical supervision (see WARNINGS, Hypotension in Volume Depleted Patients). Patients with biliary obstructive disorders or hepatic insufficiency should have treatment started under close medical supervision (see PRECAUTIONS).
Hydrochlorothiazide is effective in doses of 12.5 mg to 50 mg once daily.
To minimize dose-independent side effects, it is usually appropriate to begin combination therapy only after a patient has failed to achieve the desired effect with monotherapy.
The side effects (see WARNINGS) of telmisartan are generally rare and apparently independent of dose; those of hydrochlorothiazide are a mixture of dose-dependent phenomena (primarily hypokalemia) and dose-independent phenomena (e.g., pancreatitis), the former much more common than the latter. Therapy with any combination of telmisartan and hydrochlorothiazide will be associated with both sets of dose-independent side effects.
MICARDIS HCT tablets may be administered with other antihypertensive agents.
MICARDIS HCT tablets may be administered with or without food.

Replacement Therapy
The combination may be substituted for the titrated components.

TABLE 1 Adverse Events Occurring in ≥ 2% of Telmisartan/Hydrochlorothiazide (HCTZ) Patients*

	Telm/HCTZ (N=414) (%)	Placebo (N=74) (%)	Telm (N=209) (%)	HCTZ (N=121) (%)
Body as a whole				
Fatigue	3	1	3	3
Influenza-like symptoms	2	1	2	3
Central/peripheral nervous system				
Dizziness	5	1	4	6
Gastrointestinal system				
Diarrhea	3	0	5	2
Nausea	2	0	1	2
Respiratory system disorder				
Sinusitis	4	3	3	6
Upper respiratory tract infection	8	7	7	10

* *includes all doses of telmisartan (20–160 mg), hydrochlorothiazide (6.25–25 mg), and combinations thereof*

Dose Titration by Clinical Effect

MICARDIS HCT is available as tablets containing either telmisartan 40 mg or 80 mg and hydrochlorothiazide 12.5 mg. A patient whose blood pressure is not adequately controlled with telmisartan monotherapy 80 mg (see above) may be switched to MICARDIS HCT, telmisartan 80 mg/hydrochlorothiazide 12.5 mg once daily, and finally titrated up to 160/25 mg, if necessary.

A patient whose blood pressure is inadequately controlled by 25 mg once daily of hydrochlorothiazide, or is controlled but who experiences hypokalemia with this regimen, may be switched to MICARDIS HCT (telmisartan 80 mg/hydrochlorothiazide 12.5 mg) once daily, reducing the dose of hydrochlorothiazide without reducing the overall expected antihypertensive response. The clinical response to MICARDIS HCT should be subsequently evaluated and if blood pressure remains uncontrolled after 2–4 weeks of therapy, the dose may be titrated up to 160/25 mg, if necessary.

Patients with Renal Impairment

The usual regimens of therapy with MICARDIS HCT may be followed as long as the patient's creatinine clearance is >30 mL/min. In patients with more severe renal impairment, loop diuretics are preferred to thiazides, so MICARDIS HCT is not recommended.

Patients with Hepatic Impairment

MICARDIS HCT is not recommended for patients with severe hepatic impairment. Patients with biliary obstructive disorders or hepatic insufficiency should have treatment started under close medical supervision using the 40/12.5 mg combination (see PRECAUTIONS).

HOW SUPPLIED

MICARDIS HCT is available as bilayered, oblong-shaped, uncoated tablets containing telmisartan 40 mg or 80 mg and hydrochlorothiazide 12.5 mg. The hydrochlorothiazide layer is red and unmarked. The telmisartan layer is white to off-white, embossed with the BOEHRINGER INGELHEIM logo and either H4 for the 40/12.5 mg dose strength, or H8 for the 80/12.5 mg dose strength. Tablets are provided as follows:

MICARDIS HCT (telmisartan/hydrochlorothiazide) tablets 40 mg/12.5 mg are individually blister-sealed in cartons of 28 tablets as 4 × 7 cards (NDC 0597-0043-28).

MICARDIS HCT (telmisartan/hydrochlorothiazide) tablets 80 mg/12.5 mg are individually blister-sealed in cartons of 28 tablets as 4 × 7 cards (NDC 0597-0044-28).

Storage

Store at 25°C (77°F); excursions permitted to 15–30°C (59–86°F) (see USP Controlled Room Temperature).

Tablets should not be removed from blisters until immediately before administration.

Rx only

Manufactured by: Boehringer Ingelheim Pharma KG, Ingelheim, Germany

Marketed by: Boehringer Ingelheim Pharmaceuticals, Inc., Ridgefield, CT, USA and Abbott Laboratories, North Chicago, IL 60064

Licensed from: Boehringer Ingelheim International GmbH, Ingelheim, Germany

MC-PI-HCT (11/00)

Cell Therapeutics, Inc.

**201 ELLIOTT AVE W. #400
SEATTLE, WA 98119**

Direct Inquiries to:
Medical Information
(800) 715-0944
(510) 985-9750
Customer Service
(888) 305-2289

TRISENOX™   ℞
(arsenic trioxide) injection
**For Intravenous Use Only
10 mg/10 mL (1 mg/mL) ampule**

Rx only

WARNING

Experienced Physician and Institution: TRISENOX™ (arsenic trioxide) injection should be administered under the supervision of a physician who is experienced in the management of patients with acute leukemia.

APL Differentiation Syndrome: Some patients with APL treated with TRISENOX™ have experienced symptoms similar to a syndrome called the retinoic-acid-Acute Promyelocytic Leukemia (RA-APL) or APL differentiation syndrome, characterized by fever, dyspnea, weight gain, pulmonary infiltrates and pleural or pericardial effusions, with or without leukocytosis. This syndrome can be fatal. The management of the syndrome has not been fully studied, but high-dose steroids have been used at the first suspicion of the APL differentiation syndrome and appear to mitigate signs and symptoms. At the first signs that could suggest the syndrome (unexplained fe-

---

Adverse Events (any grade) Occurring in ≥ 5% of 40 Patients with APL who Received TRISENOX™ at a dose of 0.15 mg/kg/day

System organ class / Adverse Event	All Adverse Events, Any Grade		Grade 3 & 4 Events	
	n	%	n	%
General disorders and administration site conditions				
Fatigue	25	63	2	5
Pyrexia (Fever)	25	63	2	5
Edema—non-specific	16	40		
Rigors	15	38		
Chest pain	10	25	2	5
Injection site pain	8	20		
Pain—non specific	6	15	1	3
Injection site erythema	5	13		
Injection site edema	4	10		
Weakness	4	10	2	5
Hemorrhage	3	8		
Weight gain	5	13		
Weight loss	3	8		
Drug hypersensitivity	2	5	1	3
Gastrointestinal disorders				
Nausea	30	75		
Anorexia	9	23		
Appetite decreased	6	15		
Diarrhea	21	53		
Vomiting	23	58		
Abdominal pain (lower & upper)	23	58	4	10
Sore throat	14	35		
Constipation	11	28	1	3
Loose stools	4	10		
Dyspepsia	4	10		
Oral blistering	3	8		
Fecal incontinence	3	8		
Gastrointestinal hemorrhage	3	8		
Dry mouth	3	8		
Abdominal tenderness	3	8		
Diarrhea hemorrhagic	3	8		
Abdominal distension	3	8		
Metabolism and nutrition disorders				
Hypokalemia	20	50	5	13
Hypomagnesemia	18	45	5	13
Hyperglycemia	18	45	5	13
ALT increased	8	20	2	5
Hyperkalemia	7	18	2	5
AST increased	5	13	1	3
Hypocalcemia	4	10		
Hypoglycemia	3	8		
Acidosis	2	5		
Nervous system disorders				
Headache	24	60	1	3
Insomnia	17	43	1	3
Paresthesia	13	33	2	5
Dizziness (excluding vertigo)	9	23		
Tremor	5	13		
Convulsion	3	8	2	5

TABLE continued on next page

Trisenox—Cont.

ver, dyspnea and/or weight gain, abnormal chest auscultatory findings or radiographic abnormalities), high-dose steroids (dexamethasone 10 mg intravenously BID) should be immediately initiated, irrespective of the leukocyte count, and continued for at least 3 days or longer until signs and symptoms have abated. The majority of patients do not require termination of TRISENOX™ therapy during treatment of the APL differentiation syndrome.

ECG Abnormalities: Arsenic trioxide can cause QT interval prolongation and complete atrioventricular block. QT prolongation can lead to a torsade de pointes-type ventricular arrhythmia, which can be fatal. The risk of torsade de pointes is related to the extent of QT prolongation, concomitant administration of QT prolonging drugs, a history of torsade de pointes, preexisting QT interval prolongation, congestive heart failure, administration of potassium-wasting diuretics, or other conditions that result in hypokalemia or hypomagnesemia. One patient (also receiving amphotericin B) had torsade de pointes during induction therapy for relapsed APL with arsenic trioxide.

ECG and Electrolyte Monitoring Recommendations: Prior to initiating therapy with TRISENOX™, a 12-lead ECG should be performed and serum electrolytes (potassium, calcium, and magnesium) and creatinine should be assessed; preexisting electrolyte abnormalities should be corrected and, if possible, drugs that are known to prolong the QT interval should be discontinued. For QTc greater than 500 msec, corrective measures should be completed and the QTc reassessed with serial ECGs prior to considering using TRISENOX™. During therapy with TRISENOX™, potassium concentrations should be kept above 4 mEq/L and magnesium concentrations should be kept above 1.8 mg/dL. Patients who reach an absolute QT interval value > 500 msec should be reassessed and immediate action should be taken to correct concomitant risk factors, if any, while the risk/benefit of continuing versus suspending TRISENOX™ therapy should be considered. If syncope, rapid or irregular heartbeat develops, the patient should be hospitalized for monitoring, serum electrolytes should be assessed, TRISENOX™ therapy should be temporarily discontinued until the QTc interval regresses to below 460 msec, electrolyte abnormalities are corrected, and the syncope and irregular heartbeat cease. There are no data on the effect of TRISENOX™ on the QTc interval during the infusion.

DESCRIPTION

TRISENOX™ is a sterile injectable solution of arsenic trioxide. The molecular formula of the drug substance in the solid state is As_2O_3, with a molecular weight of 197.8 g. TRISENOX™ is available in 10 mL, single-use ampules containing 10 mg of arsenic trioxide. TRISENOX™ is formulated as a sterile, nonpyrogenic, clear solution of arsenic trioxide in water-for-injection using sodium hydroxide and dilute hydrochloric acid to adjust to pH 8. TRISENOX™ is preservative-free. Arsenic trioxide, the active ingredient, is present at a concentration of 1.0 mg/mL. Inactive ingredients and their respective approximate concentrations are sodium hydroxide (1.2 mg/mL) and hydrochloric acid, which is used to adjust the pH to 7.0–9.0.

CLINICAL PHARMACOLOGY
Mechanism of Action
The mechanism of action of TRISENOX™ is not completely understood. Arsenic trioxide causes morphological changes and DNA fragmentation characteristic of apoptosis in NB4 human promyelocytic leukemia cells *in vitro*. Arsenic trioxide also causes damage or degradation of the fusion protein PML/RAR-alpha.
Pharmacokinetics
The pharmacokinetics of trivalent arsenic, the active species of TRISENOX™, have not been characterized.
Metabolism
The metabolism of arsenic trioxide involves reduction of pentavalent arsenic to trivalent arsenic by arsenate reductase and methylation of trivalent arsenic to monomethylarsonic acid and monomethylarsonic acid to dimethylarsinic acid by methyltransferases. The main site of methylation reactions appears to be the liver. Arsenic is stored mainly in liver, kidney, heart, lung, hair and nails.
Excretion
Disposition of arsenic following intravenous administration has not been studied. Trivalent arsenic is mostly methylated in humans and excreted in urine.
Special Populations
The effects of renal or hepatic impairment or gender, age and race on the pharmacokinetics of TRISENOX™ have not been studied (see PRECAUTIONS).
Drug Interactions
No formal assessments of pharmacokinetic drug-drug interactions between TRISENOX™ and other drugs have been conducted. The methyltransferases responsible for metabolizing arsenic trioxide are not members of the cytochrome P450 family of isoenzymes (see PRECAUTIONS).

Clinical Studies
TRISENOX™ has been investigated in 40 relapsed or refractory APL patients, previously treated with an anthracycline and a retinoid regimen, in an open-label, single-arm,

Adverse Events TABLE Continued

System organ class / Adverse Event	All Adverse Events, Any Grade		Grade 3 & 4 Events	
	n	%	n	%
Somnolence	3	8		
Coma	2	5	2	5
Respiratory				
Cough	26	65		
Dyspnea	21	53	4	10
Epistaxis	10	25		
Hypoxia	9	23	4	10
Pleural effusion	8	20	1	3
Post nasal drip	5	13		
Wheezing	5	13		
Decreased breath sounds	4	10		
Crepitations	4	10		
Rales	4	10		
Hemoptysis	3	8		
Tachypnea	3	8		
Rhonchi	3	8		
Skin & subcutaneous tissue disorders				
Dermatitis	17	43		
Pruritus	13	33	1	3
Ecchymosis	8	20		
Dry Skin	6	15		
Erythema—non-specific	5	13		
Increased sweating	5	13		
Facial edema	3	8		
Night sweats	3	8		
Petechiae	3	8		
Hyperpigmentation	3	8		
Non specific skin lesions	3	8		
Urticaria	3	8		
Local exfoliation	2	5		
Eyelid edema	2	5		
Cardiac disorders				
Tachycardia	22	55		
ECG QT corrected interval prolonged > 500msec	16	40		
Palpitations	4	10		
ECG abnormal other than QT interval prolongation	3	8		
Infections and infestations				
Sinusitis	8	20		
Herpes simplex	5	13		
Upper respiratory tract infection	5	13	1	3
Bacterial infection—non-specific	3	8	1	3
Herpes zoster	3	8		
Nasopharyngitis	2	5		
Oral candidiasis	2	5		
Sepsis	2	5	2	5
Musculoskeletal, connective tissue and bone disorders				
Arthralgia	13	33	3	8
Myalgia	10	25	2	5
Bone pain	9	23	4	10
Back pain	7	18	1	3

TABLE continued on next page

Adverse Events TABLE Continued

System organ class / Adverse Event	All Adverse Events, Any Grade		Grade 3 & 4 Events	
	n	%	n	%
Neck Pain	5	13		
Pain in limb	5	13	2	5
Hematologic disorders				
Leukocytosis	20	50	1	3
Anemia	8	20	2	5
Thrombocytopenia	7	18	5	13
Febrile neutropenia	5	13	3	8
Neutropenia	4	10	4	10
Disseminated intravascular coagulation	3	8	3	8
Lymphadenopathy	3	8		
Vascular disorders				
Hypotension	10	25	2	5
Flushing	4	10		
Hypertension	4	10		
Pallor	4	10		
Psychiatric disorders				
Anxiety	12	30		
Depression	8	20		
Agitation	2	5		
Confusion	2	5		
Ocular disorders				
Eye irritation	4	10		
Blurred vision	4	10		
Dry eye	3	8		
Painful red eye	2	5		
Renal and urinary disorders				
Renal failure	3	8	1	3
Renal impairment	3	8		
Oliguria	2	5		
Incontinence	2	5		
Reproductive system disorders				
Vaginal hemorrhage	5	13		
Intermenstrual bleeding	3	8		
Ear Disorders				
Earache	3	8		
Tinnitus	2	5		

non-comparative study. Patients received 0.15 mg/kg/day intravenously over 1 to 2 hours until the bone marrow was cleared of leukemic cells or up to a maximum of 60 days. The CR (absence of visible leukemic cells in bone marrow and peripheral recovery of platelets and white blood cells with a confirmatory bone marrow ≥ 30 days later) rate in this population of previously treated patients was 28 of 40 (70%). Among the 22 patients who had relapsed less than one year after treatment with ATRA, there were 18 complete responders (82%). Of the 18 patients receiving TRISENOX™ ≥ one year from ATRA treatment, there were 10 complete responders (55%). The median time to bone marrow remission was 44 days and to onset of CR was 53 days. Three of 5 children, 5 years or older, achieved CR. No children less than 5 years old were treated.

Three to six weeks following bone marrow remission, 31 patients received consolidation therapy with TRISENOX™, at the same dose, for 25 additional days over a period up to 5 weeks. In follow-up treatment, 18 patients received further arsenic trioxide as a maintenance course. Fifteen patients had bone marrow transplants. At last follow-up, 27 of 40 patients were alive with a median follow-up time of 484 days (range 280 to 755) and 23 of 40 patients remained in complete response with a median follow-up time of 483 days (range 280 to 755).

Cytogenetic conversion to no detection of the APL chromosome rearrangement was observed in 24 of 28 (86%) patients who met the response criteria defined above, in 5 of 5

(100%) patients who met some but not all of the response criteria, and 3 of 7 (43%) of patients who did not respond Reverse Transcriptase—Polymerase Chain Reaction conversions to no detection of the APL gene rearrangement were demonstrated in 22 of 28 (79%) of patients who met the response criteria, in 3 of 5 (60%) of patients who met some but not all of the response criteria, and in 2 of 7 (29%) of patients who did not respond.

Responses were seen across all age groups tested, ranging from 6 to 72 years. The ability to achieve a CR was similar for both genders. There were insufficient patients of black, Hispanic or Asian derivation to estimate relative response rates in these groups, but responses were seen in members of each group.

Another single center study in 12 patients with relapsed or refractory APL, where patients received TRISENOX™ doses generally similar to the recommended dose, had similar results with 9 of 12 (75%) patients attaining a CR.

INDICATIONS

TRISENOX™ is indicated for induction of remission and consolidation in patients with acute promyelocytic leukemia (APL) who are refractory to, or have relapsed from, retinoid and anthracycline chemotherapy, and whose APL is characterized by the presence of the t(15;17) translocation or PML/ RAR-alpha gene expression.

The response rate of other acute myelogenous leukemia subtypes to TRISENOX™ has not been examined.

CONTRAINDICATIONS

TRISENOX™ is contraindicated in patients who are hypersensitive to arsenic.

WARNINGS (see boxed WARNING)

TRISENOX™ should be administered under the supervision of a physician who is experienced in the management of patients with acute leukemia.

APL Differentiation Syndrome (see boxed WARNING): Nine of 40 patients with APL treated with TRISENOX™, at a dose of 0.15 mg/kg, experienced the APL differentiation syndrome (see boxed WARNING and ADVERSE REACTIONS).

Hyperleukocytosis: Treatment with TRISENOX™ has been associated with the development of hyperleukocytosis ($\geq 10 \times 10^3/\mu L$) in 20 of 40 patients. A relationship did not exist between baseline WBC counts and development of hyperleukocytosis nor baseline WBC counts and peak WBC counts. Hyperleukocytosis was not treated with additional chemotherapy. WBC counts during consolidation were not as high as during induction treatment.

QT Prolongation (see boxed WARNING): QT/QTc prolongation should be expected during treatment with arsenic trioxide and torsade de pointes as well as complete heart block has been reported. Over 460 ECG tracings from 40 patients with refractory or relapsed APL treated with TRISENOX™ were evaluated for QTc prolongation. Sixteen of 40 patients (40%) had at least one ECG tracing with a QTc interval greater than 500 msec. Prolongation of the QTc was observed between 1 and 5 weeks after TRISENOX™ infusion, and then returned towards baseline by the end of 8 weeks after TRISENOX™ infusion. In these ECG evaluations, women did not experience more pronounced QT prolongation than men, and there was no correlation with age.

Complete AV block: Complete AV block has been reported with arsenic trioxide in the published literature including a case of a patient with APL.

Carcinogenesis: Carcinogenicity studies have not been conducted with TRISENOX™ by intravenous administration. The active ingredient of TRISENOX™, arsenic trioxide, is a human carcinogen.

Pregnancy: TRISENOX™ may cause fetal harm when administered to a pregnant woman. Studies in pregnant mice, rats, hamsters, and primates have shown that inorganic arsenicals cross the placental barrier when given orally or by injection. The reproductive toxicity of arsenic trioxide has been studied in a limited manner. An increase in resorptions, neural-tube defects, anophthalmia and microphthalmia were observed in rats administered 10 mg/kg of arsenic trioxide on gestation day 9 (approximately 10 times the recommended human daily dose on a mg/m^2 basis). Similar findings occurred in mice administered a 10 mg/kg dose of a related trivalent arsenic, sodium arsenite, (approximately 5 times the projected human dose on a mg/m^2 basis) on gestation days 6, 7, 8 or 9. Intravenous injection of 2 mg/kg sodium arsenite (approximately equivalent to the projected human daily dose on a mg/m^2 basis) on gestation day 7 (the lowest dose tested) resulted in neural-tube defects in hamsters.

There are no studies in pregnant women using TRISENOX™. If this drug is used during pregnancy or if the patient becomes pregnant while taking this drug, the patient should be apprised of the potential harm to the fetus. One patient who became pregnant while receiving arsenic trioxide had a miscarriage. Women of childbearing potential should be advised to avoid becoming pregnant.

PRECAUTIONS

Laboratory Tests: The patient's electrolyte, hematologic and coagulation profiles should be monitored at least twice weekly, and more frequently for clinically unstable patients during the induction phase and at least weekly during the consolidation phase. ECGs should be obtained weekly, and more frequently for clinically unstable patients, during induction and consolidation.

Drug Interactions: No formal assessments of pharmacokinetic drug-drug interactions between TRISENOX™ and other agents have been conducted. Caution is advised when TRISENOX™ is coadministered with other medications that can prolong the QT interval (e.g. certain antiarrhythmics or thioridazine) or lead to electrolyte abnormalities (such as diuretics or amphotericin B).

Carcinogenesis, Mutagenesis, Impairment of Fertility: See WARNINGS section for information on carcinogenesis. Arsenic trioxide and trivalent arsenite salts have not been demonstrated to be mutagenic to bacteria, yeast or mammalian cells. Arsenite salts are clastogenic *in vitro* (human fibroblasts, human lymphocytes, Chinese hamster ovary cells, Chinese hamster V79 lung cells). Trivalent arsenic produced an increase in the incidence of chromosome aberrations and micronuclei in bone marrow cells of mice. The effect of arsenic on fertility has not been adequately studied.

Pregnancy: Pregnancy Category D. See WARNINGS section.

Nursing Mothers: Arsenic is excreted in human milk. Because of the potential for serious adverse reactions in nursing infants from TRISENOX™, a decision should be made whether to discontinue nursing or to discontinue the drug, taking into account the importance of the drug to the mother.

Pediatric Use: There are limited clinical data on the pediatric use of TRISENOX™. Of 5 patients below the age of 18 years (age range: 5 to 16 years) treated with TRISENOX™, at the recommended dose of 0.15 mg/kg/day, 3 achieved a complete response.

Continued on next page

Trisenox—Cont.

Safety and effectiveness in pediatric patients below the age of 5 years have not been studied.

Patients with Renal or Hepatic Impairment: Safety and effectiveness of TRISENOX™ in patients with renal and hepatic impairment have not been studied. Particular caution is needed in patients with renal failure receiving TRISENOX™, as renal excretion is the main route of elimination of arsenic.

ADVERSE REACTIONS

Safety information was available for 52 patients with relapsed or refractory APL who participated in clinical trials of TRISENOX™. Forty patients in the Phase 2 study received the recommended dose of 0.15 mg/kg of which 28 completed both induction and consolidation treatment cycles. An additional 12 patients with relapsed or refractory APL received doses generally similar to the recommended dose. Most patients experienced some drug-related toxicity, most commonly leukocytosis, gastrointestinal (nausea, vomiting, diarrhea, and abdominal pain), fatigue, edema, hyperglycemia, dyspnea, cough, rash or itching, headaches, and dizziness. These adverse effects have not been observed to be permanent or irreversible nor do they usually require interruption of therapy.

Serious adverse events (SAEs), grade 3 or 4 according to version 2 of the NCI Common Toxicity Criteria, were common. Those SAEs attributed to TRISENOX™ in the Phase 2 study of 40 patients with refractory or relapsed APL included APL differentiation syndrome (n=3), hyperleukocytosis (n=3), QTc interval ≥ 500 msec (n=16, 1 with torsade de pointes), atrial dysrhythmias (n=2), and hyperglycemia (n=2).

The following table describes the adverse events that were observed in patients treated for APL with TRISENOX™ at the recommended dose at a rate of 5% or more. Similar adverse event profiles were seen in the other patient populations who received TRISENOX™.

[See table at top of page 15]

OVERDOSAGE

If symptoms suggestive of serious acute arsenic toxicity (e.g., convulsions, muscle weakness and confusion) appear, TRISENOX™ should be immediately discontinued and chelation therapy should be considered. A conventional protocol for acute arsenic intoxication includes dimercaprol administered at a dose of 3 mg/kg intramuscularly every 4 hours until immediate life-threatening toxicity has subsided. Thereafter, penicillamine at a dose of 250 mg orally, up to a maximum frequency of four times per day (≤ 1 gm per day), may be given.

DOSAGE AND ADMINISTRATION

TRISENOX™ should be diluted with 100 to 250mL 5% dextrose injection, USP or 0.9% Sodium Chloride injection, USP, using proper aseptic technique, immediately after withdrawal from the ampule. The TRISENOX™ ampule is single-use and does not contain any preservatives. Unused portions of each ampule should be discarded properly. Do not save any unused portions for later administration. Do not mix TRISENOX™ with other medications.

TRISENOX™ should be administered intravenously over 1–2 hours. The infusion duration may be extended up to 4 hours if acute vasomotor reactions are observed. A central venous catheter is not required.

Stability

After dilution, TRISENOX™ is chemically and physically stable when stored for 24 hours at room temperature and 48 hours when refrigerated.

Dosing Regimen

TRISENOX™ is recommended to be given according to the following schedule:

Induction Treatment Schedule: TRISENOX™ should be administered intravenously at a dose of 0.15 mg/kg daily until bone marrow remission. Total induction dose should not exceed 60 doses.

Consolidation Treatment Schedule: Consolidation treatment should begin 3 to 6 weeks after completion of induction therapy. TRISENOX™ should be administered intravenously at a dose of 0.15 mg/kg daily for 25 doses over a period up to 5 weeks.

HANDLING AND DISPOSAL

Procedures for proper handling and disposal of anticancer drugs should be considered. Several guidelines on this subject have been published.[1–7] There is no general agreement that all of the procedures recommended in the guidelines are necessary or appropriate.

HOW SUPPLIED

TRISENOX™ (arsenic trioxide) injection is supplied as a sterile, clear, colorless solution in 10 mL glass, single-use ampules.

NDC 60553-111-10 10 mg/10 mL (1 mg/mL) ampule in packages of ten ampules.

Store at 25°C (77°F); excursions permitted to 15–30°C (59–86°F). Do not freeze.

Do not use beyond expiration date printed on the label.

REFERENCES

1. *Recommendations for the Safe Handling of Parenteral Antineoplastic Drugs.* Publication NIH 83-2621. For sale by the Superintendent of Documents, U.S. Government Printing Office, Washington, DC 20402.
2. Council on Scientific Affairs. Guidelines for handling parenteral antineoplastics. *JAMA.* 1985;253:1590–1592.
3. National Study Commission on Cytotoxic Exposure. *Recommendations for handling cytotoxic agents.* Available from Louis P. Jeffrey, ScD, Chairman, National Study Commission on Cytotoxic Exposure, Massachusetts College of Pharmacy and Allied Health Sciences, 179 Longwood Avenue, Boston, Massachusetts 02115.
4. Clinical Oncological Society of Australia. Guidelines and recommendations for safe handling of antineoplastic agents. *Med J Australia.* 1983;1:426–428.
5. Jones RB, et al. Safe handling of chemotherapeutic agents: a report from the Mount Sinai Medical Center. *CA J Clin.* 1983;33:258–263.
6. American Society of Hospital Pharmacists Technical Assistance Bulletin on Handling Cytotoxic and Hazardous Drugs. *Am J Hosp Pharm.* 1990;47:1033–1049.
7. Controlling Occupational Exposure to Hazardous Drugs (OSHA Work-Practice Guidelines). *Am J Health-Syst Pharm.* 1996;53:1669–1685.

Rx only

For additional information, contact Cell Therapeutics, Inc. Professional Services at 1-800-715-0944
Customer Service at 1-888-305-2289.

Manufactured for:
Cell Therapeutics, Inc.
Seattle, WA 98119

AXOON 03/01 March 2001

Celltech Pharmaceuticals, Inc.

755 JEFFERSON ROAD
ROCHESTER, NY 14623

Direct Inquiries to:
Customer Service Department
P.O. Box 31766
Rochester, NY 14603
(716) 274-5300
(888) 963-3382

In Emergencies:
(800) 932-1950 (24 hours)

METADATE® CD ⒸII ℞
(methylphenidate HCl, USP)
Extended-Release Capsules
Rx Only
R549
Rev. 4/01

DESCRIPTION

METADATE CD is a central nervous system (CNS) stimulant. METADATE CD contains 20 mg of methylphenidate hydrochloride for oral administration. The extended-release capsules comprise both immediate-release (IR) and extended-release (ER) beads such that 30% of the dose (6 mg) is provided by the IR component and 70% of the dose (14 mg) is provided by the ER component.

Chemically, methylphenidate HCl is *d,l* (racemic)-*threo*-methyl α-phenyl-2-piperidineacetate hydrochloride. Its empirical formula is $C_{14}H_{19}NO_2 \cdot HCl$. Its structural formula is:

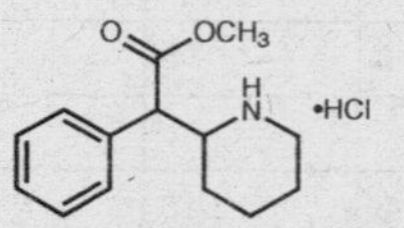

O
OCH3
H
N
•HCl

Methylphenidate HCl USP is a white, odorless, crystalline powder. Its solutions are acid to litmus. It is freely soluble in water and in methanol, soluble in alcohol, and slightly soluble in chloroform and in acetone. Its molecular weight is 269.77

METADATE CD also contains the following inert ingredients: Sugar spheres, povidone, hydroxypropylmethylcellulose and polyethylene glycol, ethylcellulose aqueous dispersion, dibutyl sebacate, gelatin, titanium dioxide, FD&C Blue No. 2.

CLINICAL PHARMACOLOGY

Pharmacodynamics: Methylphenidate HCl is a central nervous system (CNS) stimulant. The mode of therapeutic action in Attention Deficit Hyperactivity Disorder (ADHD) is not known. Methylphenidate is thought to block the reuptake of norepinephrine and dopamine into the presynaptic neuron and increase the release of these monoamines into the extraneuronal space. Methylphenidate is a racemic mixture comprised of the *d*- and *l-threo* enantiomers. The *d-threo* enantiomer is more pharmacologically active than the *l-threo* enantiomer.

Pharmacokinetics: The pharmacokinetics of the METADATE CD methylphenidate hydrochloride formulation have been studied in healthy adult volunteers and in children with attention deficit hyperactivity disorder (ADHD).

Absorption and Distribution: Methylphenidate is readily absorbed. METADATE CD has a plasma/time concentration profile showing two phases of drug release with a sharp, initial slope similar to a methylphenidate immediate-release tablet, and a second rising portion approximately three hours later, followed by a gradual decline. (See Figure 1 below.)

Comparison of Immediate Release (IR) and METADATE CD Formulations After Repeated Doses of Methylphenidate HCl in Children with ADHD: METADATE CD was administered as repeated once-daily doses of 20 mg or 40 mg to children aged 7–12 years with ADHD for one week. After a dose of 20 mg, the mean (±SD) early C_{max} was 8.6 (±2.2) ng/mL, the later C_{max} was 10.9 (±3.9)* ng/mL and AUC_{0-9h} was 63.0 (±16.8) ng•h/mL. The corresponding values after a 40 mg dose were 16.8 (±5.1) ng/mL, 15.1 (±5.8)* ng/mL and 120 (±39.6) ng•h/mL, respectively. The early peak concentrations (median) were reached about 1.5 hours after dose intake, and the second peak concentrations (median) were reached about 4.5 hours after dose intake. The means for C_{max} and AUC following a dose of 20 mg were slightly lower than those seen with 10 mg of the immediate-release formulation, dosed at 0 and 4 hours.

---

*25–30% of the subjects had only one observed peak (C_{max}) concentration of methylphenidate.

FIGURE 1

Comparison of Immediate Release (IR) and METADATE CD Formulations After Repeated Doses of Methylphenidate HCl in Children with ADHD

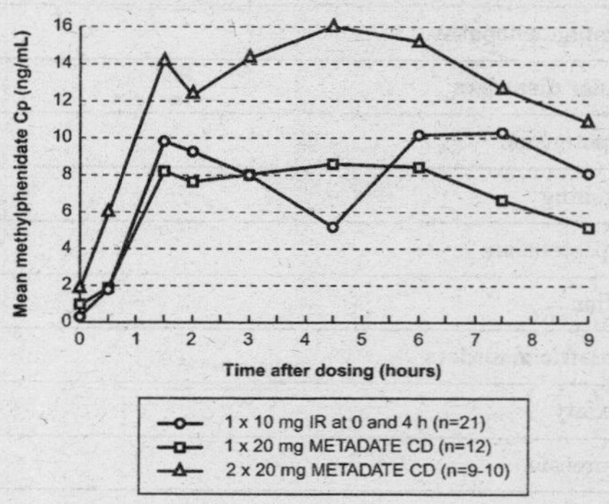

Mean methylphenidate Cp (ng/mL)
0
2
4
6
8
10
12
14
16
0
1
2
3
4
5
6
7
8
9
Time after dosing (hours)
1 x 10 mg IR at 0 and 4 h (n=21)
1 x 20 mg METADATE CD (n=12)
2 x 20 mg METADATE CD (n=9-10)

Dose Proportionality: Following single oral doses of 10–60 mg methylphenidate free base as a solution given to ten healthy male volunteers, C_{max} and AUC increased proportionally with increasing doses. After the 60 mg dose, t_{max} was reached 1.5 hours post-dose, with a mean C_{max} of 31.8 ng/mL (range 24.7–40.9 ng/mL).

Following one week of repeated once-daily doses of 20 mg or 40 mg METADATE CD to children aged 7–12 years with ADHD, C_{max} and AUC were proportional to the administered dose.

Food Effects: In a study in adult volunteers to investigate the effects of a high-fat meal on the bioavailability of a dose of 40 mg, the presence of food delayed the early peak by approximately 1 hour (range −2 to 5 hours delay). The plasma levels rose rapidly following the food-induced delay in absorption. Overall, a high-fat meal increased the C_{max} of METADATE CD by about 30% and AUC by about 17%, on average (see DOSAGE and ADMINISTRATION).

Metabolism and Excretion: In humans, methylphenidate is metabolized primarily via deesterification to alpha-phenyl-piperidine acetic acid (ritalinic acid). The metabolite has little or no pharmacologic activity.

In vitro studies showed that methylphenidate was not metabolized by cytochrome P450 isoenzymes, and did not inhibit cytochrome P450 isoenzymes at clinically observed plasma drug concentrations.

The mean terminal half-life ($t_{½}$) of methylphenidate following administration of METADATE CD ($t_{½}$=6.8h) is longer than the mean terminal $t_{½}$ following administration of methylphenidate hydrochloride immediate-release tablets ($t_{½}$=2.9h) and methylphenidate hydrochloride sustained-release tablets ($t_{½}$=3.4h) in healthy adult volunteers. This suggests that the elimination process observed for METADATE CD is controlled by the release rate of methylphenidate from the extended-release formulation, and that the drug absorption is the rate-limiting process.

Special Populations: *Gender:* The pharmacokinetics of methylphenidate after a single dose of METADATE CD were similar between adult men and women.

Race: The influence of race on the pharmacokinetics of methylphenidate after METADATE CD administration has not been studied.

Age: The pharmacokinetics of methylphenidate after METADATE CD administration have not been studied in children less than 6 years of age.

Renal and Hepatic Insufficiency: The pharmacokinetics of methylphenidate after METADATE CD administration has not been studied in patients with renal or hepatic insufficiency.

CLINICAL STUDIES

METADATE CD was evaluated in a double-blind, parallel-group, placebo-controlled trial in which 321 untreated or previously treated pediatric patients with a DSM-IV diagnosis of attention deficit hyperactivity disorder (ADHD), 6 to 15 years of age, received a single morning dose for up to 3 weeks. Patients were required to have the combined or predominantly hyperactive-impulsive subtype of ADHD; patients with the predominantly inattentive subtype were excluded. Patients randomized to the METADATE CD group received 20 mg daily for the first week. Their dosage could be increased weekly to a maximum of 60 mg by the third week, depending on individual response to treatment.

The patient's regular school teacher completed the teachers' version of the Conners' Global Index Scale (TCGIS), a scale for assessing ADHD symptoms, in the morning and again in the afternoon on three alternate days of each treatment week. The change from baseline of the overall average (i.e., an average of morning and afternoon scores over 3 days) of the total TCGIS scores during the last week of treatment was analyzed as the primary efficacy parameter. Patients treated with METADATE CD showed a statistically significant improvement in symptom scores from baseline over patients who received placebo. (See Figure 2.) Separate analyses of TCGIS scores in the morning and afternoon revealed superiority in improvement with METADATE CD over placebo during both time periods. (See Figure 3.) This demonstrates that a single morning dose of METADATE CD exerts a treatment effect in both the morning and the afternoon.

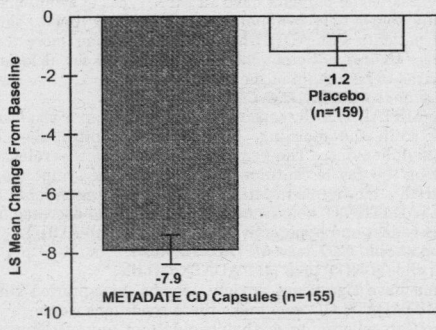

FIGURE 2

Least Squares Mean Change from Baseline in TCGIS Scores*

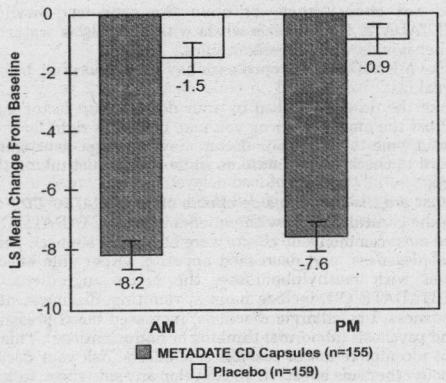

FIGURE 3

Least Squares Mean Change from Baseline in TCGIS Scores, Morning/Afternoon Groups*

* **FIGURES 2 & 3:** Last observation carried forward analysis at week 3. Error bars represent the standard error of the mean.

INDICATION AND USAGE

Attention Deficit Hyperactivity Disorder (ADHD): METADATE CD is indicated for the treatment of Attention Deficit Hyperactivity Disorder (ADHD).

The efficacy of METADATE CD in the treatment of ADHD was established in one controlled trial of children aged 6 to 15 who met DSM-IV criteria for ADHD (see CLINICAL PHARMACOLOGY).

A diagnosis of Attention Deficit Hyperactivity Disorder (ADHD; DSM-IV) implies the presence of hyperactive-impulsive or inattentive symptoms that caused impairment and were present before age 7 years. The symptoms must cause clinically significant impairment, e.g., in social, academic, or occupational functioning, and be present in two or more settings, e.g., school (or work) and at home. The symptoms must not be better accounted for by another mental disorder. For the Inattentive Type, at least six of the following symptoms must have persisted for at least 6 months: lack of attention to details/careless mistakes; lack of sustained attention; poor listener; failure to follow through on tasks; poor organization; avoids tasks requiring sustained mental effort; loses things; easily distracted; forgetful. For the Hyperactive-Impulsive Type, at least six of the following symptoms must have persisted for at least 6 months: fidgeting/squirming; leaving seat; inappropriate running/climbing; difficulty with quiet activities; "on the go;" excessive talking; blurting answers; can't wait turn; intrusive. The Combined Types requires both inattentive and hyperactive-impulsive criteria to be met.

Special Diagnostic Considerations: Specific etiology of this syndrome is unknown, and there is no single diagnostic test. Adequate diagnosis requires the use not only of medical but of special psychological, educational, and social resources. Learning may or may not be impaired. The diagnosis must be based upon a complete history and evaluation of the child

and not solely on the presence of the required number of DSM-IV characteristics.

Need for Comprehensive Treatment Program: METADATE CD is indicated as an integral part of a total treatment program for ADHD that may include other measures (psychological, educational, social) for patients with this syndrome. Drug treatment may not be indicated for all children with this syndrome. Stimulants are not intended for use in the child who exhibits symptoms secondary to environmental factors and/or other primary psychiatric disorders, including psychosis. Appropriate educational placement is essential and psychosocial intervention is often helpful. When remedial measures alone are insufficient, the decision to prescribe stimulant medication will depend upon the physician's assessment of the chronicity and severity of the child's symptoms.

Long-Term Use: The effectiveness of METADATE CD for long-term use, i.e., for more than 3 weeks, has not been systematically evaluated in controlled trials. Therefore, the physician who elects to use METADATE CD for extended periods should periodically re-evaluate the long-term usefulness of the drug for the individual patient (see DOSAGE and ADMINISTRATION).

CONTRAINDICATIONS

Agitation: METADATE CD is contraindicated in patients with marked anxiety, tension and agitation, since the drug may aggravate these symptoms.

Hypersensitivity to Methylphenidate: METADATE CD is contraindicated in patients known to be hypersensitive to methylphenidate or other components of the product.

Glaucoma: METADATE CD is contraindicated in patients with glaucoma.

Tics: METADATE CD is contraindicated in patients with motor tics or with a family history or diagnosis of Tourette's syndrome. (see ADVERSE REACTIONS).

Monoamine Oxidase Inhibitors: METADATE CD is contraindicated during treatment with monoamine oxidase inhibitors, and also within a minimum of 14 days following discontinuation of a monoamine oxidase inhibitor (hypertensive crises may result).

WARNINGS

Depression: METADATE CD should not be used to treat severe depression.

Fatigue: METADATE CD should not be used for the prevention or treatment of normal fatigue states.

Long-Term Suppression of Growth: Sufficient data on the safety of long-term use of methylphenidate in children are not yet available. Although a causal relationship has not been established, suppression of growth (i.e., weight gain, and/or height) has been reported with the long-term use of stimulants in children. Therefore, patients requiring long-term therapy should be carefully monitored. Patients who are not growing or gaining weight as expected should have their treatment interrupted.

Psychosis: Clinical experience suggests that in psychotic patients, administration of methylphenidate may exacerbate symptoms of behavior disturbance and thought disorder.

Seizures: There is some clinical evidence that methylphenidate may lower the convulsive threshold in patients with prior history of seizures, in patients with prior EEG abnormalities in absence of seizures, and, very rarely, in absence of history of seizures and no prior EEG evidence of seizures. In the presence of seizures, the drug should be discontinued.

Hypertension and other Cardiovascular Conditions: Use cautiously in patients with hypertension. Blood pressure should be monitored at appropriate intervals in patients taking METADATE CD, especially patients with hypertension. Studies of methylphenidate have shown modest increases of resting pulse and systolic and diastolic blood pressure. Therefore, caution is indicated in treating patients whose underlying medical conditions might be compromised by increases in blood pressure or heart rate, e.g., those with pre-existing hypertension, heart failure, recent myocardial infarction, or hyperthyroidism.

Visual Disturbance: Symptoms of visual disturbances have been encountered in rare cases. Difficulties with accommodation and blurring of vision have been reported.

Use in Children Under Six Years of Age: METADATE CD should not be used in children under six years, since safety and efficacy in this age group have not been established.

DRUG DEPENDENCE: METADATE® CD (methylphenidate HCl, USP), Extended-Release Capsules should be given cautiously to patients with a history of drug dependence or alcoholism. Chronic abusive use can lead to marked tolerance and psychological dependence with varying degrees of abnormal behavior. Frank psychotic episodes can occur, especially with parenteral abuse. Careful supervision is required during withdrawal from abusive use since severe depression may occur. Withdrawal following chronic therapeutic use may unmask symptoms of the underlying disorder that may require follow-up.

PRECAUTIONS

Hematologic Monitoring: Periodic CBC, differential, and platelet counts are advised during prolonged therapy.

Information for Patients: Patients should be instructed to take one dose in the morning before breakfast. They should be instructed that the capsule must be swallowed whole, and not opened, crushed, or chewed.

Patient information is printed along with this insert. To assure safe and effective use of METADATE CD, the information and instructions provided in the patient information section should be discussed with patients.

Drug Interactions: Because of possible effects on blood pressure, METADATE CD should be used cautiously with pressor agents.

Human pharmacologic studies have shown that methylphenidate may inhibit the metabolism of coumarin anticoagulants, anticonvulsants (e.g., phenobarbital, phenytoin, primidone), and some antidepressants (tricyclics and selective serotonin reuptake inhibitors). Downward dose adjustment of these drugs may be required when given concomitantly with methylphenidate. It may be necessary to adjust the dosage and monitor plasma drug concentrations (or, in the case of coumarin, coagulation times), when initiating or discontinuing concomitant methylphenidate.

Serious adverse events have been reported in concomitant use with clonidine, although no causality for the combination has been established. The safety of using methylphenidate in combination with clonidine or other centrally acting alpha-2 agonists has not been systematically evaluated.

Carcinogenesis, Mutagenesis, and Impairment of Fertility: In a lifetime carcinogenicity study carried out in B6C3F1 mice, methylphenidate caused an increase in hepatocellular adenomas and, in males only, an increase in hepatoblastomas, at a daily dose of approximately 60 mg/kg/day. This dose is approximately 30 times and 4 times the maximum recommended human dose of METADATE CD on a mg/kg and mg/m^2 basis, respectively. Hepatoblastoma is a relatively rare rodent malignant tumor type. There was no increase in total malignant hepatic tumors. The mouse strain used is sensitive to the development of hepatic tumors, and the significance of these results to humans is unknown.

Methylphenidate did not cause any increases in tumors in a lifetime carcinogenicity study carried out in F344 rats; the highest dose used was approximately 45 mg/kg/day, which is approximately 22 times and 5 times the maximum recommended human dose of METADATE CD on a mg/kg and mg/m^2 basis, respectively.

In a 24-week carcinogenicity study in the transgenic mouse strain p53+/−, which is sensitive to genotoxic carcinogens, there was no evidence of carcinogenicity. Male and female mice were fed diets containing the same concentration of methylphenidate as in the lifetime carcinogenicity study; the high-dose groups were exposed to 60 to 74 mg/kg/day of methylphenidate.

Methylphenidate was not mutagenic in the *in vitro* Ames reverse mutation assay or in the *in vitro* mouse lymphoma cell forward mutation assay. Sister chromatid exchanges and chromosome aberrations were increased, indicative of a weak clastogenic response, in an *in vitro* assay in cultured Chinese Hamster Ovary cells. Methylphenidate was negative *in vivo* in males and females in the mouse bone marrow micronucleus assay.

Methylphenidate did not impair fertility in male or female mice that were fed diets containing the drug in an 18-week Continuous Breeding study. The study was conducted at doses up to 160 mg/kg/day, approximately 80-fold and 8-fold the highest recommended human dose of METADATE CD on a mg/kg and mg/m^2 basis, respectively.

Pregnancy: Teratogenic Effects: Pregnancy Category C. Methylphenidate has been shown to have teratogenic effects in rabbits when given in doses of 200 mg/kg/day, which is approximately 100 times and 40 times the maximum recommended human dose on a mg/kg and mg/m^2 basis, respectively.

A reproduction study in rats revealed no evidence of teratogenicity at an oral dose of 58 mg/kg/day. However, this dose, which caused some maternal toxicity, resulted in decreased postnatal pup weights and survival when given to the dams from day one of gestation through the lactation period. This dose is approximately 30 fold and 6 fold the maximum recommended human dose of METADATE CD on a mg/kg and mg/m^2 basis, respectively.

There are no adequate and well-controlled studies in pregnant women. METADATE CD should be used during pregnancy only if the potential benefit justifies the potential risk to the fetus.

Nursing Mothers: It is not known whether methylphenidate is excreted in human milk. Because many drugs are excreted in human milk, caution should be exercised if METADATE CD is administered to a nursing woman.

Pediatric Use: The safety and efficacy of METADATE CD in children under 6 years old have not been established. Long-term effects of methylphenidate in children have not been well established (see WARNINGS).

ADVERSE REACTIONS

The premarketing development program for METADATE CD included exposures in a total of 228 participants in clinical trials (188 pediatric patients with ADHD, 40 healthy adult subjects). These participants received METADATE CD 20, 40, and/or 60 mg/day. The 188 patients (ages 6 to 15) were evaluated in one controlled clinical study, one controlled, crossover clinical study, and one uncontrolled clinical study. Safety data on all patients are included in the discussion that follows. Adverse reactions were assessed by collecting adverse events, results of physical examinations, vital signs, weights, laboratory analyses, and ECGs.

Adverse events during exposure were obtained primarily by general inquiry and recorded by clinical investigators using

Continued on next page

Metadate CD—Cont.

terminology of their own choosing. Consequently, it is not possible to provide a meaningful estimate of the proportion of individuals experiencing adverse events without first grouping similar types of events into a smaller number of standardized event categories. In the tables and listings that follow, COSTART terminology has been used to classify reported adverse events.

The stated frequencies of adverse events represent the proportion of individuals who experienced, at least once, a treatment-emergent adverse event of the type listed. An event was considered treatment emergent if it occurred for the first time or worsened while receiving therapy following baseline evaluation.

Adverse Findings in Clinical Trials with METADATE CD: Adverse Events Associated with Discontinuation of Treatment: In the 3-week placebo-controlled, parallel-group trial, two METADATE CD-treated patients (1%) and no placebo-treated patients discontinued due to an adverse event (rash and pruritus; and headache, abdominal pain, and dizziness, respectively).

Adverse Events Occurring at an Incidence of 5% or more Among METADATE CD-Treated Patients: Table 1 enumerates, for a pool of the three studies in pediatric patients with ADHD, at METADATE CD doses of 20, 40, or 60 mg/day, the incidence of treatment-emergent adverse events. One study was a 3-week placebo-controlled, parallel-group trial, one study was a controlled, crossover trial, and the third was an open titration trial. The table includes only those events that occurred in 5% or more of patients treated with METADATE CD where the incidence in patients treated with METADATE CD was greater than the incidence in placebo-treated patients.

The prescriber should be aware that these figures cannot be used to predict the incidence of adverse events in the course of usual medical practice where patient characteristics and other factors differ from those which prevailed in the clinical trials. Similarly, the cited frequencies cannot be compared with figures obtained from other clinical investigations involving different treatments, uses, and investigators. The cited figures, however, do provide the prescribing physician with some basis for estimating the relative contribution of drug and non-drug factors to the adverse event incidence rate in the population studied.

TABLE 1
Incidence of Treatment-Emergent Events[1]
in a Pool of 3–4 Week Clinical Trials of METADATE CD

Body System	Preferred Term	METADATE CD (n=188)	Placebo (n=190)
General	Headache	12%	8%
	Abdominal pain (stomach ache)	7%	4%
Digestive System	Anorexia (loss of appetite)	9%	2%
Nervous System	Insomnia	5%	2%

[1]: Events, regardless of causality, for which the incidence for patients treated with METADATE CD was at least 5% and greater than the incidence among placebo-treated patients. Incidence has been rounded to the nearest whole number.

Adverse Events with Other Methylphenidate HCl Products: Nervousness and insomnia are the most common adverse reactions reported with other methylphenidate products. Other reactions include hypersensitivity (including skin rash, urticaria, fever, arthralgia, exfoliative dermatitis, erythema multiforme with histopathological findings of necrotizing vasculitis, and thrombocytopenic purpura); anorexia; nausea; dizziness; palpitations; headache; dyskinesia; drowsiness; blood pressure and pulse changes, both up and down; tachycardia; angina; cardiac arrhythmia; abdominal pain; weight loss during prolonged therapy. There have been rare reports of Tourette's Syndrome. Toxic psychosis has been reported. Although a definite causal relationship has not been established, the following have been reported in patients taking this drug: instances of abnormal liver function, ranging from transaminase elevation to hepatic coma; isolated cases of cerebral arteritis and/or occlusion; leukopenia and/or anemia; transient depressed mood; a few instances of scalp hair loss. Very rare reports of neuroleptic malignant syndrome (NMS) have been reported, and, in most of these, patients were concurrently receiving therapies associated with NMS. In a single report, a ten year old boy who had been taking methylphenidate for approximately 18 months experienced an NMS-like event within 45 minutes of ingesting his first dose of venlafaxine. It is uncertain whether this case represented a drug-drug interaction, a response to either drug alone, or some other cause.

In children, loss of appetite, abdominal pain, weight loss during prolonged therapy, insomnia and tachycardia may occur more frequently; however, any of the other adverse reactions listed above may also occur.

DRUG ABUSE AND DEPENDENCE

Controlled Substance Class: METADATE CD, like other methylphenidate products, is classified as a Schedule II controlled substance by federal regulation.

Abuse, Dependence, and Tolerance: See WARNINGS for boxed warning containing drug abuse and dependence information.

OVERDOSAGE

Signs and Symptoms: Signs and symptoms of acute methylphenidate overdosage, resulting principally from overstimulation of the CNS and from excessive sympathomimetic effects, may include the following: vomiting, agitation, tremors, hyperreflexia, muscle twitching, convulsions (may be followed by coma), euphoria, confusion, hallucinations, delirium, sweating, flushing, headache, hyperpyrexia, tachycardia, palpitations, cardiac arrhythmias, hypertension, mydriasis, and dryness of mucous membranes.

Recommended Treatment: Treatment consists of appropriate supportive measures. The patient must be protected against self-injury and against external stimuli that would aggravate overstimulation already present. Gastric contents may be evacuated by gastric lavage as indicated. Before performing gastric lavage, control agitation and seizures if present and protect the airway. Other measures to detoxify the gut include administration of activated charcoal and a cathartic. Intensive care must be provided to maintain adequate circulation and respiratory exchange; external cooling procedures may be required for hyperpyrexia.

Efficacy of peritoneal dialysis or extracorporeal hemodialysis for METADATE CD overdosage has not been established.

The prolonged release of methylphenidate from METADATE CD should be considered when treating patients with overdose.

Poison Control Center: As with the management of all overdosage, the possibility of multiple drug ingestion should be considered. The physician may wish to consider contacting a poison control center for up-to-date information on the management of overdosage with methylphenidate.

DOSAGE AND ADMINISTRATION

METADATE CD is administered once daily in the morning, before breakfast.

METADATE CD must be swallowed whole with the aid of liquids, and must not be opened, crushed or chewed. (See PRECAUTIONS: Information for Patients.)

Dosage should be individualized according to the needs and responses of the patient.

Initial Treatment: The recommended starting dose of METADATE CD is 20 mg once daily. Dosage may be adjusted in weekly 20 mg increments to a maximum of 60 mg/day taken once daily in the morning, depending upon tolerability and degree of efficacy observed. Daily dosage above 60 mg is not recommended.

Maintenance/Extended Treatment: There is no body of evidence available from controlled trials to indicate how long the patient with ADHD should be treated with METADATE CD. It is generally agreed, however, that pharmacological treatment of ADHD may be needed for extended periods. Nevertheless, the physician who elects to use METADATE CD for extended periods in patients with ADHD should periodically re-evaluate the long-term usefulness of the drug for the individual patient with trials off medication to assess the patient's functioning without pharmacotherapy. Improvement may be sustained when the drug is either temporarily or permanently discontinued.

Dose Reduction and Discontinuation: If paradoxical aggravation of symptoms or other adverse events occur, the dosage should be reduced, or, if necessary, the drug should be discontinued.

If improvement is not observed after appropriate dosage adjustment over a one-month period, the drug should be discontinued.

HOW SUPPLIED

METADATE CD (methylphenidate HCl, USP) Extended-Release Capsules are available as 20 mg blue and white capsules. The capsule is printed with "MEDEVA 575" in white letters on the blue cap, and "20 mg" in black letters on the white body of the capsule.

NDC 53014-575-30   Dose Pack of 30 Capsules
PHARMACIST: Dispense only in current dose pack.
Store at 25°C (77°F): excursions permitted to 15°–30°C (59°–86°F) [See USP Controlled Room Temperature].
Keep out of the reach of children.

REFERENCE

American Psychiatric Association. *Diagnosis and Statistical Manual of Mental Disorders.* 4th ed. Washington D.C.: American Psychiatric Association 1994.
Marketed by:
CELLTECH
Celltech Pharmaceuticals, Inc.
Rochester, NY 14623 USA
Manufactured by:
Eurand America, Inc.
Vandalia, Ohio 45377 USA
® Celltech Pharma Limited
® 2001, Celltech Pharmaceuticals, Inc.
Rev. 4/01
R549

INFORMATION FOR PATIENTS TAKING METADATE® CD OR THEIR PARENTS OR CAREGIVERS

Once Daily
Metadate® CD Ⅱ
(methylphenidate HCl, USP)
Extended-Release Capsules
This information is for patients or their parents or caregivers taking METADATE CD Capsules for the treatment of Attention Deficit Hyperactivity Disorder.
Please read this before you start taking METADATE CD.
Remember, this information does not take the place of your

doctor's instructions. If you have any questions about this information or about METADATE CD, talk to your doctor or pharmacist.

What is METADATE® CD?
METADATE CD is a once-a-day treatment for Attention Deficit Hyperactivity Disorder, or ADHD. METADATE CD contains the drug methylphenidate, a central nervous system stimulant that has been used to treat ADHD for more than 30 years. METADATE CD is taken by mouth, once each day in the morning, before breakfast.

What is Attention Deficit Hyperactivity Disorder?
ADHD has three main types of symptoms: inattention, hyperactivity, and impulsiveness. Symptoms of inattention include not paying attention, making careless mistakes, not listening, not finishing tasks, not following directions, and being easily distracted. Symptoms of hyperactivity and impulsiveness include fidgeting, talking excessively, running around at inappropriate times, and interrupting others. Some patients have more symptoms of hyperactivity and impulsiveness while others have more symptoms of inattentiveness. Some patients have all three types of symptoms. Many people have symptoms like these from time to time, but patients with ADHD have these symptoms more than others their age. Symptoms must be present for at least 6 months to be certain of the diagnosis.

How does METADATE® CD work?
The METADATE CD capsule dissolves right after you swallow it in the morning, giving you an initial dose of methylphenidate. The remaining drug is slowly released during the day to continue to help lessen the symptoms of ADHD. Methylphenidate, the active ingredient in METADATE CD, helps increase attention and decrease impulsiveness and hyperactivity in patients with ADHD.

Who should NOT take METADATE® CD?
You should NOT take METADATE CD if:
• You have significant anxiety, tension, or agitation since METADATE CD may make these conditions worse.
• You are allergic to methylphenidate or any of the other ingredients in METADATE CD.
• You have glaucoma, an eye disease.
• You have tics or Tourette's Syndrome, or a family history of Tourette's Syndrome.
Talk to your doctor if you believe any of these conditions apply to you.

How should I take METADATE® CD?
Do not chew, crush, or open the capsules. Swallow METADATE CD capsules whole with the help of water or other liquids, such as milk or juice.
Take METADATE CD once each day in the morning, before breakfast.
Take the dose prescribed by your doctor. Your doctor may adjust the amount of drug you take until it is right for you. From time to time, your doctor may interrupt your treatment to check your symptoms while you are not taking the drug.

What are the possible side effects of METADATE® CD?
In the clinical studies with patients using METADATE CD, the most common side effects were headache, stomach pain, sleeplessness, and decreased appetite. Other side effects seen with methylphenidate, the active ingredient in METADATE CD, include nausea, vomiting, dizziness, nervousness, tics, allergic reactions, increased blood pressure and psychosis (abnormal thinking or hallucinations). This is not a complete list of possible side effects. Ask your doctor about other side effects. If you develop any side effect, talk to your doctor.

What must I discuss with my doctor before taking METADATE® CD?
Talk to your doctor **before** taking METADATE CD if you:
• Are being treated for depression or have symptoms of depression such as feelings of sadness, worthlessness, and hopelessness.
• Have motion tics (hard-to-control, repeated twitching of any parts of your body) or verbal tics (hard-to-control repeating of sounds or words).
• Have somebody in your family with motion tics, verbal tics, or Tourette's Syndrome.
• Have abnormal thoughts or visions, hear abnormal sounds, or have been diagnosed with psychosis.
• Have had seizures (convulsions, epilepsy) or abnormal EEGs (electoencephalograms).
• Have high blood pressure.
Tell your doctor **immediately** if you develop any of the above conditions or symptoms while taking METADATE CD.

Can I take METADATE® CD with other medicines?
Tell your doctor about **all** medicines that you are taking or intend to take. Your doctor should decide whether you can take METADATE CD with other medicines. These include:
• Other medicines that a doctor has prescribed.
• All medicines that you buy yourself without a prescription.
• Any herbal remedies that you may be taking.
You should not take METADATE CD with monoamine oxidase (MAO) inhibitors.
While on METADATE CD, do not start taking a new medicine or herbal remedy before checking with your doctor.
METADATE CD may change the way your body reacts to certain medicines. These include medicines used to treat depression, prevent seizures, or prevent blood clots (commonly called "blood thinners"). Your doctor may need to change your dose of these medicines if you are taking them with METADATE CD.

Other Important Safety Information:
Abuse of methylphenidate can lead to dependence.

Tell your doctor if you have ever abused or been dependent on alcohol or drugs, or if you are now abusing or dependent on alcohol or drugs.

Before taking METADATE CD, tell your doctor if you are pregnant or plan on becoming pregnant. If you take methylphenidate, it may be in your breast milk. Tell your doctor if you are nursing a baby.

Tell your doctor if you have blurred vision when taking METADATE CD.

Slower growth (weight gain and/or height) has been reported with long-term use of methylphenidate in children. Your doctor will be carefully watching your height and weight. If you are not growing or gaining weight as your doctor expects, your doctor may stop your METADATE CD treatment.

Call your doctor *immediately* if you take more than the amount of METADATE CD prescribed by your doctor.

What else should I know about METADATE® CD?

METADATE CD has not been studied in children under 6 years of age.

METADATE CD may be a part of your overall treatment for ADHD. Your doctor may also recommend that you have counseling or other therapy.

As with all medicines, never share METADATE CD with anyone else and take only the number of METADATE CD Capsules prescribed by your doctor.

METADATE CD should be stored in a safe place at room temperature (between 59°–86°F).

Keep out of the reach of children.

For more information call 1-888-METADATE (1-888-638-2328).

Marketed by:
CELLTECH
Celltech Pharmaceuticals, Inc.
Rochester, NY 14623 USA
Manufactured by:
Eurand America, Inc.
Vandalia, Ohio 45377 USA
® Celltech Pharma Limited
© 2001, Celltech Pharmaceuticals, Inc.
Rev. 4/01
R549

Elan Pharma
800 GATEWAY BOULEVARD
SOUTH SAN FRANCISCO, CA 94080

For Medical Information Contact:
(888) NEURO-05
(888) 638-7605
To Report Adverse Events Contact:
(877) ELAN GSS
(877) 352–6477

The products below are distributed by Elan Pharma, a business unit of Elan Pharmaceuticals, Inc.

MYOBLOC™   ℞
[mī-yō-blŏk]
(Botulinum Toxin Type B)
Injectable Solution

DESCRIPTION

MYOBLOC™ (Botulinum Toxin Type B) Injectable Solution is a sterile liquid formulation of a purified neurotoxin that acts at the neuromuscular junction to produce flaccid paralysis. The neurotoxin is produced by fermentation of the bacterium *Clostridium botulinum* type B (Bean strain) and exists in noncovalent association with hemagglutinin and non-hemagglutinin proteins as a neurotoxin complex. The neurotoxin complex is recovered from the fermentation process and purified through a series of precipitation and chromatography steps.

MYOBLOC™ is provided as a clear and colorless to light yellow sterile injectable solution in 3.5-mL glass vials. Each single use vial of formulated MYOBLOC™ contains 5000 U of Botulinum Toxin Type B per milliliter in 0.05% human serum albumin, 0.01 M sodium succinate, and 0.1 M sodium chloride at approximately pH 5.6.

One unit of MYOBLOC™ corresponds to the calculated median lethal intraperitoneal dose (LD50) in mice. The method for performing the assay is specific to Elan Pharmaceutical's manufacture of MYOBLOC™. Due to differences in specific details such as the vehicle, dilution scheme and laboratory protocols for various mouse LD50 assays, units of biological activity of MYOBLOC™ cannot be compared to or converted into units of any other botulinum toxin or any toxin assessed with any other specific assay method. Therefore, differences in species sensitivities to different botulinum neurotoxin serotypes precludes extrapolation of animal dose-activity relationships to human dose estimates. The specific activity of MYOBLOC™ ranges between 70 to 130 U/mg.

CLINICAL PHARMACOLOGY

The seven serologically distinct botulinum neurotoxins, designated A through G, share a common structural organization consisting of one Heavy Chain and one Light Chain polypeptide linked by a single disulfide bond. These toxins inhibit acetylcholine release at the neuromuscular junction via a three stage process: 1) Heavy Chain mediated neurospecific binding of the toxin, 2) internalization of the toxin

by receptor-mediated endocytosis, and 3) ATP and pH dependent translocation of the Light Chain to the neuronal cytosol where it acts as a zinc-dependent endoprotease cleaving polypeptides essential for neurotransmitter release. MYOBLOC™ specifically has been demonstrated to cleave synaptic Vesicle Associated Membrane Protein (VAMP, also known as synaptobrevin) which is a component of the protein complex responsible for docking and fusion of the synaptic vesicle to the presynaptic membrane, a necessary step to neurotransmitter release.

PHARMACOKINETICS

Though pharmacokinetic or ADME studies were not performed, MYOBLOC™ is not expected to be present in the peripheral blood at measurable levels following IM injection at the recommended doses. The recommended quantities of neurotoxin administered at each dosing session are not expected to result in systemic, distant overt clinical effects in patients without other neuromuscular dysfunction. While MYOBLOC™ has not been assessed for systemic effects, systemic effects have been shown by electromyography after IM doses of other botulinum toxins appropriate to produce clinically observable local muscle weakness.

CLINICAL STUDIES

Two phase 3, randomized, multi-center, double-blind, placebo controlled studies of the treatment of cervical dystonia were conducted. Both studies enrolled only adult patients who had a history of receiving botulinum toxin type A in an open label manner, with a perceived good response and tolerable adverse effects. Study #301 enrolled patients who were perceived as having an acceptable response to type A toxin, while Study #302 enrolled only patients who had secondarily lost responsiveness to type A toxin. Other eligibility criteria common to both studies were that all subjects had moderate or greater severity of cervical dystonia with at least 2 muscles involved, no neck contractures or other causes of decreased neck range of motion, and no history of any other neuromuscular disorder. Subjects in Study #301 were randomized to receive placebo, 5000 U or 10000 U of MYOBLOC™, and subjects in Study #302 were randomized to receive placebo or 10000 U of MYOBLOC™. Study agent was administered to subjects in a single treatment session by investigators who selected 2 to 4 muscles from any of the following: Splenius capitus, Sternocleidomastoid, Levator scapulae, Trapezius, Semispinalis capitus, and Scalene muscles. The total dose was divided between the selected muscles, and from 1 to 5 injections were made per muscle. There were 109 subjects enrolled into Study #301, and 77 into Study #302. Patient evaluations continued for 16 weeks post injection.

The primary efficacy outcome variable for both studies was the Toronto Western Spasmodic Torticollis Rating Scale (TWSTRS)-Total Score (scale range of possible scores is 0–87) at Week 4. TWSTRS is comprised of three sub-scales which examine 1) Severity—the severity of the patient's abnormal head position; 2) Pain—the severity and duration of pain due to the dystonia; and 3) Disability—the effects of the abnormal head position and pain on a patient's activities. The secondary endpoints were the Patient Global and Physician Global Assessments of change at Week 4. Both Global Assessments used a 100 point visual-analog scale (VAS).

The Patient Global Assessment allows a patient to indicate how they feel at the time of the evaluation compared to the pre-injection baseline. Likewise, the Physician Global indicates the physician's assessment of the patient's change from baseline to Week 4. Scores of 50 indicate no change, 0 much worse, and 100 much better. Results of comparisons of the primary and secondary efficacy variables are summarized in Table 1.

[See table above]

There were no statistically significant differences in results between the 5000 U and 10,000 U doses in Study #301. Exploratory analyses of these two studies suggested that the majority of patients who showed a beneficial response by Week 4 had returned to their baseline status between Weeks 12 to 16 post injection. Although there was a MYOBLOC™ associated decrease in pain, there remained many patients who experienced an increase in dystonia related neck pain irrespective of treatment group (see Adverse Reactions). TWSTRS Total Score at Week 4 and Patient Global Assessment among subgroups by gender or age showed consistent treatment associated effects across these subgroups (see also Precautions: Geriatrics). There were too few non-Caucasian patients enrolled to draw any conclusions regarding relative efficacy in racial subsets.

MYOBLOC™ was studied in two phase 2 dose ranging studies, Studies #08 and #09, that preceded the phase 3 studies. Studies #08 and #09 had a study design similar to the phase 3 studies, including eligibility criteria. Study #08 enrolled 85 subjects randomized between doses of placebo, 400 U, 1200 U, or 2400 U (21 or 22 subjects per group). Study #09 enrolled 122 subjects and randomized between doses of placebo, 2500 U, 5000 U, and 10,000 U (30 or 31 subjects per group). These studies demonstrated efficacy on the TWSTRS-Total, baseline to Week 4, at doses of 2400 U, 2500 U, 5000 U, and 10,000 U. Study #08 showed mean improvement from baseline on the Week 4 TWSTRS for placebo and 2400 U of 2.0 and 8.5 points respectively (from baselines of 42.0 and 42.4 points). Study #09 showed mean improvement from baseline to Week 4 for placebo, 2500 U, 5000 U, and 10,000 U of 3.3, 11.6, 12.5, and 16.4 points, respectively (from baselines of 45.5, 45.6, 45.2, and 47.5 points). Study #08 also indicated there is less response for doses below 2400 U.

Study #352 was an open label, intrapatient dose-escalation study of 3 treatment sessions where each patient with cervical dystonia sequentially received 10,000 U, 12,500 U and 15,000 U, at periods of 12 to 16 weeks between treatment sessions irrespective of their response to their previous dose. This study enrolled 145 patients, of whom 125 received all three treatments. Although this was an open label design where investigators and patients knew the dose at each treatment session, there were similar mean improvements on the TWSTRS-Total, from baseline to Week 4, for all three doses.

In the MYOBLOC™ injected patients (n=112) of the phase 3 studies, 19% had 2 muscles injected, 48% had 3 muscles injected, and 33% had 4 muscles injected. Table 2 indicates the frequency of use for each of the permitted muscles, and the fraction of the total dose of the treatment injected into each muscle, for those patients in whom the muscle was injected.

Table 1-Efficacy Results From Two Phase 3 MYOBLOC™ Studies

Assessments*	STUDY 301			STUDY 302	
	Placebo n = 36	5000 U n = 36	10000 U n = 37	Placebo n = 38	10000 U n = 39
TWSTRS Total					
Mean at Baseline	43.6	46.4	46.9	51.2	52.8
Change from Baseline	−4.3	−9.3	−11.7	−2.0	−11.1
95% Confidence Interval		(−8.9, −1.2)	(−11.1, −3.3)		(−12.2, −5.2)
p value		0.012	0.0004		0.0001
Patient Global					
Mean at Week Four	43.6	60.6	64.6	39.5	60.2
95% Confidence Interval		(7.0, 26.9)	(11.3, 31.1)		(11.2, 29.1)
p value		0.001	0.0001		0.0001
Physician Global					
Mean at Week Four	52.0	65.3	64.2	47.9	60.6
95% Confidence Interval		(5.5, 21.3)	(3.9, 19.7)		(7.4, 18.1)
p value		0.001	0.004		0.0001
TWSTRS-Subscales					
– Severity					
Mean at Baseline	18.4	20.2	20.2	22.1	22.6
Change from Baseline	−2.3	−3.2	−4.8	−1.2	−3.7
95% Confidence Interval		(−2.5, 0.6)	(−4.0, −1.0)		(−3.9, −1.0)
p value		0.22	0.002		0.001
– Pain					
Mean at Baseline	10.9	11.8	12.4	12.2	11.9
Change from Baseline	−0.5	−3.6	−4.2	−0.2	−3.6
95% Confidence Interval		(−4.7, −1.1)	(−5.1, −1.4)		(−5.0, −2.1)
p value		0.002	0.0008		0.0001
– Disability					
Mean at Baseline	14.3	14.4	14.4	16.9	18.3
Change from Baseline	−1.6	−2.5	−2.7	0.8	−3.8
95% Confidence Interval		(−2.7, 0.7)	(−2.8, 0.6)		(−4.1, −1.0)
p value		0.26	0.19		0.002

* 95% CI are for the differences between the active and placebo groups. The p-values are for the comparison of active dose and placebo. For TWSTRS- Total and TWSTRS-subscale scores, p-values are from ANCOVA for each variable with center and treatment in the model and the baseline value of the variable included as a convariate. For the Patient Global and Physician Global Assessments, p-values are from ANOVA for each variable with center and treatment in the model.

Continued on next page

Myobloc—Cont.

[See table below]

INDICATIONS AND USAGE

MYOBLOC™ is indicated for the treatment of patients with cervical dystonia to reduce the severity of abnormal head position and neck pain associated with cervical dystonia.

CONTRAINDICATIONS

MYOBLOC™ is contraindicated in patients with a known hypersensitivity to any ingredient in the formulation.

WARNINGS

Do not exceed the doses of MYOBLOC™, described under DOSAGE AND ADMINISTRATION. Risks resulting from administration at higher doses are not known.

Caution should be exercised when administering MYOBLOC™ to individuals with peripheral motor neuropathic diseases (e.g., amyotrophic lateral sclerosis, motor neuropathy) or neuromuscular junctional disorders (e.g., myasthenia gravis or Lambert-Eaton syndrome). Patients with neuromuscular disorders may be at increased risk of clinically significant systemic effects including severe dysphagia and respiratory compromise from typical doses of MYOBLOC™. Published medical literature has reported rare cases of administration of a botulinum toxin to patients with known or unrecognized neuromoscular disorders where the patients have shown extreme sensitivity to the systemic effects of typical clinical doses. In some cases, dysphagia has lasted months and required placement of a gastric feeding tube.

There were no documented cases of botulism resulting from the IM injection of MYOBLOC™ in patients with CD treated in clinical trials. If, however, botulism is clinically suspected, hospitalization for the monitoring of systemic weakness or paralysis and respiratory function (incipient respiratory failure) may be required.

Dysphagia is a commonly reported adverse event following treatment with all botulinum toxins in cervical dystonia patients. In the medical literature, there are reports of rare cases of dysphagia severe enough to warrant the insertion of a gastric feeding tube. There are also rare case reports where subsequent to the finding of dysphagia a patient developed aspiration pneumonia and died.

This product contains albumin, a derivative of human blood. Based on effective donor screening and product manufacturing processes, it carries an extremely remote risk for transmission of viral diseases. A theoretical risk for transmission of Creutzfeldt-Jakob disease (CJD) also is considered extremely remote. No cases of transmission of viral diseases or CJD have ever been identified for albumin.

PRECAUTIONS

Only 9 subjects without a prior history of tolerating injections of type A botulinum toxin have been studied. Treatment of botulinum toxin naïve patients should be initiated at lower doses of MYOBLOC™ (see Adverse Reactions: Overview).

DRUG INTERACTIONS

Co-administration of MYOBLOC™ and aminoglycosides or other agents interfering with neuromuscular transmission (e.g., curare-like compounds) should only be performed with caution as the effect of the toxin may be potentiated.

The effect of administering different botulinum neurotoxin serotypes at the same time or within less than 4 months of each other is unknown. However, neuromuscular paralysis may be potentiated by co-administration or overlapping administration of different botulinum toxin serotypes.

CARCINOGENESIS, MUTAGENESIS, IMPAIRMENT OF FERTILITY

No long-term carcinogenicity studies in animals have been performed.

PREGNANCY

PREGNANCY CATEGORY C. Animal reproduction studies have not been conducted with MYOBLOC™. It is also not known whether MYOBLOC™ can cause fetal harm when administered to a pregnant woman or can affect reproduction capacity. MYOBLOC™ should be given to a pregnant woman only if clearly needed.

NURSING MOTHERS

It is not known whether this drug is excreted in human milk. Because many drugs are excreted in human milk, caution should be exercised when MYOBLOC™ is administered to a nursing woman.

PEDIATRIC USE

Safety and effectiveness in pediatric patients have not been established.

GERIATRIC USE

In the controlled studies summarized in CLINICAL STUDIES, for MYOBLOC™ treated patients, 152 (74.5%) were under the age of 65, and 52 (25.5%) were aged 65 or greater. For these age groups, the most frequent reported adverse events occurred at similar rates in both age groups. Efficacy results did not suggest any large differences between these age groups. Very few patients aged 75 or greater were enrolled, therefore no conclusions regarding the safety and efficacy of MYOBLOC™ within this age group can be determined.

ADVERSE REACTIONS

Overview

The most commonly reported adverse events associated with MYOBLOC™ treatment in all studies were dry mouth, dysphagia, dyspepsia, and injection site pain. Dry mouth and dysphagia were the adverse reactions most frequently resulting in discontinuation of treatment. There was an increased incidence of dysphagia with increased dose in the sternocleidomastoid muscle. The incidence of dry mouth showed some dose-related increase with doses injected into the splenius capitis, trapezius and sternocleidomastoid muscles.

Only nine subjects without a prior history of tolerating injections of type A botulinum toxin have been studied. Adverse event rates have not been adequately evaluated in these patients, and may be higher than those described in Table 3.

Discussion

Adverse reaction rates observed in the clinical trials for a product cannot be directly compared to rates in clinical trials for another product and may not reflect the rates observed in actual clinical practice. However, adverse reaction information from clinical trials does provide a basis for identifying the adverse events that appear to be related to drug use and for approximating rates.

MYOBLOC™ was studied in both placebo controlled single treatment studies and uncontrolled repeated treatment studies; most treatment sessions and patients were in the uncontrolled studies. The data described below reflect exposure to MYOBLOC™ at varying doses in 570 subjects, including more than 300 patients with 4 or more treatment sessions. Most treatment sessions were at doses of 12,500 U or less. There were 57 patients administered a dose of 20,000 or 25,000 U. All but nine patients had a prior history of receiving Type A botulinum toxin and adequately tolerating the treatment to have received repeated doses.

The rates of adverse events and association with MYOBLOC™ are best assessed in the results from the placebo controlled studies of a single treatment session with active monitoring. The data in Table 3 reflect those adverse events occurring in at least 5% of patients exposed to MYOBLOC™ treatment in pooled placebo controlled clinical trials. Annual rates of adverse events are higher in the overall data which includes longer duration follow-up of patients with repeated treatment experience. The mean age of the population in these studies was 55 years old with approximately 66% being female. Most of the patients studied were Caucasian and all had cervical dystonia that was rated as moderate to severe in severity.

[See table below]

In the overall clinical trial experience with MYOBLOC™ (570 patients, including the uncontrolled studies), most cases of dry mouth or dysphagia were reported as mild or moderate in severity. Severe dysphagia was reported by 3% of patients, none of these requiring medical intervention. Severe dry mouth was reported by 6% of patients. Dysphagia and dry mouth were the most frequent adverse events reported as a reason for discontinuation from repeated treatment studies. These adverse events led to discontinuation from further treatments with MYOBLOC™ in some patients even when not reported as severe.

The following additional adverse events were reported in 2% or greater of patients participating in any of the clinical studies (COSTART terms, by body system):

Body as a Whole: allergic reaction, fever, headache related to injection, chest pain, chills, hernia, malaise, abscess, cyst, neoplasm, viral infection; Musculoskeletal: arthritis, joint disorder; Cardiovascular System: migraine; Respiratory: dyspnea, lung disorder, pneumonia; Nervous System: anxiety, tremor, hyperesthesia, somnolence, confusion, pain related to CD/torticollis, vertigo, vasodilation; Digestive System: gastrointestinal disorder, vomiting, glossitis, stomatitis, tooth disorder; Skin and Appendages: pruritis; Urogenital System: urinary tract infection, cystitis, vaginal moniliasis; Special Senses: amblyopia, otitis media, abnormal vision, taste perversion, tinnitus; Metabolic and Nutritional Disorders: peripheral edema, edema, hypercholesterolemia; Hemic and Lymphatic System: ecchymosis.

Immunogenicity

A two stage assay was used to test for immunogenicity and neutralizing activity induced by treatment with MYOBLOC™. In order to account for varying lengths of follow-up, life-table analysis methods were used to estimate the rates of development of immune responses and neutralizing activity. During the repeated treatment studies, 446 subjects were followed with periodic ELISA based evaluations for development of antibody responses against MYOBLOC™. Only patients who showed a positive ELISA assay were subsequently tested for the presence of neutralizing activity against MYOBLOC™ in the mouse neutralization assay (MNA). 12% of patients had positive ELISA assays at baseline. Patients began to develop new ELISA responses after a single treatment session with MYOBLOC™. By six months after initiating treatment, estimates for ELISA positive rate were 20%, which continued to rise to 36% at one year and 50% positive ELISA status at 18 months. Serum neutralizing activity was primarily not seen in patients until after 6 months. Estimated rates of development were 10% at one year and 18% at 18 months in the overall group of patients, based on analysis of samples from ELISA positive individuals. The effect of conversion to

Table 2-Studies 301 and 302 Combined Data
Fraction of Total Dose Injected into Involved Muscles

Muscle Injected	Percent Frequency Injected*	Fraction of Total Dose Injected by Percentiles		
		25th	50th	75th
Splenius Capitus	88	0.30	0.40	0.50
Sternocleidomastoid	80	0.20	0.25	0.30
Semispinalis Capitus	52	0.30	0.36	0.50
Levator Scapulae	46	0.13	0.20	0.20
Trapezius	38	0.20	0.25	0.35
Scalene Complex	13	0.20	0.25	0.30

* Percent frequency of patients in whom each muscle was injected

Table 3-Treatment-Emergent AEs Reported by at Least 5% of MYOBLOC™ Treated Patients by Dose Group, Following Single Treatment Session in Controlled Studies 09, 301 and 302

Adverse Event (COSTART Term)	Placebo (N=104)	Dosing Group 2500 U (N=31)	5000 U (N=67)	10,000 U (N=106)
Dry Mouth	3 (3%)	1 (3%)	8 (12%)	36 (34%)
Dysphagia	3 (3%)	5 (16%)	7 (10%)	27 (25%)
Neck Pain related to CD[a]	17 (16%)	0 (0%)[b]	11 (16%)	18 (17%)
Injection Site Pain	9 (9%)	5 (16%)	8 (12%)	16 (15%)
Infection	16 (15%)	4 (13%)	13 (19%)	16 (15%)
Pain	10 (10%)	2 (6%)	4 (6%)	14 (13%)
Headache	8 (8%)	3 (10%)	11 (16%)	12 (11%)
Dyspepsia	5 (5%)	1 (3%)	0 (0%)	11 (10%)
Nausea	5 (5%)	3 (10%)	2 (3%)	9 (8%)
Flu Syndrome	4 (4%)	2 (6%)	6 (9%)	9 (8%)
Torticollis	7 (7%)	0 (0%)	3 (4%)	9 (8%)
Pain Related to CD/Torticollis	4 (4%)	3 (10%)	3 (4%)	7 (7%)
Arthralgia	5 (5%)	0 (0%)	1 (1%)	7 (7%)
Back Pain	3 (3%)	1 (3%)	3 (4%)	7 (7%)
Cough Increased	3 (3%)	1 (3%)	4 (6%)	7 (7%)
Myasthenia	3 (3%)	1 (3%)	3 (4%)	6 (6%)
Asthenia	4 (4%)	1 (3%)	0 (0%)	6 (6%)
Dizziness	2 (2%)	1 (3%)	2 (3%)	6 (6%)
Accidental Injury	4 (4%)	0 (0%)	3 (4%)	5 (5%)
Rhinitis	6 (6%)	1 (3%)	1 (1%)	5 (5%)

[a] Not a COSTART term
[b] Not collected in Study –09 by special COSTART term

ELISA or MNA positive status on efficacy was not evaluated in these studies, and the clinical significance of development of antibodies has not been determined.

The data reflect the percentage of patients whose test results were considered positive for antibodies to MYOBLOC™ in both an *in vitro* and *in vivo* assay. The results of these antibody tests are highly dependent on the sensitivity and specificity of the assays. Additionally, the observed incidence of antibody positivity in an assay may be influenced by several factors including sample handling, concomitant medications, and underlying disease. For these reasons, comparison of the incidence of antibodies to MYOBLOC™ with the incidence of antibodies to other products may be misleading.

OVERDOSAGE

Symptoms of overdose are likely not to present immediately following injection(s). Should a patient ingest the product or be accidentally overdosed, they should be monitored for up to several weeks for signs and symptoms of systemic weakness or paralysis.

In the event of an overdose an antitoxin may be administered. Contact Elan Pharmaceuticals at 1-888-638-7605 for additional information and your State Health Department to process a request for antitoxin through the Centers for Disease Control and Prevention (CDC) in Atlanta, GA. The antitoxin will not reverse any botulinum toxin induced muscle weakness effects already apparent by the time of antitoxin administration.

DOSAGE AND ADMINISTRATION

The recommended initial dose of MYOBLOC™ for patients with a prior history of tolerating botulinum toxin injections is 2500 to 5000 U divided among affected muscles (see CLINICAL STUDIES). Patients without a prior history of tolerating botulinum toxin injections should receive a lower initial dose. Subsequent dosing should be optimized according to the patient's individual response. MYOBLOC™ should be administered by physicians familiar and experienced in the assessment and management of patients with CD.

The method described for performing the potency assay is specific to Elan Pharmaceutical's manufacture of MYOBLOC™. Due to differences in the specific details of this assay such as the vehicle, dilution scheme and laboratory protocols for various potency assays, Units of biological activity of MYOBLOC™ cannot be compared to or converted into units of any other botulinum toxin or any toxin assessed with any other specific assay method. Therefore, differences in species sensitivities to different botulinum neurotoxin serotypes preclude extrapolation of animal dose-activity relationship to human dose estimates.

The duration of effect in patients responding to MYOBLOC™ treatment has been observed in studies to be between 12 and 16 weeks at doses of 5000 U or 10,000 U (see CLINICAL STUDIES).

HOW SUPPLIED

MYOBLOC™ is provided as a clear and colorless to light yellow sterile injectable solution in single use 3.5-mL glass vials. Each single use vial of formulated MYOBLOC™ contains 5000 U[a] of Botulinum Toxin Type B per milliliter in 0.05% human serum albumin, 0.01 M sodium succinate, 0.1 M sodium chloride at approximately pH 5.6.

[a]See DOSAGE AND ADMINISTRATION.

MYOBLOC™ is available in the following three presentations.

Dosage Strength	Volume Per Vial	Single-Vial Carton
2500 U	0.5 mL	NDC 59075-710-10
5000 U	1.0 mL	NDC 59075-711-10
10,000 U	2.0 mL	NDC 59075-712-10

Store under refrigeration at 2°–8°C (36°–46°F).

DO NOT FREEZE. DO NOT SHAKE.

The recommended storage condition for MYOBLOC™ is refrigeration at 2–8°C for up to 21 months.

MYOBLOC™ may be diluted with normal saline. Once diluted, the product must be used within 4 hours as the formulation does not contain a preservative.

All vials of expired MYOBLOC™ and equipment used in the administration of MYOBLOC™ should be carefully discarded according to standard medical waste practices.

Do not use after the expiration date stamped on the vial.

Single use vial.

Rx only

Manufactured By:

Elan Pharmaceuticals, Inc., South San Francisco, CA 94080

U.S. License No. 1579

"MYOBLOC" and the "MYOBLOC Logo" are trademarks of Elan Pharmaceuticals, Inc.

701331

Rev. 12/00

Fujisawa Healthcare, Inc.

PARKWAY NORTH CENTER
THREE PARKWAY NORTH
DEERFIELD, IL 60015-2548

For Medical Information Contact:

Generally:

Medical and Scientific Information
(800) 727-7003

In Emergencies:

Medical and Scientific Information
(800) 727-7003

PROTOPIC® ℞

(tacrolimus)
Ointment 0.03%
Ointment 0.1%

FOR DERMATOLOGIC USE ONLY
NOT FOR OPHTHALMIC USE

DESCRIPTION

PROTOPIC (tacrolimus) Ointment contains tacrolimus, a macrolide immunosuppressant produced by *Streptomyces tsukubaensis*. It is for topical dermatologic use only. Chemically, tacrolimus is designated as [3S-[3R*[E(1S*,3S*,4S*)],4S*,5R*,8S*,9E,12R*,14R*, 15S*, 16R*,18S*,19S*,26aR*]] - 5,6,8,11,12,13,14,15,16,17,18, 19, 24,25,26,26a-hexadecahydro-5,19-dihydroxy-3-[2-(4-hydroxy-3-methoxycyclohexyl)-1-methylethenyl]-14,16-dimethoxy-4,10,12,18-tetramethyl-8-(2-propenyl)-15, 19-epoxy-3H-pyrido[2,1-*c*][1,4]oxaazacyclotricosine-1,7,20,21(4H,23H)-tetrone, monohydrate. It has the following structural formula:

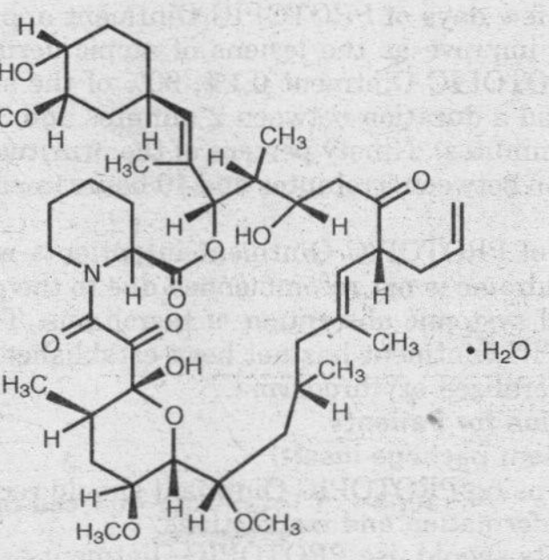

Tacrolimus has an empirical formula of $C_{44}H_{69}NO_{12} \cdot H_2O$ and a formula weight of 822.05. Each gram of PROTOPIC Ointment contains (w/w) either 0.03% or 0.1% of tacrolimus in a base of mineral oil, paraffin, propylene carbonate, white petrolatum and white wax.

CLINICAL PHARMACOLOGY

Mechanism of Action

The mechanism of action of tacrolimus in atopic dermatitis is not known. While the following have been observed, the clinical significance of these observations in atopic dermatitis is not known. It has been demonstrated that tacrolimus inhibits T-lymphocyte activation by first binding to an intracellular protein, FKBP-12. A complex of tacrolimus-FKBP-12, calcium, calmodulin, and calcineurin is then formed and the phosphatase activity of calcineurin is inhibited. This effect has been shown to prevent the dephosphorylation and translocation of nuclear factor of activated T-cells (NF-AT), a nuclear component thought to initiate gene transcription for the formation of lymphokines (such as interleukin-2, gamma interferon). Tacrolimus also inhibits the transcription for genes which encode IL-3, IL-4, IL-5, GM-CSF, and TNF-α, all of which are involved in the early stages of T-cell activation. Additionally, tacrolimus has been shown to inhibit the release of pre-formed mediators from skin mast cells and basophils, and to downregulate the expression of FcεRI on Langerhans cells.

Pharmacokinetics

The pooled results from two pharmacokinetic studies in 49 adult atopic dermatitis patients indicate that tacrolimus is absorbed after the topical application of 0.1% PROTOPIC Ointment. Peak tacrolimus blood concentrations ranged from undetectable to 20 ng/mL after single or multiple doses of 0.1% PROTOPIC Ointment, with 45 of the 49 patients having peak blood concentrations less than 5 ng/mL. The results from a pharmacokinetic study of 0.1% PROTOPIC Ointment in 20 pediatric atopic dermatitis patients (ages 6–13 years), show peak tacrolimus blood concentrations below 1.6 ng/mL in all patients.

There was no evidence based on blood concentrations that tacrolimus accumulates systemically upon intermittent topical application for periods of up to 1 year. The absolute bioavailability of topical tacrolimus is unknown. Using IV historical data for comparison, the bioavailability of tacrolimus from PROTOPIC in atopic dermatitis patients is less than 0.5%. In adults with an average of 53% BSA treated, exposure (i.e., AUC) of tacrolimus from PROTOPIC is approximately 30-fold less than that seen with oral immunosuppressive doses in kidney and liver transplant patients. The lowest tacrolimus blood level at which systemic effects can be observed is not known.

CLINICAL STUDIES

Three randomized, double-blind, vehicle-controlled, multicenter, phase 3 studies were conducted to evaluate PROTOPIC Ointment for the treatment of patients with moderate to severe atopic dermatitis. One (Pediatric) study included 351 patients 2–15 years of age, and the other two (Adult) studies included a total of 632 patients 15–79 years of age. Fifty-five percent (55%) of the patients were women and 27% were black. At baseline, 58% of the patients had severe disease and the mean body surface area (BSA) affected was 46%. Over 80% of patients had atopic dermatitis affecting the face and/or neck region. In these studies, patients applied either PROTOPIC Ointment 0.03%, PROTOPIC Ointment 0.1%, or vehicle ointment twice daily to 10%–100% of their BSA for up to 12 weeks.

In the pediatric study, a significantly greater ($p < 0.001$) percentage of patients achieved at least 90% improvement based on the physician's global evaluation of clinical response (the pre-defined primary efficacy end point) in the PROTOPIC Ointment 0.03% treatment group compared to the vehicle treatment group, but there was insufficient evidence that PROTOPIC Ointment 0.1% provided more efficacy than PROTOPIC Ointment 0.03%.

In both adult studies, a significantly greater ($p < 0.001$) percentage of patients achieved at least 90% improvement based on the physician's global evaluation of clinical response in the PROTOPIC Ointment 0.03% and PROTOPIC Ointment 0.1% treatment groups compared to the vehicle treatment group. There was evidence that PROTOPIC Ointment 0.1% may provide more efficacy than PROTOPIC Ointment 0.03%. The difference in efficacy between PROTOPIC Ointment 0.1% and 0.03% was particularly evident in adult patients with severe disease at baseline, adults with extensive BAS involvement, and black adults. Response rates for each treatment group are shown below by age groups. Because the two adult studies were identically designed, the results from these studies were pooled in this table.

[See table below]

A statistically significant difference in the percentage of adult patients with ≥ 90% improvement was achieved by week 1 for those treated with PROTOPIC Ointment 0.1%, and by week 3 for those treated with PROTOPIC Ointment 0.03%. A statistically significant difference in the percentage of pediatric patients with ≥ 90% improvement was achieved by week 2 for those treated with PROTOPIC Ointment 0.03%.

In adult patients who had achieved ≥ 90% improvement at the end of treatment, 35% of those treated with PROTOPIC Ointment 0.03% and 41% of those treated with PROTOPIC Ointment 0.1%, regressed from this state of improvement at 2 weeks after end-of-treatment. In pediatric patients who had achieved ≥ 90% improvement, 54% of those treated with PROTOPIC Ointment 0.03% regressed from this state of improvement at 2 weeks after end-of-treatment. Because patients were not followed for longer than 2 weeks after end-of-treatment, it is not known how many additional patients regressed at periods longer than 2 weeks after cessation of therapy.

In both PROTOPIC Ointment treatment groups in adults and in the PROTOPIC Ointment 0.03% treatment group in pediatric patients, a significantly greater improvement compared to vehicle ($p < 0.001$) was observed in the secondary efficacy endpoints of percent body surface area involved, patient evaluation of pruritus, erythema, edema, excoriation, oozing, scaling, and lichenification. The following two graphs depict the time course of improvement in the percent body surface area affected in adult and in pediatric patients as a result of treatment.

[See figure 1 at top of next column]

[See figure 2 at top of next column]

The following two graphs depict the time course of improvement in erythema in adult and in pediatric patients as a result of treatment.

[See figure 3 at top of next column]

[See figure 4 at top of next column]

The time course of improvement in the remaining secondary efficacy variables was similar to that of erythema, with improvement in lichenification slightly slower.

Continued on next page

Global Improvement over Baseline at the End-of-Treatment in Three Phase 3 Studies

Physician's Global Evaluation of Clinical Response (% Improvement)	Pediatric Study (2-15 Years of Age)		Adult Studies		
	Vehicle Ointment N = 116	PROTOPIC Ointment 0.03% N = 117	Vehicle Ointment N = 212	PROTOPIC Ointment 0.03% N = 211	PROTOPIC Ointment 0.1% N = 209
100%	4 (3%)	14 (12%)	2 (1%)	21 (10%)	20 (10%)
≥90%	8 (7%)	42 (36%)	14 (7%)	58 (28%)	77 (37%)
≥75%	18 (16%)	65 (56%)	30 (14%)	97 (46%)	117 (56%)
≥50%	31 (27%)	85 (73%)	42 (20%)	130 (62%)	152 (73%)

Protopic—Cont.

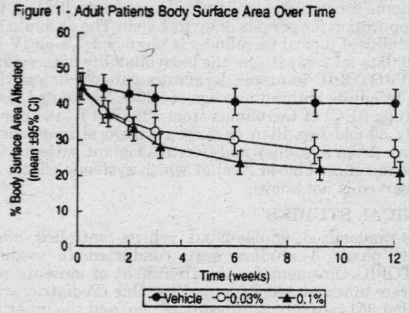

Figure 1 - Adult Patients Body Surface Area Over Time

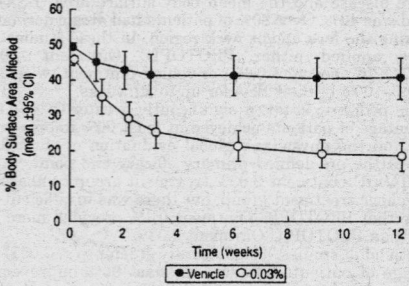

Figure 2 – Pediatric Patients Body Surface Area Over Time

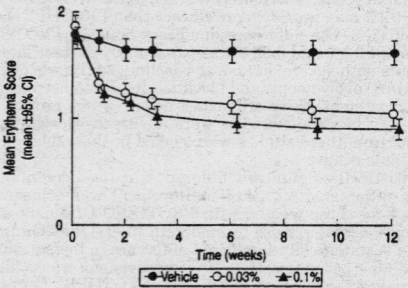

Figure 3 - Adult Patients Mean Erythema Over Time

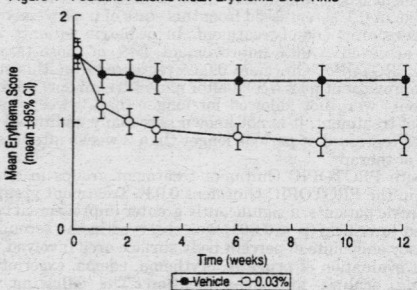

Figure 4 - Pediatric Patients Mean Erythema Over Time

A total of 571 patients applied PROTOPIC Ointment 0.1% in long-term adult and pediatric safety studies for up to one year. In the adult study, 246 patients were evaluated for at least 6 months and 68 patients for 12 months. In the pediatric study, 219 patients were evaluated for at least 6 months and 180 patients for 12 months. On average, patients received treatment for 87% of study days.

INDICATIONS AND USAGE

PROTOPIC Ointment, both 0.03% and 0.1% for adults, and only 0.03% for children aged 2 to 15 years, is indicated for short-term and intermittent long-term therapy in the treatment of patients with moderate to severe atopic dermatitis in whom the use of alternative, conventional therapies are deemed inadvisable because of potential risks, or in the treatment of patients who are not adequately responsive to or are intolerant of alternative, conventional therapies.

CONTRAINDICATIONS

PROTOPIC Ointment is contraindicated in patients with a history of hypersensitivity to tacrolimus or any other component of the preparation.

PRECAUTIONS
General

Studies have not evaluated the safety and efficacy of PROTOPIC Ointment in the treatment of clinically infected atopic dermatitis. Before commencing treatment with PROTOPIC Ointment, clinical infections at treatment sites should be cleared.

While patients with atopic dermatitis are predisposed to superficial skin infections including eczema herpeticum (Kaposi's varicelliform eruption), treatment with PROTOPIC Ointment may be associated with an increased risk of varicella zoster virus infection (chicken pox or shingles), herpes simplex virus infection, or eczema herpeticum. In the presence of these infections, the balance of risks and benefits associated with PROTOPIC Ointment use should be evaluated.

In clinical studies, 33 cases of lymphadenopathy (0.8%) were reported and were usually related to infections (particularly of the skin) and noted to resolve upon appropriate antibiotic therapy. Of these 33 cases, the majority had either a clear etiology or were known to resolve. Transplant patients receiving immunosuppressive regimens (e.g., systemic tacrolimus) are at increased risk for developing lymphoma; therefore, patients who receive PROTOPIC Ointment and who develop lymphadenopathy should have the etiology of their lymphadenopathy investigated. In the absence of a clear etiology for the lymphadenopathy, or in the presence of acute infectious mononucleosis, discontinuation of PROTOPIC Ointment should be considered. Patients who develop lymphadenopathy should be monitored to ensure that the lymphadenopathy resolves.

The enhancement of ultraviolet carcinogenicity is not necessarily dependent on phototoxic mechanisms. Despite the absence of observed phototoxicity in humans (see **ADVERSE REACTIONS**), PROTOPIC Ointment shortened the time to skin tumor formation in an animal photocarcinogenicity study (see **Carcinogenesis, Mutagenesis, Impairment of Fertility**). Therefore, it is prudent for patients to minimize or avoid natural or artificial sunlight exposure.

The use of PROTOPIC Ointment may cause local symptoms such as skin burning (burning sensation, stinging, soreness) or pruritus. Localized symptoms are most common during the first few days of PROTOPIC Ointment application and typically improve as the lesions of atopic dermatitis heal. With PROTOPIC Ointment 0.1%, 90% of the skin burning events had a duration between 2 minutes and 3 hours (median 15 minutes). Ninety percent of the pruritus events had a duration between 3 minutes and 10 hours (median 20 minutes).

The use of PROTOPIC Ointment in patients with Netherton's Syndrome is not recommended due to the potential for increased systemic absorption of tacrolimus. The safety of PROTOPIC Ointment has not been established in patients with generalized erythroderma.

Information for Patients
(See patient package insert)

Patients using PROTOPIC Ointment should receive the following information and instructions:

1. Patients should use PROTOPIC Ointment as directed by the physician. PROTOPIC Ointment is for external use only. As with any topical medication, patients or caregivers should wash hands after application if hands are not an area for treatment.
2. Patients should minimize or avoid exposure to natural or artificial sunlight (tanning beds or UVA/B treatment) while using PROTOPIC Ointment.
3. Patients should not use this medication for any disorder other than that for which it was prescribed.
4. Patients should report any signs of adverse reactions to their physician.
5. Before applying PROTOPIC Ointment after a bath or shower, be sure your skin is completely dry.

Drug Interactions

Formal topical drug interaction studies with PROTOPIC Ointment have not been conducted. Based on its minimal extent of absorption, interactions of PROTOPIC Ointment with systemically administered drugs are unlikely to occur but cannot be ruled out. The concomitant administration of known CYP3A4 inhibitors in patients with widespread and/or erythrodermic disease should be done with caution. Some examples of such drugs are erythromycin, itraconazole, ketoconazole, fluconazole, calcium channel blockers and cimetidine.

Carcinogenesis, Mutagenesis, Impairment of Fertility

No evidence of genotoxicity was seen in bacterial (*Salmonella* and *E. coli*) or mammalian (Chinese hamster lung-derived cells) *in vitro* assays of mutagenicity, the *in vitro* CHO/HGPRT assay of mutagenicity, or *in vivo* clastogenicity assays performed in mice. Tacrolimus did not cause unscheduled DNA synthesis in rodent hepatocytes.

Oral (feed) carcinogenicity studies have been carried out with systemically administered tacrolimus in male and female rats and mice. In the 80-week mouse study and in the 104-week rat study no relationship of tumor incidence to tacrolimus dosage was found at daily doses up to 3 mg/kg [9X the Maximum Recommended Human Dose (MRHD) based on AUC comparisons] and 5 mg/kg (3X the MRHD based on AUC comparisons), respectively.

A 104 week dermal carcinogenicity study was performed in mice with tacrolimus ointment (0.03%–3%), equivalent to tacrolimus doses of 1.1–118 mg/kg/day or 3.3–354 mg/m²/day. In the study, the incidence of skin tumors was minimal and the topical application of tacrolimus was not associated with skin tumor formation under ambient room lighting. However, a statistically significant elevation in the incidence of pleomorphic lymphoma in high dose male (25/50) and female animals (27/50) and in the incidence of undifferentiated lymphoma in high dose female animals (13/50) was noted in the mouse dermal carcinogenicity study. Lymphomas were noted in the mouse dermal carcinogenicity study at a daily dose of 3.5 mg/kg (0.1% tacrolimus ointment) (26X MRHD based on AUC comparisons). No drug-related tumors were noted in the mouse dermal carcinogenicity study at a daily dose of 1.1 mg/kg (0.03% tacrolimus ointment) (10X MRHD based on AUC comparisons).

In a 52-week photocarcinogenicity study, the median time to onset of skin tumor formation was decreased in hairless mice following chronic topical dosing with concurrent exposure to UV radiation (40 weeks of treatment followed by 12 weeks of observation) with tacrolimus ointment at ≥0.1% tacrolimus.

Reproductive toxicology studies were not performed with topical tacrolimus. In studies of oral tacrolimus no impairment of fertility was seen in male and female rats. Tacrolimus, given orally at 1.0 mg/kg (0.12X MRHD based on body surface area [BSA]) to male and female rats, prior to and during mating, as well as to dams during gestation and lactation, was associated with embryolethality and with adverse effects on female reproduction. Effects on female reproductive function (parturition) and embryolethal effects were indicated by a higher rate of pre-implantation loss and increased numbers of undelivered and nonviable pups. When given at 3.2 mg/kg (0.43X MRHD based on BSA), tacrolimus was associated with maternal and paternal toxicity as well as reproductive toxicity including marked adverse effects on estrus cycles, parturition, pup viability, and pup malformations.

Pregnancy
Teratogenic Effects: Pregnancy Category C

There are no adequate and well-controlled studies of topically administered tacrolimus in pregnant women. The experience with PROTOPIC Ointment when used by pregnant women is too limited to permit assessment of the safety of its use during pregnancy.

Reproduction studies were carried out with systemically administered tacrolimus in rats and rabbits. Adverse effects on the fetus were observed mainly at oral dose levels that were toxic to dams. Tacrolimus at oral doses of 0.32 and 1.0 mg/kg (0.04X–0.12X MRHD based on BSA) during organogenesis in rabbits was associated with maternal toxicity as well as an increase in incidence of abortions. At the higher dose only, an increased incidence of malformations and developmental variations was also seen. Tacrolimus, at oral doses of 3.2 mg/kg during organogenesis in rats, was associated with maternal toxicity and caused an increase in late resorptions, decreased numbers of live births, and decreased pup weight and viability. Tacrolimus, given orally at 1.0 and 3.2 mg/kg (0.04X–0.12X MRHD based on BSA) to pregnant rats after organogenesis and during lactation, was associated with reduced pup weights.

No reduction in male or female fertility was evident.

There are no adequate and well-controlled studies of systemically administered tacrolimus in pregnant women. Tacrolimus is transferred across the placenta. The use of systemically administered tacrolimus during pregnancy has been associated with neonatal hyperkalemia and renal dysfunction. PROTOPIC Ointment should be used during pregnancy only if the potential benefit to the mother justifies a potential risk to the fetus.

Nursing Mothers

Although systemic absorption of tacrolimus following topical applications of PROTOPIC Ointment is minimal relative to systemic administration, it is known that tacrolimus is excreted in human milk. Because of the potential for serious adverse reactions in nursing infants from tacrolimus, a decision should be made whether to discontinue nursing or to discontinue the drug, taking into account the importance of the drug to the mother.

Pediatric Use

PROTOPIC Ointment 0.03% may be used in pediatric patients 2 years of age and older. Two phase 3 pediatric studies were conducted involving 606 patients 2–15 years of age: one 12-week randomized vehicle-controlled study and one open-label, 1 year, long-term safety study. Three hundred and thirty (330) of these patients were 2 to 6 years of age. The most common adverse events associated with PROTOPIC Ointment application in pediatric patients were skin burning and pruritus (see **ADVERSE REACTIONS**). In addition to skin burning and pruritus, the less common events (<5%) of varicella zoster (mostly children pox), and vesiculobullous rash were more frequent in patients treated with PROTOPIC Ointment 0.03% compared to vehicle. In the long-term 1 year safety study involving 255 pediatric patients using PROTOPIC Ointment, the incidence of adverse events, including infections, did not increase with increased duration of study drug exposure or amount of ointment used. In 491 pediatric patients treated with PROTOPIC Ointment, 3(0.6%) developed eczema herpeticum. Since the safety and efficacy of PROTOPIC Ointment have not been established in pediatric patients below 2 years of age, its use in this age group is not recommended.

Geriatric Use

Twenty-five (25) patients ≥ 65 years old received PROTOPIC Ointment in phase 3 studies. The adverse event profile for these patients was consistent with that for other adult patients.

ADVERSE REACTIONS

No phototoxicity and no photoallergenicity was detected in clinical studies of 12 and 216 normal volunteers, respectively. One out of 198 normal volunteers showed evidence of sensitization in a contact sensitization study.

In three randomized vehicle-controlled studies and two long-term safety studies, 655 and 571 patients respectively, were treated with PROTOPIC Ointment.

The following table depicts the adjusted incidence of adverse events pooled across the 3 identically designed 12 week studies for patients in vehicle, PROTOPIC Ointment 0.03%, and PROTOPIC Ointment 0.1% treatment groups, and the unadjusted incidence of adverse events in two one year long-term safety studies, regardless of relationship to study drug. [See table below]

Other adverse events which occurred at an incidence greater than or equal to 1% in any clinical study include: alopecia, ALT or AST increased, anaphylactoid reaction, angina pectoris, angioedema, anorexia, anxiety, arrhythmia, arthralgia, arthritis, bilirubinemia, breast pain, cellulitis, cerebrovascular accident, cheilitis, chills, constipation, creatinine increased, dehydration, depression, dizziness, dyspnea, ear pain, ecchymosis, edema, epistaxis, exacerbation of untreated area, eye disorder, eye pain, furunculosis, gastritis, hemia, hyperglycemia, hypertension, hypoglycemia, hypoxia, laryngitis, leukocytosis, leukopenia, liver function tests abnormal, lung disorder, malaise, migraine, neck pain, neuritis, palpitations, paresthesia, peripheral vascular disorder, photosensitivity reaction, procedural complication, routine procedure, skin discoloration, sweating, taste perversion, tooth disorder, unintended pregnancy, vaginal moniliasis, vasodilatation, and vertigo.

OVERDOSAGE

PROTOPIC Ointment is not for oral use. Oral ingestion of PROTOPIC Ointment may lead to adverse effects associated with systemic administration of tacrolimus. If oral ingestion occurs, medical advice should be sought.

DOSAGE AND ADMINISTRATION

ADULT

PROTOPIC Ointment 0.03% and 0.1%

Apply a thin layer of PROTOPIC Ointment 0.03% or 0.1% to the affected skin areas twice daily and rub in gently and completely. Treatment should be continued for one week after clearing of signs and symptoms of atopic dermatitis.

The safety of PROTOPIC Ointment under occlusion which may promote systemic exposure, has not been evaluated. **PROTOPIC Ointment 0.03% and 0.1% should not be used with occlusive dressings.**

PEDIATRIC

PROTOPIC Ointment 0.03%

Apply a thin layer of PROTOPIC Ointment 0.03% to the affected skin areas twice daily and rub in gently and completely. Treatment should be continued for one week after clearing of signs and symptoms of atopic dermatitis. The safety of PROTOPIC Ointment under occlusion, which may promote systemic exposure, has not been evaluated. **PROTOPIC Ointment 0.03% should not be used with occlusive dressings.**

HOW SUPPLIED

PROTOPIC® (tacrolimus) Ointment 0.03%
NDC 0469-5201-30 Product Code 520130
30 gram laminate tube
NDC 0469-5201-60 Product Code 520160
60 gram laminate tube
PROTOPIC® (tacrolimus) Ointment 0.1%
NDC 0469-5202-30 Product Code 520230
30 gram laminate tube
NDC 0469-5202-60 Product Code 520260
60 gram laminate tube
Store at room temperature 25°C (77°F); excursions permitted to 15°–30°C (59°–86°F).
Rx only
Fujisawa Healthcare, Inc.
Deerfield, IL 60015–2548   Issued: December 2000

Patient Information About

Protopic® (tacrolimus) Ointment

Read this important information before you start using PROTOPIC [pro-TOP-ik] Ointment and each time you refill your prescription. There may be new information. This summary is not meant to take the place of your doctor's advice.

What is PROTOPIC?
PROTOPIC Ointment is a prescription medicine that is used to treat eczema (atopic dermatitis). It is for adults and children age 2 years and older. You can use PROTOPIC for short or intermittent long periods of treatment. Intermittent means starting and stopping repeatedly, as directed by your doctor. You can use it on all affected areas of your skin, including your face and neck.

Who should not use PROTOPIC?
Do not use PROTOPIC if you are
• breastfeeding
• allergic to PROTOPIC Ointment or any of its ingredients. The active ingredient is tacrolimus. Ask your doctor or pharmacist about the inactive ingredients.
Before you start using PROTOPIC, tell your doctor if you are:
• using **any** other prescription medicines, non-prescription (over-the-counter) medicines, or supplements
• receiving any form of light therapy (phototherapy, UVA or UVB) on your skin
• using any other type of skin product
• pregnant or planning to become pregnant

How do I use PROTOPIC?
Use PROTOPIC only to treat eczema that has been diagnosed by a doctor.
• Wash your hands before using PROTOPIC.
• Apply a thin layer of PROTOPIC to all skin areas that your doctor has diagnosed as eczema. Try to cover the affected areas completely. Most people find that a pea-sized amount squeezed from the tube covers an area about the size of a two-inch circle (approximately the size of a silver dollar).
• Apply the ointment twice a day, about 12 hours apart.
• Before applying PROTOPIC Ointment after a bath or shower, be sure your skin is completely dry
• Do not cover the skin being treated with bandages, dressings or wraps. Unless otherwise instructed by your doctor, do not apply another type of skin product on top of PROTOPIC Ointment. However, you can wear normal clothing
• Do not bathe, shower or swim right after applying PROTOPIC. This could wash off the ointment.
• If you are a caregiver applying PROTOPIC Ointment to a patient, or if you are a patient who is **not** treating your hands, wash your hands with soap and water after applying PROTOPIC. This should remove any ointment left on the hands.
• Use PROTOPIC only on your skin. Do **not** swallow PROTOPIC.
Because 2 strengths of PROTOPIC are available for adult patients, your doctor will decide what strength of PROTOPIC Ointment is best for you.
Many people notice that their skin starts to improve after the first few weeks of treatment. Even though your skin looks and feels better, it is important to keep using PROTOPIC as instructed by your doctor.
If you do not notice an improvement in your eczema or if your eczema gets worse within the first few weeks of treatment, tell your doctor.

What Should I Avoid While Using PROTOPIC?
• Avoid sunlight and sun lamps, tanning beds, and treatment with UVA or UVB light. If you need to be outdoors after applying PROTOPIC, wear loose fitting clothing that protects the treated area from the sun. In addition, ask your doctor what other type of protection from the sun you should use.
• Check with your doctor or pharmacist before you
  • start taking any new medicines while using PROTOPIC
  • start using any other ointment, lotions, or creams on you skin

What Are The Possible Side Effects of PROTOPIC?
The most common side effects of PROTOPIC are stinging, soreness, a burning feeling, or itching of the skin treated

Incidence Of Treatment Emergent Adverse Events

	12-Week Randomized, Double-Blind, Phase 3 Studies 12-Week Adjusted Incidence Rate (%)					Open-Label Studies (up to 1 year) 0.1% Tacrolimus Ointment Incidence(%)	
	Adult			Pediatric		Adult	Pediatric
	Vehicle n=212	0.03% Tacrolimus Ointment n=210	0.1% Tacrolimus Ointment n=209	Vehicle n=116	0.03% Tacrolimus Ointment n=118	n=316	n=255
Skin Burning†	26	46	58	29	43	47	26
Pruritus†	37	46	46	27	41	25	25
Flu-like symptoms†	19	23	31	25	28	22	35
Allergic Reaction	8	12	6	8	4	22	15
Skin Erythema	20	25	28	13	12	12	9
Headache†	11	20	19	8	5	10	18
Skin Infection	11	12	5	14	10	11	11
Fever	4	4	1	13	21	2	18
Infection	1	1	2	9	7	14	8
Cough Increased	2	1	1	14	18	3	15
Asthma	4	6	4	6	6	5	16
Herpes Simplex	4	4	4	2	0	12	5
Eczema Herpeticum	0	1	1	0	2	2	0
Pharyngitis	3	3	4	11	6	5	10
Accidental Injury	4	3	6	3	6	4	12
Pustular Rash	2	3	4	3	2	6	8
Folliculitis†	1	6	4	0	2	11	2
Rhinitis	4	3	2	2	6	5	5
Otitis Media	4	0	1	6	12	1	7
Sinusitis†	1	4	2	8	3	3	7
Diarrhea	3	3	4	2	5	4	6
Urticaria	3	3	6	1	1	5	5
Lack of Drug Effect	1	1	0	1	1	10	2
Bronchitis	0	2	2	3	3	3	6
Vomiting	0	1	1	7	6	1	5
Maculopapular Rash	2	2	2	3	0	4	2
Rash†	1	5	2	4	2	2	3
Abdominal Pain	3	1	1	2	3	1	5
Fungal Dermatitis	0	2	1	3	0	2	6
Gastroenteritis	1	2	2	3	0	4	2
Alcohol Intolerance†	0	3	7	0	0	6	0
Acne†	2	4	7	1	0	2	4
Sunburn	1	2	1	0	0	4	4
Skin Disorder	2	2	1	1	4	1	4
Conjunctivitis	0	2	2	2	1	4	2
Pain	1	2	1	0	0	4	3
Vesiculobullous Rash†	3	3	2	0	4	2	2
Lymphadenopathy	2	2	1	0	3	2	3
Nausea	4	3	2	0	1	1	2
Skin Tingling†	2	3	8	1	2	2	1
Face Edema	2	2	1	2	0	3	1
Dyspepsia†	1	1	4	0	0	1	4
Dry Skin	7	3	3	0	0	1	0
Hyperesthesia†	1	3	7	0	0	3	0
Skin Neoplasm Benign‡‡	1	1	1	0	0	2	3
Back Pain†	0	2	2	1	1	3	1
Peripheral Edema	2	4	3	0	0	2	1
Varicella Zoster/ Herpes Zoster‡‡	0	1	0	0	5	1	3
Contact Dermatitis	1	3	3	3	4	1	1
Asthenia	1	2	3	0	0	2	1
Pneumonia	0	1	1	2	0	1	2
Eczema	2	2	2	0	0	3	0
Insomnia	3	4	3	1	1	1	0
Exfoliative Dermatitis	3	3	1	0	0	0	2
Dysmenorrhea	2	4	4	0	0	0	2
Periodontal Abscess	1	0	1	0	0	3	0
Myalgia†	0	3	2	0	0	1	0
Cyst†	0	1	3	0	0	0	0

†May be reasonably associated with the use of this drug product
‡Four cases of chicken pox in the pediatric 12-week study, 1 case of "zoster of the lip" in the adult 12-week study; 7 cases of chicken pox and 1 case of shingles in the open-label pediatric study; 2 cases of herpes zoster in the open-label adult study.
‡‡Generally "warts".

Continued on next page

Protopic—Cont.

with PROTOPIC. These side effects are usually mild to moderate, are most common during the first few days of treatment, and typically lessen if your skin heals.
Less common side effects include acne, swollen or infected hair follicles, headache, increased sensitivity of the skin to hot or cold temperatures, or flu-like symptoms [common cold and congestion (stuffy nose)].
Some people may get skin tingling, upset stomach, herpes zoster (chicken pox or shingles), or muscle pain. While you are using PROTOPIC, drinking alcohol may cause the skin or face to become flushed or red and feel hot. Call your doctor if side effects continue or become a problem.

How Should I Store PROTOPIC?
Store PROTOPIC at room temperature (59° to 86°F). For instance, never leave PROTOPIC in your car in cold or hot weather. Make sure the cap on the tube is tightly closed. Keep PROTOPIC out of the reach of children.

General Advice about Prescription Medicines
Do not use PROTOPIC for a condition for which it was not prescribed. If you have any concerns about PROTOPIC, ask your doctor. Your doctor or pharmacist can give you information about PROTOPIC that was written for health care professionals. For more information, you can also visit the Fujisawa Internet site at www.fujisawa.com or call the PROTOPIC Help Line at 1-800-727-7003.

Fujisawa Healthcare, Inc.
Deerfield, IL 60015, www.fujisawa.com

Glaxo Wellcome Inc.

FIVE MOORE DRIVE
RESEARCH TRIANGLE PARK, NC 27709

For Medical Information for Healthcare Professionals Contact:
1-888-825-5249

In Emergencies:
Medical Information: 1-800-334-0089

For Consumer inquiries Contact:
1-888-825-5249

ADVAIR™ DISKUS® 100/50 ℞
(fluticasone propionate 100 mcg and salmeterol* 50 mcg inhalation powder)

ADVAIR™ DISKUS® 250/50 ℞
(fluticasone propionate 250 mcg and salmeterol* 50 mcg inhalation powder)

ADVAIR™ DISKUS® 500/50 ℞
(fluticasone propionate 500 mcg and salmeterol* 50 mcg inhalation powder)

***As salmeterol xinafoate salt 72.5 mcg, equivalent to salmeterol base 50 mcg**
FOR ORAL INHALATION ONLY

DESCRIPTION

ADVAIR DISKUS 100/50, ADVAIR DISKUS 250/50, and ADVAIR DISKUS 500/50 are combinations of fluticasone propionate and salmeterol xinafoate.
One active component of ADVAIR DISKUS is fluticasone propionate, a corticosteroid having the chemical name S-(fluoromethyl)6α,9-difluoro-11β,17-dihydroxy-16α-methyl-3-oxoandrosta-1,4-diene-17β-carbothioate, 17-propionate and the following chemical structure:

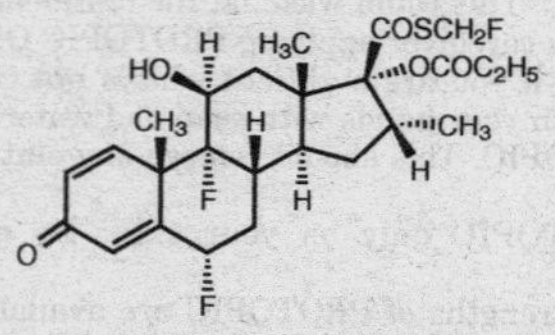

Fluticasone propionate is a white to off-white powder with a molecular weight of 500.6, and the empirical formula is $C_{25}H_{31}F_3O_5S$. It is practically insoluble in water, freely soluble in dimethyl sulfoxide and dimethylformamide, and slightly soluble in methanol and 95% ethanol.
The other active component of ADVAIR DISKUS is salmeterol xinafoate, a highly selective $beta_2$-adrenergic bronchodilator. Salmeterol xinafoate is the racemic form of the 1-hydroxy-2-naphthoic acid salt of salmeterol. The chemical name of salmeterol xinafoate is 4-hydroxy-α[1]-[[[6-(4-phenylbutoxy)-hexyl]amino]methyl]-1,3-benzenedimethanol, 1-hydroxy-2-naphthalenecarboxylate, and it has the following chemical structure:

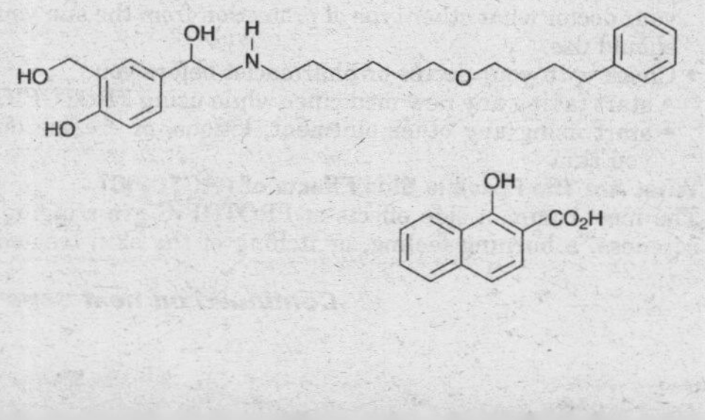

Salmeterol xinafoate is a white to off-white powder with a molecular weight of 603.8, and the empirical formula is $C_{25}H_{37}NO_4 \bullet C_{11}H_8O_3$. It is freely soluble in methanol; slightly soluble in ethanol, chloroform, and isopropanol; and sparingly soluble in water.
ADVAIR DISKUS 100/50, ADVAIR DISKUS 250/50, and ADVAIR DISKUS 500/50 are specially designed plastic devices containing a double-foil blister strip of a powder formulation of fluticasone propionate and salmeterol xinafoate intended for oral inhalation only. Each blister on the double-foil strip within the device contains 100, 250, or 500 mcg of microfine fluticasone propionate and 72.5 mcg of microfine salmeterol xinafoate salt, equivalent to 50 mcg of salmeterol base, in 12.5 mg of formulation containing lactose. Each blister contains 1 complete dose of both medications. After a blister containing medication is opened by activating the device, the medication is dispersed into the airstream created by the patient inhaling through the mouthpiece.
Under standardized in vitro test conditions, ADVAIR DISKUS delivers 93, 233, and 465 mcg of fluticasone propionate and 45 mcg of salmeterol base per blister from ADVAIR DISKUS 100/50, 250/50, and 500/50, respectively, when tested at a flow rate of 60 L/min for 2 seconds. In adult patients (n = 9) with obstructive lung disease and severely compromised lung function (mean forced expiratory volume in 1 second [FEV_1] 20% to 30% of predicted), mean peak inspiratory flow (PIF) through a DISKUS® device was 80.0 L/min (range, 46.1 to 115.3 L/min).
Inhalation profiles for adolescent (n = 13, aged 12 to 17 years) and adult (n = 17, aged 18 to 50 years) patients with asthma inhaling maximally through the DISKUS device show mean PIF of 122.2 L/min (range, 81.6 to 152.1 L/min). The actual amount of drug delivered to the lung will depend on patient factors, such as inspiratory flow profile.

CLINICAL PHARMACOLOGY

Mechanism of Action: ***ADVAIR DISKUS:*** ADVAIR DISKUS is designed to produce a greater improvement in pulmonary function and symptom control than either fluticasone propionate or salmeterol used alone at their recommended dosages. Since ADVAIR DISKUS contains both fluticasone propionate and salmeterol, the mechanisms of action described below for the individual components apply to ADVAIR DISKUS. These drugs represent 2 classes of medications (a synthetic corticosteroid and a long-acting beta-adrenergic receptor agonist) that have different effects on clinical, physiological, and inflammatory indices of asthma.
Fluticasone Propionate: Fluticasone propionate is a synthetic, trifluorinated corticosteroid with potent anti-inflammatory activity. In vitro assays using human lung cytosol preparations have established fluticasone propionate as a human glucocorticoid receptor agonist with an affinity 18 times greater than dexamethasone, almost twice that of beclomethasone-17-monopropionate (BMP), the active metabolite of beclomethasone dipropionate, and over 3 times that of budesonide. Data from the McKenzie vasoconstrictor assay in man are consistent with these results.
The precise mechanisms of fluticasone propionate action in asthma are unknown. Inflammation is recognized as an important component in the pathogenesis of asthma. Corticosteroids have been shown to inhibit multiple cell types (e.g., mast cells, eosinophils, basophils, lymphocytes, macrophages, and neutrophils) and mediator production or secretion (e.g., histamine, eicosanoids, leukotrienes, and cytokines) involved in the asthmatic response. These anti-inflammatory actions of corticosteroids contribute to their efficacy in asthma.
Salmeterol Xinafoate: Salmeterol is a long-acting beta-adrenergic agonist. In vitro studies and in vivo pharmacologic studies demonstrate that salmeterol is selective for $beta_2$-adrenoceptors compared with isoproterenol, which has approximately equal agonist activity on $beta_1$-and $beta_2$-adrenoceptors. In vitro studies show salmeterol to be at least 50 times more selective for $beta_2$-adrenoceptors than albuterol. Although $beta_2$-adrenoceptors are the predominant adrenergic receptors in bronchial smooth muscle and $beta_1$-adrenoceptors are the predominant receptors in the heart, there are also $beta_2$-adrenoceptors in the human heart comprising 10% to 50% of the total beta-adrenoceptors. The precise function of these receptors has not been established, but they raise the possibility that even highly selective $beta_2$-agonists may have cardiac effects.
The pharmacologic effects of $beta_2$-adrenoceptor agonist drugs, including salmeterol, are at least in part attributable to stimulation of intracellular adenyl cyclase, the enzyme that catalyzes the conversion of adenosine triphosphate (ATP) to cyclic-3′,5′-adenosine monophosphate (cyclic AMP). Increased cyclic AMP levels cause relaxation of bronchial smooth muscle and inhibition of release of mediators of immediate hypersensitivity from cells, especially from mast cells.
In vitro tests show that salmeterol is a potent and long-lasting inhibitor of the release of mast cell mediators, such as histamine, leukotrienes, and prostaglandin D_2, from human lung. Salmeterol inhibits histamine-induced plasma protein extravasation and inhibits platelet-activating factor-induced eosinophil accumulation in the lungs of guinea pigs when administered by the inhaled route. In humans, single doses of salmeterol administered via inhalation aerosol attenuate allergen-induced bronchial hyper-responsiveness.
Pharmacokinetics: ***ADVAIR DISKUS:*** Following administration of ADVAIR DISKUS to healthy subjects, peak plasma concentrations of fluticasone propionate were achieved in 1 to 2 hours and those of salmeterol were achieved in about 5 minutes.
In a single-dose crossover study, a higher than recommended dose of ADVAIR DISKUS was administered to 14 healthy subjects. Two inhalations of the following treatments were administered: ADVAIR DISKUS 500/50, fluticasone propionate powder 500 mcg and salmeterol powder 50 mcg given concurrently, and fluticasone propionate powder 500 mcg alone. Mean peak plasma concentrations of fluticasone propionate averaged 107, 94, and 120 pg/mL, respectively, and of salmeterol averaged 200 and 150 pg/mL, respectively, indicating no significant changes in systemic exposures of fluticasone propionate and salmeterol.
In a repeat-dose study, the highest recommended dose of ADVAIR DISKUS was administered to 45 asthmatic patients. One inhalation twice daily of the following treatments was administered: ADVAIR DISKUS 500/50, fluticasone propionate powder 500 mcg and salmeterol powder 50 mcg given concurrently, or fluticasone propionate powder 500 mcg alone. Mean peak steady-state plasma concentrations of fluticasone propionate averaged 57, 73, and 70 pg/mL, respectively, indicating no significant changes in systemic exposure of fluticasone propionate. No plasma concentrations of salmeterol were measured in this repeat-dose study.
No significant changes in excretion of fluticasone propionate or salmeterol were observed. The terminal half-life of fluticasone propionate averaged 5.33 to 7.65 hours when ADVAIR DISKUS was administered, which is similar to that reported when fluticasone propionate was given concurrently with salmeterol or when fluticasone propionate was given alone (average 5.30 to 6.91 hours). No terminal half-life of salmeterol was reported upon administration of ADVAIR DISKUS or salmeterol given concurrently with fluticasone propionate.
Special Populations: Formal pharmacokinetic studies using ADVAIR DISKUS were not conducted to examine gender differences or in special populations, such as elderly patients or patients with hepatic or renal impairment.
Drug-Drug Interactions: In the repeat- and single-dose studies, there was no evidence of significant drug interaction in systemic exposure between fluticasone propionate and salmeterol when given as ADVAIR DISKUS.
Fluticasone Propionate: Absorption: Fluticasone propionate acts locally in the lung; therefore, plasma levels do not predict therapeutic effect. Studies using oral dosing of labeled and unlabeled drug have demonstrated that the oral systemic bioavailability of fluticasone propionate is negligible (<1%), primarily due to incomplete absorption and presystemic metabolism in the gut and liver. In contrast, the majority of the fluticasone propionate delivered to the lung is systemically absorbed. The systemic bioavailability of fluticasone propionate from the DISKUS device in healthy volunteers averages 18%.
Peak steady-state fluticasone propionate plasma concentrations in adult patients (n = 11) ranged from undetectable to 266 pg/mL after a 500-mcg twice-daily dose of fluticasone propionate inhalation powder using the DISKUS device. The mean fluticasone propionate plasma concentration was 110 pg/mL.
Distribution: Following intravenous administration, the initial disposition phase for fluticasone propionate was rapid and consistent with its high lipid solubility and tissue binding. The volume of distribution averaged 4.2 L/kg.
The percentage of fluticasone propionate bound to human plasma proteins averages 91%. Fluticasone propionate is weakly and reversibly bound to erythrocytes and is not significantly bound to human transcortin.
Metabolism: The total clearance of fluticasone propionate is high (average, 1093 mL/min), with renal clearance accounting for less than 0.02% of the total. The only circulating metabolite detected in man is the 17β-carboxylic acid derivative of fluticasone propionate, which is formed through the cytochrome P450 3A4 pathway. This metabolite had less affinity (approximately 1/2000) than the parent drug for the glucocorticoid receptor of human lung cytosol in vitro and negligible pharmacological activity in animal studies. Other metabolites detected in vitro using cultured human hepatoma cells have not been detected in man.
Elimination: Following intravenous dosing, fluticasone propionate showed polyexponential kinetics and had a terminal elimination half-life of approximately 7.8 hours. Less than 5% of a radiolabeled oral dose was excreted in the urine as metabolites, with the remainder excreted in the feces as parent drug and metabolites.
Hepatic Impairment: Since fluticasone propionate is predominantly cleared by hepatic metabolism, impairment of liver function may lead to accumulation of fluticasone propionate in plasma. Therefore, patients with hepatic disease should be closely monitored.
Gender: Full pharmacokinetic profiles were obtained from 9 female and 16 male patients given fluticasone propionate inhalation powder 500 mcg twice daily using the DISKUS. No overall differences in fluticasone propionate pharmacokinetics were observed.
Special Populations: Formal pharmacokinetic studies using fluticasone propionate were not carried out in other special populations.
Drug-Drug Interactions: In a multiple-dose drug interaction study, coadministration of fluticasone propionate (500 mcg twice daily) and erythromycin (333 mg 3 times daily) did not affect fluticasone propionate pharmacokinetics. In another drug interaction study, coadministration of fluticasone propionate (1000 mcg) and ketoconazole (200 mg once daily) resulted in increased fluticasone propionate concentrations

and reduced plasma cortisol area under the plasma concentration versus time curve (AUC), but had no effect on urinary excretion of cortisol. Since fluticasone propionate is a substrate of cytochrome P450 3A4, caution should be exercised when cytochrome P450 3A4 inhibitors (e.g., ritonavir, ketoconazole) are coadministered with fluticasone propionate as this could result in increased plasma concentrations of fluticasone propionate.

Salmeterol Xinafoate: Salmeterol xinafoate, an ionic salt, dissociates in solution so that the salmeterol and 1-hydroxy-2-naphthoic acid (xinafoate) moieties are absorbed, distributed, metabolized, and eliminated independently. Salmeterol acts locally in the lung; therefore, plasma levels do not predict therapeutic effect.

Absorption: Because of the small therapeutic dose, systemic levels of salmeterol are low or undetectable after inhalation of recommended doses (50 mcg of salmeterol inhalation powder twice daily). Following chronic administration of an inhaled dose of 50 mcg of salmeterol inhalation powder twice daily, salmeterol was detected in plasma within 5 to 45 minutes in 7 asthmatic patients; plasma concentrations were very low, with mean peak concentrations of 167 pg/mL at 20 minutes and no accumulation with repeated doses.

Distribution: Binding of salmeterol to human plasma proteins averages 96% in vitro over the concentration range of 8 to 7722 ng of salmeterol base per milliliter, much higher concentrations than those achieved following therapeutic doses of salmeterol.

Metabolism: Salmeterol base is extensively metabolized by hydroxylation, with subsequent elimination predominantly in the feces. No significant amount of unchanged salmeterol base was detected in either urine or feces.

Elimination: In 2 healthy subjects who received 1 mg of radiolabeled salmeterol (as salmeterol xinafoate) orally, approximately 25% and 60% of the radiolabeled salmeterol was eliminated in urine and feces, respectively, over a period of 7 days. The terminal elimination half-life was about 5.5 hours (1 volunteer only).

The xinafoate moiety has no apparent pharmacologic activity. The xinafoate moiety is highly protein bound (>99%) and has a long elimination half-life of 11 days.

Special Populations: Formal pharmacokinetic studies of salmeterol base have not been conducted in special populations. Since salmeterol is predominantly cleared by hepatic metabolism, impairment of liver function may lead to accumulation of salmeterol in plasma. Therefore, patients with hepatic disease should be closely monitored.

Pharmacodynamics: *ADVAIR DISKUS:* Since systemic pharmacodynamic effects of salmeterol are not normally seen at the therapeutic dose, higher doses were used to produce measurable effects. Four studies were conducted in healthy subjects: (1) a single-dose crossover study using 2 inhalations of ADVAIR DISKUS 500/50, fluticasone propionate powder 500 mcg and salmeterol powder 50 mcg given concurrently, or fluticasone propionate powder 500 mcg given alone, (2) a cumulative dose study using 50 to 400 mcg of salmeterol powder given alone or as ADVAIR DISKUS 500/50, (3) a repeat-dose study for 11 days using 2 inhalations twice daily of ADVAIR DISKUS 250/50, fluticasone propionate powder 250 mcg, or salmeterol powder 50 mcg, and (4) a single-dose study using 5 inhalations of ADVAIR DISKUS 100/50, fluticasone propionate powder 100 mcg alone, or placebo. In these studies no significant differences were observed in the pharmacodynamic effects of salmeterol (pulse rate, blood pressure, QT_c interval, potassium, and glucose) whether the salmeterol was given as ADVAIR DISKUS, concurrently with fluticasone propionate from separate inhalers, or as salmeterol alone. The systemic pharmacodynamic effects of salmeterol were not altered by the presence of fluticasone propionate in ADVAIR DISKUS. The potential effect of salmeterol on the effects of fluticasone propionate on the hypothalamic-pituitary-adrenal (HPA) axis was also evaluated in these studies. No significant differences across treatments were observed in 24-hour urinary cortisol excretion and, where measured, 24-hour plasma cortisol AUC. The systemic pharmacodynamic effects of fluticasone propionate were not altered by the presence of salmeterol in ADVAIR DISKUS in healthy subjects.

In clinical studies with ADVAIR DISKUS in patients with asthma, no significant differences were observed in the systemic pharmacodynamic effects of salmeterol (pulse rate, blood pressure, QT_c interval, potassium, and glucose) whether the salmeterol was given alone or as ADVAIR DISKUS. In 72 adolescent and adult patients with asthma given either ADVAIR DISKUS 100/50 or ADVAIR DISKUS 250/50, continuous 24-hour electrocardiographic monitoring was performed after the first dose and after 12 weeks of therapy, and no clinically significant dysrhythmias were noted.

In a 28-week study in patients with asthma, ADVAIR DISKUS 500/50 twice daily was compared with the concurrent use of salmeterol powder 50 mcg plus fluticasone propionate powder 500 mcg from separate inhalers or fluticasone propionate powder 500 mcg alone. No significant differences across treatments were observed in plasma cortisol AUC after 12 weeks of dosing or in 24-hour urinary cortisol excretion after 12 and 28 weeks.

In a 12-week study in patients with asthma, ADVAIR DISKUS 250/50 twice daily was compared with fluticasone propionate powder 250 mcg alone, salmeterol powder 50 mcg alone, and placebo. For most patients, the ability to increase cortisol production in response to stress, as assessed by 30-minute cosyntropin stimulation, remained intact with ADVAIR DISKUS. One patient (3%) who received ADVAIR DISKUS 250/50 had an abnormal response (peak serum cortisol <18 mcg/dL) after dosing, compared with 2 patients (6%) who received placebo, 2 patients (6%) who received fluticasone propionate 250 mcg, and no patients who received salmeterol.

Fluticasone Propionate: In clinical trials with fluticasone propionate inhalation powder using doses up to and including 250 mcg twice daily, occasional abnormal short cosyntropin tests (peak serum cortisol <18 mcg/dL) were noted both in patients receiving fluticasone propionate and in patients receiving placebo. The incidence of abnormal tests at 500 mcg twice daily was greater than placebo. In a 2-year study carried out in 64 patients with mild, persistent asthma (mean FEV_1 91% of predicted) randomized to fluticasone propionate 500 mcg twice daily or placebo, no patient receiving fluticasone propionate had an abnormal response to 6-hour cosyntropin infusion (peak serum cortisol <18 mcg/dL). With a peak cortisol threshold of <35 mcg/dL, one patient receiving fluticasone propionate (4%) had an abnormal response at 1 year; repeat testing at 18 months and 2 years was normal. Another patient receiving fluticasone propionate (5%) had an abnormal response at 2 years. No patient on placebo had an abnormal response at 1 or 2 years.

Salmeterol Xinafoate: Inhaled salmeterol, like other beta-adrenergic agonist drugs, can in some patients produce dose-related cardiovascular effects and effects on blood glucose and/or serum potassium (see PRECAUTIONS). The cardiovascular effects (heart rate, blood pressure) associated with salmeterol occur with similar frequency, and are of similar type and severity, as those noted following albuterol administration.

The effects of rising doses of salmeterol and standard inhaled doses of albuterol were studied in volunteers and in patients with asthma. Salmeterol doses up to 84 mcg administered as inhalation aerosol resulted in heart rate increases of 3 to 16 beats/min, about the same as albuterol dosed at 180 mcg by inhalation aerosol (4 to 10 beats/min). Adolescent and adult patients receiving 50-mcg doses of salmeterol inhalation powder (n = 60) underwent continuous electrocardiographic monitoring during two 12-hour periods after the first dose and after 1 month of therapy, and no clinically significant dysrhythmias were noted.

Studies in laboratory animals (minipigs, rodents, and dogs) have demonstrated the occurrence of cardiac arrhythmias and sudden death (with histologic evidence of myocardial necrosis) when beta-agonists and methylxanthines are administered concurrently. The clinical significance of these findings is unknown.

CLINICAL TRIALS

In clinical trials comparing ADVAIR DISKUS with the individual components, improvements in most efficacy endpoints were greater with ADVAIR DISKUS than with the use of either fluticasone propionate or salmeterol alone. In addition, clinical trials showed similar results between ADVAIR DISKUS and the concurrent use of fluticasone propionate plus salmeterol at corresponding doses from separate inhalers.

Studies Comparing ADVAIR DISKUS to Fluticasone Propionate Alone or Salmeterol Alone: Three double-blind, parallel-group clinical trials were conducted with ADVAIR DISKUS in 1208 adolescent and adult patients (≥12 years, baseline FEV_1 63% to 72% of predicted normal) with asthma that was not optimally controlled on their current therapy. All treatments were inhalation powders, given as 1 inhalation from the DISKUS device twice daily, and other maintenance therapies were discontinued.

Study 1: Clinical Trial With ADVAIR DISKUS 100/50: This placebo-controlled, 12-week, US study compared ADVAIR DISKUS 100/50 with its individual components, fluticasone propionate 100 mcg and salmeterol 50 mcg. The study was stratified according to baseline asthma maintenance therapy; patients were using either inhaled corticosteroids (n = 250) (daily doses of beclomethasone dipropionate 252 to 420 mcg, flunisolide 1000 mcg, fluticasone propionate inhalation aerosol 176 mcg, or triamcinolone acetonide 600 to 1000 mcg) or salmeterol (n = 106). Baseline FEV_1 measurements were similar across treatments: ADVAIR DISKUS 100/50, 2.17 L; fluticasone propionate 100 mcg, 2.11 L; salmeterol, 2.13 L; and placebo, 2.15 L.

Predefined withdrawal criteria for lack of efficacy, an indicator of worsening asthma, were utilized for this placebo-controlled study. Worsening asthma was defined as a clinically important decrease in FEV_1 or peak expiratory flow (PEF), increase in use of VENTOLIN® (albuterol, USP) Inhalation Aerosol, increase in night awakenings due to asthma, emergency intervention or hospitalization due to asthma, or requirement for asthma medication not allowed by the protocol. As shown in Table 1, statistically significantly fewer patients receiving ADVAIR DISKUS 100/50 were withdrawn due to worsening asthma compared with fluticasone propionate, salmeterol, and placebo.

[See table below]

The FEV_1 results are displayed in Figure 1. Because this trial used predetermined criteria for worsening asthma, which caused more patients in the placebo group to be withdrawn, FEV_1 results at Endpoint (last available FEV_1 result) are also provided. Patients receiving ADVAIR DISKUS 100/50 had significantly greater improvements in FEV_1 (0.51 L, 25%) compared with fluticasone propionate 100 mcg (0.28 L, 15%), salmeterol (0.11 L, 5%), and placebo (0.01 L, 1%). These improvements in FEV_1 with ADVAIR DISKUS were achieved regardless of baseline asthma maintenance therapy (inhaled corticosteroids or salmeterol).

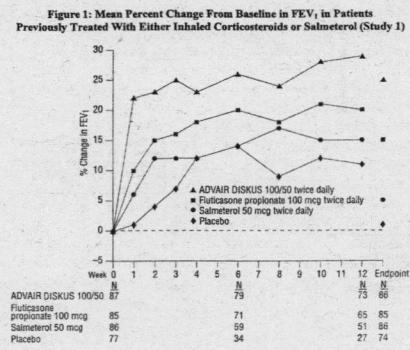

Figure 1: Mean Percent Change From Baseline in FEV_1 in Patients Previously Treated With Either Inhaled Corticosteroids or Salmeterol (Study 1)

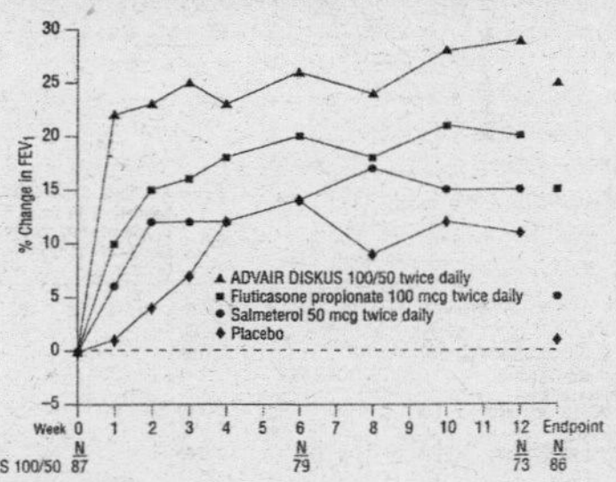

	N (Week 0)	N (Week 6)	N (Week 12)	N (Endpoint)
ADVAIR DISKUS 100/50	87	79	73	86
Fluticasone propionate 100 mcg	85	71	65	85
Salmeterol 50 mcg	86	59	51	86
Placebo	77	34	27	74

The effect of ADVAIR DISKUS 100/50 on morning and evening peak expiratory flow (PEF) endpoints is shown in Table 2.

[See table at bottom of next page]

The subjective impact of asthma on patients' perception of health was evaluated through use of an instrument called the Asthma Quality of Life Questionnaire (AQLQ) (based on a 7-point scale where 1 = maximum impairment and 7 = none). Patients receiving ADVAIR DISKUS 100/50 had clinically meaningful improvements in overall asthma-specific quality of life as defined by a difference between groups of ≥0.5 points in change from baseline AQLQ scores (difference in AQLQ score of 1.25 compared to placebo).

Study 2: Clinical Trial With ADVAIR DISKUS 250/50: This placebo-controlled, 12-week, US study compared ADVAIR DISKUS 250/50 with its individual components, fluticasone propionate 250 mcg and salmeterol 50 mcg in 349 patients using inhaled corticosteroids (daily doses of beclomethasone dipropionate 462 to 672 mcg, flunisolide 1250 to 2000 mcg, fluticasone propionate inhalation aerosol 440 mcg, or triamcinolone acetonide 1100 to 1600 mcg). Baseline FEV_1 measurements were similar across treatments: ADVAIR DISKUS 250/50, 2.23 L; fluticasone propionate 250 mcg, 2.12 L; salmeterol, 2.20 L; and placebo, 2.19 L.

Efficacy results in this study were similar to those observed in Study 1. Patients receiving ADVAIR DISKUS 250/50 had significantly greater improvements in FEV_1 (0.48 L, 23%) compared with fluticasone propionate 250 mcg (0.25 L, 13%), salmeterol (0.05 L, 4%), and placebo (decrease of 0.11 L, decrease of 5%). Statistically significantly fewer patients receiving ADVAIR DISKUS 250/50 were withdrawn from this study for worsening asthma (4%) compared with fluticasone propionate (22%), salmeterol (38%), and placebo (62%). In addition, ADVAIR DISKUS 250/50 was superior to fluticasone propionate, salmeterol, and placebo for improvements in morning and evening PEF. Patients receiving ADVAIR DISKUS 250/50 also had clinically meaningful improvements in overall asthma-specific quality of life as described in Study 1 (difference in AQLQ score of 1.29 compared to placebo).

Study 3: Clinical Trial With ADVAIR DISKUS 500/50: This 28-week, non-US study compared ADVAIR DISKUS 500/50 with fluticasone propionate 500 mcg alone and concurrent therapy (salmeterol 50 mcg plus fluticasone propionate 500 mcg administered from separate inhalers) twice daily in 503 patients using inhaled corticosteroids [daily doses of beclomethasone dipropionate 1260 to 1680 mcg, budesonide 1500 to 2000 mcg, flunisolide 1500 to 2000 mcg, or fluticasone propionate inhalation aerosol 660 to 880 mcg (750 to 1000 mcg inhalation powder)]. The primary efficacy parameter, morning PEF, was collected daily for the first 12 weeks of the study. The primary purpose of weeks 13 to 28 was to collect safety data.

Baseline PEF measurements were similar across treatments: ADVAIR DISKUS 500/50, 359 L/min; fluticasone propionate 500 mcg, 351 L/min; and concurrent therapy, 345 L/min. As shown in Figure 2, morning PEF improved significantly with ADVAIR DISKUS 500/50 compared with fluticasone propionate 500 mcg over the 12-week treatment period. Improvements in morning PEF observed with ADVAIR DISKUS 500/50 were similar to improvements observed with concurrent therapy.

[See figure at top of next column]

Onset of Action and Progression of Improvement in Asthma Control: The onset of action and progression of improvement in asthma control were evaluated in the 2 place-

Continued on next page

Table 1: Percent of Patients Withdrawn Due to Worsening Asthma in Patients Previously Treated With Either Inhaled Corticosteroids or Salmeterol (Study 1)

ADVAIR DISKUS 100/50 (n = 87)	Fluticasone Propionate 100 mcg (n = 85)	Salmeterol 50 mcg (n = 86)	Placebo (n = 77)
3%	11%	35%	49%)

Advair Diskus—Cont.

Figure 2: Mean Percent Change From Baseline in Morning Peak Expiratory Flow in Patients Previously Treated With Inhaled Corticosteroids (Study 3)

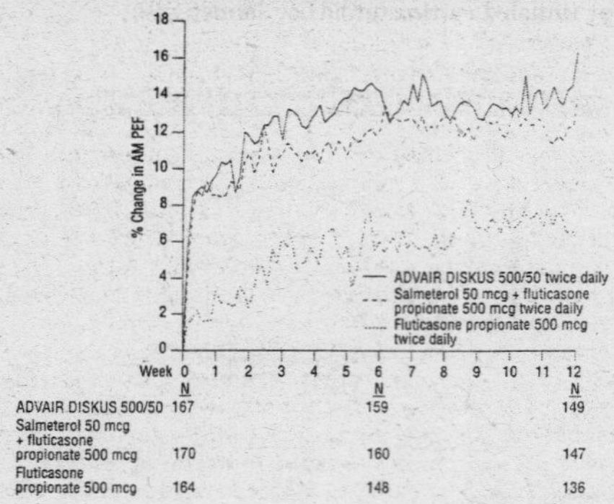

% Change in AM PEF
ADVAIR DISKUS 500/50 twice daily
Salmeterol 50 mcg + fluticasone propionate 500 mcg twice daily
Fluticasone propionate 500 mcg twice daily
Week 0 1 2 3 4 5 6 7 8 9 10 11 12
N N N
ADVAIR DISKUS 500/50 167 159 149
Salmeterol 50 mcg + fluticasone propionate 500 mcg 170 160 147
Fluticasone propionate 500 mcg 164 148 136

bo-controlled US trials. Following the first dose, the median time to onset of clinically significant bronchodilatation (≥15% improvement in FEV_1) in most patients was seen within 30 to 60 minutes. Maximum improvement in FEV_1 generally occurred within 3 hours, and clinically significant improvement was maintained for 12 hours (see Figure 3).

Following the initial dose, predose FEV_1 relative to day 1 baseline improved markedly over the first week of treatment and continued to improve over the 12 weeks of treatment in both studies.

No diminution in the 12-hour bronchodilator effect was observed with either ADVAIR DISKUS 100/50 (Figures 3 and 4) or ADVAIR DISKUS 250/50 as assessed by FEV_1 following 12 weeks of therapy.

Figure 3: Percent Change in Serial 12-hour FEV_1 in Patients Previously Using Either Inhaled Corticosteroids or Salmeterol (Study 1)

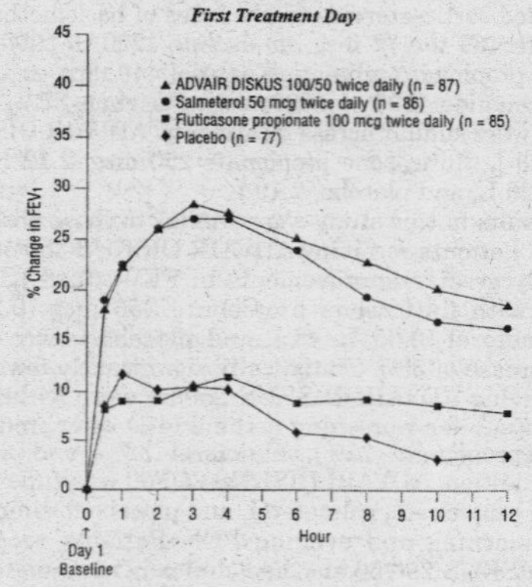

First Treatment Day
▲ ADVAIR DISKUS 100/50 twice daily (n = 87)
● Salmeterol 50 mcg twice daily (n = 86)
■ Fluticasone propionate 100 mcg twice daily (n = 85)
◆ Placebo (n = 77)
% Change in FEV1
Hour
Day 1 Baseline

[See figure at top of next column]

Reduction in asthma symptoms, use of rescue VENTOLIN Inhalation Aerosol, and improvement in morning and evening PEF also occurred within the first day of treatment with ADVAIR DISKUS, and continued to improve over the 12 weeks of therapy in both studies.

INDICATIONS AND USAGE

ADVAIR DISKUS is indicated for the long-term, twice-daily, maintenance treatment of asthma in patients 12 years of age and older.

ADVAIR DISKUS is NOT indicated for the relief of acute bronchospasm.

CONTRAINDICATIONS

ADVAIR DISKUS is contraindicated in the primary treatment of status asthmaticus or other acute episodes of asthma where intensive measures are required.

Hypersensitivity to any of the ingredients of these preparations contraindicates their use.

Figure 4: Percent Change in Serial 12-hour FEV_1 in Patients Previously Using Either Inhaled Corticosteroids or Salmeterol (Study 1)

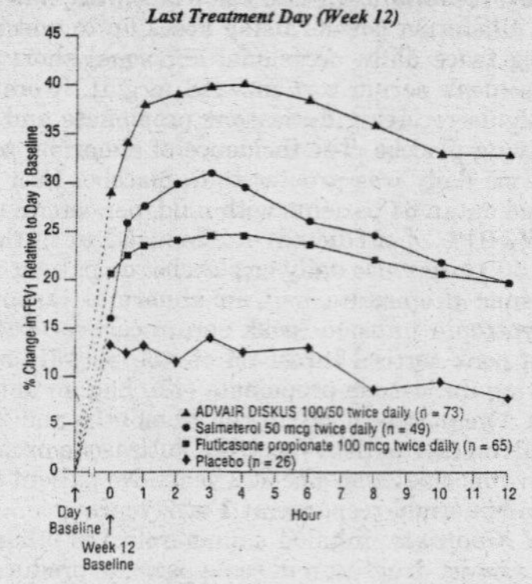

Last Treatment Day (Week 12)
% Change in FEV1 Relative to Day 1 Baseline
▲ ADVAIR DISKUS 100/50 twice daily (n = 73)
● Salmeterol 50 mcg twice daily (n = 49)
■ Fluticasone propionate 100 mcg twice daily (n = 65)
◆ Placebo (n = 26)
Hour
Day 1 Baseline
Week 12 Baseline

WARNINGS

ADVAIR DISKUS should not be used for transferring patients from systemic corticosteroid therapy.

Particular care is needed for patients who have been transferred from systemically active corticosteroids to inhaled corticosteroids because deaths due to adrenal insufficiency have occurred in patients with asthma during and after transfer from systemic corticosteroids to less systemically available inhaled corticosteroids. After withdrawal from systemic corticosteroids, a number of months are required for recovery of HPA function.

Patients who have been previously maintained on 20 mg or more per day of prednisone (or its equivalent) may be most susceptible, particularly when their systemic corticosteroids have been almost completely withdrawn. During this period of HPA suppression, patients may exhibit signs and symptoms of adrenal insufficiency when exposed to trauma, surgery, or infection (particularly gastroenteritis) or other conditions associated with severe electrolyte loss. Although inhaled corticosteroids may provide control of asthma symptoms during these episodes, in recommended doses they supply less than normal physiological amounts of glucocorticoid systemically and do NOT provide the mineralocorticoid activity that is necessary for coping with these emergencies. During periods of stress or a severe asthma attack, patients who have been withdrawn from systemic corticosteroids should be instructed to resume oral corticosteroids (in large doses) immediately and to contact their physicians for further instruction. These patients should also be instructed to carry a warning card indicating that they may need supplementary systemic corticosteroids during periods of stress or a severe asthma attack.

1. **ADVAIR DISKUS SHOULD NOT BE INITIATED IN PATIENTS DURING RAPIDLY DETERIORATING OR POTENTIALLY LIFE-THREATENING EPISODES OF ASTHMA. Serious acute respiratory events, including fatalities, have been reported both in the United States and worldwide when salmeterol, a component of ADVAIR DISKUS, has been initiated in patients with significantly worsening or acutely deteriorating asthma.** In most cases, these have occurred in patients with severe asthma (e.g., patients with a history of corticosteroid dependence, low pulmonary function, intubation, mechanical ventilation, frequent hospitalizations, or previous life-threatening acute asthma exacerbations) and/or in some patients in whom asthma has been acutely deteriorating (e.g., unresponsive to usual medications; increasing need for inhaled, short-acting $beta_2$-agonists; increasing need for systemic corticosteroids; significant increase in symptoms; recent emergency room visits; sudden or progressive deterioration in pulmonary function). However, they have occurred in a few patients with less severe asthma as well. It was not possible from these reports to determine whether salmeterol contributed to these events or simply failed to relieve the deteriorating asthma.

2. Do Not Use ADVAIR DISKUS To Treat Acute Symptoms: An inhaled, short-acting $beta_2$-agonist, not ADVAIR DISKUS, should be used to relieve acute asthma symptoms. When prescribing ADVAIR DISKUS, the physician must also provide the patient with an inhaled, short-acting $beta_2$-agonist (e.g., albuterol) for treatment of symptoms that occur acutely, despite regular twice daily (morning and evening) use of ADVAIR DISKUS.

When beginning treatment with ADVAIR DISKUS, patients who have been taking oral or inhaled, short-acting $beta_2$-agonists on a regular basis (e.g., 4 times a day) should be instructed to discontinue the regular use of these drugs. For patients on ADVAIR DISKUS, short-acting, inhaled $beta_2$ -agonists should only be used for symptomatic relief of acute asthma symptoms (see PRECAUTIONS: Information for Patients).

3. Watch for Increasing Use of Inhaled, Short-Acting $Beta_2$-agonists, Which Is a Marker of Deteriorating Asthma: Asthma may deteriorate acutely over a period of hours or chronically over several days or longer. If the patient's inhaled, short-acting $beta_2$-agonist becomes less effective, the patient needs more inhalations than usual, or the patient develops a significant decrease in PEF, these may be a marker of destabilization of asthma. In this setting, the patient requires immediate reevaluation with reassessment of the treatment regimen, giving special consideration to the possible need for replacing the current strength of ADVAIR DISKUS with a higher strength, adding additional inhaled corticosteroid, or initiating systemic corticosteroids. Patients should not use more than one inhalation twice daily (morning and evening) of ADVAIR DISKUS.

4. Do Not Use an Inhaled, Long-Acting $Beta_2$-agonist in Conjunction With ADVAIR DISKUS: Patients who are receiving ADVAIR DISKUS twice daily should not use salmeterol or other long-acting inhaled $beta_2$-agonists for prevention of exercise-induced bronchospasm or the maintenance treatment of asthma. Additional benefit would not be gained from using supplemental salmeterol for prevention of exercise-induced bronchospasm since ADVAIR DISKUS already contains salmeterol.

5. Do Not Exceed Recommended Dosage: ADVAIR DISKUS should not be used more often or at higher doses than recommended. Fatalities have been reported in association with excessive use of inhaled sympathomimetic drugs. Large doses of inhaled or oral salmeterol (12 to 20 times the recommended dose) have been associated with clinically significant prolongation of the QT_c interval, which has the potential for producing ventricular arrhythmias.

6. Paradoxical Bronchospasm: As with other inhaled asthma medications, ADVAIR DISKUS can produce paradoxical bronchospasm, which may be life threatening. If paradoxical bronchospasm occurs following dosing with ADVAIR DISKUS, it should be treated immediately with a short-acting, inhaled bronchodilator, ADVAIR DISKUS should be discontinued immediately, and alternative therapy should be instituted.

7. Immediate Hypersensitivity Reactions: Immediate hypersensitivity reactions may occur after administration of ADVAIR DISKUS, as demonstrated by cases of urticaria, angioedema, rash, and bronchospasm.

8. Upper Airway Symptoms: Symptoms of laryngeal spasm, irritation, or swelling, such as stridor and choking, have been reported in patients receiving fluticasone propionate and salmeterol, components of ADVAIR DISKUS.

9. Cardiovascular Disorders: ADVAIR DISKUS, like all products containing sympathomimetic amines, should be used with caution in patients with cardiovascular disorders, especially coronary insufficiency, cardiac arrhythmias, and hypertension. Salmeterol, a component of ADVAIR DISKUS, can produce a clinically significant cardiovascular effect in some patients as measured by pulse rate, blood pressure, and/or symptoms. Although such effects are uncommon after administration of salmeterol at recommended doses, if they occur, the drug may need to be discontinued. In addition, beta-agonists have been reported to produce electrocardiogram (ECG) changes, such as flattening of the T wave, prolongation of the QT_c interval, and ST segment depression. The clinical significance of these findings is unknown.

10. Discontinuation of Systemic Corticosteroids: Transfer of patients from systemic corticosteroid therapy to ADVAIR DISKUS may unmask conditions previously suppressed by the systemic corticosteroid therapy, e.g., rhinitis, conjunctivitis, eczema, and arthritis.

11. Immunosuppression: Persons who are using drugs that suppress the immune system are more susceptible to infections than healthy individuals. Chickenpox and measles, for example, can have a more serious or even fatal course in susceptible children or adults using corticosteroids. In such children or adults who have not had these diseases or been properly immunized, particular care should be taken to avoid exposure. How the dose, route and duration of corticosteroid administration affect the risk of developing a disseminated infection is not known. The contribution of the underlying disease and/or prior corticosteroid treatment to the risk is also not known. If exposed to chickenpox, prophylaxis with varicella zoster immune globulin (VZIG) may be indicated. If exposed to measles, prophylaxis with pooled intramuscular immunoglobulin (IG) may be indicated. (See the respective package inserts for complete VZIG and IG prescribing information.) If chickenpox develops, treatment with antiviral agents may be considered.

PRECAUTIONS

General: 1. Cardiovascular Effects: No effect on the cardiovascular system is usually seen after the administration of inhaled ADVAIR DISKUS at recommended doses. The cardiovascular and central nervous system effects seen with all sympathomimetic drugs (e.g., increased blood pressure, heart rate, excitement) can occur after use of salmeterol, a component of ADVAIR DISKUS, and may require discontinu-

Table 2: Peak Expiratory Flow Results for Patients Previously Treated With Either Inhaled Corticosteroids or Salmeterol (Study 1)

Efficacy Variable*	ADVAIR DISKUS 100/50 (n = 87)	Fluticasone Propionate 100 mcg (n = 85)	Salmeterol 50 mcg (n = 86)	Placebo (n = 77)
AM PEF (L/min)				
Baseline	393	374	369	382
Change from baseline	53	17	−2	−24
PM PEF (L/min)				
Baseline	418	390	396	398
Change from baseline	35	18	−7	−13

*Change from baseline = change from baseline at Endpoint (last available data).

ation of ADVAIR DISKUS. ADVAIR DISKUS, like all medications containing sympathomimetic amines, should be used with caution in patients with cardiovascular disorders, especially coronary insufficiency, cardiac arrhythmias, and hypertension; in patients with convulsive disorders or thyrotoxicosis; and in patients who are unusually responsive to sympathomimetic amines.

As has been described with other beta-adrenergic agonist bronchodilators, clinically significant changes in electrocardiograms have been seen infrequently in individual patients in controlled clinical studies with ADVAIR DISKUS and salmeterol. Clinically significant changes in systolic and/or diastolic blood pressure and pulse rate have been seen infrequently in individual patients in controlled clinical studies with salmeterol, a component of ADVAIR DISKUS.

2. Metabolic and Other Effects: Doses of the related beta₂-adrenoceptor agonist albuterol, when administered intravenously, have been reported to aggravate preexisting diabetes mellitus and ketoacidosis. Beta-adrenergic agonist medications may produce significant hypokalemia in some patients, possibly through intracellular shunting, which has the potential to produce adverse cardiovascular effects. The decrease in serum potassium is usually transient, not requiring supplementation.

Clinically significant changes in blood glucose and/or serum potassium were seen rarely during clinical studies with ADVAIR DISKUS at recommended doses.

During withdrawal from oral corticosteroids, some patients may experience symptoms of systemically active corticosteroid withdrawal, e.g., joint and/or muscular pain, lassitude, and depression, despite maintenance or even improvement of respiratory function.

Fluticasone propionate, a component of ADVAIR DISKUS, will often permit control of asthma symptoms with less suppression of HPA function than therapeutically equivalent oral doses of prednisone. Since fluticasone propionate is absorbed into the circulation and can be systemically active at higher doses, the beneficial effects of ADVAIR DISKUS in minimizing HPA dysfunction may be expected only when recommended dosages are not exceeded and individual patients are titrated to the lowest effective dose. A relationship between plasma levels of fluticasone propionate and inhibitory effects on stimulated cortisol production has been shown after 4 weeks of treatment with fluticasone propionate inhalation aerosol. Since individual sensitivity to effects on cortisol production exists, physicians should consider this information when prescribing ADVAIR DISKUS. Because of the possibility of systemic absorption of inhaled corticosteroids, patients treated with these drugs should be observed carefully for any evidence of systemic corticosteroid effects. Particular care should be taken in observing patients postoperatively or during periods of stress for evidence of inadequate adrenal response.

It is possible that systemic corticosteroid effects such as hypercorticism and adrenal suppression may appear in a small number of patients, particularly at higher doses. If such changes occur, the dose of fluticasone propionate should be reduced slowly, consistent with accepted procedures for reducing systemic corticosteroids and for management of asthma symptoms.

Orally inhaled corticosteroids may cause a reduction in growth velocity when administered to pediatric patients (see PRECAUTIONS: Pediatric Use). Patients should be maintained on the lowest strength of ADVAIR DISKUS that effectively controls their asthma.

The long-term effects of ADVAIR DISKUS in human subjects are not fully known. In particular, the effects resulting from chronic use of fluticasone propionate on developmental or immunologic processes in the mouth, pharynx, trachea, and lung are unknown. Some patients have received inhaled fluticasone propionate on a continuous basis for periods of 3 years or longer. In clinical studies with patients treated for 2 years with inhaled fluticasone propionate, no apparent differences in the type or severity of adverse reactions were observed after long- versus short-term treatment.

Rare instances of glaucoma, increased intraocular pressure, and cataracts have been reported following the inhaled administration of corticosteroids, including fluticasone propionate, a component of ADVAIR DISKUS.

In clinical studies with ADVAIR DISKUS, the development of localized infections of the pharynx with *Candida albicans* has occurred. When such an infection develops, it should be treated with appropriate local or systemic (i.e., oral antifungal) therapy while remaining on treatment with ADVAIR DISKUS, but at times therapy with ADVAIR DISKUS may need to be interrupted.

Inhaled corticosteroids should be used with caution, if at all, in patients with active or quiescent tuberculosis infections of the respiratory tract; untreated systemic fungal, bacterial, viral, or parasitic infections; or ocular herpes simplex.

3. Eosinophilic Conditions: In rare cases, patients on inhaled fluticasone propionate, a component of ADVAIR DISKUS, may present with systemic eosinophilic conditions, with some patients presenting with clinical features of vasculitis consistent with Churg-Strauss syndrome, a condition that is often treated with systemic corticosteroid therapy. These events usually, but not always, have been associated with the reduction and/or withdrawal of oral corticosteroid therapy following the introduction of fluticasone propionate. Cases of serious eosinophilic conditions have also been reported with other inhaled corticosteroids in this clinical setting. Physicians should be alert to eosinophilia, vasculitic rash, worsening pulmonary symptoms, cardiac complications, and/or neuropathy presenting in their pa-

tients. A causal relationship between fluticasone propionate and these underlying conditions has not been established (see ADVERSE REACTIONS).

Information for Patients: Patients being treated with ADVAIR DISKUS should receive the following information and instructions. This information is intended to aid them in the safe and effective use of this medication. It is not a disclosure of all possible adverse or intended effects.

It is important that patients understand how to use the DISKUS inhalation device appropriately and how it should be used in relation to other asthma medications they are taking. Patients should be given the following information:
1. Patients should use ADVAIR DISKUS at regular intervals as directed. Results of clinical trials indicate significant improvement may occur within the first 30 minutes of taking the first dose; however, the full benefit may not be achieved until treatment has been administered for 1 week or longer. The patient should not exceed the prescribed dosage and should contact the physician if symptoms do not improve or if the condition worsens.
2. The bronchodilation from a single dose of ADVAIR DISKUS may last up to 12 hours or longer. The recommended dosage (1 inhalation twice daily, morning and evening) should not be exceeded. Patients who are receiving ADVAIR DISKUS twice daily should not use salmeterol or other long-acting inhaled beta₂-agonists for prevention of exercise-induced bronchospasm or maintenance treatment of asthma.
3. ADVAIR DISKUS is not meant to relieve acute asthma symptoms and extra doses should not be used for that purpose. Acute symptoms should be treated with an inhaled, short-acting beta₂-agonist such as albuterol (the physician should provide the patient with such medication and instruct the patient in how it should be used).
4. The physician should be notified immediately if any of the following situations occur, which may be a sign of seriously worsening asthma:
• Decreasing effectiveness of inhaled, short-acting beta₂-agonists
• Need for more inhalations than usual of inhaled, short-acting beta₂-agonists
• Significant decrease in peak flow as outlined by the physician
5. Patients should be cautioned regarding common adverse cardiovascular effects, such as palpitations, chest pain, rapid heart rate, tremor, or nervousness.
6. When patients are prescribed ADVAIR DISKUS, other inhaled drugs and asthma medications should be used only as directed by the physician.
7. ADVAIR DISKUS should not be used with a spacer device.
8. If you are pregnant or nursing, contact your physician about the use of ADVAIR DISKUS.
9. Effective and safe use of ADVAIR DISKUS includes an understanding of the way that it should be used:
• Never exhale into the DISKUS.
• Never attempt to take the DISKUS apart.
• Always activate and use the DISKUS in a level, horizontal position.
• Never wash the mouthpiece of any part of the DISKUS. KEEP IT DRY.
• Always keep the DISKUS in a dry place.
• Discard **1 month** after removal from the moisture-protective foil overwrap pouch or after every blister has been used (when the dose indicator reads "0"), whichever comes first.
10. Patients should be warned to avoid exposure to chickenpox or measles and, if they are exposed, to consult their physicians without delay.
11. For the proper use of ADVAIR DISKUS and to attain maximum improvement, the patient should read and follow carefully the accompanying Patient's Instructions for Use.
Drug Interactions: ADVAIR DISKUS has been used concomitantly with other drugs, including short-acting beta₂-agonists, methylxanthines, and intranasal corticosteroids, commonly used in patients with asthma, without adverse drug reactions. No formal drug interaction studies have been performed with ADVAIR DISKUS.
Short-Acting Beta₂-Agonists: In clinical trials, the mean daily need for additional beta₂-agonist use in 166 patients using ADVAIR DISKUS was approximately 1.3 inhalations per day, and ranged from 0 to 9 inhalations per day. Five percent of the ADVAIR DISKUS patients in these trials averaged 6 or more inhalations per day over the course of the 12-week trials. No observed increase in frequency of cardiovascular events was noted among patients who averaged 6 or more inhalations per day.
Methylxanthines: The concurrent use of intravenously or orally administered methylxanthines (e.g., aminophylline, theophylline) by patients receiving ADVAIR DISKUS has not been completely evaluated. In clinical trials, 39 patients receiving ADVAIR DISKUS 100/50, 250/50, or 500/50 twice daily concurrently with a theophylline product had adverse event rates similar to those in 304 patients receiving ADVAIR DISKUS without theophylline. Similar results were observed in patients receiving salmeterol 50 mcg plus fluticasone propionate 500 mcg twice daily concurrently with a theophylline product (n = 39) or without theophylline (n = 132).
Fluticasone Propionate Nasal Spray: In patients taking ADVAIR DISKUS in clinical trials, no difference in the profile of adverse events or HPA axis effects was noted between patients taking FLONASE® (fluticasone propionate) Nasal Spray, 50 mcg concurrently (n = 46) and those who were not (n = 130).

Monoamine Oxidase Inhibitors and Tricyclic Antidepressants: ADVAIR DISKUS should be administered with extreme caution to patients being treated with monoamine oxidase inhibitors or tricyclic antidepressants, or within 2 weeks of discontinuation of such agents, because the action of salmeterol, a component of ADVAIR DISKUS, on the vascular system may be potentiated by these agents.
Beta-Adrenergic Receptor Blocking Agents: Beta-blockers not only block the pulmonary effect of beta-agonists, such as salmeterol, a component of ADVAIR DISKUS, but may produce severe bronchospasm in patients with asthma. Therefore, patients with asthma should not normally be treated with beta-blockers. However, under certain circumstances, there may be no acceptable alternatives to the use of beta-adrenergic blocking agents in patients with asthma. In this setting, cardioselective beta-blockers could be considered, although they should be administered with caution.
Diuretics: The ECG changes and/or hypokalemia that may result from the administration of nonpotassium-sparing diuretics (such as loop or thiazide diuretics) can be acutely worsened by beta-agonists, especially when the recommended dose of the beta-agonist is exceeded. Although the clinical significance of these effects is not known, caution is advised in the coadministration of beta-agonists with nonpotassium-sparing diuretics.
Ketoconazole and Other Inhibitors of Cytochrome P450: In a placebo-controlled, crossover study in 8 healthy volunteers, coadministration of a single dose of fluticasone propionate (1000 mcg) with multiple doses of ketoconazole (200 mg) to steady state resulted in increased mean fluticasone propionate concentrations, a reduction in plasma cortisol AUC, and no effect on urinary excretion of cortisol. This interaction may be due to an inhibition of cytochrome P450 3A4 by ketoconazole, which is also the route of metabolism of fluticasone propionate. Care should be exercised when ADVAIR DISKUS is coadministered with long-term ketoconazole and other known cytochrome P450 3A4 inhibitors.
Carcinogenesis, Mutagenesis, Impairment of Fertility: *Fluticasone Propionate:* Fluticasone propionate demonstrated no tumorigenic potential in mice at oral doses up to 1000 mcg/kg (approximately 4 times the maximum recommended daily inhalation dose in adults on a mcg/m² basis) for 78 weeks or in rats at inhalation doses up to 57 mcg/kg (less than the maximum recommended daily inhalation dose in adults on a mcg/m² basis) for 104 weeks.
Fluticasone propionate did not induce gene mutation in prokaryotic or eukaryotic cells in vitro. No significant clastogenic effect was seen in cultured human peripheral lymphocytes in vitro or in the mouse micronucleus test.
No evidence of impairment of fertility was observed in reproductive studies conducted in male and female rats at subcutaneous doses up to 500 mcg/kg (less than the maximum recommended daily inhalation dose in adults on a mcg/m² basis). Prostate weight was significantly reduced at a subcutaneous dose of 50 mcg/kg.
Salmeterol: In an 18-month carcinogenicity study in CD-mice, salmeterol at oral doses of 1.4 mg/kg and above (approximately 20 times the maximum recommended daily inhalation dose in adults based on comparison of the plasma area under the curves ([AUCs]) caused a dose-related increase in the incidence of smooth muscle hyperplasia, cystic glandular hyperplasia, leiomyomas of the uterus, and cysts in the ovaries. The incidence of leiomyosarcomas was not statistically significant. No tumors were seen at 0.2 mg/kg (approximately 3 times the maximum recommended daily inhalation doses in adults based on comparison of the AUCs).
In a 24-month oral and inhalation carcinogenicity study in Sprague Dawley rats, salmeterol caused a dose-related increase in the incidence of mesovarian leiomyomas and ovarian cysts at doses of 0.68 mg/kg and above (approximately 60 times the maximum recommended daily inhalation dose in adults on a mg/m² basis). No tumors were seen at 0.21 mg/kg (approximately 20 times the maximum recommended daily inhalation dose in adults on a mg/m² basis). These findings in rodents are similar to those reported previously for other beta-adrenergic agonist drugs. The relevance of these findings to human use is unknown.
Salmeterol produced no detectable or reproducible increases in microbial and mammalian gene mutation in vitro. No clastogenic activity occurred in vitro in human lymphocytes or in vivo in a rat micronucleus test. No effects on fertility were identified in male and female rats treated with salmeterol at oral doses up to 2 mg/kg (approximately 180 times the maximum recommended daily inhalation dose in adults on a mg/m² basis).
Pregnancy: *Teratogenic Effects: ADVAIR DISKUS:* Pregnancy Category C. From the reproduction toxicity studies in mice and rats, no evidence of enhanced toxicity was seen using combinations of fluticasone propionate and salmeterol compared to toxicity data from the components administered separately. In mice combining 150 mcg/kg subcutaneously of fluticasone propionate (less than the maximum recommended daily inhalation dose in adults on a mcg/m² basis) with 10 mg/kg orally of salmeterol (approximately 450 times the maximum recommended daily inhalation dose in adults on a mg/m² basis) were teratogenic. Cleft palate, fetal death, increased implantation loss and delayed ossification was seen. These observations are characteristic of glucocorticoids. No developmental toxicity was observed at combination doses up to 40 mcg/kg subcutaneously of fluticasone propionate (less than the maximum recommended daily inhalation dose in adults on a mcg/m² basis) and up to 1.4 mg/kg orally

Continued on next page

Advair Diskus—Cont.

of salmeterol (approximately 65 times the maximum recommended daily inhalation dose in adults on a mg/m^2 basis). In rats, no teratogenicity was observed at combination doses up to 30 mcg/kg subcutaneously of fluticasone propionate (less than the maximum recommended daily inhalation dose in adults on mcg/m^2 basis) and up to 1 mg/kg of salmeterol (approximately 90 times the maximum recommended daily inhalation dose in adults on a mg/m^2 basis). Combining 100 mcg/kg subcutaneously of fluticasone propionate (less than the maximum recommended daily inhalation dose in adults on a mcg/m^2 basis) with 10 mg/kg orally of salmeterol (approximately 900 times the maximum recommended daily inhalation dose in adults on a mg/m^2 basis) produced maternal toxicity, decreased placental weight, decreased fetal weight, umbilical hernia, delayed ossification, and changes in the occipital bone. There are no adequate and well-controlled studies with ADVAIR DISKUS in pregnant women. ADVAIR DISKUS should be used during pregnancy only if the potential benefit justifies the potential risk to the fetus.

Fluticasone Propionate: Pregnancy Category C. Subcutaneous studies in the mouse and rat at 45 and 100 mcg/kg (less than or equivalent to the maximum recommended daily inhalation dose in adults on a mcg/m^2 basis), respectively, revealed fetal toxicity characteristic of potent corticosteroid compounds, including embryonic growth retardation, omphalocele, cleft palate, and retarded cranial ossification.

In the rabbit, fetal weight reduction and cleft palate were observed at a subcutaneous dose of 4 mcg/kg (less than the maximum recommended daily inhalation dose in adults on a mcg/m^2 basis). However, no teratogenic effects were reported at oral doses up to 300 mcg/kg (approximately 5 times the maximum recommended daily inhalation dose in adults on a mcg/m^2 basis) of fluticasone propionate. No fluticasone propionate was detected in the plasma in this study, consistent with the established low bioavailability following oral administration (see CLINICAL PHARMACOLOGY).

Fluticasone propionate crossed the placenta following administration of a subcutaneous dose of 100 mcg/kg to mice (less than the maximum recommended daily inhalation dose in adults on a mcg/m^2 basis) administration of a subcutaneous or an oral dose of 100 mcg/kg to rats (approximately equivalent to the maximum recommended daily inhalation dose in adults on a mcg/m^2 basis) and an oral dose of 300 mcg/kg administered to rabbits (approximately 5 times the maximum recommended daily inhalation dose in adults on a mcg/m^2 basis).

There are no adequate and well-controlled studies in pregnant women. Fluticasone propionate should be used during pregnancy only if the potential benefit justifies the potential risk to the fetus.

Experience with oral corticosteroids since their introduction in pharmacologic, as opposed to physiologic, doses suggests that rodents are more prone to teratogenic effects from corticosteroids than humans. In addition, because there is a natural increase in corticosteroid production during pregnancy, most women will require a lower exogenous corticosteroid dose and many will not need corticosteroid treatment during pregnancy.

Salmeterol: Pregnancy Category C. No teratogenic effects occurred in rats at oral doses up to 2 mg/kg (approximately 180 times the maximum recommended daily inhalation dose in adults on a mg/m^2 basis). In pregnant Dutch rabbits administered oral doses of 1 mg/kg and above (approximately 50 times the maximum recommended daily inhalation dose in adults based on comparison of the AUCs), salmeterol exhibited fetal toxic effects characteristically resulting from beta-adrenoceptor stimulation. These included precocious eyelid openings, cleft palate, sternebral fusion, limb and paw flexures, and delayed ossification of the frontal cranial bones. No significant effects occurred at an oral dose of 0.6 mg/kg (approximately 20 times the maximum recommended daily inhalation dose in adults based on comparison of the AUCs). New Zealand White rabbits were less sensitive since only delayed ossification of the frontal bones was seen at an oral dose of 10 mg/kg (approximately 1800 times the maximum recommended daily inhalation dose in adults on a mg/m^2 basis). Extensive use of other beta-agonists has provided no evidence that these class effects in animals are relevant to their use in humans. There are no adequate and well-controlled studies with salmeterol in pregnant women. Salmeterol should be used during pregnancy only if the potential benefit justifies the potential risk to the fetus.

Salmeterol xinafoate crossed the placenta following oral administration of 10 mg/kg to mice and rats (approximately 450 and 900 times, respectively, the maximum recommended daily inhalation dose in adults on a mg/m^2 basis).

Use in Labor and Delivery: There are no well-controlled human studies that have investigated effects of ADVAIR DISKUS on preterm labor or labor at term. Because of the potential for beta-agonist interference with uterine contractility, use of ADVAIR DISKUS for management of asthma during labor should be restricted to those patients in whom the benefits clearly outweigh the risks.

Nursing Mothers: Plasma levels of salmeterol, a component of ADVAIR DISKUS, after inhaled therapeutic doses are very low. In rats, salmeterol xinafoate is excreted in the milk. There are no data from controlled trials on the use of salmeterol by nursing mothers. It is not known whether fluticasone propionate, a component of ADVAIR DISKUS, is excreted in human breast milk; however, other corticosteroids have been detected in human milk. Subcutaneous administration to lactating rats of 10 mcg/kg tritiated fluticasone propionate (less than the maximum recommended daily inhalation dose in adults on a mcg/m^2 basis) resulted in measurable radioactivity in milk.

Since there are no data from controlled trials on the use of ADVAIR DISKUS by nursing mothers, a decision should be made whether to discontinue nursing or to discontinue ADVAIR DISKUS, taking into account the importance of ADVAIR DISKUS to the mother.

Caution should be exercised when ADVAIR DISKUS is administered to a nursing woman.

Pediatric Use: The safety and effectiveness of ADVAIR DISKUS in children under 12 years of age has not been established. In one 12-week study, 257 patients 4 to 11 years inadequately controlled using inhaled corticosteroids were randomized to ADVAIR DISKUS 100/50 or concurrent therapy with fluticasone propionate inhalation powder 100 mcg plus salmeterol inhalation powder 50 mcg twice daily. The pattern of adverse events reported in patients 4 to 11 years of age was similar to that seen in patients 12 years of age and older treated with ADVAIR DISKUS.

Controlled clinical studies have shown that orally inhaled corticosteroids may cause a reduction in growth velocity in pediatric patients. This effect has been observed in the absence of laboratory evidence of HPA axis suppression, suggesting that growth velocity is a more sensitive indicator of systemic corticosteroid exposure in pediatric patients than some commonly used tests of HPA axis function. The long-term effects of this reduction in growth velocity associated with orally inhaled corticosteroids, including the impact on final adult height, are unknown. The potential for "catch up" growth following discontinuation of treatment with orally inhaled corticosteroids has not been adequately studied.

Inhaled corticosteroids, including fluticasone propionate, a component of ADVAIR DISKUS, may cause a reduction in growth velocity in children and adolescents (see PRECAUTIONS). The growth of pediatric patients receiving orally inhaled corticosteroids, including ADVAIR DISKUS, should be monitored. If a child or adolescent on any corticosteroid appears to have growth suppression, the possibility that he/she is particularly sensitive to this effect of corticosteroids should be considered. The potential growth effects of prolonged treatment should be weighed against the clinical benefits obtained. To minimize the systemic effects of orally inhaled corticosteroids, including ADVAIR DISKUS, each patient should be titrated to the lowest strength that effectively controls his/her asthma (see DOSAGE AND ADMINISTRATION).

Geriatric Use: Of the total number of patients in clinical studies of ADVAIR DISKUS, 44 were 65 years of age or older and 3 were 75 years of age or older. No overall differences in safety were observed between these patients and younger patients, and other reported clinical experience, including studies of the individual components, has not identified differences in responses between the elderly and younger patients, but greater sensitivity of some older individuals cannot be ruled out. As with other products containing beta$_2$-agonists, special caution should be observed when using ADVAIR DISKUS in geriatric patients who have concomitant cardiovascular disease that could be adversely affected by beta$_2$-agonists. Based on available data for ADVAIR DISKUS or its active components, no adjustment of dosage of ADVAIR DISKUS in geriatric patients is warranted.

ADVERSE REACTIONS

The incidence of common adverse experiences in Table 3 is based upon 2 placebo-controlled, 12-week, US clinical studies (Studies 1 and 2). A total of 705 adolescent and adult patients (349 females and 356 males) previously treated with salmeterol or inhaled corticosteroids were treated twice daily with ADVAIR DISKUS (100/50- or 250/50-mcg doses), fluticasone propionate inhalation powder (100- or 250-mcg doses), salmeterol inhalation powder 50 mcg, or placebo.

[See table below]

Table 3 includes all events (whether considered drug-related or nondrug-related by the investigator) that occurred at a rate of 3% or greater in either of the groups receiving ADVAIR DISKUS and were more common than in the placebo group. In considering these data, differences in average duration of exposure should be taken into account.

These adverse reactions were mostly mild to moderate in severity. Rare cases of immediate and delayed hypersensitivity reactions, including rash and other rare events of angioedema and bronchospasm, have been reported.

Other adverse effects that occurred in the groups receiving ADVAIR DISKUS in these studies with an incidence of 1% to 3% and that occurred at a greater incidence than with placebo were:

Blood and Lymphatic: Lymphatic signs and symptoms.

Cardiovascular: Palpitations.

Drug Interaction, Overdose, and Trauma: Muscle injuries, fractures, wounds and lacerations, contusions and hematomas, burns.

Ear, Nose, and Throat: Rhinorrhea/post nasal drip; ear, nose and throat infections; ear signs and symptoms; nasal signs and symptoms; nasal sinus disorders; rhinitis; sneezing; nasal irritation; blood in nasal mucosa.

Eye: Keratitis and conjunctivitis, viral eye infections, eye redness.

Gastrointestinal: Dental discomfort and pain, gastrointestinal signs and symptoms, gastrointestinal infections, gastroenteritis, gastrointestinal disorders, oral ulcerations, oral erythema and rashes, constipation, appendicitis, oral discomfort and pain.

Hepatobiliary Tract and Pancreas: Abnormal liver function tests.

Lower Respiratory: Lower respiratory signs and symptoms, pneumonia, lower respiratory infections.

Table 3: Overall Adverse Effects With ≥3% Incidence With ADVAIR DISKUS

Adverse Event	ADVAIR DISKUS 100/50 (n = 92) %	ADVAIR DISKUS 250/50 (n = 84) %	Fluticasone Propionate 100 mcg (n = 90) %	Fluticasone Propionate 250 mcg (n = 84) %	Salmeterol 50 mcg (n = 180) %	Placebo (n = 175) %
Ear, nose, and throat						
Upper respiratory tract infection	27	21	29	25	19	14
Pharyngitis	13	10	7	12	8	6
Upper respiratory inflammation	7	6	7	8	8	5
Sinusitis	4	5	6	1	3	4
Hoarseness/dysphonia	5	2	2	4	<1	<1
Oral candidiasis	1	4	2	2	0	0
Lower respiratory						
Viral respiratory infections	4	4	4	10	6	3
Bronchitis	2	8	1	2	2	2
Cough	3	6	0	0	3	2
Neurology						
Headaches	12	13	14	8	10	7
Gastrointestinal						
Nausea & vomiting	4	6	3	4	1	1
Gastrointestinal discomfort & pain	4	1	0	2	1	1
Diarrhea	4	2	2	2	1	1
Viral gastrointestinal infections	3	0	3	1	2	2
Non-site specific						
Candidiasis unspecified site	3	0	1	4	0	1
Musculoskeletal						
Musculoskeletal pain	4	2	1	5	3	3
Average duration of exposure (days)	77.3	78.7	72.4	70.1	60.1	42.3

Musculoskeletal: Arthralgia and articular rheumatism; muscle stiffness, tightness, and rigidity; bone and cartilage disorders.
Neurology: Sleep disorders, tremors, hypnagogic effects, compressed nerve syndromes.
Non-Site Specific: Allergies and allergic reactions, congestion, viral infections, pain, chest symptoms, fluid retention, bacterial infections, wheeze and hives, unusual taste.
Skin: Viral skin infections, urticaria, skin flakiness and acquired ichthyosis, disorders of sweat and sebum, sweating.
The incidence of common adverse experiences reported in Study 3, a 28-week, non-US clinical study of 503 patients previously treated with inhaled corticosteroids who were treated twice daily with ADVAIR DISKUS 500/50, fluticasone propionate inhalation powder 500 mcg and salmeterol inhalation powder 50 mcg used concurrently, or fluticasone propionate inhalation powder 500 mcg was similar to the incidences reported in Table 3.
Observed During Clinical Practice: In addition to adverse events reported from clinical trials, the following events have been identified during postapproval use of ADVAIR DISKUS, fluticasone propionate, and/or salmeterol. Because they are reported voluntarily from a population of unknown size, estimates of frequency cannot be made. These events have been chosen for inclusion due to a combination of their seriousness, frequency of reporting, or potential causal connection to ADVAIR DISKUS, fluticasone propionate, and/or salmeterol. In extensive US and worldwide postmarketing experience with salmeterol, a component of ADVAIR DISKUS, serious exacerbations of asthma, including some that have been fatal, have been reported. In most cases, these have occurred in patients with severe asthma and/or in some patients in whom asthma has been acutely deteriorating (see WARNINGS), but they have also occurred in a few patients with less severe asthma. It was not possible from these reports to determine whether salmeterol contributed to these events or simply failed to relieve the deteriorating asthma.
Cardiovascular: Arrhythmias (including atrial fibrillation, extrasystoles, supraventricular tachycardia), ventricular tachycardia.
Ear, Nose, and Throat: Aphonia, earache, paranasal sinus pain, throat soreness and irritation.
Endocrine and Metabolic: Cushing syndrome, Cushingoid features, growth velocity reduction in children/adolescents, hypercorticism, hyperglycemia, weight gain.
Gastrointestinal: Abdominal pain, dyspepsia, xerostomia.
Musculoskeletal: Back pain, cramps, muscle spasm, myositis.
Neurology: Paresthesia, restlessness.
Non-Site Specific: Immediate and delayed hypersensitivity reaction, pallor.
Psychiatry: Agitation, aggression, depression.
Respiratory: Chest congestion, chest tightness, dyspnea, immediate bronchospasm, influenza, paradoxical bronchospasm, tracheitis, wheezing, reports of upper respiratory symptoms of laryngeal spasm, irritation, or swelling such as stridor or choking.
Skin: Contact dermatitis, contusions, ecchymoses, photodermatitis.
Urogenital: Dysmenorrhea, irregular menstrual cycle, pelvic inflammatory disease, vaginal candidiasis, vaginitis, vulvovaginitis.
Eosinophilic Conditions: In rare cases, patients on inhaled fluticasone propionate, a component of ADVAIR DISKUS, may present with systemic eosinophilic conditions, with some patients presenting with clinical features of vasculitis consistent with Churg-Strauss syndrome, a condition that is often treated with systemic corticosteroid therapy. These events usually, but not always, have been associated with the reduction and/or withdrawal of oral corticosteroid therapy following the introduction of fluticasone propionate. Cases of serious eosinophilic conditions have also been reported with other inhaled corticosteroids in this clinical setting. While ADVAIR DISKUS should not be used for transferring patients from systemic corticosteroid therapy, physicians should be alert to eosinophilia, vasculitic rash, worsening pulmonary symptoms, cardiac complications, and/or neuropathy presenting in their patients. A causal relationship between fluticasone propionate and these underlying conditions has not been established (see PRECAUTIONS: Eosinophilic Conditions).

OVERDOSAGE

ADVAIR DISKUS: No deaths occurred in rats given combinations of salmeterol and fluticasone propionate at acute inhalation doses of 3.6 and 1.9 mg/kg, respectively (approximately 320 and 15 times the maximum recommended daily inhalation dose in adults on a mg/m^2 basis).
Fluticasone Propionate: Chronic overdosage with fluticasone propionate may result in signs/symptoms of hypercorticism (see PRECAUTIONS). Inhalation by healthy volunteers of a single dose of 4000 mcg of fluticasone propionate inhalation powder or single doses of 1760 or 3520 mcg of fluticasone propionate inhalation aerosol was well tolerated. Fluticasone propionate given by inhalation aerosol at doses of 1320 mcg twice daily for 7 to 15 days to healthy human volunteers was also well tolerated. Repeat oral doses up to 80 mg daily for 10 days in healthy volunteers and repeat oral doses up to 20 mg daily for 42 days in patients were well tolerated. Adverse reactions were of mild or moderate severity, and incidences were similar in active and placebo treatment groups. The oral and subcutaneous median lethal doses in mice and rats were >1000 mg/kg (>4300 and >8700 times, respectively, the maximum recommended daily inhalation dose in adults on a mg/m^2 basis).

Table 4: Recommended Doses of ADVAIR DISKUS for Patients Taking Inhaled Corticosteroids

Current **Daily Dose** of Inhaled Corticosteroid		Recommended Strength and Dosing Schedule of ADVAIR DISKUS
Beclomethasone dipropionate	≤420 mcg 462–840 mcg	100/50 twice daily 250/50 twice daily
Budesonide	≤400 mcg 800–1200 mcg 1600 mcg*	100/50 twice daily 250/50 twice daily 500/50 twice daily
Flunisolide	≤1000 mcg 1250–2000 mcg	100/50 twice daily 250/50 twice daily
Fluticasone propionate inhalation aerosol	≤176 mcg 440 mcg 660–880 mcg*	100/50 twice daily 250/50 twice daily 500/50 twice daily
Fluticasone propionate inhalation powder	≤200 mcg 500 mcg 1000 mcg*	100/50 twice daily 250/50 twice daily 500/50 twice daily
Triamcinolone acetonide	≤1000 mcg 1100–1600 mcg	100/50 twice daily 250/50 twice daily

*ADVAIR DISKUS should not be used for transferring patients from systemic corticosteroid therapy.

Salmeterol: The expected signs and symptoms with overdosage of salmeterol are those of excessive beta-adrenergic stimulation and/or occurrence of exaggeration of any of the signs and symptoms listed under ADVERSE REACTIONS, e.g., seizures, angina, hypertension or hypotension, tachycardia with rates up to 200 beats/min, arrhythmias, nervousness, headache, tremor, muscle cramps, dry mouth, palpitation, nausea, dizziness, fatigue, malaise, and insomnia. Overdosage with salmeterol may be expected to result in exaggeration of the pharmacologic adverse effects associated with beta-adrenoceptor agonists, including tachycardia and/or arrhythmia, tremor, headache, and muscle cramps. Overdosage with salmeterol can lead to clinically significant prolongation of the QT_c interval, which can produce ventricular arrhythmias. Other signs of overdosage may include hypokalemia and hyperglycemia.
As with all sympathomimetic medications, cardiac arrest and even death may be associated with abuse of salmeterol. Treatment consists of discontinuation of salmeterol together with appropriate symptomatic therapy. The judicious use of a cardioselective beta-receptor blocker may be considered, bearing in mind that such medication can produce bronchospasm. There is insufficient evidence to determine if dialysis is beneficial for overdosage of salmeterol. Cardiac monitoring is recommended in cases of overdosage.
No deaths were seen in rats given salmeterol at an inhalation dose of 2.9 mg/kg (approximately 250 times the maximum recommended daily inhalation dose in adults on a mg/m^2 basis) and in dogs at an inhalation dose of 0.7 mg/kg (approximately 200 times the maximum recommended daily inhalation dose in adults on a mg/m^2 basis). By the oral route, no deaths occurred in mice at 150 mg/kg (approximately 6500 times the maximum recommended daily inhalation dose in adults on a mg/m^2 basis) and in rats at 1000 mg/kg (approximately 86,000 times the maximum recommended daily inhalation dose in adults on a mg/m^2 basis).

DOSAGE AND ADMINISTRATION

ADVAIR DISKUS is available in 3 strengths, ADVAIR DISKUS 100/50, ADVAIR DISKUS 250/50, and ADVAIR DISKUS 500/50, containing 100, 250, and 500 mcg of fluticasone propionate, respectively, and 50 mcg of salmeterol per inhalation. ADVAIR DISKUS should be administered by the orally inhaled route only (see PATIENT'S INSTRUCTIONS FOR USE).
For patients 12 years of age and older, the dosage is 1 inhalation twice daily (morning and evening, approximately 12 hours apart).
The recommended starting doses for ADVAIR DISKUS are based upon patients' current asthma therapy.
- For patients who are not currently on an inhaled corticosteroid, whose disease severity warrants treatment with 2 maintenance therapies, including patients on non-corticosteroid maintenance therapy, the recommended starting dose is ADVAIR DISKUS 100/50 twice daily.
- For patients on an inhaled corticosteroid, Table 4 provides the recommended starting dose.

The maximum recommended dose is ADVAIR DISKUS 500/50 twice daily.
For all patients it is desirable to titrate to the lowest effective strength after adequate asthma stability is achieved.
[See table above]
ADVAIR DISKUS should be administered twice daily every day. More frequent administration (more than twice daily) or a higher number of inhalations (more than 1 inhalation twice daily) of the prescribed strength of ADVAIR DISKUS is not recommended as some patients are more likely to experience adverse effects with higher doses of salmeterol. The safety and efficacy of ADVAIR DISKUS when administered in excess of recommended doses have not been established.
If symptoms arise in the period between doses, an inhaled, short-acting beta$_2$-agonist should be taken for immediate relief.
Patients who are receiving ADVAIR DISKUS twice daily should not use salmeterol for prevention of exercise-induced bronchospasm, or for any other reason.
Improvement in asthma control following inhaled administration of ADVAIR DISKUS can occur within 30 minutes of beginning treatment, although maximum benefit may not be achieved for 1 week or longer after starting treatment. Individual patients will experience a variable time to onset and degree of symptom relief.
For patients who do not respond adequately to the starting dose after 2 weeks of therapy, replacing the current strength of ADVAIR DISKUS with a higher strength may provide additional asthma control.
If a previously effective dosage regimen of ADVAIR DISKUS fails to provide adequate control of asthma, the therapeutic regimen should be reevaluated and additional therapeutic options, e.g., replacing the current strength of ADVAIR DISKUS with a higher strength, adding additional inhaled corticosteroid, or initiating oral corticosteroids, should be considered.
Rinsing the mouth after inhalation is advised.
Geriatric Use: In studies where geriatric patients (65 years of age or older, see PRECAUTIONS: Geriatric Use) have been treated with ADVAIR DISKUS, efficacy and safety did not differ from that in younger patients. Based on available data for ADVAIR DISKUS and its active components, no dosage adjustment is recommended.
Directions for Use: Illustrated Patient's Instructions for Use accompany each package of ADVAIR DISKUS.

HOW SUPPLIED

ADVAIR DISKUS 100/50 is supplied as a disposable, purple-colored device containing 60 blisters. The DISKUS inhalation device is packaged within a purple-colored, plastic-coated, moisture-protective foil pouch (NDC 0173-0695-00).
ADVAIR DISKUS 100/50 is also supplied in an institutional pack of 1 purple-colored, disposable DISKUS inhalation device containing 28 blisters. The DISKUS inhalation device is packaged within a purple-colored, plastic-coated, moisture-protective foil pouch (NDC 0173-0695-02).
ADVAIR DISKUS 250/50 is supplied as a disposable, purple-colored device containing 60 blisters. The DISKUS inhalation device is packaged within a purple-colored, plastic-coated, moisture-protective foil pouch (NDC 0173-0696-00).
ADVAIR DISKUS 250/50 is also supplied in an institutional pack of 1 purple-colored, disposable DISKUS inhalation device containing 28 blisters. The DISKUS inhalation device is packaged within a purple-colored, plastic-coated, moisture-protective foil pouch (NDC 0173-0696-02).
ADVAIR DISKUS 500/50 is supplied as a disposable, purple-colored device containing 60 blisters. The DISKUS inhalation device is packaged within a purple-colored, plastic-coated, moisture-protective foil pouch (NDC 0173-0697-00).
ADVAIR DISKUS 500/50 is also supplied in an institutional pack of 1 purple-colored, disposable DISKUS inhalation device containing 28 blisters. The DISKUS inhalation device is packaged within a purple-colored, plastic-coated moisture-protective foil pouch (NDC 0173-0697-02).
Store at controlled room temperature (see USP), 20° to 25°C (68° to 77°F) in a dry place away from direct heat or sunlight. Keep out of reach of children. The DISKUS inhalation device is not reusable. The device should be discarded 1 month after removal from the moisture-protective foil overwrap pouch or after every blister has been used (when the dose indicator reads "0"), whichever comes first. Do not attempt to take the device apart.
Glaxo Wellcome Inc., Research Triangle Park, NC 27709
US Patent Nos. 4,335,121; 4,992,474; 5,225,445; 5,126,375; D342,994; 5,270,305; 5,860,419; 5,590,645; and 5,873,360

August 2000/RL-858

Continued on next page

TRIZIVIR™
[trī' zə-vir]
(abacavir sulfate, lamivudine, and zidovudine)
Tablets

> **WARNING**
> **TRIZIVIR contains 3 nucleoside analogs (abacavir sulfate, lamivudine, and zidovudine) and is intended only for patients whose regimen would otherwise include these 3 components.**
> **TRIZIVIR contains abacavir sulfate (ZIAGEN®), which has been associated with fatal hypersensitivity reactions (see WARNINGS). Patients developing signs or symptoms of hypersensitivity (which include fever; skin rash; fatigue; gastrointestinal symptoms such as nausea, vomiting, diarrhea, or abdominal pain; and respiratory symptoms such as pharyngitis, dyspnea, or cough) should discontinue TRIZIVIR as soon as a hypersensitivity reaction is suspected. To avoid a delay in diagnosis and minimize the risk of a life-threatening hypersensitivity reaction, TRIZIVIR should be permanently discontinued if hypersensitivity cannot be ruled out, even when other diagnoses are possible (e.g., acute onset respiratory diseases, gastroenteritis, or reactions to other medications).**
> **Abacavir (as TRIZIVIR OR ZIAGEN) SHOULD NOT be restarted following a hypersensitivity reaction to abacavir because more severe symptoms will recur within hours and may include life-threatening hypotension and death.**
> **Severe or fatal hypersensitivity reactions can occur within hours after reintroduction of abacavir (as TRIZIVIR OR ZIAGEN) in patients who have no identified history or unrecognized symptoms of hypersensitivity to abacavir therapy (see WARNINGS, PRECAUTIONS: Information for Patients, and ADVERSE REACTIONS).**
> **Zidovudine has been associated with hematologic toxicity including neutropenia and severe anemia, particularly in patients with advanced HIV disease (see WARNINGS). Prolonged use of zidovudine has been associated with symptomatic myopathy.**
> **Lactic acidosis and severe hepatomegaly with steatosis, including fatal cases, have been reported with the use of nucleoside analogues alone or in combination, including abacavir, lamivudine, zidovudine, and other antiretrovirals (see WARNINGS).**
> **TRIZIVIR alone or in combination with other antiretroviral agents is indicated for the treatment of HIV-1 infection. The indication for TRIZIVIR is based on analyses of surrogate markers in controlled studies with abacavir of up to 24 weeks in duration. At present, there are no results from controlled trials evaluating long-term suppression of HIV RNA or disease progression with abacavir.**
> **There are limited data on the use of this triple-combination regimen in patients with higher viral load levels (>100,000 copies/mL) at baseline.**

DESCRIPTION

TRIZIVIR: TRIZIVIR Tablets contain the following 3 synthetic nucleoside analogues: abacavir sulfate (ZIAGEN), lamivudine (also known as EPIVIR® or 3TC), and zidovudine (also known as RETROVIR®, azidothymidine, or ZDV) with inhibitory activity against human immunodeficiency virus (HIV).

TRIZIVIR Tablets are for oral administration. Each film-coated tablet contains the active ingredients 300 mg of abacavir as abacavir sulfate, 150 mg of lamivudine, and 300 mg of zidovudine, and the inactive ingredients magnesium stearate, microcrystalline cellulose, and sodium starch glycolate. The tablets are coated with a film (Opadry® green 03B11434) that is made of FD&C Blue No. 2, hydroxypropyl methylcellulose, polyethylene glycol, titanium dioxide, and yellow iron oxide.

Abacavir Sulfate: The chemical name of abacavir sulfate is *(1S,cis)*-4-[2-amino-6-(cyclopropylamino)-*9H*-purin-9-yl]-2-cyclopentene-1-methanol sulfate (salt) (2:1). Abacavir sulfate is the enantiomer with *1S, 4R* absolute configuration on the cyclopentene ring. It has a molecular formula of $(C_{14}H_{18}N_6O)_2 \bullet H_2SO_4$ and a molecular weight of 670.76 daltons. It has the following structural formula:

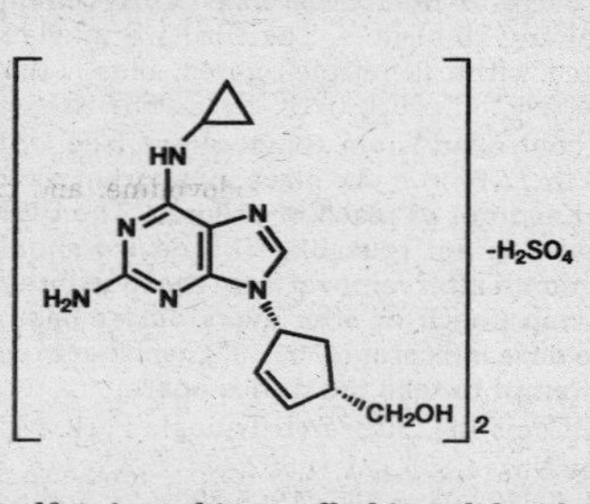

Abacavir sulfate is a white to off-white solid with a solubility of approximately 77 mg/mL in distilled water at 25°C. *In vivo,* abacavir sulfate dissociates to its free base, abacavir. In this insert, all dosages for ZIAGEN (abacavir sulfate) are expressed in terms of abacavir.

Lamivudine: The chemical name of lamivudine is (2R,cis)-4-amino-1-(2-hydroxymethyl-1,3-oxathiolan-5-yl)-(1H)-pyrimidin-2-one. Lamivudine is the (-)enantiomer of a dideoxy analogue of cytidine. Lamivudine has also been referred to as (-)2',3'-dideoxy, 3'-thiacytidine. It has a molecular formula of $C_8H_{11}N_3O_3S$ and a molecular weight of 229.3 daltons. It has the following structural formula:

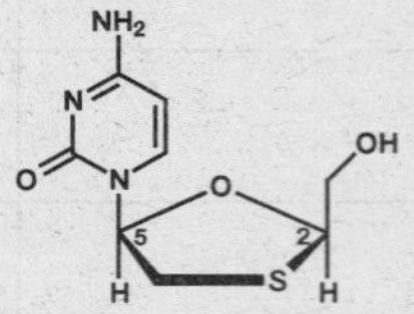

Lamivudine is a white to off-white crystalline solid with a solubility of approximately 70 mg/mL in water at 20°C.

Zidovudine: The chemical name of zidovudine is 3'-azido-3'-deoxythymidine. It has a molecular formula of $C_{10}H_{13}N_5O_4$ and a molecular weight of 267.24 daltons. It has the following structural formula:

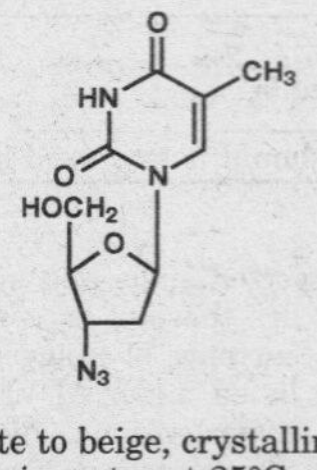

Zidovudine is a white to beige, crystalline solid with a solubility of 20.1 mg/mL in water at 25°C.

MICROBIOLOGY

Mechanism of Action:

Abacavir: Abacavir is a carbocyclic synthetic nucleoside analogue. Intracellularly, abacavir is converted by cellular enzymes to the active metabolite, carbovir triphosphate. Carbovir triphosphate is an analogue of deoxyguanosine-5'-triphosphate (dGTP). Carbovir triphosphate inhibits the activity of HIV-1 reverse transcriptase (RT) both by competing with the natural substrate dGTP and by its incorporation into viral DNA. The lack of a 3'-OH group in the incorporated nucleoside analogue prevents the formation of the 5' to 3' phosphodiester linkage essential for DNA chain elongation, and therefore, the viral DNA growth is terminated.

Lamivudine: Lamivudine is a synthetic nucleoside analogue. Intracellularly, lamivudine is phosphorylated to its active 5'-triphosphate metabolite, lamivudine triphosphate (L-TP). The principal mode of action of L-TP is inhibition of RT via DNA chain termination after incorporation of the nucleoside analogue. L-TP is a weak inhibitor of mammalian DNA polymerases-α and -β and mitochondrial DNA polymerase-γ.

Zidovudine: Zidovudine is a synthetic nucleoside analogue. Intracellularly, zidovudine is phosphorylated to its active 5'-triphosphate metabolite, zidovudine triphosphate (ZDV-TP). The principal mode of action of ZDV-TP is inhibition of RT via DNA chain termination after incorporation of the nucleoside analogue. ZDV-TP is a weak inhibitor of the mammalian DNA polymerase-α and mitochondrial DNA polymerase-γ and has been reported to be incorporated into the DNA of cells in culture.

Antiviral Activity In Vitro:

The relationship between in vitro susceptibility of HIV to abacavir, lamivudine, or zidovudine and the inhibition of HIV replication in humans has not been established.

Abacavir: The in vitro anti-HIV-1 activity of abacavir was evaluated against a T-cell tropic laboratory strain HIV-1 IIIB in lymphoblastic cell lines, a monocyte/macrophage tropic laboratory strain HIV-1 BaL in primary monocytes/macrophages, and clinical isolates in peripheral blood mononuclear cells. The concentration of drug necessary to inhibit viral replication by 50 percent (IC_{50}) ranged from 3.7 to 5.8 μM against HIV-1 IIIB, and was 0.26 ± 0.18 μM (1 μM = 0.28 mcg/mL) against 8 clinical isolates. The IC_{50} of abacavir against HIV-1 BaL varied from 0.07 to 1.0 μM. Abacavir had synergistic activity in combination with amprenavir, nevirapine, and zidovudine, and additive activity in combination with didanosine, lamivudine, stavudine, and zalcitabine in vitro. Most of these drug combinations have not been adequately studied in humans.

Lamivudine: In vitro activity of lamivudine against HIV-1 was assessed in a number of cell lines (including monocytes and fresh human peripheral blood lymphocytes). IC_{50} and IC_{90} values (50% and 90% inhibitory concentrations) for lamivudine were 0.0006 mcg/mL to 0.034 mcg/mL and 0.015 to 0.321 mcg/mL, respectively. Lamivudine had anti-HIV-1 activity in all acute virus-cell infections tested.

In HIV-1–infected MT-4 cells, lamivudine in combination with zidovudine had synergistic antiretroviral activity.

Zidovudine: In vitro activity of zidovudine against HIV-1 was assessed in a number of cell lines (including monocytes and fresh human peripheral blood lymphocytes). The IC_{50} and IC_{90} values for zidovudine were 0.003 to 0.013 mcg/mL and 0.03 to 0.13 mcg/mL, respectively. Zidovudine had anti-HIV-1 activity in all acute virus-cell infections tested. However, zidovudine activity was substantially less in chronically infected cell lines. In cell culture drug combination studies, zidovudine demonstrates synergistic activity with, delavirdine, didanosine, indinavir, nelfinavir, nevirapine, ritonavir, saquinavir, and zalcitabine, and additive activity with interferon-alpha.

Drug Resistance

HIV-1 isolates with reduced sensitivity to abacavir, lamivudine, or zidovudine have been selected in vitro and were also obtained from patients treated with abacavir, lamivudine, zidovudine, or lamivudine plus zidovudine. The clinical relevance of genotypic and phenotypic changes associated with abacavir, lamivudine, or zidovudine therapy is currently under evaluation.

Abacavir: Genetic analysis of isolates from abacavir-treated patients showed point mutations in the reverse transcriptase gene that resulted in amino acid substitutions at positions K65R, L74V, Y115F, and M184V. Mutations M184V and L74V were most frequently observed in clinical isolates. Phenotypic analysis of HIV-1 isolates that harbored abacavir-associated mutations from 17 patients after 12 weeks of abacavir monotherapy exhibited a 3-fold decrease in susceptibility to abacavir in vitro.

Lamivudine: Genotypic analysis of isolates selected in vitro and recovered from lamivudine-treated patients showed that the resistance was due to mutations in the HIV-1 reverse transcriptase gene at codon 184 from methionine to either isoleucine or valine.

Zidovudine: Genotypic analyses of the isolates selected in vitro and recovered from zidovudine-treated patients showed mutations, which result in 5 amino acid substitutions (M41L, D67N, K70R, K219Q, T215Y or F) in the HIV-1 reverse transcriptase gene. In general, higher levels of resistance were associated with greater number of mutations. In some patients harboring zidovudine-resistant virus at baseline, phenotypic sensitivity to zidovudine was restored by 12 weeks of treatment with lamivudine and zidovudine. Combination therapy with lamivudine plus zidovudine delayed the emergence of mutations conferring resistance to zidovudine.

Cross-Resistance

Cross-resistance among certain reverse transcriptase inhibitors has been recognized.

Abacavir: Recombinant laboratory strains of HIV-1 (HXB2) containing multiple reverse transcriptase mutations conferring abacavir resistance exhibited cross-resistance to lamivudine, didanosine, and zalcitabine in vitro. For clinical information in treatment-experienced patients, see INDICATIONS AND USAGE: Description of Clinical Studies and PRECAUTIONS.

Lamivudine: Cross-resistance between lamivudine and zidovudine has not been reported. Cross-resistance to didanosine and zalcitabine has been observed in some patients harboring lamivudine resistant HIV-1 isolates. In some patients treated with zidovudine plus didanosine or zalcitabine, isolates resistant to multiple drugs, including lamivudine, have emerged (see under Zidovudine below).

Zidovudine: HIV isolates with multidrug resistance to didanosine, lamivudine, stavudine, zalcitabine, and zidovudine were recovered from a small number of patients treated for ≥1 year with zidovudine plus didanosine or zidovudine plus zalcitabine. The pattern of genotypic resistant mutations with such combination therapies was different (A62V, V75I, F77L, F116Y, Q151M) from the pattern with zidovudine monotherapy, with the 151 mutation being most commonly associated with multidrug resistance. The mutation at codon 151 in combination with the mutations at 62, 75, 77, and 116 results in a virus with reduced susceptibility to, didanosine, lamivudine, stavudine, zalcitabine, and zidovudine.

CLINICAL PHARMACOLOGY

Pharmacokinetics in Adults:

TRIZIVIR In a single-dose, 3-way crossover bioavailability study of 1 TRIZIVIR tablet versus 1 ZIAGEN tablet (300 mg), 1 EPIVIR tablet (150 mg), plus 1 RETROVIR tablet (300 mg) administered simultaneously in healthy subjects (n = 24), there was no difference in the extent of absorption, as measured by the area under the plasma concentration-time curve (AUC) and maximal peak concentration (C_{max}), of all 3 components. One TRIZIVIR tablet was bioequivalent to 1 ZIAGEN tablet (300 mg), 1 EPIVIR tablet (150 mg), plus 1 RETROVIR tablet (300 mg) following single-dose administration to fasting healthy subjects (n = 24).

Abacavir Following oral administration, abacavir is rapidly absorbed and extensively distributed. Binding of abacavir to human plasma proteins is approximately 50%. Binding of abacavir to plasma proteins was independent of concentration. Total blood and plasma drug-related radioactivity concentrations are identical, demonstrating that abacavir readily distributes into erythrocytes. The primary routes of elimination of abacavir are metabolism by alcohol dehydrogenase to form the 5'-carboxylic acid and glucuronyl transferase to form the 5'-glucuronide.

Lamivudine Following oral administration, lamivudine is rapidly absorbed and extensively distributed. Binding to plasma protein is low. Approximately 70% of an intravenous dose of lamivudine is recovered as unchanged drug in the urine. Metabolism of lamivudine is a minor route of elimination. In humans, the only known metabolite is the trans-sulfoxide metabolite (approximately 5% of an oral dose after 12 hours).

Zidovudine: Following oral administration, zidovudine is rapidly absorbed and extensively distributed. Binding to plasma protein is low. Zidovudine is eliminated primarily by hepatic metabolism. The major metabolite of zidovudine is 3'-azido-3'-deoxy-5'-*O*-β-*D*-glucopyranuronosylthymidine (GZDV). GZDV area under the curve (AUC) is about 3-fold greater than the zidovudine AUC. Urinary recovery of zidovudine and GZDV accounts for 14% and 74% of the dose following oral administration, respectively. A second metabolite, 3'-amino-3'-deoxythymidine (AMT), has been identified in plasma. The AMT AUC was one fifth of the zidovudine AUC.

In humans, abacavir, lamivudine, and zidovudine are not significantly metabolized by cytochrome P450 enzymes.

The pharmacokinetic properties of abacavir, lamivudine, and zidovudine in fasting patients are summarized in Table 1.

[See table below]

Effect of Food on Absorption of TRIZIVIR

TRIZIVIR may be administered with or without food. Administration with food in a single-dose bioavailability study resulted in lower C_{max}, similar to results observed previously for the reference formulations. The average [90% CI] decrease in abacavir, lamivudine and zidovudine C_{max} was 32% [24% to 38%], 18% [10% to 25%], and 28% [13% to 40%], respectively, when administered with a high-fat meal, compared to administration under fasted conditions. Administration of TRIZIVIR with food did not alter the extent of abacavir, lamivudine, and zidovudine absorption (AUC), as compared to administration under fasted conditions (n =24).

Special Populations

Impaired Renal Function:

TRIZIVIR: Because lamivudine and zidovudine require dose adjustment in the presence of renal insufficiency, TRIZIVIR is not recommended for use in patients with creatinine clearance ≤50 mL/min (see PRECAUTIONS).

Pregnancy

See PRECAUTIONS: Pregnancy.

Zidovudine: Zidovudine pharmacokinetics have been studied in a Phase 1 study of 8 women during the last trimester of pregnancy. As pregnancy progressed, there was no evidence of drug accumulation. The pharmacokinetics of zidovudine were similar to that of nonpregnant adults. Consistent with passive transmission of the drug across the placenta, zidovudine concentrations in neonatal plasma at birth were essentially equal to those in maternal plasma at delivery. Although data are limited, methadone maintenance therapy in 5 pregnant women did not appear to alter zidovudine pharmacokinetics. In a nonpregnant adult population, a potential for interaction has been identified (see CLINICAL PHARMACOLOGY: Drug Interactions).

Abacavir and Lamivudine: No data are available on the pharmacokinetics of abacavir or lamivudine during pregnancy.

Nursing Mothers

See PRECAUTIONS: Nursing Mothers.

Zidovudine: After administration of a single dose of 200 mg zidovudine to 13 HIV-infected women, the mean concentration of zidovudine was similar in human milk and serum.

Abacavir and Lamivudine: No data are available on the pharmacokinetics of abacavir or lamivudine in nursing mothers.

Pediatric Patients

TRIZIVIR: TRIZIVIR is not intended for use in pediatric patients. TRIZIVIR should not be administered to adolescents who weigh less than 40 kg because it is a fixed-dose tablet that cannot be dose adjusted for this patient population (see PRECAUTIONS: Pediatric Use).

Geriatric Patients

The pharmacokinetics of abacavir, lamivudine, and zidovudine have not been studied in patients over 65 years of age.

Gender

Lamivudine and Zidovudine: A pharmacokinetic study in healthy male (n = 12) and female (n = 12) subjects showed no gender differences in zidovudine exposure (AUC∞) or lamivudine AUC∞ normalized for body weight.

Abacavir: The pharmacokinetics of abacavir with respect to gender have not been determined.

Race

Lamivudine: There are no significant racial differences in lamivudine pharmacokinetics.

Abacavir and Zidovudine: The pharmacokinetics of abacavir and zidovudine with respect to race have not been determined.

Drug Interactions

See PRECAUTIONS Drug Interactions.

The drug interactions described are based on studies conducted with the individual nucleoside analogues. In humans, abacavir, lamivudine, and zidovudine are not significantly metabolized by cytochrome P450 enzymes; therefore, it is unlikely that clinically significant drug interactions will occur with drugs metabolized through these pathways.

Abacavir: Due to their common metabolic pathways via glucuronyl transferase with zidovudine, 15 HIV-infected pa-

tients were enrolled in a crossover study evaluating single doses of abacavir (600 mg), lamivudine (150 mg), and zidovudine (300 mg) alone or in combination. Analysis showed no clinically relevant changes in the pharmacokinetics of abacavir with the addition of lamivudine or zidovudine or the combination of lamivudine and zidovudine. Lamivudine exposure (AUC decreased 15%) and zidovudine exposure (AUC increased 10%) did not show clinically relevant changes with concurrent abacavir.

Lamivudine and Zidovudine: No clinically significant alterations in lamivudine or zidovudine pharmacokinetics were observed in 12 asymptomatic HIV-infected adult patients given a single dose of zidovudine (200 mg) in combination with multiple doses of lamivudine (300 mg q 12 h).

[See table at bottom of next page]

INDICATIONS AND USAGE

TRIZIVIR is indicated alone or in combination with other antiretroviral agents for the treatment of HIV-1 infection. The indication for TRIZIVIR is based on analyses of surrogate markers in controlled studies with abacavir of up to 24 weeks in duration. At present, there are no results from controlled trials evaluating long-term suppression of HIV RNA or disease progression with therapy with abacavir. There are limited data on the use of this triple-combination regimen in patients with higher viral load levels (>100,000 copies/mL) at baseline (see Description of Clinical Studies for ZIAGEN).

Description of Clinical Studies:

TRIZIVIR

There have been no clinical trials conducted with TRIZIVIR (see CLINICAL PHARMACOLOGY for information about bioequivalence of TRIZIVIR).

The following studies were conducted with the individual components of TRIZIVIR.

ZIAGEN

Therapy-Naive Adults CNAAB3003 was a multicenter, double-blind, placebo-controlled study in which 173 HIV-infected, therapy-naive adults were randomized to receive either ZIAGEN (300 mg twice daily), lamivudine (150 mg twice daily), and zidovudine (300 mg twice daily) or lamivudine (150 mg twice daily) and zidovudine (300 mg twice daily). The duration of double-blind treatment was 16 weeks. Study participants were: male (76%), Caucasian (54%), African-American (28%), and Hispanic (16%). The median age was 34 years, the median pretreatment CD4 cell count was 450 cells/mm³, and median plasma HIV-1 RNA was 4.5 $\log_{10}$ copies/mL. Proportions of patients with plasma HIV-1 RNA <400 copies/mL (using Roche Amplicor HIV-1 MONITOR® Test) through 16 weeks of treatment are summarized in Figure 1.

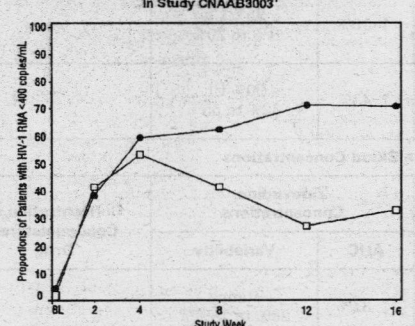

Figure 1: Proportions of Patients with HIV-1 RNA <400 copies/mL In Study CNAAB3003[†]

● ZIAGEN/Lamivudine/Zidovudine (n = 87)
□ Lamivudine/Zidovudine (n = 86)
[†]Missing data were considered as HIV-1 RNA≥400 copies/mL.

After 16 weeks of therapy, the median CD4 increases from baseline were 47 cells/mm³ in the group receiving ZIAGEN and 112 cells/mm³ in the placebo group.

Preliminary findings from a second controlled study in therapy-naive adults were supportive of the efficacy of abacavir through 16 weeks of treatment.

Therapy-Experienced Pediatric Patients A randomized, double-blind study, CNAA3006, compared ZIAGEN plus lamivudine and zidovudine versus lamivudine and zidovudine in pediatric patients, most of whom were extensively pretreated with nucleoside analogue antiretroviral agents. Patients in this study had a limited response to abacavir.

CONTRAINDICATIONS

Abacavir sulfate, one of the components of TRIZIVIR, has been associated with fatal hypersensitivity reactions. ABACAVIR (as TRIZIVIR or ZIAGEN) SHOULD NOT BE RESTARTED FOLLOWING A HYPERSENSITIVITY REACTION TO ABACAVIR (see WARNINGS, PRECAUTIONS, and ADVERSE REACTIONS).

TRIZIVIR Tablets are contraindicated in patients with previously demonstrated hypersensitivity to any of the components of the product (see WARNINGS).

WARNINGS

Hypersensitivity Reaction: TRIZIVIR contains abacavir sulfate (ZIAGEN), which has been associated with fatal hypersensitivity reactions. Patients developing signs or symptoms of hypersensitivity (which include fever; skin rash; fatigue; gastrointestinal symptoms such as nausea, vomiting, diarrhea, or abdominal pain; and respiratory symptoms such as pharyngitis, dyspnea, or cough) should discontinue TRIZIVIR as soon as a hypersensitivity reaction is first suspected, and should seek medical evaluation immediately. To avoid a delay in diagnosis and minimize the risk of a life-threatening hypersensitivity reaction, TRIZIVIR should be permanently discontinued if hypersensitivity cannot be ruled out, even when other diagnoses are possible (e.g., acute onset respiratory diseases, gastroenteritis, or reactions to other medications). Abacavir (as TRIZIVIR or ZIAGEN) SHOULD NOT be restarted following a hypersensitivity reaction to abacavir because more severe symptoms will recur within hours and may include life-threatening hypotension and death.

Severe or fatal hypersensitivity reactions can occur within hours after reintroduction of abacavir (as TRIZIVIR or ZIAGEN) in patients who have no identified history or unrecognized symptoms of hypersensitivity to abacavir therapy.

When therapy with abacavir (as TRIZIVIR or ZIAGEN) has been discontinued for reasons other than symptoms of a hypersensitivity reaction, and if reinitiation of therapy is under consideration, the reason for discontinuation should be evaluated to ensure that the patient did not have symptoms of a hypersensitivity reaction. If hypersensitivity cannot be ruled out, abacavir (as TRIZIVIR or ZIAGEN) should **NOT** be reintroduced. If symptoms consistent with hypersensitivity are not identified, reintroduction can be undertaken with continued monitoring for symptoms of a hypersensitivity reaction. Patients should be made aware that a hypersensitivity reaction can occur with reintroduction of abacavir (as TRIZIVIR or ZIAGEN), and that reintroduction of abacavir (as TRIZIVIR or ZIAGEN) should be undertaken only if medical care can be readily accessed by the patient or others (see ADVERSE REACTIONS).

In clinical trials, hypersensitivity reactions have been reported in approximately 5% of adult and pediatric patients receiving abacavir. Symptoms usually appear within the first 6 weeks of treatment with abacavir although these reactions may occur at any time during therapy (see PRECAUTIONS: Information for Patients and ADVERSE REACTIONS).

Abacavir Hypersensitivity Reaction Registry To facilitate reporting of hypersensitivity reactions and collection of information on each case, an Abacavir Hypersensitivity Registry has been established. Physicians should register patients by calling 1-800-270-0425.

Lactic Acidosis/Severe Hepatomegaly with Steatosis Lactic acidosis and severe hepatomegaly with steatosis, including fatal cases, have been reported with the use of nucleoside analogues alone or in combination, including abacavir, lamivudine, zidovudine, and other antiretrovirals. A majority of these cases have been in women. Obesity and prolonged nucleoside exposure may be risk factors. Particular caution should be exercised when administering TRIZIVIR to any patient with known risk factors for liver disease; however, cases have also been reported in patients with no known risk factors. Treatment with TRIZIVIR should be suspended in any patient who develops clinical or laboratory findings suggestive of lactic acidosis or pronounced hepatotoxicity (which may include hepatomegaly and steatosis even in the absence of marked transaminase elevations).

Bone Marrow Suppression Since TRIZIVIR contains zidovudine, TRIZIVIR should be used with caution in patients who have bone marrow compromise evidenced by granulocyte count <1000 cells/mm³ or hemoglobin <9.5 g/dL. Frequent blood counts are strongly recommended in patients with advanced HIV disease who are treated with TRIZIVIR. For HIV-infected individuals and patients with asymptomatic or early HIV disease, periodic blood counts are recommended.

Myopathy Myopathy and myositis, with pathological changes similar to that produced by HIV disease, have been associated with prolonged use of zidovudine, and therefore may occur with therapy with TRIZIVIR.

Other TRIZIVIR contains fixed doses of 3 nucleoside analogues: abacavir, lamivudine, and zidovudine and should not be administered concomitantly with abacavir, lamivudine, or zidovudine.

Because TRIZIVIR is a fixed-dose tablet, it should not be prescribed for adults or adolescents who weigh less than 40 kg or other patients requiring dosage adjustment.

The complete prescribing information for all agents being considered for use with TRIZIVIR should be consulted before combination therapy with TRIZIVIR is initiated.

Table 1: Pharmacokinetic Parameters* for Abacavir, Lamivudine, and Zidovudine in Adults						
Parameter	Abacavir		Lamivudine		Zidovudine	
Oral bioavailability (%)	86 ± 25	n = 6	86 ± 16	n = 12	64 ± 10	n = 5
Apparent volume of distribution (L/kg)	0.86 ± 0.15	n = 6	1.3 ± 0.4	n = 20	1.6 ± 0.6	n = 8
Systemic clearance (L/h/kg)	0.80 ± 0.24	n = 6	0.33 ± 0.06	n = 20	1.6 ± 0.6	n = 6
Renal clearance (L/h/kg)	.007 ± .008	n = 6	0.22 ± 0.06	n = 20	0.34 ± 0.05	n = 9
Elimination half-life (h)[†]	1.45 ± 0.32	n = 20	5 to 7		0.5 to 3	

*Data presented as mean ± standard deviation except where noted.
[†]Approximate range.

Continued on next page

Trizivir—Cont.

PRECAUTIONS

Therapy-Experienced Patients

Abacavir In clinical trials, patients with prolonged prior nucleoside reverse transcriptase inhibitor (NRTI) exposure or who had HIV-1 isolates that contained multiple mutations conferring resistance to NRTIs had limited response to abacavir. The potential for cross-resistance between abacavir and other NRTIs should be considered when choosing new therapeutic regimens in therapy-experienced patients (see MICROBIOLOGY: Cross-Resistance).

Patients with HIV and Hepatitis B Virus Coinfection

Lamivudine In clinical trials and postmarketing experience, some patients with HIV infection who have chronic liver disease due to hepatitis B virus infection experienced clinical or laboratory evidence of recurrent hepatitis upon discontinuation of lamivudine. Consequences may be more severe in patients with decompensated liver disease.

Patients with Impaired Renal Function

TRIZIVIR Since TRIZIVIR is a fixed-dose tablet and the dosage of the individual components cannot be altered, patients with creatinine clearance ≤50 mL/min should not receive TRIZIVIR.

Information for Patients

Abacavir **Patients should be advised that a Medication Guide and Warning Card summarizing the symptoms of abacavir hypersensitivity reactions should be dispensed by the pharmacist with each new prescription and refill of TRIZIVIR. The complete text of the Medication Guide is reprinted at the end of this document. Patients should be instructed to carry the Warning Card with them.**

Patients should be advised of the possibility of a hypersensitivity reaction to abacavir (as TRIZIVIR or ZIAGEN) that may result in death. Patients developing signs or symptoms of hypersensitivity (which include fever; skin rash; fatigue; gastrointestinal symptoms such as nausea, vomiting, diarrhea, or abdominal pain; and respiratory symptoms such as sore throat, shortness of breath, or cough) should discontinue treatment with TRIZIVIR and seek medical evaluation immediately. **Abacavir (as TRIZIVIR OR ZIAGEN) SHOULD NOT be restarted following a hypersensitivity reaction to abacavir because more severe symptoms will recur within hours and may include life-threatening hypotension and death.** Patients who have interrupted abacavir (as TRIZIVIR or ZIAGEN) for reactions other than symptoms of hypersensitivity (for example, those who have an interruption in drug supply) should be made aware that a severe or fatal hypersensitivity reaction can occur with reintroduction of abacavir. Patients should be instructed not to reintroduce abacavir (as TRIZIVIR or ZIAGEN) without medical consultation and that reintroduction of abacavir (as TRIZIVIR or ZIAGEN) should be undertaken only if medical care can be readily accessed by the patient or others (see ADVERSE REACTIONS and WARNINGS).

TRIZIVIR Patients should be informed that TRIZIVIR is not a cure for HIV infection and patients may continue to experience illnesses associated with HIV infection, including opportunistic infections. Patients should be advised that the use of TRIZIVIR has not been shown to reduce the risk of transmission of HIV to others through sexual contact or blood contamination.

Patients should be advised of the importance of taking TRIZIVIR as it is prescribed.

Zidovudine Patients should be informed that the important toxicities associated with zidovudine are neutropenia and/or anemia. They should be told of the extreme importance of having their blood counts followed closely while on therapy, especially for patients with advanced HIV disease.

Drug Interactions

TRIZIVIR No clinically significant changes to pharmacokinetic parameters were observed for abacavir, lamivudine, or zidovudine when administered together.

Abacavir Abacavir has no effect on the pharmacokinetic properties of ethanol. Ethanol decreases the elimination of abacavir causing an increase in overall exposure (see CLINICAL PHARMACOLOGY: Drug Interactions).

Lamivudine TMP 160 mg/SMX 800 mg once daily has been shown to increase lamivudine exposure (AUC). The effect of higher doses of TMP/SMX on lamivudine pharmacokinetics has not been investigated (see CLINICAL PHARMACOLOGY).

Table 2: Effect of Coadministered Drugs on Abacavir, Lamivudine, and Zidovudine AUC*
Note: ROUTINE DOSE MODIFICATION OF ABACAVIR, LAMIVUDINE, AND ZIDOVUDINE IS NOT WARRANTED WITH COADMINISTRATION OF THE FOLLOWING DRUGS.

Drugs That May Alter Lamivudine Blood Concentrations

Coadministered Drug and Dose	Lamivudine Dose	n	Lamivudine Concentrations		Concentration of Coadministered Drug
			AUC	Variability	
Nelfinavir 750 mg q 8 h × 7 to 10 days	single 150 mg	11	↑ 10%	95% CI: 1% to 20%	↔
Trimethoprim 160 mg/ Sulfamethoxazole 800 mg daily × 5 days	single 300 mg	14	↑ 43%	90% CI: 32% to 55%	↔

Drugs That May Alter Zidovudine Blood Concentrations

Coadministered Drug and Dose	Zidovudine Dose	n	Zidovudine Concentrations		Concentration of Coadministered Drug
			AUC	Variability	
Atovaquone 750 mg q 12 h with food	200 mg q 8 h	14	↑ 31%	Range 23% to 78%**	↔
Fluconazole 400 mg daily	200 mg q 8 h	12	↑ 74%	95% CI: 54% to 98%	Not Reported
Methadone 30 to 90 mg daily	200 mg q 4 h	9	↑ 43%	Range 16% to 64%**	↔
Nelfinavir 750 mg q 8 h × 7 to 10 days	single 200 mg	11	↓ 35%	Range 28% to 41%	↔
Probenecid 500 mg q 6 h × 2 days	2 mg/kg q 8 h × 3 days	3	↑ 106%	Range 100% to 170%**	Not Assessed
Ritonavir 300 mg q 6 h × 4 days	200 mg q 8 h × 4 days	9	↓ 25%	95% CI: 15% to 34%	↔
Valproic acid 250 mg or 500 mg q 8 h × 4 days	100 mg q 8 h × 4 days	6	↑ 80%	Range 64% to 130%**	Not Assessed

Drugs That May Alter Abacavir Blood Concentrations

Coadministered Drug and Dose	Abacavir Dose	n	Abacavir Concentrations		Concentration of Coadministered Drug
			AUC	Variability	
Ethanol 0.7 g/kg	single 600 mg	24	↑ 41%	90% CI: 35% to 48%	↔

↑ = Increase; ↓ = Decrease; ↔ = no significant change; AUC = area under the concentration versus time curve; CI = confidence interval.

* See PRECAUTIONS: Drug Interactions for additional information on drug interactions.

**Estimated range of percent difference.

Zidovudine Coadministration of ganciclovir, interferon-alpha, and other bone marrow suppressive or cytotoxic agents may increase the hematologic toxicity of zidovudine (see CLINICAL PHARMACOLOGY).

Carcinogenesis, Mutagenesis, and Impairment of Fertility

Carcinogenicity

Abacavir Carcinogenicity studies in mice and rats are ongoing with abacavir.

Lamivudine Lamivudine long-term carcinogenicity studies in mice and rats showed no evidence of carcinogenic potential at exposures up to 10 times (mice) and 58 times (rats) those observed in humans at the recommended therapeutic dose.

Zidovudine Zidovudine was administered orally at 3 dosage levels to separate groups of mice and rats (60 females and 60 males in each group). Initial single daily doses were 30, 60, and 120 mg/kg per day in mice and 80, 220, and 600 mg/kg per day in rats. The doses in mice were reduced to 20, 30, and 40 mg/kg per day after day 90 because of treatment-related anemia, whereas in rats only the high dose was reduced to 450 mg/kg per day on day 91 and then to 300 mg/kg per day on day 279.

In mice, 7 late-appearing (after 19 months) vaginal neoplasms (5 nonmetastasizing squamous cell carcinomas, 1 squamous cell papilloma, and 1 squamous polyp) occurred in animals given the highest dose. One late-appearing squamous cell papilloma occurred in the vagina of a middle-dose animal. No vaginal tumors were found at the lowest dose.

In rats, 2 late-appearing (after 20 months), nonmetastasizing vaginal squamous cell carcinomas occurred in animals given the highest dose. No vaginal tumors occurred at the low or middle dose in rats. No other drug-related tumors were observed in either sex of either species.

At doses that produced tumors in mice and rats, the estimated drug exposure (as measured by AUC) was approximately 3 times (mouse) and 24 times (rat) the estimated human exposure at the recommended therapeutic dose of 100 mg every 4 hours.

Two transplacental carcinogenicity studies were conducted in mice. One study administered zidovudine at doses of 20 mg/kg per day or 40 mg/kg per day from gestation day 10 through parturition and lactation with dosing continuing in offspring for 24 months postnatally. At these doses, exposures were approximately 3 times the estimated human exposure at the recommended doses. After 24 months, at the 40-mg/kg-per-day dose, an increase in incidence of vaginal tumors was noted with no increase in tumors in the liver or lung or any other organ in either gender. These findings are consistent with results of the standard oral carcinogenicity study in mice, as described earlier. A second study administered zidovudine at maximum tolerated doses of 12.5 mg/day or 25 mg/day (~1000 mg/kg nonpregnant body weight or ~450 mg/kg of term body weight) to pregnant mice from days 12 through 18 of gestation. There was an increase in the number of tumors in the lung, liver, and female reproductive tracts in the offspring of mice receiving the higher dose level of zidovudine.

It is not known how predictive the results of rodent carcinogenicity studies may be for humans.

Mutagenicity

Abacavir Abacavir induced chromosomal aberrations both in the presence and absence of metabolic activation in an in vitro cytogenetic study in human lymphoctyes. Abacavir was mutagenic in the absence of metabolic activation, although it was not mutagenic in the presence of metabolic activation in an L5178Y/$TK^{+/-}$ mouse lymphoma assay. At systemic exposures approximately 9 times higher than that in humans at the therapeutic dose, abacavir was clastogenic in males and not clastogenic in females in an in vivo mouse bone marrow micronucleus assay. Abacavir was not mutagenic in bacterial mutagenicity assays in the presence and absence of metabolic activation.

Lamivudine Lamivudine was mutagenic in a L5178Y/$TK^{+/-}$ mouse lymphoma assay and clastogenic in a cytogenetic assay using cultured human lymphocytes. Lamivudine was negative in a microbial mutagenicity assay, in an in vitro cell transformation assay, in a rat micronucleus test, in a rat bone marrow cytogenetic assay, and in an assay for unscheduled DNA synthesis in rat liver.

Zidovudine Zidovudine was mutagenic in a L5178Y/$TK^{+/-}$ mouse lymphoma assay, positive in an in vitro cell transformation assay, clastogenic in a cytogenetic assay using cultured human lymphocytes, and positive in mouse and rat micronucleus tests after repeated doses. It was negative in a cytogenetic study in rats given a single dose.

Impairment of Fertility

Abacavir Abacavir administered to male and female rats had no adverse effects on fertility judged by conception rates at doses up to approximately 8-fold higher than that in humans at the therapeutic dose based on body surface area comparisons.

Lamivudine In a study of reproductive performance, lamivudine, administered to male and female rats at doses up to 130 times the usual adult dose based on body surface area considerations, revealed no evidence of impaired fertility judged by conception rates and no effect on the survival, growth, and development to weaning of the offspring.

Zidovudine Zidovudine, administered to male and female rats at doses up to 7 times the usual adult dose based on body surface area considerations, had no effect on fertility judged by conception rates.

Pregnancy

Pregnancy Category C. There are no adequate and well-controlled studies of TRIZIVIR in pregnant women. Reproduction studies with abacavir, lamivudine, and zidovudine have been performed in animals (see Abacavir, Lamivudine, and Zidovudine sections below). TRIZIVIR should be used during pregnancy only if the potential benefits outweigh the risks.

Abacavir Studies in pregnant rats showed that abacavir is transferred to the fetus through the placenta. Developmental toxicity (depressed fetal body weight and reduced crown-rump length) and increased incidences of fetal anasarca and skeletal malformations were observed when rats were treated with abacavir at a dose 35 times higher than the human exposure, based on AUC (1000 mg/kg per day). In a fertility study, evidence of toxicity to the developing embryo and fetuses (increased resorptions, decreased fetal body weights) occurred only at 500 mg/kg per day. The offspring of female rats treated with abacavir at 500 mg/kg per day (beginning at embryo implantation and ending at weaning) showed increased incidence of stillbirth and lower body weights throughout life. In the rabbit, there was no evidence of drug-related developmental toxicity and no increases in fetal malformations at doses up to 8.5 times the human exposure, based on AUC.

Lamivudine Studies in pregnant rats and rabbits showed that lamivudine is transferred to the fetus through the placenta. Reproduction studies with orally administered lamivudine have been performed in rats and rabbits at 130 and 60 times, respectively, the usual adult dose (based on relative body surface area) and have revealed no evidence of teratogenicity. Some evidence of early embryolethality was seen in the rabbit at doses similar to those produced by the usual adult dose and higher, but there was no indication of this effect in the rat at orally administered doses up to 130 times the usual adult dose.

Zidovudine Reproduction studies with orally administered zidovudine in the rat and in the rabbit at doses up to 500 mg/kg per day revealed no evidence of teratogenicity with zidovudine. Zidovudine treatment resulted in embryo/fetal toxicity as evidenced by an increase in the incidence of fetal resorptions in rats given 150 or 450 mg/kg per day and rabbits given 500 mg/kg per day. The doses used in the teratology studies resulted in peak zidovudine plasma concentrations (after one-half of the daily dose) in rats 66 to 226 times, and in rabbits 12 to 87 times, mean steady-state peak human plasma concentrations (after one-sixth of the daily dose) achieved with the recommended daily dose (100 mg every 4 hours). In an additional teratology study in rats, a dose of 3000 mg/kg per day (very near the oral median lethal dose in rats of approximately 3700 mg/kg) caused marked maternal toxicity and an increase in the incidence of fetal malformations. This dose resulted in peak zidovudine plasma concentrations 350 times peak human plasma concentrations. No evidence of teratogenicity was seen in this experiment at doses of 600 mg/kg per day or less. Two rodent carcinogenicity studies were conducted (see Carcinogenesis, Mutagenesis, and Impairment of Fertility).

Antiretroviral Pregnancy Registry To monitor maternal-fetal outcomes of pregnant women exposed to TRIZIVIR or other antiretroviral agents, an Antiretroviral Pregnancy Registry has been established. Physicians are encouraged to register patients by calling 1-800-258-4263.

Nursing Mothers

The Centers for Disease Control and Prevention recommend that HIV-infected mothers not breastfeed their infants to avoid risking postnatal transmission of HIV infection.

Abacavir, Lamivudine, and Zidovudine Zidovudine is excreted in breast milk; abacavir is secreted into the milk of lactating rats; there are no data on lamivudine.

Because of both the potential for HIV transmission and the potential for serious adverse reactions in nursing infants, **mothers should be instructed not to breastfeed if they are receiving TRIZIVIR.**

Pediatric Use

TRIZIVIR is not intended for use in pediatric patients. TRIZIVIR should not be administered to adolescents who weigh less than 40 kg because it is a fixed-dose tablet that cannot be adjusted for this patient population.

Geriatric Use

Clinical studies of abacavir, lamivudine, and zidovudine did not include sufficient numbers of patients aged 65 and over to determine whether they respond differently from younger patients. In general, dose selection for an elderly patient should be cautious, reflecting the greater frequency of decreased hepatic, renal, or cardiac function, and of concomitant disease or other drug therapy. TRIZIVIR is not recommended for patients with impaired renal function (i.e., creatinine clearance ≤50 mL/min; see PRECAUTIONS: Patients with Impaired Renal Function and DOSAGE AND ADMINISTRATION).

ADVERSE REACTIONS

Abacavir **Hypersensitivity Reaction TRIZIVIR contains abacavir sulfate (ZIAGEN), which has been associated with fatal hypersensitivity reactions. Therapy with abacavir (as TRIZIVIR or ZIAGEN) SHOULD NOT be restarted following a hypersensitivity reaction because more severe symptoms will recur within hours and may include life-threatening hypotension and death. Patients developing signs or symptoms of hypersensitivity should discontinue treatment as soon as a hypersensitivity reaction is first suspected, and should seek medical evaluation immediately. To avoid a delay in diagnosis and minimize the risk of a life-threatening hypersensitivity reaction, TRIZIVIR should be permanently discontinued if hypersensitivity cannot be ruled out, even when other diagnoses are possible (e.g., acute onset respiratory diseases, gastroenteritis, or reactions to other medications).**

Severe or fatal hypersensitivity reactions can occur within hours after reintroduction of abacavir (as TRIZIVIR or ZIAGEN) in patients who have no identified history or unrecognized symptoms of hypersensitivity to abacavir therapy (see WARNINGS and PRECAUTIONS: Information for Patients).

When therapy with abacavir (as TRIZIVIR or ZIAGEN) has been discontinued for reasons other than symptoms of a hypersensitivity reaction, and if reinitiation of therapy is under consideration, the reason for discontinuation should be evaluated to ensure that the patient did not have symptoms of a hypersensitivity reaction. If hypersensitivity cannot be ruled out, abacavir (as TRIZIVIR or ZIAGEN) should **NOT** be reintroduced. If symptoms consistent with hypersensitivity are not identified, reintroduction can be undertaken with continued monitoring for symptoms of hypersensitivity reaction. Patients should be made aware that a hypersensitivity reaction can occur with reintroduction of abacavir (as TRIZIVIR or ZIAGEN), and that reintroduction of abacavir (as TRIZIVIR or ZIAGEN) should be undertaken only if medical care can be readily accessed by the patient or others (see WARNINGS).

In clinical studies, approximately 5% of adult and pediatric patients receiving abacavir developed a hypersensitivity reaction. This reaction is characterized by the appearance of symptoms indicating multi-organ/body system involvement. Symptoms usually appear within the first 6 weeks of treatment with abacavir, although these reactions may occur at any time during therapy. Frequently observed signs and symptoms include fever; skin rash; fatigue; and gastrointestinal symptoms such as nausea, vomiting, diarrhea, or abdominal pain. Other signs and symptoms include malaise, lethargy, myalgia, myolysis, arthralgia, edema, cough, dyspnea, headache, and paresthesia. Some patients who experienced a hypersensitivity reaction were initially thought to have acute onset or worsening respiratory disease. The diagnosis of hypersensitivity reaction should be carefully considered for patients presenting with symptoms of acute onset respiratory diseases, even if alternative respiratory diagnoses (pneumonia, bronchitis, flu-like illness) are possible.

Physical findings include lymphadenopathy, mucous membrane lesions (conjunctivitis and mouth ulcerations), and rash. The rash usually appears maculopapular or urticarial but may be variable in appearance. Hypersensitivity reactions have occurred without rash.

Laboratory abnormalities include elevated liver function tests, increased creatine phosphokinase or creatinine, and lymphopenia. Anaphylaxis, liver failure, renal failure, hypotension, and death have occurred in association with hypersensitivity reactions. Symptoms worsen with continued therapy but often resolve upon discontinuation of abacavir. Risk factors that may predict the occurrence or severity of hypersensitivity to abacavir have not been identified.

Selected clinical adverse events with a ≥5% frequency during therapy with ZIAGEN 300 mg twice daily and EPIVIR 150 mg twice daily and RETROVIR 300 mg twice daily compared with EPIVIR 150 mg twice daily and RETROVIR 300 mg twice daily from CNAAB3003 are listed in Table 3. [See table below]

Laboratory Abnormalities Laboratory abnormalities (anemia, neutropenia, liver function test abnormalities, and CPK elevations) were observed with similar frequencies in the 2 treatment groups in studies CNAAB3003 and CNAAB3006. Mild elevations of blood glucose were more frequent in subjects receiving abacavir. In study CNAAB3003, triglyceride elevations (all grades) were more common on the abacavir arm (25%) than on the placebo arm (11%).

Other Adverse Events In addition to adverse events in Table 3 other adverse events observed in the expanded access program for abacavir were pancreatitis and increased GGT.

Lamivudine Plus Zidovudine In 4 randomized, controlled trials of lamivudine 300 mg per day plus zidovudine 600 mg per day, the following selected clinical and laboratory adverse events were observed (see Tables 4 and 5).

Table 3: Selected Clinical Adverse Events Grades 1-4 (≥5% Frequency) in Therapy-Naive Adults (CNAAB3003) Through 16 Weeks of Treatment

Adverse Event	ZIAGEN/Lamivudine/ Zidovudine (n = 83)	Lamivudine/Zidovudine (n = 81)
Nausea	47%	41%
Nausea and vomiting	16%	11%
Diarrhea	12%	11%
Loss of appetite/anorexia	11%	10%
Insomnia and other sleep disorders	7%	5%

Table 4: Selected Clinical Adverse Events (≥5% Frequency) in 4 Controlled Clinical Trials With Lamivudine 300 mg/day and Zidovudine 600 mg/day

Adverse Event	Lamivudine plus Zidovudine (n = 251)
Body as a Whole	
Headache	35%
Malaise & fatigue	27%
Fever or chills	10%
Digestive	
Nausea	33%
Diarrhea	18%
Nausea & vomiting	13%
Anorexia and/or decreased appetite	10%
Abdominal pain	9%
Abdominal cramps	6%
Dyspepsia	5%
Nervous system	
Neuropathy	12%
Insomnia & other sleep disorders	11%
Dizziness	10%
Depressive disorders	9%
Respiratory	
Nasal signs & symptoms	20%
Cough	18%
Skin	
Skin rashes	9%
Musculoskeletal	
Musculoskeletal pain	12%
Myalgia	8%
Arthralgia	5%

Pancreatitis was observed in 3 of the 656 adult patients (<0.5%) who received lamivudine in controlled clinical trials.

Selected laboratory abnormalities observed during therapy are listed in Table 5.

Table 5: Frequencies of Selected Laboratory Abnormalities Among Adults in 4 Controlled Clinical Trials of Lamivudine 300 mg/day plus Zidovudine 600 mg/day*

Test (Abnormal Level)	Lamivudine plus Zidovudine % (n)
Neutropenia (ANC<750/mm^3)	7.2% (237)
Anemia (Hgb<8.0 g/dL)	2.9% (241)
Thrombocytopenia (platelets<50,000/mm^3)	0.4% (240)
ALT (>5.0 × ULN)	3.7% (241)
AST (>5.0 × ULN)	1.7% (241)
Bilirubin (>2.5 × ULN)	0.8% (241)
Amylase (>2.0 × ULN)	4.2% (72)

ULN = Upper limit of normal.
ANC = Absolute neutrophil count.
n = Number of patients assessed.
* Frequencies of these laboratory abnormalities were higher in patients with mild laboratory abnormalities at baseline.

Observed During Clinical Practice

Lamivudine and Zidovudine The following events have been identified during post-approval use of lamivudine and/or zidovudine. Because they are reported voluntarily from a population of unknown size, estimates of frequency cannot be made. These events have been chosen for inclusion due to a combination of their seriousness, frequency of reporting, or potential causal connection to lamivudine and/or zidovudine.

Endocrine and Metabolic Hyperglycemia.

General Sensitization reactions (including anaphylaxis), vasculitis.

Hepatobiliary Tract and Pancreas Lactic acidosis and hepatic steatosis (see WARNINGS), pancreatitis.

Musculoskeletal Muscle weakness, CPK elevation, rhabdomyolysis.

Nervous Seizures.

Skin Alopecia, erythema multiforme, Stevens-Johnson syndrome, urticaria.

OVERDOSAGE

Abacavir There is no known antidote for abacavir. It is not known whether abacavir can be removed by peritoneal dialysis or hemodialysis.

Lamivudine One case of an adult ingesting 6 grams of lamivudine was reported; there were no clinical signs or symptoms noted and hematologic tests remained normal. It is not known whether lamivudine can be removed by peritoneal dialysis or hemodialysis.

Zidovudine Acute overdoses of zidovudine have been reported in pediatric patients and adults. These involved exposures up to 50 grams. The only consistent findings were nau-

Continued on next page

Trizivir—Cont.

sea and vomiting. Other reported occurrences included headache, dizziness, drowsiness, lethargy, and confusion. Hematologic changes were transient. All patients recovered. Hemodialysis and peritoneal dialysis appear to have a negligible effect on the removal of zidovudine while elimination of its primary metabolite, GZDV, is enhanced.

DOSAGE AND ADMINISTRATION

A Medication Guide and Warning Card that provide information about recognition of hypersensitivity reactions should be dispensed with each new prescription and refill. To facilitate reporting of hypersensitivity reactions and collection of information on each case, an Abacavir Hypersensitivity Registry has been established. Physicians should register patients by calling 1-800-270-0425.

The recommended oral dose of TRIZIVIR for adults and adolescents is 1 tablet twice daily. TRIZIVIR is not recommended in adults or adolescents who weigh less than 40 kg because it is a fixed-dose tablet.

Dose Adjustment Because it is a fixed-dose tablet, TRIZIVIR should not be prescribed for patients requiring dosage adjustment such as those with creatinine clearance ≤50 mL/min or those experiencing dose-limiting adverse events.

HOW SUPPLIED

TRIZIVIR is available as tablets. Each tablet contains 300 mg of abacavir as abacavir sulfate, 150 mg of lamivudine, and 300 mg of zidovudine. The tablets are blue-green capsule-shaped, film-coated, and imprinted with GX LL1 on one side with no markings on the reverse side. They are packaged as follows:

Bottles of 60 Tablets (NDC 0173-0691-00)
Store at 25°C (77°F); excursions permitted to 15° to 30°C (59° to 86°F) [see USP Controlled Room Temperature).
Glaxo Wellcome Inc., Research Triangle Park, NC 27709
US Patent Nos. 5,047,407; 5,905,082; 4,724,232; 4,818,538; 4,833,130; 4,837,208; 5,034,394; and 5,089,500
Lamivudine is manufactured under agreement from BioChem Pharma Inc.
Laval, Quebec, Canada
©Copyright 2000, Glaxo Wellcome Inc. All rights reserved.
November 2000/RL-878

MEDICATION GUIDE

TRIZIVIR™ (TRY-zih-veer) Tablets

Generic name: abacavir sulfate, lamivudine, and zidovudine
Read the Medication Guide you get each time you fill your prescription for Trizivir. There may be new information since you filled your last prescription.

What is the most important information I should know about Trizivir?
Trizivir contains abacavir, which is also called Ziagen®. About 1 in 20 patients (5%) who take abacavir (as Trizivir or Ziagen) will have a **serious allergic reaction** (hypersensitivity reaction) that **may cause death if the drug is not stopped right away.**

You may be having this reaction if:

(1) you get a skin rash, or
(2) you get 1 or more symptoms from at least 2 of the following groups:
   • Fever
   • Nausea, vomiting, diarrhea, abdominal (stomach area) pain
   • Extreme tiredness, achiness, generally ill feeling
   • Sore throat, shortness of breath, cough

If you think you may be having a reaction, STOP taking Trizivir and call your doctor right away.

If you stop treatment with Trizivir because of this serious reaction, **NEVER take abacavir (as Trizivir or Ziagen) again.** If you take any of these medicines again after you have had this serious reaction, **you could die within hours.**

Some patients who have stopped taking abacavir (as Trizivir or Ziagen) and who have then started taking abacavir again have had serious or life-threatening allergic (hypersensitivity) reactions. If you must stop treatment with Trizivir for reasons other than symptoms of hypersensitivity, do not begin taking it again without talking to your health care provider. If your health care provider decides that you may begin taking abacavir (as Trizivir or Ziagen) again, you should do so only in a setting with other people to get access to a doctor, if needed.

A written list of these symptoms is on the Warning Card your pharmacist gives you. Carry this Warning Card with you.

Trizivir can have other serious side effects. Be sure to read the section below entitled "What are the possible side effects of Trizivir?"

What is Trizivir?
Trizivir is a medicine used to treat HIV infection. Trizivir includes 3 medicines: Ziagen (abacavir), Epivir® (lamivudine or 3TC), and Retrovir® (zidovudine, AZT, or ZDV).
All 3 of these medicines are called nucleoside analogue reverse transcriptase inhibitors (NRTIs). When used together,

they help lower the amount of HIV in your blood. This helps to keep your immune system as healthy as possible so it can fight infection.
Different combinations of medicines are used to treat HIV infection. You and your doctor should discuss which combination of medicines is best for you.
Trizivir does not cure HIV infection or AIDS. Trizivir has not been studied long enough to know if it will help you live longer or have fewer of the medical problems that are associated with HIV infection or AIDS. Therefore, you must see your health care provider regularly.

Who should not take Trizivir?
Do not take Trizivir if you have ever had a serious allergic reaction (a hypersensitivity reaction) to any of the medicines that make up Trizivir, especially Ziagen (abacavir). If you have had such a reaction, return all of your unused Trizivir to your doctor or pharmacist.
Do not take Trizivir if you weigh less than 90 pounds.

How should I take Trizivir?
To help make sure that your anti-HIV therapy is as effective as possible, take your Trizivir exactly as your doctor prescribes it. Do not skip any doses.
The usual dosage is 1 tablet twice a day. You can take Trizivir with food or on an empty stomach.
If you miss a dose of Trizivir, take the missed dose right away. Then, take the next dose at the usual scheduled time. Do not let your Trizivir run out. The amount of virus in your blood may increase if your anti-HIV drugs are stopped, even for a short time. Also, the virus in your body may become harder to treat.

What should I avoid while taking Trizivir?
Do not take Epivir, Retrovir, Combivir®, or Ziagen while taking Trizivir. These medicines are already in Trizivir.
Practice safe sex while using Trizivir. Do not use or share dirty needles. Trizivir does not reduce the risk of passing HIV to others through sexual contact or blood contamination.
Talk to your doctor if you are pregnant or if you become pregnant while taking Trizivir. Trizivir has not been studied in pregnant women. It is not known whether Trizivir will harm the unborn child.
Mothers with HIV should not breastfeed their babies because HIV is passed to the baby in breast milk. Also, Trizivir can be passed to babies in breast milk and could cause the child to have side effects.

What are the possible side effects of Trizivir?
Life-threatening allergic reaction. Trizivir contains abacavir, which is also called Ziagen. Abacavir has caused some people to have a life-threatening allergic reaction (hypersensitivity reaction) that can cause death. How to recognize a possible reaction and what to do are discussed in "What is the most important information I should know about Trizivir?" at the beginning of this Medication Guide.
Lactic acidosis and severe liver problems. The medicines in Trizivir can cause a serious condition called lactic acidosis and, in some cases, this condition can cause death. Nausea and tiredness that don't get better may be symptoms of lactic acidosis. Women are more likely than men to get this serious side effect.
Blood problems. Retrovir, one of the medicines in Trizivir, can cause serious blood cell problems. These include reduced numbers of white blood cells (neutropenia) and extremely reduced numbers of red blood cells (anemia). These blood cell problems are especially likely to happen in patients with advanced HIV disease or AIDS.
Your doctor should be checking your blood cell counts regularly while you are taking Trizivir. This is especially important if you have advanced HIV or AIDS. This is to make sure that any blood cell problems are found quickly.
Muscle weakness. Retrovir, one of the medicines in Trizivir, can cause muscle weakness. This can be a serious problem.
Other side effects. Trizivir can cause other side effects. The most common side effects of taking the medicines in Trizivir together are nausea, vomiting, diarrhea, loss of appetite, weakness or tiredness, headache, dizziness, pain or tingling of the hands or feet, and muscle and joint pain.
This listing of side effects is not complete. Your doctor or pharmacist can discuss with you a more complete list of side effects with Trizivir.
Ask a health care professional about any concerns about Trizivir. If you want more information, ask your doctor or pharmacist for the labeling for Trizivir that was written for health care professionals.
Do not use Trizivir for a condition for which it was not prescribed. Do not give Trizivir to other persons.
Glaxo Wellcome Inc. Research Triangle Park, NC 22709
This Medication Guide has been approved by the US Food and Drug Administration.

InterCure, Inc.

214 CARNEGIE CENTER SUITE 300
PRINCETON, NJ 08504

Direct Inquiries to:
Phone: 609-799-7599
Fax: 609-799-7690
Sales and Ordering:
Customer Support Center
(877) 988-9388

RESPeRATE
therapeutic device   ℞

DESCRIPTION

The RESPeRATE device is a non-invasive, non-drug therapeutic device to perform breathing exercises as an adjunctive treatment for hypertension. It includes a miniature-processing unit, headphones, and a respiration sensor on an elastic belt.

CLINICAL PHARMACOLOGY

The results of three randomized, controlled clinical studies[1-2] support the use of RESPeRATE. The studies showed that the use of the device along with prescribed hypertension medications resulted in a typical reduction of 12mm Hg systolic and 8mmHg diastolic in just six weeks of daily treatment. Pooled trial data, as well as additional trial data[3], also have shown that this blood pressure reduction increases both with age and with higher initial blood pressure[1-3]. Use of the device has been shown to lower blood pressure with patients who were taking hypertensive medications as well as in those who were not taking medication to control blood pressure. No side effects or adverse reactions were reported.

INDICATIONS AND USAGE

The RESPeRATE device is intended for use as a relaxation treatment for the reduction of stress by leading the user through interactively guided and monitored breathing exercises. The device is indicated for use only as an adjunctive treatment for high blood pressure under the direction of a physician, together with other pharmacological and/or non-pharmacological interventions as prescribed by the physician.

CONTRAINDICATIONS

None known.

PRECAUTIONS

Do not use RESPeRATE when you need to be alert, or to concentrate, or when using heavy equipment. Do not use RESPeRATE while driving. Breathe naturally throughout the exercise. Excessive deep breathing may cause dizziness and palpitations. This device has not been studied in patients with respiratory disease, diabetes, atrial fibrillation, active ischemic heart disease/unstable angina, congestive heart failure, stroke, chronic renal failure, or major organ failure.

DOSAGE AND ADMINISTRATION

Physicians should write a prescription and fax it to the mail order pharmacy @312-421-5082. Patients should call 877-988-9388 for delivery.

REFERENCES

1. Schein M, Gavish B, Herz M, et al. "Treating hypertension with a device that slows and regularizes breathing: a randomized double-blind controlled study." J Human Hypertens 2001 15(4):271–278.
2. Grossman E, Grossman A, Schein MH, et al. "Breathing control lowers blood pressure." J Human Hypertens 2001 15(4):263–269.
3. Rosenthal T, Alter A, Peleg E, Gavish B. "Device guided breathing exercises reduce blood pressure-ambulatory and home measurements." Am J Hypertension 2001:14:1:74–76.

InterCure, Inc.
214 Carnegie Center Suite 300
Princeton, NJ 08504
Direct Inquiries to:
Phone: 609-799-7599
Fax: 609-799-7690
Sales and Ordering:
Customer Support Center
(877) 988-9388

To keep your **PDR** up to date throughout the year, note these revisions on the corresponding pages of the annual volume. Simply write **"See Supplement A"** next to the product heading.

Janssen Pharmaceutica Products, L.P.

1125 TRENTON-HARBOURTON ROAD
P.O. BOX 200
TITUSVILLE, NJ 08560-0200

For Medical Information Monday through Friday 9 am-5 pm EST Contact:
(800) JANSSEN
FAX: (609) 730-2461
After Hours and Weekends:
(800) JANSSEN

REMINYL® ℞
(GALANTAMINE HBr)
TABLETS

DESCRIPTION

REMINYL® (galantamine hydrobromide), extracted from the bulbs of the daffodil, *Narcissus pseudonarcissus*, is a reversible, competitive acetylcholinesterase inhibitor. It is known chemically as (4a*S*,6*R*, 8a*S*)-4a,5,9,10,11,12-hexahydro-3-methoxy-11-methyl-6*H*-benzofuro[3a,3,2-*ef*][2]benzazepin-6-ol hydrobromide. It has an empirical formula of $C_{17}H_{21}NO_3$ •HBr and a molecular weight of 368.27. Galantamine hydrobromide is a white to almost white powder and is sparingly soluble in water. The structural formula for galantamine hydrobromide is:

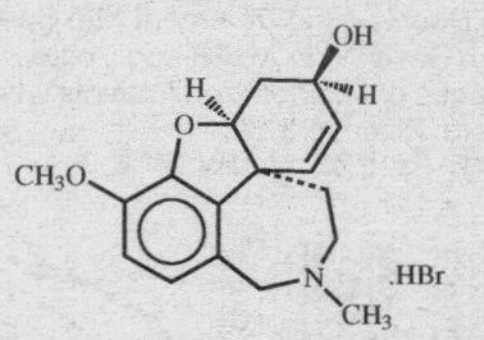

REMINYL® for oral use is available in circular biconvex film-coated tablets of 4 mg (off-white), 8 mg (pink), and 12 mg (orange-brown). Each 4, 8, and 12 mg (base equivalent) tablet contains 5.126, 10.253, and 15.379 mg of galantamine hydrobromide, respectively. Inactive ingredients include colloidal silicon dioxide, crospovidone, hydroxypropyl methylcellulose, lactose monohydrate, magnesium stearate, microcrystalline cellulose, propylene glycol, talc, and titanium dioxide. The 4 mg tablets contain yellow ferric oxide. The 8 mg tablets contain red ferric oxide. The 12 mg tablets contain red ferric oxide and FD&C yellow #6 aluminum lake.

CLINICAL PHARMACOLOGY

Mechanism of Action

Although the etiology of cognitive impairment in Alzheimer's disease (AD) is not fully understood, it has been reported that acetylcholine-producing neurons degenerate in the brains of patients with Alzheimer's disease. The degree of this cholinergic loss has been correlated with degree of cognitive impairment and density of amyloid plaques (a neuropathological hallmark of Alzheimer's disease).

Galantamine, a tertiary alkaloid, is a competitive and reversible inhibitor of acetylcholinesterase. While the precise mechanism of galantamine's action is unknown, it is postulated to exert its therapeutic effect by enhancing cholinergic function. This is accomplished by increasing the concentration of acetylcholine through reversible inhibition of its hydrolysis by cholinesterase. If this mechanism is correct, galantamine's effect may lessen as the disease process advances and fewer cholinergic neurons remain functionally intact. There is no evidence that galantamine alters the course of the underlying dementing process.

Pharmacokinetics

Galantamine is well absorbed with absolute oral bioavailability of about 90%. It has a terminal elimination half-life of about 7 hours and pharmacokinetics are linear over the range of 8–32 mg/day.

The maximum inhibition of anticholinesterase activity of about 40% was achieved about one hour after a single oral dose of 8 mg galantamine in healthy male subjects.

Absorption and Distribution

Galantamine is rapidly and completely absorbed with time to peak concentration about 1 hour. Bioavailability of the tablet was the same as the bioavailability of an oral solution. Food did not affect the AUC of galantamine but C_{max} decreased by 25% and T_{max} was delayed by 1.5 hours. The mean volume of distribution of galantamine is 175 L.

The plasma protein binding of galantamine is 18% at therapeutically relevant concentrations. In whole blood, galantamine is mainly distributed to blood cells (52.7%). The blood to plasma concentration ratio of galantamine is 1.2.

Metabolism and Elimination

Galantamine is metabolized by hepatic cytochrome P450 enzymes, glucuronidated, and excreted unchanged in the urine. *In vitro* studies indicate that cytochrome CYP2D6 and CYP3A4 were the major cytochrome P450 isoenzymes involved in the metabolism of galantamine, and inhibitors of both pathways increase oral bioavailability of galantamine modestly (See **PRECAUTIONS, Drug-Drug Interactions**). O-demethylation, mediated by CYP2D6 was greater in extensive metabolizers of CYP2D6 than in poor metabolizers. In plasma from both poor and extensive metabolizers, however, unchanged galantamine and its glucuronide accounted for most of the sample radioactivity.

In studies of oral ^{3}H-galantamine, unchanged galantamine and its glucuronide, accounted for most plasma radioactivity in poor and extensive CYP2D6 metabolizers. Up to 8 hours post-dose, unchanged galantamine accounted for 39–77% of the total radioactivity in the plasma, and galantamine glucuronide for 14–24%. By 7 days, 93–99% of the radioactivity had been recovered, with about 95% in urine and about 5% in the feces. Total urinary recovery of unchanged galantamine accounted for, on average, 32% of the dose and that of galantamine glucuronide for another 12% on average.

After i.v. or oral administration, about 20% of the dose was excreted as unchanged galantamine in the urine in 24 hours, representing a renal clearance of about 65 mL/min, about 20–25% of the total plasma clearance of about 300 mL/min.

Special Populations

CYP2D6 poor metabolizers

Approximately 7% of the normal population has a genetic variation that leads to reduced levels of activity of CYP2D6 isozyme. Such individuals have been referred to as poor metabolizers. After a single oral dose of 4 mg or 8 mg galantamine, CYP2D6 poor metabolizers demonstrated a similar C_{max} and about 35% AUC_∞ increase of unchanged galantamine compared to extensive metabolizers.

A total of 356 patients with Alzheimer's disease enrolled in two phase 3 studies were genotyped with respect to CYP2D6 (n=210 hetero-extensive metabolizers, 126 homo-extensive metabolizers, and 20 poor metabolizers). Population pharmacokinetic analysis indicated that there was a 25% decrease in median clearance in poor metabolizers compared to extensive metabolizers. Dosage adjustment is not necessary in patients identified as poor metabolizers as the dose of drug is individually titrated to tolerability.

Hepatic Impairment: Following a single 4 mg dose of galantamine, the pharmacokinetics of galantamine in subjects with mild hepatic impairment (n=8; Child-Pugh score of 5–6) were similar to those in healthy subjects. In patients with moderate hepatic impairment (n=8; Child-Pugh score of 7–9), galantamine clearance was decreased by about 25% compared to normal volunteers. Exposure would be expected to increase further with increasing degree of hepatic impairment (See **PRECAUTIONS** and **DOSAGE AND ADMINISTRATION**).

Renal Impairment: Following a single 8 mg dose of galantamine, AUC increased by 37% and 67% in moderate and severely renal-impaired patients compared to normal volunteers. (See **PRECAUTIONS** and **DOSAGE AND ADMINISTRATION**).

Elderly: Data from clinical trials in patients with Alzheimer's disease indicate that galantamine concentrations are 30–40% higher than in healthy young subjects.

Gender and Race: No specific pharmacokinetic study was conducted to investigate the effect of gender and race on the disposition of REMINYL® (galantamine hydrobromide), but a population pharmacokinetic analysis indicates (n= 539 males and 550 females) that galantamine clearance is about 20% lower in females than in males (explained by lower body weight in females) and race (n= 1029 White, 24 Black, 13 Asian and 23 other) did not affect the clearance of REMINYL®.

Drug-Drug Interactions

Multiple metabolic pathways and renal excretion are involved in the elimination of galantamine so no single pathway appears predominant. Based on *in vitro* studies, CYP2D6 and CYP3A4 were the major enzymes involved in the metabolism of galantamine. CYP2D6 was involved in the formation of O-desmethyl-galantamine, whereas CYP3A4 mediated the formation of galantamine-N-oxide. Galantamine is also glucuronidated and excreted unchanged in urine.

(A) Effect of other drugs on the metabolism of REMINYL®: Drugs that are potent inhibitors for CYP2D6 or CYP3A4 may increase the AUC of galantamine. Multiple dose pharmacokinetic studies demonstrated that the AUC of galantamine increased 30% and 40%, respectively, during coadministration of ketoconazole and paroxetine. As coadministered with erythromycin, another CYP3A4 inhibitor, the galantamine AUC increased only 10%. Population PK analysis with a database of 852 patients with Alzheimer's disease showed that the clearance of galantamine was decreased about 25–33% by concurrent administration of amitriptyline (n = 17), fluoxetine (n = 48), fluvoxamine (n = 14), and quinidine (n = 7), known inhibitors of CYP2D6.

Concurrent administration of H_2-antagonists demonstrated that ranitidine did not affect the pharmacokinetics of galantamine, and cimetidine increased the galantamine AUC by approximately 16%.

(B) Effect of REMINYL® on the metabolism of other drugs: *In vitro* studies show that galantamine did not inhibit the metabolic pathways catalyzed by CYP1A2, CYP2A6, CYP3A4, CYP4A, CYP2C, CYP2D6 and CYP2E1. This indicated that the inhibitory potential of galantamine towards the major forms of cytochrome P450 is very low. Multiple doses of galantamine (24 mg/day) had no effect on the pharmacokinetics of digoxin and warfarin (R- and S-forms). Galantamine had no effect on the increased prothrombin time induced by warfarin.

CLINICAL TRIALS

The effectiveness of REMINYL® (galantamine hydrobromide) as a treatment for Alzheimer's disease is demonstrated by the results of 4 randomized, double-blind, placebo-controlled clinical investigations in patients with probable Alzheimer's disease [diagnosed by NINCDS-ADRDA criteria, with Mini-Mental State Examination scores that were ≥ 10 and ≤ 24]. Doses studied were 8–32 mg/day given as twice daily doses. In 3 of the 4 studies patients were started on a low dose of 8 mg, then titrated weekly by 8 mg/day to 24 or 32 mg as assigned. In the fourth study (USA 4-week Dose-Escalation Fixed-Dose Study) dose escalation of 8 mg/day occurred over 4 week intervals. The mean age of patients participating in the 4 REMINYL® trials was 75 years with a range of 41 to 100. Approximately 62% of patients were women and 38% were men. The racial distribution was White 94%, Black 3% and other races 3%. Two other studies examined a three times daily dosing regimen; these also showed or suggested benefit but did not suggest an advantage over twice daily dosing.

Study Outcome Measures: In each study, the primary effectiveness of REMINYL® was evaluated using a dual outcome assessment strategy as measured by the Alzheimer's Disease Assessment Scale (ADAS-cog) and the Clinician's Interview Based Impression of Change (CIBIC-plus).

The ability of REMINYL® to improve cognitive performance was assessed with the cognitive sub-scale of the Alzheimer's Disease Assessment Scale (ADAS-cog), a multi-item instrument that has been extensively validated in longitudinal cohorts of Alzheimer's disease patients. The ADAS-cog examines selected aspects of cognitive performance including elements of memory, orientation, attention, reasoning, language and praxis. The ADAS-cog scoring range is from 0 to 70, with higher scores indicating greater cognitive impairment. Elderly normal adults may score as low as 0 or 1, but it is not unusual for non-demented adults to score slightly higher.

The patients recruited as participants in each study had mean scores on ADAS-cog of approximately 27 units, with a range from 5 to 69. Experience gained in longitudinal studies of ambulatory patients with mild to moderate Alzheimer's disease suggests that they gain 6 to 12 units a year on the ADAS-cog. Lesser degrees of change, however, are seen in patients with very mild or very advanced disease because the ADAS-cog is not uniformly sensitive to change over the course of the disease. The annualized rate of decline in the placebo patients participating in REMINYL® trials was approximately 4.5 units per year.

The ability of REMINYL® to produce an overall clinical effect was assessed using a Clinician's Interview Based Impression of Change that required the use of caregiver information, the CIBIC-plus. The CIBIC-plus is not a single instrument and is not a standardized instrument like the ADAS-cog. Clinical trials for investigational drugs have used a variety of CIBIC formats, each different in terms of depth and structure. As such, results from a CIBIC-plus reflect clinical experience from the trial or trials in which it was used and can not be compared directly with the results of CIBIC-plus evaluations from other clinical trials. The CIBIC-plus used in the trials was a semi-structured instrument based on a comprehensive evaluation at baseline and subsequent time-points of 4 major areas of patient function: general, cognitive, behavioral and activities of daily living. It represents the assessment of a skilled clinician based on his/her observation at an interview with the patient, in combination with information supplied by a caregiver familiar with the behavior of the patient over the interval rated. The CIBIC-plus is scored as a seven point categorical rating, ranging from a score of 1, indicating "markedly improved", to a score of 4, indicating "no change" to a score of 7, indicating "marked worsening". The CIBIC-plus has not been systematically compared directly to assessments not using information from caregivers (CIBIC) or other global methods.

U.S. Twenty-One-Week Fixed-Dose Study

In a study of 21 weeks duration, 978 patients were randomized to doses of 8, 16, or 24 mg of REMINYL® per day, or to placebo, each given in 2 divided doses. Treatment was initiated at 8 mg/day for all patients randomized to REMINYL®, and increased by 8 mg/day every 4 weeks. Therefore, the maximum titration phase was 8 weeks and the minimum maintenance phase was 13 weeks (in patients randomized to 24 mg/day of REMINYL®).

Effects on the ADAS-cog: Figure 1 illustrates the time course for the change from baseline in ADAS-cog scores for all four dose groups over the 21 weeks of the study. At 21 weeks of treatment, the mean differences in the ADAS-cog change scores for the REMINYL®-treated patients compared to the patients on placebo were 1.7, 3.3, and 3.6 units for the 8, 16 and 24 mg/day treatments, respectively. The 16 mg/day and 24 mg/day treatments were statistically significantly superior to placebo and to the 8 mg/day treatment. There was no statistically significant difference between the 16 mg/day and 24 mg/day dose groups.

[See figure 1 at top of next page]

Figure 2 illustrates the cumulative percentages of patients from each of the four treatment groups who had attained at least the measure of improvement in ADAS-cog score shown on the X axis. Three change scores (10-point, 7-point and 4-point reductions) and no change in score from baseline have been identified for illustrative purposes, and the percent of patients in each group achieving that result is shown in the inset table.

The curves demonstrate that both patients assigned to galantamine and placebo have a wide range of responses,

Continued on next page

Reminyl—Cont.

Figure 1: Time-course of the Change from
Baseline in ADAS-cog Score for
Patients Completing 21 Weeks (5 Months) of Treatment

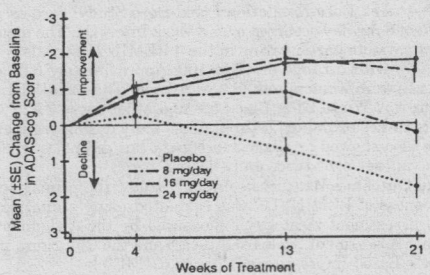

but that the REMINYL® groups are more likely to show the greater improvements.

Figure 2: Cumulative Percentage of Patients Completing
21 Weeks of Double-blind Treatment with Specified
Changes from Baseline in ADAS-cog Scores.
The Percentages of Randomized Patients who Completed
the Study were: Placebo 84%, 8 mg/day 77%,
16 mg/day 78% and 24 mg/day 78%.

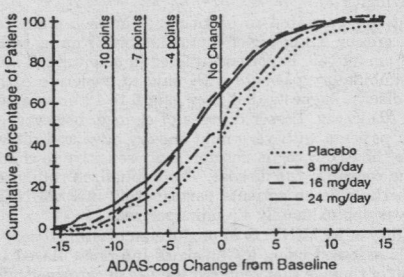

	Change in ADAS-cog			
Treatment	-10	-7	-4	0
Placebo	3.6%	7.6%	19.6%	41.8%
8 mg/day	5.9%	13.9%	25.7%	46.5%
16 mg/day	7.2%	15.9%	35.6%	65.4%
24 mg/day	10.4%	22.3%	37.0%	64.9%

Effects on the CIBIC-plus: Figure 3 is a histogram of the percentage distribution of CIBIC-plus scores attained by patients assigned to each of the four treatment groups who completed 21 weeks of treatment. The REMINYL®-placebo differences for these groups of patients in mean rating were 0.15, 0.41 and 0.44 units for the 8, 16 and 24 mg/day treatments, respectively. The 16 mg/day and 24 mg/day treatments were statistically significantly superior to placebo. The differences vs. the 8 mg/day treatment for the 16 and 24 mg/day treatments were 0.26 and 0.29, respectively. There were no statistically significant differences between the 16 mg/day and 24 mg/day dose groups.

Figure 3: Distribution of CIBIC-plus Ratings at Week 21

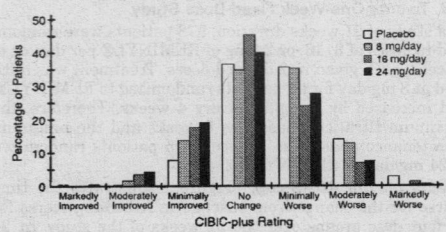

U.S. Twenty-Six-Week Fixed-Dose Study
In a study of 26 weeks duration, 636 patients were randomized to either a dose of 24 mg or 32 mg of REMINYL® per day, or to placebo, each given in two divided doses. The 26-week study was divided into a 3-week dose titration phase and a 23-week maintenance phase.
Effects on the ADAS-cog: Figure 4 illustrates the time course for the change from baseline in ADAS-cog scores for all three dose groups over the 26 weeks of the study. At 26 weeks of treatment, the mean differences in the ADAS-cog change scores for the REMINYL®-treated patients compared to the patients on placebo were 3.9 and 3.8 units for the 24 mg/day and 32 mg/day treatments, respectively. Both treatments were statistically significantly superior to placebo, but were not significantly different from each other.
[See figure at top of next column]
Figure 5 illustrates the cumulative percentages of patients from each of the three treatment groups who had attained at least the measure of improvement in ADAS-cog score shown on the X axis. Three change scores (10-point, 7-point and 4-point reductions) and no change in score from base-

Figure 4: Time-course of the Change from
Baseline in ADAS-cog Score for
Patients Completing 26 Weeks of Treatment

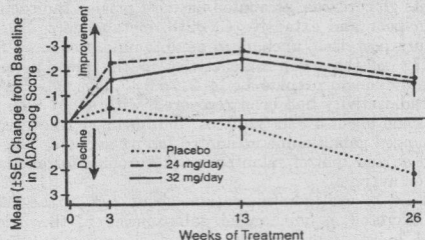

line have been identified for illustrative purposes, and the percent of patients in each group achieving that result is shown in the inset table.
The curves demonstrate that both patients assigned to REMINYL® and placebo have a wide range of responses, but that the REMINYL® groups are more likely to show the greater improvements. A curve for an effective treatment would be shifted to the left of the curve for placebo, while an ineffective or deleterious treatment would be superimposed upon, or shifted to the right of the curve for placebo, respectively.

Figure 5: Cumulative Percentage of Patients Completing
26 Weeks of Double-blind Treatment with Specified
Changes from Baseline in ADAS-cog Scores.
The Percentages of Randomized Patients who Completed
the Study were: Placebo 81%,
24 mg/day 68%, and 32 mg/day 58%.

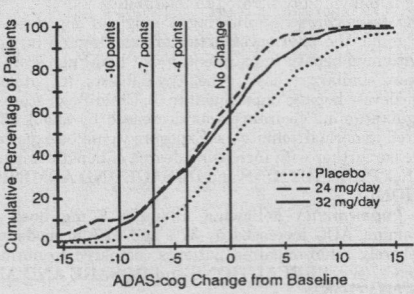

	Change in ADAS-cog			
Treatment	-10	-7	-4	0
Placebo	2.1%	5.7%	16.6%	43.9%
24 mg/day	7.6%	18.3%	33.6%	64.1%
32 mg/day	11.1%	19.7%	33.3%	58.1%

Effects on the CIBIC-plus: Figure 6 is a histogram of the percentage distribution of CIBIC-plus scores attained by patients assigned to each of the three treatment groups who completed 26 weeks of treatment. The mean REMINYL®-placebo differences for these groups of patients in the mean rating were 0.28 and 0.29 units for 24 and 32 mg/day of REMINYL®, respectively. The mean ratings for both groups were statistically significantly superior to placebo, but were not significantly different from each other.

Figure 6: Distribution of CIBIC-plus Ratings at Week 26

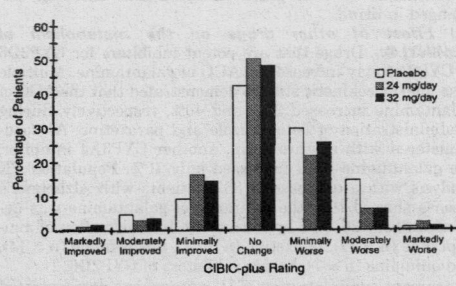

International Twenty-Six-Week Fixed-Dose Study
In a study of 26 weeks duration identical in design to the USA 26-Week Fixed-Dose Study, 653 patients were randomized to either a dose of 24 mg or 32 mg of REMINYL® per day, or to placebo, each given in two divided doses. The 26-week study was divided into a 3-week dose titration phase and a 23-week maintenance phase.
Effects on the ADAS-cog: Figure 7 illustrates the time course for the change from baseline in ADAS-cog scores for all three dose groups over the 26 weeks of the study. At 26 weeks of treatment, the mean differences in the ADAS-cog change scores for the REMINYL®-treated patients compared to the patients on placebo were 3.1 and 4.1 units for the 24 mg/day and 32 mg/day treatments, respectively. Both treatments were statistically significantly superior to placebo, but were not significantly different from each other.
[See figure 7 at top of next column]

Figure 7: Time-course of the Change from
Baseline in ADAS-cog Score for
Patients Completing 26 Weeks of Treatment

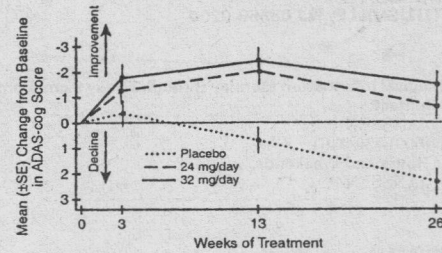

Figure 8 illustrates the cumulative percentages of patients from each of the three treatment groups who had attained at least the measure of improvement in ADAS-cog score shown on the X axis. Three change scores (10-point, 7-point and 4-point reductions) and no change in score from baseline have been identified for illustrative purposes, and the percent of patients in each group achieving that result is shown in the inset table.
The curves demonstrate that both patients assigned to REMINYL® and placebo have a wide range of responses, but that the REMINYL® groups are more likely to show the greater improvements.

Figure 8: Cumulative Percentage of Patients Completing
26 Weeks of Double-blind Treatment with Specified
Changes from Baseline in ADAS-cog Scores.
The Percentages of Randomized Patients who Completed
the Study were: Placebo 87%,
24 mg/day 80%, and 32 mg/day 75%.

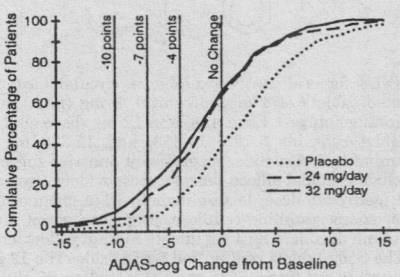

	Change in ADAS-cog			
Treatment	-10	-7	-4	0
Placebo	1.2%	5.8%	15.2%	39.8%
24 mg/day	4.5%	15.4%	30.8%	65.4%
32 mg/day	7.9%	19.7%	34.9%	63.8%

Effects on the CIBIC-plus: Figure 9 is a histogram of the percentage distribution of CIBIC-plus scores attained by patients assigned to each of the three treatment groups who completed 26 weeks of treatment. The mean REMINYL®-placebo differences for these groups of patients in the mean rating of change from baseline were 0.34 and 0.47 for 24 and 32 mg/day of REMINYL®, respectively. The mean ratings for the REMINYL® groups were statistically significantly superior to placebo, but were not significantly different from each other.

Figure 9: Distribution of CIBIC-plus Rating at Week 26

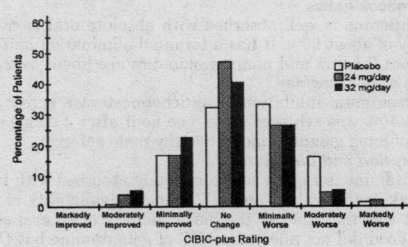

International Thirteen-Week Flexible-Dose Study
In a study of 13 weeks duration, 386 patients were randomized to either a flexible dose of 24–32 mg/day of REMINYL® or to placebo, each given in two divided doses. The 13-week study was divided into a 3-week dose titration phase and a 10-week maintenance phase. The patients in the active treatment arm of the study were maintained at either 24 mg/day or 32 mg/day at the discretion of the investigator.
Effects on the ADAS-cog: Figure 10 illustrates the time course for the change from baseline in ADAS-cog scores for both dose groups over the 13 weeks of the study. At 13 weeks of treatment, the mean difference in the ADAS-cog change scores for the treated patients compared to the patients on placebo was 1.9. REMINYL® at a dose of 24–32 mg/day was statistically significantly superior to placebo.
[See figure 10 at top of next column]

Figure 10: Time-course of the Change from Baseline in ADAS-cog Score for Patients Completing 13 Weeks of Treatment

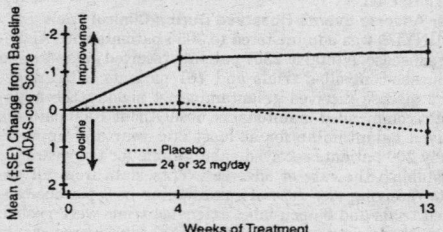

Figure 11 illustrates the cumulative percentages of patients from each of the two treatment groups who had attained at least the measure of improvement in ADAS-cog score shown on the X axis. Three change scores (10-point, 7-point and 4-point reductions) and no change in score from baseline have been identified for illustrative purposes, and the percent of patients in each group achieving that result is shown in the inset table.

The curves demonstrate that both patients assigned to REMINYL® and placebo have a wide range of responses, but that the REMINYL® group is more likely to show the greater improvement.

Figure 11: Cumulative Percentage of Patients Completing 13 Weeks of Double-blind Treatment with Specified Changes from Baseline in ADAS-cog Scores. The Percentages of Randomized Patients who Completed the Study were: Placebo 90%, 24-32 mg/day 67%.

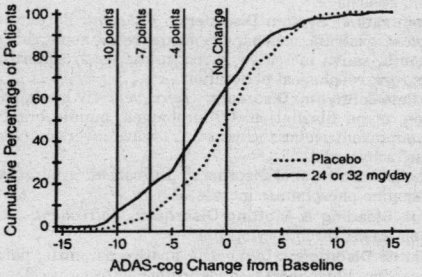

	Change in ADAS-cog			
Treatment	-10	-7	-4	0
Placebo	1.9%	5.6%	19.4%	50.0%
24 or 32 mg/day	7.1%	18.8%	32.9%	65.3%

Effects on the CIBIC-plus: Figure 12 is a histogram of the percentage distribution of CIBIC-plus scores attained by patients assigned to each of the two treatment groups who completed 13 weeks of treatment. The mean REMINYL®-placebo differences for the group of patients in the mean rating of change from baseline was 0.37 units. The mean rating for the 24–32 mg/day group was statistically significantly superior to placebo.

Figure 12: Distribution of CIBIC-plus Ratings at Week 13

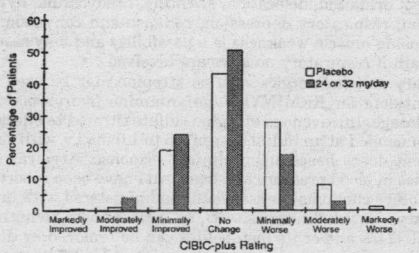

Age, gender and race: Patient's age, gender, or race did not predict clinical outcome of treatment.

INDICATIONS AND USAGE
REMINYL® (galantamine hydrobromide) is indicated for the treatment of mild to moderate dementia of the Alzheimer's type.

CONTRAINDICATIONS
REMINYL® (galantamine hydrobromide) is contraindicated in patients with known hypersensitivity to galantamine hydrobromide or to any excipients used in the formulation.

WARNINGS
Anesthesia
Galantamine, as a cholinesterase inhibitor, is likely to exaggerate the neuromuscular blockade effects of succinylcholine-type and similar neuromuscular blocking agents during anesthesia.
Cardiovascular Conditions
Because of their pharmacological action, cholinesterase inhibitors have vagotonic effects on the sinoatrial and atrio-ventricular nodes, leading to bradycardia and AV block. These actions may be particularly important to patients with supraventricular cardiac conduction disorders or to patients taking other drugs concomitantly that significantly slow heart rate. Postmarketing surveillance of marketed anticholinesterase inhibitors has shown, however, that bradycardia and all types of heart block have been reported in patients both with and without known underlying cardiac conduction abnormalities. Therefore all patients should be considered at risk for adverse effects on cardiac conduction. In randomized controlled trials, bradycardia was reported more frequently in galantamine-treated patients than in placebo-treated patients, but rarely led to treatment discontinuation. The overall frequency of this event was 2–3% for galantamine doses up to 24 mg/day compared with <1% for placebo. No increased incidence of heart block was observed at the recommended doses.

Patients treated with galantamine up to 24 mg/day using the recommended dosing schedule showed a dose-related increase in risk of syncope (placebo 0.7% [2/286]; 4 mg BID 0.4% [3/692]; 8 mg BID 1.3% [7/552]; 12 mg BID 2.2% [6/273]).

Gastrointestinal Conditions
Through their primary action, cholinomimetics may be expected to increase gastric acid secretion due to increased cholinergic activity. Therefore, patients should be monitored closely for symptoms of active or occult gastrointestinal bleeding, especially those with an increased risk for developing ulcers, e.g., those with a history of ulcer disease or patients using concurrent nonsteroidal anti-inflammatory drugs (NSAIDS). Clinical studies of REMINYL® (galantamine hydrobromide) have shown no increase, relative to placebo, in the incidence of either peptic ulcer disease or gastrointestinal bleeding.

REMINYL®, as a predictable consequence of its pharmacological properties, has been shown to produce nausea, vomiting, diarrhea, anorexia, and weight loss. (See **ADVERSE REACTIONS**)
Genitourinary
Although this was not observed in clinical trials with REMINYL®, cholinomimetics may cause bladder outflow obstruction.
Neurological Conditions
Seizures: Cholinesterase inhibitors are believed to have some potential to cause generalized convulsions. However, seizure activity may also be a manifestation of Alzheimer's disease. In clinical trials, there was no increase in the incidence of convulsions with REMINYL® compared to placebo.
Pulmonary Conditions
Because of its cholinomimetic action, galantamine should be prescribed with care to patients with a history of severe asthma or obstructive pulmonary disease.

PRECAUTIONS
Information for Patients and Caregivers: Caregivers should be instructed in the recommended administration (twice per day, preferably with morning and evening meal) and dose escalation (dose increases should follow minimum of four weeks at prior dose).

Patients and caregivers should be advised that the most frequent adverse events associated with use of the drug can be minimized by following the recommended dosage and administration.

Patients and caregivers should be informed that if therapy has been interrupted for several days or longer, the patient should be restarted at the lowest dose and the dose escalated to the current dose.
Special Populations
Hepatic Impairment
In patients with moderately impaired hepatic function, dose titration should proceed cautiously (See **CLINICAL PHARMACOLOGY** and **DOSAGE AND ADMINISTRATION**). The use of REMINYL® (galantamine hydrobromide) in patients with severe hepatic impairment is not recommended.
Renal Impairment
In patients with moderately impaired renal function, dose titration should proceed cautiously (See **CLINICAL PHARMACOLOGY** and **DOSAGE AND ADMINISTRATION**). In patients with severely impaired renal function (CL_{cr} < 9 mL/min) the use of REMINYL® is not recommended.
Drug-Drug Interactions
Use with Anticholinergics
REMINYL® has the potential to interfere with the activity of anticholinergic medications.
Use with Cholinomimetics and Other Cholinesterase Inhibitors
A synergistic effect is expected when cholinesterase inhibitors are given concurrently with succinylcholine, other cholinesterase inhibitors, similar neuromuscular blocking agents or cholinergic agonists such as bethanechol.
A) Effect of Other Drugs on Galantamine
In vitro
CYP3A4 and CYP2D6 are the major enzymes involved in the metabolism of galantamine. CYP3A4 mediates the formation of galantamine-N-oxide; CYP2D6 leads to the formation of O-desmethyl-galantamine. Because galantamine is also glucuronidated and excreted unchanged, no single pathway appears predominant.
In vivo
Cimetidine and Ranitidine: Galantamine was administered as a single dose of 4 mg on day 2 of a 3-day treatment with either cimetidine (800 mg daily) or ranitidine (300 mg daily). Cimetidine increased the bioavailability of galantamine by approximately 16%. Ranitidine had no effect on the PK of galantamine.

Ketoconazole: Ketoconazole, a strong inhibitor of CYP3A4 and an inhibitor of CYP2D6, at a dose of 200 mg BID for 4 days, increased the AUC of galantamine by 30%.
Erythromycin: Erythromycin, a moderate inhibitor of CYP3A4, at a dose of 500 mg QID for 4 days, affected the AUC of galantamine minimally (10% increase).
Paroxetine: Paroxetine, a strong inhibitor of CYP2D6, at 20 mg/day for 16 days, increased the oral bioavailability of galantamine by about 40%.
B) Effect of Galantamine on Other Drugs
In vitro
Galantamine did not inhibit the metabolic pathways catalyzed by CYP1A2, CYP2A6, CYP3A4, CYP4A, CYP2C, CYP2D6 or CYP2E1. This indicates that the inhibitory potential of galantamine towards the major forms of cytochrome P450 is very low.
In vivo
Warfarin: Galantamine at 24 mg/day had no effect on the pharmacokinetics of R-and-S-warfarin (25 mg single dose) or on the prothrombin time. The protein binding of warfarin was unaffected by galantamine.
Digoxin: Galantamine at 24 mg/day had no effect on the steady-state pharmacokinetics of digoxin (0.375 mg once daily) when they were coadministered. In this study, however, one healthy subject was hospitalized for 2nd and 3rd degree heart block and bradycardia.
Carcinogenesis, Mutagenesis and Impairment of Fertility
In a 24-month oral carcinogenicity study in rats, a slight increase in endometrial adenocarcinomas was observed at 10 mg/kg/day (4 times the Maximum Recommended Human Dose [MRHD] on a mg/m² basis or 6 times on an exposure [AUC] basis and 30 mg/kg/day (12 times MRHD on a mg/m² basis or 19 times on an AUC basis). No increase in neoplastic changes was observed in females at 2.5 mg/kg/day (equivalent to the MRHD on a mg/m² basis or 2 times on an AUC basis) or in males up to the highest dose tested of 30 mg/kg/day (12 times the MRHD on a mg/m² and AUC basis).

Galantamine was not carcinogenic in a 6-month oral carcinogenicity study in transgenic (P 53-deficient) mice up to 20 mg/kg/day, or in a 24-month oral carcinogenicity study in male and female mice up to 10 mg/kg/day (2 times the MRHD on a mg/m² basis and equivalent on an AUC basis). Galantamine produced no evidence of genotoxic potential when evaluated in the *in vitro* Ames *S. typhimurium* or *E. coli* reverse mutation assay, *in vitro* mouse lymphoma assay, *in vivo* micronucleus test in mice, or *in vitro* chromosome aberration assay in Chinese hamster ovary cells.

No impairment of fertility was seen in rats given up to 16 mg/kg/day (7 times the MRHD on a mg/m² basis) for 14 days prior to mating in females and for 60 days prior to mating in males.
Pregnancy
Pregnancy Category B: In a study in which rats were dosed from day 14 (females) or day 60 (males) prior to mating through the period of organogenesis, a slightly increased incidence of skeletal variations was observed at doses of 8 mg/kg/day (3 times the Maximum Recommended Human Dose [MRHD] on a mg/m² basis) and 16 mg/kg/day. In a study in which pregnant rats were dosed from the beginning of organogenesis through day 21 post-partum, pup weights were decreased at 8 and 16 mg/kg/day, but no adverse effects on other postnatal developmental parameters were seen. The doses causing the above effects in rats produced slight maternal toxicity. No major malformations were caused in rats given up to 16 mg/kg/day. No drug related teratogenic effects were observed in rabbits given up to 40 mg/kg/day (32 times the MRHD on a mg/m² basis) during the period of organogenesis.

There are no adequate and well-controlled studies of REMINYL® in pregnant women. REMINYL® should be used during pregnancy only if the potential benefit justifies the potential risk to the fetus.
Nursing Mothers
It is not known whether galantamine is excreted in human breast milk. REMINYL® has no indication for use in nursing mothers.
Pediatric Use
There are no adequate and well-controlled trials documenting the safety and efficacy of galantamine in any illness occurring in children. Therefore, use of REMINYL® in children is not recommended.

ADVERSE REACTIONS
Adverse Events Leading to Discontinuation: In two large scale, placebo-controlled trials of 6 months duration, in which patients were titrated weekly from 8 to 16 to 24, and to 32 mg/day, the risk of discontinuation because of an adverse event in the galantamine group exceeded that in the placebo group by about threefold. In contrast, in a 5-month trial with escalation of the dose by 8 mg/day every 4 weeks, the overall risk of discontinuation because of an adverse event was 7%, 7%, and 10% for the placebo, galantamine 16 mg/day, and galantamine 24 mg/day groups, respectively, with gastrointestinal adverse effects the principle reason for discontinuing galantamine. Table 1 shows the most frequent adverse events leading to discontinuation in this study.

Continued on next page

Reminyl—Cont.

Table 1: Most Frequent Adverse Events Leading to Discontinuation in a Placebo-controlled, Double-blind Trial with a 4-Week Dose Escalation Schedule

	4-week Escalation		
	Placebo	16 mg/day	24 mg/day
Adverse Event	N=286	N=279	N=273
Nausea	<1%	2%	4%
Vomiting	0%	1%	3%
Anorexia	<1%	1%	<1%
Dizziness	<1%	2%	1%
Syncope	0%	0%	1%

Adverse Events Reported in Controlled Trials: The reported adverse events in REMINYL® (galantamine hydrobromide) trials reflect experience gained under closely monitored conditions in a highly selected patient population. In actual practice or in other clinical trials, these frequency estimates may not apply, as the conditions of use, reporting behavior and the types of patients treated may differ.

The majority of these adverse events occurred during the dose-escalation period. In those patients who experienced the most frequent adverse event, nausea, the median duration of the nausea was 5–7 days.

Administration of REMINYL® with food, the use of anti-emetic medication, and ensuring adequate fluid intake may reduce the impact of these events.

The most frequent adverse events, defined as those occurring at a frequency of at least 5% and at least twice the rate on placebo with the recommended maintenance dose of either 16 or 24 mg/day of REMINYL® under conditions of every 4 week dose-escalation for each dose increment of 8 mg/day, are shown in Table 2. These events were primarily gastrointestinal and tended to be less frequent with the 16 mg/kg recommended initial maintenance dose.

Table 2: The Most Frequent Adverse Events in the Placebo-controlled Trial with Dose Escalation Every 4 Weeks Occurring in at Least 5% of Patients Receiving REMINYL® and at Least Twice the Rate on Placebo

	Placebo	REMINYL® 16 mg/day	REMINYL® 24 mg/day
Adverse Event	N=286	N=279	N=273
Nausea	5%	13%	17%
Vomiting	1%	6%	10%
Diarrhea	6%	12%	6%
Anorexia	3%	7%	9%
Weight decrease	1%	5%	5%

Table 3: The most common adverse events (adverse events occurring with an incidence of at least 2% with REMINYL® treatment and in which the incidence was greater than with placebo treatment) are listed in Table 3 for four placebo-controlled trials for patients treated with 16 or 24 mg/day of REMINYL®.

[See table below]

Adverse events occurring with an incidence of at least 2% in placebo-treated patients that was either equal to or greater than with REMINYL® treatment were constipation, agitation, confusion, anxiety, hallucination, injury, back pain, peripheral edema, asthenia, chest pain, urinary incontinence, upper respiratory tract infection, bronchitis, coughing, hypertension, fall, and purpura.

There were no important differences in adverse event rate related to dose or sex. There were too few non-Caucasian patients to assess the effects of race on adverse event rates. No clinically relevant abnormalities in laboratory values were observed.

Other Adverse Events Observed During Clinical Trials
REMINYL® was administered to 3055 patients with Alzheimer's disease. A total of 2357 patients received galantamine in placebo-controlled trials and 761 patients with Alzheimer's disease received galantamine 24 mg/day, the maximum recommended maintenance dose. About 1000 patients received galantamine for at least one year and approximately 200 patients received galantamine for two years. To establish the rate of adverse events, data from all patients receiving any dose of galantamine in 8 placebo-controlled trials and 6 open-label extension trials were pooled. The methodology to gather and codify these adverse events was standardized across trials, using WHO terminology. All adverse events occurring in approximately 0.1% are included, except for those already listed elsewhere in labeling, WHO terms too general to be informative, or events unlikely to be drug caused. Events are classified by body system and listed using the following definitions: frequent adverse events—those occurring in at least 1/100 patients; infrequent adverse events—those occurring in 1/100 to 1/1000 patients; rare adverse events—those occurring in fewer than 1/1000 patients. These adverse events are not necessarily related to REMINYL® treatment and in most cases were observed at a similar frequency in placebo-treated patients in the controlled studies.

Body As a Whole—General Disorders: *Frequent:* chest pain

Cardiovascular System Disorders: *Infrequent:* postural hypotension, hypotension, dependent edema, cardiac failure

Central & Peripheral Nervous System Disorders: *Infrequent:* vertigo, hypertonia, convulsions, involuntary muscle contractions, paresthesia, ataxia, hypokinesia, hyperkinesia, apraxia, aphasia

Gastrointestinal System Disorders: *Frequent:* flatulence; *Infrequent:* gastritis, melena, dysphagia, rectal hemorrhage, dry mouth, saliva increased, diverticulitis, gastroenteritis, hiccup; *rare:* esophageal perforation

Heart Rate & Rhythm Disorders: *Infrequent:* AV block, palpitation, atrial fibrillation, QT prolonged, bundle branch block, supraventricular tachycardia, T-wave inversion, ventricular tachycardia

Metabolic & Nutritional Disorders: *Infrequent:* hyperglycemia, alkaline phosphatase increased

Platelet, Bleeding & Clotting Disorders: *Infrequent:* purpura, epistaxis, thrombocytopenia

Psychiatric Disorders: *Infrequent:* apathy, paroniria, paranoid reaction, libido increased, delirium

Urinary System Disorders: *Frequent:* incontinence; *Infrequent:* hematuria, micturition frequency, cystitis, urinary retention, nocturia, renal calculi

OVERDOSAGE

Because strategies for the management of overdose are continually evolving, it is advisable to contact a poison control center to determine the latest recommendations for the management of an overdose of any drug.

As in any case of overdose, general supportive measures should be utilized. Signs and symptoms of significant overdosing of galantamine are predicted to be similar to those of overdosing of other cholinomimetics. These effects generally involve the central nervous system, the parasympathetic nervous system, and the neuromuscular junction. In addition to muscle weakness or fasciculations, some or all of the following signs of cholinergic crisis may develop: severe nausea, vomiting, gastrointestinal cramping, salivation, lacrimation, urination, defecation, sweating, bradycardia, hypotension, respiratory depression, collapse and convulsions. Increasing muscle weakness is a possibility and may result in death if respiratory muscles are involved.

Tertiary anticholinergics such as atropine may be used as an antidote for REMINYL® (galantamine hydrobromide) overdosage. Intravenous atropine sulfate titrated to effect is recommended at an initial dose of 0.5 to 1.0 mg i.v. with subsequent doses based upon clinical response. Atypical responses in blood pressure and heart rate have been reported with other cholinomimetics when coadministered with quaternary anticholinergics. It is not known whether REMINYL® and/or its metabolites can be removed by dialysis (hemodialysis, peritoneal dialysis, or hemofiltration). Dose-related signs of toxicity in animals included hypoactivity, tremors, clonic convulsions, salivation, lacrimation, chromodacryorrhea, mucoid feces, and dyspnea.

DOSAGE AND ADMINISTRATION

The dosage of REMINYL® (galantamine hydrobromide) shown to be effective in controlled clinical trials is 16–32 mg/day given as twice daily dosing. As the dose of 32 mg/day is less well tolerated than lower doses and does not provide increased effectiveness, the recommended dose range is 16–24 mg/day given in a BID regimen. The dose of 24 mg/day did not provide a statistically significant greater clinical benefit than 16 mg/day. It is possible, however, that a daily dose of 24 mg of REMINYL® might provide additional benefit for some patients.

The recommended starting dose of REMINYL® is 4 mg twice a day (8 mg/day). After a minimum of 4 weeks of treatment, if this dose is well tolerated, the dose should be increased to 8 mg twice a day (16 mg/day). A further increase to 12 mg twice a day (24 mg/day) should be attempted only after a minimum of 4 weeks at the previous dose.

Table 3: Adverse Events Reported in at Least 2% of Patients with Alzheimer's Disease Administered REMINYL® and at a Frequency Greater than with Placebo

Body System Adverse Event	Placebo (N=801)	REMINYL®[a] (N=1040)
Body as a whole - general disorders		
Fatigue	3%	5%
Syncope	1%	2%
Central & peripheral nervous system disorders		
Dizziness	6%	9%
Headache	5%	8%
Tremor	2%	3%
Gastrointestinal system disorders		
Nausea	9%	24%
Vomiting	4%	13%
Diarrhea	7%	9%
Abdominal pain	4%	5%
Dyspepsia	2%	5%
Heart rate and rhythm disorders		
Bradycardia	1%	2%
Metabolic and nutritional disorders		
Weight decrease	2%	7%
Psychiatric disorders		
Anorexia	3%	9%
Depression	5%	7%
Insomnia	4%	5%
Somnolence	3%	4%
Red blood cell disorders		
Anemia	2%	3%
Respiratory system disorders		
Rhinitis	3%	4%
Urinary system disorders		
Urinary tract infection	7%	8%
Hematuria	2%	3%

a: Adverse events in patients treated with 16 or 24 mg/day of REMINYL® in four placebo-controlled trials are included.

REMINYL® should be administered twice a day, preferably with morning and evening meals.

Patients and caregivers should be informed that if therapy has been interrupted for several days or longer, the patient should be restarted at the lowest dose and the dose escalated to the current dose.

The abrupt withdrawal of REMINYL® in those patients who had been receiving doses in the effective range was not associated with an increased frequency of adverse events in comparison with those continuing to receive the same doses of that drug. The beneficial effects of REMINYL® are lost, however, when the drug is discontinued.

Doses in Special Populations

Galantamine plasma concentrations may be increased in patients with moderate to severe hepatic impairment. In patients with moderately impaired hepatic function (Child-Pugh score of 7–9), the dose should generally not exceed 16 mg/day. The use of REMINYL® in patients with severe hepatic impairment (Child-Pugh score of 10–15) is not recommended.

For patients with moderate renal impairment the dose should generally not exceed 16 mg/day. In patients with severe renal impairment (creatinine clearance <9 mL/min), the use of REMINYL® is not recommended.

HOW SUPPLIED

REMINYL® (galantamine hydrobromide) tablets are imprinted "JANSSEN" on one side, and "G" and the strength "4", "8", or "12" on the other.

4 mg off-white tablet: bottles of 60 NDC 50458-390-60
8 mg pink tablet: bottles of 60 NDC 50458-391-60
12 mg orange-brown tablet: bottles of 60 NDC 50458-392-60

Storage and Handling

REMINYL® tablets should be stored at 25°C (77°F); excursions permitted to 15–30°C (59–86°F) [see USP Controlled Room Temperature].

Keep out of reach of children.

7517303
March 2001
US Patent No. 4,663,318
© Janssen 2001

Manufactured by: Janssen-Cilag SpA, Latina, Italy
Distributed by: Janssen Pharmaceutica Products, L.P., Titusville, NJ 08560

Eli Lilly and Company

LILLY CORPORATE CENTER
INDIANAPOLIS, IN 46285

Direct Inquiries to:
Lilly Corporate Center
Indianapolis, IN 46285
(317) 276-2000
www.lilly.com

For Medical Information Contact:
Lilly Research Laboratories
Lilly Corporate Center
Indianapolis, IN 46285
(800) 545-5979

PROZAC® ℞

[*prō 'zăk*]
(fluoxetine hydrochloride)

DESCRIPTION

Prozac® (fluoxetine hydrochloride) is an antidepressant for oral administration; it is also marketed for the treatment of premenstrual dysphoric disorder (Sarafem™, fluoxetine hydrochloride). It is chemically unrelated to tricyclic, tetracyclic, or other available antidepressant agents. It is designated (±)-N-methyl-3-phenyl-3-[(α,α,α-trifluoro-*p*-tolyl)oxy]propylamine hydrochloride and has the empirical formula of $C_{17}H_{18}F_3NO \bullet HCl$. Its molecular weight is 345.79. The structural formula is:

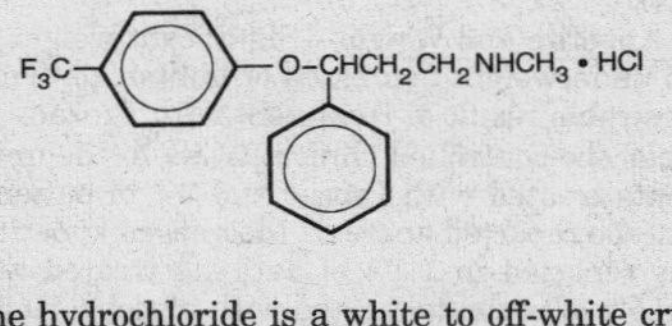

Fluoxetine hydrochloride is a white to off-white crystalline solid with a solubility of 14 mg/mL in water.

Each Pulvule® contains fluoxetine hydrochloride equivalent to 10 mg (32.3 µmol), 20 mg (64.7 µmol), or 40 mg (129.3 µmol) of fluoxetine. The Pulvules also contain starch, gelatin, silicone, titanium dioxide, iron oxide, and other inactive ingredients. The 10-mg and 20-mg Pulvules also contain F D & C Blue No. 1, and the 40-mg Pulvule also contains F D & C Blue No. 1 and F D & C Yellow No.6.

Each tablet contains fluoxetine hydrochloride equivalent to 10 mg (32.3 µmol) of fluoxetine. The tablets also contain microcrystalline cellulose, magnesium stearate, crospovidone, hydroxypropyl methylcellulose, titanium dioxide, polyethylene glycol, and yellow iron oxide. In addition to the above ingredients, the 10-mg tablet contains F D & C Blue No.1 aluminum lake, and polysorbate 80.

The oral solution contains fluoxetine hydrochloride equivalent to 20 mg/5 mL (64.7 µmol) of fluoxetine. It also contains alcohol 0.23%, benzoic acid, flavoring agent, glycerin, purified water, and sucrose.

Prozac Weekly™ capsules, a delayed release formulation, contain enteric-coated pellets of fluoxetine hydrochloride equivalent to 90 mg (291 µmol) of fluoxetine. The capsules also contain F D & C Yellow No. 10, F D & C Blue No. 2, gelatin, hydroxypropyl methylcellulose, hydroxypropyl methylcellulose acetate succinate, sodium lauryl sulfate, sucrose, sugar spheres, talc, titanium dioxide, triethyl citrate, and other inactive ingredients.

CLINICAL PHARMACOLOGY

Pharmacodynamics: The antidepressant, antiobsessive-compulsive, and antibulimic actions of fluoxetine are presumed to be linked to its inhibition of CNS neuronal uptake of serotonin. Studies at clinically relevant doses in man have demonstrated that fluoxetine blocks the uptake of serotonin into human platelets. Studies in animals also suggest that fluoxetine is a much more potent uptake inhibitor of serotonin than of norepinephrine.

Antagonism of muscarinic, histaminergic, and α_1-adrenergic receptors has been hypothesized to be associated with various anticholinergic, sedative, and cardiovascular effects of classical tricyclic antidepressant (TCA) drugs. Fluoxetine binds to these and other membrane receptors from brain tissue much less potently in vitro than do the tricyclic drugs.

Absorption, Distribution, Metabolism, and Excretion: Systemic Bioavailability—In man, following a single oral 40-mg dose, peak plasma concentrations of fluoxetine from 15 to 55 ng/mL are observed after 6 to 8 hours.

The Pulvule, tablet, oral solution, and Prozac Weekly capsule dosage forms of fluoxetine are bioequivalent. Food does not appear to affect the systemic bioavailability of fluoxetine, although it may delay its absorption by 1 to 2 hours, which is probably not clinically significant. Thus, fluoxetine may be administered with or without food. Prozac Weekly capsules, a delayed release formulation, contain enteric-coated pellets that resist dissolution until reaching a segment of the gastrointestinal tract where the pH exceeds 5.5. The enteric coating delays the onset of absorption of fluoxetine 1 to 2 hours relative to the immediate release formulations.

Protein Binding—Over the concentration range from 200 to 1,000 ng/mL, approximately 94.5% of fluoxetine is bound in vitro to human serum proteins, including albumin and α_1-glycoprotein. The interaction between fluoxetine and other highly protein-bound drugs has not been fully evaluated, but may be important (*see* PRECAUTIONS).

Enantiomers—Fluoxetine is a racemic mixture (50/50) of *R*-fluoxetine and *S*-fluoxetine enantiomers. In animal models, both enantiomers are specific and potent serotonin uptake inhibitors with essentially equivalent pharmacologic activity. The *S*-fluoxetine enantiomer is eliminated more slowly and is the predominant enantiomer present in plasma at steady state.

Metabolism—Fluoxetine is extensively metabolized in the liver to norfluoxetine and a number of other unidentified metabolites. The only identified active metabolite, norfluoxetine, is formed by demethylation of fluoxetine. In animal models, *S*-norfluoxetine is a potent and selective inhibitor of serotonin uptake and has activity essentially equivalent to *R*- or *S*-fluoxetine. *R*-norfluoxetine is significantly less potent than the parent drug in the inhibition of serotonin uptake. The primary route of elimination appears to be hepatic metabolism to inactive metabolites excreted by the kidney.

Clinical Issues Related to Metabolism/Elimination—The complexity of the metabolism of fluoxetine has several consequences that may potentially affect fluoxetine's clinical use.

Variability in Metabolism—A subset (about 7%) of the population has reduced activity of the drug metabolizing enzyme cytochrome P450IID6. Such individuals are referred to as "poor metabolizers" of drugs such as debrisoquin, dextromethorphan, and the TCAs. In a study involving labeled and unlabeled enantiomers administered as a racemate, these individuals metabolized *S*-fluoxetine at a slower rate and thus achieved higher concentrations of *S*-fluoxetine. Consequently, concentrations of *S*-norfluoxetine at steady state were lower. The metabolism of *R*-fluoxetine in these poor metabolizers appears normal. When compared with normal metabolizers, the total sum at steady state of the plasma concentrations of the four active enantiomers was not significantly greater among poor metabolizers. Thus, the net pharmacodynamic activities were essentially the same. Alternative, nonsaturable pathways (non-IID6) also contribute to the metabolism of fluoxetine. This explains how fluoxetine achieves a steady-state concentration rather than increasing without limit.

Because fluoxetine's metabolism, like that of a number of other compounds including tricyclic and other selective serotonin antidepressants, involves the P450IID6 system, concomitant therapy with drugs also metabolized by this enzyme system (such as the TCAs) may lead to drug interactions (*see* Drug Interactions *under* PRECAUTIONS).

Accumulation and Slow Elimination—The relatively slow elimination of fluoxetine (elimination half-life of 1 to 3 days after acute administration and 4 to 6 days after chronic administration) and its active metabolite, norfluoxetine (elimination half-life of 4 to 16 days after acute and chronic administration), leads to significant accumulation of these active species in chronic use and delayed attainment of steady state, even when a fixed dose is used. After 30 days of dosing at 40 mg/day, plasma concentrations of fluoxetine in the range of 91 to 302 ng/mL and norfluoxetine in the range of 72 to 258 ng/mL have been observed. Plasma concentrations of fluoxetine were higher than those predicted by single-dose studies, because fluoxetine's metabolism is not proportional to dose. Norfluoxetine, however, appears to have linear pharmacokinetics. Its mean terminal half-life after a single dose was 8.6 days and after multiple dosing was 9.3 days. Steady-state levels after prolonged dosing are similar to levels seen at 4 to 5 weeks.

The long elimination half-lives of fluoxetine and norfluoxetine assure that, even when dosing is stopped, active drug substance will persist in the body for weeks (primarily depending on individual patient characteristics, previous dosing regimen, and length of previous therapy at discontinuation). This is of potential consequence when drug discontinuation is required or when drugs are prescribed that might interact with fluoxetine and norfluoxetine following the discontinuation of Prozac.

Weekly Dosing—Administration of Prozac Weekly once-weekly results in increased fluctuation between peak and trough concentrations of fluoxetine and norfluoxetine compared to once-daily dosing (for fluoxetine: 24% [daily] to 164% [weekly] and for norfluoxetine: 17% [daily] to 43% [weekly]). Plasma concentrations may not necessarily be predictive of clinical response. Peak concentrations from once-weekly doses of Prozac Weekly capsules of fluoxetine are in the range of the average concentration for 20 mg once-daily dosing. Average trough concentrations are 76% lower for fluoxetine and 47% lower for norfluoxetine than the concentrations maintained by 20 mg once-daily dosing. Average steady-state concentrations of either once-daily or once-weekly dosing are in relative proportion to the total dose administered. Average steady-state fluoxetine concentrations are approximately 50% lower following the once-weekly regimen compared to the once-daily regimen.

C_{max} for fluoxetine following the 90 mg dose was approximately 1.7 fold higher than the C_{max} value for the established 20 mg once-daily regimen following transition the next day to the once-weekly regimen. In contrast, when the first 90 mg once-weekly dose and the last 20 mg once-daily dose were separated by one week, C_{max} values were similar. Also, there was a transient increase in the average steady-state concentrations of fluoxetine observed following transition the next day to the once-weekly regimen. From a pharmacokinetic perspective, it may be better to separate the first 90 mg weekly dose and the last 20 mg once-daily dose by one week (*see* DOSAGE AND ADMINISTRATION).

Liver Disease—As might be predicted from its primary site of metabolism, liver impairment can affect the elimination of fluoxetine. The elimination half-life of fluoxetine was prolonged in a study of cirrhotic patients, with a mean of 7.6 days compared to the range of 2 to 3 days seen in subjects without liver disease; norfluoxetine elimination was also delayed, with a mean duration of 12 days for cirrhotic patients compared to the range of 7 to 9 days in normal subjects. This suggests that the use of fluoxetine in patients with liver disease must be approached with caution. If fluoxetine is administered to patients with liver disease, a lower or less frequent dose should be used (*see* PRECAUTIONS *and* DOSAGE AND ADMINISTRATION).

Renal Disease—In depressed patients on dialysis (N=12), fluoxetine administered as 20 mg once daily for two months produced steady-state fluoxetine and norfluoxetine plasma concentrations comparable to those seen in patients with normal renal function. While the possibility exists that renally excreted metabolites of fluoxetine may accumulate to higher levels in patients with severe renal dysfunction, use of a lower or less frequent dose is not routinely necessary in renally impaired patients (*see* Use in Patients With Concomitant Illness *under* PRECAUTIONS *and* DOSAGE AND ADMINISTRATION).

Age—The disposition of single doses of fluoxetine in healthy elderly subjects (greater than 65 years of age) did not differ significantly from that in younger normal subjects. However, given the long half-life and nonlinear disposition of the drug, a single-dose study is not adequate to rule out the possibility of altered pharmacokinetics in the elderly, particularly if they have systemic illness or are receiving multiple drugs for concomitant diseases. The effects of age upon the metabolism of fluoxetine have been investigated in 260 elderly but otherwise healthy depressed patients (≥60 years of age) who received 20 mg fluoxetine for 6 weeks. Combined fluoxetine plus norfluoxetine plasma concentrations were 209.3 ± 85.7 ng/mL at the end of 6 weeks. No unusual age-associated pattern of adverse events was observed in those elderly patients.

Clinical Trials:

Depression—Daily Dosing: The efficacy of Prozac for the treatment of patients with depression (≥ 18 years of age) has been studied in 5- and 6-week placebo-controlled trials. Prozac was shown to be significantly more effective than placebo as measured by the Hamilton Depression Rating Scale (HAM-D). Prozac was also significantly more effective than placebo on the HAM-D subscores for depressed mood, sleep disturbance, and the anxiety subfactor.

Two 6-week controlled studies (N=671, randomized) comparing Prozac 20 mg and placebo have shown Prozac 20 mg daily to be effective in the treatment of elderly patients (≥ 60 years of age) with depression. In these studies, Prozac produced a significantly higher rate of response and remission as defined respectively by a 50% decrease in the HAM-D score and a total endpoint HAM-D score of ≤ 8.

Continued on next page

Prozac Weekly—Cont.

Prozac was well tolerated and the rate of treatment discontinuations due to adverse events did not differ between Prozac (12%) and placebo (9%).

A study was conducted involving depressed outpatients who had responded (modified HAMD-17 score of ≤ 7 during each of the last 3 weeks of open-label treatment and absence of major depression by DSM-III-R criteria) by the end of an initial 12-week open treatment phase on Prozac 20 mg/day. These patients (N=298) were randomized to continuation on double-blind Prozac 20 mg/day or placebo. At 38 weeks (50 weeks total), a statistically significantly lower relapse rate (defined as symptoms sufficient to meet a diagnosis of major depression for 2 weeks or a modified HAMD-17 score of ≥ 14 for 3 weeks) was observed for patients taking Prozac compared to those on placebo.

Weekly dosing for maintenance/continuation treatment: A longer-term study was conducted involving adult outpatients meeting DSM-IV criteria for major depressive disorder who had responded (defined as having a modified HAMD-17 score of ≤9, a CGI-Severity rating of ≤2, and no longer meeting criteria for major depression) for 3 consecutive weeks at the end of 13 weeks of open-label treatment with Prozac 20 mg once-daily. These patients were randomized to double-blind, once-weekly continuation treatment with Prozac Weekly, Prozac 20 mg once-daily, or placebo. Prozac Weekly once-weekly and Prozac 20 mg once-daily demonstrated superior efficacy (having a significantly longer time to relapse of depressive symptoms) compared to placebo for a period of 25 weeks. However, the equivalence of these two treatments during continuation therapy has not been established.

Obsessive-Compulsive Disorder—The effectiveness of Prozac for the treatment for obsessive-compulsive disorder (OCD) was demonstrated in two 13-week, multicenter, parallel group studies (Studies 1 and 2) of adult outpatients who received fixed Prozac doses of 20, 40, or 60 mg/day (on a once a day schedule, in the morning) or placebo. Patients in both studies had moderate to severe OCD (DSM-III-R), with mean baseline ratings on the Yale-Brown Obsessive Compulsive Scale (YBOCS, total score) ranging from 22 to 26. In Study 1, patients receiving Prozac experienced mean reductions of approximately 4 to 6 units on the YBOCS total score, compared to a 1-unit reduction for placebo patients. In Study 2, patients receiving Prozac experienced mean reductions of approximately 4 to 9 units on the YBOCS total score, compared to a 1-unit reduction for placebo patients. While there was no indication of a dose response relationship for effectiveness in Study 1, a dose response relationship was observed in Study 2, with numerically better responses in the two higher dose groups. The following table provides the outcome classification by treatment group on the Clinical Global Impression (CGI) improvement scale for Studies 1 and 2 combined:

Outcome Classification (%) on CGI Improvement Scale for Completers in Pool of Two OCD Studies

		Prozac		
Outcome Classification	Placebo	20 mg	40 mg	60 mg
Worse	8%	0%	0%	0%
No Change	64%	41%	33%	29%
Minimally Improved	17%	23%	28%	24%
Much Improved	8%	28%	27%	28%
Very Much Improved	3%	8%	12%	19%

Exploratory analyses for age and gender effects on outcome did not suggest any differential responsiveness on the basis of age or sex.

Bulimia Nervosa—The effectiveness of Prozac for the treatment of bulimia was demonstrated in two 8-week and one 16-week, multicenter, parallel group studies of adult outpatients meeting DSM-III-R criteria for bulimia. Patients in the 8-week studies received either 20 or 60 mg/day of Prozac or placebo in the morning. Patients in the 16-week study received a fixed Prozac dose of 60 mg/day (once a day) or placebo. Patients in these three studies had moderate to severe bulimia with median binge-eating and vomiting frequencies ranging from 7 to 10 per week and 5 to 9 per week, respectively. In these 3 studies, Prozac 60 mg, but not 20 mg, was statistically significantly superior to placebo in reducing the number of binge-eating and vomiting episodes per week. The statistically significantly superior effect of 60 mg vs placebo was present as early as Week 1 and persisted throughout each study. The Prozac related reduction in bulimic episodes appeared to be independent of baseline depression as assessed by the Hamilton Depression Rating Scale. In each of these 3 studies, the treatment effect, as measured by differences between Prozac 60 mg, and placebo on median reduction from baseline in frequency of bulimic behaviors at endpoint, ranged from one to two episodes per week for binge-eating and two to four episodes per week for vomiting. The size of the effect was related to baseline frequency, with greater reductions seen in patients with higher baseline frequencies. Although some patients achieved freedom from binge-eating and purging as a result of treatment, for the majority, the benefit was a partial reduction in the frequency of binge-eating and purging.

INDICATIONS AND USAGE

Depression—Prozac is indicated for the treatment of depression. The efficacy of Prozac was established in 5- and 6-week trials with depressed adult and geriatric outpatients (≥ 18 years of age) whose diagnoses corresponded most closely to the DSM-III (currently DSM-IV) category of major depressive disorder (*see* Clinical Trials *under* CLINICAL PHARMACOLOGY).

A major depressive episode (DSM-IV) implies a prominent and relatively persistent (nearly every day for at least 2 weeks) depressed or dysphoric mood that usually interferes with daily functioning, and includes at least five of the following nine symptoms: depressed mood; loss of interest in usual activities; significant change in weight and/or appetite; insomnia or hypersomnia; psychomotor agitation or retardation; increased fatigue; feelings of guilt or worthlessness; slowed thinking or impaired concentration; a suicide attempt or suicidal ideation.

The antidepressant action of Prozac in hospitalized depressed patients has not been adequately studied.

The efficacy of Prozac 20 mg once-daily in maintaining an antidepressant response for up to 38 weeks following 12 weeks of open-label acute treatment (50 weeks total) was demonstrated in a placebo-controlled trial (*see* Clinical Trials *under* CLINICAL PHARMACOLOGY).

The efficacy of Prozac Weekly once-weekly in maintaining an antidepressant response has been demonstrated in a placebo-controlled trial for up to 25 weeks following open-label acute treatment of 13 weeks with Prozac 20 mg daily for a total antidepressant treatment of 38 weeks. However, it is unknown whether or not Prozac Weekly given on a once-weekly basis provides the same level of protection from relapse as that provided by Prozac 20 mg daily (*see* Clinical Trials *under* CLINICAL PHARMACOLOGY).

The usefulness of the drug in patients receiving fluoxetine for extended periods should be reevaluated periodically.

Obsessive-Compulsive Disorder—Prozac is indicated for the treatment of obsessions and compulsions in patients with obsessive-compulsive disorder (OCD), as defined in the DSM-III-R; ie, the obsessions or compulsions cause marked distress, are time-consuming, or significantly interfere with social or occupational functioning.

The efficacy of Prozac was established in 13-week trials with obsessive-compulsive outpatients whose diagnoses corresponded most closely to the DSM-III-R category of obsessive-compulsive disorder (*see* Clinical Trials *under* CLINICAL PHARMACOLOGY).

Obsessive-compulsive disorder is characterized by recurrent and persistent ideas, thoughts, impulses, or images (obsessions) that are ego-dystonic and/or repetitive, purposeful, and intentional behaviors (compulsions) that are recognized by the person as excessive or unreasonable.

The effectiveness of Prozac in long-term use, ie, for more than 13 weeks, has not been systematically evaluated in placebo-controlled trials. Therefore, the physician who elects to use Prozac for extended periods should periodically reevaluate the long-term usefulness of the drug for the individual patient (*see* DOSAGE AND ADMINISTRATION).

Bulimia Nervosa—Prozac is indicated for the treatment of binge-eating and vomiting behaviors in patients with moderate to severe bulimia nervosa.

The efficacy of Prozac was established in 8 to 16 week trials for adult outpatients with moderate to severe bulimia nervosa, ie, at least three bulimic episodes per week for 6 months (*see* Clinical Trials *under* CLINICAL PHARMACOLOGY).

The effectiveness of Prozac in long-term use, ie, for more than 16 weeks, has not been systematically evaluated in placebo-controlled trials. Therefore, the physician who elects to use Prozac for extended periods should periodically reevaluate the long-term usefulness of the drug for the individual patient (*see* DOSAGE AND ADMINISTRATION).

CONTRAINDICATIONS

Prozac is contraindicated in patients known to be hypersensitive to it.

Monoamine Oxidase Inhibitors—There have been reports of serious, sometimes fatal, reactions (including hyperthermia, rigidity, myoclonus, autonomic instability with possible rapid fluctuations of vital signs, and mental status changes that include extreme agitation progressing to delirium and coma) in patients receiving fluoxetine in combination with a monoamine oxidase inhibitor (MAOI), and in patients who have recently discontinued fluoxetine and are then started on an MAOI. Some cases presented with features resembling neuroleptic malignant syndrome. Therefore, Prozac should not be used in combination with an MAOI, or within a minimum of 14 days of discontinuing therapy with an MAOI. Since fluoxetine and its major metabolite have very long elimination half-lives, at least 5 weeks (perhaps longer, especially if fluoxetine has been prescribed chronically and/or at higher doses [*see* Accumulation and Slow Elimination *under* CLINICAL PHARMACOLOGY]) should be allowed after stopping Prozac before starting an MAOI.

Thioridazine—Thioridazine should not be administered with Prozac or within a minimum of 5 weeks after Prozac has been discontinued (*see* WARNINGS).

WARNINGS

Rash and Possibly Allergic Events—In US fluoxetine clinical trials, 7% of 10,782 patients developed various types of rashes and/or urticaria. Among the cases of rash and/or urticaria reported in premarketing clinical trials, almost a third were withdrawn from treatment because of the rash and/or systemic signs or symptoms associated with the rash. Clinical findings reported in association with rash include fever, leukocytosis, arthralgias, edema, carpal tunnel syndrome, respiratory distress, lymphadenopathy, proteinuria, and mild transaminase elevation. Most patients improved promptly with discontinuation of fluoxetine and/or adjunctive treatment with antihistamines or steroids, and all patients experiencing these events were reported to recover completely.

In premarketing clinical trials, two patients are known to have developed a serious cutaneous systemic illness. In neither patient was there an unequivocal diagnosis, but one was considered to have a leukocytoclastic vasculitis, and the other, a severe desquamating syndrome that was considered variously to be a vasculitis or erythema multiforme. Other patients have had systemic syndromes suggestive of serum sickness.

Since the introduction of Prozac, systemic events, possibly related to vasculitis and including lupus-like syndrome, have developed in patients with rash. Although these events are rare, they may be serious, involving the lung, kidney, or liver. Death has been reported to occur in association with these systemic events.

Anaphylactoid events, including bronchospasm, angioedema, laryngospasm, and urticaria alone and in combination, have been reported.

Pulmonary events, including inflammatory processes of varying histopathology and/or fibrosis, have been reported rarely. These events have occurred with dyspnea as the only preceding symptom.

Whether these systemic events and rash have a common underlying cause or are due to different etiologies or pathogenic processes is not known. Furthermore, a specific underlying immunologic basis for these events has not been identified. Upon the appearance of rash or of other possibly allergic phenomena for which an alternative etiology cannot be identified, Prozac should be discontinued.

Potential Interaction With Thioridazine—In a study of 19 healthy male subjects, which included 6 slow and 13 rapid hydroxylators of debrisoquin, a single 25-mg oral dose of thioridazine produced a 2.4-fold higher C_{max} and a 4.5-fold higher AUC for thioridazine in the slow hydroxylators compared to the rapid hydroxylators. The rate of debrisoquin hydroxylation is felt to depend on the level of cytochrome P450IID6 isozyme activity. Thus, this study suggests that drugs which inhibit P450IID6, such as certain SSRIs, including fluoxetine, will produce elevated plasma levels of thioridazine (*see* PRECAUTIONS).

Thioridazine administration produces a dose-related prolongation of the QTc interval, which is associated with serious ventricular arrhythmias, such as torsades de pointes-type arrhythmias, and sudden death. This risk is expected to increase with fluoxetine-induced inhibition of thioridazine metabolism (*see* CONTRAINDICATIONS).

PRECAUTIONS

General—Anxiety and Insomnia—In US placebo-controlled clinical trials for depression, 12% to 16% of patients treated with Prozac and 7% to 9% of patients treated with placebo reported anxiety, nervousness, or insomnia.

In US placebo-controlled clinical trials for OCD, insomnia was reported in 28% of patients treated with Prozac and in 22% of patients treated with placebo. Anxiety was reported in 14% of patients treated with Prozac and in 7% of patients treated with placebo.

In US placebo-controlled clinical trials for bulimia nervosa, insomnia was reported in 33% of patients treated with Prozac 60 mg, and 13% of patients treated with placebo. Anxiety and nervousness were reported respectively in 15% and 11% of patients treated with Prozac 60 mg, and in 9% and 5% of patients treated with placebo.

Among the most common adverse events associated with discontinuation (incidence at least twice that for placebo and at least 1% for Prozac in clinical trials collecting only a primary event associated with discontinuation) in US placebo-controlled fluoxetine clinical trials were anxiety (2% in OCD), insomnia (1% in combined indications and 2% in bulimia), and nervousness (1% in depression) (*see* Table 3, below).

Altered Appetite and Weight—Significant weight loss, especially in underweight depressed or bulimic patients, may be an undesirable result of treatment with Prozac.

In US placebo-controlled clinical trials for depression, 11% of patients treated with Prozac and 2% of patients treated with placebo reported anorexia (decreased appetite). Weight loss was reported in 1.4% of patients treated with Prozac and in 0.5% of patients treated with placebo. However, only rarely have patients discontinued treatment with Prozac because of anorexia or weight loss.

In US placebo-controlled clinical trials for OCD, 17% of patients treated with Prozac and 10% of patients treated with placebo reported anorexia (decreased appetite). One patient discontinued treatment with Prozac because of anorexia.

In US placebo-controlled clinical trials for bulimia nervosa, 8% of patients treated with Prozac 60 mg, and 4% of patients treated with placebo reported anorexia (decreased appetite). Patients treated with Prozac 60 mg, on average lost 0.45 kg compared with a gain of 0.16 kg by patients treated with placebo in the 16-week double-blind trial. Weight change should be monitored during therapy.

Activation of Mania/Hypomania—In US placebo-controlled clinical trials for depression, mania/hypomania was reported in 0.1% of patients treated with Prozac and 0.1% of patients treated with placebo. Activation of mania/hypomania has also been reported in a small proportion of patients with Major Affective Disorder treated with other marketed antidepressants.

In US placebo-controlled clinical trials for OCD, mania/hypomania was reported in 0.8% of patients treated with Prozac and no patients treated with placebo. No patients reported mania/hypomania in US placebo-controlled clinical trials for bulimia. In all US Prozac clinical trials, 0.7% of 10,782 patients reported mania/hypomania.

Seizures—In US placebo-controlled clinical trials for depression, convulsions (or events described as possibly having been seizures) were reported in 0.1% of patients treated with Prozac and 0.2% of patients treated with placebo. No patients reported convulsions in US placebo-controlled clinical trials for either OCD or bulimia. In all US Prozac clinical trials, 0.2% of 10,782 patients reported convulsions. The percentage appears to be similar to that associated with other marketed antidepressants. Prozac should be introduced with care in patients with a history of seizures.

Suicide—The possibility of a suicide attempt is inherent in depression and may persist until significant remission occurs. Close supervision of high-risk patients should accompany initial drug therapy. Prescriptions for Prozac should be written for the smallest quantity of capsules consistent with good patient management, in order to reduce the risk of overdose.

Because of well-established comorbidity between OCD and depression and bulimia and depression, the same precautions observed when treating patients with depression should be observed when treating patients with OCD or bulimia.

The Long Elimination Half-Lives of Fluoxetine and Its Metabolites—Because of the long elimination half-lives of the parent drug and its major active metabolite, changes in dose will not be fully reflected in plasma for several weeks, affecting both strategies for titration to final dose and withdrawal from treatment (see CLINICAL PHARMACOLOGY and DOSAGE AND ADMINISTRATION).

Use in Patients With Concomitant Illness—Clinical experience with Prozac in patients with concomitant systemic illness is limited. Caution is advisable in using Prozac in patients with diseases or conditions that could affect metabolism or hemodynamic responses.

Fluoxetine has not been evaluated or used to any appreciable extent in patients with a recent history of myocardial infarction or unstable heart disease. Patients with these diagnoses were systematically excluded from clinical studies during the product's premarket testing. However, the electrocardiograms of 312 patients who received Prozac in double-blind trials were retrospectively evaluated; no conduction abnormalities that resulted in heart block were observed. The mean heart rate was reduced by approximately 3 beats/min.

In subjects with cirrhosis of the liver, the clearances of fluoxetine and its active metabolite, norfluoxetine, were decreased, thus increasing the elimination half-lives of these substances. A lower or less frequent dose should be used in patients with cirrhosis.

Studies in depressed patients on dialysis did not reveal excessive accumulation of fluoxetine or norfluoxetine in plasma (see Renal Disease under CLINICAL PHARMACOLOGY). Use of a lower or less frequent dose for renally impaired patients is not routinely necessary (see DOSAGE AND ADMINISTRATION).

In patients with diabetes, Prozac may alter glycemic control. Hypoglycemia has occurred during therapy with Prozac, and hyperglycemia has developed following discontinuation of the drug. As is true with many other types of medication when taken concurrently by patients with diabetes, insulin and/or oral hypoglycemic dosage may need to be adjusted when therapy with Prozac is instituted or discontinued.

Interference With Cognitive and Motor Performance—Any psychoactive drug may impair judgment, thinking, or motor skills, and patients should be cautioned about operating hazardous machinery, including automobiles, until they are reasonably certain that the drug treatment does not affect them adversely.

Information for Patients—Physicians are advised to discuss the following issues with patients for whom they prescribe Prozac:

Because Prozac may impair judgment, thinking, or motor skills, patients should be advised to avoid driving a car or operating hazardous machinery until they are reasonably certain that their performance is not affected.

Patients should be advised to inform their physician if they are taking or plan to take any prescription or over-the-counter drugs, or alcohol.

Patients should be advised to notify their physician if they become pregnant or intend to become pregnant during therapy.

Patients should be advised to notify their physician if they are breast feeding an infant.

Patients should be advised to notify their physician if they develop a rash or hives.

Laboratory Tests—There are no specific laboratory tests recommended.

Drug Interactions—As with all drugs, the potential for interaction by a variety of mechanisms (eg, pharmacodynamic, pharmacokinetic drug inhibition or enhancement, etc) is a possibility (see Accumulation and Slow Elimination under CLINICAL PHARMACOLOGY).

Drugs Metabolized by P450IID6—Approximately 7% of the normal population has a genetic defect that leads to reduced levels of activity of the cytochrome P450 isoenzyme P450IID6. Such individuals have been referred to as "poor metabolizers" of drugs such as debrisoquin, dextromethorphan, and TCAs. Many drugs, such as most antidepressants, including fluoxetine and other selective uptake inhibitors of serotonin, are metabolized by this isoenzyme; thus, both the pharmacokinetic properties and relative proportion of metabolites are altered in poor metabolizers. However, for fluoxetine and its metabolite the sum of the plasma concentrations of the four active enantiomers is comparable between poor and extensive metabolizers (see Variability in Metabolism under CLINICAL PHARMACOLOGY).

Fluoxetine, like other agents that are metabolized by P450IID6, inhibits the activity of this isoenzyme, and thus may make normal metabolizers resemble "poor metabolizers." Therapy with medications that are predominantly metabolized by the P450IID6 system and that have a relatively narrow therapeutic index (see list below), should be initiated at the low end of the dose range if a patient is receiving fluoxetine concurrently or has taken it in the previous 5 weeks. Thus, his/her dosing requirements resemble those of "poor metabolizers." If fluoxetine is added to the treatment regimen of a patient already receiving a drug metabolized by P450IID6, the need for decreased dose of the original medication should be considered. Drugs with a narrow therapeutic index represent the greatest concern (eg, flecainide, vinblastine, and TCAs). Due to the risk of serious ventricular arrhythmias and sudden death potentially associated with elevated plasma levels of thioridazine, thioridazine should not be administered with fluoxetine or within a minimum of 5 weeks after fluoxetine has been discontinued (see CONTRAINDICATIONS and WARNINGS).

Drugs Metabolized by Cytochrome P450IIIA4—In an in vivo interaction study involving co-administration of fluoxetine with single doses of terfenadine (a cytochrome P450IIIA4 substrate), no increase in plasma terfenadine concentrations occurred with concomitant fluoxetine. In addition, in vitro studies have shown ketoconazole, a potent inhibitor of P450IIIA4 activity, to be at least 100 times more potent than fluoxetine or norfluoxetine as an inhibitor of the metabolism of several substrates for this enzyme, including astemizole, cisapride, and midazolam. These data indicate that fluoxetine's extent of inhibition of cytochrome P450IIIA4 activity is not likely to be of clinical significance.

CNS Active Drugs—The risk of using Prozac in combination with other CNS active drugs has not been systematically evaluated. Nonetheless, caution is advised if the concomitant administration of Prozac and such drugs is required. In evaluating individual cases, consideration should be given to using lower initial doses of the concomitantly administered drugs, using conservative titration schedules, and monitoring of clinical status (see Accumulation and Slow Elimination under CLINICAL PHARMACOLOGY).

Anticonvulsants—Patients on stable doses of phenytoin and carbamazepine have developed elevated plasma anticonvulsant concentrations and clinical anticonvulsant toxicity following initiation of concomitant fluoxetine treatment.

Antipsychotics—Some clinical data suggests a possible pharmacodynamic and/or pharmacokinetic interaction between serotonin specific reuptake inhibitors (SSRIs) and antipsychotics. Elevation of blood levels of haloperidol and clozapine has been observed in patients receiving concomitant fluoxetine. A single case report has suggested possible additive effects of pimozide and fluoxetine leading to bradycardia. For thioridazine, see CONTRAINDICATIONS and WARNINGS.

Benzodiazepines—The half-life of concurrently administered diazepam may be prolonged in some patients (see Accumulation and Slow Elimination under CLINICAL PHARMACOLOGY). Coadministration of alprazolam and fluoxetine has resulted in increased alprazolam plasma concentrations and in further psychomotor performance decrement due to increased alprazolam levels.

Lithium—There have been reports of both increased and decreased lithium levels when lithium was used concomitantly with fluoxetine. Cases of lithium toxicity and increased serotonergic effects have been reported. Lithium levels should be monitored when these drugs are administered concomitantly.

Tryptophan—Five patients receiving Prozac in combination with tryptophan experienced adverse reactions, including agitation, restlessness, and gastrointestinal distress.

Monoamine Oxidase Inhibitors—See CONTRAINDICATIONS.

Other Antidepressants—In two studies, previously stable plasma levels of imipramine and desipramine have increased greater than 2 to 10-fold when fluoxetine has been administered in combination. This influence may persist for three weeks or longer after fluoxetine is discontinued. Thus, the dose of TCA may need to be reduced and plasma TCA concentrations may need to be monitored temporarily when fluoxetine is coadministered or has been recently discontinued (see Accumulation and Slow Elimination under CLINICAL PHARMACOLOGY, and Drugs Metabolized by P450IID6 under Drug Interactions).

Sumatriptan—There have been rare postmarketing reports describing patients with weakness, hyperreflexia, and incoordination following the use of an SSRI and sumatriptan. If concomitant treatment with sumatriptan and an SSRI (eg, fluoxetine, fluvoxamine, paroxetine, sertraline, or citalopram) is clinically warranted, appropriate observation of the patient is advised.

Potential Effects of Coadministration of Drugs Tightly Bound to Plasma Proteins—Because fluoxetine is tightly bound to plasma protein, the administration of fluoxetine to a patient taking another drug that is tightly bound to protein (eg, Coumadin, digitoxin) may cause a shift in plasma concentrations potentially resulting in an adverse effect. Conversely, adverse effects may result from displacement of protein-bound fluoxetine by other tightly bound drugs (see Accumulation and Slow Elimination under CLINICAL PHARMACOLOGY).

Warfarin—Altered anti-coagulant effects, including increased bleeding, have been reported when fluoxetine is coadministered with warfarin. Patients receiving warfarin therapy should receive careful coagulation monitoring when fluoxetine is initiated or stopped.

Electroconvulsive Therapy—There are no clinical studies establishing the benefit of the combined use of ECT and fluoxetine. There have been rare reports of prolonged seizures in patients on fluoxetine receiving ECT treatment.

Carcinogenesis, Mutagenesis, Impairment of Fertility—There is no evidence of carcinogenicity, mutagenicity, or impairment of fertility with Prozac.

Carcinogenicity—The dietary administration of fluoxetine to rats and mice for 2 years at doses of up to 10 and 12 mg/kg/day, respectively (approximately 1.2 and 0.7 times, respectively, the maximum recommended human dose [MRHD] of 80 mg on a mg/m^2 basis), produced no evidence of carcinogenicity.

Mutagenicity—Fluoxetine and norfluoxetine have been shown to have no genotoxic effects based on the following assays: bacterial mutation assay, DNA repair assay in cultured rat hepatocytes, mouse lymphoma assay, and in vivo sister chromatid exchange assay in Chinese hamster bone marrow cells.

Impairment of Fertility—Two fertility studies conducted in rats at doses of up to 7.5 and 12.5 mg/kg/day (approximately 0.9 and 1.5 times the MRHD on a mg/m^2 basis) indicated that fluoxetine had no adverse effects on fertility.

Pregnancy—Pregnancy Category C: In embryo-fetal development studies in rats and rabbits, there was no evidence of teratogenicity following administration of up to 12.5 and 15 mg/kg/day, respectively (1.5 and 3.6 times, respectively, the maximum recommended human dose [MRHD] of 80 mg on a mg/m^2 basis), throughout organogenesis. However, in rat reproduction studies, an increase in stillborn pups, a decrease in pup weight, and an increase in pup deaths during the first 7 days postpartum occurred following maternal exposure to 12 mg/kg/day (1.5 times the MRHD on a mg/m^2 basis) during gestation or 7.5 mg/kg/day (0.9 times the MRHD on a mg/m^2 basis) during gestation and lactation. There was no evidence of developmental neurotoxicity in the surviving offspring of rats treated with 12 mg/kg/day during gestation. The no-effect dose for rat pup mortality was 5 mg/kg/day (0.6 times the MRHD on a mg/m^2 basis). Prozac should be used during pregnancy only if the potential benefit justifies the potential risk to the fetus.

Labor and Delivery—The effect of Prozac on labor and delivery in humans is unknown. However, because fluoxetine crosses the placenta and because of the possibility that fluoxetine may have adverse effects on the newborn, fluoxetine should be used during labor and delivery only if the potential benefit justifies the potential risk to the fetus.

Nursing Mothers—Because Prozac is excreted in human milk, nursing while on Prozac is not recommended. In one breast milk sample, the concentration of fluoxetine plus norfluoxetine was 70.4 ng/mL. The concentration in the mother's plasma was 295.0 ng/mL. No adverse effects on the infant were reported. In another case, an infant nursed by a mother on Prozac developed crying, sleep disturbance, vomiting, and watery stools. The infant's plasma drug levels were 340 ng/mL of fluoxetine and 208 ng/mL of norfluoxetine on the second day of feeding.

Pediatric Use—Safety and effectiveness in pediatric patients have not been established.

Geriatric Use—US fluoxetine clinical trials (10,782 patients) included 687 patients ≥65 years of age and 93 patients ≥75 years of age. The efficacy in geriatric patients has been established (see Clinical Trials under CLINICAL PHARMACOLOGY. For pharmacokinetic information in geriatric patients, see Age under CLINICAL PHARMACOLOGY. No overall differences in safety or effectiveness were observed between these subjects and younger subjects, and other reported clinical experience has not identified differences in responses between the elderly and younger patients, but greater sensitivity of some older individuals cannot be ruled out. As with other SSRIs, fluoxetine has been associated with cases of clinically significant hyponatremia in elderly patients (see Hyponatremia under PRECAUTIONS).

Hyponatremia—Cases of hyponatremia (some with serum sodium lower than 110 mmol/L) have been reported. The hyponatremia appeared to be reversible when Prozac was discontinued. Although these cases were complex with varying possible etiologies, some were possibly due to the syndrome of inappropriate antidiuretic hormone secretion (SIADH). The majority of these occurrences have been in older patients and in patients taking diuretics or who were otherwise volume depleted. In two 6-week controlled studies in patients ≥60 years of age, 10 of 323 fluoxetine patients and 6 of 327 placebo recipients had a lowering of serum sodium below the reference range; this difference was not statistically significant. The lowest observed concentration was 129 mmol/L. The observed decreases were not clinically significant.

Continued on next page

Prozac Weekly—Cont.

Platelet Function—There have been rare reports of altered platelet function and/or abnormal results from laboratory studies in patients taking fluoxetine. While there have been reports of abnormal bleeding in several patients taking fluoxetine, it is unclear whether fluoxetine had a causative role.

Adverse Reactions: Multiple doses of Prozac had been administered to 10,782 patients with various diagnoses in US clinical trials as of May 8, 1995. Adverse events were recorded by clinical investigators using descriptive terminology of their own choosing. Consequently, it is not possible to provide a meaningful estimate of the proportion of individuals experiencing adverse events without first grouping similar types of events into a limited (ie, reduced) number of standardized event categories.

In the tables and tabulations that follow, COSTART Dictionary terminology has been used to classify reported adverse events. The stated frequencies represent the proportion of individuals who experienced, at least once, a treatment-emergent adverse event of the type listed. An event was considered treatment-emergent if it occurred for the first time or worsened while receiving therapy following baseline evaluation. It is important to emphasize that events reported during therapy were not necessarily caused by it.

The prescriber should be aware that the figures in the tables and tabulations cannot be used to predict the incidence of side effects in the course of usual medical practice where patient characteristics and other factors differ from those that prevailed in the clinical trials. Similarly, the cited frequencies cannot be compared with figures obtained from other clinical investigations involving different treatments, uses, and investigators. The cited figures, however, do provide the prescribing physician with some basis for estimating the relative contribution of drug and nondrug factors to the side effect incidence rate in the population studied.

Incidence in US Placebo-Controlled Clinical Trials (excluding data from extensions of trials)—Table 1 enumerates the most common treatment-emergent adverse events associated with the use of Prozac (incidence of at least 5% for Prozac and at least twice that for placebo within at least one of the indications) for the treatment of depression, OCD, and bulimia in US controlled clinical trials. Table 2 enumerates treatment-emergent adverse events that occurred in 2% or more patients treated with Prozac and with incidence greater than placebo who participated in US controlled clinical trials comparing Prozac with placebo in the treatment of depression, OCD, or bulimia. Table 2 provides combined data for the pool of studies that are provided separately by indication in Table 1.

[See table below]

Table 2.
TREATMENT-EMERGENT ADVERSE EVENTS: INCIDENCE IN US DEPRESSION, OCD, AND BULIMIA PLACEBO-CONTROLLED CLINICAL TRIALS

Body System/ Adverse Event*	Percentage of patients reporting event	
	Depression, OCD, and bulimia combined	
	Prozac (N=2444)	Placebo (N=1331)
Body as a Whole		
Headache	21	20
Asthenia	12	6
Flu Syndrome	5	4
Fever	2	1
Cardiovascular System		
Vasodilatation	3	1
Palpitation	2	1
Digestive System		
Nausea	23	10
Diarrhea	12	8
Anorexia	11	3
Dry mouth	10	7
Dyspepsia	8	5
Flatulence	3	2
Vomiting	3	2
Metabolic and Nutritional disorders		
Weight loss	2	1
Nervous System		
Insomnia	20	11
Anxiety	13	8
Nervousness	13	9
Somnolence	13	6
Dizziness	10	7
Tremor	10	3
Libido decreased	4	—
Respiratory System		
Pharyngitis	5	4
Yawn	3	—
Skin and Appendages		
Sweating	8	3
Rash	4	3
Pruritus	3	2
Special Senses		
Abnormal vision	3	1

* Included are events reported by at least 2% of patients taking Prozac, except the following events, which had an incidence on placebo ≥ Prozac (depression, OCD, and bulimia combined): abdominal pain, abnormal dreams, accidental injury, back pain, chest pain, constipation, cough increased, depression (includes suicidal thoughts), dysmenorrhea, gastrointestinal disorder, infection, myalgia, pain, paresthesia, rhinitis, sinusitis, thinking abnormal. —Incidence less than 1%.

Associated with Discontinuation in US Placebo-Controlled Clinical Trials (excluding data from extensions of trials)—Table 3 lists the adverse events associated with discontinuation of Prozac treatment (incidence at least twice that for placebo and at least 1% for Prozac in clinical trials collecting only a primary event associated with discontinuation) in depression, OCD, and bulimia.

Table 3.
MOST COMMON ADVERSE EVENTS ASSOCIATED WITH DISCONTINUATION IN US DEPRESSION, OCD, AND BULIMIA PLACEBO-CONTROLLED CLINICAL TRIALS

Depression, OCD, and bulimia combined (N=1108)	Depression (N=392)	OCD (N=266)	Bulimia (N=450)
—		Anxiety (2%)	—
Insomnia (1%)	—	—	Insomnia (2%)
—	Nervousness (1%)	—	—
—	—	Rash (1%)	—

Events Observed in Prozac Weekly Clinical Trials—Treatment-emergent adverse events in clinical trials with Prozac Weekly were similar to the adverse events reported by patients in clinical trials with Prozac daily. In a placebo-controlled clinical trial, more patients taking Prozac Weekly reported diarrhea than patients taking placebo (10% vs. 3%, respectively) or taking Prozac 20 mg daily (10% vs. 5%, respectively).

Male and Female Sexual Dysfunction with SSRIs—Although changes in sexual desire, sexual performance, and sexual satisfaction often occur as manifestations of a psychiatric disorder, they may also be a consequence of pharmacologic treatment. In particular, some evidence suggests that SSRIs can cause such untoward sexual experiences. Reliable estimates of the incidence and severity of untoward experiences involving sexual desire, performance, and satisfaction are difficult to obtain, however, in part because patients and physicians may be reluctant to discuss them. Accordingly, estimates of the incidence of untoward sexual experience and performance, cited in product labeling, are likely to underestimate their actual incidence. In patients enrolled in US depression, OCD, and bulimia placebo-controlled clinical trials, decreased libido was the only sexual side effect reported by at least 2% of patients taking fluoxetine (4% fluoxetine, <1% placebo). There have been spontaneous reports in women taking fluoxetine of orgasmic dysfunction, including anorgasmia.

There are no adequate and well-controlled studies examining sexual dysfunction with fluoxetine treatment.

Priapism has been reported with all SSRIs.

While it is difficult to know the precise risk of sexual dysfunction associated with the use of SSRIs, physicians should routinely inquire about such possible side effects.

Other Events Observed In All US Clinical Trials—Following is a list of all treatment-emergent adverse events reported at anytime by individuals taking fluoxetine in US clinical trials (10,782 patients) except (1) those listed in the body or footnotes of Tables 1 or 2 above or elsewhere in labeling; (2) those for which the COSTART terms were uninformative or misleading; (3) those events for which a causal relationship to Prozac use was considered remote; and (4) events occurring in only one patient treated with Prozac and which did not have a substantial probability of being acutely life-threatening.

Events are classified within body system categories using the following definitions: frequent adverse events are defined as those occurring on one or more occasions in at least 1/100 patients; infrequent adverse events are those occurring in 1/100 to 1/1,000 patients; rare events are those occurring in less than 1/1,000 patients.

Body as a Whole—*Frequent:* chills; *Infrequent:* chills and fever, face edema, intentional overdose, malaise, pelvic pain, suicide attempt; *Rare:* abdominal syndrome acute, hypothermia, intentional injury, neuroleptic malignant syndrome*, photosensitivity reaction.

Cardiovascular System—*Frequent:* hemorrhage, hypertension; *Infrequent:* angina pectoris, arrhythmia, congestive heart failure, hypotension, migraine, myocardial infarct, postural hypotension, syncope, tachycardia, vascular headache; *Rare:* atrial fibrillation, bradycardia, cerebral embolism, cerebral ischemia, cerebrovascular accident, extrasystoles, heart arrest, heart block, pallor, peripheral vascular disorder, phlebitis, shock, thrombophlebitis, thrombosis, vasospasm, ventricular arrhythmia, ventricular extrasystoles, ventricular fibrillation.

Digestive System—*Frequent:* increased appetite, nausea and vomiting; *Infrequent:* aphthous stomatitis, cholelithiasis, colitis, dysphagia, eructation, esophagitis, gastritis, gastroenteritis, glossitis, gum hemorrhage, hyperchlorhydria, increased salivation, liver function tests abnormal, melena, mouth ulceration, nausea/vomiting/diarrhea, stomach ulcer, stomatitis, thirst; *Rare:* biliary pain, bloody diarrhea, chole-

Table 1.
MOST COMMON TREATMENT-EMERGENT ADVERSE EVENTS: INCIDENCE IN US DEPRESSION, OCD, AND BULIMIA PLACEBO-CONTROLLED CLINICAL TRIALS

Body System/ Adverse Event	Percentage of patients reporting event					
	Depression		OCD		Bulimia	
	Prozac (N=1728)	Placebo (N=975)	Prozac (N=266)	Placebo (N=89)	Prozac (N=450)	Placebo (N=267)
Body as a Whole						
Asthenia	9	5	15	11	21	9
Flu syndrome	3	4	10	7	8	3
Cardiovascular System						
Vasodilatation	3	2	5	—	2	1
Digestive System						
Nausea	21	9	26	13	29	11
Anorexia	11	2	17	10	8	4
Dry mouth	10	7	12	3	9	6
Dyspepsia	7	5	10	4	10	6
Nervous System						
Insomnia	16	9	28	22	33	13
Anxiety	12	7	14	7	15	9
Nervousness	14	9	14	15	11	5
Somnolence	13	6	17	7	13	5
Tremor	10	3	9	1	13	1
Libido decreased	3	—	11	2	5	1
Abnormal dreams	1	1	5	2	5	3
Respiratory System						
Pharyngitis	3	3	11	9	10	5
Sinusitis	1	4	5	2	6	4
Yawn	—	—	7	—	11	—
Skin and Appendages						
Sweating	8	3	7	—	8	3
Rash	4	3	6	3	4	4
Urogenital System						
Impotence†	2	—			7	
Abnormal ejaculation†	—	—	7		7	

† Denominator used was for males only (N= 690 Prozac depression; N=410 placebo depression; N=116 Prozac OCD; N=43 placebo OCD; N=14 Prozac bulimia; N=1 placebo bulimia).
—Incidence less than 1%.

cystitis, duodenal ulcer, enteritis, esophageal ulcer, fecal incontinence, gastrointestinal hemorrhage, hematemesis, hemorrhage of colon, hepatitis, intestinal obstruction, liver fatty deposit, pancreatitis, peptic ulcer, rectal hemorrhage, salivary gland enlargement, stomach ulcer hemorrhage, tongue edema.

Endocrine System—*Infrequent:* hypothyroidism; *Rare:* diabetic acidosis, diabetes mellitus.

Hemic and Lymphatic System—*Infrequent:* anemia, ecchymosis; *Rare:* blood dyscrasia, hypochromic anemia, leukopenia, lymphedema, lymphocytosis, petechia, purpura, thrombocythemia, thrombocytopenia.

Metabolic and Nutritional—*Frequent:* weight gain; *Infrequent:* dehydration, generalized edema, gout, hypercholesteremia, hyperlipemia, hypokalemia, peripheral edema; *Rare:* alcohol intolerance, alkaline phosphatase increased, BUN increased, creatine phosphokinase increased, hyperkalemia, hyperuricemia, hypocalcemia, iron deficiency anemia, SGPT increased.

Musculoskeletal System—*Infrequent:* arthritis, bone pain, bursitis, leg cramps, tenosynovitis; *Rare:* arthrosis, chondrodystrophy, myasthenia, myopathy, myositis, osteomyelitis, osteoporosis, rheumatoid arthritis.

Nervous System—*Frequent:* agitation, amnesia, confusion, emotional lability, sleep disorder; *Infrequent:* abnormal gait, acute brain syndrome, akathisia, apathy, ataxia, buccoglossal syndrome, CNS depression, CNS stimulation, depersonalization, euphoria, hallucinations, hostility, hyperkinesia, hypertonia, hypesthesia, incoordination, libido increased, myoclonus, neuralgia, neuropathy, neurosis, paranoid reaction, personality disorder†, psychosis, vertigo; *Rare:* abnormal electroencephalogram, antisocial reaction, circumoral paresthesia, coma, delusions, dysarthria, dystonia, extrapyramidal syndrome, foot drop, hyperesthesia, neuritis, paralysis, reflexes decreased, reflexes increased, stupor.

Respiratory System—*Infrequent:* asthma, epistaxis, hiccup, hyperventilation; *Rare:* apnea, atelectasis, cough decreased, emphysema, hemoptysis, hypoventilation, hypoxia, larynx edema, lung edema, pneumothorax, stridor.

Skin and Appendages—*Infrequent:* acne, alopecia, contact dermatitis, eczema, maculopapular rash, skin discoloration, skin ulcer, vesiculobullous rash; *Rare:* furunculosis, herpes zoster, hirsutism, petechial rash, psoriasis, purpuric rash, pustular rash, seborrhea.

Special Senses—*Frequent:* ear pain, taste perversion, tinnitus; *Infrequent:* conjunctivitis, dry eyes, mydriasis, photophobia; *Rare:* blepharitis, deafness, diplopia, exophthalmos, eye hemorrhage, glaucoma, hyperacusis, iritis, parosmia, scleritis, strabismus, taste loss, visual field defect.

Urogenital System—*Frequent:* urinary frequency; *Infrequent:* abortion‡, albuminuria, amenorrhea, anorgasmia, breast enlargement, breast pain, cystitis, dysuria, female lactation‡, fibrocystic breast‡, hematuria, leukorrhea‡, menorrhagia‡, metrorrhagia‡, nocturia, polyuria, urinary incontinence, urinary retention, urinary urgency, vaginal hemorrhage‡; *Rare:* breast engorgement, glycosuria, hypomenorrhea‡, kidney pain, oliguria, priapism‡, uterine hemorrhage‡, uterine fibroids enlarged‡.

---

* Neuroleptic malignant syndrome is the COSTART term that best captures serotonin syndrome.
† Personality disorder is the COSTART term for designating nonaggressive objectionable behavior.
‡ Adjusted for gender.

Postintroduction Reports—Voluntary reports of adverse events temporally associated with Prozac that have been received since market introduction and that may have no causal relationship with the drug include the following: aplastic anemia, atrial fibrillation, cataract, cerebral vascular accident, cholestatic jaundice, confusion, dyskinesia (including, for example, a case of buccal-lingual-masticatory syndrome with involuntary tongue protrusion reported to develop in a 77-year-old female after 5 weeks of fluoxetine therapy and which completely resolved over the next few months following drug discontinuation), eosinophilic pneumonia, epidermal necrolysis, erythema nodosum, exfoliative dermatitis, gynecomastia, heart arrest, hepatic failure/necrosis, hyperprolactinemia, hypoglycemia, immune-related hemolytic anemia, kidney failure, misuse/abuse, movement disorders developing in patients with risk factors including drugs associated with such events and worsening of preexisting movement disorders, neuroleptic malignant syndrome-like events, optic neuritis, pancreatitis, pancytopenia, priapism, pulmonary embolism, pulmonary hypertension, QT prolongation, serotonin syndrome (a range of signs and symptoms that can rarely, in its most severe form, resemble neuroleptic malignant syndrome), Stevens-Johnson syndrome, sudden unexpected death, suicidal ideation, thrombocytopenia, thrombocytopenic purpura, vaginal bleeding after drug withdrawal, ventricular tachycardia (including torsades de pointes-type arrhythmias), and violent behaviors.

DRUG ABUSE AND DEPENDENCE

Controlled Substance Class—Prozac is not a controlled substance.

Physical and Psychological Dependence—Prozac has not been systematically studied, in animals or humans, for its potential for abuse, tolerance, or physical dependence. While the premarketing clinical experience with Prozac did not reveal any tendency for a withdrawal syndrome or any drug-seeking behavior, these observations were not systematic and it is not possible to predict on the basis of this limited experience the extent to which a CNS-active drug will be misused, diverted, and/or abused once marketed. Consequently, physicians should carefully evaluate patients for

history of drug abuse and follow such patients closely, observing them for signs of misuse or abuse of Prozac (eg, development of tolerance, incrementation of dose, drug-seeking behavior).

Overdosage: *Human Experience*—Worldwide exposure to fluoxetine hydrochloride is estimated to be over 38 million patients (circa 1999). Of the 1578 cases of overdose involving fluoxetine hydrochloride, alone or with other drugs, reported from this population there were 195 deaths.

Among 633 adult patients who overdosed on fluoxetine hydrochloride alone, 34 resulted in a fatal outcome, 378 completely recovered, and 15 patients experienced sequelae after overdosage, including abnormal accommodation, abnormal gait, confusion, unresponsiveness, nervousness, pulmonary dysfunction, vertigo, tremor, elevated blood pressure, impotence, movement disorder, and hypomania. The remaining 206 patients had an unknown outcome. The most common signs and symptoms associated with non-fatal overdosage were seizures, somnolence, nausea, tachycardia, and vomiting. The largest known ingestion of fluoxetine hydrochloride in adult patients was 8 grams in a patient who took fluoxetine alone and who subsequently recovered. However, in an adult patient who took fluoxetine alone, an ingestion as low as 520 mg has been associated with lethal outcome, but causality has not been established.

Among pediatric patients (ages 3 months to 17 years), there were 156 cases of overdose involving fluoxetine alone or in combination with other drugs. Six patients died, 127 patients completely recovered, 1 patient experienced renal failure, and 22 patients had an unknown outcome. One of the six fatalities was a 9-year-old boy who had a history of OCD, Tourette's syndrome with tics, attention deficit disorder, and fetal alcohol syndrome. He had been receiving 100 mg of fluoxetine daily for 6 months in addition to clonidine, methylphenidate, and promethazine. Mixed-drug ingestion or other methods of suicide complicated all six overdoses in children that resulted in fatalities. The largest ingestion in pediatric patients was 3 grams which was nonlethal.

Other important adverse events reported with fluoxetine overdose (single or multiple drugs) include coma, delirium, ECG abnormalities (such as QT interval prolongation and ventricular tachycardia, including torsades de pointes-type arrhythmias), hypotension, mania, neuroleptic malignant syndrome-like events, pyrexia, stupor, and syncope.

Animal Experience—Studies in animals do not provide precise or necessarily valid information about the treatment of human overdose. However, animal experiments can provide useful insights into possible treatment strategies.

The oral median lethal dose in rats and mice was found to be 452 and 248 mg/kg respectively. Acute high oral doses produced hyperirritability and convulsions in several animal species.

Among six dogs purposely overdosed with oral fluoxetine, five experienced grand mal seizures. Seizures stopped immediately upon the bolus intravenous administration of a standard veterinary dose of diazepam. In this short-term study, the lowest plasma concentration at which a seizure occurred was only twice the maximum plasma concentration seen in humans taking 80 mg/day, chronically.

In a separate single-dose study, the ECG of dogs given high doses did not reveal prolongation of the PR, QRS, or QT intervals. Tachycardia and an increase in blood pressure were observed. Consequently, the value of the ECG in predicting cardiac toxicity is unknown. Nonetheless, the ECG should ordinarily be monitored in cases of human overdose (see Management of Overdose).

Management of Overdose—Treatment should consist of those general measures employed in the management of overdosage with any antidepressant. Ensure an adequate airway, oxygenation, and ventilation. Monitor cardiac rhythm and vital signs. General supportive and symptomatic measures are also recommended. Induction of emesis is not recommended. Gastric lavage with a large-bore orogastric tube with appropriate airway protection, if needed, may be indicated if performed soon after ingestion, or in symptomatic patients.

Activated charcoal should be administered. Due to the large volume of distribution of this drug, forced diuresis, dialysis, hemoperfusion, and exchange transfusion are unlikely to be of benefit. No specific antidotes for fluoxetine are known.

A specific caution involves patients who are taking or have recently taken fluoxetine and might ingest excessive quantities of a TCA. In such a case, accumulation of the parent tricyclic and/or an active metabolite may increase the possibility of clinically significant sequelae and extend the time needed for close medical observation (see Other Antidepressants *under* PRECAUTIONS).

Based on experience in animals, which may not be relevant to humans, fluoxetine-induced seizures that fail to remit spontaneously may respond to diazepam.

In managing overdosage, consider the possibility of multiple drug involvement. The physician should consider contacting a poison control center for additional information on the treatment of any overdose. Telephone numbers for certified poison control centers are listed in the *Physicians' Desk Reference (PDR).*

Dosage and Administration: *Depression: Initial Treatment*—In controlled trials used to support the efficacy of fluoxetine, patients were administered morning doses ranging from 20 to 80 mg/day. Studies comparing fluoxetine 20, 40, and 60 mg/day to placebo indicate that 20 mg/day is suf-

ficient to obtain a satisfactory antidepressant response in most cases. Consequently, a dose of 20 mg/day, administered in the morning, is recommended as the initial dose.

A dose increase may be considered after several weeks if no clinical improvement is observed. Doses above 20 mg/day may be administered on a once a day (morning) or b.i.d. schedule (ie, morning and noon) and should not exceed a maximum dose of 80 mg/day.

As with other antidepressants, the full antidepressant effect may be delayed until 4 weeks of treatment or longer.

As with many other medications, a lower or less frequent dosage should be used in patients with hepatic impairment. A lower or less frequent dosage should also be considered for the elderly (see Geriatric Use *under* PRECAUTIONS), and for patients with concurrent disease or on multiple concomitant medications. Dosage adjustments for renal impairment are not routinely necessary (see Liver Disease *and* Renal Disease *under* CLINICAL PHARMACOLOGY, *and* Use in Patients with Concomitant Illness *under* PRECAUTIONS).

Maintenance/Continuation/Extended Treatment—It is generally agreed that acute episodes of depression require several months or longer of sustained pharmacologic therapy. Whether the dose of antidepressant needed to induce remission is identical to the dose needed to maintain and/or sustain euthymia is unknown.

Daily Dosing—Systematic evaluation of Prozac has shown that its antidepressant efficacy is maintained for periods of up to 38 weeks following 12 weeks of open-label acute treatment (50 weeks total) at a dose of 20 mg/day (see Clinical Trials *under* CLINICAL PHARMACOLOGY).

Weekly Dosing—Systematic evaluation of Prozac Weekly has shown that its antidepressant efficacy is maintained for periods of up to 25 weeks with once-weekly dosing following 13 weeks of open-label treatment with Prozac 20 mg once-daily. However, therapeutic equivalence of Prozac Weekly given on a once-weekly basis with Prozac 20 mg given daily for delaying time to relapse has not been established (see Clinical Trials *under* CLINICAL PHARMACOLOGY).

Weekly dosing with Prozac Weekly capsule is recommended to be initiated 7 days after the last daily dose of Prozac 20 mg (see CLINICAL PHARMACOLOGY).

If satisfactory response is not maintained with Prozac Weekly, consider reestablishing a daily dosing regimen (see Clinical Trials *under* CLINICAL PHARMACOLOGY).

Obsessive-Compulsive Disorder:

Initial Treatment—In the controlled clinical trials of fluoxetine supporting its effectiveness in the treatment of obsessive-compulsive disorder, patients were administered fixed daily doses of 20, 40, or 60 mg of fluoxetine or placebo (see Clinical Trials *under* CLINICAL PHARMACOLOGY). In one of these studies, no dose response-relationship for effectiveness was demonstrated. Consequently, a dose of 20 mg/day, administered in the morning, is recommended as the initial dose. Since there was a suggestion of a possible dose response relationship for effectiveness in the second study, a dose increase may be considered after several weeks if insufficient clinical improvement is observed. The full therapeutic effect may be delayed until 5 weeks of treatment or longer.

Doses above 20 mg/day may be administered on a once a day (ie, morning) or b.i.d. schedule (ie, morning and noon). A dose range of 20 to 60 mg/day is recommended, however, doses of up to 80 mg/day have been well tolerated in open studies of OCD. The maximum fluoxetine dose should not exceed 80 mg/day.

As with the use of Prozac in depression, a lower or less frequent dosage should be used in patients with hepatic impairment. A lower or less frequent dosage should also be considered for the elderly (see Geriatric Use *under* PRECAUTIONS), and for patients with concurrent disease or on multiple concomitant medications. Dosage adjustments for renal impairment are not routinely necessary (see Liver Disease *and* Renal Disease *under* CLINICAL PHARMACOLOGY, *and* Use in Patients with Concomitant Illness *under* PRECAUTIONS).

Maintenance/Continuation Treatment—While there are no systematic studies that answer the question of how long to continue Prozac, OCD is a chronic condition and it is reasonable to consider continuation for a responding patient. Although the efficacy of Prozac after 13 weeks has not been documented in controlled trials, patients have been continued in therapy under double-blind conditions for up to an additional 6 months without loss of benefit. However, dosage adjustments should be made to maintain the patient on the lowest effective dosage, and patients should be periodically reassessed to determine the need for treatment.

Bulimia Nervosa:

Initial Treatment—In the controlled clinical trials of fluoxetine supporting its effectiveness in the treatment of bulimia nervosa, patients were administered fixed daily fluoxetine doses of 20 or 60 mg, or placebo (see Clinical Trials *under* CLINICAL PHARMACOLOGY). Only the 60 mg dose was statistically significantly superior to placebo in reducing the frequency of binge-eating and vomiting. Consequently, the recommended dose is 60 mg/day, administered in the morning. For some patients it may be advisable to titrate up to this target dose over several days. Fluoxetine doses above 60 mg/day have not been systematically studied in patients with bulimia.

As with the use of Prozac in depression and OCD, a lower or less frequent dosage should be used in patients with hepatic

Continued on next page

Prozac Weekly—Cont.

impairment. A lower or less frequent dosage should also be considered for the elderly (*see* Geriatric Use *under* PRECAUTIONS), and for patients with concurrent disease or on multiple concomitant medications. Dosage adjustments for renal impairment are not routinely necessary (*see* Liver Disease *and* Renal Disease *under* CLINICAL PHARMACOLOGY, *and* Use in Patients with Concomitant Illness *under* PRECAUTIONS).

Maintenance/Continuation Treatment—While there are no systematic studies that answer the question of how long to continue Prozac, bulimia is a chronic condition and it is reasonable to consider continuation for a responding patient. Although the efficacy of Prozac after 16 weeks has not been documented in controlled trials, some patients have been continued in therapy under double-blind conditions for up to an additional 6 months without loss of benefit. However, patients should be periodically reassessed to determine the need for continued treatment.

Switching Patients to a Tricyclic Antidepressant (TCA)—Dosage of a TCA may need to be reduced, and plasma TCA concentrations may need to be monitored temporarily when fluoxetine is coadministered or has been recently discontinued (*see* Other Antidepressants *under* Drug Interactions).

Switching Patients to or from a Monoamine Oxidase Inhibitor—At least 14 days should elapse between discontinuation of an MAOI and initiation of therapy with Prozac. In addition, at least 5 weeks, perhaps longer, should be allowed after stopping Prozac before starting an MAOI (*see* CONTRAINDICATIONS *and* PRECAUTIONS).

How Supplied:

The following products are manufactured by Eli Lilly and Company for Dista Products Company.

Prozac® Pulvules®, USP, are available in:

The 10-mg* Pulvule is opaque green and green, imprinted with DISTA 3104 on the cap and Prozac 10 mg on the body:

NDC 0777-3104-02(PU3104**) Bottles of 100
NDC 0777-3104-07(PU3104**) Bottles of 2000
NDC 0777-3104-82(PU3104**) - 20 FlexPak™§ blister cards of 31

The 20-mg* Pulvule is an opaque green cap and off-white body, imprinted with DISTA 3105 on the cap and Prozac 20 mg on the body:

NDC 0777-3105-30(PU3105**) Bottles of 30
NDC 0777-3105-02(PU3105**) Bottles of 100
NDC 0777-3105-07(PU3105**) Bottles of 2000
NDC 0777-3105-33(PU3105**) (ID† 100) Blisters
NDC 0777-3105-82(PU3105**) - 20 FlexPak™§ blister cards of 31

The 40-mg* Pulvule is an opaque green cap and opaque orange body, imprinted with DISTA 3107 on the cap and Prozac 40 mg on the body:

NDC 0777-3107-30(PU3107**) - Bottles of 30

Liquid, Oral Solution is available in:

20 mg* per 5 mL with mint flavor:

NDC 0777-5120-58(MS-5120‡) - Bottles of 120 mL

The following products are manufactured and distributed by Eli Lilly and Company. Prozac® Tablets are available in:

The 10-mg* tablet is green, elliptical shaped, and scored, with PROZAC 10 debossed on opposite side of score.

NDC 0002-4006-30(TA4006)-Bottles of 30
NDC 0002-4006-02(TA4006)-Bottles of 100

Prozac® Weekly™ Capsules are available in:

The 90 mg* capsule is an opaque green cap and clear body containing discretely visible white pellets through the clear body of the capsule, imprinted with Lilly on the cap, and 3004 and 90 mg on the body.

NDC 0002-3004-75(PU3004)-Blister package of 4

---

*Fluoxetine base equivalent.
**Protect from light.
†Identi-Dose® (unit dose medication, Lilly).
‡Dispense in a tight, light-resistant container.
§FlexPak™ (flexible blister card, Lilly).
Store at controlled room temperature, 59° to 86°F (15° to 30°C).

ANIMAL TOXICOLOGY

Phospholipids are increased in some tissues of mice, rats, and dogs given fluoxetine chronically. This effect is reversible after cessation of fluoxetine treatment. Phospholipid accumulation in animals has been observed with many cationic amphiphilic drugs, including fenfluramine, imipramine, and ranitidine. The significance of this effect in humans is unknown.

Literature revised February 28, 2001

PV 3451 DPP   [22801]
www.lilly.com   PRINTED IN USA
Eli Lilly and Company
Indianapolis, IN 46285
USA
Prozac® (fluoxetine hydrochloride)

To keep your **PDR** up to date throughout the year, note these revisions on the corresponding pages of the annual volume. Simply write **"See Supplement A"** next to the product heading.

3M Pharmaceuticals

3M CENTER, BLDG. 275-6W-13
ST. PAUL, MN 55133-3275

Commercial Customers:
Orders, Returns, Accounting
(800) 447-4537

Trade and Government:
(800) 328-6523

For Medical Information Contact:
Drug Surveillance & Information
3M Pharmaceuticals
3M Center, Bldg. 275-6W-13
St. Paul, MN 55133-3275
(800) 328-0255
For Aldara™:
(800) 814-1795
In Emergencies:
(651) 736-4930 (all hours)

Website:
www.3M.com/pharma

QVAR™   ℞
(beclomethasone dipropionate HFA)
Inhalation Aerosol

DESCRIPTION

The active component of QVAR 40 mcg Inhalation Aerosol and QVAR 80 mcg Inhalation Aerosol is beclomethasone dipropionate, USP, an anti-inflammatory corticosteroid having the chemical name 9-chloro-11β,17,21-trihydroxy-16β-methylpregna-1,4-diene-3,20-dione 17,21-dipropionate. Beclomethasone dipropionate is a diester of beclomethasone, a synthetic corticosteroid chemically related to dexamethasone. Beclomethasone differs from dexamethasone in having a chlorine at the 9-alpha carbon in place of a fluorine, and in having a 16 beta-methyl group instead of a 16 alpha-methyl group. Beclomethasone dipropionate is a white to creamy white, odorless powder with a molecular formula of $C_{28}H_{37}ClO_7$ and a molecular weight of 521.1. Its chemical structure is:

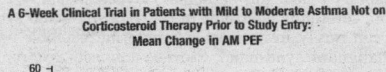

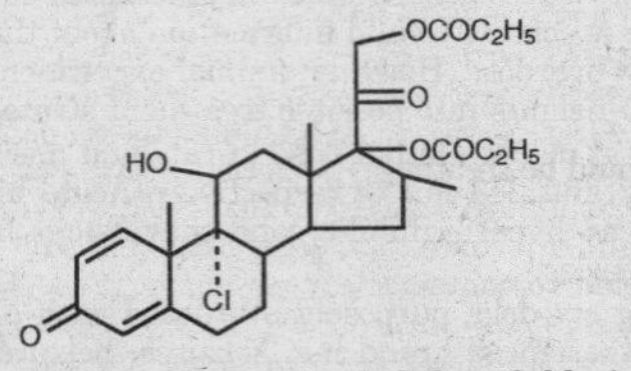

Beclomethasone dipropionate is slightly soluble in water, very soluble in chloroform and freely soluble in acetone and in alcohol.

QVAR is a pressurized, metered-dose aerosol intended for oral inhalation only. Each unit contains a solution of beclomethasone dipropionate in propellant HFA-134a (1,1,1,2 tetrafluoroethane) and ethanol. QVAR 40 mcg delivers 40 mcg of beclomethasone dipropionate from the actuator and 50 mcg from the valve. QVAR 80 mcg delivers 80 mcg of beclomethasone dipropionate from the actuator and 100 mcg from the valve. This product delivers 50 microliters (59 milligrams) of solution formulation from the valve with each actuation. Each canister provides 100 inhalations. QVAR should be "primed" or actuated twice prior to taking the first dose from a new canister, or when the inhaler has not been used for more than ten days. Avoid spraying in the eyes or face while priming QVAR.

This product does not contain chlorofluorocarbons (CFCs).

CLINICAL PHARMACOLOGY

Airway inflammation is known to be an important component in the pathogenesis of asthma. Inflammation occurs in both large and small airways. Corticosteroids have multiple anti-inflammatory effects, inhibiting both inflammatory cells and release of inflammatory mediators. It is presumed that these anti-inflammatory actions play an important role in the efficacy of beclomethasone dipropionate in controlling symptoms and improving lung function in asthma. Inhaled beclomethasone dipropionate probably acts topically at the site of deposition in the bronchial tree after inhalation.

Pharmacokinetics

Bioavailability information on beclomethasone dipropionate (BDP) after inhaled administration is not available in adults. BDP undergoes rapid and extensive conversion to beclomethasone-17-monopropionate (17-BMP) during absorption. The pharmacokinetics of 17-BMP have been studied in asthmatics given single doses.

Absorption: The mean peak plasma concentration (C_{max}) of BDP was 88 pg/ml at 0.5 hour after inhalation of 320 mcg using QVAR (four actuations of the 80 mcg/actuation strength). The mean peak plasma concentration of the major and most active metabolite, 17-BMP, was 1419 pg/ml at 0.7 hour after inhalation of 320 mcg of QVAR. When the same nominal dose is provided by the two QVAR strengths (40 and 80 mcg/actuation), equivalent systemic pharmacokinetics can be expected. The C_{max} of 17-BMP increased dose proportionally in the dose range of 80 and 320 mcg.

Metabolism: Three major metabolites are formed via cytochrome P450 3A catalyzed biotransformation—

---

beclomethasone-17-monopropionate (17-BMP), beclomethasone-21-monopropionate (21-BMP) and beclomethasone (BOH). Lung slices metabolize BDP rapidly to 17-BMP and more slowly to BOH. 17-BMP is the most active metabolite.

Distribution: There is no evidence of tissue storage of BDP or its metabolites.

Elimination: The major route of elimination of inhaled BDP appears to be via metabolism. More than 90% of inhaled BDP is found as 17-BMP in the systemic circulation. The mean elimination half-life of 17-BMP is 2.8 hours. Irrespective of the route of administration (injection, oral or inhalation), BDP and its metabolites are mainly excreted in the feces. Less than 10% of the drug and its metabolites are excreted in the urine.

Special Populations: Formal pharmacokinetic studies using QVAR were not conducted in any special populations.

Pharmacodynamics

Improvement in asthma control following inhalation can occur within 24 hours of beginning treatment in some patients, although maximum benefit may not be achieved for 1 to 2 weeks, or longer. The effects of QVAR on the hypothalamic-pituitary-adrenal (HPA) axis were studied in 40 corticosteroid naive patients. QVAR, at doses of 80, 160 or 320 mcg twice daily was compared with placebo and 336 mcg twice daily of beclomethasone dipropionate in a CFC propellant based formulation (CFC-BDP). Active treatment groups showed an expected dose-related reduction in 24-hour urinary free cortisol (a sensitive marker of adrenal production of cortisol). Patients treated with the highest recommended dose of QVAR (320 mcg twice daily) had a 37.3% reduction in 24-hour urinary free cortisol compared to a reduction of 47.3% produced by treatment with 336 mcg twice daily of CFC-BDP. There was a 12.2% reduction in 24 hour urinary free cortisol seen in the group of patients that received 80 mcg twice daily of QVAR and a 24.6% reduction in the group of patients that received 160 mcg twice daily. An open label study of 354 asthma patients given QVAR at recommended doses for one year assessed the effect of QVAR treatment on the HPA axis (as measured by both morning and stimulated plasma cortisol). Less than 1% of patients treated for one year with QVAR had an abnormal response (peak less than 18 mcg/dL) to short-cosyntropin test.

CLINICAL TRIALS

Blinded, randomized, parallel, placebo-controlled and active-controlled clinical studies were conducted in 940 adult asthma patients to assess the efficacy and safety of QVAR in the treatment of asthma. Fixed doses ranging from 40 mcg to 160 mcg twice daily were compared to placebo, and doses ranging from 40 mcg to 320 mcg twice daily were compared with doses of 42 mcg to 336 mcg twice daily of an active CFC-BDP comparator. These studies provided information about appropriate dosing through a range of asthma severity. In all efficacy trials, at the doses studied, measures of pulmonary function [forced expiratory volume in 1 second (FEV_1) and morning peak expiratory flow (AM PEF)] and asthma symptoms were significantly improved with QVAR treatment when compared to placebo.

In controlled clinical trials with patients not adequately controlled with beta-agonist alone, QVAR was effective at improving asthma control at doses as low as 40 mcg twice daily (80 mcg/day). Comparable asthma control was achieved at lower daily doses of QVAR than with CFC-BDP. Treatment with increasing doses of both QVAR and CFC-BDP generally resulted in increased improvement in FEV_1. In this trial the improvement in FEV_1 across doses was greater for QVAR than for CFC-BDP, indicating a shift in the dose response curve for QVAR. For this reason, when considering QVAR dosing selection for patients currently using CFC-BDP, it is important to consult the dosing recommendations specifically for QVAR (see DOSAGE AND ADMINISTRATION).

Patients Not Previously Receiving Corticosteroid Therapy

In a 6 week clinical trial, 270 steroid naive patients with symptomatic asthma being treated with as-needed beta-agonist bronchodilators, were randomized to receive either 40 mcg twice daily of QVAR, 80 mcg twice daily of QVAR, or placebo. Both doses of QVAR were effective in improving asthma control with significantly greater improvements in FEV_1, AM PEF, and asthma symptoms than with placebo. Shown below is the change from baseline in AM PEF during this trial.

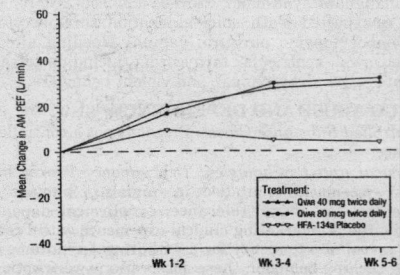

A 6-Week Clinical Trial in Patients with Mild to Moderate Asthma Not on Corticosteroid Therapy Prior to Study Entry: Mean Change in AM PEF

In a 6-week clinical trial, 256 patients with symptomatic asthma being treated with as-needed beta-agonist bronchodilators, were randomized to receive either 160 mcg twice daily of QVAR (delivered as either 40 mcg/actuation or 80 mcg/actuation) or placebo. Treatment with QVAR significantly improved asthma control, as assessed by FEV$_1$, AM PEF, and asthma symptoms, when compared to treatment with placebo. Comparable improvement in AM PEF was seen for patients receiving 160 mcg twice daily QVAR from the 40 mcg and 80 mcg strength products.

Patients Responsive to a Short Course of Oral Corticosteroids

In another clinical trial, 347 patients with symptomatic asthma, being treated with as-needed inhaled beta-agonist bronchodilators and, in some cases, inhaled corticosteroids, were given a 7–12 day course of oral corticosteroids and then randomized to receive either 320 mcg daily of QVAR, 672 mcg of CFC-BDP, or placebo. Patients treated with either QVAR or CFC-BDP had significantly better asthma control, as assessed by AM PEF, FEV$_1$ and asthma symptoms, and fewer study withdrawals due to asthma symptoms, than those treated with placebo over 12 weeks of treatment. A daily dose of 320 mcg QVAR administered in divided doses provided comparable control of AM PEF and FEV$_1$ as 672 mcg of CFC-BDP. Shown below are the mean AM PEF results from this trial.

A 12-Week Clinical Trial in Moderate Symptomatic Patients with Asthma Responding to Oral Corticosteroid Therapy: Mean AM PEF by Study Week

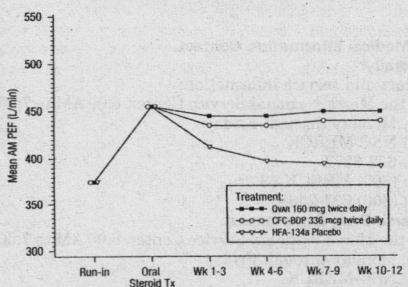

Patients Previously on Inhaled Corticosteroids

In a 6-week clinical trial, 323 patients, who exhibited a deterioration in asthma control during an inhaled corticosteroid washout period, were randomized to daily treatment with either 40, 160, or 320 mcg twice daily QVAR or 42, 168, or 336 mcg twice daily CFC-BDP. Treatment with increasing doses of both QVAR and CFC-BDP resulted in increased improvement in FEV$_1$, FEF$_{25-75\%}$ (forced expiratory flow over 25–75% of the vital capacity), and asthma symptoms. Shown below is the change from baseline in FEV$_1$ as percent predicted after 6 weeks of treatment.

A 6-Week Dose Response Clinical Trial in Patients with Inhaled Corticosteroid Dependent Asthma: Mean Change in FEV$_1$ as Percent of Predicted

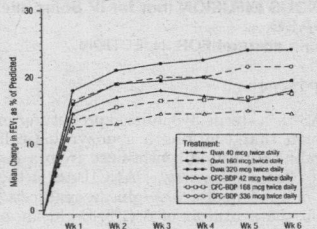

Patients Previously Maintained on Oral Corticosteroids

Clinical experience has shown that some patients with asthma who require oral corticosteroid therapy for control of symptoms can be partially or completely withdrawn from oral corticosteroids if therapy with beclomethasone dipropionate aerosol is substituted. Inhaled corticosteroids may not be effective for all patients with asthma or at all stages of the disease in a given patient.

INDICATIONS AND USAGE

QVAR is indicated in the maintenance treatment of asthma as prophylactic therapy. QVAR is also indicated for asthma patients who require systemic corticosteroid administration, where adding QVAR may reduce or eliminate the need for the systemic corticosteroids.
Beclomethasone dipropionate is NOT indicated for the relief of acute bronchospasm.

CONTRAINDICATIONS

QVAR is contraindicated in the primary treatment of status asthmaticus or other acute episodes of asthma where intensive measures are required.
Hypersensitivity to any of the ingredients of this preparation contraindicates its use.

WARNINGS

Particular care is needed in patients who are transferred from systemically active corticosteroids to QVAR because deaths due to adrenal insufficiency have occurred in asthmatic patients during and after transfer from systemic corticosteroids to less systemically available inhaled corticosteroids. After withdrawal from systemic corticosteroids, a number of months are required for recovery of hypothalamic-pituitary-adrenal (HPA) function.

Patients who have been previously maintained on 20 mg or more per day of prednisone (or its equivalent) may be most susceptible, particularly when their systemic corticosteroids have been almost completely withdrawn. During this period of HPA suppression, patients may exhibit signs and symptoms of adrenal insufficiency when exposed to trauma, surgery, or infections (particularly gastroenteritis) or other conditions with severe electrolyte loss. Although QVAR may provide control of asthmatic symptoms during these episodes, in recommended doses it supplies less than normal physiological amounts of glucocorticoid systemically and does NOT provide the mineralocorticoid that is necessary for coping with these emergencies.
During periods of stress or a severe asthmatic attack, patients who have been withdrawn from systemic corticosteroids should be instructed to resume oral corticosteroids (in large doses) immediately and to contact their physician for further instruction. These patients should also be instructed to carry a warning card indicating that they may need supplementary systemic steroids during periods of stress or a severe asthma attack.

Transfer of patients from systemic steroid therapy to QVAR may unmask allergic conditions previously suppressed by the systemic steroid therapy, e.g., rhinitis, conjunctivitis, and eczema.
Persons who are on drugs which suppress the immune system are more susceptible to infections than healthy individuals. Chickenpox and measles, for example, can have a more serious or even fatal course in non-immune children or adults on corticosteroids. In such children or adults who have not had these diseases or been properly immunized, particular care should be taken to avoid exposure. It is not known how the dose, route and duration of corticosteroid administration affects the risk of developing a disseminated infection. Nor is the contribution of the underlying disease and/or prior corticosteroid treatment known. If exposed to chickenpox, prophylaxis with varicella-zoster immune globulin (VZIG) may be indicated. If exposed to measles, prophylaxis with pooled intramuscular immunoglobulin (IG) may be indicated. (See the respective package inserts for complete VZIG and IG prescribing information.) If chickenpox develops, treatment with antiviral agents may be considered.
QVAR is not a bronchodilator and is not indicated for rapid relief of bronchospasm.
As with other inhaled asthma medications, bronchospasm, with an immediate increase in wheezing, may occur after dosing. If bronchospasm occurs following dosing with QVAR, it should be treated immediately with a short acting inhaled bronchodilator. Treatment with QVAR should be discontinued and alternate therapy instituted. Patients should be instructed to contact their physician immediately when episodes of asthma, which are not responsive to bronchodilators, occur during the course of treatment with QVAR. During such episodes, patients may require therapy with oral corticosteroids.

PRECAUTIONS

General: During withdrawal from oral corticosteroids, some patients may experience symptoms of systemically active corticosteroid withdrawal, e.g., joint and/or muscular pain, lassitude and depression, despite maintenance or even improvement of respiratory function. Although suppression of HPA function below the clinical normal range did not occur with doses of QVAR up to and including 640 mcg/day, a dose dependent reduction of adrenal cortisol production was observed. Since inhaled beclomethasone dipropionate is absorbed into the circulation and can be systemically active, HPA axis suppression by QVAR could occur when recommended doses are exceeded or in particularly sensitive individuals. Since individual sensitivity to effects on cortisol production exist, physicians should consider this information when prescribing QVAR. Because of the possibility of systemic absorption of inhaled corticosteroids, patients treated with these drugs should be observed carefully for any evidence of systemic corticosteroid effect. Particular care should be taken in observing patients postoperatively or during periods of stress for evidence of inadequate adrenal response. It is possible that systemic corticosteroid effects, such as hypercorticism and adrenal suppression, may appear in a small number of patients, particularly at higher doses. If such changes occur, QVAR should be reduced slowly, consistent with accepted procedures for management of asthma symptoms and for tapering of systemic steroids.
A reduction in growth velocity in growing children may occur as a result of inadequate control of chronic diseases such as asthma or from use of corticosteroids for treatment. Physicians should closely follow the growth of all pediatric patients taking corticosteroids by any route and weigh the benefits of corticosteroid therapy and asthma control against the possibility of growth suppression.
The long-term and systemic effects of QVAR in humans are still not fully known. In particular, the effects resulting from chronic use of the agent on developmental or immunologic processes in the mouth, pharynx, trachea, and lung are unknown.
Inhaled corticosteroids should be used with caution, if at all, in patients with active or quiescent tuberculosis infection of the respiratory tract; untreated systemic fungal, bacterial, parasitic or viral infections; or ocular herpes simplex.
Rare instances of glaucoma, increased intraocular pressure, and cataracts have been reported following the inhaled administration of corticosteroids.

Information for Patients: Patients being treated with QVAR should receive the following information and instructions. This information is intended to aid them in the safe and effective use of this medication. It is not a disclosure of all possible adverse or intended effects.
Persons who are on immunosuppressant doses of corticosteroids should be warned to avoid exposure to chickenpox or measles. Patients should also be advised that if they are exposed to these diseases, medical advice should be sought without delay.
Patients should use QVAR at regular intervals as directed. Results of clinical trials indicated significant improvements may occur within the first 24 hours of treatment in some patients; however, the full benefit may not be achieved until treatment has been administered for 1 to 2 weeks, or longer. The patient should not increase the prescribed dosage but should contact their physician if symptoms do not improve or if the condition worsens.
Patients should be advised that QVAR is not intended for use in the treatment of acute asthma. The patient should be instructed to contact their physician immediately if there is any deterioration of their asthma.
Patients should be instructed on the proper use of their inhaler. Patients may wish to rinse their mouth after QVAR use. The patient should also be advised that QVAR may have a different taste and inhalation sensation than that of an inhaler containing CFC propellant.
QVAR use should not be stopped abruptly. The patient should contact their physician immediately if use of QVAR is discontinued.
For the proper use of QVAR, the patient should read and carefully follow the Patient's Instructions which accompany each package of QVAR.

Carcinogenesis, Mutagenesis, Impairment of Fertility: The carcinogenicity of beclomethasone dipropionate was evaluated in rats which were exposed for a total of 95 weeks, 13 weeks at inhalation doses up to 0.4 mg/kg/day and the remaining 82 weeks at combined oral and inhalation doses up to 2.4 mg/kg/day. There was no evidence of carcinogenicity in this study at the highest dose, which is approximately 30 times the maximum recommended human daily inhalation dose on a mg/m^2 basis.
Beclomethasone dipropionate did not induce gene mutation in the bacterial cells or mammalian Chinese Hamster ovary (CHO) cells *in vitro*. No significant clastogenic effect was seen in cultured CHO cells *in vitro* or in the mouse micronucleus test *in vivo*.
In rats, beclomethasone dipropionate caused decreased conception rates at an oral dose of 16 mg/kg/day (approximately 200 times the maximum recommended human daily inhalation dose on a mg/m^2 basis). Impairment of fertility, as evidence by inhibition of the estrous cycle in dogs, was observed following treatment by the oral route at a dose of 0.5 mg/kg/day (approximately 20 times the maximum recommended human daily inhalation dose on a mg/m^2 basis). No inhibition of the estrous cycle in dogs was seen following 12 months of exposure to beclomethasone dipropionate by the inhalation route at an estimated daily dose of 0.33 mg/kg (approximately 15 times the maximum recommended human daily inhalation dose on a mg/m^2 basis).
Pregnancy: Teratogenic Effects: Pregnancy Category C: Like other corticosteroids, parenteral (subcutaneous) beclomethasone dipropionate was teratogenic and embryocidal in the mouse and rabbit when given at a dose of 0.1 mg/kg/day in mice or at a dose of 0.025 mg/kg/day in rabbits. These doses in mice and rabbits were approximately one-half the maximum recommended human daily inhalation dose on a mg/m^2 basis. No teratogenicity or embryocidal effects were seen in rats when exposed to an inhalation dose of 15 mg/kg/day (approximately 190 times the maximum recommended human daily inhalation dose on a mg/m^2 basis). There are no adequate and well controlled studies in pregnant women. Beclomethasone dipropionate should be used during pregnancy only if the potential benefit justifies the potential risk to the fetus.
Non-teratogenic Effects: Findings of drug-related adrenal toxicity in fetuses following administration of beclomethasone dipropionate to rats suggest that infants born of mothers receiving substantial doses of QVAR during pregnancy should be observed for adrenal suppression.
Nursing Mothers: Corticosteroids are secreted in human milk. Because of the potential for serious adverse reactions in nursing infants from QVAR, a decision should be made whether to discontinue nursing or to discontinue the drug, taking into account the importance of the drug to the mother.
Pediatric Use: Eighty (80) patients between the ages of 12 and 16 years were treated with QVAR in clinical trials (16 in US pivotal clinical trials and 64 in a trial conducted outside the US). The safety and effectiveness of QVAR in children below 12 years of age have not been established. Oral corticosteroids have been shown to cause a reduction in growth velocity in children and teenagers with extended use. If a child or teenager on any corticosteroid appears to have growth suppression, the possibility that they are particularly sensitive to this effect of corticosteroids should be considered (see PRECAUTIONS, General).
Geriatric Use: Clinical studies of QVAR did not include sufficient numbers of subjects aged 65 and over to determine whether they respond differently from younger subjects. Other reported clinical experience has not identified differences in responses between the elderly and younger patients. In general, dose selection for an elderly patient should be

Continued on next page

Qvar—Cont.

cautious, usually starting at the low end of the dosing range, reflecting the greater frequency of decreased hepatic, renal, or cardiac function, and of concomitant disease or other drug therapy.

ADVERSE REACTIONS

The following reporting rates of common adverse experiences are based upon four clinical trials in which 1196 Patients (671 female and 525 male adults previously treated with as-needed bronchodilators and/or inhaled corticosteroids) were treated with QVAR (doses of 40, 80, 160, or 320 mcg twice daily) or CFC-BDP (doses of 42, 168, or 336 mcg twice daily) or placebo. The table below includes all events reported by patients taking QVAR (whether considered drug related or not) that occurred at a rate over 3% for either QVAR or CFC-BDP. In considering these data, difference in average duration of exposure and clinical trial design should be taken into account.
[See table below]
Other adverse events that occurred in these clinical trials using QVAR with an incidence of 1% to 3% and which occurred at a greater incidence than placebo were: dysphonia, dysmenorrhea and coughing.
No patients treated with QVAR in the clinical development program developed symptomatic oropharyngeal candidiasis. If such an infection develops, treatment with appropriate antifungal therapy or discontinuance of treatment with QVAR may be required.
Rare cases of immediate and delayed hypersensitivity reactions, including urticaria, angioedema, rash, and bronchospasm, have been reported following the oral and intranasal inhalation of beclomethasone dipropionate.

OVERDOSAGE

There were no deaths over 15 days following the oral administration of a single dose of 3000 mg/kg in mice, 2000 mg/kg in rats, and 1000 mg/kg in rabbits. The doses in mice, rats, and rabbits were 19,000, 25,000, and 25,000 times, respectively, the maximum recommended human daily inhalation dose on a mg/m^2 basis.

DOSAGE AND ADMINISTRATION

Patients should prime QVAR by actuating into the air twice before using for the first time or if QVAR has not been used for over ten days. Avoid spraying in the eyes or face when priming QVAR. QVAR is a solution aerosol, which does not require shaking. Consistent dose delivery is achieved, whether using the 40 or 80 mcg strengths, due to proportionality of the two products (i.e., two actuations of 40 mcg strength should provide a dose comparable to one actuation of the 80 mcg strength).
QVAR should be administered by the oral inhaled route in patients 12 years of age and older. The onset and degree of symptom relief will vary in individual patients. Improvement in asthma symptoms should be expected within the first or second week of starting treatment, but maximum benefit should not be expected until 3–4 weeks of therapy. For patients who do not respond adequately to the starting dose after 3–4 weeks of therapy, higher doses may provide additional asthma control. The safety and efficacy of QVAR when administered in excess of recommended doses has not been established.
[See table below]
The recommended dosage of QVAR relative to CFC-based beclomethasone dipropionate (CFC-BDP) inhalation aerosols is lower due to differences in delivery characteristics between the products. Recognizing that a definitive comparative therapeutic ratio between QVAR and CFC-BDP has not been demonstrated, any patient who is switched from CFC-BDP to QVAR should be dosed appropriately, taking into ac-

count the dosing recommendations above, and should be monitored to ensure that the dose of QVAR selected is safe and efficacious. As with any inhaled corticosteroid, physicians are advised to titrate the dose of QVAR downward over time to the lowest level that maintains proper asthma control.
Patients should be instructed on the proper use of their inhaler. Patients should be advised that QVAR may have a different taste and inhalation sensation than that of an inhaler containing CFC propellant.
Pediatric Use: Safety and effectiveness of QVAR have not been demonstrated in pediatric patients less than 12 years of age.
Patients Not Receiving Systemic Corticosteroids
Patients who require maintenance therapy of their asthma may benefit from treatment with QVAR at the doses recommended above. In patients who respond to QVAR, improvement in pulmonary function is usually apparent within 1 to 4 weeks after the start of therapy. Once the desired effect is achieved, consideration should be given to tapering to the lowest effective dose.
Patients Maintained on Systemic Corticosteroids
QVAR may be effective in the management of asthmatics maintained on systemic corticosteroids and may permit replacement or significant reduction in the dosage of systemic corticosteroids.
The patient's asthma should be reasonably stable before treatment with QVAR is started. Initially, QVAR should be used concurrently with the patient's usual maintenance dose of systemic corticosteroids. After approximately one week, gradual withdrawal of the systemic corticosteroids is started by reducing the daily or alternate daily dose. Reductions may be made after an interval of one or two weeks, depending on the response of the patient. A slow rate of withdrawal is strongly recommended. Generally these decrements should not exceed 2.5 mg of prednisone or its equivalent. During withdrawal, some patients may experience symptoms of systemic corticosteroid withdrawal, e.g. joint and/or muscular pain, lassitude and depression, despite maintenance or even improvement in pulmonary function. Such patients should be encouraged to continue with the inhaler but should be monitored for objective signs of adrenal insufficiency. If evidence of adrenal insufficiency occurs, the systemic corticosteroid doses should be increased temporarily and thereafter withdrawal should continue more slowly. During periods of stress or a severe asthma attack, transfer patients may require supplementary treatment with systemic corticosteroids.

DIRECTIONS FOR USE

Illustrated Patient's Instructions for proper use accompany each package of QVAR.

HOW SUPPLIED

QVAR is supplied in two strengths:
QVAR 40 mcg is supplied in a 7.3 g canister containing 100 actuations with a beige plastic actuator and gray dust cap, and Patient's Instructions; box of one; 100 Actuations—NDC 50580-175-40
QVAR 80 mcg is supplied in a 7.3 g canister containing 100 actuations with a dark mauve plastic actuator and gray dust cap, and Patient's Instructions; box of one; 100 Actuations—NDC 50580-177-80
The correct amount of medication in each inhalation cannot be assured after 100 actuations from the 7.3 g canister even though the canister is not completely empty. The canister should be discarded when the labeled number of actuations have been used.
Store QVAR Inhalation Aerosol when not being used, so that the product rests on the concave end of the canister with the plastic actuator on top.
Store at 25°C (77°F).

Excursions between 15° and 30°C (59° and 86°F) are permitted (see USP). For optimal results, the canister should be at room temperature when used. QVAR Inhalation Aerosol canister should only be used with the QVAR Inhalation Aerosol actuator and the actuator should not be used with any other inhalation drug product.
CONTENTS UNDER PRESSURE
Do not puncture. Do not use or store near heat or open flame. Exposure to temperatures above 49°C (120°F) may cause bursting. Never throw container into fire or incinerator.
Keep out of reach of children.
Rx only
Developed and Manufactured by:
3M Pharmaceuticals   OR   3M Health Care, Ltd.
Northridge, CA 91324   Loughborough, UK
For:
McNeil Consumer Healthcare
Fort Washington, PA 19034
November 2000
3M, McNeil and QVAR are trademarks

Merck & Co., Inc.
WEST POINT, PA 19486

For Medical Information Contact:
Generally:
Product and service information:
Call the Merck National Service Center, 8:00 AM to 7:00 PM (ET), Monday through Friday:
(800) NSC-MERCK
(800) 672-6372
FAX: (800) MERCK-68
FAX: (800) 637-2568
Adverse Drug Experiences:
Call the Merck National Service Center, 8:00 AM to 7:00 PM (ET), Monday through Friday:
(800) NSC-MERCK
(800) 672-6372
In Emergencies:
24-hour emergency information for healthcare professionals:
(800) NSC-MERCK
(800) 672-6372

Sales and Ordering:
For product orders and direct account inquiries only, call the Order Management Center,
8:00 AM to 7:00 PM (ET), Monday through Friday:
(800) MERCK RX
(800) 637-2579

INTRAVENOUS INFUSION (not for IV Bolus Injection)
CANCIDAS®   ℞
(caspofungin acetate) FOR INJECTION

DESCRIPTION

CANCIDAS* is a sterile, lyophilized product for intravenous (IV) infusion that contains a semisynthetic lipopeptide (echinocandin) compound synthesized from a fermentation product of *Glarea lozoyensis*. CANCIDAS is the first of a new class of antifungal drugs (glucan synthesis inhibitors) that inhibit the synthesis of β (1,3)-D-glucan, an integral component of the fungal cell wall.
CANCIDAS (caspofungin acetate) is 1-[(4R,5S)-5-[(2-amino-ethyl)amino]-N^2-(10,12-dimethyl-1-oxotetradecyl)-4-hydroxy-L-ornithine]-5-[(3R)-3-hydroxy-L-ornithine] pneumocandin B$_0$ diacetate (salt). In addition to the active ingredient caspofungin acetate, CANCIDAS contains the following inactive ingredients: sucrose, mannitol, acetic acid, and sodium hydroxide. Caspofungin acetate is a hygroscopic, white to off-white powder. It is freely soluble in water and methanol, and slightly soluble in ethanol. The pH of a saturated aqueous solution of caspofungin acetate is approximately 6.6. The empirical formula is $C_{52}H_{88}N_{10}O_{15} \cdot 2C_2H_4O_2$ and the formula weight is 1213.42. The structural formula is:

Adverse Events Reported by at Least 3% of the Patients for Either QVAR or CFC-BDP by Treatment and Daily Dose

Adverse Events	Placebo (N=289) %	QVAR Total (N=624) %	QVAR 80–160 mcg (N=233) %	QVAR 320 mcg (N=335) %	QVAR 640 mcg (N=56) %	CFC-BDP Total (N=283) %	CFC-BDP 84 mcg (N=59) %	CFC-BDP 336 mcg (N=55) %	CFC-BDP 672 mcg (N=169) %
HEADACHE	9	12	15	8	25	15	14	11	17
PHARYNGITIS	4	8	6	5	27	10	12	9	10
UPPER RESP TRACT INFECTION	11	9	7	11	5	12	3	9	17
RHINITIS	9	6	8	3	7	11	15	9	10
INCREASED ASTHMA SYMPTOMS	18	3	2	4	0	8	14	5	7
ORAL SYMPTOMS INHALATION ROUTE	2	3	3	3	2	6	7	5	5
SINUSITIS	2	3	3	3	0	4	7	2	4
PAIN	<1	2	1	2	5	3	3	5	2
BACK PAIN	1	1	2	<1	4	4	2	4	4
NAUSEA	0	1	<1	1	2	3	5	5	1
DYSPHONIA	2	<1	1	0	4	4	0	0	6

Recommended Dosage for QVAR:

Previous Therapy	Recommended Starting Dose	Highest Recommended Dose
Bronchodilators Alone	40 to 80 mcg twice daily	320 mcg twice daily
Inhaled Corticosteroids	40 to 160 mcg twice daily	320 mcg twice daily

*Registered trademark of MERCK & CO., Inc.

CLINICAL PHARMACOLOGY

Pharmacokinetics

Distribution

Plasma concentrations of caspofungin decline in a polyphasic manner following single 1-hour IV infusions. A short α-phase occurs immediately postinfusion, followed by a β-phase (half-life of 9 to 11 hours) that characterizes much of the profile and exhibits clear log-linear behavior from 6 to 48 hours postdose during which the plasma concentration decreases 10-fold. An additional, longer half-life phase, γ-phase, (half-life of 40-50 hours), also occurs. Distribution, rather than excretion or biotransformation, is the dominant mechanism influencing plasma clearance. Caspofungin is extensively bound to albumin (~97%), and distribution into red blood cells is minimal. Mass balance results showed that approximately 92% of the administered radioactivity was distributed to tissues by 36 to 48 hours after a single 70-mg dose of [³H] caspofungin acetate. There is little excretion or biotransformation of caspofungin during the first 30 hours after administration.

Metabolism

Caspofungin is slowly metabolized by hydrolysis and N-acetylation. Caspofungin also undergoes spontaneous chemical degradation to an open-ring peptide compound, L-747969. At later time points (5 to 20 days postdose), there is a low level (3 to 7 picomoles/mg protein, or 0.6 to 1.3% of administered dose) of covalent binding of radiolabel in plasma following single-dose administration of [³H] caspofungin acetate, which may be due to two reactive intermediates formed during the chemical degradation of caspofungin to L-747969. Additional metabolism involves hydrolysis into constitutive amino acids and their degradates, including dihydroxyhomotyrosine and N-acetyl-dihydroxyhomotyrosine. These two tyrosine derivatives are found only in urine, suggesting rapid clearance of these derivatives by the kidneys.

Excretion

In a single-dose radiolabeled pharmacokinetic study, plasma, urine, and feces were collected over 27 days. Plasma concentrations of radioactivity and of caspofungin were similar during the first 24 to 48 hours postdose; thereafter drug levels fell more rapidly. Radiolabel remained quantifiable through Day 27, whereas caspofungin concentrations fell below the limit of quantitation after 6 to 8 days postdose. After single intravenous administration of [³H] caspofungin acetate, excretion of caspofungin and its metabolites in humans were 35% of dose in feces and 41% of dose in urine. A small amount of caspofungin is excreted unchanged in urine (~1.4% of dose). Renal clearance of parent drug is low (~0.15 mL/min) and total clearance of caspofungin is 12 mL/min.

Special Populations

Gender

Plasma concentrations of caspofungin in healthy men and women were similar following a single 70-mg dose. After 13 daily 50-mg doses, caspofungin plasma concentrations in women were elevated slightly (approximately 22% in area under the curve [AUC]) relative to men. No dosage adjustment is necessary based on gender.

Geriatric

Plasma concentrations of caspofungin in healthy older men and women (≥65 years of age) were increased slightly (approximately 28% in area under the curve [AUC]) compared to young healthy men after a single 70-mg dose of caspofungin. Age is not a significant determinant of caspofungin pharmacokinetics in patients with fungal infections. No dosage adjustment is necessary for the elderly (see PRECAUTIONS, *Geriatric Use*).

Race

Regression analyses of patient pharmacokinetic data indicated that no clinically significant differences in the pharmacokinetics of caspofungin were seen among Caucasians, Blacks, and Hispanics. No dosage adjustment is necessary on the basis of race.

Renal Insufficiency

In a clinical study of single 70-mg doses, caspofungin pharmacokinetics were similar in volunteers with mild renal insufficiency (creatinine clearance 50 to 80 mL/min) and control subjects. Moderate (creatinine clearance 31 to 49 mL/min), advanced (creatinine clearance 5 to 30 mL/min), and end-stage (creatinine clearance <10 mL/min and dialysis dependent) renal insufficiency moderately increased caspofungin plasma concentrations after single-dose administration (range: 30 to 49% for AUC). However, in patients with invasive aspergillosis who received multiple daily doses of CANCIDAS 50 mg, there was no significant effect of mild to advanced renal impairment on caspofungin trough concentrations. No dosage adjustment is necessary for patients with renal insufficiency. Caspofungin is not dialyzable, thus supplementary dosing is not required following hemodialysis.

Hepatic Insufficiency

Plasma concentrations of caspofungin after a single 70-mg dose in patients with mild hepatic insufficiency (Child-Pugh score 5 to 6) were increased by approximately 55% in AUC compared to healthy control subjects. In a 14-day multiple-dose study (70 mg on Day 1 followed by 50 mg daily thereafter), plasma concentrations in patients with mild hepatic insufficiency were increased modestly (19 to 25% in AUC) on Days 7 and 14 relative to healthy control subjects. No dosage adjustment is recommended for patients with mild he-

patic insufficiency. Patients with moderate hepatic insufficiency (Child-Pugh score 7 to 9) who received a single 70-mg dose of CANCIDAS had an average plasma caspofungin increase of 76% in AUC compared to control subjects. A dosage reduction is recommended for patients with moderate hepatic insufficiency (see DOSAGE AND ADMINISTRATION). There is no clinical experience in patients with severe hepatic insufficiency (Child-Pugh score >9).

Pediatric Patients

CANCIDAS has not been adequately studied in patients under 18 years of age.

MICROBIOLOGY

Mechanism of Action

Caspofungin acetate, the active ingredient of CANCIDAS, inhibits the synthesis of β (1,3)-D-glucan, an essential component of the cell wall of susceptible filamentous fungi. β (1,3)-D-glucan is not present in mammalian cells. Caspofungin has shown activity in regions of active cell growth of the hyphae of *Aspergillus fumigatus*.

Activity in vitro

Caspofungin exhibits *in vitro* activity against *Aspergillus fumigatus*, *Aspergillus flavus*, and *Aspergillus terreus*. Susceptibility testing was performed according to the National Committee for Clinical Laboratory Standards (NCCLS) proposed method (M38-P). Standardized susceptibility testing methods for β (1,3)-D-glucan synthesis inhibitors have not been established, and results of susceptibility studies do not correlate with clinical outcome.

Activity in vivo

Caspofungin, administered parenterally to immunocompetent and immunosuppressed rodents, as long as 24 hours after disseminated or pulmonary infection with *Aspergillus fumigatus*, has shown prolonged survival, which has not been consistently associated with a reduction in mycological burden.

Drug Resistance

In vitro resistance development to caspofungin by *Aspergillus* species has not been studied. In limited clinical experience, drug resistance in patients with invasive aspergillosis has not been observed. The incidence of drug resistance by various clinical isolates of *Aspergillus* species is unknown.

Drug Interactions

Studies *in vitro* and *in vivo* of caspofungin, in combination with amphotericin B, suggest no antagonism of antifungal activity against *A. fumigatus*. The clinical significance of these results is unknown.

CLINICAL STUDIES

Invasive Aspergillosis

Sixty-nine patients between the ages of 18 and 80 with invasive aspergillosis were enrolled in an open-label, noncomparative study to evaluate the safety, tolerability, and efficacy of CANCIDAS. Enrolled patients had previously been refractory to or intolerant of other antifungal therapy(ies). Refractory patients were classified as those who had disease progression or failed to improve despite therapy for at least 7 days with amphotericin B, lipid formulations of amphotericin B, itraconazole, or an investigational azole with reported activity against *Aspergillus*. Intolerance to previous therapy was defined as a doubling of creatinine (or creatinine ≥2.5 mg/dL while on therapy), other acute reactions, or infusion-related toxicity. To be included in the study, patients with pulmonary disease must have had definite (positive tissue histopathology or positive culture from tissue obtained by an invasive procedure) or probable (positive radiographic or computed tomography evidence with supporting culture from bronchoalveolar lavage or sputum, galactomannan enzyme-linked immunosorbent assay, and/or polymerase chain reaction) invasive aspergillosis. Patients with extrapulmonary disease had to have definite invasive aspergillosis. The definitions were modeled after the Mycoses Study Group Criteria.[1] Patients were administered a single 70-mg loading dose of CANCIDAS and subsequently dosed with 50 mg daily. The mean duration of therapy was 33.7 days, with a range of 1 to 162 days.

---

[1] Denning DW, Lee JY, Hostetler JS, et al. NIAID Mycoses Study Group multicenter trial of oral itraconazole therapy for invasive aspergillosis. *Am J Med* 1994; 97:135-144.

An independent expert panel evaluated patient data, including diagnosis of invasive aspergillosis, response and tolerability to previous antifungal therapy, treatment course on CANCIDAS, and clinical outcome.

A favorable response was defined as either complete resolution (complete response) or clinically meaningful improvement (partial response) of all signs and symptoms and attributable radiographic findings. Stable, nonprogressive disease was considered to be an unfavorable response.

Among the 69 patients enrolled in the study, 63 met entry diagnostic criteria and had outcome data; and of these, 52 patients received treatment for >7 days. Fifty-three (84%) were refractory to previous antifungal therapy and 10 (16%) were intolerant. Forty-five patients had pulmonary disease and 18 had extrapulmonary disease. Underlying conditions were hematologic malignancy (N=24), allogeneic bone marrow transplant or stem cell transplant (N=18), organ transplant (N=8), solid tumor (N=3), or other conditions (N=10). All patients in the study received concomitant therapies for their other underlying conditions. Eighteen patients received tacrolimus and CANCIDAS concomitantly, of whom 8 also received mycophenolate mofetil.

Overall, the expert panel determined that 41% (26/63) of patients receiving at least one dose of CANCIDAS had a favorable response. For those patients who received >7 days of

therapy with CANCIDAS, 50% (26/52) had a favorable response. The favorable response rates for patients who were either refractory to or intolerant of previous therapies were 36% (19/53) and 70% (7/10), respectively. The response rates among patients with pulmonary disease and extrapulmonary disease were 47% (21/45) and 28% (5/18), respectively. Among patients with extrapulmonary disease, 2 of 8 patients who also had definite, probable, or possible CNS involvement had a favorable response. Two of these 8 patients had progression of disease and manifested CNS involvement while on therapy.

There is substantial evidence that CANCIDAS is well tolerated and effective for the treatment of invasive aspergillosis in patients who are refractory to or intolerant of itraconazole, amphotericin B, and/or lipid formulations of amphotericin B. However, the efficacy of CANCIDAS has not been evaluated in concurrently controlled clinical studies, with other antifungal therapies.

INDICATIONS AND USAGE

CANCIDAS is indicated for the treatment of invasive aspergillosis in patients who are refractory to or intolerant of other therapies (i.e., amphotericin B, lipid formulations of amphotericin B, and/or itraconazole).

CANCIDAS has not been studied as initial therapy for invasive aspergillosis.

CONTRAINDICATIONS

CANCIDAS is contraindicated in patients with hypersensitivity to any component of this product.

WARNINGS

Concomitant use of CANCIDAS with cyclosporine is not recommended unless the potential benefit outweighs the potential risk to the patient. In one clinical study, 3 of 4 healthy subjects who received CANCIDAS 70 mg on Days 1 through 10, and also received two 3 mg/kg doses of cyclosporine 12 hours apart on Day 10, developed transient elevations of alanine transaminase (ALT) on Day 11 that were 2 to 3 times the upper limit of normal (ULN). In a separate panel of subjects in the same study, 2 of 8 who received CANCIDAS 35 mg daily for 3 days and cyclosporine (two 3 mg/kg doses administered 12 hours apart) on Day 1 had small increases in ALT (slightly above the ULN) on Day 2. In both groups, elevations in aspartate transaminase (AST) paralleled ALT elevations, but were of lesser magnitude (see ADVERSE REACTIONS, *Laboratory Abnormalities*.) Hence, concomitant use of CANCIDAS with cyclosporine is not recommended until multiple-dose use in patients is studied.

PRECAUTIONS

General

The efficacy of a 70-mg dose regimen in patients who are not clinically responding to the 50 mg daily dose is not known. Limited safety data suggest that an increase in dose to 70 mg daily is well tolerated. The safety and efficacy of doses above 70 mg have not been adequately studied.

The safety information on treatment durations longer than 2 weeks is limited, however, available data suggest that CANCIDAS continues to be well tolerated with longer courses of therapy (68 patients received from 15 to 60 days of therapy; 12 patients received from 61 to 162 days of therapy).

Drug Interactions

Studies *in vitro* show that caspofungin acetate is not an inhibitor of any enzyme in the cytochrome P450 (CYP) system. In clinical studies, caspofungin did not induce the CYP3A4 metabolism of other drugs. Caspofungin is not a substrate for P-glycoprotein and is a poor substrate for cytochrome P450 enzymes.

Clinical studies in healthy volunteers show that the pharmacokinetics of CANCIDAS are not altered by itraconazole, amphotericin B, mycophenolate, or tacrolimus. CANCIDAS has no effect on the pharmacokinetics of itraconazole, amphotericin B, or the active metabolite of mycophenolate.

CANCIDAS reduced the blood AUC_{0-12} of tacrolimus (FK-506, Prograf®[2]) by approximately 20%, peak blood concentration (C_{max}) by 16%, and 12-hour blood concentration (C_{12hr}) by 26% in healthy subjects when tacrolimus (2 doses of 0.1 mg/kg 12 hours apart) was administered on the 10th day of CANCIDAS 70 mg daily, as compared to results from a control period in which tacrolimus was administered alone. For patients receiving both therapies, standard monitoring of tacrolimus blood concentrations and appropriate tacrolimus dosage adjustments are recommended.

---

[2] Registered trademark of Fujisawa Healthcare, Inc.

In two clinical studies, cyclosporine (one 4 mg/kg dose or two 3 mg/kg doses) increased the AUC of caspofungin by approximately 35%. CANCIDAS did not increase the plasma levels of cyclosporine. There were transient increases in liver ALT and AST when CANCIDAS and cyclosporine were coadministered (see WARNINGS and ADVERSE EFFECTS, *Laboratory Abnormalities*).

The results from regression analyses of patient pharmacokinetic data suggest that coadministration of inducers of

Continued on next page

Information on the Merck & Co. products listed on these pages is from the full prescribing information in use April 1, 2001.

Cancidas—Cont.

drug clearance and/or mixed inducer/inhibitors with CANCIDAS may result in clinically meaningful reductions in caspofungin concentrations. This is based on results from a small number of patients who were administered the inducers and/or mixed inducer/inhibitors efavirenz, nelfinavir, nevirapine, phenytoin, rifampin, dexamethasone, or carbamazepine prior to and/or concomitant with caspofungin. There are presently no data from formal drug interaction studies to evaluate these regression analyses of patient pharmacokinetic data, and it is not known which drug clearance mechanism involved in caspofungin disposition may be inducible. When coadministering CANCIDAS with efavirenz, nelfinavir, nevirapine, phenytoin, rifampin, dexamethasone, or carbamazepine, an increase in the daily dose of CANCIDAS to 70 mg, following the usual 70-mg loading dose, should be considered in patients who are not clinically responding.

Carcinogenesis, Mutagenesis, and Impairment of Fertility
No long-term studies in animals have been performed to evaluate the carcinogenic potential of caspofungin.
Caspofungin did not show evidence of mutagenic or genotoxic potential when evaluated in the following *in vitro* assays: bacterial (Ames) and mammalian cell (V79 Chinese hamster lung fibroblasts) mutagenesis assays, the alkaline elution/rat hepatocyte DNA strand break test, and the chromosome aberration assay in Chinese hamster ovary cells. Caspofungin was not genotoxic when assessed in the mouse bone marrow chromosomal test at doses up to 12.5 mg/kg (equivalent to a human dose of 1 mg/kg based on body surface area comparisons), administered intravenously.
Fertility and reproductive performance were not affected by the intravenous administration of caspofungin to rats at doses up to 5 mg/kg. At 5 mg/kg exposures were similar to those seen in patients treated with the 70-mg dose.

Pregnancy
Pregnancy Category C. CANCIDAS was shown to be embryotoxic in rats and rabbits. Findings included incomplete ossification of the skull and torso and an increased incidence of cervical rib in rats.
An increased incidence of incomplete ossifications of the talus/calcaneus was seen in rabbits. Caspofungin also produced increases in resorptions in rats and rabbits and peri-implantation losses in rats. These findings were observed at doses which produced exposures similar to those seen in patients treated with a 70-mg dose. Caspofungin crossed the placental barrier in rats and rabbits and was detected in the plasma of fetuses of pregnant animals dosed with CANCIDAS. There are no adequate and well-controlled studies in pregnant women. CANCIDAS should be used during pregnancy only if the potential benefit justifies the potential risk to the fetus.

Nursing Mothers
Caspofungin was found in the milk of lactating, drug-treated rats. It is not known whether caspofungin is excreted in human milk. Because many drugs are excreted in human milk, caution should be exercised when caspofungin is administered to a nursing woman.

Patients with Hepatic Insufficiency
Patients with mild hepatic insufficiency (Child-Pugh score 5 to 6) do not need a dosage adjustment. For patients with moderate hepatic insufficiency (Child-Pugh score 7 to 9), after the initial 70-mg loading dose, CANCIDAS 35 mg daily is recommended. There is no clinical experience in patients with severe hepatic insufficiency (Child-Pugh score >9).

Pediatric Use
Safety and effectiveness in pediatric patients have not been established.

Geriatric Use
Clinical studies of CANCIDAS did not include sufficient numbers of patients aged 65 and over to determine whether they respond differently from younger patients. Although the number of elderly patients was not large enough for a statistical analysis, no overall differences in safety or efficacy were observed between these and younger patients. Plasma concentrations of caspofungin in healthy older men and women (≥65 years of age) were increased slightly (approximately 28% in AUC) compared to young healthy men. No dose adjustment is recommended for the elderly; however, greater sensitivity of some older individuals cannot be ruled out.

ADVERSE REACTIONS

General
Possible histamine-mediated symptoms have been reported in clinical studies including isolated reports of rash, facial swelling, pruritus, or sensation of warmth. One case of anaphylaxis characterized by dyspnea, stridor, and worsening of rash during initial administration of CANCIDAS was reported.

Clinical Adverse Experiences
The overall safety of caspofungin was assessed in 623 individuals who received single or multiple doses of caspofungin acetate. Of the 623 individuals, 349 patients were enrolled in phase II and phase III clinical studies. Patients in clinical studies often had serious underlying medical conditions (e.g., HIV, bone marrow transplant, hematologic malignancy) requiring multiple concomitant medications. Sixty-nine patients with invasive aspergillosis were enrolled in an open-label noncomparative study; the majority of these patients had underlying hematologic malignancies.
Clinical adverse experiences with an incidence ≥2%, reported in patients treated with CANCIDAS in the noncomparative aspergillosis study are presented in Table 1.

TABLE 1
Drug-related Clinical Adverse Experiences in Patients with Invasive Aspergillosis (open-label, noncomparative study)*
Incidence ≥2% by Body System

	CANCIDAS 50 mg N=69 (percent)
Body as a Whole	
Fever	2.9
Peripheral Vascular System	
Infused vein complications	2.9
Digestive System	
Nausea	2.9
Vomiting	2.9
Skin & Skin Appendage	
Flushing	2.9

*Relationship to drug was determined by the investigator to be possibly, probably, or definitely drug-related. Patients received CANCIDAS 70 mg on Day 1, then 50 mg daily for the remainder of their treatment.

Also reported infrequently in this patient population were pulmonary edema, ARDS, and radiographic infiltrates.
Laboratory abnormalities with an incidence ≥2%, reported in patients treated with CANCIDAS in the noncomparative aspergillosis study are presented in Table 2.

TABLE 2
Drug-related Laboratory Abnormalities Reported Among Patients with Invasive Aspergillosis (open-label, noncomparative study)*
Incidence ≥2% by Body System

	CANCIDAS 50 mg N=69 (percent)
Blood Chemistry	
Serum alkaline phosphatase increased	2.9
Serum potassium decreased	2.9
Hematology	
Eosinophils increased	3.2
Urinalysis	
Urine protein increased	4.9
Urine RBCs increased	2.2

*Relationship to drug was determined by the investigator to be possibly, probably, or definitely drug-related. Patients received CANCIDAS 70 mg on Day 1, then 50 mg daily for the remainder of their treatment.

Drug-related clinical adverse experiences occurring in ≥2% of patients in 3 active-control studies for investigational indications other than aspergillosis are presented in Table 3. [See table 3 at left]
Laboratory abnormalities occurring in ≥2% of patients in 3 active-control studies for investigational indications other than aspergillosis are presented in Table 4. [See table 4 on next page]
In one clinical study, 3 of 4 subjects who received CANCIDAS 70 mg daily on Days 1 through 10, and also received two 3 mg/kg doses of cyclosporine 12 hours apart on Day 10, developed transient elevations of ALT on Day 11 that were 2 to 3 times the upper limit of normal (ULN). In a separate panel of subjects in the same study, 2 of 8 subjects who received CANCIDAS 35 mg daily for 3 days and cyclosporine (two 3 mg/kg doses administered 12 hours apart) on Day 1 had small increases in ALT (slightly above the ULN) on Day 2. In another clinical study, 2 of 8 healthy men developed transient ALT elevations of less than 2X ULN. In this study, cyclosporine (4 mg/kg) was administered on Days 1 and 12, and CANCIDAS was administered (70 mg) daily on Days 3 through 13. In one subject, the ALT elevation occurred on Days 7 and 9 and, in the other subject, the ALT elevation occurred on Day 19. These elevations returned to normal by Day 27. In all groups, elevations in AST paralleled ALT elevations but were of lesser magnitude. In these clinical studies, cyclosporine (one 4 mg/kg dose or two 3 mg/kg doses) increased the AUC of caspofungin by approximately 35% (see WARNINGS).

TABLE 3
Drug-related Clinical Adverse Experiences Among Patients Treated for Investigational Indications Other than Aspergillosis*
Incidence ≥2% for at least one treatment dose (per comparison) by Body System

	CANCIDAS 50 mg[†] N=83 (percent)	CANCIDAS 50 mg[††] N=80 (percent)	CANCIDAS 70 mg[††] N=65 (percent)	Amphotericin B 0.5 mg/Kg[††] N=89 (percent)
Body as a Whole				
Asthenia/fatigue	**	0.0	0.0	6.7
Chills	**	2.5	1.5	75.3
Edema/swelling	**	0.0	0.0	5.6
Edema, facial	**	0.0	3.1	0.0
Fever	3.6	21.3	26.2	69.7
Flu-like illness	**	0.0	3.1	0.0
Malaise	**	0.0	0.0	5.6
Pain	**	1.3	4.6	5.6
Pain, abdominal	3.6	2.5	0.0	9.0
Warm sensation	**	0.0	1.5	4.5
Peripheral Vascular System				
Infused vein complication	12.0	2.5	1.5	0.0
Phlebitis/thrombophlebitis	15.7	11.3	13.8	22.5
Cardiovascular System				
Tachycardia	**	1.3	0.0	4.5
Vasculitis	**	0.0	0.0	3.4
Digestive System				
Anorexia	**	1.3	0.0	3.4
Diarrhea	3.6	1.3	3.1	11.2
Nausea	6.0	2.5	3.1	21.3
Vomiting	1.2	1.3	3.1	13.5
Hemic & Lymphatic System				
Anemia	**	3.8	0.0	9.0
Metabolic/Nutritional/Immune				
Anaphylaxis	**	0.0	0.0	2.2
Musculoskeletal System				
Myalgia	**	0.0	3.1	2.2
Pain, back	**	0.0	0.0	2.2
Pain, musculoskeletal	**	1.3	0.0	4.5
Nervous System & Psychiatric				
Headache	6.0	11.3	7.7	19.1
Insomnia	**	0.0	0.0	2.2
Paresthesia	**	1.3	3.1	1.1
Tremor	**	0.0	0.0	7.9
Respiratory System				
Tachypnea	**	1.3	0.0	4.5
Skin & Skin Appendage				
Erythema	**	1.3	1.5	7.9
Induration	**	0.0	3.1	6.7
Pruritus	**	2.5	1.5	0.0
Rash	**	1.3	4.6	3.4
Sweating	**	1.3	0.0	3.4

*Relationship to drug was determined by the investigator to be possibly, probably or definitely drug-related.
**Incidence <2%
[†]Derived from a Phase III comparator-controlled clinical study.
[††]Derived from Phase II comparator-controlled clinical studies.

OVERDOSAGE

In clinical studies the highest dose was 100 mg, administered as a single dose to 5 patients. This dose was generally well tolerated. No overdosages have been reported. Caspofungin is not dialyzable. The minimum lethal dose of caspofungin in rats was 50 mg/kg, a dose which is equivalent to 10 times the recommended daily dose based on relative body surface area comparison.

ANIMAL PHARMACOLOGY AND TOXICOLOGY

In one 5-week study in monkeys at doses which produced exposures approximately 4 to 6 times those seen in patients treated with a 70-mg dose, scattered small foci of subcapsular necrosis were observed microscopically in the livers of some animals (2/8 monkeys at 5 mg/kg and 4/8 monkeys at 8 mg/kg); however, this histopathological finding was not seen in another study of 27 weeks duration at similar doses.

DOSAGE AND ADMINISTRATION

General Recommendations
A single 70-mg loading dose should be administered on Day 1, followed by 50 mg daily thereafter. CANCIDAS should be administered by slow IV infusion of approximately 1 hour. Duration of treatment should be based upon the severity of the patient's underlying disease, recovery from immunosuppression, and clinical response. Do not mix or co-infuse CANCIDAS with other medications. DO NOT USE DILUENTS CONTAINING DEXTROSE (α-D-GLUCOSE). The efficacy of a 70 mg dose regimen in patients who are not clinically responding to the 50 mg daily dose is not known. Limited safety data suggests that an increase in dose to 70 mg daily is well tolerated. The safety and efficacy of doses above 70 mg have not been adequately studied.
Hepatic Insufficiency
Patients with mild hepatic insufficiency (Child-Pugh score 5 to 6) do not need a dosage adjustment. However, for patients with moderate hepatic insufficiency (Child-Pugh score 7 to 9), after the initial 70-mg loading dose, CANCIDAS 35 mg daily is recommended. There is no clinical experience in patients with severe hepatic insufficiency (Child-Pugh score >9) (see CLINICAL PHARMACOLOGY, *Pharmacokinetics, Special Populations*).

Preparation of the 70-mg Day 1 loading-dose infusion
1. Equilibrate the refrigerated vial of CANCIDAS to room temperature.
2. Aseptically add 10.5 mL of 0.9% Sodium Chloride Injection to the vial.[a] This reconstituted solution may be stored for up to one hour at ≤25°C (≤77°F).[b]
3. Aseptically transfer 10 mL[c] of reconstituted CANCIDAS to an IV bag (or bottle) containing 250 mL 0.9% Sodium Chloride Injection.[d] (If a 70-mg vial is unavailable, see below: *Alternative Infusion Preparation Methods, Preparation of 70-mg Day 1 loading dose from two 50-mg vials.*)
Preparation of the daily 50-mg infusion
1. Equilibrate the refrigerated vial of CANCIDAS to room temperature.
2. Aseptically add 10.5 mL of 0.9% Sodium Chloride Injection to the vial.[a] This reconstituted solution may be stored for up to one hour at ≤25°C (≤77°F).[b]
3. Aseptically transfer 10 mL[c] of reconstituted CANCIDAS to an IV bag (or bottle) containing 250 mL 0.9% Sodium Chloride Injection.[d] (If a reduced infusion volume is medically necessary, see below: *Alternative Infusion Preparation Methods, Preparation of 50-mg daily doses at reduced volume.*)
Alternative Infusion Preparation Methods
Preparation of 70-mg Day 1 loading dose from two 50-mg vials
Reconstitute two 50-mg vials with 10.5 mL of diluent each (see *Preparation of the daily 50-mg infusion*). Aseptically transfer a total of 14 mL of the reconstituted CANCIDAS from the two vials to 250 mL of 0.9% Sodium Chloride Injection.
Preparation of 50-mg daily doses at reduced volume
When medically necessary, the 50-mg daily doses can be prepared by adding 10 mL of reconstituted CANCIDAS to 100 mL of 0.9% Sodium Chloride Injection (see *Preparation of the daily 50-mg infusion*).
Preparation of a 35-mg daily dose for patients with moderate Hepatic Insufficiency
Reconstitute one 50-mg vial (see above: *Preparation of the daily 50-mg infusion*). Aseptically transfer 7 mL of the reconstituted CANCIDAS from the vial to 250 mL of 0.9% Sodium Chloride Injection or, if medically necessary, to 100 mL of 0.9% Sodium Chloride Injection.

Preparation notes:
[a]The white to off-white cake will dissolve completely. Mix gently until a clear solution is obtained.
[b]Visually inspect the reconstituted solution for particulate matter or discoloration during reconstitution and prior to infusion. Do not use if the solution is cloudy or has precipitated.
[c]CANCIDAS is formulated to provide the full labeled vial dose (70 mg or 50 mg) when 10 mL is withdrawn from the vial.
[d]This infusion solution must be used within 24 hours, during which time it should be kept at ≤25°C (≤77°F).

[See table 5 below]

HOW SUPPLIED

No. 3822 — CANCIDAS 50 mg is a white to off-white powder/cake for infusion in a vial labeled with a red aluminum band and a plastic cap.
NDC 0006-3822-10 one single-use vial.
No. 3823 — CANCIDAS 70 mg is a white to off-white powder/cake for infusion in a vial with a yellow/orange aluminum band and a plastic cap.
NDC 0006-3823-10 one single-use vial.
Storage
Vials
The lyophilized vials should be stored refrigerated at 2° to 8°C (36° to 46°F).
Reconstituted Concentrate
Reconstituted CANCIDAS may be stored at ≤25°C (≤77°F) for one hour prior to the preparation of the patient infusion solution.
Diluted Product
The final patient infusion solution in the IV bag or bottle can be stored at ≤25°C (≤77°F) for 24 hours.

9344300   Issued January 2001
COPYRIGHT ©MERCK & CO., INC., Whitehouse Station, NJ 08889, USA
All rights reserved

TABLE 4
Drug-related Laboratory Abnormalities Reported Among Patients Treated for Investigational Indications Other than Aspergillosis*
Incidence ≥2% (for at least one treatment dose) by Laboratory Test Category

	CANCIDAS 50 mg[†] N=163 (percent)	CANCIDAS 70 mg[††] N=65 (percent)	Amphotericin B 0.5 mg/Kg[††] N=89 (percent)
Blood Chemistry			
ALT increased	10.6	10.8	22.7
AST increased	13.0	10.8	22.7
Blood urea increased	0.0	0.0	10.3
Direct serum bilirubin increased	0.6	0.0	2.5
Serum albumin decreased	8.6	4.6	14.9
Serum alkaline phosphatase increased	10.5	7.7	19.3
Serum bicarbonate decreased	0.9	0.0	6.6
Serum creatinine increased	0.0	1.5	28.1
Serum potassium decreased	3.7	10.8	31.5
Serum uric acid increased	0.6	0.0	3.4
Total serum bilirubin increased	0.0	0.0	4.5
Total serum protein decreased	3.1	0.0	3.4
Hematology			
Eosinophils increased	3.1	3.1	1.1
Hematocrit decreased	11.1	1.5	32.6
Hemoglobin decreased	12.3	3.1	37.1
Neutrophils decreased	1.9	3.1	1.1
Platelet count decreased	3.1	1.5	3.4
Prothrombin time increased	1.3	1.5	2.3
WBC count decreased	6.2	4.6	7.9
Urinalysis			
Urine blood increased	0.0	0.0	4.0
Urine casts increased	0.0	0.0	8.0
Urine pH increased	0.8	0.0	3.6
Urine protein increased	1.2	0.0	4.5
Urine RBCs increased	1.1	3.8	12.0
Urine WBCs increased	0.0	7.7	24.0

*Relationship to drug was determined by the investigator to be possibly, probably or definitely drug-related.
[†]Derived from Phase II and Phase III comparator-controlled clinical studies.
[††]Derived from Phase II comparator-controlled clinical studies.

TABLE 5
CANCIDAS Concentrations

Dose	Reconstituted Solution Concentration	Infusion Volume	Infusion Solution Concentration
70-mg initial dose	7.2 mg/mL	260 mL	0.28 mg/mL
50-mg daily dose	5.2 mg/mL	260 mL	0.20 mg/mL
70-mg initial dose* (from two 50 mg vials)	5.2 mg/mL	264 mL	0.28 mg/mL
50-mg daily dose* (reduced volume)	5.2 mg/mL	110 mL	0.47 mg/mL
35-mg daily dose* (from one 50 mg vial) for Moderate Hepatic Insufficiency	5.2 mg/mL or 5.2 mg/mL	257 mL or 107 mL	0.14 mg/mL or 0.34 mg/mL

*See following text for these special situations

Novartis Pharmaceuticals Corporation

NOVARTIS PHARMACEUTICALS CORPORATION
59 Route 10
East Hanover, NJ 07936
(for branded products)

GENEVA PHARMACEUTICALS, INC.
A NOVARTIS COMPANY
2655 West Midway Boulevard
PO Box 446
Broomfield, CO 80038-0446
(for branded generic product listing refer to Geneva Pharmaceuticals, Inc.)

For Information Contact *(branded products):*

Customer Response Department
(888) NOW-NOVARTIS [888-669-6682]

Global Internet Address:
http://www.novartis.com

For Information Contact *(branded generic products):*

Customer Support Department
(800) 525-8747
(303) 466-2400
FAX: (303) 438-4600

DENAVIR®   ℞
[děn 'ă-vĭr]
brand of
penciclovir cream, 1%
For Dermatologic Use Only
Rx only

Prescribing information for this product, which appears on pages 3051–3052 of the 2001 PDR, has been completely revised as follows. Please write "See Supplement A" next to the product heading.

DESCRIPTION

Denavir contains penciclovir, an antiviral agent active against herpes viruses. *Denavir* is available for topical administration as a 1% white cream. Each gram of *Denavir* contains 10 mg of penciclovir and the following inactive ingredients: cetomacrogol 1000 BP, cetostearyl alcohol, mineral oil, propylene glycol, purified water and white petrolatum.
Chemically, penciclovir is known as 9-[4-hydroxy-3-(hydroxymethyl) butyl]guanine. Its molecular formula is $C_{10}H_{15}N_5O_3$; its molecular weight is 253.26. It is a synthetic acyclic guanine derivative and has the following structure:
[See chemical structure at top of next column]

Continued on next page

Denavir—Cont.

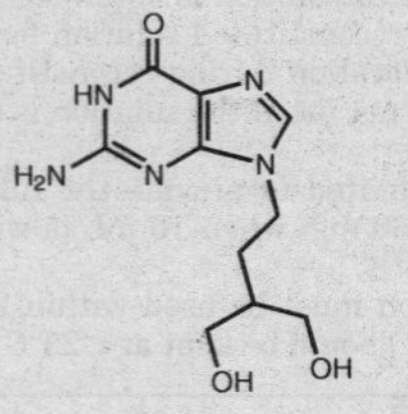

penciclovir

Penciclovir is a white to pale yellow solid. At 20°C it has a solubility of 0.2 mg/mL in methanol, 1.3 mg/mL in propylene glycol, and 1.7 mg/mL in water. In aqueous buffer (pH 2) the solubility is 10.0 mg/mL. Penciclovir is not hygroscopic. Its partition coefficient in n-octanol/water at pH 7.5 is 0.024 (logP= -1.62).

CLINICAL PHARMACOLOGY

Microbiology

Mechanism of Antiviral Activity: The antiviral compound penciclovir has *in vitro* inhibitory activity against herpes simplex virus types 1 (HSV-1) and 2 (HSV-2). In cells infected with HSV-1 or HSV-2, viral thymidine kinase phosphorylates penciclovir to a monophosphate form which, in turn, is converted to penciclovir triphosphate by cellular kinases. *In vitro* studies demonstrate that penciclovir triphosphate inhibits HSV polymerase competitively with deoxyguanosine triphosphate. Consequently, herpes viral DNA synthesis and, therefore, replication are selectively inhibited.

Antiviral Activity *In Vitro* and *In Vivo*: In cell culture studies, penciclovir has antiviral activity against HSV-1 and HSV-2. Sensitivity test results, expressed as the concentration of the drug required to inhibit growth of the virus by 50% (IC_{50}) or 99% (IC_{99}) in cell culture, vary depending upon a number of factors, including the assay protocols. See Table 1.

[See table below]

Drug Resistance: Penciclovir-resistant mutants of HSV can result from qualitative changes in viral thymidine kinase or DNA polymerase. The most commonly encountered acyclovir-resistant mutants that are deficient in viral thymidine kinase are also resistant to penciclovir.

Pharmacokinetics

Measurable penciclovir concentrations were not detected in plasma or urine of healthy male volunteers (n=12) following single or repeat application of the 1% cream at a dose of 180 mg penciclovir daily (approximately 67 times the estimated usual clinical dose).

Pediatric Patients: The systemic absorption of penciclovir following topical administration has not been evaluated in patients <18 years of age.

CLINICAL TRIALS

Denavir was studied in two double-blind, placebo (vehicle)-controlled trials for the treatment of recurrent herpes labialis in which otherwise healthy adults were randomized to either *Denavir* or placebo. Therapy was to be initiated by the subjects within 1 hour of noticing signs or symptoms and continued for 4 days, with application of study medication every 2 hours while awake. In both studies, the mean duration of lesions was approximately one-half-day shorter in the subjects treated with *Denavir* (N=1,516) as compared to subjects treated with placebo (N=1,541) (approximately 4.5 days versus 5 days, respectively). The mean duration of lesion pain was also approximately one-half-day shorter in the *Denavir* group compared to the placebo group.

INDICATIONS AND USAGE

Denavir (penciclovir cream) is indicated for the treatment of recurrent herpes labialis (cold sores) in adults.

CONTRAINDICATIONS

Denavir is contraindicated in patients with known hypersensitivity to the product or any of its components.

PRECAUTIONS

General

Denavir should only be used on herpes labialis on the lips and face. Because no data are available, application to human mucous membranes is not recommended. Particular care should be taken to avoid application in or near the eyes since it may cause irritation. The effect of *Denavir* has not been established in immunocompromised patients.

Carcinogenesis, Mutagenesis, Impairment of Fertility

In clinical trials, systemic drug exposure following the topical administration of penciclovir cream was negligible, as the penciclovir content of all plasma and urine samples was below the limit of assay detection (0.1 mcg/mL and 10 mcg/mL, respectively). However, for the purpose of inter-species dose comparisons presented in the following sections, an assumption of 100% absorption of penciclovir from the topically applied product has been used. Based on use of the maximal recommended topical dose of penciclovir of 0.05 mg/kg/day and an assumption of 100% absorption, the maximum theoretical plasma $AUC_{0\text{-}24\ hrs}$ for penciclovir is approximately 0.129 mcg.hr/mL.

Carcinogenesis: Two-year carcinogenicity studies were conducted with famciclovir (the oral prodrug of penciclovir) in rats and mice. An increase in the incidence of mammary adenocarcinoma (a common tumor in female rats of the strain used) was seen in female rats receiving 600 mg/kg/day (approximately 395× the maximum theoretical human exposure to penciclovir following application of the topical product, based on area under the plasma concentration curve comparisons [24 hr. AUC]). No increases in tumor incidence were seen among male rats treated at doses up to 240 mg/kg/day (approximately 190× the maximum theoretical human AUC for penciclovir), or in male and female mice at doses up to 600 mg/kg/day (approximately 100× the maximum theoretical human AUC for penciclovir).

Mutagenesis: When tested *in vitro*, penciclovir did not cause an increase in gene mutation in the Ames assay using multiple strains of *S. typhimurium* or *E. coli* (at up to 20,000 mcg/plate), nor did it cause an increase in unscheduled DNA repair in mammalian HeLa S3 cells (at up to 5,000 mcg/mL). However, an increase in clastogenic responses was seen with penciclovir in the L5178Y mouse lymphoma cell assay (at doses ≥1000 mcg/mL) and, in human lymphocytes incubated *in vitro* at doses ≥250 mcg/mL. When tested *in vivo*, penciclovir caused an increase in micronuclei in mouse bone marrow following the intravenous administration of doses ≥500 mg/kg (≥810× the maximum human dose, based on body surface area conversion).

Impairment of Fertility: Testicular toxicity was observed in multiple animal species (rats and dogs) following repeated intravenous administration of penciclovir (160 mg/kg/day and 100 mg/kg/day, respectively, approximately 1155 and 3255× the maximum theoretical human AUC). Testicular changes seen in both species included atrophy of the seminiferous tubules and reductions in epididymal sperm counts and/or an increased incidence of sperm with abnormal morphology or reduced motility. Adverse testicular effects were related to an increasing dose or duration of exposure to penciclovir. No adverse testicular or reproductive effects (fertility and reproductive function) were observed in rats after 10 to 13 weeks dosing at 80 mg/kg/day, or testicular effects in dogs after 13 weeks dosing at 30 mg/kg/day (575 and 845× the maximum theoretical human AUC, respectively). Intravenously administered penciclovir had no effect on fertility or reproductive performance in female rats at doses of up to 80 mg/kg/day (260× the maximum human dose [BSA]).

There was no evidence of any clinically significant effects on sperm count, motility or morphology in 2 placebo-controlled clinical trials of Famvir® (famciclovir [the oral prodrug of penciclovir], 250 mg b.i.d.; n=66) in immunocompetent men with recurrent genital herpes, when dosing and follow-up were maintained for 18 and 8 weeks, respectively (approximately 2 and 1 spermatogenic cycles in the human).

Pregnancy

Teratogenic Effects-Pregnancy Category B. No adverse effects on the course and outcome of pregnancy or on fetal development were noted in rats and rabbits following the intravenous administration of penciclovir at doses of 80 and 60 mg/kg/day, respectively (estimated human equivalent doses of 13 and 18 mg/kg/day for the rat and rabbit, respectively, based on body surface area conversion; the body surface area doses being 260 and 355× the maximum recommended dose following topical application of the penciclovir cream). There are, however, no adequate and well-controlled studies in pregnant women. Because animal reproduction studies are not always predictive of human response, penciclovir should be used during pregnancy only if clearly needed.

Nursing Mothers

There is no information on whether penciclovir is excreted in human milk after topical administration. However, following oral administration of famciclovir (the oral prodrug of penciclovir) to lactating rats, penciclovir was excreted in breast milk at concentrations higher than those seen in the plasma. Therefore, a decision should be made whether to discontinue the drug, taking into account the importance of the drug to the mother. There are no data on the safety of penciclovir in newborns.

Pediatric Use

Safety and effectiveness in pediatric patients have not been established.

Geriatric Use

In 74 patients ≥65 years of age, the adverse events profile was comparable to that observed in younger patients.

ADVERSE REACTIONS

In two double-blind, placebo-controlled trials, 1516 patients were treated with Denavir (penciclovir cream) and 1541 with placebo. The most frequently reported adverse event was headache, which occurred in 5.3% of the patients treated with *Denavir* and 5.8% of the placebo-treated patients. The rates of reported local adverse reactions are shown in Table 2 below. One or more local adverse reactions were reported by 2.7% of the patients treated with *Denavir* and 3.9% of placebo-treated patients.

Table 2—Local Adverse Reactions Reported in Phase III Trials

	Penciclovir n=1516 %	Placebo n=1541 %
Application site reaction	1.3	1.8
Hypesthesia/Local anesthesia	0.9	1.4
Taste perversion	0.2	0.3
Pruritus	0.0	0.3
Pain	0.0	0.1
Rash (erythematous)	0.1	0.1
Allergic reaction	0.0	0.1

Two studies, enrolling 108 healthy subjects, were conducted to evaluate the dermal tolerance of 5% penciclovir cream (a 5-fold higher concentration than the commercial formulation) compared to vehicle using repeated occluded patch testing methodology. The 5% penciclovir cream induced mild erythema in approximately one-half of the subjects exposed, an irritancy profile similar to the vehicle control in terms of severity and proportion of subjects with a response. No evidence of sensitization was observed.

OVERDOSAGE

Since penciclovir is poorly absorbed following oral administration, adverse reactions related to penciclovir ingestion are unlikely. There is no information on overdose.

DOSAGE AND ADMINISTRATION

Denavir should be applied every 2 hours during waking hours for a period of 4 days. Treatment should be started as early as possible (i.e., during the prodrome or when lesions appear).

HOW SUPPLIED

Denavir is supplied in a 1.5 gram tube containing 10 mg of penciclovir per gram.

NDC 0078-0369-64

Store at controlled room temperature, 20°-25°C (68°-77°F) [see USP]

Rx only

JANUARY 2001 T2000-71

89011301

Manufactured in Cidra, PR by **SmithKline Beecham Pharmaceuticals**, for

Novartis Pharmaceuticals Corporation

East Hanover, NJ 07936

Table 1

Method of Assay	Virus Type	Cell Type	IC50 (mcg/mL)	IC99 (mcg/mL)
Plaque Reduction	HSV-1 (c.i.)	MRC-5	0.2-0.6	
	HSV-1 (c.i.)	WISH	0.04-0.5	
	HSV-2 (c.i.)	MRC-5	0.9-2.1	
	HSV-2 (c.i.)	WISH	0.1-0.8	
Virus Yield Reduction	HSV-1 (c.i.)	MRC-5		0.4-0.5
	HSV-2 (c.i.)	MRC-5		0.6-0.7
DNA Synthesis Inhibition	HSV-1 (SC16)	MRC-5	0.04	
	HSV-2 (MS)	MRC-5	0.05	

(c.i.) = clinical isolates. The latent stage of any herpes virus is not known to respond to any antiviral therapy.

FAMVIR® ℞

[fam'-vir]

brand of famciclovir

Tablets

Prescribing information for this product, which appears on pages 3091–3094 of the 2001 PDR, has been revised as follows. Please write "See Supplement A" next to the product heading.

DESCRIPTION

Famvir contains famciclovir, an orally administered prodrug of the antiviral agent penciclovir. Chemically, famciclovir is known as 2-[2-(2-amino-9*H*-purin-9-yl)ethyl]-1,3-propanediol diacetate. Its molecular formula is $C_{14}H_{19}N_5O_4$; its molecular weight is 321.3. It is a synthetic acyclic guanine derivative and has the following structure:

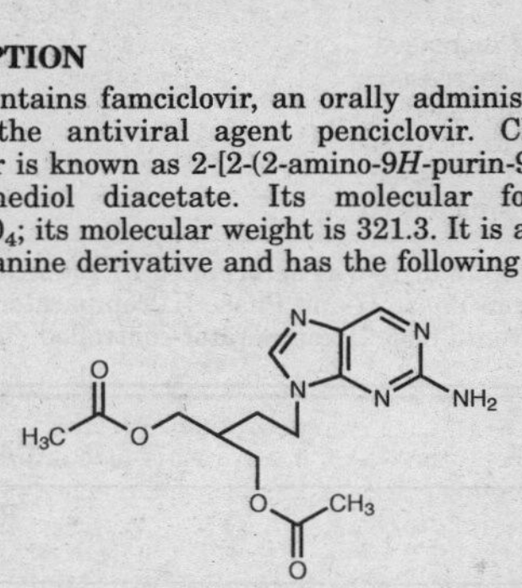

famciclovir

Famciclovir is a white to pale yellow solid. It is freely soluble in acetone and methanol, and sparingly soluble in ethanol and isopropanol. At 25°C famciclovir is freely soluble (>25% w/v) in water initially, but rapidly precipitates as the sparingly soluble (2-3% w/v) monohydrate. Famciclovir is not hygroscopic below 85% relative humidity. Partition coefficients are: octanol/water (pH 4.8) *P*=1.09 and octanol/phosphate buffer (pH 7.4) *P*=2.08.

Tablets for Oral Administration: Each white, film-coated tablet contains famciclovir. The 125 mg and 250 mg tablets

Table 1

Method of Assay	Virus Type	Cell Type	IC_{50} (mcg/mL)	IC_{99}
Plaque Reduction	VZV (c.i.)	MRC-5	5.0 ± 3.0	
	VZV (c.i.)	Hs68	0.9 ± 0.4	
	HSV-1 (c.i.)	MRC-5	0.2 – 0.6	
	HSV-1 (c.i.)	WISH	0.04 – 0.5	
	HSV-2 (c.i.)	MRC-5	0.9 – 2.1	
	HSV-2 (c.i.)	WISH	0.1 – 0.8	
Virus Yield	HSV-1 (c.i.)	MRC-5		0.4 – 0.5
Reduction	HSV-2 (c.i.)	MRC-5		0.6 – 0.7
DNA Synthesis	VZV (Ellen)	MRC-5	0.1	
Inhibition	HSV-1 (SC16)	MRC-5	0.04	
	HSV-2 (MS)	MRC-5	0.05	

(c.i.) = clinical isolates.

are round; the 500 mg tablets are oval. Inactive ingredients consist of hydroxypropyl cellulose, hydroxypropyl methylcellulose, lactose, magnesium stearate, polyethylene glycols, sodium starch glycolate and titanium dioxide.

MICROBIOLOGY

Mechanism of Antiviral Activity: Famciclovir undergoes rapid biotransformation to the active antiviral compound penciclovir, which has inhibitory activity against herpes simplex virus types 1 (HSV-1) and 2 (HSV-2) and varicella zoster virus (VZV). In cells infected with HSV-1, HSV-2 or VZV, viral thymidine kinase phosphorylates penciclovir to a monophosphate form that, in turn, is converted to penciclovir triphosphate by cellular kinases. *In vitro* studies demonstrate that penciclovir triphosphate inhibits HSV-2 DNA polymerase competitively with deoxyguanosine triphosphate. Consequently, herpes viral DNA synthesis and, therefore, replication are selectively inhibited.

Penciclovir triphosphate has an intracellular half-life of 10 hours in HSV-1-, 20 hours in HSV-2- and 7 hours in VZV-infected cells cultured *in vitro*; however, the clinical significance is unknown.

Antiviral Activity *In Vitro* and *In Vivo*: In cell culture studies, penciclovir has antiviral activity against the following herpesviruses (listed in decreasing order of potency): HSV-1, HSV-2 and VZV. Sensitivity test results, expressed as the concentration of the drug required to inhibit the growth of the virus by 50% (IC_{50}) or 99% (IC_{99}) in cell culture, vary greatly depending upon a number of factors, including the assay protocols, and in particular the cell type used. See Table 1.

[See table above]

Drug Resistance: Resistance of HSV and VZV to antiviral nucleoside analogs can result from mutations in the viral thymidine kinase (TK) and DNA polymerase genes. Mutations in the viral TK gene may lead to complete loss of viral TK activity (TK negative), reduced levels of TK activity (TK partial) or alteration in the ability of viral TK to phosphorylate the drug without an equivalent loss in the ability to phosphorylate thymidine (TK altered). The most commonly encountered acyclovir-resistant mutants are TK negative and they are also resistant to penciclovir. The possibility of viral resistance to penciclovir should be considered in patients who fail to respond or experience recurrent viral infections during therapy.

CLINICAL PHARMACOLOGY

Pharmacokinetics

Absorption and Bioavailability: Famciclovir is the diacetyl 6-deoxy analog of the active antiviral compound penciclovir. Following oral administration, little or no famciclovir is detected in plasma or urine.

The absolute bioavailability of famciclovir is 77±8% as determined following the administration of a 500 mg famciclovir oral dose and a 400 mg penciclovir intravenous dose to 12 healthy male subjects.

Penciclovir concentrations increased in proportion to dose over a famciclovir dose range of 125 mg to 750 mg administered as a single dose. Single oral dose administration of 125 mg, 250 mg or 500 mg famciclovir to healthy male volunteers across 17 studies gave the following pharmacokinetic parameters:

Table 2

Dose	AUC (0-inf)† (mcg.hr./mL)	C_{max}‡ (mcg/mL)	T_{max}§ (h)
125 mg	2.24	0.8	0.9
250 mg	4.48	1.6	0.9
500 mg	8.95	3.3	0.9

†AUC (0-inf) (mcg.hr./mL)=area under the plasma concentration-time profile extrapolated to infinity.
‡C_{max} (mcg/mL)=maximum observed plasma concentration.
§T_{max} (h)= time to C_{max}.

Following single oral-dose administration of 500 mg famciclovir to seven patients with herpes zoster, the mean ± SD AUC, C_{max}, and T_{max} were 12.1±1.7 mcg.hr./mL, 4.0±0.7 mcg/mL, and 0.7±0.2 hours, respectively. The AUC of penciclovir was approximately 35% greater in patients with herpes zoster as compared to healthy volunteers. Some of this difference may be due to differences in renal function between the two groups.

There is no accumulation of penciclovir after the administration of 500 mg famciclovir t.i.d. for 7 days.

Penciclovir C_{max} decreased approximately 50% and T_{max} was delayed by 1.5 hours when a capsule formulation of famciclovir was administered with food (nutritional content was approximately 910 Kcal and 26% fat). There was no effect on the extent of availability (AUC) of penciclovir. There was an 18% decrease in C_{max} and a delay in T_{max} of about 1 hour when famciclovir was given 2 hours after a meal as compared to its administration 2 hours before a meal. Because there was no effect on the extent of systemic availability of penciclovir, it appears that *Famvir* can be taken without regard to meals.

Distribution: The volume of distribution (Vd_{β}) was 1.08±0.17 L/kg in 12 healthy male subjects following a single intravenous dose of penciclovir at 400 mg administered as a 1-hour intravenous infusion.

Penciclovir is <20% bound to plasma proteins over the concentration range of 0.1 to 20 mcg/mL. The blood/plasma ratio of penciclovir is approximately 1.

Metabolism: Following oral administration, famciclovir is deacetylated and oxidized to form penciclovir. Metabolites that are inactive include 6-deoxy penciclovir, monoacetylated penciclovir, and 6-deoxy monoacetylated penciclovir (5%, <0.5% and <0.5% of the dose in the urine, respectively). Little or no famciclovir is detected in plasma or urine.

An *in vitro* study using human liver microsomes demonstrated that cytochrome P450 does not play an important role in famciclovir metabolism. The conversion of 6-deoxy penciclovir to penciclovir is catalyzed by aldehyde oxidase.

Elimination: Approximately 94% of administered radioactivity was recovered in urine over 24 hours (83% of the dose was excreted in the first 6 hours) after the administration of 5 mg/kg radiolabeled penciclovir as a 1-hour infusion to three healthy male volunteers. Penciclovir accounted for 91% of the radioactivity excreted in the urine.

Following the oral administration of a single 500 mg dose of radiolabeled famciclovir to three healthy male volunteers, 73% and 27% of administered radioactivity were recovered in urine and feces over 72 hours, respectively. Penciclovir accounted for 82% and 6-deoxy penciclovir accounted for 7% of the radioactivity excreted in the urine. Approximately 60% of the administered radiolabeled dose was collected in urine in the first 6 hours.

After intravenous administration of penciclovir in 48 healthy male volunteers, mean ± S.D. total plasma clearance of penciclovir was 36.6±6.3 L/hr (0.48±0.09 L/hr/kg). Penciclovir renal clearance accounted for 74.5±8.8% of total plasma clearance.

Renal clearance of penciclovir following the oral administration of a single 500 mg dose of famciclovir to 109 healthy male volunteers was 27.7±7.6 L/hr.

The plasma elimination half-life of penciclovir was 2.0±0.3 hours after intravenous administration of penciclovir to 48 healthy male volunteers and 2.3±0.4 hours after oral administration of 500 mg famciclovir to 124 healthy male volunteers. The half-life in seven patients with herpes zoster was 3.0±1.1 hours.

HIV-Infected Patients: Following oral administration of a single dose of 500 mg famciclovir (the oral prodrug of penciclovir) to HIV-positive patients, the pharmacokinetic parameters of penciclovir were comparable to those observed in healthy subjects.

Renal Insufficiency: Apparent plasma clearance, renal clearance, and the plasma-elimination rate constant of penciclovir decreased linearly with reductions in renal function. After the administration of a single 500 mg famciclovir oral dose (n=27) to healthy volunteers and to volunteers with varying degrees of renal insufficiency (CL_{CR} ranged from 6.4 to 138.8 mL/min.), the following results were obtained (Table 3):

[See table below]

In a multiple dose study of famciclovir conducted in subjects with varying degrees of renal impairment (n=18), the pharmacokinetics of penciclovir were comparable to those after single doses.

Table 3

Parameter (mean ± S.D.)	CL_{CR}† ≥ 60 (mL/min.)	CL_{CR} 40-59 (mL/min.)	CL_{CR} 20-39 (mL/min.)	CL_{CR} <20 (mL/min.)
CL_{CR} (mL/min)	88.1 ± 20.6	49.3 ± 5.9	26.5 ± 5.3	12.7 ± 5.9
CL_R (L/hr)	30.1 ± 10.6	13.0 ± 1.3‡	4.2 ± 0.9	1.6 ± 1.0
CL/F§ (L/hr)	66.9 ± 27.5	27.3 ± 2.8	12.8 ± 1.3	5.8 ± 2.8
Half-life (hr)	2.3 ± 0.5	3.4 ± 0.7	6.2 ± 1.6	13.4 ± 10.2
n	15	5	4	3

† CL_{CR} is measured creatinine clearance.
‡ n=4.
§ CL/F consists of bioavailability factor and famciclovir to penciclovir conversion factor.

A dosage adjustment is recommended for patients with renal insufficiency (see DOSAGE AND ADMINISTRATION).

Hepatic Insufficiency: Well-compensated chronic liver disease (chronic hepatitis [n=6], chronic ethanol abuse [n=8], or primary biliary cirrhosis [n=1]) had no effect on the extent of availability (AUC) of penciclovir following a single dose of 500 mg famciclovir. However, there was a 44% decrease in penciclovir mean maximum plasma concentration and the time to maximum plasma concentration was increased by 0.75 hours in patients with hepatic insufficiency compared to normal volunteers. No dosage adjustment is recommended for patients with well-compensated hepatic impairment. The pharmacokinetics of penciclovir have not been evaluated in patients with severe uncompensated hepatic impairment.

Elderly Subjects: Based on cross-study comparisons, mean penciclovir AUC was 40% larger and penciclovir renal clearance was 22% lower after the oral administration of famciclovir in elderly volunteers (n=18, age 65 to 79 years) compared to younger volunteers. Some of this difference may be due to differences in renal function between the two groups.

Gender: The pharmacokinetics of penciclovir were evaluated in 18 healthy male and 18 healthy female volunteers after single-dose oral administration of 500 mg famciclovir. AUC of penciclovir was 9.3±1.9 mcg.hr./mL and 11.1±2.1 mcg.hr./mL in males and females, respectively. Penciclovir renal clearance was 28.5±8.9 L/hr and 21.8±4.3 L/hr, respectively. These differences were attributed to differences in renal function between the two groups. No famciclovir dosage adjustment based on gender is recommended.

Pediatric Patients: The pharmacokinetics of famciclovir or penciclovir have not been evaluated in patients <18 years of age.

Race: The pharmacokinetics of famciclovir or penciclovir with respect to race have not been evaluated.

Drug Interactions

Effects on penciclovir

No clinically significant alterations in penciclovir pharmacokinetics were observed following single-dose administration of 500 mg famciclovir after pre-treatment with multiple doses of allopurinol, cimetidine, theophylline, or zidovudine. No clinically significant effect on penciclovir pharmacokinetics was observed following multiple-dose (t.i.d.) administration of famciclovir (500 mg) with multiple doses of digoxin.

Effects of famciclovir on co-administered drugs

The steady-state pharmacokinetics of digoxin were not altered by concomitant administration of multiple doses of famciclovir (500 mg t.i.d.). No clinically significant effect on the pharmacokinetics of zidovudine or zidovudine glucuronide was observed following a single oral dose of 500 mg famciclovir.

CLINICAL TRIALS

Herpes Zoster

Famvir (famciclovir) was studied in a placebo-controlled, double-blind trial of 419 immunocompetent adults with uncomplicated herpes zoster. Comparisons included *Famvir* 500 mg t.i.d., *Famvir* 750 mg t.i.d., or placebo. Treatment was begun within 72 hours of initial lesion appearance and therapy was continued for 7 days.

The median time to full crusting in *Famvir*-treated patients was 5 days compared to 7 days in placebo-treated patients. The times to full crusting, loss of vesicles, loss of ulcers, and loss of crusts were shorter for *Famvir* 500 mg-treated patients than for placebo-treated patients in the overall study population. The effects of *Famvir* were greater when therapy was initiated within 48 hours of rash onset; it was also more pronounced in patients 50 years of age or older. Among the 65.2% of patients with at least one positive viral culture, *Famvir*-treated patients had a shorter median duration of viral shedding than placebo-treated patients (1 day and 2 days, respectively).

There were no overall differences in the duration of pain before rash healing between *Famvir* and placebo-treated groups. In addition, there was no difference in the incidence of pain after rash healing (postherpetic neuralgia) between the treatment groups. In the 186 patients (44.4% of total study population) who did develop postherpetic neuralgia, the median duration of postherpetic neuralgia was shorter in patients treated with *Famvir* 500 mg than in those treated with placebo (63 days and 119 days, respectively). No additional efficacy was demonstrated with higher doses of *Famvir*.

A double-blind controlled trial in 545 immunocompetent adults with uncomplicated herpes zoster treated within 72 hours of initial lesion appearance compared three doses of *Famvir* to acyclovir 800 mg 5 times per day. Times to full lesion crusting and times to loss of acute pain were compa-

Continued on next page

Famvir—Cont.

rable for all groups and there were no statistically significant differences in the time to loss of postherpetic neuralgia between *Famvir* and acyclovir-treated groups.

Herpes Simplex Infections

Recurrent Genital Herpes: In two placebo-controlled trials, 626 immunocompetent adults with a recurrence of genital herpes were treated with *Famvir* 125 mg b.i.d. (n=160), *Famvir* 250 mg b.i.d. (n=169), *Famvir* 500 mg b.i.d. (n=154) or placebo (n=143) for 5 days. Treatment was initiated within 6 hours of either symptom onset or lesion appearance. In the two studies combined, the median time to healing in *Famvir* 125 mg-treated patients was 4 days compared to 5 days in placebo-treated patients and the median time to cessation of viral shedding was 1.8 vs. 3.4 days in *Famvir* 125 mg and placebo recipients, respectively. The median time to loss of all symptoms was 3.2 days in *Famvir* 125 mg-treated patients vs. 3.8 days in placebo-treated patients. No additional efficacy was demonstrated with higher doses of *Famvir*.

Suppression of Recurrent Genital Herpes: 934 immunocompetent adults with a history of 6 or more recurrences per year were randomized into two double-blind, 1-year, placebo-controlled trials. Comparisons included *Famvir* 125 mg t.i.d., 250 mg b.i.d., 250 mg t.i.d. and placebo. At one-year, 60% to 65% of patients were still receiving *Famvir* and 25% were receiving placebo treatment. Patient reported recurrence rates for the 250 mg b.i.d. dose at 6 and 12 months are shown in Table 4.

Table 4

	Recurrence Rates at 6 Months		Recurrence Rates at 12 Months	
	***Famvir* 250 mg b.i.d.**	**Placebo**	***Famvir* 250 mg b.i.d.**	**Placebo**
n	236	233	236	233
Recurrence-free	39%	10%	29%	6%
Recurrences†	47%	74%	53%	78%
Lost to Follow-up‡	14%	16%	17%	16%

†Based on patient reported data; not necessarily confirmed by a physician.

‡Patients recurrence-free at time of last contact prior to withdrawal.

Famvir-treated patients had approximately 1/5 the median number of recurrences as compared to placebo-treated patients.

Higher doses of *Famvir* were not associated with an increase in efficacy.

Recurrent Mucocutaneous Herpes Simplex Infection in HIV-Infected Patients

A randomized, double-blind, multicenter study compared famciclovir 500 mg twice daily for 7 days (n=150) with oral acyclovir 400 mg 5 times daily for 7 days (n=143) in HIV-infected patients with recurrent mucocutaneous HSV infection treated within 48 hours of lesion onset. Approximately 40% of patients had a CD_4 count below 200 cells/mm^3, 54% of patients had anogenital lesions and 35% had orolabial lesions. Famciclovir therapy was comparable to oral acyclovir in reducing new lesion formation and in time to complete healing.

INDICATIONS AND USAGE

Herpes Zoster: Famvir (famciclovir) is indicated for the treatment of acute herpes zoster (shingles).

Herpes Simplex Infections: *Famvir* is indicated for:
- treatment or suppression of recurrent genital herpes in immunocompetent patients
- treatment of recurrent mucocutaneous herpes simplex infections in HIV-infected patients.

CONTRAINDICATIONS

Famvir (famciclovir) is contraindicated in patients with known hypersensitivity to the product, its components, and Denavir® (penciclovir cream).

PRECAUTIONS

General

The efficacy of *Famvir* has not been established for initial episode genital herpes infection, ophthalmic zoster, disseminated zoster or in immunocompromised patients with herpes zoster.

Dosage adjustment is recommended when administering *Famvir* to patients with creatinine clearance values <60 mL/min. (see DOSAGE AND ADMINISTRATION). In patients with underlying renal disease who have received inappropriately high doses of *Famvir* for their level of renal function, acute renal failure has been reported.

Information for Patients

Patients should be informed that *Famvir* is not a cure for genital herpes. There are no data evaluating whether *Famvir* will prevent transmission of infection to others. As genital herpes is a sexually transmitted disease, patients should avoid contact with lesions or intercourse when lesions and/or symptoms are present to avoid infecting partners. Genital herpes can also be transmitted in the absence of symptoms through asymptomatic viral shedding. If medical management of recurrent episodes is indicated, patients should be advised to initiate therapy at the first sign or symptom.

Drug Interactions

Concurrent use with probenecid or other drugs significantly eliminated by active renal tubular secretion may result in increased plasma concentrations of penciclovir.

The conversion of 6-deoxy penciclovir to penciclovir is catalyzed by aldehyde oxidase. Interactions with other drugs metabolized by this enzyme could potentially occur.

Carcinogenesis, Mutagenesis, Impairment of Fertility

Famciclovir was administered orally unless otherwise stated.

Carcinogenesis: Two-year dietary carcinogenicity studies with famciclovir were conducted in rats and mice. An increase in the incidence of mammary adenocarcinoma (a common tumor in animals of this strain) was seen in female rats receiving the high dose of 600 mg/kg/day (1.5 to 9.0× the human systemic exposure at the recommended daily oral doses of 500 mg t.i.d., 250 mg b.i.d., or 125 mg b.i.d. based on area under the plasma concentration curve comparisons [24 hr AUC] for penciclovir). No increases in tumor incidence were reported in male rats treated at doses up to 240 mg/kg/day (0.9 to 5.4× the human AUC), or in male and female mice at doses up to 600 mg/kg/day (0.4 to 2.4× the human AUC).

Mutagenesis: Famciclovir and penciclovir (the active metabolite of famciclovir) were tested for genotoxic potential in a battery of *in vitro* and *in vivo* assays. Famciclovir and penciclovir were negative in *in vitro* tests for gene mutations in bacteria (*S. typhimurium* and *E. coli*) and unscheduled DNA synthesis in mammalian HeLa 83 cells (at doses up to 10,000 and 5000 mcg/plate, respectively). Famciclovir was also negative in the L5178Y mouse lymphoma assay (5000 mcg/mL), the *in vivo* mouse micronucleus test (4800 mg/kg), and rat dominant lethal study (5000 mg/kg). Famciclovir induced increases in polyploidy in human lymphocytes *in vitro* in the absence of chromosomal damage (1200 mcg/mL). Penciclovir was positive in the L5178Y mouse lymphoma assay for gene mutation/chromosomal aberrations, with and without metabolic activation (1000 mcg/mL). In human lymphocytes, penciclovir caused chromosomal aberrations in the absence of metabolic activation (250 mcg/ mL). Penciclovir caused an increased incidence of micronuclei in mouse bone marrow *in vivo* when administered intravenously at doses highly toxic to bone marrow (500 mg/kg), but not when administered orally.

Impairment of Fertility: Testicular toxicity was observed in rats, mice, and dogs following repeated administration of famciclovir or penciclovir. Testicular changes included atrophy of the seminiferous tubules, reduction in sperm count, and/or increased incidence of sperm with abnormal morphology or reduced motility. The degree of toxicity to male reproduction was related to dose and duration of exposure. In male rats, decreased fertility was observed after 10 weeks of dosing at 500 mg/kg/day (1.9 to 11.4× the human AUC). The no observable effect level for sperm and testicular toxicity in rats following chronic administration (26 weeks) was 50 mg/kg/day (0.2 to 1.2× the human systemic exposure based on AUC comparisons). Testicular toxicity was observed following chronic administration to mice (104 weeks) and dogs (26 weeks) at doses of 600 mg/kg/day (0.4 to 2.4× the human AUC) and 150 mg/kg/day (1.7 to 10.2× the human AUC), respectively.

Famciclovir had no effect on general reproductive performance or fertility in female rats at doses up to 1000 mg/kg/day (3.6 to 21.6× the human AUC).

Two placebo-controlled studies in a total of 130 otherwise healthy men with a normal sperm profile over an 8-week baseline period and recurrent genital herpes receiving oral *Famvir* (250 mg b.i.d.) (n=66) or placebo (n=64) therapy for 18 weeks showed no evidence of significant effects on sperm count, motility or morphology during treatment or during an 8-week follow-up.

Pregnancy

Teratogenic Effects–Pregnancy Category B. Famciclovir was tested for effects on embryo-fetal development in rats and rabbits at oral doses up to 1000 mg/kg/day (approximately 3.6 to 21.6× and 1.8 to 10.8× the human systemic exposure to penciclovir based on AUC comparisons for the rat and rabbit, respectively) and intravenous doses of 360 mg/kg/day in rats (2 to 12× the human dose based on body surface area [BSA] comparisons) or 120 mg/kg/day in rabbits (1.5 to 9.0× the human dose [BSA]). No adverse effects were observed on embryo-fetal development. Similarly, no adverse effects were observed following intravenous administration of penciclovir to rats (80 mg/kg/day, 0.4 to 2.6× the human dose [BSA]) or rabbits (60 mg/kg/day, 0.7 to 4.2× the human dose [BSA]). There are, however, no adequate and well-controlled studies in pregnant women. Because animal reproduction studies are not always predictive of human response, famciclovir should be used during pregnancy only if the benefit to the patient clearly exceeds the potential risk to the fetus.

Pregnancy Exposure Registry: To monitor maternal-fetal outcomes of pregnant women exposed to *Famvir*, Novartis Pharmaceuticals Corporation maintains a *Famvir* Pregnancy Registry. Physicians are encouraged to register their patients by calling (888) 669-6682.

Nursing Mothers

Following oral administration of famciclovir to lactating rats, penciclovir was excreted in breast milk at concentrations higher than those seen in the plasma. It is not known whether it is excreted in human milk. There are no data on the safety of *Famvir* in infants.

Usage in Children

Safety and efficacy in children under the age of 18 years have not been established.

Geriatric Use

Of 816 patients with herpes zoster in clinical studies who were treated with *Famvir*, 248 (30.4%) were ≥65 years of age and 103 (13%) were ≥75 years of age. No overall differences were observed in the incidence or types of adverse events between younger and older patients.

ADVERSE REACTIONS

Immunocompetent Patients

The safety of *Famvir* has been evaluated in clinical studies involving 816 *Famvir*-treated patients with herpes zoster (*Famvir*, 250 mg t.i.d. to 750 mg t.i.d.); 528 *Famvir*-treated patients with recurrent genital herpes (*Famvir*, 125 mg b.i.d. to 500 mg t.i.d.); and 1,197 patients with recurrent genital herpes treated with *Famvir* as suppressive therapy (125 mg q.d. to 250 mg t.i.d.) of which 570 patients received *Famvir* (open-labeled and/or double-blind) for at least 10 months. Table 5 lists selected adverse events.

[See table 5 at left]

Table 5
Selected Adverse Events Reported by ≥2% of Patients in Placebo-controlled Famvir (famciclovir) Trials*

	Incidence					
	Herpes Zoster		Recurrent Genital Herpes		Genital Herpes-Suppression	
Event	***Famvir* (n=273) %**	**Placebo (n=146) %**	***Famvir* (n=640) %**	**Placebo (n=225) %**	***Famvir* (n=458) %**	**Placebo (n=63) %**
Nervous System						
Headache	22.7	17.8	23.6	16.4	39.3	42.9
Paresthesia	2.6	0.0	1.3	0.0	0.9	0.0
Migraine	0.7	0.7	1.3	0.4	3.1	0.0
Gastrointestinal						
Nausea	12.5	11.6	10.0	8.0	7.2	9.5
Diarrhea	7.7	4.8	4.5	7.6	9.0	9.5
Vomiting	4.8	3.4	1.3	0.9	3.1	1.6
Flatulence	1.5	0.7	1.9	2.2	4.8	1.6
Abdominal Pain	1.1	3.4	3.9	5.8	7.9	7.9
Body as a Whole						
Fatigue	4.4	3.4	6.3	4.4	4.8	3.2
Skin and Appendages						
Pruritus	3.7	2.7	0.9	0.0	2.2	0.0
Rash	0.4	0.7	0.6	0.4	3.3	1.6
Reproductive Female						
Dysmenorrhea	0.0	0.7	2.2	1.3	7.6	6.3

*Patients may have entered into more than one clinical trial.

The following adverse events have been reported during post-approval use of *Famvir:* urticaria, hallucinations and confusion (including delirium, disorientation, confusional state, occurring predominantly in the elderly). Because these adverse events are reported voluntarily from a population of unknown size, estimates of frequency cannot be made.

Table 6 lists selected laboratory abnormalities in genital herpes suppression trials.

Table 6
Selected Laboratory Abnormalities in Genital Herpes Suppression Studies*

Parameter	***Famvir* (n = 660)† %**	**Placebo (n = 210)† %**
Anemia (<0.8 × NRL)	0.1	0.0
Leukopenia (<0.75 × NRL)	1.3	0.9
Neutropenia (<0.8 × NRL)	3.2	1.5
AST (SGOT) (>2 × NRH)	2.3	1.2
ALT (SGPT) (>2 × NRH)	3.2	1.5
Total Bilirubin (>1.5 × NRH)	1.9	1.2

Serum Creatinine (>1.5 × NRH)	0.2	0.3
Amylase (>1.5 × NRH)	1.5	1.9
Lipase (>1.5 × NRH)	4.9	4.7

*Percentage of patients with laboratory abnormalities that were increased or decreased from baseline and were outside of specified ranges.
†n values represent the minimum number of patients assessed for each laboratory parameter.
NRH = Normal Range High.
NRL = Normal Range Low.

HIV-Infected Patients
In HIV-infected patients, the most frequently reported adverse events for famciclovir (500 mg twice daily; n=150) and acyclovir (400 mg, 5×/day; n=143), respectively, were headache (16.7 vs 15.4%), nausea (10.7 vs 12.6%), diarrhea (6.7 vs 10.5%), vomiting (4.7 vs 3.5%), fatigue (4.0 vs 2.1%), and abdominal pain (3.3 vs 5.6%).

OVERDOSAGE

Appropriate symptomatic and supportive therapy should be given. Penciclovir is removed by hemodialysis (see PRECAUTIONS, General).

DOSAGE AND ADMINISTRATION

Herpes Zoster
The recommended dosage is 500 mg every 8 hours for 7 days. Therapy should be initiated promptly as soon as herpes zoster is diagnosed. No data are available on efficacy of treatment started greater than 72 hours after rash onset.
Herpes Simplex Infections
Recurrent genital herpes: The recommended dosage is 125 mg twice daily for 5 days. Initiate therapy at the first sign or symptom if medical management of a genital herpes recurrence is indicated. The efficacy of *Famvir* has not been established when treatment is initiated more than 6 hours after onset of symptoms or lesions.
Suppression of recurrent genital herpes: The recommended dosage is 250 mg twice daily for up to 1 year. The safety and efficacy of *Famvir* therapy beyond 1 year of treatment have not been established.
HIV-Infected Patients
For recurrent orolabial or genital herpes simplex infection, the recommended dosage is 500 mg twice daily for 7 days.
In patients with reduced renal function, dosage reduction is recommended (see PRECAUTIONS, General).
[See table above]
Administration with Food
When famciclovir was administered with food, penciclovir C_{max} decreased approximately 50%. Because the systemic availability of penciclovir (AUC) was not altered, it appears that *Famvir* may be taken without regard to meals.

HOW SUPPLIED

Famvir is supplied as film-coated tablets as follows: 125 mg in bottles of 30; 250 mg in bottles of 30; and 500 mg in bottles of 30 and Single Unit Packages of 50 (intended for institutional use only).
Famvir 125 mg tablets are white, round, debossed with FAMVIR on one side and 125 on the other.
125 mg 30's .... NDC 0078-0366-15
Famvir 250 mg tablets are white, round, debossed with FAMVIR on one side and 250 on the other.
250 mg 30's .... NDC 0078-0367-15
Famvir 500 mg tablets are white, oval, debossed with FAMVIR on one side and 500 on the other.
500 mg 30's .... NDC 0078-0368-15
500 mg SUP 50's .... NDC 0078-0368-64
Store between 15°C and 30°C (59°F and 86°F).
January 2001
Manufactured in Crawley, UK
by **SmithKline Beecham Pharmaceuticals**
for Novartis Pharmaceuticals Corporation T2000-72
East Hanover, New Jersey 07936 89011401

FORADIL® AEROLIZER™ ℞
[fŏr 'ă-dĭl]
(formoterol fumarate inhalation powder)
FOR ORAL INHALATION ONLY

Rx only
Prescribing Information

DESCRIPTION

FORADIL® AEROLIZER™ consists of a capsule dosage form containing a dry powder formulation of Foradil (formoterol fumarate) intended for oral inhalation only with the Aerolizer™ Inhaler.
Each clear, hard gelatin capsule contains a dry powder blend of 12 mcg of formoterol fumarate and 25 mg of lactose as a carrier.
The active component of Foradil is formoterol fumarate, a racemate. Formoterol fumarate is a selective beta$_2$-adrenergic bronchodilator. Its chemical name is (±)-2-hydroxy-5-[(1RS)-1-hydroxy-2-[[(1RS)-2-(4-methoxyphenyl)-1-methylethyl]-amino]ethyl]formanilide fumarate dihydrate; its structural formula is
[See chemical structure at top of next column]
Formoterol fumarate has a molecular weight of 840.9, and its empirical formula is $(C_{19}H_{24}N_2O_4)_2 \cdot C_4H_4O_4 \cdot 2H_2O$. Formoterol fumarate is a white to yellowish crystalline powder, which is freely soluble in glacial acetic acid, soluble in

Table 7

Indication and Normal Dosage Regimen	Creatinine Clearance (mL/min.)	Adjusted Dosage Regimen Dose (mg)	Dosing Interval
Herpes Zoster 500 mg every 8 hours	>60	500	every 8 hours
	40–59	500	every 12 hours
	20–39	500	every 24 hours
	<20	250	every 24 hours
	HD*	250	following each dialysis
Recurrent Genital Herpes 125 mg every 12 hours	≥40	125	every 12 hours
	20–39	125	every 24 hours
	<20	125	every 24 hours
	HD*	125	following each dialysis
Suppression of Recurrent Genital Herpes 250 mg every 12 hours	≥40	250	every 12 hours
	20–39	125	every 12 hours
	<20	125	every 24 hours
	HD*	125	following each dialysis
Recurrent Orolabial and Genital Herpes Simplex Infection in HIV-Infected Patients 500 mg every 12 hours	≥40	500	every 12 hours
	20–39	500	every 24 hours
	<20	250	every 24 hours
	HD*	250	following each dialysis

*Hemodialysis

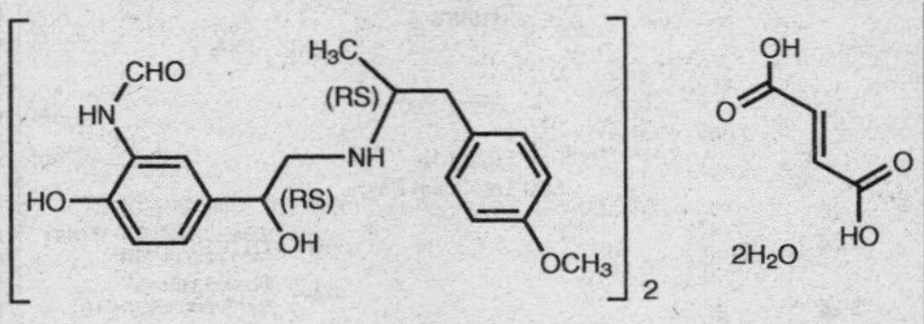

methanol, sparingly soluble in ethanol and isopropanol, slightly soluble in water, and practically insoluble in acetone, ethyl acetate, and diethyl ether.
The Aerolizer Inhaler is a plastic device used for inhaling Foradil. The amount of drug delivered to the lung will depend on patient factors, such as inspiratory flow rate and inspiratory time. Under standardized in vitro testing at a fixed flow rate of 60 L/min for 2 seconds, the Aerolizer Inhaler delivered 10 mcg of formoterol fumarate from the mouthpiece. Peak inspiratory flow rates (PIFR) achievable through the Aerolizer Inhaler were evaluated in 33 adult and adolescent patients and 32 pediatric patients with mild-to-moderate asthma. Mean PIFR was 117.82 L/min (range 34-188 L/min) for adult and adolescent patients, and 99.66 L/min (range 43-187 L/min) for pediatric patients. Approximately ninety percent of each population studied generated a PIFR through the device exceeding 60 L/min.
To use the delivery system, a Foradil capsule is placed in the well of the Aerolizer Inhaler, and the capsule is pierced by pressing and releasing the buttons on the side of the device. The formoterol fumarate formulation is dispersed into the air stream when the patient inhales rapidly and deeply through the mouthpiece.

CLINICAL PHARMACOLOGY

Mechanism of Action
Formoterol fumarate is a long-acting selective beta$_2$-adrenergic receptor agonist (beta$_2$-agonist). Inhaled formoterol fumarate acts locally in the lung as a bronchodilator. In vitro studies have shown that formoterol has more than 200-fold greater agonist activity at beta$_2$-receptors than at beta$_1$-receptors. Although beta$_2$-receptors are the predominant adrenergic receptors in bronchial smooth muscle and beta$_1$-receptors are the predominant receptors in the heart, there are also beta$_2$-receptors in the human heart comprising 10%-50% of the total beta-adrenergic receptors. The precise function of these receptors has not been established, but they raise the possibility that even highly selective beta$_2$-agonists may have some effect on the cardiovascular system.
The pharmacologic effects of beta$_2$-adrenoceptor agonist drugs, including formoterol, are at least in part attributable to stimulation of intracellular adenyl cyclase, the enzyme that catalyzes the conversion of adenosine triphosphate (ATP) to cyclic-3′, 5′-adenosine monophosphate (cyclic AMP). Increased cyclic AMP levels cause relaxation of bronchial smooth muscle and inhibition of release of mediators of immediate hypersensitivity from cells, especially from mast cells.
In vitro tests show that formoterol is an inhibitor of the release of mast cell mediators, such as histamine and leukotrienes, from the human lung. Formoterol also inhibits histamine-induced plasma albumin extravasation in anesthetized guinea pigs and inhibits allergen-induced eosinophil influx in dogs with airway hyper-responsiveness. The relevance of these in vitro and animal findings to humans is unknown.
Animal Pharmacology
Studies in laboratory animals (minipigs, rodents, and dogs) have demonstrated the occurrence of cardiac arrhythmias and sudden death (with histologic evidence of myocardial necrosis) when beta-agonists and methylxanthines are administered concurrently. The clinical significance of these findings is unknown.

Pharmacokinetics
Information on the pharmacokinetics of formoterol in plasma has been obtained by oral inhalation of doses higher than the recommended range. Urinary excretion of unchanged formoterol was used as an indirect measure of systemic exposure. Plasma drug disposition data parallel urinary excretion, and the elimination half-lives calculated for urine and plasma are similar.
Absorption
Following inhalation of a single 120 mcg dose of formoterol fumarate by 12 healthy subjects, formoterol was rapidly absorbed into plasma, reaching a maximum drug concentration of 92 pg/mL within 5 minutes of dosing.
Following inhalation of 12 to 96 mcg of formoterol fumarate by 10 healthy males, urinary excretion of both (R,R)- and (S,S)-enantiomers of formoterol increased proportionally to the dose. Thus, absorption of formoterol following inhalation appeared linear over the dose range studied.
In a study in patients with asthma, when formoterol 12 or 24 mcg twice daily was given by oral inhalation to steady-state, the accumulation index ranged from 1.67 to 2.08, based on the urinary excretion of unchanged formoterol. This suggests some accumulation of formoterol in plasma with multiple dosing. The excreted amounts of formoterol at steady-state were close to those predicted based on single-dose kinetics.
As with many drug products for oral inhalation, it is likely that the majority of the inhaled formoterol fumarate delivered is swallowed and then absorbed from the gastrointestinal tract.
Distribution
The binding of formoterol to human plasma proteins in vitro was 61%–64% at concentrations from 0.1 to 100 ng/mL. Binding to human serum albumin in vitro was 31%-38% over a range of 5 to 500 ng/mL. The concentrations of formoterol used to assess the plasma protein binding were higher than those achieved in plasma following inhalation of a single 120 mcg dose.
Metabolism
Formoterol is metabolized primarily by direct glucuronidation at either the phenolic or aliphatic hydroxyl group and O-demethylation followed by glucuronide conjugation at either phenolic hydroxyl groups. The most prominent pathway involves direct conjugation at the phenolic hydroxyl group. The second major pathway involves O-demethylation followed by conjugation at the phenolic 2′-hydroxyl group. Four cytochrome P450 isozymes (CYP2D6, CYP2C19, CYP2C9 and CYP2A6) are involved in the O-demethylation of formoterol. Formoterol did not inhibit CYP450 enzymes at therapeutically relevant concentrations.
Excretion
Following oral administration of 80 mcg of radiolabeled formoterol fumarate to 2 healthy subjects, 59%-62% of the radioactivity was eliminated in the urine and 32%-34% in the feces over a period of 104 hours. Renal clearance of formoterol from blood in these subjects was about 150 mL/min. Following inhalation of a 12 mcg or 24 mcg dose by 16 patients with asthma, about 10% and 15%-18% of the total dose was excreted in the urine as unchanged formoterol and direct glucuronide conjugates of formoterol, respectively.
Based on plasma concentrations measured following inhalation of a single 120 mcg dose by 12 healthy subjects, the mean terminal elimination half-life was determined to be 10 hours. From urinary excretion rates measured in these subjects, the mean terminal elimination half-lives for the (R,R)- and (S,S)-enantiomers were determined to be 13.9 and 12.3 hours, respectively. The (R,R)- and (S,S)-enantiomers represented about 40% and 60% of unchanged drug excreted in the urine, respectively, following single inhaled doses between 12 and 120 mcg in healthy volunteers and single and repeated doses of 12 and 24 mcg in patients with

Continued on next page

Foradil Aerolizer—Cont.

asthma. Thus, the relative proportion of the two enantiomers remained constant over the dose range studied and there was no evidence of relative accumulation of one enantiomer over the other after repeated dosing.

Special Populations

Gender: After correction for body weight, formoterol pharmacokinetics did not differ significantly between males and females.

Geriatric and Pediatric: The pharmacokinetics of formoterol have not been studied in the elderly population, and limited data are available in pediatric patients.

In a study of children with asthma who were 5 to12 years of age, when formoterol fumarate 12 or 24 mcg was given twice daily by oral inhalation for 12 weeks, the accumulation index ranged from 1.18 to 1.84 based on urinary excretion of unchanged formoterol. Hence, the accumulation in children did not exceed that in adults, where the accumulation index ranged from 1.67 to 2.08 (see above). Approximately 6% and 6.5% to 9% of the dose was recovered in the urine of the children as unchanged and conjugated formoterol, respectively.

Hepatic/Renal Impairment: The pharmacokinetics of formoterol have not been studied in patients with hepatic or renal impairment.

Pharmacodynamics

Systemic Safety and Pharmacokinetic/Pharmacodynamic Relationships

The major adverse effects of inhaled beta$_2$-agonists occur as a result of excessive activation of the systemic beta-adrenergic receptors. The most common adverse effects in adults and adolescents include skeletal muscle tremor and cramps, insomnia, tachycardia, decreases in plasma potassium, and increases in plasma glucose.

Pharmacokinetic/pharmacodynamic (PK/PD) relationships between heart rate, ECG parameters, and serum potassium levels and the urinary excretion of formoterol were evaluated in 10 healthy volunteers following inhalation of single doses containing 12, 24, 48, or 96 mcg of formoterol fumarate. There was a linear relationship between urinary formoterol excretion and decreases in serum potassium, increases in plasma glucose, and increases in heart rate.

In a second study, PK/PD relationships between plasma formoterol levels and heart rate, ECG parameters, and plasma potassium levels were evaluated in 12 healthy volunteers following inhalation of a single 120 mcg dose of formoterol fumarate (10 times the recommended clinical dose). Reductions of plasma potassium concentration were observed in all subjects. Maximum reductions from baseline ranged from 0.55 to 1.52 mmol/L with a median maximum reduction of 1.01 mmol/L. The formoterol plasma concentration was highly correlated with the reduction in plasma potassium concentration. Generally, the maximum effect on plasma potassium was noted 1 to 3 hours after peak formoterol plasma concentrations were achieved. An increase of heart rate of about 30% was observed 6 hours post-dose. An average increase of corrected QT interval (QTc) of about 25.1 msec was observed 6 hours post-dose. The QTc returned to baseline within 24 hours post-dose. Formoterol plasma concentrations were weakly correlated with heart rate and increase of QTc duration.

The electrocardiographic and cardiovascular effects of FORADIL AEROLIZER were compared with those of albuterol and placebo in two pivotal 12-week double-blind studies. A subset of patients underwent continuous electrocardiographic monitoring during three 24-hour periods. No important differences in ventricular or supraventricular ectopy between treatment groups were observed. In these two studies, the total number of patients exposed to any dose of FORADIL AEROLIZER who had continuous electrocardiographic monitoring was about 200.

Tachyphylaxis/Tolerance

In a clinical study in 19 adult patients with mild asthma, the bronchoprotective effect of formoterol, as assessed by methacholine challenge, was studied following an initial dose of 24 mcg (twice the recommended dose) and after 2 weeks of 24 mcg twice daily. Tolerance to the bronchoprotective effects of formoterol was observed as evidenced by a diminished bronchoprotective effect on FEV$_1$ after 2 weeks of dosing, with loss of protection at the end of the 12 hour dosing period.

Rebound bronchial hyper-responsiveness after cessation of chronic formoterol therapy has not been observed.

In three large clinical trials, while efficacy of formoterol versus placebo was maintained, a slightly reduced bronchodilatory response (as measured by 12-hour FEV$_1$ AUC) was observed within the formoterol arms over time, particularly with the 24 mcg twice daily dose (twice the daily recommended dose). A similarly reduced FEV$_1$ AUC over time was also noted in the albuterol treatment arms (180 mcg four times daily by metered-dose inhaler).

CLINICAL TRIALS

Adolescent and Adult Asthma Trials

In a placebo-controlled, single-dose clinical trial, the onset of bronchodilation (defined as a 15% or greater increase from baseline in FEV$_1$) was similar for FORADIL AEROLIZER 12 mcg and albuterol 180 mcg by metered-dose inhaler.

In single-dose and multiple-dose clinical trials, the maximum improvement in FEV$_1$ for FORADIL AEROLIZER 12 mcg generally occurred within 1 to 3 hours, and an increase in FEV$_1$ above baseline was observed for 12 hours in most patients.

FORADIL AEROLIZER was compared to albuterol 180 mcg four times daily by metered-dose inhaler, and placebo in a total of 1095 adult and adolescent patients 12 years of age and above with mild-to-moderate asthma (defined as FEV$_1$ 40%-80% of the patients predicted normal value) who participated in two pivotal, 12-week, multi-center, randomized, double-blind, parallel group studies.

The results of both studies showed that FORADIL AEROLIZER 12 mcg twice daily resulted in significantly greater post-dose bronchodilation (as measured by serial FEV$_1$ for 12 hours post-dose) throughout the 12-week treatment period. Mean FEV$_1$ measurements from both studies are shown below for the first and last treatment days (see Figures 1 and 2).

Figures 1a and 1b: Mean FEV$_1$ from Clinical Trial A

Figure 1a
First Treatment Day

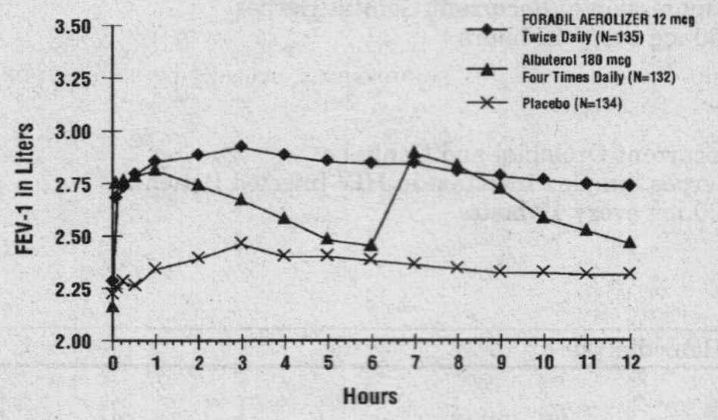
FORADIL AEROLIZER 12 mcg Twice Daily (N=135)
Albuterol 180 mcg Four Times Daily (N=132)
Placebo (N=134)
FEV-1 in Liters
Hours
3.50
3.25
3.00
2.75
2.50
2.25
2.00
0 1 2 3 4 5 6 7 8 9 10 11 12

Figure 1b
Last Treatment Day

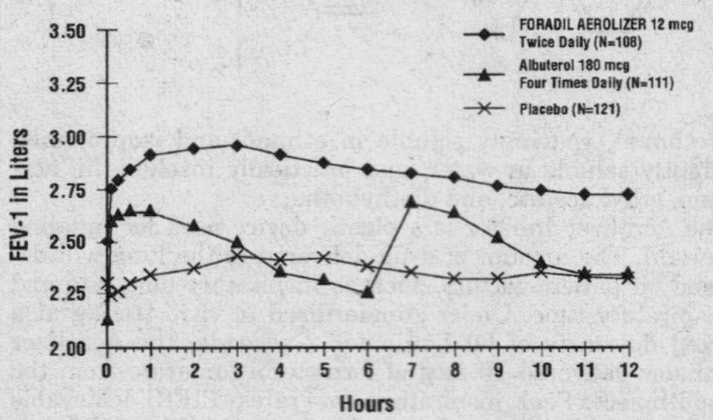
FORADIL AEROLIZER 12 mcg Twice Daily (N=108)
Albuterol 180 mcg Four Times Daily (N=111)
Placebo (N=121)
FEV-1 in Liters
Hours
3.50
3.25
3.00
2.75
2.50
2.25
2.00
0 1 2 3 4 5 6 7 8 9 10 11 12

Figures 2a and 2b: Mean FEV$_1$ from Clinical Trial B

Figure 2a
First Treatment Day

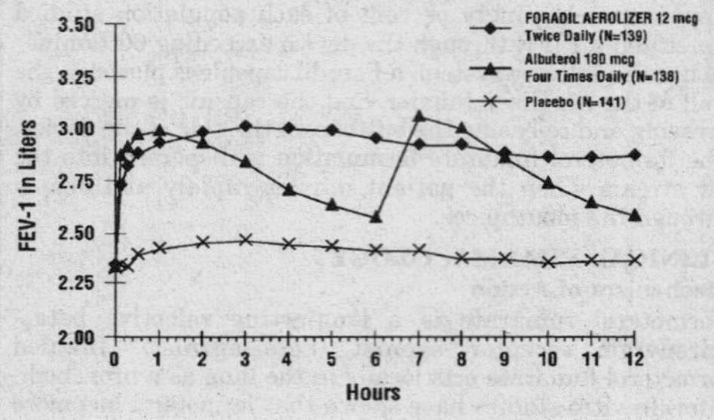
FORADIL AEROLIZER 12 mcg Twice Daily (N=139)
Albuterol 180 mcg Four Times Daily (N=138)
Placebo (N=141)
FEV-1 in Liters
Hours
3.50
3.25
3.00
2.75
2.50
2.25
2.00
0 1 2 3 4 5 6 7 8 9 10 11 12

Figure 2b
Last Treatment Day

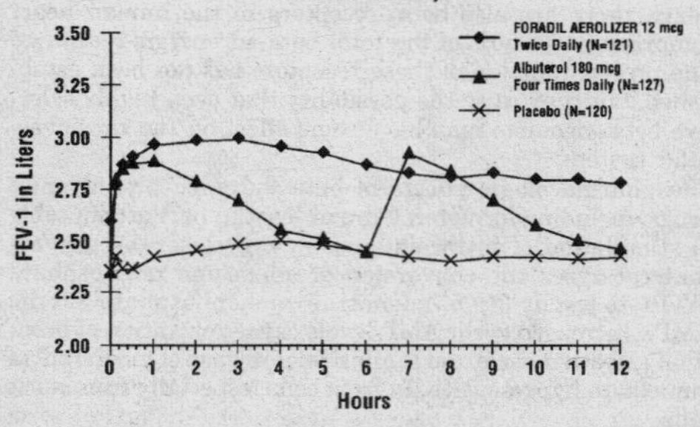
FORADIL AEROLIZER 12 mcg Twice Daily (N=121)
Albuterol 180 mcg Four Times Daily (N=127)
Placebo (N=120)
FEV-1 in Liters
Hours
3.50
3.25
3.00
2.75
2.50
2.25
2.00
0 1 2 3 4 5 6 7 8 9 10 11 12

Compared with placebo and albuterol, patients treated with FORADIL AEROLIZER 12 mcg demonstrated improvement in many secondary efficacy endpoints, including improved combined and nocturnal asthma symptom scores, fewer nighttime awakenings, fewer nights in which patients used rescue medication, and higher morning and evening peak flow rates.

Pediatric Asthma Trial

A 12-month, multi-center, randomized, double-blind, parallel-group, study compared FORADIL AEROLIZER and placebo in a total of 518 children with asthma (ages 5-12 years) who required daily bronchodilators and anti-inflammatory treatment. Efficacy was evaluated on the first day of treatment, at Week 12, and at the end of treatment.

FORADIL AEROLIZER 12 mcg twice daily demonstrated a greater 12-hour FEV$_1$ AUC compared to placebo on the first day of treatment, after twelve weeks of treatment, and after one year of treatment.

Adolescent and Adult Exercise-Induced Bronchospasm Trials

The effect of FORADIL AEROLIZER on exercise-induced bronchospasm (defined as >20% fall in FEV$_1$) was examined in two randomized, single-dose, double-blind, crossover studies in a total of 38 patients 13 to 41 years of age with exercise-induced bronchospasm. Exercise challenge testing was conducted 15 minutes, and 4, 8, and 12 hours following administration of a single dose of study drug (FORADIL AEROLIZER 12 mcg, albuterol 180 mcg by metered-dose inhaler, or placebo) on separate test days. FORADIL AEROLIZER 12 mcg and albuterol 180 mcg were each superior to placebo for FEV$_1$ measurements obtained 15 minutes after study drug administration. FORADIL AEROLIZER 12 mcg maintained superiority over placebo at 4, 8, and 12 hours after administration. The efficacy of FORADIL AEROLIZER in the prevention of exercise-induced bronchospasm when dosed on a regular twice daily regimen has not been studied.

INDICATIONS AND USAGE

FORADIL AEROLIZER is indicated for long-term, twice-daily (morning and evening) administration in the maintenance treatment of asthma and in the prevention of bronchospasm in adults and children 5 years of age and older with reversible obstructive airways disease, including patients with symptoms of nocturnal asthma, who require regular treatment with inhaled, short-acting, beta$_2$-agonists. It is not indicated for patients whose asthma can be managed by occasional use of inhaled, short-acting, beta$_2$-agonists.

FORADIL AEROLIZER is also indicated for the acute prevention of exercise-induced bronchospasm (EIB) in adults and children 12 years of age and older, when administered on an occasional, as needed basis.

FORADIL AEROLIZER can be used concomitantly with short-acting beta$_2$-agonists, inhaled or systemic corticosteroids, and theophylline therapy (see PRECAUTIONS, Drug Interactions). A satisfactory clinical response to FORADIL AEROLIZER does not eliminate the need for continued treatment with an anti-inflammatory agent.

CONTRAINDICATIONS

Foradil (formoterol fumarate) is contraindicated in patients with a history of hypersensitivity to formoterol fumarate or to any components of this product.

WARNINGS

IMPORTANT INFORMATION: FORADIL AEROLIZER SHOULD NOT BE INITIATED IN PATIENTS WITH SIGNIFICANTLY WORSENING OR ACUTELY DETERIORATING ASTHMA, WHICH MAY BE A LIFE-THREATENING CONDITION. The use of FORADIL AEROLIZER in this setting is inappropriate.

FORADIL AEROLIZER IS NOT A SUBSTITUTE FOR INHALED OR ORAL CORTICOSTEROIDS. Corticosteroids should not be stopped or reduced at the time FORADIL AEROLIZER is initiated. (See PRECAUTIONS, Information for Patients and the accompanying Patient Instructions For Use.)

When beginning treatment with FORADIL AEROLIZER, patients who have been taking inhaled, short-acting beta$_2$-agonists on a regular basis (e.g., four times a day) should be instructed to discontinue the regular use of these drugs and use them only for symptomatic relief of acute asthma symptoms (see PRECAUTIONS, Information for Patients).

Paradoxical Bronchospasm

As with other inhaled beta$_2$-agonists, formoterol can produce paradoxical bronchospasm, that may be life-threatening. If paradoxical bronchospasm occurs, FORADIL AEROLIZER should be discontinued immediately and alternative therapy instituted.

Deterioration of Asthma

Asthma may deteriorate acutely over a period of hours or chronically over several days or longer. If the usual dose of FORADIL AEROLIZER no longer controls the symptoms of bronchoconstriction, and the patient's inhaled, short-acting beta$_2$-agonist becomes less effective or the patient needs more inhalation of short-acting beta$_2$-agonist than usual, these may be markers of deterioration of asthma. In this setting, a re-evaluation of the patient and the asthma treatment regimen should be undertaken at once, giving special consideration to the possible need for anti-inflammatory treatment, e.g., corticosteroids. Increasing the daily dosage of FORADIL AEROLIZER beyond the recommended dose in this situation is not appropriate. FORADIL AEROLIZER should not be used more frequently than twice daily (morning and evening) at the recommended dose.

Use of Anti-inflammatory Agents

The use of beta$_2$-agonists alone may not be adequate to control asthma in many patients. Early consideration should be given to adding anti-inflammatory agents, e.g., corticosteroids. There are no data demonstrating that Foradil has any clinical anti-inflammatory effect and therefore it cannot be expected to take the place of corticosteroids. Patients who already require oral or inhaled corticosteroids for treatment of asthma should be continued on this type of treatment even if they feel better as a result of initiating or increasing the dose of FORADIL AEROLIZER. Any change in corticosteroid dosage, in particular a reduction, should be made ONLY after clinical evaluation (see PRECAUTIONS, Information for Patients).

Cardiovascular Effects

Formoterol fumarate, like other beta$_2$-agonists, can produce a clinically significant cardiovascular effect in some patients as measured by increases in pulse rate, blood pressure, and/or symptoms. Although such effects are uncommon after administration of FORADIL AEROLIZER at recommended doses, if they occur, the drug may need to be discontinued. In addition, beta-agonists have been reported to produce ECG changes, such as flattening of the T wave, prolongation of the QTc interval, and ST segment depression. The clinical significance of these findings is unknown. Therefore, formoterol fumarate, like other sympathomimetic amines, should be used with caution in patients with cardiovascular disorders, especially coronary insufficiency, cardiac arrhythmias, and hypertension (see PRECAUTIONS, General).

Immediate Hypersensitivity Reactions

Immediate hypersensitivity reactions may occur after administration of FORADIL AEROLIZER, as demonstrated by cases of anaphylactic reactions, urticaria, angioedema, rash, and bronchospasm.

Do Not Exceed Recommended Dose

Fatalities have been reported in association with excessive use of inhaled sympathomimetic drugs in patients with asthma. The exact cause of death is unknown, but cardiac arrest following an unexpected development of a severe acute asthmatic crisis and subsequent hypoxia is suspected.

PRECAUTIONS

General

FORADIL AEROLIZER should not be used to treat acute symptoms of asthma. FORADIL AEROLIZER has not been studied in the relief of acute asthma symptoms and extra doses should not be used for that purpose. When prescribing FORADIL AEROLIZER, the physician should also provide the patient with an inhaled, short-acting beta$_2$-agonist for treatment of symptoms that occur acutely, despite regular twice-daily (morning and evening) use of FORADIL AEROLIZER. Patients should also be cautioned that increasing inhaled beta$_2$-agonist use is a signal of deteriorating asthma. (See Information for Patients and the accompanying Patient Instructions For Use.)

Formoterol fumarate, like other sympathomimetic amines, should be used with caution in patients with cardiovascular disorders, especially coronary insufficiency, cardiac arrhythmias, and hypertension; in patients with convulsive disorders or thyrotoxicosis; and in patients who are unusually responsive to sympathomimetic amines. Clinically significant changes in systolic and/or diastolic blood pressure, pulse rate and electrocardiograms have been seen infrequently in individual patients in controlled clinical studies with formoterol. Doses of the related beta$_2$-agonist albuterol, when administered intravenously, have been reported to aggravate preexisting diabetes mellitus and ketoacidosis.

Beta-agonist medications may produce significant hypokalemia in some patients, possibly through intracellular shunting, which has the potential to produce adverse cardiovascular effects. The decrease in serum potassium is usually transient, not requiring supplementation.

Clinically significant changes in blood glucose and/or serum potassium were infrequent during clinical studies with long-term administration of FORADIL AEROLIZER at the recommended dose.

Foradil® capsules should ONLY be used with the Aerolizer™ Inhaler and SHOULD NOT be taken orally.

Foradil® capsules should always be stored in the blister, and only removed IMMEDIATELY before use.

Information for Patients

It is important that patients understand how to use the Aerolizer Inhaler appropriately and how it should be used in relation to other asthma medications they are taking (see the accompanying Patient Instructions For Use).

The active ingredient of Foradil (formoterol fumarate) is a long-acting, bronchodilator used for the treatment of asthma, including nocturnal asthma, and for the prevention of exercise-induced bronchospasm. FORADIL AEROLIZER provides bronchodilation for up to 12 hours. Patients should be advised not to increase the dose or frequency of FORADIL AEROLIZER without consulting the prescribing physician. Patients should be warned not to stop or reduce concomitant asthma therapy without medical advice.

FORADIL AEROLIZER is not indicated to relieve acute asthma symptoms and extra doses should not be used for that purpose. Acute symptoms should be treated with an inhaled, short-acting, beta$_2$-agonist (the health-care provider should prescribe the patient with such medication and instruct the patient in how it should be used). Patients should be instructed to seek medical attention if their symptoms worsen, if FORADIL AEROLIZER treatment becomes less effective, or if they need more inhalations of a short-acting beta$_2$-agonist than usual. Patients should not inhale more than the contents of the prescribed number of capsules at any one time. The daily dosage of FORADIL AEROLIZER should not exceed one capsule twice daily (24 mcg total daily dose).

When FORADIL AEROLIZER is used for the prevention of EIB, the contents of one capsule should be taken at least 15 minutes prior to exercise. Additional doses of FORADIL AEROLIZER should not be used for 12 hours. Prevention of EIB has not been studied in patients who are receiving chronic FORADIL AEROLIZER administration twice daily and these patients should not use additional FORADIL AEROLIZER for prevention of EIB.

FORADIL AEROLIZER should not be used as a substitute for oral or inhaled corticosteroids. The dosage of these medications should not be changed and they should not be stopped without consulting the physician, even if the patient feels better after initiating treatment with FORADIL AEROLIZER.

Patients should be informed that treatment with beta$_2$-agonists may lead to adverse events which include palpitations, chest pain, rapid heart rate, tremor or nervousness. Patients should be informed never to use FORADIL AEROLIZER with a spacer and never to exhale into the device.

Patients should avoid exposing the Foradil capsules to moisture and should handle the capsules with dry hands. The Aerolizer™ Inhaler should never be washed and should be kept dry. The patient should always use the new Aerolizer Inhaler that comes with each refill.

Women should be advised to contact their physician if they become pregnant or if they are nursing.

Patients should be told that in rare cases, the gelatin capsule might break into small pieces. These pieces should be retained by the screen built into the Aerolizer Inhaler. However, it remains possible that rarely, tiny pieces of gelatin might reach the mouth or throat after inhalation. The capsule is less likely to shatter when pierced if: storage conditions are strictly followed, capsules are removed from the blister immediately before use, and the capsules are only pierced once.

Drug Interactions

If additional adrenergic drugs are to be administered by any route, they should be used with caution because the pharmacologically predictable sympathetic effects of formoterol may be potentiated.

Concomitant treatment with xanthine derivatives, steroids, or diuretics may potentiate any hypokalemic effect of adrenergic agonists.

The ECG changes and/or hypokalemia that may result from the administration of non-potassium sparing diuretics (such as loop or thiazide diuretics) can be acutely worsened by beta-agonists, especially when the recommended dose of the beta-agonist is exceeded. Although the clinical significance of these effects is not known, caution is advised in the co-administration of beta-agonist with non-potassium sparing diuretics.

Formoterol, as with other beta$_2$-agonists, should be administered with extreme caution to patients being treated with monamine oxidase inhibitors, tricyclic antidepressants, or drugs known to prolong the QTc interval because the action of adrenergic agonists on the cardiovascular system may be potentiated by these agents. Drugs that are known to prolong the QTc interval have an increased risk of ventricular arrhythmias.

Beta-adrenergic receptor antagonists (beta-blockers) and formoterol may inhibit the effect of each other when administered concurrently. Beta-blockers not only block the therapeutic effects of beta-agonists, such as formoterol, but may produce severe bronchospasm in asthmatic patients. Therefore, patients with asthma should not normally be treated with beta-blockers. However, under certain circumstances, e.g., as prophylaxis after myocardial infarction, there may be no acceptable alternatives to the use of beta-blockers in patients with asthma. In this setting, cardioselective beta-blockers could be considered, although they should be administered with caution.

Carcinogenesis, Mutagenesis, Impairment of Fertility

The carcinogenic potential of formoterol fumarate has been evaluated in 2-year drinking water and dietary studies in both rats and mice. In rats, the incidence of ovarian leiomyomas was increased at doses of 15 mg/kg and above in the drinking water study and at 20 mg/kg in the dietary study, but not at dietary doses up to 5 mg/kg (AUC exposure approximately 450 times human exposure at the maximum recommended daily inhalation dose). In the dietary study, the incidence of benign ovarian theca-cell tumors was increased at doses of 0.5 mg/kg and above (AUC exposure at the low dose of 0.5 mg/kg was approximately 45 times human exposure at the maximum recommended daily inhalation dose). This finding was not observed in the drinking water study, nor was it seen in mice (see below).

In mice, the incidence of adrenal subcapsular adenomas and carcinomas was increased in males at doses of 69 mg/kg and above in the drinking water study, but not at doses up to 50 mg/kg (AUC exposure approximately 590 times human exposure at the maximum recommended daily inhalation dose) in the dietary study. The incidence of hepatocarcinomas was increased in the dietary study at doses of 20 and 50 mg/kg in females and 50 mg/kg in males, but not at doses up to 5 mg/kg in either males or females (AUC exposure approximately 60 times human exposure at the maximum recommended daily inhalation dose). Also in the dietary study, the incidence of uterine leiomyomas and leiomyosarcomas was increased at doses of 2 mg/kg and above (AUC exposure at the low dose of 2 mg/kg was approximately 25 times human exposure at the maximum recommended daily inhalation dose). Increases in leiomyomas of the rodent female genital tract have been similarly demonstrated with other beta-agonist drugs.

Formoterol fumarate was not mutagenic or clastogenic in the following tests: mutagenicity tests in bacterial and mammalian cells, chromosomal analyses in mammalian cells, unscheduled DNA synthesis repair tests in rat hepatocytes and human fibroblasts, transformation assay in mammalian fibroblasts and micronucleus tests in mice and rats.

Reproduction studies in rats revealed no impairment of fertility at oral doses up to 3 mg/kg (approximately 1000 times the maximum recommended daily inhalation dose in humans on a mg/m^2 basis).

Pregnancy, Teratogenic Effects, Pregnancy Category C

Formoterol fumarate has been shown to cause stillbirth and neonatal mortality at oral doses of 6 mg/kg (approximately 2000 times the maximum recommended daily inhalation dose in humans on a mg/m^2 basis) and above in rats receiving the drug during the late stage of pregnancy. These effects, however, were not produced at a dose of 0.2 mg/kg (approximately 70 times the maximum recommended daily inhalation dose in humans on a mg/m^2 basis). When given to rats throughout organogenesis, oral doses of 0.2 mg/kg and above delayed ossification of the fetus, and doses of 6 mg/kg and above decreased fetal weight. Formoterol fumarate did not cause malformations in rats or rabbits following oral administration. Because there are no adequate and well-controlled studies in pregnant women, FORADIL AEROLIZER should be used during pregnancy only if the potential benefit justifies the potential risk to the fetus.

Use in Labor and Delivery

Formoterol fumarate has been shown to cause stillbirth and neonatal mortality at oral doses of 6 mg/kg (approximately 2000 times the maximum recommended daily inhalation dose in humans on a mg/m^2 basis) and above in rats receiving the drug for several days at the end of pregnancy. These effects were not produced at a dose of 0.2 mg/kg (approximately 70 times the maximum recommended daily inhalation dose in humans on a mg/m^2 basis). There are no adequate and well-controlled human studies that have investigated the effects of FORADIL AEROLIZER during labor and delivery.

Because beta-agonists may potentially interfere with uterine contractility, FORADIL AEROLIZER should be used during labor only if the potential benefit justifies the potential risk.

Nursing Mothers

In reproductive studies in rats, formoterol was excreted in the milk. It is not known whether formoterol is excreted in human milk, but because many drugs are excreted in human milk, caution should be exercised if FORADIL AEROLIZER is administered to nursing women. There are no well-controlled human studies of the use of FORADIL AEROLIZER in nursing mothers.

Pediatric Use

Asthma

A total of 776 children 5 years of age and older with asthma were studied in three multiple-dose controlled clinical trials. Of the 512 children who received formoterol, 508 were 5-12 years of age, and approximately one third were 5-8 years of age.

Exercise Induced Bronchoconstriction

A total of 20 adolescent patients, 12-16 years of age, were studied in three well-controlled single-dose clinical trials. The safety and effectiveness of FORADIL AEROLIZER in pediatric patients below 5 years of age has not been established. (See CLINICAL TRIALS, Pediatric Asthma Trial, and ADVERSE REACTIONS, Experience in Pediatric, Adolescent and Adult Patients.)

Geriatric Use

Of the total number of patients who received FORADIL AEROLIZER in adolescent and adult chronic dosing clinical trials, 318 were 65 years of age or older and 39 were 75 years of age and older. No overall differences in safety or effectiveness were observed between these subjects and younger subjects. A slightly higher frequency of chest infection was reported in the 39 patients 75 years of age and older, although a causal relationship with Foradil has not been established. Other reported clinical experience has not identified differences in responses between the elderly and younger adult patients, but greater sensitivity of some older individuals cannot be ruled out. (See PRECAUTIONS, Drug Interactions.)

ADVERSE REACTIONS

Adverse reactions to Foradil are similar in nature to other selective beta$_2$-adrenoceptor agonists; e.g., angina, hypertension or hypotension, tachycardia, arrhythmias, nervousness, headache, tremor, dry mouth, palpitation, muscle cramps, nausea, dizziness, fatigue, malaise, hypokalemia, hyperglycemia, metabolic acidosis and insomnia.

Experience in Pediatric, Adolescent and Adult Patients

Of the 5,824 patients in multiple-dose controlled clinical trials, 1,985 were treated with FORADIL AEROLIZER at the recommended dose of 12 mcg twice daily. The following table shows adverse events where the frequency was greater than or equal to 1% in the Foradil 12 mcg twice daily group and where the rates in the Foradil group exceeded placebo. Three adverse events showed dose ordering among tested doses of 6, 12 and 24 mcg administered twice daily; tremor, dizziness and dysphonia.

NUMBER AND FREQUENCY OF ADVERSE EXPERIENCES IN PATIENTS 5 YEARS OF AGE AND OLDER FROM MULTIPLE-DOSE CONTROLLED CLINICAL TRIALS

Adverse Event	Foradil Aerolizer 12 mcg twice daily		Placebo	
	n	(%)	n	(%)
Total Patients	1985	(100)	969	(100)
Infection viral	341	(17.2)	166	(17.1)

Continued on next page

Foradil Aerolizer—Cont.

Bronchitis	92	(4.6)	42	(4.3)
Chest infection	54	(2.7)	4	(0.4)
Dyspnea	42	(2.1)	16	(1.7)
Chest pain	37	(1.9)	13	(1.3)
Tremor	37	(1.9)	4	(0.4)
Dizziness	31	(1.6)	15	(1.5)
Insomnia	29	(1.5)	8	(0.8)
Tonsilitis	23	(1.2)	7	(0.7)
Rash	22	(1.1)	7	(0.7)
Dysphonia	19	(1.0)	9	(0.9)

Experience in Children

The safety of FORADIL AEROLIZER compared to placebo was investigated in one large, multicenter, randomized, double-blind clinical trial in 518 children with asthma (ages 5-12 years) in need of daily bronchodilators and anti-inflammatory treatment. The numbers and percent of patients who reported adverse events were comparable in the 12 mcg twice daily and placebo groups. In general, the pattern of the adverse events observed in children differed from the usual pattern seen in adults. The adverse events that were more frequent in the formoterol group than in the placebo group reflected infection/inflammation (viral infection, rhinitis, tonsilitis, gastroenteritis) or abdominal complaints (abdominal pain, nausea, dyspepsia).

Post Marketing Experience

In extensive worldwide marketing experience with Foradil, serious exacerbations of asthma, including some that have been fatal, have been reported. While most of these cases have been in patients with severe or acutely deteriorating asthma (see WARNINGS), a few have occurred in patients with less severe asthma. The contribution of Foradil to these cases could not be determined.

Rare reports of anaphylactic reactions, including severe hypotension and angioedema, have also been received in association with the use of formoterol fumarate inhalation powder.

DRUG ABUSE AND DEPENDENCE

There was no evidence in clinical trials of drug dependence with the use of Foradil.

OVERDOSAGE

The expected signs and symptoms with overdosage of FORADIL AEROLIZER are those of excessive beta-adrenergic stimulation and/or occurrence or exaggeration of any of the signs and symptoms listed under ADVERSE REACTIONS, e.g., angina, hypertension or hypotension, tachycardia, with rates up to 200 beats/min., arrhythmias, nervousness, headache, tremor, seizures, muscle cramps, dry mouth, palpitation, nausea, dizziness, fatigue, malaise, hypokalemia, hyperglycemia, and insomnia. Metabolic acidosis may also occur. As with all inhaled sympathomimetic medications, cardiac arrest and even death may be associated with an overdose of FORADIL AEROLIZER.

Treatment of overdosage consists of discontinuation of FORADIL AEROLIZER together with institution of appropriate symptomatic and/or supportive therapy. The judicious use of a cardioselective beta-receptor blocker may be considered, bearing in mind that such medication can produce bronchospasm. There is insufficient evidence to determine if dialysis is beneficial for overdosage of FORADIL AEROLIZER. Cardiac monitoring is recommended in cases of overdosage.

The minimum acute lethal inhalation dose of formoterol fumarate in rats is 156 mg/kg, 53,000 and 25,000 times the maximum recommended daily inhalation dose in adults and children, respectively, on a mg/m^2 basis. The median lethal oral doses in Chinese hamsters, rats, and mice provide even higher multiples of the maximum recommended daily inhalation dose in humans.

DOSAGE AND ADMINISTRATION

Foradil capsules should be administered only by the oral inhalation route (see the accompanying Patient Instructions for Use) and only using the Aerolizer Inhaler. Foradil capsules should not be ingested (i.e., swallowed) orally. Foradil capsules should always be stored in the blister, and only removed IMMEDIATELY BEFORE USE.

For Maintenance Treatment of Asthma

For adults and children 5 years of age and older, the usual dosage is the inhalation of the contents of one 12-mcg Foradil capsule every 12 hours using the Aerolizer™ Inhaler. The patient must not exhale into the device. The total daily dose of Foradil should not exceed one capsule twice daily (24 mcg total daily dose). More frequent administration or administration of a larger number of inhalations is not recommended. If symptoms arise between doses, an inhaled short-acting beta$_2$-agonist should be taken for immediate relief.

If a previously effective dosage regimen fails to provide the usual response, medical advice should be sought immediately as this is often a sign of destabilization of asthma. Under these circumstances, the therapeutic regimen should be reevaluated and additional therapeutic options, such as inhaled or systemic corticosteroids, should be considered.

For Prevention of Exercise-Induced Bronchospasm (EIB)

For adults and adolescents 12 years of age or older, the usual dosage is the inhalation of the contents of one 12-mcg Foradil capsule at least 15 minutes before exercise administered on an occasional as-needed basis.

Additional doses of FORADIL AEROLIZER should not be used for 12 hours after the administration of this drug. Regular, twice-daily dosing has not been studied in preventing EIB. Patients who are receiving FORADIL AEROLIZER twice daily for maintenance treatment of their asthma should not use additional doses for prevention of EIB and may require a short-acting bronchodilator.

HOW SUPPLIED

FORADIL® AEROLIZER™ contains: 60 aluminum blister-packaged 12-mcg Foradil (formoterol fumarate) clear gelatin capsules with "CG" printed on one end and "FXF" printed on the opposite end; one Aerolizer™ Inhaler; and Patient Instructions for Use .... **(NDC 0083-0167-74)**.

Foradil® capsules should be used with the Aerolizer™ Inhaler only. The Aerolizer™ Inhaler should not be used with any other capsules.

Prior to dispensing: Store in a refrigerator, 2°C-8°C (36°F-46°F)

After dispensing to patient: Store at 20°C to 25°C (68°F to 77°F) [see USP Controlled Room Temperature]. Protect from heat and moisture. CAPSULES SHOULD ALWAYS BE STORED IN THE BLISTER AND ONLY REMOVED FROM THE BLISTER IMMEDIATELY BEFORE USE.

Always discard the Foradil® capsules and Aerolizer™ Inhaler by the "Use by" date and always use the new Aerolizer Inhaler provided with each new prescription.

Keep out of the reach of children.

T2001-11
FEBRUARY 2001 Printed in U.S.A. 89012201
Distributed by:
Novartis Pharmaceuticals Corporation
East Hanover, NJ 07936

STARLIX® ℞

[stăr-līks']

(nateglinide) tablets

Rx only

DESCRIPTION

Starlix® (nateglinide) is an oral antidiabetic agent used in the management of Type 2 diabetes mellitus [also known as non-insulin dependent diabetes mellitus (NIDDM) or adult-onset diabetes]. Starlix, (-)-N-[(trans-4-isopropylcyclohexane)carbonyl]-D- phenylalanine, is structurally unrelated to the oral sulfonylurea insulin secretagogues.

The structural formula is as shown

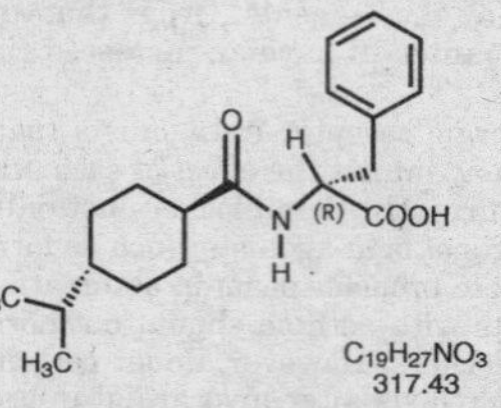

$C_{19}H_{27}NO_3$
317.43

Nateglinide is a white powder with a molecular weight of 317.43. It is freely soluble in methanol, ethanol, and chloroform, soluble in ether, sparingly soluble in acetonitrile and octanol, and practically insoluble in water. Starlix biconvex tablets contain 60 mg, or 120 mg, of nateglinide for oral administration.

Inactive ingredients: colloidal silicon dioxide, croscarmellose sodium, hydroxypropyl methylcellulose, iron oxides (red or yellow), lactose monohydrate, magnesium stearate, microcrystalline cellulose, polyethylene glycol, povidone, talc, and titanium dioxide.

CLINICAL PHARMACOLOGY

Mechanism of Action

Nateglinide is an amino-acid derivative that lowers blood glucose levels by stimulating insulin secretion from the pancreas. This action is dependent upon functioning beta-cells in the pancreatic islets. Nateglinide interacts with the ATP-sensitive potassium (K^+_{ATP}) channel on pancreatic beta-cells. The subsequent depolarization of the beta cell opens the calcium channel, producing calcium influx and insulin secretion. The extent of insulin release is glucose dependent and diminishes at low glucose levels. Nateglinide is highly tissue selective with low affinity for heart and skeletal muscle.

Pharmacokinetics

Absorption

Following oral administration immediately prior to a meal, nateglinide is rapidly absorbed with mean peak plasma drug concentrations (C_{max}) generally occurring within 1 hour (T_{max}) after dosing. When administered to patients with Type 2 diabetes over the dosage range 60 mg to 240 mg three times a day for one week, nateglinide demonstrated linear pharmacokinetics for both AUC (area under the time/plasma concentration curve) and C_{max}. T_{max} was also found to be independent of dose in this patient population. Absolute bioavailability is estimated to be approximately 73%. When given with or after meals, the extent of nateglinide absorption (AUC) remains unaffected. However, there is a delay in the rate of absorption characterized by a decrease in C_{max} and a delay in time to peak plasma concentration (T_{max}). Plasma profiles are characterized by multiple plasma concentration peaks when nateglinide is administered under fasting conditions. This effect is diminished when nateglinide is taken prior to a meal.

Distribution

Based on data following intravenous (IV) administration of nateglinide, the steady-state volume of distribution of nateglinide is estimated to be approximately 10 liters in healthy subjects. Nateglinide is extensively bound (98%) to serum proteins, primarily serum albumin, and to a lesser extent α_1 acid glycoprotein. The extent of serum protein binding is independent of drug concentration over the test range of 0.1-10 μg/mL.

Metabolism

Nateglinide is metabolized by the mixed-function oxidase system prior to elimination. The major routes of metabolism are hydroxylation followed by glucuronide conjugation. The major metabolites are less potent antidiabetic agents than nateglinide. The isoprene minor metabolite possesses potency similar to that of the parent compound nateglinide.

In vitro data demonstrate that nateglinide is predominantly metabolized by cytochrome P450 isoenzymes CYP2C9 (70%) and CYP3A4 (30%).

Excretion

Nateglinide and its metabolites are rapidly and completely eliminated following oral administration. Within 6 hours after dosing, approximately 75% of the administered ^{14}C-nateglinide was recovered in the urine. Eighty-three percent of the ^{14}C-nateglinide was excreted in the urine with an additional 10% eliminated in the feces. Approximately 16% of the ^{14}C-nateglinide was excreted in the urine as parent compound. In all studies of healthy volunteers and patients with Type 2 diabetes, nateglinide plasma concentrations declined rapidly with an average elimination half-life of approximately 1.5 hours. Consistent with this short elimination half-life, there was no apparent accumulation of nateglinide upon multiple dosing of up to 240 mg three times daily for 7 days.

Special Populations

Geriatric: Age did not influence the pharmacokinetic properties of nateglinide. Therefore, no dose adjustments are necessary for elderly patients.

Gender: No clinically significant differences in nateglinide pharmacokinetics were observed between men and women. Therefore, no dose adjustment based on gender is necessary.

Race: Results of a population pharmacokinetic analysis including subjects of Caucasian, Black, and other ethnic origins suggest that race has little influence on the pharmacokinetics of nateglinide.

Renal Impairment: Compared to healthy matched subjects, patients with Type 2 diabetes and moderate-to-severe renal insufficiency (CrCl 15-50 mL/min) not on dialysis displayed similar apparent clearance, AUC, and C_{max}. Patients with Type 2 diabetes and renal failure on dialysis exhibited reduced overall drug exposure. However, hemodialysis patients also experienced reductions in plasma protein binding compared to the matched healthy volunteers.

Hepatic Impairment: The peak and total exposure of nateglinide in non-diabetic subjects with mild hepatic insufficiency were increased by 30% compared to matched healthy subjects. Starlix® (nateglinide) should be used with caution in patients with chronic liver disease. (See PRECAUTIONS, Hepatic Impairment.)

Pharmacodynamics

Starlix is rapidly absorbed and stimulates pancreatic insulin secretion within 20 minutes of oral administration. When Starlix is dosed three times daily before meals there is a rapid rise in plasma insulin, with peak levels approximately 1 hour after dosing and a fall to baseline by 4 hours after dosing.

In a double-blind, controlled clinical trial in which Starlix was administered before each of three meals, plasma glucose levels were determined over a 12-hour, daytime period after 7 weeks of treatment. Starlix was administered 10 minutes before meals. The meals were based on standard diabetic weight maintenance menus with the total caloric content based on each subject's height. Starlix produced statistically significant decreases in fasting and postprandial glycemia compared to placebo.

CLINICAL STUDIES

A total of 3164 patients were randomized in eight double-blind, placebo- or active-controlled studies 8 to 24 weeks in duration to evaluate the safety and efficacy of Starlix® (nateglinide). 3118 patients had efficacy values beyond baseline. In these studies Starlix was administered up to 30 minutes before each of three main meals daily.

Starlix® Monotherapy Compared to Placebo

In a randomized, double-blind, placebo-controlled, 24-week study, patients with Type 2 diabetes with $HbA_{1C} \geq 6.8\%$ on diet alone were randomized to receive either Starlix (60 mg or 120 mg three times daily before meals) or placebo. Baseline HbA_{1C} ranged from 7.9% to 8.1% and 77.8% of patients were previously untreated with oral antidiabetic therapy. Patients previously treated with antidiabetic medications were required to discontinue that medication for at least 2 months before randomization. The addition of Starlix before meals resulted in statistically significant reductions in mean HbA_{1C} and mean fasting plasma glucose (FPG) compared to placebo (see Table 1). The reductions in HbA_{1C} and FPG were similar for patients naïve to, and those previously exposed to, antidiabetic medications.

In this study, one episode of severe hypoglycemia (plasma glucose < 36 mg/dL) was reported in a patient treated with Starlix 120 mg three times daily before meals. No patients experienced hypoglycemia that required third party assistance. Patients treated with Starlix had statistically significant mean increases in weight compared to placebo (see Table 1).

In another randomized, double-blind, 24-week, active- and placebo-controlled study, patients with Type 2 diabetes were

Table 1 Endpoint results for a 24-week, fixed dose study of Starlix® monotherapy

	Placebo	Starlix 60 mg three times daily before meals	Starlix 120 mg three times daily before meals
HbA$_{1c}$ (%)	N=168	N=167	N=168
Baseline (mean)	8.0	7.9	8.1
Change from baseline (mean)	+0.2	−0.3	−0.5
Difference from placebo (mean)		−0.5[a]	−0.7[a]
FPG (mg/dL)	N=172	N=171	N=169
Baseline (mean)	167.9	161.0	166.5
Change from baseline (mean)	+9.1	+0.4	−4.5
Difference from placebo (mean)		−8.7[a]	−13.6[a]
Weight (kg)	N=170	N=169	N=166
Baseline (mean)	85.8	83.7	86.3
Change from baseline (mean)	−0.7	+0.3	+0.9
Difference from placebo (mean)		+1.0[a]	+1.6[a]

[a] p-value ≤ 0.004

Table 2 Endpoint results for a 24-week study of Starlix® monotherapy and combination with metformin

	Placebo	Starlix 120 mg three times daily before meals	Metformin 500 mg three times daily	Starlix 120 mg before meals plus Metformin*
HbA$_{1c}$ (%) All	N=160	N=171	N=172	N=162
Baseline (mean)	8.3	8.3	8.4	8.4
Change from baseline (mean)	+0.4	−0.4[bc]	−0.8[c]	−1.5
Difference from placebo		−0.8[a]	−1.2[a]	−1.9[a]
Naïve	N=98	N=99	N=98	N=81
Baseline (mean)	8.2	8.1	8.3	8.2
Change from baseline (mean)	+0.3	−0.7[c]	−0.8[c]	−1.6
Difference from placebo		−1.0[a]	−1.1[a]	−1.9[a]
Non-Naïve	N=62	N=72	N=74	N=81
Baseline (mean)	8.3	8.5	8.7	8.7
Change from baseline (mean)	+0.6	+0.004[bc]	−0.8[c]	−1.4
Difference from placebo		−0.6[a]	−1.4[a]	−2.0[a]
FPG (mg/dL) All	N=166	N=173	N=174	N=167
Baseline (mean)	194.0	196.5	196.0	197.7
Change from baseline (mean)	+8.0	−13.1[bc]	−30.0[c]	−44.9
Difference from placebo		−21.1[a]	−38.0[a]	−52.9[a]
Weight (kg) All	N=160	N=169	N=169	N=160
Baseline (mean)	85.0	85.0	86.0	87.4
Change from baseline (mean)	−0.4	+0.9[bc]	−0.1	+0.2
Difference from placebo		+1.3[a]	+0.3	+0.6

[a] p-value ≤ 0.05 vs. placebo
[b] p-value ≤ 0.03 vs. metformin
[c] p-value ≤ 0.05 vs. combination
*Metformin was administered three times daily

randomized to receive Starlix (120 mg three times daily before meals), metformin 500 mg (three times daily), a combination of Starlix 120 mg (three times daily before meals) and metformin 500 mg (three times daily), or placebo. Baseline HbA$_{1c}$ ranged from 8.3% to 8.4%. Fifty-seven percent of patients were previously untreated with oral antidiabetic therapy. Starlix monotherapy resulted in significant reductions in mean HbA$_{1c}$ and mean FPG compared to placebo that were similar to the results of the study reported above (see Table 2).
[See table 1 above]

Starlix® Monotherapy Compared to Other Oral Antidiabetic Agents
Glyburide
In a 24-week, double-blind, active-controlled trial, patients with Type 2 diabetes who had been on a sulfonylurea for ≥ 3 months and who had a baseline HbA$_{1c}$ ≥ 6.5% were randomized to receive Starlix (60 mg or 120 mg three times daily before meals) or glyburide 10 mg once daily. Patients randomized to Starlix had significant increases in mean HbA$_{1c}$ and mean FPG at endpoint compared to patients randomized to glyburide.
Metformin
In another randomized, double-blind, 24-week, active- and placebo-controlled study, patients with Type 2 diabetes were randomized to receive Starlix (120 mg three times daily before meals), metformin 500 mg (three times daily), a combination of Starlix 120 mg (three times daily before meals) and metformin 500 mg (three times daily), or placebo. Baseline HbA$_{1c}$ ranged from 8.3% to 8.4%. Fifty-seven percent of patients were previously untreated with oral antidiabetic therapy. The reductions in mean HbA$_{1c}$ and mean FPG at endpoint with metformin monotherapy were significantly greater than the reductions in these variables with Starlix

monotherapy (see Table 2). Relative to placebo, Starlix monotherapy was associated with significant increases in mean weight whereas metformin monotherapy was associated with significant decreases in mean weight. Among the subset of patients naïve to antidiabetic therapy, the reductions in mean HbA$_{1c}$ and mean FPG for Starlix monotherapy were similar to those for metformin monotherapy (see Table 2). Among the subset of patients previously treated with other antidiabetic agents, primarily glyburide, HbA$_{1c}$ in the Starlix monotherapy group increased slightly from baseline, whereas HbA$_{1c}$ was reduced in the metformin monotherapy group (see Table 2).

Starlix® Combination Therapy
Metformin
In another randomized, double-blind, 24-week, active- and placebo-controlled study, patients with Type 2 diabetes were randomized to receive Starlix (120 mg three times daily before meals), metformin 500 mg (three times daily), a combination of Starlix 120 mg (three times daily before meals) and metformin 500 mg (three times daily), or placebo. Baseline HbA$_{1c}$ ranged from 8.3% to 8.4%. Fifty-seven percent of patients were previously untreated with oral antidiabetic therapy. Patients previously treated with antidiabetic medications were required to discontinue medication for at least 2 months before randomization. The combination of Starlix and metformin resulted in statistically significantly greater reductions in HbA$_{1c}$ and FPG compared to either Starlix or metformin monotherapy (see Table 2). Starlix, alone or in combination with metformin, significantly reduced the prandial glucose elevation from pre-meal to 2-hours post-meal compared to placebo and metformin alone.
In this study, one episode of severe hypoglycemia (plasma glucose ≤ 36 mg/dL) was reported in a patient receiving the combination of Starlix and metformin and four episodes of

severe hypoglycemia were reported in a single patient in the metformin treatment arm. No patient experienced an episode of hypoglycemia that required third party assistance. Compared to placebo, Starlix monotherapy was associated with a statistically significant increase in weight, while no significant change in weight was observed with combined Starlix and metformin therapy (see Table 2).
In another 24-week, double-blind, placebo-controlled trial, patients with Type 2 diabetes with HbA$_{1c}$ ≥ 6.8% after treatment with metformin (≥ 1500 mg daily for ≥ 1 month) were first entered into a four week run-in period of metformin monotherapy (2000 mg daily) and then randomized to receive Starlix (60 mg or 120 mg three times daily before meals) or placebo in addition to metformin. Combination therapy with Starlix and metformin was associated with statistically significantly greater reductions in HbA$_{1c}$ compared to metformin monotherapy (-0.4% and -0.6% for Starlix 60 mg and Starlix 120 mg plus metformin, respectively).
[See table 2 at left]
Glyburide
In a 12-week study of patients with Type 2 diabetes inadequately controlled on glyburide 10 mg once daily, the addition of Starlix (60 mg or 120 mg three times daily before meals) did not produce any additional benefit.

INDICATIONS AND USAGE

Starlix® (nateglinide) is indicated as monotherapy to lower blood glucose in patients with Type 2 diabetes (non-insulin dependent diabetes mellitus, NIDDM) whose hyperglycemia cannot be adequately controlled by diet and physical exercise and who have not been chronically treated with other anti-diabetic agents.
Starlix is also indicated for use in combination with metformin. In patients whose hyperglycemia is inadequately controlled with metformin, Starlix may be added to, but not substituted for, metformin.
Patients whose hyperglycemia is not adequately controlled with glyburide or other insulin secretagogues should not be switched to Starlix, nor should Starlix be added to their treatment regimen.

CONTRAINDICATIONS

Starlix® (nateglinide) is contraindicated in patients with:
1. Known hypersensitivity to the drug or its inactive ingredients.
2. Type 1 diabetes.
3. Diabetic ketoacidosis. This condition should be treated with insulin.

PRECAUTIONS

Hypoglycemia: All oral blood glucose lowering drugs that are absorbed systemically are capable of producing hypoglycemia. The frequency of hypoglycemia is related to the severity of the diabetes, the level of glycemic control, and other patient characteristics. Geriatric patients, malnourished patients, and those with adrenal or pituitary insufficiency are more susceptible to the glucose lowering effect of these treatments. The risk of hypoglycemia may be increased by strenuous physical exercise, ingestion of alcohol, insufficient caloric intake on an acute or chronic basis, or combinations with other oral antidiabetic agents. Hypoglycemia may be difficult to recognize in patients with autonomic neuropathy and/or those who use beta-blockers. Starlix® (nateglinide) should be administered prior to meals to reduce the risk of hypoglycemia. Patients who skip meals should also skip their scheduled dose of Starlix to reduce the risk of hypoglycemia.
Hepatic Impairment: Starlix should be used with caution in patients with moderate-to-severe liver disease because such patients have not been studied.
Loss of Glycemic Control
Transient loss of glycemic control may occur with fever, infection, trauma, or surgery. Insulin therapy may be needed instead of Starlix therapy at such times. Secondary failure, or reduced effectiveness of Starlix over a period of time, may occur.
Information for Patients
Patients should be informed of the potential risks and benefits of Starlix and of alternative modes of therapy. The risks and management of hypoglycemia should be explained. Patients should be instructed to take Starlix 1 to 30 minutes before ingesting a meal, but to skip their scheduled dose if they skip the meal so that the risk of hypoglycemia will be reduced. Drug interactions should be discussed with patients. Patients should be informed of potential drug-drug interactions with Starlix.
Laboratory Tests
Response to therapies should be periodically assessed with glucose values and HbA$_{1c}$ levels.
Drug Interactions
In vitro drug metabolism studies indicate that Starlix is predominantly metabolized by the cytochrome P450 isozyme CYP2C9 (70%) and to a lesser extent CYP3A4 (30%). Starlix is a potential inhibitor of the CYP2C9 isoenzyme *in vivo* as indicated by its ability to inhibit the *in vitro* metabolism of tolbutamide. Inhibition of CYP3A4 metabolic reactions was not detected in *in vitro* experiments.
Glyburide: In a randomized, multiple-dose crossover study, patients with Type 2 diabetes were administered 120 mg Starlix three times a day before meals for 1 day in combination with glyburide 10 mg daily. There were no clinically relevant alterations in the pharmacokinetics of either agent.
Metformin: When Starlix 120 mg three times daily before meals was administered in combination with metformin

Continued on next page

Starlix—Cont.

500 mg three times daily to patients with Type 2 diabetes, there were no clinically relevant changes in the pharmacokinetics of either agent.

Digoxin: When Starlix 120 mg before meals was administered in combination with a single 1-mg dose of digoxin to healthy volunteers, there were no clinically relevant changes in the pharmacokinetics of either agent.

Warfarin: When healthy subjects were administered Starlix 120 mg three times daily before meals for four days in combination with a single dose of warfarin 30 mg on day 2, there were no alterations in the pharmacokinetics of either agent. Prothrombin time was not affected.

Diclofenac: Administration of morning and lunch doses of Starlix 120 mg in combination with a single 75-mg dose of diclofenac in healthy volunteers resulted in no significant changes to the pharmacokinetics of either agent.

Nateglinide is highly bound to plasma proteins (98%), mainly albumin. *In vitro* displacement studies with highly protein-bound drugs such as furosemide, propranolol, captopril, nicardipine, pravastatin, glyburide, warfarin, phenytoin, acetylsalicylic acid, tolbutamide, and metformin showed no influence on the extent of nateglinide protein binding. Similarly, nateglinide had no influence on the serum protein binding of propranolol, glyburide, nicardipine, warfarin, phenytoin, acetylsalicylic acid, and tolbutamide *in vitro*. However, prudent evaluation of individual cases is warranted in the clinical setting.

Certain drugs, including nonsteroidal anti-inflammatory agents (NSAIDs), salicylates, monoamine oxidase inhibitors, and non-selective beta-adrenergic-blocking agents may potentiate the hypoglycemic action of Starlix and other oral antidiabetic drugs.

Certain drugs including thiazides, corticosteroids, thyroid products, and sympathomimetics may reduce the hypoglycemic action of Starlix and other oral antidiabetic drugs. When these drugs are administered to or withdrawn from patients receiving Starlix, the patient should be observed closely for changes in glycemic control.

Drug/Food Interactions

The pharmacokinetics of nateglinide were not affected by the composition of a meal (high protein, fat, or carbohydrate). However, peak plasma levels were significantly reduced when Starlix was administered 10 minutes prior to a liquid meal. Starlix did not have any effect on gastric emptying in healthy subjects as assessed by acetaminophen testing.

Carcinogenesis/Mutagenesis/Impairment of Fertility

Carcinogenicity: A two-year carcinogenicity study in Sprague-Dawley rats was performed with oral doses of nateglinide up to 900 mg/kg/day, which produced AUC exposures in male and female rats approximately 30 and 40 times the human therapeutic exposure respectively with a recommended Starlix dose of 120 mg, three times daily before meals. A two-year carcinogenicity study in B6C3F1 mice was performed with oral doses of nateglinide up to 400 mg/kg/day, which produced AUC exposures in male and female mice approximately 10 and 30 times the human therapeutic exposure with a recommended Starlix dose of 120 mg, three times daily before meals. No evidence of a tumorigenic response was found in either rats or mice.

Mutagenesis: Nateglinide was not genotoxic in the *in vitro* Ames test, mouse lymphoma assay, chromosome aberration assay in Chinese hamster lung cells, or in the *in vivo* mouse micronucleus test.

Impairment of Fertility: Fertility was unaffected by administration of nateglinide to rats at doses up to 600 mg/kg (approximately 16 times the human therapeutic exposure with a recommended Starlix dose of 120 mg three times daily before meals).

Pregnancy

Pregnancy Category C

Nateglinide was not teratogenic in rats at doses up to 1000 mg/kg (approximately 60 times the human therapeutic exposure with a recommended Starlix dose of 120 mg three times daily before meals). In the rabbit, embryonic development was adversely affected and the incidence of gallbladder agenesis or small gallbladder was increased at a dose of 500 mg/kg (approximately 40 times the human therapeutic exposure with a recommended Starlix dose of 120 mg, three times daily before meals). There are no adequate and well-controlled studies in pregnant women. Starlix should not be used during pregnancy.

Labor and Delivery

The effect of Starlix on labor and delivery in humans is not known.

Nursing Mothers

Studies in lactating rats showed that nateglinide is excreted in the milk; the AUC_{0-48h} ratio in milk to plasma was approximately 1:4. During the peri- and postnatal period body weights were lower in offspring of rats administered nateglinide at 1000 mg/kg (approximately 60 times the human therapeutic exposure with a recommended Starlix dose of 120 mg, three times daily before meals). It is not known whether Starlix is excreted in human milk. Because many drugs are excreted in human milk, Starlix should not be administered to a nursing woman.

Pediatric Use

The safety and effectiveness of Starlix in pediatric patients have not been established.

Geriatric Use

No differences were observed in safety or efficacy of Starlix between patients age 65 and over, and those under age 65. However, greater sensitivity of some older individuals to Starlix therapy cannot be ruled out.

ADVERSE REACTIONS

In clinical trials, approximately 2400 patients with Type 2 diabetes were treated with Starlix® (nateglinide). Of these, approximately 1200 patients were treated for 6 months or longer and approximately 190 patients for one year or longer.

Hypoglycemia was relatively uncommon in all treatment arms of the clinical trials. Only 0.3% of Starlix patients discontinued due to hypoglycemia. Gastrointestinal symptoms, especially diarrhea and nausea, were no more common in patients using the combination of Starlix and metformin than in patients receiving metformin alone. The following table lists events that occurred more frequently in Starlix patients than placebo patients in controlled clinical trials.

Common Adverse Events (≥ 2% in Starlix® patients) in Starlix® Monotherapy Trials (% of patients)

	Placebo N=458	Starlix N=1441
Preferred Term		
Upper Respiratory Infection	8.1	10.5
Back Pain	3.7	4.0
Flu Symptoms	2.6	3.6
Dizziness	2.2	3.6
Arthropathy	2.2	3.3
Diarrhea	3.1	3.2
Accidental Trauma	1.7	2.9
Bronchitis	2.6	2.7
Coughing	2.2	2.4
Hypoglycemia	0.4	2.4

Laboratory Abnormalities

Uric acid: There were increases in mean uric acid levels for patients treated with Starlix alone, Starlix in combination with metformin, metformin alone, and glyburide alone. The respective differences from placebo were 0.29 mg/dL, 0.45 mg/dL, 0.28 mg/dL, and 0.19 mg/dL. The clinical significance of these findings is unknown.

OVERDOSAGE

In a clinical study in patients with Type 2 diabetes, Starlix® (nateglinide) was administered in increasing doses up to 720 mg a day for 7 days and there were no clinically significant adverse events reported. There have been no instances of overdose with Starlix in clinical trials. However, an overdose may result in an exaggerated glucose-lowering effect with the development of hypoglycemic symptoms. Hypoglycemic symptoms without loss of consciousness or neurological findings should be treated with oral glucose and adjustments in dosage and/or meal patterns. Severe hypoglycemic reactions with coma, seizure, or other neurological symptoms should be treated with intravenous glucose. As nateglinide is highly protein bound, dialysis is not an efficient means of removing it from the blood.

DOSAGE AND ADMINISTRATION

Starlix® (nateglinide) should be taken 1 to 30 minutes prior to meals.

Monotherapy and Combination with Metformin

The recommended starting and maintenance dose of Starlix, alone or in combination with metformin, is 120 mg three times daily before meals.

The 60-mg dose of Starlix, either alone or in combination with metformin, may be used in patients who are near goal HbA_{1C} when treatment is initiated.

Dosage in Geriatric Patients

No special dose adjustments are usually necessary. However, greater sensitivity of some individuals to Starlix therapy cannot be ruled out.

Dosage in Renal and Hepatic Impairment

No dosage adjustment is necessary in patients with mild-to-severe renal insufficiency or in patients with mild hepatic insufficiency. Dosing of patients with moderate-to-severe hepatic dysfunction has not been studied. Therefore, Starlix should be used with caution in patients with moderate-to-severe liver disease (see PRECAUTIONS, Hepatic Impairment).

HOW SUPPLIED

Starlix® (nateglinide) tablets

60 mg

Pink, round, beveled edge tablet with "STARLIX" debossed on one side and "60" on the other.

Bottles of 100	NDC 0078-0351-05
Bottles of 500	NDC 0078-0351-08

120 mg

Yellow, ovaloid tablet with "STARLIX" debossed on one side and "120" on the other.

Bottles of 100	NDC 0078-0352-05
Bottles of 500	NDC 0078-0352-08

Storage

Store at 25°C (77°F); excursions permitted to 15°C-30°C (59°F-86°F).

Dispense in a tight container, USP.

T2000-41
DECEMBER 2000   Printed in U.S.A.   89010101

Organon Inc.

**375 MT. PLEASANT AVE.
WEST ORANGE, NJ 07052**

Direct Inquiries to:
(973) 325-4500

REMERON®SOLTAB™   ℞
(mirtazapine)
Orally Disintegrating Tablets

DESCRIPTION

REMERON®SolTab™ (mirtazapine) Orally Disintegrating Tablets are an antidepressant for oral administration. Mirtazapine has a tetracyclic chemical structure unrelated to selective serotonin reuptake inhibitors, tricyclics or monoamine oxidase inhibitors (MAOI). Mirtazapine belongs to the piperazino-azepine group of compounds. It is designated 1,2,3,4,10,14b-hexahydro-2-methyl-pyrazino [2,1-a] pyrido [2,3-c] benzazepine and has the empirical formula of $C_{17}H_{19}N_3$. Its molecular weight is 265.36. The structural formula is the following and it is the racemic mixture:

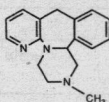

Mirtazapine is a white to creamy white crystalline powder which is slightly soluble in water.

REMERON®SolTab™ is available for oral administration as an orally disintegrating tablet containing 15, 30, or 45 mg of mirtazapine. It disintegrates in the mouth within seconds after placement on the tongue allowing its contents to be subsequently swallowed with or without water.

REMERON®SolTab™ also contains the following inactive ingredients: aspartame, citric acid, crospovidone, hydroxypropyl methylcellulose, magnesium stearate, mannitol, microcrystalline cellulose, natural and artificial orange flavor, polymethacrylate, povidone, sodium bicarbonate, starch, sucrose.

CLINICAL PHARMACOLOGY

Pharmacodynamics

The mechanism of action of REMERON®SolTab™ (mirtazapine) Orally Disintegrating Tablets, as with other antidepressants, is unknown.

Evidence gathered in preclinical studies suggests that mirtazapine enhances central noradrenergic and serotonergic activity. These studies have shown that mirtazapine acts as an antagonist at central presynaptic α_2 adrenergic inhibitory autoreceptors and heteroreceptors, an action that is postulated to result in an increase in central noradrenergic and serotonergic activity.

Mirtazapine is a potent antagonist of $5\text{-}HT_2$ and $5\text{-}HT_3$ receptors. Mirtazapine has no significant affinity for the $5\text{-}HT_{1A}$ and $5\text{-}HT_{1B}$ receptors.

Mirtazapine is a potent antagonist of histamine (H_1) receptors, a property that may explain its prominent sedative effects.

Mirtazapine is a moderate peripheral α_1 adrenergic antagonist, a property that may explain the occasional orthostatic hypotension reported in association with its use.

Mirtazapine is a moderate antagonist at muscarinic receptors, a property that may explain the relatively low incidence of anticholinergic side effects associated with its use.

Pharmacokinetics

REMERON®SolTab™ (mirtazapine) Orally Disintegrating Tablets are rapidly and completely absorbed following oral administration and have a half-life of about 20–40 hours. Peak plasma concentrations are reached within about 2 hours following an oral dose. The presence of food in the stomach has a minimal effect on both the rate and extent of absorption and does not require a dosage adjustment. REMERON®SolTab™ Orally Disintegrating Tablets are bioequivalent to REMERON® (mirtazapine) Tablets.

Mirtazapine is extensively metabolized after oral administration. Major pathways of biotransformation are demethylation and hydroxylation followed by glucuronide conjugation. *In vitro* data from human liver microsomes indicate that cytochrome 2D6 and 1A2 are involved in the formation of the 8-hydroxy metabolite of mirtazapine, whereas cytochrome 3A is considered to be responsible for the formation of the N-desmethyl and N-oxide metabolite. Mirtazapine has an absolute bioavailability of about 50%. It is eliminated predominantly via urine (75%) with 15% in feces. Several unconjugated metabolites possess pharmacological activity but are present in the plasma at very low levels. The (−) enantiomer has an elimination half-life that is approximately twice as long as the (+) enantiomer and therefore achieves plasma levels that are about three times as high as that of the (+) enantiomer.

Plasma levels are linearly related to dose over a dose range of 15 to 80 mg. The mean elimination half-life of mirtazapine after oral administration ranges from approximately 20–40 hours across age and gender subgroups, with females of all ages exhibiting significantly longer elimination half-lives than males (mean half-life of 37 hours for females vs. 26 hours for males). Steady state plasma levels of mirtazapine are attained within 5 days, with about 50% accumulation (accumulation ratio = 1.5).

Mirtazapine is approximately 85% bound to plasma proteins over a concentration of 0.01 to 10 µg/mL.

Special Populations

Geriatric

Following oral administration of REMERON® (mirtazapine) Tablets 20 mg/day for 7 days to subjects of varying ages (range, 25–74), oral clearance of mirtazapine was reduced in the elderly compared to the younger subjects. The differences were most striking in males, with a 40% lower clearance in elderly males compared to younger males, while the clearance in elderly females was only 10% lower compared to younger females. Caution is indicated in administering REMERON®SolTab™ (mirtazapine) Orally Disintegrating Tablets to elderly patients (see PRECAUTIONS and DOSAGE AND ADMINISTRATION).

Pediatrics

Safety and effectiveness of mirtazapine in the pediatric population have not been established (see PRECAUTIONS).

Gender

The mean elimination half-life of mirtazapine after oral administration ranges from approximately 20–40 hours across age and gender subgroups, with females of all ages exhibiting significantly longer elimination half-lives than males (mean half-life of 37 hours for females vs. 26 hours for males) (see Pharmacokinetics).

Race

There have been no clinical studies to evaluate the effect of race on the pharmacokinetics of REMERON®SolTab™.

Renal Insufficiency

The disposition of mirtazapine was studied in patients with varying degrees of renal function. Elimination of mirtazapine is correlated with creatinine clearance. Total body clearance of mirtazapine was reduced approximately 30% in patients with moderate (Clcr = 11–39 mL/min/1.73 m^2) and approximately 50% in patients with severe (Clcr = < 10 mL/min/1.73 m^2) renal impairment with compared to normal subjects. Caution is indicated in administering REMERON®SolTab™ to patients with compromised renal function (see PRECAUTIONS and DOSAGE AND ADMINISTRATION).

Hepatic Insufficiency

Following a single 15 mg oral dose of REMERON®, the oral clearance of mirtazapine was decreased by approximately 30% in hepatically impaired patients compared to subjects with normal hepatic function. Caution is indicated in administering REMERON®SolTab™ to patients with compromised hepatic function (see PRECAUTIONS and DOSAGE AND ADMINISTRATION).

Clinical Trials Showing Effectiveness

The efficacy of REMERON® (mirtazapine) Tablets as a treatment for depression was established in four placebo-controlled, 6-week trials in adult outpatients meeting DSM-III criteria for major depression. Patients were titrated with mirtazapine from a dose range of 5 mg up to 35 mg/day. Overall, these studies demonstrated mirtazapine to be superior to placebo on at least three of the following four measures: 21-Item Hamilton Depression Rating Scale (HDRS) total score; HDRS Depressed Mood Item; CGI Severity score; and Montgomery and Asberg Depression Rating Scale (MADRS). Superiority of mirtazapine over placebo was also found for certain factors of the HDRS, including anxiety/somatization factor and sleep disturbance factor. The mean mirtazapine dose for patients who completed these four studies ranged from 21 to 32 mg/day. A fifth study of similar design utilized a higher dose (up to 50 mg) per day and also showed effectiveness.

Examination of age and gender subsets of the population did not reveal any differential responsiveness on the basis of these subgroupings.

INDICATIONS AND USAGE

REMERON®SolTab™ (mirtazapine) Orally Disintegrating Tablets are indicated for the treatment of depression.

The efficacy of REMERON® (mirtazapine) Tablets in the treatment of depression was established in six week controlled trials of outpatients whose diagnoses corresponded most closely to the Diagnostic and Statistical Manual of Mental Disorders—3rd edition (DSM-III) category of major depressive disorder (see CLINICAL PHARMACOLOGY).

A major depressive episode (DSM-IV) implies a prominent and relatively persistent (nearly every day for at least 2 weeks) depressed or dysphoric mood that usually interferes with daily functioning, and includes at least five of the following nine symptoms: depressed mood, loss of interest in usual activities, significant change in weight and/or appetite, insomnia or hypersomnia, psychomotor agitation or retardation, increased fatigue, feelings of guilt or worthlessness, slowed thinking or impaired concentration, a suicide attempt or suicidal ideation.

The antidepressant effectiveness of REMERON®SolTab™ in hospitalized depressed patients has not been adequately studied.

The effectiveness of REMERON®SolTab™ in long-term use, that is, for more than 6 weeks, has not been systematically evaluated in controlled trials. Therefore, the physician who elects to use REMERON®SolTab™ for extended periods should periodically evaluate the long-term usefulness of the drug for the individual patient.

CONTRAINDICATIONS

REMERON®SolTab™ (mirtazapine) Orally Disintegrating Tablets are contraindicated in patients with a known hypersensitivity to mirtazapine.

WARNINGS

Agranulocytosis

In premarketing clinical trials, two (one with Sjögren's Syndrome) out of 2796 patients treated with REMERON® (mirtazapine) Tablets developed agranulocytosis [absolute neutrophil count (ANC) <500/mm^3 with associated signs and symptoms, e.g., fever, infection, etc.] and a third patient developed severe neutropenia (ANC < 500/mm^3 without any associated symptoms). For these three patients, onset of severe neutropenia was detected on days 61, 9, and 14 of treatment, respectively. All three patients recovered after REMERON® was stopped. These three cases yield a crude incidence of severe neutropenia (with or without associated infection) of approximately 1.1 per thousand patients exposed, with a very wide 95% confidence interval, i.e., 2.2 cases per 10,000 to 3.1 cases per 1000. If a patient develops a sore throat, fever, stomatitis or other signs of infection, along with a low WBC count, treatment with REMERON®SolTab™ (mirtazapine) Orally Disintegrating Tablets should be discontinued and the patient should be closely monitored.

MAO Inhibitors

In patients receiving other antidepressants in combination with a monoamine oxidase inhibitor (MAOI) and in patients who have recently discontinued an antidepressant drug and then are started on an MAOI, there have been reports of serious, and sometimes fatal, reactions, including nausea, vomiting, flushing, dizziness, tremor, myoclonus, rigidity, diaphoresis, hyperthermia, autonomic instability with rapid fluctuations of vital signs, seizures, and mental status changes ranging from agitation to coma. Although there are no human data pertinent to such an interaction with REMERON®SolTab™ (mirtazapine) Orally Disintegrating Tablets, it is recommended that REMERON®SolTab™ not be used in combination with an MAOI, or within 14 days of initiating or discontinuing therapy with an MAOI.

PRECAUTIONS

General

Somnolence

In US controlled studies, somnolence was reported in 54% of patients treated with REMERON® (mirtazapine) Tablets, compared to 18% for placebo and 60% for amitriptyline. In these studies, somnolence resulted in discontinuation for 10.4% of REMERON® treated patients, compared to 2.2% for placebo. It is unclear whether or not tolerance develops to the somnolent effects of REMERON®. Because of REMERON®'s potentially significant effects on impairment of performance, patients should be cautioned about engaging in activities requiring alertness until they have been able to assess the drug's effect on their own psychomotor performance (see Information for Patients).

Dizziness

In US controlled studies, dizziness was reported in 7% of patients treated with REMERON®, compared to 3% for placebo and 14% for amitriptyline. It is unclear whether or not tolerance develops to the dizziness observed in association with the use of REMERON®.

Increased Appetite/Weight Gain

In US controlled studies, appetite increase was reported in 17% of patients treated with REMERON®, compared to 2% for placebo and 6% for amitriptyline. In these same trials, weight gain of ≥ 7% of body weight was reported in 7.5% of patients treated with mirtazapine, compared to 0% for placebo and 5.9% for amitriptyline. In a pool of premarketing US studies, including many patients for long-term, open label treatment, 8% of patients receiving REMERON® discontinued for weight gain.

Cholesterol/Triglycerides

In US controlled trials, nonfasting cholesterol increases to ≥ 20% above the upper limits of normal were observed in 15% of patients treated with REMERON®, compared to 7% for placebo and 8% for amitriptyline. In these same studies, nonfasting triglyceride increases to ≥ 500 mg/dL were observed in 6% of patients treated with mirtazapine, compared to 3% for placebo and 3% for amitriptyline.

Transaminase Elevations

Clinically significant ALT (SGPT) elevations (≥ 3 times the upper limit of the normal range) were observed in 2.0% (8/424) of patients exposed to REMERON® in a pool of short-term US controlled trials, compared to 0.3% (1/328) of placebo patients and 2.0% (3/181) of amitriptyline patients. Most of these patients with ALT increases did not develop signs or symptoms associated with compromised liver function. While some patients were discontinued for the ALT increases, in other cases, the enzyme levels returned to normal despite continued REMERON® treatment. REMERON®SolTab™ should be used with caution in patients with impaired hepatic function (see CLINICAL PHARMACOLOGY and DOSAGE AND ADMINISTRATION).

Activation of Mania/Hypomania

Mania/hypomania occurred in approximately 0.2% (3/1299 patients) or REMERON®-treated patients in US studies. Although the incidence of mania/hypomania was very low during treatment with mirtazapine, it should be used carefully in patients with a history of mania/hypomania.

Seizure

In premarketing clinical trials only one seizure was reported among the 2796 US and non-US patients treated with REMERON®. However, no controlled studies have been carried out in patients with a history of seizures. Therefore, care should be exercised when mirtazapine is used in these patients.

Suicide

Suicide ideation is inherent in depression and may persist until significant remission occurs. As with any patient receiving antidepressants, high-risk patients should be closely supervised during initial drug therapy. Prescriptions of REMERON®SolTab™ should be written for the smallest quantity consistent with good patient management, in order to reduce the risk of overdose.

Use in Patients with Concomitant Illness

Clinical experience with REMERON®SolTab™ in patients with concomitant systemic illness is limited. Accordingly, care is advisable in prescribing mirtazapine for patients with diseases or conditions that affect metabolism or hemodynamic responses.

REMERON®SolTab™ has not been systematically evaluated or used to any appreciable extent in patients with a recent history of myocardial infarction or other significant heart disease. REMERON® was associated with significant orthostatic hypotension in early clinical pharmacology trials with normal volunteers. Orthostatic hypotension was infrequently observed in clinical trials with depressed patients. REMERON®SolTab™ should be used with caution in patients with known cardiovascular or cerebrovascular disease that could be exacerbated by hypotension (history of myocardial infarction, angina, or ischemic stroke) and conditions that would predispose patients to hypotension (dehydration, hypovolemia, and treatment with antihypertensive medication).

Mirtazapine clearance is decreased in patients with moderate [glomerular filtration rate (GFR) = 11–39 mL/min/1.73 m^2] and severe [GFR < 10 mL/min/1.73 m^2 renal impairment, and also in patients with hepatic impairment. Caution is indicated in administering REMERON®SolTab™ to such patients (see CLINICAL PHARMACOLOGY and DOSAGE AND ADMINISTRATION).

Information for Patients

Physicians are advised to discuss the following issues with patients for whom they prescribe REMERON®SolTab™ (mirtazapine) Orally Disintegrating Tablets:

Agranulocytosis

Patients who are to receive REMERON®SolTab™ should be warned about the risk of developing agranulocytosis. Patients should be advised to contact their physician if they experience any indication of infection such as fever, chills, sore throat, mucous membrane ulceration or other possible signs of infection. Particular attention should be paid to any flu-like complaints or other symptoms that might suggest infection.

Interference with Cognitive and Motor Performance

REMERON®SolTab™ may impair judgement, thinking, and particularly, motor skills, because of its prominent sedative effect. The drowsiness associated with mirtazapine use may impair a patient's ability to drive, use machines or perform tasks that require alertness. Thus, patients should be cautioned about engaging in hazardous activities until they are reasonably certain that REMERON®SolTab™ therapy does not adversely affect their ability to engage in such activities.

Completing Course of Therapy

While patients may notice improvement with REMERON®SolTab™ therapy in 1 to 4 weeks, they should be advised to continue therapy as directed.

Concomitant Medication

Patients should be advised to inform their physician if they are taking, or intend to take, any prescription or over-the-counter drugs since there is a potential for REMERON®SolTab™ to interact with other drugs.

Alcohol

The impairment of cognitive and motor skills produced by REMERON® has been shown to be additive with those produced by alcohol. Accordingly, patients should be advised to avoid alcohol while taking any dosage form of mirtazapine.

Phenylketonurics

Phenylketonuric patients should be informed that REMERON®SolTab™ contains phenylalanine 2.6 mg per 15 mg tablet, 5.2 mg per 30 mg tablet, and 7.8 mg per 45 mg tablet.

Pregnancy

Patients should be advised to notify their physician if they become pregnant or intend to become pregnant during REMERON®SolTab™ therapy.

Nursing

Patients should be advised to notify their physician if they are breast-feeding an infant.

Laboratory Tests

There are no routine laboratory tests recommended.

Drug Interactions

As with other drugs, the potential for interaction by a variety of mechanisms (e.g., pharmacodynamic, pharmacokinetic inhibition or enhancement, etc.) is a possibility (see CLINICAL PHARMACOLOGY).

Drugs Affecting Hepatic Metabolism

The metabolism and pharmacokinetics of REMERON®SolTab™ (mirtazapine) Orally Disintegrating Tablets may be affected by the induction or inhibition of drug-metabolizing enzymes.

Drugs that are Metabolized by and/or Inhibit Cytochrome P450 Enzymes

Many drugs are metabolized by and/or inhibit various cytochrome P450 enzymes, e.g., 2D6, 1A2, 3A4, etc. *In vitro* studies have shown that mirtazapine is a substrate for several of these enzymes, including 2D6, 1A2, and 3A4. While *in vitro* studies have shown that mirtazapine is not a potent inhibitor of any of these enzymes, an indication that mirtazapine is not likely to have a clinically significant inhibitory effect on the metabolism of other drugs that are substrates for these cytochrome P450 enzymes, the concomitant

Continued on next page

Remeron Soltab—Cont.

use of REMERON®SolTab™ with most other drugs metabolized by these enzymes has not been formally studied. Consequently, it is not possible to make any definitive statements about the risks of coadministration of REMERON®SolTab™ with such drugs.

Alcohol

Concomitant administration of alcohol (equivalent to 60 g) had a minimal effect on plasma levels of mirtazapine (15 mg) in 6 healthy male subjects. However, the impairment of cognitive and motor skills produced by REMERON® were shown to be additive with those produced by alcohol. Accordingly, patients should be advised to avoid alcohol while taking REMERON®SolTab™.

Diazepam

Concomitant administration of diazepam (15 mg) had a minimal effect on plasma levels of mirtazapine (15 mg) in 12 healthy subjects. However, the impairment of motor skills produced by REMERON® has been shown to be additive with those caused by diazepam. Accordingly, patients should be advised to avoid diazepam and other similar drugs while taking REMERON®SolTab™.

Carcinogenesis, Mutagenesis, Impairment of Fertility

Carcinogenesis

Carcinogenicity studies were conducted with mirtazapine given in the diet at doses of 2, 20, and 200 mg/kg/day to mice and 2, 20, and 60 mg/kg/day to rats. The highest doses used are approximately 20 and 12 times the maximum recommended human dose (MRHD) of 45 mg/day on a mg/m^2 basis in mice and rats, respectively. There was an increased incidence of hepatocellular adenoma and carcinoma in male mice at the high dose. In rats, there was an increase in hepatocellular adenoma in females at the mid and high doses and in hepatocellular tumors and thyroid follicular adenoma/cystadenoma and carcinoma in males at the high dose. The data suggest that the above effects could possibly be mediated by non-genotoxic mechanisms, the relevance of which to humans is not known.

The doses used in the mouse study may not have been high enough to fully characterize the carcinogenic potential of REMERON® (mirtazapine) Tablets.

Mutagenesis

Mirtazapine was not mutagenic or clastogenic and did not induce general DNA damage as determined in several genotoxicity tests: Ames test, *in vitro* gene mutation assay in Chinese hamster V 79 cells, *in vitro* sister chromatid exchange assay in cultured rabbit/lymphocytes, *in vivo* bone marrow micronucleus test in rats, and unscheduled DNA synthesis assay in HeLa cells.

Impairment of Fertility

In a fertility study in rats, mirtazapine was given at doses up to 100 mg/kg [20 times the maximum recommended human dose (MRHD) on a mg/m^2 basis]. Mating and conception were not affected by the drug, but estrous cycling was disrupted at doses that were 3 or more times the MRHD and pre-implantation losses occurred at 20 times the MRHD.

Pregnancy

Teratogenic Effects—Pregnancy Category C

Reproduction studies in pregnant rats and rabbits at doses up to 100 mg/kg and 40 mg/kg, respectively [20 and 17 times the maximum recommended human dose (MRHD) on a mg/m^2 basis, respectively], have revealed no evidence of teratogenic effects. However, in rats, there was an increase in post-implantation losses in dams treated with mirtazapine. There was an increase in pup deaths during the first 3 days of lactation and a decrease in pup birth weights. The cause of these deaths is not known. The effects occurred at doses that were 20 times the MRHD, but not at 3 times the MRHD, on a mg/m^2 basis. There are no adequate and well controlled studies in pregnant women. Because animal reproduction studies are not always predictive of human response, this drug should be used during pregnancy only if clearly needed.

Nursing Mothers

It is not known whether mirtazapine is excreted in human milk. Because many drugs are excreted in human milk, caution should be exercised when REMERON®SolTab™ (mirtazapine) Orally Disintegrating Tablets are administered to nursing women.

Pediatric Use

Safety and effectiveness in children have not been established.

Geriatric Use

Approximately 190 elderly individuals (≥ 65 years of age) participated in clinical studies with REMERON® (mirtazapine) Tablets. This drug is known to be substantially excreted by the kidney (75%), and the risk of decreased clearance of this drug is greater in patients with impaired renal function. Because elderly patients are more likely to have decreased renal function, care should be taken in dose selection. Sedating drugs may cause confusion and over-sedation in the elderly. No unusual adverse age-related phenomena were identified in this group. Pharmacokinetic studies revealed a decreased clearance in the elderly. Caution is indicated in administering REMERON®SolTab™ (mirtazapine) Orally Disintegrating Tablets to elderly patients (see CLINICAL PHARMACOLOGY and DOSAGE AND ADMINISTRATION).

ADVERSE REACTIONS

Associated with Discontinuation of Treatment

Approximately 16 percent of the 453 patients who received REMERON® (mirtazapine) Tablets in US 6-week controlled clinical trials discontinued treatment due to an adverse experience, compared to 7 percent of the 361 placebo-treated patients in those studies. The most common events (≥ 1%) associated with discontinuation and considered to be drug related (i.e., those events associated with dropout at a rate at least twice that of placebo included:

Common Adverse Events Associated with Discontinuation of Treatment in 6-Week U.S. REMERON® Trials

Adverse Event	Percentage of Patients Discontinuing with Adverse Event	
	REMERON® (n=453)	Placebo (n=361)
Somnolence	10.4%	2.2%
Nausea	1.5%	0%

Commonly Observed Adverse Events in US Controlled Clinical Trials

The most commonly observed adverse events associated with the use of REMERON® (mirtazapine) Tablets (incidence of 5% of greater) and not observed at an equivalent incidence among placebo-treated patients (REMERON® incidence at least twice that for placebo) were:

Common Treatment-Emergent Adverse Events Associated with the Use of REMERON® in 6-Week U.S. Trials

Adverse Event	Percentage of Patients Reporting Adverse Event	
	REMERON® (n=453)	Placebo (n=361)
Somnolence	54%	18%
Increased Appetite	17%	2%
Weight Gain	12%	2%
Dizziness	7%	3%

Adverse Events Occurring at an Incidence of 1% or More Among REMERON®-Treated Patients

The table that follows enumerates adverse events that occurred at an incidence of 1% or more, and were more frequent than in the placebo group, among REMERON® (mirtazapine) Tablets-treated patients who participated in short-term US placebo-controlled trials in which patients were dosed in a range of 5 to 60 mg/day. This table shows the percentage of patients in each group who had at least one episode of an event at some time during their treatment. Reported adverse events were classified using a standard COSTART-based dictionary terminology.

The prescriber should be aware that these figures cannot be used to predict the incidence of side effects in the course of usual medical practice where patient characteristics and other factors differ from those which prevailed in the clinical trials. Similarly, the cited frequencies cannot be compared with figures obtained from other investigations involving different treatments, uses and investigators. The cited figures, however, do provide the prescribing physician with some basis for estimating the relative contribution of drug and non-drug factors to the side effect incidence rate in the population studied.

INCIDENCE OF ADVERSE CLINICAL EXPERIENCES[1] (≥ 1%) IN SHORT-TERM U.S. CONTROLLED STUDIES

Body System Adverse Clinical Experience	REMERON® (n=453)	Placebo (n=361)
Body as a Whole		
Asthenia	8%	5%
Flu Syndrome	5%	3%
Back Pain	2%	1%
Digestive System		
Dry Mouth	25%	15%
Increased Appetite	17%	2%
Constipation	13%	7%
Metabolic and Nutritional Disorders		
Weight Gain	12%	2%
Peripheral Edema	2%	1%
Edema	1%	0%
Musculoskeletal System		
Myalgia	2%	1%
Nervous System		
Somnolence	54%	18%
Dizziness	7%	3%
Abnormal Dreams	4%	1%
Thinking Abnormal	3%	1%
Tremor	2%	1%
Confusion	2%	0%
Respiratory System		
Dyspnea	1%	0%
Urogenital System		
Urinary Frequency	2%	1%

[1] Events reported by at least 1% of patients treated with REMERON® are included, except the following events which had an incidence on placebo ≥ REMERON®: headache, infection, pain, chest pain, palpitation, tachycardia, postural hypotension, nausea, dyspepsia, diarrhea, flatulence, insomnia, nervousness, libido decreased, hypertonia, pharyngitis, rhinitis, sweating, amblyopia, tinnitus, taste perversion.

ECG Changes

The electrocardiograms for 338 patients who received REMERON® and 261 patients who received placebo in 6-week, placebo-controlled trials were analyzed. Prolongation in QTc ≥ 500 msec was not observed among mirtazapine-treated patients; mean change in QTc was +1.6 msec for mirtazapine and −3.1 msec for placebo. Mirtazapine was associated with a mean increase in heart rate of 3.4 bpm, compared to 0.8 bpm for placebo. The clinical significance of these changes is unknown.

Other Adverse Events Observed During the Premarketing Evaluation of REMERON®

During its premarketing assessment, multiple doses of REMERON® (mirtazapine) Tablets were administered to 2796 patients in clinical studies. The conditions and duration of exposure to mirtazapine varied greatly, and included (in overlapping categories) open and double-blind studies, uncontrolled and controlled studies, inpatient and outpatient studies, fixed dose and titration studies. Untoward events associated with this exposure were recorded by clinical investigators using terminology of their own choosing. Consequently, it is not possible to provide a meaningful estimate of the proportion of individuals experiencing adverse events without first grouping similar types of untoward events into a smaller number of standardized event categories.

In the tabulations that follow, reported adverse events were classified using a COSTART-based dictionary terminology. The frequencies presented, therefore, represent the proportion of the 2796 patients exposed to multiple doses of REMERON® who experienced an event of the type cited on at least one occasion while receiving REMERON®. All reported events are included except those already listed in the previous table, those adverse experiences subsumed under COSTART terms that are either overly general or excessively specific so as to be uninformative, and those events for which a drug cause was very remote.

It is important to emphasize that, although the events reported occurred during treatment with REMERON®, they were not necessarily caused by it.

Events are further categorized by body system and listed in order of decreasing frequency according to the following definitions: frequent adverse events are those occurring on one or more occasions in at least 1/100 patients; infrequent adverse events are those occurring in 1/100 to 1/1000 patients; rare events are those occurring in fewer than 1/1000 patients. Only those events not already listed in the previous table appear in this listing. Events of major clinical importance are also described in the WARNINGS and PRECAUTIONS sections.

Body as a Whole: *frequent*: malaise, abdominal pain, abdominal syndrome acute; *infrequent*: chills, fever, face edema, ulcer, photosensitivity reaction, neck rigidity, neck pain, abdomen enlarged; *rare*: cellulitis, chest pain substernal.

Cardiovascular System: *frequent*: hypertension, vasodilatation; *infrequent*: angina pectoris, myocardial infarction, bradycardia, ventricular extrasystoles, syncope, migraine, hypotension; *rare*: atrial arrhythmia, bigeminy, vascular headache, pulmonary embolus, cerebral ischemia, cardiomegaly, phlebitis, left heart failure.

Digestive System: *frequent*: vomiting, anorexia; *infrequent*: eructation, glossitis, cholecystitis, nausea and vomiting, gum hemorrhage, stomatitis, colitis, liver function tests abnormal; *rare*: tongue discoloration, ulcerative stomatitis, salivary gland enlargement, increased salivation, intestinal obstruction, pancreatitis, aphthous stomatitis, cirrhosis of liver, gastritis, gastroenteritis, oral moniliasis, tongue edema.

Endocrine System: *rare*: goiter, hypothyroidism.

Hemic and Lymphatic System: *rare*: lymphadenopathy, leukopenia, petechia, anemia, thrombocytopenia, lymphocytosis, pancytopenia.

Metabolic and Nutritional Disorders: *frequent*: thirst; *infrequent*: dehydration, weight loss; *rare*: gout, SGOT increased, healing abnormal, acid phosphatase increased, SGPT increased, diabetes mellitus.
Musculoskeletal System: *frequent*: myasthenia, arthraliga; *infrequent*: arthritis, tenosynovitis; *rare*: pathologic fracture, osteoporosis fracture, bone pain, myositis, tendon rupture, arthrosis, bursitis.
Nervous System: *frequent*: hypesthesia, apathy, depression, hypokinesia, vertigo, twitching, agitation, anxiety, amnesia, hyperkinesia, paresthesia; *infrequent*: ataxia, delirium, delusions, depersonalization, dyskinesia, extrapyramidal syndrome, libido increased, coordination abnormal, dysarthria, hallucinations, manic reaction, neurosis, dystonia, hostility, reflexes increased, emotional lability, euphoria, paranoid reaction; *rare*: aphasia, nystagmus, akathisia, stupor, dementia, diplopia, drug dependence, paralysis, grand mal convulsion, hypotonia, myoclonus, psychotic depression, withdrawal syndrome.
Respiratory System: *frequent*: cough increased, sinusitis; *infrequent*: epistaxis, bronchitis, asthma, pneumonia; *rare*: asphyxia, laryngitis, pneumothorax, hiccup.
Skin and Appendages: *frequent*: pruritus, rash; *infrequent*: acne, exfoliative dermatitis, dry skin, herpes simplex, alopecia; *rare*: urticaria, herpes zoster, skin hypertrophy, seborrhea, skin ulcer.
Special Senses: *infrequent*: eye pain, abnormality of accommodation, conjunctivitis, deafness, keratoconjunctivitis, lacrimation disorder, glaucoma, hyperacusis, ear pain, *rare*: blepharitis, partial transitory deafness, otitis media, taste loss, parosmia.
Urogenital System: *frequent*: urinary tract infection; *infrequent*: kidney calculus, cystitis, dysuria, urinary incontinence, urinary retention, vaginitis, hematuria, breast pain, amenorrhea, dysmenorrhea, leukorrhea, impotence; *rare*: polyuria, urethritis, metrorrhagia, menorrhagia, abnormal ejaculation, breast engorgement, breast enlargement, urinary urgency.

Other Adverse Events Observed During Postmarketing Evaluation of REMERON®

Adverse events reported since market introduction, which were temporally (but not necessarily causally) related to mirtazapine therapy, include four cases of the ventricular arrhythmia torsades de pointes. In three of the four cases, however, concomitant drugs were implicated. All patients recovered.

DRUG ABUSE AND DEPENDENCE

Controlled Substance Class

REMERON®SolTab™ (mirtazapine) Orally Disintegrating Tablets are not a controlled substance.

Physical and Psychologic Dependence

REMERON®SolTab™ (mirtazapine) Orally Disintegrating Tablets have not been systematically studied in animals or humans for its potential for abuse, tolerance or physical dependence. While the clinical trials did not reveal any tendency for any drug-seeking behavior, these observations were not systematic and it is not possible to predict on the basis of this limited experience the extent to which a CNS-active drug will be misused, diverted and/or abused once marketed. Consequently, patients should be evaluated carefully for history of drug abuse, and such patients should be observed closely for signs of REMERON®SolTab™ misuse or abuse (e.g., development of tolerance, incrementations of dose, drug-seeking behavior).

OVERDOSAGE

Human Experience

There is very limited experience with REMERON®SolTab™ (mirtazapine) Orally Disintegrating Tablets overdose. In premarketing clinical studies, there were eight reports of REMERON® overdose alone or in combination with other pharmacological agents. The only drug overdose death reported while taking REMERON® was in combination with amitriptyline and chlorprothixene in a non-US clinical study. Based on plasma levels, the REMERON® dose taken was 30–45 mg, while plasma levels of amitriptyline and chlorprothixene were found to be at toxic levels. All other premarketing overdose cases resulted in full recovery. Signs and symptoms reported in association with overdose included disorientation, drowsiness, impaired memory, and tachycardia. There were no reports of ECG abnormalities, coma or convulsions following overdose with REMERON® alone.

Overdose Management

Treatment should consist of those general measures employed in the management of overdose with any antidepressant. Ensure an adequate airway, oxygenation, and ventilation. Monitor cardiac rhythm and vital signs. General supportive and symptomatic measures are also recommended. Induction of emesis is not recommended. Gastric lavage with a large-bore orogastric tube with appropriate airway protection, if needed, may be indicated if performed soon after ingestion, or in symptomatic patients. Because of the rapid disintegration of REMERON®SolTab™ (mirtazapine) Orally Disintegrating Tablets, pill fragments may not appear in gastric contents obtained with lavage.
Activated charcoal should be administered. There is no experience with the use of forced diuresis, dialysis, hemoperfusion or exchange transfusion in the treatment of mirtazapine overdosage. No specific antidotes for mirtazapine are known.
In managing overdosage, consider the possibility of multiple-drug involvement. The physician should consider contacting a poison control center for additional information on the treatment of any overdose. Telephone numbers for certified poison control centers are listed in the *Physicians' Desk Reference* (PDR).

DOSAGE AND ADMINISTRATION

Initial Treatment

The recommended starting dose for REMERON®SolTab™ (mirtazapine) Orally Disintegrating Tablets is 15 mg/day, administered in a single dose, preferably in the evening prior to sleep. In the controlled clinical trials establishing the antidepressant efficacy of REMERON®, the effective dose range was generally 15–45 mg/day. While the relationship between dose and antidepressant response for REMERON® has not been adequately explored, patients not responding to the initial 15 mg dose may benefit from dose increases up to a maximum of 45 mg/day. REMERON® has an elimination half-life of approximately 20–40 hours; therefore, dose changes should not be made at intervals of less than one to two weeks in order to allow sufficient time for evaluation of the therapeutic response to a given dose.

Administration of REMERON®SolTab™ (mirtazapine) Orally Disintegrating Tablets

Patients should be instructed to open tablet blister pack with dry hands and place the tablet on the tongue. The tablet should be used immediately after removal from its blister; once removed, it cannot be stored. REMERON®SolTab™ (mirtazapine) Orally Disintegrating Tablets will disintegrate rapidly on the tongue and can be swallowed with saliva. No water is needed for taking the tablet. Patients should not attempt to split the tablet.

Elderly and Patients with Renal or Hepatic Impairment

The clearance of mirtazapine is reduced in elderly patients and in patients with moderate to severe renal or hepatic impairment. Consequently, the prescriber should be aware that plasma mirtazapine levels may be increased in these patient groups, compared to levels observed in younger adults without renal or hepatic impairment (see PRECAUTIONS and CLINICAL PHARMACOLOGY).

Maintenance/Extended Treatment

There is no body of evidence available from controlled trials to indicate how long the depressed patient should be treated with REMERON®SolTab™ (mirtazapine) Orally Disintegrating Tablets. It is generally agreed, however, that pharmacological treatment for acute episodes of depression should continue for up to six months or longer. Whether the dose of antidepressant needed to induce remission is identical to the dose needed to maintain euthymia is unknown.

Switching Patients To or From a Monoamine Oxidase Inhibitor

At least 14 days should elapse between discontinuation of an MAOI and initiation of therapy with REMERON®SolTab™ (mirtazapine) Orally Disintegrating Tablets. In addition, at least 14 days should be allowed after stopping REMERON®SolTab™ before starting an MAOI.

HOW SUPPLIED

REMERON®SolTab™ (mirtazapine) Orally Disintegrating Tablets are supplied as:

15 mg Tablets—round, white with "T_1Z" debossed on one side.
Box of 30 5 × 6 Unit Dose Blisters NDC 0052-0106-30
Box of 90 15 × 6 Unit Dose Blisters NDC 0052-0106-90
Long Term Care Carton
Box of 30 5 × 6 Unit Dose Blisters NDC 0052-0106-93

30 mg Tablets—round, white with "T_2Z" debossed on one side.
Box of 30 5 × 6 Unit Dose Blisters NDC 0052-0108-30
Box of 90 15 × 6 Unit Dose Blisters NDC 0052-0108-90
Long Term Care Carton
Box of 30 5 × 6 Unit Dose Blisters NDC 0052-0108-93

45 mg Tablets—round, white with "T_4Z" debossed on one side.
Box of 30 5 × 6 Unit Dose Blisters NDC 0052-0110-30
Box of 90 15 × 6 Unit Dose Blisters NDC 0052-0110-90

Storage

Store at 25°C (77°F); excursions permitted to 15–30°C (59–86°F) [see USP Controlled Room Temperature]. Protect from light and moisture. Use immediately upon opening individual tablet blister.

℞ only

Manufactured for Organon Inc., West Orange, NJ 07052
by CIMA Labs Inc., Eden Prairie, MN 55344
5310216 12/00 04

In the PDR annual,
the **Brand and Generic Name Index**
(PINK section)
alphabetizes drugs under both
brand and generic names.

Pfizer Inc.

235 EAST 42nd STREET
NEW YORK, NY 10017–5755

For Medical Information Contact:
(800) 438-1985
24 hours a day, seven days a week.

GEODON™ ℞
(ziprasidone HCl)

DESCRIPTION

GEODON™ is available as GEODON Capsules (ziprasidone hydrochloride) for oral administration. Ziprasidone is an antipsychotic agent that is chemically unrelated to phenothiazine or butyrophenone antipsychotic agents. It has a molecular weight of 412.94 (free base), with the following chemical name: 5-[2-[4-(1,2-benzisothiazol-3-yl)-1-piperazinyl]ethyl]-6-chloro-1,3-dihydro-2*H*-indol-2-one. The empirical formula of $C_{21}H_{21}ClN_4OS$ (free base of ziprasidone) represents the following structural formula:

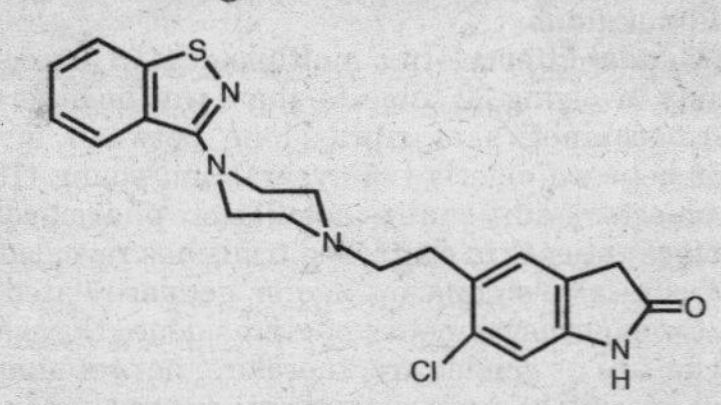

GEODON Capsules contain a monohydrochloride, monohydrate salt of ziprasidone. Chemically, ziprasidone hydrochloride monohydrate is 5-[2-[4-(1,2-benzisothiazol-3-yl)-1-piperazinyl]ethyl]-6-chloro-1,3-dihydro-2*H*-indol-2-one, monohydrochloride, monohydrate. The empirical formula is $C_{21}H_{21}ClN_4OS \cdot HCl \cdot H_2O$ and its molecular weight is 467.42. Ziprasidone hydrochloride monohydrate is a white to slightly pink powder.
GEODON Capsules are supplied for oral administration in 20 mg (blue/white), 40 mg (blue/blue), 60 mg (white/white), and 80 mg (blue/white) capsules. GEODON Capsules contain ziprasidone hydrochloride monohydrate, lactose, pregelatinized starch, and magnesium stearate.

CLINICAL PHARMACOLOGY

Pharmacodynamics

Ziprasidone exhibited high *in vitro* binding affinity for the dopamine D_2 and D_3, the serotonin $5HT_{2A}$, $5HT_{2C}$, $5HT_{1A}$, $5HT_{1D}$, and α_1-adrenergic receptors (K_i's of 4.8, 7.2, 0.4, 1.3, 3.4, 2, and 10 nM, respectively), and moderate affinity for the histamine H_1 receptor (K_i=47 nM). Ziprasidone functioned as an antagonist at the D_2, $5HT_{2A}$, and $5HT_{1D}$ receptors, and as an agonist at the $5HT_{1A}$ receptor. Ziprasidone inhibited synaptic reuptake of serotonin and norepinephrine. No appreciable affinity was exhibited for other receptor/binding sites tested, including the cholinergic muscarinic receptor (IC_{50} >1 μM).
The mechanism of action of ziprasidone, as with other drugs having efficacy in schizophrenia, is unknown. However, it has been proposed that this drug's efficacy in schizophrenia is mediated through a combination of dopamine type 2 (D_2) and serotonin type 2 ($5HT_2$) antagonism. Antagonism at receptors other than dopamine and $5HT_2$ with similar receptor affinities may explain some of the other therapeutic and side effects of ziprasidone.
Ziprasidone's antagonism of histamine H_1 receptors may explain the somnolence observed with this drug.
Ziprasidone's antagonism of α_1-adrenergic receptors may explain the orthostatic hypotension observed with this drug.

Pharmacokinetics

Ziprasidone's activity is primarily due to the parent drug. The multiple-dose pharmacokinetics of ziprasidone are dose-proportional within the proposed clinical dose range, and ziprasidone accumulation is predictable with multiple dosing. Elimination of ziprasidone is mainly via hepatic metabolism with a mean terminal half-life of about 7 hours within the proposed clinical dose range. Steady-state concentrations are achieved within one to three days of dosing. The mean apparent systemic clearance is 7.5 mL/min/kg. Ziprasidone is unlikely to interfere with the metabolism of drugs metabolized by cytochrome P450 enzymes.
Absorption: Ziprasidone is well absorbed after oral administration, reaching peak plasma concentrations in 6 to 8 hours. The absolute bioavailability of a 20 mg dose under fed conditions is approximately 60%. The absorption of ziprasidone is increased up to two-fold in the presence of food.
Distribution: Ziprasidone has a mean apparent volume of distribution of 1.5 L/kg. It is greater than 99% bound to plasma proteins, binding primarily to albumin and α_1-acid glycoprotein. The *in vitro* plasma protein binding of ziprasidone was not altered by warfarin or propranolol, two highly protein-bound drugs, nor did ziprasidone alter the binding of these drugs in human plasma. Thus, the potential for drug interactions with ziprasidone due to displacement is minimal.
Metabolism and Elimination: Ziprasidone is extensively metabolized after oral administration with only a small

Continued on next page

Geodon—Cont.

amount excreted in the urine (<1%) or feces (<4%) as unchanged drug. Ziprasidone is primarily cleared via three metabolic routes to yield four major circulating metabolites, benzisothiazole (BITP) sulphoxide, BITP-sulphone, ziprasidone sulphoxide, and S-methyl-dihydroziprasidone. Approximately 20% of the dose is excreted in the urine, with approximately 66% being eliminated in the feces. Unchanged ziprasidone represents about 44% of total drug-related material in serum. In vitro studies using human liver subcellular fractions indicate that S-methyl-dihydroziprasidone is generated in two steps. The data indicate that the reduction reaction is mediated by aldehyde oxidase and the subsequent methylation is mediated by thiol methyltransferase. In vitro studies using human liver microsomes and recombinant enzymes indicate that CYP3A4 is the major CYP contributing to the oxidative metabolism of ziprasidone. CYP1A2 may contribute to a much lesser extent. Based on in vivo abundance of excretory metabolites, less than one-third of ziprasidone metabolic clearance is mediated by cytochrome P450 catalyzed oxidation and approximately two-thirds via reduction by aldehyde oxidase. There are no known clinically relevant inhibitors or inducers of aldehyde oxidase.

Special Populations

Age and Gender Effects—In a multiple-dose (8 days of treatment) study involving 32 subjects, there was no difference in the pharmacokinetics of ziprasidone between men and women or between elderly (>65 years) and young (18 to 45 years) subjects. Additionally, population pharmacokinetic evaluation of patients in controlled trials has revealed no evidence of clinically significant age or gender-related differences in the pharmacokinetics of ziprasidone. Dosage modifications for age or gender are, therefore, not recommended.

Race—No specific pharmacokinetic study was conducted to investigate the effects of race. Population pharmacokinetic evaluation has revealed no evidence of clinically significant race-related differences in the pharmacokinetics of ziprasidone. Dosage modifications for race are, therefore, not recommended.

Smoking—Based on in vitro studies utilizing human liver enzymes, ziprasidone is not a substrate for CYP1A2; smoking should therefore not have an effect on the pharmacokinetics of ziprasidone. Consistent with these in vitro results, population pharmacokinetic evaluation has not revealed any significant pharmacokinetic differences between smokers and nonsmokers.

Renal Impairment—Because ziprasidone is highly metabolized, with less than 1% of the drug excreted unchanged, renal impairment alone is unlikely to have a major impact on the pharmacokinetics of ziprasidone. The pharmacokinetics of ziprasidone following 8 days of 20 mg BID dosing were similar among subjects with varying degrees of renal impairment (n=27), and subjects with normal renal function, indicating that dosage adjustment based upon the degree of renal impairment is not required. Ziprasidone is not removed by hemodialysis.

Hepatic Impairment—As ziprasidone is cleared substantially by the liver, the presence of hepatic impairment would be expected to increase the AUC of ziprasidone; a multiple-dose study at 20 mg BID for 5 days in subjects (n=13) with clinically significant (Childs-Pugh Class A and B) cirrhosis revealed an increase in AUC_{0-12} of 13% and 34% in Childs-Pugh Class A and B, respectively, compared to a matched control group (n=14). A half-life of 7.1 hours was observed in subjects with cirrhosis compared to 4.8 hours in the control group.

Drug-Drug Interactions

An in vitro enzyme inhibition study utilizing human liver microsomes showed that ziprasidone had little inhibitory effect on CYP1A2, CYP2C9, CYP2C19, CYP2D6 and CYP3A4, and thus would not likely interfere with the metabolism of drugs primarily metabolized by these enzymes. In vivo studies have revealed no effect of ziprasidone on the pharmacokinetics of dextromethorphan, estrogen, progesterone, or lithium (see **Drug Interactions** under **PRECAUTIONS**).

In vivo studies have revealed an approximately 35% decrease in ziprasidone AUC by concomitantly administered carbamazepine, an approximately 35–40% increase in ziprasidone AUC by concomitantly administered ketoconazole, but no effect on ziprasidone's pharmacokinetics by cimetidine or antacid (see **Drug Interactions** under **PRECAUTIONS**).

Clinical Trials

The efficacy of ziprasidone in the treatment of schizophrenia was evaluated in 5 placebo-controlled studies, 4 short-term (4- and 6-week) trials and one long-term (52-week) trial. All trials were in inpatients, most of whom met DSM III-R criteria for schizophrenia. Each study included 2 to 3 fixed doses of ziprasidone as well as placebo. Four of the 5 trials were able to distinguish ziprasidone from placebo; one short-term study did not. Although a single fixed-dose haloperidol arm was included as a comparative treatment in one of the three short-term trials, this single study was inadequate to provide a reliable and valid comparison of ziprasidone and haloperidol.

Several instruments were used for assessing psychiatric signs and symptoms in these studies. The Brief Psychiatric Rating Scale (BPRS) and the Positive and Negative Syndrome Scale (PANSS) are both multi-item inventories of general psychopathology usually used to evaluate the effects of drug treatment in schizophrenia. The BPRS psychosis cluster (conceptual disorganization, hallucinatory behavior, suspiciousness, and unusual thought content) is considered

a particularly useful subset for assessing actively psychotic schizophrenic patients. A second widely used assessment, the Clinical Global Impression (CGI), reflects the impression of a skilled observer, fully familiar with the manifestations of schizophrenia, about the overall clinical state of the patient. In addition, the Scale for Assessing Negative Symptoms (SANS) was employed for assessing negative symptoms in one trial.

The results of the trials follow:

(1) In a 4-week, placebo-controlled trial (n=139) comparing 2 fixed doses of ziprasidone (20 and 60 mg BID) with placebo, only the 60 mg BID dose was superior to placebo on the BPRS total score and the CGI severity score. This higher dose group was not superior to placebo on the BPRS psychosis cluster or on the SANS.

(2) In a 6-week, placebo-controlled trial (n=302) comparing 2 fixed doses of ziprasidone (40 and 80 mg BID) with placebo, both dose groups were superior to placebo on the BPRS total score, the BPRS psychosis cluster, the CGI severity score and the PANSS total and negative subscale scores. Although 80 mg BID had a numerically greater effect than 40 mg BID, the difference was not statistically significant.

(3) In a 6-week, placebo-controlled trial (n=419) comparing 3 fixed doses of ziprasidone (20, 60, and 100 mg BID) with placebo, all three dose groups were superior to placebo on the PANSS total score, the BPRS total score, the BPRS psychosis cluster, and the CGI severity score. Only the 100 mg BID dose group was superior to placebo on the PANSS negative subscale score. There was no clear evidence for a dose-response relationship within the 20 mg BID to 100 mg BID dose range.

(4) In a 4-week, placebo-controlled trial (n=200) comparing 3 fixed doses of ziprasidone (5, 20 and 40 mg BID), none of the dose groups was statistically superior to placebo on any outcome of interest.

(5) A study was conducted in chronic, symptomatically stable schizophrenic inpatients (n=294) randomized to 3 fixed doses of ziprasidone (20, 40, or 80 mg BID) or placebo and followed for 52 weeks. Patients were observed for "impending psychotic relapse", defined as CGI-improvement score of ≥ 6 (much worse or very much worse) and/or scores ≥ 6 (moderately severe) on the hostility or uncooperativeness items of the PANSS on two consecutive days. Ziprasidone was significantly superior to placebo in both time to relapse and rate of relapse, with no significant difference between the different dose groups.

There were insufficient data to examine population subsets based on age and race. Examination of population subsets based on gender did not reveal any differential responsiveness.

INDICATIONS AND USAGE

Ziprasidone is indicated for the treatment of schizophrenia. When deciding among the alternative treatments available for this condition, the prescriber should consider the finding of ziprasidone's greater capacity to prolong the QT/QTc interval compared to several other antipsychotic drugs (see **WARNINGS**). Prolongation of the QTc interval is associated in some other drugs with the ability to cause torsade de pointes-type arrhythmia, a potentially fatal polymorphic ventricular tachycardia, and sudden death. In many cases this would lead to the conclusion that other drugs should be tried first. Whether ziprasidone will cause torsade de pointes or increase the rate of sudden death is not yet known (see **WARNINGS**).

The efficacy of ziprasidone was established in short-term (4- and 6-week) controlled trials of schizophrenic inpatients (see **CLINICAL PHARMACOLOGY**).

In a placebo-controlled trial involving the follow-up for up to 52 weeks of stable schizophrenic inpatients, GEODON was demonstrated to delay the time to and rate of relapse. The physician who elects to use GEODON for extended periods should periodically reevaluate the long-term usefulness of the drug for the individual patient.

CONTRAINDICATIONS

QT Prolongation

Because of ziprasidone's dose-related prolongation of the QT interval and the known association of fatal arrhythmias with QT prolongation by some other drugs (see **WARNINGS**), ziprasidone should not be used with other drugs that prolong the QT interval, including (not a complete list) quinidine, dofetilide, pimozide, sotalol, thioridazine, moxifloxacin, and sparfloxacin.

Because ziprasidone prolongs the QT interval, it is contraindicated in patients with a known history of QT prolongation (including congenital long QT syndrome), with recent acute myocardial infarction, or with uncompensated heart failure (see **WARNINGS**).

Hypersensitivity

Ziprasidone is contraindicated in individuals with a known hypersensitivity to the product.

WARNINGS

QT Prolongation and Risk of Sudden Death

A study directly comparing the QT/QTc prolonging effect of ziprasidone with several other drugs effective in the treatment of schizophrenia was conducted in patient volunteers. In the first phase of the trial, ECGs were obtained at the time of maximum plasma concentration when the drug was administered alone. In the second phase of the trial, ECGs were obtained at the time of maximum plasma concentration while the drug was coadministered with an inhibitor of the CYP4503A4 metabolism of the drug.

In the first phase of the study, the mean change in QTc from baseline was calculated for each drug, using a sample-based correction that removes the effect of heart rate on

the QT interval. The mean increase in QTc from baseline for ziprasidone ranged from approximately 9 to 14 msec greater than for four of the comparator drugs (risperidone, olanzapine, quetiapine, and haloperidol), but was approximately 14 msec less than the prolongation observed for thioridazine.

In the second phase of the study, the effect of ziprasidone on QTc length was not augmented by the presence of a metabolic inhibitor (ketoconazole 200 mg BID).

In placebo-controlled trials, ziprasidone increased the QTc interval compared to placebo by approximately 10 msec at the highest recommended daily dose of 160 mg. In clinical trials with ziprasidone, the electrocardiograms of 2/2988 (0.06%) patients who received GEODON and 1/440 (0.23%) patients who received placebo revealed QTc intervals exceeding the potentially clinically relevant threshold of 500 msec. In the ziprasidone-treated patients, neither case suggested a role of ziprasidone. One patient had a history of prolonged QTc and a screening measurement of 489 msec; QTc was 503 msec during ziprasidone treatment. The other patient had a QTc of 391 msec at the end of treatment with ziprasidone and upon switching to thioridazine experienced QTc measurements of 518 and 593 msec.

Some drugs that prolong the QT/QTc interval have been associated with the occurrence of torsade de pointes and with sudden unexplained death. The relationship of QT prolongation to torsade de pointes is clearest for larger increases (20 msec and greater) but it is possible that smaller QT/QTc prolongations may also increase risk, or increase it in susceptible individuals, such as those with hypokalemia, hypomagnesemia, or genetic predisposition. Although torsade de pointes has not been observed in association with the use of ziprasidone at recommended doses in premarketing studies, experience is too limited to rule out an increased risk.

As with other antipsychotic drugs and placebo, sudden unexplained deaths have been reported in patients taking ziprasidone at recommended doses. The premarketing experience for ziprasidone did not reveal an excess risk of mortality for ziprasidone compared to other antipsychotic drugs or placebo, but the extent of exposure was limited, especially for the drugs used as active controls and placebo. Nevertheless, ziprasidone's larger prolongation of QTc length compared to several other antipsychotic drugs raises the possibility that the risk of sudden death may be greater for ziprasidone than for other available drugs for treating schizophrenia. This possibility needs to be considered in deciding among alternative drug products (see INDICATIONS AND USAGE).

Certain circumstances may increase the risk of the occurrence of torsade de pointes and/or sudden death in association with the use of drugs that prolong the QTc interval, including (1) bradycardia; (2) hypokalemia or hypomagnesemia; (3) concomitant use of other drugs that prolong the QTc interval; and (4) presence of congenital prolongation of the QT interval.

Ziprasidone use should be avoided in combination with other drugs that are known to prolong the QTc interval. Ziprasidone should also be avoided in patients with congenital long QT syndrome and in patients with a history of cardiac arrhythmias (see CONTRAINDICATIONS, and see Drug Interactions under PRECAUTIONS).

It is recommended that patients being considered for ziprasidone treatment who are at risk for significant electrolyte disturbances, hypokalemia in particular, have baseline serum potassium and magnesium measurements. Hypokalemia (and/or hypomagnesemia) may increase the risk of QT prolongation and arrhythmia. Hypokalemia may result from diuretic therapy, diarrhea, and other causes. Patients with low serum potassium and/or magnesium should be repleted with those electrolytes before proceeding with treatment. It is essential to periodically monitor serum electrolytes in patients for whom diuretic therapy is introduced during ziprasidone treatment. Persistently prolonged QTc intervals may also increase the risk of further prolongation and arrhythmia, but it is not clear that routine screening ECG measures are effective in detecting such patients. Rather, ziprasidone should be avoided in patients with histories of significant cardiovascular illness, e.g., QT prolongation, recent acute myocardial infarction, uncompensated heart failure, or cardiac arrhythmia. Ziprasidone should be discontinued in patients who are found to have persistent QTc measurements >500 msec.

For patients taking ziprasidone who experience symptoms that could indicate the occurrence of torsade de pointes, e.g., dizziness, palpitations, or syncope, the prescriber should initiate further evaluation, e.g., Holter monitoring may be useful.

Neuroleptic Malignant Syndrome (NMS)

A potentially fatal symptom complex sometimes referred to as Neuroleptic Malignant Syndrome (NMS) has been reported in association with administration of antipsychotic drugs. Clinical manifestations of NMS are hyperpyrexia, muscle rigidity, altered mental status and evidence of autonomic instability (irregular pulse or blood pressure, tachycardia, diaphoresis, and cardiac dysrhythmia). Additional signs may include elevated creatinine phosphokinase, myoglobinuria (rhabdomyolysis), and acute renal failure.

The diagnostic evaluation of patients with this syndrome is complicated. In arriving at a diagnosis, it is important to exclude cases where the clinical presentation includes both serious medical illness (e.g., pneumonia, systemic infection, etc.) and untreated or inadequately treated extrapyramidal signs and symptoms (EPS). Other important considerations in the differential diagnosis include central anticholinergic toxicity, heat stroke, drug fever, and primary central nervous system (CNS) pathology.

The management of NMS should include: (1) immediate discontinuation of antipsychotic drugs and other drugs not essential to concurrent therapy; (2) intensive symptomatic treatment and medical monitoring; and (3) treatment of any concomitant serious medical problems for which specific treatments are available. There is no general agreement about specific pharmacological treatment regimens for NMS.

If a patient requires antipsychotic drug treatment after recovery from NMS, the potential reintroduction of drug therapy should be carefully considered. The patient should be carefully monitored, since recurrences of NMS have been reported.

Tardive Dyskinesia

A syndrome of potentially irreversible, involuntary, dyskinetic movements may develop in patients undergoing treatment with antipsychotic drugs. Although the prevalence of the syndrome appears to be highest among the elderly, especially elderly women, it is impossible to rely upon prevalence estimates to predict, at the inception of antipsychotic treatment, which patients are likely to develop the syndrome. Whether antipsychotic drug products differ in their potential to cause tardive dyskinesia is unknown.

The risk of developing tardive dyskinesia and the likelihood that it will become irreversible are believed to increase as the duration of treatment and the total cumulative dose of antipsychotic drugs administered to the patient increase. However, the syndrome can develop, although much less commonly, after relatively brief treatment periods at low doses.

There is no known treatment for established cases of tardive dyskinesia, although the syndrome may remit, partially or completely, if antipsychotic treatment is withdrawn. Antipsychotic treatment itself, however, may suppress (or partially suppress) the signs and symptoms of the syndrome and thereby may possibly mask the underlying process. The effect that symptomatic suppression has upon the long-term course of the syndrome is unknown.

Given these considerations, ziprasidone should be prescribed in a manner that is most likely to minimize the occurrence of tardive dyskinesia. Chronic antipsychotic treatment should generally be reserved for patients who suffer from a chronic illness that (1) is known to respond to antipsychotic drugs, and (2) for whom alternative, equally effective, but potentially less harmful treatments are not available or appropriate. In patients who do require chronic treatment, the smallest dose and the shortest duration of treatment producing a satisfactory clinical response should be sought. The need for continued treatment should be reassessed periodically.

If signs and symptoms of tardive dyskinesia appear in a patient on ziprasidone, drug discontinuation should be considered. However, some patients may require treatment with ziprasidone despite the presence of the syndrome.

PRECAUTIONS
General
Rash—In premarketing trials with ziprasidone, about 5% of patients developed rash and/or urticaria, with discontinuation of treatment in about one-sixth of these cases. The occurrence of rash was related to dose of ziprasidone, although the finding might also be explained by the longer exposure time in the higher dose patients. Several patients with rash had signs and symptoms of associated systemic illness, e.g., elevated WBCs. Most patients improved promptly with adjunctive treatment with antihistamines or steroids and/or upon discontinuation of ziprasidone, and all patients experiencing these events were reported to recover completely. Upon appearance of rash for which an alternative etiology cannot be identified, ziprasidone should be discontinued.
Orthostatic Hypotension—Ziprasidone may induce orthostatic hypotension associated with dizziness, tachycardia, and, in some patients, syncope, especially during the initial dose-titration period, probably reflecting its α_1-adrenergic antagonist properties. Syncope was reported in 0.6% of the patients treated with ziprasidone.

Ziprasidone should be used with particular caution in patients with known cardiovascular disease (history of myocardial infarction or ischemic heart disease, heart failure or conduction abnormalities), cerebrovascular disease or conditions which would predispose patients to hypotension (dehydration, hypovolemia, and treatment with antihypertensive medications).
Seizures—During clinical trials, seizures occurred in 0.4% of patients treated with ziprasidone. There were confounding factors that may have contributed to the occurrence of seizures in many of these cases. As with other antipsychotic drugs, ziprasidone should be used cautiously in patients with a history of seizures or with conditions that potentially lower the seizure threshold, e.g., Alzheimer's dementia. Conditions that lower the seizure threshold may be more prevalent in a population of 65 years or older.
Hyperprolactinemia—As with other drugs that antagonize dopamine D_2 receptors, ziprasidone elevates prolactin levels in humans. Increased prolactin levels were also observed in animal studies with this compound, and were associated with an increase in mammary gland neoplasia in mice (a similar effect was not observed in rats (see **Carcinogenesis**). Tissue culture experiments indicate that approximately one-third of human breast cancers are prolactin-dependent *in vitro*, a factor of potential importance if the prescription of these drugs is contemplated in a patient with previously de-

tected breast cancer. Although disturbances such as galactorrhea, amenorrhea, gynecomastia, and impotence have been reported with prolactin-elevating compounds, the clinical significance of elevated serum prolactin levels is unknown for most patients. Neither clinical studies nor epidemiologic studies conducted to date have shown an association between chronic administration of this class of drugs and tumorigenesis in humans; the available evidence is considered too limited to be conclusive at this time.
Potential for Cognitive and Motor Impairment—Somnolence was a commonly reported adverse event in patients treated with ziprasidone. In the 4- and 6-week placebo-controlled trials, somnolence was reported in 14% of patients on ziprasidone compared to 7% of placebo patients. Somnolence led to discontinuation in 0.3% of patients in short-term clinical trials. Since ziprasidone has the potential to impair judgment, thinking, or motor skills, patients should be cautioned about performing activities requiring mental alertness, such as operating a motor vehicle (including automobiles) or operating hazardous machinery until they are reasonably certain that ziprasidone therapy does not affect them adversely.
Priapism—One case of priapism was reported in the premarketing database. While the relationship of the event to ziprasidone use has not been established, other drugs with alpha-adrenergic blocking effects have been reported to induce priapism, and it is possible that ziprasidone may share this capacity. Severe priapism may require surgical intervention.
Body Temperature Regulation—Although not reported with ziprasidone in premarketing trials, disruption of the body's ability to reduce core body temperature has been attributed to antipsychotic agents. Appropriate care is advised when prescribing ziprasidone for patients who will be experiencing conditions which may contribute to an elevation in core body temperature, e.g., exercising strenuously, exposure to extreme heat, receiving concomitant medication with anticholinergic activity, or being subject to dehydration.
Dysphagia—Esophageal dysmotility and aspiration have been associated with antipsychotic drug use. Aspiration pneumonia is a common cause of morbidity and mortality in elderly patients, in particular those with advanced Alzheimer's dementia. Ziprasidone and other antipsychotic drugs should be used cautiously in patients at risk for aspiration pneumonia.
Suicide—The possibility of a suicide attempt is inherent in psychotic illness and close supervision of high-risk patients should accompany drug therapy. Prescriptions for ziprasidone should be written for the smallest quantity of capsules consistent with good patient management in order to reduce the risk of overdose.
Use in Patients with Concomitant Illness—Clinical experience with ziprasidone in patients with certain concomitant systemic illnesses (see **Renal Impairment** and **Hepatic Impairment** under **CLINICAL PHARMACOLOGY, Special Populations**) is limited.

Ziprasidone has not been evaluated or used to any appreciable extent in patients with a recent history of myocardial infarction or unstable heart disease. Patients with these diagnoses were excluded from premarketing clinical studies. Because of the risk of QTc prolongation and orthostatic hypotension with ziprasidone, caution should be observed in cardiac patients (see **QTc Prolongation** under **WARNINGS** and **Orthostatic Hypotension** under **PRECAUTIONS**).
Information for Patients
Please refer to the patient package insert. To assure safe and effective use of GEODON, the information and instructions provided in the patient information should be discussed with patients.
Laboratory Tests
Patients being considered for ziprasidone treatment that are at risk of significant electrolyte disturbances should have baseline serum potassium and magnesium measurements. Low serum potassium and magnesium should be repleted before proceeding with treatment. Patients who are started on diuretics during ziprasidone therapy need periodic monitoring of serum potassium and magnesium. Ziprasidone should be discontinued in patients who are found to have persistent QTc measurements >500 msec (see **WARNINGS**).
Drug Interactions
Drug-drug interactions can be pharmacodynamic (combined pharmacologic effects) or pharmacokinetic (alteration of plasma levels). The risks of using ziprasidone in combination with other drugs have been evaluated as described below. Based upon the pharmacodynamic and pharmacokinetic profile of ziprasidone, possible interactions could be anticipated:
Pharmacodynamic Interactions
(1) Ziprasidone should not be used with any drug that prolongs the QT interval (see **CONTRAINDICATIONS**).
(2) Given the primary CNS effects of ziprasidone, caution should be used when it is taken in combination with other centrally acting drugs.
(3) Because of its potential for inducing hypotension, ziprasidone may enhance the effects of certain antihypertensive agents.
(4) Ziprasidone may antagonize the effects of levodopa and dopamine agonists.
Pharmacokinetic Interactions
The Effect of Other Drugs on Ziprasidone
Carbamazepine—Carbamazepine is an inducer of CYP3A4; administration of 200 mg BID for 21 days resulted in a decrease of approximately 35% in the AUC of ziprasidone. This

effect may be greater when higher doses of carbamazepine are administered.
Ketoconazole—Ketoconazole, a potent inhibitor of CYP3A4, at a dose of 400 mg QD for 5 days, increased the AUC and C_{max} of ziprasidone by about 35–40%. Other inhibitors of CYP3A4 would be expected to have similar effects.
Cimetidine—Cimetidine at a dose of 800 mg QD for 2 days did not affect ziprasidone pharmacokinetics.
Antacid—The coadministration of 30 mL of MAALOX with ziprasidone did not affect the pharmacokinetics of ziprasidone.

In addition, population pharmacokinetic analysis of schizophrenic patients enrolled in controlled clinical trials has not revealed evidence of any clinically significant pharmacokinetic interactions with benztropine, propranolol, or lorazepam.
Effect of Ziprasidone on Other Drugs
In vitro studies revealed little potential for ziprasidone to interfere with the metabolism of drugs cleared primarily by CYP1A2, CYP2C9, CYP2C19, CYP2D6, and CYP3A4, and little potential for drug interactions with ziprasidone due to displacement (see **CLINICAL PHARMACOLOGY, Pharmacokinetics**).
Lithium—Ziprasidone at a dose of 40 mg BID administered concomitantly with lithium at a dose of 450 mg BID for 7 days did not affect the steady-state level or renal clearance of lithium.
Oral Contraceptives—Ziprasidone at a dose of 20 mg BID did not affect the pharmacokinetics of concomitantly administered oral contraceptives, ethinylestradiol (0.03 mg) and levonorgestrel (0.15 mg).
Dextromethorphan—Consistent with *in vitro* results, a study in normal healthy volunteers showed that ziprasidone did not alter the metabolism of dextromethorphan, a CYP2D6 model substrate, to its major metabolite, dextrorphan. There was no statistically significant change in the urinary dextromethorphan/dextrorphan ratio.
Carcinogenesis, Mutagenesis, Impairment of Fertility
Carcinogenesis—Lifetime carcinogenicity studies were conducted with ziprasidone in Long Evans rats and CD-1 mice. Ziprasidone was administered for 24 months in the diet at doses of 2, 6, or 12 mg/kg/day to rats, and 50, 100, or 200 mg/kg/day to mice (0.1 to 0.6 and 1 to 5 times the maximum recommended human dose [MRHD] of 200 mg/day on a mg/m² basis, respectively). In the rat study, there was no evidence of an increased incidence of tumors compared to controls. In male mice, there was no increase in incidence of tumors relative to controls. In female mice, there were dose-related increases in the incidences of pituitary gland adenoma and carcinoma, and mammary gland adenocarcinoma at all doses tested (50 to 200 mg/kg/day or 1 to 5 times the MRHD on a mg/m² basis). Proliferative changes in the pituitary and mammary glands of rodents have been observed following chronic administration of other antipsychotic agents and are considered to be prolactin-mediated. Increases in serum prolactin were observed in a 1-month dietary study in female, but not male, mice at 100 and 200 mg/kg/day (or 2.5 and 5 times the MRHD on a mg/m² basis). Ziprasidone had no effect on serum prolactin in rats in a 5-week dietary study at the doses that were used in the carcinogenicity study. The relevance for human risk of the findings of prolactin-mediated endocrine tumors in rodents is unknown (see **Hyperprolactinemia** under **PRECAUTIONS, General**).
Mutagenesis—Ziprasidone was tested in the Ames bacterial mutation assay, the *in vitro* mammalian cell gene mutation mouse lymphoma assay, the *in vitro* chromosomal aberration assay in human lymphocytes, and the *in vivo* chromosomal aberration assay in mouse bone marrow. There was a reproducible mutagenic response in the Ames assay in one strain of *S. typhimurium* in the absence of metabolic activation. Positive results were obtained in both the *in vitro* mammalian cell gene mutation assay and the *in vitro* chromosomal aberration assay in human lymphocytes.
Impairment of Fertility—Ziprasidone was shown to increase time to copulation in Sprague-Dawley rats in two fertility and early embryonic development studies at doses of 10 to 160 mg/kg/day (0.5 to 8 times the MRHD of 200 mg/day on a mg/m² basis). Fertility rate was reduced at 160 mg/kg/day (8 times the MRHD on a mg/m² basis). There was no effect on fertility at 40 mg/kg/day (2 times the MRHD on a mg/m² basis). The effect on fertility appeared to be in the female since fertility was not impaired when males given 160 mg/kg/day (8 times the MRHD on a mg/m² basis) were mated with untreated females. In a 6-month study in male rats given 200 mg/kg/day (10 times the MRHD on a mg/m² basis) there were no treatment-related findings observed in the testes.
Pregnancy—**Pregnancy Category C**—In animal studies ziprasidone demonstrated developmental toxicity, including possible teratogenic effects at doses similar to human therapeutic doses. When ziprasidone was administered to pregnant rabbits during the period of organogenesis, an increased incidence of fetal structural abnormalities (ventricular septal defects and other cardiovascular malformations and kidney alterations) was observed at a dose of 30 mg/kg/day (3 times the MRHD of 200 mg/day on a mg/m² basis). There was no evidence to suggest that these developmental effects were secondary to maternal toxicity. The developmental no-effect dose was 10 mg/kg/day (equivalent to the MRHD on a mg/m² basis). In rats, embryofetal toxicity (decreased fetal weights, delayed skeletal ossification) was observed following administration of 10 to 160 mg/kg/day (0.5 to 8 times the MRHD on

Continued on next page

Geodon—Cont.

a mg/m² basis) during organogenesis or throughout gestation, but there was no evidence of teratogenicity. Doses of 40 and 160 mg/kg/day (2 and 8 times the MRHD on a mg/m² basis) were associated with maternal toxicity. The developmental no-effect dose was 5 mg/kg/day (0.2 times the MRHD on a mg/m² basis).

There was an increase in the number of pups born dead and a decrease in postnatal survival through the first 4 days of lactation among the offspring of female rats treated during gestation and lactation with doses of 10 mg/kg/day (0.5 times the MRHD on a mg/m² basis) or greater. Offspring developmental delays and neurobehavioral functional impairment were observed at doses of 5 mg/kg/day (0.2 times the MRHD on a mg/m² basis) or greater. A no-effect level was not established for these effects.

There are no adequate and well-controlled studies in pregnant women. Ziprasidone should be used during pregnancy only if the potential benefit justifies the potential risk to the fetus.

Labor and Delivery—The effect of ziprasidone on labor and delivery in humans is unknown.

Nursing Mothers—It is not known whether, and if so in what amount, ziprasidone or its metabolites are excreted in human milk. It is recommended that women receiving ziprasidone should not breast feed.

Pediatric Use—The safety and effectiveness of ziprasidone in pediatric patients have not been established.

Geriatric Use—Of the approximately 4500 patients treated with ziprasidone in clinical studies, 2.4% (109) were 65 years of age or over. In general, there was no indication of any different tolerability of ziprasidone or for reduced clearance of ziprasidone in the elderly compared to younger adults. Nevertheless, the presence of multiple factors that might increase the pharmacodynamic response to ziprasidone, or cause poorer tolerance or orthostasis, should lead to consideration of a lower starting dose, slower titration, and careful monitoring during the initial dosing period for some elderly patients.

ADVERSE REACTIONS

The premarketing development program for ziprasidone included over 5400 patients and/or normal subjects exposed to one or more doses of ziprasidone. Of these 5400 subjects, over 4500 were patients who participated in multiple-dose effectiveness trials, and their experience corresponded to approximately 1733 patient years. The conditions and duration of treatment with ziprasidone included open-label and double-blind studies, inpatient and outpatient studies, and short-term and longer-term exposure.

Adverse events during exposure were obtained by collecting voluntarily reported adverse experiences, as well as results of physical examinations, vital signs, weights, laboratory analyses, ECGs, and results of ophthalmologic examinations. Adverse experiences were recorded by clinical investigators using terminology of their own choosing. Consequently, it is not possible to provide a meaningful estimate of the proportion of individuals experiencing adverse events without first grouping similar types of events into a smaller number of standardized event categories. In the table and tabulations that follow, standard COSTART dictionary terminology has been used to classify reported adverse events.

The stated frequencies of adverse events represent the proportion of individuals who experienced, at least once, a treatment-emergent adverse event of the type listed. An event was considered treatment emergent if it occurred for the first time or worsened while receiving therapy following baseline evaluation.

Adverse Findings Observed in Short-Term, Placebo-Controlled Trials

The following findings are based on a pool of two 6-week, and two 4-week placebo-controlled trials in which ziprasidone was administered in doses ranging from 10 to 200 mg/day.

Adverse Events Associated with Discontinuation of Treatment in Short-Term, Placebo-Controlled Trials

Approximately 4.1% (29/702) of ziprasidone-treated patients in short-term, placebo-controlled studies discontinued treatment due to an adverse event, compared with about 2.2% (6/273) on placebo. The most common event associated with dropout was rash, including 7 dropouts for rash among ziprasidone patients (1%) compared to no placebo patients (see **PRECAUTIONS**).

Adverse Events Occurring at an Incidence of 1% or More Among Ziprasidone-Treated Patients in Short-Term, Placebo-Controlled Trials

Table 1 enumerates the incidence, rounded to the nearest percent, of treatment-emergent adverse events that occurred during acute therapy (up to 6 weeks) in predominantly schizophrenic patients, including only those events that occurred in 1% or more of patients treated with ziprasidone and for which the incidence in patients treated with ziprasidone was greater than the incidence in placebo-treated patients.

The prescriber should be aware that these figures cannot be used to predict the incidence of side effects in the course of usual medical practice where patient characteristics and other factors differ from those which prevailed in the clinical trials. Similarly, the cited frequencies cannot be compared with figures obtained from other clinical investigations involving different treatments, uses, and investigators. The cited figures, however, do provide the prescribing physician

with some basis for estimating the relative contribution of drug and non-drug factors to the side effect incidence rate in the population studied.

In these studies, the most commonly observed adverse events associated with the use of ziprasidone (incidence of 5% or greater) and observed at a rate on ziprasidone at least twice that of placebo were somnolence (14%), extrapyramidal syndrome (5%), and respiratory disorder (8%).

Table 1. Treatment-Emergent Adverse Event Incidence in Short-Term Placebo-Controlled Trials

Body System/Adverse Event	Percentage of Patients Reporting Event	
	Ziprasidone (N=702)	Placebo (N=273)
Body as a Whole		
Asthenia	5	3
Accidental Injury	4	2
Cardiovascular		
Tachycardia	2	1
Postural Hypotension	1	0
Digestive		
Nausea	10	7
Constipation	9	8
Dyspepsia	8	7
Diarrhea	5	4
Dry Mouth	4	2
Anorexia	2	1
Musculoskeletal		
Myalgia	1	0
Nervous		
Somnolence	14	7
Akathisia	8	7
Dizziness	8	6
Extrapyramidal Syndrome	5	1
Dystonia	4	2
Hypertonia	3	2
Respiratory		
Respiratory Disorder*	8	3
Rhinitis	4	2
Cough Increased	3	1
Skin and Appendages		
Rash	4	3
Fungal Dermatitis	2	1
Special Senses		
Abnormal Vision	3	2

*Cold symptoms and upper respiratory infection account for >90% of investigator terms pointing to "respiratory disorder".

Explorations for interactions on the basis of gender did not reveal any clinically meaningful differences in the adverse event occurrence on the basis of this demographic factor.

Dose Dependency of Adverse Events in Short-Term, Placebo-Controlled Trials

An analysis for dose response in this 4-study pool revealed an apparent relation of adverse event to dose for the following events: asthenia, postural hypotension, anorexia, dry mouth, increased salivation, arthralgia, anxiety, dizziness, dystonia, hypertonia, somnolence, tremor, rhinitis, rash, and abnormal vision.

Extrapyramidal Symptoms (EPS)—The incidence of reported EPS for ziprasidone-treated patients in the short-term, placebo-controlled trials was 5% vs. 1% for placebo. Objectively collected data from those trials on the Simpson Angus Rating Scale (for EPS) and the Barnes Akathisia Scale (for akathisia) did not generally show a difference between ziprasidone and placebo.

Vital Sign Changes—Ziprasidone is associated with orthostatic hypotension (see **PRECAUTIONS**).

Weight Gain—The proportions of patients meeting a weight gain criterion of ≥7% of body weight were compared in a pool of four 4- and 6-week placebo-controlled clinical trials, revealing a statistically significantly greater incidence of

weight gain for ziprasidone (10%) compared to placebo (4%). A median weight gain of 0.5 kg was observed in ziprasidone patients compared to no median weight change in placebo patients. In this set of clinical trials, weight gain was reported as an adverse event in 0.4% and 0.4% of ziprasidone and placebo patients, respectively. During long-term therapy with ziprasidone, a categorization of patients at baseline on the basis of body mass index (BMI) revealed the greatest mean weight gain and highest incidence of clinically significant weight gain (>7% of body weight) in patients with low BMI (<23) compared to normal (23–27) or overweight patients (>27). There was a mean weight gain of 1.4 kg for those patients with a "low" baseline BMI, no mean change for patients with a "normal" BMI, and a 1.3 kg mean weight loss for patients who entered the program with a "high" BMI.

ECG Changes—Ziprasidone is associated with an increase in the QTc interval (see **WARNINGS**). Ziprasidone was associated with a mean increase in heart rate of 1.4 beats per minute compared to a 0.2 beats per minute decrease among placebo patients.

Other Adverse Events Observed During the Premarketing Evaluation of Ziprasidone

Following is a list of COSTART terms that reflect treatment-emergent adverse events as defined in the introduction to the **ADVERSE REACTIONS** section reported by patients treated with ziprasidone at multiple doses >4 mg/day within the database of 3834 patients. All reported events are included except those already listed in Table 1 or elsewhere in labeling, those event terms that were so general as to be uninformative, events reported only once and that did not have a substantial probability of being acutely life-threatening, events that are part of the illness being treated or are otherwise common as background events, and events considered unlikely to be drug-related. It is important to emphasize that, although the events reported occurred during treatment with ziprasidone, they were not necessarily caused by it.

Events are further categorized by body system and listed in order of decreasing frequency according to the following definitions: frequent adverse events are those occurring in at least 1/100 patients (only those not already listed in the tabulated results from placebo-controlled trials appear in this listing); infrequent adverse events are those occurring in 1/100 to 1/1000 patients; rare events are those occurring in fewer than 1/1000 patients.

Body as a Whole: *Frequent:* abdominal pain, flu syndrome, fever, accidental fall, face edema, chills, photosensitivity reaction, flank pain, hypothermia, motor vehicle accident.

Cardiovascular System: *Frequent:* hypertension; *Infrequent:* bradycardia, angina pectoris, atrial fibrillation; *Rare:* first degree AV block, bundle branch block, phlebitis, pulmonary embolus, cardiomegaly, cerebral infarct, cerebrovascular accident, deep thrombophlebitis, myocarditis, thrombophlebitis.

Digestive System: *Frequent:* vomiting; *Infrequent:* rectal hemorrhage, dysphagia, tongue edema; *Rare:* gum hemorrhage, jaundice, fecal impaction, gamma glutamyl transpeptidase increased, hematemesis, cholestatic jaundice, hepatitis, hepatomegaly, leukoplakia of mouth, fatty liver deposit, melena.

Endocrine: *Rare:* hypothyroidism, hyperthyroidism, thyroiditis.

Hemic and Lymphatic System: *Infrequent:* anemia, ecchymosis, leukocytosis, leukopenia, eosinophilia, lymphadenopathy; *Rare:* thrombocytopenia, hypochromic anemia, lymphocytosis, monocytosis, basophilia, lymphedema, polycythemia, thrombocythemia.

Metabolic and Nutritional Disorders: *Infrequent:* thirst, transaminase increased, peripheral edema, hyperglycemia, creatine phosphokinase increased, alkaline phosphatase increased, hypercholesteremia, dehydration, lactic dehydrogenase increased, albuminuria, hypokalemia; *Rare:* BUN increased, creatinine increased, hyperlipemia, hypocholesteremia, hyperkalemia, hypochloremia, hypoglycemia, hyponatremia, hypoproteinemia, glucose tolerance decreased, gout, hyperchloremia, hyperuricemia, hypocalcemia, hypoglycemic reaction, hypomagnesemia, ketosis, respiratory alkalosis.

Musculoskeletal System: *Infrequent:* tenosynovitis; *Rare:* myopathy.

Nervous System: *Frequent:* agitation, tremor, dyskinesia, hostility, paresthesia, confusion, vertigo, hypokinesia, hyperkinesia, abnormal gait, oculogyric crisis, hypesthesia, ataxia, amnesia, cogwheel rigidity, delirium, hypotonia, akinesia, dysarthria, withdrawal syndrome, buccoglossal syndrome, choreoathetosis, diplopia, incoordination, neuropathy; *Rare:* myoclonus, nystagmus, torticollis, circumoral paresthesia, opisthotonos, reflexes increased, trismus.

Respiratory System: *Frequent:* dyspnea; *Infrequent:* pneumonia, epistaxis; *Rare:* hemoptysis, laryngismus.

Skin and Appendages: *Infrequent:* maculopapular rash, urticaria, alopecia, eczema, exfoliative dermatitis, contact dermatitis, vesiculobullous rash.

Special Senses: *Infrequent:* conjunctivitis, dry eyes, tinnitus, blepharitis, cataract, photophobia; *Rare:* eye hemorrhage, visual field defect, keratitis, keratoconjunctivitis.

Urogenital System: *Infrequent:* impotence, abnormal ejaculation, amenorrhea, hematuria, menorrhagia, female lactation, polyuria, urinary retention, metrorrhagia, male sexual dysfunction, anorgasmia, glycosuria; *Rare:* gynecomastia, vaginal hemorrhage, nocturia, oliguria, female sexual dysfunction, uterine hemorrhage.

DRUG ABUSE AND DEPENDENCE

Controlled Substance Class—Ziprasidone is not a controlled substance.

Physical and Psychological Dependence—Ziprasidone has not been systematically studied, in animals or humans, for its potential for abuse, tolerance, or physical dependence. While the clinical trials did not reveal any tendency for drug-seeking behavior, these observations were not systematic and it is not possible to predict on the basis of this limited experience the extent to which ziprasidone will be misused, diverted, and/or abused once marketed. Consequently, patients should be evaluated carefully for a history of drug abuse, and such patients should be observed closely for signs of ziprasidone misuse or abuse (e.g., development of tolerance, increases in dose, drug-seeking behavior).

OVERDOSAGE

Human Experience—In premarketing trials involving more than 5400 patients and/or normal subjects, accidental or intentional overdosage of ziprasidone was documented in 10 patients. All of these patients survived without sequelae. In the patient taking the largest confirmed amount, 3240 mg, the only symptoms reported were minimal sedation, slurring of speech, and transitory hypertension (200/95).

Management of Overdosage—In case of acute overdosage, establish and maintain an airway and ensure adequate oxygenation and ventilation. Intravenous access should be established and gastric lavage (after intubation, if patient is unconscious) and administration of activated charcoal together with a laxative should be considered. The possibility of obtundation, seizure, or dystonic reaction of the head and neck following overdose may create a risk of aspiration with induced emesis.

Cardiovascular monitoring should commence immediately and should include continuous electrocardiographic monitoring to detect possible arrhythmias. If antiarrhythmic therapy is administered, disopyramide, procainamide, and quinidine carry a theoretical hazard of additive QT- prolonging effects that might be additive to those of ziprasidone.

Hypotension and circulatory collapse should be treated with appropriate measures such as intravenous fluids. If sympathomimetic agents are used for vascular support, epinephrine and dopamine should not be used, since beta stimulation combined with α_1 antagonism associated with ziprasidone may worsen hypotension. Similarly, it is reasonable to expect that the alpha-adrenergic-blocking properties of bretylium might be additive to those of ziprasidone, resulting in problematic hypotension.

In cases of severe extrapyramidal symptoms, anticholinergic medication should be administered. There is no specific antidote to ziprasidone, and it is not dialyzable. The possibility of multiple drug involvement should be considered. Close medical supervision and monitoring should continue until the patient recovers.

DOSAGE AND ADMINISTRATION

When deciding among the alternative treatments available for schizophrenia, the prescriber should consider the finding of ziprasidone's greater capacity to prolong the QT/QTc interval compared to several other antipsychotic drugs (see **WARNINGS**).

Initial Treatment

GEODON Capsules should be administered at an initial daily dose of 20 mg BID with food. In some patients, daily dosage may subsequently be adjusted on the basis of individual clinical status up to 80 mg BID. Dosage adjustments, if indicated, should generally occur at intervals of not less than 2 days, as steady-state is achieved within 1 to 3 days. In order to ensure use of the lowest effective dose, ordinarily patients should be observed for improvement for several weeks before upward dosage adjustment.

Efficacy in schizophrenia was demonstrated in a dose range of 20 to 100 mg BID in short-term, placebo-controlled clinical trials. There were trends toward dose response within the range of 20 to 80 mg BID, but results were not consistent. An increase to a dose greater than 80 mg BID is not generally recommended. The safety of doses above 100 mg BID has not been systematically evaluated in clinical trials.

Dosing in Special Populations

Dosage adjustments are generally not required on the basis of age, gender, race, or renal or hepatic impairment.

Maintenance Treatment

While there is no body of evidence available to answer the question of how long a patient treated with ziprasidone should remain on it, systematic evaluation of ziprasidone has shown that its efficacy in schizophrenia is maintained for periods of up to 52 weeks at a dose of 20 to 80 mg BID (see **CLINICAL PHARMACOLOGY**). No additional benefit was demonstrated for doses above 20 mg BID. Patients should be periodically reassessed to determine the need for maintenance treatment.

HOW SUPPLIED

GEODON™ Capsules are differentiated by capsule color/size and are imprinted in black ink with "Pfizer" and a unique number. GEODON™ Capsules are supplied for oral administration in 20 mg (blue/white), 40 mg (blue/blue), 60 mg (white/white), and 80 mg (blue/white) capsules.They are supplied in the following strengths and package configurations:

GEODON™ Capsules

Package Configuration	Capsule Strength (mg)	NDC Code	Imprint
Bottles of 60	20	NDC-0049-3960-60	396
Bottles of 60	40	NDC-0049-3970-60	397
Bottles of 60	60	NDC-0049-3980-60	398
Bottles of 60	80	NDC-0049-3990-60	399

Storage and Handling—GEODON Capsules should be stored at controlled room temperature, 15°–30°C (59°–86°F).

Rx only

Pharmacia & Upjohn

100 ROUTE 206 NORTH
PEAPACK, NEW JERSEY 07977

Direct Inquiries to:
1-888-768-5501

For Medical and Pharmaceutical Information, Including Emergencies, Contact:
(616) 833-8244

DETROL® LA ℞

tolterodine tartrate
extended release capsules

DESCRIPTION

DETROL LA Capsules contain tolterodine tartrate. The active moiety, tolterodine, is a muscarinic receptor antagonist. The chemical name of tolterodine tartrate is (R)-N,N-diisopropyl-3-(2-hydroxy-5-methylphenyl)-3-phenylpropanamine L-hydrogen tartrate. The empirical formula of tolterodine tartrate is $C_{26}H_{37}NO_7$, and its molecular weight is 475.6. The structural formula of tolterodine tartrate is represented below.

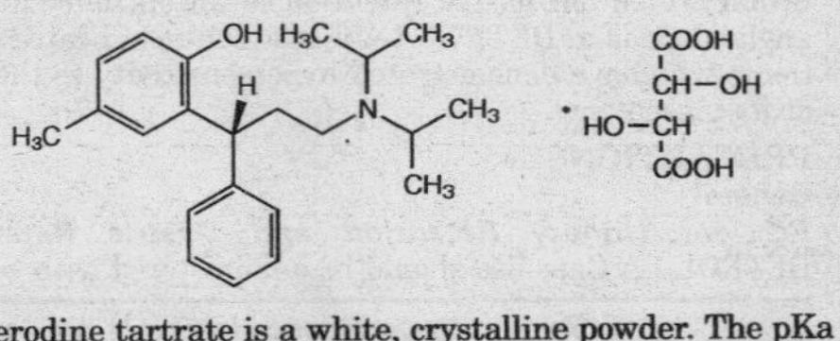

Tolterodine tartrate is a white, crystalline powder. The pKa value is 9.87 and the solubility in water is 12 mg/mL. It is soluble in methanol, slightly soluble in ethanol, and practically insoluble in toluene. The partition coefficient (Log D) between n-octanol and water is 1.83 at pH 7.3.

DETROL LA for oral administration contains 2 mg or 4 mg of tolterodine tartrate. Inactive ingredients are sucrose, starch, hydroxypropyl methylcellulose, ethylcellulose, ammonium hydroxide, medium chain triglycerides, oleic acid, gelatin, and FD&C Blue #2. The 2 mg capsules also contain yellow iron oxide. Both capsule strengths are imprinted with a pharmaceutical grade printing ink that contains shellac glaze, titanium dioxide, ammonium hydroxide, propylene glycol, and simethicone.

CLINICAL PHARMACOLOGY

Tolterodine is a competitive muscarinic receptor antagonist. Both urinary bladder contraction and salivation are mediated via cholinergic muscarinic receptors.

After oral administration, tolterodine is metabolized in the liver, resulting in the formation of the 5-hydroxymethyl derivative, a major pharmacologically active metabolite. The 5-hydroxymethyl metabolite, which exhibits an antimuscarinic activity similar to that of tolterodine, contributes significantly to the therapeutic effect. Both tolterodine and the 5-hydroxymethyl metabolite exhibit a high specificity for muscarinic receptors, since both show negligible activity or affinity for other neurotransmitter receptors and other potential cellular targets, such as calcium channels.

Tolterodine has a pronounced effect on bladder function. Effects on urodynamic parameters before and 1 and 5 hours after a single 6.4-mg dose of tolterodine immediate release were determined in healthy volunteers. The main effects of tolterodine at 1 and 5 hours were an increase in residual urine, reflecting an incomplete emptying of the bladder, and a decrease in detrusor pressure. These findings are consistent with an antimuscarinic action on the lower urinary tract.

Pharmacokinetics

Absorption: In a study with ^{14}C-tolterodine solution in healthy volunteers who received a 5-mg oral dose, at least 77% of the radiolabeled dose was absorbed. C_{max} and area under the concentration-time curve (AUC) determined after dosage of tolterodine immediate release are dose-proportional over the range of 1 to 4 mg. Based on the sum of unbound serum concentrations of tolterodine and the 5-hydroxymethyl metabolite ("active moiety"), the AUC of tolterodine extended release 4 mg daily is equivalent to tolterodine immediate release 4 mg (2 mg bid). C_{max} and C_{min} levels of tolterodine extended release are about 75% and 150% of tolterodine immediate release, respectively. Maximum serum concentrations of tolterodine extended release are observed 2 to 6 hours after dose administration.

Effect of Food: There is no effect of food on the pharmacokinetics of tolterodine extended release.

Distribution: Tolterodine is highly bound to plasma proteins, primarily α_1-acid glycoprotein. Unbound concentrations of tolterodine average 3.7% ± 0.13% over the concentration range achieved in clinical studies. The 5-hydroxymethyl metabolite is not extensively protein bound, with unbound fraction concentrations averaging 36% ± 4.0%. The blood to serum ratio of tolterodine and the 5-hydroxymethyl metabolite averages 0.6 and 0.8, respectively, indicating that these compounds do not distribute extensively into erythrocytes. The volume of distribution of tolterodine following administration of a 1.28-mg intravenous dose is 113 ± 26.7 L.

Metabolism: Tolterodine is extensively metabolized by the liver following oral dosing. The primary metabolic route involves the oxidation of the 5-methyl group and is mediated by the cytochrome P450 2D6 (CYP2D6) and leads to the formation of a pharmacologically active 5-hydroxymethyl metabolite. Further metabolism leads to formation of the 5-carboxylic acid and *N*-dealkylated 5-carboxylic acid metabolites, which account for 51% ± 14% and 29% ± 6.3% of the metabolites recovered in the urine, respectively.

Variability in Metabolism: A subset (about 7%) of the Caucasian population is devoid of CYP2D6, the enzyme responsible for the formation of the 5-hydroxymethyl metabolite of tolterodine. The identified pathway of metabolism for these individuals ("poor metabolizers") is dealkylation via cytochrome P450 3A4 (CYP3A4) to *N*-dealkylated tolterodine. The remainder of the population is referred to as "extensive metabolizers." Pharmacokinetic studies revealed that tolterodine is metabolized at a slower rate in poor metabolizers than in extensive metabolizers; this results in significantly higher serum concentrations of tolterodine and in negligible concentrations of the 5-hydroxymethyl metabolite.

Excretion: Following administration of a 5-mg oral dose of ^{14}C-tolterodine solution to healthy volunteers, 77% of radioactivity was recovered in urine and 17% was recovered in feces in 7 days. Less than 1% (<2.5% in poor metabolizers) of the dose was recovered as intact tolterodine, and 5% to 14% (<1% in poor metabolizers) was recovered as the active 5-hydroxymethyl metabolite.

A summary of mean (± standard deviation) pharmacokinetic parameters of tolterodine extended release and the 5-hydroxymethyl metabolite in extensive (EM) and poor (PM) metabolizers is provided in Table 1. These data were obtained following single and multiple doses of tolterodine extended release administered daily to 17 healthy male volunteers (13 EM, 4 PM).

[See table below]

Pharmacokinetics in Special Populations

Age: In Phase 1, multiple-dose studies in which tolterodine immediate release 4 mg (2 mg bid) was administered, serum concentrations of tolterodine and of the 5-hydroxymethyl metabolite were similar in healthy elderly volunteers (aged 64 through 80 years) and healthy young volunteers (aged less than 40 years). In another Phase 1 study, elderly volunteers (aged 71 through 81 years) were given tolterodine immediate release 2 or 4 mg (1 or 2 mg bid). Mean serum concentrations of tolterodine and the 5-hydroxymethyl metabolite in these elderly volunteers were approximately 20% and 50% higher,

Continued on next page

Table 1. Summary of Mean (±SD) Pharmacokinetic Parameters of Tolterodine Extended Release and its Active Metabolite (5-hydroxymethyl metabolite) in Healthy Volunteers

	Tolterodine				5-hydroxymethyl metabolite			
	t_{max}† (h)	C_{max} (μg/L)	C_{avg} (μg/L)	$t^1/_2$ (h)	t_{max}† (h)	C_{max} (μg/L)	C_{avg} (μg/L)	$t^1/_2$ (h)
Single dose 4 mg* EM	4 (2 – 6)	1.3 (0.8)	0.8 (0.57)	8.4 (3.2)	4 (3 – 6)	1.6 (0.5)	1.0 (0.32)	8.8 (5.9)
Multiple dose 4 mg EM	4 (2 – 6)	3.4 (4.9)	1.7 (2.8)	6.9 (3.5)	4 (2 – 6)	2.7 (0.90)	1.4 (0.6)	9.9 (4.0)
PM	4 (3 – 6)	19 (16)	13 (11)	18 (16)	–‡	–	–	–

*Parameter dose-normalized from 8 to 4 mg for the single-dose data
C_{max} = Maximum serum concentration; t_{max} = Time of occurrence of C_{max};
C_{avg} = Average serum concentration; $t^1/_2$ = Terminal elimination half-life
†Data presented as median (range)
‡ = not applicable

Detrol LA—Cont.

respectively, than reported in young healthy volunteers. However, no overall differences were observed in safety between older and younger patients on tolterodine in the Phase 3, 12-week, controlled clinical studies; therefore, no tolterodine dosage adjustment for elderly patients is recommended (see **PRECAUTIONS, Geriatric Use**).

Pediatric: The pharmacokinetics of tolterodine has not been established in pediatric patients.

Gender: The pharmacokinetics of tolterodine immediate release and the 5-hydroxymethyl metabolite are not influenced by gender. Mean C_{max} of tolterodine immediate release (1.6 µg/L in males versus 2.2 µg/L in females) and the active 5-hydroxymethyl metabolite (2.2 µg/L in males versus 2.5 µg/L in females) are similar in males and females who were administered tolterodine immediate release 2 mg. Mean AUC values of tolterodine (6.7 µg·h/L in males versus 7.8 µg·h/L in females) and the 5-hydroxymethyl metabolite (10 µg·h/L in males versus 11 µg·h/L in females) are also similar. The elimination half-life of tolterodine immediate release for both males and females is 2.4 hours, and the half-life of the 5-hydroxymethyl metabolite is 3.0 hours in females and 3.3 hours in males.

Race: Pharmacokinetic differences due to race have not been established.

Renal Insufficiency: Renal impairment can significantly alter the disposition of tolterodine immediate release and its metabolites. In a study conducted in patients with creatinine clearance between 10 and 30 mL/min, tolterodine immediate release and the 5-hydroxymethyl metabolite levels were approximately 2-3 fold higher in patients with renal impairment than in healthy volunteers. Exposure levels of other metabolites of tolterodine (e.g., tolterodine acid, N-dealkylated tolterodine acid, N-dealkylated tolterodine and N-dealkylated hydroxy tolterodine) were significantly higher (10-30 fold) in renally impaired patients as compared to the healthy volunteers. The recommended dose for patients with significantly reduced renal function is tolterodine 2 mg daily (see **PRECAUTIONS, General**).

Hepatic Insufficiency: Liver impairment can significantly alter the disposition of tolterodine immediate release. In a study of tolterodine immediate release conducted in cirrhotic patients, the elimination half-life of tolterodine immediate release was longer in cirrhotic patients (mean, 8.7 hours) than in healthy, young and elderly volunteers (mean, 2 to 4 hours). The clearance of orally administered tolterodine immediate release was substantially lower in cirrhotic patients (1.1 ± 1.7 L/h/kg) than in the healthy volunteers (5.7 ± 3.8 L/h/kg). The recommended dose for patients with significantly reduced hepatic function is tolterodine 2 mg daily (see **PRECAUTIONS, General**).

Drug-Drug Interactions

Fluoxetine: Fluoxetine is a selective serotonin reuptake inhibitor and a potent inhibitor of CYP2D6 activity. In a study to assess the effect of fluoxetine on the pharmacokinetics of tolterodine immediate release and its metabolites, it was observed that fluoxetine significantly inhibited the metabolism of tolterodine immediate release in extensive metabolizers, resulting in a 4.8-fold increase in tolterodine AUC. There was a 52% decrease in C_{max} and a 20% decrease in AUC of the 5-hydroxymethyl metabolite. Fluoxetine thus alters the pharmacokinetics in patients who would otherwise be extensive metabolizers of tolterodine immediate release to resemble the pharmacokinetic profile in poor metabolizers. The sums of unbound serum concentrations of tolterodine immediate release and the 5-hydroxymethyl metabolite are only 25% higher during the interaction. No dose adjustment is required when tolterodine and fluoxetine are coadministered.

Other Drugs Metabolized by Cytochrome P450 Isoenzymes: Tolterodine immediate release does not cause clinically significant interactions with other drugs metabolized by the major drug metabolizing CYP enzymes. In vivo drug-interaction data show that tolterodine immediate release does not result in clinically relevant inhibition of CYPIA2, 2D6, 2C9, 2C19, or 3A4 as evidenced by lack of influence on the marker drugs caffeine, debrisoquine, S-warfarin, and omeprazole. In vitro data show that tolterodine immediate release is a competitive inhibitor of CYP2D6 at high concentrations (Ki 1.05 µM), while tolterodine immediate release as well as the 5-hydroxymethyl metabolite are devoid of any significant inhibitory potential regarding the other isoenzymes.

CYP3A4 Inhibitors: The effect of 200 mg daily dose of ketoconazole on the pharmacokinetics of tolterodine immediate release was studied in 8 healthy volunteers, all of whom were poor metabolizers (see **Pharmacokinetics**, Variability in Metabolism for discussion of poor metabolizers). In the presence of ketoconazole, the mean C_{max} and AUC of tolterodine increased by 2 and 2.5 fold, respectively. Based on these findings, other potent CYP3A4 inhibitors such as other azole antifungals (e.g., itraconazole, miconazole) or macrolide antibiotics (e.g., erythromycin, clarithromycin) or cyclosporine or vinblastine may also lead to increases of tolterodine plasma concentrations (see **PRECAUTIONS** and **DOSAGE AND ADMINISTRATION**).

Warfarin: In healthy volunteers, coadministration of tolterodine immediate release 4 mg (2 mg bid) for 7 days and a single dose of warfarin 25 mg on day 4 had no effect on prothrombin time, Factor VII suppression, or on the pharmacokinetics of warfarin.

Oral Contraceptives: Tolterodine immediate release 4 mg (2 mg bid) had no effect on the pharmacokinetics of an oral contraceptive (ethinyl estradiol 30 µg/levonorgestrel 150 µg) as evidenced by the monitoring of ethinyl estradiol and

levonorgestrel over a 2-month period in healthy female volunteers.

Diuretics: Coadministration of tolterodine immediate release up to 8 mg (4 mg bid) for up to 12 weeks with diuretic agents, such as indapamide, hydrochlorothiazide, triamterene, bendroflumethiazide, chlorothiazide, methylchlorothiazide, or furosemide, did not cause any adverse electrocardiographic (ECG) effects.

CLINICAL STUDIES

DETROL LA Capsules 2 mg were evaluated in 29 patients in a Phase 2 dose-effect study. DETROL LA 4 mg was evaluated for the treatment of overactive bladder with symptoms of urge urinary incontinence and frequency in a randomized, placebo-controlled, multicenter, double-blind, Phase 3, 12-week study. A total of 507 patients received DETROL LA 4 mg once daily in the morning and 508 received placebo. The majority of patients were Caucasian (95%) and female (81%), with a mean age of 61 years (range, 20 to 93 years). In the study, 642 patients (42%) were 65 to 93 years of age. The study included patients known to be responsive to tolterodine immediate release and other anticholinergic medications, however, 47% of patients never received prior pharmacotherapy for overactive bladder. At study entry, 97% of patients had at least 5 urge incontinence episodes per week and 91% of patients had 8 or more micturitions per day. The primary efficacy endpoint was change in mean number of incontinence episodes per week at week 12 from baseline. Secondary efficacy endpoints included change in mean number of micturitions per day and mean volume voided per micturition at week 12 from baseline.
[See table below]

INDICATIONS AND USAGE

DETROL LA Capsules are once daily extended release capsules indicated for the treatment of overactive bladder with symptoms of urge urinary incontinence, urgency, and frequency.

CONTRAINDICATIONS

DETROL LA Capsules are contraindicated in patients with urinary retention, gastric retention, or uncontrolled narrow-angle glaucoma. DETROL LA is also contraindicated in patients who have demonstrated hypersensitivity to the drug or its ingredients.

PRECAUTIONS

General

Risk of Urinary Retention and Gastric Retention: DETROL LA Capsules should be administered with caution

to patients with clinically significant bladder outflow obstruction because of the risk of urinary retention and to patients with gastrointestinal obstructive disorders, such as pyloric stenosis, because of the risk of gastric retention (see **CONTRAINDICATIONS**).

Controlled Narrow-Angle Glaucoma: DETROL LA should be used with caution in patients being treated for narrow-angle glaucoma.

Reduced Hepatic and Renal Function: For patients with significantly reduced hepatic function or renal function, the recommended dose for DETROL LA is 2 mg daily (see **CLINICAL PHARMACOLOGY, Pharmacokinetics in Special Populations**).

Information for Patients

Patients should be informed that antimuscarinic agents such as DETROL LA may produce blurred vision.

Drug Interactions

CYP3A4 Inhibitors: Ketoconazole, an inhibitor of the drug metabolizing enzyme CYP3A4, significantly increased plasma concentrations of tolterodine when coadministered to subjects who were poor metabolizers (see **CLINICAL PHARMACOLOGY**, Variability in Metabolism and **Drug-Drug Interactions**). For patients receiving ketoconazole or other potent CYP3A4 inhibitors such as other azole antifungals (e.g., itraconazole, miconazole) or macrolide antibiotics (e.g., erythromycin, clarithromycin) or cyclosporine or vinblastine, the recommended dose of DETROL LA is 2 mg daily.

Drug-Laboratory-Test Interactions

Interactions between tolterodine and laboratory tests have not been studied.

Carcinogenesis, Mutagenesis, Impairment of Fertility

Carcinogenicity studies with tolterodine immediate release were conducted in mice and rats. At the maximum tolerated dose in mice (30 mg/kg/day), female rats (20 mg/kg/day), and male rats (30 mg/kg/day), AUC values obtained for tolterodine were 355, 291, and 462 µg·h/L, respectively. In comparison, the human AUC value for a 2-mg dose administered twice daily is estimated at 34 µg·h/L. Thus, tolterodine exposure in the carcinogenicity studies was 9- to 14-fold higher than expected in humans. No increase in tumors was found in either mice or rats.

No mutagenic effects of tolterodine were detected in a battery of in vitro tests, including bacterial mutation assays (Ames test) in four strains of *Salmonella typhimurium* and in two strains of *Escherichia coli*, a gene mutation assay in L5178Y mouse lymphoma cells, and chromosomal aberration tests in human lymphocytes. Tolterodine was also negative in vivo in the bone marrow micronucleus test in the mouse.

Table 2. 95% Confidence Intervals (CI) for the Difference between DETROL LA (4 mg daily) and Placebo for Mean Change at Week 12 from Baseline*

	DETROL LA (n=507)	Placebo (n=508)†	Treatment Difference, vs. Placebo (95% CI)
Number of incontinence episodes/week			
Mean Baseline	22.1	23.3	−4.8‡
Mean Change from Baseline	−11.8 (SD 17.8)	−6.9 (SD 15.4)	(−6.9, −2.8)
Number of micturitions/day			
Mean Baseline	10.9	11.3	
Mean Change from Baseline	−1.8 (SD 3.4)	−1.2 (SD 2.9)	−0.6‡ (−1.0, −0.2)
Volume Voided per micturition (mL)			
Mean Baseline	141	136	
Mean Change from Baseline	34 (SD 51)	14 (SD 41)	20‡ (14, 26)

SD=Standard Deviation
* Intent-to-treat analysis
† 1 to 2 patients missing in placebo group for each efficacy parameter
‡ The difference between DETROL LA and placebo was statistically significant

Table 3. Incidence* (%) of Adverse Events Exceeding Placebo Rate and Reported in ≥1% of Patients Treated with DETROL LA (4 mg daily) in a 12-week, Phase 3 Clinical Trial

Body System	Adverse Event	% DETROL LA n=505	% Placebo n=507
Autonomic Nervous	dry mouth	23	8
General	headache	6	4
	fatigue	2	1
Central/Peripheral Nervous	dizziness	2	1
Gastrointestinal	constipation	6	4
	abdominal pain	4	2
	dyspepsia	3	1
Vision	xerophthalmia	3	2
	vision abnormal	1	0
Psychiatric	somnolence	3	2
	anxiety	1	0
Respiratory	sinusitis	2	1
Urinary	dysuria	1	0

* in nearest integer

In female mice treated for 2 weeks before mating and during gestation with 20 mg/kg/day (corresponding to AUC value of about 500 µg·h/L), neither effects on reproductive performance or fertility were seen. Based on AUC values, the systemic exposure was about 15-fold higher in animals than in humans. In male mice, a dose of 30 mg/kg/day did not induce any adverse effects on fertility.

Pregnancy
Pregnancy Category C. At oral doses of 20 mg/kg/day (approximately 14 times the human exposure), no anomalies or malformations were observed in mice. When given at doses of 30 to 40 mg/kg/day, tolterodine has been shown to cause embryolethality, reduce fetal weight, and increase the incidence of fetal abnormalities (cleft palate, digital abnormalities, intra-abdominal hemorrhage, and various skeletal abnormalities, primarily reduced ossification) in mice. At these doses, the AUC values were about 20- to 25-fold higher than in humans. Rabbits treated subcutaneously at a dose of 0.8 mg/kg/day achieved an AUC of 100 µg·h/L, which is about three-fold higher than that resulting from the human dose. This dose did not result in any embryotoxicity or teratogenicity. There are no studies of tolterodine in pregnant women. Therefore, DETROL LA should be used during pregnancy only if the potential benefit for the mother justifies the potential risk to the fetus.

Nursing Mothers
Tolterodine immediate release is excreted into the milk in mice. Offspring of female mice treated with tolterodine 20 mg/kg/day during the lactation period had slightly reduced body-weight gain. The offspring regained the weight during the maturation phase. It is not known whether tolterodine is excreted in human milk; therefore, DETROL LA should not be administered during nursing. A decision should be made whether to discontinue nursing or to discontinue DETROL LA in nursing mothers.

Pediatric Use
The safety and effectiveness of tolterodine in pediatric patients has not been established.

Geriatric Use
No overall differences in safety were observed between the older and younger patients treated with tolterodine (see **CLINICAL PHARMACOLOGY, Pharmacokinetics in Special Populations**).

ADVERSE REACTIONS
The Phase 2 and 3 clinical trial program for DETROL LA Capsules included 1073 patients who were treated with DETROL LA (n=537) or placebo (n=536). The patients were treated with 2, 4, 6, or 8 mg/day for up to 15 months. Because clinical trials are conducted under widely varying conditions, adverse reaction rates observed in the clinical trials of a drug cannot be directly compared to rates in the clinical trials of another drug and may not reflect the rates observed in practice. The adverse reaction information from clinical trials does, however, provide a basis for identifying the adverse events that appear to be related to drug use and for approximating rates. The data described below reflect exposure to DETROL LA 4 mg once daily every morning in 505 patients and to placebo in 507 patients exposed for 12 weeks in the Phase 3, controlled clinical study.

Adverse events were reported in 52% (n=263) of patients receiving DETROL LA and in 49% (n=247) of patients receiving placebo. The most common adverse events reported by patients receiving DETROL LA were dry mouth, headache, constipation, and abdominal pain. Dry mouth was the most frequently reported adverse event for patients treated with DETROL LA occurring in 23.4% of patients treated with DETROL LA and 7.7% of placebo-treated patients. Dry mouth, constipation, abnormal vision (accommodation abnormalities), urinary retention, and dry eyes are expected side effects of antimuscarinic agents. A serious adverse event was reported by 1.4% (n=7) of patients receiving DETROL LA and by 3.6% (n=18) of patients receiving placebo. The frequency of discontinuation due to adverse events was highest during the first 4 weeks of treatment. Similar percentages of patients treated with DETROL LA or placebo discontinued treatment due to adverse events. Treatment was discontinued due to adverse events and dry mouth was reported as an adverse event in 2.4% (n=12) of patients treated with DETROL LA and in 1.2% (n=6) of patients treated with placebo.

Table 3 lists the adverse events reported in 1% or more of patients treated with DETROL LA 4 mg once daily in the 12-week study. The adverse events were reported regardless of causality.

[See table at bottom of previous page]

OVERDOSAGE
A 27-month-old child who ingested 5 to 7 tolterodine immediate release tablets 2 mg was treated with a suspension of activated charcoal and was hospitalized overnight with symptoms of dry mouth. The child fully recovered.

Management of Overdosage
Overdosage with DETROL LA Capsules can potentially result in severe central anticholinergic effects and should be treated accordingly.
ECG monitoring is recommended in the event of overdosage. In dogs, changes in the QT interval (slight prolongation of 10% to 20%) were observed at a suprapharmacologic dose of 4.5 mg/kg, which is about 68 times higher than the recommended human dose. In clinical trials of normal volunteers and patients, QT interval prolongation was not observed with tolterodine immediate release at doses up to 8 mg (4 mg bid) and higher doses were not evaluated.

DOSAGE AND ADMINISTRATION
The recommended dose of DETROL LA Capsules are 4 mg daily. DETROL LA should be taken once daily with liquids and swallowed whole. The dose may be lowered to 2 mg daily based on individual response and tolerability, however, limited efficacy data is available for DETROL LA 2 mg (see **CLINICAL STUDIES**).
For patients with significantly reduced hepatic or renal function or who are currently taking drugs that are potent inhibitors of CYP3A4, the recommended dose of DETROL LA is 2 mg daily (see **CLINICAL PHARMACOLOGY** and **PRECAUTIONS, Drug Interactions**).

HOW SUPPLIED
DETROL LA Capsules 2 mg are blue-green with symbol and 2 printed in white ink. DETROL LA Capsules 4 mg are blue with symbol and 4 printed in white ink. DETROL LA Capsules are supplied as follows:

Bottles of 30	
2 mg Capsules	NDC 0009-5190-01
4 mg Capsules	NDC 0009-5191-01
Bottles of 90	
2 mg Capsules	NDC 0009-5190-02
4 mg Capsules	NDC 0009-5191-02
Bottles of 500	
2 mg Capsules	NDC 0009-5190-03
4 mg Capsules	NDC 0009-5191-03
Unit Dose Blisters	
2 mg Capsules	NDC 0009-5190-04
4 mg Capsules	NDC 0009-5191-04

Store at 25°C (77°F); excursions permitted to 15-30°C (59-86°F) [see USP Controlled Room Temperature]. Protect from light.

Rx only
US Patent No. 5,382,600
Manufactured for
Pharmacia & Upjohn Company
Kalamazoo, MI 49001, USA
By
International Processing Corporation
Winchester, Kentucky 40391, USA
December 2000   818 229 000

LUNELLE™ Monthly Contraceptive Injection   ℞
medroxyprogesterone acetate and estradiol cypionate injectable suspension

Patients should be counseled that this product does not protect against HIV infection (AIDS) and other sexually transmitted diseases.

DESCRIPTION
LUNELLE™ Monthly Contraceptive Injection contains medroxyprogesterone acetate and estradiol cypionate as its active ingredients. The chemical name for medroxyprogesterone acetate is pregn-4-ene-3,20-dione,17-(acetyloxy)-6-methyl-(6α)-. The empirical formula is $C_{24}H_{34}O_4$ and its molecular weight is 386.53. Medroxyprogesterone acetate is a white to off-white, odorless crystalline powder that is stable in air and melts between 200°C and 210°C. It is freely soluble in chloroform, soluble in acetone and dioxane, sparingly soluble in alcohol and methanol, slightly soluble in ether, and practically insoluble in water. The chemical name for estradiol cypionate is estra-1,3,5,(10)-triene-3,17-diol,(17β)-,17-cyclopentanepropanoate. Estradiol cypionate is a white to off-white crystalline powder that melts between 149°C and 153°C. It is soluble in alcohol, acetone, chloroform, and dioxane; sparingly soluble in vegetable oils; and practically insoluble in water. The empirical formula is $C_{26}H_{36}O_3$ and its molecular weight is 396.57. The structural formulas for these ingredients are represented below:
[See chemical structures at top of next column]
LUNELLE™ Monthly Contraceptive Injection is available as a 0.5 mL aqueous suspension and contains 25 mg medroxyprogesterone acetate and 5 mg estradiol cypionate. Inactive ingredients are 0.9 mg methylparaben, 14.28 mg polyethylene glycol, 0.95 mg polysorbate 80, 0.1 mg propylparaben, 4.28 mg sodium chloride, and sterile water for injection.

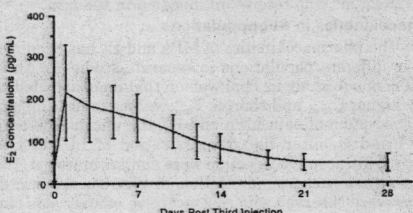

Medroxyprogesterone Acetate

Estradiol Cypionate

CLINICAL PHARMACOLOGY
LUNELLE™ Monthly Contraceptive Injection (medroxyprogesterone acetate and estradiol cypionate injectable suspension) when administered at the recommended dose to women every month inhibits the secretion of gonadotropins, which, in turn, prevents follicular maturation and ovulation. Although the primary mechanism of this action is inhibition of ovulation, other possible mechanisms of action include thickening and a reduction in volume of cervical mucus (which decrease sperm penetration) and thinning of the endometrium (which may reduce the likelihood of implantation).

Pharmacokinetics
Steady-state pharmacokinetic parameters of medroxyprogesterone acetate (MPA) and 17β-estradiol (E_2), the parent active moiety of estradiol cypionate (E_2C), following the third monthly injection of LUNELLE™ Monthly Contraceptive Injection are shown in Table 1.
[See table below]
Absorption: Absorption of MPA and E_2 from the injection site is prolonged after an intramuscular injection of LUNELLE™ Monthly Contraceptive Injection. The time to maximum plasma concentration (T_{max}) typically occurs within 1 to 10 days postinjection for MPA and 1 to 7 days postinjection for E_2. The peak concentrations (C_{max}) generally range from 0.94 to 2.17 ng/mL for MPA and from 140 to 480 pg/mL for E_2. The PK profile of E_2 following administration of LUNELLE™ Monthly Contraceptive Injection is shown in Figure 1a.

Figure 1a. Mean (SD) Serum Concentration-Time Profile of 17β-Estradiol (E_2) after the 3rd Monthly IM Injection of LUNELLE™ Monthly Contraceptive Injection to Surgically Sterile Females

[See figure at top of next column]
Berne RM, Levy MN, 1988.
Effect of Injection Site: AUC_{0-28} for MPA values were statistically significantly higher following injection of LUNELLE™ Monthly Contraceptive Injection into the arm as compared to the anterior thigh (average increase was approximately 25%). The mean MPA C_{max} was higher but not

Continued on next page

Table 1. Pharmacokinetic Parameters of Medroxyprogesterone Acetate (MPA) and Estradiol (17β-E_2) after the 3rd Monthly Injection of LUNELLE™ Monthly Contraceptive Injection in 14 Surgically Sterile Women

		C_{max} (ng/mL)	T_{max} (day)	AUC_{0-28} (ng•day/mL)	$AUC_{0-\infty}$ (ng•day/mL)	$t_{1/2}$ (day)
MPA	Mean	1.25	3.5	21.51	33.65	14.7
	Min	0.94	1.0	14.44	22.02	6.2
	Max	2.17	10.0	27.00	49.09	36.0
17β-E_2	Mean	0.25	2.1	2.74	2.99	8.4
	Min	0.14	1.0	1.65	1.65	2.6
	Max	0.48	7.0	3.56	3.89	20.4

C_{max} = peak serum concentration; T_{max} = time when C_{max} is observed; AUC_{0-28} = area under the concentration-time curve over 28 days; $t_{1/2}$ = terminal half-life; 1 nanogram = 10^3 picogram.

Lunelle—Cont.

Figure 1b. Plasma E_2 Hormone Profile of the Normal Menstrual Cycle

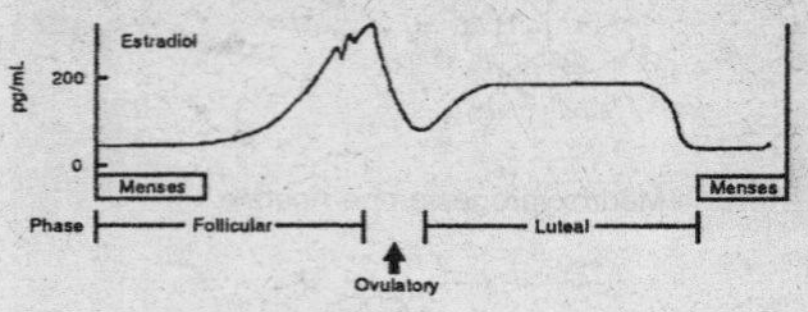

statistically significant (average increase 6 to 12%) when LUNELLE™ Monthly Contraceptive Injection was injected into the arm compared with the C_{max} observed after injection into the hip or the anterior thigh. However, the average MPA trough (C_{min}) concentrations and the half-lives were comparable for the three injection sites. E_2 concentrations were not measured.

Distribution: Plasma protein binding of MPA averages 86%. MPA binding occurs primarily to serum albumin; no binding of MPA occurs with sex-hormone-binding globulin (SHBG). Estrogens circulate in blood bound to albumin, SHBG, α1-glycoproteins, and transcortin. Estradiol is primarily bound to SHBG and albumin and approximately 3% remains unbound. Unbound estrogens are known to modulate pharmacologic response.

Metabolism: MPA is extensively metabolized. Its metabolism primarily involves ring A and/or side-chain reduction, loss of the acetyl group, hydroxylation in the 2-, 6-, and 21-positions or a combination of these positions, resulting in numerous derivatives. E_2C undergoes ester hydrolysis after intramuscular injection of LUNELLE™ Monthly Contraceptive Injection, releasing the parent, active compound E_2. Exogenously delivered or endogenously derived E_2 is primarily metabolized to estrone and estriol, both of which are metabolized to their sulfate and glucuronide forms.

Elimination: Residual MPA concentrations at the end of a monthly injection of LUNELLE™ Monthly Contraceptive Injection are generally below 0.5 ng/mL, consistent with its apparent elimination half-life of 15 days. Most MPA metabolites are excreted in the urine as glucuronide conjugates with only small amounts excreted as sulfates. Following the peak concentration, serum E_2 levels typically decline to 100 pg/mL by day 14 and are consistent with the apparent elimination half-life of 7 to 8 days. Estrogen metabolites are primarily excreted in the urine as glucuronides and sulfates.

Return of Ovulation: Return of ovulation correlated to some extent with MPA AUC_{0-84} days. Additionally, body weight and site of injection affected the AUC of MPA. AUC_{0-28} values are significantly higher when LUNELLE™ Monthly Contraceptive Injection is injected into the arm compared to the anterior thigh muscle and into women with BMI ≤28 kg/m^2 compared to those with BMI >28 kg/m^2. Consequently, return of ovulation may be delayed in women with BMI ≤28 kg/m^2 who receive an injection in the arm.

Pharmacokinetics in Subpopulations

Race: The pharmacokinetics of MPA and E_2 has been evaluated in different populations in separate studies. With the exception of one study in Thai women that demonstrated relatively higher C_{max} and shorter T_{max} values indicating more rapid absorption of both MPA and E_2, the pharmacokinetics of MPA and E_2 after the administration of LUNELLE™ Monthly Contraceptive Injection were similar in women from various ethnic backgrounds. Although pharmacokinetic differences were observed, the contraceptive efficacy was similar among all women of all ethnic backgrounds studied. Following discontinuation, ovulation returned earlier in Thai women.

Pediatric: Safety and efficacy of LUNELLE™ Monthly Contraceptive Injection have been established in women of reproductive age. Safety and efficacy are expected to be the same for postpubertal adolescents under 16 years of age and users 16 years of age and older. Use of this product before menarche is not indicated.

Geriatric: LUNELLE™ Monthly Contraceptive Injection is intended for use in healthy women desiring contraception; studies in geriatric women have not been conducted.

Effect of Body Weight: No dosage adjustment is necessary based on body weight. The effect of body weight on the pharmacokinetics of MPA was assessed in a subset of women (n = 77, body mass index ranged from 18 to 45.5 kg/m^2) enrolled in a Phase 3 trial. AUC_{0-28} values for MPA were significantly higher in thinner women with body mass index ≤28 kg/m^2 (average increase was approximately 20%) when compared to that in heavier women with body mass index >28 kg/m^2. The mean MPA C_{max} was higher (average increase 42%) in thin/normal women with body mass index ≤28 kg/m^2 compared with heavier women with body mass index >28 kg/m^2. The range of MPA trough (C_{min}) concentrations and the half-lives were comparable for both groups.

Hepatic Insufficiency: No formal studies have evaluated the effect of hepatic disease on the disposition of LUNELLE™ Monthly Contraceptive Injection. However, steroid hormones may be poorly metabolized in patients with impaired liver function. (See CONTRAINDICATIONS.)

Renal Insufficiency: No formal studies have evaluated the effect of renal disease on the pharmacokinetics of LUNELLE™ Monthly Contraceptive Injection. However, since both steroidal components of LUNELLE™ Monthly Contraceptive Injection are almost exclusively eliminated by hepatic metabolism, no dosage adjustment is necessary in women with renal dysfunction.

Drug-Drug Interactions

No formal drug-drug interaction studies were conducted with LUNELLE™ Monthly Contraceptive Injection. Aminoglutethimide administered concomitantly with LUNELLE™ Monthly Contraceptive Injection may significantly depress the serum concentrations of MPA. Users of LUNELLE™ Monthly Contraceptive Injection should be warned of the possibility of decreased efficacy with the use of this or any related drugs. (See PRECAUTIONS, DRUG INTERACTIONS.)

CLINICAL STUDIES

LUNELLE™ Monthly Contraceptive Injection has been studied for safety and efficacy in various comparative and introductory clinical trials around the world. One US study was performed with the goal of describing bleeding patterns in women using LUNELLE™ Monthly Contraceptive Injection compared to women using a standard oral contraceptive product. The group of LUNELLE™ Monthly Contraceptive Injection users in this study was 67.9% White, 15.5% Hispanic, 13.6% Black, 2.4% Asian, and 0.6% other.

In the clinical trials, reported 12-month pregnancy rates have been low (≤0.2%). Due to certain limitations of the available data (loss to follow-up, lack of pregnancy testing, use of barrier contraceptive products, and concomitant medications, etc.), a precise estimate of the failure rate is not possible, but is likely in the range of 0.1 to 1%.

The bleeding pattern over one year of use for LUNELLE™ Monthly Contraceptive Injection was examined in the US trial. Bleeding patterns during the last three months (months 9–12) of LUNELLE™ Monthly Contraceptive Injection use were compared with a concurrent group of standard oral contraceptive users. During this last three-month reference period, 58.6% of women using LUNELLE™ Monthly Contraceptive Injection experienced altered bleeding patterns (compared to 23.7% in the comparison group). See also WARNINGS, BLEEDING IRREGULARITIES. The one-year Life Table bleeding-related discontinuation rate for LUNELLE™ Monthly Contraceptive Injection was 6.1% for 782 participants in a US trial of up to 15 months duration. Bleeding patterns did not predict discontinuation from this large clinical trial.

Bleeding data from the US trial was re-analyzed based on injection intervals of 23 to 33 days. During the first injection interval, withdrawal bleeding lasted for more than 7 days in 42% of women, including 16% whose bleeding exceeded 10 days. The remaining 58% experienced bleeding for 7 days or less. Withdrawal bleeding began between days 20 and 25 (median 21) after initial injection in 48% of women using LUNELLE™ Monthly Contraceptive Injection.

At the end of one year of treatment, withdrawal bleeding lasted for more than 7 days in 29% of women, including 7% whose bleeding exceeded 10 days. The remaining 71% experienced bleeding 7 days or less in duration. Fifty percent of patients experienced withdrawal bleeding that began within 21–25 days (median 22) after their previous injection.

In any given injection interval, approximately 75% of women experienced a single withdrawal bleeding episode, without additional breakthrough bleeding or spotting, during that interval. In any given injection interval, approximately 15% of women experienced no bleeding and 10% experienced bleeding or spotting at various times in that injection interval.

In the US trial, weight gain was the most common adverse event leading to discontinuation of LUNELLE™ Monthly Contraceptive Injection (5.7% LUNELLE™ Monthly Contraceptive Injection group vs. 0.9% in the oral contraceptive comparator group). Weight change over 12 months in the LUNELLE™ Monthly Contraceptive Injection group ranged from 48 pounds lost to 49 pounds gained. Mean body weight change in the LUNELLE™ Monthly Contraceptive Injection group was a gain of 4 pounds after 13 injections and a gain of 5 pounds after 15 injections. Wide variability in individual weight gain or loss was observed; however, an increasing percentage of LUNELLE™ Monthly Contraceptive Injection users exhibited weight change in excess of 10 and 20 pounds with continued treatment. See also PRECAUTIONS, Weight Change.

INDICATIONS AND USAGE

LUNELLE™ Monthly Contraceptive Injection is indicated for the prevention of pregnancy.

The efficacy of LUNELLE™ Monthly Contraceptive Injection is dependent on adherence to the recommended dosage schedule (e.g., intramuscular injections every 28 to 30 days, not to exceed 33 days). To ensure that LUNELLE™ Monthly Contraceptive Injection is not administered inadvertently to a pregnant woman, the first injection should be given during the first 5 days of a normal menstrual period. LUNELLE™ Monthly Contraceptive Injection should be administered no earlier than 4 weeks after delivery if not breastfeeding or 6 weeks after delivery if breastfeeding (see NURSING MOTHERS).

Several clinical trials of LUNELLE™ Monthly Contraceptive Injection have reported 12-month failure rates of <1% by Life Table analysis (see also CLINICAL STUDIES). Pregnancy rates for various contraceptive methods are typically reported for the first year of use and are shown in Table 2.

[See table 2 at middle of next page]

CONTRAINDICATIONS

The information contained in this package insert is based not only on information specific to LUNELLE™ Monthly Contraceptive Injection, but also on studies carried out in women who used injectable progestin-only contraceptives (medroxyprogesterone acetate) or oral contraceptives with higher doses of both estrogens and progestogens than those in common use today. The effect of long-term use of hormonal contraceptives with formulations having lower doses of both estrogens and progestogens remains to be determined.

LUNELLE™ Monthly Contraceptive Injection should not be used in women with any of the following conditions or circumstances.

- Known or suspected pregnancy.
- Thrombophlebitis or thromboembolic disorders.
- A past history of deep-vein thrombophlebitis or thromboembolic disorders.
- Cerebral vascular or coronary artery disease.
- Undiagnosed abnormal genital bleeding.
- Liver dysfunction or disease, such as history of hepatic adenoma or carcinoma; history of cholestatic jaundice of pregnancy or jaundice with prior hormonal contraceptive use including severe pruritus of pregnancy.
- Carcinoma of the endometrium, breast, or other known or suspected estrogen-dependent neoplasia.
- Known hypersensitivity to any of the ingredients contained in LUNELLE™ Monthly Contraceptive Injection.
- Heavy smoking (≥15 cigarettes per day) and over age 35.
- Severe hypertension.
- Diabetes with vascular involvement.
- Headaches with focal neurological symptoms.
- Valvular heart disease with complications.

WARNINGS

Cigarette smoking increases the risk of serious cardiovascular side effects from contraceptives containing estrogen. This risk increases with age and with heavy smoking (15 or more cigarettes per day) and is quite marked in women over 35 years of age. Women who use LUNELLE™ Monthly Contraceptive Injection should be strongly advised not to smoke.

The use of oral contraceptives is associated with increased risks of several serious conditions including myocardial infarction, thromboembolism, stroke, hepatic neoplasia, and gallbladder disease, although the risk of serious morbidity or mortality is very small in healthy women without underlying risk factors. The risk of morbidity and mortality increases significantly in the presence of other underlying risk factors such as hypertension, hyperlipidemias, obesity, and diabetes.

Practitioners prescribing LUNELLE™ Monthly Contraceptive Injection should be familiar with the following information relating to these risks.

Throughout this labeling, epidemiological studies reported are of two types: retrospective or case control studies and prospective or cohort studies. Case control studies provide a measure of the relative risk of a disease, namely, a ratio of the incidence of a disease among oral contraceptive users to that among non-users. The relative risk does not provide information on the actual clinical occurrence of a disease. Cohort studies provide a measure of attributable risk, which is the difference in the incidence of disease between oral contraceptive users and non-users. The attributable risk does provide information about the actual occurrence of a disease in the population. For further information, the reader is referred to a text on epidemiological methods.

1. THROMBOEMBOLIC DISORDERS AND OTHER VASCULAR PROBLEMS

a. Myocardial Infarction

An increased risk of myocardial infarction has been attributed to oral contraceptive use. This risk is primarily in smokers or women with other underlying risk factors for coronary artery disease such as hypertension, hypercholesterolemia, morbid obesity, and diabetes. The relative risk of heart attack for current oral contraceptive users has been estimated to be two to six. The risk is very low in women under the age of 30.

Smoking in combination with oral contraceptive use has been shown to contribute substantially to the incidence of myocardial infarctions in women in their mid-thirties or older with smoking accounting for the majority of excess cases. Mortality rates associated with circulatory disease have been shown to increase substantially in smokers over 35 years of age and older and non-smokers over 40 years of age who use oral contraceptives (see Table 3).

[See table 3 at bottom of next page]

Oral contraceptives may compound the effects of well-known risk factors, such as hypertension, diabetes, hyperlipidemias, age, and obesity. In particular, some progestogens are known to decrease high density lipoproteins (HDL) cholesterol and cause glucose intolerance, while estrogens may create a state of hyperinsulinism. Oral contraceptives have been shown to increase blood pressure among users (see WARNINGS, No. 9). Similar effects on risk factors have been associated with an increased risk of heart disease. LUNELLE™ Monthly Contraceptive Injection must be used with caution in women with cardiovascular disease risk factors.

b. Thromboembolism

An increased risk of thromboembolic and thrombotic diseases associated with the use of oral contraceptives is well established. Case control studies have found the relative risk of users compared with non-users to be 3 for the first episode of superficial venous thrombosis, 4 to 11 for deep vein thrombosis or pulmonary embolism, and 1.5 to 6 for women with predisposing conditions for venous thromboembolic disease. Cohort studies have shown the relative risk to be somewhat lower, about 3 for new cases and about 4.5 for new cases requiring hospitalization. The risk of thromboembolic disease due to oral contraceptives is not related to length of use and disappears after pill use is stopped.

A two- to four-fold increase in relative risk of post-operative thromboembolic complications has been reported with the use of oral contraceptives. The relative risk of venous thrombosis in women who have predisposing conditions is twice that of women without such medical conditions. If feasible, oral contraceptives should be discontinued at least 4 weeks prior to and for 2 weeks after elective surgery of a type associated with an increase in risk of thromboembolism and during and following prolonged immobilization. Since the immediate postpartum period is also associated with an increased risk of thromboembolism, oral contraceptives and other combined hormonal contraceptives such as LUNELLE™ Monthly Contraceptive Injection, should be started no earlier than 4 weeks after delivery.

The clinician should be alert to the earliest manifestations of thrombotic disorders (thrombophlebitis, pulmonary embolism, cerebrovascular disorders, and retinal thrombosis). Should any of these occur or be suspected, LUNELLE™ Monthly Contraceptive Injection should not be readministered.

c. Cerebrovascular Disease

Oral contraceptives have been shown to increase both the relative and attributable risks of cerebrovascular events (thrombotic and hemorrhagic strokes), although, in general, the risk is greatest among older (>35 years), hypertensive women who also smoke. Hypertension was found to be a risk factor for both users and non-users, for both types of strokes, while smoking interacted to increase the risk for hemorrhagic stroke.

The relative risk of thrombotic strokes has been shown to range from 3 for normotensive users to 14 for users with severe hypertension. The relative risk of hemorrhagic stroke is reported to be 1.2 for non-smokers who used oral contraceptives, 2.6 for smokers who did not use oral contraceptives, 7.6 for smokers who used oral contraceptives, 1.8 for normotensive users, and 25.7 for users with severe hypertension. The attributable risk is also greater in older women.

d. Dose-related Risk of Vascular Disease

A positive association has been observed between the amount of estrogen and progestogen in oral contraceptives and the risk of vascular disease. A decline in serum HDL has been reported with many progestational agents. A decline in serum HDL has been associated with an increased incidence of ischemic heart disease. Because estrogens increase HDL cholesterol, the net effect of an oral contraceptive depends on a balance achieved between doses of estrogen and progestogen and the type of progestogens used in the contraceptives. The activity and amount of both hormones should be considered in the choice of a hormonal contraceptive.

e. Persistence of Risk of Vascular Disease

There are two studies which have shown persistence of risk of vascular disease for ever-users of oral contraceptives. In a study in the United States, the risk of developing myocardial infarction after discontinuing oral contraceptives persists for at least 9 years for women 40–49 years who had used oral contraceptives for five or more years, but this increased risk was not demonstrated in other age groups. In another study in Great Britain, the risk of developing cerebrovascular disease persisted for at least 6 years after discontinuation of oral contraceptives, although excess risk was very small. However, both studies were performed with oral contraceptive formulations containing 50 micrograms or more of estrogen.

2. ESTIMATES OF MORTALITY FROM CONTRACEPTIVE USE

One study gathered data from a variety of sources that have estimated the mortality rate associated with different methods of contraception at different ages (see Table 4). These estimates include the combined risk of death associated with contraceptive methods plus the risk attributable to pregnancy in the event of method failure. Each method of contraception has its specific benefits and risks. The study concluded that with the exception of oral contraceptive users 35 years and older who smoke, and oral contraceptive users 40 years and older who do not smoke, mortality associated with all methods of birth control is low and below that associated with childbirth.

The observation of a possible increase in risk of mortality with age for oral contraceptive users is based on data gathered in the 1970s, but not reported until 1983. However, current clinical practice involves the use of lower estrogen-dose formulations combined with careful restriction of oral contraceptive use to women who do not have the various risk factors listed in this labeling.

Because of these changes in practice and because of some limited new data that suggest the risk of cardiovascular disease with the use of oral contraceptives may now be less than previously observed, the Fertility and Maternal Health Drugs Advisory Committee was asked to review the topic in 1989. The Committee concluded that although cardiovascular disease risk may be increased with oral contraceptive use after age 40 in healthy non-smoking women (even with the newer low-dose formulations), there are also greater potential health risks associated with pregnancy in older women and with the alternative surgical and medical procedures that may be necessary if such women do not have access to effective and acceptable means of contraception. Therefore, the Committee recommended that the benefits of oral contraceptive use by healthy non-smoking women over age 40 may outweigh the possible risks. Women of all ages who take oral contraceptives should take a product which contains the lowest amount of estrogen and progestogen that is effective.

[See table 4 at bottom of next page]

3. CARCINOMA OF THE REPRODUCTIVE ORGANS AND BREASTS

Numerous epidemiological studies have been performed on the incidence of breast, endometrial, ovarian, and cervical cancer in women using oral contraceptives. Although the risk of breast cancer may be slightly increased among current and recent users of combined oral contraceptives, this excess risk decreases over time after product discontinuation, and by 10 years after cessation the increased risk disappears. In addition, breast cancers diagnosed in current or ever-oral contraceptive users tend to be less invasive than in non-users.

The risk of breast cancer does not increase with duration of use, and no relationships have been found with dose or type of steroid. The patterns of risk are also similar regardless of a woman's reproductive history or her family breast cancer history. The sub-group for whom risk has been found to be significantly elevated is women who first used combined oral contraceptives before age 20, but because breast cancer is so rare at these young ages, the number of cases attributable to this early combined oral contraceptive use is extremely small.

Table 2. Percentage of Women Experiencing an Unintended Pregnancy During the First Year of Typical Use and the First Year of Perfect Use of Contraception and the Percentage Continuing Use at the End of the First Year: United States

Method	% of Women Experiencing an Unintended Pregnancy within the First Year of Use		% of Women Continuing Use at 1 Year[3]
	Typical Use[1]	Perfect Use[2]	
Chance[4]	85	85	
Spermicides[5]	26	6	40
Periodic Abstinence	25		63
Calendar		9	
Ovulation Method		3	
Symptothermal[6]		2	
Post-ovulation		1	
Cap[7]			
Parous Women	40	26	42
Nulliparous Women	20	9	56
Sponge			
Parous Women	40	20	42
Nulliparous Women	20	9	56
Diaphragm[7]	20	6	56
Withdrawal	19	4	
Condom[8]			
Female (Reality)	21	5	56
Male	14	3	61
Pill	5		71
Progestin only		0.5	
Combined		0.1	
IUD			
Progesterone T	2.0	1.5	81
Copper T 380A	0.8	0.6	78
LNg 20	0.1	0.1	81
Depo-Provera	0.3	0.3	70
Norplant and Norplant-2	0.05	0.05	88
Female Sterilization	0.5	0.5	100
Male Sterilization	0.15	0.10	100

Emergency Contraceptive Pills: Treatment initiated within 72 hours after unprotected intercourse reduces the risk of pregnancy by at least 75%.[9]

Lactational Amenorrhea Method: LAM is a highly effective, temporary method of contraception.[10]

Adapted from Hatcher et al., 1998.

[1] Among typical couples who initiate use of a method (not necessarily for the first time), the percentage who experience an accidental pregnancy during the first year if they do not stop use for any other reason.

[2] Among couples who initiate use of a method (not necessarily for the first time) and who use it perfectly (both consistently and correctly), the percentage who experience an accidental pregnancy during the first year if they do not stop use for any other reason.

[3] Among couples attempting to avoid pregnancy, the percentage who continue to use a method for 1 year.

[4] The percentages becoming pregnant in columns (2) and (3) are based on data from populations where contraception is not used and from women who cease using contraception in order to become pregnant. Among such populations, about 89% become pregnant within 1 year. This estimate was lowered slightly (to 85%) to represent the percentages who would become pregnant within 1 year among women now relying on reversible methods of contraception if they abandoned contraception altogether.

[5] Foams, creams, gels, vaginal suppositories, and vaginal film.

[6] Cervical mucus (ovulation) method supplemented by calendar in the pre-ovulatory and basal body temperature in the post-ovulatory phases.

[7] With spermicidal cream or jelly.

[8] Without spermicides.

[9] The treatment schedule is one dose within 72 hours after unprotected intercourse, and a second dose 12 hours after the first dose. The Food and Drug Administration has declared the following brands of oral contraceptives to be safe and effective for emergency contraception: Ovral (1 dose is 2 white pills), Alesse (1 dose is 5 pink pills), Nordette or Levlen (1 dose is 4 light-orange pills), Lo/Ovral (1 dose is 4 white pills), Triphasil or Tri-Levlen (1 dose is 4 yellow pills).

[10] However, to maintain effective protection against pregnancy, another method of contraception must be used as soon as menstruation resumes, the frequency or duration of breastfeeds is reduced, bottle feeds are introduced, or the baby reaches 6 months of age.

Table 3. Circulatory Disease Mortality Rates per 100,000 Women Years by Age, Smoking Status and Oral Contraceptive Use

Age (y)	Ever-Users Non-smokers	Ever-Users Smokers	Controls Non-smokers	Controls Smokers
15–24	0.0	10.5	0.0	0.0
25–34	4.4	14.2	2.7	4.2
35–44	21.5	63.4	6.4	15.2
45+	52.4	206.7	11.4	27.9

Adapted from Layde PM, Beral V., 1981.

Continued on next page

Lunelle—Cont.

Women who currently have or have had breast cancer should not use combined hormonal contraceptives because breast cancer is a hormonally sensitive tumor.

Long-term case-controlled surveillance of users of depot medroxyprogesterone acetate (DMPA) found slight or no increased overall risk of breast cancer. A pooled analysis from two case-control studies, the World Health Organization (WHO) Study and the New Zealand Study, reported the relative risk of breast cancer for women who had ever used DMPA as 1.1. Overall, there was no increase in risk with increasing duration of use of DMPA. The relative risk of breast cancer for women of all ages who had initiated use of DMPA within the previous 5 years was estimated to be 2.0. The WHO Study, a component of the pooled analysis described above, showed an increased relative risk of 2.19 of breast cancer associated with use of DMPA in women whose first exposure to drug was within the previous 4 years and who were under 35 years of age. However, the overall relative risk for ever-users of DMPA was only 1.2.

Some studies suggest that oral contraceptive use has been associated with an increase in the risk of cervical intraepithelial neoplasia in some populations of women. However, there continues to be controversy about the extent to which such findings may be due to differences in sexual behavior and other factors.

A statistically insignificant increase in relative risk estimates of invasive squamous-cell cervical cancer has been associated with the use of DMPA in women who were first exposed before the age of 35 years. The overall, non-significant relative rate of invasive squamous-cell cervical cancer in women who ever used DMPA was estimated to be 1.11. No trends in risk with duration of use or times since initial or most recent exposure were observed.

In spite of many studies of the relationship between oral contraceptive use and breast and cervical cancers, a cause and effect relationship has not been established. No long-term studies have been conducted with LUNELLE™ Monthly Contraceptive Injection to evaluate risk for carcinoma of the reproductive organs.

4. HEPATIC NEOPLASIA

Benign hepatic adenomas are associated with oral contraceptive use, although the incidence of benign tumors is rare in the United States. Indirect calculations have estimated the attributable risk to be in the range of 3.3 cases per 100,000 cases for users, a risk that increases after 4 or more years of use. Rupture of benign, hepatic adenomas may cause death through intra-abdominal hemorrhage.

Studies from Britain have shown an increased risk of developing hepatocellular carcinoma in long-term (>8 years) oral contraceptive users. However, these cancers are extremely rare in the United States and the attributable risk (the excess incidence) of liver cancers in oral contraceptive users approaches less than one per million users.

5. OCULAR LESIONS

There have been clinical case reports of retinal thrombosis associated with the use of oral contraceptives. LUNELLE™ Monthly Contraceptive Injection should be discontinued if there is unexplained partial or complete loss of vision, onset of proptosis or diplopia, papilledema, or retinal vascular lesions. Appropriate diagnostic and therapeutic measures should be undertaken immediately.

6. HORMONAL CONTRACEPTIVE USE BEFORE OR DURING PREGNANCY

The use of hormonal contraceptives during pregnancy is not indicated.

Extensive epidemiological studies have revealed no increased risk of birth defects in women who have used oral contraceptives prior to pregnancy. Studies also do not suggest a teratogenic effect, particularly in so far as cardiac anomalies and limb reduction defects are concerned, when oral contraceptives are taken inadvertently during early pregnancy.

Pregnancies occurring in women receiving injectable progestin-only contraceptives are uncommon. Neonates from unexpected pregnancies that occurred 1 to 2 months after injection of DMPA may be at an increased risk of low birth weight, which, in turn, is associated with an increased risk of neonatal death. A significant increase in incidence of polysyndactyly and chromosomal anomalies was observed among infants of users of DMPA, the former being most pronounced in women under 30 years of age. The unrelated nature of these defects, the lack of confirmation from other studies, the distant preconceptual exposure to DMPA, and the chance effects due to multiple statistical comparisons, make a causal association unlikely.

Neonates exposed to MPA in utero and followed to adolescence, showed no evidence of any adverse effects on their health including their physical, intellectual, sexual or social development.

Several reports suggest an association between intrauterine exposure to progestational drugs in the first trimester of pregnancy and genital abnormalities in male and female fetuses. The risk of hypospadias (five to eight per 1,000 male births in the general population) may be approximately doubled with exposure to these drugs. There are insufficient data to quantify the risk to exposed female fetuses, but because some of these drugs induce mild virilization of the external genitalia of the female fetus and because of the increased association of hypospadias in the male fetus, these drugs should be avoided during pregnancy.

Unexpected pregnancies occurring in women receiving LUNELLE™ Monthly Contraceptive Injection are uncommon and have not shown congenital malformations or other adverse events.

The administration of combined hormonal contraceptives, such as LUNELLE™ Monthly Contraceptive Injection, to induce withdrawal bleeding should not be used as a test for pregnancy. LUNELLE™ Monthly Contraceptive Injection should not be used during pregnancy to treat threatened or habitual abortion. It is recommended that for any patient who has missed two consecutive periods, pregnancy should be considered before initiating or continuing LUNELLE™ Monthly Contraceptive Injection. If the patient has exceeded the prescribed injection interval (>33 days) for LUNELLE™ Monthly Contraceptive Injection, the possibility of pregnancy should be ruled out before another injection is administered.

7. GALLBLADDER DISEASE

Combined hormonal contraceptives may worsen existing gallbladder disease and may accelerate the development of this disease in previously asymptomatic women. Women with a history of combined hormonal contraceptive-related cholestasis are more likely to have the condition recur with subsequent combined hormonal contraceptive use.

In a study of 782 women taking LUNELLE™ Monthly Contraceptive Injection for up to 15 cycles, cholecystitis and cholelithiasis were the only serious adverse events judged to be possibly related to the study drug. They were reported as an adverse event in five subjects, and three subjects required cholecystectomy.

8. CARBOHYDRATE AND LIPID METABOLIC EFFECTS

Combined hormonal or progestin-only contraceptives have been shown to cause glucose intolerance in some users. However, in the non-diabetic woman, combined hormonal contraceptives appear to have no effect on fasting blood glucose. Pre-diabetic and diabetic patients should be carefully observed while receiving therapy with LUNELLE™ Monthly Contraceptive Injection.

A small proportion of women may have persistent hypertriglyceridemia while using oral contraceptives. Changes in serum triglycerides and lipoprotein levels have been reported in oral contraceptive users.

9. ELEVATED BLOOD PRESSURE

An increase in blood pressure has been reported in women taking oral contraceptives and this increase is more likely in older oral contraceptive users and with continued use. Data from the Royal College of General Practitioners and subsequent randomized trials have shown that the incidence of hypertension increases with increasing concentrations of progestogens. In a US clinical study, no increase in mean blood pressure was observed over 15 months use of LUNELLE™ Monthly Contraceptive Injection.

Women with a history of hypertension or hypertension-related diseases, or renal disease should be encouraged to use another method of contraception. If women elect to use combined hormonal contraceptives such as LUNELLE™ Monthly Contraceptive Injection, they should be monitored closely and if significant elevation of blood pressure occurs, LUNELLE™ Monthly Contraceptive Injection should be discontinued. For most women, elevated blood pressure will return to normal after stopping oral contraceptives, and there is no difference in the occurrence of hypertension among former and never-users.

10. HEADACHE

The onset or exacerbation of migraine or development of headache with a new pattern which is recurrent, persistent, or severe requires evaluation of the cause before further injections of LUNELLE™ Monthly Contraceptive Injection are given.

11. BLEEDING IRREGULARITIES

Most women using LUNELLE™ Monthly Contraceptive Injection (58.6%) experienced alteration of menstrual bleeding patterns, including 4.1% amenorrhea, after one year of use. Altered bleeding patterns include frequent bleeding, irregular bleeding, prolonged bleeding, infrequent bleeding, and amenorrhea. As women continued using LUNELLE™ Monthly Contraceptive Injection, the percent experiencing frequent or prolonged bleeding decreased, while the percent experiencing amenorrhea increased. The percent of women experiencing irregular bleeding remained fairly constant at approximately 30% throughout the first year of use.

Regardless of the bleeding pattern, subsequent injections should be given 1 month (28 to 30 days, not to exceed 33 days) after the previous injection, unless discontinuation is medically indicated.

If abnormal bleeding associated with LUNELLE™ Monthly Contraceptive Injection persists or is severe, appropriate investigation should be instituted to rule out the possibility of organic pathology, and appropriate treatment should be instituted when necessary. In the event of amenorrhea, pregnancy should be ruled out.

12. BONE MINERAL DENSITY CHANGES

Use of injectable progestogen-only methods may be considered among the risk factors for development of osteoporosis. The rate of bone loss is greatest in the early years of use and then subsequently approaches the normal rate of age-related fall. Formal studies on the effect of bone mineral density changes in women receiving LUNELLE™ Monthly Contraceptive Injection have not been conducted.

13. ANAPHYLAXIS AND ANAPHYLACTOID REACTION

Anaphylaxis and anaphylactoid reactions have been reported with the components of LUNELLE™ Monthly Contraceptive Injection. Allergic reactions occurring in women using LUNELLE™ Monthly Contraceptive Injection have been mainly dermatologic, not respiratory, in nature. If an anaphylactic reaction occurs, appropriate therapy should be instituted. Serious anaphylactic reactions require emergency medical treatment.

PRECAUTIONS

1. **General. Patients should be counseled that this product does not protect against HIV infection (AIDS) and other sexually transmitted diseases.**
2. **Physical Examination.** It is good medical practice for all women to have an annual history and physical examination, including women using combined hormonal contraceptives. The physical examination should include special reference to blood pressure, breasts, abdomen and pelvic organs, including cervical cytology, and relevant laboratory tests. In case of undiagnosed, persistent, or recurrent abnormal vaginal bleeding, appropriate measures should be conducted to rule out malignancy. Women with a strong family history of breast cancer or who have breast nodules should be monitored with particular care.
3. **Weight Change.** In a study of 782 women using LUNELLE™ Monthly Contraceptive Injection for up to 15 cycles, 5.7% of participants discontinued due to weight gain. Weight gain was the most common adverse event leading to discontinuation of the drug. Women gained an average of 4 pounds during the first year, and an additional 2 pounds during the second year, of LUNELLE™ Monthly Contraceptive Injection use. The range of weight change during the first year of LUNELLE™ Monthly Contraceptive Injection use was 48 pounds lost to 49 pounds gained. The following table shows the range of weight changes seen for women continuing use up to 24 cycles.

Weight Change	12 Cycles (n=469)	15 Cycles (n=433)	24 Cycles (n=111)
Lost >20 pounds	1%	2%	5%
Lost >10 to 20 pounds	6%	6%	7%
Gained >10 to 20 pounds	19%	24%	14%
Gained >20 pounds	5%	7%	23%

4. **Lipid Disorders.** Women who are being treated for hyperlipidemias should be followed closely if they use combined hormonal contraceptives. Some progestogens may elevate LDL levels and may render the control of hyperlipidemias more difficult.
5. **Liver Function.** If jaundice develops in any woman receiving combined hormonal contraceptives, the medication should be discontinued. Steroid hormones may be poorly metabolized in patients with impaired liver function.

Table 4. Annual Number of Birth-Related or Method-Related Deaths Associated with Control of Fertility per 100,000 Non-sterile Women, by Fertility Control Method According to Age

Method of Control & Outcome	Range of Ages (years)					
	15–19	20–24	25–29	30–34	35–39	40–44
No fertility control*	7.0	7.4	9.1	14.8	25.7	28.2
Oral hormonal contraceptives** (non-smoker)	0.3	0.5	0.9	1.9	13.8	31.6
Oral hormonal contraceptives** (smoker)	2.2	3.4	6.6	13.5	51.1	117.2
IUD**	0.8	0.8	1.0	1.0	1.4	1.4
Condom*	1.1	1.6	0.7	0.2	0.3	0.4
Diaphragm/spermicide*	1.9	1.2	1.2	1.3	2.2	2.8
Periodic abstinence	2.5	1.6	1.6	1.7	2.9	3.6

Adapted from Ory HW. 1983.

* Deaths are birth-related

**Deaths are method-related

6. **Fluid Retention.** Progestogens and/or estrogens may cause some degree of fluid retention; therefore, caution should be used in treating any patient with a pre-existing medical condition that might be adversely affected by fluid retention.
7. **Contact Lenses.** Contact lens wearers who develop visual changes or changes in lens tolerance should be assessed by an ophthalmologist.
8. **Emotional Disorders.** Patients becoming significantly depressed while taking combined hormonal contraceptives should stop the medication and use an alternative method of contraception in an attempt to determine whether the symptom is drug-related. Women with a history of depression should be carefully observed and consideration should be given to the discontinuation of LUNELLE™ Monthly Contraceptive Injection if depression recurs to a serious degree.

DRUG INTERACTIONS

1. Effects of Other Drugs on MPA

Aminoglutethamide may decrease the serum concentration of MPA. Users of LUNELLE™ Monthly Contraceptive Injection should be informed of the possibility of decreased effectiveness with the use of this or any related drug. (See CLINICAL PHARMACOLOGY, Drug-Drug Interactions.)

2. Effects of Other Drugs on Combined Hormonal Contraceptives

Rifampin. Metabolism of some synthetic estrogens (e.g., ethinyl estradiol) and progestins (e.g., norethindrone) is increased by rifampin. A reduction in contraceptive effectiveness and an increase in menstrual irregularities have been associated with concomitant use of rifampin.

Anticonvulsants. Anticonvulsants such as phenobarbital, phenytoin, and carbamazepine have been shown to increase the metabolism of some synthetic estrogens and progestins, which could result in a reduction of contraceptive effectiveness.

Antibiotics. Pregnancy while taking oral contraceptives has been reported when the oral contraceptives were administered with antimicrobials such as ampicillin, tetracycline, and griseofulvin. However, clinical pharmacokinetic studies have not demonstrated any consistent effects of antibiotics (other than rifampin) on plasma concentrations of synthetic steroids.

Herbal products. Herbal products containing St. John's Wort (hypericum perforatum) may induce hepatic enzymes (cytochrome P450) and p-glycoprotein transporter and may reduce the effectiveness of contraceptive steroids. This may also result in breakthrough bleeding.

Other. Ascorbic acid and acetominophen may increase plasma concentrations of some synthetic estrogens, possibly by inhibition of conjugation. A reduction in contraceptive effectiveness and an increased incidence of menstrual irregularities has been suggested with phenylbutazone.

3. Effects of Combined Hormonal Contraceptives on Other Drugs

Combined hormonal contraceptives containing some synthetic estrogens (e.g., ethinyl estradiol) may inhibit the metabolism of other compounds. Increased plasma concentrations of cyclosporine, prednisolone and theophylline have been reported with concomitant administration of oral contraceptives. In addition, oral contraceptives may induce the conjugation of other compounds. Decreased plasma concentrations of acetominophen and increased clearance of temazepam, salicylic acid, morphine and clofibric acid have been noted when these drugs were administered with oral contraceptives.

4. Drug Interactions with Laboratory Tests

Certain endocrine and liver function tests and blood components may be affected by combined hormonal contraceptives:

a. Increased prothrombin and factors VII, VIII, IX, and X; decreased antithrombin 3; increased norepinephrine-induced platelet aggregability.
b. Increased thyroid binding globulin (TBG) leading to increased circulating total thyroid hormone, as measured by protein-bound iodine (PBI). T4 by column or by radioimmunoassay. Free T3 resin uptake is decreased, reflecting the elevated TBG, free T4 concentration is unaltered.
c. Other binding proteins may be elevated in serum.
d. Sex-hormone-binding-globulins are increased and result in elevated levels of total circulating sex steroids and corticoids; however, free or biologically active levels remain unchanged.
e. Triglycerides may be increased.
f. Glucose tolerance may be decreased.
g. Serum folate levels may be depressed by combined hormonal contraceptive therapy. This may be of clinical significance if a woman becomes pregnant shortly after discontinuing combined hormonal contraceptives.

The pathologist should be advised of progestogen and estrogen therapy when relevant tissue specimens are submitted.

The following laboratory tests may be affected by progestins including LUNELLE™ Monthly Contraceptive Injection:

a. Plasma and urinary steroid levels are decreased (e.g., progesterone, estradiol, pregnanediol, testosterone, cortisol).
b. Gonadotropin levels are decreased.
c. Sex-hormone-binding-globulin concentrations are decreased.
d. Sulfobromophthalein and other liver function test values may be increased.

CARCINOGENESIS, MUTAGENESIS, IMPAIRMENT OF FERTILITY

See WARNINGS section.

PREGNANCY

Pregnancy Category X. See CONTRAINDICATIONS and WARNINGS.

Return of Ovulation and Fertility

Ovulation (signaled by a rise in serum progesterone concentrations ≥4.7 ng/mL) was observed 63 to 112 days after the third monthly injection of LUNELLE™ Monthly Contraceptive Injection in 11 of 14 women participating in a pharmacodynamic study. The remaining three women had not ovulated by day 85 and were lost to follow-up.

In a study of 21 women who received LUNELLE™ Monthly Contraceptive Injection for 3 months, 52% ovulated during the first post-treatment month, and 71% during the second post-treatment month. In another study of 10 women receiving long-term administration (2 years of treatment) of LUNELLE™ Monthly Contraceptive Injection, 60% ovulated by the third post-treatment month.

A study of 70 women who discontinued LUNELLE™ Monthly Contraceptive Injection to become pregnant demonstrated that more than 50% achieved fertility within 6 months after discontinuation, and 83% did so by 1 year.

NURSING MOTHERS

The effects of LUNELLE™ Monthly Contraceptive Injection in nursing mothers have not been evaluated and are unknown. However, estrogen administration to nursing mothers has been shown to decrease the quantity and quality of breast milk. Small amounts of combined hormonal contraceptive steroids have been identified in the milk of nursing mothers and a few adverse effects on the child have been reported, including jaundice and breast enlargement. Long-term follow-up of children whose mothers used combined hormonal contraceptives while breastfeeding has shown no deleterious effects. However, women who are breastfeeding should not start taking combined hormonal contraceptives until six weeks postpartum.

PEDIATRIC USE

Safety and efficacy of LUNELLE™ Monthly Contraceptive Injection have been established in women of reproductive age. Safety and efficacy are expected to be the same for post-pubertal adolescents under 16 years of age and users 16 years of age and older. Use of this product before menarche is not indicated.

INFORMATION FOR PATIENTS

Patients should be given a copy of the patient labeling prior to administration of LUNELLE™ Monthly Contraceptive Injection.

Patients should be advised that the contraceptive efficacy of LUNELLE™ Monthly Contraceptive Injection depends on receiving injections monthly (28 to 30 days, not to exceed 33 days). The injection schedule must be measured by the number of days, not by bleeding episodes. It is recommended that for any patient who has missed two consecutive menstrual periods, pregnancy should be considered before initiating or continuing LUNELLE™ Monthly Contraceptive Injection. Thereafter, a woman who has continued amenorrhea while using LUNELLE™ Monthly Contraceptive Injection and who has received her injections according to the recommended dosing schedule may continue to receive subsequent injections each month after the previous injection (not to exceed 33 days), unless discontinuation is medically indicated. All patients presenting for a follow-up injection of LUNELLE™ Monthly Contraceptive Injection after day 33 should use a barrier method of contraception and should not receive another injection of LUNELLE™ Monthly Contraceptive Injection until pregnancy has been ruled out.

Patients should be advised that menstrual bleeding patterns are likely to be disrupted with use of LUNELLE™ Monthly Contraceptive Injection. A few patients may experience amenorrhea. Irregular bleeding that occurs after a regular bleeding pattern has emerged should be investigated. In the presence of excessive or prolonged bleeding, other causes should be investigated and consideration should be given to alternative methods of contraception.

Patients should be counseled that this product does not protect against HIV infection (AIDS) and other sexually transmitted diseases.

ADVERSE REACTIONS

An increased risk of the following serious adverse reactions has been associated with the use of combined hormonal contraceptives (see CONTRAINDICATIONS and WARNINGS).

- Arterial thromboembolism
- Cerebral hemorrhage
- Cerebral thrombosis
- Gallbladder disease
- Hepatic adenomas or benign liver tumors
- Hypertension
- Myocardial infarction
- Pulmonary embolism
- Thrombophlebitis

The following adverse reactions have been reported in patients receiving LUNELLE™ Monthly Contraceptive Injection and are believed to be drug-related:

- Abdominal pain
- Acne
- Alopecia
- Amenorrhea
- Asthenia
- Breast tenderness/pain
- Decreased libido
- Depression
- Dizziness
- Dysmenorrhea
- Emotional lability
- Enlarged abdomen
- Headache
- Menorrhagia
- Metrorrhagia
- Nausea
- Nervousness
- Vaginal moniliasis
- Vulvovaginal disorder
- Weight gain

There is evidence of an association between the following conditions and the use of combined hormonal contraceptives, although additional confirmatory studies are needed:

- Mesenteric thrombosis
- Retinal thrombosis

The following additional adverse reactions have been reported in users of combined hormonal contraceptives, and are believed to be drug-related:

- Anaphylactic reactions
- Breast changes: enlargement, secretion
- Cervical changes
- Cholestatic jaundice
- Corneal curvature changes (i.e., steepening)
- Diminution in lactation when given immediately postpartum
- Edema
- Intolerance to contact lenses
- Melasma that may persist
- Migraine
- Rash (allergic)
- Reduced carbohydrate tolerance
- Temporary infertility after treatment discontinuation
- Weight decrease

The following additional adverse reactions have been reported in users of combined hormonal contraceptives, and the association has been neither confirmed nor refuted:

- Budd-Chiari syndrome
- Cataracts
- Changes in appetite
- Changes in libido
- Colitis
- Cystitis-like syndrome
- Erythema multiforme
- Erythema nodosum
- Hemolytic uremic syndrome
- Hemorrhagic eruption
- Hirsutism
- Impaired renal function
- Premenstrual syndrome
- Porphyria
- Vaginitis

The most frequent adverse events (reported by 1% or more patients) leading to discontinuation in various trials of women using LUNELLE™ Monthly Contraceptive Injection were weight gain, menorrhagia, amenorrhea, metrorrhagia, vaginal spotting, emotional lability, acne, breast tenderness/pain, headache, dysmenorrhea, nausea, and depression.

OVERDOSAGE

Overdosage of a progestin/estrogen drug combination may cause nausea and vomiting, and vaginal bleeding or other menstrual irregularities in females.

DOSAGE AND ADMINISTRATION

LUNELLE™ Monthly Contraceptive Injection is effective for contraception during the first cycle of use when administered as recommended.

The recommended dose of LUNELLE™ Monthly Contraceptive Injection is 0.5 mL administered by intramuscular injection, into the deltoid, gluteus maximus, or anterior thigh. The aqueous suspension must be vigorously shaken just before use to ensure a uniform suspension of 25 mg medroxyprogesterone acetate and 5 mg estradiol cypionate.

First Injection

- Within first 5 days of the onset of a normal menstrual period, **or**
- Within 5 days of a complete first trimester abortion, **or**
- No earlier than 4 weeks postpartum if not breastfeeding.
- No earlier than 6 weeks postpartum if breastfeeding.

Second and Subsequent Injections

- Monthly (28 to 30 days) after previous injection, not to exceed 33 days.
- If the patient has not adhered to the prescribed schedule (greater than 33 days since last injection), pregnancy should be considered and she should not receive another injection until pregnancy is ruled out.
- Shortening the injection interval could lead to a change in menstrual pattern.
- Do not use bleeding episodes to guide the injection schedule.

Switching from other Methods of Contraception

When switching from other contraceptive methods, LUNELLE™ Monthly Contraceptive Injection should be given in a manner that ensures continuous contraceptive coverage based upon the mechanism of action of both methods, e.g., patients switching from oral contraceptives should have their first injection of LUNELLE™ Monthly Contraceptive Injection within 7 days after taking their last active pill.

HOW SUPPLIED

LUNELLE™ Monthly Contraceptive Injection (25 mg medroxyprogesterone acetate and 5 mg estradiol cypionate

Continued on next page

Lunelle—Cont.

per 0.5 mL sterile aqueous injectable suspension) is available in a vial containing enough product to deliver 0.5 mL for single-dose administration (NDC 0009-3484-04).

Store at 25°C (77°F); excursions permitted to 15–30°C (59–86°F) [see USP Controlled Room Temperature].

℞ only

References available upon request.

Manufactured by:
Pharmacia & Upjohn Company
Kalamazoo, MI 49001, USA
October 2000

817 821 000
692804
3484-04

LUNELLE™ Monthly Contraceptive Injection (like all hormonal contraceptives) is intended to prevent pregnancy. It does not protect against HIV infection (AIDS) and other sexually transmitted diseases.

Every woman who considers using hormonal contraceptives must understand the benefits and risks of this type of birth control. This sheet contains important information about hormonal contraceptives that you need in order to decide if LUNELLE™ Monthly Contraceptive Injection is a good type of birth control for you. Please read this sheet carefully and ask your health care provider to help you compare LUNELLE™ Monthly Contraceptive Injection with other methods of birth control. This sheet is not meant to take the

place of careful discussions with your health care provider. You should discuss the information provided in this sheet with him or her, both when you first start taking LUNELLE™ Monthly Contraceptive Injection and during your revisits. You should also follow your health care provider's advice with regard to regular check-ups while you are on LUNELLE™ Monthly Contraceptive Injection.

WHAT IS LUNELLE™ MONTHLY CONTRACEPTIVE INJECTION?

LUNELLE™ Monthly Contraceptive Injection is a type of hormonal birth control that is given as an injection (a shot) in your arm, thigh, or buttock once a month to prevent pregnancy. It contains hormones which have effects similar to the natural hormones, estrogen and progesterone, produced in your body. Similar combinations of hormones are found in some oral contraceptives also known as "birth control pills" or "the pill." When you receive your injections once a month as prescribed, LUNELLE™ Monthly Contraceptive Injection is as effective as birth control pills. When given according to the prescribed schedule, LUNELLE™ Monthly Contraceptive Injection is effective in preventing pregnancy during the cycle in which it is given. Clinical studies have shown that when women receive LUNELLE™ Monthly Contraceptive Injection according to the recommended schedule, the failure rate of this method of birth control is less than 1% per year.

The following table shows the typical failure rates for other methods of birth control during the first year of use:

[See table below]

WHO SHOULD NOT TAKE LUNELLE™ MONTHLY CONTRACEPTIVE INJECTION

Cigarette smoking increases the risk of serious cardiovascular side effects from hormonal contraceptive use. This risk increases with age and with heavy smoking (15 or more cigarettes per day) and is quite marked in women over 35 years of age. Women who use hormonal contraceptives are strongly advised not to smoke.

Some women should not use hormonal contraceptives. For example, you should not take LUNELLE™ Monthly Contraceptive Injection if you are pregnant or think you may be pregnant. You should also not use LUNELLE™ Monthly Contraceptive Injection if you have any of the following conditions:

- A history of heart attack or stroke
- Blood clots in the legs (thrombophlebitis), lungs (pulmonary embolism), or eyes
- A history of blood clots in the deep veins of your legs
- Chest pain (angina pectoris)
- Known or suspected breast cancer or cancer of the lining of the uterus, cervix or vagina
- Unexplained vaginal bleeding (until a diagnosis is reached by your doctor)
- Yellowing of the whites of the eyes or of the skin (jaundice) during pregnancy or during previous use of the pill or other hormonal contraceptives
- Liver tumor (benign or cancerous)
- Known or suspected pregnancy
- Allergy to any of the ingredients contained in LUNELLE™ Monthly Contraceptive Injection
- Over age 35 and smoke 15 or more cigarettes per day

Tell your health care provider if you have ever had any of these conditions. Your health care provider can recommend a safer method of birth control.

OTHER CONSIDERATIONS BEFORE TAKING LUNELLE™ MONTHLY CONTRACEPTIVE INJECTION

For the majority of women, hormonal contraceptives can be taken safely. But there are some women who are at high risk of developing certain serious diseases that can be life-threatening or may cause temporary or permanent disability. Tell your health care provider if you have:

- Breast nodules, fibrocystic disease of the breast, an abnormal breast x-ray or mammogram, strong family history of breast cancer
- Diabetes
- Elevated cholesterol or triglycerides
- High blood pressure
- Migraine or other headaches or epilepsy
- Mental depression
- Gallbladder, heart or kidney disease
- History of scanty or irregular menstrual periods
- Smoke, especially if 35 years or older

Women with any of these conditions should be checked often by their health care provider if they choose to use LUNELLE™ Monthly Contraceptive Injection.

Also, be sure to inform your doctor or health care provider if you smoke or are on any medications.

RISKS OF TAKING HORMONAL CONTRACEPTIVES

1. Risk of developing blood clots, heart attacks, and strokes

Blood clots and blockage of blood vessels are the most serious side effects of taking hormonal contraceptives. In particular, blood clots can occur in the legs and can travel to the lungs and can cause sudden blocking of the vessel carrying blood to the lungs. Rarely, clots occur in the blood vessels of the eye and may cause blindness, double vision, or impaired vision.

If you take hormonal contraceptives such as LUNELLE™ Monthly Contraceptive Injection and need elective surgery, need to stay in bed for a prolonged illness, or have recently had a baby, you may be at risk of developing blood clots. You should consult your doctor about stopping hormonal contraceptives three to four weeks before surgery and not taking hormonal contraceptives for two weeks after surgery or during bed rest. You should also not take hormonal contraceptives soon after delivery of a baby. It is advisable to wait for at least four weeks after delivery before using hormonal contraceptives such as LUNELLE™ Monthly Contraceptive Injection. (See also the section on Breast Feeding in GENERAL PRECAUTIONS.)

Hormonal contraceptives may also increase the tendency to develop strokes (stoppage or rupture of blood vessels in the brain) and angina pectoris and heart attacks (blockage of blood vessels in the heart). Any of these conditions can cause death or disability.

Smoking greatly increases the possibility of developing blood clots or suffering heart attacks and strokes. Furthermore, smoking and the use of hormonal contraceptives greatly increase the chances of developing and dying of heart disease, particularly if you are over 35 years of age.

2. Gallbladder disease

Hormonal contraceptive users probably have a greater risk than non-users of having gallbladder disease.

3. Liver tumors

In rare cases, hormonal contraceptives can cause benign but dangerous liver tumors. These benign liver tumors can rupture and cause fatal internal bleeding. In addition, a possible but not definite association has been found with hormonal contraceptives and liver cancers in two studies, in which a few women who developed these very rare cancers were found to have used hormonal contraceptives for long

---

Percentage of Women Experiencing an Unintended Pregnancy During the First Year of Typical Use and the First Year of Perfect Use of Contraception and the Percentage Continuing Use at the End of the First Year: United States

Method	% of Women Experiencing an Unintended Pregnancy within the First Year of Use		% of Women Continuing Use at 1 Year[3]
	Typical Use[1]	Perfect Use[2]	
Chance[4]	85	85	
Spermicides[5]	26	6	40
Periodic Abstinence	25		63
Calendar		9	
Ovulation Method		3	
Symptothermal[6]		2	
Post-ovulation		1	
Cap[7]			
Parous Women	40	26	42
Nulliparous Women	20	9	56
Sponge			
Parous Women	40	20	42
Nulliparous Women	20	9	56
Diaphragm[7]	20	6	56
Withdrawal	19	4	
Condom[8]			
Female (Reality)	21	5	56
Male	14	3	61
Pill	5		71
Progestin only		0.5	
Combined		0.1	
IUD			
Progesterone T	2.0	1.5	81
Copper T 380A	0.8	0.6	78
LNg 20	0.1	0.1	81
Depo-Provera	0.3	0.3	70
Norplant and			
Norplant-2	0.05	0.05	88
Female Sterilization	0.5	0.5	100
Male Sterilization	0.15	0.10	100

Emergency Contraceptive Pills: Treatment initiated within 72 hours after unprotected intercourse reduces the risk of pregnancy by at least 75%.[9]

Lactation Amenorrhea Method: LAM is a highly effective, temporary method of contraception.[10]

Adapted from Hatcher et al., 1998.

[1] Among *typical* couples who initiate use of a method (not necessarily for the first time), the percentage who experience an accidental pregnancy during the first year if they do not stop use for any other reason.

[2] Among couples who initiate use of a method (not necessarily for the first time) and who use it *perfectly* (both consistently and correctly), the percentage who experience an accidental pregnancy during the first year if they do not stop use for any other reason.

[3] Among couples attempting to avoid pregnancy, the percentage who continue to use a method for 1 year.

[4] The percentages becoming pregnant in columns (2) and (3) are based on data from populations where contraception is not used and from women who cease using contraception in order to become pregnant. Among such populations, about 89% become pregnant within 1 year. This estimate was lowered slightly (to 85%) to represent the percentages who would become pregnant within 1 year among women now relying on reversible methods of contraception if they abandoned contraception altogether.

[5] Foams, creams, gels, vaginal suppositories, and vaginal film.

[6] Cervical mucus (ovulation) method supplemented by calendar in the pre-ovulatory and basal body temperature in the post-ovulatory phases.

[7] With spermicidal cream or jelly.

[8] Without spermicides.

[9] The treatment schedule is one dose within 72 hours after unprotected intercourse, and a second dose 12 hours after the first dose. The Food and Drug Administration has declared the following brands of oral contraceptives to be safe and effective for emergency contraception: Ovral (1 dose is 2 white pills), Alesse (1 dose is 5 pink pills), Nordette or Levlen (1 dose is 4 light-orange pills), Lo/Ovral (1 dose is 4 white pills), Triphasil or Tri-Levlen (1 dose is 4 yellow pills).

[10] However, to maintain effective protection against pregnancy, another method of contraception must be used as soon as menstruation resumes, the frequency or duration of breastfeeds is reduced, bottle feeds are introduced, or the baby reaches 6 months of age.

periods. However, liver cancers are extremely rare. The chance of developing liver cancer from using hormonal contraceptives is thus even rarer.

4. Cancer of the reproductive organs and breasts

There is, at present, no confirmed evidence that oral hormonal contraceptives increase the risk of cancer of the reproductive organs in human studies. Studies to date of women taking the pill have reported conflicting findings on whether pill use increases the risk of developing cancer of the breast. Most of the studies on breast cancer and pill use have found no overall increase in the risk of developing breast cancer, although some studies have reported an increased risk of developing breast cancer in certain groups of women.

Some studies have found an increase in the incidence of cancer of the cervix in women who use oral hormonal contraceptives. However, this finding may be related to factors other than the use of oral hormonal contraceptives.

Studies have found that women who used injectable hormonal contraceptives (Depo-Provera Contraceptive Injection) had no increased overall risk of developing cancer of the breast, ovary, uterus, or cervix. However, women under 35 years of age whose first exposure to Depo-Provera Contraceptive Injection was within the previous 4 to 5 years may have a slightly increased risk of developing breast cancer similar to that seen with oral contraceptives.

Women who use hormonal contraceptives and have a strong family history of breast cancer or who have breast nodules or abnormal mammogram should be closely followed by their doctors.

5. Changes in bone mineral density

Use of injectable hormonal contraceptives containing the progesterone-type hormone found in LUNELLE™ Monthly Contraceptive Injection may be associated with a decrease in the amount of mineral stored in your bones. This could increase your risk of developing bone fractures. The rate of bone mineral loss is greatest in the early years of use of this type of contraceptive, but after that, it begins to resemble the normal rate of age-related bone mineral loss.

Formal studies on the effect of bone mineral density changes in women receiving LUNELLE™ Monthly Contraceptive Injection have not been conducted.

6. Allergic reactions

Severe allergic reactions have been reported in some women using injectable hormonal contraceptives containing the progesterone-type hormone found in LUNELLE™ Monthly Contraceptive Injection. Allergic reactions occurring in women using LUNELLE™ Monthly Contraceptive Injection have been mainly skin reactions, and not respiratory in nature. Serious allergic reactions require emergency medical treatment.

ESTIMATED RISK OF DEATH FROM A BIRTH CONTROL METHOD OR PREGNANCY

All methods of birth control and pregnancy are associated with a risk of developing certain diseases that may lead to disability or death. An estimate of the number of deaths associated with different methods of birth control and pregnancy has been calculated and is shown in the following table.

[See table below]

In the above table, the risk of death from any birth control method is less than the risk of childbirth, except for oral hormonal contraceptive users over the age of 35 who smoke and oral hormonal contraceptive users over the age of 40 even if they do not smoke. It can be seen in the table that for women aged 15 to 39, the risk of death was highest with pregnancy (7–26 deaths per 100,000 women, depending on age). Among oral hormonal contraceptive users who do not smoke, the risk of death is always lower than that associated with pregnancy for any age group, although over the age of 40, the risk increases to 32 deaths per 100,000 women, compared to 28 associated with pregnancy at that age. However, for oral hormonal contraceptive users who smoke and are over the age of 35, the estimated number of deaths exceeds those for other methods of birth control. If a woman is over the age of 40 and smokes, her estimated risk of death is four times higher (117/100,000 women) than the estimated risk associated with pregnancy (28/100,000 women) in that age group.

An Advisory Committee of the FDA discussed this issue in 1989 and recommended that the benefits of oral contraceptive use by healthy, non-smoking women over 40 years of age may outweigh the possible risks. However, women of all ages are cautioned to use the lowest dose oral contraceptive that is effective, and are strongly advised not to smoke.

WARNING SIGNALS

If any of these adverse effects occur while you are taking LUNELLE™ Monthly Contraceptive Injection, call your doctor immediately:

- Sharp chest pain, coughing of blood, or sudden shortness of breath (indicating a possible clot in the lung)
- Pain in the calf (indicating a possible clot in the leg)
- Crushing chest pain or heaviness in the chest (indicating a possible heart attack)
- Sudden severe headache or vomiting, dizziness or fainting, disturbances of vision or speech, weakness, or numbness in an arm or leg (indicating a possible stroke)
- Sudden partial or complete loss of vision (indicating a possible clot in the eye)
- Breast lumps (indicating possible breast cancer or fibrocystic disease of the breast; ask your doctor or health care provider to show you how to examine your breasts)
- Severe pain or tenderness in the abdominal area (indicating a possibly ruptured liver tumor, ovarian cyst, or pregnancy outside the uterus)
- Difficulty in sleeping, weakness, lack of energy, fatigue, or change in mood (possibly indicating severe depression)
- Jaundice or a yellowing of the skin or eyeballs, accompanied frequently by fever, fatigue, loss of appetitie, dark-colored urine, or light-colored bowel movements (indicating possible liver problems)
- Persistent pain, pus, or bleeding at the injection site
- Unusually heavy vaginal bleeding

SIDE EFFECTS OF LUNELLE™ MONTHLY CONTRACEPTIVE INJECTION

1. Vaginal bleeding

Most women using LUNELLE™ Monthly Contraceptive Injection experience alteration of menstrual bleeding. Bleeding patterns may vary from a single monthly bleed to no bleeding at all or slight staining between menstrual periods to frequent, prolonged, and/or unpredictable bleeding. In any given injection interval, approximately 50% of women using LUNELLE™ Monthly Contraceptive Injection experience withdrawal bleeding that begins 20–25 days after the injection. Withdrawal bleeding lasts more than 7 days in 42% of women during the first month of use and in 29% of women at the end of one year of use. In any given injection interval, approximately 15% of women may have no bleeding at all and 10% may experience bleeding or spotting at various times in the cycle. Irregular bleeding often occurs during the first few months of LUNELLE™ Monthly Contraceptive Injection use and may persist with continued use in up to one third of women. Your menstrual blood flow may be heavier or lighter, and there may be no bleeding, fewer days of bleeding, or more days of bleeding than what you have previously experienced. Such bleeding usually does not indicate any serious problems. If an altered bleeding pattern persists or the bleeding is severe, discuss it with your health care provider. There is also a small risk that (painful) cramps may be associated with bleeding.

2. Weight change

Weight gain is a common side effect in women using LUNELLE™ Monthly Contraceptive Injection. The average expected weight gain is 4 pounds in the first year of use. Some women gain more than 10 to 20 pounds in the first year. Women have gained as much as 49 pounds or lost as much as 48 pounds in one year of use. Clinical trials showed wide variability in individual weight change with an increasing percentage of LUNELLE™ Monthly Contraceptive Injection users experiencing weight change in excess of 10 to 20 pounds with continued treatment.

3. Contact lenses

If you wear contact lenses and notice a change in vision or an inability to wear your lenses, contact your doctor or health care provider.

4. Fluid retention

Hormonal contraceptives may cause edema (fluid retention) with swelling of the fingers or ankles and may raise your blood pressure. If you experience fluid retention, contact your doctor or health care provider.

5. Other side effects

Other side effects may include breast pain or tenderness, acne, change in appetite, nausea, headache, nervousness, depression, mood changes, changes in sexual desire, dizziness, loss of scalp hair, rash, and vaginal infections.

If any of these side effects bother you, call your health care provider.

GENERAL PRECAUTIONS

1. Missed periods and use of hormonal contraceptives before or during early pregnancy.

You may not menstruate regularly after you receive an injection of LUNELLE™ Monthly Contraceptive Injection. If you have received your injections regularly and miss one menstrual period, be sure to inform your health care provider. The risk of unexpected pregnancy for women receiving injectable contraceptives as scheduled is very low. If you have not received your injections as scheduled and missed a menstrual period, or if you missed two consecutive menstrual periods, you may be pregnant. Check with your health care provider immediately to determine whether you are pregnant. Do not continue the injections until you are sure you are not pregnant, but use another method of contraception.

There is no conclusive evidence that oral hormonal contraceptive use is associated with an increase in birth defects, when taken inadvertently during early pregnancy. Nevertheless, hormonal contraceptives should not be used during pregnancy.

With Depo-Provera Contraceptive Injection, there have been reports of an increased risk of low birth weight and neonatal infant death or other health problems in infants conceived close to the time of injection. However, these pregnancies are uncommon. Children exposed in the womb to one of the hormones found in LUNELLE™ Monthly Contraceptive Injection (MPA), and followed to adolescence, showed no evidence of any adverse effects on their health including their physical, mental, sexual or social development.

If you think you may have become pregnant while using LUNELLE™ Monthly Contraceptive Injection, see your health care provider as soon as possible. You should check with your health care provider about risks to your unborn child from any medication taken during pregnancy.

2. While breast feeding

If you are breast feeding, consult your health care provider before starting hormonal contraceptives, including LUNELLE™ Monthly Contraceptive Injection. Some of the drugs in hormonal contraceptives are passed on to the child in breast milk. A few adverse effects on the child have been reported, including yellowing of the skin (jaundice) and breast enlargement. In addition, hormonal contraceptives may decrease the amount and quality of your milk. To insure the best quantity and quality of your breast milk, you should wait until 6 weeks after childbirth before you start using LUNELLE™ Monthly Contraceptive Injection. If possible, do not use hormonal contraceptives while breast feeding.

Breast feeding provides only partial protection from becoming pregnant and this partial protection decreases significantly as you breast feed for longer periods of time. You should use another method of contraception while breast feeding and consider starting hormonal contraceptives only after you have weaned your child completely.

3. Laboratory tests

If you are scheduled for any laboratory tests, tell your doctor you are taking a hormonal contraceptive. Certain blood tests may be affected by hormonal contraceptives.

4. Drug interactions

Certain drugs may interact with hormonal contraceptives to make them less effective in preventing pregnancy or cause a change in bleeding patterns. Such drugs include aminoglutethimide, rifampin, drugs used for epilepsy such as barbiturates (for example, phenobarbital), carbamazepine, and phenytoin (Dilantin is one brand of this drug), phenylbutazone (Butazolidin is one brand), herbal products containing St. John's Wort (hypericum perforatum), and possible certain antibiotics. You may need to use an additional contraception method when you take drugs which can make hormonal contraceptives less effective. Drug interaction studies have not been conducted with LUNELLE™ Monthly Contraceptive Injection.

5. Sexually transmitted diseases

This product (like all hormonal contraceptives) is intended to prevent pregnancy. It does not protect against transmission of HIV (AIDS) and other sexually transmitted diseases such as chlamydia, genital herpes, genital warts, gonorrhea, hepatitis B, and syphilis.

6. Weight change

LUNELLE™ Monthly Contraceptive Injection may cause weight gain of more than 10 pounds.

WHEN DO I GET MY LUNELLE™ MONTHLY CONTRACEPTIVE INJECTION?

LUNELLE™ Monthly Contraceptive Injection can only be effective if you receive your injections at the proper times.

First Injection

- Within the first 5 days of the start of your normal menstrual period.
- If you are presently using another type of birth control, your health care provider will decide the best time for you to start LUNELLE™ Monthly Contraceptive Injection. This will help make sure you have continued contraceptive coverage.

Continued on next page

Annual Number of Birth-Related or Method-Related Deaths Associated with Control of Fertility per 100,000 Non-sterile Women, by Fertility Control Method According to Age

Method of Control & Outcome	Range of Ages (years)					
	15–19	20–24	25–29	30–34	35–39	40–44
No fertility control*	7.0	7.4	9.1	14.8	25.7	28.2
Oral hormonal contraceptives** (non-smoker)	0.3	0.5	0.9	1.9	13.8	31.6
Oral hormonal contraceptives** (smoker)	2.2	3.4	6.6	13.5	51.1	117.2
IUD**	0.8	0.8	1.0	1.0	1.4	1.4
Condom*	1.1	1.6	0.7	0.2	0.3	0.4
Diaphragm/spermicide*	1.9	1.2	1.2	1.3	2.2	2.8
Periodic abstinence	2.5	1.6	1.6	1.7	2.9	3.6

* Deaths are birth-related
**Deaths are method-related

Lunelle—Cont.

- If you have recently been pregnant or had a baby, discuss with your health care provider the best time for you to start LUNELLE™ Monthly Contraceptive Injection.

Next Injections

- LUNELLE™ Monthly Contraceptive Injection must be given monthly, every 28 to 30 days and no later than 33 days after your last injection.
  The time for your next injection is determined by the number of days since your previous injection, and not by the timing or amount of your menstrual bleeding.
  Even if you do not have any menstrual bleeding, you should still return once a month for your injection of LUNELLE™ Monthly Contraceptive Injection.
- It is important that you receive each of your next injections at the right time. If you cannot receive your injection on time, contact your health care provider to receive an earlier injection.

What Happens if I Miss an Injection or Wait Longer than 33 Days Between Injections?

- You could become pregnant if you miss your injection or wait longer than 33 days between injections. The more days you wait, the greater the risk that you could become pregnant.
- Ask your health care provider to recommend another type of birth control (such as condoms or a spermicide) for you to use.
- Talk with your health care provider to find out when you should receive your next injection of LUNELLE™ Monthly Contraceptive Injection.
- Your health care provider may do a test to make sure you are not pregnant before giving you your next injection of LUNELLE™ Monthly Contraceptive Injection.

Pregnancy Due to Failure with LUNELLE™ Monthly Contraceptive Injection

The incidence of failure with LUNELLE™ Monthly Contraceptive Injection in pregnancy is less than 1 percent (i.e., one pregnancy per 100 women per year) if given every month as directed. If you think that you may be pregnant, be sure to call your health care provider.

What If I Want to Become Pregnant?

You will need to stop your monthly injections of LUNELLE™ Monthly Contraceptive Injection. Most women begin to produce eggs again (and could become pregnant) about two to three months after their last injection.

There may be some delay in becoming pregnant after you stop using hormonal contraceptives, including LUNELLE™ Monthly Contraceptive Injection, especially if you had irregular menstrual cycles before you started using hormonal contraceptives. There does not appear to be any increase in birth defects in newborn babies when pregnancy occurs soon after stopping hormonal contraceptives.

OVERDOSAGE

Serious ill effects have not been reported following ingestion of large doses of oral hormonal contraceptives by young children. Overdosage may cause nausea and withdrawal bleeding in females. In case of overdosage, contact your health care provider or pharmacist.

OTHER INFORMATION

Your health care provider will take a medical and family history before prescribing hormonal contraceptives. You should receive yearly physical examinations by your health care provider. Be sure to inform your health care provider if there is a family history of any of the conditions listed previously in this leaflet. Be sure to keep all appointments with your health care provider, because this is a time to determine if there are early signs of side effects of hormonal contraceptive use. If you want more information about hormonal contraceptives, ask your health care provider or pharmacist for a more technical leaflet called the Prescribing Information that you may wish to read.

Each 0.5 mL dose of LUNELLE™ Monthly Contraceptive Injection contains:

Active Ingredients: medroxyprogesterone acetate (25 mg), estradiol cypionate (5 mg)

Inactive ingredients: methylparaben (0.9 mg), polyethylene glycol (14.28 mg), polysorbate 80 (0.95 mg), propylparaben (0.1 mg), sodium chloride (4.28 mg), sterile water for injection

Manufactured by:
Pharmacia & Upjohn Company
Kalamazoo, MI 49001, USA
October 2000

817 821 000
692804
3484-04

To keep your **PDR** up to date throughout the year, note these revisions on the corresponding pages of the annual volume. Simply write **"See Supplement A"** next to the product heading.

Roche Pharmaceuticals

Roche Laboratories Inc.
340 Kingsland Street
Nutley, NJ 07110-1199

Please note that there has been a change in the Medical Needs Program toll-free telephone number, which appears on page 2721 of the 2001 PDR.

For Medical Information
(Including routine inquiries, adverse drug events and product complaints)
Call: (800) 526-6367
In Emergencies: 24-hour service
For the Medical Needs Program:
Call: (800) 285-4484
Write: Professional Product Information

KYTRIL® ℞
(granisetron hydrochloride)
INJECTION

DESCRIPTION

KYTRIL (granisetron hydrochloride) Injection is an antinauseant and antiemetic agent. Chemically it is *endo*-N-(9-methyl-9-azabicyclo [3.3.1] non-3-yl)-1-methyl-1H-indazole-3-carboxamide hydrochloride with a molecular weight of 348.9 (312.4 free base). Its empirical formula is $C_{18}H_{24}N_4O \bullet HCl$, while its chemical structure is:

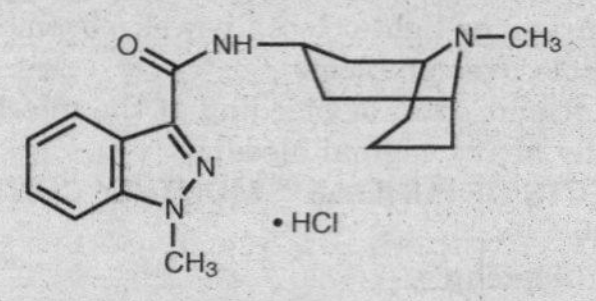

granisetron hydrochloride

Granisetron hydrochloride is a white to off-white solid that is readily soluble in water and normal saline at 20°C. KYTRIL Injection is a clear, colorless, sterile, nonpyrogenic, aqueous solution for intravenous administration.

KYTRIL is available in 1 mL single-dose and 4 mL multi-dose vials.

Single-Dose Vials: Each 1 mL of preservative-free aqueous solution contains 1.12 mg granisetron hydrochloride equivalent to granisetron, 1 mg and sodium chloride, 9 mg. The solution's pH ranges from 4.7 to 7.3.

Multi-Dose Vials: Each 1 mL contains 1.12 mg granisetron hydrochloride equivalent to granisetron, 1 mg; sodium chloride, 9 mg; citric acid, 2 mg; benzyl alcohol, 10 mg, as a preservative. The solution's pH ranges from 4.0 to 6.0.

CLINICAL PHARMACOLOGY

Granisetron is a selective 5-hydroxytryptamine$_3$ (5-HT$_3$) receptor antagonist with little or no affinity for other serotonin receptors, including 5-HT$_1$; 5-HT$_{1A}$; 5-HT$_{1B/C}$; 5-HT$_2$; for alpha$_1$-, alpha$_2$- or beta-adrenoreceptors; for dopamine-D$_2$; or for histamine-H$_1$; benzodiazepine; picrotoxin, or opioid receptors.

Serotonin receptors of the 5-HT$_3$ type are located peripherally on vagal nerve terminals and centrally in the chemoreceptor trigger zone of the area postrema. During chemotherapy-induced vomiting, mucosal enterochromaffin cells release serotonin, which stimulates 5-HT$_3$ receptors. This evokes vagal afferent discharge, inducing vomiting. Animal studies demonstrate that, in binding to 5-HT$_3$ receptors, granisetron blocks serotonin stimulation and subsequent vomiting after emetogenic stimuli such as cisplatin. In the ferret animal model, a single granisetron injection prevented vomiting due to high-dose cisplatin or arrested vomiting within 5 to 30 seconds.

In most human studies, granisetron has had little effect on blood pressure, heart rate or ECG. No evidence of an effect on plasma prolactin or aldosterone concentrations has been found in other studies.

KYTRIL Injection exhibited no effect on oro-cecal transit time in normal volunteers given a single intravenous infusion of 50 mcg/kg or 200 mcg/kg. Single and multiple oral doses slowed colonic transit in normal volunteers.

Pharmacokinetics: In adult cancer patients undergoing chemotherapy and in volunteers, infusion of a single 40 mcg/kg dose of KYTRIL Injection produced the following mean pharmacokinetic data:

[See table 1 below]

There was high inter and intrasubject variability noted in these studies. No difference in mean AUC was found between males and females, although males had a higher C_{max} generally.

Granisetron metabolism involves N-demethylation and aromatic ring oxidation followed by conjugation. Animal studies suggest that some of the metabolites may also have 5-HT$_3$ receptor antagonist activity.

Clearance is predominantly by hepatic metabolism. In normal volunteers, approximately 12% of the administered dose is eliminated unchanged in the urine in 48 hours. The remainder of the dose is excreted as metabolites, 49% in the urine and 34% in the feces.

In vitro liver microsomal studies show that granisetron's major route of metabolism is inhibited by ketoconazole, suggestive of metabolism mediated by the cytochrome P-450 3A subfamily.

Plasma protein binding is approximately 65% and granisetron distributes freely between plasma and red blood cells.

Elderly: The ranges of the pharmacokinetic parameters in elderly volunteers (mean age 71 years), given a single 40 mcg/kg intravenous dose of KYTRIL Injection, were generally similar to those in younger healthy volunteers; mean values were lower for clearance and longer for half-life in the elderly (see Table 1).

Pediatric Patients: A pharmacokinetic study in pediatric cancer patients (2 to 16 years of age), given a single 40 mcg/kg intravenous dose of KYTRIL Injection, showed that volume of distribution and total clearance increased with age. No relationship with age was observed for peak plasma concentration or terminal phase plasma half-life. When volume of distribution and total clearance are adjusted for body weight, the pharmacokinetics of granisetron are similar in pediatric and adult cancer patients.

Renal Failure Patients: Total clearance of granisetron was not affected in patients with severe renal failure who received a single 40 mcg/kg intravenous dose of KYTRIL Injection.

Hepatically Impaired Patients: A pharmacokinetic study in patients with hepatic impairment due to neoplastic liver involvement showed that total clearance was approximately halved compared to patients without hepatic impairment. Given the wide variability in pharmacokinetic parameters noted in patients and the good tolerance of doses well above the recommended 10 mcg/kg dose, dosage adjustment in patients with possible hepatic functional impairment is not necessary.

CLINICAL TRIALS

KYTRIL Injection has been shown to prevent nausea and vomiting associated with single-day and repeat cycle cancer chemotherapy.

Single-Day Chemotherapy: Cisplatin-Based Chemotherapy: In a double-blind, placebo-controlled study in 28 cancer patients, KYTRIL Injection, administered as a single intravenous infusion of 40 mcg/kg, was significantly more effective than placebo in preventing nausea and vomiting induced by cisplatin chemotherapy (see Table 2).

[See table 2 at top of next page]

KYTRIL Injection was also evaluated in a randomized dose response study of cancer patients receiving cisplatin ≥ 75 mg/m². Additional chemotherapeutic agents included: anthracyclines, carboplatin, cytostatic antibiotics, folic acid derivatives, methylhydrazine, nitrogen mustard analogs, podophyllotoxin derivatives, pyrimidine analogs and vinca alkaloids. KYTRIL Injection doses of 10 and 40 mcg/kg were superior to 2 mcg/kg in preventing cisplatin-induced nausea and vomiting, but 40 mcg/kg was not significantly superior to 10 mcg/kg (see Table 3).

[See table 3 at top of next page]

KYTRIL (granisetron hydrochloride) Injection was also evaluated in a double-blind, randomized dose response study of 353 patients stratified for high (≥ 80 to 120 mg/m²) or low (50 to 79 mg/m²) cisplatin dose. Response rates of patients for both cisplatin strata are given in Table 4.

[See table 4 at middle of next page]

Table 1. Pharmacokinetic Parameters in Adult Cancer Patients Undergoing Chemotherapy and in Volunteers, Following a Single Intravenous 40 mcg/kg Dose of KYTRIL (granisetron hydrochloride) Injection

	Peak Plasma Concentration (ng/mL)	Terminal Phase Plasma Half-Life (h)	Total Clearance (L/h/kg)	Volume of Distribution (L/kg)
Cancer Patients				
Mean	63.8*	8.95*	0.38*	3.07*
Range	18.0 to 176	0.90 to 31.1	0.14 to 1.54	0.85 to 10.4
Volunteers				
21 to 42 years				
Mean	64.3†	4.91†	0.79†	3.04†
Range	11.2 to 182	0.88 to 15.2	0.20 to 2.56	1.68 to 6.13
65 to 81 years				
Mean	57.0†	7.69†	0.44†	3.97†
Range	14.6 to 153	2.65 to 17.7	0.17 to 1.06	1.75 to 7.01

*5-minute infusion.
†3-minute infusion.

Table 2. Prevention of Chemotherapy-Induced Nausea and Vomiting—Single-Day Cisplatin Therapy[1]

	KYTRIL Injection	Placebo	P-Value
Number of Patients	14	14	
Response Over 24 Hours			
Complete Response[2]	93%	7%	<0.001
No Vomiting	93%	14%	<0.001
No More Than Mild Nausea	93%	7%	<0.001

1. Cisplatin administration began within 10 minutes of KYTRIL Injection infusion and continued for 1.5 to 3.0 hours. Mean cisplatin dose was 86 mg/m² in the KYTRIL Injection group and 80 mg/m² in the placebo group.
2. No vomiting and no moderate or severe nausea.

Table 3. Prevention of Chemotherapy-Induced Nausea and Vomiting—Single-Day High-Dose Cisplatin Therapy[1]

	KYTRIL Injection (mcg/kg)			P-Value (vs. 2 mcg/kg)	
	2	10	40	10	40
Number of Patients	52	52	53		
Response Over 24 Hours					
Complete Response[2]	31%	62%	68%	<0.002	<0.001
No Vomiting	38%	65%	74%	<0.001	<0.001
No More Than Mild Nausea	58%	75%	79%	NS	0.007

1. Cisplatin administration began within 10 minutes of KYTRIL Injection infusion and continued for 2.6 hours (mean). Mean cisplatin doses were 96 to 99 mg/m².
2. No vomiting and no moderate or severe nausea.

Table 4. Prevention of Chemotherapy-Induced Nausea and Vomiting—Single-Day High-Dose and Low-Dose Cisplatin Therapy[1]

	KYTRIL Injection (mcg/kg)				P-Value (vs. 5 mcg/kg)		
	5	10	20	40	10	20	40
High-Dose Cisplatin							
Number of Patients	40	49	48	47			
Response Over 24 Hours							
Complete Response[2]	18%	41%	40%	47%	0.018	0.025	0.004
No Vomiting	28%	47%	44%	53%	NS	NS	0.016
No Nausea	15%	35%	38%	43%	0.036	0.019	0.005
Low-Dose Cisplatin							
Number of Patients	42	41	40	46			
Response Over 24 Hours							
Complete Response[2]	29%	56%	58%	41%	0.012	0.009	NS
No Vomiting	36%	63%	65%	43%	0.012	0.008	NS
No Nausea	29%	56%	38%	33%	0.012	NS	NS

1. Cisplatin administration began within 10 minutes of KYTRIL Injection infusion and continued for 2 hours (mean). Mean cisplatin doses were 64 and 98 mg/m² for low and high strata.
2. No vomiting and no use of rescue antiemetic.

Table 5. Prevention of Chemotherapy-Induced Nausea and Vomiting—Single-Day Moderately Emetogenic Chemotherapy

	KYTRIL Injection	Chlorpromazine[1]	P-Value
Number of Patients	133	133	
Response Over 24 Hours			
Complete Response[2]	68%	47%	<0.001
No Vomiting	73%	53%	<0.001
No More Than Mild Nausea	77%	59%	<0.001

1. Patients also received dexamethasone, 12 mg.
2. No vomiting and no moderate or severe nausea.

Table 6. Prevention of Chemotherapy-Induced Nausea and Vomiting in Pediatric Patients

	KYTRIL Injection Dose (mcg/kg)		
	10	20	40
Number of Patients	29	26	25
Median Number of Vomiting Episodes	2	3	1
Complete Response Over 24 Hours[1]	21%	31%	32%

1. No vomiting and no moderate or severe nausea.

For both the low and high cisplatin strata, the 10, 20 and 40 mcg/kg doses were more effective than the 5 mcg/kg dose in preventing nausea and vomiting within 24 hours of chemotherapy administration. The 10 mcg/kg dose was at least as effective as the higher doses.

Moderately Emetogenic Chemotherapy: KYTRIL Injection, 40 mcg/kg, was compared with the combination of chlorpromazine (50 to 200 mg/24 hours) and dexamethasone (12 mg) in patients treated with moderately emetogenic chemotherapy, including primarily carboplatin >300 mg/m², cisplatin 20 to 50 mg/m² and cyclophosphamide >600 mg/m². KYTRIL Injection was superior to the chlorpromazine regimen in preventing nausea and vomiting (see Table 5).
[See table 5 above]
In other studies of moderately emetogenic chemotherapy, no significant difference in efficacy was found between KYTRIL doses of 40 mcg/kg and 160 mcg/kg doses.

Repeat-Cycle Chemotherapy: In an uncontrolled trial, 512 cancer patients received KYTRIL Injection, 40 mcg/kg, prophylactically, for two cycles of chemotherapy, 224 patients received it for at least four cycles and 108 patients received it for at least six cycles. KYTRIL Injection efficacy remained relatively constant over the first six repeat cycles, with complete response rates (no vomiting and no moderate or severe nausea in 24 hours) of 60% to 69%. No patients were studied for more than 15 cycles.

Pediatric Studies: A randomized double-blind study evaluated the 24-hour response of 80 pediatric cancer patients (age 2 to 16 years) to KYTRIL Injection 10, 20 or 40 mcg/kg. Patients were treated with cisplatin ≥ 60 mg/m², cytarabine ≥ 3 g/m², cyclophosphamide ≥ 1 g/m² or nitrogen mustard ≥ 6 mg/m² (see Table 6).
[See table 6 above]
A second pediatric study compared KYTRIL Injection 20 mcg/kg to chlorpromazine plus dexamethasone in 88 pa-

tients treated with ifosfamide ≥ 3 g/m²/day for two or three days. KYTRIL Injection was administered on each day of ifosfamide treatment. At 24 hours, 22% of KYTRIL Injection patients achieved complete response (no vomiting and no moderate or severe nausea in 24 hours) compared with 10% on the chlorpromazine regimen. The median number of vomiting episodes with KYTRIL Injection was 1.5; with chlorpromazine it was 7.0.

INDICATIONS AND USAGE

KYTRIL (granisetron hydrochloride) Injection is indicated for the prevention of nausea and vomiting associated with initial and repeat courses of emetogenic cancer therapy, including high-dose cisplatin.

CONTRAINDICATIONS

KYTRIL Injection is contraindicated in patients with known hypersensitivity to the drug or to any of its components.

PRECAUTIONS

Drug Interactions: Granisetron does not induce or inhibit the cytochrome P-450 drug-metabolizing enzyme system. There have been no definitive drug-drug interaction studies to examine pharmacokinetic or pharmacodynamic interaction with other drugs, but in humans, KYTRIL Injection has been safely administered with drugs representing benzodiazepines, neuroleptics and anti-ulcer medications commonly prescribed with antiemetic treatments. KYTRIL Injection also does not appear to interact with emetogenic cancer chemotherapies. Because granisetron is metabolized by hepatic cytochrome P-450 drug-metabolizing enzymes, inducers or inhibitors of these enzymes may change the clearance and, hence, the half-life of granisetron.

Carcinogenesis, Mutagenesis, Impairment of Fertility: In a 24-month carcinogenicity study, rats were treated orally with granisetron 1, 5 or 50 mg/kg/day (6, 30 or 300 mg/m²/day). The 50 mg/kg/day dose was reduced to 25 mg/kg/day (150 mg/m²/day) during week 59 due to toxicity. For a 50 kg person of average height (1.46 m² body surface area), these doses represent 16, 81 and 405 times the recommended clinical dose (0.37 mg/m², iv) on a body surface area basis. There was a statistically significant increase in the incidence of hepatocellular carcinomas and adenomas in males treated with 5 mg/kg/day (30 mg/m²/day, 81 times the recommended human dose based on body surface area) and above, and in females treated with 25 mg/kg/day (150 mg/m²/day, 405 times the recommended human dose based on body surface area). No increase in liver tumors was observed at a dose of 1 mg/kg/day (6 mg/m²/day, 16 times the recommended human dose based on body surface area) in males and 5 mg/kg/day (30 mg/m²/day, 81 times the recommended human dose based on body surface area) in females. In a 12-month oral toxicity study, treatment with granisetron 100 mg/kg/day (600 mg/m²/day, 1622 times the recommended human dose based on body surface area) produced hepatocellular adenomas in male and female rats while no such tumors were found in the control rats. A 24-month mouse carcinogenicity study of granisetron did not show a statistically significant increase in tumor incidence, but the study was not conclusive.

Because of the tumor findings in rat studies, KYTRIL (granisetron hydrochloride) Injection should be prescribed only at the dose and for the indication recommended (see INDICATIONS AND USAGE and DOSAGE AND ADMINISTRATION).

Granisetron was not mutagenic in in vitro Ames test and mouse lymphoma cell forward mutation assay, and in vivo mouse micronucleus test and in vitro and ex vivo rat hepatocyte UDS assays. It, however, produced a significant increase in UDS in HeLa cells in vitro and a significant increased incidence of cells with polyploidy in an in vitro human lymphocyte chromosomal aberration test.

Granisetron at subcutaneous doses up to 6 mg/kg/day (36 mg/m²/day, 97 times the recommended human dose based on body surface area) was found to have no effect on fertility and reproductive performance of male and female rats.

Pregnancy: Teratogenic Effects. Pregnancy Category B. Reproduction studies have been performed in pregnant rats at intravenous doses up to 9 mg/kg/day (54 mg/m²/day, 146 times the recommended human dose based on body surface area) and pregnant rabbits at intravenous doses up to 3 mg/kg/day (35.4 mg/m²/day, 96 times the recommended human dose based on body surface area) and have revealed no evidence of impaired fertility or harm to the fetus due to granisetron. There are, however, no adequate and well-controlled studies in pregnant women. Because animal reproduction studies are not always predictive of human response, this drug should be used during pregnancy only if clearly needed.

Nursing Mothers: It is not known whether granisetron is excreted in human milk. Because many drugs are excreted in human milk, caution should be exercised when KYTRIL Injection is administered to a nursing woman.

Pediatric Use: See DOSAGE AND ADMINISTRATION for use in children 2 to 16 years of age. Safety and effectiveness in children under 2 years of age have not been established.

Geriatric Use: During clinical trials, 713 patients 65 years of age or older received KYTRIL (granisetron HCl) Injection. Effectiveness and safety were similar in patients of various ages.

ADVERSE REACTIONS

The following have been reported during controlled clinical trials or in the routine management of patients. The per-

Continued on next page

Kytril Injection—Cont.

centage figures are based on clinical trial experience only. Table 7 gives the comparative frequencies of the five most commonly reported adverse events (≥ 3%) in patients receiving KYTRIL Injection, in single-day chemotherapy trials. These patients received chemotherapy, primarily cisplatin, and intravenous fluids during the 24-hour period following KYTRIL Injection administration. Events were generally recorded over seven days post-KYTRIL Injection administration. In the absence of a placebo group, there is uncertainty as to how many of these events should be attributed to KYTRIL, except for headache, which was clearly more frequent than in comparison groups.

Table 7. Principal Adverse Events in Clinical Trials—Single-Day Chemotherapy

	Percent of Patients with Event	
	KYTRIL Injection 40 mcg/kg (n=1268)	Comparator[1] (n=422)
Headache	14%	6%
Asthenia	5%	6%
Somnolence	4%	15%
Diarrhea	4%	6%
Constipation	3%	3%

1. Metoclopramide/dexamethasone and phenothiazines/dexamethasone.

In over 3,000 patients receiving KYTRIL Injection (2 to 160 mcg/kg) in single-day and multiple-day clinical trials with emetogenic cancer therapies, adverse events, other than those in Table 7, were observed; attribution of many of these events to KYTRIL is uncertain.

Hepatic: In comparative trials, mainly with cisplatin regimens, elevations of AST and ALT (>2 times the upper limit of normal) following administration of KYTRIL Injection occurred in 2.8% and 3.3% of patients, respectively. These frequencies were not significantly different from those seen with comparators (AST: 2.1%; ALT: 2.4%).

Cardiovascular: Hypertension (2%); hypotension, arrhythmias such as sinus bradycardia, atrial fibrillation, varying degrees of A-V block, ventricular ectopy including non-sustained tachycardia, and ECG abnormalities have been observed rarely.

Central Nervous System: Agitation, anxiety, CNS stimulation and insomnia were seen in less than 2% of patients. Extrapyramidal syndrome occurred rarely and only in the presence of other drugs associated with this syndrome.

Hypersensitivity: Rare cases of hypersensitivity reactions, sometimes severe (eg, anaphylaxis, shortness of breath, hypotension, urticaria) have been reported.

Other: Fever (3%), taste disorder (2%), skin rashes (1%). In multiple-day comparative studies, fever occurred more frequently with KYTRIL Injection (8.6%) than with comparative drugs (3.4%, $P<0.014$), which usually included dexamethasone.

OVERDOSAGE

There is no specific antidote for KYTRIL (granisetron hydrochloride) Injection overdosage. In case of overdosage, symptomatic treatment should be given. Overdosage of up to 38.5 mg of granisetron hydrochloride injection has been reported without symptoms or only the occurrence of a slight headache.

DOSAGE AND ADMINISTRATION

The recommended dosage for KYTRIL Injection is 10 mcg/kg administered intravenously within 30 minutes before initiation of chemotherapy, and only on the day(s) chemotherapy is given. KYTRIL Injection may be administered intravenously either undiluted over 30 seconds, or diluted with 0.9% Sodium Chloride or 5% Dextrose and infused over 5 minutes.

Pediatric Use: The recommended dose in children 2 to 16 years of age is 10 mcg/kg (see CLINICAL TRIALS). Children under 2 years of age have not been studied.

Use in the Elderly, Renal Failure Patients or Hepatically Impaired Patients: No dosage adjustment is recommended. (See CLINICAL PHARMACOLOGY: Pharmacokinetics.)

Infusion Preparation: KYTRIL Injection, administered as a 5-minute infusion, should be diluted in 0.9% Sodium Chloride or 5% Dextrose to a total volume of 20 to 50 mL.

Stability: Intravenous infusion of KYTRIL Injection should be prepared at the time of administration. However, KYTRIL Injection has been shown to be stable for at least 24 hours when diluted in 0.9% Sodium Chloride or 5% Dextrose and stored at room temperature under normal lighting conditions.

As a general precaution, KYTRIL Injection should not be mixed in solution with other drugs. Parenteral drug products should be inspected visually for particulate matter and discoloration before administration whenever solution and container permit.

HOW SUPPLIED

KYTRIL (granisetron hydrochloride) Injection, 1 mg/mL (free base), is supplied in 1 mL Single-Use Vials and 4 mL Multi-Dose Vials.

NDC 0004-0239-09 (package of 1 Single-Dose Vial)
NDC 0004-0240-09 (package of 1 Multi-Dose Vial)

Store single-dose vials and multi-dose vials at 25°C (77°F); excursions permitted to 15° to 30°C (59° to 86°F).

Once the multi-dose vial is penetrated, its contents should be used within 30 days.

Do not freeze. Protect from light.

Rx only

Distributed by:
Roche Pharmaceuticals
Roche Laboratories Inc.
340 Kingsland Street
Nutley, New Jersey 07110-1199

Revised: November 2000

KYTRIL®
(granisetron hydrochloride)
TABLETS ℞

DESCRIPTION

KYTRIL Tablets contain granisetron hydrochloride, an antinauseant and antiemetic agent. Chemically it is *endo*-N-(9-methyl-9-azabicyclo [3.3.1] non-3-yl)-1-methyl-1H-indazole-3-carboxamide hydrochloride with a molecular weight of 348.9 (312.4 free base). Its empirical formula is $C_{18}H_{24}N_4O \bullet HCl$, while its chemical structure is:

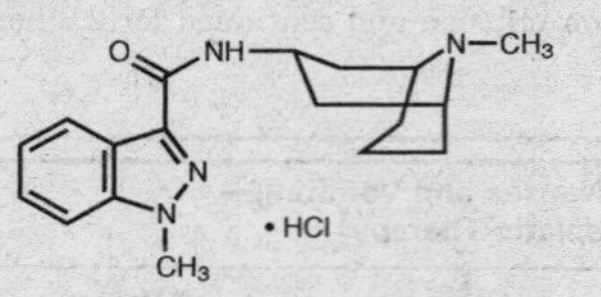

granisetron hydrochloride

Granisetron hydrochloride is a white to off-white solid that is readily soluble in water and normal saline at 20°C.

Tablets for Oral Administration: Each white, triangular, biconvex, film-coated KYTRIL Tablet contains 1.12 mg granisetron hydrochloride equivalent to granisetron, 1 mg. Inactive ingredients are: hydroxypropyl methylcellulose, lactose, magnesium stearate, microcrystalline cellulose, polyethylene glycol, polysorbate 80, sodium starch glycolate and titanium dioxide.

CLINICAL PHARMACOLOGY

Granisetron is a selective 5-hydroxytryptamine$_3$ (5-HT_3) receptor antagonist with little or no affinity for other serotonin receptors, including 5-HT_1; 5-HT_{1A}; 5-$HT_{1B/C}$; 5-HT_2; for alpha$_1$-, alpha$_2$-, or beta-adrenoreceptors; for dopamine-D_2; or for histamine-H_1; benzodiazepine; picrotoxin, or opioid receptors.

Serotonin receptors of the 5-HT_3 type are located peripherally on vagal nerve terminals and centrally in the chemoreceptor trigger zone of the area postrema. During chemotherapy that induces vomiting, mucosal enterochromaffin cells release serotonin, which stimulates 5-HT_3 receptors. This evokes vagal afferent discharge, inducing vomiting. Animal studies demonstrate that, in binding to 5-HT_3 receptors, granisetron blocks serotonin stimulation and subsequent vomiting after emetogenic stimuli such as cisplatin. In the ferret animal model, a single granisetron injection prevented vomiting due to high-dose cisplatin or arrested vomiting within 5 to 30 seconds.

In most human studies, granisetron has had little effect on blood pressure, heart rate or ECG. No evidence of an effect on plasma prolactin or aldosterone concentrations has been found in other studies.

Following single and multiple oral doses, KYTRIL slowed colonic transit in normal volunteers. However, KYTRIL had no effect on oro-cecal transit time in normal volunteers when given as a single intravenous (IV) infusion of 50 mcg/kg or 200 mcg/kg.

Pharmacokinetics: In healthy volunteers and adult cancer patients undergoing chemotherapy, administration of oral KYTRIL produced the following mean pharmacokinetic data:

[See table below]

The effects of gender on the pharmacokinetics of oral KYTRIL have not been studied. However, after intravenous infusion of KYTRIL, no difference in mean AUC was found between males and females, although males had a higher C_{max} generally.

When oral KYTRIL was administered with food, AUC was decreased by 5% and C_{max} increased by 30% in non-fasted healthy volunteers who received a single dose of 10 mg.

Granisetron metabolism involves N-demethylation and aromatic ring oxidation followed by conjugation. Animal studies suggest that some of the metabolites may also have 5-HT_3 receptor antagonist activity.

Clearance is predominantly by hepatic metabolism. In normal volunteers, approximately 11% of the orally administered dose is eliminated unchanged in the urine in 48 hours. The remainder of the dose is excreted as metabolites, 48% in the urine and 38% in the feces.

In vitro liver microsomal studies show that granisetron's major route of metabolism is inhibited by ketoconazole, suggestive of metabolism mediated by the cytochrome P-450 3A subfamily.

Plasma protein binding is approximately 65% and granisetron distributes freely between plasma and red blood cells.

In elderly and pediatric patients and in patients with renal failure or hepatic impairment, the pharmacokinetics of granisetron was determined following administration of intravenous KYTRIL:

Elderly: The ranges of the pharmacokinetic parameters in elderly volunteers (mean age 71 years), given a single 40 mcg/kg intravenous dose of KYTRIL Injection, were generally similar to those in younger healthy volunteers; mean values were lower for clearance and longer for half-life in the elderly.

Renal Failure Patients: Total clearance of granisetron was not affected in patients with severe renal failure who received a single 40 mcg/kg intravenous dose of KYTRIL Injection.

Hepatically Impaired Patients: A pharmacokinetic study with intravenous KYTRIL in patients with hepatic impairment due to neoplastic liver involvement showed that total clearance was approximately halved compared to patients without hepatic impairment. Given the wide variability in pharmacokinetic parameters noted in patients and the good tolerance of doses well above the recommended dose, dosage adjustment in patients with possible hepatic functional impairment is not necessary.

Pediatric Patients: A pharmacokinetic study in pediatric cancer patients (2 to 16 years of age), given a single 40 mcg/kg intravenous dose of KYTRIL Injection, showed that volume of distribution and total clearance increased with age. No relationship with age was observed for peak plasma concentration or terminal phase plasma half-life. When volume of distribution and total clearance are adjusted for body weight, the pharmacokinetics of granisetron are similar in pediatric and adult cancer patients.

CLINICAL TRIALS

Chemotherapy-induced Nausea and Vomiting: Oral KYTRIL prevents nausea and vomiting associated with initial and repeat courses of emetogenic cancer therapy, as shown by 24-hour efficacy data from studies using both moderately- and highly-emetogenic chemotherapy.

Moderately Emetogenic Chemotherapy: The first trial compared oral KYTRIL doses of 0.25 mg to 2 mg bid, in 930 cancer patients receiving, principally, cyclophosphamide, carboplatin and cisplatin (20 mg/m^2 to 50 mg/m^2). Efficacy was based on: complete response (ie, no vomiting, no moderate or severe nausea, no rescue medication), no vomiting and no nausea. Table 2 summarizes the results of this study.

[See table 2 at middle of next page]

Results from a second double-blind, randomized trial evaluating KYTRIL 2 mg qd and KYTRIL 1 mg bid were compared to prochlorperazine 10 mg bid derived from a historical control. At 24 hours, there was no statistically significant difference in efficacy between the two oral KYTRIL regimens. Both regimens were statistically superior to the prochlorperazine control regimen (see Table 3).

[See table 3 at bottom of next page]

Results from a KYTRIL 2 mg qd alone treatment arm in a third double-blind, randomized trial, were compared to prochlorperazine (PCPZ), 10 mg bid, derived from a historical control. The 24-hour results for KYTRIL 2 mg qd were statistically superior to PCPZ for all efficacy parameters: complete response (58%), no vomiting (79%), no nausea (51%), total control (49%). The PCPZ rates are shown in Table 3.

Cisplatin-based Chemotherapy: The first double-blind trial compared oral KYTRIL 1 mg bid, relative to placebo (historical control), in 119 cancer patients receiving high-dose cisplatin (mean dose 80 mg/m^2). At 24 hours, oral KYTRIL 1 mg bid was significantly ($P<0.001$) superior to placebo (historical control) in all efficacy parameters: complete response (52%), no vomiting (56%) and no nausea

Table 1. Pharmacokinetic Parameters (Median [range]) Following Oral KYTRIL (granisetron hydrochloride)

	Peak Plasma Concentration (ng/mL)	Terminal Phase Plasma Half-Life (h)	Volume of Distribution (L/kg)	Total Clearance (L/h/kg)
Cancer Patients 1 mg bid, 7 days (n=27)	5.99 [0.63 to 30.9]	N.D.*	N.D.	0.52 [0.09 to 7.37]
Volunteers single 1 mg dose (n=39)	3.63 [0.27 to 9.14]	6.23 [0.96 to 19.9]	3.94 [1.89 to 39.4]	0.41 [0.11 to 24.6]

* Not determined after oral administration; following a single intravenous dose of 40 mcg/kg, terminal phase half-life was determined to be 8.95 hours.

N.D. Not determined.

(45%). The placebo rates were 7%, 14% and 7%, respectively, for the three efficacy parameters.

Results from a KYTRIL 2 mg qd alone treatment arm in a second double-blind, randomized trial, were compared to both KYTRIL 1 mg bid and placebo historical controls. The 24-hour results for KYTRIL 2 mg qd were: complete response (44%), no vomiting (58%), no nausea (46%), total control (40%). The efficacy of KYTRIL 2 mg qd was comparable to KYTRIL 1 mg bid and statistically superior to placebo. The placebo rates were 7%, 14%, 7%, 7%, respectively, for the four parameters.

No controlled study comparing granisetron injection with the oral formulation to prevent chemotherapy-induced nausea and vomiting has been performed.

Radiation-Induced Nausea and Vomiting: Total Body Irradiation: In a double-blind randomized study, 18 patients receiving KYTRIL Tablets, 2 mg daily, experienced significantly greater antiemetic protection compared to patients in a historical negative control group who received conventional (non-5-HT_3 antagonist) antiemetics. Total body irradiation consisted of 11 fractions of 120 cGy administered over 4 days, with three fractions on each of the first 3 days, and two fractions on the fourth day. KYTRIL Tablets were given one hour before the first radiation fraction of each day.

Twenty-two percent (22%) of patients treated with KYTRIL Tablets did not experience vomiting or receive rescue antiemetics over the entire 4-day dosing period, compared to 0% of patients in the historical negative control group ($P<0.01$). In addition, patients who received KYTRIL Tablets also experienced significantly fewer emetic episodes during the first day of radiation and over the 4-day treatment period, compared to patients in the historical negative control group. The median time to the first emetic episode was 36 hours for patients who received KYTRIL Tablets.

Fractionated Abdominal Radiation: The efficacy of KYTRIL, 2 mg daily, was evaluated in a double-blind, placebo-controlled randomized trial of 260 patients. KYTRIL Tablets were given 1 hour before radiation, composed of up to 20 daily fractions of 180 to 300 cGy each. The exceptions were patients with seminoma or those receiving whole abdomen irradiation who initially received 150 cGy per fraction. Radiation was administered to the upper abdomen with a field size of at least 100 cm^2.

The proportion of patients without emesis and those without nausea for KYTRIL Tablets, compared to placebo, were statistically significant ($P<0.0001$) at 24 hours after radiation, irrespective of the radiation dose. KYTRIL was superior to placebo in patients receiving up to 10 daily fractions of radiation, but was not superior to placebo in patients receiving 20 fractions.

Patients treated with KYTRIL Tablets (n=134) had a significantly longer time to the first episode of vomiting (35 vs. 9 days, $P<0.001$) relative to those patients who received placebo (n=126), and a significantly longer time to the first episode of nausea (11 vs. 1 day, $P<0.001$). KYTRIL provided significantly greater protection from nausea and vomiting than placebo.

INDICATIONS AND USAGE

KYTRIL (granisetron hydrochloride) is indicated for the prevention of:

1) nausea and vomiting associated with initial and repeat courses of emetogenic cancer therapy, including high-dose cisplatin.
2) nausea and vomiting associated with radiation, including total body irradiation and fractionated abdominal radiation.

CONTRAINDICATIONS

KYTRIL is contraindicated in patients with known hypersensitivity to the drug or any of its components.

PRECAUTIONS

Drug Interactions: Granisetron does not induce or inhibit the cytochrome P-450 drug-metabolizing enzyme system. There have been no definitive drug-drug interaction studies to examine pharmacokinetic or pharmacodynamic interaction with other drugs but, in humans, KYTRIL Injection has been safely administered with drugs representing benzodiazepines, neuroleptics and anti-ulcer medications commonly prescribed with antiemetic treatments. KYTRIL Injection also does not appear to interact with emetogenic cancer chemotherapies. Because granisetron is metabolized by hepatic cytochrome P-450 drug-metabolizing enzymes, inducers or inhibitors of these enzymes may change the clearance and, hence, the half-life of granisetron.

Carcinogenesis, Mutagenesis, Impairment of Fertility: In a 24-month carcinogenicity study, rats were treated orally with granisetron 1, 5 or 50 mg/kg/day (6, 30 or 300 mg/m^2/day). The 50 mg/kg/day dose was reduced to 25 mg/kg/day (150 mg/m^2/day) during week 59 due to toxicity. For a 50 kg person of average height (1.46m^2 body surface area), these doses represent 4, 20 and 101 times the recommended clinical dose (1.48 mg/m^2, oral) on a body surface area basis. There was a statistically significant increase in the incidence of hepatocellular carcinomas and adenomas in males treated with 5 mg/kg/day (30 mg/m^2/day, 20 times the recommended human dose based on body surface area) and above, and in females treated with 25 mg/kg/day (150 mg/m^2/day, 101 times the recommended human dose based on body surface area). No increase in liver tumors was observed at a dose of 1 mg/kg/day (6 mg/m^2/day, 4 times the recommended human dose based on body surface area) in males and 5 mg/kg/day (30 mg/m^2/day, 20 times the recommended human dose based on body surface area) in females. In a 12-month oral toxicity study, treatment with granisetron 100 mg/kg/day (600 mg/m^2/day, 405 times the recommended human dose based on body surface area) produced hepatocellular adenomas in male and female rats while no such tumors were found in the control rats. A 24-month mouse carcinogenicity study of granisetron did not show a statistically significant increase in tumor incidence, but the study was not conclusive.

Because of the tumor findings in rat studies, KYTRIL (granisetron hydrochloride) Tablets should be prescribed only at the dose and for the indication recommended (see INDICATIONS AND USAGE, and DOSAGE AND ADMINISTRATION).

Granisetron was not mutagenic in in vitro Ames test and mouse lymphoma cell forward mutation assay, and in vivo mouse micronucleus test and in vitro and ex vivo rat hepatocyte UDS assays. It, however, produced a significant increase in UDS in HeLa cells in vitro and a significant increased incidence of cells with polyploidy in an in vitro human lymphocyte chromosomal aberration test.

Granisetron at oral doses up to 100 mg/kg/day (600 mg/m^2/day, 405 times the recommended human dose based on body surface area) was found to have no effect on fertility and reproductive performance of male and female rats.

Pregnancy: Teratogenic Effects: Pregnancy Category B. Reproduction studies have been performed in pregnant rats at oral doses up to 125 mg/kg/day (750 mg/m^2/day, 507 times the recommended human dose based on body surface area) and pregnant rabbits at oral doses up to 32 mg/kg/day (378 mg/m^2/day, 255 times the recommended human dose based on body surface area) and have revealed no evidence of impaired fertility or harm to the fetus due to granisetron. There are, however, no adequate and well-controlled studies in pregnant women. Because animal reproduction studies are not always predictive of human response, this drug should be used during pregnancy only if clearly needed.

Nursing Mothers: It is not known whether granisetron is excreted in human milk. Because many drugs are excreted in human milk, caution should be exercised when KYTRIL is administered to a nursing woman.

Pediatric Use: Safety and effectiveness in children have not been established.

Geriatric Use: During clinical trials, 325 patients 65 years of age or older received oral KYTRIL; 298 were 65 to 74 years of age and 27 were 75 years of age or older. Efficacy and safety were maintained with increasing age.

ADVERSE REACTIONS

Chemotherapy-induced Nausea and Vomiting: Over 3,700 patients have received oral KYTRIL in clinical trials with emetogenic cancer therapies consisting primarily of cyclophosphamide or cisplatin regimens.

In patients receiving oral KYTRIL 1 mg bid for 1, 7 or 14 days, or 2 mg qd for 1 day, the following table lists adverse experiences reported in more than 5% of the patients with comparator and placebo incidences.

[See table 4 below]

Other adverse events reported in clinical trials were:

Gastrointestinal: In single-day dosing studies in which adverse events were collected for 7 days, nausea (20%) and vomiting (12%) were recorded as adverse events after the 24-hour efficacy assessment period.

Hepatic: In comparative trials, elevation of AST and ALT (>2 times the upper limit of normal) following the administration of oral KYTRIL occurred in 5% and 6% of patients, respectively. These frequencies were not significantly different from those seen with comparators (AST: 2%; ALT: 9%).

Cardiovascular: Hypertension (1%); hypotension, angina pectoris, atrial fibrillation and syncope have been observed rarely.

Central Nervous System: Dizziness (5%), insomnia (5%), anxiety (2%), somnolence (1%). One case compatible with but not diagnostic of extrapyramidal symptoms has been reported in a patient treated with oral KYTRIL.

Hypersensitivity: Rare cases of hypersensitivity reactions, sometimes severe (eg, anaphylaxis, shortness of breath, hypotension, urticaria) have been reported.

Other: Fever (5%). Events often associated with chemotherapy also have been reported: leukopenia (9%), decreased appetite (6%), anemia (4%), alopecia (3%), thrombocytopenia (2%).

Over 5,000 patients have received injectable KYTRIL in clinical trials.

Table 5 gives the comparative frequencies of the five commonly reported adverse events (≥ 3%) in patients receiving KYTRIL Injection, 40 mcg/kg, in single-day chemotherapy trials. These patients received chemotherapy, primarily cisplatin, and intravenous fluids during the 24-hour period following KYTRIL Injection administration.

Continued on next page

Table 2. Prevention of Nausea and Vomiting 24 Hours Post-Chemotherapy[1]

Efficacy Measures	Percentages of Patients Oral KYTRIL Dose			
	0.25 mg bid (n=229) %	0.5 mg bid (n=235) %	1 mg bid (n=233) %	2 mg bid (n=233) %
Complete Response[2]	61	70*	81*†	72*
No Vomiting	66	77*	88*	79*
No Nausea	48	57	63*	54

1. Chemotherapy included oral and injectable cyclophosphamide, carboplatin, cisplatin (20 mg/m^2 to 50 mg/m^2), dacarbazine, doxorubicin, epirubicin.
2. No vomiting, no moderate or severe nausea, no rescue medication.
* Statistically significant ($P<0.01$) vs. 0.25 mg bid.
† Statistically significant ($P<0.01$) vs. 0.5 mg bid.

Table 3. Prevention of Nausea and Vomiting 24 Hours Post-Chemotherapy[1]

Efficacy Measures	Percentages of Patients		
	Oral KYTRIL 1 mg bid (n=354) %	Oral KYTRIL 2 mg qd (n=343) %	Prochlorperazine[2] 10 mg bid (n=111) %
Complete Response[3]	69*	64*	41
No Vomiting	82*	77*	48
No Nausea	51*	53*	35
Total Control[4]	51*	50*	33

1. Moderately emetogenic chemotherapeutic agents included cisplatin (20 mg/m^2 to 50 mg/m^2), oral and intravenous cyclophosphamide, carboplatin, dacarbazine, doxorubicin.
2. Historical control from a previous double-blind KYTRIL trial.
3. No vomiting, no moderate or severe nausea, no rescue medication.
4. No vomiting, no nausea, no rescue medication.
* Statistically significant ($P<0.05$) vs. prochlorperazine historical control.

Table 4. Principal Adverse Events in Clinical Trials

	Percent of Patients with Event			
	Oral KYTRIL[1] 1 mg bid (n=978)	Oral KYTRIL[1] 2 mg qd (n=1450)	Comparator[2] (n=599)	Placebo (n=185)
Headache[3]	21%	20%	13%	12%
Constipation	18%	14%	16%	8%
Asthenia	14%	18%	10%	4%
Diarrhea	8%	9%	10%	4%
Abdominal pain	6%	4%	6%	3%
Dyspepsia	4%	6%	5%	4%

1. Adverse events were recorded for 7 days when oral KYTRIL was given on a single day and for up to 28 days when oral KYTRIL was administered for 7 or 14 days.
2. Metoclopramide/dexamethasone; phenothiazines/dexamethasone; dexamethasone alone; prochlorperazine.
3. Usually mild to moderate in severity.

Kytril Tablets—Cont.

Table 5. Principal Adverse Events in Clinical Trials-Single-Day Chemotherapy

	Percent of Patients with Event	
	KYTRIL Injection[1] 40 mcg/kg (n=1,268)	Comparator[2] (n=422)
Headache	14%	6%
Asthenia	5%	6%
Somnolence	4%	15%
Diarrhea	4%	6%
Constipation	3%	3%

1. Adverse events were generally recorded over 7 days post-KYTRIL Injection administration.
2. Metoclopramide/dexamethasone and phenothiazines/dexamethasone.

In the absence of a placebo group, there is uncertainty as to how many of these events should be attributed to KYTRIL, except for headache, which was clearly more frequent than in comparison groups.

Radiation-induced Nausea and Vomiting: In controlled clinical trials, the adverse events reported by patients receiving KYTRIL tablets and concurrent radiation were similar to those reported by patients receiving KYTRIL tablets prior to chemotherapy. The most frequently reported adverse events were diarrhea, asthenia and constipation. Headache, however, was less prevalent in this patient population.

OVERDOSAGE

There is no specific treatment for granisetron hydrochloride overdosage. In case of overdosage, symptomatic treatment should be given. Overdosage of up to 38.5 mg of granisetron hydrochloride injection has been reported without symptoms or only the occurrence of a slight headache.

DOSAGE AND ADMINISTRATION

Emetogenic Chemotherapy: The recommended adult dosage of oral KYTRIL (granisetron hydrochloride) is 2 mg once daily or 1 mg twice daily. In the 2 mg once-daily regimen, two 1 mg tablets are given up to 1 hour before chemotherapy. In the 1 mg twice-daily regimen, the first 1 mg tablet is given up to 1 hour before chemotherapy, and the second tablet, 12 hours after the first. Either regimen is administered only on the day(s) chemotherapy is given. Continued treatment, while not on chemotherapy, has not been found to be useful. Use in the Elderly, Pediatric Patients, Renal Failure Patients or Hepatically Impaired Patients: No dosage adjustment is recommended (see CLINICAL PHARMACOLOGY: Pharmacokinetics).

Radiation (either Total Body Irradiation or Fractionated Abdominal Radiation): The recommended adult dosage of oral KYTRIL is 2 mg once daily. Two 1 mg tablets are taken within 1 hour of radiation.

Pediatric Use: There is no experience with oral KYTRIL in the prevention of radiation-induced nausea and vomiting in pediatric patients.

Use in the Elderly: No dosage adjustment is recommended.

HOW SUPPLIED

Tablets: White, triangular, biconvex, film-coated tablets; tablets are debossed K1 on one face.

1 mg Unit of Use 2's: NDC 0004-0241-33

1 mg SUP 20's: NDC 0004-0241-26 (intended for institutional use only)

Store between 15° and 30°C (59° and 86°F). Protect from light.

Rx only

Distributed by:
Roche Pharmaceuticals
Roche Laboratories Inc.
340 Kingsland Street
Nutley, New Jersey 07110-1199

Revised: December 2000
Copyright © 1999-2000 by Roche Laboratories Inc. All rights reserved.

VALCYTE™ ℞
(valganciclovir hydrochloride tablets)

DESCRIPTION

Valcyte (valganciclovir HCl tablets) contains valganciclovir hydrochloride (valganciclovir HCl), a hydrochloride salt of the L-valyl ester of ganciclovir that exists as a mixture of two diastereomers. Ganciclovir is a synthetic guanine derivative active against cytomegalovirus (CMV).

Valganciclovir is available as a 450 mg tablet for oral administration. Each tablet contains 496.3 mg of valganciclovir HCl (corresponding to 450 mg of valganciclovir), and the inactive ingredients microcrystalline cellulose, povidone K-30, crospovidone, and stearic acid. The film-coat applied to the tablets contains Opadry Pink®.

Valganciclovir HCl is a white to off-white crystalline powder with a molecular formula of $C_{14}H_{22}N_6O_5 \cdot HCl$ and a molecular weight of 390.83. The chemical name for valganciclovir HCl is L-Valine, 2-[(2-amino-1,6-dihydro-6-oxo-9H-purin-9-yl)methoxy]-3-hydroxypropyl ester, monohydrochloride. Valganciclovir HCl is a polar hydrophilic compound with a solubility of 70 mg/mL in water at 25°C at a pH of 7.0 and an n-octanol/water partition coefficient of 0.0095 at pH 7.0. The pKa for valganciclovir is 7.6.

The chemical structure of valganciclovir HCl is:

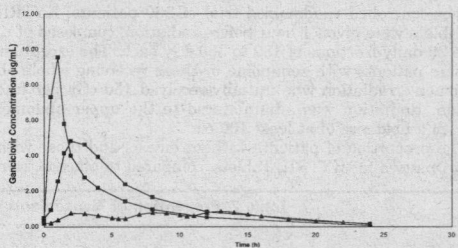

All doses in this insert are specified in terms of valganciclovir.

VIROLOGY

Mechanism of Action

Valganciclovir is an L-valyl ester (prodrug) of ganciclovir that exists as a mixture of two diastereomers. After oral administration, both diastereomers are rapidly converted to ganciclovir by intestinal and hepatic esterases. Ganciclovir is a synthetic analogue of 2'-deoxyguanosine, which inhibits replication of human cytomegalovirus in vitro and in vivo.

In CMV-infected cells ganciclovir is initially phosphorylated to ganciclovir monophosphate by the viral protein kinase, pUL97. Further phosphorylation occurs by cellular kinases to produce ganciclovir triphosphate, which is then slowly metabolized intracellularly (half-life 18 hours). As the phosphorylation is largely dependent on the viral kinase, phosphorylation of ganciclovir occurs preferentially in virus-infected cells. The virustatic activity of ganciclovir is due to inhibition of viral DNA synthesis by ganciclovir triphosphate.

Antiviral Activity

The quantitative relationship between the in vitro susceptibility of human herpesviruses to antivirals and clinical response to antiviral therapy has not been established, and virus sensitivity testing has not been standardized. Sensitivity test results, expressed as the concentration of drug required to inhibit the growth of virus in cell culture by 50% (IC_{50}), vary greatly depending upon a number of factors. Thus the IC_{50} of ganciclovir that inhibits human CMV replication in vitro (laboratory and clinical isolates) has ranged from 0.02 to 5.75 μg/mL (0.08 to 22.94 μM). Ganciclovir inhibits mammalian cell proliferation (CIC_{50}) in vitro at higher concentrations ranging from 10.21 to >250 μg/mL (40 to >1000 μM). Bone marrow-derived colony-forming cells are more sensitive (CIC_{50} = 0.69 to 3.06 μg/mL: 2.7 to 12 μM).

Viral Resistance

Viruses resistant to ganciclovir can arise after prolonged treatment with valganciclovir by selection of mutations in either the viral protein kinase gene (UL97) responsible for ganciclovir monophosphorylation and/or in the viral polymerase gene (UL54). Virus with mutations in the UL97 gene is resistant to ganciclovir alone, whereas virus with mutations in the UL54 gene may show cross-resistance to other antivirals with a similar mechanism of action.

The current working definition of CMV resistance to ganciclovir in in vitro assays is $IC_{50} \geq 1.5$ μg/mL (≥ 6.0 μM). CMV resistance to ganciclovir has been observed in individuals with AIDS and CMV retinitis who have never received ganciclovir therapy. Viral resistance has also been observed in patients receiving prolonged treatment for CMV retinitis with ganciclovir. The possibility of viral resistance should be considered in patients who show poor clinical response or experience persistent viral excretion during therapy.

CLINICAL PHARMACOLOGY

Pharmacokinetics
BECAUSE THE MAJOR ELIMINATION PATHWAY FOR GANCICLOVIR IS RENAL, DOSAGE REDUCTIONS ACCORDING TO CREATININE CLEARANCE ARE REQUIRED FOR VALCYTE TABLETS. FOR DOSING INSTRUCTIONS IN PATIENTS WITH RENAL IMPAIRMENT, REFER TO DOSAGE AND ADMINISTRATION.

The ganciclovir pharmacokinetic measures following administration of 900 mg valganciclovir and 5 mg/kg intravenous ganciclovir and 1000 mg three times daily oral ganciclovir are summarized in Table 1.
[See table below]

The area under the plasma concentration-time curve (AUC) for ganciclovir administered as Valcyte tablets is comparable to the ganciclovir AUC for intravenous ganciclovir. Ganciclovir C_{max} following valganciclovir administration is 40% lower than following intravenous ganciclovir administration. During maintenance dosing, ganciclovir $AUC_{0-24 hr}$ and C_{max} following oral ganciclovir administration (1000 mg three times daily) are lower relative to valganciclovir and intravenous ganciclovir. The ganciclovir C_{min} following intravenous ganciclovir and valganciclovir administration are less than the ganciclovir C_{min} following oral ganciclovir administration. The clinical significance of the differences in ganciclovir pharmacokinetics for these three ganciclovir delivery systems is unknown.

Figure 1. Ganciclovir Plasma Concentration Time Profiles in HIV-positive/CMV-positive Patients*

*Plasma concentration-time profiles for ganciclovir (GCV) from valganciclovir (VGCV) and intravenous ganciclovir were obtained from a multiple dose study (WV15376 n=21 and n=18, respectively) in HIV-positive/CMV-positive patients with CMV retinitis. The plasma concentration-time profile for oral ganciclovir was obtained from a multiple dose study (GAN2230 n=24) in HIV-positive/CMV-positive patients without CMV retinitis.

Absorption
Valganciclovir, a prodrug of ganciclovir, is well absorbed from the gastrointestinal tract and rapidly metabolized in the intestinal wall and liver to ganciclovir. The absolute bioavailability of ganciclovir from Valcyte tablets following administration with food was approximately 60% (3 studies, n=18; n=16; n=28). Ganciclovir median T_{max} following administration of 450 mg to 2625 mg valganciclovir tablets ranged from 1 to 3 hours. Dose proportionality with respect to ganciclovir AUC following administration of valganciclovir tablets was demonstrated only under fed conditions. Systemic exposure to the prodrug, valganciclovir, is transient and low, and the AUC_{24} and C_{max} values are approximately 1% and 3% of those of ganciclovir, respectively.

Table 1. Mean Ganciclovir Pharmacokinetic* Measures in Healthy Volunteers and HIV-positive/CMV-positive Adults at Maintenance Dosage

Formulation	Valcyte Tablets	Cytovene®-IV	Cytovene®
Dosage	900 mg once daily with food	5 mg/kg once daily	1000 mg three times daily with food
$AUC_{0-24 hr}$ (μg•h/mL)	29.1 ± 9.7 (3 studies, n=57)	26.5 ± 5.9 (4 studies, n=68)	Range of means 12.3 to 19.2 (6 studies, n=94)
C_{max} (μg/mL)	5.61 ± 1.52 (3 studies, n=58)	9.46 ± 2.02 (4 studies, n=68)	Range of means 0.955 to 1.40 (6 studies, n=94)
Absolute oral bioavailability (%)	59.4 ± 6.1 (2 studies, n=32)	Not Applicable	Range of means 6.22± 1.29 to 8.53 ± 1.53 (2 studies, n=32)
Elimination half-life (hr)	4.08 ± 0.76 (4 studies, n=73)	3.81 ± 0.71 (4 studies, n=69)	Range of means 3.86 to 5.03 (4 studies, n=61)
Renal clearance (mL/min/kg)	3.21 ± 0.75 (1 study, n=20)	2.99 ± 0.67 (1 study, n=16)	Range of means 2.67 to 3.98 (3 studies, n=30)

* Data were obtained from single and multiple dose studies in healthy volunteers, HIV-positive patients, and HIV-positive/CMV-positive patients with and without retinitis. Patients with CMV retinitis tended to have higher ganciclovir plasma concentrations than patients without CMV retinitis.

Food Effects

When valganciclovir tablets were administered with a high fat meal containing approximately 600 total calories (31.1 g fat, 51.6 g carbohydrates, and 22.2 g protein) at a dose of 875 mg once daily to 16 HIV-positive subjects, the steady-state ganciclovir AUC increased by 30% (95% CI 12-51%), and the C_{max} increased by 14% (95% CI -5–36%), without any prolongation in time to peak plasma concentrations (T_{max}). Valcyte tablets should be administered with food (see DOSAGE AND ADMINISTRATION).

Distribution

Due to the rapid conversion of valganciclovir to ganciclovir, plasma protein binding of valganciclovir was not determined. Plasma protein binding of ganciclovir is 1% to 2% over concentrations of 0.5 and 51 µg/ml. When ganciclovir was administered intravenously, the steady state volume of distribution of ganciclovir was 0.703 ± 0.134 L/kg (n=69). After administration of valganciclovir tablets, no correlation was observed between ganciclovir AUC and reciprocal weight; oral dosing of valganciclovir tablets according to weight is not required.

Metabolism

Valganciclovir is rapidly hydrolyzed to ganciclovir; no other metabolites have been detected. No metabolite of orally-administered radiolabeled ganciclovir (1000 mg single dose) accounted for more than 1% to 2% of the radioactivity recovered in the feces or urine.

Elimination

The major route of elimination of valganciclovir is by renal excretion as ganciclovir through glomerular filtration and active tubular secretion. Systemic clearance of intravenously administered ganciclovir was 3.07 ± 0.64 mL/min/kg (n=68) while renal clearance was 2.99± 0.67 mL/min/kg (n=16).

The terminal half-life ($t_{1/2}$) of ganciclovir following oral administration of valganciclovir tablets to either healthy or HIV-positive/CMV-positive subjects was 4.08 ± 0.76 hours (n=73), and that following administration of intravenous ganciclovir was 3.81 ± 0.71 hours (n=69).

Special Populations

Renal Impairment

The pharmacokinetics of ganciclovir from a single oral dose of 900 mg Valcyte tablets were evaluated in 24 otherwise healthy individuals with renal impairment.

[See table 2 above]

Decreased renal function results in decreased clearance of ganciclovir from valganciclovir, and a corresponding increase in terminal half-life. Therefore, dosage adjustment is required for patients with impaired renal function (see PRECAUTIONS: General).

Hemodialysis

Hemodialysis reduces plasma concentrations of ganciclovir by about 50% following valganciclovir administration. Patients receiving hemodialysis (CrCl <10 ml/min) cannot use Valcyte tablets because the daily dose of Valcyte tablets required for these patients is less than 450 mg (see PRECAUTIONS: General and DOSAGE AND ADMINISTRATION: Hemodialysis Patients).

Liver Transplant Patients

In liver transplant patients, the ganciclovir $AUC_{0-24 hr}$ achieved with 900 mg valganciclovir was 41.7 ± 9.9 µg•h/mL (n=28) and the $AUC_{0-24 hr}$ achieved with the approved dosage of 5 mg/kg intravenous ganciclovir was 48.2 ± 17.3 µg•h/mL (n=27).

Race/Ethnicity and Gender

Insufficient data are available to demonstrate any effect of race or gender on the pharmacokinetics of valganciclovir.

Pediatrics

Valcyte tablets have not been studied in pediatric patients; the pharmacokinetic characteristics of Valcyte tablets in these patients have not been established (see PRECAUTIONS: Pediatric Use).

Geriatrics

No studies of Valcyte tablets have been conducted in adults older than 65 years of age (see PRECAUTIONS: Geriatric Use).

INDICATIONS AND USAGE

Valcyte tablets are indicated for the treatment of cytomegalovirus (CMV) retinitis in patients with acquired immunodeficiency syndrome (AIDS) (see CLINICAL TRIALS).

CLINICAL TRIALS

Induction Therapy of CMV Retinitis

Study WV15376

In a randomized, open-label controlled study, 160 patients with AIDS and newly diagnosed CMV retinitis were randomized to receive treatment with either Valcyte tablets (900 mg twice daily for 21 days, then 900 mg once daily for 7 days) or with intravenous ganciclovir solution (5 mg/kg twice daily for 21 days, then 5 mg/kg once daily for 7 days). Study participants were: male (91%), White (53%), Hispanic (31%), and Black (11%). The median age was 39 years, the median baseline HIV-1 RNA 4.9 $\log_{10}$, and the median CD4 cell count was 23 cells/mm³. A determination of CMV retinitis progression by the masked review of retinal photographs taken at baseline and week 4 was the primary outcome measurement of the three week induction therapy. Table 3 provides the outcomes at four weeks.

[See table 3 above]

Maintenance Therapy of CMV Retinitis

No comparative clinical data are available on the efficacy of Valcyte for the maintenance therapy of CMV retinitis because all patients in study WV15376 received open-label Valcyte after week 4. However, the AUC for ganciclovir is similar following administration of 900 mg valganciclovir

Table 2. Pharmacokinetics of Ganciclovir From a Single Oral Dose of 900 mg Valcyte Tablets

Estimated Creatinine Clearance (mL/min)	N	Apparent Clearance (mL/min) Mean ± SD	AUC_{last} (µg·h/mL) Mean ± SD	Half-life (hours) Mean± SD
51–70	6	249 ± 99	49.5 ± 22.4	4.85 ± 1.4
21–50	6	136 ± 64	91.9 ± 43.9	10.2 ± 4.4
11–20	6	45 ± 11	223 ± 46	21.8 ± 5.2
≤10	6	12.8 ± 8	366 ± 66	67.5 ± 34

Table 3. Week 4 Masked Review of Retinal Photographs in Study WV15376

	Cytovene-IV	Valcyte
Determination of CMV retinitis progression at Week 4	N=80	N=80
Progressor	7	7
Non-progressor	63	64
Death	2	1
Discontinuations due to Adverse Events	1	2
Failed to return	1	1
CMV not confirmed at baseline or no interpretable baseline photos	6	5

Table 4. Results of Drug Interaction Studies with Ganciclovir: Effects of Co-administered Drug on Ganciclovir Plasma AUC and C_{max} Values

Co-administered Drug	Ganciclovir Dosage	n	Ganciclovir Pharmacokinetic (PK) Parameter	Clinical Comment
Zidovudine 100 mg every 4 hours	1000 mg every 8 hours	12	AUC ↓ 17 ± 25% (range: −52% to 23%)	Zidovudine and Valcyte each have the potential to cause neutropenia and anemia. Some patients may not tolerate concomitant therapy at full dosage.
Didanosine 200 mg every 12 hours administered 2 hours before ganciclovir	1000 mg every 8 hours	12	AUC ↓ 21 ± 17% (range: −44% to 5%)	Effect not likely to be clinically significant.
Didanosine 200 mg every 12 hours stimultaneously administered with ganciclovir	1000 mg every 8 hours	12	No effect on ganciclovir PK parameters observed	No effect expected.
	IV ganciclovir 5 mg/kg twice daily	11	No effect on ganciclovir PK parameters observed	No effect expected.
	IV ganciclovir 5 mg/kg once daily	11	No effect on ganciclovir PK parameters observed	No effect expected.
Probenecid 500 mg every 6 hours	1000 mg every 8 hours	10	AUC ↑ 53 ± 91% (range: −14% to 299%) Ganciclovir renal clearance ↓ 22 ± 20% (Range: −54% to −4%)	Patients taking probenecid and Valcyte should be monitored for evidence of ganciclovir toxicity.
Zalcitabine 0.75 mg every 8 hours administered 2 hours before ganciclovir	1000 mg every 8 hours	10	AUC ↑ 13%	Effect not likely to be clinically significant.
Trimethoprim 200 mg once daily	1000 mg every 8 hours	12	Ganciclovir renal clearance ↓ 16.3% Half-life ↑ 15%	Effect not likely to be clinically significant.
Mycophenolate Mofetil 1.5 g single dose	IV ganciclovir 5 mg/kg single dose	12	No effect on ganciclovir PK parameters observed (patients with normal renal function)	Patients with renal impairment should be monitored carefully as levels of metabolites of both drugs may increase.

once daily and 5 mg/kg intravenous ganciclovir once daily. Although the ganciclovir C_{max} is lower following valganciclovir administration compared to intravenous ganciclovir, it is higher than the C_{max} obtained following oral ganciclovir administration (see Figure 1 in CLINICAL PHARMACOLOGY). Therefore, use of valganciclovir as maintenance therapy is supported by a plasma concentration-time profile similar to that of two approved products for maintenance therapy of CMV retinitis.

CONTRAINDICATIONS

Valcyte tablets are contraindicated in patients with hypersensitivity to valganciclovir or ganciclovir.

WARNINGS

THE CLINICAL TOXICITY OF VALCYTE, WHICH IS METABOLIZED TO GANCICLOVIR, INCLUDES GRANULOCYTOPENIA, ANEMIA AND THROMBOCYTOPENIA. IN ANIMAL STUDIES GANCICLOVIR WAS CARCINOGENIC, TERATOGENIC AND CAUSED ASPERMATOGENESIS.

Hematologic

Valcyte tablets should not be administered if the absolute neutrophil count is less than 500 cells/µL, the platelet count is less than 25,000/µL, or the hemoglobin is less than 8 g/dL.

Severe leukopenia, neutropenia, anemia, thrombocytopenia, pancytopenia, bone marrow depression and aplastic anemia

have been observed in patients treated with Valcyte tablets (and ganciclovir) (see PRECAUTIONS: Laboratory Testing and ADVERSE EVENTS).

Valcyte tablets should, therefore, be used with caution in patients with pre-existing cytopenias, or who have received or who are receiving myelosuppressive drugs or irradiation. Cytopenia may occur at any time during treatment and may increase with continued dosing. Cell counts usually begin to recover within 3 to 7 days of discontinuing drug.

Impairment of Fertility

Animal data indicate that administration of ganciclovir causes inhibition of spermatogenesis and subsequent infertility. These effects were reversible at lower doses and irreversible at higher doses (see PRECAUTIONS: Carcinogenesis, Mutagenesis and Impairment of Fertility). It is considered probable that in humans, valganciclovir at the recommended doses may cause temporary or permanent inhibition of spermatogenesis. Animal data also indicate that suppression of fertility in females may occur.

Teratogenesis, Carcinogenesis and Mutagenesis

Because of the mutagenic and teratogenic potential of ganciclovir, women of childbearing potential should be advised to use effective contraception during treatment. Similarly, men should be advised to practice barrier contraception dur-

Continued on next page

Valcyte—Cont.

ing, and for at least 90 days following, treatment with Valcyte tablets (see PRECAUTIONS: Carcinogenesis, Mutagenesis and Pregnancy: Category C).
In animal studies, ganciclovir was found to be mutagenic and carcinogenic. Valganciclovir should, therefore, be considered a potential teratogen and carcinogen in humans with the potential to cause birth defects and cancers (see DOSAGE AND ADMINISTRATION: Handling and Disposal).

PRECAUTIONS

General

Strict adherence to dosage recommendations is essential to avoid overdose.
The bioavailability of ganciclovir from Valcyte tablets is significantly higher than from ganciclovir capsules. Patients switching from ganciclovir capsules should be advised of the risk of overdosage if they take more than the prescribed number of Valcyte tablets. **Valcyte tablets cannot be substituted for Cytovene capsules on a one-to-one basis** (see OVERDOSAGE and DOSAGE AND ADMINISTRATION).
Since ganciclovir is excreted by the kidneys, normal clearance depends on adequate renal function. **IF RENAL FUNCTION IS IMPAIRED, DOSAGE ADJUSTMENTS ARE REQUIRED FOR VALCYTE TABLETS.** Such adjustments should be based on measured or estimated creatinine clearance values (see DOSAGE AND ADMINISTRATION: Renal Impairment).
For patients on hemodialysis (CrCl <10 mL/min) it is recommended that ganciclovir be used (in accordance with the dose-reduction algorithm cited in the Cytovene®-IV and Cytovene® Package Insert section on DOSAGE AND ADMINISTRATION: Renal Impairment) rather than Valcyte tablets (see DOSAGE AND ADMINISTRATION: Hemodialysis and CLINICAL PHARMACOLOGY: Special Populations: *Hemodialysis*).

Information for Patients (see Patient Package Insert)

Valcyte tablets cannot be substituted for ganciclovir capsules on a one-to-one basis. Patients switching from ganciclovir capsules should be advised of the risk of overdosage if they take more than the prescribed number of Valcyte tablets (see OVERDOSAGE and DOSAGE AND ADMINISTRATION).
Valcyte is changed to ganciclovir once it is absorbed into the body. All patients should be informed that the major toxicities of ganciclovir include granulocytopenia (neutropenia), anemia and thrombocytopenia and that dose modifications may be required, including discontinuation. The importance of close monitoring of blood counts while on therapy should be emphasized. Patients should be informed that ganciclovir has been associated with elevations in serum creatinine.
Patients should be instructed to take Valcyte tablets with food to maximize bioavailability.
Patients should be advised that ganciclovir has caused decreased sperm production in animals and may cause decreased fertility in humans. Women of childbearing potential should be advised that ganciclovir causes birth defects in animals and should not be used during pregnancy. Because of the potential for serious adverse events in nursing infants, mothers should be instructed not to breastfeed if they are receiving Valcyte tablets. Women of childbearing potential should be advised to use effective contraception during treatment with Valcyte tablets. Similarly, men should be advised to practice barrier contraception during and for at least 90 days following treatment with Valcyte tablets.
Although there is no information from human studies, patients should be advised that ganciclovir should be considered a potential carcinogen.
Convulsions, sedation, dizziness, ataxia and/or confusion have been reported with the use of Valcyte tablets and/or ganciclovir. If they occur, such effects may affect tasks requiring alertness including the patient's ability to drive and operate machinery.
Patients should be told that ganciclovir is not a cure for CMV retinitis, and that they may continue to experience progression of retinitis during or following treatment. Patients should be advised to have ophthalmologic follow-up examinations at a minimum of every 4 to 6 weeks while being treated with Valcyte tablets. Some patients will require more frequent follow-up.

Laboratory Testing

Due to the frequency of neutropenia, anemia and thrombocytopenia in patients receiving Valcyte tablets (see ADVERSE EVENTS), it is recommended that complete blood counts and platelet counts be performed frequently, especially in patients in whom ganciclovir or other nucleoside analogues have previously resulted in leukopenia, or in whom neutrophil counts are less than 1000 cells/μL at the beginning of treatment. Increased monitoring for cytopenias may be warranted if therapy with oral ganciclovir is changed to oral valganciclovir, because of increased plasma concentrations of ganciclovir after valganciclovir administration (see CLINICAL PHARMACOLOGY).
Increased serum creatinine levels have been observed in trials evaluating Valcyte tablets. Patients should have serum creatinine or creatinine clearance values monitored carefully to allow for dosage adjustments in renally impaired patients (see DOSAGE AND ADMINISTRATION: Renal Impairment). The mechanism of impairment of renal function is not known.

Drug Interactions

Drug Interaction Studies Conducted With Valganciclovir:
No in vivo drug-drug interaction studies were conducted with valganciclovir. However, because valganciclovir is rapidly and extensively converted to ganciclovir, interactions associated with ganciclovir will be expected for Valcyte tablets.
Drug Interaction Studies Conducted With Ganciclovir:
Binding of ganciclovir to plasma proteins is only about 1% to 2%, and drug interactions involving binding site displacement are not anticipated.
Drug-drug interaction studies were conducted in patients with normal renal function. Patients with impaired renal function may have increased concentrations of ganciclovir and the coadministered drug following concomitant administration of Valcyte tablets and drugs excreted by the same pathway as ganciclovir. Therefore, these patients should be closely monitored for toxicity of ganciclovir and the coadministered drug.
[See table 4 on previous page]
[See table 5 below]

Carcinogenesis, Mutagenesis and Impairment of Fertility‡

No long-term carcinogenicity studies have been conducted with valganciclovir. However, upon oral administration, valganciclovir is rapidly and extensively converted to ganciclovir. Therefore, like ganciclovir, valganciclovir is a potential carcinogen.
Ganciclovir was carcinogenic in the mouse at oral doses of 20 and 1000 mg/kg/day (approximately 0.1× and 1.4×, respectively, the mean drug exposure in humans following the recommended intravenous dose of 5 mg/kg, based on area under the plasma concentration curve [AUC] comparisons). At the dose of 1000 mg/kg/day there was a significant increase in the incidence of tumors of the preputial gland in males, forestomach (nonglandular mucosa) in males and females, and reproductive tissues (ovaries, uterus, mammary gland, clitoral gland and vagina) and liver in females. At the dose of 20 mg/kg/day, a slightly increased incidence of tumors was noted in the preputial and harderian glands in males, forestomach in males and females, and liver in females. No carcinogenic effect was observed in mice administered ganciclovir at 1 mg/kg/day (estimated as 0.01× the human dose based on AUC comparison). Ganciclovir should be considered a potential carcinogen in humans.
Valganciclovir increases mutations in mouse lymphoma cells. In the mouse micronucleus assay, valganciclovir was clastogenic at a dose of 1500 mg/kg (60× human mean exposure for ganciclovir based upon AUC). Valganciclovir was not mutagenic in the Ames Salmonella assay. Ganciclovir increased mutations in mouse lymphoma cells and DNA damage in human lymphocytes in vitro. In the mouse micronucleus assay, ganciclovir was clastogenic at doses of 150 and 500 mg/kg (IV) (2.8 to 10x human exposure based on AUC) but not 50 mg/kg (exposure approximately comparable to the human based on AUC). Ganciclovir was not mutagenic in the Ames Salmonella assay.
Valganciclovir is converted to ganciclovir and therefore is expected to have similar reproductive toxicity effects as ganciclovir (see WARNINGS: Impairment of Fertility). Ganciclovir caused decreased mating behavior, decreased fertility, and an increased incidence of embryolethality in female mice following intravenous doses of 90 mg/kg/day (approximately 1.7× the mean drug exposure in humans following the dose of 5 mg/kg, based on AUC comparisons). Ganciclovir caused decreased fertility in male mice and hypospermatogenesis in mice and dogs following daily oral or intravenous administration of doses ranging from 0.2 to 10 mg/kg. Systemic drug exposure (AUC) at the lowest dose showing toxicity in each species ranged from 0.03 to 0.1× the AUC of the recommended human intravenous dose. Valganciclovir caused similar effects on spermatogenesis in mice, rats, and dogs. It is considered likely that ganciclovir (and valganciclovir) could cause inhibition of human spermatogenesis.

Pregnancy

Category C‡
Valganciclovir is converted to ganciclovir and therefore is expected to have reproductive toxicity effects similar to ganciclovir. Ganciclovir has been shown to be embryotoxic in rabbits and mice following intravenous administration, and teratogenic in rabbits. Fetal resorptions were present in at least 85% of rabbits and mice administered 60 mg/kg/day and 108 mg/kg/day (2× the human exposure based on AUC comparisons), respectively. Effects observed in rabbits included: fetal growth retardation, embryolethality, teratogenicity and/or maternal toxicity. Teratogenic changes included cleft palate, anophthalmia/microphthalmia, aplastic organs (kidney and pancreas), hydrocephaly and brachygnathia. In mice, effects observed were maternal/fetal toxicity and embryolethality.
Daily intravenous doses of 90 mg/kg administered to female mice prior to mating, during gestation, and during lactation caused hypoplasia of the testes and seminal vesicles in the month-old male offspring, as well as pathologic changes in the nonglandular region of the stomach (see Teratogenesis, Carcinogenesis and Mutagenesis). The drug exposure in mice as estimated by the AUC was approximately 1.7× the human AUC.
Data obtained using an ex vivo human placental model show that ganciclovir crosses the placenta and that simple diffusion is the most likely mechanism of transfer. The transfer was not saturable over a concentration range of 1 to 10 mg/mL and occurred by passive diffusion.
Valganciclovir may be teratogenic or embryotoxic at dose levels recommended for human use. There are no adequate and well-controlled studies in pregnant women. Valcyte tablets should be used during pregnancy only if the potential benefit justifies the potential risk to the fetus.

‡ **Footnote:** All dose comparisons presented in the Carcinogenesis, Mutagenesis, Impairment of Fertility, and Pregnancy subsections are based on the human AUC following administration of a single 5 mg/kg infusion of intravenous ganciclovir.

Nursing Mothers

It is not known whether ganciclovir or valganciclovir is excreted in human milk. Because valganciclovir caused granulocytopenia, anemia and thrombocytopenia in clinical trials and ganciclovir was mutagenic and carcinogenic in animal studies, the possibility of serious adverse events from ganciclovir in nursing infants is possible (see WARNINGS).

Table 5. Results of Drug Interaction Studies with ganciclovir: Effects of ganciclovir on Plasma AUC and C_{max} Values of Co-administered Drug

Co-administered Drug	Ganciclovir Dosage	n	Co-administered Drug Pharmacokinetic (PK) Parameter	Clinical Comment
Zidovudine 100 mg every 4 hours	1000 mg every 8 hours	12	AUC_{0-4} ↑ 19 ± 27% (range: −11% to 74%)	Zidovudine and Valcyte each have the potential to cause neutropenia and anemia. Some patients may not tolerate concomitant therapy at full dosage.
Didanosine 200 mg every 12 hours when administered 2 hours prior to or concurrent with ganciclovir	1000 mg every 8 hours	12	AUC_{0-12} ↑ 111 ± 114% (range: 10% to 493%)	Patients should be closely monitored for didanosine toxicity.
Didanosine 200 mg every 12 hours	IV ganciclovir 5 mg/kg twice daily	11	AUC_{0-12} ↑ 70 ± 40% (range: 3% to 121%) C_{max} ↑ 49 ± 48% (range: −28% to 125%)	Patients should be closely monitored for didanosine toxicity.
Didanosine 200 mg every 12 hours	IV ganciclovir 5 mg/kg once daily	11	AUC_{0-12} ↑ 50 ± 26% (range: 22% to 110%) C_{max} ↑ 36 ± 36% (range: −27% to 94%)	Patients should be closely monitored for didanosine toxicity.
Zalcitabine 0.75 mg every 8 hours administered 2 hours before ganciclovir	1000 mg every 8 hours	10	No clinically relevant PK parameter changes	No effect expected.
Trimethoprim 200 mg once daily	1000 mg every 8 hours	12	Increase in C_{min}	Effect not likely to be clinically significant.
Mycophenolate Mofetil 1.5 g single dose	IV ganciclovir 5 mg/kg single dose	12	No PK interaction observed (patients with normal renal function)	Patients with renal impairment should be monitored carefully as levels of metabolites of both drugs may increase.

Table 6. Percentage of Selected Adverse Events Occurring During the Randomized Phase of Study WV15376

Adverse Event	Valganciclovir Arm N=79	Intravenous Ganciclovir Arm N=79
Diarrhea	16%	10%
Neutropenia	11%	13%
Nausea	8%	14%
Headache	9%	5%
Anemia	8%	8%
Catheter-related infection	3%	11%

Because of potential for serious adverse events in nursing infants, **mothers should be instructed not to breastfeed if they are receiving Valcyte tablets.** In addition, the Centers for Disease Control and Prevention recommend that HIV-infected mothers not breastfeed their infants to avoid risking postnatal transmission of HIV.

Pediatric Use
Safety and effectiveness of Valcyte tablets in pediatric patients have not been established.

Geriatric Use
The pharmacokinetic characteristics of Valcyte in elderly patients have not been established. Since elderly individuals frequently have a reduced glomerular filtration rate, particular attention should be paid to assessing renal function before and during administration of Valcyte (see DOSAGE AND ADMINISTRATION).

Clinical studies of Valcyte did not include sufficient numbers of subjects aged 65 and over to determine whether they respond differently from younger subjects. In general, dose selection for an elderly patient should be cautious, reflecting the greater frequency of decreased hepatic, renal, or cardiac function, and of concomitant disease or other drug therapy. Valcyte is known to be substantially excreted by the kidney, and the risk of toxic reactions to this drug may be greater in patients with impaired renal function. Because elderly patients are more likely to have decreased renal function, care should be taken in dose selection. In addition, renal function should be monitored and dosage adjustments should be made accordingly (see PRECAUTIONS: General, CLINICAL PHARMACOLOGY: Special Populations: *Renal Impairment*, and DOSAGE AND ADMINISTRATION: Renal Impairment).

ADVERSE EVENTS
Experience With Valcyte Tablets
Valganciclovir, a prodrug of ganciclovir, is rapidly converted to ganciclovir after oral administration. Adverse events known to be associated with ganciclovir usage can therefore be expected to occur with Valcyte tablets.

As shown in Table 6, the safety profiles of Valcyte tablets and intravenous ganciclovir during 28 days of randomized therapy (21 days induction dose and 7 days maintenance dose) in 158 patients were comparable, with the exception of catheter-related infection, which occurred with greater frequency in patients randomized to receive IV ganciclovir (see Table 6).

[See table 6 above]

Tables 7 and 8 show the pooled adverse event data and abnormal laboratory values from two single arm, open-label clinical trials, WV15376 (after the initial four weeks of randomized therapy) and WV15705. A total of 370 patients received maintenance therapy with valganciclovir tablets 900 mg q day. Approximately 252 (68%) of these patients received Valcyte tablets for more than nine months (maximum duration was 36 months).

Table 7. Pooled Selected Adverse Events Reported in • 5% of Patients in Two Clinical Studies

Adverse Events According to Body System	% Patients N=370
Gastrointestinal system	
Diarrhea	41%
Nausea	30%
Vomiting	21%
Abdominal pain	15%
Body as a whole	
Pyrexia	31%
Headache	22%
Hemic and lymphatic system	
Neutropenia	27%
Anemia	26%
Thrombocytopenia	6%
Central and peripheral nervous system	
Insomnia	16%
Peripheral neuropathy	9%
Parethesia	8%
Special senses	
Retinal detachment	15%

Serious adverse events reported from these two clinical trials (N=370) with a frequency of less than 5% and which are not mentioned in the two tables above, are listed below:

Hemic and lymphatic system: pancytopenia, bone marrow depression, aplastic anemia
Urogenital system: decreased creatinine clearance
Infections: local and systemic infections and sepsis
Bleeding complications: potentially life-threatening bleeding associated with thrombocytopenia
Central and peripheral nervous system: convulsion, psychosis, hallucinations, confusion, agitation
Body as a whole: valganciclovir hypersensitivity
Laboratory abnormalities reported with Valcyte tablets are listed below:

Table 8. Pooled Laboratory Abnormalities Reported in Two Clinical Studies

Laboratory Abnormalities	N=370
Neutropenia: AUC /µL	
<500	19%
500 – <750	17%
750 – <1000	17%
Anemia: Hemoglobin g/dL	
<6.5	7%
6.5 – <8.0	13%
8.0 – <9.5	16%
Thrombocytopenia: Platelets /µL	
<25000	4%
25000 – <50000	6%
50000 – <100000	22%
Serum Creatinine: mg/dL	
>2.5	3%
>1.5 – 2.5	12%

Experience with Ganciclovir
Valganciclovir is rapidly converted to ganciclovir upon oral administration. Adverse events reported with Valcyte in general were similar to those reported with ganciclovir (Cytovene). Please refer to the Cytovene label for more information on post-marketing adverse events associated with ganciclovir.

OVERDOSAGE
Overdose Experience With Valcyte Tablets
One adult developed fatal bone marrow depression (medullary aplasia) after several days of dosing that was at least 10-fold greater than recommended for the patient's estimated degree of renal impairment.

It is expected that an overdose of Valcyte tablets could also possibly result in increased renal toxicity (see PRECAUTIONS: General and DOSAGE AND ADMINISTRATION: Renal Impairment).

Since ganciclovir is dialyzable, dialysis may be useful in reducing serum concentrations in patients who have received an overdose of Valcyte tablets (see CLINICAL PHARMACOLOGY: Special Populations: *Hemodialysis*). Adequate hydration should be maintained. The use of hematopoietic growth factors should be considered (see CLINICAL PHARMACOLOGY: Special Populations: *Hemodialysis*).

Overdose Experience With Intravenous Ganciclovir
Reports of overdoses with intravenous ganciclovir have been received from clinical trials and during postmarketing experience. The majority of patients experienced one or more of the following adverse events:

Hematological toxicity: pancytopenia, bone marrow depression, medullary aplasia, leukopenia, neutropenia, granulocytopenia
Hepatotoxicity: hepatitis, liver function disorder
Renal toxicity: worsening of hematuria in a patient with pre-existing renal impairment, acute renal failure, elevated creatinine
Gastrointestinal toxicity: abdominal pain, diarrhea, vomiting
Neurotoxicity: generalized tremor, convulsion

DOSAGE AND ADMINISTRATION
Strict adherence to dosage recommendations is essential to avoid overdose. Valcyte tablets cannot be substituted for Cytovene capsules on a one-to-one basis.

Valcyte tablets are administered orally, and should be taken with food (see CLINICAL PHARMACOLOGY: Absorption). After oral administration, valganciclovir is rapidly and extensively converted into ganciclovir. The bioavailability of ganciclovir from Valcyte tablets is significantly higher than from ganciclovir capsules. Therefore the dosage and administration of Valcyte tablets as described below should be closely followed (see PRECAUTIONS: General and OVERDOSAGE).

For the Treatment of CMV Retinitis in Patients With Normal Renal Function

Induction:
For patients with active CMV retinitis, the recommended dosage is 900 mg (two 450 mg tablets) twice a day for 21 days with food.
Maintenance:
Following induction treatment, or in patients with inactive CMV retinitis, the recommended dosage is 900 mg (two 450 mg tablets) once daily with food.

Renal Impairment
Serum creatinine or creatinine clearance levels should be monitored carefully. Dosage adjustment is required according to creatinine clearance as shown in the table below (see PRECAUTIONS: General and CLINICAL PHARMACOLOGY: Special Populations: *Renal Impairment*). Increased monitoring for cytopenias may be warranted in patients with renal impairment (see PRECAUTIONS: Laboratory Testing).

[See table 9 below]

Hemodialysis Patients
Valcyte should not be prescribed to patients receiving hemodialysis (see CLINICAL PHARMACOLOGY: Special Populations: *Hemodialysis* and PRECAUTIONS: General).

Handling and Disposal
Caution should be exercised in the handling of Valcyte tablets. Tablets should not be broken or crushed. Since valganciclovir is considered a potential teratogen and carcinogen in humans, caution should be observed in handling broken tablets (see WARNINGS: Teratogenesis, Carcinogenesis and Mutagenesis). Avoid direct contact of broken or crushed tablets with skin or mucous membranes. If such contact occurs, wash thoroughly with soap and water, and rinse eyes thoroughly with plain water.

Because ganciclovir shares some of the properties of antitumor agents (ie, carcinogenicity and mutagenicity), consideration should be given to handling and disposal according to guidelines issued for antineoplastic drugs. Several guidelines on this subject have been published (see REFERENCES).

There is no general agreement that all of the procedures recommended in the guidelines are necessary or appropriate.

HOW SUPPLIED
Valcyte (valganciclovir HCl tablets) is available as 450 mg pink convex oval tablets with "VGC" on one side and "450" on the other side. Each tablet contains valganciclovir HCl equivalent to 450 mg valganciclovir. Valcyte is supplied in bottles of 60 tablets (NDC 0004-0038-22).

Store at 25°C (77°F); excursions permitted to 15°C to 30°C (59°F to 86°F) [See USP controlled room temperature].

REFERENCES
1. Recommendations for the Safe Handling of Cytotoxic Drugs. US Department of Health and Human Services, National Institutes of Health, Bethesda, MD, September 1992. NIH Publication No. 92–2621
2. American Society of Hospital Pharmacists technical assistance bulletin on handling cytotoxic and hazardous drugs. *Am J Hosp Pharm.* 1990; 47:1033-1049
3. Controlling Occupational Exposures to Hazardous Drugs.

Continued on next page

Table 9. Dose Modifications for Patients with Impaired Renal Function

CrCl* (mL/min)	Induction Dose	Maintenance Dose
≥ 60	900 mg twice daily	900 mg once daily
40 – 59	450 mg twice daily	450 mg once daily
25 – 39	450 mg once daily	450 mg every 2 days
10 – 24	450 mg every 2 days	450 mg twice weekly

*An estimated creatinine clearance can be related to serum creatinine by the following formulas:

$$\text{For males} = \frac{(140 - \text{age [years]}) \times \text{body weight [kg]}}{(72) \times \text{(serum creatinine [mg/dL])}}$$

For females = 0.85 × male value

Valcyte—Cont.

US Department of Labor. Occupational Health and Safety Administration. OSHA Technical Manual. Section VI – Chapter 2, January 20, 1999

Cytovene is a registered trademark of Syntex (U.S.A.) LLC.
Valcyte tablets are manufactured by Patheon Inc., Mississauga, Ontario, Canada L5N 7K9

℞ only

Distributed by:
Roche Pharmaceuticals
Roche Laboratories Inc.
340 Kingsland Street
Nutley, New Jersey 07110-1199

Issued: March 2001

Copyright © 2001 by Roche Laboratories Inc. All rights reserved.

Schering Corporation

a wholly-owned subsidiary of Schering-Plough Corporation
GALLOPING HILL ROAD
KENILWORTH, NJ 07033

Direct Inquiries to:
(908) 298-4000
CUSTOMER SERVICE:
(800) 222-7579
FAX: (908) 820-6400

For Medical Information Contact:
Schering Laboratories
Drug Information Services
2000 Galloping Hill Road
Kenilworth, NJ 07033
(800) 526-4099
FAX: (908) 298-2188

PEG-Intron™ ℞
(Peginterferon alfa-2b)
Powder for Injection

> **WARNING**
> Alpha interferons, including PEG-Intron, cause or aggravate fatal or life-threatening neuropsychiatric, autoimmune, ischemic, and infectious disorders. Patients should be monitored closely with periodic clinical and laboratory evaluations. Patients with persistently severe or worsening signs or symptoms of these conditions should be withdrawn from therapy. In many but not all cases these disorders resolve after stopping PEG-Intron therapy. See **WARNINGS, ADVERSE REACTIONS.**

DESCRIPTION

PEG-Intron™, peginterferon alfa-2b Powder for Injection, is a covalent conjugate of recombinant alfa interferon with monomethoxy polyethylene glycol (PEG). The molecular weight of the PEG portion of the molecule is 12,000 daltons. The average molecular weight of the PEG-Intron molecule is approximately 31,000 daltons. The specific activity of pegylated interferon alfa-2b is approximately 0.7×10^8 IU/mg protein.

Interferon alfa-2b, the starting material used to manufacture PEG-Intron, is a water-soluble protein with a molecular weight of 19,271 daltons produced by recombinant DNA techniques. It is obtained from the bacterial fermentation of a strain of *Escherichia coli* bearing a genetically engineered plasmid containing an interferon gene from human leukocytes.

PEG-Intron is a white to off-white lyophilized powder supplied in 2-mL vials for subcutaneous use. Each vial contains either 74 µg, 118.4 µg, 177.6 µg, or 222 µg of PEG-Intron, and 1.11 mg dibasic sodium phosphate anhydrous, 1.11 mg monobasic sodium phosphate dihydrate, 59.2 mg sucrose and 0.074 mg polysorbate 80. Following reconstitution with 0.7 mL of the supplied diluent (Sterile Water for Injection, USP), each vial contains PEG-Intron at strengths of either 100 µg/mL, 160 µg/mL, 240 µg/mL or 300 µg/mL.

CLINICAL PHARMACOLOGY

General: The biological activity of PEG-Intron is derived from its interferon alfa-2b moiety. Interferons exert their cellular activities by binding to specific membrane receptors on the cell surface and initiate a complex sequence of intracellular events. These include the induction of certain enzymes, suppression of cell proliferation, immunomodulating activities such as enhancement of the phagocytic activity of macrophages and augmentation of the specific cytotoxicity of lymphocytes for target cells, and inhibition of virus replication in virus-infected cells. Interferon alfa upregulates the Th1 T-helper cell subset in *in vitro* studies. The clinical relevance of these findings is not known.

Pharmacodynamics: PEG-Intron raises concentrations of effector proteins such as serum neopterin and 2*5* oligoadenylate synthetase, raises body temperature, and causes reversible decreases in leukocyte and platelet counts. The correlation between the *in vitro* and *in vivo* pharmacologic and pharmacodynamic and clinical effects is unknown.

Pharmacokinetics: Following a single subcutaneous dose of PEG-Intron, the mean absorption half-life ($t\ ^1/_2\ k_a$) was 4.6 hours. Maximal serum concentrations (C_{max}) occur between 15–44 hours post-dose, and are sustained for up to 48–72 hours. The C_{max} and AUC measurements of PEG-Intron increase in a dose-related manner. After multiple dosing, there is an increase in bioavailability of PEG-Intron. Week 48 mean trough concentrations (320 pg/mL; range 0, 2960) are approximately 3-fold higher than Week 4 mean trough concentrations (94 pg/mL; range 0, 416). The mean PEG-Intron elimination half-life is approximately 40 hours (range 22 to 60 hours) in patients with HCV infection. The apparent clearance of PEG-Intron is estimated to be approximately 22.0 mL/hr•kg. Renal elimination accounts for 30% of the clearance. Single dose peginterferon alfa-2b pharmacokinetics following a subcutaneous 1.0 µg/kg dose suggest the clearance of peginterferon alfa-2b is reduced by approximately half in patients with impaired renal function (creatinine clearance <50 mL/minute).

Pegylation of interferon alfa-2b produces a product (PEG-Intron) whose clearance is lower than that of non-pegylated interferon alfa-2b. When compared to INTRON A, PEG-Intron (1.0 µg/kg) has approximately a seven-fold lower mean apparent clearance and a five-fold greater mean half-life permitting a reduced dosing frequency. At effective therapeutic doses, PEG-Intron has approximately ten-fold greater C_{max} and 50-fold greater AUC than interferon alfa-2b.

Pharmacokinetic data from geriatric patients (> 65 years of age) treated with a single subcutaneous dose of 1.0 µg/kg of PEG-Intron showed no remarkable differences in C_{max}, AUC, clearance, or elimination half-life from those obtained in younger patients.

During the 48 week treatment period with PEG-Intron no differences in the pharmacokinetic profiles were observed between male and female patients with chronic hepatitis C infection.

Drug Interactions: It is not known if PEG-Intron therapy causes clinically significant drug-drug interactions with drugs metabolized by the liver in patients with hepatitis C. In 12 healthy subjects known to be CYP2D6 extensive metabolizers, a single subcutaneous dose of 1 µg/kg PEG-Intron did not inhibit CYP1A2, 2C8/9, 2D6, hepatic 3A4 or N-acetyltransferase; the effects of PEG-Intron on CYP2C19 were not assessed.

CLINICAL STUDIES

A randomized study compared treatment with PEG-Intron (0.5, 1.0, or 1.5 µg/kg once weekly SC) to treatment with INTRON A, (3 million units three times weekly SC) in 1219 adults with chronic hepatitis from HCV infection. The patients were not previously treated with interferon alfa, had compensated liver disease, detectable HCV RNA, elevated ALT, and liver histopathology consistent with chronic hepatitis. Patients were treated for 48 weeks and were followed for 24 weeks post-treatment. Seventy percent of all patients were infected with HCV genotype 1, and 74% of all patients had high baseline levels of HCV RNA (more than 2 million copies per mL of serum), two factors known to predict poor response to treatment.

Response to treatment was defined as undetectable HCV RNA and normalization of ALT at 24 weeks post-treatment. The response rates to the 1.0 and 1.5 µg/kg PEG-Intron doses were similar to each other and were both higher than response rates to INTRON A. (See **Table 1**)

[See table below]

TABLE 1. Rates of Response to Treatment

	A PEG-Intron 0.5 µg/kg (N=315)	B PEG-Intron 1.0 µg/kg (N=298)	C INTRON A 3 MIU TIW (N=307)	B-C (95% CI) Difference between PEG-Intron 1.0 µg/kg and INTRON A
Treatment Response (Combined Virologic Response and ALT Normalization)	17%	24%	12%	11 (5, 18)
Virologic Response[a]	18%	25%	12%	12 (6, 9)
ALT Normalization	24%	29%	18%	11 (5, 18)

[a]Serum HCV RNA is measured by a research-based quantitive polymerase chain reaction with a lower limit of detection of 100 copies/mL at the National Genetics Institute, Culver City, CA.

Patients with both viral genotype 1 and high serum levels of HCV RNA at baseline were less likely to respond to treatment with PEG-Intron. Among patients with the two unfavorable prognostic variables, 8% (12/157) responded to PEG-Intron treatment and 2% (4/169) responded to INTRON A. Doses of PEG-Intron higher than the recommended dose did not result in higher response rates in these patients.

Patients receiving PEG-Intron with viral genotype 1 had a response rate of 14% (28/199) while patients with other viral genotypes had a 45% (43/96) response rate.

Ninety-six percent of the responders in the PEG-Intron groups and 100% of responders in the INTRON A group first cleared their viral RNA by week 24 of treatment. See **DOSAGE AND ADMINISTRATION.**

The treatment response rates were similar in men and women. Response rates were lower in African American and Hispanic patients and higher in Asians compared to Caucasians. Although African Americans had a higher proportion of poor prognostic factors compared to Caucasians the number of non-Caucasians studied (9% of the total) was insufficient to allow meaningful conclusions about differences in response rates after adjusting for prognostic factors.

Liver biopsies were obtained before and after treatment in 60% of patients. A modest reduction in inflammation compared to baseline that was similar in all four treatment groups was observed.

INDICATIONS AND USAGE

PEG-Intron, peginterferon alfa-2b, monotherapy is indicated for the treatment of chronic hepatitis C in patients not previously treated with interferon alpha who have compensated liver disease and are at least 18 years of age. The safety and efficacy of peginterferon alfa-2b (PEG-Intron) in combination with ribavirin (REBETOL) for the treatment of chronic hepatitis C have not been established.

CONTRAINDICATIONS

PEG-Intron is contraindicated in patients with:
- hypersensitivity to PEG-Intron or any component of the product
- autoimmune hepatitis
- decompensated liver disease

WARNINGS

Patients should be monitored for the following serious conditions, some of which may become life threatening. Patients with persistently severe or worsening signs or symptoms should be withdrawn from therapy.

Neuropsychiatric events

Life-threatening or fatal neuropsychiatric events, including suicide, suicidal and homicidal ideation, depression, relapse of drug addiction/overdose, and aggressive behavior have occurred in patients with and without a previous psychiatric disorder during PEG-Intron treatment and follow-up. Psychoses and hallucinations have been observed in patients treated with alpha interferons. PEG-Intron should be used with extreme caution in patients with a history of psychiatric disorders. Patients should be advised to report immediately any symptoms of depression and/or suicidal ideation to their prescribing physicians. Physicians should monitor all patients for evidence of depression and other psychiatric symptoms. In severe cases, PEG-Intron should be stopped immediately and psychiatric intervention instituted.

Bone marrow toxicity

PEG-Intron suppresses bone marrow function, sometimes resulting in severe cytopenias. PEG-Intron should be discontinued in patients who develop severe decreases in neutrophil or platelet counts. Very rarely alpha interferons may be associated with aplastic anemia. (See **DOSAGE AND ADMINISTRATION**)

Endocrine disorders

PEG-Intron causes or aggravates hypothyroidism and hyperthyroidism. Hyperglycemia has been observed in patients treated with PEG-Intron. Diabetes mellitus has been observed in patients treated with alpha interferons. Patients with these conditions who cannot be effectively treated by medication should not begin PEG-Intron therapy. Patients who develop these conditions during treatment and cannot be controlled with medication should not continue PEG-Intron therapy.

Cardiovascular events

Cardiovascular events, which include hypotension, arrhythmia, tachycardia, cardiomyopathy, and myocardial infarction have been observed in patients treated with PEG-Intron. PEG-Intron should be used cautiously in patients with cardiovascular disease. Patients with a history of myocardial infarction and arrhythmic disorder who require PEG-Intron therapy should be closely monitored (see **Laboratory tests**).

Colitis

Fatal and nonfatal ulcerative and hemorrhagic colitis has been observed within 12 weeks of the start of alpha interferon treatment. Abdominal pain, bloody diarrhea, and fever are the typical manifestations. PEG-Intron treatment should be discontinued immediately in patients who develop these symptoms and signs. The colitis usually resolves within 1–3 weeks of discontinuation of alpha interferons.

Pancreatitis
Fatal and nonfatal pancreatitis has been observed in patients treated with alpha interferon. PEG-Intron therapy should be suspended in patients with signs and symptoms suggestive of pancreatitis and discontinued in patients diagnosed with pancreatitis.
Autoimmune disorders
Development or exacerbation of autoimmune disorders (e.g., thyroiditis, thrombocytopenia, rheumatoid arthritis, interstitial nephritis, systemic lupus erythematosus, psoriasis) have been observed in patients receiving PEG-Intron. PEG-Intron should be used with caution in patients with autoimmune disorders.
Pulmonary disorders
Dyspnea, pulmonary infiltrates, pneumonitis and pneumonia, some resulting in patient deaths, have been associated with PEG-Intron or alpha interferon therapy. Patients with pulmonary infiltrates or pulmonary function impairment should be closely monitored.
Hypersensitivity
Serious, acute hypersensitivity reactions (e.g., urticaria, angioedema, bronchoconstriction, anaphylaxis) have been rarely observed during alpha interferon therapy. If such a reaction develops during treatment with PEG-Intron, discontinue treatment and institute appropriate medical therapy immediately. Transient rashes do not necessitate interruption of treatment.

PRECAUTIONS

- PEG-Intron has not been studied in patients who have failed other alpha interferon treatments.
- The safety and efficacy of PEG-Intron for the treatment of hepatitis C in patients who have received liver or other organ transplant recipients have not been studied.
- The safety and efficacy of PEG-Intron for the treatment of patients with HCV coinfected with HIV or HBV have not been established.

Ophthalmologic disorders: Retinal hemorrhages, cotton wool spots, and retinal artery or vein obstruction have been observed after treatment with PEG-Intron or alpha interferons. Patients who have diabetes mellitus or hypertension should have eye examinations before the start of PEG-Intron treatment.
Patients with renal failure: Patients with impairment of renal function should be closely monitored for signs and symptoms of interferon toxicity and doses of PEG-Intron should be adjusted accordingly. PEG-Intron should be used with caution in patients with creatinine clearance <50 mL/min. See **DOSAGE AND ADMINISTRATION.**
Immunogenicity: One percent of patients (7/734) receiving PEG-Intron developed low-titer (≤64) neutralizing antibodies to INTRON A. The clinical and pathological significance of the appearance of serum neutralizing antibodies is unknown. No apparent correlation of antibody development to clinical response or adverse events was observed. The incidence of post-treatment binding antibody was approximately 10% for patients receiving PEG-Intron and approximately 15% for patients receiving INTRON A. The data reflect the percentage of patients whose test results were considered positive for antibodies to PEG-Intron in a Biacore assay that is used to measure binding antibodies, and in an antiviral neutralization assay which measures serum neutralizing antibodies. The percentage of patients whose test results were considered positive for antibodies is highly dependent on the sensitivity and specificity of the assays. Additionally the observed incidence of antibody positivity in these assays may be influenced by several factors including sample timing and handling, concomitant medications, and underlying disease. For these reasons, comparison of the incidence of antibodies to PEG-Intron with the incidence of antibodies to other products may be misleading.
Laboratory Tests: PEG-Intron may cause severe decreases in neutrophil and platelet counts, and abnormality of TSH. In 10% of patients treated with PEG-Intron ALT levels rose 2 to 5-fold above baseline. The elevations were transient and were not associated with deterioration of other liver functions.
Patients on PEG-Intron therapy should have hematology and blood chemistry testing before the start of treatment and then periodically thereafter. In the clinical trial CBC (including neutrophil and platelet counts) and chemistries (including AST, ALT, and bilirubin) were measured during the treatment period at weeks 2, 4, 8, 12, and then at 6-week intervals or more frequently if abnormalities developed. TSH levels were measured every 12 weeks during the treatment period.
Patients who have pre-existing cardiac abnormalities should have electrocardiograms administered before treatment with PEG-Intron.
Information for Patients: Patients receiving PEG-Intron should be directed in its appropriate use, informed of the benefits and risks associated with treatment, and referred to the **MEDICATION GUIDE.**
A puncture-resistant container for the disposal of used syringes and needles should be supplied to the patient for at home use. Patients should be thoroughly instructed in the importance of proper disposal and cautioned against any reuse of needles and syringes. The full container should be disposed of according to the directions provided by the physician (see **MEDICATION GUIDE**).
Patients should be informed that there are no data evaluating whether PEG-Intron therapy will prevent transmission of HCV infection to others. Also, it is not known if treatment with PEG-Intron will cure hepatitis C or prevent cirrhosis, liver failure, or liver cancer that may be the result of infection with the hepatitis C virus.
Patients should be advised that laboratory evaluations are required before starting therapy and periodically thereafter (see **Laboratory Tests**). It is advised that patients be well-hydrated, especially during the initial stages of treatment. "Flu-like" symptoms associated with administration of PEG-Intron may be minimized by bedtime administration of PEG-Intron or by use of antipyretics.
Carcinogenesis, Mutagenesis, Impairment of Fertility
Carcinogenesis: PEG-Intron has not been tested for its carcinogenic potential.
Mutagenesis: Neither PEG-Intron, nor its components interferon or methoxypolyethylene glycol caused damage to DNA when tested in the standard battery of mutagenesis assays, in the presence and absence of metabolic activation.
Impairment of Fertility: Irregular menstrual cycles were observed in female cynomolgus monkeys given subcutaneous injections of 4239 μg/m^2 PEG-Intron every other day for one month, at approximately 345 times the recommended weekly human dose (based upon body surface area). These effects included transiently decreased serum levels of estradiol and progesterone, suggestive of anovulation. Normal menstrual cycles and serum hormone levels resumed in these animals 2 to 3 months following cessation of PEG-Intron treatment. Every other day dosing with 262 μg/m^2 (approximately 21 times the weekly human dose) had no effects on cycle duration or reproductive hormone status. The effects of PEG-Intron on male fertility have not been studied.
Pregnancy Category C: Non-pegylated Interferon alfa-2b, has been shown to have abortifacient effects in *Macaca mulatta* (rhesus monkeys) at 15 and 30 million IU/kg (estimated human equivalent of 5 and 10 million IU/kg, based on body surface area adjustment for a 60 kg adult). PEG-Intron should be assumed to also have abortifacient potential. There are no adequate and well-controlled studies in pregnant women. PEG-Intron therapy is to be used during pregnancy only if the potential benefit justifies the potential risk to the fetus. Therefore, PEG-Intron is recommended for use in fertile women only when they are using effective contraception during the treatment period.
Nursing Mothers: It is not known whether the components of PEG-Intron are excreted in human milk. Because of the potential for adverse reactions from the drug in nursing infants, a decision must be made whether to discontinue nursing or discontinue the treatment, taking into account the importance of the product to the mother.
Pediatric Use Safety and effectiveness in pediatric patients below the age of 18 years have not been established.
Geriatric Patients Clinical studies of PEG-Intron did not include sufficient numbers of subjects aged 65 and over to determine whether they respond differently than younger subjects. Other reported clinical experience has not identified differences in responses between the elderly and younger patients. However, treatment with alpha interferons, including PEG-Intron, is associated with CNS, cardiac, and systemic (flu-like) adverse effects. Because these adverse reactions may be more severe in the elderly, caution should be exercised in use of PEG-Intron in this population. This drug is known to be substantially excreted by the kidney. Because elderly patients are more likely to have decreased renal function, the risk of toxic reactions to this drug may be greater in patients with impaired renal function.

ADVERSE REACTIONS

Nearly all study patients experienced one or more adverse events. The incidence of serious adverse events was similar (about 12%) in all treatment groups. In many but not all cases, events resolve after stopping PEG-Intron therapy. Some patients continued to experience adverse events for several months after discontinuation of therapy. There was one patient death, a suicide, among patients receiving PEG-Intron and two patient deaths in the INTRON A group (1 murder/suicide and 1 sudden death). Overall, 10% of patients in the PEG-Intron groups discontinued therapy due to adverse events compared to 6% in the INTRON A group. Fourteen percent of patients in the PEG-Intron groups required dose reduction compared to 6% in the INTRON A group.
The most common adverse events associated with PEG-Intron were "flu-like" symptoms which occurred in approximately 50% of patients, and may decrease in severity as treatment continues. Application site disorders occurred frequently (47%) and included injection site inflammation, and reaction (i.e. bruise, itchiness, irritation). Injection site pain was reported in 2% of patients receiving PEG-Intron. Alopecia (thinning of the hair) is also often associated with PEG-Intron.
Fifty-seven percent of patients treated with PEG-Intron experienced psychiatric adverse events, most commonly depression (29%). Suicidal behavior (ideation, attempts, and suicides) occurred in 1% of all patients during or shortly after treatment with PEG-Intron. (See **WARNINGS**).
Patients receiving PEG-Intron appeared to experience a greater number of adverse events (e.g., injection site reaction, fever, rigors, nausea) compared to patients receiving INTRON A. The number of adverse events in all body systems in general was higher in patients receiving the higher PEG-Intron dosages.
Adverse events that occurred in the Phase 3 clinical trial at ≥5% incidence are provided in **Table 2** by treatment group.

TABLE 2. Adverse Events Occurring in ≥5% of Patients

Adverse Events	PEG-Intron 1.0 μg/kg (N=297)	INTRON A 3 MIU (N=303)
	Percentage of Patients Reporting Adverse Events*	
Application Site Disorders		
Injection Site Inflammation/Reaction	47	20
Autonomic Nervous System Disorders		
Flushing	6	3
Sweating Increased	6	7
Body as a Whole—General Disorders		
Headache	56	52
Fatigue	52	54
Influenza-Like Symptoms	46	38
Rigors	23	19
Fever	22	12
Weight Decrease	11	13
RUQ pain	8	8
Malaise	7	6
Central and Peripheral Nervous System Disorders		
Dizziness	12	10
Hypertonia	5	3
Endocrine Disorders		
Hypothyrodism	5	3
Gastro-intestinal System Disorders		
Nausea	26	20
Anorexia	20	17
Diarrhea	18	16
Abdominal Pain	15	11
Vomiting	7	6
Dyspepsia	6	7
Hematologic Disorders		
Neutropenia	6	2
Thrombocytopenia	7	<1
Infectious Disorders		
Infection Viral	11	10
Liver and Biliary System Disorders		
Hepatomegaly	6	5
Musculoskeletal System Disorders		
Musculoskeletal Pain	56	58
Psychiatric Disorders		
Depression	29	25
Insomnia	23	23
Anxiety/Emotional Lability/Irritability	28	34
Respiratory System Disorders		
Pharyngitis	10	7
Sinusitis	7	7
Coughing	6	5
Skin and Appendages Disorders		
Alopecia	22	22
Pruritus	12	8
Dry skin	11	9
Rash	6	7

*Patients reporting one or more adverse events. A patient may have reported more than one adverse event within a body system/organ class category.

Numerous adverse events were observed at a frequency <5%. In the absence of a non-treatment control group the relationship to study drug could not be determined.
Individual serious adverse events occurred at a frequency ≤1% and included suicide attempt, suicidal ideation, severe depression; relapse of drug addiction/overdose; nerve palsy (facial, oculomotor); cardiomyopathy, myocardial infarction, retinal ischemia, retinal vein thrombosis, transient ischemic attack, supraventricular arrhythmias, loss of consciousness; neutropenia, infection (pneumonia, abscess); autoimmune thrombocytopenia, hyperthyroidism, rheumatoid arthritis, interstitial nephritis, lupus-like syndrome, aggravated psoriasis; urticaria.
Laboratory Values
Neutrophils Neutrophil counts decreased in 70% of patients. Severe potentially life-threatening neutropenia ($<0.5 \times 10^9$/L) occurred in 1% of patients.
Platelets Platelet counts decreased in 20% of patients. Treatment with PEG-Intron resulted in severe decreases in platelet counts (<50,000/mm^3) in 1% of patients.
The incidence and severity of thrombocytopenia and neutropenia were greater in the PEG-Intron groups compared to

Continued on next page

PEG Intron—Cont.

the interferon alfa group. Platelet and neutrophil counts generally returned to pretreatment levels within 4 weeks of the cessation of therapy.

Thyroid Function   TSH abnormalities developed in 16% of patients and were associated with clinically apparent hypothyroidism (5%) or hyperthyroidism (1%). Subjects developed new onset TSH abnormalities while on treatment and during the follow-up period. At the end of the follow-up period 7% of subjects still had abnormal TSH values.

OVERDOSAGE

There is limited experience with overdosage. In the clinical study, 13 patients accidentally received a dose greater than that prescribed. There were no instances in which a patient received more than 2.5 times the intended dose. The maximum dose received by any patient was 3.45 µg/kg weekly over a period of approximately 12 weeks. There were no serious reactions attributed to these overdosages.

DOSAGE AND ADMINISTRATION

A patient should self-inject only if the physician determines that it is appropriate and the patient agrees to medical follow-up as necessary and training in proper injection technique has been given to him/her. (See illustrated **MEDICATION GUIDE** for instructions.)

PEG-Intron is administered subcutaneously once weekly for one year. The dose should be administered on the same day of each week. Initial dosing should be based on weight as described in **Table 3.**

[See table 3 below]

Serum HCV RNA levels should be assessed after 24 weeks of treatment. Discontinuation of treatment should be considered in any patient who has not achieved an HCV RNA below the limit of detection of the assay after 24 weeks of therapy with PEG-Intron. (See **CLINICAL STUDIES**.)

There are no safety and efficacy data for treatment longer than 48 weeks or for re-treatment of patients who relapse following PEG-Intron therapy.

Dose Reduction

If a serious adverse reaction develops during the course of treatment (see **WARNINGS**) discontinue or modify the dosage of PEG-Intron to one-half the starting dosage until the adverse event abates or decreases in severity. If persistent or recurrent intolerance develops despite adequate dosage adjustment, discontinue treatment with PEG-Intron. For dose modification in the event of neutropenia and thrombocytopenia see **Table 4.**

TABLE 4. Guidelines for Dose Modifications for Neutropenia and Thrombocytopenia

	Dose Reduction	Permanent Discontinuation
Neutrophil Count	$<0.75 \times 10^9/L$	$<0.50 \times 10^9/L$
Platelet Count	$<80 \times 10^9/L$	$<50 \times 10^9/L$

Preparation and Administration

Two B-D Safety Lok™ syringes are provided in the package; one syringe is for the reconstitution steps and one for the patient injection. There is a plastic safety sleeve to be pulled over the needle after use. The syringe locks with an audible click when the green stripe on the safety sleeve covers the red stripe on the needle. Brief instructions for the preparation and administration of PEG-Intron Powder for Injection are provided below. Please refer to the **MEDICATION GUIDE** for detailed, step by step instructions.

Reconstitute the PEG-Intron lyophilized product with only 0.7 mL of supplied diluent (Sterile Water for Injection, USP). **The diluent vial is for single use only. The remaining diluent should be discarded.** No other medications should be added to solutions containing PEG-Intron, and PEG-Intron should not be reconstituted with other diluents. Swirl gently to hasten complete dissolution of the powder. The reconstituted solution should be clear and colorless. Visually inspect the solution for particulate matter and discoloration prior to administration. The solution should not be used if discolored or cloudy, or if particulates are present. (See **MEDICATION GUIDE** for detailed instructions).

The reconstituted solution should be used immediately and cannot be stored for more than 24 hours at 2°–8°C (see **Storage**). The appropriate PEG-Intron dose should be withdrawn and injected subcutaneously. (See **MEDICATION GUIDE** for detailed instructions.) The PEG-Intron vial is a single use vial and does not contain a preservative. **DO NOT REENTER VIAL. DISCARD UNUSED PORTION.** Once the dose from a single dose vial has been withdrawn, the sterility of any remaining product can no longer be guaranteed. Pooling of unused portions of some medications has been linked to bacterial contamination and morbidity.

After preparation and administration of the PEG-Intron injection, it is essential to follow the procedure for proper disposal of syringes and needles. A puncture-resistant container should be used for disposal of syringes. Patients should be instructed in the technique and importance of proper syringe disposal and be cautioned against reuse of these items (see **MEDICATION GUIDE** for detailed instructions.)

Storage

PEG-Intron, should be stored at 25°C (77°F): excursions permitted to 15–30°C (59–86°F)[see USP Controlled Room Temperature]. After reconstitution with supplied Diluent the solution should be used immediately, but may be stored up to 24 hours at 2° to 8°C (36° to 46°F). The reconstituted solution contains no preservative, is clear and colorless. **Do not freeze.**

HOW SUPPLIED

PEG-Intron is a white to off-white lyophilized powder supplied in 2-mL vials. The PEG-Intron Powder for Injection should be reconstituted with 0.7 mL of the supplied Diluent (Sterile Water for Injection, USP) prior to use.

[See table below]

Schering Corporation
Kenilworth, NJ 07033 USA
Copyright © 2001, Schering Corporation. All rights reserved.

1/01   24564703

TABLE 3. Recommended Dosing

Vial Strength* to Use (µg/mL)	Weight (kg)	Amount of PEG-Intron to Administer (µg)	Volume of PEG-Intron* to Administer (mL)
100	37–45	40	0.4
	46–56	50	0.5
160	57–72	64	0.4
	73–88	80	0.5
240	89–106	96	0.4
	107–136	120	0.5
300	137–160	150	0.5

* When reconstituted as directed

	Each PEG-Intron Package Contains:	
For Patients 37–56 kg	A box containing one 100 µg/mL vial of PEG-Intron Powder for Injection and one 5 mL vial of Diluent (Sterile Water for Injection, USP), 2 B-D Safety Lok™ syringes with a safety sleeve and 2 alcohol swabs.	(NDC 0085-1368-01)
For Patients 57–88 kg	A box containing one 160 µg/mL vial of PEG-Intron Powder for Injection and one 5 mL vial of Diluent (Sterile Water for Injection, USP), 2 B-D Safety Lok™ syringes with a safety sleeve and 2 alcohol swabs.	(NDC 0085-1291-01)
For Patients 89–136 kg	A box containing one 240 µg/mL vial of PEG-Intron Powder for Injection and one 5 mL vial of Diluent (Sterile Water for Injection, USP), 2 B-D Safety Lok™ syringes with a safety sleeve and 2 alcohol swabs.	(NDC 0085-1304-01)
For Patients 137–160 kg	A box containing one 300 µg/mL vial of PEG-Intron Powder for Injection and one 5 mL vial of Diluent (Sterile Water for Injection, USP), 2 B-D Safety Lok™ syringes with a safety sleeve and 2 alcohol swabs.	(NDC 0085-1279-01)

Schwarz Pharma, Inc.
6140 W. EXECUTIVE DRIVE
MEQUON, WI 53092

For Medical Information Contact:
Schwarz Pharma, Inc.
Professional Services
(262) 238-9994
(800) 558-5114

NULEV™   ℞
[nū' lěv]
(hyoscyamine sulfate orally disintegrating tablets)
0.125 mg
Rx Only

DESCRIPTION

NuLev™ (hyoscyamine sulfate orally disintegrating tablets) 0.125 mg is formulated for oral administration using patented DuraSolv™ technology. NuLev disintegrates within seconds after placement on the tongue, allowing it to be swallowed with or without water.

Hyoscyamine sulfate is one of the principal anticholinergic/antispasmodic components of belladonna alkaloids. The empirical formula is $(C_{17}H_{23}NO_3)_2 \cdot H_2SO_4 \cdot 2H_2O$ and the molecular weight is 712.85. Chemically, it is benzeneacetic acid, α-(hydroxymethyl)-, 8-methyl-8-azabicyclo [3.2.1.] oct-3-yl ester, [3(S)-endo]-, sulfate (2:1), dihydrate with the following structure:

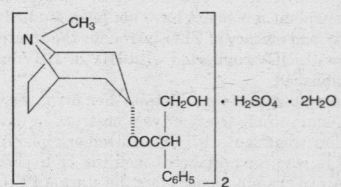

Each tablet also contains as inactive ingredients: aspartame, colloidal silicon dioxide, crospovidone, flavor, magnesium stearate, mannitol, microcrystalline cellulose.

CLINICAL PHARMACOLOGY

Hyoscyamine sulfate inhibits specifically the actions of acetylcholine on structures innervated by postganglionic cholinergic nerves and on smooth muscles that respond to acetylcholine but lack cholinergic innervation. These peripheral cholinergic receptors are present in the autonomic effector cells of the smooth muscle, cardiac muscle, the sino-atrial node, the atrioventricular node, and the exocrine glands. At therapeutic doses, it is completely devoid of any action on autonomic ganglia. Hyoscyamine sulfate inhibits gastrointestinal propulsive motility and decreases gastric acid secretion. Hyoscyamine sulfate also controls excessive pharyngeal, tracheal and bronchial secretions.

Hyoscyamine sulfate is absorbed totally and completely by oral administration. Once absorbed, hyoscyamine sulfate disappears rapidly from the blood and is distributed throughout the entire body. The half-life of hyoscyamine sulfate is 2 to 3½ hours. Hyoscyamine sulfate is partly hydrolyzed to tropic acid and tropine but the majority of the drug is excreted in the urine unchanged within the first 12 hours. Only traces of this drug are found in breast milk. Hyoscyamine sulfate passes the blood brain barrier and the placental barrier.

INDICATIONS AND USAGE

NuLev is effective as adjunctive therapy in the treatment of peptic ulcer. It can also be used to control gastric secretion, visceral spasm and hypermotility in spastic colitis, spastic bladder, cystitis, pylorospasm, and associated abdominal cramps. May be used in functional intestinal disorders to reduce symptoms such as those seen in mild dysenteries, diverticulitis, and acute enterocolitis. For use as adjunctive therapy in the treatment of irritable bowel syndrome (irritable colon, spastic colon, mucous colitis) and functional gastrointestinal disorders. Also used as adjunctive therapy in the treatment of neurogenic bladder and neurogenic bowel disturbances (including the splenic flexure syndrome and neurogenic colon). NuLev is indicated along with morphine or other narcotics in symptomatic relief of biliary and renal colic; as a "drying agent" in the relief of symptoms of acute rhinitis; in the therapy of parkinsonism to reduce rigidity and tremors and to control associated sialorrhea and hyperhidrosis. May be used in the therapy of poisoning by anticholinesterase agents.

CONTRAINDICATIONS

Glaucoma; obstructive uropathy (for example, bladder neck obstruction due to prostatic hypertrophy); obstructive disease of the gastrointestinal tract (as in achalasia, pyloroduodenal stenosis): paralytic ileus, intestinal atony of elderly or debilitated patients; unstable cardiovascular status in acute hemorrhage; severe ulcerative colitis; toxic megacolon complicating ulcerative colitis; myasthenia gravis.

WARNINGS

In the presence of high environmental temperature, heat prostration can occur with drug use (fever and heat stroke due to decreased sweating). Diarrhea may be an early symptom of incomplete intestinal obstruction, especially in patients with ileostomy or colostomy. In this instance, treatment with this drug would be inappropriate and possibly harmful. Like other anticholinergic agents, NuLev may produce drowsiness, dizziness or blurred vision. In this event, the patient should be warned not to engage in activities requiring mental alertness such as operating a motor vehicle or other machinery or to perform hazardous work while taking this drug.

Psychosis has been reported in sensitive individuals given anticholinergic drugs. CNS signs and symptoms include confusion, disorientation, short term memory loss, hallucinations, dysarthria, ataxia, coma, euphoria, decreased anxiety, fatigue, insomnia, agitation and mannerisms, and inappropriate affect. These CNS signs and symptoms usually resolve within 12 to 48 hours after discontinuation of the drug.

PRECAUTIONS

General:

Use with caution in patients with: autonomic neuropathy, hyperthyroidism, coronary heart disease, congestive heart failure, cardiac arrhythmias, hypertension, and renal disease. Investigate any tachycardia before giving any anticholinergic drug since they may increase the heart rate. Use with caution in patients with hiatal hernia associated with reflux esophagitis.

Information for Patients:

Like other anticholinergic agents, NuLev may produce drowsiness, dizziness, or blurred vision. In this event, the patient should be warned not to engage in activities requiring mental alertness such as operating a motor vehicle or other machinery or to perform hazardous work while taking this drug.

Use of NuLev may decrease sweating resulting in heat prostration, fever or heat stroke; febrile patients or those who may be exposed to elevated environmental temperatures should use caution.

Phenylketonurics: Phenylketonuric patients should be informed that NuLev contains phenylalanine 1.7 mg per orally disintegrating tablet.

Drug Interactions: Additive adverse effects resulting from cholinergic blockade may occur when NuLev is administered concomitantly with other antimuscarinics, amantadine, haloperidol, phenothiazines, monoamine oxidase (MAO) inhibitors, tricyclic antidepressants or some antihistamines.

Antacids may interfere with the absorption of hyoscyamine sulfate. Administer NuLev before meals; antacids after meals.

Carcinogenesis, Mutagenesis, Impairment of Fertility: No long-term studies in animals have been performed to determine the carcinogenic, mutagenic or impairment of fertility potential of hyoscyamine sulfate; however 40 years of marketing experience with hyoscyamine sulfate shows no demonstrable evidence of a problem.

Pregnancy—Pregnancy Category C: Animal reproduction studies have not been conducted with hyoscyamine sulfate. It is also not known whether hyoscyamine sulfate can cause fetal harm when administered to a pregnant woman or can affect reproduction capacity. NuLev should be given to a pregnant woman only if clearly needed.

Nursing Mothers: Hyoscyamine sulfate is excreted in human milk. Caution should be exercised when NuLev is administered to a nursing woman.

ADVERSE REACTIONS

Not all of the following adverse reactions have been reported with hyoscyamine sulfate. The following adverse reactions have been reported for pharmacologically similar drugs with anticholinergic/antispasmodic action. Adverse reactions may include dryness of the mouth; urinary hesitancy and retention; blurred vision; tachycardia; palpitations; mydriasis; cycloplegia; increased ocular tension; loss of taste; headache; nervousness; drowsiness; weakness; dizziness; insomnia; nausea; vomiting; impotence; suppression of lactation; constipation; bloated feeling; allergic reactions or drug idiosyncrasies; urticaria and other dermal manifestations; ataxia; speech disturbance; some degree of mental confusion and/or excitement (especially in elderly persons); and deceased sweating.

OVERDOSAGE

The signs and symptoms of overdose are headache, nausea, vomiting, blurred vision, dilated pupils, hot dry skin, dizziness, dryness of the mouth, difficulty in swallowing, and CNS stimulation.

Measures to be taken are immediate lavage of the stomach and injection of physostigmine 0.5 to 2 mg intravenously and repeated as necessary up to a total of 5 mg. Fever may be treated symptomatically (tepid water sponge baths, hypothermic blanket). Excitement to a degree which demands attention may be managed with sodium thiopental 2% solution given slowly intravenously or chloral hydrate (100–200 mL of a 2% solution) by rectal infusion. In the event of progression of the curare-like effect to paralysis of the respiratory muscles, artificial respiration should be instituted and maintained until effective respiratory action returns.

In rats, the LD_{50} for hyoscyamine is 375 mg/kg. Hyoscyamine sulfate is dialyzable.

DOSAGE AND ADMINISTRATION

Dosage may be adjusted according to the conditions and severity of symptoms. Place NuLev on tongue, allowing the tablet to rapidly disintegrate and be swallowed. May be taken with or without water.

Adults and pediatric patients 12 years of age and older: 1 to 2 tablets every four hours or as needed. Do not exceed 12 tablets in 24 hours.

Pediatric patients 2 to under 12 years of age: ½ to 1 tablet every four hours or as needed. Do not exceed 6 tablets in 24 hours.

HOW SUPPLIED

NuLev™ (hyoscyamine sulfate orally disintegrating tablets) 0.125 mg are white, mint-flavored, round and imprinted with SP and 111.

Bottles of 100 tablets NDC 0091-3111-01

Store at 25°C (77°F); excursions permitted to 15–30°C (59–86°F).

Protect from moisture.

Dispense in tight, light-resistant container as defined in USP.

Manufactured for

SCHWARZ PHARMA

Milwaukee, Wisconsin 53201

By:

CIMA™

Eden Prairie, MN 55344

NuLev™ uses CIMA's DuraSolv™ technology.

Patent No. 6,024,981

Printed in USA

PC4205 7/2000

Watson Laboratories, Inc.

311 BONNIE CIRCLE
CORONA, CA 92880

Direct Inquiries to:
Customer Service Department
Telephone: 800/272-5525
FAX: 909/735-2871
For Medical Information Contact:
Telephone: 800/272-5525

Maxidone™ TABLETS Ⓒ℞

Rx only

DESCRIPTION

Maxidone™ (Hydrocodone bitartrate and acetaminophen) is supplied in tablet form for oral administration.

Hydrocodone bitartrate is an opioid analgesic and antitussive and occurs as fine, white crystals or as a crystalline powder. It is affected by light. The chemical name is 4,5α-epoxy-3-methoxy-17-methylmorphinan-6-one tartrate (1:1) hydrate (2:5). It has the following structural formula:

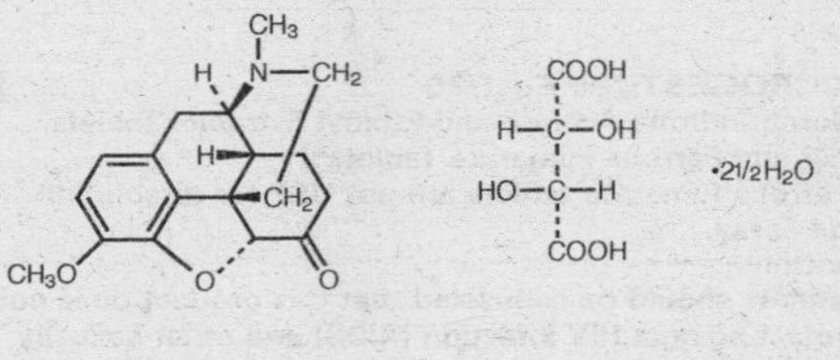

$C_{18}H_{21}NO_3 \cdot C_4H_6O_6 \cdot 2\frac{1}{2}H_2O$ MW=494.50

Acetaminophen, 4[1]-hydroxyacetanilide, a slightly bitter, white, odorless, crystalline powder, is a non-opiate, non-salicylate analgesic and antipyretic. It has the following structural formula:

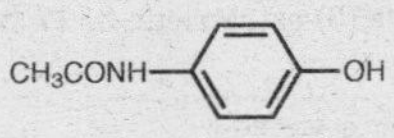

$C_8H_9NO_2$ MW=151.17

Each Maxidone™ tablet contains:

Hydrocodone Bitartrate	10 mg
Acetaminophen	750 mg

In addition, each tablet contains the following inactive ingredients: anhydrous lactose, croscarmellose sodium, crospovidone, magnesium stearate, microcrystalline cellulose, povidone, pregelatinized starch, stearic acid, and D&C Yellow #10 Alluminum Lake.

CLINICAL PHARMACOLOGY

Hydrocodone is a semisynthetic narcotic analgesic and antitussive with multiple actions qualitatively similar to those of codeine. Most of these involve the central nervous system and smooth muscle. The precise mechanism of action of hydrocodone and other opiates is not known, although it is believed to relate to the existence of opiate receptors in the central nervous system. In addition to analgesia, narcotics may produce drowsiness, changes in mood and mental clouding.

The analgesic action of acetaminophen involves peripheral influences, but the specific mechanism is as yet undetermined. Antipyretic activity is mediated through hypothalamic heat regulating centers. Acetaminophen inhibits prostaglandin synthetase. Therapeutic doses of acetaminophen have negligible effects on the cardiovascular or respiratory systems; however, toxic doses may cause circulatory failure and rapid, shallow breathing.

Pharmacokinetics: The behavior of the individual components is described below.

Hydrocodone: Following a 10 mg oral dose of hydrocodone administered to five adult male subjects, the mean peak concentration was 23.6 ± 5.2 ng/mL. Maximum serum levels were achieved at 1.3 ± 0.3 hours and the half-life was determined to be 3.8 ± 0.3 hours. Hydrocodone exhibits a complex pattern of metabolism including O-demethylation, N-demethylation and 6-keto reduction to the corresponding 6-α- and 6-β-hydroxymetabolites.

See **OVERDOSAGE** for toxicity information.

Acetaminophen: Acetaminophen is rapidly absorbed from the gastrointestinal tract and is distributed throughout most body tissues. The plasma half-life is 1.25 to 3 hours, but may be increased by liver damage and following overdosage. Elimination of acetaminophen is principally by liver metabolism (conjugation) and subsequent renal excretion of metabolites. Approximately 85% of an oral dose appears in the urine within 24 hours of administration, most as the glucuronide conjugate, with small amounts of other conjugates and unchanged drug.

See **OVERDOSAGE** for toxicity information.

INDICATIONS AND USAGE

Maxidone™ Tablets are indicated for the relief of moderate to moderately severe pain.

CONTRAINDICATIONS

Maxidone™ Tablets should not be administered to patients who have previously exhibited hypersensitivity to hydrocodone or acetaminophen.

WARNINGS

Respiratory Depression: At high doses or in sensitive patients, hydrocodone may produce dose-related respiratory depression by acting directly on the brain stem respiratory center. Hydrocodone also affects the center that controls respiratory rhythm, and may produce irregular and periodic breathing.

Head Injury and Increased Intracranial Pressure: The respiratory depressant effects of narcotics and their capacity to elevate cerebrospinal fluid pressure may be markedly exaggerated in the presence of head injury, other intracranial lesions or a pre-existing increase in intracranial pressure. Furthermore, narcotics produce adverse reactions which may obscure the clinical course of patients with head injuries.

Acute Abdominal Conditions: The administration of narcotics may obscure the diagnosis or clinical course of patients with acute abdominal conditions.

PRECAUTIONS

General: Special Risk Patients: As with any narcotic analgesic agent, Maxidone™ Tablets should be used with caution in elderly or debilitated patients, and those with severe impairment of hepatic or renal function, hypothyroidism, Addison's disease, prostatic hypertrophy or urethral stricture. The usual precautions should be observed and the possibility of respiratory depression should be kept in mind.

Cough reflex: Hydrocodone suppresses the cough reflex; as with all narcotics, caution should be exercised when Maxidone™ Tablets are used postoperatively and in patients with pulmonary disease.

Information for Patients: Maxidone™ Tablets, like all narcotics, may impair mental and/or physical abilities required for the performance of potentially hazardous tasks such as driving a car or operating machinery; patients should be cautioned accordingly.

Alcohol and other CNS depressants may produce an additive CNS depression, when taken with this combination product, and should be avoided.

Hydrocodone may be habit-forming. Patients should take the drug only for as long as it is prescribed, in the amounts prescribed, and no more frequently than prescribed.

Laboratory Tests: In patients with severe hepatic or renal disease, effects of therapy should be monitored with serial liver and/or renal function tests.

Drug Interactions: Patients receiving narcotics, antihistamines, antipsychotics, antianxiety agents, or other CNS depressants (including alcohol) concomitantly with Maxidone™ Tablets may exhibit an additive CNS depression. When combined therapy is contemplated, the dose of one or both agents should be reduced.

The use of MAO inhibitors or tricyclic antidepressants with hydrocodone preparations may increase the effect of either the antidepressant or hydrocodone.

Drug/Laboratory Test Interactions: Acetaminophen may produce false-positive test results for urinary 5-hydroxyindoleacetic acid.

Carcinogenesis, Mutagenesis, Impairment of Fertility: No adequate studies have been conducted in animals to determine whether hydrocodone or acetaminophen have a potential for carcinogenesis, mutagenesis, or impairment of fertility.

Pregnancy:

Teratogenic Effects: Pregnancy Category C: There are no adequate and well-controlled studies in pregnant women. Maxidone™ Tablets should be used during pregnancy only it the potential benefit justifies the potential risk to the fetus.

Nonteratogenic Effects: Babies born to mothers who have been taking opioids regularly prior to deliver will be physically dependent. The withdrawal signs include irritability and excessive crying, tremors, hyperactive reflexes, increased respiratory rate, increased stools, sneezing, yawning, vomiting and fever. The intensity of the syndrome does

Continued on next page

Maxidone—Cont.

not always correlate with the duration of maternal opioid use or dose. There is no consensus on the best method of managing withdrawal.

Labor and Delivery: As with all narcotics, administration of Maxidone™ Tablets to the mother shortly before delivery may result in some degree of respiratory depression in the newborn, especially if higher doses are used.

Nursing Mothers: Acetaminophen is excreted in breast milk in small amounts, but the significance of its effects on nursing infants is not known. It is not known whether hydrocodone is excreted in human milk. Because many drugs are excreted in human milk and because of the potential for serious adverse reactions in nursing infants from Maxidone™ Tablets, a decision should be made whether to discontinue nursing or to discontinue the drug, taking into account the importance of the drug to the mother.

Pediatric Use: Safety and effectiveness in pediatric patients have not been established.

ADVERSE REACTIONS

The most frequently reported adverse reactions are lightheadedness, dizziness, sedation, nausea and vomiting. These effects seem to be more prominent in ambulatory than in nonambulatory patients, and some of these adverse reactions may be alleviated if the patient lies down.

Other adverse reactions include:

Central Nervous System: Drowsiness, mental clouding, lethargy, impairment of mental and physical performance, anxiety, fear, dysphoria, psychic dependence, mood changes.

Gastrointestinal System: Prolonged administration of Maxidone™ Tablets may produce constipation.

Genitourinary System: Ureteral spasm, spasm of vesical sphincters and urinary retention have been reported with opiates.

Respiratory Depression: Hydrocodone bitartrate may produce dose-related respiratory depression by acting directly on brain stem respiratory centers (see **OVERDOSAGE**).

Dermatological: Skin rash, pruritus.

The following adverse drug events may be borne in mind as potential effects of acetaminophen: allergic reactions, rash, thrombocytopenia, agranulocytosis.

Potential effects of high dosage are listed in the **OVERDOSAGE** section.

DRUG ABUSE AND DEPENDENCE

Controlled Substance: Maxidone™ Tablets are classified as a Schedule III controlled substance.

Abuse and Dependence: Psychic dependence, physical dependence, and tolerance may develop upon repeated administration of narcotics; therefore, Maxidone™ Tablets should be prescribed and administered with caution. However, psychic dependence is unlikely to develop when Maxidone™ Tablets are used for a short time for the treatment of pain.

Physical dependence, the condition in which continued administration of the drug is required to prevent the appearance of a withdrawal syndrome, assumes clinically significant proportions only after several weeks, of continued narcotic use, although some mild degree of physical dependence may develop after a few days of narcotic therapy. Tolerance, in which increasingly large doses are required in order to produce the same degree of analgesia, is manifested initially by a shortened duration of analgesic effect, and subsequently by decreases in the intensity of analgesia. The rate of development of tolerance varies among patients.

OVERDOSAGE

Following an acute overdosage, toxicity may result from hydrocodone or acetaminophen.

Signs and Symptoms

Hydrocodone: Serious overdose with hydrocodone is characterized by respiratory depression (a decrease in respiratory rate and/or tidal volume, Cheyne-Stokes respiration, cyanosis), extreme somnolence progressing to stupor or coma, skeletal muscle flaccidity, cold and clammy skin, and sometimes bradycardia and hypotension. In severe overdosage, apnea, circulatory collapse, cardiac arrest and death may occur.

Acetaminophen: In acetaminophen overdosage: dose-dependent, potentially fatal hepatic necrosis is the most serious adverse effect. Renal tubular necrosis, hypoglycemic coma and thrombocytopenia may also occur.

F[illegible]ptoms following a potentially hepatotoxic over-[illegible] include: nausea, vomiting, diaphoresis and gen-[illegible]aise. Clinical and laboratory evidence of hepatic toxicity may not be apparent until 48 to 72 hours post-ingestion.

In adults, hepatic toxicity has rarely been reported with acute overdoses of less than 10 grams, or fatalities with less than 15 grams.

Treatment: A single or multiple overdose with hydrocodone and acetaminophen is a potentially lethal polydrug overdose, and consultation with a regional poison control center is recommended.

Immediate treatment includes support of cardiorespiratory function and measures to reduce drug absorption. Vomiting should be induced mechanically, or with syrup of ipecac, if the patient is alert (adequate pharyngeal and laryngeal reflexes). Oral activated charcoal (1 g/kg) should follow gastric emptying. The first dose should be accompanied by an appropriate cathartic. If repeated doses are used, the cathartic might be included with alternate doses as required. Hypotension is usually hypovolemic and should respond to fluids. Vasopressors and other supportive measures should be employed as indicated. A cuffed endo-tracheal tube should be inserted before gastric lavage of the unconscious patient and, when necessary, to provide assisted respiration.

Meticulous attention should be given to maintaining adequate pulmonary ventilation. In severe cases of intoxication, peritoneal dialysis, or preferably hemodialysis may be considered. If hypoprothrombinemia occurs due to acetaminophen overdose, vitamin K should be administered intravenously

Naloxone, a narcotic antagonist, can reverse respiratory depression and coma associated with opioid overdose. Naloxone hydrochloride 0.4 mg to 2 mg is given parenterally. Since the duration of action of hydrocodone may exceed that of the naloxone, the patient should be kept under continuous surveillance and repeated doses of the antagonist should be administered as needed to maintain adequate respiration. A narcotic antagonist should not be administered in the absence of clinically significant respiratory or cardiovascular depression.

If the dose of acetaminophen may have exceeded 140 mg/kg, acetylcysteine should be administered as early as possible. Serum acetaminophen levels should be obtained, since levels four or more hours following ingestion help predict acetaminophen toxicity. Do not await acetaminophen assay results before initiating treatment. Hepatic enzymes should be obtained initially, and repeated at 24-hour intervals.

Methemoglobinemia over 30% should be treated with methylene blue by slow intravenous administration.

The toxic dose for adults for acetaminophen is 10 g.

DOSAGE AND ADMINISTRATION

Dosage should be adjusted according to the severity of the pain and the response of the patient. However, it should be kept in mind that tolerance to hydrocodone can develop with continued use and that the incidence of untoward effects is dose related.

The usual adult dosage is one tablet every four to six hours as needed for pain. The total daily dose should not exceed 5 tablets.

HOW SUPPLIED

Maxidone™ is supplied as a yellow, capsule-shaped tablet containing 10 mg hydrocodone bitartrate and 750 mg acetaminophen, bisected on one side and debossed with "Maxidone 634" on the other side.

Bottles of 100	NDC 52544-634-01
Bottles of 500	NDC 52544-634-05

Store at controlled room temperature, 15°C to 30°C (59°F to 86°F).

Dispense in a tight, light-resistant container with a child-resistant closure.

Rx only

WATSON PHARMA, INC. 13790
a subsidiary of Watson Laboratories, Inc.
Revised May 1999
Corona, CA 92880

MICROGESTIN™ Fe 1/20 ℞

(Norethindrone Acetate and Ethinyl Estradiol Tablets, USP and Ferrous Fumarate Tablets*)

***Ferrous fumarate tablets are not USP for dissolution and assay.**

Rx Only

Patients should be counseled that this product does not protect against HIV infection (AIDS) and other sexually transmitted diseases.

DESCRIPTION

Microgestin Fe 1/20 is a progestogen-estrogen combination. The structural formula of norethindrone acetate (17 alpha-ethinyl-19-nortestosterone acetate) and ethinyl estradiol (17 alpha-ethinyl-1, 3, 5(10)-estratriene-3, 17 beta-diol) are as follows:

Norethindrone Acetate

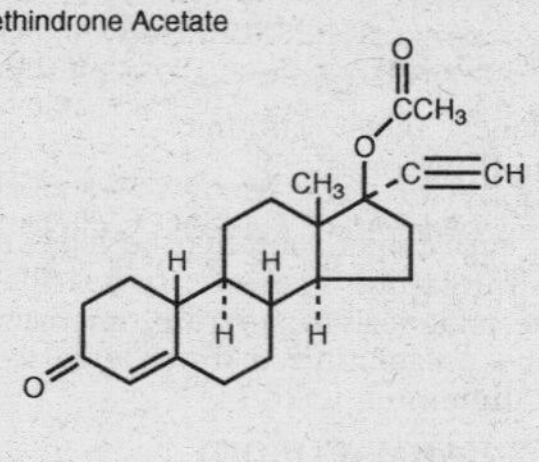

$C_{22}H_{28}O_3$ MW=340.46

Ethinyl Estradiol

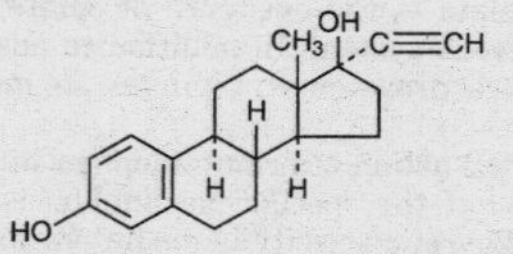

$C_{20}H_{24}O_2$ MW=296.40

Microgestin Fe 1/20 provides a continuous dosage regimen consisting of 21 white oral contraceptive tablets and 7 brown ferrous fumarate tablets. The ferrous fumarate tablets are present to facilitate ease of drug administration via a 28-day regimen, are non-hormonal, and do not serve any therapeutic purpose.

Each white tablet, for oral administration, contains 1 mg norethindrone acetate and 20 mcg ethinyl estradiol. It also contains the following inactive ingredients: anhydrous lactose, ethyl alcohol, magnesium stearate, microcrystalline cellulose, polacrilin potassium, and povidone.

Each brown tablet for oral administration contains 75 mg ferrous fumarate and anhydrous lactose, crospovidone, magnesium stearate, and pregelatinized starch.

CLINICAL PHARMACOLOGY

Combination oral contraceptives act by suppression of gonadotropins. Although the primary mechanism of this action is inhibition of ovulation, other alterations include changes in the cervical mucus (which increase the difficulty of sperm entry into the uterus) and the endometrium (which reduce the likelihood of implantation).

Pharmacokinetics

The pharmacokinetics of norethindrone acetate and ethinyl estradiol have not been characterized; however, the following pharmacokinetic information regarding norethindrone acetate and ethinyl estradiol is taken from the literature.

Absorption

Norethindrone acetate appears to be completely and rapidly deacetylated to norethindrone after oral administration, since the disposition of norethindrone acetate is indistinguishable from that of orally administered norethindrone (1). Norethindrone acetate and ethinyl estradiol are subject to first-pass metabolism after oral dosing, resulting in an absolute bioavailability of approximately 64% for norethindrone and 43% for ethinyl estradiol (1–3).

Distribution

Volume of distribution of norethindrone and ethinyl estradiol ranges from 2 to 4 L/kg (1–3). Plasma protein binding of both steroids is extensive (>95%); norethindrone binds to both albumin and sex hormone binding globulin, whereas ethinyl estradiol binds only to albumin (4).

Metabolism

Norethindrone undergoes extensive biotransformation, primarily via reduction, followed by sulfate and glucuronide conjugation. The majority of metabolites in the circulation are sulfates, with glucuronides accounting for most of the urinary metabolites (5). A small amount of norethindrone acetate is metabolically converted to ethinyl estradiol. Ethinyl estradiol is also extensively metabolized, both by oxidation and by conjugation with sulfate and glucuronide. Sulfates are the major circulating conjugates of ethinyl estradiol and glucuronides predominate in urine. The primary oxidative metabolite is 2-hydroxy ethinyl estradiol, formed by the CYP3A4 isoform of cytochrome P450. Part of the first-pass metabolism of ethinyl estradiol is believed to occur in gastrointestinal mucosa. Ethinyl estradiol may undergo enterohepatic circulation (6).

Excretion

Norethindrone and ethinyl estradiol are excreted in both urine and feces, primarily as metabolites (5,6). Plasma clearance values for norethindrone and ethinyl estradiol are similar (approximately 0.4 L/hr/kg) (1–3).

Special Population

Race:

The effect of race on the disposition of norethindrone acetate and ethinyl estradiol has not been evaluated.

Renal Insufficiency

The effect of renal disease on the disposition of norethindrone acetate and ethinyl estradiol has not been evaluated. In premenopausal women with chronic renal failure undergoing peritoneal dialysis who received multiple doses of an oral contraceptive containing ethinyl estradiol and norethindrone, plasma ethinyl estradiol concentrations were higher and norethindrone concentrations were unchanged compared to concentrations in premenopausal women with normal renal function.

Hepatic Insufficiency

The effect of hepatic disease on the disposition of norethindrone acetate and ethinyl estradiol has not been evaluated. However, ethinyl estradiol and norethindrone may be poorly metabolized in patients with impaired liver function.

Drug-Drug Interactions

Numerous drug-drug interactions have been reported for oral contraceptives. A summary of these is found under **PRECAUTIONS, Drug Interactions.**

INDICATIONS AND USAGE

Microgestin Fe 1/20 is indicated for the prevention of pregnancy in women who elect to use oral contraceptives as a method of contraception.

Oral contraceptives are highly effective. Table I lists the typical accidental pregnancy rates for users of combination oral contraceptives and other methods of contraception. The efficacy of these contraceptive methods, except sterilization, depends upon the reliability with which they are used. Correct and consistent use of methods can result in lower failure rates.

Table I
LOWEST EXPECTED AND TYPICAL FAILURE RATES DURING THE FIRST YEAR OF CONTINUOUS USE OF A METHOD
% of Women Experiencing An Unintended Pregnancy in the First Year Of Continuous Use.

Method	Lowest Expected*	Typical**
(No contraception)	(85)	(85)
Oral contraceptives	—	3
combined	0.1	N/A***
progestin only	0.5	N/A***

Diaphragm with spermicidal cream or jelly	6	20
Spermicides alone (foam, creams, gels, and vaginal suppositories, and vaginal film)	6	26
Vaginal Sponge		
nulliparous	9	20
parous	20	40
Implant	0.05	0.05
Injection:		
depot medroxyprogesterone acetate	0.3	0.3
IUD		
progesterone T	1.5	2.0
copper T 380A	0.6	0.8
LNg 20	0.1	0.1
Condom without spermicides		
female	5	21
male	3	14
Cervical Cap with spermicidal cream or jelly		
nulliparous	9	20
parous	26	40
Periodic abstinence		
(all methods)	1–9	25
Withdrawal	4	19
Female sterilization	0.5	0.5
Male sterilization	0.10	0.15

Adapted from R.A. Hatcher et al. Reference 7

*The authors' best guess of the percentage of women expected to experience an accidental pregnancy among couples who initiate a method (not necessarily for the first time) and who use it consistently and correctly during the first year if they do not stop for any other reason.

**This term represents "typical" couples who initiate use of a method (not necessarily for the first time), who experience an accidental pregnancy during the first year if they do not stop for any other reason.

*** N/A—Data not available

CONTRAINDICATIONS

Oral contraceptives should not be used in women who currently have the following conditions:
• Thrombophlebitis or thromboembolic disorders
• A past history of deep vein thrombophlebitis or thromboembolic disorders
• Cerebral vascular or coronary artery disease
• Known or suspected carcinoma of the breast
• Carcinoma of the endometrium or other known or suspected estrogen-dependent neoplasia
• Undiagnosed abnormal genital bleeding
• Cholestatic jaundice of pregnancy or jaundice with prior pill use
• Hepatic adenomas or carcinomas
• Known or suspected pregnancy

WARNINGS

Cigarette smoking increases the risk of serious cardiovascular side effects from oral contraceptive use. This risk increases with age and with heavy smoking (15 or more cigarettes per day) and is quite marked in women over 35 years of age. Women who use oral contraceptives should be strongly advised not to smoke.

The use of oral contraceptives is associated with increased risks of several serious conditions including myocardial infarction, thromboembolism, stroke, hepatic neoplasia, and gallbladder disease, although the risk of serious morbidity or mortality is very small in healthy women without underlying risk factors. The risk of morbidity and mortality increases significantly in the presence of other underlying risk factors such as hypertension, hyperlipidemias, obesity, and diabetes.

Practitioners prescribing oral contraceptives should be familiar with the following information relating to these risks. The information contained in this package insert is principally based on studies carried out in patients who used oral contraceptives with higher formulations of estrogens and progestogens than those in common use today. The effect of long-term use of the oral contraceptives with lower formulations of both estrogens and progestogens remains to be determined.

Throughout this labeling, epidemiological studies reported are of two types: retrospective or case control studies and prospective or cohort studies. Case control studies provide a measure of the relative risk of a disease, namely, a *ratio* of the incidence of a disease among oral contraceptive users to that among nonusers. The relative risk does not provide information on the actual clinical occurrence of a disease. Cohort studies provide a measure of attributable risk, which is the *difference* in the incidence of disease between oral contraceptive users and nonusers. The attributable risk does provide information about the actual occurrence of a disease in the population (adapted from References 8 and 9 with the authors permission). For further information, the reader is referred to a text on epidemiological methods.

1. Thromboembolic Disorders and Other Vascular Problems

a. Myocardial Infarction

An increased risk of myocardial infarction has been attributed to oral contraceptive use. This risk is primarily in smokers or women with other underlying risk factors for coronary artery disease such as hypertension, hypercholesterolemia, morbid obesity, and diabetes. The relative risk of heart attack for current oral contraceptive users has been estimated to be two to six (10–16). The risk is very low under the age of 30.

Smoking in combination with oral contraceptive use has been shown to contribute substantially to the incidence of myocardial infarctions in women in their mid-thirties or older with smoking accounting for the majority of excess cases (17). Mortality rates associated with circulatory disease have been shown to increase substantially in smokers over the age of 35 and non-smokers over the age of 40 (Table II) among women who use oral contraceptives.

TABLE II
CIRCULATORY DISEASE MORTALITY RATES PER 100,000 WOMEN YEARS BY AGE, SMOKING STATUS AND ORAL CONTRACEPTIVE USE

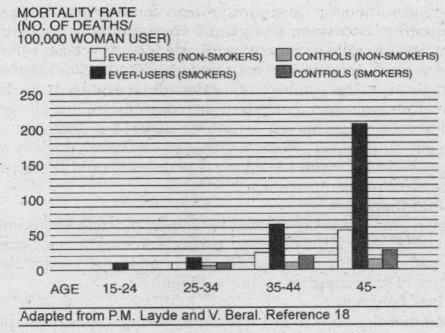

Adapted from P.M. Layde and V. Beral. Reference 18

Oral contraceptives may compound the effects of well-known risk factors, such as hypertension, diabetes, hyperlipidemias, age and obesity (19). In particular, some progestogens are known to decrease HDL cholesterol and cause glucose intolerance, while estrogens may create a state of hyperinsulinism (20-24). Oral contraceptives have been shown to increase blood pressure among users (see section 9 in WARNINGS). Similar effects on risk factors have been associated with an increased risk of heart disease. Oral contraceptives must be used with caution in women with cardiovascular disease risk factors.

b. Thromboembolism

An increased risk of thromboembolic and thrombotic disease associated with the use of oral contraceptives is well established. Case control studies have found the relative risk of users compared to nonusers to be 3 for the first episode of superficial venous thrombosis, 4 to 11 for deep vein thrombosis or pulmonary embolism, and 1.5 to 6 for women with predisposing conditions for venous thromboembolic disease (9, 10, 25–30). Cohort studies have shown the relative risk to be somewhat lower, about 3 for new cases and about 4.5 for new cases requiring hospitalization (31). The risk of thromboembolic disease due to oral contraceptives is not related to length of use and disappears after pill use is stopped (8).

A two- to four-fold increase in relative risk of postoperative thromboembolic complications has been reported with the use of oral contraceptives (15,32). The relative risk of venous thrombosis in women who have predisposing conditions is twice that of women without such medical conditions (15,32). If feasible, oral contraceptives should be discontinued at least four weeks prior to and for two weeks after elective surgery of a type associated with an increase in risk of thromboembolism and during and following prolonged immobilization. Since the immediate post-partum period is also associated with an increased risk of thromboembolism, oral contraceptives should be started no earlier than four to six weeks after delivery in women who elect not to breast feed.

c. Cerebrovascular Disease

Oral contraceptives have been shown to increase both the relative and attributable risks of cerebrovascular events (thrombotic and hemorrhagic strokes), although, in general, the risk is greatest among older (>35 years), hypertensive women who also smoke. Hypertension was found to be a risk factor for both users and non-users, for both types of strokes, while smoking interacted to increase the risk for hemorrhagic strokes (33–35).

In a large study, the relative risk of thrombotic strokes has been shown to range from 3 for normotensive users to 14 for users with severe hypertension (36). The relative risk of hemorrhagic stroke is reported to be 1.2 for non-smokers who used oral contraceptives, 2.6 for smokers who did not use oral contraceptives, 7.6 for smokers who used oral contraceptives, 1.8 for normotensive users and 25.7 for users with severe hypertension (36). The attributable risk is also greater in older women (9).

d. Dose-Related Risk of Vascular Disease from Oral Contraceptives

A positive association has been observed between the amount of estrogen and progestogen in oral contraceptives and the risk of vascular disease (37–39). A decline in serum high-density lipoproteins (HDL) has been reported with many progestational agents (20–22). A decline in serum high-density lipoproteins has been associated with an increased incidence of ischemic heart disease. Because estrogens increase HDL cholesterol, the net effect of an oral contraceptive depends on a balance achieved between doses of estrogen and progestin and the nature of the progestin used in the contraceptives. The amount and activity of both hormones should be considered in the choice of an oral contraceptive.

Minimizing exposure to estrogen and progestogen is in keeping with good principles of therapeutics. For any particular oral contraceptive, the dosage regimen prescribed should be one which contains the least amount of estrogen and progestogen that is compatible with the needs of the individual patient. New acceptors of oral contraceptive agents should be started on preparations containing the lowest dose of estrogen which produces satisfactory results for the patient.

e. Persistence of Risk of Vascular Disease

There are two studies which have shown persistence of risk of vascular disease for ever-users of oral contraceptives. In a study in the United States, the risk of developing myocardial infarction after discontinuing oral contraceptives persists for at least 9 years for women 40 to 49 years who had used oral contraceptives for 5 or more years, but this increased risk was not demonstrated in other age groups (14). In another study in Great Britain, the risk of developing cerebrovascular disease persisted for at least 6 years after discontinuation of oral contraceptives, although excess risk was very small (40). However, both studies were performed with oral contraceptive formulations containing 50 mcg or higher of estrogens.

2. Estimates of Mortality from Contraceptive Use

One study gathered data from a variety of sources which have estimated the mortality rate associated with different methods of contraception at different ages (Table III). These estimates include the combined risk of death associated with contraceptive methods plus the risk attributable to pregnancy in the event of method failure. Each method of contraception has its specific benefits and risks. The study concluded that with the exception of oral contraceptive users 35 and older who smoke and 40 and older who do not smoke, mortality associated with all methods of birth control is low and below that associated with childbirth. The observation of a possible increase in risk of mortality with age for oral contraceptive users is based on data gathered in the 1970s but not reported until 1983 (41). However, current clinical practice involves the use of lower estrogen dose formulations combined with careful restriction of oral contraceptive use to women who do not have the various risk factors listed in this labeling.

Because of these changes in practice and, also, because of some limited new data which suggest that the risk of cardiovascular disease with the use of oral contraceptives may now be less than previously observed (Porter JB, Hunter J, Jick H, et al. Oral contraceptives and nonfatal vascular disease. Obstet Gynecol 1985;66:1–4 and Porter JB, Hershel J, Walker AM. Mortality among oral contraceptive users. Obstet Gynecol 1987;70:29–32), the Fertility and Maternal Health Drugs Advisory Committee was asked to review the topic in 1989. The Committee concluded that although cardiovascular disease risks may be increased with oral contraceptive use after age 40 in healthy non-smoking women (even with the newer low-dose formulations), there are greater potential health risks associated with pregnancy in older women and with the alternative surgical and medical procedures which may be necessary if such women do not have access to effective and acceptable means of contraception.

Therefore, the Committee recommended that the benefits of oral contraceptive use by healthy non-smoking women over 40 may outweigh the possible risks. Of course, older women, as all women who take oral contraceptives, should take the lowest possible dose formulation that is effective.
[See table III at top of next page]

3. Carcinoma of the Reproductive Organs

Numerous epidemiological studies have been performed on the incidence of breast, endometrial, ovarian, and cervical cancer in women using oral contraceptives. Most of the studies on breast cancer and oral contraceptive use report that the use of oral contraceptives is not associated with an increase in the risk of developing breast cancer (42,44,89). Some studies have reported an increased risk of developing breast cancer in certain subgroups of oral contraceptive users, but the findings reported in these studies are not consistent (43,45–49,85–88).

Some studies suggest that oral contraceptive use has been associated with an increase in the risk of cervical intraepithelial neoplasia in some populations of women (51–54). However, there continues to be controversy about the extent to which such findings may be due to differences in sexual behavior and other factors.

In spite of many studies of the relationship between oral contraceptive use and breast and cervical cancers, a cause and effect relationship has not been established.

4. Hepatic Neoplasia

Benign hepatic adenomas are associated with oral contraceptive use, although the incidence of benign tumors is rare in the United States. Indirect calculations have estimated the attributable risk to be in the range of 3.3 cases/100,000 for users, a risk that increases after four or more years of use (55). Rupture of rare, benign, hepatic adenomas may cause death through intra-abdominal hemorrhage (56,57). Studies from Britain have shown an increased risk of developing hepatocellular carcinoma (58–60) in long-term

Continued on next page

Microgestin Fe 1/20—Cont.

(>8 years) oral contraceptive users. However, these cancers are extremely rare in the U.S., and the attributable risk (the excess incidence) of liver cancers in oral contraceptive users approaches less than one per million users.

5. Ocular Lesions
There have been clinical case reports of retinal thrombosis associated with the use of oral contraceptives. Oral contraceptives should be discontinued if there is unexplained partial or complete loss of vision; onset of proptosis or diplopia; papilledema; or retinal vascular lesions. Appropriate diagnostic and therapeutic measures should be undertaken immediately.

6. Oral Contraceptive Use Before and During Early Pregnancy
Extensive epidemiological studies have revealed no increased risk of birth defects in women who have used oral contraceptives prior to pregnancy (61-63). Studies also do not suggest a teratogenic effect, particularly insofar as cardiac anomalies and limb reduction defects are concerned (61,62,64,65), when taken inadvertently during early pregnancy.
The administration of oral contraceptives to induce withdrawal bleeding should not be used as a test for pregnancy. Oral contraceptives should not be used during pregnancy to treat threatened or habitual abortion.
It is recommended that for any patient who has missed two consecutive periods, pregnancy should be ruled out before continuing oral contraceptive use. If the patient has not adhered to the prescribed schedule, the possibility of pregnancy should be considered at the time of the first missed period. Oral contraceptive use should be discontinued if pregnancy is confirmed.

7. Gallbladder Disease
Earlier studies have reported an increased lifetime relative risk of gallbladder surgery in users of oral contraceptives and estrogens (66,67). More recent studies, however, have shown that the relative risk of developing gallbladder disease among oral contraceptive users may be minimal (68–70). The recent findings of minimal risk may be related to the use of oral contraceptive formulations containing lower hormonal doses of estrogens and progestogens.

8. Carbohydrate and Lipid Metabolic Effects
Oral contraceptives have been shown to cause glucose intolerance in a significant percentage of users (23). Oral contraceptives containing greater than 75 mcg of estrogens cause hyperinsulinism, while lower doses of estrogen cause less glucose intolerance (71). Progestogens increase insulin secretion and create insulin resistance, this effect varying with different progestational agents (23,72). However, in the non-diabetic woman, oral contraceptives appear to have no effect on fasting blood glucose (73). Because of these demonstrated effects, prediabetic and diabetic women should be carefully observed while taking oral contraceptives.
A small proportion of women will have persistent hypertriglyceridemia while on the pill. As discussed earlier (see WARNINGS 1a. and 1d.), changes in serum triglycerides and lipoprotein levels have been reported in oral contraceptive users.

9. Elevated Blood Pressure
An increase in blood pressure has been reported in women taking oral contraceptives (74) and this increase is more likely in older oral contraceptive users (75) and with continued use (74). Data from the Royal College of General Practitioners (18) and subsequent randomized trials have shown that the incidence of hypertension increases with increasing concentrations of progestogens.
Women with a history of hypertension or hypertension-related diseases, or renal disease (76) should be encouraged to use another method of contraception. If women elect to use oral contraceptives, they should be monitored closely and if significant elevation of blood pressure occurs, oral contraceptives should be discontinued. For most women, elevated blood pressure will return to normal after stopping oral contraceptives (75), and there is no difference in the occurrence of hypertension among ever and never users (74,76,77).

10. Headache
The onset or exacerbation of migraine or development of headache with a new pattern which is recurrent, persistent, or severe requires discontinuation of oral contraceptives and evaluation of the cause.

11. Bleeding Irregularities
Breakthrough bleeding and spotting are sometimes encountered in patients on oral contraceptives, especially during the first three months of use. Non-hormonal causes should be considered, and adequate diagnostic measures taken to rule out malignancy or pregnancy in the event of breakthrough bleeding, as in the case of any abnormal vaginal bleeding. If pathology has been excluded, time or a change to another formulation may solve the problem. In the event of amenorrhea, pregnancy should be ruled out.
Some women may encounter post-pill amenorrhea or oligomenorrhea, especially when such a condition was preexistent.

TABLE III
ANNUAL NUMBER OF BIRTH-RELATED OR METHOD-RELATED DEATHS ASSOCIATED WITH CONTROL OF FERTILITY PER 100,000 NONSTERILE WOMEN, BY FERTILITY CONTROL METHOD ACORDING TO AGE

Method of control and outocme	15–19	20–24	25–29	30–34	35–39	40–44
No fertility control methods*	7.0	7.4	9.1	14.8	25.7	28.2
Oral contraceptives nonsmoker**	0.3	0.5	0.9	1.9	13.8	31.6
Oral contraceptives smoker**	2.2	3.4	6.6	13.5	51.1	117.2
IUD**	0.8	0.8	1.0	1.0	1.4	1.4
Condom*	1.1	1.6	0.7	0.2	0.3	0.4
Diaphragm/spermicide*	1.9	1.2	1.2	1.3	2.2	2.8
Periodic abstinence*	2.5	1.6	1.6	1.7	2.9	3.6

* Deaths are birth related
** Deaths are method related

Adapted from H.W. Ory. Reference 41

PRECAUTIONS

1. Patients should be counseled that this product does not protect against HIV infection (AIDS) and other sexually transmitted diseases.

2. Physical Examination and Follow-Up
It is good medical practice for all women to have annual history and physical examinations, including women using oral contraceptives. The physical examination, however, may be deferred until after initiation of oral contraceptives if requested by the woman and judged appropriate by the clinician. The physical examination should include special reference to blood pressure, breasts, abdomen, and pelvic organs, including cervical cytology, and relevant laboratory tests. In case of undiagnosed, persistent or recurrent abnormal vaginal bleeding, appropriate measures should be conducted to rule out malignancy. Women with a strong family history of breast cancer or who have breast nodules should be monitored with particular care.

3. Lipid Disorders
Women who are being treated for hyperlipidemia should be followed closely if they elect to use oral contraceptives. Some progestogens may elevate LDL levels and may render the control of hyperlipidemias more difficult.

4. Liver Function
If jaundice develops in any woman receiving such drugs, the medication should be discontinued. Steroid hormones may be poorly metabolized in patients with impaired liver function.

5. Fluid Retention
Oral contraceptives may cause some degree of fluid retention. They should be prescribed with caution, and only with careful monitoring, in patients with conditions which might be aggravated by fluid retention.

6. Emotional Disorders
Women with a history of depression should be carefully observed and the drug discontinued if depression recurs to a serious degree.

7. Contact Lenses
Contact lens wearers who develop visual changes or changes in lens tolerance should be assessed by an ophthalmologist.

8. Drug Interactions
Effects of Other Drugs on Oral Contraceptives (78)
Rifampin: Metabolism of both norethindrone and ethinyl estradiol is increased by rifampin. A reduction in contraceptive effectiveness and increased incidence of breakthrough bleeding and menstrual irregularities have been associated with concomitant use of rifampin.
Anticonvulsants: Anticonvulsants such as phenobarbital, phenytoin, and carbamazepine, have been shown to increase the metabolism of ethinyl estradiol and/or norethindrone, which could result in a reduction in contraceptive effectiveness.
Troglitazone: Administration of troglitazone with an oral contraceptive containing ethinyl estradiol and norethindrone reduced the plasma concentrations of both by approximately 30%, which could result in a reduction of contraceptive effectiveness.
Antibiotics: Pregnancy while taking oral contraceptives has been reported when the oral contraceptives were administered with antimicrobials such as ampicillin, tetracycline, and griseofulvin. However, clinical pharmacokinetic studies have not demonstrated any consistent effect of antibiotics (other than rifampin) on plasma concentrations of synthetic steroids.
Atorvastatin: Coadministration of atorvastatin and an oral contraceptive increased AUC values for norethindrone and ethinyl estradiol by approximately 30% and 20%, respectively.
Other: Ascorbic acid and acetaminophen may increase plasma ethinyl estradiol concentrations, possibly by inhibition of conjugation. A reduction in contraceptive effectiveness and increased incidence of breakthrough bleeding has been suggested with phenylbutazone.
Effects of Oral Contraceptives on Other Drugs
Oral contraceptive combinations containing ethinyl estradiol may inhibit the metabolism of other compounds. Increased plasma concentrations of cyclosporine, prednisolone, and theophylline have been reported with concomitant administration of oral contraceptives. In addition, oral contraceptives may induce the conjugation of other compounds. Decreased plasma concentrations of acetaminophen and increased clearance of temazepam, salicylic acid, morphine, and clofibric acid have been noted when these drugs were administered with oral contraceptives.

9. Interactions With Laboratory Tests
Certain endocrine and liver function tests and blood components may be affected by oral contraceptives:

a. Increased prothrombin and factors VII, VIII, IX and X; decreased antithrombin 3; increased norepinephrine-induced platelet aggregability.
b. Increased thyroid binding globulin (TBG) leading to increased circulating total thyroid hormone, as measured by protein-bound iodine (PBI), T_4 by column or by radioimmunoassay. Free T_3 resin uptake is decreased, reflecting the elevated TBG; free T_4 concentration is unaltered.
c. Other binding proteins may be elevated in serum.
d. Sex-binding globulins are increased and result in elevated levels of total circulating sex steroids and corticoids; however, free or biologically active levels remain unchanged.
e. Triglycerides may be increased.
f. Glucose tolerance may be decreased.
g. Serum folate levels may be depressed by oral contraceptive therapy. This may be of clinical significance if a woman becomes pregnant shortly after discontinuing oral contraceptives.

10. Carcinogenesis
See **WARNINGS** section.

11. Pregnancy
Pregnancy Category X.
See **CONTRAINDICATIONS** and **WARNINGS** sections.

12. Nursing Mothers
Small amounts of oral contraceptive steroids have been identified in the milk of nursing mothers, and a few adverse effects on the child have been reported, including jaundice and breast enlargement. In addition, oral contraceptives given in the postpartum period may interfere with lactation by decreasing the quantity and quality of breast milk. If possible, the nursing mother should be advised not to use oral contraceptives but to use other forms of contraception until she has completely weaned her child.

13. Pediatric Use
Safety and efficacy of norethindrone acetate and ethinyl estradiol has been established in women of reproductive age. Safety and efficacy are expected to be the same for postpubertal adolescents under the age of 16 and for users 16 years and older. Use of this product before menarche is not indicated.

INFORMATION FOR THE PATIENT
See patient labeling printed below.

ADVERSE REACTIONS

An increased risk of the following serious adverse reactions has been associated with the use of oral contraceptives (see **WARNINGS** section):
- Thrombophlebitis
- Arterial thromboembolism
- Pulmonary embolism
- Myocardial infarction
- Cerebral hemorrhage
- Cerebral thrombosis
- Hypertension
- Gallbladder disease
- Hepatic adenomas or benign liver tumors

There is evidence of an association between the following conditions and the use of oral contraceptives, although additional confirmatory studies are needed:
- Mesenteric thrombosis
- Retinal thrombosis

The following adverse reactions have been reported in patients receiving oral contraceptives and are believed to be drug-related:
- Nausea
- Vomiting
- Gastrointestinal symptoms (such as abdominal cramps and bloating)
- Breakthrough bleeding
- Spotting
- Change in menstrual flow
- Amenorrhea
- Temporary infertility after discontinuation of treatment
- Edema
- Melasma which may persist
- Breast changes: tenderness, enlargement, secretion
- Change in weight (increase or decrease)
- Change in cervical erosion or secretion
- Diminution in lactation when given immediately postpartum
- Cholestatic jaundice
- Migraine
- Rash (allergic)
- Mental depression
- Reduced tolerance to carbohydrates
- Vaginal candidiasis

- Change in corneal curvature (steepening)
- Intolerance to contact lenses

The following adverse reactions have been reported in users of oral contraceptives and the association has been neither confirmed nor refuted:

- Pre-menstrual syndrome
- Cataracts
- Changes in appetite
- Cystitis-like syndrome
- Headache
- Nervousness
- Dizziness
- Hirsutism
- Loss of scalp hair
- Erythema multiforme
- Erythema nodosum
- Hemorrhagic eruption
- Vaginitis
- Porphyria
- Impaired renal function
- Hemolytic uremic syndrome
- Budd-Chiari syndrome
- Acne
- Changes in libido
- Colitis

OVERDOSAGE

Serious ill effects have not been reported following acute ingestion of large doses of oral contraceptives by young children. Overdosage may cause nausea, and withdrawal bleeding may occur in females.

NON-CONTRACEPTIVE HEALTH BENEFITS

The following non-contraceptive health benefits related to the use of oral contraceptives are supported by epidemiological studies which largely utilized oral contraceptive formulations containing estrogen doses exceeding 0.035 mg of ethinyl estradiol or 0.05 mg of mestranol (79–84).

Effects on Menses:
- Increased menstrual cycle regularity
- Decreased blood loss and decreased incidence of iron deficiency anemia
- Decreased incidence of dysmenorrhea

Effects Related to Inhibition of Ovulation:
- Decreased incidence of functional ovarian cysts
- Decreased incidence of ectopic pregnancies

Effects From Long-Term Use:
- Decreased incidence of fibroadenomas and fibrocystic disease of the breast
- Decreased incidence of acute pelvic inflammatory disease
- Decreased incidence of endometrial cancer
- Decreased incidence of ovarian cancer

DOSAGE AND ADMINISTRATION

The tablet dispenser has been designed to make oral contraceptive dosing as easy and as convenient as possible. The tablets are arranged in four rows of seven tablets each, with the days of the week appearing on the tablet dispenser below the last row of tablets.

Important: The patient should be instructed to use an additional method of protection until after the first week of administration in the initial cycle when utilizing the Sunday-Start Regimen.

The possibility of ovulation and conception prior to initiation of use should be considered.

Dosage and Administration for 28-Day Dosage Regimen

To achieve maximum contraceptive effectiveness, Microgestin Fe should be taken exactly as directed and at intervals not exceeding 24 hours.

Microgestin Fe provides a continuous administration regimen consisting of 21 white tablets of Microgestin and 7 brown non-hormone containing tablets of ferrous fumarate. The ferrous fumarate tablets are present to facilitate ease of drug administration via a 28-day regimen and do not serve any therapeutic purpose. There is no need for the patient to count days between cycles because there are no "off-tablet days."

A. Sunday-Start Regimen:

The patient begins taking the first white tablet from the top row of the dispenser (labeled Sunday) on the first Sunday after menstrual flow begins. When menstrual flow begins on Sunday, the first white tablet is taken on the same day. The patient takes one white tablet daily for 21 days. The last white tablet will be taken on a Saturday. Upon completion of all 21 white tablets, and without interruption, the patient takes one brown tablet daily for 7 days. Upon completion of this first course of tablets, the patient begins a second course of 28-day tablets, without interruption, the next day, Sunday, starting with the Sunday white tablet in the top row. Adhering to this regimen of one white tablet daily for 21 days, followed without interruption by one brown tablet daily for 7 days, the patient will start all subsequent cycles on a Sunday.

B. Day-1 Start Regimen:

The first day of menstrual flow is Day 1. The patient starts taking one white tablet daily, beginning with the first white tablet in the top row. After the last white tablet (Saturday) has been taken, if any white tablets remain in the top row, the patient takes the remaining white tablets starting with the Sunday white tablets in the top row, followed by the brown tablets for a week (7 days). For all subsequent cycles, the patient begins a new 28 tablet regimen on the eighth day after taking her last white tablet, again starting with the first tablet in the top row. Following this regimen of 21

white tablets and 7 brown tablets, the patient will start all subsequent cycles on the same day of the week as the first course.

Tablets should be taken regularly with a meal or at bedtime. It should be stressed that efficacy of medication depends on strict adherence to the dosage schedule.

Special Notes on Administration

Menstruation usually begins two or three days, but may begin as late as the fourth or fifth day, after the brown tablets have been started. In any event, the next course of tablets should be started without interruption. If spotting occurs while the patient is taking white tablets, continue medication without interruption.

If the patient forgets to take one or more white tablets, the following is suggested:

One tablet is missed
- take tablet as soon as remembered
- take next tablet at the regular time

Two consecutive tablets are missed (week 1 or week 2)
- take *two* tablets as soon as remembered
- take *two* tablets the next day
- use another birth control method for seven days following the missed tablets

Two consecutive tablets are missed (week 3)

Sunday-Start Regimen:
- take *one* tablet daily until Sunday
- discard remaining tablets
- start new pack of tablets immediately (Sunday)
- use another birth control method for seven days following the missed tablets

Day-1 Start Regimen:
- discard remaining tablets
- start new pack of tablets that same day
- use another birth control method for seven days following the missed tablets

Three (or more) consecutive tablets are missed

Sunday-Start Regimen:
- take *one* tablet daily until Sunday
- discard remaining tablets
- start new pack of tablets immediately (Sunday)
- use another birth control method for seven days following the missed tablets

Day-1 Start Regimen:
- discard remaining tablets
- start new pack of tablets that same day
- use another birth control method for seven days following the missed tablets

The possibility of ovulation occurring increases with each successive day that scheduled white tablets are missed. While there is little likelihood of ovulation occurring if only one white tablet is missed, the possibility of spotting or bleeding is increased. This is particularly likely to occur if two or more consecutive white tablets are missed.

If the patient forgets to take any of the seven brown tablets in week four, those brown tablets that were missed are discarded and one brown tablet is taken each day until the pack is empty. A back up birth control method is not required during this time. A new pack of tablets should be started no later than the eighth day after the last white tablet was taken.

In the rare case of bleeding which resembles menstruation, the patient should be advised to discontinue medication and then begin taking tablets from a new tablet dispenser on the next Sunday or the first day (Day-1), depending on her regimen. Persistent bleeding which is not controlled by this method indicates the need for reexamination of the patient, at which time nonfunctional causes should be considered.

Use of Oral Contraceptives in the Event of a Missed Menstrual Period

1. If the patient has not adhered to the prescribed dosage regimen, the possibility of pregnancy should be considered after the first missed period and oral contraceptives should be withheld until pregnancy has been ruled out.

2. If the patient has adhered to the prescribed regimen and misses two consecutive periods, pregnancy should be ruled out before continuing the contraceptive regimen.

After several months on treatment, bleeding may be reduced to a point of virtual absence. This reduced flow may occur as a result of medication, in which event it is not indicative of pregnancy.

HOW SUPPLIED

Microgestin Fe 1/20 is available in cartons of six (6) dispensers. Each dispenser contains 21 norethindrone acetate and ethinyl estradiol tablets and 7 ferrous fumarate tablets. Microgestin are available as round white tablets debossed with "WATSON 630" on one side and plain on the other side. Each tablet contains 1 mg of norethindrone acetate and 20 mcg of ethinyl estradiol. They are supplied as follows:

Blister package of 28's   NDC-52544-630-28

Ferrous fumarate tablets are available as round brown tablets debossed with "WATSON 632" on one side and plain on the other side. Each tablet contains 75 mg ferrous fumarate.

Store at controlled room temperature 15°C to 30°C (59°F to 86°F).

REFERENCES

1. Back DJ, et al.: Kinetics of norethindrone in women II. Single-dose kinetics. Clin Pharmacol Ther 1978;24:448–453. 2. Humpel M, et al.: Investigations of pharmacokinetics of ethinyloestradiol to specific consideration of a possible first-pass effect in women. Contraception 1979;19:421–432. 3. Back DJ, et al. An investigation of the pharmacokinetics of ethynylestradiol in women using radioimmunoassay. Con-

traception 1979;20:263–273. 4. Hammond GL, et al. Distribution and percentages of non-protein bound contraceptive steroids in human serum. J Steroid Biochem 1982;17:375–380. 5. Fotherby K. Pharmacokinetics and metabolism of progestins in humans, in Pharmacology of the contraceptive steroids, Goldzieher JW, Fotherby K (eds), Raven Press, Ltd., New York, 1994, 99–126. 6. Goldzieher JW. Pharmacokinetics and metabolism of ethynyl estrogens, in Pharmacology of the contraceptive steroids, Goldzieher JW, Fotherby K (eds), Raven Press Ltd., New York, 1994, 127–151. 7. Hatcher, RA, et al. 1998. Contraceptive Technology, Seventeenth Edition. New York: Irvington Publishers. 8. Stadel, B.V.: Oral contraceptives and cardiovascular disease. (Pt. 1). *New England Journal of Medicine*, 305:612–618, 1981. 9. Stadel, B.V.: Oral contraceptives and cardiovascular disease. (Pt. 2). *New England Journal of Medicine*, 305:672–677, 1981. 10. Adam, S.A., and M. Thorogood: Oral contraception and myocardial infarction revisited: The effects of new preparations and prescribing patterns. *Brit. J. Obstet. and Gynec.*, 88:838–845, 1981. 11. Mann, J.I., and W.H. Inman: Oral contraceptives and death from myocardial infarction. *Brit. Med. J.*, 2(5965): 245–248, 1975. 12. Mann, J.I., et al.: Myocardial infarction in young women with special reference to oral contraceptive practice. *Brit. Med. J.*, 2(5956):241–245, 1975. 13. Royal College of General Practitioners' Oral Contraception Study: Further analyses of mortality in oral contraceptive users. *Lancet*, 1:541–546, 1981. 14. Slone, D., et al.: Risk of myocardial infarction in relation to current and discontinued use of oral contraceptives. *N.E.J.M.*, 305:420–424, 1981. 15. Vessey, M.P.: Female hormones and vascular disease: An epidemiological overview. *Brit. J. Fam. Plann.*, 6:1–12, 1980. 16. Russell-Briefel, R.G., et al.: Cardiovascular risk status and oral contraceptive use, United States, 1976-80. *Preventive Medicine*, 15:352–362, 1986. 17. Goldbaum, G.M., et al.: The relative impact of smoking and oral contraceptive use on women in the United States. *J.A.M.A.*, 258:1339–1342, 1987. 18. Layde, P.M., and V. Beral: Further analyses of mortality in oral contraceptive users: Royal College General Practitioners' Oral Contraception Study. (Table 5) *Lancet*, 1:541–546, 1981. 19. Knopp, R.H.: Arteriosclerosis risk: The roles of oral contraceptives and postmenopausal estrogens. *J. of Reprod. Med.*, 31(9)(Supplement): 913–921, 1986. 20. Krauss, R.M., et al.: Effects of two low-dose oral contraceptives on serum lipids and lipoproteins: Differential changes in high-density lipoproteins subclasses. *Am. J. Obstet. Gyn.*, 145:446–452, 1983. 21. Wahl, P., et al.: Effect of estrogen/progestin potency on lipid/lipoprotein cholesterol. *N.E.J.M.*, 308:862–867, 1983. 22. Wynn, V., and R. Niththyananthan: The effect of progestin in combined oral contraceptives on serum lipids with special reference to high-density lipoproteins. *Am. J. Obstet. and Gyn.*, 142:766–771, 1982. 23. Wynn, V., and I. Godsland: Effects of oral contraceptives on carbohydrate metabolism. *J Reprod. Medicine*, 31 (9)(Supplement): 892–897, 1986. 24. LaRosa, J.C.: Atherosclerotic risk factors in cardiovascular disease. *J. Reprod. Med.*, 31(9)(Supplement): 906–912, 1986. 25. Inman, W.H., and M.P. Vessey: Investigations of death from pulmonary, coronary, and cerebral thrombosis and embolism in women of child-bearing age. *Brit. Med. J.*, 2(5599): 193–199, 1968. 26. Maguire, M.G., et al.: Increased risk of thrombosis due to oral contraceptives: A further report. *Am. J. Epidemiology*, 110(2): 188–195, 1979. 27. Pettiti, D.B., et al.: Risk of vascular disease in women: Smoking, oral contraceptives, noncontraceptive estrogens, and other factors. *J.A.M.A.*, 242:1150–1154, 1979. 28. Vessey, M.P., and R. Doll: Investigation of relation between use of oral contraceptives and thromboembolic disease. *Brit. Med. J.*, 2(5599): 199–205, 1968. 29. Vessey, M.P. and R. Doll: Investigation of relation between use of oral contraceptives and thromboembolic disease: A further report. *Brit. Med. J.*, 2(5658): 651–657, 1969. 30. Porter, J.B., et al.: Oral contraceptives and non-fatal vascular disease: Recent experience. *Obstet. and Gyn.*, 59(3):299–302, 1982. 31. Vessey, M., et al.: A long-term follow-up study of women using different methods of contraception: An interim report. *J. Biosocial. Sci.*, 8:375–427, 1976. 32. Royal College of General Practitioners: Oral contraceptives, venous thrombosis, and varicose veins. *J. of Royal College of General Practitioners*, 28:393–399, 1978. 33. Collaborative Group for the study of stroke in young women: Oral contraception and increased risk of cerebral ischemia or thrombosis. *N.E.J.M.* 288: 871–878, 1973. 34. Petitti, D.B., and J. Wingerd: Use of oral contraceptives, cigarette smoking, and risk of subarachnoid hemorrhage. *Lancet*, 2:234–236, 1978. 35. Inman, W.H.: Oral contraceptives and fatal subarachnoid hemorrhage. *Brit. Med. J.*, 2(6203): 1468–1470, 1979. 36. Collaborative Group for the study of stroke in young women: Oral contraceptives and stroke in young women: Associated risk factors. *J.A.M.A.*, 231:718–722, 1975. 37. Inman, W.H., et al.: Thromboembolic disease and the steroidal content of oral contraceptives. A report to the Committee on Safety of Drugs. *Brit. Med. J.*, 2:203–209, 1970. 38. Meade, T.W., et al.: Progestogens and cardiovascular reactions associated with oral contraceptives and a comparison of the safety of 50- and 35-mcg oestrogen preparations. *Brit. Med. J.*, 280(6224): 1157–1161, 1980. 39. Kay, C.R.: Progestogens and arterial disease: Evidence from the Royal College of General Practitioners' study. *Amer. J. Obstet. Gyn.*, 142:762–765, 1982. 40. Royal College of General Practitioners: Incidence of arterial disease among oral contraceptive users. *J. Coll. Gen. Pract.*, 33:75–82, 1983. 41. Ory, H.W: Mortality associated with fertility and fertility control: 1983. *Family Planning Perspectives*, 15:50–56, 1983. 42. The Cancer and Steroid Hormone Study of the Centers for Disease Control and the National Institute of Child Health and Human De-

Continued on next page

Microgestin Fe 1/20—Cont.

velopment: Oral-contraceptive use and the risk of breast cancer. *N.E.J.M.*, 315: 405–411, 1986. **43.** Pike, M.C., et al.: Breast cancer in young women and use of oral contraceptives: Possible modifying effect of formulation and age at use. *Lancet*, 2:926–929, 1983. **44.** Paul, C., et al.: Oral contraceptives and breast cancer: A national study. *Brit. Med. J.*, 293:723–725, 1986. **45.** Miller, D.R., et al.: Breast cancer risk in relation to early oral contraceptive use. *Obstet. Gynec.*, 68:863–868, 1986. **46.** Olson, H., et al.: Oral contraceptive use and breast cancer in young women in Sweden (letter). *Lancet*, 2:748–749, 1985. **47.** McPherson, K., et al.: Early contraceptive use and breast cancer: Results of another case-control study. *Brit. J. Cancer*, 56: 653–660, 1987. **48.** Huggins, G.R., and P.F. Zucker: Oral contraceptives and neoplasia: 1987 update. *Fertil. Steril.*, 47:733–761, 1987. **49.** McPherson, K., and J.O. Drife: The pill and breast cancer: Why the uncertainty? *Brit. Med. J.*, 293:709–710, 1986. **50.** Shapiro, S.: Oral contraceptives: Time to take stock. *N.E.J.M.*, 315:450–451, 1987. **51.** Ory, H., et al.: Contraceptive choice and prevalence of cervical dysplasia and carcinoma in situ. *Am. J. Obstet. Gynec.*, 124:573–577, 1976. **52.** Vessey, M.P., et al.: Neoplasia of the cervix uteri and contraception: A possible adverse effect of the pill. *Lancet*, 2: 930, 1983. **53.** Brinton, L.A., et al.: Long-term use of oral contraceptives and risk of invasive cervical cancer. *Int. J. Cancer*, 38:339–344, 1986. **54.** WHO Collaborative Study of Neoplasia and Steroid Contraceptives: Invasive cervical cancer and combined oral contraceptives. *Brit. Med. J.*, 290:961–965, 1985. **55.** Rooks, J.B., et al.: Epidemiology of hepatocellular adenoma: The role of oral contraceptive use. *J.A.M.A.*, 242:644–648, 1979. **56.** Bein, N.N., and H.S. Goldsmith: Recurrent massive hemorrhage from benign hepatic tumors secondary to oral contraceptives. *Brit. J. Surg.*, 64:433–435, 1977. **57.** Klatskin, G.: Hepatic tumors: Possible relationship to use of oral contraceptives. *Gastroenterology*, 73:386–394, 1977. **58.** Henderson, B.E., et al.: Hepatocellular carcinoma and oral contraceptives. *Brit. J. Cancer*, 48:437–440, 1983. **59.** Neuberger, J., D. Forman, et al.: Oral contraceptives and hepatocellular carcinoma. *Brit. Med. J.*, 292:1355–1357, 1986. **60.** Forman, D., et al.: Cancer of the liver and oral contraceptives. *Brit. Med. J.*, 292: 1357–1361, 1986. **61.** Harlap, S., and J. Eldor. Births following oral contraceptive failures. *Obstet. Gynec.*, 55:447–452, 1980. **62.** Savolainen, E., et al.: Teratogenic hazards of oral contraceptives analyzed in a national malformation register. *Amer. J. Obstet Gynec.*, 140:521–524, 1981. **63.** Janerich, D.T., et al.: Oral contraceptives and birth defects. *Am. J. Epidemiology*, 112:73–79, 1980. **64.** Ferencz, C., et al.: Maternal hormone therapy and congenital heart disease. *Teratology*, 21:225–239, 1980. **65.** Rothman, K.J., et al.: Exogenous hormones and other drug exposures of children with congenital heart disease. *Am. J. Epidemiology*, 109:433–439, 1979. **66.** Boston Collaborative Drug Surveillance Program: Oral contraceptives and venous thromboembolic disease, surgically confirmed gallbladder disease, and breast tumors. *Lancet*, 1:1399–1404, 1973. **67.** Royal College of General Practitioners: *Oral Contraceptives and Health.* New York, Pittman, 1974, 100p. **68.** Layde, P.M., et al.: Risk of gallbladder disease: A cohort study of young women attending family planning clinics. *J. Epidemiol. and Comm. Health*, 36: 274–278, 1982. **69.** Rome Group for the Epidemiology and Prevention of Cholelithiasis (GREPCO): Prevalence of gallstone disease in an Italian adult female population. *Am. J. Epidemiol.*, 119:796–805, 1984. **70.** Strom, B.L., et al.: Oral contraceptives and other risk factors for gallbladder disease. *Clin. Pharmacol. Ther.*, 39:335–341, 1986. **71.** Wynn, V., et al.: Comparison of effects of different combined oral-contraceptive formulations on carbohydrate and lipid metabolism. *Lancet*, 1:1045–1049, 1979. **72.** Wynn, V.: Effect of progesterone and progestins on carbohydrate metabolism. In *Progesterone and Progestin.* Edited by C.W. Bardin, E. Milgrom, P. Mauvis-Jarvis. New York, Raven Press, 395–410, 1983. **73.** Perlman, J.A., et al.: Oral glucose tolerance and the potency of oral contraceptive progestogens. *J. Chronic Dis.*, 38:857–864, 1985. **74.** Royal College of General Practitioners' Oral Contraception Study: Effect on hypertension and benign breast disease of progestogen component in combined oral contraceptives. *Lancet*, 1:624, 1977. **75.** Fisch, I.R., and J. Frank: Oral contraceptives and blood pressure. *J.A.M.A.*, 237:2499–2503, 1977. **76.** Laragh, A.J.: Oral contraceptive induced hypertension: Nine years later. *Amer. J. Obstet. Gynecol.*, 126:141–147, 1976. **77.** Ramcharan, S., et al.: Incidence of hypertension in the Walnut Creek Contraceptive Drug Study cohort. In *Pharmacology of Steroid Contraceptive Drugs.* Edited by S. Garattini and H.W. Berendes. New York, Raven Press, 277–288, 1977. (Monographs of the Mario Negri Institute for Pharmacological Research, Milan.) **78.** Back DJ, et al. Drug interactions, in Pharmacology of the contraceptive steroids, Goldzieher JW, Fotherby K (eds), Raven Press, Ltd., New York, 1994, 407–425. **79.** The Cancer and Steroid Hormone Study of the Centers for Disease Control and the National Institute of Child Health and Human Development: Oral contraceptive use and the risk of ovarian cancer. *J.A.M.A.*, 249:1596–1599, 1983. **80.** The Cancer and Steroid Hormone Study of the Centers for Disease Control and the National Institute of Child Health and Human Development: Combination oral contraceptive use and the risk of endometrial cancer. *J.A.M.A.*, 257:796–800, 1987. **81.** Ory, H.W.: Functional ovarian cysts and oral contraceptives: Negative association confirmed surgically. *J.A.M.A.*, 228:68–69, 1974. **82.** Ory, H.W., et al.: Oral contraceptives and reduced risk of benign breast disease, *N.E.J.M.*, 294:

41–422, 1976. **83.** Ory, H.W.: The noncontraceptive health benefits from oral contraceptive use. *Fam. Plann. Perspectives*, 14:182–184, 1982. **84.** Ory, H.W., et al.: Making Choices: Evaluating the health risks and benefits of birth control methods. New York, The Alan Guttmacher Institute, 1, 1983. **85.** Miller, D.R., et al.: Breast cancer before age 45 and oral contraceptive use: new findings. *Am. J. Epidemiol.*, 129:269–280, 1989. **86.** Kay, C.R., and P.C. Hannaford: Breast cancer and the pill: a further report from the Royal College of General Practitioners Oral Contraception Study. *Br. J. Cancer*, 58:675–680, 1988. **87.** Stadel, B.V., et al.: Oral contraceptives and premenopausal breast cancer in nulliparous women. *Contraception*, 38:287–299, 1988. **88.** UK National Case-Control Study Group: Oral contraceptive use and breast cancer risk in young women. *Lancet*, 973–982, 1989. **89.** Romieu, I., et al.: Prospective study of oral contraceptive use and risk of breast cancer in women. *J. Natl. Cancer Inst.*, 81:1313–1321, 1989.

The patient labeling for oral contraceptive drug products is set forth below:

This product (like all oral contraceptives) is intended to prevent pregnancy. It does not protect against HIV infection (AIDS) and other sexually transmitted diseases.

BRIEF SUMMARY PATIENT PACKAGE INSERT

Oral contraceptives, also known as "birth control pills" or "the pill," are taken to prevent pregnancy and, when taken correctly, have a failure rate of about 1% per year when used without missing any pills. The typical failure rate of large numbers of pill users is less than 3% per year when women who miss pills are included. For most women oral contraceptives are also free of serious or unpleasant side effects. However, forgetting to take pills considerably increases the chances of pregnancy.

For the majority of women, oral contraceptives can be taken safely. But there are some women who are at high risk of developing certain serious diseases that can be life-threatening or may cause temporary or permanent disability. The risks associated with taking oral contraceptives increase significantly if you:

- Smoke
- Have high blood pressure, diabetes, high cholesterol
- Have or have had clotting disorders, heart attack, stroke, angina pectoris, cancer of the breast or sex organs, jaundice, or malignant or benign liver tumors.

You should not take the pill if you suspect you are pregnant or have unexplained vaginal bleeding.

> **Cigarette smoking increases the risk of serious cardiovascular side effects from oral contraceptive use. This risk increases with age and with heavy smoking (15 or more cigarettes per day) and is quite marked in women over 35 years of age. Women who use oral contraceptives are strongly advised not to smoke.**

Most side effects of the pill are not serious. The most common side effects are nausea, vomiting, bleeding between menstrual periods, weight gain, breast tenderness, and difficulty wearing contact lenses. These side effects, especially nausea, vomiting, and breakthrough bleeding, may subside within the first three months of use.

The serious side effects of the pill occur very infrequently, especially if you are in good health and are young. However, you should know that the following medical conditions have been associated with or made worse by the pill:

1. Blood clots in the legs (thrombophlebitis), lungs (pulmonary embolism), stoppage or rupture of a blood vessel in the brain (stroke), blockage of blood vessels in the heart (heart attack or angina pectoris) or other organs of the body. As mentioned above, smoking increases the risk of heart attacks and strokes and subsequent serious medical consequences.
2. Liver tumors, which may rupture and cause severe bleeding. A possible but not definite association has been found with the pill and liver cancer. However, liver cancers are extremely rare. The chance of developing liver cancer from using the pill is thus even rarer.
3. High blood pressure, although blood pressure usually returns to normal when the pill is stopped.

The symptoms associated with these serious side effects are discussed in the detailed leaflet given to you with your supply of pills. Notify your doctor or health care provider if you notice any unusual physical disturbances while taking the pill. In addition, drugs such as rifampin, as well as some anticonvulsants and some antibiotics, may decrease oral contraceptive effectiveness.

Most of the studies to date on breast cancer and pill use have found no increase in the risk of developing breast cancer, although some studies have reported an increased risk of developing breast cancer in certain groups of women. However, some studies have found an increase in the risk of developing cancer of the cervix in women taking the pill, but this finding may be related to differences in sexual behavior or other factors not related to use of the pill. Therefore, there is insufficient evidence to rule out the possibility that the pill may cause cancer of the breast or cervix.

Taking the pill provides some important non-contraceptive benefits. These include less painful menstruation, less menstrual blood loss and anemia, fewer pelvic infections, and fewer cancers of the ovary and the lining of the uterus.

Be sure to discuss any medical condition you may have with your health care provider. Your health care provider will

take a medical and family history and examine you before prescribing oral contraceptives. The physical examination may be delayed to another time if you request it and your health care provider believes that it is a good medical practice to postpone it. You should be reexamined at least once a year while taking oral contraceptives. The detailed patient information leaflet gives you further information which you should read and discuss with your health care provider.

This product (like all oral contraceptives) is intended to prevent pregnancy. It does not protect against transmission of HIV (AIDS) and other sexually transmitted diseases such as chlamydia, genital herpes, genital warts, gonorrhea, hepatitis B, and syphilis.

INSTRUCTIONS TO PATIENT

Tablet Dispenser

The Microgestin tablet dispenser has been designed to make oral contraceptive dosing as easy and as convenient as possible. The tablets are arranged in four rows of seven tablets each, with the days of the week appearing on the tablet dispenser below the last row of tablets.

Each white tablet contains 1 mg norethindrone acetate and 20 mcg ethinyl estradiol.

Each brown tablet contains 75 mg ferrous fumarate, and is intended to help you remember to take the tablets correctly. These brown tablets are not intended to have any health benefit.

Directions

To remove a tablet, press down on it with your thumb or finger. The tablet will drop through the back of the tablet dispenser. Do not press with your thumbnail, fingernail, or any other sharp object.

HOW TO TAKE THE PILL

IMPORTANT POINTS TO REMEMBER

BEFORE YOU START TAKING YOUR PILLS:
1. BE SURE TO READ THESE DIRECTIONS:
   Before you start taking your pills.
   Anytime you are not sure what to do.
2. THE RIGHT WAY TO TAKE THE PILL IS TO TAKE ONE PILL EVERY DAY AT THE SAME TIME. If you miss pills you could get pregnant. This includes starting the pack late. The more pills you miss, the more likely you are to get pregnant.
3. MANY WOMEN HAVE SPOTTING OR LIGHT BLEEDING, OR MAY FEEL SICK TO THEIR STOMACH, DURING THE FIRST 1-3 PACKS OF PILLS. If you do have spotting or light bleeding or feel sick to your stomach, do not stop taking the pill. The problem will usually go away. If it doesnt go away, check with your doctor or clinic.
4. MISSING PILLS CAN ALSO CAUSE SPOTTING OR LIGHT BLEEDING, even when you make up these missed pills. On the days you take 2 pills to make up for missed pills, you could also feel a little sick to your stomach.
5. IF YOU HAVE VOMITING OR DIARRHEA, for any reason, or IF YOU TAKE SOME MEDICINES, including some antibiotics, your birth control pills may not work as well. Use a back-up birth control method (such as condoms or foam) until you check with your doctor or clinic.
6. IF YOU HAVE TROUBLE REMEMBERING TO TAKE THE PILL, talk to your doctor or clinic about how to make pill-taking easier or about using another method of birth control.
7. IF YOU HAVE ANY QUESTIONS OR ARE UNSURE ABOUT THE INFORMATION IN THIS LEAFLET, call your doctor or clinic.

BEFORE YOU START TAKING YOUR PILLS

1. DECIDE WHAT TIME OF DAY YOU WANT TO TAKE YOUR PILL. It is important to take it at about the same time every day.
2. BE SURE YOUR PILL PACK HAS 28 PILLS: The 28-pill pack has 21 "active" white pills (with hormones) to take for 3 weeks, followed by 1 week of reminder brown pills (without hormones).
3. ALSO FIND:
   1) where on the pack to start taking pills,
   2) in what order to take the pills (follow the arrows), and
   3) the week numbers as shown in the following picture:

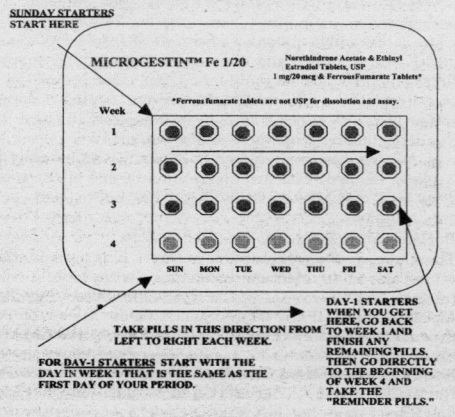

Microgestin Fe 1/20 will contain: 21 WHITE PILLS for WEEKS 1, 2, and 3. WEEK 4 will contain BROWN PILLS ONLY.

4. BE SURE YOU HAVE READY AT ALL TIMES: ANOTHER KIND OF BIRTH CONTROL (such as condoms or foam) to use as a back-up in case you miss pills.
An EXTRA, FULL PILL PACK.

WHEN TO START THE FIRST PACK OF PILLS

You have a choice of which day to start taking your first pack of pills. Decide with your doctor or clinic which is the best day for you. Pick a time of day which will be easy to remember.

Day-1 Start:
1. Take the first "active" white pill of the first pack during the first 24 hours of your period.
2. You will not need to use a back-up method of birth control, since you are starting the pill at the beginning of your period.

Sunday Start:
1. Take the first "active" white pill of the first pack on the Sunday after your period starts, even if you are still bleeding. If your period begins on Sunday, start the pack that same day.
2. Use another method of birth control as a back-up method if you have sex anytime from the Sunday you start your first pack until the next Sunday (7 days). Condoms or foam are good back-up methods of birth control.

WHAT TO DO DURING THE MONTH

1. TAKE ONE PILL AT THE SAME TIME EVERY DAY UNTIL THE PACK IS EMPTY.
Do not skip pills even if you are spotting or bleeding between monthly periods or feel sick to your stomach (nausea).
Do not skip pills even if you do not have sex very often.
2. WHEN YOU FINISH A PACK OR SWITCH YOUR BRAND OF PILLS:
Start the next pack on the day after your last "reminder" pill. Do not wait any days between packs.

WHAT TO DO IF YOU MISS PILLS

If you MISS 1 white "active" pill:
1. Take it as soon as you remember. Take the next pill at your regular time. This means you may take 2 pills in 1 day.
2. You do not need to use a back-up birth control method if you have sex.

If you MISS 2 white "active" pills in a row in WEEK 1 or WEEK 2 of your pack:
1. Take 2 pills on the day you remember and 2 pills the next day.
2. Then take 1 pill a day until you finish the pack.
3. You COULD GET PREGNANT if you have sex in the 7 days after you miss pills. You MUST use another birth control method (such as condoms or foam) as a back-up method of birth control until you have taken a white "active" pill every day for 7 days.

If you MISS 2 white "active" pills in a row in THE 3RD WEEK:
1. If you are a Day-1 Starter:
THROW OUT the rest of the pill pack and start a new pack that same day.
If you are a Sunday Starter:
Keep taking 1 pill every day until Sunday. On Sunday, THROW OUT the rest of the pack and start a new pack of pills that same day.
2. You may not have your period this month, but this is expected. However, if you miss your period 2 months in a row, call your doctor or clinic because you might be pregnant.
3. You COULD GET PREGNANT if you have sex in the 7 days after you miss pills. You MUST use another birth control method (such as condoms or foam) as a back-up method of birth control until you have taken a white "active" pill every day for 7 days.

If you MISS 3 OR MORE white "active" pills in a row (during the first 3 weeks):
1. If you are a Day-1 Starter:
THROW OUT the rest of the pill pack and start a new pack that same day.
If you are a Sunday Starter:
Keep taking 1 pill every day until Sunday. On Sunday, THROW OUT the rest of the pack and start a new pack of pills that same day.
2. You may not have your period this month, but this is expected. However, if you miss your period 2 months in a row, call your doctor or clinic because you might be pregnant.
3. You COULD GET PREGNANT if you have sex in the 7 days after you miss pills. You MUST use another birth control method (such as condoms or foam) as a back-up method of birth control until you have taken a white "active" pill every day for 7 days.

A REMINDER:
IF YOU FORGET ANY OF THE 7 BROWN "REMINDER" PILLS IN WEEK 4:
THROW AWAY THE PILLS YOU MISSED.
KEEP TAKING 1 PILL EACH DAY UNTIL THE PACK IS EMPTY.
YOU DO NOT NEED A BACK-UP METHOD.

FINALLY, IF YOU ARE STILL NOT SURE WHAT TO DO ABOUT THE PILLS YOU HAVE MISSED:
Use a BACK-UP METHOD anytime you have sex. KEEP TAKING ONE white "ACTIVE" PILL EACH DAY until you can reach your doctor or clinic.

Based on his or her assessment of your medical needs, your doctor or health care provider has prescribed this drug for you. Do not give this drug to anyone else.
Keep this and all drugs out of the reach of children.
Store at controlled room temperature 15°C to 30°C (59°F to 86°F).
This product (like all oral contraceptives) is intended to prevent pregnancy. It does not protect against HIV infection (AIDS) and other sexually transmitted diseases.

DETAILED PATIENT PACKAGE INSERT
What You Should Know About Oral Contraceptives

Any woman who considers using oral contraceptives (the "birth control pill" or "the pill") should understand the benefits and risks of using this form of birth control. This leaflet will give you much of the information you will need to make this decision and will also help you determine if you are at risk of developing any of the serious side effects of the pill. It will tell you how to use the pill properly so that it will be as effective as possible. However, this leaflet is not a replacement for a careful discussion between you and your health care provider. You should discuss the information provided in this leaflet with him or her, both when you first start taking the pill and during your revisits. You should also follow your health care providers advice with regard to regular check-ups while you are on the pill.

EFFECTIVENESS OF ORAL CONTRACEPTIVES

Oral contraceptives or "birth control pills" or "the pill" are used to prevent pregnancy and are more effective than other non-surgical methods of birth control. When they are taken correctly, the chance of becoming pregnant is less than 1% (1 pregnancy per 100 women per year of use) when used perfectly, without missing any pills. Typical failure rates are actually 3% per year. The chance of becoming pregnant increases with each missed pill during a menstrual cycle.
In comparison, typical failure rates for other methods of birth control during the first year of use are as follows:
Implant: <1%
Injection: <1%
IUD: <1 to 2%
Diaphragm with Spermicides: 20%
Spermicides alone: 26%
Vaginal Sponge: 20 to 40%
Female sterilization: <1%
Male sterilization: <1%
Cervical Cap: 20 to 40%
Condom alone (male): 14%
Condom alone (female): 21%
Periodic abstinence: 25%
Withdrawal: 19%
No method: 85%

WHO SHOULD NOT TAKE ORAL CONTRACEPTIVES

Cigarette smoking increases the risk of serious cardiovascular side effects from oral contraceptive use. This risk increases with age and with heavy smoking (15 or more cigarettes per day) and is quite marked in women over 35 years of age. Women who use oral contraceptives are strongly advised not to smoke.

Some women should not use the pill. For example, you should not take the pill if you are pregnant or think you may be pregnant. You should also not use the pill if you have any of the following conditions:
• A history of heart attack or stroke
• Blood clots in the legs (thrombophlebitis), lungs (pulmonary embolism), or eyes
• A history of blood clots in the deep veins of your legs
• Chest pain (angina pectoris)
• Known or suspected breast cancer or cancer of the lining of the uterus, cervix or vagina
• Unexplained vaginal bleeding (until a diagnosis is reached by your doctor)
• Yellowing of the whites of the eyes or of the skin (jaundice) during pregnancy or during previous use of the pill
• Liver tumor (benign or cancerous)
• Known or suspected pregnancy
Tell your health care provider if you have ever had any of these conditions. Your health care provider can recommend a safer method of birth control.

OTHER CONSIDERATIONS BEFORE TAKING ORAL CONTRACEPTIVES

Tell your health care provider if you have:
• Breast nodules, fibrocystic disease of the breast, an abnormal breast x-ray or mammogram
• Diabetes
• Elevated cholesterol or triglycerides
• High blood pressure
• Migraine or other headaches or epilepsy
• Mental depression
• Gallbladder, heart, or kidney disease
• History of scanty or irregular menstrual periods
Women with any of these conditions should be checked often by their health care provider if they choose to use oral contraceptives.
Also, be sure to inform your doctor or health care provider if you smoke or are on any medications.

RISKS OF TAKING ORAL CONTRACEPTIVES
1. Risk of Developing Blood Clots

Blood clots and blockage of blood vessels are the most serious side effects of taking oral contraceptives; in particular, a clot in the legs can cause thrombophlebitis and a clot that travels to the lungs can cause a sudden blocking of the vessel carrying blood to the lungs. Rarely, clots occur in the blood vessels of the eye and may cause blindness, double vision, or impaired vision.
If you take oral contraceptives and need elective surgery, need to stay in bed for a prolonged illness, or have recently delivered a baby, you may be at risk of developing blood clots. You should consult your doctor about stopping oral contraceptives three to four weeks before surgery and not taking oral contraceptives for two weeks after surgery or during bed rest. You should also not take oral contraceptives soon after delivery of a baby. It is advisable to wait for at least four weeks after delivery if you are not breast feeding. If you are breast feeding, you should wait until you have weaned your child before using the pill. (See also the section on **Breast Feeding** in **GENERAL PRECAUTIONS**.)

2. Heart Attacks and Strokes

Oral contraceptives may increase the tendency to develop strokes (stoppage or rupture of blood vessels in the brain) and angina pectoris and heart attacks (blockage of blood vessels in the heart). Any of these conditions can cause death or disability.
Smoking greatly increases the possibility of suffering heart attacks and strokes. Furthermore, smoking and the use of oral contraceptives greatly increase the chances of developing and dying of heart disease.

3. Gallbladder Disease

Oral contraceptive users probably have a greater risk than nonusers of having gallbladder disease, although this risk may be related to pills containing high doses of estrogens.

4. Liver Tumors

In rare cases, oral contraceptives can cause benign but dangerous liver tumors. These benign liver tumors can rupture and cause fatal internal bleeding. In addition, a possible but not definite association has been found with the pill and liver cancers in two studies, in which a few women who developed these very rare cancers were found to have used oral contraceptives for long periods. However, liver cancers are extremely rare. The chance of developing liver cancer from using the pill is thus even rarer.

5. Cancer of the Reproductive Organs and Breasts

There is, at present, no confirmed evidence that oral contraceptive use increases the risk of developing cancer of the reproductive organs. Studies to date of women taking the pill have reported conflicting findings on whether pill use increases the risk of developing cancer of the breast or cervix. Most of the studies on breast cancer and pill use have found no overall increase in the risk of developing breast cancer, although some studies have reported an increased risk of developing breast cancer in certain groups of women. Women who use oral contraceptives and have a strong family history of breast cancer or who have breast nodules or abnormal mammograms should be closely followed by their doctors.
Some studies have found an increase in the incidence of cancer of the cervix in women who use oral contraceptives. However, this finding may be related to factors other than the use of oral contraceptives.

ESTIMATED RISK OF DEATH FROM A BIRTH CONTROL METHOD OR PREGNANCY

All methods of birth control and pregnancy are associated with a risk of developing certain diseases which may lead to disability or death. An estimate of the number of deaths associated with different methods of birth control and pregnancy has been calculated and is shown in the following table.
[See table at top of next page]
In the above table, the risk of death from any birth control method is less than the risk of childbirth, except for oral contraceptive users over the age of 35 who smoke and pill users over the age of 40 even if they do not smoke. It can be seen in the table that for women aged 15 to 39, the risk of death was highest with pregnancy (7–26 deaths per 100,000 women, depending on age). Among pill users who do not smoke, the risk of death was always lower than that associated with pregnancy for any age group, although over the age of 40, the risk increases to 32 deaths per 100,000 women, compared to 28 associated with pregnancy at that age. However, for pill users who smoke and are over the age of 35, the estimated number of deaths exceeds those for other methods of birth control. If a woman is over the age of 40 and smokes, her estimated risk of death is four times higher (117/100,000 women) than the estimated risk associated with pregnancy (28/100,000 women) in that age group.
The suggestion that women over 40 who dont smoke should not take oral contraceptives is based on information from older higher dose pills and on less selective use of pills than is practiced today. An Advisory Committee of the FDA discussed this issue in 1989 and recommended that the benefits of oral contraceptive use by healthy, non-smoking women over 40 years of age may outweigh the possible risks. However, all women, especially older women, are cautioned to use the lowest dose pill that is effective.

WARNING SIGNALS

If any of these adverse effects occur while you are taking oral contraceptives, call your doctor immediately:

Continued on next page

Microgestin Fe 1/20—Cont.

- Sharp chest pain, coughing of blood, or sudden shortness of breath (indicating a possible clot in the lung)
- Pain in the calf (indicating a possible clot in the leg)
- Crushing chest pain or heaviness in the chest (indicating a possible heart attack)
- Sudden severe headache or vomiting, dizziness or fainting, disturbances of vision or speech, weakness, or numbness in an arm or leg (indicating a possible stroke)
- Sudden partial or complete loss of vision (indicating a possible clot in the eye)
- Breast lumps (indicating possible breast cancer or fibrocystic disease of the breast; ask your doctor or health care provider to show you how to examine your breasts)
- Severe pain or tenderness in the stomach area (indicating a possibly ruptured liver tumor)
- Difficulty in sleeping, weakness, lack of energy, fatigue, or change in mood (possibly indicating severe depression)
- Jaundice or a yellowing of the skin or eyeballs, accompanied frequently by fever, fatigue, loss of appetite, dark colored urine, or light colored bowel movements (indicating possible liver problems)

SIDE EFFECTS OF ORAL CONTRACEPTIVES

1. Vaginal Bleeding

Irregular vaginal bleeding or spotting may occur while you are taking the pills. Irregular bleeding may vary from slight staining between menstrual periods to breakthrough bleeding which is a flow much like a regular period. Irregular bleeding occurs most often during the first few months of oral contraceptive use, but may also occur after you have been taking the pill for some time. Such bleeding may be temporary and usually does not indicate serious problems. It is important to continue taking your pills on schedule. If the bleeding occurs in more than one cycle or lasts for more than a few days, talk to your doctor or health care provider.

2. Contact Lenses

If you wear contact lenses and notice a change in vision or an inability to wear your lenses, contact your doctor or health care provider.

3. Fluid Retention

Oral contraceptives may cause edema (fluid retention) with swelling of the fingers or ankles and may raise your blood pressure. If you experience fluid retention, contact your doctor or health care provider.

4. Melasma

A spotty darkening of the skin is possible, particularly of the face.

5. Other Side Effects

Other side effects may include change in appetite, headache, nervousness, depression, dizziness, loss of scalp hair, rash, and vaginal infections.

If any of these side effects bother you, call your doctor or health care provider.

GENERAL PRECAUTIONS

1. Missed Periods and Use of Oral Contraceptives Before or During Early Pregnancy

There may be times when you may not menstruate regularly after you have completed taking a cycle of pills. If you have taken your pills regularly and miss one menstrual period, continue taking your pills for the next cycle but be sure to inform your health care provider before doing so. If you have not taken the pills daily as instructed and missed a menstrual period, or if you missed two consecutive menstrual periods, you may be pregnant. Check with your health care provider immediately to determine whether you are pregnant. Do not continue to take oral contraceptives until you are sure you are not pregnant, but continue to use another method of contraception.

There is no conclusive evidence that oral contraceptive use is associated with an increase in birth defects, when taken inadvertently during early pregnancy. Previously, a few studies had reported that oral contraceptives might be associated with birth defects, but these studies have not been confirmed. Nevertheless, oral contraceptives or any other drugs should not be used during pregnancy unless clearly necessary and prescribed by your doctor. You should check with your doctor about risks to your unborn child of any medication taken during pregnancy.

2. While Breast Feeding

If you are breast feeding, consult your doctor before starting oral contraceptives. Some of the drug will be passed on to the child in the milk. A few adverse effects on the child have been reported, including yellowing of the skin (jaundice) and breast enlargement. In addition, oral contraceptives may decrease the amount and quality of your milk. If possible, do not use oral contraceptives while breast feeding. You should use another method of contraception since breast feeding provides only partial protection from becoming pregnant and this partial protection decreases significantly as you breast feed for longer periods of time. You should consider starting oral contraceptives only after you have weaned your child completely.

3. Laboratory Tests

If you are scheduled for any laboratory tests, tell your doctor you are taking birth control pills. Certain blood tests may be affected by birth control pills.

4. Drug Interactions

Certain drugs may interact with birth control pills to make them less effective in preventing pregnancy or cause an increase in breakthrough bleeding. Such drugs include rifampin; drugs used for epilepsy such as barbiturates (for example, phenobarbital), carbamazepine, and phenytoin (Dilantin® is one brand of this drug); troglitazone; phenylbutazone; and possibly certain antibiotics. You may need to use additional contraception when you take drugs which can make oral contraceptives less effective.

ANNUAL NUMBER OF BIRTH-RELATED OR METHOD-RELATED DEATHS ASSOCIATED WITH CONTROL OF FERTILITY PER 100,000 NONSTERILE WOMEN, BY FERTILITY CONTROL METHOD ACCORDING TO AGE.

Method of control and outcome	15–19	20–24	25–29	30–34	35–39	40–44
No fertility control methods*	7.0	7.4	9.1	14.8	25.7	28.2
Oral contraceptives nonsmoker**	0.3	0.5	0.9	1.9	13.8	31.6
Oral contraceptives smoker**	2.2	3.4	6.6	13.5	51.1	117.2
IUD**	0.8	0.8	1.0	1.0	1.4	1.4
Condom*	1.1	1.6	0.7	0.2	0.3	0.4
Diaphragm/spermicide*	1.9	1.2	1.2	1.3	2.2	2.8
Periodic abstinence*	2.5	1.6	1.6	1.7	2.9	3.6

* Deaths are birth related
** Deaths are method related

Birth control pills interact with certain drugs. These drugs include acetaminophen, clofibric acid, cyclosporine, morphine, prednisolone, salicylic acid, temazepam, and theophylline. You should tell your doctor if you are taking any of these medications.

5. This product (like all oral contraceptives) is intended to prevent pregnancy. It does not protect against transmission of HIV (AIDS) and other sexually transmitted diseases such as chlamydia, genital herpes, genital warts, gonorrhea, hepatitis B, and syphilis.

INSTRUCTIONS TO PATIENT

Tablet Dispenser

The Microgestin tablet dispenser has been designed to make oral contraceptive dosing as easy and as convenient as possible. The tablets are arranged in four rows of seven tablets each, with the days of the week appearing on the tablet dispenser below the last row of tablets.

Each *white* tablet contains 1 mg norethindrone acetate and 20 mcg ethinyl estradiol.

Each *brown* tablet contains 75 mg ferrous fumarate and is intended to help you remember to take the tablets correctly. These brown tablets are not intended to have any health benefit.

Directions

To remove a tablet, press down on it with your thumb or finger. The tablet will drop through the back of the tablet dispenser. Do not press with your thumbnail, fingernail, or any other sharp object.

HOW TO TAKE THE PILL

IMPORTANT POINTS TO REMEMBER

BEFORE YOU START TAKING YOUR PILLS:

1. BE SURE TO READ THESE DIRECTIONS:
   Before you start taking your pills.
   Anytime you are not sure what to do.
2. THE RIGHT WAY TO TAKE THE PILL IS TO TAKE ONE PILL EVERY DAY AT THE SAME TIME. If you miss pills you could get pregnant. This includes starting the pack late. The more pills you miss, the more likely you are to get pregnant.
3. MANY WOMEN HAVE SPOTTING OR LIGHT BLEEDING, OR MAY FEEL SICK TO THEIR STOMACH, DURING THE FIRST 1–3 PACKS OF PILLS. If you do have spotting or light bleeding or feel sick to your stomach, do not stop taking the pill. The problem will usually go away. If it doesnt go away, check with your doctor or clinic.
4. MISSING PILLS CAN ALSO CAUSE SPOTTING OR LIGHT BLEEDING, even when you make up these missed pills. On the days you take 2 pills to make up for missed pills, you could also feel a little sick to your stomach.
5. IF YOU HAVE VOMITING OR DIARRHEA, for any reason, or IF YOU TAKE SOME MEDICINES, including some antibiotics, your birth control pills may not work as well. Use a back-up birth control method (such as condoms or foam) until you check with your doctor or clinic.
6. IF YOU HAVE TROUBLE REMEMBERING TO TAKE THE PILL, talk to your doctor or clinic about how to make pill-taking easier or about using another method of birth control.
7. IF YOU HAVE ANY QUESTIONS OR ARE UNSURE ABOUT THE INFORMATION IN THIS LEAFLET, call your doctor or clinic.

BEFORE YOU START TAKING YOUR PILLS

1. DECIDE WHAT TIME OF DAY YOU WANT TO TAKE YOUR PILL. It is important to take it at about the same time every day.
2. BE SURE YOUR PILL PACK HAS 28 PILLS:
   The pill pack has 21 "active" white pills (with hormones) to take for 3 weeks, followed by 1 week of reminder brown pills (without hormones).
3. ALSO FIND:
   1) where on the pack to start taking pills,
   2) in what order to take the pills (follow the arrows), and
   3) the week numbers as shown in the following picture:

[See figure at top of next column]

Microgestin Fe 1/20 will contain: 21 WHITE PILLS for WEEKS 1, 2, and 3. WEEK 4 will contain BROWN PILLS ONLY.

4. BE SURE YOU HAVE READY AT ALL TIMES:
   ANOTHER KIND OF BIRTH CONTROL (such as condoms or foam) to use as a back-up in case you miss pills.
   An EXTRA, FULL PILL PACK.

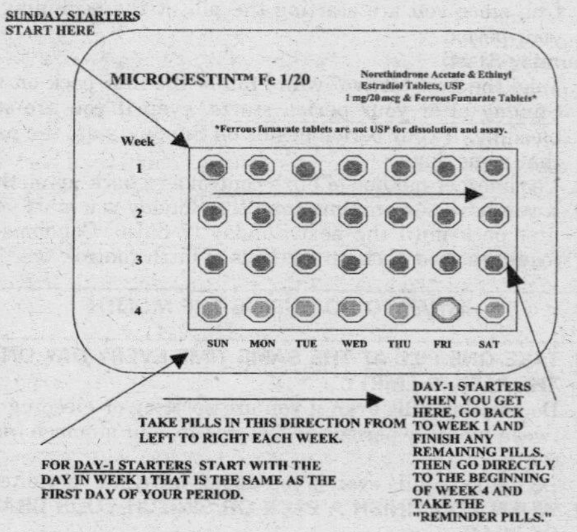
SUNDAY STARTERS
START HERE
MICROGESTIN™ Fe 1/20
Norethindrone Acetate & Ethinyl Estradiol Tablets, USP
1 mg/20 mcg & FerrousFumarate Tablets*
*Ferrous fumarate tablets are not USP for dissolution and assay.
Week
1
2
3
4
SUN
MON
TUE
WED
THU
FRI
SAT
TAKE PILLS IN THIS DIRECTION FROM LEFT TO RIGHT EACH WEEK.
FOR DAY-1 STARTERS START WITH THE DAY IN WEEK 1 THAT IS THE SAME AS THE FIRST DAY OF YOUR PERIOD.
DAY-1 STARTERS WHEN YOU GET HERE, GO BACK TO WEEK 1 AND FINISH ANY REMAINING PILLS. THEN GO DIRECTLY TO THE BEGINNING OF WEEK 4 AND TAKE THE "REMINDER PILLS."

WHEN TO START THE FIRST PACK OF PILLS

You have a choice of which day to start taking your first pack of pills. Decide with your doctor or clinic which is the best day for you. Pick a time of day which will be easy to remember.

DAY-1 START:

1. Take the first "active" white pill of the first pack during the first 24 hours of your period.
2. You will not need to use a back-up method of birth control, since you are starting the pill at the beginning of your period.

SUNDAY START:

1. Take the first "active" white pill of the first pack on the Sunday after your period starts, even if you are still bleeding. If your period begins on Sunday, start the pack that same day.
2. Use another method of birth control as a back-up method if you have sex anytime from the Sunday you start your first pack until the next Sunday (7 days). Condoms or foam are good back-up methods of birth control.

WHAT TO DO DURING THE MONTH

1. **TAKE ONE PILL AT THE SAME TIME EVERY DAY UNTIL THE PACK IS EMPTY.**
   Do not skip pills even if you are spotting or bleeding between monthly periods or feel sick to your stomach (nausea).
   Do not skip pills even if you do not have sex very often.
2. **WHEN YOU FINISH A PACK OR SWITCH YOUR BRAND OF PILLS:**
   Start the next pack on the day after your last "reminder" pill. Do not wait any days between packs.

WHAT TO DO IF YOU MISS PILLS

If you MISS 1 white "active" pill:

1. Take it as soon as you remember. Take the next pill at your regular time. This means you may take 2 pills in 1 day.
2. You do not need to use a back-up birth control method if you have sex.

If you MISS 2 white "active" pills in a row in WEEK 1 or WEEK 2 of your pack:

1. Take 2 pills on the day you remember and 2 pills the next day.
2. Then take 1 pill a day until you finish the pack.
3. You COULD GET PREGNANT if you have sex in the 7 days after you miss pills. You MUST use another birth control method (such as condoms or foam) as a back-up method of birth control until you have taken a white "active pill" every day for 7 days.

If you MISS 2 white "active" pills in a row in THE 3rd WEEK:

1. **If you are a Day-1 Starter:**
   THROW OUT the rest of the pill pack and start a new pack that same day.
   If you are a Sunday Starter:
   Keep taking 1 pill every day until Sunday. On Sunday, THROW OUT the rest of the pack and start a new pack of pills that same day.

2. You may not have your period this month, but this is expected. However, if you miss your period 2 months in a row, call your doctor or clinic because you might be pregnant.
3. You COULD GET PREGNANT if you have sex in the 7 days after you miss pills. You MUST use another birth control method (such as condoms or foam) as a back-up method of birth control until you have taken a white "active" pill every day for 7 days.

If you MISS 3 OR MORE white "active" pills in a row (during the first 3 weeks):

1. **If you are a Day-1 Starter:**
THROW OUT the rest of the pill pack and start a new pack that same day.
If you are a Sunday Starter:
Keep taking 1 pill every day until Sunday. On Sunday, THROW OUT the rest of the pack and start a new pack of pills that same day.
2. You may not have your period this month, but this is expected. However, if you miss your period 2 months in a row, call your doctor or clinic because you might be pregnant.
3. You COULD GET PREGNANT if you have sex in the 7 days after you miss pills. You MUST use another birth control method (such as condoms or foam) as a back-up method of birth control until you have taken a white "active" pill every day for 7 days.

A REMINDER:
IF YOU FORGET ANY OF THE 7 BROWN "REMINDER" PILLS IN WEEK 4:
THROW AWAY THE PILLS YOU MISSED.
KEEP TAKING 1 PILL EACH DAY UNTIL THE PACK IS EMPTY.
YOU DO NOT NEED A BACK-UP METHOD.

FINALLY, IF YOU ARE STILL NOT SURE WHAT TO DO ABOUT THE PILLS YOU HAVE MISSED:
Use a BACK-UP METHOD anytime you have sex. KEEP TAKING ONE WHITE "ACTIVE" PILL EACH DAY until you can reach your doctor or clinic.

PREGNANCY DUE TO PILL FAILURE

The incidence of pill failure resulting in pregnancy is approximately 1% (ie, one pregnancy per 100 women per year) if taken every day as directed, but more typical failure rates are about 3%. If failure does occur, the risk to the fetus is minimal.

PREGNANCY AFTER STOPPING THE PILL

There may be some delay in becoming pregnant after you stop using oral contraceptives, especially if you had irregular menstrual cycles before you used oral contraceptives. It may be advisable to postpone conception until you begin menstruating regularly once you have stopped taking the pill and desire pregnancy.
There does not appear to be any increase in birth defects in newborn babies when pregnancy occurs soon after stopping the pill.

OVERDOSAGE

Serious ill effects have not been reported following ingestion of large doses of oral contraceptives by young children. Overdosage may cause nausea and withdrawal bleeding in females. In case of overdosage, contact your health care provider or pharmacist.

OTHER INFORMATION

Your health care provider will take a medical and family history and examine you before prescribing oral contraceptives. The physical examination may be delayed to another time if you request it and your health care provider believes that it is a good medical practice to postpone it. You should be reexamined at least once a year. Be sure to inform your health care provider if there is a family history of any of the conditions listed previously in this leaflet. Be sure to keep all appointments with your health care provider, because this is a time to determine if there are early signs of side effects of oral contraceptive use.
Do not use the drug for any condition other than the one for which it was prescribed. This drug has been prescribed specifically for you; do not give it to others who may want birth control pills.

HEALTH BENEFITS FROM ORAL CONTRACEPTIVES

In addition to preventing pregnancy, use of oral contraceptives may provide certain benefits. They are:

- Menstrual cycles may become more regular
- Blood flow during menstruation may be lighter and less iron may be lost. Therefore, anemia due to iron deficiency is less likely to occur
- Pain or other symptoms during menstruation may be encountered less frequently
- Ectopic (tubal) pregnancy may occur less frequently
- Noncancerous cysts or lumps in the breast may occur less frequently
- Acute pelvic inflammatory disease may occur less frequently
- Oral contraceptive use may provide some protection against developing two forms of cancer: cancer of the ovaries and cancer of the lining of the uterus.

If you want more information about birth control pills, ask your doctor or pharmacist. They have a more technical leaflet called the "Physician Insert," which you may wish to read.
Remembering to take tablets according to schedule is stressed because of its importance in providing you the greatest degree of protection.

MISSED MENSTRUAL PERIODS FOR THIS DOSAGE REGIMEN

At times there may be no menstrual period after a cycle of pills. Therefore, if you miss one menstrual period but have taken the pills *exactly as you were supposed to*, continue as usual into the next cycle. If you have not taken the pills correctly and miss a menstrual period, *you may be pregnant* and should stop taking oral contraceptives until your doctor or health care provider determines whether or not you are pregnant. Until you can get to your doctor or health care provider, use another form of contraception. If two consecutive menstrual periods are missed, you should stop taking pills until it is determined whether or not you are pregnant. Although there does not appear to be any increase in birth defects in newborn babies, if you become pregnant while using oral contraceptives, you should discuss the situation with your doctor or health care provider.

Periodic Examination

Your doctor or health care provider will take a complete medical and family history before prescribing oral contraceptives. At that time and about once a year thereafter, he or she will generally examine your blood pressure, breasts, abdomen, and pelvic organs (including a Papanicolaou smear, ie, test for cancer).

Keep this and all drugs out of the reach of children.
Store at controlled room temperature 15°–30°C (59°– 86°F).
WATSON PHARMA®
Watson Pharma, Inc.
a subsidiary of
Watson Laboratories, Inc. 14038
Corona, CA 92880 March 2001

MICROGESTIN™ Fe 1.5/30 ℞

(Norethindrone Acetate and Ethinyl Estradiol Tablets, USP and Ferrous Fumarate Tablets*)
***Ferrous fumarate tablets are not USP for dissolution and assay.**
Rx Only
Patients should be counseled that this product does not protect against HIV infection (AIDS) and other sexually transmitted diseases.

DESCRIPTION

Microgestin Fe 1.5/30 is a progestogen-estrogen combination.
The structural formula of norethindrone acetate (17 alpha-ethinyl-19-nortestosterone acetate) and ethinyl estradiol (17 alpha-ethinyl-1, 3, 5(10)-estratriene-3, 17 beta-diol) are as follows:

Norethindrone Acetate

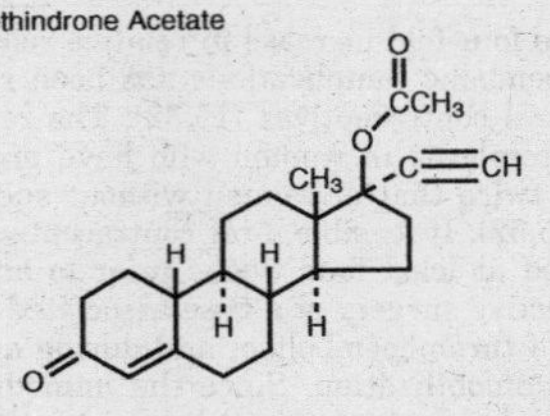

$C_{22}H_{28}O_3$ MW=340.46

Ethinyl Estradiol

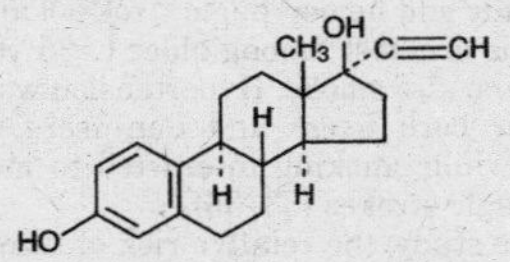

$C_{20}H_{24}O_2$ MW=296.40

Microgestin Fe 1.5/30 provides a continuous dosage regimen consisting of 21 green oral contraceptive tablets and 7 brown ferrous fumarate tablets. The ferrous fumarate tablets are present to facilitate ease of drug administration via a 28-day regimen, are non-hormonal, and do not serve any therapeutic purpose.
Each green tablet, for oral administration, contains 1.5 mg norethindrone acetate and 30 mcg ethinyl estradiol. It also contains the following inactive ingredients: anhydrous lactose, ethyl alcohol, FD&C green (a composite of D&C yellow No. 10 and FD&C blue No. 1), magnesium stearate, microcrystalline cellulose, polacrilin potassium, and povidone.
Each brown tablet for oral administration contains 75 mg ferrous fumarate and anhydrous lactose, crospovidone, magnesium stearate, and pregelatinized starch.

CLINICAL PHARMACOLOGY

Combination oral contraceptives act by suppression of gonadotropins. Although the primary mechanism of this action is inhibition of ovulation, other alterations include changes in the cervical mucus (which increase the difficulty of sperm entry into the uterus) and the endometrium (which reduce the likelihood of implantation).

Pharmacokinetics

The pharmacokinetics of norethindrone acetate and ethinyl estradiol have not been characterized; however, the following pharmacokinetic information regarding norethindrone acetate and ethinyl estradiol is taken from the literature.

Absorption

Norethindrone acetate appears to be completely and rapidly deacetylated to norethindrone after oral administration, since the disposition of norethindrone acetate is indistinguishable from that of orally administered norethindrone (1). Norethindrone acetate and ethinyl estradiol are subject to first-pass metabolism after oral dosing, resulting in an absolute bioavailability of approximately 64% for norethindrone and 43% for ethinyl estradiol (1–3).

Distribution

Volume of distribution of norethindrone and ethinyl estradiol ranges from 2 to 4 L/kg (1–3). Plasma protein binding of both steroids is extensive (>95%); norethindrone binds to both albumin and sex hormone binding globulin, whereas ethinyl estradiol binds only to albumin (4).

Metabolism

Norethindrone undergoes extensive biotransformation, primarily via reduction, followed by sulfate and glucuronide conjugation. The majority of metabolites in the circulation are sulfates, with glucuronides accounting for most of the urinary metabolites (5). A small amount of norethindrone acetate is metabolically converted to ethinyl estradiol. Ethinyl estradiol is also extensively metabolized, both by oxidation and by conjugation with sulfate and glucuronide. Sulfates are the major circulating conjugates of ethinyl estradiol and glucuronides predominate in urine. The primary oxidative metabolite is 2-hydroxy ethinyl estradiol, formed by the CYP3A4 isoform of cytochrome P450. Part of the first-pass metabolism of ethinyl estradiol is believed to occur in gastrointestinal mucosa. Ethinyl estradiol may undergo enterohepatic circulation (6).

Excretion

Norethindrone and ethinyl estradiol are excreted in both urine and feces, primarily as metabolites (5,6). Plasma clearance values for norethindrone and ethinyl estradiol are similar (approximately 0.4 L/hr/kg) (1–3).

Special Population

Race:
The effect of race on the disposition of norethindrone acetate and ethinyl estradiol has not been evaluated.

Renal Insufficiency
The effect of renal disease on the disposition of norethindrone acetate and ethinyl estradiol has not been evaluated. In premenopausal women with chronic renal failure undergoing peritoneal dialysis who received multiple doses of an oral contraceptive containing ethinyl estradiol and norethindrone, plasma ethinyl estradiol concentrations were higher and norethindrone concentrations were unchanged compared to concentrations in premenopausal women with normal renal function.

Hepatic Insufficiency
The effect of hepatic disease on the disposition of norethindrone acetate and ethinyl estradiol has not been evaluated. However, ethinyl estradiol and norethindrone may be poorly metabolized in patients with impaired liver function.

Drug-Drug Interactions
Numerous drug-drug interactions have been reported for oral contraceptives. A summary of these is found under **PRECAUTIONS, Drug Interactions.**

INDICATIONS AND USAGE

Microgestin Fe 1.5/30 is indicated for the prevention of pregnancy in women who elect to use oral contraceptives as a method of contraception.
Oral contraceptives are highly effective. Table I lists the typical accidental pregnancy rates for users of combination oral contraceptives and other methods of contraception. The efficacy of these contraceptive methods, except sterilization, depends upon the reliability with which they are used. Correct and consistent use of methods can result in lower failure rates.

TABLE I
LOWEST EXPECTED AND TYPICAL FAILURE RATES DURING THE FIRST YEAR OF CONTINUOUS USE OF A METHOD
% of Women Experiencing an Unintended Pregnancy in the First Year of Continuous Use.

Method	Lowest Expected*	Typical**
(No contraception)	(85)	(85)
Oral contraceptives	-	3
combined	0.1	N/A***
progestin only	0.5	N/A***
Diaphragm with spermicidal cream or jelly	6	20
Spermicides alone (foam, creams, gels, vaginal suppositories, and vaginal film)	6	26
Vaginal Sponge		
nulliparous	9	20
parous	20	40
Implant	0.05	0.05
Injection:		
depot medroxyprogesterone acetate	0.3	0.3

Continued on next page

Microgestin Fe 1.5/30—Cont.

IUD

progesterone T	1.5	2.0
copper T 380A	0.6	0.8
LNg 20	0.1	0.1
Condom without spermicides		
female	5	21
male	3	14
Cervical Cap with spermicidal cream or jelly		
nulliparous	9	20
parous	26	40
Periodic abstinence		
(all methods)	1–9	25
Withdrawal	4	19
Female sterilization	0.5	0.5
Male sterilization	0.10	0.15

Adapted from RA Hatcher et al. Reference 7.

*The authors' best guess of the percentage of women expected to experience an accidental pregnancy among couples who initiate a method (not necessarily for the first time) and who use it consistently and correctly during the first year if they do not stop for any other reason.
**This term represents "typical" couples who initiate use of a method (not necessarily for the first time), who experience an accidental pregnancy during the first year if they do not stop for any other reason.
***N/A—Data not available

CONTRAINDICATIONS

Oral contraceptives should not be used in women who currently have the following conditions:

- Thrombophlebitis or thromboembolic disorders
- A past history of deep vein thrombophlebitis or thromboembolic disorders
- Cerebral vascular or coronary artery disease
- Known or suspected carcinoma of the breast
- Carcinoma of the endometrium or other known or suspected estrogen-dependent neoplasia
- Undiagnosed abnormal genital bleeding
- Cholestatic jaundice of pregnancy or jaundice with prior pill use
- Hepatic adenomas or carcinomas
- Known or suspected pregnancy

WARNINGS

> **Cigarette smoking increases the risk of serious cardiovascular side effects from oral contraceptive use. This risk increases with age and with heavy smoking (15 or more cigarettes per day) and is quite marked in women over 35 years of age. Women who use oral contraceptives should be strongly advised not to smoke.**

The use of oral contraceptives is associated with increased risks of several serious conditions including myocardial infarction, thromboembolism, stroke, hepatic neoplasia, and gallbladder disease, although the risk of serious morbidity or mortality is very small in healthy women without underlying risk factors. The risk of morbidity and mortality increases significantly in the presence of other underlying risk factors such as hypertension, hyperlipidemias, obesity, and diabetes.

Practitioners prescribing oral contraceptives should be familiar with the following information relating to these risks. The information contained in this package insert is principally based on studies carried out in patients who used oral contraceptives with higher formulations of estrogens and progestogens than those in common use today. The effect of long-term use of the oral contraceptives with lower formulations of both estrogens and progestogens remains to be determined.

Throughout this labeling, epidemiological studies reported are of two types: retrospective or case control studies and prospective or cohort studies. Case control studies provide a measure of the relative risk of a disease, namely, a *ratio* of the incidence of a disease among oral contraceptive users to that among nonusers. The relative risk does not provide information on the actual clinical occurrence of a disease. Cohort studies provide a measure of attributable risk, which is the *difference* in the incidence of disease between oral contraceptive users and nonusers. The attributable risk does provide information about the actual occurrence of a disease in the population (adapted from References 8 and 9 with the author's permission). For further information, the reader is referred to a text on epidemiological methods.

1. Thromboembolic Disorders and Other Vascular Problems

a. Myocardial Infarction

An increased risk of myocardial infarction has been attributed to oral contraceptive use. This risk is primarily in smokers or women with other underlying risk factors for coronary artery disease such as hypertension, hypercholesterolemia, morbid obesity, and diabetes. The relative risk of heart attack for current oral contraceptive users has been estimated to be two to six (10–16). The risk is very low under the age of 30.

Smoking in combination with oral contraceptive use has been shown to contribute substantially to the incidence of myocardial infarctions in women in their mid-thirties or older with smoking accounting for the majority of excess

cases (17). Mortality rates associated with circulatory disease have been shown to increase substantially in smokers over the age of 35 and non-smokers over the age of 40 (Table II) among women who use oral contraceptives.

TABLE II
CIRCULATORY DISEASE MORTALITY RATES PER 100,000 WOMEN YEARS BY AGE, SMOKING STATUS AND ORAL CONTRACEPTIVE USE

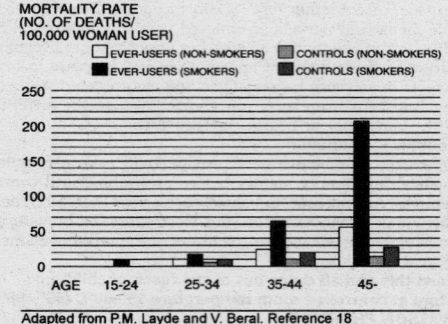

Adapted from P.M. Layde and V. Beral. Reference 18

Oral contraceptives may compound the effects of well-known risk factors, such as hypertension, diabetes, hyperlipidemias, age and obesity (19). In particular, some progestogens are known to decrease HDL cholesterol and cause glucose intolerance, while estrogens may create a state of hyperinsulinism (20–24). Oral contraceptives have been shown to increase blood pressure among users (see section **9** in **WARNINGS**). Similar effects on risk factors have been associated with an increased risk of heart disease. Oral contraceptives must be used with caution in women with cardiovascular disease risk factors.

b. Thromboembolism

An increased risk of thromboembolic and thrombotic disease associated with the use of oral contraceptives is well established. Case control studies have found the relative risk of users compared to nonusers to be 3 for the first episode of superficial venous thrombosis, 4 to 11 for deep vein thrombosis or pulmonary embolism, and 1.5 to 6 for women with predisposing conditions for venous thromboembolic disease (9, 10, 25–30). Cohort studies have shown the relative risk to be somewhat lower, about 3 for new cases and about 4.5 for new cases requiring hospitalization (31). The risk of thromboembolic disease due to oral contraceptives is not related to length of use and disappears after pill use is stopped (8).

A two- to four-fold increase in relative risk of postoperative thromboembolic complications has been reported with the use of oral contraceptives (15,32). The relative risk of venous thrombosis in women who have predisposing conditions is twice that of women without such medical conditions (15,32). If feasible, oral contraceptives should be discontinued at least four weeks prior to and for two weeks after elective surgery of a type associated with an increase in risk of thromboembolism and during and following prolonged immobilization. Since the immediate post-partum period is also associated with an increased risk of thromboembolism, oral contraceptives should be started no earlier than four to six weeks after delivery in women who elect not to breast feed.

c. Cerebrovascular Disease

Oral contraceptives have been shown to increase both the relative and attributable risks of cerebrovascular events (thrombotic and hemorrhagic strokes), although, in general, the risk is greatest among older (>35 years), hypertensive women who also smoke. Hypertension was found to be a risk factor for both users and non-users, for both types of strokes, while smoking interacted to increase the risk for hemorrhagic strokes (33–35).

In a large study, the relative risk of thrombotic strokes has been shown to range from 3 for normotensive users to 14 for users with severe hypertension (36). The relative risk of hemorrhagic stroke is reported to be 1.2 for non-smokers who used oral contraceptives, 2.6 for smokers who did not use oral contraceptives, 7.6 for smokers who used oral contraceptives, 1.8 for normotensive users and 25.7 for users with severe hypertension (36). The attributable risk is also greater in older women (9).

d. Dose-Related Risk of Vascular Disease from Oral Contraceptives

A positive association has been observed between the amount of estrogen and progestogen in oral contraceptives and the risk of vascular disease (37–39). A decline in serum high-density lipoproteins (HDL) has been reported with many progestational agents (20–22). A decline in serum high-density lipoproteins has been associated with an increased incidence of ischemic heart disease. Because estrogens increase HDL cholesterol, the net effect of an oral contraceptive depends on a balance achieved between doses of estrogen and progestin and the nature of the progestin used in the contraceptives. The amount and activity of both hormones should be considered in the choice of an oral contraceptive.

Minimizing exposure to estrogen and progestogen is in keeping with good principles of therapeutics. For any particular oral contraceptive, the dosage regimen prescribed should be one which contains the least amount of estrogen and progestogen that is compatible with the needs of the in-

dividual patient. New acceptors of oral contraceptive agents should be started on preparations containing the lowest dose of estrogen which produces satisfactory results for the patient.

e. Persistence of Risk of Vascular Disease

There are two studies which have shown persistence of risk of vascular disease for ever-users of oral contraceptives. In a study in the United States, the risk of developing myocardial infarction after discontinuing oral contraceptives persists for at least 9 years for women 40 to 49 years who had used oral contraceptives for 5 or more years, but this increased risk was not demonstrated in other age groups (14). In another study in Great Britain, the risk of developing cerebrovascular disease persisted for at least 6 years after discontinuation of oral contraceptives, although excess risk was very small (40). However, both studies were performed with oral contraceptive formulations containing 50 mcg or higher of estrogens.

2. Estimates of Mortality from Contraceptive Use

One study gathered data from a variety of sources which have estimated the mortality rate associated with different methods of contraception at different ages (Table III). These estimates include the combined risk of death associated with contraceptive methods plus the risk attributable to pregnancy in the event of method failure. Each method of contraception has its specific benefits and risks. The study concluded that with the exception of oral contraceptive users 35 and older who smoke and 40 and older who do not smoke, mortality associated with all methods of birth control is low and below that associated with childbirth. The observation of a possible increase in risk of mortality with age for oral contraceptive users is based on data gathered in the 1970's but not reported until 1983 (41). However, current clinical practice involves the use of lower estrogen dose formulations combined with careful restriction of oral contraceptive use to women who do not have the various risk factors listed in this labeling.

Because of these changes in practice and, also, because of some limited new data which suggest that the risk of cardiovascular disease with the use of oral contraceptives may now be less than previously observed (Porter JB, Hunter J, Jick H, et al. Oral contraceptives and nonfatal vascular disease. Obstet Gynecol 1985;66:1–4 and Porter JB, Hershel J, Walker AM. Mortality among oral contraceptive users. Obstet Gynecol 1987;70:29–32), the Fertility and Maternal Health Drugs Advisory Committee was asked to review the topic in 1989. The Committee concluded that although cardiovascular disease risks may be increased with oral contraceptive use after age 40 in healthy non-smoking women (even with the newer low-dose formulations), there are greater potential health risks associated with pregnancy in older women and with the alternative surgical and medical procedures which may be necessary if such women do not have access to effective and acceptable means of contraception.

Therefore, the Committee recommended that the benefits of oral contraceptive use by healthy non-smoking women over 40 may outweigh the possible risks. Of course, older women, as all women who take oral contraceptives, should take the lowest possible dose formulation that is effective.
[See table III at bottom of next page]

3. Carcinoma of the Reproductive Organs

Numerous epidemiological studies have been performed on the incidence of breast, endometrial, ovarian, and cervical cancer in women using oral contraceptives. Most of the studies on breast cancer and oral contraceptive use report that the use of oral contraceptives is not associated with an increase in the risk of developing breast cancer (42,44,89). Some studies have reported an increased risk of developing breast cancer in certain subgroups of oral contraceptive users, but the findings reported in these studies are not consistent (43,45–49,85–88).

Some studies suggest that oral contraceptive use has been associated with an increase in the risk of cervical intraepithelial neoplasia in some populations of women (51–54). However, there continues to be controversy about the extent to which such findings may be due to differences in sexual behavior and other factors.

In spite of many studies of the relationship between oral contraceptive use and breast and cervical cancers, a cause and effect relationship has not been established.

4. Hepatic Neoplasia

Benign hepatic adenomas are associated with oral contraceptive use, although the incidence of benign tumors is rare in the United States. Indirect calculations have estimated the attributable risk to be in the range of 3.3 cases/100,000 for users, a risk that increases after four or more years of use (55). Rupture of rare, benign, hepatic adenomas may cause death through intra-abdominal hemorrhage (56,57).

Studies from Britain have shown an increased risk of developing hepatocellular carcinoma (58–60) in long-term (>8 years) oral contraceptive users. However, these cancers are extremely rare in the U.S., and the attributable risk (the excess incidence) of liver cancers in oral contraceptive users approaches less than one per million users.

5. Ocular Lesions

There have been clinical case reports of retinal thrombosis associated with the use of oral contraceptives. Oral contraceptives should be discontinued if there is unexplained partial or complete loss of vision; onset of proptosis or diplopia; papilledema; or retinal vascular lesions. Appropriate diagnostic and therapeutic measures should be undertaken immediately.

6. Oral Contraceptive Use Before and During Early Pregnancy

Extensive epidemiological studies have revealed no increased risk of birth defects in women who have used oral contraceptives prior to pregnancy (61–63). Studies also do not suggest a teratogenic effect, particularly insofar as cardiac anomalies and limb reduction defects are concerned (61,62,64,65), when taken inadvertently during early pregnancy.

The administration of oral contraceptives to induce withdrawal bleeding should not be used as a test for pregnancy. Oral contraceptives should not be used during pregnancy to treat threatened or habitual abortion.

It is recommended that for any patient who has missed two consecutive periods, pregnancy should be ruled out before continuing oral contraceptive use. If the patient has not adhered to the prescribed schedule, the possibility of pregnancy should be considered at the time of the first missed period. Oral contraceptive use should be discontinued if pregnancy is confirmed.

7. Gallbladder Disease
Earlier studies have reported an increased lifetime relative risk of gallbladder surgery in users of oral contraceptives and estrogens (66,67). More recent studies, however, have shown that the relative risk of developing gallbladder disease among oral contraceptive users may be minimal (68–70). The recent findings of minimal risk may be related to the use of oral contraceptive formulations containing lower hormonal doses of estrogens and progestogens.

8. Carbohydrate and Lipid Metabolic Effects
Oral contraceptives have been shown to cause glucose intolerance in a significant percentage of users (23). Oral contraceptives containing greater than 75 mcg of estrogens cause hyperinsulinism, while lower doses of estrogen cause less glucose intolerance (71). Progestogens increase insulin secretion and create insulin resistance, this effect varying with different progestational agents (23,72). However, in the non-diabetic woman, oral contraceptives appear to have no effect on fasting blood glucose (73). Because of these demonstrated effects, prediabetic and diabetic women should be carefully observed while taking oral contraceptives.

A small proportion of women will have persistent hypertriglyceridemia while on the pill. As discussed earlier (see **WARNINGS** 1a. and 1d.), changes in serum triglycerides and lipoprotein levels have been reported in oral contraceptive users.

9. Elevated Blood Pressure
An increase in blood pressure has been reported in women taking oral contraceptives (74) and this increase is more likely in older oral contraceptive users (75) and with continued use (74). Data from the Royal College of General Practitioners (18) and subsequent randomized trials have shown that the incidence of hypertension increases with increasing concentrations of progestogens.

Women with a history of hypertension or hypertension-related diseases, or renal disease (76) should be encouraged to use another method of contraception. If women elect to use oral contraceptives, they should be monitored closely and if significant elevation of blood pressure occurs, oral contraceptives should be discontinued. For most women, elevated blood pressure will return to normal after stopping oral contraceptives (75), and there is no difference in the occurrence of hypertension among ever and never users (74,76,77).

10. Headache
The onset or exacerbation of migraine or development of headache with a new pattern which is recurrent, persistent, or severe requires discontinuation of oral contraceptives and evaluation of the cause.

11. Bleeding Irregularities
Breakthrough bleeding and spotting are sometimes encountered in patients on oral contraceptives, especially during the first three months of use. Non-hormonal causes should be considered, and adequate diagnostic measures taken to rule out malignancy or pregnancy in the event of breakthrough bleeding, as in the case of any abnormal vaginal bleeding. If pathology has been excluded, time or a change to another formulation may solve the problem. In the event of amenorrhea, pregnancy should be ruled out.

Some women may encounter post-pill amenorrhea or oligomenorrhea, especially when such a condition was preexistent.

PRECAUTIONS
1. Patients should be counseled that this product does not protect against HIV infection (AIDS) and other sexually transmitted diseases.

2. Physical Examination and Follow-Up
It is good medical practice for all women to have annual history and physical examinations, including women using oral contraceptives. The physical examination, however, may be deferred until after initiation of oral contraceptives if requested by the woman and judged appropriate by the clinician. The physical examination should include special reference to blood pressure, breasts, abdomen, and pelvic organs, including cervical cytology, and relevant laboratory tests. In case of undiagnosed, persistent or recurrent abnormal vaginal bleeding, appropriate measures should be conducted to rule out malignancy. Women with a strong family history of breast cancer or who have breast nodules should be monitored with particular care.

3. Lipid Disorders
Women who are being treated for hyperlipidemia should be followed closely if they elect to use oral contraceptives. Some progestogens may elevate LDL levels and may render the control of hyperlipidemias more difficult.

4. Liver Function
If jaundice develops in any woman receiving such drugs, the medication should be discontinued. Steroid hormones may be poorly metabolized in patients with impaired liver function.

5. Fluid Retention
Oral contraceptives may cause some degree of fluid retention. They should be prescribed with caution, and only with careful monitoring, in patients with conditions which might be aggravated by fluid retention.

6. Emotional Disorders
Women with a history of depression should be carefully observed and the drug discontinued if depression recurs to a serious degree.

7. Contact Lenses
Contact lens wearers who develop visual changes or changes in lens tolerance should be assessed by an ophthalmologist.

8. Drug Interactions
Effects of Other Drugs on Oral Contraceptives (78)

Rifampin: Metabolism of both norethindrone and ethinyl estradiol is increased by rifampin. A reduction in contraceptive effectiveness and increased incidence of breakthrough bleeding and menstrual irregularities have been associated with concomitant use of rifampin.

Anticonvulsants: Anticonvulsants such as phenobarbital, phenytoin, and carbamazepine, have been shown to increase the metabolism of ethinyl estradiol and/or norethindrone, which could result in a reduction in contraceptive effectiveness.

Troglitazone: Administration of troglitazone with an oral contraceptive containing ethinyl estradiol and norethindrone reduced the plasma concentrations of both by approximately 30%, which could result in a reduction of contraceptive effectiveness.

Antibiotics: Pregnancy while taking oral contraceptives has been reported when the oral contraceptives were administered with antimicrobials such as ampicillin, tetracycline, and griseofulvin. However, clinical pharmacokinetic studies have not demonstrated any consistent effect of antibiotics (other than rifampin) on plasma concentrations of synthetic steroids.

Atorvastatin: Coadministration of atorvastatin and an oral contraceptive increased AUC values for norethindrone and ethinyl estradiol by approximately 30% and 20%, respectively.

Other: Ascorbic acid and acetaminophen may increase plasma ethinyl estradiol concentrations, possibly by inhibition of conjugation. A reduction in contraceptive effectiveness and increased incidence of breakthrough bleeding has been suggested with phenylbutazone.

Effects of Oral Contraceptives on Other Drugs

Oral contraceptive combinations containing ethinyl estradiol may inhibit the metabolism of other compounds. Increased plasma concentrations of cyclosporine, prednisolone, and theophylline have been reported with concomitant administration of oral contraceptives. In addition, oral contraceptives may induce the conjugation of other compounds. Decreased plasma concentrations of acetaminophen and increased clearance of temazepam, salicylic acid, morphine, and clofibric acid have been noted when these drugs were administered with oral contraceptives.

9. Interactions With Laboratory Tests
Certain endocrine and liver function tests and blood components may be affected by oral contraceptives:

a. Increased prothrombin and factors VII, VIII, IX and X; decreased antithrombin 3; increased norepinephrine-induced platelet aggregability.

b. Increased thyroid binding globulin (TBG) leading to increased circulating total thyroid hormone, as measured by protein-bound iodine (PBI), T_4 by column or by radioimmunoassay. Free T_3 resin uptake is decreased, reflecting the elevated TBG; free T_4 concentration is unaltered.

c. Other binding proteins may be elevated in serum.

d. Sex-binding globulins are increased and result in elevated levels of total circulating sex steroids and corticoids; however, free or biologically active levels remain unchanged.

e. Triglycerides may be increased.

f. Glucose tolerance may be decreased.

g. Serum folate levels may be depressed by oral contraceptive therapy. This may be of clinical significance if a woman becomes pregnant shortly after discontinuing oral contraceptives.

10. Carcinogenesis
See **WARNINGS** section.

11. Pregnancy
Pregnancy Category X.
See **CONTRAINDICATIONS** and **WARNINGS** sections.

12. Nursing Mothers
Small amounts of oral contraceptive steroids have been identified in the milk of nursing mothers, and a few adverse effects on the child have been reported, including jaundice and breast enlargement. In addition, oral contraceptives given in the postpartum period may interfere with lactation by decreasing the quantity and quality of breast milk. If possible, the nursing mother should be advised not to use oral contraceptives but to use other forms of contraception until she has completely weaned her child.

13. Pediatric Use
Safety and efficacy of norethindrone acetate and ethinyl estradiol has been established in women of reproductive age. Safety and efficacy are expected to be the same for postpubertal adolescents under the age of 16 and for users 16 years and older. Use of this product before menarche is not indicated.

INFORMATION FOR THE PATIENT
See patient labeling printed below.

ADVERSE REACTIONS
An increased risk of the following serious adverse reactions has been associated with the use of oral contraceptives (see **WARNINGS** section):
- Thrombophlebitis
- Arterial thromboembolism
- Pulmonary embolism
- Myocardial infarction
- Cerebral hemorrhage
- Cerebral thrombosis
- Hypertension
- Gallbladder disease
- Hepatic adenomas or benign liver tumors

There is evidence of an association between the following conditions and the use of oral contraceptives, although additional confirmatory studies are needed:
- Mesenteric thrombosis
- Retinal thrombosis

The following adverse reactions have been reported in patients receiving oral contraceptives and are believed to be drug-related:
- Nausea
- Vomiting
- Gastrointestinal symptoms (such as abdominal cramps and bloating)
- Breakthrough bleeding
- Spotting
- Change in menstrual flow
- Amenorrhea
- Temporary infertility after discontinuation of treatment
- Edema
- Melasma which may persist
- Breast changes: tenderness, enlargement, secretion
- Change in weight (increase or decrease)
- Change in cervical erosion or secretion
- Diminution in lactation when given immediately postpartum
- Cholestatic jaundice
- Migraine
- Rash (allergic)
- Mental depression
- Reduced tolerance to carbohydrates
- Vaginal candidiasis
- Change in corneal curvature (steepening)
- Intolerance to contact lenses

The following adverse reactions have been reported in users of oral contraceptives and the association has been neither confirmed nor refuted:
- Pre-menstrual syndrome
- Cataracts
- Changes in appetite
- Cystitis-like syndrome

TABLE III
ANNUAL NUMBER OF BIRTH-RELATED OR METHOD-RELATED DEATHS ASSOCIATED WITH CONTROL OF FERTILITY PER 100,000 NONSTERILE WOMEN, BY FERTILITY CONTROL METHOD ACCORDING TO AGE

Method of control and outcome	15–19	20–24	25–29	30–34	35–39	40–44
No fertility control methods*	7.0	7.4	9.1	14.8	25.7	28.2
Oral contraceptives non-smoker**	0.3	0.5	0.9	1.9	13.8	31.6
Oral contraceptives smoker**	2.2	3.4	6.6	13.5	51.1	117.2
IUD**	0.8	0.8	1.0	1.0	1.4	1.4
Condom*	1.1	1.6	0.7	0.2	0.3	0.4
Diaphragm/spermicide*	1.9	1.2	1.2	1.3	2.2	2.8
Periodic abstinence*	2.5	1.6	1.6	1.7	2.9	3.6

*Deaths are birth related.
**Deaths are method related.

Adapted from H.W. Ory, Reference 41.

Continued on next page

Microgestin Fe 1.5/30—Cont.

- Headache
- Nervousness
- Dizziness
- Hirsutism
- Loss of scalp hair
- Erythema multiforme
- Erythema nodosum
- Hemorrhagic eruption
- Vaginitis
- Porphyria
- Impaired renal function
- Hemolytic uremic syndrome
- Budd-Chiari syndrome
- Acne
- Changes in libido
- Colitis

OVERDOSAGE

Serious ill effects have not been reported following acute ingestion of large doses of oral contraceptives by young children. Overdosage may cause nausea, and withdrawal bleeding may occur in females.

NON-CONTRACEPTIVE HEALTH BENEFITS

The following non-contraceptive health benefits related to the use of oral contraceptives are supported by epidemiological studies which largely utilized oral contraceptive formulations containing estrogen doses exceeding 0.035 mg of ethinyl estradiol or 0.05 mg of mestranol (79–84).

Effects on Menses:
- Increased menstrual cycle regularity
- Decreased blood loss and decreased incidence of iron deficiency anemia
- Decreased incidence of dysmenorrhea

Effects Related to Inhibition of Ovulation:
- Decreased incidence of functional ovarian cysts
- Decreased incidence of ectopic pregnancies

Effects From Long-Term Use:
- Decreased incidence of fibroadenomas and fibrocystic disease of the breast
- Decreased incidence of acute pelvic inflammatory disease
- Decreased incidence of endometrial cancer
- Decreased incidence of ovarian cancer

DOSAGE AND ADMINISTRATION

The tablet dispenser has been designed to make oral contraceptive dosing as easy and as convenient as possible. The tablets are arranged in four rows of seven tablets each, with the days of the week appearing on the tablet dispenser below the last row of tablets.

Important: The patient should be instructed to use an additional method of protection until after the first week of administration in the initial cycle when utilizing the Sunday-Start Regimen.

The possibility of ovulation and conception prior to initiation of use should be considered.

Dosage and Administration for 28-Day Dosage Regimen

To achieve maximum contraceptive effectiveness, Microgestin Fe should be taken exactly as directed and at intervals not exceeding 24 hours.

Microgestin Fe provides a continuous administration regimen consisting of 21 green tablets of Microgestin and 7 brown non-hormone containing tablets of ferrous fumarate. The ferrous fumarate tablets are present to facilitate ease of drug administration via a 28-day regimen and do not serve any therapeutic purpose. There is no need for the patient to count days between cycles because there are no "off-tablet days."

A. Sunday-Start Regimen:

The patient begins taking the first green tablet from the top row of the dispenser (labeled Sunday) on the first Sunday after menstrual flow begins. When menstrual flow begins on Sunday, the first green tablet is taken on the same day. The patient takes one green tablet daily for 21 days. The last green tablet will be taken on a Saturday. Upon completion of all 21 green tablets, and without interruption, the patient takes one brown tablet daily for 7 days. Upon completion of this first course of tablets, the patient begins a second course of 28-day tablets, without interruption, the next day, Sunday, starting with the Sunday green tablet in the top row. Adhering to this regimen of one green tablet daily for 21 days, followed without interruption by one brown tablet daily for 7 days, the patient will start all subsequent cycles on a Sunday.

B. Day-1 Start Regimen:

The first day of menstrual flow is Day 1. The patient starts taking one green tablet daily, beginning with the first green tablet in the top row. After the last green tablet (Saturday) has been taken, if any green tablets remain in the top row, the patient takes the remaining green tablets starting with the Sunday green tablets in the top row, followed by the brown tablets for a week (7 days). For all subsequent cycles, the patient begins a new 28 tablet regimen on the eighth day after taking her last green tablet, again starting with the first tablet in the top row. Following this regimen of 21 green tablets and 7 brown tablets, the patient will start all subsequent cycles on the same day of the week as the first course.

Tablets should be taken regularly with a meal or at bedtime. It should be stressed that efficacy of medication depends on strict adherence to the dosage schedule.

Special Notes on Administration

Menstruation usually begins two or three days, but may begin as late as the fourth or fifth day, after the brown tablets have been started. In any event, the next course of tablets should be started without interruption. If spotting occurs while the patient is taking green tablets, continue medication without interruption.

If the patient forgets to take one or more green tablets, the following is suggested:

One tablet is missed
- take tablet as soon as remembered
- take next tablet at the regular time

Two consecutive tablets are missed (week 1 or week 2)
- take *two* tablets as soon as remembered
- take *two* tablets the next day
- use another birth control method for seven days following the missed tablets

Two consecutive tablets are missed (week 3)

Sunday-Start Regimen:
- take *one* tablet daily until Sunday
- discard remaining tablets
- start new pack of tablets immediately (Sunday)
- use another birth control method for seven days following the missed tablets

Day-1 Start Regimen:
- discard remaining tablets
- start new pack of tablets that same day
- use another birth control method for seven days following the missed tablets

Three (or more) consecutive tablets are missed

Sunday-Start Regimen:
- take *one* tablet daily until Sunday
- discard remaining tablets
- start new pack of tablets immediately (Sunday)
- use another birth control method for seven days following the missed tablets

Day-1 Start Regimen:
- discard remaining tablets
- start new pack of tablets that same day
- use another birth control method for seven days following the missed tablets

The possibility of ovulation occurring increases with each successive day that scheduled green tablets are missed. While there is little likelihood of ovulation occurring if only one green tablet is missed, the possibility of spotting or bleeding is increased. This is particularly likely to occur if two or more consecutive green tablets are missed.

If the patient forgets to take any of the seven brown tablets in week four, those brown tablets that were missed are discarded and one brown tablet is taken each day until the pack is empty. A back up birth control method is not required during this time. A new pack of tablets should be started no later than the eighth day after the last green tablet was taken.

In the rare case of bleeding which resembles menstruation, the patient should be advised to discontinue medication and then begin taking tablets from a new tablet dispenser on the next Sunday or the first day (Day-1), depending on her regimen. Persistent bleeding which is not controlled by this method indicates the need for reexamination of the patient, at which time nonfunctional causes should be considered.

Use of Oral Contraceptives in the Event of a Missed Menstrual Period

1. If the patient has not adhered to the prescribed dosage regimen, the possibility of pregnancy should be considered after the first missed period and oral contraceptives should be withheld until pregnancy has been ruled out.
2. If the patient has adhered to the prescribed regimen and misses two consecutive periods, pregnancy should be ruled out before continuing the contraceptive regimen.

After several months on treatment, bleeding may be reduced to a point of virtual absence. This reduced flow may occur as a result of medication, in which event it is not indicative of pregnancy.

HOW SUPPLIED

Microgestin Fe 1.5/30 is available in cartons of six (6) dispensers. Each dispenser contains 21 norethindrone acetate and ethinyl estradiol tablets and 7 ferrous fumarate tablets. Microgestin are available as round green tablets debossed with **"WATSON 631"** on one side and plain on the other side. Each tablet contains 1.5 mg of norethindrone acetate and 30 mcg of ethinyl estradiol. They are supplied as follows:

Blister package of 28's   NDC-52544-631-28

Ferrous fumarate tablets are available as round brown tablets debossed with **"WATSON 632"** on one side and plain on the other side. Each tablet contains 75 mg ferrous fumarate.

Store at controlled room temperature 15°–30°C (59°–86°F).

REFERENCES

1. Back DJ, et al.: Kinetics of norethindrone in women II. Single-dose kinetics. Clin Pharmacol Ther 1978;24:448–453. 2. Humpel M, et al.: Investigations of pharmacokinetics of ethinyloestradiol to specific consideration of a possible first-pass effect in women. Contraception 1979;19:421–432. 3. Back DJ, et al. An investigation of the pharmacokinetics of ethynylestradiol in women using radioimmunoassay. Contraception 1979;20:263–273. 4. Hammond GL, et al. Distribution and percentages of non-protein bound contraceptive steroids in human serum. J Steroid Biochem 1982;17:375–380. 5. Fotherby K. Pharmacokinetics and metabolism of progestins in humans, in Pharmacology of the contraceptive steroids, Goldzieher JW, Fotherby K (eds), Raven Press, Ltd., New York, 1994, 99–126. 6. Goldzieher JW. Pharmacokinetics and metabolism of ethynyl estrogens, in Pharmacology of the contraceptive steroids, Goldzieher JW, Fotherby K (eds), Raven Press Ltd., New York, 1994, 127–151. 7. Hatcher, RA, et al. 1998. Contraceptive Technology, Seventeenth Edition. New York: Irvington Publishers. 8. Stadel, B.V.: Oral contraceptives and cardiovascular disease. (Pt. 1). New England Journal of Medicine, 305:612–618, 1981. 9. Stadel, B.V.: Oral contraceptives and cardiovascular disease. (Pt. 2). New England Journal of Medicine, 305:672–677, 1981. 10. Adam, S.A., and M. Thorogood: Oral contraception and myocardial infarction revisited: The effects of new preparations and prescribing patterns. Brit. J. Obstet. and Gynec., 88:838–845, 1981. 11. Mann, J.I., and W.H. Inman: Oral contraceptives and death from myocardial infarction. Brit. Med. J., 2(5965): 245–248, 1975. 12. Mann, J.I., et al.: Myocardial infarction in young women with special reference to oral contraceptive practice. Brit. Med. J., 2(5956):241–245, 1975. 13. Royal College of General Practitioners' Oral Contraception Study: Further analyses of mortality in oral contraceptive users. Lancet, 1:541–546, 1981. 14. Slone, D., et al.: Risk of myocardial infarction in relation to current and discontinued use of oral contraceptives. N.E.J.M., 305:420–424, 1981. 15. Vessey, M.P.: Female hormones and vascular disease: An epidemiological overview. Brit. J. Fam. Plann., 6:1–12, 1980. 16. Russell-Briefel, R.G., et al.: Cardiovascular risk status and oral contraceptive use, United States, 1976–80. Preventive Medicine, 15:352–362, 1986. 17. Goldbaum, G.M., et al.: The relative impact of smoking and oral contraceptive use on women in the United States. J.A.M.A., 258:1339–1342, 1987. 18. Layde, P.M., and V. Beral: Further analyses of mortality in oral contraceptive users: Royal College General Practitioners' Oral Contraception Study. (Table 5) Lancet, 1:541–546, 1981. 19. Knopp, R.H.: Arteriosclerosis risk: The roles of oral contraceptives and postmenopausal estrogens. J. of Reprod. Med., 31(9)(Supplement): 913–921, 1986. 20. Krauss, R.M., et al.: Effects of two low-dose oral contraceptives on serum lipids and lipoproteins: Differential changes in high-density lipoproteins subclasses. Am. J. Obstet. Gyn., 145:446–452, 1983. 21. Wahl, P., et al.: Effect of estrogen/progestin potency on lipid/lipoprotein cholesterol. N.E.J.M., 308:862–867, 1983. 22. Wynn, V., and R. Niththyananthan: The effect of progestin in combined oral contraceptives on serum lipids with special reference to high-density lipoproteins. Am. J. Obstet. and Gyn., 142:766–771, 1982. 23. Wynn, V., and I. Godsland: Effects of oral contraceptives on carbohydrate metabolism. J Reprod. Medicine, 31 (9)(Supplement): 892–897, 1986. 24. LaRosa, J.C.: Atherosclerotic risk factors in cardiovascular disease. J. Reprod. Med., 31(9)(Supplement): 906–912, 1986. 25. Inman, W.H., and M.P. Vessey: Investigations of death from pulmonary, coronary, and cerebral thrombosis and embolism in women of child-bearing age. Brit. Med. J., 2(5599): 193–199, 1968. 26. Maguire, M.G., et al.: Increased risk of thrombosis due to oral contraceptives: A further report. Am. J. Epidemiology, 110(2): 188–195, 1979. 27. Pettiti, D.B., et al.: Risk of vascular disease in women: Smoking, oral contraceptives, noncontraceptive estrogens, and other factors. J.A.M.A., 242:1150–1154, 1979. 28. Vessey, M.P., and R. Doll: Investigation of relation between use of oral contraceptives and thromboembolic disease. Brit. Med. J., 2(5599): 199–205, 1968. 29. Vessey, M.P. and R. Doll: Investigation of relation between use of oral contraceptives and thromboembolic disease: A further report. Brit. Med. J., 2(5658): 651–657, 1969. 30. Porter, J.B., et al.: Oral contraceptives and non-fatal vascular disease: Recent experience. Obstet. and Gyn., 59(3):299–302, 1982. 31. Vessey, M., et al.: A long-term follow-up study of women using different methods of contraception: An interim report. J. Biosocial. Sci., 8:375–427, 1976. 32. Royal College of General Practitioners: Oral contraceptives, venous thrombosis, and varicose veins. J. of Royal College of General Practitioners, 28:393–399, 1978. 33. Collaborative Group for the study of stroke in young women: Oral contraception and increased risk of cerebral ischemia or thrombosis. N.E.J.M. 288: 871–878, 1973. 34. Petitti, D.B., and J. Wingerd: Use of oral contraceptives, cigarette smoking, and risk of subarachnoid hemorrhage. Lancet, 2:234–236, 1978. 35. Inman, W.H.: Oral contraceptives and fatal subarachnoid hemorrhage. Brit. Med. J., 2(6203): 1468–1470, 1979. 36. Collaborative Group for the study of stroke in young women: Oral contraceptives and stroke in young women: Associated risk factors. J.A.M.A., 231:718–722, 1975. 37. Inman, W.H., et al.: Thromboembolic disease and the steroidal content of oral contraceptives. A report to the Committee on Safety of Drugs. Brit. Med. J., 2:203–209, 1970. 38. Meade, T.W., et al.: Progestogens and cardiovascular reactions associated with oral contraceptives and a comparison of the safety of 50- and 35-mcg oestrogen preparations. Brit. Med. J., 280(6224): 1157–1161, 1980. 39. Kay, C.R.: Progestogens and arterial disease: Evidence from the Royal College of General Practitioners' study. Amer. J. Obstet. Gyn., 142:762–765, 1982. 40. Royal College of General Practitioners: Incidence of arterial disease among oral contraceptive users. J. Coll. Gen. Pract., 33:75–82, 1983. 41. Ory, H.W: Mortality associated with fertility and fertility control: 1983. Family Planning Perspectives, 15:50–56, 1983. 42. The Cancer and Steroid Hormone Study of the Centers for Disease Control and the National Institute of Child Health and Human Development: Oral-contraceptive use and the risk of breast cancer. N.E.J.M., 315: 405–411, 1986. 43. Pike, M.C., et al.: Breast cancer in young women and use of oral contraceptives: Possible modifying effect of formulation and age at use. Lancet, 2:926–929, 1983. 44. Paul, C., et al.: Oral contraceptives and breast cancer: A national study. Brit. Med. J., 293:723–725, 1986. 45. Miller, D.R., et al.: Breast cancer risk in relation to early oral contraceptive use. Obstet. Gynec., 68:863–868, 1986. 46. Olson, H., et al.: Oral contraceptive use and breast cancer in young women in Sweden (let-

ter). *Lancet*, 2:748–749, 1985. **47.** McPherson, K., et al.: Early contraceptive use and breast cancer: Results of another case-control study. *Brit. J. Cancer*, 56: 653–660, 1987. **48.** Huggins, G.R., and P.F. Zucker: Oral contraceptives and neoplasia: 1987 update. *Fertil. Steril.*, 47:733–761, 1987. **49.** McPherson, K., and J.O. Drife: The pill and breast cancer: Why the uncertainty? *Brit. Med. J.*, 293:709–710, 1986. **50.** Shapiro, S.: Oral contraceptives: Time to take stock. *N.E.J.M.*, 315:450–451, 1987. **51.** Ory, H., et al.: Contraceptive choice and prevalence of cervical dysplasia and carcinoma in situ. *Am. J. Obstet. Gynec.*, 124:573–577, 1976. **52.** Vessey, M.P., et al.: Neoplasia of the cervix uteri and contraception: A possible adverse effect of the pill. *Lancet*, 2: 930, 1983. **53.** Brinton, L.A., et al.: Long-term use of oral contraceptives and risk of invasive cervical cancer. *Int. J. Cancer*, 38:339–344, 1986. **54.** WHO Collaborative Study of Neoplasia and Steroid Contraceptives: Invasive cervical cancer and combined oral contraceptives. *Brit. Med. J.*, 290:961–965, 1985. **55.** Rooks, J.B., et al.: Epidemiology of hepatocellular adenoma: The role of oral contraceptive use. *J.A.M.A.*, 242:644–648, 1979. **56.** Bein, N.N., and H.S. Goldsmith: Recurrent massive hemorrhage from benign hepatic tumors secondary to oral contraceptives. *Brit. J. Surg.*, 64:433–435, 1977. **57.** Klatskin, G.: Hepatic tumors: Possible relationship to use of oral contraceptives. *Gastroenterology*, 73:386–394, 1977. **58.** Henderson, B.E., et al.: Hepatocellular carcinoma and oral contraceptives. *Brit. J. Cancer*, 48:437–440, 1983. **59.** Neuberger, J., D. Forman, et al.: Oral contraceptives and hepatocellular carcinoma. *Brit. Med. J.*, 292:1355–1357, 1986. **60.** Forman, D., et al.: Cancer of the liver and oral contraceptives. *Brit. Med. J.*, 292: 1357–1361, 1986. **61.** Harlap, S., and J. Eldor. Births following oral contraceptive failures. *Obstet. Gynec.*, 55:447–452, 1980. **62.** Savolainen, E., et al.: Teratogenic hazards of oral contraceptives analyzed in a national malformation register. *Amer. J. Obstet Gynec.*, 140:521–524, 1981. **63.** Janerich, D.T., et al.: Oral contraceptives and birth defects. *Am. J. Epidemiology*, 112:73–79, 1980. **64.** Ferencz, C., et al.: Maternal hormone therapy and congenital heart disease. *Teratology*, 21:225–239, 1980. **65.** Rothman, K.J., et al.: Exogenous hormones and other drug exposures of children with congenital heart disease. *Am. J. Epidemiology*, 109:433–439, 1979. **66.** Boston Collaborative Drug Surveillance Program: Oral contraceptives and venous thromboembolic disease, surgically confirmed gallbladder disease, and breast tumors. *Lancet*, 1:1399–1404, 1973. **67.** Royal College of General Practitioners: *Oral Contraceptives and Health*. New York, Pittman, 1974, 100p. **68.** Layde, P.M., et al.: Risk of gallbladder disease: A cohort study of young women attending family planning clinics. *J. Epidemiol. and Comm. Health*, 36: 274–278, 1982. **69.** Rome Group for the Epidemiology and Prevention of Cholelithiasis (GREPCO): Prevalence of gallstone disease in an Italian adult female population. *Am. J. Epidemiol.*, 119:796–805, 1984. **70.** Strom, B.L., et al.: Oral contraceptives and other risk factors for gallbladder disease. *Clin. Pharmacol. Ther.*, 39:335–341, 1986. **71.** Wynn, V., et al.: Comparison of effects of different combined oral-contraceptive formulations on carbohydrate and lipid metabolism. *Lancet*, 1:1045–1049, 1979. **72.** Wynn, V.: Effect of progesterone and progestins on carbohydrate metabolism. In *Progesterone and Progestin*. Edited by C.W. Bardin, E. Milgrom, P. Mauvis-Jarvis. New York, Raven Press, 395–410, 1983. **73.** Perlman, J.A., et al.: Oral glucose tolerance and the potency of oral contraceptive progestogens. *J. Chronic Dis.*, 38:857–864, 1985. **74.** Royal College of General Practitioners' Oral Contraception Study: Effect on hypertension and benign breast disease of progestogen component in combined oral contraceptives. *Lancet*, 1:624, 1977. **75.** Fisch, I.R., and J. Frank: Oral contraceptives and blood pressure. *J.A.M.A.*, 237:2499-2503, 1977. **76.** Laragh, A.J.: Oral contraceptive induced hypertension: Nine years later. *Amer. J. Obstet. Gynecol.*, 126:141–147, 1976. **77.** Ramcharan, S., et al.: Incidence of hypertension in the Walnut Creek Contraceptive Drug Study cohort. In *Pharmacology of Steroid Contraceptive Drugs*. Edited by S. Garattini and H.W. Berendes. New York, Raven Press, 277–288, 1977. (Monographs of the Mario Negri Institute for Pharmacological Research, Milan.) **78.** Back DJ, et al. Drug interactions, in Pharmacology of the contraceptive steroids, Goldzieher JW, Fotherby K (eds), Raven Press, Ltd., New York, 1994, 407–425. **79.** The Cancer and Steroid Hormone Study of the Centers for Disease Control and the National Institute of Child Health and Human Development: Oral contraceptive use and the risk of ovarian cancer. *J.A.M.A.*, 249:1596–1599, 1983. **80.** The Cancer and Steroid Hormone Study of the Centers for Disease Control and the National Institute of Child Health and Human Development: Combination oral contraceptive use and the risk of endometrial cancer. *J.A.M.A.*, 257:796–800, 1987. **81.** Ory, H.W.: Functional ovarian cysts and oral contraceptives: Negative association confirmed surgically. *J.A.M.A.*, 228:68–69, 1974. **82.** Ory, H.W., et al.: Oral contraceptives and reduced risk of benign breast disease. *N.E.J.M.*, 294: 41–422, 1976. **83.** Ory, H.W.: The noncontraceptive health benefits from oral contraceptive use. *Fam. Plann. Perspectives*, 14:182–184, 1982. **84.** Ory, H.W., et al.: Making Choices: Evaluating the health risks and benefits of birth control methods. New York, The Alan Guttmacher Institute, 1, 1983. **85.** Miller, D.R., et al.: Breast cancer before age 45 and oral contraceptive use: new findings. *Am. J. Epidemiol.*, 129:269–280, 1989. **86.** Kay, C.R., and P.C. Hannaford: Breast cancer and the pill: a further report from the Royal College of General Practitioners Oral Contraception Study. *Br. J. Cancer*, 58:675–680, 1988. **87.** Stadel, B.V., et al.: Oral contraceptives and premenopausal breast cancer in nulliparous women. *Contraception*, 38:287–299, 1988. **88.** UK National Case-Control Study Group: Oral contraceptive use and breast cancer risk in young women. *Lancet*, 973–982, 1989. **89.** Romieu, I., et al.: Prospective study of oral contraceptive use and risk of breast cancer in women. *J. Natl. Cancer Inst.*, 81:1313–1321, 1989.

The patient labeling for oral contraceptive drug products is set forth below:

This product (like all oral contraceptives) is intended to prevent pregnancy. It does not protect against HIV infection (AIDS) and other sexually transmitted diseases.

BRIEF SUMMARY PATIENT PACKAGE INSERT

Oral contraceptives, also known as "birth control pills" or "the pill," are taken to prevent pregnancy and, when taken correctly, have a failure rate of about 1% per year when used without missing any pills. The typical failure rate of large numbers of pill users is less than 3% per year when women who miss pills are included. For most women oral contraceptives are also free of serious or unpleasant side effects. However, forgetting to take pills considerably increases the chances of pregnancy.

For the majority of women, oral contraceptives can be taken safely. But there are some women who are at high risk of developing certain serious diseases that can be life-threatening or may cause temporary or permanent disability. The risks associated with taking oral contraceptives increase significantly if you:

- Smoke
- Have high blood pressure, diabetes, high cholesterol
- Have or have had clotting disorders, heart attack, stroke, angina pectoris, cancer of the breast or sex organs, jaundice, or malignant or benign liver tumors.

You should not take the pill if you suspect you are pregnant or have unexplained vaginal bleeding.

Cigarette smoking increases the risk of serious cardiovascular side effects from oral contraceptive use. This risk increases with age and with heavy smoking (15 or more cigarettes per day) and is quite marked in women over 35 years of age. Women who use oral contraceptives are strongly advised not to smoke.

Most side effects of the pill are not serious. The most common side effects are nausea, vomiting, bleeding between menstrual periods, weight gain, breast tenderness, and difficulty wearing contact lenses. These side effects, especially nausea, vomiting, and breakthrough bleeding, may subside within the first three months of use.

The serious side effects of the pill occur very infrequently, especially if you are in good health and are young. However, you should know that the following medical conditions have been associated with or made worse by the pill:

1. Blood clots in the legs (thrombophlebitis), lungs (pulmonary embolism), stoppage or rupture of a blood vessel in the brain (stroke), blockage of blood vessels in the heart (heart attack or angina pectoris) or other organs of the body. As mentioned above, smoking increases the risk of heart attacks and strokes and subsequent serious medical consequences.
2. Liver tumors, which may rupture and cause severe bleeding. A possible but not definite association has been found with the pill and liver cancer. However, liver cancers are extremely rare. The chance of developing liver cancer from using the pill is thus even rarer.
3. High blood pressure, although blood pressure usually returns to normal when the pill is stopped.

The symptoms associated with these serious side effects are discussed in the detailed leaflet given to you with your supply of pills. Notify your doctor or health care provider if you notice any unusual physical disturbances while taking the pill. In addition, drugs such as rifampin, as well as some anticonvulsants and some antibiotics, may decrease oral contraceptive effectiveness.

Most of the studies to date on breast cancer and pill use have found no increase in the risk of developing breast cancer, although some studies have reported an increased risk of developing breast cancer in certain groups of women. However, some studies have found an increase in the risk of developing cancer of the cervix in women taking the pill, but this finding may be related to differences in sexual behavior or other factors not related to use of the pill. Therefore, there is insufficient evidence to rule out the possibility that the pill may cause cancer of the breast or cervix.

Taking the pill provides some important non-contraceptive benefits. These include less painful menstruation, less menstrual blood loss and anemia, fewer pelvic infections, and fewer cancers of the ovary and the lining of the uterus.

Be sure to discuss any medical condition you may have with your health care provider. Your health care provider will take a medical and family history and examine you before prescribing oral contraceptives. The physical examination may be delayed to another time if you request it and your health care provider believes that it is a good medical practice to postpone it. You should be reexamined at least once a year while taking oral contraceptives. The detailed patient information leaflet gives you further information which you should read and discuss with your health care provider.

This product (like all oral contraceptives) is intended to prevent pregnancy. It does not protect against transmission of HIV (AIDS) and other sexually transmitted diseases such as chlamydia, genital herpes, genital warts, gonorrhea, hepatitis B, and syphilis.

INSTRUCTIONS TO PATIENT

Tablet Dispenser

The Microgestin tablet dispenser has been designed to make oral contraceptive dosing as easy and as convenient as possible. The tablets are arranged in four rows of seven tablets each, with the days of the week appearing on the tablet dispenser below the last row of tablets.

Each green tablet contains 1.5 mg norethindrone acetate and 30 mcg ethinyl estradiol.

Each brown tablet contains 75 mg ferrous fumarate, and is intended to help you remember to take the tablets correctly. These brown tablets are not intended to have any health benefit.

Directions

To remove a tablet, press down on it with your thumb or finger. The tablet will drop through the back of the tablet dispenser. Do not press with your thumbnail, fingernail, or any other sharp object.

HOW TO TAKE THE PILL

IMPORTANT POINTS TO REMEMBER

BEFORE YOU START TAKING YOUR PILLS:

1. BE SURE TO READ THESE DIRECTIONS:
   Before you start taking your pills.
   Anytime you are not sure what to do.
2. THE RIGHT WAY TO TAKE THE PILL IS TO TAKE ONE PILL EVERY DAY AT THE SAME TIME. If you miss pills you could get pregnant. This includes starting the pack late. The more pills you miss, the more likely you are to get pregnant.
3. MANY WOMEN HAVE SPOTTING OR LIGHT BLEEDING, OR MAY FEEL SICK TO THEIR STOMACH, DURING THE FIRST 1–3 PACKS OF PILLS. If you do have spotting or light bleeding or feel sick to your stomach, do not stop taking the pill. The problem will usually go away. If it doesn't go away, check with your doctor or clinic.
4. MISSING PILLS CAN ALSO CAUSE SPOTTING OR LIGHT BLEEDING, even when you make up these missed pills. On the days you take 2 pills to make up for missed pills, you could also feel a little sick to your stomach.
5. IF YOU HAVE VOMITING OR DIARRHEA, for any reason, or IF YOU TAKE SOME MEDICINES, including some antibiotics, your birth control pills may not work as well. Use a back-up birth control method (such as condoms or foam) until you check with your doctor or clinic.
6. IF YOU HAVE TROUBLE REMEMBERING TO TAKE THE PILL, talk to your doctor or clinic about how to make pill-taking easier or about using another method of birth control.
7. IF YOU HAVE ANY QUESTIONS OR ARE UNSURE ABOUT THE INFORMATION IN THIS LEAFLET, call your doctor or clinic.

BEFORE YOU START TAKING YOUR PILLS

1. DECIDE WHAT TIME OF DAY YOU WANT TO TAKE YOUR PILL. It is important to take it at about the same time every day.
2. BE SURE YOUR PILL PACK HAS 28 PILLS: The pill pack has 21 "active" green pills (with hormones) to take for 3 weeks, followed by 1 week of reminder brown pills (without hormones).
3. ALSO FIND:
   1) where on the pack to start taking pills,
   2) in what order to take the pills (follow the arrows), and
   3) the week numbers as shown in the following picture:

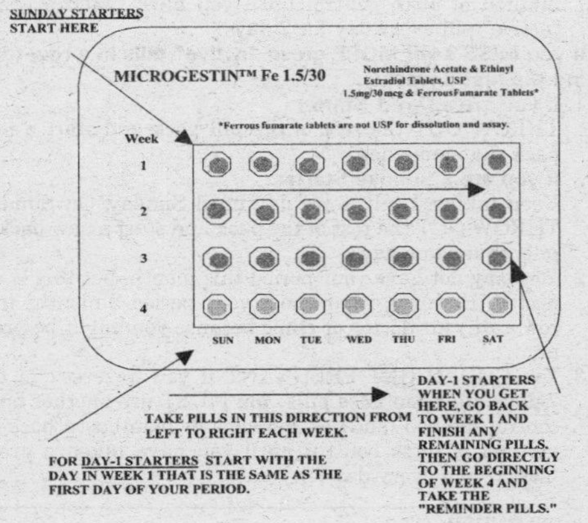
SUNDAY STARTERS
START HERE
MICROGESTIN™ Fe 1.5/30
Norethindrone Acetate & Ethinyl Estradiol Tablets, USP 1.5mg/30mcg & FerrousFumarate Tablets*
*Ferrous fumarate tablets are not USP for dissolution and assay.
Week
1
2
3
4
SUN MON TUE WED THU FRI SAT
TAKE PILLS IN THIS DIRECTION FROM LEFT TO RIGHT EACH WEEK.
FOR DAY-1 STARTERS START WITH THE DAY IN WEEK 1 THAT IS THE SAME AS THE FIRST DAY OF YOUR PERIOD.
DAY-1 STARTERS WHEN YOU GET HERE, GO BACK TO WEEK 1 AND FINISH ANY REMAINING PILLS. THEN GO DIRECTLY TO THE BEGINNING OF WEEK 4 AND TAKE THE "REMINDER PILLS."

Microgestin Fe 1.5/30 will contain: 21 GREEN PILLS for WEEKS 1, 2, and 3. WEEK 4 will contain BROWN PILLS ONLY.

4. BE SURE YOU HAVE READY AT ALL TIMES: ANOTHER KIND OF BIRTH CONTROL (such as condoms or foam) to use as a back-up in case you miss pills.
   An EXTRA, FULL PILL PACK.

Continued on next page

Microgestin Fe 1.5/30—Cont.

WHEN TO START THE FIRST PACK OF PILLS

You have a choice of which day to start taking your first pack of pills. Decide with your doctor or clinic which is the best day for you. Pick a time of day which will be easy to remember.

Day-1 Start:
1. Take the first "active" green pill of the first pack during the first 24 hours of your period.
2. You will not need to use a back-up method of birth control, since you are starting the pill at the beginning of your period.

Sunday Start:
1. Take the first "active" green pill of the first pack on the Sunday after your period starts, even if you are still bleeding. If your period begins on Sunday, start the pack that same day.
2. Use another method of birth control as a back-up method if you have sex anytime from the Sunday you start your first pack until the next Sunday (7 days). Condoms or foam are good back-up methods of birth control.

WHAT TO DO DURING THE MONTH

1. **TAKE ONE PILL AT THE SAME TIME EVERY DAY UNTIL THE PACK IS EMPTY.**
   Do not skip pills even if you are spotting or bleeding between monthly periods or feel sick to your stomach (nausea).
   Do not skip pills even if you do not have sex very often.
2. **WHEN YOU FINISH A PACK OR SWITCH YOUR BRAND OF PILLS:**
   Start the next pack on the day after your last "reminder" pill. Do not wait any days between packs.

WHAT TO DO IF YOU MISS PILLS

If you MISS 1 green "active" pill:
1. Take it as soon as you remember. Take the next pill at your regular time. This means you may take 2 pills in 1 day.
2. You do not need to use a back-up birth control method if you have sex.

If you MISS 2 green "active" pills in a row in WEEK 1 or WEEK 2 of your pack:
1. Take 2 pills on the day you remember and 2 pills the next day.
2. Then take 1 pill a day until you finish the pack.
3. You COULD GET PREGNANT if you have sex in the 7 days after you miss pills. You MUST use another birth control method (such as condoms or foam) as a back-up method of birth control until you have taken a green "active" pill every day for 7 days.

If you MISS 2 green "active" pills in a row in THE 3RD WEEK:
1. **If you are a Day-1 Starter:**
   THROW OUT the rest of the pill pack and start a new pack that same day.
   If you are a Sunday Starter:
   Keep taking 1 pill every day until Sunday. On Sunday, THROW OUT the rest of the pack and start a new pack of pills that same day.
2. You may not have your period this month, but this is expected. However, if you miss your period 2 months in a row, call your doctor or clinic because you might be pregnant.
3. You COULD GET PREGNANT if you have sex in the 7 days after you miss pills. You MUST use another birth control method (such as condoms or foam) as a back-up method of birth control until you have taken a green "active" pill every day for 7 days.

If you MISS 3 OR MORE green "active" pills in a row (during the first 3 weeks):
1. **If you are a Day-1 Starter:**
   THROW OUT the rest of the pill pack and start a new pack that same day.
   If you are a Sunday Starter:
   Keep taking 1 pill every day until Sunday. On Sunday, THROW OUT the rest of the pack and start a new pack of pills that same day.
2. You may not have your period this month, but this is expected. However, if you miss your period 2 months in a row, call your doctor or clinic because you might be pregnant.
3. You COULD GET PREGNANT if you have sex in the 7 days after you miss pills. You MUST use another birth control method (such as condoms or foam) as a back-up method of birth control until you have taken a green "active" pill every day for 7 days.

A REMINDER:
IF YOU FORGET ANY OF THE 7 BROWN "REMINDER" PILLS IN WEEK 4:
THROW AWAY THE PILLS YOU MISSED.
KEEP TAKING 1 PILL EACH DAY UNTIL THE PACK IS EMPTY.
YOU DO NOT NEED A BACK-UP METHOD.

FINALLY, IF YOU ARE STILL NOT SURE WHAT TO DO ABOUT THE PILLS YOU HAVE MISSED:
Use a BACK-UP METHOD anytime you have sex.
KEEP TAKING ONE GREEN "ACTIVE" PILL EACH DAY until you can reach your doctor or clinic.

Based on his or her assessment of your medical needs, your doctor or health care provider has prescribed this drug for you. Do not give this drug to anyone else.
Keep this and all drugs out of the reach of children.
Store at controlled room temperature 15°–30°C (59°–86°F).
This product (like all oral contraceptives) is intended to prevent pregnancy. It does not protect against HIV infection (AIDS) and other sexually transmitted diseases.

DETAILED PATIENT PACKAGE INSERT

What You Should Know About Oral Contraceptives
Any woman who considers using oral contraceptives (the "birth control pill" or "the pill") should understand the benefits and risks of using this form of birth control. This leaflet will give you much of the information you will need to make this decision and will also help you determine if you are at risk of developing any of the serious side effects of the pill. It will tell you how to use the pill properly so that it will be as effective as possible. However, this leaflet is not a replacement for a careful discussion between you and your health care provider. You should discuss the information provided in this leaflet with him or her, both when you first start taking the pill and during your revisits. You should also follow your health care provider's advice with regard to regular check-ups while you are on the pill.

EFFECTIVENESS OF ORAL CONTRACEPTIVES
Oral contraceptives or "birth control pills" or "the pill" are used to prevent pregnancy and are more effective than other non-surgical methods of birth control. When they are taken correctly, the chance of becoming pregnant is less than 1% (1 pregnancy per 100 women per year of use) when used perfectly, without missing any pills. Typical failure rates are actually 3% per year. The chance of becoming pregnant increases with each missed pill during a menstrual cycle.
In comparison, typical failure rates for other methods of birth control during the first year of use are as follows:
Implant: <1%
Injection: <1%
IUD: <1 to 2%
Diaphragm with Spermicides: 20%
Spermicides alone: 26%
Vaginal Sponge: 20 to 40%
Female sterilization: <1%
Male sterilization: <1%
Cervical Cap: 20 to 40%
Condom alone (male): 14%
Condom alone (female): 21%
Periodic abstinence: 25%
Withdrawal: 19%
No method: 85%

WHO SHOULD NOT TAKE ORAL CONTRACEPTIVES

Cigarette smoking increases the risk of serious cardiovascular side effects from oral contraceptive use. This risk increases with age and with heavy smoking (15 or more cigarettes per day) and is quite marked in women over 35 years of age. Women who use oral contraceptives are strongly advised not to smoke.

Some women should not use the pill. For example, you should not take the pill if you are pregnant or think you may be pregnant. You should also not use the pill if you have any of the following conditions:
- A history of heart attack or stroke
- Blood clots in the legs (thrombophlebitis), lungs (pulmonary embolism), or eyes
- A history of blood clots in the deep veins of your legs
- Chest pain (angina pectoris)
- Known or suspected breast cancer or cancer of the lining of the uterus, cervix or vagina
- Unexplained vaginal bleeding (until a diagnosis is reached by your doctor)
- Yellowing of the whites of the eyes or of the skin (jaundice) during pregnancy or during previous use of the pill
- Liver tumor (benign or cancerous)
- Known or suspected pregnancy

Tell your health care provider if you have ever had any of these conditions. Your health care provider can recommend a safer method of birth control.

OTHER CONSIDERATIONS BEFORE TAKING ORAL CONTRACEPTIVES
Tell your health care provider if you have:
- Breast nodules, fibrocystic disease of the breast, an abnormal breast x-ray or mammogram
- Diabetes
- Elevated cholesterol or triglycerides
- High blood pressure
- Migraine or other headaches or epilepsy
- Mental depression
- Gallbladder, heart, or kidney disease
- History of scanty or irregular menstrual periods

Women with any of these conditions should be checked often by their health care provider if they choose to use oral contraceptives.
Also, be sure to inform your doctor or health care provider if you smoke or are on any medications.

RISKS OF TAKING ORAL CONTRACEPTIVES
1. Risk of Developing Blood Clots
Blood clots and blockage of blood vessels are the most serious side effects of taking oral contraceptives; in particular, a clot in the legs can cause thrombophlebitis and a clot that travels to the lungs can cause a sudden blocking of the vessel carrying blood to the lungs. Rarely, clots occur in the blood vessels of the eye and may cause blindness, double vision, or impaired vision.
If you take oral contraceptives and need elective surgery, need to stay in bed for a prolonged illness, or have recently delivered a baby, you may be at risk of developing blood clots. You should consult your doctor about stopping oral contraceptives three to four weeks before surgery and not taking oral contraceptives for two weeks after surgery or during bed rest. You should also not take oral contraceptives soon after delivery of a baby. It is advisable to wait for at least four weeks after delivery if you are not breast feeding. If you are breast feeding, you should wait until you have weaned your child before using the pill. (See also the section on **Breast Feeding** in **GENERAL PRECAUTIONS**.)
2. Heart Attacks and Strokes
Oral contraceptives may increase the tendency to develop strokes (stoppage or rupture of blood vessels in the brain) and angina pectoris and heart attacks (blockage of blood vessels in the heart). Any of these conditions can cause death or disability.
Smoking greatly increases the possibility of suffering heart attacks and strokes. Furthermore, smoking and the use of oral contraceptives greatly increase the chances of developing and dying of heart disease.
3. Gallbladder Disease
Oral contraceptive users probably have a greater risk than nonusers of having gallbladder disease, although this risk may be related to pills containing high doses of estrogens.
4. Liver Tumors
In rare cases, oral contraceptives can cause benign but dangerous liver tumors. These benign liver tumors can rupture and cause fatal internal bleeding. In addition, a possible but not definite association has been found with the pill and liver cancers in two studies, in which a few women who developed these very rare cancers were found to have used oral contraceptives for long periods. However, liver cancers are extremely rare. The chance of developing liver cancer from using the pill is thus even rarer.
5. Cancer of the Reproductive Organs and Breasts
There is, at present, no confirmed evidence that oral contraceptive use increases the risk of developing cancer of the reproductive organs. Studies to date of women taking the pill have reported conflicting findings on whether pill use increases the risk of developing cancer of the breast or cervix.
Most of the studies on breast cancer and pill use have found no overall increase in the risk of developing breast cancer, although some studies have reported an increased risk of developing breast cancer in certain groups of women. Women who use oral contraceptives and have a strong family history of breast cancer or who have breast nodules or abnormal mammograms should be closely followed by their doctors.
Some studies have found an increase in the incidence of cancer of the cervix in women who use oral contraceptives. However, this finding may be related to factors other than the use of oral contraceptives.

ESTIMATED RISK OF DEATH FROM A BIRTH CONTROL METHOD OR PREGNANCY
All methods of birth control and pregnancy are associated with a risk of developing certain diseases which may lead to disability or death. An estimate of the number of deaths associated with different methods of birth control and pregnancy has been calculated and is shown in the following table.
[See table III at bottom of next page]
In the above table, the risk of death from any birth control method is less than the risk of childbirth, except for oral contraceptive users over the age of 35 who smoke and pill users over the age of 40 even if they do not smoke. It can be seen in the table that for women aged 15 to 39, the risk of death was highest with pregnancy (7–26 deaths per 100,000 women, depending on age). Among pill users who do not smoke, the risk of death was always lower than that associated with pregnancy for any age group, although over the age of 40, the risk increases to 32 deaths per 100,000 women, compared to 28 associated with pregnancy at that age. However, for pill users who smoke and are over the age of 35, the estimated number of deaths exceeds those for other methods of birth control. If a woman is over the age of 40 and smokes, her estimated risk of death is four times higher (117/100,000 women) than the estimated risk associated with pregnancy (28/100,000 women) in that age group.
The suggestion that women over 40 who don't smoke should not take oral contraceptives is based on information from older higher dose pills and on less selective use of pills than is practiced today. An Advisory Committee of the FDA discussed this issue in 1989 and recommended that the benefits of oral contraceptive use by healthy, non-smoking women over 40 years of age may outweigh the possible risks. However, all women, especially older women, are cautioned to use the lowest dose pill that is effective.

WARNING SIGNALS
If any of these adverse effects occur while you are taking oral contraceptives, call your doctor immediately:
- Sharp chest pain, coughing of blood, or sudden shortness of breath (indicating a possible clot in the lung)
- Pain in the calf (indicating a possible clot in the leg)
- Crushing chest pain or heaviness in the chest (indicating a possible heart attack)
- Sudden severe headache or vomiting, dizziness or fainting, disturbances of vision or speech, weakness, or numbness in an arm or leg (indicating a possible stroke)

- Sudden partial or complete loss of vision (indicating a possible clot in the eye)
- Breast lumps (indicating possible breast cancer or fibrocystic disease of the breast; ask your doctor or health care provider to show you how to examine your breasts)
- Severe pain or tenderness in the stomach area (indicating a possibly ruptured liver tumor)
- Difficulty in sleeping, weakness, lack of energy, fatigue, or change in mood (possibly indicating severe depression)
- Jaundice or a yellowing of the skin or eyeballs, accompanied frequently by fever, fatigue, loss of appetite, dark colored urine, or light colored bowel movements (indicating possible liver problems)

SIDE EFFECTS OF ORAL CONTRACEPTIVES

1. Vaginal Bleeding

Irregular vaginal bleeding or spotting may occur while you are taking the pills. Irregular bleeding may vary from slight staining between menstrual periods to breakthrough bleeding which is a flow much like a regular period. Irregular bleeding occurs most often during the first few months of oral contraceptive use, but may also occur after you have been taking the pill for some time. Such bleeding may be temporary and usually does not indicate serious problems. It is important to continue taking your pills on schedule. If the bleeding occurs in more than one cycle or lasts for more than a few days, talk to your doctor or health care provider.

2. Contact Lenses

If you wear contact lenses and notice a change in vision or an inability to wear your lenses, contact your doctor or health care provider.

3. Fluid Retention

Oral contraceptives may cause edema (fluid retention) with swelling of the fingers or ankles and may raise your blood pressure. If you experience fluid retention, contact your doctor or health care provider.

4. Melasma

A spotty darkening of the skin is possible, particularly on the face.

5. Other Side Effects

Other side effects may include change in appetite, headache, nervousness, depression, dizziness, loss of scalp hair, rash, and vaginal infections.

If any of these side effects bother you, call your doctor or health care provider.

GENERAL PRECAUTIONS

1. Missed Periods and Use of Oral Contraceptives Before or During Early Pregnancy

There may be times when you may not menstruate regularly after you have completed taking a cycle of pills. If you have taken your pills regularly and miss one menstrual period, continue taking your pills for the next cycle but be sure to inform your health care provider before doing so. If you have not taken the pills daily as instructed and missed a menstrual period, or if you missed two consecutive menstrual periods, you may be pregnant. Check with your health care provider immediately to determine whether you are pregnant. Do not continue to take oral contraceptives until you are sure you are not pregnant, but continue to use another method of contraception.

There is no conclusive evidence that oral contraceptive use is associated with an increase in birth defects, when taken inadvertently during early pregnancy. Previously, a few studies had reported that oral contraceptives might be associated with birth defects, but these studies have not been confirmed. Nevertheless, oral contraceptives or any other drugs should not be used during pregnancy unless clearly necessary and prescribed by your doctor. You should check with your doctor about risks to your unborn child of any medication taken during pregnancy.

2. While Breast Feeding

If you are breast feeding, consult your doctor before starting oral contraceptives. Some of the drug will be passed on to the child in the milk. A few adverse effects on the child have been reported, including yellowing of the skin (jaundice) and breast enlargement. In addition, oral contraceptives may decrease the amount and quality of your milk. If possible, do not use oral contraceptives while breast feeding. You should use another method of contraception since breast feeding provides only partial protection from becoming pregnant and this partial protection decreases significantly as you breast feed for longer periods of time. You should consider starting oral contraceptives only after you have weaned your child completely.

3. Laboratory Tests

If you are scheduled for any laboratory tests, tell your doctor you are taking birth control pills. Certain blood tests may be affected by birth control pills.

4. Drug Interactions

Certain drugs may interact with birth control pills to make them less effective in preventing pregnancy or cause an increase in breakthrough bleeding. Such drugs include rifampin; drugs used for epilepsy such as barbiturates (for example, phenobarbital), carbamazepine, and phenytoin (Dilantin® is one brand of this drug); troglitazone; phenylbutazone; and possibly certain antibiotics. You may need to use additional contraception when you take drugs which can make oral contraceptives less effective.

Birth control pills interact with certain drugs. These drugs include acetaminophen, clofibric acid, cyclosporine, morphine, prednisolone, salicylic acid, temazepam, and theophylline. You should tell your doctor if you are taking any of these medications.

5. This product (like all oral contraceptives) is intended to prevent pregnancy. It does not protect against transmission of HIV (AIDS) and other sexually transmitted diseases such as chlamydia, genital herpes, genital warts, gonorrhea, hepatitis B, and syphilis.

INSTRUCTIONS TO PATIENT

Tablet Dispenser

The Microgestin tablet dispenser has been designed to make oral contraceptive dosing as easy and as convenient as possible. The tablets are arranged in four rows of seven tablets each, with the days of the week appearing on the tablet dispenser below the last row of tablets.

Each *green* tablet contains 1.5 mg norethindrone acetate and 30 mcg ethinyl estradiol.

Each *brown* tablet contains 75 mg ferrous fumarate and is intended to help you remember to take the tablets correctly. These brown tablets are not intended to have any health benefit.

Directions

To remove a tablet, press down on it with your thumb or finger. The tablet will drop through the back of the tablet dispenser. Do not press with your thumbnail, fingernail, or any other sharp object.

HOW TO TAKE THE PILL

IMPORTANT POINTS TO REMEMBER

BEFORE YOU START TAKING YOUR PILLS:
1. BE SURE TO READ THESE DIRECTIONS:
   Before you start taking your pills.
   Anytime you are not sure what to do.
2. THE RIGHT WAY TO TAKE THE PILL IS TO TAKE ONE PILL EVERY DAY AT THE SAME TIME. If you miss pills you could get pregnant. This includes starting the pack late. The more pills you miss, the more likely you are to get pregnant.
3. MANY WOMEN HAVE SPOTTING OR LIGHT BLEEDING, OR MAY FEEL SICK TO THEIR STOMACH, DURING THE FIRST 1–3 PACKS OF PILLS. If you do have spotting or light bleeding or feel sick to your stomach, do not stop taking the pill. The problem will usually go away. If it doesn't go away, check with your doctor or clinic.
4. MISSING PILLS CAN ALSO CAUSE SPOTTING OR LIGHT BLEEDING, even when you make up these missed pills. On the days you take 2 pills to make up for missed pills, you could also feel a little sick to your stomach.
5. IF YOU HAVE VOMITING OR DIARRHEA, for any reason, or IF YOU TAKE SOME MEDICINES, including some antibiotics, your birth control pills may not work as well. Use a back-up birth control method (such as condoms or foam) until you check with your doctor or clinic.
6. IF YOU HAVE TROUBLE REMEMBERING TO TAKE THE PILL, talk to your doctor or clinic about how to make pill-taking easier or about using another method of birth control.
7. IF YOU HAVE ANY QUESTIONS OR ARE UNSURE ABOUT THE INFORMATION IN THIS LEAFLET, call your doctor or clinic.

BEFORE YOU START TAKING YOUR PILLS

1. DECIDE WHAT TIME OF DAY YOU WANT TO TAKE YOUR PILL. It is important to take it at about the same time every day.
2. BE SURE YOUR PILL PACK HAS 28 PILLS: The pill pack has 21 "active" green pills (with hormones) to take for 3 weeks, followed by 1 week of reminder brown pills (without hormones).
3. ALSO FIND:
   1) where on the pack to start taking pills,
   2) in what order to take the pills (follow the arrows), and
   3) the week numbers as shown in the following picture:

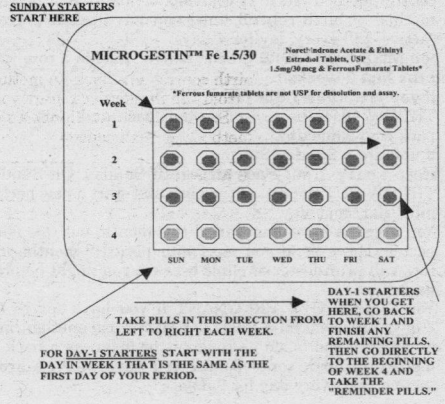

Microgestin Fe 1.5/30 will contain: 21 GREEN PILLS for WEEKS 1, 2, and 3. WEEK 4 will contain BROWN PILLS ONLY.
4. BE SURE YOU HAVE READY AT ALL TIMES: ANOTHER KIND OF BIRTH CONTROL (such as condoms or foam) to use as a back-up in case you miss pills. An EXTRA, FULL PILL PACK.

WHEN TO START THE FIRST PACK OF PILLS

You have a choice of which day to start taking your first pack of pills. Decide with your doctor or clinic which is the best day for you. Pick a time of day which will be easy to remember.

DAY-1 START:
1. Take the first "active" green pill of the first pack during the first 24 hours of your period.
2. You will not need to use a back-up method of birth control, since you are starting the pill at the beginning of your period.

SUNDAY START:
1. Take the first "active" green pill of the first pack on the Sunday after your period starts, even if you are still bleeding. If your period begins on Sunday, start the pack that same day.
2. Use another method of birth control as a back-up method if you have sex anytime from the Sunday you start your first pack until the next Sunday (7 days). Condoms or foam are good back-up methods of birth control.

WHAT TO DO DURING THE MONTH

1. TAKE ONE PILL AT THE SAME TIME EVERY DAY UNTIL THE PACK IS EMPTY.
   Do not skip pills even if you are spotting or bleeding between monthly periods or feel sick to your stomach (nausea).
   Do not skip pills even if you do not have sex very often.
2. WHEN YOU FINISH A PACK OR SWITCH YOUR BRAND OF PILLS:
   Start the next pack on the day after your last "reminder" pill. Do not wait any days between packs.

WHAT TO DO IF YOU MISS PILLS

If you MISS 1 green "active" pill:
1. Take it as soon as you remember. Take the next pill at your regular time. This means you may take 2 pills in 1 day.
2. You do not need to use a back-up birth control method if you have sex.

If you MISS 2 green "active" pills in a row in WEEK 1 or WEEK 2 of your pack:
1. Take 2 pills on the day you remember and 2 pills the next day.
2. Then take 1 pill a day until you finish the pack.
3. You COULD GET PREGNANT if you have sex in the 7 days after you miss pills. You MUST use another birth control method (such as condoms or foam) as a back-up method of birth control until you have taken a green "active" pill every day for 7 days.

ANNUAL NUMBER OF BIRTH-RELATED OR METHOD-RELATED DEATHS ASSOCIATED WITH CONTROL OF FERTILITY PER 100,000 NONSTERILE WOMEN, BY FERTILITY CONTROL METHOD ACCORDING TO AGE

Method of control and outcome	15–19	20–24	25–29	30–34	35–39	40–44
No fertility control methods*	7.0	7.4	9.1	14.8	25.7	28.2
Oral contraceptives non-smoker**	0.3	0.5	0.9	1.9	13.8	31.6
Oral contraceptives smoker**	2.2	3.4	6.6	13.5	51.1	117.2
IUD**	0.8	0.8	1.0	1.0	1.4	1.4
Condom*	1.1	1.6	0.7	0.2	0.3	0.4
Diaphragm/ spermicide*	1.9	1.2	1.2	1.3	2.2	2.8
Periodic abstinence*	2.5	1.6	1.6	1.7	2.9	3.6

*Deaths are birth related.
**Deaths are method related.

Continued on next page

Microgestin Fe 1.5/30—Cont.

If you MISS 2 green "active" pills in a row in THE 3rd WEEK:

1. **If you are a Day-1 Starter:**
   THROW OUT the rest of the pill pack and start a new pack that same day.
   If you are a Sunday Starter:
   Keep taking 1 pill every day until Sunday. On Sunday, THROW OUT the rest of the pack and start a new pack of pills that same day.
2. You may not have your period this month, but this is expected. However, if you miss your period 2 months in a row, call your doctor or clinic because you might be pregnant.
3. You COULD GET PREGNANT if you have sex in the 7 days after you miss pills. You MUST use another birth control method (such as condoms or foam) as a back-up method of birth control until you have taken a green "active" pill every day for 7 days.

If you MISS 3 OR MORE green "active" pills in a row (during the first 3 weeks):

1. **If you are a Day-1 Starter:**
   THROW OUT the rest of the pill pack and start a new pack that same day.
   If you are a Sunday Starter:
   Keep taking 1 pill every day until Sunday. On Sunday, THROW OUT the rest of the pack and start a new pack of pills that same day.
2. You may not have your period this month, but this is expected. However, if you miss your period 2 months in a row, call your doctor or clinic because you might be pregnant.
3. You COULD GET PREGNANT if you have sex in the 7 days after you miss pills. You MUST use another birth control method (such as condoms or foam) as a back-up method of birth control until you have taken a green "active" pill every day for 7 days.

A REMINDER:
IF YOU FORGET ANY OF THE 7 BROWN "REMINDER" PILLS IN WEEK 4:
THROW AWAY THE PILLS YOU MISSED.
KEEP TAKING 1 PILL EACH DAY UNTIL THE PACK IS EMPTY.
YOU DO NOT NEED A BACK-UP METHOD.

FINALLY, IF YOU ARE STILL NOT SURE WHAT TO DO ABOUT THE PILLS YOU HAVE MISSED:
Use a BACK-UP METHOD anytime you have sex. KEEP TAKING ONE GREEN "ACTIVE" PILL EACH DAY until you can reach your doctor or clinic.

PREGNANCY DUE TO PILL FAILURE
The incidence of pill failure resulting in pregnancy is approximately 1% (ie, one pregnancy per 100 women per year) if taken every day as directed, but more typical failure rates are about 3%. If failure does occur, the risk to the fetus is minimal.
PREGNANCY AFTER STOPPING THE PILL
There may be some delay in becoming pregnant after you stop using oral contraceptives, especially if you had irregular menstrual cycles before you used oral contraceptives. It may be advisable to postpone conception until you begin menstruating regularly once you have stopped taking the pill and desire pregnancy.
There does not appear to be any increase in birth defects in newborn babies when pregnancy occurs soon after stopping the pill.
OVERDOSAGE
Serious ill effects have not been reported following ingestion of large doses of oral contraceptives by young children. Overdosage may cause nausea and withdrawal bleeding in females. In case of overdosage, contact your health care provider or pharmacist.
OTHER INFORMATION
Your health care provider will take a medical and family history and examine you before prescribing oral contraceptives. The physical examination may be delayed to another time if you request it and your health care provider believes that it is a good medical practice to postpone it. You should be reexamined at least once a year. Be sure to inform your health care provider if there is a family history of any of the conditions listed previously in this leaflet. Be sure to keep all appointments with your health care provider, because this is a time to determine if there are early signs of side effects of oral contraceptive use.
Do not use the drug for any condition other than the one for which it was prescribed. This drug has been prescribed specifically for you; do not give it to others who may want birth control pills.
HEALTH BENEFITS FROM ORAL CONTRACEPTIVES
In addition to preventing pregnancy, use of oral contraceptives may provide certain benefits. They are:

- Menstrual cycles may become more regular
- Blood flow during menstruation may be lighter and less iron may be lost. Therefore, anemia due to iron deficiency is less likely to occur
- Pain or other symptoms during menstruation may be encountered less frequently
- Ectopic (tubal) pregnancy may occur less frequently
- Noncancerous cysts or lumps in the breast may occur less frequently
- Acute pelvic inflammatory disease may occur less frequently
- Oral contraceptive use may provide some protection against developing two forms of cancer: cancer of the ovaries and cancer of the lining of the uterus.

If you want more information about birth control pills, ask your doctor or pharmacist. They have a more technical leaflet called the "Physician Insert," which you may wish to read.
Remembering to take tablets according to schedule is stressed because of its importance in providing you the greatest degree of protection.
MISSED MENSTRUAL PERIODS FOR THIS DOSAGE REGIMEN
At times there may be no menstrual period after a cycle of pills. Therefore, if you miss one menstrual period but have taken the pills *exactly as you were supposed to*, continue as usual into the next cycle. If you have not taken the pills correctly and miss a menstrual period, *you may be pregnant* and should stop taking oral contraceptives until your doctor or health care provider determines whether or not you are pregnant. Until you can get to your doctor or health care provider, use another form of contraception. If two consecutive menstrual periods are missed, you should stop taking pills until it is determined whether or not you are pregnant. Although there does not appear to be any increase in birth defects in newborn babies, if you become pregnant while using oral contraceptives, you should discuss the situation with your doctor or health care provider.
Periodic Examination
Your doctor or health care provider will take a complete medical and family history before prescribing oral contraceptives. At that time and about once a year thereafter, he or she will generally examine your blood pressure, breasts, abdomen, and pelvic organs (including a Papanicolaou smear, ie, test for cancer).
Keep this and all drugs out of the reach of children.
Store at controlled room temperature 15°– 30°C (59°–86°F).
WATSON PHARMA®
Watson Pharma, Inc.
a subsidiary of
Watson Laboratories, Inc. 14039
Corona, CA 92880 March 2001

NORCO® 5/325 ℂⅢ ℞
HYDROCODONE BITARTRATE AND ACETAMINOPHEN TABLETS, USP
5 mg/325 mg

Rx only

DESCRIPTION
Hydrocodone bitartrate and acetaminophen is supplied in tablet form for oral administration. **WARNING: May be habit forming** (see PRECAUTIONS, Information for Patients, and DRUG ABUSE AND DEPENDENCE). Hydrocodone bitartrate is an opioid analgesic and antitussive and occurs as fine, white crystals or as a crystalline powder. It is affected by light. The chemical name is 4,5α-epoxy-3-methoxy-17-methylmorphinan-6-one tartrate (1:1) hydrate (2:5). It has the following structural formula:

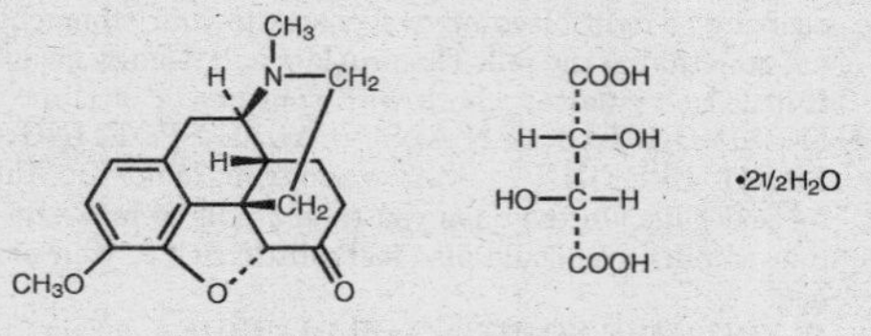

$C_{18}H_{21}NO_3 \cdot C_4H_6O_6 \cdot 2\frac{1}{2}H_2O$
MW = 494.490

Acetaminophen, 4′-hydroxyacetanilide, a slightly bitter, white, odorless, crystalline powder, is a non-opiate, non-salicylate analgesic and antipyretic. It has the following structural formula:

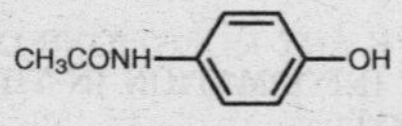

$C_8H_9NO_2$
MW = 151.16

Each Norco® 5/325 tablet contains:

Hydrocodone Bitartrate	5 mg
Acetaminophen	325 mg

In addition, each tablet contains the following inactive ingredients: colloidal silicon dioxide, croscarmellose sodium, crospovidone, microcrystalline cellulose, povidone, pregelatinized starch, stearic acid and sugar spheres which are composed of starch derived from corn, sucrose, and FD&C Yellow #6.

CLINICAL PHARMACOLOGY
Hydrocodone is a semisynthetic narcotic analgesic and antitussive with multiple actions qualitatively similar to those of codeine. Most of these involve the central nervous system and smooth muscle. The precise mechanism of action of hydrocodone and other opiates is not known, although it is believed to relate to the existence of opiate receptors in the central nervous system. In addition to analgesia, narcotics may produce drowsiness, changes in mood and mental clouding.
The analgesic action of acetaminophen involves peripheral influences, but the specific mechanism is as yet undetermined. Antipyretic activity is mediated through hypothalamic heat regulating centers. Acetaminophen inhibits prostaglandin synthetase. Therapeutic doses of acetaminophen have negligible effects on the cardiovascular or respiratory systems; however, toxic doses may cause circulatory failure and rapid, shallow breathing.
Pharmacokinetics: The behavior of the individual components is described below.
Hydrocodone: Following a 10 mg oral dose of hydrocodone administered to five adult male subjects, the mean peak concentration was 23.6 ± 5.2 ng/mL. Maximum serum levels were achieved at 1.3 ± 0.3 hours and the half-life was determined to be 3.8 ± 0.3 hours. Hydrocodone exhibits a complex pattern of metabolism including O-demethylation, N-demethylation and 6-keto reduction to the corresponding 6-α- and 6-β-hydroxymetabolites.
See OVERDOSAGE for toxicity information.
Acetaminophen: Acetaminophen is rapidly absorbed from the gastrointestinal tract and is distributed throughout most body tissues. The plasma half-life is 1.25 to 3 hours, but may be increased by liver damage and following overdosage. Elimination of acetaminophen is principally by liver metabolism (conjugation) and subsequent renal excretion of metabolites. Approximately 85% of an oral dose appears in the urine within 24 hours of administration, most as the glucuronide conjugate, with small amounts of other conjugates and unchanged drug. See OVERDOSAGE for toxicity information.

INDICATIONS AND USAGE
Norco® 5/325 tablets (Hydrocodone Bitartrate and Acetaminophen Tablets, USP, 5 mg/325 mg) are indicated for the relief of moderate to moderately severe pain.

CONTRAINDICATIONS
This product should not be administered to patients who have previously exhibited hypersensitivity to hydrocodone or acetaminophen.

WARNINGS
Respiratory Depression: At high doses or in sensitive patients, hydrocodone may produce dose-related respiratory depression by acting directly on the brain stem respiratory center. Hydrocodone also affects the center that controls respiratory rhythm, and may produce irregular and periodic breathing.
Head Injury and Increased Intracranial Pressure: The respiratory depressant effects of narcotics and their capacity to elevate cerebrospinal fluid pressure may be markedly exaggerated in the presence of head injury, other intracranial lesions or a preexisting increase in intracranial pressure. Furthermore, narcotics produce adverse reactions which may obscure the clinical course of patients with head injuries.
Acute Abdominal Conditions: The administration of narcotics may obscure the diagnosis or clinical course of patients with acute abdominal conditions.

PRECAUTIONS
General: Special Risk Patients: As with any narcotic analgesic agent, Norco® 5/325 tablets should be used with caution in elderly or debilitated patients, and those with severe impairment of hepatic or renal function, hypothyroidism, Addison's disease, prostatic hypertrophy or urethral stricture. The usual precautions should be observed and the possibility of respiratory depression should be kept in mind.
Cough Reflex: Hydrocodone suppresses the cough reflex; as with all narcotics, caution should be exercised when Norco® 5/325 tablets are used postoperatively and in patients with pulmonary disease.
Information for Patients: Hydrocodone, like all narcotics, may impair mental and/or physical abilities required for the performance of potentially hazardous tasks such as driving a car or operating machinery; patients should be cautioned accordingly. Alcohol and other CNS depressants may produce an additive CNS depression, when taken with the combination product, and should be avoided.
Hydrocodone may be habit-forming. Patients should take the drug only for as long as it is prescribed, in the amounts prescribed, and no more frequently than prescribed.
Laboratory Tests: In patients with severe hepatic or renal disease, effects of therapy should be monitored with serial liver and/or renal function tests.
Drug Interactions: Patients receiving narcotics, antihistamines, antipsychotics, antianxiety agents, or other CNS depressants (including alcohol) concomitantly with Norco® 5/325 tablets may exhibit an additive CNS depression. When combined therapy is contemplated, the dose of one or both agents should be reduced.
The use of MAO inhibitors or tricyclic antidepressants with hydrocodone preparations may increase the effect of either the antidepressant or hydrocodone.
Drug/Laboratory Test Interactions: Acetaminophen may produce false-positive test results for urinary 5-hydroxyindoleacetic acid.
Carcinogenesis, Mutagenesis, Impairment of Fertility: No adequate studies have been conducted in animals to determine whether hydrocodone or acetaminophen have a potential for carcinogenesis, mutagenesis, or impairment of fertility.
Pregnancy: *Teratogenic Effects:* Pregnancy Category C: There are no adequate and well-controlled studies in pregnant women. Norco® 5/325 tablets should be used during pregnancy only if the potential benefit justifies the potential risk to the fetus.

Nonteratogenic Effects: Babies born to mothers who have been taking opioids regularly prior to delivery will be physically dependent. The withdrawal signs include irritability and excessive crying, tremors, hyperactive reflexes, increased respiratory rate, increased stools, sneezing, yawning, vomiting and fever. The intensity of the syndrome does not always correlate with the duration of maternal opioid use or dose. There is no consensus on the best method of managing withdrawal.

Labor and Delivery: As with all narcotics, administration of Norco® 5/325 tablets to the mother shortly before delivery may result in some degree of respiratory depression in the newborn, especially if higher doses are used.

Nursing Mothers: Acetaminophen is excreted in breast milk in small amounts, but the significance of its effects on nursing infants is not known. It is not known whether hydrocodone is excreted in human milk. Because many drugs are excreted in human milk and because of the potential for serious adverse reactions in nursing infants from hydrocodone and acetaminophen, a decision should be made whether to discontinue nursing or to discontinue the drug, taking into account the importance of the drug to the mother.

Pediatric Use: Safety and effectiveness in pediatric patients have not been established.

ADVERSE REACTIONS

The most frequently reported adverse reactions are lightheadedness, dizziness, sedation, nausea and vomiting. These effects seem to be more prominent in ambulatory than in non-ambulatory patients, and some of these adverse reactions may be alleviated if the patient lies down.

Other adverse reactions include:

Central Nervous System: Drowsiness, mental clouding, lethargy, impairment of mental and physical performance, anxiety, fear, dysphoria, psychic dependence, mood changes.

Gastrointestinal System: Prolonged administration of Norco® 5/325 tablets may produce constipation.

Genitourinary System: Ureteral spasm, spasm of vesical sphincters and urinary retention have been reported with opiates.

Respiratory Depression: Hydrocodone bitartrate may produce dose-related respiratory depression by acting directly on brain stem respiratory centers (see OVERDOSAGE).

Dermatological: Skin rash, pruritus.

The following adverse drug events may be borne in mind as potential effects of acetaminophen: allergic reactions, rash, thrombocytopenia, agranulocytosis.

Potential effects of high dosage are listed in the OVERDOSAGE section.

DRUG ABUSE AND DEPENDENCE

Controlled Substance: Norco® 5/325 tablets (Hydrocodone Bitartrate and Acetaminophen Tablets, USP, 5 mg/325 mg) are classified as a Schedule III controlled substance.

Abuse and Dependence: Psychic dependence, physical dependence, and tolerance may develop upon repeated administration of narcotics; therefore, Norco® 5/325 tablets should be prescribed and administered with caution. However, psychic dependence is unlikely to develop when Norco® 5/325 tablets are used for a short time for the treatment of pain.

Physical dependence, the condition in which continued administration of the drug is required to prevent the appearance of a withdrawal syndrome, assumes clinically significant proportions only after several weeks of continued narcotic use, although some mild degree of physical dependence may develop after a few days of narcotic therapy. Tolerance, in which increasingly large doses are required in order to produce the same degree of analgesia, is manifested initially by a shortened duration of analgesic effect, and subsequently by decreases in the intensity of analgesia. The rate of development of tolerance varies among patients.

OVERDOSAGE

Following an acute overdosage, toxicity may result from hydrocodone or acetaminophen.

Signs and Symptoms: Hydrocodone: Serious overdose with hydrocodone is characterized by respiratory depression (a decrease in respiratory rate and/or tidal volume, Cheyne-Stokes respiration, cyanosis), extreme somnolence progressing to stupor or coma, skeletal muscle flaccidity, cold and clammy skin, and sometimes bradycardia and hypotension. In severe overdosage, apnea, circulatory collapse, cardiac arrest and death may occur.

Acetaminophen: In acetaminophen overdosage: dose-dependent, potentially fatal hepatic necrosis is the most serious adverse effect. Renal tubular necrosis, hypoglycemic coma and thrombocytopenia may also occur.

Early symptoms following a potentially hepatotoxic overdose may include: nausea, vomiting, diaphoresis and general malaise. Clinical and laboratory evidence of hepatic toxicity may not be apparent until 48 to 72 hours post-ingestion.

In adults, hepatic toxicity has rarely been reported with acute overdoses of less than 10 grams, or fatalities with less than 15 grams.

Treatment: A single or multiple overdose with hydrocodone and acetaminophen is a potentially lethal polydrug overdose, and consultation with a regional poison control center is recommended.

Immediate treatment includes support of cardiorespiratory function and measures to reduce drug absorption. Vomiting should be induced mechanically, or with syrup of ipecac, if the patient is alert (adequate pharyngeal and laryngeal reflexes). Oral activated charcoal (1 g/kg) should follow gastric emptying. The first dose should be accompanied by an appropriate cathartic. If repeated doses are used, the cathartic might be included with alternate doses as required. Hypotension is usually hypovolemic and should respond to fluids. Vasopressors and other supportive measures should be employed as indicated. A cuffed endo-tracheal tube should be inserted before gastric lavage of the unconscious patient and, when necessary, to provide assisted respiration.

Meticulous attention should be given to maintaining adequate pulmonary ventilation. In severe cases of intoxication, peritoneal dialysis, or preferably hemodialysis may be considered. If hypoprothrombinemia occurs due to acetaminophen overdose, vitamin K should be administered intravenously.

Naloxone, a narcotic antagonist, can reverse respiratory depression and coma associated with opioid overdose. Naloxone hydrochloride 0.4 mg to 2 mg is given parenterally. Since the duration of action of hydrocodone may exceed that of the naloxone, the patient should be kept under continuous surveillance and repeated doses of the antagonist should be administered as needed to maintain adequate respiration. A narcotic antagonist should not be administered in the absence of clinically significant respiratory or cardiovascular depression.

If the dose of acetaminophen may have exceeded 140 mg/kg, acetylcysteine should be administered as early as possible. Serum acetaminophen levels should be obtained, since levels four or more hours following ingestion help predict acetaminophen toxicity. Do not await acetaminophen assay results before initiating treatment. Hepatic enzymes should be obtained initially, and repeated at 24-hour intervals.

Methemoglobinemia over 30% should be treated with methylene blue by slow intravenous administration.

The toxic dose for adults for acetaminophen is 10 g.

DOSAGE AND ADMINISTRATION

Dosage should be adjusted according to severity of pain and response of the patient. However, it should be kept in mind that tolerance to hydrocodone can develop with continued use and that the incidence of untoward effects is dose related.

The usual adult dosage is one or two tablets every four to six hours as needed for pain.

HOW SUPPLIED

Norco® 5/325 tablets (Hydrocodone Bitartrate and Acetaminophen Tablets, USP, 5 mg/325 mg) contain hydrocodone bitartrate 5 mg and acetaminophen 325 mg. They are supplied as white with orange specks, capsule-shaped, bisected tablets, debossed Watson on one side and 913 on the other side, in containers of 100 tablets, NDC 52544-913-01, in containers of 500 tablets, NDC 52544-913-05.

Storage: Store at controlled room temperature, 15°C to 30°C (59°F to 86°F).

Dispense in a tight, light-resistant container with a child-resistant closure.

A Schedule CIII Narcotic.

Rx Only

Manufactured for

WATSON PHARMA, INC.

A subsidiary of

Watson Laboratories, Inc.

Corona, CA 92880

Rev 12/00

UNITHROID™ ℞

(levothyroxine sodium tablets, USP)

DESCRIPTION

UNITHROID™ (levothyroxine sodium tablets, USP) contains synthetic crystalline L-3,3′,5,5′-tetraiodothyronine sodium salt [levothyroxine (T_4) sodium]. Synthetic T_4 is identical to that produced in the human thyroid gland. Levothyroxine (T_4) sodium has an empirical formula of $C_{15}H_{10}I_4N\ NaO_4 \times H_2O$, molecular weight of 798.86 g/mol (anhydrous), and structural formula as shown:

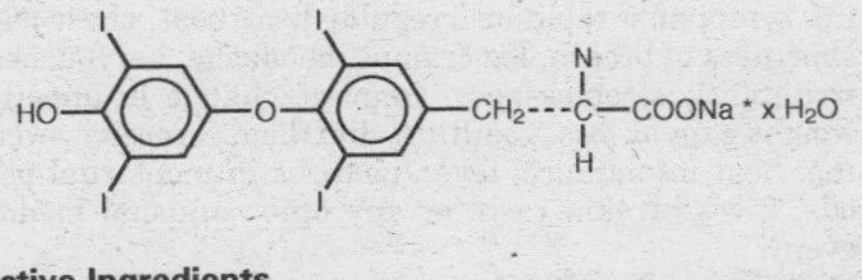

Inactive Ingredients

Colloidal silicon dioxide, lactose, magnesium stearate, microcrystalline cellulose, corn starch, acacia and sodium starch glycolate. The following are the coloring additives per tablet strength:

Strength (mcg)	Color Additive(s)
25	FD&C Yellow No. 6 Aluminum Lake
50	None
75	FD&C Red No. 40 Aluminum Lake, FD&C Blue No. 2 Aluminum Lake
88	D&C Yellow No. 10 Aluminum Lake, FD&C Yellow No. 6 Aluminum Lake, FD&C Blue No. 1 Aluminum Lake
100	D&C Yellow No. 10 Aluminum Lake, FD&C Yellow No. 6 Aluminum Lake
112	D&C Red No. 27 Aluminum Lake
125	FD&C Yellow No. 6 Aluminum Lake, FD&C Red No. 40 Aluminum Lake, FD&C Blue No. 1 Aluminum Lake
150	FD&C Blue No. 2 Aluminum Lake
175	FD&C Blue No. 1 Aluminum Lake, D&C Red No. 27 Aluminum Lake
200	FD&C Red No. 40 Aluminum Lake
300	D&C Yellow No. 10 Aluminum Lake, FD&C Yellow No. 6 Aluminum Lake, FD&C Blue No. 1 Aluminum Lake

CLINICAL PHARMACOLOGY

Thyroid hormone synthesis and secretion is regulated by the hypothalamic-pituitary-thyroid axis. Thyrotropin-releasing hormone (TRH) released from the hypothalamus stimulates secretion of thyrotropin-stimulating hormone, TSH, from the anterior pituitary. TSH, in turn, is the physiologic stimulus for the synthesis and secretion of thyroid hormones, L-thyroxine (T_4) and L-triiodothyronine (T_3), by the thyroid gland. Circulating serum T_3 and T_4 levels exert a feedback effect on both TRH and TSH secretion. When serum T_3 and T_4 levels increase, TRH and TSH secretion decrease. When thyroid hormone levels decrease, TRH and TSH secretion increase.

The mechanisms by which thyroid hormones exert their physiologic actions are not completely understood, but it is thought that their principal effects are exerted through control of DNA transcription and protein synthesis. T_3 and T_4 diffuse into the cell nucleus and bind to thyroid receptor proteins attached to DNA. This hormone nuclear receptor complex activates gene transcription and synthesis of messenger RNA and cytoplasmic proteins.

Thyroid hormones regulate multiple metabolic processes and play an essential role in normal growth and development, and normal maturation of the central nervous system and bone. The metabolic actions of thyroid hormones include augmentation of cellular respiration and thermogenesis, as well as metabolism of proteins, carbohydrates and lipids. The protein anabolic effects of thyroid hormones are essential to normal growth and development.

The physiologic actions of thyroid hormones are produced predominately by T_3, the majority of which (approximately 80%) is derived from T_4 by deiodination in peripheral tissues.

Levothyroxine, at doses individualized according to patient response, is effective as replacement or supplemental therapy in hypothyroidism of any etiology, except transient hypothyroidism during the recovery phase of subacute thyroiditis.

Levothyroxine is also effective in the suppression of pituitary TSH secretion in the treatment or prevention of various types of euthyroid goiters, including thyroid nodules, Hashimoto's thyroiditis, multinodular goiter and, as adjunctive therapy in the management of thyrotropin-dependent well-differentiated thyroid cancer (see **INDICATIONS AND USAGE, PRECAUTIONS, DOSAGE AND ADMINISTRATION**).

PHARMACOKINETICS

Absorption—Absorption of orally administered T_4 from the gastrointestinal (GI) tract ranges from 40% to 80%. The majority of the levothyroxine dose is absorbed from the jejunum and upper ileum. The relative bioavailability of UNITHROID tablets, compared to an equal nominal dose of oral levothyroxine sodium solution, is approximately 99%. T_4 absorption is increased by fasting, and decreased in malabsorption syndromes and by certain foods such as soybean infant formula. Dietary fiber decreases bioavailability of T_4. Absorption may also decrease with age. In addition, many drugs and foods affect T_4 absorption (see **PRECAUTIONS, Drug Interactions** and **Drug-Food Interactions**).

Distribution—Circulating thyroid hormones are greater than 99% bound to plasma proteins, including thyroxine-binding globulin (TBG), thyroxine-binding prealbumin (TBPA), and albumin (TBA), whose capacities and affinities vary for each hormone. The higher affinity of both TBG and TBPA for T_4 partially explains the higher serum levels, slower metabolic clearance, and longer half-life of T_4 compared to T_3. Protein-bound thyroid hormones exist in reverse equilibrium with small amounts of free hormone. Only unbound hormone is metabolically active. Many drugs and physiologic conditions affect the binding of thyroid hormones to serum proteins (see **PRECAUTIONS, Drug Interactions** and **Drug-Laboratory Test Interactions**). Thyroid hormones do not readily cross the placental barrier (see **PRECAUTIONS, Pregnancy**).

Metabolism—T_4 is slowly eliminated (see **TABLE 1**). The major pathway of thyroid hormone metabolism is through sequential deiodination. Approximately eighty-percent of circulating T_3 is derived from peripheral T_4 by monodeiodination. The liver is the major site of degradation for both T_4 and T_3;

Continued on next page

Unithroid—Cont.

with T_4 deiodination also occurring at a number of additional sites, including the kidney and other tissues. Approximately 80% of the daily dose of T_4 is deiodinated to yield equal amounts of T_3 and reverse T_3 (rT_3). T_3 and rT_3 are further deiodinated to diiodothyronine. Thyroid hormones are also metabolized via conjugation with glucuronides and sulfates and excreted directly into the bile and gut where they undergo enterohepatic recirculation.

Elimination—Thyroid hormones are primarily eliminated by the kidneys. A portion of the conjugated hormone reaches the colon unchanged and is eliminated in the feces. Approximately 20% of T_4 is eliminated in the stool. Urinary excretion of T_4 decreases with age.

[See table below]

Table 1: Pharmacokinetic Parameters of Thyroid Hormones in Euthyroid Patients

Hormone	Ratio Released from Thyroid Gland	Biologic Potency	$t_{½}$ (days)	Protein Binding (%)[2]
Levothyroxine (T_4)	20	1	6–7[1]	99.96
Liothyronine (T_3)	1	4	≤ 2	99.5

[1] 3 to 4 days in hyperthyroidism. 9 to 10 days in hypothyroidism;
[2] Includes TBG, TBPA and TBA

INDICATIONS AND USAGE

Levothyroxine sodium is used for the following indications:

Hypothyroidism—As replacement or supplemental therapy in congenital or acquired hypothyroidism of any etiology, except transient hypothyroidism during the recovery phase of subacute thyroiditis. Specific indications include: primary (thyroidal), secondary (pituitary), and tertiary (hypothalamic) hypothyroidism and subclinical hypothyroidism. Primary hypothyroidism may result from functional deficiency, primary atrophy, partial or total congenital absence of the thyroid gland, or from the effects of surgery, radiation, or drugs, with or without the presence of goiter.

Pituitary TSH Suppression—In the treatment or prevention of various types of euthyroid goiters (see **PRECAUTIONS**), including thyroid nodules (see **PRECAUTIONS**), subacute or chronic lymphocytic thyroiditis (Hashimoto's thyroiditis), multinodular goiter and, as an adjunct to surgery and radioiodine therapy in the management of thyrotropin-dependent well-differentiated thyroid cancer.

CONTRAINDICATIONS

Levothyroxine is contraindicated in patients with untreated thyrotoxicosis of any etiology and in patients with acute myocardial infarction. Levothyroxine is contraindicated in patients with uncorrected adrenal insufficiency since thyroid hormones may precipitate an acute adrenal crisis by increasing the metabolic clearance of glucocorticoids (see **PRECAUTIONS**). UNITHROID is contraindicated in patients with hypersensitivity to any of the inactive ingredients in UNITHROID tablets. (See **DESCRIPTION, Inactive Ingredients**).

WARNINGS

WARNING: Thyroid hormones, including UNITHROID, either alone or with other therapeutic agents, should not be used for the treatment of obesity. In euthyroid patients, doses within the range of daily hormonal requirements are ineffective for weight reduction. Larger doses may produce serious or even life threatening manifestations of toxicity, particularly when given in association with sympathomimetic amines such as those used for their anorectic effects.

Levothyroxine sodium should not be used in the treatment of male or female infertility unless this condition is associated with hypothyroidism.

PRECAUTIONS

General

Levothyroxine has a narrow therapeutic index. Regardless of the indication for use, careful dosage titration is necessary to avoid the consequences of over- or under-treatment. These consequences include, among others, effects on growth and development, cardiovascular function, bone metabolism, reproductive function, cognitive function, emotional state, gastrointestinal function, and on glucose and lipid metabolism.

Effects on bone mineral density—In women, long-term levothyroxine sodium therapy has been associated with decreased bone mineral density, especially in postmenopausal women on greater than replacement doses or in women who are receiving suppressive doses of levothyroxine sodium. Therefore, it is recommended that patients receiving levothyroxine sodium be given the minimum dose necessary to achieve the desired clinical and biochemical response.

Patients with underlying cardiovascular disease—Exercise caution when administering levothyroxine to patients with cardiovascular disorders and to the elderly in whom there is an increased risk of occult cardiac disease. In these patients, levothyroxine therapy should be initiated at lower doses than those recommended in younger individuals or in patients without cardiac disease (see **PRECAUTIONS, Geriatric Use** and **DOSAGE AND ADMINISTRATION**). If cardiac symptoms develop or worsen, the levothyroxine dose should be reduced or withheld for one week and then cautiously restated at a lower dose. Overtreatment with levothyroxine sodium may have adverse cardiovascular effects such as an increase in heart rate, cardiac wall thickness, and cardiac contractility and may precipitate angina or arrhythmias. Patients with coronary artery disease who are receiving levothyroxine therapy should be monitored closely during surgical procedures, since the possibility of precipitating cardiac arrhythmias may be greater in those treated with levothyroxine. Concomitant administration of levothyroxine and sympathomimetic agents to patients with coronary artery disease may precipitate coronary insufficiency.

Patients with autonomous thyroid tissue—Exercise caution when administering levothyroxine to patients with autonomous thyroid tissue in order to prevent precipitation of thyrotoxicosis.

Associated endocrine disorders

Hypothalamic/pituitary hormone deficiencies—In patients with secondary or tertiary hypothyroidism, additional hypothalamic/pituitary hormone deficiencies should be considered, and, if diagnosed, treated (see **PRECAUTIONS, Autoimmune polyglandular syndrome** for adrenal insufficiency).

Autoimmune polyglandular syndrome—Occasionally, chronic autoimmune thyroiditis may occur in association with other autoimmune disorders such as adrenal insufficiency, pernicious anemia, and insulin-dependent diabetes mellitus. Patients with concomitant adrenal insufficiency should be treated with replacement glucocorticoids prior to initiation of treatment with levothyroxine sodium. Failure to do so may precipitate an acute adrenal crisis when thyroid hormone therapy is initiated, due to increased metabolic clearance of glucocorticoids by thyroid hormone. Patients with diabetes mellitus may require upward adjustments of their antidiabetic therapeutic regimens when treated with levothyroxine (see **PRECAUTIONS, Drug Interactions**).

Other associated medical conditions

Infants with congenital hypothyroidism appear to be at increased risk for other congenital anomalies, with cardiovascular anomalies (pulmonary stenosis, atrial septal defect, and ventricular septal defect,) being the most common association.

Information for Patients

Patients should be informed of the following information to aid in the safe and effective use of UNITHROID:

1. Notify your physician if you are allergic to any foods or medicines, are pregnant or intend to become pregnant, are breast-feeding or are taking any other medications, including prescription and over-the-counter preparations.
2. Notify your physician of any other medical conditions you may have, particularly heart disease, diabetes, clotting disorders, and adrenal or pituitary gland problems. Your dose of medications used to control these other conditions may need to be adjusted while you are taking UNITHROID. If you have diabetes, monitor your blood and/or urinary glucose levels as directed by your physician and immediately report any changes to your physician. If you are taking anticoagulants (blood thinners), your clotting status should be checked frequently.
3. Use UNITHROID only as prescribed by your physician. Do not discontinue or change the amount you take or how often you take it, unless directed to do so by your physician.
4. The levothyroxine in UNITHROID is intended to replace a hormone that is normally produced by your thyroid gland. Generally, replacement therapy is to be taken for life, except in cases of transient hypothyroidism, which is usually associated with an inflammation of the thyroid gland (thyroiditis).
5. Take UNITHROID as a single dose, preferably on an empty stomach, one-half to one hour before breakfast. Levothyroxine absorption is increased on an empty stomach.
6. It may take several weeks before you notice an improvement in your symptoms.
7. Notify your physician if you experience any of the following symptoms: rapid or irregular heartbeat, chest pain, shortness of breath, leg cramps, headache, nervousness, irritability, sleeplessness, tremors, change in appetite, weight gain or loss, vomiting, diarrhea, excessive sweating, heat intolerance, fever, changes in menstrual periods, hives or skin rash, or any other unusual medical event.
8. Notify your physician if you become pregnant while taking UNITHROID. It is likely that your dose of UNITHROID will need to be increased while you are pregnant.
9. Notify your physician or dentist that you are taking UNITHROID prior to any surgery.
10. Partial hair loss may occur rarely during the first few months of UNITHROID therapy, but this is usually temporary.
11. UNITHROID should not be used as a primary or adjunctive therapy in a weight control program.
12. Keep UNITHROID out of the reach of children. Store UNITHROID away from heat, moisture, and light.

Laboratory Tests

General

The diagnosis of hypothyroidism is confirmed by measuring TSH levels using a sensitive assay (second generation assay sensitivity ≤ 0.1 mIU/L or third generation assay sensitivity ≤ 0.01 mIU/L) and measurement of free-T_4.

The adequacy of therapy is determined by periodic assessment of appropriate laboratory tests and clinical evaluation. The choice of laboratory tests depends on various factors including the etiology of the underlying thyroid disease, the presence of concomitant medical conditions, including pregnancy, and the use of concomitant medications (see **PRECAUTIONS, Drug Interactions** and **Drug-Laboratory Test Interactions**). Persistent clinical and laboratory evidence of hypothyroidism despite an apparent adequate replacement dose of UNITHROID may be evidence of inadequate absorption, poor compliance, drug interactions, or decreased T_4 potency of the drug product.

Adults

In adult patients with primary (thyroidal) hypothyroidism, serum TSH levels (using a sensitive assay) alone may be used to monitor therapy. The frequency of TSH monitoring during levothyroxine dose titration depends on the clinical situation but it is generally recommended at 6–8 week intervals until normalization. For patients who have recently initiated levothyroxine therapy and whose serum TSH has normalized or in patients who have had their dosage or brand of levothyroxine changed, the serum TSH concentration should be measured after 8–12 weeks. When the optimum replacement dose has been attained, clinical (physical examination) and biochemical monitoring may be performed every 6–12 months, depending on the clinical situation, and whenever there is a change in the patient's status. It is recommended that a physical examination and a serum TSH measurement be performed at least annually in patients receiving UNITHROID. (see **PRECAUTIONS** and **DOSAGE AND ADMINISTRATION**).

Pediatrics

In patients with congenital hypothyroidism, the adequacy of replacement therapy should be assessed by measuring both serum TSH (using a sensitive assay) and total- or free-T_4. During the first three years of life, the serum total- or free-T_4 should be maintained at all times in the upper half of the normal range. While the aim of therapy is to also normalize the serum TSH level, this is not always possible in a small percentage of patients, particularly in the first few months of therapy. TSH may not normalize due to a resetting of the pituitary-thyroid feedback threshold as a result of *in utero* hypothyroidism. Failure of the serum T_4 to increase into the upper half of the normal range within 2 weeks of initiation of UNITHROID therapy and/or of the serum TSH to decrease below 20 mU/L within 4 weeks should alert the physician to the possibility that the child is not receiving adequate therapy. Careful inquiry should then be made regarding compliance, dose of medication administered, and method of administration prior to raising the dose of UNITHROID.

The recommended frequency of monitoring of TSH and total or free T_4 in children is as follows: at 2 and 4 weeks after the initiation of treatment; every 1–2 months during the first year of life; every 2–3 months between 1 and 3 years of age; and every 3 to 12 months thereafter until growth is completed. More frequent intervals of monitoring may be necessary if poor compliance is suspected or abnormal values are obtained. It is recommended that TSH and T_4 levels, and a physical examination, if indicated, be performed 2 weeks after any change in UNITHROID dosage. Routine clinical examination, including assessment of mental and physical growth and development, and bone maturation should be performed at regular intervals (see **PRECAUTIONS, Pediatric Use** and **DOSAGE AND ADMINISTRATION**).

Secondary (pituitary) and tertiary (hypothalamic) hypothyroidism

Adequacy of therapy should be assessed by measuring serum free-T4 levels, which should be maintained in the upper half of the normal range in these patients.

Drug Interactions

Many drugs affect thyroid hormone pharmacokinetics and metabolism (e.g., absorption, synthesis, secretion, catabolism, protein binding, and target tissue response) and may alter the therapeutic response to UNITHROID. In addition, thyroid hormones and thyroid status have varied effects on the pharmacokinetics and action of other drugs. A listing of drug-thyroidal axis interactions is contained in **Table 2**.

The list of drug-thyroidal axis interactions in **Table 2** may not be comprehensive due to the introduction of new drugs that interact with the thyroidal axis or the discovery of previously unknown interactions. The prescriber should be aware of this fact and should consult appropriate reference sources (e.g., package inserts of newly approved drugs, medical literature) for additional information if a drug-drug interaction with levothyroxine is suspected.

Table 2: Drug-Thyroidal Axis Interactions

Drug or Drug Class	Effect
Drugs that may reduce TSH secretion—the redution is not sustained; therefore, hypothyroidism does not occur	
Dopamine/Dopamine Agonists Glucocorticoids Octreotide	Use of these agents may result in a transient reduction in TSH secretion when administered at the following doses: dopamine ($\geq$ 1µg•kg/min); Glucocorticoids (hydrocortisone $\geq$ 100 mg/day or equivalent); Octreotide (> 100 ug/day).

Drugs that alter thyroid hormone secretion

Drugs that may decrease thyroid hormone secretion, which may result in hypothyroidism

Drug	Effect
Aminoglutethimide Amiodarone Iodide (including iodine-combining radiographic contrast agents) Lithium Methimazole Propylthiouracil (PTU) Sulfonamides Tolbutamide	Long-term lithium therapy can result in goiter in up to 50% of patients, and either subclinical or overt hypothyroidism, each in up to 20% of patients. The fetus, neonate, elderly and euthyroid patients with underlying thyroid disease (e.g., Hashimoto's thyroiditis or with Grave's disease previously treated with radioiodine or surgery) are among those individuals who are particularly susceptible to iodine-induced hypothyroidism. Oral cholecystographic agents and amiodarone are slowly excreted, producing more prolonged hypothyroidism than parenterally administered iodinated contrast agents. Long-term aminoglutethimide therapy may minimally decrease T_4 and T_3 levels and increase TSH, although all values remain within normal limits in most patients.

Drugs that may increase thyroid hormone secretion, which may result in hyperthyroidism

Drug	Effect
Amiodarone Iodide (including iodine-containing radiographic contrast agents)	Iodide and drugs that contain pharmacologic amounts of iodide may cause hypothyroidism in euthyroid patients with Grave's disease previously treated with antithyroid drugs or in euthyroid patients with thyroid autonomy (e.g., multinodular goiter or hyper functioning thyroid adenoma). Hyperthyroidism may develop over several weeks and may persist for several months after therapy discontinuation. Amiodarone may induce hyperthyroidism by causing thyroiditis.

Drugs that may decrease T_4 absorption, which may result in hypothyroidism

Drug	Effect
Antacids —Aluminum & Magnesium Hydroxides —Simethicone Bile Acid Sequestrants —Cholestyramine —Colestipol Calcium Carbonate Cation Exchange Resins —Kayexalate Ferrous Sulfate Sucralfate	Concurrent use may reduce the efficacy of levothyroxine by binding and delaying or preventing absorption, potentially resulting in hypothyroidism. Calcium carbonate may form an insoluble chelate with levothyroxine, and ferrous sulfate likely forms a ferric-thyroxine complex. Administer levothyroxine at least 4 hours apart from these agents.

Drugs that may alter T_4 and T_3 serum transport (changes in total T_4)—but FT_4 concentrations remain normal; and, therefore, hyperthyroidism does not occur

Drugs that may increase serum TBG concentration	Drugs that may decrease serum TBG concentration
Clofibrate Estrogen-containing oral contraceptives Estrogens (oral)	Androgens/Anabolic Steroids Asparaginase Glucocorticoids Slow-Release Nicotinic Acid

Heroin/Methadone 5-Fluorouracil Mitotane Tamoxifen	

Drugs that may cause protein-binding site displacement

Drug	Effect
Furosemide (> 80 mg IV) Heparin Hydantoins Non Steroidal Anti-Inflammatory Drugs —Fenamates —Phenylbutazone Salicylates (> 2 g/day)	Administration of these agents with levothyroxine results in an intitial transient increase in FT_4. Continued administration results in a decrease in serum T4 and normal FT_4 and TSH concentrations and, therefore, patients are clinically euthyroid. Salicylates inhibit binding of T_4 and T_3 to TBG and transthyrelin. An initial increase in serum FT_4, is followed by return of FT_4 to normal levels with sustained therapeutic serum salicylate concentrations, although total-T_4 levels may decrease by as much as 30%.

Drugs that may alter T_4 and T_3 metabolism

Drugs that may increase hepatic metabolism, which may result in hypothyroidism

Drug	Effect
Carbamazepine Hydantoins Phenobarbital Rifampin	Stimulation of hepatic microsomal drug-metabolizing enzyme activity may cause increased hepatic degradation of levothyroxine, resulting in increased levothyroxine requirements. Phenytoin and carbamazepine reduce serum protein binding of levothyroxine, and total- and free-T_4 may be reduced by 20% to 40%, but most patients have normal serum TSH levels and are clinically euthyroid.

Drugs that may decrease T_4 5'—deiodinase activity

Drug	Effect
Amiodarone Beta-adrenergic antagonists –(e.g., Propranolol > 160 mg/day) Glucocorticoids –(e.g., Dexamethasone $\geq$ 4 mg/day) Propylthiouracil (PTU)	Administration of these enzyme inhibitors decrease the peripheral conversion of T_4 to T_3, leading to decreased T3 levels. However, serum T_4 levels are usually normal but may occasionally be slightly increased. In patients treated with large doses of propranolol (> 160 mg/day), T_3 and T_4 levels change slightly, TSH levels remain normal, and patients are clinically euthyroid. It should be noted that actions of particular beta-adrenergic antagonists may be impaired when the hypothyroid patient is converted to the euthyroid state. Short-term administration of large doses of glucocorticoids may decrease serum T_3 concentrations by 30% with minimal change in serum T_4 levels. However, long-term glucocorticoid therapy may result in slightly decreased T_3 and T_4 levels due to decreased TBG production (see above).

Miscellanous

Drug	Effect
Anticoagulants (oral) —Coumarin Derivatives —Indandione Derivatives	Thyroid hormones appear to increase the catabolism of vitamin K-dependent clotting factors, thereby increasing the anticoagulant activity of oral anticoagulants. Concomitant use of these agents impairs the compensatory increases in clotting factor synthesis. Prothrombin time should be carefully monitored in patients taking levothyroxine and oral anticoagulants and the dose of anticoagulant therapy adjusted accordingly.
Antidepressants –Tricyclics (e.g., Amitriptyline) –Tetracyclics (e.g., Maprotiline)	Concurrent use of tri/tetracyclic antidepressants and levothyroxine may increase the therapeutic and toxic effects of both drugs,
–Selective Serotonin Reuptake Inhibitors (SSRIs; e.g., Sertraline)	possibly due to increased receptor sensitivity to catecholamines. Toxic effects may include increased risk of cardiac arrhythmias and CNS stimulation; onset of action of tricyclics may be accelerated. Administration of sertraline in patients stabilized on levothyroxine may result in increased levothyroxine requirements.
Antidiabetic Agents –Biguanides –Meglitinides –Sulfonylureas –Thiazolidediones –Insulin	Addition of levothyroxine to antidiabetic or insulin therapy may result in increased antidiabetic agent or insulin requirements. Careful monitoring of diabetic control is recommended, especially when thyroid therapy is started, changed, or discontinued.
Cardiac Glycosides	Serum digitalis glycoside levels may be reduced in hyperthyroidism or when the hypothyroid patient is converted to the euthyroid state. Therapeutic effect of digitalis glycosides may be reduced.
Cytokines –Interferon-α –Interleukin-2	Therapy with interferon-α has been associated with the development of antithyroid microsomal antibodies in 20% of patients and some have transient hypothyroidism, hyperthyroidism, or both. Patients who have antithyroid antibodies before treatment are at higher risk for thyroid dysfunction during treatment. Interleukin-2 has been associated with transient painless thyroiditis in 20% of patients. Interferon-$\beta\sim$ and -γ have not been reported to cause thyroid dysfunction.
Growth Hormones –Somatrem –Somatropin	Excessive use of thyroid hormones with growth hormones may accelerate epiphyseal closure. However, untreated hypothyroidism may interfere with growth response to growth hormone.
Ketamine	Concurrent use may produce marked hypertension and tachycardia; cautious administration to patients receiving thyroid hormone therapy is recommended.
Methylxanthine Bronchodilators –(e.g., Theophylline)	Decreased theophylline clearance may occur in hypothyroid patients; clearance returns to normal when the euthyroid state is achieved.
Radiographic Agents	Thyroid hormones may reduce the uptake of ^{123}I, ^{131}I, and ^{99m}Tc.
Sympathomimetics	Concurrent use may increase the effects of sympathomimetics or thyroid hormone. Thyroid hormones may increase the risk of coronary insufficiency when sympathomimetic agents are administered to patients with coronary artery disease.
Chloral Hydrate Diazepam Ethionamide Lovastatin Metoclopramide 6-Mercaptopurine Nitroprusside Para-aminosalicylate sodium Perphenazine Resorcinol (excessive topical use) Thiazide Diuretics	These agents have been associated with thyroid hormone and/or TSH level alterations by various mechanisms.

Continued on next page

Unithroid—Cont.

Strength (mcg)	Color	NDC# for bottles of 100	NDC# for bottles of 1000
25	Peach	NDC 52544-902-01	NDC 52544-902-10
50	White	NDC 52544-903-01	NDC 52544-903-10
75	Purple	NDC 52544-904-01	NDC 52544-904-10
88	Olive	NDC 52544-905-01	NDC 52544-905-10
100	Yellow	NDC 52544-906-01	NDC 52544-906-10
112	Rose	NDC 52544-907-01	NDC 52544-907-10
125	Tan	NDC 52544-908-01	NDC 52544-908-10
150	Blue	NDC 52544-909-01	NDC 52544-909-10
175	Lilac	NDC 52544-910-01	NDC 52544-910-10
200	Pink	NDC 52544-911-01	NDC 52544-911-10
300	Green	NDC 52544-912-01	NDC 52544-912-10

Oral anticoagulants—Levothyroxine increases the response to oral anticoagulant therapy. Therefore, a decrease in the dose of anticoagulant may be warranted with correction of the hypothyroid state or when the UNITHROID dose is increased. Prothrombin time should be closely monitored to permit appropriate and timely dosage adjustments (see **Table 2**).

Digitalis glycosides—The therapeutic effects of digitalis glycosides may be reduced by levothyroxine. Serum digitalis glycoside levels may be decreased when a hypothyroid patient becomes euthyroid, necessitating an increase in the dose of digitalis glycosides (see **Table 2**).

Drug-Food Interactions—Consumption of certain foods may affect levothyroxine absorption thereby necessitating adjustments in dosing. Soybean flour (infant formula), cotton seed meal, walnuts, and dietary fiber may bind and decrease the absorption of levothyroxine sodium from the GI tract.

Drug-Laboratory Test Interactions—Changes in TBG concentration must be considered when interpreting T_4 and T_3 values, which necessitates measurement and evaluation of unbound (free) hormone and/or determination of the free T_4 index (FT_4I). Pregnancy, infectious hepatitis, estrogens, estrogen-containing oral contraceptives, and acute intermittent porphyria increase TBG concentrations. Decreases in TBG concentrations are observed in nephrosis, severe hypoproteinemia, severe liver disease, acromegaly, and after androgen or corticosteroid therapy (see also **Table 2**). Familial hyper- or hypo-thyroxine binding globulinemias have been described, with the incidence of TBG deficiency approximating 1 in 9000.

Carcinogenesis, Mutagenesis, and Impairment of Fertility—Animal studies have not been performed to evaluate the carcinogenic potential, mutagenic potential or effects on fertility of levothyroxine. The synthetic T_4 in UNITHROID is identical to that produced naturally by the human thyroid gland. Although there has been a reported association between prolonged thyroid hormone therapy and breast cancer, this has not been confirmed. Patients receiving UNITHROID for appropriate clinical indications should be titrated to the lowest effective replacement dose.

Pregnancy—Category A—Studies in women taking levothyroxine sodium during pregnancy have not shown an increased risk of congenital abnormalities. Therefore, the possibility of fetal harm appears remote. UNITHROID should not be discontinued during pregnancy and hypothyroidism diagnosed during pregnancy should be promptly treated.

Hypothyroidism during pregnancy is associated with a higher rate of complications, including spontaneous abortion, pre-eclampsia, stillbirth and premature delivery. Maternal hypothyroidism may have an adverse effect on fetal and childhood growth and development. During pregnancy, serum T_4 levels may decrease and serum TSH levels increase to values outside the normal range. Since elevations in serum TSH may occur as early as 4 weeks gestation, pregnant women taking UNITHROID should have their TSH measured during each trimester. An elevated serum TSH level should be corrected by an increase in the dose of UNITHROID. Since postpartum TSH levels are similar to preconception values, the UNITHROID dosage should return to the pre-pregnancy dose immediately after delivery. A serum TSH level should be obtained 6–8 weeks postpartum.

Thyroid hormones do not readily cross the placental barrier; however, some transfer does occur as evidenced by levels in cord blood of athyroceotic fetuses being approximately one-third maternal levels. Transfer of thyroid hormone from the mother to the fetus; however, may not be adequate to prevent *in utero* hypothyroidism.

Nursing Mothers—Although thyroid hormones are excreted only minimally in human milk, caution should be exercised when UNITHROID is administered to a nursing woman. However, adequate replacement doses of levothyroxine are generally needed to maintain normal lactation.

Pediatric Use

General

The goal of treatment in pediatric patients with hypothyroidism is to achieve and maintain normal intellectual and physical growth and development.

The initial dose of levothyroxine varies with age and body weight (see **DOSAGE AND ADMINISTRATION, Table 3**). Dosing adjustments are based on an assessment of the individual patient's clinical and laboratory parameters (see **PRECAUTIONS, Laboratory Tests**).

In children in whom a diagnosis of permanent hypothyroidism has not been established, it is recommended that levothyroxine administration be discontinued for a 30-day trial period, but only after the child is at least 3 years of age. Serum T_4 and TSH levels should then be obtained. If the T_4 is low and the TSH high, the diagnosis of permanent hypothyroidism is established, and levothyroxine therapy should be reinstituted. If the T_4 and TSH are normal, euthyroidism may be assumed and, therefore, the hypothyroidism can be considered to have been transient. In this instance, however, the physician should carefully monitor the child and repeat the thyroid function tests if any signs or symptoms of hypothyroidism develop. In this setting, the clinician should have a high index of suspicion of relapse. If the results of the levothyroxine withdrawal test are inconclusive, careful follow-up and subsequent testing will be necessary.

Since some more severely affected children may become clinically hypothyroid when treatment is discontinued for 30 days, an alternate approach is reduce the replacement dose of levothyroxine by half during the 30-day trial period. If, after 30 days, the serum TSH is elevated above 20 mU/L, the diagnosis permanent hypothyroidism is confirmed and full replacement therapy should be resumed. However, if the serum TSH has not risen to greater than 20 mU/L, levothyroxine treatment should be discontinued for another 30-day trial period followed by repeat serum T_4 and TSH.

The presence of concomitant medical conditions should be considered in certain clinical circumstances and, if present, appropriately treated (see **PRECAUTIONS**).

Congenital Hypothyroidism (see **PRECAUTIONS, Laboratory Tests** and **DOSAGE AND ADMINISTRATION**)

Rapid restoration of normal serum T_4 concentrations is essential for preventing the adverse effects of congenital hypothyroidism on intellectual development as well as on overall physical growth and maturation. Therefore, UNITHROID therapy should be initiated immediately upon diagnosis and is generally continued for life.

During the first 2 weeks of UNITHROID therapy, infants should be closely monitored for cardiac overload, arrhythmias, and aspiration from avid suckling.

The patient should be monitored closely to avoid undertreatment or overtreatment. Undertreatment may have deleterious effects on intellectual development and linear growth. Overtreatment has been associated with craniosynostosis in infants, and may adversely affect the tempo of brain maturation and accelerate the bone age with resultant premature closure of the epiphyses and compromised adult stature.

Acquired Hypothyroidism in Pediatric Patients

The patient should be monitored closely to avoid undertreatment and overtreatment. Undertreatment may result in poor school performance due to impaired concentration and slowed mentation and in reduced adult height. Overtreatment may accelerate the bone age and result in premature epiphyseal closure and compromised adult stature.

Treated children may manifest a period of catch-up growth, which may be adequate in some cases to normalize adult height. In children with severe or prolonged hypothyroidism, catch-up growth may not be adequate to normalize adult height.

Geriatric Use

Because of the increased prevalence of cardiovascular disease among the elderly, levothyroxine therapy should not be initiated at the full replacement dose (see **PRECAUTIONS** and **DOSAGE AND ADMINISTRATION**).

ADVERSE REACTIONS

Adverse reactions associated with levothyroxine therapy are primarily those of hyperthyroidism due to therapeutic overdosage. They include the following:

General: fatigue, increased appetite, weight loss, heat intolerance, fever, excessive sweating;

Central nervous system: headache, hyperactivity, nervousness, anxiety, irritability, emotional lability, insomnia;

Musculoskeletal: tremors, muscle weakness;

Cardiac: palpitations, tachycardia, arrhythmias, increased pulse and blood pressure, heart failure, angina, myocardial infarction, cardiac arrest;

Pulmonary: dyspnea;

GI: diarrhea, vomiting, abdominal cramps;

Dermatologic: hair loss;

Reproductive: menstrual irregularities, infertility.

Pseudotumor cerebri has been reported in children receiving levothyroxine therapy.

Seizures have been reported rarely with the institution of levothyroxine therapy.

Inadequate levothyroxine dosage will produce or fail to ameliorate the signs and symptoms of hypothyroidism.

Hypersensitivity reactions to inactive ingredients have occurred in patients treated with thyroid hormone products. These include urticaria, pruritus, skin rash, flushing, angioedema, various GI symptoms (abdominal pain, nausea, vomiting and diarrhea), fever, arthralgia, serum sickness and wheezing. Hypersensitivity to levothyroxine itself is not known to occur.

OVERDOSAGE

The signs and symptoms of overdosage are those of hyperthyroidism (see **PRECAUTIONS** and **ADVERSE REACTIONS**). In addition, confusion and disorientation may occur. Cerebral embolism, shock, coma, and death have been reported. Seizures have occurred in a child ingesting approximately 20 mg of levothyroxine. Symptoms may not necessarily be evident or may not appear until several days after ingestion of levothyroxine sodium.

Acute Massive Overdosage—This may be a life-threatening emergency, therefore, symptomatic and supportive therapy should be instituted immediately. If not contraindicated (e.g., by seizures, coma, or loss of the gag reflex), the stomach should be emptied by emesis or gastric lavage to decrease gastrointestinal absorption. Activated charcoal or cholestyramine may also be used to decrease absorption. Central and peripheral increased sympathetic activity may be treated by administering B-receptor antagonists, e.g., propranolol (1 to 3 mg intravenously over a 10 minute period, or orally, 80 to 160 mg/day). Provide respiratory support as needed; control congestive heart failure; control fever, hypoglycemia, and fluid loss as necessary. Glucocorticoids may be given to inhibit the conversion of T_4 to T_3. Because T_4 is highly protein bound, very little drug will be removed by dialysis.

DOSAGE AND ADMINISTRATION

General Principles:

The goal of replacement therapy is to achieve and maintain a clinical and biochemical euthyroid state. The goal of suppressive therapy is to inhibit growth and/or function of abnormal thyroid tissue. The dose of UNITHROID that is adequate to achieve these goals depends on a variety of factors including the patient's age, body weight, cardiovascular status, concomitant medical conditions, including pregnancy, concomitant medications, and the specific nature of the condition being treated (see **PRECAUTIONS**). Hence, the following recommendations serve only as dosing guidelines. Dosing must be individualized and adjustments made based on periodic assessment of the patient's clinical response and laboratory parameters (see **PRECAUTIONS, Laboratory Tests**).

UNITHROID is administered as a single daily dose, preferably one-half to one-hour before breakfast. UNITHROID should be taken at least 4 hours apart from drugs that are known to interfere with its absorption (see **PRECAUTIONS, Drug Interactions**).

Due to the long half-life of levothyroxine, the peak therapeutic effect at a given dose of levothyroxine may not be attained for 4–6 weeks.

Caution should be exercised when administering UNITHROID to patients with underlying cardiovascular disease, to the elderly, and to those with concomitant adrenal insufficiency (see **PRECAUTIONS**).

Specific Patient Populations:

Hypothyroidism in Adults and in Children in Whom Growth and Puberty are Complete (see **PRECAUTIONS, Laboratory Tests**).

Therapy may begin at full replacement doses in otherwise healthy individuals less than 50 years old and in those older than 50 years who have been recently treated for hyperthyroidism or who have been hypothyroid for only a short time (such as a few months). The average full replacement dose of levothyroxine is approximately 1.7 mcg/kg/day (e.g., **100–125 mcg/day** for a 70 kg adult). Older patients may require less than 1 mcg/kg/day. Levothyroxine doses greater than 200 mcg/day are seldom required. An inadequate response to daily doses ≥ 300 mcg/day is rare and may indicate poor compliance, malabsorption, and/or drug interactions.

For most patients older than 50 years or for patients under 50 years of age with underlying cardiac disease, an initial starting dose of **25–50 mcg/day** of levothyroxine is recommended, with gradual increments in dose at 6–8 week intervals. The recommended starting dose of levothyroxine in elderly patients with cardiac disease is **12.5–25 mcg/day**, with gradual dose increments at 4–6 week intervals. The levothyroxine dose is generally adjusted in 12.5–25 mcg increments until the patient with primary hypothyroidism is clinically euthyroid and the serum TSH has normalized.

In patients with severe hypothyroidism, the recommended initial levothyroxine dose is **12.5–25 mcg/day** with increases of 25 mcg/day every 2–4 weeks, accompanied by clinical and laboratory assessment, until the TSH level is normalized.

In patients with secondary (pituitary) or tertiary (hypothalamic) hypothyroidism, the levothyroxine dose should be titrated until the patient is clinically euthyroid and the serum free-T_4 level is restored to the upper half of the normal range.

Pediatric Dosage—Congenital or Acquired Hypothyroidism (see **PRECAUTIONS, Laboratory Tests**)

General Principles

In general, levothyroxine therapy should be instituted at full replacement doses as soon as possible. Delays in diagnosis and institution of therapy may have deleterious effects on the child's intellectual and physical growth and development. Undertreatment and overtreatment should be avoided (see **PRECAUTIONS, Pediatric Use**).

UNITHROID may be administered to infants and children who cannot swallow intact tablets by crushing the tablet and suspending the freshly crushed tablet in a small amount (5–10 mL or 1–2 teaspoons) of water. This suspension can be administered by spoon or dropper. **DO NOT STORE THE SUSPENSION.** Foods that decrease absorption of levothyroxine such as soybean infant formula, should not be used for administering levothyroxine. (see **PRECAUTIONS, Drug-Food Interactions**).

Newborns

The recommended starting dose of levothyroxine in newborn infants is **10–15 mcg/kg/day**. A lower starting dose (e.g., 25 mcg/day) should be considered in infants at risk for cardiac failure, and the dose should be increased in 4–6 weeks as needed based on clinical and laboratory response to treatment. In infants with very low (<5 mcg/dl) or undetectable serum T_4 concentrations, the recommended initial starting dose is **50 mcg/day** of levothyroxine.

Infants and Children

Levothyroxine therapy is usually initiated at full replacement doses, with the recommended dose per body weight decreasing with age (see **TABLE 3**). However, in children with chronic or severe hypothyroidism, an initial dose of **25 mcg/day** of levothyroxine is recommended with increments of 25 mcg every 2–4 weeks until the desired effect is achieved.

Hyperactivity in an older child can be minimized if the starting dose is one-fourth of the recommended full replacement dose, and the dose is then increased on a weekly basis by an amount equal to one-fourth the full recommended replacement dose until the full recommended replacement dose is reached.

Table 3: Levothyroxine Dosing Guidelines for Pediatric Hypothyroidism

AGE	Daily Dose Per Kg Body Weight[a]
0–3 months	10–15 mcg/kg/day
3–6 months	8–10 mcg/kg/day
6–12 months	6–8 mcg/kg/day
1–5 years	5–6 mcg/kg/day
6–12 years	4–5 mcg/kg/day
>12 years	2–3 mcg/kg/day
Growth and puberty complete	1.7 mcg/kg/day

[a] The dose should be adjusted based on clinical response and laboratory parameters (see **PRECAUTIONS, Laboratory Tests** and **Pediatric Use**).

Pregnancy—Pregnancy may increase levothyroxine requirements (see **PREGNANCY**).

Subclinical Hypothyroidism—If this condition is treated, lower levothyroxine doses (e.g. **1 mcg/kg/day**) than that used for full replacement may be adequate to normalize the serum TSH level. Patients who are not treated should be monitored yearly for changes in clinical status and thyroid laboratory parameters.

TSH Suppression in Well-differentiated Thyroid Cancer and Thyroid Nodules—Levothyroxine is used as an adjunct to surgery and radioiodine therapy in the treatment of well-differentiated (papillary and follicular) thyroid cancer. Generally, TSH is suppressed to <0.1 mU/L, and this usually requires a levothyroxine dose of **greater than 2 mcg/kg/day**. In the treatment of benign nodules and nontoxic multinodular goiter, TSH is generally suppressed to a higher target (0.1–0.3 mU/L) than that used for the treatment of thyroid cancer. Exercise caution when administering levothyroxine to patients with autonomous thyroid tissue (see **PRECAUTIONS**).

Myxedema Coma—Myxedema coma is a life-threatening emergency characterized by poor circulation and hypometabolism, and may result in unpredictable absorption of levothyroxine sodium from the gastrointestinal tract. Therefore, oral levothyroxine is not recommended to treat this condition. Intravenous levothyroxine sodium should be administered.

HOW SUPPLIED

UNITHROID™ (levothyroxine sodium tablets, USP) are round, color coded, partial bisected tablets debossed with JSP and ID Number:

[See table at top of previous page]

STORAGE CONDITIONS

20°C to 25°C (68°F to 77°F) with excursions between 15°C to 30°C (59°F to 86°F)

Rx only

Manufactured for:
Watson Pharma, Inc.
A Subsidiary of Watson Laboratories, Inc.
Corona, CA 92880

Manufactured by:
Jerome Stevens Pharmaceuticals, Inc.
Bohemia, NY 11716

Rev. 10/00

MG #15532

REVISED INFORMATION

As new research data and clinical findings become available, the product information in *PDR* is revised accordingly. Revisions submitted since the 2001 edition went to press can be found below. To remind yourself of a revision, write "See Supplement A" next to the product's heading in the book.

AstraZeneca LP
WILMINGTON, DE 19850-5437

For Medical Information,
Adverse Drug Experiences,
and Customer Service
Contact: (800) 236-9933

ATACAND® ℞
(candesartan cilexetil)
TABLETS

Prescribing information for this product, which appears on page(s) 564–566 of the 2001 PDR, has been completely revised as follows. Please write "See Supplement A" next to the product heading.

USE IN PREGNANCY
When used in pregnancy during the second and third trimesters, drugs that act directly on the renin-angiotensin system can cause injury and even death to the developing fetus. When pregnancy is detected, ATACAND should be discontinued as soon as possible. See WARNINGS, Fetal/Neonatal Morbidity and Mortality.

DESCRIPTION
ATACAND* (candesartan cilexetil), a prodrug, is hydrolyzed to candesartan during absorption from the gastrointestinal tract. Candesartan is a selective AT$_1$ subtype angiotensin II receptor antagonist.

Candesartan cilexetil, a nonpeptide, is chemically described as (±)-1-[[(cyclohexyloxy)carbonyl]oxy]ethyl 2-ethoxy-1-[[2'-(1H-tetrazol-5-yl) [1,1'-biphenyl]-4-yl]methyl]-1H-benzimidazole-7-carboxylate.

Its empirical formula is $C_{33}H_{34}N_6O_6$, and its structural formula is

⬇ site of ester hydrolysis.

Candesartan cilexetil is a white to off-white powder with a molecular weight of 610.67. It is practically insoluble in water and sparingly soluble in methanol. Candesartan cilexetil is a racemic mixture containing one chiral center at the cyclohexyloxycarbonyloxy ethyl ester group. Following oral administration, candesartan cilexetil undergoes hydrolysis at the ester link to form the active drug, candesartan, which is achiral.

ATACAND is available for oral use as tablets containing either 4 mg, 8 mg, 16 mg, or 32 mg of candesartan cilexetil and the following inactive ingredients: hydroxypropyl cellulose, polyethylene glycol, lactose, corn starch, carboxymethylcellulose calcium, and magnesium stearate. Ferric oxide (reddish brown) is added to the 8-mg, 16-mg, and 32-mg tablets as a colorant.

CLINICAL PHARMACOLOGY
Mechanism of Action
Angiotensin II is formed from angiotensin I in a reaction catalyzed by angiotensin-converting enzyme (ACE, kininase II). Angiotensin II is the principal pressor agent of the renin-angiotensin system, with effects that include vasoconstriction, stimulation of synthesis and release of aldosterone, cardiac stimulation, and renal reabsorption of sodium. Candesartan blocks the vasoconstrictor and aldosterone-secreting effects of angiotensin II by selectively blocking the binding of angiotensin II to the AT$_1$ receptor in many tissues, such as vascular smooth muscle and the adrenal gland. Its action is, therefore, independent of the pathways for angiotensin II synthesis.

There is also an AT$_2$ receptor found in many tissues, but AT$_2$ is not known to be associated with cardiovascular homeostasis. Candesartan has much greater affinity (>10,000-fold) for the AT$_1$ receptor than for the AT$_2$ receptor.

Blockade of the renin-angiotensin system with ACE inhibitors, which inhibit the biosynthesis of angiotensin II from angiotensin I, is widely used in the treatment of hypertension. ACE inhibitors also inhibit the degradation of bradykinin, a reaction also catalyzed by ACE. Because candesartan does not inhibit ACE (kininase II), it does not affect the response to bradykinin. Whether this difference has clinical relevance is not yet known. Candesartan does not bind to or block other hormone receptors or ion channels known to be important in cardiovascular regulation.

Blockade of the angiotensin II receptor inhibits the negative regulatory feedback of angiotensin II on renin secretion, but the resulting increased plasma renin activity and angiotensin II circulating levels do not overcome the effect of candesartan on blood pressure.

Pharmacokinetics
General
Candesartan cilexetil is rapidly and completely bioactivated by ester hydrolysis during absorption from the gastrointestinal tract to candesartan, a selective AT$_1$ subtype angiotensin II receptor antagonist. Candesartan is mainly excreted unchanged in urine and feces (via bile). It undergoes minor hepatic metabolism by O-deethylation to an inactive metabolite. The elimination half-life of candesartan is approximately 9 hours. After single and repeated administration, the pharmacokinetics of candesartan are linear for oral doses up to 32 mg of candesartan cilexetil. Candesartan and its inactive metabolite do not accumulate in serum upon repeated once-daily dosing.

Following administration of candesartan cilexetil, the absolute bioavailability of candesartan was estimated to be 15%. After tablet ingestion, the peak serum concentration (C_{max}) is reached after 3 to 4 hours. Food with a high fat content does not affect the bioavailability of candesartan after candesartan cilexetil administration.

Metabolism and Excretion
Total plasma clearance of candesartan is 0.37 mL/min/kg, with a renal clearance of 0.19 mL/min/kg. When candesartan is administered orally, about 26% of the dose is excreted unchanged in urine. Following an oral dose of ^{14}C-labeled candesartan cilexetil, approximately 33% of radioactivity is recovered in urine and approximately 67% in feces. Following an intravenous dose of ^{14}C-labeled candesartan, approximately 59% of radioactivity is recovered in urine and approximately 36% in feces. Biliary excretion contributes to the elimination of candesartan.

Distribution
The volume of distribution of candesartan is 0.13 L/kg. Candesartan is highly bound to plasma proteins (>99%) and does not penetrate red blood cells. The protein binding is constant at candesartan plasma concentrations well above the range achieved with recommended doses. In rats, it has been demonstrated that candesartan crosses the blood-brain barrier poorly, if at all. It has also been demonstrated in rats that candesartan passes across the placental barrier and is distributed in the fetus.

Special Populations
Pediatric: The pharmacokinetics of candesartan cilexetil have not been investigated in patients <18 years of age.

Geriatric and Gender: The pharmacokinetics of candesartan have been studied in the elderly (≥65 years) and in both sexes. The plasma concentration of candesartan was higher in the elderly (C_{max} was approximately 50% higher, and AUC was approximately 80% higher) compared to younger subjects administered the same dose. The pharmacokinetics of candesartan were linear in the elderly, and candesartan and its inactive metabolite did not accumulate in the serum of these subjects upon repeated, once-daily administration. No initial dosage adjustment is necessary. (See DOSAGE AND ADMINISTRATION.) There is no difference in the pharmacokinetics of candesartan between male and female subjects.

Renal Insufficiency: In hypertensive patients with renal insufficiency, serum concentrations of candesartan were elevated. After repeated dosing, the AUC and C_{max} were approximately doubled in patients with severe renal impairment (creatinine clearance <30 mL/min/1.73m^2) compared to patients with normal kidney function. The pharmacokinetics of candesartan in hypertensive patients undergoing hemodialysis are similar to those in hypertensive patients with severe renal impairment. Candesartan cannot be removed by hemodialysis. No initial dosage adjustment is necessary in patients with renal insufficiency. (See DOSAGE AND ADMINISTRATION.)

Hepatic Insufficiency: No differences in the pharmacokinetics of candesartan were observed in patients with mild to moderate chronic liver disease. The pharmacokinetics after candesartan cilexetil administration have not been investigated in patients with severe hepatic insufficiency. No initial dosage adjustment is necessary in patients with mild hepatic disease. (See DOSAGE AND ADMINISTRATION.)

Drug Interactions
See PRECAUTIONS, Drug Interactions.

Pharmacodynamics
Candesartan inhibits the pressor effects of angiotensin II infusion in a dose-dependent manner. After 1 week of once-daily dosing with 8 mg of candesartan cilexetil, the pressor effect was inhibited by approximately 90% at peak with approximately 50% inhibition persisting for 24 hours.

Plasma concentrations of angiotensin I and angiotensin II, and plasma renin activity (PRA), increased in a dose-dependent manner after single and repeated administration of candesartan cilexetil to healthy subjects and hypertensive patients. ACE activity was not altered in healthy subjects after repeated candesartan cilexetil administration. The once-daily administration of up to 16 mg of candesartan cilexetil to healthy subjects did not influence plasma aldosterone concentrations, but a decrease in the plasma concentration of aldosterone was observed when 32 mg of candesartan cilexetil was administered to hypertensive patients. In spite of the effect of candesartan cilexetil on aldosterone secretion, very little effect on serum potassium was observed.

In multiple-dose studies with hypertensive patients, there were no clinically significant changes in metabolic function, including serum levels of total cholesterol, triglycerides, glucose, or uric acid. In a 12-week study of 161 patients with non-insulin-dependent (type 2) diabetes mellitus and hypertension, there was no change in the level of HbA$_{1c}$.

Clinical Trials
The antihypertensive effects of ATACAND were examined in 14 placebo-controlled trials of 4- to 12-weeks duration, primarily at daily doses of 2 to 32 mg per day in patients with baseline diastolic blood pressures of 95 to 114 mm Hg. Most of the trials were of candesartan cilexetil as a single agent, but it was also studied as add-on to hydrochlorothiazide and amlodipine. These studies included a total of 2350 patients randomized to one of several doses of candesartan cilexetil and 1027 to placebo. Except for a study in diabetics, all studies showed significant effects, generally dose related, of 2 to

Continued on next page

Atacand—Cont.

32 mg on trough (24 hour) systolic and diastolic pressures compared to placebo, with doses of 8 to 32 mg giving effects of about 8–12/4–8 mm Hg. There were no exaggerated first-dose effects in these patients. Most of the antihypertensive effect was seen within 2 weeks of initial dosing, and the full effect in 4 weeks. With once-daily dosing, blood pressure effect was maintained over 24 hours, with trough to peak ratios of blood pressure effect generally over 80%. Candesartan cilexetil had an additional blood pressure lowering effect when added to hydrochlorothiazide.

The antihypertensive effect was similar in men and women and in patients older and younger than 65. Candesartan was effective in reducing blood pressure regardless of race, although the effect was somewhat less in blacks (usually a low-renin population). This has been generally true for angiotensin II antagonists and ACE inhibitors.

In long-term studies of up to 1 year, the antihypertensive effectiveness of candesartan cilexetil was maintained, and there was no rebound after abrupt withdrawal.

There were no changes in the heart rate of patients treated with candesartan cilexetil in controlled trials.

INDICATIONS AND USAGE

ATACAND is indicated for the treatment of hypertension. It may be used alone or in combination with other antihypertensive agents.

CONTRAINDICATIONS

ATACAND is contraindicated in patients who are hypersensitive to any component of this product.

WARNINGS

Fetal/Neonatal Morbidity and Mortality

Drugs that act directly on the renin-angiotensin system can cause fetal and neonatal morbidity and death when administered to pregnant women. Several dozen cases have been reported in the world literature in patients who were taking angiotensin-converting enzyme inhibitors. When pregnancy is detected, ATACAND should be discontinued as soon as possible.

The use of drugs that act directly on the renin-angiotensin system during the second and third trimesters of pregnancy has been associated with fetal and neonatal injury, including hypotension, neonatal skull hypoplasia, anuria, reversible or irreversible renal failure, and death. Oligohydramnios has also been reported, presumably resulting from decreased fetal renal function; oligohydramnios in this setting has been associated with fetal limb contractures, craniofacial deformation, and hypoplastic lung development. Prematurity, intrauterine growth retardation, and patent ductus arteriosus have also been reported, although it is not clear whether these occurrences were due to exposure to the drug. These adverse effects do not appear to have resulted from intrauterine drug exposure that has been limited to the first trimester. Mothers whose embryos and fetuses are exposed to an angiotensin II receptor antagonist only during the first trimester should be so informed. Nonetheless, when patients become pregnant, physicians should have the patient discontinue the use of ATACAND as soon as possible.

Rarely (probably less often than once in every thousand pregnancies), no alternative to a drug acting on the renin-angiotensin system will be found. In these rare cases, the mothers should be apprised of the potential hazards to their fetuses, and serial ultrasound examinations should be performed to assess the intra-amniotic environment.

If oligohydramnios is observed, ATACAND should be discontinued unless it is considered life saving for the mother. Contraction stress testing (CST), a nonstress test (NST), or biophysical profiling (BPP) may be appropriate, depending upon the week of pregnancy. Patients and physicians should be aware, however, that oligohydramnios may not appear until after the fetus has sustained irreversible injury.

Infants with histories of *in utero* exposure to an angiotensin II receptor antagonist should be closely observed for hypotension, oliguria, and hyperkalemia. If oliguria occurs, attention should be directed toward support of blood pressure and renal perfusion. Exchange transfusion or dialysis may be required as means of reversing hypotension and/or substituting for disordered renal function.

There is no clinical experience with the use of ATACAND in pregnant women. Oral doses $\geq$ 10 mg of candesartan cilexetil/kg/day administered to pregnant rats during late gestation and continued through lactation were associated with reduced survival and an increased incidence of hydronephrosis in the offspring. The 10-mg/kg/day dose in rats is approximately 2.8 times the maximum recommended daily human dose (MRHD) of 32 mg on a mg/m² basis (comparison assumes human body weight of 50 kg). Candesartan cilexetil given to pregnant rabbits at an oral dose of 3 mg/kg/day (approximately 1.7 times the MRHD on a mg/m² basis) caused maternal toxicity (decreased body weight and death) but, in surviving dams, had no adverse effects on fetal survival, fetal weight, or external, visceral, or skeletal development. No maternal toxicity or adverse effects on fetal development were observed when oral doses up to 1000 mg of candesartan cilexetil/kg/day (approximately 138 times the MRHD on a mg/m² basis) were administered to pregnant mice.

Hypotension in Volume- and Salt-Depleted Patients

In patients with an activated renin-angiotensin system, such as volume- and/or salt-depleted patients (e.g., those being treated with diuretics), symptomatic hypotension may occur. These conditions should be corrected prior to admin-

istration of ATACAND, or the treatment should start under close medical supervision (see DOSAGE AND ADMINISTRATION).

If hypotension occurs, the patients should be placed in the supine position and, if necessary, given an intravenous infusion of normal saline. A transient hypotensive response is not a contraindication to further treatment which usually can be continued without difficulty once the blood pressure has stabilized.

PRECAUTIONS
General

Impaired Renal Function: As a consequence of inhibiting the renin-angiotensin-aldosterone system, changes in renal function may be anticipated in susceptible individuals treated with ATACAND. In patients whose renal function may depend upon the activity of the renin-angiotensin-aldosterone system (e.g., patients with severe congestive heart failure), treatment with angiotensin-converting enzyme inhibitors and angiotensin receptor antagonists has been associated with oliguria and/or progressive azotemia and (rarely) with acute renal failure and/or death. Similar results may be anticipated in patients treated with ATACAND. (See CLINICAL PHARMACOLOGY, Special Populations.)

In studies of ACE inhibitors in patients with unilateral or bilateral renal artery stenosis, increases in serum creatinine or blood urea nitrogen (BUN) have been reported. There has been no long-term use of ATACAND in patients with unilateral or bilateral renal artery stenosis, but similar results may be expected.

Information for Patients

Pregnancy: Female patients of childbearing age should be told about the consequences of second- and third-trimester exposure to drugs that act on the renin-angiotensin system, and they should also be told that these consequences do not appear to have resulted from intrauterine drug exposure that has been limited to the first trimester. These patients should be asked to report pregnancies to their physicians as soon as possible.

Drug Interactions

No significant drug interactions have been reported in studies of candesartan cilexetil given with other drugs such as glyburide, nifedipine, digoxin, warfarin, hydrochlorothiazide, and oral contraceptives in healthy volunteers. Because candesartan is not significantly metabolized by the cytochrome P450 system and at therapeutic concentrations has no effects on P450 enzymes, interactions with drugs that inhibit or are metabolized by those enzymes would not be expected.

Carcinogenesis, Mutagenesis, Impairment of Fertility

There was no evidence of carcinogenicity when candesartan cilexetil was orally administered to mice and rats for up to 104 weeks at doses up to 100 and 1000 mg/kg/day, respectively. Rats received the drug by gavage, whereas mice received the drug by dietary administration. These (maximally-tolerated) doses of candesartan cilexetil provided systemic exposures to candesartan (AUCs) that were, in mice, approximately 7 times and, in rats, more than 70 times the exposure in man at the maximum recommended daily human dose (32 mg).

Candesartan cilexetil was not genotoxic in the microbial mutagenesis and mammalian cell mutagenesis assays and in the *in vivo* chromosomal aberration and rat unscheduled DNA synthesis assays. In addition, candesartan was not genotoxic in the microbial mutagenesis, mammalian cell mutagenesis, and *in vitro* and *in vivo* chromosome aberration assays.

Fertility and reproductive performance were not affected in studies with male and female rats given oral doses of up to 300 mg/kg/day (83-times the maximum daily human dose of 32 mg on a body surface area basis).

Pregnancy

Pregnancy Categories C (first trimester) *and D* (second and third trimesters). See WARNINGS, Fetal/Neonatal Morbidity and Mortality.

Nursing Mothers

It is not known whether candesartan is excreted in human milk, but candesartan has been shown to be present in rat milk. Because of the potential for adverse effects on the nursing infant, a decision should be made whether to discontinue nursing or discontinue the drug, taking into account the importance of the drug to the mother.

Pediatric Use

Safety and effectiveness in pediatric patients have not been established.

Geriatric Use

Of the total number of subjects in clinical studies of ATACAND, 21% were 65 and over, while 3% were 75 and over. No overall differences in safety or effectiveness were observed between these subjects and younger subjects, and other reported clinical experience has not identified differences in responses between the elderly and younger patients, but greater sensitivity of some older individuals cannot be ruled out. In a placebo-controlled trial of about 200 elderly hypertensive patients (ages 65 to 87 years), administration of candesartan cilexetil was well tolerated and lowered blood pressure by about 12/6 mm Hg more than placebo.

ADVERSE REACTIONS

ATACAND has been evaluated for safety in more than 3600 patients/subjects, including more than 3200 patients treated for hypertension. About 600 of these patients were studied for at least 6 months and about 200 for at least 1

year. In general, treatment with ATACAND was well tolerated. The overall incidence of adverse events reported with ATACAND was similar to placebo.

The rate of withdrawals due to adverse events in all trials in patients (7510 total) was 3.3% (ie. 108 of 3260) of patients treated with candesartan cilexetil as monotherapy and 3.5% (ie. 39 of 1106) of patients treated with placebo. In placebo-controlled trials, discontinuation of therapy due to clinical adverse events occurred in 2.4% (ie. 57 of 2350) of patients treated with ATACAND and 3.4% (ie. 35 of 1027) of patients treated with placebo.

The most common reasons for discontinuation of therapy with ATACAND were headache (0.6%) and dizziness (0.3%). The adverse events that occurred in placebo-controlled clinical trials in at least 1% of patients treated with ATACAND and at a higher incidence in candesartan cilexetil (n=2350) than placebo (n=1027) patients included back pain (3% vs 2%), dizziness (4% vs 3%), upper respiratory tract infection (6% vs 4%), pharyngitis (2% vs 1%), and rhinitis (2% vs 1%). The following adverse events occurred in placebo-controlled clinical trials at a more than 1% rate but at about the same or greater incidence in patients receiving placebo compared to candesartan cilexetil: fatigue, peripheral edema, chest pain, headache, bronchitis, coughing, sinusitis, nausea, abdominal pain, diarrhea, vomiting, arthralgia, albuminuria.

Other potentially important adverse events that have been reported, whether or not attributed to treatment, with an incidence of 0.5% or greater from the more than 3200 patients worldwide treated with ATACAND are listed below. It cannot be determined whether these events were causally related to ATACAND. **Body as a Whole:** asthenia, fever; **Central and Peripheral Nervous System:** paresthesia, vertigo; **Gastrointestinal System Disorder:** dyspepsia, gastroenteritis; **Heart Rate and Rhythm Disorders:** tachycardia, palpitation; **Metabolic and Nutritional Disorders:** creatine phosphokinase increased, hyperglycemia, hypertriglyceridemia, hyperuricemia; **Musculoskeletal System Disorders:** myalgia; **Platelet/Bleeding-Clotting Disorders:** epistaxis; **Psychiatric Disorders:** anxiety, depression, somnolence; **Respiratory System Disorders:** dyspnea; **Skin and Appendages Disorders:** rash, sweating increased; **Urinary System Disorders:** hematuria.

Other reported events seen less frequently included angina pectoris, myocardial infarction, and angioedema.

Adverse events occurred at about the same rates in men and women, older and younger patients, and black and nonblack patients.

Post-Marketing Experience

Other adverse events reported for candesartan cilexetil where a causal relationship could not be established include very rare cases of neutropenia, leukopenia and agranulocytosis.

Laboratory Test Findings

In controlled clinical trials, clinically important changes in standard laboratory parameters were rarely associated with the administration of ATACAND.

Creatinine, Blood Urea Nitrogen: Minor increases in blood urea nitrogen (BUN) and serum creatinine were observed infrequently.

Hyperuricemia: Hyperuricemia was rarely found (19 or 0.6% of 3260 patients treated with candesartan cilexetil and 5 or 0.5% of 1106 patients treated with placebo).

Hemoglobin and Hematocrit: Small decreases in hemoglobin and hematocrit (mean decreases of approximately 0.2 grams/dL and 0.5 volume percent, respectively) were observed in patients treated with ATACAND alone but were rarely of clinical importance. Anemia, leukopenia, and thrombocytopenia were associated with withdrawal of one patient each from clinical trials.

Potassium: A small increase (mean increase of 0.1 mEq/L) was observed in patients treated with ATACAND alone but was rarely of clinical importance. One patient from a congestive heart failure trial was withdrawn for hyperkalemia (serum potassium = 7.5 mEq/L). This patient was also receiving spironolactone.

Liver Function Tests: Elevations of liver enzymes and/or serum bilirubin were observed infrequently. Five patients assigned to candesartan cilexetil in clinical trials were withdrawn because of abnormal liver chemistries. All had elevated transaminases. Two had mildly elevated total bilirubin, but one of these patients was diagnosed with Hepatitis A.

OVERDOSAGE

No lethality was observed in acute toxicity studies in mice, rats, and dogs given single oral doses of up to 2000 mg/kg of candesartan cilexetil. In mice given single oral doses of the primary metabolite, candesartan, the minimum lethal dose was greater than 1000 mg/kg but less than 2000 mg/kg. Limited data are available in regard to overdosage in humans. In one recorded case of an intentional overdose, a 43-year-old female patient (Body Mass Index of 31 kg/m²) ingested an estimated 160 mg of candesartan cilexetil in conjunction with multiple other pharmaceutical agents (ibuprofen, naproxen sodium, diphenhydramine hydrochloride, and ketoprofen). Gastric lavage was performed; the patient was monitored in hospital for several days and was discharged without sequelae.

Candesartan cannot be removed by hemodialysis.

Treatment: To obtain up-to-date information about the treatment of overdose, consult your Regional Poison Control Center. Telephone numbers of certified poison control centers are listed in the *Physicians' Desk Reference (PDR)*. In managing overdose, consider the possibilities of multiple-drug overdoses, drug-drug interactions, and altered pharmacokinetics in your patient.

The most likely manifestation of overdosage with ATACAND would be hypotension, dizziness, and tachycardia; bradycardia could occur from parasympathetic (vagal) stimulation. If symptomatic hypotension should occur, supportive treatment should be instituted.

DOSAGE AND ADMINISTRATION

Dosage must be individualized. Blood pressure response is dose related over the range of 2 to 32 mg. The usual recommended starting dose of ATACAND is 16 mg once daily when it is used as monotherapy in patients who are not volume depleted. ATACAND can be administered once or twice daily with total daily doses ranging from 8 mg to 32 mg. Larger doses do not appear to have a greater effect, and there is relatively little experience with such doses. Most of the antihypertensive effect is present within 2 weeks, and maximal blood pressure reduction is generally obtained within 4 to 6 weeks of treatment with ATACAND.

No initial dosage adjustment is necessary for elderly patients, for patients with mildly impaired renal function, or for patients with mildly impaired hepatic function (see CLINICAL PHARMACOLOGY, Special Populations). For patients with possible depletion of intravascular volume (e.g., patients treated with diuretics, particularly those with impaired renal function), ATACAND should be initiated under close medical supervision and consideration should be given to administration of a lower dose (see WARNINGS, Hypotension in Volume- and Salt-Depleted Patients).

ATACAND may be administered with or without food.

If blood pressure is not controlled by ATACAND alone, a diuretic may be added. ATACAND may be administered with other antihypertensive agents.

HOW SUPPLIED

No. 3782—Tablets ATACAND, 4 mg, are white to off-white, circular/biconvex-shaped, non-film-coated tablets, coded ACF on one side and 004 on the other. They are supplied as follows:

NDC 0186-0004-31 unit of use bottles of 30.

No. 3780—Tablets ATACAND, 8 mg, are light pink, circular/biconvex-shaped, non-film-coated tablets, coded ACG on one side and 008 on the other. They are supplied as follows:

NDC 0186-0008-31 unit of use bottles of 30.

No. 3781—Tablets ATACAND, 16 mg, are pink, circular/biconvex-shaped, non-film-coated tablets, coded ACH on one side and 016 on the other. They are supplied as follows:

NDC 0186-0016-31 unit of use bottles of 30
NDC 0186-0016-54 unit of use bottles of 90
NDC 0186-0016-28 unit dose packages of 100.

No. 3791—Tablets ATACAND, 32 mg, are pink, circular/biconvex-shaped, non-film-coated tablets, coded ACL on one side and 032 on the other. They are supplied as follows:

NDC 0186-0032-31 unit of use bottles of 30
NDC 0186-0032-54 unit of use bottles of 90
NDC 0186-0032-28 unit dose packages of 100.

Storage

Store at 25°C (77°F); excursions permitted to 15–30°C (59–86°F) [see USP Controlled Room Temperature]. Keep container tightly closed.

ATACAND is a trademark of the AstraZeneca Group of Companies

© AstraZeneca 2000

* Trademark of the AstraZeneca Group of Companies
© AstraZeneca 2000
All rights reverved
Revised June 2000
Manufactured under the license
from Takeda Chemical Industries, Ltd.
by: AstraZeneca AB, S-151 85 Södertälje, Sweden
for: AstraZeneca LP, Wilmington, DE 19850
Made in Sweden
9174306
610002-06

EMLA® Anesthetic Disc ℞

(lidocaine 2.5% and prilocaine 2.5% cream)
Topical Adhesive System

EMLA® Cream

(lidocaine 2.5% and prilocaine 2.5%)

Prescribing information for this product, which appears on pages 568–571 of the 2001 PDR, has been completely revised as follows. Please write "See Supplement A" next to the product heading.

DESCRIPTION

EMLA Cream (lidocaine 2.5% and prilocaine 2.5%) is an emulsion in which the oil phase is a eutectic mixture of lidocaine and prilocaine in a ratio of 1:1 by weight. This eutectic mixture has a melting point below room temperature and therefore both local anesthetics exist as a liquid oil rather than as crystals. It is packaged in 5 gram and 30 gram tubes. It is also packaged in the Anesthetic Disc, which is a single-dose unit of EMLA contained within an occlusive dressing. The Anesthetic Disc is composed of a laminate backing, an absorbent cellulose disc, and an adhesive tape ring. The disc contains 1 gram of EMLA emulsion, the active contact surface being approximately 10 cm^2. The surface area of the entire anesthetic disc is approximately 40 cm^2.

TABLE 1
Absorption of Lidocaine and Prilocaine from EMLA Cream: Normal Volunteers (N=16)

EMLA (g)	Area (cm^2)	Time on (hrs)	Drug Content (mg)	Absorbed (mg)	C_{max} (μg/mL)	T_{max} (hr)
60	400	3	lidocaine 1500	54	0.12	4
			prilocaine 1500	92	0.07	4
60	400	24*	lidocaine 1500	243	0.28	10
			prilocaine 1500	503	0.14	10

*Maximum recommended duration of exposure is 4 hours.

Lidocaine is chemically designated as acetamide, 2-(diethylamino)-N- (2,6-dimethylphenyl), has an octanol:water partition ratio of 43 at pH 7.4, and has the following structure:

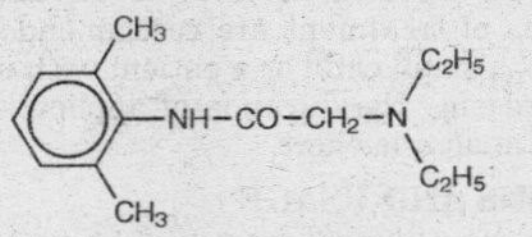

$C_{14}H_{22}N_2O$ M.W. 234.3

Prilocaine is chemically designated as propanamide, N-(2-methylphenyl)-2-(propylamino), has an octanol:water partition ratio of 25 at pH 7.4, and has the following structure:

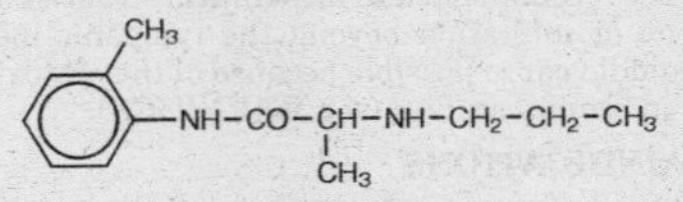

$C_{13}H_{20}N_2O$ M.W. 220.3

Each gram of EMLA contains lidocaine 25 mg, prilocaine 25 mg, polyoxyethylene fatty acid esters (as emulsifiers), carboxypolymethylene (as a thickening agent), sodium hydroxide to adjust to a pH approximating 9, and purified water to 1 gram. EMLA contains no preservative, however it passes the USP antimicrobial effectiveness test due to the pH. The specific gravity of EMLA Cream is 1.00.

CLINICAL PHARMACOLOGY

Mechanism of Action: EMLA (lidocaine 2.5% and prilocaine 2.5%), applied to intact skin under occlusive dressing, provides dermal analgesia by the release of lidocaine and prilocaine from the cream into the epidermal and dermal layers of the skin and by the accumulation of lidocaine and prilocaine in the vicinity of dermal pain receptors and nerve endings. Lidocaine and prilocaine are amide-type local anesthetic agents. Both lidocaine and prilocaine stabilize neuronal membranes by inhibiting the ionic fluxes required for the initiation and conduction of impulses, thereby effecting local anesthetic action.

The onset, depth and duration of dermal analgesia on intact skin provided by EMLA depends primarily on the duration of application. To provide sufficient analgesia for clinical procedures such as intravenous catheter placement and venipuncture, EMLA should be applied under an occlusive dressing for at least 1 hour. To provide dermal analgesia for clinical procedures such as split skin graft harvesting, EMLA should be applied under occlusive dressing for at least 2 hours. Satisfactory dermal analgesia is achieved 1 hour after application, reaches maximum at 2 to 3 hours, and persists for 1 to 2 hours after removal. Absorption from the genital mucosa is more rapid and onset time is shorter (5 to 10 minutes) than after application to intact skin. After a 5 to 10 minute application of EMLA to female genital mucosa, the average duration of effective analgesia to an argon laser stimulus (which produced a sharp, pricking pain) was 15 to 20 minutes (individual variations in the range of 5 to 45 minutes).

Dermal application of EMLA may cause a transient, local blanching followed by a transient, local redness or erythema.

Pharmacokinetics: EMLA is a eutectic mixture of lidocaine 2.5% and prilocaine 2.5% formulated as an oil in water emulsion. In this eutectic mixture, both anesthetics are liquid at room temperature (see DESCRIPTION) and the penetration and subsequent systemic absorption of both prilocaine and lidocaine are enhanced over that which would be seen if each component in crystalline form was applied separately as a 2.5% topical cream.

Absorption: The amount of lidocaine and prilocaine systemically absorbed from EMLA is directly related to both the duration of application and to the area over which it is applied. In two pharmacokinetic studies, 60 g of EMLA Cream (1.5 g lidocaine and 1.5 g prilocaine) was applied to 400 cm^2 of intact skin on the lateral thigh and then covered by an occlusive dressing. The subjects were then randomized such that one-half of the subjects had the occlusive dressing and residual cream removed after 3 hours, while the remainder left the dressing in place for 24 hours. The results from these studies are summarized below.

[See table above]

When 60 g of EMLA Cream was applied over 400 cm^2 for 24 hours, peak blood levels of lidocaine are approximately 1/20 the systemic toxic level. Likewise, the maximum prilocaine level is about 1/36 the toxic level. In a pharmacokinetic study, EMLA Cream was applied to penile skin in 20 adult male patients in doses ranging from 0.5 g to 3.3 g for 15 minutes. Plasma concentrations of lidocaine and prilocaine following EMLA Cream application in this study were consistently low (2.5–16 ng/mL for lidocaine and 2.5–7 ng/mL for prilocaine). The application of EMLA to broken or inflamed skin, or to 2,000 cm^2 or more of skin where more of both anesthetics are absorbed, could result in higher plasma levels that could, in susceptible individuals, produce a systemic pharmacologic response.

The absorption of EMLA Cream applied to genital mucous membranes was studied in two open-label clinical trials. Twenty-nine patients received 10 g of EMLA Cream applied for 10 to 60 minutes in the vaginal fornices. Plasma concentrations of lidocaine and prilocaine following EMLA Cream application in these studies ranged from 148 to 641 ng/mL for lidocaine and 40 to 346 ng/mL for prilocaine and time to reach maximum concentration (t_{max}) ranged from 21 to 125 minutes for lidocaine and from 21 to 95 minutes for prilocaine. These levels are well below the concentrations anticipated to give rise to systemic toxicity (approximately 5000 ng/mL for lidocaine and prilocaine).

Distribution: When each drug is administered intravenously, the steady-state volume of distribution is 1.1 to 2.1 L/kg (mean 1.5, ±0.3 SD, n=13) for lidocaine and is 0.7 to 4.4 L/kg (mean 2.6, ±1.3 SD, n=13) for prilocaine. The larger distribution volume for prilocaine produces the lower plasma concentrations of prilocaine observed when equal amounts of prilocaine and lidocaine are administered. At concentrations produced by application of EMLA, lidocaine is approximately 70% bound to plasma proteins, primarily alpha-1-acid glycoprotein. At much higher plasma concentrations (1 to 4 μg/mL of free base) the plasma protein binding of lidocaine is concentration dependent. Prilocaine is 55% bound to plasma proteins. Both lidocaine and prilocaine cross the placental and blood brain barrier, presumably by passive diffusion.

Metabolism: It is not known if lidocaine or prilocaine are metabolized in the skin. Lidocaine is metabolized rapidly by the liver to a number of metabolites including monoethylglycinexylidide (MEGX) and glycinexylidide (GX), both of which have pharmacologic activity similar to, but less potent than that of lidocaine. The metabolite, 2,6-xylidine, has unknown pharmacologic activity. Following intravenous administration, MEGX and GX concentrations in serum range from 11 to 36% and from 5 to 11% of lidocaine concentrations, respectively. Prilocaine is metabolized in both the liver and kidneys by amidases to various metabolites including *ortho*-toluidine and N-n-propylalanine. It is not metabolized by plasma esterases. The *ortho*-toluidine metabolite has been shown to be carcinogenic in several animal models (see Carcinogenesis subsection of PRECAUTIONS). In addition, *ortho*-toluidine can produce methemoglobinemia following systemic doses of prilocaine approximating 8 mg/kg (see ADVERSE REACTIONS). Very young patients, patients with glucose-6-phosphate deficiencies and patients taking oxidizing drugs such as antimalarials and sulfonamides are more susceptible to methemoglobinemia (see Methemoglobinemia subsection of PRECAUTIONS).

Elimination: The half-life of lidocaine elimination from the plasma following IV administration is approximately 65 to 150 minutes (mean 110, ±24 SD, n=13). More than 98% of an absorbed dose of lidocaine can be recovered in the urine as metabolites or parent drug. The systemic clearance is 10 to 20 mL/min/kg (mean 13, ±3 SD, n=13). The elimination half-life of prilocaine is approximately 10 to 150 minutes (mean 70, ±48 SD, n=13). The systemic clearance is 18 to 64 mL/min/kg (mean 38, ±15 SD, n=13). During intravenous studies, the elimination half-life of lidocaine was statistically significantly longer in elderly patients (2.5 hours) than in younger patients (1.5 hours). No studies are available on the intravenous pharmacokinetics of prilocaine in elderly patients.

Pediatrics: Some pharmacokinetic (PK) data are available in infants (1 month to <2 years old) and children (2 to <12 years old). One PK study was conducted in 9 full-term neonates (mean age: 7 days and mean gestational age: 38.8 weeks). The study results show that neonates had comparable plasma lidocaine and prilocaine concentrations and blood methemoglobin concentrations as those found in previous pediatric PK studies and clinical trials. There was a tendency towards an increase in methemoglobin formation. However, due to assay limitations and very little amount of blood that could be collected from neonates, large variations in the above reported concentrations were found.

Special Populations: No specific PK studies were conducted. The half-life may be increased in cardiac or hepatic dysfunction. Prilocaine's half-life also may be increased in hepatic or renal dysfunction since both of these organs are involved in prilocaine metabolism.

Continued on next page

EMLA—Cont.

CLINICAL STUDIES

EMLA Cream application in adults prior to IV cannulation or venipuncture was studied in 200 patients in four clinical studies in Europe. Application for at least 1 hour provided significantly more dermal analgesia than placebo cream or ethyl chloride. EMLA Cream was comparable to subcutaneous lidocaine, but was less efficacious than intradermal lidocaine. Most patients found EMLA Cream treatment preferable to lidocaine infiltration or ethyl chloride spray.

EMLA Cream was compared with 0.5% lidocaine infiltration prior to skin graft harvesting in one open label study in 80 adult patients in England. Application of EMLA Cream for 2 to 5 hours provided dermal analgesia comparable to lidocaine infiltration.

EMLA Cream application in children was studied in seven non-US studies (320 patients) and one US study (100 patients). In controlled studies, application of EMLA Cream for at least 1 hour with or without presurgical medication prior to needle insertion provided significantly more pain reduction than placebo. In children under the age of seven years, EMLA Cream was less effective than in older children or adults.

EMLA Cream was compared with placebo in the laser treatment of facial port-wine stains in 72 pediatric patients (ages 5–16). EMLA Cream was effective in providing pain relief during laser treatment.

EMLA Cream alone was compared to EMLA Cream followed by lidocaine infiltration and lidocaine infiltration alone prior to cryotherapy for the removal of male genital warts. The data from 121 patients demonstrated that EMLA Cream was not effective as a sole anesthetic agent in managing the pain from the surgical procedure. The administration of EMLA Cream prior to lidocaine infiltration provided significant relief of discomfort associated with local anesthetic infiltration and thus was effective in the overall reduction of pain from the procedure only when used in conjunction with local anesthetic infiltration of lidocaine.

Emla Cream was studied in 105 full term neonates (gestational age: 37 weeks) for blood drawing and circumcision procedures. When considering the use of EMLA in neonates, the primary concerns are the systemic absorption of the active ingredients and the subsequent formation of methemoglobin. In clinical studies performed in neonates, the plasma levels of lidocaine, prilocaine, and methemoglobin were not reported in a range expected to cause clinical symptoms.

Local dermal effects associated with EMLA Cream application in these studies on intact skin included paleness, redness and edema and were transient in nature (see ADVERSE REACTIONS).

The application of EMLA Cream on genital mucous membranes for minor, superficial surgical procedures (eg, removal of condylomata acuminata) was studied in 80 patients in a placebo-controlled clinical trial (60 patients received EMLA and 20 patients received placebo). EMLA Cream (5 to 10g) applied between 1 and 75 minutes before surgery, with a median time of 15 minutes, provided effective local anesthesia for minor superficial surgical procedures. The best quality of anesthesia was achieved after 5 to 15 minutes' application. The application of EMLA Cream to genital mucous membranes as pretreatment for local anesthetic infiltration was studied in a double-blind, placebo-controlled study in 44 female patients (21 patients received EMLA cream and 23 patients received placebo) scheduled for infiltration prior to a surgical procedure of the external vulva or genital mucosa. EMLA Cream applied to the genital mucous membranes for 5 to 10 minutes resulted in adequate topical anesthesia for local anesthetic injection.

Individualization of Dose: The dose of EMLA which provides effective analgesia depends on the duration of the application over the treated area.

All pharmacokinetic and clinical studies employed a thick layer of EMLA Cream (1–2 g/10 cm^2). The duration of application prior to venipuncture was 1 hour. The duration of application prior to taking split thickness skin grafts was

2 hours. Although a thinner application may be efficacious, such has not been studied and may result in less complete analgesia or a shorter duration of adequate analgesia.

The systemic absorption of lidocaine and prilocaine is a side effect of the desired local effect. The amount of drug absorbed depends on surface area and duration of application. The systemic blood levels depend on the amount absorbed and patient size (weight) and rate of systemic drug elimination. Long duration of application, large treatment area, small patients, or impaired elimination may result in high blood levels. The systemic blood levels are typically a small fraction (1/20 to 1/36) of the blood levels which produce toxicity. Table 2 which follows gives maximum recommended doses, application areas and application times for infants and children.

[See table below]

An IV antiarrhythmic dose of lidocaine is 1 mg/kg (70 mg/70 kg) and gives a blood level of about 1 µg/mL. Toxicity would be expected at blood levels above 5 µg/mL. Smaller areas of treatment are recommended in a debilitated patient, a small child or a patient with impaired elimination. Decreasing the duration of application is likely to decrease the analgesic effect.

INDICATIONS AND USAGE

EMLA (a eutectic mixture of lidocaine 2.5% and prilocaine 2.5%) is indicated as a topical anesthetic for use on:
— **normal intact skin** for local analgesia.
— **genital mucous membranes** for superficial minor surgery and as pretreatment for infiltration anesthesia.

EMLA is not recommended in any clinical situation in which penetration or migration beyond the tympanic membrane into the middle ear is possible because of the ototoxic effects observed in animal studies (see WARNINGS).

CONTRAINDICATIONS

EMLA (lidocaine 2.5% and prilocaine 2.5%) is contraindicated in patients with a known history of sensitivity to local anesthetics of the amide type or to any other component of the product.

WARNINGS

Application of EMLA to larger areas or for longer times than those recommended could result in sufficient absorption of lidocaine and prilocaine resulting in serious adverse effects (see Individualization of Dose).

Studies in laboratory animals (guinea pigs) have shown that EMLA has an ototoxic effect when instilled into the middle ear. In these same studies, animals exposed to EMLA Cream in the external auditory canal only, showed no abnormality. EMLA should not be used in any clinical situation in which its penetration or migration beyond the tympanic membrane into the middle ear is possible.

Methemoglobinemia: EMLA should not be used in those rare patients with congenital or idiopathic methemoglobinemia and in infants under the age of twelve months who are receiving treatment with methemoglobin-inducing agents.

Very young patients or patients with glucose-6-phosphatatase dehydrogenase deficiency are more susceptible to methemoglobinemia.

Patients taking drugs associated with drug-induced methemoglobinemia such as sulfonamides, acetaminophen, acetanilid, aniline dyes, benzocaine, chloroquine, dapsone, naphthalene, nitrates and nitrites, nitrofurantoin, nitroglycerin, nitroprusside, pamaquine, para-aminosalicylic acid, phenacetin, phenobarbital, phenytoin, primaquine, quinine, are also at greater risk for developing methemoglobinemia.

There have been reports of significant methemoglobinemia (20–30%) in infants and children following excessive applications of EMLA Cream. These cases involved the use of large doses, larger than recommended areas of application, or infants under the age of 3 months who did not have fully mature enzyme systems. In addition, a few of these cases involved the concomitant administration of methemoglobin-inducing agents. Most patients recovered spontaneously after removal of the cream. Treatment with IV methylene blue may be effective if required.

Physicians are cautioned to make sure that parents or other caregivers understand the need for careful application of EMLA, to ensure that the doses and areas of application recommended in Table 2 are not exceeded (especially in children under the age of 3 months) and to limit the period of application to the minimum required to achieve the desired anesthesia.

Neonates and infants up to 3 months of age should be monitored for Met-Hb levels before, during, and after the application of EMLA, provided the test results can be obtained quickly.

PRECAUTIONS

General: Repeated doses of EMLA may increase blood levels of lidocaine and prilocaine. EMLA should be used with caution in patients who may be more sensitive to the systemic effects of lidocaine and prilocaine including acutely ill, debilitated, or elderly patients.

EMLA coming in contact with the eye should be avoided because animal studies have demonstrated severe eye irritation. Also the loss of protective reflexes can permit corneal irritation and potential abrasion. Absorption of EMLA in conjunctival tissues has not been determined. If eye contact occurs, immediately wash out the eye with water or saline and protect the eye until sensation returns.

Patients allergic to paraaminobenzoic acid derivatives (procaine, tetracaine, benzocaine, etc.) have not shown cross sensitivity to lidocaine and/or prilocaine, however, EMLA should be used with caution in patients with a history of drug sensitivities, especially if the etiologic agent is uncertain.

Patients with severe hepatic disease, because of their inability to metabolize local anesthetics normally, are at greater risk of developing toxic plasma concentrations of lidocaine and prilocaine.

Lidocaine and prilocaine have been shown to inhibit viral and bacterial growth. The effect of EMLA on **intradermal** injections of **live** vaccines has not been determined.

Information for Patients: When EMLA is used, the patient should be aware that the production of dermal analgesia may be accompanied by the block of all sensations in the treated skin. For this reason, the patient should avoid inadvertent trauma to the treated area by scratching, rubbing, or exposure to extreme hot or cold temperatures until complete sensation has returned.

Drug Interactions: EMLA should be used with caution in patients receiving Class I antiarrhythmic drugs (such as tocainide and mexiletine) since the toxic effects are additive and potentially synergistic.

Prilocaine may contribute to the formation of methemoglobin in patients treated with other drugs known to cause this condition (see Methemoglobinemia subsection of WARNINGS).

Carcinogenesis, Mutagenesis, Impairment of Fertility

Carcinogenesis: Metabolites of prilocaine have been shown to be carcinogenic in laboratory animals. In the animal studies reported below, doses or blood levels are compared to the Single Dermal Administration (SDA) of 60 g of EMLA Cream to 400 cm^2 for 3 hours to a small person (50 kg). The typical application of EMLA Cream for one or two treatments for venipuncture sites (2.5 or 5 g) would be 1/24 or 1/12 of that dose in an adult or about the same mg/kg dose in an infant. The typical application of EMLA Anesthetic Disc for one or two treatments for venipuncture sites (1 or 2 g) would be 1/60 or 1/30 of that dose in an adult or about half the mg/kg dose in an infant.

Chronic oral toxicity studies of *ortho*-toluidine, a metabolite of prilocaine, in mice (900 to 14,400 mg/m^2; 60 to 960 times SDA) and rats (900 to 4,800 mg/m^2; 60 to 320 times SDA) have shown that *ortho*-toluidine is a carcinogen in both species. The tumors included hepatocarcinomas/adenomas in female mice, multiple occurrences of hemangiosarcomas/hemangiomas in both sexes of mice, sarcomas of multiple organs, transitional-cell carcinomas/papillomas of urinary bladder in both sexes of rats, subcutaneous fibromas/fibrosarcomas and mesotheliomas in male rats, and mammary gland fibroadenomas/adenomas in female rats. The lowest dose tested (900 mg/m^2; 60 times SDA) was carcinogenic in both species. Thus the no-effect dose must be less than 60 times SDA. The animal studies were conducted at 150 to 2,400 mg/kg in mice and at 150 to 800 mg/kg in rats. The dosages have been converted to mg/m^2 for the SDA calculations above.

Mutagenesis: The mutagenic potential of lidocaine HCl has been tested in the Ames Salmonella/mammalian microsome test and by analysis of structural chromosome aberrations in human lymphocytes *in vitro*, and by the mouse micronucleus test *in vivo*. There was no indication in these three tests of any mutagenic effects.

Ortho-toluidine, a metabolite of prilocaine, (0.5 µg/mL) showed positive results in *Escherichia coli* DNA repair and phage-induction assays. Urine concentrates from rats treated with *ortho*-toluidine (300 mg/kg orally; 300 times SDA) were mutagenic for *Salmonella typhimurium* with metabolic activation. Several other tests on *ortho*-toluidine, including reverse mutations in five different *Salmonella typhimurium* strains with or without metabolic activation and with single strand breaks in DNA of V79 Chinese hamster cells, were negative.

Impairment of Fertility: See Use in Pregnancy.

Use in Pregnancy: Teratogenic Effects: Pregnancy Category B.

Reproduction studies with lidocaine have been performed in rats and have revealed no evidence of harm to the fetus

TABLE 2
EMLA MAXIMUM RECOMMENDED DOSE, APPLICATION AREA, AND APPLICATION TIME BY AGE AND WEIGHT*
For Infants and Children
Based on Application to Intact Skin

Age and Body Weight Requirements	Maximum Total Dose of EMLA	Maximum Application Area**	Maximum Application Time
0 up to 3 months or < 5 kg	1 g	10 cm^2	1 hour
3 up to 12 months and > 5 kg	2 g	20 cm^2	4 hours
1 to 6 years and > 10 kg	10 g	100 cm^2	4 hours
7 to 12 years and > 20 kg	20 g	200 cm^2	4 hours

Please note: If a patient greater than 3 months old does not meet the minimum weight requirement, the maximum total dose of EMLA should be restricted to that which corresponds to the patient's **weight**.

* These are broad guidelines for avoiding systemic toxicity in applying EMLA to patients with normal intact skin and with normal renal and hepatic function.

**For more individualized calculation of how much lidocaine and prilocaine may be absorbed, physicians can use the following estimates of lidocaine and prilocaine absorption for children and adults:

The estimated mean (±SD) absorption of lidocaine is 0.045 (±0.016) mg/cm^2/hr.

The estimated mean (±SD) absorption of prilocaine is 0.077 (±0.036) mg/cm^2/hr.

(30 mg/kg subcutaneously; 22 times SDA). Reproduction studies with prilocaine have been performed in rats and have revealed no evidence of impaired fertility or harm to the fetus (300 mg/kg intramuscularly; 188 times SDA). There are, however, no adequate and well-controlled studies in pregnant women. Because animal reproduction studies are not always predictive of human response, EMLA should be used during pregnancy only if clearly needed.

Reproduction studies have been performed in rats receiving subcutaneous administration of an aqueous mixture containing lidocaine HCl and prilocaine HCl at 1:1 (w/w). At 40 mg/kg each, a dose equivalent to 29 times SDA lidocaine and 25 times SDA prilocaine, no teratogenic, embryotoxic or fetotoxic effects were observed.

Labor and Delivery: Neither lidocaine nor prilocaine are contraindicated in labor and delivery. Should EMLA be used concomitantly with other products containing lidocaine and/or prilocaine, total doses contributed by all formulations must be considered.

Nursing Mothers: Lidocaine, and probably prilocaine, are excreted in human milk. Therefore, caution should be exercised when EMLA is administered to a nursing mother since the milk:plasma ratio of lidocaine is 0.4 and is not determined for prilocaine.

Pediatric Use: Controlled studies of EMLA Cream in children under the age of seven years have shown less overall benefit than in older children or adults. These results illustrate the importance of emotional and psychological support of younger children undergoing medical or surgical procedures.

EMLA should be used with care in patients with conditions or therapy associated with methemoglobinemia (see Methemoglobinemia subsection of WARNINGS).

When using EMLA in young children, especially infants under the age of 3 months, care must be taken to insure that the caregiver understands the need to limit the dose and area of application, and to prevent accidental ingestion (see DOSAGE AND ADMINISTRATION and Methemoglobinemia).

In neonates (minimum gestation age: 37 weeks) and children weighing less than 20 kg, the area and duration of application should be limited (see TABLE 2 in Individualization of Dose).

Geriatric Use
Of the total number of patients in clinical studies of EMLA, 180 were age 65 to 74 and 138 were 75 and over. No overall differences in safety or efficacy were observed between these patients and younger patients. Other reported clinical experience has not identified differences in responses between the elderly and younger patients, but greater sensitivity of some older individuals cannot be ruled out.

Plasma levels of lidocaine and prilocaine in geriatric and non-geriatric patients following application of a thick layer of EMLA are very low and well below potentially toxic levels. However, there are no sufficient data to evaluate quantitative differences in systemic plasma levels of lidocaine and prilocaine between geriatric and non-geriatric patients following application of EMLA. Consideration should be given for those elderly patients who have enhanced sensitivity to systemic absorption. (See PRECAUTIONS.)

After intravenous dosing, the elimination half-life of lidocaine is significantly longer in elderly patients (2.5 hours) than in younger patients (1.5 hours). (See CLINICAL PHARMACOLOGY.)

ADVERSE REACTIONS
Localized Reactions: During or immediately after treatment with EMLA on intact skin, the skin at the site of treatment may develop erythema or edema or may be the locus of abnormal sensation. Rare cases of discrete purpuric or petechial reactions at the application site have been reported. Rare cases of hyperpigmentation following the use of EMLA Cream have been reported. The relationship to EMLA Cream or the underlying procedure has not been established. In clinical studies on intact skin involving over 1,300 EMLA Cream-treated subjects, one or more such local reactions were noted in 56% of patients, and were generally mild and transient, resolving spontaneously within 1 or 2 hours. There were no serious reactions which were ascribed to EMLA Cream.

Two recent reports describe blistering on the foreskin in neonates about to undergo circumcision. Both neonates received 1.0 g of EMLA.

In patients treated with EMLA Cream on intact skin, local effects observed in the trials included: paleness (pallor or blanching) 37%, redness (erythema) 30%, alterations in temperature sensations 7%, edema 6%, itching 2% and rash, less than 1%.

In clinical studies on genital mucous membranes involving 378 EMLA Cream-treated patients, one or more application site reactions, usually mild and transient, were noted in 41% of patients. The most common application site reactions were redness (21%), burning sensation (17%) and edema (10%).

Allergic Reactions: Allergic and anaphylactoid reactions associated with lidocaine or prilocaine can occur. They are characterized by urticaria, angioedema, bronchospasm, and shock. If they occur they should be managed by conventional means. The detection of sensitivity by skin testing is of doubtful value.

Systemic (Dose Related) Reactions: Systemic adverse reactions following appropriate use of EMLA are unlikely due to the small dose absorbed (see Pharmacokinetics subsection of CLINICAL PHARMACOLOGY). Systemic adverse effects of lidocaine and/or prilocaine are similar in nature to those observed with other amide local anesthetics including

CNS excitation and/or depression (light-headedness, nervousness, apprehension, euphoria, confusion, dizziness, drowsiness, tinnitus, blurred or double vision, vomiting, sensations of heat, cold or numbness, twitching, tremors, convulsions, unconsciousness, respiratory depression and arrest). Excitatory CNS reactions may be brief or not occur at all, in which case the first manifestation may be drowsiness merging into unconsciousness. Cardiovascular manifestations may include bradycardia, hypotension and cardiovascular collapse leading to arrest.

OVERDOSAGE
Peak blood levels following a 60 g application to 400 cm² of intact skin for 3 hours are 0.05 to 0.16 µg/mL for lidocaine and 0.02 to 0.10 µg/mL for prilocaine. Toxic levels of lidocaine (>5 µg/mL) and/or prilocaine (>6 µg/mL) cause decreases in cardiac output, total peripheral resistance and mean arterial pressure. These changes may be attributable to direct depressant effects of these local anesthetic agents on the cardiovascular system. In the absence of massive topical overdose or oral ingestion, evaluation should include evaluation of other etiologies for the clinical effects or overdosage from other sources of lidocaine, prilocaine or other local anesthetics. Consult the package inserts for parenteral Xylocaine (lidocaine HCl) or Citanest (prilocaine HCl) for further information for the management of overdose.

DOSAGE AND ADMINISTRATION
Adult Patients—Intact Skin
EMLA Cream and Anesthetic Disc
A thick layer of EMLA Cream is applied to intact skin and covered with an occlusive dressing, or alternatively, an EMLA Anesthetic Disc is applied to intact skin:

Minor Dermal Procedures: For minor procedures such as intravenous cannulation and venipuncture, apply 2.5 grams of EMLA Cream (1/2 the 5 g tube) over 20 to 25 cm² of skin surface, or 1 EMLA Anesthetic Disc (1g over 10 cm²) for at least 1 hour. In controlled clinical trials using EMLA Cream, two sites were usually prepared in case there was a technical problem with cannulation or venipuncture at the first site.

EMLA Cream
A thick layer of EMLA Cream is applied to intact skin and covered with an occlusive dressing:

Major Dermal Procedures: For more painful dermatological procedures involving a larger skin area such as split thickness skin graft harvesting, apply 2 grams of EMLA Cream per 10 cm² of skin and allow to remain in contact with the skin for at least 2 hours.

Adult Male Genital Skin: As an adjunct prior to local anesthetic infiltration, apply a thick layer of EMLA Cream (1 g/10 cm²) to the skin surface for 15 minutes. Local anesthetic infiltration should be performed immediately after removal of EMLA Cream.

Dermal analgesia can be expected to increase for up to 3 hours under occlusive dressing and persist for 1 to 2 hours after removal of the cream. The amount of lidocaine and prilocaine absorbed during the period of application can be estimated from the information in Table 2, ** footnote, in Individualization of Dose.

Adult Female Patients—Genital Mucous Membranes
For minor procedures on the female external genitalia, such as removal of condylomata acuminata, as well as for use as pretreatment for anesthetic infiltration, apply a thick layer (5–10 grams) of EMLA Cream for 5 to 10 minutes. Occlusion is not necessary for absorption, but may be helpful to keep the cream in place. Patients should be lying down during the EMLA Cream application, especially if no occlusion is used. The procedure or the local anesthetic infiltration should be performed immediately after the removal of EMLA Cream.

Pediatric Patients—Intact Skin
The following are the maximum recommended doses, application areas and application times for EMLA based on a child's age and weight:

[See table above]

Please note: If a patient greater than 3 months old does not meet the minimum weight requirement, the maximum total dose of EMLA should be restricted to that which corresponds to the patient's **weight**.

Practitioners should carefully instruct caregivers to avoid application of excessive amounts of EMLA (see PRECAUTIONS).

When applying EMLA to the skin of young children, care must be taken to maintain careful observation of the child to prevent accidental ingestion of EMLA, the occlusive dressing, or the anesthetic disc. A secondary protective covering to prevent inadvertent disruption of the application site may be useful.

EMLA should not be used in neonates with a gestational age less than 37 weeks nor in infants under the age of twelve months who are receiving treatment with methemoglobin-inducing agents (see Methemoglobinemia subsection of WARNINGS).

When EMLA (lidocaine 2.5% and prilocaine 2.5%) is used concomitantly with other products containing local anes-

thetic agents, the amount absorbed from all formulations must be considered (see Individualization of Dose). The amount absorbed in the case of EMLA is determined by the area over which it is applied and the duration of application under occlusion (see Table 2, ** footnote, in Individualization of Dose).

Although the incidence of systemic adverse reactions with EMLA is very low, caution should be exercised, particularly when applying it over large areas and leaving it on for longer than 2 hours. The incidence of systemic adverse reactions can be expected to be directly proportional to the area and time of exposure (see Individualization of Dose).

HOW SUPPLIED
EMLA Cream is available as the following:
NDC 0186-1515-01   5 gram tube,   box of 1, contains 2 Tegaderm® dressings (6 cm × 7 cm)
NDC 0186-1515-01
Product No. 0186-1515-03   5 gram tube,   box of 5, contains 12 Tegaderm® dressings (6 cm × 7 cm)
NDC 0186-1516-01   30 gram tube,   box of 1
EMLA Anesthetic Disc is available in the following:
NDC 0186-1512-70   1 gram Anesthetic Disc,   box of 2
NDC 0186-1512-70
Product No. 0186-1512-71 1 gram Anesthetic Disc, box of 10
NOT FOR OPHTHALMIC USE.
KEEP CONTAINER TIGHTLY CLOSED AT ALL TIMES WHEN NOT IN USE.
Store at controlled room temperature 15–30°C (59–86°F).
EMLA is a trademark of the AstraZeneca group
© AstraZeneca 2001
EMLA Anesthetic Disc manufactured for: AstraZeneca LP, Wilmington, DE 19850
by: AstraZeneca, AB Södertälje, Sweden
EMLA Cream manufactured by: AstraZeneca LP, Wilmington, DE 19850
721700-06   Rev. 1/01

INSTRUCTIONS FOR APPLICATION
EMLA®
CREAM (lidocaine 2.5% and prilocaine 2.5%)

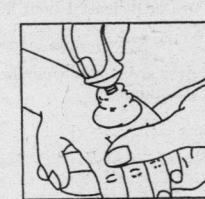

1. In adults, apply 2.5 g of cream (1/2 the 5 g tube) per 20 to 25 cm² (approx. 2 in. by 2 in.) of skin in a thick layer at the site of the procedure. For pediatric patients, apply ONLY as prescribed by your physician. If your child is below the age of 3 months or small for their age, please inform your doctor before applying EMLA, which can be harmful, if applied over too much skin at one time in young children.

If your child becomes very sleepy, excessively sleepy, or develops duskiness of the face or lips after applying EMLA, remove the cream and contact your physician at once.

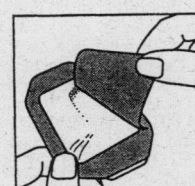

2. Take an occlusive dressing (provided with the 5 g tubes only) and remove the center cut-out piece.

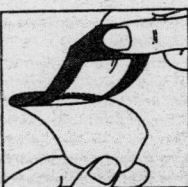

3. Peel the paper liner from the paper framed dressing. (Instructions contained on reverse side.)

Continued on next page

Age and Body Weight Requirements	Maximum Total Dose of EMLA	Maximum Application Area	Maximum Application Time
0 up to 3 months or < 5 kg	1 g	10 cm²	1 hour
3 up to 12 months and > 5 kg	2 g	20 cm²	4 hours
1 to 6 years and > 10 kg	10 g	100 cm²	4 hours
7 to 12 years and > 20 kg	20 g	200 cm²	4 hours

EMLA—Cont.

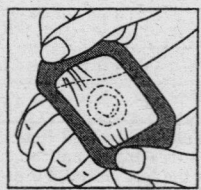

4. Cover the EMLA® Cream so that you get a thick layer underneath. Do not spread out the cream. Smooth down the dressing edges carefully and ensure it is secure to avoid leakage. (This is especially important when the patient is a child.)

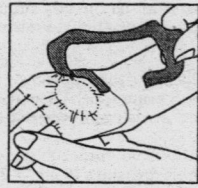

5. Remove the paper frame. The time of application can easily be marked directly on the occlusive dressing. EMLA® must be applied at least 1 hour before the start of a routine procedure and for 2 hours before the start of a painful procedure.

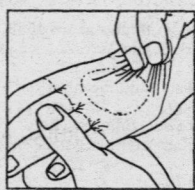

6. Remove the occlusive dressing, wipe off the EMLA® Cream, clean the entire area with an antiseptic solution and prepare the patient for the procedure. The duration of effective skin anesthesia will be at least 1 hour after removal of the occlusive dressing.

PRECAUTIONS

1. Do not apply near eyes or on open wounds.
2. Keep out of reach of children.
AstraZeneca LP
Wilmington, DE 19850
721700-06   Rev 1/01

LEXXEL®   ℞
(enalapril maleate-felodipine ER)
TABLETS

Prescribing information for this product, which appears on pages 575–578 of the 2001 PDR, has been revised. Please write "See Supplement A" next to the product heading.
Revisions occurred to the following sections:

• PRECAUTIONS, Drug Interactions—add 5 new paragraphs after the fifth paragraph in the subsection as follows:
CYP3A4 Inhibitors—Felodipine is metabolized by CYP3A4. Co-administration of CYP3A4 inhibitors (eg, ketoconazole, itraconazole, erythromycin, grapefruit juice, cimetidine) with felodipine may lead to severalfold increases in the plasma levels of felodipine, either due to an increase in bioavailability or due to a decrease in metabolism. These increases in concentration may lead to increased effects, (lower blood pressure and increased heart rate). These effects have been observed with co-administration of itraconazole (a potent CYP3A4 inhibitor). Caution should be used when CYP3A4 inhibitors are co-administered with felodipine. A conservative approach to dosing felodipine should be taken. The following specific interactions have been reported:
Itraconazole—Co-administration of another extended release formulation of felodipine with itraconazole resulted in approximately 8-fold increase in the AUC, more than 6-fold increase in the C_{max}, and 2-fold prolongation in the half-life of felodipine.
Erythromycin—Co-administration of felodipine (PLENDIL) with erythromycin resulted in approximately 2.5-fold increase in the AUC and C_{max}, and about 2-fold prolongation in the half-life of felodipine.
Grapefruit juice—Co-administration of felodipine with grapefruit juice resulted in more than 2-fold increase in the AUC and C_{max}, but no prolongation in the half-life of felodipine.
Cimetidine—Co-administration of felodipine with cimetidine (a non-specific CYP-450 inhibitor) resulted in an increase of approximately 50% in the AUC and the C_{max} of felodipine.

Delete the entire original 8th paragraph beginning with Cimetidine and ending with cimetidine.
• PRECAUTIONS, Carcinogenesis, Mutagenesis, Impairment of Fertility—last sentence of the subsection, insert the words "(up to 24 times the maximum recommended human dose on a mg/m² basis)" after 26.9 mg/kg/day and before the word showed.
• PRECAUTIONS, Pregnancy—second paragraph, second line, change "0.5 to 5 times" to read "0.8 to 8 times". In the 5th paragraph, 3rd line, at the beginning of the parentheses change "(1.4" to "(2.1".
• ADVERSE REACTIONS, subheading Felodipine as an Extended-Release Formulation, sub-subheading Skin add Angioedema, and after urticaria, add leukocytoclastic vasculitis

---

NAROPIN®   ℞
[nă-rōpin]
(ropivacaine HCl Injection)

Prescribing information for this product, which appears on pages 579–582 of the 2001 PDR, has been completely revised as follows. Please write "See Supplement A" next to the product heading.

DESCRIPTION

Naropin® Injection contains ropivacine HCl which is a member of the amino amide class of local anesthetics. Naropin Injection is a sterile, isotonic solution that contains the enantiomerically pure drug substance, sodium chloride for isotonicity and Water for Injection. Sodium hydroxide and/or hydrochloric acid may be used for pH adjustment. It is administered parenterally.
Ropivacaine HCl is chemically described as S-(-)-1-propyl-2',6'-pipecoloxylidide hydrochloride monohydrate. The drug substance is a white crystalline powder, with a molecular formula of $C_{17}H_{26}N_2O \cdot HCl \cdot H_2O$, molecular weight of 328.89 and the following structural formula:

At 25°C ropivacaine HCl has a solubility of 53.8 mg/mL in water, a distribution ratio between n-octanol and phosphate buffer at pH 7.4 of 14:1 and a pKa of 8.07 in 0.1 M KCl solution. The pKa of ropivacaine is approximately the same as bupivacaine (8.1) and is similar to that of mepivacaine (7.7). However, ropivacaine has an intermediate degree of lipid solubility compared to bupivacaine and mepivacaine.
Naropin Injection is preservative-free and is available in single dose containers in 2.0 (0.2%), 5.0 (0.5%), 7.5 (0.75%) and 10.0 mg/mL (1.0%) concentrations. The specific gravity of Naropin Injection solutions range from 1.002 to 1.005 at 25°C.

CLINICAL PHARMACOLOGY
Mechanism of Action
Ropivacaine is a member of the amino amide class of local anesthetics and is supplied as the pure S-(-)-enantiomer. Local anesthetics block the generation and the conduction of nerve impulses, presumably by increasing the threshold for electrical excitation in the nerve, by slowing the propagation of the nerve impulse, and by reducing the rate of rise of the action potential. In general, the progression of anesthesia is related to the diameter, myelination and conduction velocity

---

of affected nerve fibers. Clinically, the order of loss of nerve function is as follows: (1) pain, (2) temperature, (3) touch, (4) proprioception, and (5) skeletal muscle tone.

PHARMACOKINETICS
Absorption
The systemic concentration of ropivacaine is dependent on the total dose and concentration of drug administered, the route of administration, the patient's hemodynamic/circulatory condition, and the vascularity of the administration site.
From the epidural space, ropivacaine shows complete and biphasic absorption. The half-lives of the 2 phases, (mean ± SD) are 14 ± 7 minutes and 4.2 ± 0.9 h, respectively. The slow absorption is the rate limiting factor in the elimination of ropivacaine which explains why the terminal half-life is longer after epidural than after intravenous administration. Ropivacaine shows dose-proportionality up to the highest intravenous dose studied, 80 mg, corresponding to a mean ± SD peak plasma concentration of 1.9 ± 0.3 µg/mL.
[See table below]
In some patients after a 300 mg dose for brachial plexus block, free plasma concentrations of ropivacaine may approach the threshold for CNS toxicity. (See PRECAUTIONS.) At a dose of greater than 300 mg, for local infiltration, the terminal half-life may be longer (>30 hours).

Distribution
After intravascular infusion, ropivacaine has a steady state volume of distribution of 41 ± 7 liters. Ropivacaine is 94% protein bound, mainly to α₁-acid glycoprotein. An increase in total plasma concentrations during continuous epidural infusion has been observed, related to a postoperative increase of α₁-acid glycoprotein. Variations in unbound, ie, pharmacologically active, concentrations have been less than in total plasma concentration. Ropivacaine readily crosses the placenta and equilibrium in regard to unbound concentration will be rapidly reached. (See PRECAUTIONS, Labor and Delivery.)

Metabolism
Ropivacaine is extensively metabolized in the liver, predominantly by aromatic hydroxylation mediated by cytochrome P4501A to 3-hydroxy ropivacaine. After a single IV dose approximately 37% of the total dose is excreted in the urine as both free and conjugated 3-hydroxy ropivacaine. Low concentrations of 3-hydroxy ropivacaine have been found in the plasma. Urinary excretion of the 4-hydroxy ropivacaine, and both the 3-hydroxy N-de-alkylated (3-OH-PPX) and 4-hydroxy N-de-alkylated (4-OH-PPX) metabolites account for less than 3% of the dose. An additional metabolite, 2-hydroxy-methyl-ropivacaine, has been identified but not quantified in the urine. The N-de-alkylated metabolite of ropivacaine (PPX) and 3-OH-ropivacaine are the major metabolites excreted in the urine during epidural infusion. Total PPX concentration in the plasma was about half as that of total ropivacaine; however, mean unbound concentrations of PPX were about 7 to 9 times higher than that of unbound ropivacaine following continuous epidural infusion up to 72 hours. Unbound PPX, 3-hydroxy and 4-hydroxy ropivacaine, have a pharmacological activity in animal models less than that of ropivacaine. There is no evidence of *in vivo* racemization in urine of ropivacaine.

Elimination
The kidney is the main excretory organ for most local anesthetic metabolites. In total, 86% of the ropivacaine dose is excreted in the urine after intravenous administration of which only 1% relates to unchanged drug. Ropivacaine has a mean ± SD total plasma clearance of 387 ± 107 mL/min, an unbound plasma clearance of 7.2 ± 1.6 L/min, and a renal clearance of 1 mL/min. The mean ± SD terminal half-life is 1.8 ± 0.7 h after intravascular administration and 4.2 ± 1.0 h after epidural administration (see Absorption).

Pharmacodynamics
Studies in humans have demonstrated that, unlike most other local anesthetics, the presence of epinephrine has no major effect on either the time of onset or duration of action of ropivacaine. Likewise, addition of epinephrine to ropivacaine has no effect on limiting systemic absorption of ropivacaine.

Table 1
Pharmacokinetic (plasma concentration-time) data from clinical trials

Route	Epidural Infusion[a]	Epidural Infusion[a]	Epidural Block[b]	Epidural Block[b]	Epidural Block[b]	Plexus Block[c]	IV Infusion[d]
Dose (mg)	1493±10	2075±206	1217±277	150	187.5	300	40
N	12	12	11	8	8	10	12
C_{max} (mg/L)	2.4±1[e]	2.8±0.5[e]	2.3±1.1[e]	1.1±0.2	1.6±0.6	2.3±0.8	1.2±0.2[f]
T_{max} (min)	n/a[h]	n/a	n/a	43±14	34±9	54±22	n/a
AUC_0 (mg.h/L)	135.5±50	145±34	161±90	7.2±2	11.3±4	13±3.3	1.8±0.6
CL (L/h)	11.03	13.7	n/a	5.5±2	5±2.6	n/a	21.2±7
t_{1/2} (hr)[g]	5±2.5	5.7±3	6.0±3	5.7±2	7.1±3	6.8±3.2	1.9±0.5

a Continuous 72 hour epidural infusion after an epidural block with 5 or 10 mg/mL.
b Epidural anesthesia with 7.5 mg/mL (0.75%) for cesarean delivery.
c Brachial plexus block with 7.5 mg/mL (0.75%) ropivacaine.
d 20 minute IV infusion to volunteers (40 mg).
e C_{max} measured at the end of infusion (ie, at 72 hr).
f C_{max} measured at the end of infusion (ie, at 20 minutes).
g t_{1/2} is the true terminal elimination half-life. On the other hand, t_{1/2} follows absorption-dependent elimination (flip-flop) after non-intravenous administration.
h n/a=not applicable

Systemic absorption of local anesthetics can produce effects on the central nervous and cardiovascular systems. At blood concentrations achieved with therapeutic doses, changes in cardiac conduction, excitability, refractoriness, contractility, and peripheral vascular resistance have been reported. Toxic blood concentrations depress cardiac conduction and excitability, which may lead to atrioventricular block, ventricular arrhythmias and to cardiac arrest, sometimes resulting in fatalities. In addition, myocardial contractility is depressed and peripheral vasodilation occurs, leading to decreased cardiac output and arterial blood pressure.

Following systemic absorption, local anesthetics can produce central nervous system stimulation, depression or both. Apparent central stimulation is usually manifested as restlessness, tremors and shivering, progressing to convulsions, followed by depression and coma, progressing ultimately to respiratory arrest. However, the local anesthetics have a primary depressant effect on the medulla and on higher centers. The depressed stage may occur without a prior excited stage.

In 2 clinical pharmacology studies (total n=24) ropivacaine and bupivacaine were infused (10 mg/min) in human volunteers until the appearance of CNS symptoms, eg, visual or hearing disturbances, perioral numbness, tingling and others. Similar symptoms were seen with both drugs. In 1 study, the mean ± SD maximum tolerated intravenous dose of ropivacaine infused (124 ± 38 mg) was significantly higher than that of bupivacaine (99 ± 30 mg) while in the other study the doses were not different (115 ± 29 mg of ropivacaine and 103 ± 30 mg of bupivacaine). In the latter study, the number of subjects reporting each symptom was similar for both drugs with the exception of muscle twitching which was reported by more subjects with bupivacaine than ropivacaine at comparable intravenous doses. At the end of the infusion, ropivacaine in both studies caused significantly less depression of cardiac conductivity (less QRS widening) than bupivacaine. Ropivacaine and bupivacaine caused evidence of depression of cardiac contractility, but there were no changes in cardiac output.

Clinical data in one published article indicate that differences in various pharmacodynamic measures were observed with increasing age. In one study, the upper level of analgesia increased with age, the maximum decrease of mean arterial pressure (MAP) declined with age during the first hour after epidural administration, and the intensity of motor blockade increased with age. However, no pharmacokinetic differences were observed between elderly and younger patients.

In non-clinical pharmacology studies comparing ropivacaine and bupivacaine in several animal species, the cardiac toxicity of ropivacaine was less than that of bupivacaine, although both were considerably more toxic than lidocaine. Arrhythmogenic and cardio-depressant effects were seen in animals at significantly higher doses of ropivacaine than bupivacaine. The incidence of successful resuscitation was not significantly different between the ropivacaine and bupivacaine groups.

Clinical Trials

Ropivacaine was studied as a local anesthetic both for surgical anesthesia and for acute pain management. (See Dosage and Administration.)

The onset, depth and duration of sensory block are, in general, similar to bupivacaine. However, the depth and duration of motor block, in general, are less than that with bupivacaine.

Epidural Administration In Surgery

There were 25 clinical studies performed in 900 patients to evaluate Naropin epidural injection for general surgery. Naropin was used in doses ranging from 75 to 250 mg. In doses of 100–200 mg, the median (1st–3rd quartile) onset time to achieve a T10 sensory block was 10 (5–13) minutes and the median (1st–3rd quartile) duration at the T10 level was 4 (3–5) hours. (See DOSAGE AND ADMINISTRATION.) Higher doses produced a more profound block with a greater duration of effect.

Epidural Administration In Cesarean Section

A total of 12 studies were performed with epidural administration of Naropin for cesarean section. Eight of these studies involved 218 patients using the concentration of 5 mg/mL (0.5%) in doses up to 150 mg. Median onset measured at T6 ranged from 11 to 26 minutes. Median duration of sensory block at T6 ranged from 1.7 to 3.2 h, and duration of motor block ranged from 1.4 to 2.9 h. Naropin provided adequate muscle relaxation for surgery in all cases.

In addition, 4 active controlled studies for cesarean section were performed in 264 patients at a concentration of 7.5 mg/mL (0.75%) in doses up to 187.5 mg. Median onset measured at T6 ranged from 4 to 15 minutes. Seventy-seven to 96% of Naropin-exposed patients reported no pain at delivery. Some patients received other anesthetic, analgesic, or sedative modalities during the course of the operative procedure.

Epidural Administration In Labor And Delivery

A total of 9 double-blind clinical studies, involving 240 patients were performed to evaluate Naropin for epidural block for management of labor pain. When administered in doses up to 278 mg as intermittent injections or as a continuous infusion, Naropin produced adequate pain relief.

A prospective meta-analysis on 6 of these studies provided detailed evaluation of the delivered newborns and showed no difference in clinical outcomes compared to bupivacaine. There were significantly fewer instrumental deliveries in mothers receiving ropivacaine as compared to bupivacaine.

Table 2
LABOR AND DELIVERY META-ANALYSIS: MODE OF DELIVERY

Delivery Mode	Naropin n=199		Bupivacaine n=188	
	n	%	n	%
Spontaneous Vertex	116	58	92	49
Vacuum Extractor	26	}27*	33	}40
Forceps	28		42	
Cesarean Section	29	15	21	11

*p=0.004 versus bupivacaine

Epidural Administration In Postoperative Pain Management

There were 8 clinical studies performed in 382 patients to evaluate Naropin 2 mg/mL (0.2%) for postoperative pain management after upper and lower abdominal surgery and after orthopedic surgery. The studies utilized intravascular morphine via PCA as a rescue medication and quantified as an efficacy variable.

Epidural anesthesia with Naropin 5 mg/mL, (0.5%) was used intraoperatively for each of these procedures prior to initiation of postoperative Naropin. The incidence and intensity of the motor block were dependent on the dose rate of Naropin and the site of injection. Cumulative doses of up to 770 mg of ropivacaine were administered over 24 hours (intraoperative block plus postoperative continuous infusion). The overall quality of pain relief, as judged by the patients, in the ropivacaine groups was rated as good or excellent (73% to 100%). The frequency of motor block was greatest at 4 hours and decreased during the infusion period in all groups. At least 80% of patients in the upper and lower abdominal studies and 42% in the orthopedic studies had no motor block at the end of the 21-hour infusion period. Sensory block was also dose rate-dependent and a decrease in spread was observed during the infusion period.

A double blind, randomized, clinical trial compared lumbar epidural infusion of Naropin (n=26) and bupivacaine (n=26) at 2 mg/mL (8 mL/h), for 24 hours after knee replacement. In this study, the pain scores were higher in the Naropin group, but the incidence and the intensity of motor block were lower.

Continuous epidural infusion of Naropin 2 mg/mL (0.2%) during up to 72 hours for postoperative pain management after major abdominal surgery was studied in 2 multicenter, double-blind studies. A total of 391 patients received a low thoracic epidural catheter, and Naropin 7.5 mg/L (0.75%) was given for surgery, in combination with GA. Postoperatively, Naropin 2 mg/mL (0.2%), 4–14 mL/h, alone or with fentanyl 1, 2, or 4 μg/mL was infused through the epidural catheter and adjusted according to the patient's needs. These studies support the use of Naropin 2 mg/mL (0.2%) for epidural infusion at 6–14 mL/h (12–28 mg) for up to 72 hours and demonstrated adequate analgesia with only slight and nonprogressive motor block in cases of moderate to severe postoperative pain.

Clinical studies with 2 mg/mL (0.2%) Naropin have demonstrated that infusion rates of 6–14 mL (12–28 mg) per hour provide adequate analgesia with nonprogressive motor block in cases of moderate to severe postoperative pain. In these studies, this technique resulted in a significant reduction in patients' morphine rescue dose requirement. Clinical experience supports the use of Naropin epidural infusions for up to 72 hours.

Peripheral Nerve Block

Naropin, 5 mg/mL (0.5%), was evaluated for its ability to provide anesthesia for surgery using the techniques of Peripheral Nerve Block. There were 13 studies performed including a series of 4 pharmacodynamic and pharmacokinetic studies performed on minor nerve blocks. From these, 235 Naropin treated patients were evaluable for efficacy. Naropin was used in doses up to 275 mg. When used for brachial plexus block, onset depended on technique used. Supraclavicular blocks were consistently more successful than axillary blocks. The median onset of sensory block (anesthesia) produced by ropivacaine 0.5% via axillary block ranged from 10 minutes (medial brachial cutaneous nerve) to 45 minutes (musculocutaneous nerve). Median duration ranged from 3.7 hours (medial brachial cutaneous nerve) to 8.7 hours (ulnar nerve). The 5 mg/mL (0.5%) Naropin solution gave success rates from 56% to 86% for axillary blocks, compared with 92% for supraclavicular blocks.

In addition, Naropin, 7.5 mg/mL (0.75%), was evaluated in 99 Naropin treated patients, in 2 double-blind studies, performed to provide anesthesia for surgery using the techniques of Brachial Plexus Block. Naropin 7.5 mg/mL was compared to bupivacaine 5 mg/mL. In 1 study, patients underwent axillary brachial plexus block using injections of 40 mL (300 mg) of Naropin, 7.5 mg/mL (0.75%) or 40 mL injections of bupivacaine, 5 mg/mL (200 mg). In a second study, patients underwent subclavian perivascular brachial plexus block using 30 mL (225 mg) of Naropin, 7.5 mg/mL (0.75%) or 30 mL of bupivacaine 5 mg/mL (150 mg). There was no significant difference between the Naropin and bupivacaine groups in either study with regard to onset of anesthesia, duration of sensory blockade, or duration of anesthesia.

The median duration of anesthesia varied between 11.4 and 14.4 hours with both techniques. In one study, using the axillary technique, the quality of analgesia and muscle relaxation in the Naropin group was judged to be significantly superior to bupivacaine by both investigator and surgeon. However, using the subclavian perivascular technique, no statistically significant difference was found in the quality of analgesia and muscle relaxation as judged by both the investigator and surgeon. The use of Naropin 7.5 mg/mL for block of the brachial plexus via either the subclavian perivascular approach using 30 mL (225 mg) or via the axillary approach using 40 mL (300 mg) both provided effective and reliable anesthesia.

Local Infiltration

A total of 7 clinical studies were performed to evaluate the local infiltration of Naropin to produce anesthesia for surgery and analgesia in postoperative pain management. In these studies 297 patients who received Naropin in doses up to 200 mg (concentrations up to 5 mg/mL, 0.5%) were evaluable for efficacy. With infiltration of 100–200 mg Naropin, the time to first request for analgesic was 2–6 hours. When compared to placebo, Naropin produced lower pain scores and a reduction of analgesic consumption.

INDICATIONS AND USAGE

Naropin is indicated for the production of local or regional anesthesia for surgery and for acute pain management.

Surgical Anesthesia:	epidural block for surgery including cesarean section; major nerve block; local infiltration
Acute Pain Management:	epidural continuous infusion or intermittent bolus eg, postoperative or labor; local infiltration

CONTRAINDICATIONS

Naropin is contraindicated in patients with a known hypersensitivity to ropivacaine or to any local anesthetic agent of the amide type.

WARNINGS

IN PERFORMING NAROPIN BLOCKS, UNINTENDED INTRAVENOUS INJECTION IS POSSIBLE AND MAY RESULT IN CARDIAC ARRHYTHMIA OR CARDIAC ARREST. THE POTENTIAL FOR SUCCESSFUL RESUSCITATION HAS NOT BEEN STUDIED IN HUMANS. NAROPIN SHOULD BE ADMINISTERED IN INCREMENTAL DOSES. IT IS NOT RECOMMENDED FOR EMERGENCY SITUATIONS, WHERE A FAST ONSET OF SURGICAL ANESTHESIA IS NECESSARY. HISTORICALLY, PREGNANT PATIENTS WERE REPORTED TO HAVE A HIGH RISK FOR CARDIAC ARRHYTHMIAS, CARDIAC/CIRCULATORY ARREST AND DEATH WHEN 0.75% BUPIVACAINE (ANOTHER MEMBER OF THE AMINO AMIDE CLASS OF LOCAL ANESTHETICS) WAS INADVERTENTLY RAPIDLY INJECTED INTRAVENOUSLY.

LOCAL ANESTHETICS SHOULD ONLY BE ADMINISTERED BY CLINICIANS WHO ARE WELL VERSED IN THE DIAGNOSIS AND MANAGEMENT OF DOSE-RELATED TOXICITY AND OTHER ACUTE EMERGENCIES WHICH MIGHT ARISE FROM THE BLOCK TO BE EMPLOYED, AND THEN ONLY AFTER INSURING THE **IMMEDIATE (WITHOUT DELAY)** AVAILABILITY OF OXYGEN, OTHER RESUSCITATIVE DRUGS, CARDIOPULMONARY RESUSCITATIVE EQUIPMENT, AND THE PERSONNEL RESOURCES NEEDED FOR PROPER MANAGEMENT OF TOXIC REACTIONS AND RELATED EMERGENCIES (See also ADVERSE REACTIONS and PRECAUTIONS). DELAY IN PROPER MANAGEMENT OF DOSE-RELATED TOXICITY, UNDERVENTILATION FROM ANY CAUSE, AND/OR ALTERED SENSITIVITY MAY LEAD TO THE DEVELOPMENT OF ACIDOSIS, CARDIAC ARREST AND, POSSIBLY, DEATH. SOLUTIONS OF NAROPIN SHOULD NOT BE USED FOR THE PRODUCTION OF OBSTETRICAL PARACERVICAL BLOCK ANESTHESIA, RETROBULBAR BLOCK, OR SPINAL ANESTHESIA (SUBARACHNOID BLOCK) DUE TO INSUFFICIENT DATA TO SUPPORT SUCH USE. INTRAVENOUS REGIONAL ANESTHESIA (BIER BLOCK) SHOULD NOT BE PERFORMED DUE TO A LACK OF CLINICAL EXPERIENCE AND THE RISK OF ATTAINING TOXIC BLOOD LEVELS OF ROPIVACAINE.

It is essential that aspiration for blood, or cerebrospinal fluid (where applicable), be done prior to injecting any local anesthetic, both the original dose and all subsequent doses, to avoid intravascular or subarachnoid injection. However, a negative aspiration does *not* ensure against an intravascular or subarachnoid injection.

A well-known risk of epidural anesthesia may be an unintentional subarachnoid injection of local anesthetic. Two clinical studies have been performed to verify the safety of Naropin at a volume of 3 mL injected into the subarachnoid space since this dose represents an incremental epidural volume that could be unintentionally injected. The 15 and 22.5 mg doses injected resulted in sensory levels as high as T5 and T4, respectively. Anesthesia to pinprick started in the sacral dermatomes in 2–3 minutes, extended to the T10 level in 10–13 minutes and lasted for approximately 2 hours. The results of these two clinical studies showed that a 3 mL dose did not produce any serious adverse events when spinal anesthesia blockade was achieved.

Naropin should be used with caution in patients receiving other local anesthetics or agents structurally related to amide-type local anesthetics, since the toxic effects of these drugs are additive.

PRECAUTIONS

General

The safe and effective use of local anesthetics depends on proper dosage, correct technique, adequate precautions and readiness for emergencies.

Continued on next page

Naropin—Cont.

Resuscitative equipment, oxygen and other resuscitative drugs should be available for immediate use. (See WARNINGS and ADVERSE REACTIONS.) The lowest dosage that results in effective anesthesia should be used to avoid high plasma levels and serious adverse events. Injections should be made slowly and incrementally, with frequent aspirations before and during the injection to avoid intravascular injection. When a continuous catheter technique is used, syringe aspirations should also be performed before and during each supplemental injection. During the administration of epidural anesthesia, it is recommended that a test dose of a local anesthetic with a fast onset be administered initially and that the patient be monitored for central nervous system and cardiovascular toxicity, as well as for signs of unintended intrathecal administration before proceeding. When clinical conditions permit, consideration should be given to employing local anesthetic solutions, which contain epinephrine for the test dose because circulatory changes compatible with epinephrine may also serve as a warning sign of unintended intravascular injection. An intravascular injection is still possible even if aspirations for blood are negative. Administration of higher than recommended doses of Naropin to achieve greater motor blockade or increased duration of sensory blockade may result in cardiovascular depression, particularly in the event of inadvertent intravascular injection. Tolerance to elevated blood levels varies with the physical condition of the patient. Debilitated, elderly patients and acutely ill patients should be given reduced doses commensurate with their age and physical condition. Local anesthetics should also be used with caution in patients with hypotension, hypovolemia or heart block.

Careful and constant monitoring of cardiovascular and respiratory vital signs (adequacy of ventilation) and the patient's state of consciousness should be performed after each local anesthetic injection. It should be kept in mind at such times that restlessness, anxiety, incoherent speech, lightheadedness, numbness and tingling of the mouth and lips, metallic taste, tinnitus, dizziness, blurred vision, tremors, twitching, depression, or drowsiness may be early warning signs of central nervous system toxicity. Because amide-type local anesthetics such as ropivacaine are metabolized by the liver, these drugs, especially repeat doses, should be used cautiously in patients with hepatic disease. Patients with severe hepatic disease, because of their inability to metabolize local anesthetics normally, are at a greater risk of developing toxic plasma concentrations. Local anesthetics should also be used with caution in patients with impaired cardiovascular function because they may be less able to compensate for functional changes associated with the prolongation of A-V conduction produced by these drugs.

Many drugs used during the conduct of anesthesia are considered potential triggering agents for malignant hyperthermia (MH). Amide-type local anesthetics are not known to trigger this reaction. However, since the need for supplemental general anesthesia cannot be predicted in advance, it is suggested that a standard protocol for MH management should be available.

Epidural Anesthesia

During epidural administration, Naropin should be administered in incremental doses of 3 to 5 mL with sufficient time between doses to detect toxic manifestations of unintentional intravascular or intrathecal injection. Syringe aspirations should also be performed before and during each supplemental injection in continuous (intermittent) catheter techniques. An intravascular injection is still possible even if aspirations for blood are negative. During the administration of epidural anesthesia, it is recommended that a test dose be administered initially and the effects monitored before the full dose is given. When clinical conditions permit, the test dose should contain an appropriate dose of epinephrine to serve as a warning of unintentional intravascular injection. If injected into a blood vessel, this amount of epinephrine is likely to produce a transient "epinephrine response" within 45 seconds, consisting of an increase in heart rate and systolic blood pressure, circumoral pallor, palpitations and nervousness in the unsedated patient. The sedated patient may exhibit only a pulse rate increase of 20 or more beats per minute for 15 or more seconds. Therefore, following the test dose, the heart should be continuously monitored for a heart rate increase. Patients on beta-blockers may not manifest changes in heart rate, but blood pressure monitoring can detect a rise in systolic blood pressure. A test dose of a short-acting amide anesthetic such as lidocaine is recommended to detect an unintentional intrathecal administration. This will be manifested within a few minutes by signs of spinal block (eg, decreased sensation of the buttocks, paresis of the legs, or, in the sedated patient, absent knee jerk). An intravascular or subarachnoid injection is still possible even if results of the test dose are negative. The test dose itself may produce a systemic toxic reaction, high spinal or epinephrine-induced cardiovascular effects.

Use in Brachial Plexus Block

Ropivacaine plasma concentrations may approach the threshold for central nervous system toxicity after the administration of 300 mg of ropivacaine for brachial plexus block. Caution should be exercised when using the 300 mg dose. (See OVERDOSAGE.)

Use in Head and Neck Area

Small doses of local anesthetics injected into the head and neck area may produce adverse reactions similar to systemic toxicity seen with unintentional intravascular injections of larger doses. The injection procedures require the utmost care. Confusion, convulsions, respiratory depression, and/or respiratory arrest, and cardiovascular stimulation or depression have been reported. These reactions may be due to intra-arterial injection of the local anesthetic with retrograde flow to the cerebral circulation. Patients receiving these blocks should have their circulation and respiration monitored and be constantly observed. Resuscitative equipment and personnel for treating adverse reactions should be immediately available. Dosage recommendations should not be exceeded. (See DOSAGE AND ADMINISTRATION.)

Use in Ophthalmic Surgery

The use of Naropin in retrobulbar blocks for ophthalmic surgery has not been studied. Until appropriate experience is gained, the use of Naropin for such surgery is not recommended.

Information for Patients

When appropriate, patients should be informed in advance that they may experience temporary loss of sensation and motor activity in the anesthetized part of the body following proper administration of lumbar epidural anesthesia. Also, when appropriate, the physician should discuss other information including adverse reactions in the Naropin package insert.

Drug Interactions

Naropin should be used with caution in patients receiving other local anesthetics or agents structurally related to amide-type local anesthetics, since the toxic effects of these drugs are additive. Cytochrome P4501A2 is involved in the formation of 3-hydroxy ropivacaine, the major metabolite. In vivo, the plasma clearance of ropivacaine was reduced by 70% during coadministration of fluvoxamine (25 mg bid for 2 days), a selective and potent CYP1A2 inhibitor. Thus strong inhibitors of cytochrome P4501A2, such as fluvoxamine, given concomitantly during administration of Naropin, can interact with Naropin leading to increased ropivacaine plasma levels. Caution should be exercised when CYP1A2 inhibitors are coadministered. Possible interactions with drugs known to be metabolized by CYP1A2 via competitive inhibition such as theophylline and imipramine may also occur. Coadministration of a selective and potent inhibitor of CYP3A4, ketoconazole (100 mg bid for 2 days with ropivacaine infusion administered 1 hour after ketoconazole) caused a 15% reduction in in-vivo plasma clearance of ropivacaine.

Carcinogenesis, Mutagenesis, Impairment of Fertility

Long term studies in animals of most local anesthetics, including ropivacaine, to evaluate the carcinogenic potential have not been conducted.

Weak mutagenic activity was seen in the mouse lymphoma test. Mutagenicity was not noted in the other assays, demonstrating that the weak signs of in vitro activity in the mouse lymphoma test were not manifest under diverse in vivo conditions.

Studies performed with ropivacaine in rats did not demonstrate an effect on fertility or general reproductive performance over 2 generations.

Pregnancy Category B

Reproduction toxicity studies have been performed in pregnant New Zealand white rabbits and Sprague-Dawley rats. During gestation days 6–18, rabbits received 1.3, 4.2, or 13 mg/kg/day subcutaneously. In rats, subcutaneous doses of 5.3, 11 and 26 mg/kg/day were administered during gestation days 6–15. No teratogenic effects were observed in rats and rabbits at the highest doses tested. The highest doses of 13 mg/kg/day (rabbits) and 26 mg/kg/day (rats) are approximately 1/3 of the maximum recommended human dose (epidural, 770 mg/24 hours) based on a mg/m² basis. In 2 prenatal and postnatal studies, the female rats were dosed daily from day 15 of gestation to day 20 postpartum. The doses were 5.3, 11 and 26 mg/kg/day subcutaneously. There were no treatment-related effects on late fetal development, parturition, lactation, neonatal viability, or growth of the offspring.

In another study with rats, the males were dosed daily for 9 weeks before mating and during mating. The females were dosed daily for 2 weeks before mating and then during the mating, pregnancy, and lactation, up to day 42 post coitus. At 23 mg/kg/day, an increased loss of pups was observed during the first 3 days postpartum. The effect was considered secondary to impaired maternal care due to maternal toxicity.

There are no adequate or well-controlled studies in pregnant women of the effects of Naropin on the developing fetus. Naropin should only be used during pregnancy if the benefits outweigh the risk.

Teratogenicity studies in rats and rabbits did not show evidence of any adverse effects on organogenesis or early fetal development in rats (26 mg/kg sc) or rabbits (13 mg/kg). The doses used were approximately equal to total daily dose based on body surface area. There were no treatment-related effects on late fetal development, parturition, lactation, neonatal viability, or growth of the offspring in 2 perinatal and postnatal studies in rats, at dose levels equivalent to the maximum recommended human dose based on body surface area. In another study at 23 mg/kg, an increased pup loss was seen during the first 3 days postpartum, which was considered secondary to impaired maternal care due to maternal toxicity.

Labor and Delivery

Local anesthetics, including ropivacaine, rapidly cross the placenta, and when used for epidural block can cause varying degrees of maternal, fetal and neonatal toxicity (see CLINICAL PHARMACOLOGY, PHARMACOKINETICS). The incidence and degree of toxicity depend upon the procedure performed, the type and amount of drug used, and the technique of drug administration. Adverse reactions in the parturient, fetus and neonate involve alterations of the central nervous system, peripheral vascular tone and cardiac function.

Maternal hypotension has resulted from regional anesthesia with Naropin for obstetrical pain relief. Local anesthetics produce vasodilation by blocking sympathetic nerves. Elevating the patient's legs and positioning her on her left side will help prevent decreases in blood pressure. The fetal heart rate also should be monitored continuously, and electronic fetal monitoring is highly advisable. Epidural anesthesia has been reported to prolong the second stage of labor by removing the patient's reflex urge to bear down or by interfering with motor function. Spontaneous vertex delivery occurred more frequently in patients receiving Naropin than in those receiving bupivacaine.

Nursing Mothers

Some local anesthetic drugs are excreted in human milk and caution should be exercised when they are administered to a nursing woman. The excretion of ropivacaine or its metabolites in human milk has not been studied. Based on the milk/plasma concentration ratio in rats, the estimated daily dose to a pup will be about 4% of the dose given to the mother. Assuming that the milk/plasma concentration in humans is of the same order, the total Naropin dose to which the baby is exposed by breast-feeding is far lower than by exposure in utero in pregnant women at term (see Precautions).

Pediatric Use

The safety and efficacy of Naropin in pediatric patients have not been established.

Geriatric Use

Of the 2,978 subjects that were administered Naropin Injection in 71 controlled and uncontrolled clinical studies, 803 patients (27%) were 65 years of age or older which includes 127 patients (4%) 75 years of age and over. Naropin Injection was found to be safe and effective in the patients in these studies. Clinical data in one published article indicate that differences in various pharmacodynamic measures were observed with increasing age. In one study, the upper level of analgesia increased with age, the maximum decrease of mean arterial pressure (MAP) declined with age during the first hour after epidural administration, and the intensity of motor blockade increased with age.

This drug and its metabolites are known to be excreted by the kidney, and the risk of toxic reactions to this drug may be greater in patients with impaired renal function. Elderly patients are more likely to have decreased hepatic, renal, or cardiac function, as well as concomitant disease. Therefore, care should be taken in dose selection, starting at the low end of the dosage range, and it may be useful to monitor renal function. (See PHARMACOKINETICS, Elimination.)

ADVERSE REACTIONS

Reactions to ropivacaine are characteristic of those associated with other amide-type local anesthetics. A major cause of adverse reactions to this group of drugs may be associated with excessive plasma levels, which may be due to overdosage, unintentional intravascular injection or slow metabolic degradation.

The reported adverse events are derived from clinical studies conducted in the U.S. and other countries. The reference drug was usually bupivacaine. The studies used a variety of premedications, sedatives, and surgical procedures of varying length. A total of 3988 patients have been exposed to Naropin at concentrations up to 1.0% in clinical trials. Each patient was counted once for each type of adverse event.

Incidence ≥5%

For the indications of epidural administration in surgery, cesarean section, post-operative pain management, peripheral nerve block, and local infiltration, the following treatment-emergent adverse events were reported with an incidence of ≥5% in all clinical studies (N=3988): hypotension (37.0%), nausea (24.8%), vomiting (11.6%), bradycardia (9.3%), fever (9.2%), pain (8.0%), postoperative complications (7.1%), anemia (6.1%), paresthesia (5.6%), headache (5.1%), pruritus (5.1%), and back pain (5.0%).

Incidence 1–5%

Urinary retention, dizziness, rigors, hypertension, tachycardia, anxiety, oliguria, hypoesthesia, chest pain, hypokalemia, dyspnea, cramps, and urinary tract infection.

Incidence in Controlled Clinical Trials

The reported adverse events are derived from controlled clinical studies with Naropin (concentrations ranged from 0.125% to 1.0% for Naropin and 0.25% to 0.75% for bupivacaine) in the U.S. and other countries involving 3094 patients. Table 3A and 3B list adverse events (number and percentage) that occurred in at least 1% of Naropin-treated patients in these studies. The majority of patients receiving concentrations higher than 5.0 mg/mL (0.5%) were treated with Naropin.

Table 3A
Adverse Events Reported in ≥1% of Adult Patients Receiving Regional or Local Anesthesia (Surgery, Labor, Cesarean Section, Post-Operative Pain Management, Peripheral Nerve Block and Local Infiltration)

Adverse Reaction	Naropin total N=1661		Bupivacaine total N=1433	
	N	(%)	N	(%)
Hypotension	536	(32.3)	408	(28.5)
Nausea	283	(17.0)	207	(14.4)
Vomiting	117	(7.0)	88	(6.1)

Bradycardia	96	(5.8)	73	(5.1)
Headache	84	(5.1)	68	(4.7)
Paresthesia	82	(4.9)	57	(4.0)
Back pain	73	(4.4)	75	(5.2)
Pain	71	(4.3)	71	(5.0)
Pruritus	63	(3.8)	40	(2.8)
Fever	61	(3.7)	37	(2.6)
Dizziness	42	(2.5)	23	(1.6)
Rigors (Chills)	42	(2.5)	24	(1.7)
Postoperative complications	41	(2.5)	44	(3.1)
Hypoesthesia	27	(1.6)	24	(1.7)
Urinary retention	23	(1.4)	20	(1.4)
Progression of labor poor/failed	23	(1.4)	22	(1.5)
Anxiety	21	(1.3)	11	(0.8)
Breast disorder, breast-feeding	21	(1.3)	12	(0.8)
Rhinitis	18	(1.1)	13	(0.9)

Table 3B
Adverse Events Reported in ≥1% of Fetuses or Neonates of Mothers Who Received Regional Anesthesia (Cesarean Section and Labor Studies)

Adverse Reaction	Naropin total N=639		Bupivacaine total N=573	
	N	(%)	N	(%)
Fetal bradycardia	77	(12.1)	68	(11.9)
Neonatal jaundice	49	(7.7)	47	(8.2)
Neonatal complication-NOS	42	(6.6)	38	(6.6)
Apgar score low	18	(2.8)	14	(2.4)
Neonatal respiratory disorder	17	(2.7)	18	(3.1)
Neonatal tachypnea	14	(2.2)	15	(2.6)
Neonatal fever	13	(2.0)	14	(2.4)
Fetal tachycardia	13	(2.0)	12	(2.1)
Fetal distress	11	(1.7)	10	(1.7)
Neonatal infection	10	(1.6)	8	(1.4)
Neonatal hypoglycemia	8	(1.3)	16	(2.8)

Incidence <1%
The following adverse events were reported during the Naropin clinical program in more than one patient (N=3988), occurred at an overall incidence of <1%, and were considered relevant:
Application Site Reactions—injection site pain
Cardiovascular System—vasovagal reaction, syncope, postural hypotension, non-specific ECG abnormalities
Female Reproductive—poor progression of labor, uterine atony
Gastrointestinal System—fecal incontinence, tenesmus, neonatal vomiting
General and Other Disorders—hypothermia, malaise, asthenia, accident and/or injury
Hearing and Vestibular—tinnitus, hearing abnormalities
Heart Rate and Rhythm—extrasystoles, non-specific arrhythmias, atrial fibrillation
Liver and Biliary System—jaundice
Metabolic Disorders—hypomagnesemia
Musculoskeletal System—myalgia
Myo/Endo/Pericardium—ST segment changes, myocardial infarction
Nervous System—tremor, Horner's syndrome, paresis, dyskinesia, neuropathy, vertigo, coma, convulsion, hypokinesia, hypotonia, ptosis, stupor
Psychiatric Disorders—agitation, confusion, somnolence, nervousness, amnesia, hallucination, emotional lability, insomnia, nightmares
Respiratory System—bronchospasm, coughing
Skin Disorders—rash, urticaria
Urinary System Disorders—urinary incontinence, micturition disorder
Vascular—deep vein thrombosis, phlebitis, pulmonary embolism
Vision—vision abnormalities
For the indication epidural anesthesia for surgery, the 15 most common adverse events were compared between different concentrations of Naropin and bupivacaine. Table 4 is based on data from trials in the U.S. and other countries where Naropin was administered as an epidural anesthetic for surgery.
[See table 4 at right]
Using data from the same studies, the number (%) of patients experiencing hypotension is displayed by patient age, drug and concentration in Table 5. In Table 6, the adverse events for Naropin are broken down by gender.
[See table 5 at right]

Table 6
Most Common Adverse Events by Gender (Epidural Administration)
Total N: Females = 405, Males = 355

Adverse Reaction	Female		Male	
	N	(%)	N	(%)
hypotension	220	(54.3)	138	(38.9)
nausea	119	(29.4)	23	(6.5)
bradycardia	65	(16.0)	56	(15.8)
vomiting	59	(14.6)	8	(2.3)

back pain	41	(10.1)	23	(6.5)
headache	33	(8.1)	17	(4.8)
chills	18	(4.4)	5	(1.4)
fever	16	(4.0)	3	(0.8)
pruritus	16	(4.0)	1	(0.3)
pain	12	(3.0)	4	(1.1)
urinary retention	11	(2.7)	7	(2.0)
dizziness	9	(2.2)	4	(1.1)
hypoesthesia	8	(2.0)	2	(0.6)
paresthesia	8	(2.0)	10	(2.8)

Systemic Reactions
The most commonly encountered acute adverse experiences that demand immediate countermeasures are related to the central nervous system and the cardiovascular system. These adverse experiences are generally dose-related and due to high plasma levels which may result from overdosage, rapid absorption from the injection site, diminished tolerance or from unintentional intravascular injection of the local anesthetic solution. In addition to systemic dose-related toxicity, unintentional subarachnoid injection of drug during the intended performance of lumbar epidural block or nerve blocks near the vertebral column (especially in the head and neck region) may result in underventilation or apnea ("Total or High Spinal"). Also, hypotension due to loss of sympathetic tone and respiratory paralysis or underventilation due to cephalad extension of the motor level of anesthesia may occur. This may lead to secondary cardiac arrest if untreated. Factors influencing plasma protein binding, such as acidosis, systemic diseases that alter protein production or competition with other drugs for protein binding sites, may diminish individual tolerance.
Epidural administration of Naropin has, in some cases, as with other local anesthetics, been associated with transient increases in temperature to >38.5°C. This occurred more frequently at doses of Naropin >16 mg/h.
Neurologic Reactions
These are characterized by excitation and/or depression. Restlessness, anxiety, dizziness, tinnitus, blurred vision or tremors may occur, possibly proceeding to convulsions. However, excitement may be transient or absent, with depression being the first manifestation of an adverse reaction. This may quickly be followed by drowsiness merging into unconsciousness and respiratory arrest. Other central nervous system effects may be nausea, vomiting, chills, and constriction of the pupils.
The incidence of convulsions associated with the use of local anesthetics varies with the route of administration and the total dose administered. In a survey of studies of epidural anesthesia, overt toxicity progressing to convulsions occurred in approximately 0.1% of local anesthetic administrations.
The incidence of adverse neurological reactions associated with the use of local anesthetics may be related to the total dose and concentration of local anesthetic administered and are also dependent upon the particular drug used, the route of administration, and the physical status of the patient. Many of these observations may be related to local anes-

thetic techniques, with or without a contribution from the drug. During lumbar epidural block, occasional unintentional penetration of the subarachnoid space by the catheter or needle may occur. Subsequent adverse effects may depend partially on the amount of drug administered intrathecally as well as the physiological and physical effects of a dural puncture. These observations may include spinal block of varying magnitude (including high or total spinal block), hypotension secondary to spinal block, urinary retention, loss of bladder and bowel control (fecal and urinary incontinence), and loss of perineal sensation and sexual function. Signs and symptoms of subarachnoid block typically start within 2–3 minutes of injection. Doses of 15 and 22.5 mg of Naropin resulted in sensory levels as high as T5 and T4, respectively. Analgesia started in the upper dermatomes in 2–3 minutes and extended to the T10 level in 10–13 minutes and lasted for approximately 2 hours. Other neurological effects following unintentional subarachnoid administration during epidural anesthesia may include persistent anesthesia, paresthesia, weakness, paralysis of the lower extremities, and loss of sphincter control; all of which may have slow, incomplete or no recovery. Headache, septic meningitis, meningismus, slowing of labor, increased incidence of forceps delivery, or cranial nerve palsies due to traction on nerves from loss of cerebrospinal fluid have been reported (see DOSAGE AND ADMINISTRATION discussion of Lumbar Epidural Block). A high spinal is characterized by paralysis of the arms, loss of consciousness, respiratory paralysis and bradycardia.
Cardiovascular System Reactions
High doses or unintentional intravascular injection may lead to high plasma levels and related depression of the myocardium, decreased cardiac output, heart block, hypotension, bradycardia, ventricular arrhythmias, including ventricular tachycardia and ventricular fibrillation, and possibly cardiac arrest. (See WARNINGS, PRECAUTIONS, and OVERDOSAGE sections.)
Allergic Reactions
Allergic type reactions are rare and may occur as a result of sensitivity to the local anesthetic (see WARNINGS). These reactions are characterized by signs such as urticaria, pruritus, erythema, angioneurotic edema (including laryngeal edema), tachycardia, sneezing, nausea, vomiting, dizziness, syncope, excessive sweating, elevated temperature, and possibly, anaphylactoid symptomatology (including severe hypotension). Cross sensitivity among members of the amide-type local anesthetic group has been reported. The usefulness of screening for sensitivity has not been definitively established.

OVERDOSAGE

Acute emergencies from local anesthetics are generally related to high plasma levels encountered, or large doses administered, during therapeutic use of local anesthetics or to unintended subarachnoid or intravascular injection of local anesthetic solution. (See ADVERSE REACTIONS, WARNINGS, and PRECAUTIONS.)
MANAGEMENT OF LOCAL ANESTHETIC EMERGENCIES
Therapy with Naropin should be discontinued at the first sign of toxicity. No specific information is available for the

Continued on next page

Table 4
Common Events (Epidural Administration)

Adverse Reaction	Naropin						Bupivacaine			
	5 mg/mL total N=256		7.5 mg/mL total N=297		10 mg/mL total N=207		5 mg/mL total N=236		7.5 mg/mL total N=174	
	N	(%)	N	(%)	N	(%)	N	(%)	N	(%)
hypotension	99	(38.7)	146	(49.2)	113	(54.6)	91	(38.6)	89	(51.1)
nausea	34	(13.3)	68	(22.9)			41	(17.4)	36	(20.7)
bradycardia	29	(11.3)	58	(19.5)	40	(19.3)	32	(13.6)	25	(14.4)
back pain	18	(7.0)	23	(7.7)	34	(16.4)	21	(8.9)	23	(13.2)
vomiting	18	(7.0)	33	(11.1)	23	(11.1)	19	(8.1)	14	(8.0)
headache	12	(4.7)	20	(6.7)	16	(7.7)	13	(5.5)	9	(5.2)
fever	8	(3.1)	5	(1.7)	18	(8.7)	11	(4.7)		
chills	6	(2.3)	7	(2.4)	6	(2.9)	4	(1.7)	3	(1.7)
urinary retention	5	(2.0)	8	(2.7)	10	(4.8)	10	(4.2)		
paresthesia	5	(2.0)	10	(3.4)	5	(2.4)	7	(3.0)		
pruritus			14	(4.7)	3	(1.4)			7	(4.0)

Table 5
Effects of Age on Hypotension (Epidural Administration)
Total N: Naropin = 760, bupivacaine = 410

	Naropin						Bupivacaine			
AGE	5 mg/mL		7.5 mg/mL		10 mg/mL		5 mg/mL		7.5 mg/mL	
	N	(%)	N	(%)	N	(%)	N	(%)	N	(%)
<65	68	(32.2)	99	(43.2)	87	(51.5)	64	(33.5)	73	(48.3)
≥65	31	(68.9)	47	(69.1)	26	(68.4)	27	(60.0)	16	(69.6)

Naropin—Cont.

treatment of toxicity with Naropin; therefore, treatment should be symptomatic and supportive. The first consideration is prevention, best accomplished by incremental injection of Naropin, careful and constant monitoring of cardiovascular and respiratory vital signs and the patient's state of consciousness after each local anesthetic and during continuous infusion. At the first sign of change in mental status, oxygen should be administered.

The first step in the management of systemic toxic reactions, as well as underventilation or apnea due to unintentional subarachnoid injection of drug solution, consists of immediate attention to the establishment and maintenance of a patent airway and effective assisted or controlled ventilation with 100% oxygen with a delivery system capable of permitting immediate positive airway pressure by mask. Circulation should be assisted as necessary. This may prevent convulsions if they have not already occurred.

If necessary, use drugs to control convulsions. Intravenous barbiturates, anticonvulsant agents, or muscle relaxants should only be administered by those familiar with their use. Immediately after the institution of these ventilatory measures, the adequacy of the circulation should be evaluated. Supportive treatment of circulatory depression may require administration of intravenous fluids, and, when appropriate, a vasopressor dictated by the clinical situation (such as ephedrine or epinephrine to enhance myocardial contractile force).

The mean dosages of ropivacaine producing seizures, after intravenous infusion in dogs, nonpregnant and pregnant sheep were 4.9, 6.1 and 5.9 mg/kg, respectively. These doses were associated with peak arterial total plasma concentrations of 11.4, 4.3 and 5.0 µg/mL, respectively.

In human volunteers given intravenous Naropin, the mean maximum tolerated total and free arterial plasma concentrations were 4.3 and 0.6 µg/mL respectively, at which time moderate CNS symptoms (muscle twitching) were noted.

Clinical data from patients experiencing local anesthetic induced convulsions demonstrated rapid development of hypoxia, hypercarbia and acidosis within a minute of the onset of convulsions. These observations suggest that oxygen consumption and carbon dioxide production are greatly increased during local anesthetic convulsions and emphasize the importance of immediate and effective ventilation with oxygen which may avoid cardiac arrest.

If difficulty is encountered in the maintenance of a patent airway or if prolonged ventilatory support (assisted or controlled) is indicated, endotracheal intubation, employing drugs and techniques familiar to the clinician, may be indicated after initial administration of oxygen by mask.

The supine position is dangerous in pregnant women at term because of aorta-caval compression by the gravid uterus. Therefore, during treatment of systemic toxicity, maternal hypotension or fetal bradycardia following regional block, the parturient should be maintained in the left lateral decubitus position if possible, or manual displacement of the uterus off the great vessels should be accomplished. Resuscitation of obstetrical patients may take longer than resuscitation of non-pregnant patients and closed-chest cardiac compression may be ineffective. Rapid delivery of the fetus may improve the response to resuscitative efforts.

DOSAGE AND ADMINISTRATION

The rapid injection of a large volume of local anesthetic solution should be avoided and fractional (incremental) doses should always be used. The smallest dose and concentration required to produce the desired result should be administered.

The dose of any local anesthetic administered varies with the anesthetic procedure, the area to be anesthetized, the vascularity of the tissues, the number of neuronal segments to be blocked, the depth of anesthesia and degree of muscle relaxation required, the duration of anesthesia desired, individual tolerance, and the physical condition of the patient. Patients in poor general condition due to aging or other compromising factors such as partial or complete heart conduction block, advanced liver disease or severe renal dysfunction require special attention although regional anesthesia is frequently indicated in these patients. To reduce the risk of potentially serious adverse reactions, attempts should be made to optimize the patient's condition before major blocks are performed, and the dosage should be adjusted accordingly.

Use an adequate test dose (3–5 mL of a short acting local anesthetic solution containing epinephrine) prior to induction of complete block. This test dose should be repeated if the patient is moved in such a fashion as to have displaced the epidural catheter. Allow adequate time for onset of anesthesia following administration of each test dose.

Parenteral drug products should be inspected visually for particulate matter and discoloration prior to administration, whenever solution and container permit. Solutions which are discolored or which contain particulate matter should not be administered.

[See table 7 above]

The doses in the table are those considered to be necessary to produce a successful block and should be regarded as guidelines for use in adults. Individual variations in onset and duration occur. The figures reflect the expected average dose range needed. For other local anesthetic techniques standard current textbooks should be consulted.

Table 7
Dosage Recommendations

	Conc. mg/mL	(%)	Volume mL	Dose mg	Onset min	Duration hours
SURGICAL ANESTHESIA						
Lumbar Epidural	5.0	(0.5%)	15–30	75–150	15–30	2–4
Administration	7.5	(0.75%)	15–25	113–188	10–20	3–5
Surgery	10.0	(1.0%)	15–20	150–200	10–20	4–6
Lumbar Epidural	5.0	(0.5%)	20–30	100–150	15–25	2–4
Administration	7.5	(0.75%)	15–20	113–150	10–20	3–5
Cesarean Section						
Thoracic Epidural	5.0	(0.5%)	5–15	25–75	10–20	n/a[1]
Administration	7.5	(0.75%)	5–15	38–113	10–20	n/a[1]
Surgery						
Major Nerve Block	5.0	(0.5%)	35–50	175–250	15–30	5–8
(eg, brachial plexus block)	7.5	(0.75%)	10–40	75–300	10–25	6–10
Field Block	5.0	(0.5%)	1–40	5–200	1–15	2–6
(eg, minor nerve blocks and infiltration)						
LABOR PAIN MANAGEMENT						
Lumbar Epidural Administration						
Initial Dose	2.0	(0.2%)	10–20	20–40	10–15	0.5–1.5
Continuous infusion[2]	2.0	(0.2%)	6–14 mL/h	12–28 mg/h	n/a[1]	n/a[1]
Incremental injections (top-up)[2]	2.0	(0.2%)	10–15 mL/h	20–30 mg/h	n/a[1]	n/a[1]
POSTOPERATIVE PAIN MANAGEMENT						
Lumbar Epidural Administration						
Continuous infusion[3]	2.0	(0.2%)	6–14 mL/h	12–28 mg/h	n/a[1]	n/a[1]
Thoracic Epidural Administration	2.0	(0.2%)	6–14 mL/h	12–28 mg/h	n/a[1]	n/a[1]
Continuous infusion[3]						
Infiltration	2.0	(0.2%)	1–100	2–200	1–5	2–6
(eg, minor nerve block)	5.0	(0.5%)	1–40	5–200	1–5	2–6

1 = Not Applicable
2 = Median dose of 21 mg per hour was administered by continuous infusion or by incremental injections (top-ups) over a median delivery time of 5.5 hours.
3 = Cumulative doses up to 770 mg of Naropin over 24 hours (intraoperative block plus postoperative infusion); Continuous epidural infusion at rates up to 28 mg per hour for 72 hours have been well tolerated in adults, ie, 2016 mg plus surgical dose of approximately 100–150 mg as top-up.

Naropin® Polyamp DuoFit™ Sterile Pak:
Boxes of 5
polypropylene ampules fitting both Luer-lock and Luer-slip (tapered) syringes

2.0 mg/mL (0.2%)	10 mL	NDC 0186-0859-47	
		Product No. 0186-0859-44	
2.0 mg/mL (0.2%)	20 mL	NDC 0186-0859-57	
		Product No. 0186-0859-54	
5.0 mg/mL (0.5%)	10 mL	NDC 0186-0863-47	
		Product No. 0186-0863-44	
5.0 mg/mL (0.5%)	20 mL	NDC 0186-0863-57	
		Product No. 0186-0863-54	
7.5 mg/mL (0.75%)	10 mL	NDC 0186-0867-47	
		Product No. 0186-0867-44	
7.5 mg/mL (0.75%)	20 mL	NDC 0186-0867-57	
		Product No. 0186-0867-54	
10.0 mg/mL (1.0%)	10 mL	NDC 0186-0868-47	
		Product No. 0186-0868-44	
10.0 mg/mL (1.0%)	20 mL	NDC 0186-0868-57	
		Product No. 0186-0868-54	

Naropin® Single Dose Vials:

2.0 mg/mL (0.2%)	20 mL	NDC 0186-0859-51
5.0 mg/mL (0.5%)	30 mL	NDC 0186-0863-61
7.5 mg/mL (0.75%)	20 mL	NDC 0186-0867-51
10.0 mg/mL (1.0%)	20 mL	NDC 0186-0868-51

Naropin® E-Z OFF® Single Dose Vials:

7.5 mg/mL (0.75%)	10 mL	NDC 0186-0867-41
10.0 mg/mL (1.0%)	10 mL	NDC 0186-0868-41

Naropin® Single Dose Ampules:

2.0 mg/mL (0.2%)	20 mL	NDC 0186-0859-52
5.0 mg/mL (0.5%)	30 mL	NDC 0186-0863-62
7.5 mg/mL (0.75%)	20 mL	NDC 0186-0867-52
10.0 mg/mL (1.0%)	20 mL	NDC 0186-0868-52

Naropin® Single Dose Infusion Bottles:

2.0 mg/mL (0.2%)	100 mL	NDC 0186-0859-81
2.0 mg/mL (0.2%)	200 mL	NDC 0186-0859-91

Naropin® Sterile-Pak Single Dose Vials:
Boxes of 5:

2.0 mg/mL (0.2%)	20 mL	NDC 0186-0859-51
		Product No. 0186-0859-59
5.0 mg/mL (0.5%)	30 mL	NDC 0186-0863-61
		Product No. 0186-0863-69
7.5 mg/mL (0.75%)	20 mL	NDC 0186-0867-51
		Product No. 0186-0867-59
10.0 mg/mL (1.0%)	20 mL	NDC 0186-0868-51
		Product No. 0186-0868-59

When prolonged blocks are used, either through continuous infusion or through repeated bolus administration, the risks of reaching a toxic plasma concentration or inducing local neural injury must be considered. Experience to date indicates that a cumulative dose of up to 770 mg Naropin administered over 24 hours is well tolerated in adults when used for postoperative pain management: ie, 2016 mg. Caution should be exercised when administering Naropin for prolonged periods of time, eg, >70 hours in debilitated patients.

For treatment of postoperative pain, the following technique can be recommended: If regional anesthesia was not used intraoperatively, then an initial epidural block with 5–7 mL Naropin is induced via an epidural catheter. Analgesia is maintained with an infusion of Naropin, 2 mg/mL (0.2%). Clinical studies have demonstrated that infusion rates of 6–14 mL (12–28 mg) per hour provide adequate analgesia with nonprogressive motor block. With this technique a significant reduction in the need for opioids was demonstrated. Clinical experience supports the use of Naropin epidural infusions for up to 72 hours.

HOW SUPPLIED

[See table at bottom of previous page]
The solubility of ropivacaine is limited at pH above 6. Thus care must be taken as precipitation may occur if Naropin is mixed with alkaline solutions.

Disinfecting agents containing heavy metals, which cause release of respective ions (mercury, zinc, copper, etc.) should not be used for skin or mucous membrane disinfection since they have been related to incidents of swelling and edema. When chemical disinfection of the container surface is desired, either isopropyl alcohol (91%) or ethyl alcohol (70%) is recommended. It is recommended that chemical disinfection be accomplished by wiping the ampule or vial stopper thoroughly with cotton or gauze that has been moistened with the recommended alcohol just prior to use. When a container is required to have a sterile outside, a Sterile-Pak should be chosen. Glass containers may, as an alternative, be autoclaved once. Stability has been demonstrated using a targeted F_0 of 7 minutes at 121°C.

Solutions should be stored at controlled room temperature 20–25°C (68–77°F) [see USP].

These products are intended for single use and are free from preservatives. Any solution remaining from an opened container should be discarded promptly. In addition, continuous infusion bottles should not be left in place for more than 24 hours.

All trademarks are the property of the AstraZeneca group
©AstraZeneca 2001
AstraZeneca LP, Wilmington, DE 19850

TABLETS
PLENDIL®
(Felodipine)
EXTENDED-RELEASE TABLETS

℞

Prescribing information for this product, which appears on pages 585–587 of the 2001 PDR, has been revised as follows. Please write "See Supplement A" next to the product heading.

- PRECAUTIONS, Carcinogenesis, Mutagenesis, Impairment of Fertility—fifth paragraph, second line, insert the words " (up to 24 times the maximum recommended human dose on a mg/m^2 basis)" after 26.9 mg/kg/day and before the word showed.
- PRECAUTIONS, Pregnancy—first paragraph, second line, change "0.5 to 5 times" to read "0.8 to 8 times". In the 3rd paragraph, 3rd line, at the beginning of the parentheses change "(1.4" to "(2.1".

POLOCAINE®

℞

[pō'-lō-caine"]
(Mepivacaine Hydrochloride Injection, USP)

POLOCAINE®-MPF
(Mepivacaine Hydrochloride Injection, USP)
THESE SOLUTIONS ARE NOT INTENDED FOR SPINAL ANESTHESIA OR DENTAL USE
Rx only

Prescribing information for this product, which appears on pages 587 of the 2001 PDR, has been completely revised as follows. Please write "See Supplement A" next to the product heading.

DESCRIPTION

Mepivacaine hydrochloride is 2-Piperidinecarboxamide, N-(2,6-dimethylphenyl)-1-methyl-, monohydrochloride and has the following structural formula:

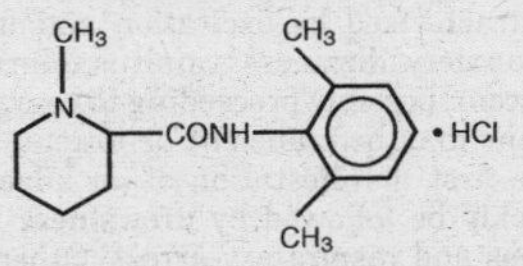

The molecular formula is $C_{15}H_{22}N_2O \cdot HCl$.
It is a white, crystalline odorless, powder, soluble in water, but very resistant to both acid and alkaline hydrolysis.
Mepivacaine hydrochloride is a local anesthetic available as sterile isotonic solutions (clear, colorless) in concentrations of 1%, 1.5% and 2% for injection via local infiltration, peripheral nerve block, and caudal and lumbar epidural blocks.

Mepivacaine hydrochloride is related chemically and pharmacologically to the amide-type local anesthetics. It contains an amide linkage between the aromatic nucleus and the amino group.
[See table above]
The pH of the solution is adjusted between 4.5 and 6.8 with sodium hydroxide or hydrochloric acid.

CLINICAL PHARMACOLOGY

Local anesthetics block the generation and the conduction of nerve impulses, presumably by increasing the threshold for electrical excitation in the nerve, by slowing the propagation of the nerve impulse, and by reducing the rate of rise of the action potential. In general, the progression of anesthesia is related to the diameter, myelination, and conduction velocity of affected nerve fibers. Clinically, the order of loss of nerve function is as follows: pain, temperature, touch, proprioception, and skeletal muscle tone.

Systemic absorption of local anesthetics produces effects on the cardiovascular and central nervous systems. At blood concentrations achieved with normal therapeutic doses, changes in cardiac conduction, excitability, refractoriness, contractility, and peripheral vascular resistance are minimal. However, toxic blood concentrations depress cardiac conduction and excitability, which may lead to atrioventricular block and ultimately to cardiac arrest. In addition, myocardial contractility is depressed and peripheral vasodilation occurs, leading to decreased cardiac output and arterial blood pressure.

Following systemic absorption, local anesthetics can produce central nervous system stimulation, depression, or both. Apparent central stimulation is manifested as restlessness, tremors, and shivering, progressing to convulsions, followed by depression and coma progressing ultimately to respiratory arrest. However, the local anesthetics have a primary depressant effect on the medulla and on higher centers. The depressed stage may occur without a prior excited stage.

A clinical study using 15 mL of 2% epidural mepivacaine at the T 9-10 interspace in 62 patients, 20–79 years of age, demonstrated a 40% decrease in the amount of mepivacaine required to block a given number of dermatomes in the elderly (60–79 years, N=13) as compared to young adults 20–39 years).

Another study using 10 mL of 2% lumbar epidural mepivacaine in 161 patients, 19–75 years of age, demonstrated a strong inverse relationship between patient age and the number of dermatomes blocked per cc of mepivacaine injected.

Pharmacokinetics

The rate of systemic absorption of local anesthetics is dependent upon the total dose and concentration of drug administered, the route of administration, the vascularity of the administration site, and the presence or absence of epinephrine in the anesthetic solution. A dilute concentration of epinephrine (1:200,000 or 5µg/mL) usually reduces the rate of absorption and plasma concentration of mepivacaine, however, it has been reported that vasoconstrictors do not significantly prolong anesthesia with mepivacaine.

Onset of anesthesia with mepivacaine is rapid, the time of onset for sensory block ranging from about 3 to 20 minutes depending upon such factors as the anesthetic technique, the type of block, the concentration of the solution, and the individual patient. The degree of motor blockade produced is dependent on the concentration of the solution. A 0.5% solution will be effective in small superficial nerve blocks while the 1% concentration will block sensory and sympathetic conduction without loss of motor function. The 1.5% solution will provide extensive and often complete motor block and the 2% concentration of mepivacaine hydrochloride will produce complete sensory and motor block of any nerve group. The duration of anesthesia also varies depending upon the technique and type of block, the concentration, and the individual. Mepivacaine will normally provide anesthesia which is adequate for 2 to 2½ hours of surgery. Local anesthetics are bound to plasma proteins in varying degrees. Generally, the lower the plasma concentration of drug, the higher the percentage of drug bound to plasma.

Local anesthetics appear to cross the placenta by passive diffusion. The rate and degree of diffusion is governed by the degree of plasma protein binding, the degree of ionization, and the degree of lipid solubility. Fetal/maternal ratios of local anesthetics appear to be inversely related to the degree of plasma protein binding, because only the free, unbound drug is available for placental transfer. Mepivacaine is approximately 75% bound to plasma proteins. The extent of placental transfer is also determined by the degree of ionization and lipid solubility of the drug. Lipid soluble, nonionized drugs readily enter the fetal blood from the maternal circulation. Depending upon the route of administration, local anesthetics are distributed to some extent to all body tissues, with high concentrations found in highly perfused organs such as the liver, lungs, heart, and brain.

Various pharmacokinetic parameters of the local anesthetics can be significantly altered by the presence of hepatic or renal disease, addition of epinephrine, factors affecting urinary pH, renal blood flow, the route of drug administration, and the age of the patient. The half-life of mepivacaine in adults is 1.9 to 3.2 hours and in neonates 8.7 to 9 hours.

Mepivacaine, because of its amide structure, is not detoxified by the circulating plasma esterases. It is rapidly metabolized, with only a small percentage of the anesthetic (5 percent to 10 percent) being excreted unchanged in the urine. The liver is the principal site of metabolism, with over 50% of the administered dose being excreted into the bile as metabolites. Most of the metabolized mepivacaine is probably resorbed in the intestine and then excreted into the urine since only a small percentage is found in the feces. The principal route of excretion is via the kidney. Most of the anesthetic and its metabolites are eliminated within 30 hours. It has been shown that hydroxylation and N-demethylation, which are detoxification reactions, play important roles in the metabolism of the anesthetic. Three metabolites of mepivacaine have been identified from human adults: two phenols, which are excreted almost exclusively as their glucuronide conjugates, and the N-demethylated compound (2',6'-pipecoloxylidide).

Mepivacaine does not ordinarily produce irritation or tissue damage, and does not cause methemoglobinemia when administered in recommended doses and concentrations.

INDICATIONS AND USAGE

POLOCAINE (Mepivacaine HCl Injection, USP), is indicated for production of local or regional analgesia and anesthesia by local infiltration, peripheral nerve block techniques, and central neural techniques including epidural and caudal blocks.

The routes of administration and indicated concentrations for mepivacaine are:

local infiltration	0.5% (via dilution) or 1%
peripheral nerve blocks	1% and 2%
epidural block	1%, 1.5%, 2%
caudal block	1%, 1.5%, 2%

See DOSAGE AND ADMINISTRATION for additional information. Standard textbooks should be consulted to determine the accepted procedures and techniques for the administration of mepivacaine.

CONTRAINDICATIONS

Mepivacaine is contraindicated in patients with a known hypersensitivity to it or to any local anesthetic agent of the amide-type or to other components of mepivacaine solutions.

WARNINGS

LOCAL ANESTHETICS SHOULD ONLY BE EMPLOYED BY CLINICIANS WHO ARE WELL VERSED IN DIAGNOSIS AND MANAGEMENT OF DOSE-RELATED TOXICITY AND OTHER ACUTE EMERGENCIES WHICH MIGHT ARISE FROM THE BLOCK TO BE EMPLOYED, AND THEN ONLY AFTER INSURING THE IMMEDIATE AVAILABILITY OF OXYGEN, OTHER RESUSCITATIVE DRUGS, CARDIOPULMONARY RESUSCITATIVE EQUIPMENT, AND THE PERSONNEL RESOURCES NEEDED FOR PROPER MANAGEMENT OF TOXIC REACTIONS AND RELATED EMERGENCIES. (See also ADVERSE REACTIONS and PRECAUTIONS.) DELAY IN PROPER MANAGEMENT OF DOSE-RELATED TOXICITY, UNDERVENTILATION FROM ANY CAUSE, AND/OR ALTERED SENSITIVITY MAY LEAD TO THE DEVELOPMENT OF ACIDOSIS, CARDIAC ARREST AND, POSSIBLY, DEATH.

Local anesthetic solutions containing antimicrobial preservatives (ie, those supplied in multiple-dose vials) should not be used for epidural or caudal anesthesia because safety has not been established with regard to intrathecal injection, either intentionally or inadvertently, of such preservatives.

It is essential that aspiration for blood or cerebrospinal fluid (where applicable) be done prior to injecting any local anesthetic, both the original dose and all subsequent doses, to avoid intravascular or subarachnoid injection. However, a negative aspiration does not ensure against an intravascular or subarachnoid injection.

Reactions resulting in fatality have occurred on rare occasions with the use of local anesthetics.

Mepivacaine with epinephrine or other vasopressors should not be used concomitantly with ergot-type oxytocic drugs, because a severe persistent hypertension may result. Likewise, solutions of mepivacaine containing a vasoconstrictor, such as epinephrine, should be used with extreme caution in patients receiving monoamine oxidase inhibitors (MAOI) or antidepressants of the triptyline or imipramine types, because severe prolonged hypertension may result.

Local anesthetic procedures should be used with caution when there is inflammation and/or sepsis in the region of the proposed injection.

Continued on next page

Composition of Available Solutions*

	1% Single Dose 30 mL Vial mg/mL	1% Multiple Dose 50 mL Vial mg/mL	1.5% Single Dose 30 mL Vial mg/mL	2% Single Dose 20 mL Vial mg/mL	2% Multiple Dose 50 mL Vial mg/mL
Mepivacaine hychrochloride	10	10	15	20	20
Sodium chloride	6.6	7	5.6	4.6	5
Potassium chloride	0.3		0.3	0.3	
Calcium chloride	0.33		0.33	0.33	
Methylparaben		1			1

*In Water For Injection

Polocaine—Cont.

Mixing or the prior or intercurrent use of any local anesthetic with mepivacaine cannot be recommended because of insufficient data on the clinical use of such mixtures.

PRECAUTIONS

General

The safety and effectiveness of local anesthetics depend on proper dosage, correct technique, adequate precautions, and readiness for emergencies. Resuscitative equipment, oxygen, and other resuscitative drugs should be available for immediate use. (See WARNINGS and ADVERSE REACTIONS.) During major regional nerve blocks, the patient should have IV fluids running via an indwelling catheter to assure a functioning intravenous pathway. The lowest dosage of local anesthetic that results in effective anesthesia should be used to avoid high plasma levels and serious adverse effects. Injections should be made slowly, with frequent aspirations before and during the injection to avoid intravascular injection. Current opinion favors fractional administration with constant attention to the patient, rather than rapid bolus injection. Syringe aspirations should also be performed before and during each supplemental injection in continuous (intermittent) catheter techniques. An intravascular injection is still possible even if aspirations for blood are negative.

During the administration of epidural anesthesia, it is recommended that a test dose be administered initially and the effects monitored before the full dose is given. When using a "continuous" catheter technique, test doses should be given prior to both the original and all reinforcing doses, because plastic tubing in the epidural space can migrate into a blood vessel or through the dura. When the clinical conditions permit, an effective test dose should contain epinephrine (10 µg to 15 µg have been suggested) to serve as a warning of unintended intravascular injection. If injected into a blood vessel, this amount of epinephrine is likely to produce an "epinephrine response" within 45 seconds, consisting of an increase of pulse and blood pressure, circumoral pallor, palpitations, and nervousness in the unsedated patient. The sedated patient may exhibit only a pulse rate increase of 20 or more beats per minute for 15 or more seconds. Therefore, following the test dose, the heart rate should be monitored for a heart rate increase. The test dose should also contain 45 mg to 50 mg of mepivacaine hydrochloride to detect an unintended intrathecal administration. This will be evidenced within a few minutes by signs of spinal block (eg, decreased sensation of the buttocks, paresis of the legs, or, in the sedated patient, absent knee jerk).

Injection of repeated doses of local anesthetics may cause significant increases in plasma levels with each repeated dose due to slow accumulation of the drug or its metabolites or to slow metabolic degradation. Tolerance to elevated blood levels varies with the status of the patient. Debilitated, elderly patients, and acutely ill patients should be given reduced doses commensurate with their age and physical status. Local anesthetics should also be used with caution in patients with severe disturbances of cardiac rhythm, shock, heart block, or hypotension.

Careful and constant monitoring of cardiovascular and respiratory (adequacy of ventilation) vital signs, and the patient's state of consciousness should be performed after each local anesthetic injection. It should be kept in mind at such times that restlessness, anxiety, incoherent speech, lightheadedness, numbness and tingling of the mouth and lips, metallic taste, tinnitus, dizziness, blurred vision, tremors, twitching, depression, or drowsiness may be early warning signs of central nervous system toxicity.

Local anesthetic solutions containing a vasoconstrictor should be used cautiously and in carefully restricted quantities in areas of the body supplied by end arteries or having otherwise compromised blood supply such as digits, nose, external ear, penis. Patients with hypertensive vascular disease may exhibit exaggerated vasoconstrictor response. Ischemic injury or necrosis may result.

Mepivacaine should be used with caution in patients with known allergies and sensitivities.

Because amide-type local anesthetics such as mepivacaine are metabolized by the liver and excreted by the kidneys, these drugs, especially repeat doses, should be used cautiously in patients with hepatic and renal disease. Patients with severe hepatic disease, because of their inability to metabolize local anesthetics normally, are at greater risk of developing toxic plasma concentrations. Local anesthetics should also be used with caution in patients with impaired cardiovascular function because they may be less able to compensate for functional changes associated with the prolongation of AV conduction produced by these drugs.

Serious dose-related cardiac arrhythmias may occur if preparations containing a vasoconstrictor such as epinephrine are employed in patients during or following the administration of potent inhalation anesthetics. In deciding whether to use these products concurrently in the same patient, the combined action of both agents upon the myocardium, the concentration and volume of vasoconstrictor used, and the time since injection, when applicable, should be taken into account.

Many drugs used during the conduct of anesthesia are considered potential triggering agents for familial malignant hyperthermia. Because it is not known whether amide-type local anesthetics may trigger this reaction and because the need for supplemental general anesthesia cannot be predicted in advance, it is suggested that a standard protocol for management should be available. Early unexplained signs of tachycardia, tachypnea, labile blood pressure, and metabolic acidosis may precede temperature elevation. Successful outcome is dependent on early diagnosis, prompt discontinuance of the suspect triggering agent(s), and institution of treatment, including oxygen therapy, indicated supportive measures, and dantrolene. (Consult dantrolene sodium intravenous package insert before using.)

Use in Head and Neck Area

Small doses of local anesthetics injected into the head and neck area may produce adverse reactions similar to systemic toxicity seen with unintentional intravascular injections of larger doses. The injection procedures require the utmost care.

Confusion, convulsions, respiratory depression, and/or respiratory arrest, and cardiovascular stimulation or depression have been reported. These reactions may be due to intra-arterial injection of the local anesthetic with retrograde flow to the cerebral circulation. Patients receiving these blocks should have their circulation and respiration monitored and be constantly observed. Resuscitative equipment and personnel for treating adverse reactions should be immediately available. Dosage recommendations should not be exceeded.

Information for Patients

When appropriate, patients should be informed in advance that they may experience temporary loss of sensation and motor activity, usually in the lower half of the body, following proper administration of caudal or epidural anesthesia. Also, when appropriate, the physician should discuss other information including adverse reactions listed in this package insert.

Clinically Significant Drug Interactions

The administration of local anesthetic solutions containing epinephrine or norepinephrine to patients receiving monoamine oxidase inhibitors or tricyclic antidepressants may produce severe, prolonged hypertension. Concurrent use of these agents should generally be avoided. In situations when concurrent therapy is necessary, careful patient monitoring is essential.

Concurrent administration of vasopressor drugs and of ergot-type oxytocic drugs may cause severe, persistent hypertension or cerebrovascular accidents.

Phenothiazines and butyrophenones may reduce or reverse the pressor effect of epinephrine.

Carcinogenesis, Mutagenesis, and Impairment of Fertility

Long-term studies in animals of most local anesthetics including mepivacaine to evaluate the carcinogenic potential have not been conducted. Mutagenic potential or the effect on fertility have not been determined. There is no evidence from human data that mepivacaine may be carcinogenic or mutagenic or that it impairs fertility.

Pregnancy Category C

Animal reproduction studies have not been conducted with mepivacaine. There are no adequate and well-controlled studies in pregnant women of the effect of mepivacaine on the developing fetus. Mepivacaine hydrochloride should be used during pregnancy only if the potential benefit justifies the potential risk to the fetus. This does not preclude the use of mepivacaine at term for obstetrical anesthesia or analgesia. (See Labor and Delivery.)

Mepivacaine has been used for obstetrical analgesia by the epidural, caudal, and paracervical routes without evidence of adverse effects on the fetus when no more than the maximum safe dosages are used and strict adherence to technique is followed.

Labor and Delivery

Local anesthetics rapidly cross the placenta, and when used for epidural, paracervical, caudal, or pudendal block anesthesia, can cause varying degrees of maternal, fetal, and neonatal toxicity. (See Pharmacokinetics—CLINICAL PHARMACOLOGY.) The incidence and degree of toxicity depend upon the procedure performed, the type and amount of drug used, and the technique of drug administration. Adverse reactions in the parturient, fetus, and neonate involve alterations of the central nervous system, peripheral vascular tone, and cardiac function.

Maternal hypotension has resulted from regional anesthesia. Local anesthetics produce vasodilation by blocking sympathetic nerves. Elevating the patient's legs and positioning her on her left side will help prevent decreases in blood pressure. The fetal heart rate also should be monitored continuously and electronic fetal monitoring is highly advisable.

Epidural, paracervical, caudal, or pudendal anesthesia may alter the forces of parturition through changes in uterine contractility or maternal expulsive efforts. In one study, paracervical block anesthesia was associated with a decrease in the mean duration of first stage labor and facilitation of cervical dilation. Epidural anesthesia has been reported to prolong the second stage of labor by removing the parturient's reflex urge to bear down or by interfering with motor function. The use of obstetrical anesthesia may increase the need for forceps assistance.

The use of some local anesthetic drug products during labor and delivery may be followed by diminished muscle strength and tone for the first day or two of life. The long-term significance of these observations is unknown.

Fetal bradycardia may occur in 20 to 30 percent of patients receiving paracervical block anesthesia with the amide-type local anesthetics and may be associated with fetal acidosis. Fetal heart rate should always be monitored during paracervical anesthesia. Added risk appears to be present in prematurity, postmaturity, toxemia of pregnancy, and fetal distress. The physician should weigh the possible advantages against dangers when considering paracervical block in these conditions. Careful adherence to recommended dosage is of the utmost importance in obstetrical paracervical block. Failure to achieve adequate analgesia with recommended doses should arouse suspicion of intravascular or fetal intracranial injection.

Cases compatible with unintended fetal intracranial injection of local anesthetic solution have been reported following intended paracervical or pudendal block or both. Babies so affected present with unexplained neonatal depression at birth which correlates with high local anesthetic serum levels and usually manifest seizures within six hours. Prompt use of supportive measures combined with forced urinary excretion of the local anesthetic has been used successfully to manage this complication.

Case reports of maternal convulsions and cardiovascular collapse following use of some local anesthetics for paracervical block in early pregnancy (as anesthesia for elective abortion) suggest that systemic absorption under these circumstances may be rapid. The recommended maximum dose of the local anesthetic should not be exceeded. Injection should be made slowly and with frequent aspiration. Allow a five-minute interval between sides.

It is extremely important to avoid aortocaval compression by the gravid uterus during administration of regional block to parturients. To do this, the patient must be maintained in the left lateral decubitus position or a blanket roll or sandbag may be placed beneath the right hip and the gravid uterus displaced to the left.

Nursing Mothers

It is not known whether local anesthetic drugs are excreted in human milk. Because many drugs are excreted in human milk, caution should be exercised when local anesthetics are administered to a nursing woman.

Pediatric Use

Guidelines for the administration of mepivacaine to pediatric patients are presented in DOSAGE AND ADMINISTRATION.

Geriatric Use

Clinical studies and other reported clinical experience indicates that use of the drug in elderly patients requires a decreased dosage. (See CLINICAL PHARMACOLOGY, PRECAUTIONS, General, and DOSAGE AND ADMINISTRATION).

Mepivacaine and mepivacaine metabolites are known to be substantially excreted by the kidney, and the risk of toxic reactions to this drug may be greater in patients with impaired renal function. Because elderly patients are more likely to have decreased renal function, care should be taken in dose selection, and it may be useful to monitor renal function.

ADVERSE REACTIONS

Reactions to mepivacaine are characteristic of those associated with other amide-type local anesthetics. A major cause of adverse reactions to this group of drugs is excessive plasma levels, which may be due to overdosage, inadvertent intravascular injection, or slow metabolic degradation.

Systemic

The most commonly encountered acute adverse experiences which demand immediate countermeasures are related to the central nervous system and the cardiovascular system. These adverse experiences are generally dose related and due to high plasma levels which may result from overdosage, rapid absorption from the injection site, diminished tolerance, or from unintentional intravascular injection of the local anesthetic solution. In addition to systemic dose-related toxicity, unintentional subarachnoid injection of drug during the intended performance of caudal or lumbar epidural block or nerve blocks near the vertebral column (especially in the head and neck region) may result in underventilation or apnea ("Total or High Spinal"). Also, hypotension due to loss of sympathetic tone and respiratory paralysis or underventilation due to cephalad extension of the motor level of anesthesia may occur. This may lead to secondary cardiac arrest if untreated. Factors influencing plasma protein binding, such as acidosis, systemic diseases which alter protein production, or competition of other drugs for protein binding sites, may diminish individual tolerance.

Central Nervous System Reactions

These are characterized by excitation and/or depression. Restlessness, anxiety, dizziness, tinnitus, blurred vision, or tremors may occur, possibly proceeding to convulsions. However, excitement may be transient or absent, with depression being the first manifestation of an adverse reaction. This may quickly be followed by drowsiness merging into unconsciousness and respiratory arrest. Other central nervous system effects may be nausea, vomiting, chills, and constriction of the pupils.

The incidence of convulsions associated with the use of local anesthetics varies with the procedure used and the total dose administered. In a survey of studies of epidural anesthesia, overt toxicity progressing to convulsions occurred in approximately 0.1% of local anesthetic administrations.

Cardiovascular Reactions

High doses or, inadvertent intravascular injection, may lead to high plasma levels and related depression of the myocardium, decreased cardiac output, heart block, hypotension (or sometimes hypertension), bradycardia, ventricular arrhythmias, and possibly cardiac arrest. (See WARNINGS, PRECAUTIONS, and OVERDOSAGE sections.)

Allergic

Allergic-type reactions are rare and may occur as a result of sensitivity to the local anesthetic or to other formulation ingredients, such as the antimicrobial preservative methylparaben, contained in multiple-dose vials. These reactions are characterized by signs such as urticaria, pruritus, erythema, angioneurotic edema (including laryngeal edema), tachycardia, sneezing, nausea, vomiting, dizziness, syncope, excessive sweating, elevated temperature, and possibly, anaphylactoid-like symptomatology (including severe hypotension). Cross sensitivity among members of the amide-type local anesthetic group has been reported. The usefulness of screening for sensitivity has not been definitely established.

Neurologic

The incidences of adverse neurologic reactions associated with the use of local anesthetics may be related to the total dose of local anesthetic administered and are also dependent upon the particular drug used, the route of administration, and the physical status of the patient. Many of these effects may be related to local anesthetic techniques, with or without a contribution from the drug.

In the practice of caudal or lumbar epidural block, occasional unintentional penetration of the subarachnoid space by the catheter or needle may occur. Subsequent adverse effects may depend partially on the amount of drug administered intrathecally and the physiological and physical effects of a dural puncture. A high spinal is characterized by paralysis of the legs, loss of consciousness, respiratory paralysis, and bradycardia.

Neurologic effects following epidural or caudal anesthesia may include spinal block of varying magnitude (including high or total spinal block); hypotension secondary to spinal block; urinary retention; fecal and urinary incontinence; loss of perineal sensation and sexual function; persistent anesthesia, paresthesia, weakness, paralysis of the lower extremities, and loss of sphincter control all of which may have slow, incomplete, or no recovery; headache; backache; septic meningitis; meningismus; slowing of labor; increased incidence of forceps delivery; cranial nerve palsies due to traction on nerves from loss of cerebrospinal fluid.

Neurologic effects following other procedures or routes of administration may include persistent anesthesia, paresthesia, weakness, paralysis, all of which may have slow, incomplete or no recovery.

OVERDOSAGE

Acute emergencies from local anesthetics are generally related to high plasma levels encountered during therapeutic use of local anesthetics or to unintended subarachnoid injection of local anesthetic solution. (See ADVERSE REACTIONS, WARNINGS, and PRECAUTIONS.)

Management of Local Anesthetic Emergencies

The first consideration is prevention, best accomplished by careful and constant monitoring of cardiovascular and respiratory vital signs and the patients state of consciousness after each local anesthetic injection. At the first sign of change, oxygen should be administered.

The first step in the management of systemic toxic reactions, as well as underventilation or apnea due to unintentional subarachnoid injection of drug solution, consists of immediate attention to the establishment and maintenance of a patent airway and effective assisted or controlled ventilation with a delivery system capable of permitting immediate positive airway pressure by mask. This may prevent convulsions if they have not already occurred. If necessary, use drugs to control the convulsions. A 50 mg to 100 mg bolus IV injection of succinylcholine will paralyze the patient without depressing the central nervous or cardiovascular systems and facilitate ventilation. A bolus IV dose of 5 mg to 10 mg of diazepam or 50 mg to 100 mg of thiopental will permit ventilation and counteract central nervous system stimulation, but these drugs also depress central nervous system, respiratory, and cardiac function, add to postictal depression and may result in apnea. Intravenous barbiturates, anticonvulsant agents, or muscle relaxants should only be administered by those familiar with their use. Immediately after the institution of these ventilatory measures, the adequacy of the circulation should be evaluated. Supportive treatment of circulatory depression may require administration of intravenous fluids, and when appropriate, a vasopressor dictated by the clinical situation (such as ephedrine or epinephrine to enhance myocardial contractile force).

Endotracheal intubation, employing drugs and techniques familiar to the clinician may be indicated after initial administration of oxygen by mask, if difficulty is encountered in the maintenance of patent airway or if prolonged ventilatory support (assisted or controlled) is indicated.

Recent clinical data from patients experiencing local anesthetic induced convulsions demonstrated rapid development of hypoxia, hypercarbia, and acidosis within a minute of the onset of convulsions. These observations suggest that oxygen consumption and carbon dioxide production are greatly increased during local anesthetic convulsions and emphasize the importance of immediate and effective ventilation with oxygen which may avoid cardiac arrest.

If not treated immediately, convulsions with simultaneous hypoxia, hypercarbia, and acidosis, plus myocardial depression from the direct effects of the local anesthetic may result in cardiac arrhythmias, bradycardia, asystole, ventricular fibrillation, or cardiac arrest. Respiratory abnormalities, including apnea, may occur. Underventilation or apnea due to unintentional subarachnoid injection of local anesthetic solution may produce these same signs and also lead to cardiac arrest if ventilatory support is not instituted. If cardiac arrest should occur, standard cardiopulmonary resuscitative measures should be instituted and maintained for a prolonged period if necessary. Recovery has been reported after prolonged resuscitative efforts.

The supine position is dangerous in pregnant women at term because of aortocaval compression by the gravid uterus. Therefore, during treatment of systemic toxicity, maternal hypotension, or fetal bradycardia following regional block, the parturient should be maintained in the left lateral decubitus position if possible, or manual displacement of the uterus off the great vessels should be accomplished.

The mean seizure dosage of mepivacaine in rhesus monkeys was found to be 18.8 mg/kg with mean arterial plasma concentration of 24.4 μg/mL. The intravenous and subcutaneous LD_{50} in mice is 23 mg/kg to 35 mg/kg and 280 mg/kg respectively.

DOSAGE AND ADMINISTRATION

The dose of any local anesthetic administered varies with the anesthetic procedure, the area to be anesthetized, the vascularity of the tissues, the number of neuronal segments to be blocked, the depth of anesthesia and degree of muscle relaxation required, the duration of anesthesia desired, individual tolerance and the physical condition of the patient. The smallest dose and concentration required to produce the desired result should be administered. Dosages of mepivacaine hydrochloride should be reduced for elderly and debilitated patients and patients with cardiac and/or liver disease. The rapid injection of a large volume of local anesthetic solution should be avoided and fractional doses should be used when feasible.

For specific techniques and procedures, refer to standard textbooks.

The recommended single *adult* dose (or the total of a series of doses given in one procedure) of mepivacaine hydrochloride for unsedated, healthy, normal-sized individuals should not usually exceed 400 mg. The recommended dosage is based on requirements for the average adult and should be reduced for elderly or debilitated patients.

While maximum doses of 7 mg/kg (550 mg) have been administered without adverse effect, these are not recommended, except in exceptional circumstances and under no circumstances should the administration be repeated at intervals of less than 1½ hours. The total dose for any 24-hour period should not exceed 1,000 mg because of a slow accumulation of the anesthetic or its derivatives or slower than normal metabolic degradation or detoxification with repeat administration. (See CLINICAL PHARMACOLOGY and PRECAUTIONS.)

Pediatric patients tolerate the local anesthetic as well as adults. However, the pediatric dose should be *carefully measured* as a percentage of the total adult dose *based on weight*, and should not exceed 5 mg/kg to 6 mg/kg (2.5 mg/lb to 3 mg/lb) in pediatric patients, especially those weighing less than 30 lbs. In pediatric patients *under 3 years of age or weighing less than 30 lbs* concentrations less than 2% (eg, 0.5% to 1.5%) should be employed.

Unused portions of solutions not containing preservatives, ie, those supplied in single-dose vials, should be discarded following initial use. This product should be inspected visually for particulate matter and discoloration prior to administration whenever solution and container permit. Solutions which are discolored or which contain particulate matter should not be administered.
[See table above]

HOW SUPPLIED

Single-dose vials and multiple-dose vials of POLOCAINE may be sterilized by autoclaving at 15 pound pressure, 121°C (250°F) for 15 minutes. Solutions of POLOCAINE may be reautoclaved when necessary. Do not administer solutions which are discolored or which contain particulate matter.

THESE SOLUTIONS ARE NOT INTENDED FOR SPINAL ANESTHESIA OR DENTAL USE.

POLOCAINE-MPF (Mepivacaine HCl Injection, USP) without preservatives is available as follows:
1%   Single-dose vials of 30 mL (NDC 0186-0412-01)
1.5% Single-dose vials of 30 mL (NDC 0186-0418-01)
2%   Single-dose vials of 20 mL (NDC 0186-0422-01)
POLOCAINE (Mepivacaine HCl Injection, USP) with preservatives is available as follows:
1%   Multiple-dose vials of 50 mL (NDC 0186-0410-01)
2%   Multiple-dose vials of 50 mL (NDC 0186-0420-01)
Store at controlled room temperature 15–30°C (59–86°F); brief exposure up to 40°C (104°F) does not adversely affect the product.
All trademarks are the property of the AstraZeneca group
© AstraZeneca 2000
AstraZeneca LP, Wilmington, DE 19850
721668-01
Rev. 11/00

SENSORCAINE®   ℞
[sén-sor-caine]
(bupivacaine HCl Injection, USP)

SENSORCAINE®–MPF
(bupivacaine HCl Injection, USP)

SENSORCAINE® with Epinephrine
(bupivacaine HCl and epinephrine Injection, USP)
1:200,000 (as bitartrate)

SENSORCAINE®–MPF with Epinephrine
(bupivacaine HCl and epinephrine Injection, USP)
1:200,000 (as bitartrate)

Prescribing information for this product, which appears on pages 599–602 of the 2001 PDR, has been completely revised as follows. Please write "See Supplement A" next to the product heading.
Rx only

Continued on next page

Recommended Concentrations and Doses of Mepivacaine Hydrochloride

Procedure	Concentration	Total Dose mL	mg	Comments
Cervical, branchial, intercostal, pudendal nerve block	1%	5–40	50–400	Pudendal block: one half of total dose injected each side.
	2%	5–20	100–400	
Transvaginal block (paracervical plus pudendal)	1%	up to 30 (both sides)	up to 300 (both sides)	One half of total dose injected each side. See PRECAUTIONS.
Paracervical block	1%	up to 20 (both sides)	up to 200 (both sides)	One half of total dose injected each side. This is maximum recommended dose per 90-minute period in obstetrical and non-obstetrical patients. Inject slowly, 5 minutes between sides. See PRECAUTIONS.
Caudal and Epidural block	1%	15–30	150–300	*Use only single-dose vials which do not contain a preservative.
	1.5%	10–25	150–375	
	2%	10–20	200–400	
Infiltration	1%	up to 40	up to 400	An equivalent amount of a 0.5% solution (prepared by diluting the 1% solution with Sodium Chloride Injection, USP) may be used for large areas.
Therapeutic block (pain management)	1%	1–5	10–50	
	2%	1–5	20–100	

Unused portions of solutions not containing preservatives should be discarded

*Dosage forms listed as POLOCAINE-MPF (Mepivacaine HCl Injection, USP) are single-dose solutions which do not contain a preservative.

Sensorcaine—Cont.

DESCRIPTION

Sensorcaine® (bupivacaine HCl) injections are sterile isotonic solutions that contain a local anesthetic agent with and without epinephrine (as bitartrate) 1:200,000 and are administered parenterally by injection. See INDICATIONS AND USAGE for specific uses. Solutions of bupivacaine HCl may be autoclaved if they do not contain epinephrine.
Sensorcaine injections contain bupivacaine HCl which is chemically designated as 2-piperidinecarboxamide, 1-butyl-N-(2,6-dimethylphenyl)-, monohydrochloride, monohydrate and has the following structure:

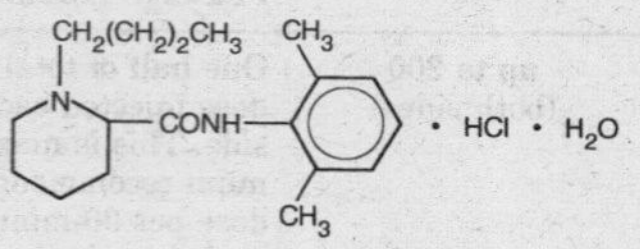

Epinephrine is (-)-3,4-Dihydroxy-α [(methylamino)methyl] benzyl alcohol. It has the following structural formula:

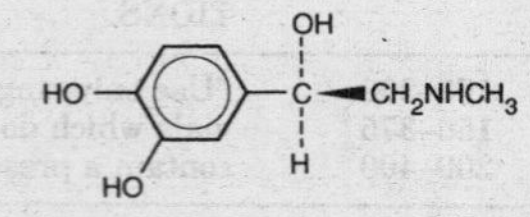

The pK_a of bupivacaine (8.1) is similar to that of lidocaine (7.86). However, bupivacaine possesses a greater degree of lipid solubility and is protein bound to a greater extent than lidocaine.
Bupivacaine is related chemically and pharmacologically to the aminoacyl local anesthetics. It is a homologue of mepivacaine and is chemically related to lidocaine. All three of these anesthetics contain an amide linkage between the aromatic nucleus and the amino or piperidine group. They differ in this respect from the procaine-type local anesthetics, which have an ester linkage.
Dosage forms listed as Sensorcaine-MPF indicates single dose solutions that are Methyl Paraben Free (MPF).
Sensorcaine-MPF is a sterile isotonic solution containing sodium chloride. Sensorcaine in multiple dose vials, each mL also contains 1 mg methylparaben as antiseptic preservative. The pH of these solutions is adjusted to between 4.0 and 6.5 with sodium hydroxide and/or hydrochloric acid.
Sensorcaine-MPF with Epinephrine 1:200,000 (as bitartrate) is a sterile isotonic solution containing sodium chloride. Each mL contains bupivacaine hydrochloride and 0.005 mg epinephrine, with 0.5 mg sodium metabisulfite as an antioxidant and 0.2 mg citric acid (anhydrous) as stabilizer. Sensorcaine with Epinephrine 1:200,000 (as bitartrate) in multiple dose vials, each mL also contains 1 mg methylparaben as antiseptic preservative. The pH of these solutions is adjusted to between 3.3 to 5.5 with sodium hydroxide and/or hydrochloric acid. Filled under nitrogen.
Note: The user should have an appreciation and awareness of the formulations and their intended uses. (See DOSAGE AND ADMINISTRATION.)

CLINICAL PHARMACOLOGY

Local anesthetics block the generation and the conduction of nerve impulses, presumably by increasing the threshold for electrical excitation in the nerve, by slowing the propagation of the nerve impulse, and by reducing the rate of rise of the action potential. In general, the progression of anesthesia is related to the diameter, myelination and conduction velocity of affected nerve fibers. Clinically, the order of loss of nerve function is as follows: (1) pain, (2) temperature, (3) touch, (4) proprioception, and (5) skeletal muscle tone.
Systemic absorption of local anesthetics produces effects on the cardiovascular and central nervous systems. At blood concentrations achieved with therapeutic doses, changes in cardiac conduction, excitability, refractoriness, contractility, and peripheral vascular resistance are minimal. However, toxic blood concentrations depress cardiac conduction and excitability, which may lead to atrioventricular block, ventricular arrhythmias and to cardiac arrest, sometimes resulting in fatalities. In addition, myocardial contractility is depressed and peripheral vasodilation occurs, leading to decreased cardiac output and arterial blood pressure. Recent clinical reports and animal research suggest that these cardiovascular changes are more likely to occur after unintended intravascular injection of bupivacaine. Therefore, incremental dosing is necessary.
Following systemic absorption, local anesthetics can produce central nervous system stimulation, depression or both. Apparent central stimulation is usually manifested as restlessness, tremors and shivering, progressing to convulsions, followed by depression and coma, progressing ultimately to respiratory arrest. However, the local anesthetics have a primary depressant effect on the medulla and on higher centers. The depressed stage may occur without a prior excited stage.
Pharmacokinetics: The rate of systemic absorption of local anesthetics is dependent upon the total dose and concentration of drug administered, the route of administration, the vascularity of the administration site, and the presence or absence of epinephrine in the anesthetic solution. A dilute concentration of epinephrine (1:200,000 or 5 µg/mL) usually reduces the rate of absorption and peak plasma concentration of bupivacaine, permitting the use of moderately larger total doses and sometimes prolonging the duration of action. The onset of action with bupivacaine is rapid and anesthesia is long-lasting. The duration of anesthesia is significantly longer with bupivacaine than with any other commonly used local anesthetic. It has also been noted that there is a period of analgesia that persists after the return of sensation, during which time the need for potent analgesics is reduced.
Local anesthetics are bound to plasma proteins in varying degrees. Generally, the lower the plasma concentration of drug, the higher the percentage of drug bound to plasma proteins.
Local anesthetics appear to cross the placenta by passive diffusion. The rate and degree of diffusion is governed by: (1) the degree of plasma protein binding, (2) the degree of ionization, and (3) the degree of lipid solubility. Fetal/maternal ratios of local anesthetics appear to be inversely related to the degree of plasma protein binding, because only the free, unbound drug is available for placental transfer. Bupivacaine, with a high protein binding capacity (95%), has a low fetal/maternal ratio (0.2–0.4). The extent of placental transfer is also determined by the degree of ionization and lipid solubility of the drug. Lipid soluble, nonionized drugs readily enter the fetal blood from the maternal circulation.
Depending upon the route of administration, local anesthetics are distributed to some extent to all body tissues, with high concentrations found in highly perfused organs such as the liver, lungs, heart, and brain.
Pharmacokinetic studies on the plasma profile of bupivacaine after direct intravenous injection suggest a three-compartment open model. The first compartment is represented by the rapid intravascular distribution of the drug. The second compartment represents the equilibration of the drug throughout the highly perfused organs such as the brain, myocardium, lungs, kidneys, and liver. The third compartment represents an equilibration of the drug with poorly perfused tissues, such as muscle and fat. The elimination of drug from tissue depends largely upon the ability of binding sites in the circulation to carry it to the liver where it is metabolized.
After injection of Sensorcaine (bupivacaine HCl) for caudal, epidural or peripheral nerve block in man, peak levels of bupivacaine in the blood are reached in 30 to 45 minutes, followed by a decline to insignificant levels during the next 3 to 6 hours.
Various pharmacokinetic parameters of the local anesthetics can be significantly altered by the presence of hepatic or renal disease, addition of epinephrine, factors affecting urinary pH, renal blood flow, the route of drug administration, and the age of the patient. The half-life of bupivacaine in adults is 2.7 hours and in neonates 8.1 hours.
In clinical studies, elderly patients reached the maximal spread of analgesia and maximal motor blockade more rapidly than younger patients. Elderly patients also exhibited higher peak plasma concentrations following administration of this product. The total plasma clearance was decreased in these patients.
Amide-type local anesthetics such as bupivacaine are metabolized primarily in the liver via conjugation with glucuronic acid.
Patients with hepatic disease, especially those with severe hepatic disease, may be more susceptible to the potential toxicities of the amide-type local anesthetics. The major metabolite of bupivacaine is 2,6-pipecoloxylidine.
The kidney is the main excretory organ for most local anesthetics and their metabolites. Urinary excretion is affected by renal perfusion and factors affecting urinary pH. Only 5% of bupivacaine is excreted unchanged in the urine.
When administered in recommended doses and concentrations, Sensorcaine (bupivacaine HCl) does not ordinarily produce irritation or tissue damage and does not cause methemoglobinemia.

INDICATIONS AND USAGE

Sensorcaine (bupivacaine HCl) is indicated for the production of local or regional anesthesia or analgesia for surgery, for oral surgery procedures, for diagnostic and therapeutic procedures, and for obstetrical procedures. Only the 0.25% and 0.5% concentrations are indicated for obstetrical anesthesia. (See WARNINGS.)
Experience with non-obstetrical surgical procedures in pregnant patients is not sufficient to recommend use of the 0.75% concentration in these patients. Sensorcaine is not recommended for intravenous regional anesthesia (Bier Block). (See WARNINGS.)
The routes of administration and indicated Sensorcaine concentrations are:

local infiltration	0.25%
peripheral nerve block	0.25%, 0.5%
retrobulbar block	0.75%
sympathetic block	0.25%
lumbar epidural	0.25%, 0.5% and 0.75% (non-obstetrical)
caudal	0.25%, 0.5%
epidural test dose	(see PRECAUTIONS)

(See DOSAGE AND ADMINISTRATION for additional information.) Standard textbooks should be consulted to determine the accepted procedures and techniques for the administration of Sensorcaine.
Use only the single dose ampules and single dose vials for caudal or epidural anesthesia; the multiple dose vials contain a preservative and, therefore, should not be used for these procedures.

CONTRAINDICATIONS

Sensorcaine (bupivacaine HCl) is contraindicated in obstetrical paracervical block anesthesia. Its use by this technique has resulted in fetal bradycardia and death.
Sensorcaine is contraindicated in patients with a known hypersensitivity to it or to any local anesthetic agent of the amide type or to other components of bupivacaine solutions.

WARNINGS

THE 0.75% CONCENTRATION OF SENSORCAINE INJECTION IS NOT RECOMMENDED FOR OBSTETRICAL ANESTHESIA. THERE HAVE BEEN REPORTS OF CARDIAC ARREST WITH DIFFICULT RESUSCITATION OR DEATH DURING USE OF BUPIVACAINE FOR EPIDURAL ANESTHESIA IN OBSTETRICAL PATIENTS. IN MOST CASES, THIS HAS FOLLOWED USE OF THE 0.75% CONCENTRATION. RESUSCITATION HAS BEEN DIFFICULT OR IMPOSSIBLE DESPITE APPARENTLY ADEQUATE PREPARATION AND APPROPRIATE MANAGEMENT. CARDIAC ARREST HAS OCCURRED AFTER CONVULSIONS RESULTING FROM SYSTEMIC TOXICITY, PRESUMABLY FOLLOWING UNINTENTIONAL INTRAVASCULAR INJECTION. THE 0.75% CONCENTRATION SHOULD BE RESERVED FOR SURGICAL PROCEDURES WHERE A HIGH DEGREE OF MUSCLE RELAXATION AND PROLONGED EFFECT ARE NECESSARY.

LOCAL ANESTHETICS SHOULD ONLY BE EMPLOYED BY CLINICIANS WHO ARE WELL VERSED IN DIAGNOSIS AND MANAGEMENT OF DOSE-RELATED TOXICITY AND OTHER ACUTE EMERGENCIES WHICH MIGHT ARISE FROM THE BLOCK TO BE EMPLOYED, AND THEN ONLY AFTER INSURING THE *IMMEDIATE* AVAILABILITY OF OXYGEN, OTHER RESUSCITATIVE DRUGS, CARDIOPULMONARY RESUSCITATIVE EQUIPMENT, AND THE PERSONNEL RESOURCES NEEDED FOR PROPER MANAGEMENT OF TOXIC REACTIONS AND RELATED EMERGENCIES. (See also ADVERSE REACTIONS, PRECAUTIONS, and OVERDOSAGE.) DELAY IN PROPER MANAGEMENT OF DOSE-RELATED TOXICITY, UNDERVENTILATION FROM ANY CAUSE AND/OR ALTERED SENSITIVITY MAY LEAD TO THE DEVELOPMENT OF ACIDOSIS, CARDIAC ARREST AND, POSSIBLY, DEATH.
Local anesthetic solutions containing antimicrobial preservatives, ie, those supplied in multiple dose vials, should not be used for epidural or caudal anesthesia because safety has not been established with regard to intrathecal injection, either intentional or unintentional, of such preservatives.
It is essential that aspiration for blood or cerebrospinal fluid (where applicable) be done prior to injecting any local anesthetic, both the original dose and all subsequent doses, to avoid intravascular or subarachnoid injection. However, a negative aspiration does *not* ensure against an intravascular or subarachnoid injection.
Bupivacaine and Epinephrine Injection or other vasopressors should not be used concomitantly with ergot-type oxytocic drugs, because a severe persistent hypertension may occur. Likewise, solutions of bupivacaine containing a vasoconstrictor, such as epinephrine, should be used with extreme caution in patients receiving monoamine oxidase (MAO) inhibitors or antidepressants of the triptyline or imipramine types, because severe prolonged hypertension may result.
Until further experience is gained in children younger than 12 years, administration of bupivacaine in this age group is not recommended.
Mixing of the prior or intercurrent use of any local anesthetic with bupivacaine cannot be recommended because of insufficient data on the clinical use of such mixtures.
There have been reports of cardiac arrest and death during the use of bupivacaine for intravenous regional anesthesia (Bier Block). Information on safe dosages and techniques of administration of bupivacaine in this procedure is lacking. Therefore, bupivacaine is not recommended for use in this technique.
Sensorcaine with epinephrine solutions contain sodium metabisulfite, a sulfite that may cause allergic-type reactions including anaphylactic symptoms and life-threatening or less severe asthmatic episodes in certain susceptible people. The overall prevalence of sulfite sensitivity in the general population is unknown and probably low. Sulfite sensitivity is seen more frequently in asthmatic than in nonasthmatic people.

PRECAUTIONS

General: The safety and effectiveness of local anesthetics depend on proper dosage, correct technique, adequate precautions, and readiness for emergencies. Resuscitative equipment, oxygen, and other resuscitative drugs should be available for immediate use. (See WARNINGS, ADVERSE REACTIONS, and OVERDOSAGE.) During major regional nerve blocks, the patient should have I.V. fluids running via an indwelling catheter to assure a functioning intravenous pathway. The lowest dosage of local anesthetic that results in effective anesthesia should be used to avoid high plasma levels and serious adverse effects. The rapid injection of a large volume of local anesthetic solution should be avoided and fractional (incremental) doses should be used when feasible.
Epidural Anesthesia: During epidural administration of Sensorcaine (bupivacaine HCl), concentrated solutions (0.5–0.75%) should be administered in incremental doses of 3 to 5 mL with sufficient time between doses to detect toxic manifestations of unintentional intravascular or intrathecal injection. Syringe aspirations should also be performed before and during each supplemental injection in continuous

(intermittent) catheter techniques. An intravascular injection is still possible even if aspirations for blood are negative. During the administration of epidural anesthesia, it is recommended that a test dose be administered initially and the effects monitored before the full dose is given. When using a "continuous" catheter technique, test doses should be given prior to both the original and all reinforcing doses, because plastic tubing in the epidural space can migrate into a blood vessel or through the dura. When clinical conditions permit, the test dose should contain epinephrine (10 to 15 µg have been suggested) to serve as a warning of unintentional intravascular injection. If injected into a blood vessel, this amount of epinephrine is likely to produce a transient "epinephrine response" within 45 seconds, consisting of an increase in heart rate and systolic blood pressure, circumoral pallor, palpitations and nervousness in the unsedated patient. The sedated patient may exhibit only a pulse rate increase of 20 or more beats per minute for 15 or more seconds. Therefore, following the test dose, the heart rate should be monitored for a heart rate increase. Patients on beta-blockers may not manifest changes in heart rate, but blood pressure monitoring can detect an evanescent rise in systolic blood pressure. The test dose should also contain 10 to 15 mg of Sensorcaine or an equivalent dose of a short-acting amide anesthetic such as 30 to 40 mg of lidocaine, to detect an unintentional intrathecal administration. This will be manifested within a few minutes by signs of spinal block (eg, decreased sensation of the buttocks, paresis of the legs, or, in the sedated patient, absent knee jerk). An intravascular or subarachnoid injection is still possible even if results of the test dose are negative. The test dose itself may produce a systemic toxic reaction, high spinal or epinephrine-induced cardiovascular effects.

Injection of repeated doses of local anesthetics may cause significant increases in plasma levels with each repeated dose due to slow accumulation of the drug or its metabolites or to slow metabolic degradation. Tolerance to elevated blood levels varies with the physical condition of the patient. Debilitated, elderly patients, acutely ill patients and children should be given reduced doses commensurate with their age and physical condition. Local anesthetics should also be used with caution in patients with hypotension or heart block.

Careful and constant monitoring of cardiovascular and respiratory vital signs (adequacy of ventilation) and the patient's state of consciousness should be performed after each local anesthetic injection. It should be kept in mind at such times that restlessness, anxiety, incoherent speech, lightheadedness, numbness and tingling of the mouth and lips, metallic taste, tinnitus, dizziness, blurred vision, tremors, twitching, depression, or drowsiness may be early warning signs of central nervous system toxicity.

Local anesthetic solutions containing a vasoconstrictor should be used cautiously and in carefully restricted quantities in areas of the body supplied by end arteries or having otherwise compromised blood supply such as digits, nose, external ear, penis, etc. Patients with hypertensive vascular disease may exhibit exaggerated vasoconstrictor response. Ischemic injury or necrosis may result.

Because amide-type local anesthetics such as bupivacaine are metabolized by the liver, these drugs, especially repeat doses, should be used cautiously in patients with hepatic disease. Patients with severe hepatic disease, because of their inability to metabolize local anesthetics normally, are at a greater risk of developing toxic plasma concentrations. Local anesthetics should also be used with caution in patients with impaired cardiovascular function because they may be less able to compensate for functional changes associated with the prolongation of A-V conduction produced by these drugs.

Serious dose-related cardiac arrhythmias may occur if preparations containing a vasoconstrictor such as epinephrine are employed in patients during or following the administration of potent inhalation anesthetics. In deciding whether to use these products concurrently in the same patient, the combined action of both agents upon the myocardium, the concentration and volume of vasoconstrictor used, and the time since injection, when applicable, should be taken into account.

Many drugs used during the conduct of anesthesia are considered potential triggering agents for familial malignant hyperthermia. Because it is not known whether amide-type local anesthetics may trigger this reaction and because the need for supplemental general anesthesia cannot be predicted in advance, it is suggested that a standard protocol for management should be available. Early unexplained signs of tachycardia, tachypnea, labile blood pressure and metabolic acidosis may precede temperature elevation. Successful outcome is dependent on early diagnosis, prompt discontinuance of the suspect triggering agent(s) and prompt treatment, including oxygen therapy, dantrolene (consult dantrolene sodium intravenous package insert before using) and other supportive measures.

Use in Head and Neck Area: Small doses of local anesthetics injected into the head and neck area, including retrobulbar, dental and stellate ganglion blocks, may produce adverse reactions similar to systemic toxicity seen with unintentional intravascular injections of larger doses. The injection procedures require the utmost care. Confusion, convulsions, respiratory depression, and/or respiratory arrest, and cardiovascular stimulation or depression have been reported. These reactions may be due to intra-arterial injection of the local anesthetic with retrograde flow to the cerebral circulation. They may also be due to puncture of the dural sheath of the optic nerve during retrobulbar block with dif-

fusion of any local anesthetic along the subdural space to the midbrain. Patients receiving these blocks should have their circulation and respiration monitored and be constantly observed. Resuscitative equipment and personnel for treating adverse reactions should be immediately available. Dosage recommendations should not be exceeded (see DOSAGE AND ADMINISTRATION).

Use in Ophthalmic Surgery: Clinicians who perform retrobulbar blocks should be aware that there have been reports of respiratory arrest following local anesthetic injection. Prior to retrobulbar block, as with all other regional procedures, the immediate availability of equipment, drugs, and personnel to manage respiratory arrest or depression, convulsions, and cardiac stimulation or depression should be assured (see also WARNINGS and Use in Head and Neck Area, above). As with other anesthetic procedures, patients should be constantly monitored following ophthalmic blocks for signs of these adverse reactions, which may occur following relatively low total doses. A concentration of 0.75% bupivacaine is indicated for retrobulbar block; however, this concentration is not indicated for any other peripheral nerve block, including the facial nerve and not indicated for local infiltration, including the conjunctiva (see INDICATIONS and PRECAUTIONS, General). Mixing Sensorcaine (bupivacaine HCl) with other local anesthetics is not recommended because of insufficient data on the clinical use of such mixtures.

When Sensorcaine (bupivacaine HCl) 0.75% is used for retrobulbar block, complete corneal anesthesia usually precedes onset of clinically acceptable external ocular muscle akinesia. Therefore, presence of akinesia rather than anesthesia alone should determine readiness of the patient for surgery.

Information for Patients: When appropriate, patients should be informed in advance that they may experience temporary loss of sensation and motor activity, usually in the lower half of the body following proper administration of caudal or lumbar epidural anesthesia. Also, when appropriate, the physician should discuss other information including adverse reactions in the Sensorcaine package insert.

Clinically Significant Drug Interactions: The administration of local anesthetic solutions containing epinephrine or norepinephrine to patients receiving monoamine oxidase inhibitors or tricyclic antidepressants may produce severe, prolonged hypertension. Concurrent use of these agents should generally be avoided. In situations in which concurrent therapy is necessary, careful patient monitoring is essential.

Concurrent administration of vasopressor drugs and of ergot-type oxytocic drugs may cause severe, persistent hypertension or cerebrovascular accidents.

Phenothiazines and butyrophenones may reduce or reverse the pressor effect of epinephrine.

Carcinogenesis, Mutagenesis, and Impairment of Fertility: Long-term studies in animals of most local anesthetics, including bupivacaine, to evaluate the carcinogenic potential have not been conducted. Mutagenic potential or the effect on fertility has not been determined. There is no evidence from human data that Sensorcaine (bupivacaine HCl) may be carcinogenic or mutagenic or that it impairs fertility.

Pregnancy Category C: Decreased pup survival in rats and embryocidal effect in rabbits have been observed when bupivacaine HCl was administered to these species in doses comparable to nine and five times, respectively, the maximum recommended daily human dose (400 mg). There are no adequate and well-controlled studies in pregnant women of the effect of bupivacaine on the developing fetus. Sensorcaine should be used during pregnancy only if the potential benefit justifies the potential risk to the fetus. This does not exclude the use of Sensorcaine (0.25% and 0.5% concentrations) at term for obstetrical anesthesia or analgesia. (See Labor and Delivery.)

Labor and Delivery: See Box WARNINGS regarding obstetrical use in 0.75% concentration.

Sensorcaine is contraindicated in obstetrical paracervical block anesthesia.

Local anesthetics rapidly cross the placenta, and when used for epidural, caudal or pudendal block anesthesia, can cause varying degrees of maternal, fetal and neonatal toxicity. (See Pharmacokinetics in CLINICAL PHARMACOLOGY.) The incidence and degree of toxicity depend upon the procedure performed, the type and amount of drug used, and the technique of drug administration. Adverse reactions in the parturient, fetus and neonate involve alterations of the central nervous system, peripheral vascular tone and cardiac function.

Maternal hypotension has resulted from regional anesthesia. Local anesthetics produce vasodilation by blocking sympathetic nerves. Elevating the patient's legs and positioning her on her left side will help prevent decreases in blood pressure. The fetal heart rate also should be monitored continuously, and electronic fetal monitoring is highly advisable. Epidural, caudal, or pudendal anesthesia may alter the forces of parturition through changes in uterine contractility or maternal expulsive efforts. Epidural anesthesia has been reported to prolong the second stage of labor by removing the parturient's reflex urge to bear down or by interfering with motor function. The use of obstetrical anesthesia may increase the need for forceps assistance. The use of some local anesthetic drug products during labor and delivery may be followed by diminished muscle strength and tone for the first day or two of life. This has not been reported with Sensorcaine.

It is extremely important to avoid aortocaval compression by the gravid uterus during administration of regional block to parturients. To do this, the patient must be maintained in

the left lateral decubitus position or a blanket roll or sandbag may be placed beneath the right hip and the gravid uterus displaced to the left.

Nursing Mothers: Bupivacaine has been reported to be excreted in human milk suggesting that the nursing infant could be theoretically exposed to a dose of the drug. Because of the potential for serious adverse reactions in nursing infants from bupivacaine, a decision should be made whether to discontinue nursing or not administer bupivacaine, taking into account the importance of the drug to the mother.

Pediatric Use: Until further experience is gained in children younger than 12 years, administration of Sensorcaine (bupivacaine HCl) Injection in this age group is not recommended. Continuous infusions of bupivacaine in children have been reported to result in high systemic levels of bupivacaine and seizures; high plasma levels may also be associated with cardiovascular abnormalities. (See WARNINGS, PRECAUTIONS, AND OVERDOSAGE.)

Geriatric Use: Patients over 65 years, particularly those with hypertension, may be at increased risk for developing hypotension while undergoing anesthesia with bupivacaine. (See ADVERSE REACTIONS.)

Elderly patients may require lower doses of bupivacaine. (See PRECAUTIONS, Epidural Anesthesia, and DOSAGE AND ADMINISTRATION.)

In clinical studies, differences in various pharmacokinetic parameters have been observed between elderly and younger patients. (See CLINICAL PHARMACOLOGY.)

This product is known to be substantially excreted by the kidney, and the risk of toxic reactions to this drug may be greater in patients with impaired renal function. Because elderly patients are more likely to have decreased renal function, care should be taken in dose selection, and it may be useful to monitor renal function. (See CLINICAL PHARMACOLOGY.)

ADVERSE REACTIONS

Reactions to Sensorcaine (bupivacaine HCl) are characteristic of those associated with other amide-type local anesthetics. A major cause of adverse reactions to this group of drugs may be associated with its excessive plasma levels, which may be due to overdosage, unintentional intravascular injection or slow metabolic degradation.

Systemic: The most commonly encountered acute adverse experiences that demand immediate countermeasures are related to the central nervous system and the cardiovascular system. These adverse experiences are generally dose related and due to high plasma levels which may result from overdosage, rapid absorption from the injection site, diminished tolerance or from unintentional intravascular injection of the local anesthetic solution. In addition to systemic dose-related toxicity, unintentional subarachnoid injection of drug during the intended performance of caudal or lumbar epidural block or nerve blocks near the vertebral column (especially in the head and neck region) may result in underventilation or apnea ("Total or High Spinal"). Also, hypotension due to loss of sympathetic tone and respiratory paralysis or underventilation due to cephalad extension of the motor level of anesthesia may occur. This may lead to secondary cardiac arrest if untreated. Patients over 65 years, particularly those with hypertension, may be at increased risk for experiencing the hypotensive effects of bupivacaine. Factors influencing plasma protein binding, such as acidosis, systemic diseases that alter protein production or competition with other drugs for protein binding sites, may diminish individual tolerance.

Central Nervous System Reactions: These are characterized by excitation and/or depression. Restlessness, anxiety, dizziness, tinnitus, blurred vision or tremors may occur, possibly proceeding to convulsions. However, excitement may be transient or absent, with depression being the first manifestation of an adverse reaction. This may quickly be followed by drowsiness merging into unconsciousness and respiratory arrest. Other central nervous system effects may be nausea, vomiting, chills, and constriction of the pupils.

The incidence of convulsions associated with the use of local anesthetics varies with the procedure used and the total dose administered. In a survey of studies of epidural anesthesia, overt toxicity progressing to convulsions occurred in approximately 0.1% of local anesthetic administrations.

Cardiovascular System Reactions: High doses or unintentional intravascular injection may lead to high plasma levels and related depression of the myocardium, decreased cardiac output, heart block, hypotension, bradycardia, ventricular arrhythmias, including ventricular tachycardia and ventricular fibrillation, and cardiac arrest. (See WARNINGS, PRECAUTIONS, and OVERDOSAGE sections.)

Allergic: Allergic type reactions are rare and may occur as a result of sensitivity to the local anesthetic or to other formulation ingredients, such as the antimicrobial preservative methylparaben contained in multiple dose vials or sulfites in epinephrine-containing solutions (see WARNINGS). These reactions are characterized by signs such as urticaria, pruritus, erythema, angioneurotic edema (including laryngeal edema), tachycardia, sneezing, nausea, vomiting, dizziness, syncope, excessive sweating, elevated temperature, and possibly, anaphylactoid symptomatology (including severe hypotension). Cross sensitivity among members of the amide-type local anesthetic group has been reported. The usefulness of screening for sensitivity has not been definitely established.

Neurologic: The incidence of adverse neurologic reactions associated with the use of local anesthetics may be related to the total dose of local anesthetic administered and are also dependent upon the particular drug used, the route of admin-

Continued on next page

Sensorcaine—Cont.

istration and the physical status of the patient. Many of these effects may be related to local anesthetic techniques, with or without a contribution from the drug.

In the practice of caudal or lumbar epidural block, occasional unintentional penetration of the subarachnoid space by the catheter or needle may occur. Subsequent adverse effects may depend partially on the amount of drug administered intrathecally and the physiological and physical effects of a dural puncture. A high spinal is characterized by paralysis of the legs, loss of consciousness, respiratory paralysis and bradycardia.

Neurologic effects following epidural or caudal anesthesia may include spinal block of varying magnitude (including high or total spinal block); hypotension secondary to spinal block; urinary retention; fecal and urinary incontinence; loss of perineal sensation and sexual function; persistent anesthesia, paresthesia, weakness, paralysis of the lower extremities and loss of sphincter control, all of which may have slow, incomplete or no recovery; headache; backache; septic meningitis; meningismus; slowing of labor; increased incidence of forceps delivery; or cranial nerve palsies due to traction on nerves from loss of cerebrospinal fluid.

Neurologic effects following other procedures or routes of administration may include persistent anesthesia, paresthesia, weakness, paralysis, all of which may have slow, incomplete, or no recovery.

OVERDOSAGE

Acute emergencies from local anesthetics are generally related to high plasma levels encountered during therapeutic use of local anesthetics or to unintended subarachnoid injection of local anesthetic solution. (See ADVERSE REACTIONS, WARNINGS, and PRECAUTIONS.)

Management of Local Anesthetic Emergencies: The first consideration is prevention, best accomplished by careful and constant monitoring of cardiovascular and respiratory vital signs and the patient's state of consciousness after each local anesthetic injection. At the first sign of change, oxygen should be administered.

The first step in the management of systemic toxic reactions, as well as underventilation or apnea due to unintentional subarachnoid injection of drug solution, consists of ***immediate*** *attention to the establishment and maintenance of a patent airway and effective assisted or controlled ventilation with 100% oxygen with a delivery system capable of permitting immediate positive airway pressure by mask.* This may prevent convulsions if they have not already occurred.

If necessary, use drugs to control the convulsions. A 50 to 100 mg bolus I.V. injection of succinylcholine will paralyze the patient without depressing the central nervous or cardiovascular systems and facilitate ventilation. A bolus I.V. dose of 5 to 10 mg of diazepam or 50 to 100 mg of thiopental will permit ventilation and counteract central nervous system stimulation, but these drugs also depress the central nervous system, respiratory and cardiac function, add to postictal depression, and may result in apnea. Intravenous barbiturates, anticonvulsant agents, or muscle relaxants should only be administered by those familiar with their use. Immediately after the institution of these ventilatory measures, the adequacy of the circulation should be evaluated. Supportive treatment of circulatory depression may require administration of intravenous fluids, and, when appropriate, a vasopressor dictated by the clinical situation (such as ephedrine or epinephrine to enhance myocardial contractile force).

Endotracheal intubation, employing drugs and techniques familiar to the clinician, may be indicated after initial administration of oxygen by mask, if difficulty is encountered in the maintenance of a patent airway or if prolonged ventilatory support (assisted or controlled) is indicated.

Recent clinical data from patients experiencing local anesthetic induced convulsions demonstrated rapid development of hypoxia, hypercarbia, and acidosis with bupivacaine within a minute of the onset of convulsions. These observations suggest that oxygen consumption and carbon dioxide production are greatly increased during local anesthetic convulsions and emphasize the importance of immediate and effective ventilation with oxygen which may avoid cardiac arrest.

If not treated immediately, convulsions with simultaneous hypoxia, hypercarbia and acidosis, plus myocardial depression from the direct effects of the local anesthetic may result in cardiac arrhythmias, bradycardia, asystole, ventricular fibrillation, or cardiac arrest. Respiratory abnormalities, including apnea, may occur. Underventilation or apnea due to unintentional subarachnoid injection of local anesthetic solution may produce these same signs and also lead to cardiac arrest if ventilatory support is not instituted.

If cardiac arrest should occur, a successful outcome may require prolonged resuscitative efforts.

The supine position is dangerous in pregnant women at term because of aortocaval compression by the gravid uterus. Therefore, during treatment of systemic toxicity, maternal hypotension or fetal bradycardia following regional block, the parturient should be maintained in the left lateral decubitus position if possible, or manual displacement of the uterus off the great vessels should be accomplished.

The mean seizure dosage of bupivacaine in rhesus monkeys was found to be 4.4 mg/kg with mean arterial plasma concentration of 4.5 mcg/mL. The intravenous and subcutaneous LD_{50} in mice is 6 to 8 mg/kg and 38 to 54 mg/kg respectively.

TABLE 1. DOSAGE RECOMMENDATIONS— SENSORCAINE (bupivacaine HCl) INJECTIONS

Type of Block	Conc.	Each Dose (mL)	Each Dose (mg)	Motor Block[1]
Local Infiltration	0.25%[4]	up to max.	up to max.	—
Epidural	0.75%[2,4]	10–20	75–150	complete
	0.5%[4]	10–20	50–100	moderate to complete
	0.25%[4]	10–20	25–50	partial to moderate
Caudal	0.5%[4]	15–30	75–150	moderate to complete
	0.25%[4]	15–30	37.5–75	moderate
Peripheral Nerves	0.5%[4]	5 to max.	25 to max.	moderate to complete
	0.25%[4]	5 to max.	12.5 to max.	moderate to complete
Retrobulbar[3]	0.75%[4]	2–4	15–30	complete
Sympathetic	0.25%	20–50	50–125	—
Epidural[3]	0.5%	2–3	10–15	—
Test Dose	w/epi		10–15 µg epinephrine (See PRECAUTIONS)	

[1]With continuous (intermittent) techniques, repeat doses increase the degree of motor block. The first repeat dose of 0.5% may produce complete motor block. Intercostal nerve block with 0.25% may also produce complete motor block for intra-abdominal surgery.

[2]For single dose use, not for intermittent epidural technique. Not for obstetric anesthesia.

[3]See PRECAUTIONS.

[4]Solutions with or without epinephrine.

Sensorcaine-MPF (methylparaben free) is available in the following forms:	
Single Dose Ampules:	
5 mL	0.5% with epinephrine 1:200,000
30 mL	0.75% without epinephrine
Single Dose Vials:	
10 mL with E-Z Off® vial closure;	0.25%, 0.5% and 0.75% without epinephrine 0.25% and 0.5% with epinephrine 1:200,000
30 mL	0.25%, 0.5% and 0.75% without epinephrine 0.25% and 0.5% with epinephrine 1:200,000
Sensorcaine is available in the following forms:	
Multiple Dose Vials:	
50 mL	0.25% and 0.5% without epinephrine 0.25% and 0.5% with epinephrine 1:200,000

DOSAGE AND ADMINISTRATION

The dose of any local anesthetic administered varies with the anesthetic procedure, the area to be anesthetized, the vascularity of the tissues, the number of neuronal segments to be blocked, the depth of anesthesia and degree of muscle relaxation required, the duration of anesthesia desired, individual tolerance, and the physical condition of the patient. The smallest dose and concentration required to produce the desired result should be administered. Dosages of Sensorcaine should be reduced for young, elderly and/or debilitated patients and patients with cardiac and/or liver disease. The rapid injection of a large volume of local anesthetic solution should be avoided and fractional (incremental) doses should be used when feasible.

For specific techniques and procedures, refer to standard textbooks.

In recommended doses, Sensorcaine (bupivacaine HCl) produces complete sensory block, but the effect on motor function differs among the three concentrations.

0.25%—when used for caudal, epidural, or peripheral nerve block, produces incomplete motor block. Should be used for operations in which muscle relaxation is not important, or when another means of providing muscle relaxation is used concurrently. Onset of action may be slower than with the 0.5% or 0.75% solutions.

0.5%—provides motor blockade for caudal, epidural, or nerve block, but muscle relaxation may be inadequate for operations in which complete muscle relaxation is essential.

0.75%—produces complete motor block. Most useful for epidural block in abdominal operations requiring complete muscle relaxation, and for retrobulbar anesthesia. Not for obstetrical anesthesia.

The duration of anesthesia with Sensorcaine is such that for most indications, a single dose is sufficient.

Maximum dosage limit must be individualized in each case after evaluating the size and physical status of the patient, as well as the usual rate of systemic absorption from a particular injection site. Most experience to date is with single doses of Sensorcaine up to 225 mg with epinephrine 1:200,000 and 175 mg without epinephrine; more or less drug may be used depending on individualization of each case.

These doses may be repeated up to once every three hours. In clinical studies to date, total daily doses up to 400 mg have been reported. Until further experience is gained, this dose should not be exceeded in 24 hours. The duration of anesthetic effect may be prolonged by the addition of epinephrine.

The dosages in Table 1 have generally proved satisfactory and are recommended as a guide for use in the average adult. These dosages should be reduced for young, elderly or debilitated patients. Until further experience is gained Sensorcaine is not recommended for children younger than 12 years. Sensorcaine is contraindicated for obstetrical paracervical blocks, and is not recommended for intravenous regional anesthesia (Bier Block).

Use in Epidural Anesthesia: During epidural administration of Sensorcaine, 0.5% and 0.75% solutions should be administered in incremental doses of 3 mL to 5 mL with sufficient time between doses to detect toxic manifestations of unintentional intravascular or intrathecal injection. In obstetrics, only the 0.5% and 0.25% concentrations should be used; incremental doses of 3 mL to 5 mL of the 0.5% solution not exceeding 50 mg to 100 mg at any dosing interval are recommended. Repeat doses should be preceded by a test dose containing epinephrine if not contraindicated. Use only the single dose ampules and single dose vials for caudal or epidural anesthesia; the multiple dose vials contain a preservative and therefore should not be used for these procedures.

Test Dose for Caudal and Lumbar Epidural Blocks: See PRECAUTIONS.

Unused portions of solutions in single dose containers should be discarded, since this product form contains no preservatives.

[See table 1 above]

NOTE: Parenteral drug products should be inspected visually for particulate matter and discoloration prior to administration whenever the solution and container permit. The Injection is not to be used if its color is pinkish or darker than slightly yellow or if it contains a precipitate.

HOW SUPPLIED

SOLUTIONS OF SENSORCAINE (BUPIVACAINE HYDROCHLORIDE) SHOULD NOT BE USED FOR THE PRODUCTION OF SPINAL ANESTHESIA (SUBARACHNOID BLOCK) BECAUSE OF INSUFFICIENT DATA TO SUPPORT SUCH USE.

[See second table above]

Disinfecting agents containing heavy metals, which cause release of respective ions (mercury, zinc, copper, etc.), should not be used for skin or mucous membrane disinfection since they have been related to incidents of swelling and edema. When chemical disinfection of the container surface is desired, either isopropyl alcohol (91%) or ethyl alcohol (70%) is recommended. It is recommended that chemical disinfection be accomplished by wiping the ampule or vial stopper thoroughly with cotton or gauze that has been moistened with the recommended alcohol just prior to use.

Solutions should be stored at controlled room temperature 15–30°C (59–86°F) [See USP].

Solutions containing epinephrine should be protected from light.

All trademarks are the property of the AstraZeneca group
© AstraZeneca 2000

AstraZeneca LP, Wilmington, DE 19850 721680-07
Rev. 10/00

TABLETS
TONOCARD®
(tocainide HCl) ℞

Prescribing information for this product, which appears on pages 604–607 of the 2001 PDR, has been revised. Please write "See Supplement A" next to the product heading.

Revisions occurred to the following sections:

PRECAUTIONS, Nursing Mothers—Delete the following words from the first sentence, "It is not known whether".

Capitalize the letter t in Tocainide. Delete the following words from the second sentence, "Because many drugs are secreted in human milk and". Capitalize the letter b in because.

TOPROL-XL® TABLETS ℞
(metoprolol succinate)
Extended Release Tablets
Tablets: 50 mg, 100 mg, and 200 mg

Prescribing information for this product, which appears on pages 606–607 of the 2001 PDR, has been completely revised as follows. Please write "See Supplement A" next to the product heading.

DESCRIPTION

Toprol-XL, metoprolol succinate, is a $beta_1$-selective (cardioselective) adrenoceptor blocking agent, for oral administration, available as extended release tablets. Toprol-XL has been formulated to provide a controlled and predictable release of metoprolol for once daily administration. The tablets comprise a multiple unit system containing metoprolol succinate in a multitude of controlled release pellets. Each pellet acts as a separate drug delivery unit and is designed to deliver metoprolol continuously over the dosage interval. The tablets contain 23.75, 47.5, 95 and 190 mg of metoprolol succinate equivalent to 25, 50, 100 and 200 mg of metoprolol tartrate, USP, respectively. Its chemical name is (±)1-(isopropylamino)-3-[p-(2-methoxyethyl) phenoxy]-2-propanol succinate (2:1) (salt). Its structural formula is:

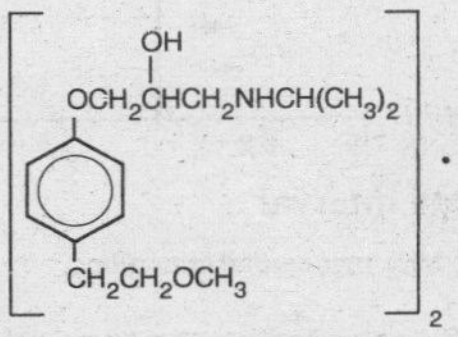

Metoprolol succinate is a white crystalline powder with a molecular weight of 652.8. It is freely soluble in water; soluble in methanol; sparingly soluble in ethanol; slightly soluble in dichloromethane and 2-propanol; practically insoluble in ethyl-acetate, acetone, diethylether and heptane. Inactive ingredients: silicon dioxide, cellulose compounds, sodium stearyl fumarate, polyethylene glycol, titanium dioxide, paraffin.

CLINICAL PHARMACOLOGY

General

Metoprolol is a $beta_1$-selective (cardioselective) adrenergic receptor blocking agent. This preferential effect is not absolute, however, and at higher plasma concentrations, metoprolol also inhibits $beta_2$-adrenoreceptors, chiefly located in the bronchial and vascular musculature. Metoprolol has no intrinsic sympathomimetic activity, and membrane-stabilizing activity is detectable only at plasma concentrations much greater than required for beta-blockade. Animal and human experiments indicate that metoprolol slows the sinus rate and decreases AV nodal conduction.

Clinical pharmacology studies have confirmed the beta-blocking activity of metoprolol in man, as shown by (1) reduction in heart rate and cardiac output at rest and upon exercise, (2) reduction of systolic blood pressure upon exercise, (3) inhibition of isoproterenol-induced tachycardia, and (4) reduction of reflex orthostatic tachycardia.

The relative $beta_1$-selectivity of metoprolol has been confirmed by the following: (1) In normal subjects, metoprolol is unable to reverse the $beta_2$-mediated vasodilating effects of epinephrine. This contrasts with the effect of nonselective beta-blockers, which completely reverse the vasodilating effects of epinephrine. (2) In asthmatic patients, metoprolol reduces FEV_1 and FVC significantly less than a nonselective beta-blocker, propranolol, at equivalent $beta_1$-receptor blocking doses.

In five controlled studies in normal healthy subjects, the same daily doses of Toprol-XL and immediate release metoprolol were compared in terms of the extent and duration of $beta_1$-blockade produced. Both formulations were given in a dose range equivalent to 100–400 mg of immediate release metoprolol per day. In these studies, Toprol-XL was administered once a day and immediate release metoprolol was administered once to four times a day. A sixth controlled study compared the $beta_1$-blocking effects of a 50 mg daily dose of the two formulations. In each study, $beta_1$-blockade was expressed as the percent change from baseline in exercise heart rate following standardized submaximal exercise tolerance tests at steady state. Toprol-XL administered once a day, and immediate release metoprolol administered once to four times a day, provided comparable total $beta_1$-blockade over 24 hours (area under the $beta_1$-blockade versus time curve) in the dose range 100–400 mg. At a dosage of 50 mg once daily, Toprol-XL produced significantly higher total $beta_1$-blockade over 24 hours than immediate release metoprolol. For Toprol-XL, the percent reduction in exercise heart rate was relatively stable throughout the entire dosage interval and the level of $beta_1$-blockade increased with increasing doses from 50 to 300 mg daily. The effects at peak/trough (i.e. at 24 hours post dosing) were; 14/9, 16/10, 24/14, 27/22 and 27/20% reduction in exercise heart rate for doses of 50, 100, 200, 300 and 400 mg Toprol-XL once a day, respectively. In contrast to Toprol-XL, immediate release metoprolol given at a dose of 50–100 mg once a day, produced a significantly larger peak effect on exercise tachycardia, but the effect was not evident at 24 hours. To match the peak to trough ratio obtained with Toprol-XL over the dosing range of 200 to 400 mg, a t.i.d. to q.i.d. divided dosing regimen was required for immediate release metoprolol. A controlled crossover study in heart failure patients compared the plasma concentrations and $beta_1$-blocking effects of 50 mg immediate release metoprolol administered t.i.d., 100 mg and 200 mg Toprol-XL once daily. A 50 mg dose of immediate release metoprolol t.i.d. produced a peak plasma level of metoprolol similar to the peak level observed with 200 mg of Toprol-XL. A 200 mg dose of Toprol-XL produced a larger effect on suppression of exercised-induced and Holter-monitored heart rate over 24 hours compared to 50 mg t.i.d. of immediate release metoprolol.

The relationship between plasma metoprolol levels and reduction in exercise heart rate is independent of the pharmaceutical formulation. Using the E_{max} model, the maximal $beta_1$-blocking effect has been estimated to produce a 30% reduction in exercise heart rate. $Beta_1$-blocking effects in the range of 30–80% of the maximal effect (corresponding to approximately 8–23% reduction in exercise heart rate) are expected to occur at metoprolol plasma concentrations ranging from 30–540 nmol/L. The concentration-effect curve begins reaching a plateau between 200–300 nmol/L, and higher plasma levels produce little additional $beta_1$-blocking effect. The relative $beta_1$-selectivity of metoprolol diminishes and blockade of $beta_2$-adrenoceptors increases at higher plasma concentrations.

Although beta-adrenergic receptor blockade is useful in the treatment of angina, hypertension, and heart failure there are situations in which sympathetic stimulation is vital. In patients with severely damaged hearts, adequate ventricular function may depend on sympathetic drive. In the presence of AV block, beta-blockade may prevent the necessary facilitating effect of sympathetic activity on conduction. $Beta_2$-adrenergic blockade results in passive bronchial constriction by interfering with endogenous adrenergic bronchodilator activity in patients subject to bronchospasm and may also interfere with exogenous bronchodilators in such patients.

In other studies, treatment with Toprol-XL produced an improvement in left ventricular ejection fraction. Toprol-XL was also shown to delay the increase in left ventricular end-systolic and end-diastolic volumes after 6 months of treatment.

Hypertension

The mechanism of the antihypertensive effects of beta-blocking agents has not been elucidated. However, several possible mechanisms have been proposed: (1) competitive antagonism of catecholamines at peripheral (especially cardiac) adrenergic neuron sites, leading to decreased cardiac output; (2) a central effect leading to reduced sympathetic outflow to the periphery; and (3) suppression of renin activity.

Clinical Trials

In controlled clinical studies, an immediate release dosage form of metoprolol has been shown to be an effective antihypertensive agent when used alone or as concomitant therapy with thiazide-type diuretics at dosages of 100–450 mg daily. Toprol-XL, in dosages of 100 to 400 mg once daily, has been shown to possess comparable β_1-blockade as conventional metoprolol tablets administered two to four times daily. In addition, Toprol-XL administered at a dose of 50 mg once daily has been shown to lower blood pressure 24-hours post-dosing in placebo controlled studies. In controlled, comparative, clinical studies, immediate release metoprolol appeared comparable as an antihypertensive agent to propranolol, methyldopa, and thiazide-type diuretics, and affected both supine and standing blood pressure. Because of variable plasma levels attained with a given dose and lack of a consistent relationship of antihypertensive activity to drug plasma concentration, selection of proper dosage requires individual titration.

Angina Pectoris

By blocking catecholamine-induced increases in heart rate, in velocity and extent of myocardial contraction, and in blood pressure, metoprolol reduces the oxygen requirements of the heart at any given level of effort, thus making it useful in the long-term management of angina pectoris.

Clinical Trials

In controlled clinical trials, an immediate release formulation of metoprolol has been shown to be an effective antianginal agent, reducing the number of angina attacks and increasing exercise tolerance. The dosage used in these studies ranged from 100 to 400 mg daily. Toprol-XL, in dosages of 100 to 400 mg once daily, has been shown to possess beta-blockade similar to conventional metoprolol tablets administered two to four times daily.

Heart Failure

The precise mechanism for the beneficial effects of beta-blockers in heart failure has not been elucidated.

Clinical Trials

MERIT-HF was a double-blind, placebo-controlled study of Toprol-XL conducted in 14 countries including the US. It randomized 3991 patients (1990 to Toprol-XL) with ejection fraction ≤ 0.40 and NYHA Class II-IV heart failure attributable to ischemia, hypertension, or cardiomyopathy. The protocol excluded patients with contraindications to beta-blocker use, those expected to undergo heart surgery, and those within 28 days of myocardial infarction or unstable angina. The primary endpoints of the trial were (1) all-cause mortality plus all-cause hospitalization (time to first event), and (2) all-cause mortality. Patients were stabilized on optimal concomitant therapy for heart failure, including diuretics, ACE inhibitors, cardiac glycosides, and nitrates. At randomization, 41% of patients were NYHA Class II, 55% NYHA Class III; 65% of patients had heart failure attributed to ischemic heart disease; 44% had a history of hypertension; 25% had diabetes mellitus; 48% had a history of myocardial infarction. Among patients in the trial, 90% were on diuretics, 89% were on ACE inhibitors, 64% were on digitalis, 27% were on a lipid-lowering agent, 37% were on an oral-anticoagulant, and the mean ejection fraction was 0.28. The mean duration of follow-up was one year. At the end of the study, the mean daily dose of Toprol-XL was 159 mg.

The trial was terminated early for a statistically significant reduction in all-cause mortality (34%, nominal p=0.00009). The risk of all-cause mortality plus all-cause hospitalization was reduced by 19% (p=0.00012). The trial also showed improvements in heart failure-related mortality and heart failure-related hospitalizations, and NYHA functional class.

The table below shows the principal results for the overall study population. The figure below illustrates principal results for a wide variety of subgroup comparisons, including US vs. non-US populations (the latter of which was not pre-specified). The combined endpoints of all-cause mortality plus all-cause hospitalization and of mortality plus heart failure hospitalization showed consistent effects in the overall study population and the subgroups, including women and the US population. However, in the US subgroup and women, overall mortality and cardiovascular mortality appeared less affected. Analyses of female and US patients were carried out because they each represented about 25% of the overall population. Nonetheless, subgroup analyses can be difficult to interpret and it is not known whether these represent true differences or chance effects.

Clinical Endpoints in the MERIT-HF Study

Clinical Endpoint	Number of Patients: Placebo n=2001	Number of Patients: Toprol-XL n=1990	Relative Risk (95% CI)	Risk Reduction w/Toprol-XL	Nominal P-value
All-cause mortality plus all-cause hospitalization†	767	641	0.81 (0.73-0.90)	19%	0.00012
All-cause mortality	217	145	0.66 (0.53-0.81)	34%	0.00009
All-cause mortality plus heart failure hospitalization†	439	311	0.69 (0.60-0.80)	31%	0.0000008
Cardiovascular mortality	203	128	0.62 (0.50-0.78)	38%	0.000022
Sudden death	132	79	0.59 (0.45-0.78)	41%	0.0002
Death due to worsening heart failure	58	30	0.51 (0.33-0.79)	49%	0.0023
Hospitalizations due to worsening heart failure‡	451	317	N/A	N/A	0.0000076
Cardiovascular hospitalization‡	773	649	N/A	N/A	0.00028

†Time to first event
‡Comparison of treatment groups examines the number of hospitalizations (Wilcoxon test); relative risk and risk reduction are not applicable.

[See table above]
[See figure at top of next page]

Pharmacokinetics

In man, absorption of metoprolol is rapid and complete. Plasma levels following oral administration of conventional metoprolol tablets, however, approximate 50% of levels following intravenous administration, indicating about 50% first-pass metabolism. Metoprolol crosses the blood-brain barrier and has been reported in the CSF in a concentration 78% of the simultaneous plasma concentration.

Continued on next page

Toprol-XL—Cont.

Plasma levels achieved are highly variable after oral administration. Only a small fraction of the drug (about 12%) is bound to human serum albumin. Metoprolol is a racemic mixture of R-, and S- enantiomers, and is primarily metabolized by CYP2D6. When administered orally, it exhibits stereoselective metabolism that is dependent on oxidation phenotype. Elimination is mainly by biotransformation in the liver, and the plasma half-life ranges from approximately 3 to 7 hours. Less than 5% of an oral dose of metoprolol is recovered unchanged in the urine; the rest is excreted by the kidneys as metabolites that appear to have no beta blocking activity. Following intravenous administration of metoprolol, the urinary recovery of unchanged drug is approximately 10%. The systemic availability and half-life of metoprolol in patients with renal failure do not differ to a clinically significant degree from those in normal subjects. Consequently, no reduction in dosage is usually needed in patients with chronic renal failure.

Metoprolol is metabolized predominantly by CYP2D6, an enzyme that is absent in about 8% of Caucasians (poor metabolizers) and about 2% of most other populations. CYP2D6 can be inhibited by a number of drugs. Concomitant use of inhibiting drugs in poor metabolizers will increase blood levels of metoprolol several fold, decreasing metoprolol's cardioselectivity. (See PRECAUTIONS, Drug Interactions.)

In comparison to conventional metoprolol, the plasma metoprolol levels following administration of Toprol-XL are characterized by lower peaks, longer time to peak and significantly lower peak to trough variation. The peak plasma levels following once daily administration of Toprol-XL average one-fourth to one-half the peak plasma levels obtained following a corresponding dose of conventional metoprolol, administered once daily or in divided doses. At steady state the average bioavailability of metoprolol following administration of Toprol-XL, across the dosage range of 50 to 400 mg once daily, was 77% relative to the corresponding single or divided doses of conventional metoprolol. Nevertheless, over the 24 hour dosing interval, β_1-blockade is comparable and dose-related (see CLINICAL PHARMACOLOGY). The bioavailability of metoprolol shows a dose-related, although not directly proportional, increase with dose and is not significantly affected by food following Toprol-XL administration.

INDICATIONS AND USAGE

Hypertension
Toprol-XL is indicated for the treatment of hypertension. It may be used alone or in combination with other antihypertensive agents.

Angina Pectoris
Toprol-XL is indicated in the long-term treatment of angina pectoris.

Heart Failure
Toprol-XL is indicated for the treatment of stable, symptomatic (NYHA Class II or III) heart failure of ischemic, hypertensive, or cardiomyopathic origin. It was studied in patients already receiving ACE inhibitors, diuretics, and, in the majority of cases, digitalis. In this population, Toprol-XL decreased the rate of mortality plus hospitalization, largely through a reduction in cardiovascular mortality and hospitalizations for heart failure.

CONTRAINDICATIONS

Toprol-XL is contraindicated in severe bradycardia, heart block greater than first degree, cardiogenic shock, decompensated cardiac failure, and sick sinus syndrome (unless a permanent pacemaker is in place) (see WARNINGS).

WARNINGS

Ischemic Heart Disease: Following abrupt cessation of therapy with certain beta-blocking agents, exacerbations of angina pectoris and, in some cases, myocardial infarction have occurred. When discontinuing chronically administered Toprol-XL, particularly in patients with ischemic heart disease, the dosage should be gradually reduced over a period of 1–2 weeks and the patient should be carefully monitored. If angina markedly worsens or acute coronary insufficiency develops, Toprol-XL administration should be reinstated promptly, at least temporarily, and other measures appropriate for the management of unstable angina should be taken. Patients should be warned against interruption or discontinuation of therapy without the physicians advice. Because coronary artery disease is common and may be unrecognized, it may be prudent not to discontinue Toprol-XL therapy abruptly even in patients treated only for hypertension.

Bronchospastic Diseases: PATIENTS WITH BRONCHOSPASTIC DISEASES SHOULD, IN GENERAL, NOT RECEIVE BETA-BLOCKERS. Because of its relative beta$_1$-selectivity, however, Toprol-XL may be used with caution in patients with bronchospastic disease who do not respond to, or cannot tolerate, other antihypertensive treatment. Since beta$_1$-selectivity is not absolute, a beta$_2$-stimulating agent should be administered concomitantly, and the lowest possible dose of Toprol-XL should be used (see DOSAGE AND ADMINISTRATION).

Major Surgery: The necessity or desirability of withdrawing beta-blocking therapy prior to major surgery is controversial; the impaired ability of the heart to respond to reflex adrenergic stimuli may augment the risks of general anesthesia and surgical procedures.

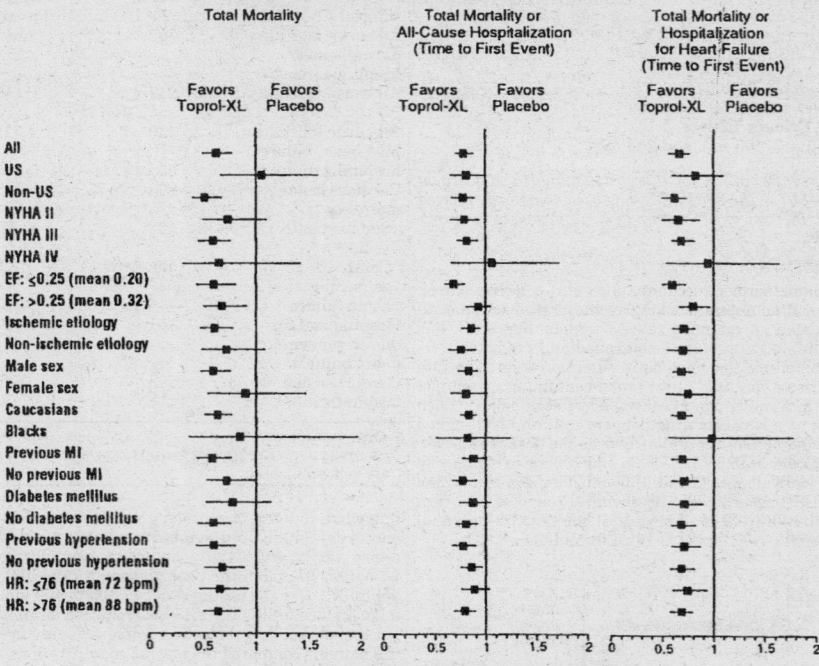

Results for Subgroups in MERIT-HF

US = United States; NYHA = New York Heart Association; EF = ejection fraction; MI = myocardial infarction; HR = heart rate.

Toprol-XL like other beta-blockers, is a competitive inhibitor of beta-receptor agonists, and its effects can be reversed by administration of such agents, e.g., dobutamine or isoproterenol. However, such patients may be subject to protracted severe hypotension. Difficulty in restarting and maintaining the heart beat has also been reported with beta-blockers.

Diabetes and Hypoglycemia: Toprol-XL should be used with caution in diabetic patients if a beta-blocking agent is required. Beta-blockers may mask tachycardia occurring with hypoglycemia, but other manifestations such as dizziness and sweating may not be significantly affected.

Thyrotoxicosis: Beta-adrenergic blockade may mask certain clinical signs (e.g., tachycardia) of hyperthyroidism. Patients suspected of developing thyrotoxicosis should be managed carefully to avoid abrupt withdrawal of beta-blockade, which might precipitate a thyroid storm.

PRECAUTIONS

General
Toprol-XL should be used with caution in patients with impaired hepatic function.
Worsening cardiac failure may occur during up-titration of Toprol-XL. If such symptoms occur, diuretics should be increased and the dose of Toprol-XL should not be advanced until clinical stability is restored (see DOSAGE AND ADMINISTRATION). It may be necessary to lower the dose of Toprol-XL or temporarily discontinue it. Such episodes do not preclude subsequent successful titration of Toprol-XL.

Information for Patients
Patients should be advised to take Toprol-XL regularly and continuously, as directed, preferably with or immediately following meals. If a dose should be missed, the patient should take only the next scheduled dose (without doubling it). Patients should not interrupt or discontinue Toprol-XL without consulting the physician.
Patients should be advised (1) to avoid operating automobiles and machinery or engaging in other tasks requiring alertness until the patient's response to therapy with Toprol-XL has been determined; (2) to contact the physician if any difficulty in breathing occurs; (3) to inform the physician or dentist before any type of surgery that he or she is taking Toprol-XL.
Heart failure patients should be advised to consult their physician if they experience signs or symptoms of worsening heart failure such as weight gain or increasing shortness of breath.

Laboratory Tests
Clinical laboratory findings may include elevated levels of serum transaminase, alkaline phosphatase, and lactate dehydrogenase.

Drug Interactions
Catecholamine-depleting drugs (e.g., reserpine) may have an additive effect when given with beta-blocking agents. Patients treated with Toprol-XL plus a catecholamine depletor should therefore be closely observed for evidence of hypotension or marked bradycardia, which may produce vertigo, syncope, or postural hypotension.
Drugs that inhibit CYP2D6 such as quinidine, fluoxetine, paroxetine, and propafenone are likely to increase metoprolol concentration. In healthy subjects with CYP2D6 extensive metabolizer phenotype, coadministration of quinidine 100 mg and immediate release metoprolol 200 mg, tripled the concentration of S-metoprolol and doubled the metoprolol elimination half-life. In four patients with cardi-

ovascular disease, coadministration of propafenone 150 mg t.i.d. with immediate release metoprolol 50 mg t.i.d. resulted in two- to five-fold increases in the steady-state concentration of metoprolol. These increases in plasma concentration would decrease the cardioselectivity of metoprolol.

Carcinogenesis, Mutagenesis, Impairment of Fertility
Long-term studies in animals have been conducted to evaluate the carcinogenic potential of metoprolol tartrate. In 2-year studies in rats at three oral dosage levels of up to 800 mg/kg/day (41 times, on a mg/m^2 basis, the daily dose of 200 mg for a 60-kg patient), there was no increase in the development of spontaneously occurring benign or malignant neoplasms of any type. The only histologic changes that appeared to be drug related were an increased incidence of generally mild focal accumulation of foamy macrophages in pulmonary alveoli and a slight increase in biliary hyperplasia. In a 21-month study in Swiss albino mice at three oral dosage levels of up to 750 mg/kg/day (18 times, on a mg/m^2 basis, the daily dose of 200 mg for 60-kg patient), benign lung tumors (small adenomas) occurred more frequently in female mice receiving the highest dose than in untreated control animals. There was no increase in malignant or total (benign plus malignant) lung tumors, nor in the overall incidence of tumors or malignant tumors. This 21-month study was repeated in CD-1 mice, and no statistically or biologically significant differences were observed between treated and control mice of either sex for any type of tumor.
All genotoxicity tests performed on metoprolol tartrate (a dominant lethal study in mice, chromosome studies in somatic cells, a Salmonella/mammalian-microsome mutagenicity test, and a nucleus anomaly test in somatic interphase nuclei) and metoprolol succinate (a Salmonella/mammalian-microsome mutagenicity test) were negative.
No evidence of impaired fertility due to metoprolol tartrate was observed in a study performed in rats at doses up to 22 times, on a mg/m^2 basis, the daily dose of 200 mg in a 60-kg patient.

Pregnancy Category C
Metoprolol tartrate has been shown to increase post-implantation loss and decrease neonatal survival in rats at doses up to 22 times, on a mg/m^2 basis, the daily dose of 200 mg in a 60-kg patient. Distribution studies in mice confirm exposure of the fetus when metoprolol tartrate is administered to the pregnant animal. These studies have revealed no evidence of impaired fertility or teratogenicity. There are no adequate and well-controlled studies in pregnant women. Because animal reproduction studies are not always predictive of human response, this drug should be used during pregnancy only if clearly needed.

Nursing Mothers
Metoprolol is excreted in breast milk in very small quantities. An infant consuming 1 liter of breast milk daily would receive a dose of less than 1 mg of the drug. Caution should be exercised when Toprol-XL is administered to a nursing woman.

Pediatric Use
Safety and effectiveness in pediatric patients have not been established.

Geriatric Use
Clinical studies of Toprol-XL in hypertension did not include sufficient numbers of subjects aged 65 and over to determine whether they respond differently from younger subjects.

Other reported clinical experience in hypertensive patients has not identified differences in responses between elderly and younger patients.

Of the 1,990 patients with heart failure randomized to Toprol-XL in the MERIT-HF trial, 50% (990) were 65 years of age and older and 12% (238) were 75 years of age and older. There were no notable differences in efficacy or the rate of adverse events between older and younger patients. In general, dose selection for an elderly patient should be cautious, usually starting at the low end of the dosing range, reflecting greater frequency of decreased hepatic, renal, or cardiac function, and of concomitant disease or other drug therapy.

Risk of Anaphylactic Reactions
While taking beta-blockers, patients with a history of severe anaphylactic reactions to a variety of allergens may be more reactive to repeated challenge, either accidental, diagnostic or therapeutic. Such patients may be unresponsive to the usual doses of epinephrine used to treat allergic reaction.

ADVERSE REACTIONS
Hypertension and Angina
Most adverse effects have been mild and transient. The following adverse reactions have been reported for metoprolol tartrate.
Central Nervous System: Tiredness and dizziness have occurred in about 10 of 100 patients. Depression has been reported in about 5 of 100 patients. Mental confusion and short-term memory loss have been reported. Headache, somnolence, nightmares, and insomnia have also been reported.
Cardiovascular: Shortness of breath and bradycardia have occurred in approximately 3 of 100 patients. Cold extremities; arterial insufficiency, usually of the Raynaud type; palpitations; congestive heart failure; peripheral edema; syncope; chest pain; and hypotension have been reported in about 1 of 100 patients (see CONTRAINDICATIONS, WARNINGS and PRECAUTIONS).
Respiratory: Wheezing (bronchospasm) and dyspnea have been reported in about 1 of 100 patients (see WARNINGS).
Gastrointestinal: Diarrhea has occurred in about 5 of 100 patients. Nausea, dry mouth, gastric pain, constipation, flatulence, digestive tract disorders and heartburn have been reported in about 1 of 100 patients.
Hypersensitive Reactions: Pruritus or rash have occurred in about 5 of 100 patients. Worsening of psoriasis has also been reported.
Miscellaneous: Peyronie's disease has been reported in fewer than 1 of 100,000 patients. Musculoskeletal pain, blurred vision, decreased libido and tinnitus have also been reported.

There have been rare reports of reversible alopecia, agranulocytosis, and dry eyes. Discontinuation of the drug should be considered if any such reaction is not otherwise explicable. The oculomucocutaneous syndrome associated with the beta-blocker practolol has not been reported with metoprolol.

Potential Adverse Reactions
A variety of adverse reactions not listed above have been reported with other beta-adrenergic blocking agents and should be considered potential adverse reactions to Toprol-XL.
Central Nervous System: Reversible mental depression progressing to catatonia; an acute reversible syndrome characterized by disorientation for time and place, short-term memory loss, emotional lability, slightly clouded sensorium, and decreased performance on neuropsychometrics.
Cardiovascular: Intensification of AV block (see CONTRAINDICATIONS).
Hematologic: Agranulocytosis, nonthrombocytopenic purpura, thrombocytopenic purpura.
Hypersensitive Reactions: Fever combined with aching and sore throat, laryngospasm, and respiratory distress.
Heart Failure
In the MERIT-HF study, serious adverse events and adverse events leading to discontinuation of study medication were systematically collected. In the MERIT-HF study comparing Toprol-XL in daily doses up to 200 mg (mean dose 159 mg once-daily) (n=1990) to placebo (n=2001), 10.3% of Toprol-XL patients discontinued for adverse events vs. 12.2% of placebo patients.
The table below lists adverse events in the MERIT-HF study that occurred at an incidence of equal to or greater than 1% in the Toprol-XL group and greater than placebo by more than 0.5%, regardless of the assessment of causality.

Adverse Events Occurring in the MERIT-HF Study at an Incidence ≥ 1% in the Toprol-XL Group and Greater than Placebo by More Than 0.5%		
	Toprol-XL n=1990 % of patients	Placebo n=2001 % of patients
Dizziness/vertigo	1.8	1.0
Bradycardia	1.5	0.4
Accident and/or injury	1.4	0.8

Other adverse events with an incidence of > 1% on Toprol-XL and as common on placebo (within 0.5%) included myocardial infarction, pneumonia, cerebrovascular disorder, chest pain, dyspnea/dyspnea aggravated, syncope, coronary artery disorder, ventricular tachycardia/arrhythmia aggravated, hypotension, diabetes mellitus/diabetes mellitus aggravated, abdominal pain, and fatigue.

OVERDOSAGE
Acute Toxicity
There have been a few reports of overdosage with Toprol-XL and no specific overdosage information was obtained with this drug, with the exception of animal toxicology data. However, since Toprol-XL (metoprolol succinate salt) contains the same active moiety, metoprolol, as conventional metoprolol tablets (metoprolol tartrate salt), the recommendations on overdosage for metoprolol conventional tablets are applicable to Toprol-XL.
Signs and Symptoms
Overdosage of Toprol-XL may lead to severe hypotension, sinus bradycardia, atrioventricular block, heart failure, cardiogenic shock, cardiac arrest, bronchospasm, impairment of consciousness/coma, nausea, vomiting, and cyanosis.
Treatment
In general, patients with acute or recent myocardial infarction or congestive heart failure may be more hemodynamically unstable than other patients and should be treated accordingly. When possible the patient should be treated under intensive care conditions. On the basis of the pharmacologic actions of metoprolol, the following general measures should be employed.
Elimination of the Drug: Gastric lavage should be performed.
Bradycardia: Atropine should be administered. If there is no response to vagal blockade, isoproterenol should be administered cautiously.
Hypotension: A vasopressor should be administered, e.g., levarterenol or dopamine.
Bronchospasm: A beta$_2$-stimulating agent and/or a theophylline derivative should be administered.
Cardiac Failure: A digitalis glycoside and diuretics should be administered. In shock resulting from inadequate cardiac contractility, administration of dobutamine, isoproterenol or glucagon may be considered.

DOSAGE AND ADMINISTRATION
Toprol-XL is an extended release tablet intended for once-a-day administration. When switching from immediate release metoprolol tablet to Toprol-XL, the same total daily dose of Toprol-XL should be used.
As with immediate release metoprolol, dosages of Toprol-XL should be individualized and titration may be needed in some patients.
Toprol-XL tablets are scored and can be divided; however, the whole or half tablet should be swallowed whole and not chewed or crushed.
Hypertension
The usual initial dosage is 50 to 100 mg daily in a single dose, whether used alone or added to a diuretic. The dosage may be increased at weekly (or longer) intervals until optimum blood pressure reduction is achieved. In general, the maximum effect of any given dosage level will be apparent after 1 week of therapy. Dosages above 400 mg per day have not been studied.
Angina Pectoris
The dosage of Toprol-XL should be individualized. The usual initial dosage is 100 mg daily, given in a single dose. The dosage may be gradually increased at weekly intervals until optimum clinical response has been obtained or there is a pronounced slowing of the heart rate. Dosages above 400 mg per day have not been studied. If treatment is to be discontinued, the dosage should be reduced gradually over a period of 1–2 weeks (see WARNINGS).
Heart Failure
Dosage must be individualized and closely monitored during up-titration. Prior to initiation of Toprol-XL, the dosing of diuretics, ACE inhibitors, and digitalis (if used) should be stabilized. The recommended starting dose of Toprol-XL is 25 mg once daily for two weeks in patients with NYHA class II heart failure and 12.5 mg once daily in patients with more severe heart failure. The dose should then be doubled every two weeks to the highest dosage level tolerated by the patient or up to 200 mg of Toprol-XL. If transient worsening of heart failure occurs, it may be treated with increased doses of diuretics, and it may also be necessary to lower the dose of Toprol-XL or temporarily discontinue it. The dose of Toprol-XL should not be increased until symptoms of worsening heart failure have been stabilized. Initial difficulty with titration should not preclude later attempts to introduce Toprol-XL. If heart failure patients experience symptomatic bradycardia, the dose of Toprol-XL should be reduced.

HOW SUPPLIED
Tablets containing metoprolol succinate equivalent to the indicated weight of metoprolol tartrate, USP, are white, biconvex, film-coated, and scored.

Tablet	Shape	Engraving	Bottle of 100 NDC 0186-
25 mg*	Oval	A β	1088-05
50 mg	Round	A mo	1090-05
100 mg	Round	A ms	1092-05
200 mg	Oval	A my	1094-05

* The 25-mg tablet is scored on both sides.
Store at 25°C (77°F). Excursions permitted to 15–30°C (59-86°F). (See USP Controlled Room Temperature.)

All trademarks are the property of the AstraZeneca group
©AstraZeneca 2001
Manufactured for: AstraZeneca LP
Wilmington, DE 19850
By: AstraZeneca AB
S-151 85 Södertälje, Sweden
Made in Sweden
64175-00
Rev 01/01

AstraZeneca Pharmaceuticals LP
1800 CONCORD PIKE
WILMINGTON, DE 19850-5437 USA

For Product and Business Information, and Adverse Drug Experiences:
Information Center
1-800-236-9933

For Product Ordering:
Trade Customer Service
1-800-842-9920

Internet: www.astrazeneca-us.com

ARIMIDEX® ℞
anastrozole
TABLETS

Prescribing information for this product, which appears on pages 613–615 of the 2001 PDR, has been completely revised as follows. Please write "See Supplement A" next to the product heading.

DESCRIPTION
ARIMIDEX® (anastrozole) tablets for oral administration contain 1 mg of anastrozole, a non-steroidal aromatase inhibitor. It is chemically described as 1,3-Benzenediacetonitrile, α, α, α', α'-tetramethyl-5-(1H-1,2,4-triazol-1-yl-methyl). Its molecular formula is $C_{17}H_{19}N_5$ and its structural formula is:

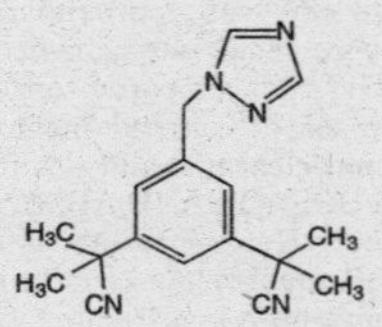

Anastrozole is an off-white powder with a molecular weight of 293.4. Anastrozole has moderate aqueous solubility (0.5 mg/mL at 25°C); solubility is independent of pH in the physiological range. Anastrozole is freely soluble in methanol, acetone, ethanol, and tetrahydrofuran, and very soluble in acetonitrile.
Each tablet contains as inactive ingredients: lactose, magnesium stearate, hydroxypropylmethylcellulose, polyethylene glycol, povidone, sodium starch glycolate, and titanium dioxide.

CLINICAL PHARMACOLOGY
Mechanism of Action
Many breast cancers have estrogen receptors and growth of these tumors can be stimulated by estrogen. In post-menopausal women, the principal source of circulating estrogen (primarily estradiol) is conversion of adrenally-generated androstenedione to estrone by aromatase in peripheral tissues, such as adipose tissue, with further conversion of estrone to estradiol. Many breast cancers also contain aromatase; the importance of tumor-generated estrogens is uncertain.
Treatment of breast cancer has included efforts to decrease estrogen levels, by ovariectomy premenopausally and by use of anti-estrogens and progestational agents both pre- and post-menopausally; and these interventions lead to decreased tumor mass or delayed progression of tumor growth in some women.
Anastrozole is a potent and selective non-steroidal aromatase inhibitor. It significantly lowers serum estradiol concentrations and has no detectable effect on formation of adrenal corticosteriods or aldosterone.
Pharmacokinetics
Inhibition of aromatase activity is primarily due to anastrozole, the parent drug. Studies with radiolabeled drug have demonstrated that orally administered anastrozole is well absorbed into the systemic circulation with 83 to 85% of the radiolabel recovered in urine and feces. Food does not affect the extent of absorption. Elimination of anastrozole is primarily via hepatic metabolism (approximately 85%) and to a lesser extent, renal excretion (approximately 11%), and anastrozole has a mean terminal elimination half-life of approximately 50 hours in postmenopausal women. The major circulating metabolite of anastrozole, triazole, lacks pharmacologic activity. The pharmacokinetic parameters are similar in patients and in healthy postmenopausal volun-

Continued on next page

Arimidex—Cont.

teers. The pharmacokinetics of anastrozole are linear over the dose range of 1 to 20 mg and do not change with repeated dosing. Consistent with the approximately 2-day terminal elimination half-life, plasma concentrations approach steady-state levels at about 7 days of once daily dosing and steady-state levels are approximately three- to four-fold higher than levels observed after a single dose of ARIMIDEX. Anastrozole is 40% bound to plasma proteins in the therapeutic range.

Metabolism and Excretion: Studies in postmenopausal women demonstrated that anastrozole is extensively metabolized with about 10% of the dose excreted in the urine as unchanged drug within 72 hours of dosing, and the remainder (about 60% of the dose) is excreted in urine as metabolites. Metabolism of anastrozole occurs by N-dealkylation, hydroxylation and glucuronidation. Three metabolites of anastrozole have been identified in human plasma and urine. The known metabolites are triazole, a glucuronide conjugate of hydroxy-anastrozole, and a glucuronide of anastrozole itself. Several minor (less than 5% of the radioactive dose) metabolites have not been identified.

Because renal elimination is not a significant pathway of elimination, total body clearance of anastrozole is unchanged even in severe (creatinine clearance less than 30 mL/min/1.73m^2) renal impairment, dosing adjustment in patients with renal dysfunction is not necessary (see Special Populations and DOSAGE AND ADMINISTRATION sections). Dosage adjustment is also unnecessary in patients with stable hepatic cirrhosis (see Special Populations and DOSAGE AND ADMINISTRATION sections).

Special Populations:

Geriatric: Anastrozole pharmacokinetics have been investigated in postmenopausal female volunteers and patients with breast cancer. No age related effects were seen over the range <50 to >80 years.

Race: Estradiol and estrone sulfate levels were similar between Japanese and Caucasian postmenopausal women who received 1 mg of anastrozole daily for 16 days. Anastrozole mean steady state minimum plasma concentrations in Caucasian and Japanese postmenopausal women were 25.7 and 30.4 ng/mL, respectively.

Renal Insufficiency: Anastrozole pharmacokinetics have been investigated in subjects with renal insufficiency. Anastrozole renal clearance decreased proportionally with creatinine clearance and was approximately 50% lower in volunteers with severe renal impairment (creatinine clearance < 30 mL/min/1.73m^2) compared to controls. Since only about 10% of anastrozole is excreted unchanged in the urine, the reduction in renal clearance did not influence the total body clearance (see DOSAGE AND ADMINISTRATION).

Hepatic Insufficiency: Hepatic metabolism accounts for approximately 85% of anastrozole elimination. Anastrozole pharmacokinetics have been investigated in subjects with hepatic cirrhosis related to alcohol abuse. The apparent oral clearance (CL/F) of anastrozole was approximately 30% lower in subjects with stable hepatic cirrhosis than in control subjects with normal liver function. However, plasma anastrozole concentrations in the subjects with hepatic cirrhosis were within the range of concentrations seen in normal subjects across all clinical trials (see DOSAGE AND ADMINISTRATION), so that no dosage adjustment is needed.

Drug-Drug Interactions: Anastrozole inhibited reactions catalyzed by cytochrome P450 1A2, 2C8/9, and 3A4 *in vitro* with Ki values which were approximately 30 times higher than the mean steady-state C_{max} values observed following a 1 mg daily dose. Anastrozole had no inhibitory effect on reactions catalyzed by cytochrome P450 2A6 or 2D6 *in vitro*. Administration of a single 30 mg/kg or multiple 10 mg/kg doses of anastrozole to subjects had no effect on the clearance of antipyrine or urinary recovery of antipyrine metabolites. Based on these *in vitro* and *in vivo* results, it is unlikely that co-administration of ARIMIDEX 1 mg with other drugs will result in clinically significant inhibition of cytochrome P450 mediated metabolism.

In a study conducted in 16 male volunteers, anastrozole did not alter the pharmacokinetics as measured by C_{max} and AUC, and anticoagulant activity as measured by prothrombin time, activated partial thromboplastine time, and thrombin time of both R- and S-warfarin.

Pharmacodynamics

Effect on Estradiol: Mean serum concentrations of estradiol were evaluated in multiple daily dosing trials with 0.5, 1, 3, 5, and 10 mg of ARIMIDEX in postmenopausal women with advanced breast cancer. Clinically significant suppression of serum estradiol was seen with all doses. Doses of 1 mg and higher resulted in suppression of mean serum concentrations of estradiol to the lower limit of detection (3.7 pmol/L). The recommended daily dose, ARIMIDEX 1 mg, reduced estradiol by approximately 70% within 24 hours and by approximately 80% after 14 days of daily dosing. Suppression of serum estradiol was maintained for up to 6 days after cessation of daily dosing with ARIMIDEX 1 mg.

Effect on Corticosteroids: In multiple daily dosing trials with 3, 5, and 10 mg, the selectivity of anastrozole was assessed by examining effects on corticosteroid synthesis. For all doses, anastrozole did not affect cortisol or aldosterone secretion at baseline or in response to ACTH. No glucocorticoid or mineralocorticoid replacement therapy is necessary with anastrozole.

Other Endocrine Effects: In multiple daily dosing trials with 5 and 10 mg, thyroid stimulating hormone (TSH) was measured; there was no increase in TSH during the administration of ARIMIDEX. ARIMIDEX does not possess direct progestogenic, androgenic, or estrogenic activity in animals, but does perturb the circulating levels of progesterone, androgens, and estrogens.

Table 1
Number (%) of subjects

Receptor status	Trial 0030 ARIMIDEX 1 mg (n=171)	Trial 0030 Tamoxifen 20 mg (n=182)	Trial 0027 ARIMIDEX 1 mg (n=340)	Trial 0027 Tamoxifen 20 mg (n=328)
ER+ and/or PR+	151 (88.3)	162 (89.0)	154 (45.3)	144 (43.9)
ER unknown, PR unknown	19 (11.1)	20 (11.0)	185 (54.4)	183 (55.8)

ER = Estrogen receptor
PR = Progesterone receptor

Table 2
Number (%) of subjects

End Point	Trial 0030 ARIMIDEX 1 mg (n=171)	Trial 0030 Tamoxifen 20 mg (n=182)	Trial 0027 ARIMIDEX 1 mg (n=340)	Trial 0027 Tamoxifen 20 mg (n=328)
Time to progression (TTP)				
Median TTP (months)	11.1	5.6	8.2	8.3
Number (%) of subjects who progressed	114 (67%)	138 (76%)	249 (73%)	247 (75%)
Hazard ratio (LCL)[1]	1.42 (1.15)		1.01 (0.87)	
2-sided 95% CI	(1.11, 1.82)		(0.85, 1.20)	
p-value[2]	0.006		0.920	
Best objective response rate				
Number (%) of subjects with CR + PR	36 (21.1%)	31 (17.0%)	112 (32.9%)	107 (32.6%)
Odds Ratio (LCL)[3]	1.30 (0.83)		1.01 (0.77)	

CR = Complete Response
PR = Partial Response
CI = Confidence Interval
LCL = Lower Confidence Limit
[1] Tamoxifen:ARIMIDEX
[2] Two-sided Log Rank
[3] ARIMIDEX:Tamoxifen

Clinical Studies - First Line Therapy in Postmenopausal Women with Advanced Breast Cancer: Two double-blind, well-controlled clinical studies of similar design (0030, a North American study and 0027, a predominately European study) were conducted to assess the efficacy of ARIMIDEX compared with tamoxifen as first-line therapy for hormone receptor positive or hormone receptor unknown locally advanced or metastatic breast cancer in postmenopausal women. A total of 1021 patients between the ages of 30 and 92 years old were randomized to receive trial treatment. Patients were randomized to receive 1 mg of ARIMIDEX once daily or 20 mg of tamoxifen once daily. The primary end points for both trials were time to tumor progression, objective tumor response rate, and safety.

Demographics and other baseline characteristics, including patients who had measurable and no measurable disease, patients who were given previous adjuvant therapy, the site of metastatic disease and ethnic origin were similar for the two treatment groups for both trials. The following table summarizes the hormone receptor status at entry for all randomized patients in trials 0030 and 0027.

[See table 1 above]

For the primary endpoints, trial 0030 showed ARIMIDEX was at least as effective as tamoxifen for objective tumor response rate. ARIMIDEX had a statistically significant advantage over tamoxifen (p=0.006) for time to tumor progression (see Table 2 and Figure 1). Trial 0027 showed ARIMIDEX was at least as effective as tamoxifen for objective tumor response rate and time to tumor progression (See Table 2 and Figure 2).

Table 2 below summarizes the results of trial 0030 and trial 0027 for the primary efficacy endpoints.

[See table 2 above]

Figure 1 - Kaplan-Meier probability of time to disease progression for all randomized patients (intent-to-treat) in Trial 0030

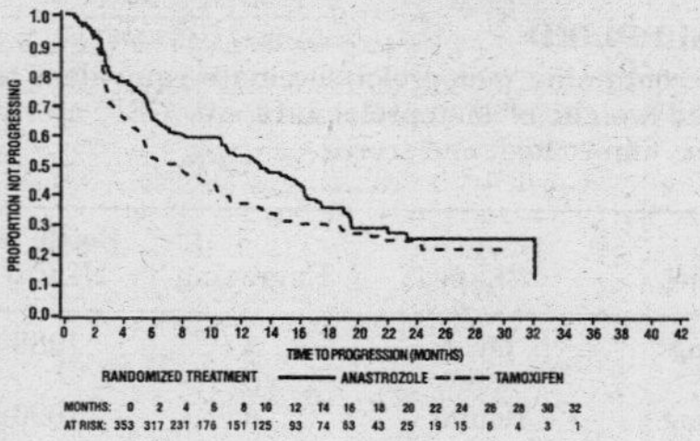

[See figure 2 at top of next column]

Results from the secondary endpoints of time to treatment failure, duration of tumor response, and duration of clinical benefit were supportive of the results of the primary efficacy endpoints. There were too few deaths occurring across treatment groups of both trials to draw conclusions on overall survival differences.

Figure 2 - Kaplan-Meier probability of time to progression for all randomized patients (intent-to-treat) in Trial 0027

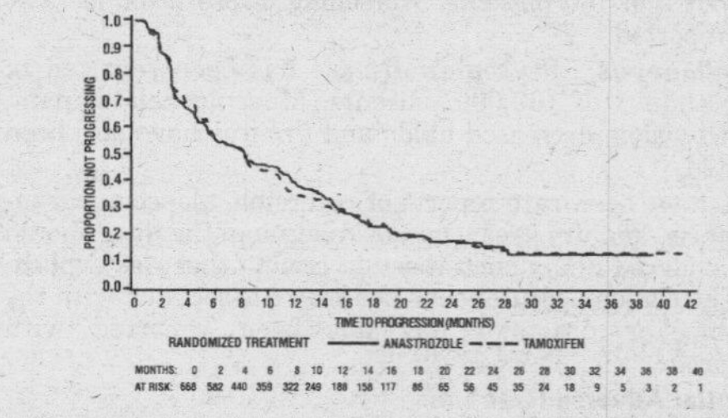

Clinical Studies - Second Line Therapy in Postmenopausal Women with Advanced Breast Cancer who had Disease Progression following Tamoxifen Therapy: Anastrozole was studied in two well-controlled clinical trials (0004, a North American study; 0005, a predominately European study) in postmenopausal women with advanced breast cancer who had disease progression following tamoxifen therapy for either advanced or early breast cancer. Some of the patients had also received previous cytotoxic treatment. Most patients were ER-positive; a smaller fraction were ER-unknown or ER-negative; the ER-negative patients were eligible only if they had had a positive response to tamoxifen. Eligible patients with measurable and non-measurable disease were randomized to receive either a single daily dose of 1 mg or 10 mg of ARIMIDEX or megestrol acetate 40 mg four times a day. The studies were double-blinded with respect to ARIMIDEX. Time to progression and objective response (only patients with measurable disease could be considered partial responders) rates were the primary efficacy variables. Objective response rates were calculated based on the Union Internationale Contre le Cancer (UICC) criteria. The rate of prolonged (more than 24 weeks) stable disease, the rate of progression, and survival were also calculated.

Both trials included over 375 patients; demographics and other baseline characteristics were similar for the three treatment groups in each trial. Patients in the 0005 trial had responded better to prior tamoxifen treatment. Of the patients entered who had prior tamoxifen therapy for advanced disease (58% in Trial 0004; 57% in Trial 0005), 18% of these patients in Trial 0004 and 42% in Trial 0005 were reported by the primary investigator to have responded. In Trial 0004, 81% of patients were ER-positive, 13% were ER-unknown, and 6% were ER-negative. In Trial 0005, 58% of patients were ER-positive, 37% were ER-unknown, and 5% were ER-negative. In Trial 0004, 62% of patients had measurable disease compared to 79% in Trial 0005. The sites of metastatic disease were similar among treatment groups for each trial. On average, 40% of the patients had soft tissue metastases; 60% had bone metastases; and 40% had visceral (15% liver) metastases.

As shown in the table below, similar results were observed among treatment groups and between the two trials. None of the within trial differences were statistically significant.

[See table 3 at top of next page]

More than 1/3 of the patients in each treatment group in both studies had either an objective response or stabilization of their disease for greater than 24 weeks. Among the 263 patients who received ARIMIDEX 1 mg, there were 11

Table 3

	ARIMIDEX 1 mg	ARIMIDEX 10 mg	Megestrol Acetate 160 mg
Trial 0004			
(N. America)	(n=128)	(n=130)	(n=128)
Median Follow-up (months)*	31.3	30.9	32.9
Median Time to Death (months)	29.6	25.7	26.7
2 Year Survival Probability (%)	62.0	58.0	53.1
Median Time to Progression (months)	5.7	5.3	5.1
Objective Response (all patients) (%)	12.5	10.0	10.2
Stable Disease for >24 weeks (%)	35.2	29.2	32.8
Progression (%)	86.7	85.4	90.6
Trial 0005			
(Europe, Australia, S. Africa)	(n=135)	(n=118)	(n=125)
Median Follow-up (months)*	31.0	30.9	31.5
Median Time to Death (months)	24.3	24.8	19.8
2 Year Survival Probability (%)	50.5	50.9	39.1
Median Time to Progression (months)	4.4	5.3	3.9
Objective Response (all patients) (%)	12.6	15.3	14.4
Stable Disease for >24 weeks (%)	24.4	25.4	23.2
Progression (%)	91.9	89.8	92.0

*Surviving Patients

Table 4

Trials 0004 & 0005 (Pooled Data)	ARIMIDEX 1 mg N=263	ARIMIDEX 10 mg N=248	Megestrol Acetate 160 mg N=253
Median Time to Death (months)	26.7	25.5	22.5
2 Year Survival Probability (%)	56.1	54.6	46.3
Median Time to Progression (months)	4.8	5.3	4.6
Objective Response (all patients) (%)	12.5	12.5	12.3

complete responders and 22 partial responders. In patients who had an objective response, more than 80% were still responding at 6 months from randomization and more than 45% were still responding at 12 months from randomization.

When data from the two controlled trials are pooled, the objective response rates and median times to progression and death were similar for patients randomized to ARIMIDEX 1 mg and megestrol acetate. There is, in this data, no indication that ARIMIDEX 10 mg is superior to ARIMIDEX 1 mg.

[See table 4 above]

Objective response rates and median times to progression and death for ARIMIDEX 1 mg were similar to megestrol acetate for women over or under 65. There were too few non-white patients studied to draw conclusions about racial differences in response.

INDICATIONS AND USAGE

ARIMIDEX is indicated for the first-line treatment of postmenopausal women with hormone receptor positive or hormone receptor unknown locally advanced or metastatic breast cancer.

ARIMIDEX is indicated for the treatment of advanced breast cancer in postmenopausal women with disease progression following tamoxifen therapy.

Patients with ER-negative disease and patients who did not respond to previous tamoxifen therapy rarely responded to ARIMIDEX.

CONTRAINDICATIONS

None known.

WARNINGS

ARIMIDEX can cause fetal harm when administered to a pregnant woman. Anastrozole has been found to cross the placenta following oral administration of 0.1 mg/kg in rats and rabbits (about 3/4 and 1.5 times the recommended human dose, respectively, on a mg/m^2 basis). Studies in both rats and rabbits at doses equal to or greater than 0.1 and 0.02 mg/kg/day, respectively (about 3/4 and 1/3, respectively, the recommended human dose on a mg/m^2 basis), administered during the period of organogenesis showed that anastrozole increased pregnancy loss (increased pre- and/or post-implantation loss, increased resorption, and decreased numbers of live fetuses); effects were dose related in rats. Placental weights were significantly increased in rats at doses of 0.1 mg/kg/day or more.

Evidence of fetotoxicity, including delayed fetal development (i.e., incomplete ossification and depressed fetal body weights), was observed in rats administered doses of 1 mg/kg/day (which produced plasma anastrozole C_{ssmax} and AUC_{0-24} hr that were 19 times and 9 times higher than the respective values found in healthy postmenopausal humans at the recommended dose). There was no evidence of teratogenicity in rats administered doses up to 1.0 mg/kg/day. In rabbits, anastrozole caused pregnancy failure at doses equal to or greater than 1.0 mg/kg/day (about 16 times the recommended human dose on a mg/m^2 basis); there was no evidence of teratogenicity in rabbits administered 0.2 mg/kg/day (about 3 times the recommended human dose on a mg/m^2 basis).

There are no adequate and well-controlled studies in pregnant women using ARIMIDEX. If ARIMIDEX is used during pregnancy, or if the patient becomes pregnant while receiving this drug, the patient should be apprised of the potential hazard to the fetus or potential risk for loss of the pregnancy.

PRECAUTIONS

General: Before starting treatment with ARIMIDEX, pregnancy must be excluded (see WARNINGS).

ARIMIDEX should be administered under the supervision of a qualified physician experienced in the use of anticancer agents.

Laboratory Tests: Three-fold elevations of mean serum gamma glutamyl transferase (GT) levels have been observed among patients with liver metastases receiving ARIMIDEX or megestrol acetate. These changes were likely related to the progression of liver metastases in these patients, although other contributing factors could not be ruled out.

Drug Interactions: (See CLINICAL PHARMACOLOGY) Anastrozole inhibited *in vitro* metabolic reactions catalyzed by cytochromes P450 1A2, 2C8/9, and 3A4 but only at relatively high concentrations. Anastrozole did not inhibit P450 2A6 or the polymorphic P450 2D6 in human liver microsomes. Anastrozole did not alter the pharmacokinetics of antipyrine. Although there have been no formal interaction studies other than with antipyrine, based on these *in vivo* and *in vitro* studies, it is unlikely that co-administration of a 1 mg dose of ARIMIDEX with other drugs will result in clinically significant drug inhibition of cytochrome P450-mediated metabolism of the other drugs.

An interaction study with warfarin showed no clinically significant effect of anastrozole on warfarin pharmacokinetics or anticoagulant activity.

Drug/Laboratory Test Interactions: No clinically significant changes in the results of clinical laboratory tests have been observed.

Carcinogenesis: A conventional carcinogenesis study in rats at doses of 1.0 to 25 mg/kg/day (about 8 to 200 times the daily maximum recommended human dose on a mg/m^2 basis) administered by oral gavage for up to 2 years revealed an increase in the incidence of hepatocellular adenoma and carcinoma and uterine stromal polyps in females and thyroid adenoma in males at the high dose. A dose related increase was observed in the incidence of ovarian and uterine hyperplasia in females. At 25 mg/kg/day, plasma $AUC_{0-24\ hr.}$ levels in rats were 110 to 125 times higher than the level exhibited in post-menopausal volunteers at the recommended dose. A separate carcinogenicity study in mice at oral doses of 5 to 50 mg/kg/day (about 20 to 200 times the daily maximum recommended human dose on a mg/m^2 basis) for up to 2 years produced an increase in the incidence of benign ovarian stromal, epithelial and granulosa cell tumors at all dose levels. A dose related increase in the incidence of ovarian hyperplasia was also observed in female mice. These ovarian changes are considered to be rodent-specific effects of aromatase inhibition and are of questionable significance to humans. The incidence of lymphosarcoma was increased in males and females at the high dose. At 50 mg/kg/day, plasma AUC levels in mice were 35 to 40 times higher than the level exhibited in post-menopausal volunteers at the recommended dose.

Mutagenesis: ARIMIDEX has not been shown to be mutagenic in *in vitro* tests (Ames and E. coli bacterial tests, CHO-K1 gene mutation assay) or clastogenic either *in vitro* (chromosome aberrations in human lymphocytes) or *in vivo* (micronucleus test in rats).

Impairment of Fertility: Studies to investigate the effect of ARIMIDEX on fertility have not been conducted; however, chronic studies indicated hypertrophy of the ovaries and the presence of follicular cysts in rats administered doses equal to or greater than 1 mg/kg/day (which produced plasma anastrozole C_{ssmax} and $AUC_{0-24\ hr}$ that were 19 and 9 times higher than the respective values found in healthy post-menopausal humans at the recommended dose). In addition, hyperplastic uteri were observed in chronic studies of female dogs administered doses equal to or greater than 1 mg/kg/day (which produced plasma anastrozole C_{ssmax} and $AUC_{0-24\ hr}$ that were 22 times and 16 times higher than the respective values found in post-menopausal humans at the recommended dose). It is not known whether these effects on the reproductive organs of animals are associated with impaired fertility in humans.

Pregnancy: Pregnancy Category D: (See WARNINGS).

Nursing Mothers: It is not known if anastrozole is excreted in human milk. Because many drugs are excreted in human milk, caution should be exercised when ARIMIDEX is administered to a nursing woman. (See WARNINGS and PRECAUTIONS.)

Pediatric Use: The safety and efficacy of ARIMIDEX in pediatric patients have not been established.

Geriatric Use: In studies 0027 and 0030 about 50% of patients were 65 or older. Patients ≥ 65 years of age had moderately better tumor response and time to tumor progression than patients < 65 years of age regardless of randomized treatment. In studies 0004 and 0005 fifty percent of patients were 65 or older. Response rates and time to progression were similar for the over 65 and younger patients.

ADVERSE REACTIONS

First Line Therapy: ARIMIDEX was generally well tolerated in two well-controlled clinical trials (i.e., Trials 0030 and 0027). Adverse events occurring with an incidence of at least 5% in either treatment group of trials 0030 and 0027 during or within 2 weeks of the end of treatment are shown in Table 5.

Table 5

Body system Adverse event[a]	Number (%) of subjects ARIMIDEX (n=506)		Tamoxifen (n=511)	
Whole body				
Asthenia	83	(16.4)	81	(15.9)
Pain	70	(13.8)	73	(14.3)
Back pain	60	(11.9)	68	(13.3)
Headache	47	(9.3)	40	(7.8)
Abdominal pain	40	(7.9)	38	(7.4)
Chest pain	37	(7.3)	37	(7.2)
Flu syndrome	35	(6.9)	30	(5.9)
Pelvic pain	23	(4.5)	30	(5.9)
Cardiovascular				
Vasodilation	128	(25.3)	106	(20.7)
Hypertension	25	(4.9)	36	(7.0)
Digestive				
Nausea	94	(18.6)	106	(20.7)
Constipation	47	(9.3)	66	(12.9)
Diarrhea	40	(7.9)	33	(6.5)
Vomiting	38	(7.5)	36	(7.0)
Anorexia	26	(5.1)	46	(9.0)
Metabolic and nutritional				
Peripheral edema	51	(10.1)	41	(8.0)
Musculoskeletal				
Bone pain	54	(10.7)	52	(10.2)
Nervous				
Dizziness	30	(5.9)	22	(4.3)
Insomnia	30	(5.9)	38	(5.5)
Depression	23	(4.5)	32	(6.3)
Hypertonia	16	(3.2)	26	(5.1)
Respiratory				
Cough increased	55	(10.9)	52	(10.2)
Dyspnea	51	(10.1)	47	(9.2)
Pharyngitis	49	(9.7)	68	(13.3)
Skin and appendages				
Rash	38	(7.5)	34	(7.6)
Urogenital				
Leukorrhea	9	(1.8)	31	(6.1)

[a]A patient may have had more than 1 adverse event.

Less frequent adverse experiences reported in patients receiving ARIMIDEX 1 mg in either Trial 0030 or Trial 0027 were similar to those reported for second-line therapy.

Based on results from second-line therapy and the established safety profile of tamoxifen, the incidences of 9 prespecified adverse event categories potentially causally related to one or both of the therapies because of their pharmacology were statistically analyzed. No significant differences were seen between treatment groups.

Table 6

Adverse Event Group[a]	Number (n) and Percentage of Patients: ARIMIDEX 1 mg (n = 506) n	(%)	NOLVADEX 20 mg (n = 511) n	(%)
Depression	23	(4.5)	32	(6.3)
Tumor Flare	15	(3.0)	18	(3.5)
Thromboembolic Disease[a]	18	(3.5)	33	(6.5)
Venous[b]	5		15	
Coronary and Cerebral[c]	13		19	
Gastrointestinal Disturbance	170	(33.6)	196	(38.4)
Hot Flushes	134	(26.5)	118	(23.1)
Vaginal Dryness	9	(1.7)	3	(0.6)

Continued on next page

Arimidex—Cont.

Lethargy	6	(1.2)	15	(2.9)		
Vaginal Bleeding	5	(1.0)	11	(2.2)		
Weight Gain	11	(2.2)	8	(1.6)		

[a] A patient may have had more than 1 adverse event
[b] Includes pulmonary embolus, thrombophlebitis, retinal vein thrombosis
[c] Includes myocardial infarction, myocardial ischemia, angina pectoris, cerebrovascular accident, cerebral ischemia and cerebral infarct

Despite the lack of estrogenic activity for ARIMIDEX, there was no increase in myocardial infarction or fracture when compared with tamoxifen.

Second Line Therapy: ARIMIDEX was generally well tolerated in two well-controlled clinical trials (i.e., Trials 0004 and 0005), with less than 3.3% of the ARIMIDEX-treated patients and 4.0% of the megestrol acetate-treated patients withdrawing due to an adverse event.

The principal adverse event more common with ARIMIDEX than megestrol acetate was diarrhea. Adverse events reported in greater than 5% of the patients in any of the treatment groups in these two well-controlled clinical trials, regardless of causality, are presented below:

Table 7
Number (n) and Percentage of Patients with Adverse Event†

Adverse Event	ARIMIDEX 1 mg (n = 262) n	%	ARIMIDEX 10 mg (n = 246) n	%	Megestrol Acetate 160 mg (n=253) n	%
Asthenia	42	(16.0)	33	(13.4)	47	(18.6)
Nausea	41	(15.6)	48	(19.5)	28	(11.1)
Headache	34	(13.0)	44	(17.9)	24	(9.5)
Hot Flushes	32	(12.2)	29	(10.6)	21	(8.3)
Pain	28	(10.7)	38	(15.4)	29	(11.5)
Back Pain	28	(10.7)	26	(10.6)	19	(7.5)
Dyspnea	24	(9.2)	27	(11.0)	53	(20.9)
Vomiting	24	(9.2)	26	(10.6)	16	(6.3)
Cough Increased	22	(8.4)	18	(7.3)	19	(7.5)
Diarrhea	22	(8.4)	18	(7.3)	7	(2.8)
Constipation	18	(6.9)	18	(7.3)	21	(8.3)
Abdominal Pain	18	(6.9)	14	(5.7)	18	(7.1)
Anorexia	18	(6.9)	19	(7.7)	11	(4.3)
Bone Pain	17	(6.5)	26	(11.8)	19	(7.5)
Pharyngitis	16	(6.1)	23	(9.3)	15	(5.9)
Dizziness	16	(6.1)	12	(4.9)	15	(5.9)
Rash	15	(5.7)	15	(6.1)	19	(7.5)
Dry Mouth	15	(5.7)	11	(4.5)	13	(5.1)
Peripheral Edema	14	(5.3)	21	(8.5)	28	(11.1)
Pelvic Pain	14	(5.3)	17	(6.9)	13	(5.1)
Depression	14	(5.3)	6	(2.4)	5	(2.0)
Chest Pain	13	(5.0)	18	(7.3)	13	(5.1)
Paresthesia	12	(4.6)	15	(6.1)	9	(3.6)
Vaginal Hemorrhage	6	(2.3)	4	(1.6)	13	(5.1)
Weight Gain	4	(1.5)	9	(3.7)	30	(11.9)
Sweating	4	(1.5)	3	(1.2)	16	(6.3)
Increased Appetite	0	(0)	1	(0.4)	13	(5.1)

†A patient may have more than one adverse event.

Other less frequent (2% to 5%) adverse experiences reported in patients receiving ARIMIDEX 1 mg in either Trial 0004 or Trial 0005 are listed below. These adverse experiences are listed by body system and are in order of decreasing frequency within each body system regardless of assessed causality.

Body as a Whole: Flu syndrome; fever; neck pain; malaise; accidental injury; infection
Cardiovascular: Hypertension; thrombophlebitis
Hepatic: Gamma GT increased; SGOT increased; SGPT increased
Hematologic: Anemia; leukopenia
Metabolic and Nutritional: Alkaline phosphatase increased; weight loss
Mean serum total cholesterol levels increased by 0.5 mmol/L among patients receiving ARIMIDEX. Increases in LDL cholesterol have been shown to contribute to these changes.
Musculoskeletal: Myalgia; arthralgia; pathological fracture
Nervous: Somnolence; confusion; insomnia; anxiety; nervousness
Respiratory: Sinusitis; bronchitis; rhinitis
Skin and Appendages: Hair thinning; pruritus
Urogenital: Urinary tract infection; breast pain
Vaginal bleeding has been reported infrequently, mainly in patients during the first few weeks after changing from existing hormonal therapy to treatment with ARIMIDEX. If bleeding persists, further evaluation should be considered.
During clinical trials and postmarketing experience joint pain/stiffness has been reported in association with the use of ARIMIDEX.
The incidences of the following adverse event groups potentially causally related to one or both of the therapies because of their pharmacology, were statistically analyzed: weight gain, edema, thromboembolic disease, gastrointestinal disturbance, hot flushes, and vaginal dryness. These six groups, and the adverse events captured in the groups, were prospectively defined. The results are shown in the table below.

Table 8
Number (n) and Percentage of Patients

Adverse Event Group	ARIMIDEX 1 mg (n = 262) n	(%)	ARIMIDEX 10 mg (n = 246) n	(%)	Megestrol Acetate 160 mg (n = 253) n	(%)
Gastrointestinal Disturbance	77	(29.4)	81	(32.9)	54	(21.3)
Hot Flushes	33	(12.6)	29	(11.8)	35	(13.8)
Edema	19	(7.3)	28	(11.4)	35	(13.8)
Thromboembolic Disease	9	(3.4)	4	(1.6)	12	(4.7)
Vaginal Dryness	5	(1.9)	3	(1.2)	2	(0.8)
Weight Gain	4	(1.5)	10	(4.1)	30	(11.9)

More patients treated with megestrol acetate reported weight gain as an adverse event compared to patients treated with ARIMIDEX 1 mg ($p<0.0001$). Other differences were not statistically significant.
An examination of the magnitude of change in weight in all patients was also conducted. Thirty-four percent (87/253) of the patients treated with megestrol acetate experienced weight gain of 5% or more and 11% (27/253) of the patients treated with megestrol acetate experienced weight gain of 10% or more. Among patients treated with ARIMIDEX 1 mg, 13% [33/262] experienced weight gain of 5% or more and 3% [6/262] experienced weight gain of 10% or more. On average, this 5 to 10% weight gain represented between 6 and 12 pounds.
No patients receiving ARIMIDEX or megestrol acetate discontinued treatment due to drug-related weight gain.

OVERDOSAGE

Clinical trials have been conducted with ARIMIDEX, up to 60 mg in a single dose given to healthy male volunteers and up to 10 mg daily given to postmenopausal women with advanced breast cancer; these dosages were well tolerated. A single dose of ARIMIDEX that results in life threatening symptoms has not been established. In rats, lethality was observed after single oral doses that were greater than 100 mg/kg (about 800 times the recommended human dose on a mg/m^2 basis) and was associated with severe irritation to the stomach (necrosis, gastritis, ulceration, and hemorrhage).
In an oral acute toxicity study in the dog the median lethal dose was greater than 45 mg/kg/day.
There is no specific antidote to overdosage and treatment must be symptomatic. In the management of an overdose, consider that multiple agents may have been taken. Vomiting may be induced if the patient is alert. Dialysis may be helpful because ARIMIDEX is not highly protein bound. General supportive care, including frequent monitoring of vital signs and close observation of the patient, is indicated.

DOSAGE AND ADMINISTRATION

First-line Therapy: The dose of ARIMIDEX is one 1 mg tablet taken once a day. Treatment with ARIMIDEX should continue until tumor progression is evident.
Second-line Therapy: The dose of ARIMIDEX is one 1 mg tablet taken once a day.
Patients treated with ARIMIDEX do not require glucocorticoid or mineralocorticoid replacement therapy.
Patients with Hepatic Impairment: (See CLINICAL PHARMACOLOGY.) Hepatic metabolism accounts for approximately 85% of anastrozole elimination. Although clearance of anastrozole was decreased in patients with cirrhosis due to alcohol abuse, plasma anastrozole concentrations stayed in the usual range seen in patients without liver disease. Therefore, no changes in dose are recommended for patients with mild-to-moderate hepatic impairment, although patients should be monitored for side effects. ARIMIDEX has not been studied in patients with severe hepatic impairment.
Patients with Renal Impairment: No changes in dose are necessary for patients with renal impairment.
Use in the Elderly: No dosage adjustment is necessary.

HOW SUPPLIED

White, biconvex, film-coated tablets containing 1 mg of anastrozole. The tablets are impressed on one side with a logo consisting of a letter "A" (upper case) with an arrowhead attached to the foot of the extended right leg of the "A" and on the reverse with the tablet strength marking "Adx 1". These tablets are supplied in bottles of 30 tablets (NDC 0310-0201-30).
Store at controlled room temperature, 20°–25°C (68°–77°F) [see USP].

AstraZeneca
AstraZeneca Pharmaceuticals LP
1800 Concord Pike PO Box 15437
Wilmington DE 19850-5437

AI1077 Rev H 08/00

CASODEX® ℞
bicalutamide tablets

Prescribing information for this product, which appears on pages 615–617 of the 2001 PDR, has been completely revised as follows. Please write "See Supplement A" next to the product heading.

DESCRIPTION

CASODEX® (bicalutamide) Tablets for oral administration contain 50 mg of bicalutamide, a non-steroidal antiandrogen with no other known endocrine activity. The chemical name is propanamide, N-[4-cyano-3-(trifluoromethyl)phenyl]-3-[(4-fluorophenyl)sulfonyl]-2-hydroxy-2-methyl-,(+-). The structural and empirical formulas are:

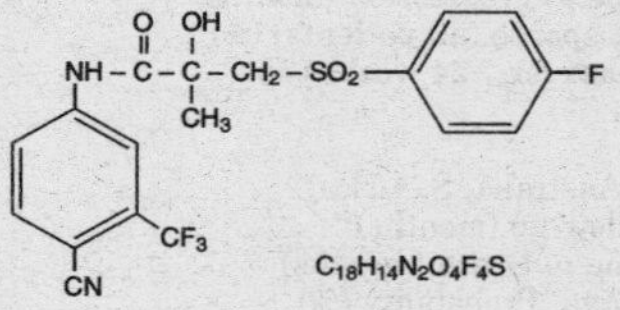

$C_{18}H_{14}N_2O_4F_4S$

Bicalutamide has a molecular weight of 430.37. The pKa' is approximately 12. Bicalutamide is a fine white to off-white powder which is practically insoluble in water at 37°C (5 mg per 1000 mL), slightly soluble in chloroform and absolute ethanol, sparingly soluble in methanol, and soluble in acetone and tetrahydrofuran.
CASODEX is a racemate with its antiandrogenic activity being almost exclusively exhibited by the R-enantiomer of bicalutamide; the S-enantiomer is essentially inactive.
The inactive ingredients of CASODEX Tablets are lactose, magnesium stearate, methylhydroxypropylcellulose, polyethylene glycol, polyvidone, sodium starch glycolate, and titanium dioxide.

CLINICAL PHARMACOLOGY

Mechanism of Action: CASODEX is a non-steroidal antiandrogen. It competitively inhibits the action of androgens by binding to cytosol androgen receptors in the target tissue. Prostatic carcinoma is known to be androgen sensitive and responds to treatment that counteracts the effect of androgen and/or removes the source of androgen.
When CASODEX is combined with luteinizing hormone-releasing hormone (LHRH) analogue therapy, the suppression of serum testosterone induced by the LHRH analogue is not affected. However, in clinical trials with CASODEX as a single agent for prostate cancer, rises in serum testosterone and estradiol have been noted.

Pharmacokinetics

Absorption: Bicalutamide is well-absorbed following oral administration, although the absolute bioavailability is unknown. Co-administration of bicalutamide with food has no clinically significant effect on rate or extent of absorption.
Distribution: Bicalutamide is highly protein-bound (96%). See Drug-Drug Interactions below.
Metabolism/Elimination: Bicalutamide undergoes stereospecific metabolism. The S (inactive) isomer is metabolized primarily by glucuronidation. The R (active) isomer also undergoes glucuronidation but is predominantly oxidized to an inactive metabolite followed by glucuronidation. Both the parent and metabolite glucuronides are eliminated in the urine and feces. The S-enantiomer is rapidly cleared relative to the R-enantiomer, with the R-enantiomer accounting for about 99% of total steady-state plasma levels.

Special Populations

Geriatric: In two studies in patients given 50 or 150 mg daily, no significant relationship between age and steady-state levels of total bicalutamide or the active R-enantiomer has been shown.
Hepatic Insufficiency: No clinically significant difference in the pharmacokinetics of either enantiomer of bicalutamide was noted in patients with mild-to-moderate hepatic disease as compared to healthy controls. However, the half-life of the R-enantiomer was increased approximately 76% (5.9 and 10.4 days for normal and impaired patients, respectively) in patients with severe liver disease (n=4).
Renal Insufficiency: Renal impairment (as measured by creatinine clearance) had no significant effect on the elimination of total bicalutamide or the active R-enantiomer.
Women, Pediatrics: Bicalutamide has not been studied in women or pediatric subjects.
Drug-Drug Interactions: Clinical studies have not shown any drug interactions between bicalutamide and LHRH analogues (goserelin or leuprolide). There is no evidence that bicalutamide induces hepatic enzymes. *In vitro* protein-binding studies have shown that bicalutamide can displace coumarin anticoagulants from binding sites. Prothrombin times should be closely monitored in patients already receiving coumarin anticoagulants who are started on CASODEX.
Pharmacokinetics of the active enantiomer of CASODEX in normal males and patients with prostate cancer are presented in Table 1.

Table 1

Parameter	Mean	Standard Deviation
Normal Males (n=30)		
Apparent Oral Clearance (L/hr)	0.320	0.103
Single Dose Peak Concentration (μg/mL)	0.768	0.178
Single Dose Time to Peak Concentration (hours)	31.3	14.6
Half-Life (days)	5.8	2.29

Patients with Prostate Cancer (n=40)		
C_{ss} (µg/mL)	8.939	3.504

C_{ss} = Mean Steady-State Concentration

Clinical Studies

In a multicenter, double-blind, controlled clinical trial, 813 patients with previously untreated advanced prostate cancer were randomized to receive CASODEX 50 mg once daily (404 patients) or flutamide 250 mg (409 patients) three times a day, each in combination with LHRH analogues (either goserelin acetate implant or leuprolide acetate depot).

In an analysis conducted after a median follow-up of 160 weeks was reached, 213 (52.7%) patients treated with CASODEX-LHRH analogue therapy and 235 (57.5%) patients treated with flutamide-LHRH analogue therapy had died. There was no significant difference in survival between treatment groups (see Figure 1). The hazard ratio for time to death (survival) was 0.87 (95% confidence interval 0.72 to 1.05).

Figure 1
The Kaplan-Meier Probability of Death For Both Antiandrogen Treatment Groups

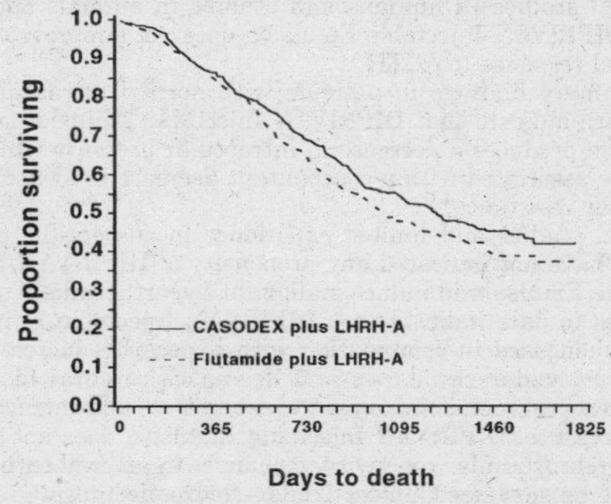

There was no significant difference in time to objective tumor progression between treatment groups (see Figure 2). Objective tumor progression was defined as the appearance of any bone metastases or the worsening of any existing bone metastases on bone scan attributable to metastatic disease, or an increase by 25% or more of any existing measurable extraskeletal metastases. The hazard ratio for time to progression of CASODEX plus LHRH analogue to that of flutamide plus LHRH analogue was 0.93 (95% confidence interval, 0.79 to 1.10).

Figure 2
The Kaplan-Meier Curve For Time to Progression For Both Antiandrogen Treatment Groups

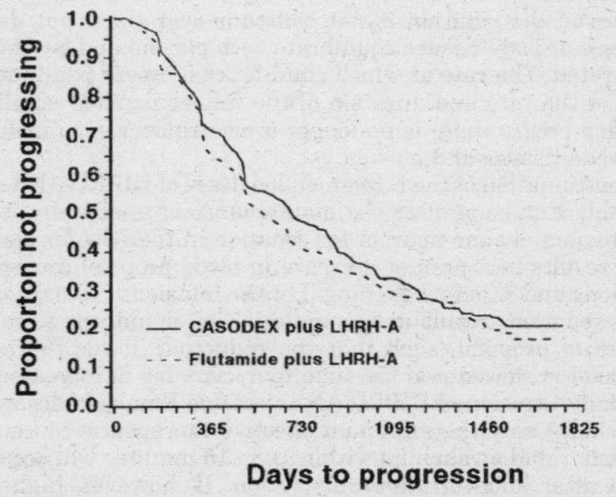

Quality of life was assessed with self-administered patient questionnaires on pain, social functioning, emotional well-being, vitality, activity limitation, bed disability, overall health, physical capacity, general symptoms, and treatment related symptoms. Assessment of the Quality of Life questionnaires did not indicate consistent significant differences between the two treatment groups.

INDICATIONS AND USAGE

CASODEX is indicated for use in combination therapy with a luteinizing hormone-releasing hormone (LHRH) analogue for the treatment of Stage D_2 metastatic carcinoma of the prostate.

CONTRAINDICATIONS

CASODEX is contraindicated in any patient who has shown a hypersensitivity reaction to the drug or any of the tablet's components.

CASODEX has no indication for women, and should not be used in this population, particularly for non-serious or non-life threatening conditions. Further, CASODEX should not be used by women who are or may become pregnant. If this drug is used during pregnancy, or if the patient becomes pregnant while taking this drug, the patient should be apprised of the potential hazard to the fetus. CASODEX may cause fetal harm when administered to pregnant women. The male offspring of rats receiving doses of 10 mg/kg/day (plasma drug concentrations in rats equal to approximately 2/3 human therapeutic concentrations*) and above were observed to have reduced anogenital distance and hypospadias in reproductive toxicology studies. These pharmacological effects have been observed with other antiandrogens. No other teratogenic effects were observed in rabbits receiving doses up to 200 mg/kg/day (approximately 1/3 human therapeutic concentrations*) or rats receiving doses up to 250 mg/kg/day (approximately 2 times human therapeutic concentrations*).

*Based on a maximum dose of 50 mg/day of bicalutamide for an average 70 kg patient.

WARNINGS

Hepatitis: Rare cases of death or hospitalization due to severe liver injury have been reported post-marketing in association with the use of CASODEX. Hepatotoxicity in these reports generally occurred within the first three to four months of treatment. Hepatitis or marked increases in liver enzymes leading to drug discontinuation occurred in approximately 1% of CASODEX patients in controlled clinical trials. Serum transaminase levels should be measured prior to starting treatment with CASODEX, at regular intervals for the first four months of treatment, and periodically thereafter. If clinical symptoms or signs suggestive of liver dysfunction occur (e.g., nausea, vomiting, abdominal pain, fatigue, anorexia, "flu-like" symptoms, dark urine, jaundice, or right upper quadrant tenderness), the serum transaminases, in particular the serum ALT, should be measured immediately. If at any time a patient has jaundice, or their ALT rises above two times the upper limit of normal, CASODEX should be immediately discontinued with close follow-up of liver function.

PRECAUTIONS

General:

1. CASODEX should be used with caution in patients with moderate-to-severe hepatic impairment. CASODEX is extensively metabolized by the liver. Limited data in subjects with severe hepatic impairment suggest that excretion of CASODEX may be delayed and could lead to further accumulation. Periodic liver function tests should be considered for hepatic-impaired patients on long-term therapy (see WARNINGS).
2. In clinical trials with CASODEX as a single agent for prostate cancer, gynecomastia and breast pain have been reported in up to 38% and 39% of patients, respectively.
3. Regular assessments of serum Prostate Specific Antigen (PSA) may be helpful in monitoring the patient's response. If PSA levels rise during CASODEX therapy, the patient should be evaluated for clinical progression. For patients who have objective progression of disease together with an elevated PSA, a treatment-free period of antiandrogen, while continuing the LHRH analogue, may be considered.

Information for Patients: Patients should be informed that therapy with CASODEX and the LHRH analogue should be initiated concomitantly, and that they should not interrupt or stop taking these medications without consulting their physician. Treatment with CASODEX should be started at the same time as treatment with an LHRH analogue.

Drug Interactions: *In vitro* studies have shown CASODEX can displace coumarin anticoagulants, such as warfarin, from their protein-binding sites. It is recommended that if CASODEX is started in patients already receiving coumarin anticoagulants, prothrombin times should be closely monitored and adjustment of the anticoagulant dose may be necessary (see CLINICAL PHARMACOLOGY, Drug-Drug Interactions).

Carcinogenesis, Mutagenesis, Impairment of Fertility: Two-year oral carcinogenicity studies were conducted in both male and female rats and mice at doses of 5, 15 or 75 mg/kg/day of bicalutamide. A variety of tumor target organ effects were identified and were attributed to the antiandrogenicity of bicalutamide, namely, testicular benign interstitial (Leydig) cell tumors in male rats at all dose levels (the steady-state plasma concentration with the 5 mg/kg/day dose is approximately 2/3 human therapeutic concentrations*) and uterine adenocarcinoma in female rats at 75 mg/kg/day (approximately 1 1/2 times the human therapeutic concentrations*). There is no evidence of Leydig cell hyperplasia in patients; uterine tumors are not relevant to the indicated patient population.

A small increase in the incidence of hepatocellular carcinoma in male mice given 75 mg/kg/day of bicalutamide (approximately 4 times human therapeutic concentrations*) and an increased incidence of benign thyroid follicular cell adenomas in rats given 5 mg/kg/day (approximately 2/3 human therapeutic concentrations*) and above were recorded. These neoplastic changes were progressions of non-neoplastic changes related to hepatic enzyme induction observed in animal toxicity studies. Enzyme induction has not been observed following bicalutamide administration in man. There were no tumorigenic effects suggestive of genotoxic carcinogenesis.

A comprehensive battery of both *in vitro* and *in vivo* genotoxicity tests (yeast gene conversion, Ames, *E. coli*, CHO/HGPRT, human lymphocyte cytogenetic, mouse micronucleus, and rat bone marrow cytogenetic tests) has demonstrated that CASODEX does not have genotoxic activity.

Administration of CASODEX may lead to inhibition of spermatogenesis. The long-term effects of CASODEX on male fertility have not been studied.

In male rats dosed at 250 mg/kg/day (approximately 2 times human therapeutic concentrations*), the precoital interval and time to successful mating were increased in the first pairing but no effects on fertility following successful mating were seen. These effects were reversed by 7 weeks after the end of an 11-week period of dosing.

No effects on female rats dosed at 10, 50 and 250 mg/kg/day (approximately 2/3, 1 and 2 times human therapeutic concentrations, respectively*) or their female offspring were observed. Administration of bicalutamide to pregnant females resulted in feminization of the male offspring leading to hypospadias at all dose levels. Affected male offspring were also impotent.

*Based on a maximum dose of 50 mg/day of bicalutamide for an average 70 kg patient.

Pregnancy: Pregnancy Category X (see CONTRAINDICATIONS).

Nursing Mothers: CASODEX is not indicated for use in women. It is not known whether this drug is excreted in human milk. Because many drugs are excreted in human milk, caution should be exercised when CASODEX is administered to a nursing woman.

Pediatric Use: Safety and effectiveness of CASODEX in pediatric patients have not been established.

ADVERSE REACTIONS

In patients with advanced prostate cancer treated with CASODEX in combination with an LHRH analogue, the most frequent adverse experience was hot flashes (53%).

In the multicenter, double-blind, controlled clinical trial comparing CASODEX 50 mg once daily with flutamide 250 mg three times a day, each in combination with an LHRH analogue, the following adverse experiences with an incidence of 5% or greater, regardless of causality, have been reported.

Table 2 - Incidence of Adverse Events (≥ 5% in Either Treatment Group) Regardless of Causality

Body System Adverse Event	Treatment Group Number of Patients (%)	
	CASODEX Plus LHRH Analogue (n=401)	Flutamide Plus LHRH Analogue (n=407)
Body as a Whole		
Pain (General)	142 (35)	127 (31)
Back Pain	102 (25)	105 (26)
Asthenia	89 (22)	87 (21)
Pelvic Pain	85 (21)	70 (17)
Infection	71 (18)	57 (14)
Abdominal Pain	46 (11)	46 (11)
Chest Pain	34 (8)	34 (8)
Headache	29 (7)	27 (7)
Flu Syndrome	28 (7)	30 (7)
Cardiovascular		
Hot Flashes	211 (53)	217 (53)
Hypertension	34 (8)	29 (7)
Digestive		
Constipation	87 (22)	69 (17)
Nausea	62 (15)	58 (14)
Diarrhea	49 (12)	107 (26)
Increased Liver Enzyme Test †	30 (7)	46 (11)
Dyspepsia	30 (7)	23 (6)
Flatulence	26 (6)	22 (5)
Anorexia	25 (6)	29 (7)
Vomiting	24 (6)	32 (8)
Hemic and Lymphatic		
Anemia ††	45 (11)	53 (13)
Metabolic and Nutritional		
Peripheral Edema	53 (13)	42 (10)
Weight Loss	30 (7)	39 (10)
Hyperglycemia	26 (6)	27 (7)
Alkaline Phosphatase Increased	22 (5)	24 (6)
Weight Gain	22 (5)	18 (4)
Musculoskeletal		
Bone Pain	37 (9)	43 (11)
Myasthenia	27 (7)	19 (5)
Arthritis	21 (5)	29 (7)
Pathological Fracture	17 (4)	32 (8)
Nervous System		
Dizziness	41 (10)	35 (9)
Paresthesia	31 (8)	40 (10)
Insomnia	27 (7)	39 (10)
Anxiety	20 (5)	9 (2)
Depression	16 (4)	33 (8)
Respiratory System		
Dyspnea	51 (13)	32 (8)
Cough Increased	33 (8)	24 (6)
Pharyngitis	32 (8)	23 (6)
Bronchitis	24 (6)	22 (3)
Pneumonia	18 (4)	19 (5)
Rhinitis	15 (4)	22 (5)
Skin and Appendages		
Rash	35 (9)	30 (7)
Sweating	25 (6)	20 (5)

Continued on next page

Casodex—Cont.

Urogenital		
Nocturia	49 (12)	55 (14)
Hematuria	48 (12)	26 (6)
Urinary Tract Infection	35 (9)	36 (9)
Gynecomastia	36 (9)	30 (7)
Impotence	27 (7)	35 (9)
Breast Pain	23 (6)	15 (4)
Urinary Frequency	23 (6)	29 (7)
Urinary Retention	20 (5)	14 (3)
Urination Impaired	19 (5)	15 (4)
Urinary Incontinence	15 (4)	32 (8)

† Increased liver enzyme test includes increases in AST, ALT or both.
†† Anemia includes anemia, hypochromic- and iron deficiency anemia.

Other adverse experiences (greater than or equal to 2%, but less than 5%) reported in the CASODEX-LHRH analogue treatment group are listed below by body system and are in order of decreasing frequency within each body system regardless of causality.
Body as a Whole: Neoplasm; Neck pain; Fever; Chills; Sepsis; Hernia; Cyst
Cardiovascular: Angina pectoris; Congestive heart failure; Myocardial infarction, Heart arrest; Coronary artery disorder; Syncope
Digestive: Melena; Rectal hemorrhage; Dry mouth; Dysphagia; Gastrointestinal disorder; Periodontal abscess; Gastrointestinal carcinoma
Metabolic and Nutritional: Edema; BUN increased; Creatinine increased; Dehydration; Gout; Hypercholesteremia
Musculoskeletal: Myalgia; Leg cramps
Nervous: Hypertonia; Confusion; Somnolence; Libido decreased; Neuropathy; Nervousness
Respiratory: Lung disorder; Asthma; Epistaxis; Sinusitis
Skin and Appendages: Dry skin; Alopecia; Pruritus; Herpes zoster; Skin carcinoma; Skin disorder
Special Senses: Cataract specified
Urogenital: Dysuria; Urinary urgency; Hydronephrosis; Urinary tract disorder
Abnormal Laboratory Test Values: Laboratory abnormalities including elevated AST, ALT, bilirubin, BUN, and creatinine and decreased hemoglobin and white cell count have been reported in both CASODEX-LHRH analogue treated and flutamide-LHRH analogue treated patients.
Postmarketing Experience: Rare cases of interstitial pneumonitis and pulmonary fibrosis have been reported with CASODEX.

OVERDOSAGE

Long-term clinical trials have been conducted with dosages up to 200 mg of CASODEX daily and these dosages have been well tolerated. A single dose of CASODEX that results in symptoms of an overdose considered to be life-threatening has not been established.
There is no specific antidote; treatment of an overdose should be symptomatic.
In the management of an overdose with CASODEX, vomiting may be induced if the patient is alert. It should be remembered that, in this patient population, multiple drugs may have been taken. Dialysis is not likely to be helpful since CASODEX is highly protein bound and is extensively metabolized. General supportive care, including frequent monitoring of vital signs and close observation of the patient, is indicated.

DOSAGE AND ADMINISTRATION

The recommended dose for CASODEX therapy in combination with an LHRH analogue is one 50 mg tablet once daily (morning or evening), with or without food. It is recommended that CASODEX be taken at the same time each day. Treatment with CASODEX should be started at the same time as treatment with an LHRH analogue.
Dosage Adjustment in Renal Impairment: No dosage adjustment is necessary for patients with renal impairment (see CLINICAL PHARMACOLOGY, Special Populations, Renal Insufficiency).
Dosage Adjustment in Hepatic Impairment: No dosage adjustment is necessary for patients with mild to moderate hepatic impairment. Although there is a 76% (5.9 and 10.4 days for normal and impaired patients, respectively) increase in the half-life of the active enantiomer of bicalutamide in patients with severe liver impairment (n=4), no dosage adjustment is necessary (see CLINICAL PHARMACOLOGY, Special Populations, Hepatic Impairment, PRECAUTIONS and WARNINGS sections).

HOW SUPPLIED

50 mg Tablets. (NDC 0310-0705) White, film-coated tablets (identified on one side with "CDX50" and on the reverse with the "CASODEX logo") are supplied in unit dose blisters of 30 tablets per carton (0310-0705-39), bottles of 30 tablets (0310-0705-30) and bottles of 100 tablets (0310-0705-10).
Store at controlled room temperature, 20–25°C (68–77°F).
64145-01 Rev L 09/00
Manufactured for
ZENECA
Pharmaceuticals
A Business Unit of Zeneca Inc.
Wilmington, Delaware 19850-5437 USA
by Zeneca GmbH, Plankstadt, Germany

DIPRIVAN® 1% ℞
INJECTABLE EMULSION
10 mg/mL propofol
FOR I.V. ADMINISTRATION

Prescribing information for this product, which appears on pages 620–626 of the 2001 PDR, has been completely revised as follows. Please write "See Supplement A" next to the product heading.

DESCRIPTION

DIPRIVAN® (propofol) Injectable Emulsion is a sterile, nonpyrogenic emulsion containing 10 mg/mL of propofol suitable for intravenous administration. Propofol is chemically described as 2,6-diisopropylphenol and has a molecular weight of 178.27. The structural and molecular formulas are:

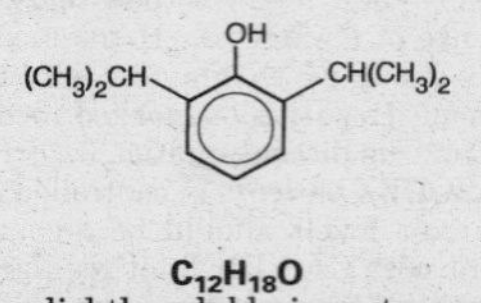

$C_{12}H_{18}O$

Propofol is very slightly soluble in water and, thus, is formulated in a white, oil-in-water emulsion. The pKa is 11. The octanol/water partition coefficient for propofol is 6761:1 at a pH of 6–8.5. In addition to the active component, propofol, the formulation also contains soybean oil (100 mg/mL), glycerol (22.5 mg/mL), egg lecithin (12 mg/mL), and disodium edetate (0.005%); with sodium hydroxide to adjust pH. The DIPRIVAN Injectable Emulsion is isotonic and has a pH of 7–8.5.
STRICT ASEPTIC TECHNIQUE MUST ALWAYS BE MAINTAINED DURING HANDLING. DIPRIVAN INJECTABLE EMULSION IS A SINGLE-USE PARENTERAL PRODUCT WHICH CONTAINS 0.005% DISODIUM EDETATE TO RETARD THE RATE OF GROWTH OF MICROORGANISMS IN THE EVENT OF ACCIDENTAL EXTRINSIC CONTAMINATION. HOWEVER, DIPRIVAN INJECTABLE EMULSION CAN STILL SUPPORT THE GROWTH OF MICROORGANISMS AS IT IS NOT AN ANTIMICROBIALLY PRESERVED PRODUCT UNDER USP STANDARDS. ACCORDINGLY, STRICT ASEPTIC TECHNIQUE MUST STILL BE ADHERED TO. DO NOT USE IF CONTAMINATION IS SUSPECTED. DISCARD UNUSED PORTIONS AS DIRECTED WITHIN THE REQUIRED TIME LIMITS (SEE DOSAGE AND ADMINISTRATION, HANDLING PROCEDURES). THERE HAVE BEEN REPORTS IN WHICH FAILURE TO USE ASEPTIC TECHNIQUE WHEN HANDLING DIPRIVAN INJECTABLE EMULSION WAS ASSOCIATED WITH MICROBIAL CONTAMINATION OF THE PRODUCT AND WITH FEVER, INFECTION/SEPSIS, OTHER LIFE-THREATENING ILLNESS, AND/OR DEATH.

CLINICAL PHARMACOLOGY

General
DIPRIVAN Injectable Emulsion is an intravenous sedative-hypnotic agent for use in the induction and maintenance of anesthesia or sedation. Intravenous injection of a therapeutic dose of propofol produces hypnosis rapidly with minimal excitation, usually within 40 seconds from the start of an injection (the time for one arm-brain circulation). As with other rapidly acting intravenous anesthetic agents, the half-time of the blood-brain equilibration is approximately 1 to 3 minutes, and this accounts for the rapid induction of anesthesia.
Pharmacodynamics
Pharmacodynamic properties of propofol are dependent upon the therapeutic blood propofol concentrations. Steady state propofol blood concentrations are generally proportional to infusion rates, especially within an individual patient. Undesirable side effects such as cardiorespiratory depression are likely to occur at higher blood concentrations which result from bolus dosing or rapid increase in infusion rate. An adequate interval (3 to 5 minutes) must be allowed between clinical dosage adjustments in order to assess drug effects.
The hemodynamic effects of DIPRIVAN Injectable Emulsion during induction of anesthesia vary. If spontaneous ventilation is maintained, the major cardiovascular effects are arterial hypotension (sometimes greater than a 30% decrease) with little or no change in heart rate and no appreciable decrease in cardiac output. If ventilation is assisted or controlled (positive pressure ventilation), the degree and incidence of decrease in cardiac output are accentuated. Addition of a potent opioid (e.g., fentanyl) when used as a premedicant further decreases cardiac output and respiratory drive.
If anesthesia is continued by infusion of DIPRIVAN Injectable Emulsion, the stimulation of endotracheal intubation and surgery may return arterial pressure towards normal. However, cardiac output may remain depressed. Comparative clinical studies have shown that the hemodynamic effects of DIPRIVAN Injectable Emulsion during induction of anesthesia are generally more pronounced than with other IV induction agents traditionally used for this purpose.
Clinical and preclinical studies suggest that DIPRIVAN Injectable Emulsion is rarely associated with elevation of plasma histamine levels.
Induction of anesthesia with DIPRIVAN Injectable Emulsion is frequently associated with apnea in both adults and pediatric patients. In 1573 adult patients who received DIPRIVAN Injectable Emulsion (2 to 2.5 mg/kg), apnea lasted less than 30 seconds in 7% of patients, 30–60 seconds in 24% of patients, and more than 60 seconds in 12% of patients. In 218 pediatric patients from birth through 16 years of age assessable for apnea who received bolus doses of DIPRIVAN Injectable Emulsion (1 to 3.6 mg/kg), apnea lasted less than 30 seconds in 12% of patients, 30–60 seconds in 10% of patients, and more than 60 seconds in 5% of patients.
During maintenance, DIPRIVAN Injectable Emulsion causes a decrease in ventilation usually associated with an increase in carbon dioxide tension which may be marked depending upon the rate of administration and other concurrent medications (e.g., opioids, sedatives, etc.).
During monitored anesthesia care (MAC) sedation, attention must be given to the cardiorespiratory effects of DIPRIVAN Injectable Emulsion. Hypotension, oxyhemoglobin desaturation, apnea, airway obstruction, and/or oxygen desaturation can occur, especially following a rapid bolus of DIPRIVAN Injectable Emulsion. During initiation of MAC sedation, slow infusion or slow injection techniques are preferable over rapid bolus administration, and during maintenance of MAC sedation, a variable rate infusion is preferable over intermittent bolus administration in order to minimize undesirable cardiorespiratory effects. In the elderly, debilitated, or ASA III/IV patients, rapid (single or repeated) bolus dose administration should not be used for MAC sedation. (See WARNINGS.)
Clinical studies in humans and studies in animals show that DIPRIVAN Injectable Emulsion does not suppress the adrenal response to ACTH.
Preliminary findings in patients with normal intraocular pressure indicate that DIPRIVAN Injectable Emulsion anesthesia produces a decrease in intraocular pressure which may be associated with a concomitant decrease in systemic vascular resistance.
Animal studies and limited experience in susceptible patients have not indicated any propensity of DIPRIVAN Injectable Emulsion to induce malignant hyperthermia.
Studies to date indicate that DIPRIVAN Injectable Emulsion when used in combination with hypocarbia increases cerebrovascular resistance and decreases cerebral blood flow, cerebral metabolic oxygen consumption, and intracranial pressure. DIPRIVAN Injectable Emulsion does not affect cerebrovascular reactivity to changes in arterial carbon dioxide tension (see Clinical Trials—Neuroanesthesia).
Hemosiderin deposits have been observed in the livers of dogs receiving DIPRIVAN Injectable Emulsion containing 0.005% disodium edetate over a four week period; the clinical significance is unknown.
Pharmacokinetics
The proper use of DIPRIVAN Injectable Emulsion requires an understanding of the disposition and elimination characteristics of propofol.
The pharmacokinetics of propofol are well described by a three compartment linear model with compartments representing the plasma, rapidly equilibrating tissues, and slowly equilibrating tissues.
Following an IV bolus dose, there is rapid equilibration between the plasma and the highly perfused tissue of the brain, thus accounting for the rapid onset of anesthesia. Plasma levels initially decline rapidly as a result of both rapid distribution and high metabolic clearance. Distribution accounts for about half of this decline following a bolus of propofol.
However, distribution is not constant over time, but decreases as body tissues equilibrate with plasma and become saturated. The rate at which equilibration occurs is a function of the rate and duration of the infusion. When equilibration occurs there is no longer a net transfer of propofol between tissues and plasma.
Discontinuation of the recommended doses of DIPRIVAN Injectable Emulsion after the maintenance of anesthesia for approximately one-hour, or for sedation in the ICU for one-day, results in a prompt decrease in blood propofol concentrations and rapid awakening. Longer infusions (10 days of ICU sedation) result in accumulation of significant tissue stores of propofol, such that the reduction in circulating propofol is slowed and the time to awakening is increased.
By daily titration of DIPRIVAN Injectable Emulsion dosage to achieve only the minimum effective therapeutic concentration, rapid awakening within 10 to 15 minutes will occur even after long-term administration. If, however, higher than necessary infusion levels have been maintained for a long time, propofol will be redistributed from fat and muscle to the plasma, and this return of propofol from peripheral tissues will slow recovery.
The figure below illustrates the fall of plasma propofol levels following ICU sedation infusions of various durations.

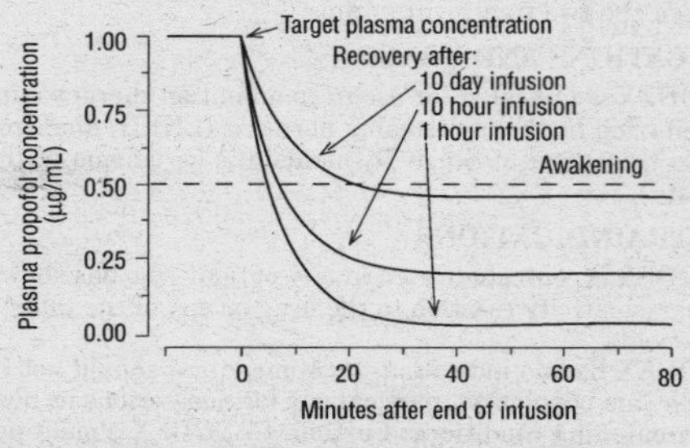

The large contribution of distribution (about 50%) to the fall of propofol plasma levels following brief infusions means that after very long infusions (at steady state), about half the initial rate will maintain the same plasma levels. Failure to reduce the infusion rate in patients receiving DIPRIVAN Injectable Emulsion for extended periods may result in excessively high blood concentrations of the drug. Thus, titration to clinical response and daily evaluation of sedation levels are important during use of DIPRIVAN Injectable Emulsion infusion for ICU sedation, especially of long duration.

Adults: Propofol clearance ranges from 23–50 mL/kg/min (1.6 to 3.4 L/min in 70 kg adults). It is chiefly eliminated by hepatic conjugation to inactive metabolites which are excreted by the kidney. A glucuronide conjugate accounts for about 50% of the administered dose. Propofol has a steady state volume of distribution (10-day infusion) approaching 60 L/kg in healthy adults. A difference in pharmacokinetics due to gender has not been observed. The terminal half-life of propofol after a 10-day infusion is 1 to 3 days.

Geriatrics: With increasing patient age, the dose of propofol needed to achieve a defined anesthetic end point (dose-requirement) decreases. This does not appear to be an age-related change of pharmacodynamics or brain sensitivity, as measured by EEG burst suppression. With increasing patient age pharmacokinetic changes are such that for a given IV bolus dose, higher peak plasma concentrations occur, which can explain the decreased dose requirement. These higher peak plasma concentrations in the elderly can predispose patients to cardiorespiratory effects including hypotension, apnea, airway obstruction, and/or oxygen desaturation. The higher plasma levels reflect an age-related decrease in volume of distribution and reduced intercompartmental clearance. Lower doses are thus recommended for initiation and maintenance of sedation/anesthesia in elderly patients. (See CLINICAL PHARMACOLOGY—Individualization of Dosage.)

Pediatrics: The pharmacokinetics of propofol were studied in 53 children between the ages of 3 and 12 years who received DIPRIVAN Injectable Emulsion for periods of approximately 1–2 hours. The observed distribution and clearance of propofol in these children were similar to adults.

Organ Failure: The pharmacokinetics of propofol do not appear to be different in people with chronic hepatic cirrhosis or chronic renal impairment compared to adults with normal hepatic and renal function. The effects of acute hepatic or renal failure on the pharmacokinetics of propofol have not been studied.

Clinical Trials

Anesthesia and Monitored Anesthesia Care (MAC) Sedation

DIPRIVAN Injectable Emulsion was compared to intravenous and inhalational anesthetic or sedative agents in 91 trials involving a total of 5,135 patients. Of these, 3,354 received DIPRIVAN Injectable Emulsion and comprised the overall safety database for anesthesia and MAC sedation. Fifty-five of these trials, 20 for anesthesia induction and 35 for induction and maintenance of anesthesia or MAC sedation, were carried out in the US or Canada and provided the basis for dosage recommendations and the adverse event profile during anesthesia or MAC sedation.

Pediatric Anesthesia

DIPRIVAN Injectable Emulsion was studied in 14 clinical trials involving 691 pediatric patients, including 42 cardiac surgical patients. Of the total 691 patients, 90 were less than 3 years of age and 601 were 3 years of age or older. Of these, 506 were from US/Canadian clinical trials and comprised the overall safety and efficacy database for Pediatric Anesthesia. The majority of the remaining patients were healthy ASA I/II patients. (See Table 1)

[See table 1 above]

[See table 2 above]

Also includes all time following induction dose.

Neuroanesthesia

DIPRIVAN Injectable Emulsion was studied in 50 patients undergoing craniotomy for supratentorial tumors in two clinical trials. The mean lesion size (anterior/posterior and lateral) was 31 mm and 32 mm in one trial and 55 mm and 42 mm in the other trial respectively.

[See table 3 above]

In ten of these patients, DIPRIVAN Injectable Emulsion was administered by infusion in a controlled clinical trial to evaluate the effect of DIPRIVAN Injectable Emulsion on cerebrospinal fluid pressure (CSFP). The mean arterial pressure was maintained relatively constant over 25 minutes with a change from baseline of −4% ± 17% (mean ± SD), whereas the percent change in cerebrospinal fluid pressure (CSFP) was −46% ± 14%. As CSFP is an indirect measure of intracranial pressure (ICP), when given by infusion or slow bolus, DIPRIVAN Injectable Emulsion, in combination with hypocarbia, is capable of decreasing ICP independent of changes in arterial pressure.

Intensive Care Unit (ICU) Sedation

Adult Patients:

DIPRIVAN Injectable Emulsion was compared to benzodiazepines and/or opioids in 14 clinical trials involving a total of 550 ICU patients. Of these, 302 received DIPRIVAN Injectable Emulsion and comprise the overall safety database for ICU sedation. Six of these studies were carried out in the US or Canada and provide the basis for dosage recommendations and the adverse event profile.

Information from 193 literature reports of DIPRIVAN Injectable Emulsion used for ICU sedation in over 950 patients and information from the clinical trials are summarized below:

[See table 4 above]

TABLE 1. PEDIATRIC INDUCTION OF ANESTHESIA

Patients Receiving DIPRIVAN Injectable Emulsion Median and (Range)

Age Range	No. of Patients	Induction Dose	Injection Duration
Birth through 16 years	353	2.5 mg/kg (1–3.6)	20 sec. (6–45)

TABLE 2. PEDIATRIC MAINTENANCE OF ANESTHESIA

Patients Receiving DIPRIVAN Injectable Emulsion Median and (Range)

Age Range	No. of Patients	Maintenance Dosage µg/kg/min	Duration minutes
2 months to 2 years	68	199 (82–394)	65 (12 - 282)
2 to 12 years	165	188 (12–1041)	69 (23 - 374)
>12 through 16 years	27	161 (84–359)	69 (26 - 251)

TABLE 3. NEUROANESTHESIA CLINICAL TRIALS

Patients Receiving DIPRIVAN Injectable Emulsion Median and (Range)

Patient Type	No. of Patients	Induction Bolus Dosages (mg/kg)	Maintenance Dosage (µg/kg/min)	Maintenance Duration (min)
Craniotomy patients	50	1.36 (0.9–6.9)	146 (68–425)	285 (48–622)

TABLE 4. ADULT ICU SEDATION CLINICAL TRIALS AND LITERATURE

Patients receiving DIPRIVAN Injectable Emulsion Median and (Range)

	Number of Patients		Sedation Dose		Sedation Duration
ICU Patient Type	Trials	Literature	µg/kg/min	mg/kg/h	Hours
Post-CABG	41	—	11 (0.1–30)	0.66 (0.006–1.8)	10 (2–14)
	—	334	(5–100)	(0.3–6)	(4–24)
Post-Surgical	60	—	20 (6–53)	1.2 (0.4–3.2)	18 (0.3–187)
	—	142	(23–82)	(1.4–4.9)	(6–96)
Neuro/Head Trauma	7	—	25 (13–37)	1.5 (0.8–2.2)	168 (112–282)
	—	184	(8.3–87)	(0.5–5.2)	(8 hr–5 days)
Medical	49	—	41 (9–131)	2.5 (0.5–7.9)	72 (0.4–337)
	—	76	(3.3–62)	(0.2–3.7)	(4–96)
Special Patients					
ARDS/Resp. Failure	—	56	(10–142)	(0.6–8.5)	(1 hr–8 days)
COPD/Asthma	—	49	(17–75)	(1–4.5)	(1–8 days)
Status Epilepticus	—	15	(25–167)	(1.5–10)	(1–21 days)
Tetanus	—	11	(5–100)	(0.3–6)	(1–25 days)

Trials (Individual patients from clinical studies)
Literature (Individual patients from published reports)
CABG (Coronary Artery Bypass Graft)
ARDS (Adult Respiratory Distress Syndrome)

Cardiac Anesthesia

DIPRIVAN Injectable Emulsion was evaluated in 5 clinical trials conducted in the US and Canada, involving a total of 569 patients undergoing coronary artery bypass graft (CABG). Of these, 301 patients received DIPRIVAN Injectable Emulsion. They comprise the safety database for cardiac anesthesia and provide the basis for dosage recommendations in this patient population, in conjunction with reports in the published literature.

Individualization of Dosage

General: STRICT ASEPTIC TECHNIQUE MUST ALWAYS BE MAINTAINED DURING HANDLING. DIPRIVAN INJECTABLE EMULSION IS A SINGLE-USE PARENTERAL PRODUCT WHICH CONTAINS 0.005% DISODIUM EDETATE TO RETARD THE RATE OF GROWTH OF MICROORGANISMS IN THE EVENT OF ACCIDENTAL EXTRINSIC CONTAMINATION. HOWEVER, DIPRIVAN INJECTABLE EMULSION CAN STILL SUPPORT THE GROWTH OF MICROORGANISMS AS IT IS NOT AN ANTIMICROBIALLY PRESERVED PRODUCT UNDER USP STANDARDS. ACCORDINGLY, STRICT ASEPTIC TECHNIQUE MUST STILL BE ADHERED TO. DO NOT USE IF CONTAMINATION IS SUSPECTED. DISCARD UNUSED PORTIONS AS DIRECTED WITHIN THE REQUIRED TIME LIMITS (SEE DOSAGE AND ADMINISTRATION, HANDLING PROCEDURES). THERE HAVE BEEN REPORTS IN WHICH FAILURE TO USE ASEPTIC TECHNIQUE WHEN HANDLING DIPRIVAN INJECTABLE EMULSION WAS ASSOCIATED WITH MICROBIAL CONTAMINATION OF THE PRODUCT AND WITH FEVER, INFECTION/SEPSIS, OTHER LIFE-THREATENING ILLNESS, AND/OR DEATH.

Propofol blood concentrations at steady state are generally proportional to infusion rates, especially in individual patients. Undesirable effects such as cardiorespiratory depression are likely to occur at higher blood concentrations which result from bolus dosing or rapid increases in the infusion rate. An adequate interval (3 to 5 minutes) must be allowed between clinical dosage adjustments in order to assess drug effects.

When administering DIPRIVAN Injectable Emulsion by infusion, syringe pumps or volumetric pumps are recommended to provide controlled infusion rates. When infusing DIPRIVAN Injectable Emulsion to patients undergoing magnetic resonance imaging, metered control devices may be utilized if mechanical pumps are impractical.

Changes in vital signs (increases in pulse rate, blood pressure, sweating and/or tearing) that indicate a response to surgical stimulation or lightening of anesthesia may be controlled by the administration of DIPRIVAN Injectable Emulsion 25 mg (2.5 mL) to 50 mg (5 mL) incremental boluses and/or by increasing the infusion rate.

For minor surgical procedures (e.g., body surface) nitrous oxide (60%–70%) can be combined with a variable rate DIPRIVAN Injectable Emulsion infusion to provide satisfactory anesthesia. With more stimulating surgical procedures (e.g., intra-abdominal), or if supplementation with nitrous oxide is not provided, administration rate(s) of DIPRIVAN Injectable Emulsion and/or opioids should be increased in order to provide adequate anesthesia.

Infusion rates should always be titrated downward in the absence of clinical signs of light anesthesia until a mild response to surgical stimulation is obtained in order to avoid administration of DIPRIVAN Injectable Emulsion at rates higher than are clinically necessary. Generally, rates of 50 to 100 µg/kg/min in adults should be achieved during maintenance in order to optimize recovery times.

Other drugs that cause CNS depression (hypnotics/sedatives, inhalational anesthetics, and opioids) can increase CNS depression induced by propofol. Morphine premedication (0.15 mg/kg) with nitrous oxide 67% in oxygen has been shown to decrease the necessary propofol injection maintenance infusion rate and therapeutic blood concentrations when compared to non-narcotic (lorazepam) premedication.

Induction of General Anesthesia

Adult Patients: Most adult patients under 55 years of age and classified ASA I/II require 2 to 2.5 mg/kg of DIPRIVAN Injectable Emulsion for induction when unpremedicated or when premedicated with oral benzodiazepines or intramuscular opioids. For induction, DIPRIVAN Injectable Emulsion should be titrated (approximately 40 mg every 10 seconds) against the response of the patient until the clinical signs show the onset of anesthesia. As with other sedative-hypnotic agents, the amount of intravenous opioid and/or benzodiazepine premedication will influence the response of the patient to an induction dose of DIPRIVAN Injectable Emulsion.

Elderly, Debilitated, or ASA III/IV Patients: It is important to be familiar and experienced with the intravenous use of DIPRIVAN Injectable Emulsion before treating elderly, debilitated, or ASA III/IV patients. Due to the reduced clearance and higher blood concentrations, most of these patients require approximately 1 to 1.5 mg/kg (approximately 20 mg every 10 seconds) of DIPRIVAN Injectable Emulsion for induction of anesthesia according to their condition and responses. A rapid bolus should not be used, as this will increase the likelihood of undesirable cardiorespiratory depression including hypotension, apnea, airway obstruction, and/or oxygen desaturation. (See DOSAGE AND ADMINISTRATION.)

Pediatric Patients: Most patients aged 3 years through 16 years and classified ASA I or II require 2.5 to 3.5 mg/kg of DIPRIVAN Injectable Emulsion for induction when unpremedicated or when lightly premedicated with oral benzodiazepines or intramuscular opioids. Within this dosage range,

Continued on next page

Diprivan—Cont.

younger pediatric patients may require higher induction doses than older pediatric patients. As with other sedative-hypnotic agents, the amount of intravenous opioid and/or benzodiazepine premedication will influence the response of the patient to an induction dose of DIPRIVAN Injectable Emulsion. A lower dosage is recommended for pediatric patients classified as ASA III or IV. Attention should be paid to minimize pain on injection when administering DIPRIVAN Injectable Emulsion to pediatric patients. Boluses of DIPRIVAN Injectable Emulsion may be administered via small veins if pretreated with lidocaine or via antecubital or larger veins (See PRECAUTIONS—General).

Neurosurgical Patients: Slower induction is recommended using boluses of 20 mg every 10 seconds. Slower boluses or infusions of DIPRIVAN Injectable Emulsion for induction of anesthesia, titrated to clinical responses, will generally result in reduced induction dosage requirements (1 to 2 mg/kg). (See PRECAUTIONS and DOSAGE AND ADMINISTRATION.)

Cardiac Anesthesia: DIPRIVAN Injectable Emulsion has been well-studied in patients with coronary artery disease, but experience in patients with hemodynamically significant valvular or congenital heart disease is limited. As with other anesthetic and sedative-hypnotic agents, DIPRIVAN Injectable Emulsion in healthy patients causes a decrease in blood pressure that is secondary to decreases in preload (ventricular filling volume at the end of the diastole) and afterload (arterial resistance at the beginning of the systole). The magnitude of these changes is proportional to the blood and effect site concentrations achieved. These concentrations depend upon the dose and speed of the induction and maintenance infusion rates.

In addition, lower heart rates are observed during maintenance with DIPRIVAN Injectable Emulsion, possibly due to reduction of the sympathetic activity and/or resetting of the baroreceptor reflexes. Therefore, anticholinergic agents should be administered when increases in vagal tone are anticipated.

As with other anesthetic agents, DIPRIVAN Injectable Emulsion reduces myocardial oxygen consumption. Further studies are needed to confirm and delineate the extent of these effects on the myocardium and the coronary vascular system.

Morphine premedication (0.15 mg/kg) with nitrous oxide 67% in oxygen has been shown to decrease the necessary DIPRIVAN Injectable Emulsion maintenance infusion rates and therapeutic blood concentrations when compared to non-narcotic (lorazepam) premedication. The rate of DIPRIVAN Injectable Emulsion administration should be determined based on the patient's premedication and adjusted according to clinical responses.

A rapid bolus induction should be avoided. A slow rate of approximately 20 mg every 10 seconds until induction onset (0.5 to 1.5 mg/kg) should be used. In order to assure adequate anesthesia, when DIPRIVAN Injectable Emulsion is used as the primary agent, maintenance infusion rates should not be less than 100 μg/kg/min and should be supplemented with analgesic levels of continuous opioid administration. When an opioid is used as the primary agent, DIPRIVAN Injectable Emulsion maintenance rates should not be less than 50 μg/kg/min and care should be taken to ensure amnesia with concomitant benzodiazepines. Higher doses of DIPRIVAN Injectable Emulsion will reduce the opioid requirements (see Table 5). When DIPRIVAN Injectable Emulsion is used as the primary anesthetic, it should not be administered with the high-dose opioid technique as this may increase the likelihood of hypotension (see PRECAUTIONS—Cardiac Anesthesia).

[See table below]

Maintenance of General Anesthesia

Adult Patients:

In adults, anesthesia can be maintained by administering DIPRIVAN Injectable Emulsion by infusion or intermittent IV bolus injection. The patient's clinical response will determine the infusion rate or the amount and frequency of incremental injections.

Continuous Infusion: DIPRIVAN Injectable Emulsion 100 to 200 μg/kg/min administered in a variable rate infusion with 60%–70% nitrous oxide and oxygen provides anesthesia for patients undergoing general surgery. Maintenance by infusion of DIPRIVAN Injectable Emulsion should immediately follow the induction dose in order to provide satisfactory or continuous anesthesia during the induction phase. During this initial period following the induction dose, higher rates of infusion are generally required (150 to 200 μg/kg/min) for the first 10 to 15 minutes. Infusion rates should subsequently be decreased 30%–50% during the first half-hour of maintenance. Generally, rates of 50–100 μg/kg/min in adults should be achieved during maintenance in order to optimize recovery times.

Other drugs that cause CNS depression (hypnotics/sedatives, inhalational anesthetics, and opioids) can increase the CNS depression induced by propofol.

Intermittent Bolus: Increments of DIPRIVAN Injectable Emulsion 25 mg (2.5 mL) to 50 mg (5 mL) may be administered with nitrous oxide in adult patients undergoing general surgery. The incremental boluses should be administered when changes in vital signs indicate a response to surgical stimulation or light anesthesia.

Pediatric Patients: DIPRIVAN Injectable Emulsion administered as a variable rate infusion supplemented with nitrous oxide 60%–70% provides satisfactory anesthesia for most children 2 months of age or older, ASA class I or II, undergoing general anesthesia.

In general, for the pediatric population, maintenance by infusion of DIPRIVAN Injectable Emulsion at a rate of 200–300 μg/kg/min should immediately follow the induction dose. Following the first half-hour of maintenance, infusion rates of 125–150 μg/kg/min are typically needed. DIPRIVAN Injectable Emulsion SHOULD BE TITRATED TO ACHIEVE THE DESIRED CLINICAL EFFECT. Younger pediatric patients may require higher maintenance infusion rates than older pediatric patients. (See Table 2 Clinical Trials.)

DIPRIVAN Injectable Emulsion has been used with a variety of agents commonly used in anesthesia such as atropine, scopolamine, glycopyrrolate, diazepam, depolarizing and nondepolarizing muscle relaxants, and opioid analgesics, as well as with inhalational and regional anesthetic agents.

In the elderly, debilitated, or ASA III/IV patients, rapid bolus doses should not be used as this will increase cardiorespiratory effects including hypotension, apnea, airway obstruction, and/or oxygen desaturation.

Monitored Anesthesia Care (MAC) Sedation

Adult Patients:

When DIPRIVAN Injectable Emulsion is administered for MAC sedation, rates of administration should be individualized and titrated to clinical response. In most patients, the rates of DIPRIVAN Injectable Emulsion administration will be in the range of 25–75 μg/kg/min.

During initiation of MAC sedation, slow infusion or slow injection techniques are preferable over rapid bolus administration. During maintenance of MAC sedation, a variable rate infusion is preferable over intermittent bolus dose administration. In the elderly, debilitated, or ASA III/IV patients, rapid (single or repeated) bolus dose administration should not be used for MAC sedation. (See WARNINGS.) **A rapid bolus injection can result in undesirable cardiorespiratory depression including hypotension, apnea, airway obstruction, and/or oxygen desaturation.**

Initiation of MAC Sedation: For initiation of MAC sedation, either an infusion or a slow injection method may be utilized while closely monitoring cardiorespiratory function. With the infusion method, sedation may be initiated by infusing DIPRIVAN Injectable Emulsion at 100 to 150 μg/kg/min (6 to 9 mg/kg/h) for a period of 3 to 5 minutes and titrating to the desired clinical effect while closely monitoring respiratory function. With the slow injection method for initiation, patients will require approximately 0.5 mg/kg administered over 3 to 5 minutes and titrated to clinical responses. When DIPRIVAN Injectable Emulsion is administered slowly over 3 to 5 minutes, most patients will be adequately sedated, and the peak drug effect can be achieved while minimizing undesirable cardiorespiratory effects occurring at high plasma levels.

In the elderly, debilitated, or ASA III/IV patients, rapid (single or repeated) bolus dose administration should not be used for MAC sedation. (See WARNINGS.) The rate of administration should be over 3–5 minutes and the dosage of DIPRIVAN Injectable Emulsion should be reduced to approximately 80% of the usual adult dosage in these patients according to their condition, responses, and changes in vital signs. (See DOSAGE AND ADMINISTRATION.)

TABLE 5. CARDIAC ANESTHESIA TECHNIQUES

Primary Agent	Rate	Secondary Agent/Rate (Following Induction with Primary Agent)
DIPRIVAN Injectable Emulsion		OPIOID[a]/0.05–0.075 μg/kg/min (no bolus)
Preinduction anxiolysis	25 μg/kg/min	
Induction	0.5–1.5 mg/kg over 60 sec	
Maintenance (Titrated to Clinical Response)	100–150 μg/kg/min	
OPIOID[b]		DIPRIVAN Injectable Emulsion/ 50–100 μg/kg/min (no bolus)
Induction	25–50 μg/kg	
Maintenance	0.2–0.3 μg/kg/min	

[a]OPIOID is defined in terms of fentanyl equivalents, i.e.,
1 μg of fentanyl = 5 μg of alfentanil (for bolus)
= 10 μg of alfentanil (for maintenance)
or
= 0.1 μg of sufentanil

[b]Care should be taken to ensure amnesia with concomitant benzodiazepine therapy

Maintenance of MAC Sedation: For maintenance of sedation, a variable rate infusion method is preferable over an intermittent bolus dose method. With the variable rate infusion method, patients will generally require maintenance rates of 25 to 75 μg/kg/min (1.5 to 4.5 mg/kg/h) during the first 10 to 15 minutes of sedation maintenance. Infusion rates should subsequently be decreased over time to 25 to 50 μg/kg/min and adjusted to clinical responses. In titrating to clinical effect, allow approximately 2 minutes for onset of peak drug effect.

Infusion rates should always be titrated downward in the absence of clinical signs of light sedation until mild responses to stimulation are obtained in order to avoid sedative administration of DIPRIVAN Injectable Emulsion at rates higher than are clinically necessary.

If the intermittent bolus dose method is used, increments of DIPRIVAN Injectable Emulsion 10 mg (1 mL) or 20 mg (2 mL) can be administered and titrated to desired clinical effect. With the intermittent bolus method of sedation maintenance, there is the potential for respiratory depression, transient increases in sedation depth, and/or prolongation of recovery.

In the elderly, debilitated, or ASA III/IV patients, rapid (single or repeated) bolus dose administration should not be used for MAC sedation. (See WARNINGS.) The rate of administration and the dosage of DIPRIVAN Injectable Emulsion should be reduced to approximately 80% of the usual adult dosage in these patients according to their condition, responses, and changes in vital signs. (See DOSAGE AND ADMINISTRATION.)

DIPRIVAN Injectable Emulsion can be administered as the sole agent for maintenance of MAC sedation during surgical/diagnostic procedures. When DIPRIVAN Injectable Emulsion sedation is supplemented with opioid and/or benzodiazepine medications, these agents increase the sedative and respiratory effects of DIPRIVAN Injectable Emulsion and may also result in a slower recovery profile. (See PRECAUTIONS, Drug Interactions.)

ICU Sedation: (See WARNINGS and DOSAGE AND ADMINISTRATION, Handling Procedures.)

Adult Patients: For intubated, mechanically ventilated adult patients, Intensive Care Unit (ICU) sedation should be initiated slowly with a continuous infusion in order to titrate to desired clinical effect and minimize hypotension. (See DOSAGE AND ADMINISTRATION.)

Across all 6 US/Canadian clinical studies, the mean infusion maintenance rate for all DIPRIVAN Injectable Emulsion patients was 27 ± 21 μg/kg/min. The maintenance infusion rates required to maintain adequate sedation ranged from 2.8 μg/kg/min to 130 μg/kg/min. The infusion rate was lower in patients over 55 years of age (approximately 20 μg/kg/min) compared to patients under 55 years of age (approximately 38 μg/kg/min). In these studies, morphine or fentanyl was used as needed for analgesia.

Most adult ICU patients recovering from the effects of general anesthesia or deep sedation will require maintenance rates of 5 to 50 μg/kg/min (0.3 to 3 mg/kg/h) individualized and titrated to clinical response. (See DOSAGE AND ADMINISTRATION.) With medical ICU patients or patients who have recovered from the effects of general anesthesia or deep sedation, the rate of administration of 50 μg/kg/min or higher may be required to achieve adequate sedation. These higher rates of administration may increase the likelihood of patients developing hypotension.

Although there are reports of reduced analgesic requirements, most patients received opioids for analgesia during maintenance of ICU sedation. Some patients also received benzodiazepines and/or neuromuscular blocking agents. During long-term maintenance of sedation, some ICU patients were awakened once or twice every 24 hours for assessment of neurologic or respiratory function. (See Clinical Trials, Table 4.)

In post-CABG (coronary artery bypass graft) patients, the maintenance rate of propofol administration was usually low (median 11 μg/kg/min) due to the intraoperative administration of high opioid doses. Patients receiving DIPRIVAN Injectable Emulsion required 35% less nitroprusside than midazolam patients; this difference was statistically significant ($P<0.05$). During initiation of sedation in post-CABG patients, a 15% to 20% decrease in blood pressure was seen in the first 60 minutes. It was not possible to determine cardiovascular effects in patients with severely compromised ventricular function (See Clinical Trials, Table 4).

In Medical or Postsurgical ICU studies comparing DIPRIVAN Injectable Emulsion to benzodiazepine infusion or bolus, there were no apparent differences in maintenance of adequate sedation, mean arterial pressure, or laboratory findings. Like the comparators, DIPRIVAN Injectable Emulsion reduced blood cortisol during sedation while maintaining responsivity to challenges with adrenocorticotropic hormone (ACTH). Case reports from the published literature generally reflect that DIPRIVAN Injectable Emulsion has been used safely in patients with a history of porphyria or malignant hyperthermia.

In hemodynamically stable head trauma patients ranging in age from 19–43 years, adequate sedation was maintained with DIPRIVAN Injectable Emulsion or morphine (N=7 in each group). There were no apparent differences in adequacy of sedation, intracranial pressure, cerebral perfusion pressure, or neurologic recovery between the treatment groups. In literature reports from Neurosurgical ICU and severely head-injured patients DIPRIVAN Injectable Emulsion infusion with or without diuretics and hyperventilation controlled intracranial pressure while maintaining cerebral

perfusion pressure. In some patients, bolus doses resulted in decreased blood pressure and compromised cerebral perfusion pressure. (See Clinical Trials, Table 4.)
DIPRIVAN Injectable Emulsion was found to be effective in status epilepticus which was refractory to the standard anticonvulsant therapies. For these patients as well as for ARDS/respiratory failure and tetanus patients, sedation maintenance dosages were generally higher than those for other critically ill patient populations. (See Clinical Trials, Table 4.)
Abrupt discontinuation of DIPRIVAN Injectable Emulsion prior to weaning or for daily evaluation of sedation levels should be avoided. This may result in rapid awakening with associated anxiety, agitation, and resistance to mechanical ventilation. Infusions of DIPRIVAN Injectable Emulsion should be adjusted to maintain a light level of sedation through the weaning process or evaluation of sedation level. (See PRECAUTIONS.)

INDICATIONS AND USAGE

DIPRIVAN Injectable Emulsion is an IV sedative-hypnotic agent that can be used for both induction and/or maintenance of anesthesia as part of a balanced anesthetic technique for inpatient and outpatient surgery in adult patients and pediatric patients greater than 3 years of age. DIPRIVAN Injectable Emulsion can also be used for maintenance of anesthesia as part of a balanced anesthetic technique for inpatient and outpatient surgery in adult patients and in pediatric patients greater than 2 months of age.
DIPRIVAN Injectable Emulsion is not recommended for induction of anesthesia below the age of 3 years or for maintenance of anesthesia below the age of 2 months because its safety and effectiveness have not been established in those populations.
In adult patients, DIPRIVAN Injectable Emulsion, when administered intravenously as directed, can be used to initiate and maintain monitored anesthesia care (MAC) sedation during diagnostic procedures. DIPRIVAN Injectable Emulsion may also be used for MAC sedation in conjunction with local/regional anesthesia in patients undergoing surgical procedures. (See PRECAUTIONS.)
Safety, effectiveness and dosing guidelines for DIPRIVAN Injectable Emulsion have not been established for MAC Sedation/light general anesthesia in the pediatric population undergoing diagnostic or nonsurgical procedures and therefore it is not recommended for this use. (See PRECAUTIONS, Pediatric Use).
DIPRIVAN Injectable Emulsion should only be administered to intubated, mechanically ventilated adult patients in the Intensive Care Unit (ICU) to provide continuous sedation and control of stress responses. In this setting, DIPRIVAN Injectable Emulsion should be administered only by persons skilled in the medical management of critically ill patients and trained in cardiovascular resuscitation and airway management.
DIPRIVAN Injectable Emulsion is not indicated for use in Pediatric ICU sedation since the safety of this regimen has not been established. (See PRECAUTIONS, Pediatric Use).
DIPRIVAN Injectable Emulsion is not recommended for obstetrics, including cesarean section deliveries. DIPRIVAN Injectable Emulsion crosses the placenta, and as with other general anesthetic agents, the administration of DIPRIVAN Injectable Emulsion may be associated with neonatal depression. (See PRECAUTIONS.)
DIPRIVAN Injectable Emulsion is not recommended for use in nursing mothers because DIPRIVAN Injectable Emulsion has been reported to be excreted in human milk and the effects of oral absorption of small amounts of propofol are not known. (See PRECAUTIONS.)

CONTRAINDICATIONS

DIPRIVAN Injectable Emulsion is contraindicated in patients with a known hypersensitivity to DIPRIVAN Injectable Emulsion or its components, or when general anesthesia or sedation are contraindicated.

WARNINGS

For general anesthesia or monitored anesthesia care (MAC) sedation, DIPRIVAN Injectable Emulsion should be administered only by persons trained in the administration of general anesthesia and not involved in the conduct of the surgical/diagnostic procedure. Patients should be continuously monitored, and facilities for maintenance of a patent airway, artificial ventilation, and oxygen enrichment and circulatory resuscitation must be immediately available.
For sedation of intubated, mechanically ventilated adult patients in the Intensive Care Unit (ICU), DIPRIVAN Injectable Emulsion should be administered only by persons skilled in the management of critically ill patients and trained in cardiovascular resuscitation and airway management.
In the elderly, debilitated, or ASA III/IV patients, rapid (single or repeated) bolus administration should not be used during general anesthesia or MAC sedation in order to minimize undesirable cardiorespiratory depression including hypotension, apnea, airway obstruction, and/or oxygen desaturation.
MAC sedation patients should be continuously monitored by persons not involved in the conduct of the surgical or diagnostic procedure; oxygen supplementation should be immediately available and provided where clinically indicated; and oxygen saturation should be monitored in all patients. Patients should be continuously monitored for early signs of hypotension, apnea, airway obstruction, and/or oxygen desaturation. These cardiorespiratory effects are more likely to occur following rapid initiation (loading) boluses or during supplemental maintenance boluses, especially in the elderly, debilitated, or ASA III/IV patients.
DIPRIVAN Injectable Emulsion should not be coadministered through the same IV catheter with blood or plasma because compatibility has not been established. *In vitro* tests have shown that aggregates of the globular component of the emulsion vehicle have occurred with blood/plasma/serum from humans and animals. The clinical significance is not known.
STRICT ASEPTIC TECHNIQUE MUST ALWAYS BE MAINTAINED DURING HANDLING. DIPRIVAN INJECTABLE EMULSION IS A SINGLE-USE PARENTERAL PRODUCT WHICH CONTAINS 0.005% DISODIUM EDETATE TO RETARD THE RATE OF GROWTH OF MICROORGANISMS IN THE EVENT OF ACCIDENTAL EXTRINSIC CONTAMINATION. HOWEVER, DIPRIVAN INJECTABLE EMULSION CAN STILL SUPPORT THE GROWTH OF MICROORGANISMS AS IT IS NOT AN ANTIMICROBIALLY PRESERVED PRODUCT UNDER USP STANDARDS. ACCORDINGLY, STRICT ASEPTIC TECHNIQUE MUST STILL BE ADHERED TO. DO NOT USE IF CONTAMINATION IS SUSPECTED. DISCARD UNUSED PORTIONS AS DIRECTED WITHIN THE REQUIRED TIME LIMITS (SEE DOSAGE AND ADMINISTRATION, HANDLING PROCEDURES). THERE HAVE BEEN REPORTS IN WHICH FAILURE TO USE ASEPTIC TECHNIQUE WHEN HANDLING DIPRIVAN INJECTABLE EMULSION WAS ASSOCIATED WITH MICROBIAL CONTAMINATION OF THE PRODUCT AND WITH FEVER, INFECTION/SEPSIS, OTHER LIFE-THREATENING ILLNESS, AND/OR DEATH.

PRECAUTIONS

General

Adult and Pediatric Patients: A lower induction dose and a slower maintenance rate of administration should be used in elderly, debilitated, or ASA III/IV patients. (See CLINICAL PHARMACOLOGY—Individualization of Dosage.) Patients should be continuously monitored for early signs of significant hypotension and/or bradycardia. Treatment may include increasing the rate of intravenous fluid, elevation of lower extremities, use of pressor agents, or administration of atropine. Apnea often occurs during induction and may persist for more than 60 seconds. Ventilatory support may be required. Because DIPRIVAN Injectable Emulsion is an emulsion, caution should be exercised in patients with disorders of lipid metabolism such as primary hyperlipoproteinemia, diabetic hyperlipemia, and pancreatitis.
Very rarely the use of DIPRIVAN may be associated with the development of a period of postoperative unconsciousness which may be accompanied by an increase in muscle tone. This may or may not be preceded by a brief period of wakefulness. Recovery is spontaneous. The clinical criteria for discharge from the recovery/day surgery area established for each institution should be satisfied before discharge of the patient from the care of the anesthesiologist.
When DIPRIVAN Injectable Emulsion is administered to an epileptic patient, there may be a risk of seizure during the recovery phase.
Attention should be paid to minimize pain on administration of DIPRIVAN Injectable Emulsion. Transient local pain can be minimized if the larger veins of the forearm or antecubital fossa are used. Pain during intravenous injection may also be reduced by prior injection of IV lidocaine (1 mL of a 1% solution). Pain on injection occurred frequently in pediatric patients (45%) when a small vein of the hand was utilized without lidocaine pretreatment. With lidocaine pretreatment or when antecubital veins were utilized, pain was minimal (incidence less than 10%) and well-tolerated.
Venous sequelae (phlebitis or thrombosis) have been reported rarely (<1%). In two well-controlled clinical studies using dedicated intravenous catheters, no instances of venous sequelae were observed up to 14 days following induction.
Intra-arterial injection in animals did not induce local tissue effects. Accidental intra-arterial injection has been reported in patients, and, other than pain, there were no major sequelae.
Intentional injection into subcutaneous or perivascular tissues of animals caused minimal tissue reaction. During the post-marketing period, there have been rare reports of local pain, swelling, blisters, and/or tissue necrosis following accidental extravasation of DIPRIVAN Injectable Emulsion.
Perioperative myoclonia, rarely including convulsions and opisthotonos, has occurred in temporal relationship in cases in which DIPRIVAN Injectable Emulsion has been administered.
Clinical features of anaphylaxis, which may include angioedema, bronchospasm, erythema, and hypotension, occur rarely following DIPRIVAN Injectable Emulsion administration, although use of other drugs in most instances makes the relationship to DIPRIVAN Injectable Emulsion unclear.
There have been rare reports of pulmonary edema in temporal relationship to the administration of DIPRIVAN Injectable Emulsion, although a causal relationship is unknown.
Very rarely, cases of unexplained postoperative pancreatitis (requiring hospital admission) have been reported after anesthesia in which DIPRIVAN Injectable Emulsion was one of the induction agents used. Due to a variety of confounding factors in these cases, including concomitant medications, a causal relationship to DIPRIVAN Injectable Emulsion is unclear.
DIPRIVAN Injectable Emulsion has no vagolytic activity. Reports of bradycardia, asystole, and rarely, cardiac arrest have been associated with DIPRIVAN Injectable Emulsion. Pediatric patients are susceptible to this effect, particularly when fentanyl is given concomitantly. The intravenous administration of anticholinergic agents (e.g., atropine or glycopyrrolate) should be considered to modify potential increases in vagal tone due to concomitant agents (e.g., succinylcholine) or surgical stimuli.

Intensive Care Unit Sedation

Adult Patients (See WARNINGS and DOSAGE AND ADMINISTRATION, Handling Procedures.) The administration of DIPRIVAN Injectable Emulsion should be initiated as a continuous infusion and changes in the rate of administration made slowly (>5 min) in order to minimize hypotension and avoid acute overdosage. (See CLINICAL PHARMACOLOGY—Individualization of Dosage.)
Patients should be monitored for early signs of significant hypotension and/or cardiovascular depression, which may be profound. These effects are responsive to discontinuation of DIPRIVAN Injectable Emulsion, IV fluid administration, and/or vasopressor therapy.
As with other sedative medications, there is wide interpatient variability in DIPRIVAN Injectable Emulsion dosage requirements, and these requirements may change with time.
Failure to reduce the infusion rate in patients receiving DIPRIVAN Injectable Emulsion for extended periods may result in excessively high blood concentrations of the drug. Thus, titration to clinical response and daily evaluation of sedation levels are important during use of DIPRIVAN Injectable Emulsion infusion for ICU sedation, especially of long duration.
Opioids and paralytic agents should be discontinued and respiratory function optimized prior to weaning patients from mechanical ventilation. Infusions of DIPRIVAN Injectable Emulsion should be adjusted to maintain a light level of sedation prior to weaning patients from mechanical ventilatory support. Throughout the weaning process, this level of sedation may be maintained in the absence of respiratory depression. Because of the rapid clearance of DIPRIVAN Injectable Emulsion, abrupt discontinuation of a patient's infusion may result in rapid awakening of the patient with associated anxiety, agitation, and resistance to mechanical ventilation, making weaning from mechanical ventilation difficult. It is therefore recommended that administration of DIPRIVAN Injectable Emulsion be continued in order to maintain a light level of sedation throughout the weaning process until 10–15 minutes prior to extubation, at which time the infusion can be discontinued.
There have been very rare reports of rhabdomyolysis associated with the administration of DIPRIVAN Injectable Emulsion for ICU sedation.
Since DIPRIVAN Injectable Emulsion is formulated in an oil-in-water emulsion, elevations in serum triglycerides may occur when DIPRIVAN Injectable Emulsion is administered for extended periods of time. Patients at risk of hyperlipidemia should be monitored for increases in serum triglycerides or serum turbidity. Administration of DIPRIVAN Injectable Emulsion should be adjusted if fat is being inadequately cleared from the body. A reduction in the quantity of concurrently administered lipids is indicated to compensate for the amount of lipid infused as part of the DIPRIVAN Injectable Emulsion formulation; 1 mL of DIPRIVAN Injectable Emulsion contains approximately 0.1 g of fat (1.1 kcal).
EDTA is a strong chelator of trace metals—including zinc. Although with DIPRIVAN Injectable Emulsion there are no reports of decreased zinc levels or zinc deficiency-related adverse events, DIPRIVAN Injectable Emulsion should not be infused for longer than 5 days without providing a drug holiday to safely replace estimated or measured urine zinc losses.
In clinical trials mean urinary zinc loss was approximately 2.5 to 3.0 mg/day in adult patients and 1.5 to 2.0 mg/day in pediatric patients.
In patients who are predisposed to zinc deficiency, such as those with burns, diarrhea, and/or major sepsis, the need for supplemental zinc should be considered during prolonged therapy with DIPRIVAN Injectable Emulsion.
At high doses (2–3 grams per day), EDTA has been reported, on rare occasions, to be toxic to the renal tubules. Studies to-date, in patients with normal or impaired renal function have not shown any alteration in renal function with DIPRIVAN Injectable Emulsion containing 0.005% disodium edetate. In patients at risk for renal impairment, urinalysis and urine sediment should be checked before initiation of sedation and then be monitored on alternate days during sedation.
The long-term administration of DIPRIVAN Injectable Emulsion to patients with renal failure and/or hepatic insufficiency has not been evaluated.
Neurosurgical Anesthesia: When DIPRIVAN Injectable Emulsion is used in patients with increased intracranial pressure or impaired cerebral circulation, significant decreases in mean arterial pressure should be avoided because of the resultant decreases in cerebral perfusion pressure. To avoid significant hypotension and decreases in cerebral perfusion pressure, an infusion or slow bolus of approximately 20 mg every 10 seconds should be utilized instead of rapid, more frequent, and/or larger boluses of DIPRIVAN Injectable Emulsion. Slower induction titrated to clinical responses, will generally result in reduced induction dosage requirements (1 to 2 mg/kg). When increased ICP is suspected, hyperventilation and hypocarbia should accompany the administration of DIPRIVAN Injectable Emulsion. (See DOSAGE AND ADMINISTRATION.)
Cardiac Anesthesia: Slower rates of administration should be utilized in premedicated patients, geriatric patients, pa-

Continued on next page

Diprivan—Cont.

tients with recent fluid shifts, or patients who are hemodynamically unstable. Any fluid deficits should be corrected prior to administration of DIPRIVAN Injectable Emulsion. In those patients where additional fluid therapy may be contraindicated, other measures, e.g., elevation of lower extremities, or use of pressor agents, may be useful to offset the hypotension which is associated with the induction of anesthesia with DIPRIVAN Injectable Emulsion.

Information for Patients: Patients should be advised that performance of activities requiring mental alertness, such as operating a motor vehicle, or hazardous machinery or signing legal documents may be impaired for some time after general anesthesia or sedation.

Drug Interactions: The induction dose requirements of DIPRIVAN Injectable Emulsion may be reduced in patients with intramuscular or intravenous premedication, particularly with narcotics (e.g., morphine, meperidine, and fentanyl, etc.) and combinations of opioids and sedatives (e.g., benzodiazepines, barbiturates, chloral hydrate, droperidol, etc.). These agents may increase the anesthetic or sedative effects of DIPRIVAN Injectable Emulsion and may also result in more pronounced decreases in systolic, diastolic, and mean arterial pressures and cardiac output.

During maintenance of anesthesia or sedation, the rate of DIPRIVAN Injectable Emulsion administration should be adjusted according to the desired level of anesthesia or sedation and may be reduced in the presence of supplemental analgesic agents (e.g., nitrous oxide or opioids). The concurrent administration of potent inhalational agents (e.g., isoflurane, enflurane, and halothane) during maintenance with DIPRIVAN Injectable Emulsion has not been extensively evaluated. These inhalational agents can also be expected to increase the anesthetic or sedative and cardiorespiratory effects of DIPRIVAN Injectable Emulsion.

DIPRIVAN Injectable Emulsion does not cause a clinically significant change in onset, intensity or duration of action of the commonly used neuromuscular blocking agents (e.g., succinylcholine and nondepolarizing muscle relaxants).

No significant adverse interactions with commonly used premedications or drugs used during anesthesia or sedation (including a range of muscle relaxants, inhalational agents, analgesic agents, and local anesthetic agents) have been observed in adults. In pediatric patients, administration of fentanyl concomitantly with DIPRIVAN Injectable Emulsion may result in serious bradycardia.

Carcinogenesis, Mutagenesis, Impairment of Fertility: Animal carcinogenicity studies have not been performed with propofol.

In vitro and *in vivo* animal tests failed to show any potential for mutagenicity by propofol. Tests for mutagenicity included the Ames (using *Salmonella* sp) mutation test, gene mutation/gene conversion using *Saccharomyces cerevisiae*, *in vitro* cytogenetic studies in Chinese hamsters and a mouse micronucleus test.

Studies in female rats at intravenous doses up to 15 mg/kg/day (approximately equivalent to the recommended human induction dose on a mg/m^2 basis) for 2 weeks before pregnancy to day 7 of gestation did not show impaired fertility. Male fertility in rats was not affected in a dominant lethal study at intravenous doses up to 15 mg/kg/day for 5 days.

Pregnancy Category B: Reproduction studies have been performed in rats and rabbits at intravenous doses of 15 mg/kg/day (approximately equivalent to the recommended human induction dose on a mg/m^2 basis) and have revealed no evidence of impaired fertility or harm to the fetus due to propofol. Propofol, however, has been shown to cause maternal deaths in rats and rabbits and decreased pup survival during the lactating period in dams treated with 15 mg/kg/day (approximately equivalent to the recommended human induction dose on a mg/m^2 basis). The pharmacological activity (anesthesia) of the drug on the mother is probably responsible for the adverse effects seen in the offspring. There are, however, no adequate and well-controlled studies in pregnant women. Because animal reproduction studies are not always predictive of human responses, this drug should be used during pregnancy only if clearly needed.

Labor and Delivery: DIPRIVAN Injectable Emulsion is not recommended for obstetrics, including cesarean section deliveries. DIPRIVAN Injectable Emulsion crosses the placenta, and as with other general anesthetic agents, the administration of DIPRIVAN Injectable Emulsion may be associated with neonatal depression.

Nursing Mothers: DIPRIVAN Injectable Emulsion is not recommended for use in nursing mothers because DIPRIVAN Injectable Emulsion has been reported to be excreted in human milk and the effects of oral absorption of small amounts of propofol are not known.

Pediatric Use: The safety and effectiveness of DIPRIVAN Injectable Emulsion have been established for induction of anesthesia in pediatric patients aged 3 years and older and for the maintenance of anesthesia aged 2 months and older. DIPRIVAN Injectable Emulsion is not recommended for the induction of anesthesia in patients younger than 3 years of age and for the maintenance of anesthesia in patients younger than 2 months of age as safety and effectiveness have not been established.

In pediatric patients, administration of fentanyl concomitantly with DIPRIVAN Injectable Emulsion may result in serious bradycardia (see PRECAUTIONS—General).

DIPRIVAN Injectable Emulsion is not indicated for use in pediatric patients for ICU sedation or for MAC sedation for surgical, nonsurgical or diagnostic procedures as safety and effectiveness have not been established.

There have been anecdotal reports of serious adverse events and death in pediatric patients with upper respiratory tract infections receiving DIPRIVAN Injectable Emulsion for ICU sedation.

In one multicenter clinical trial of ICU sedation in critically ill pediatric patients that excluded patients with upper respiratory tract infections, the incidence of mortality observed in patients who received DIPRIVAN Injectable Emulsion (n=222) was 9%, while that for patients who received standard sedative agents (n=105) was 4%. While causality has not been established, DIPRIVAN Injectable Emulsion is not indicated for sedation in pediatric patients until further studies have been performed to document its safety in that population. (See CLINICAL PHARMACOLOGY—Pediatric Patients: and Dosage and Administration).

In pediatric patients, abrupt discontinuation following prolonged infusion may result in flushing of the hands and feet, agitation, tremulousness and hyperirritability. Increased incidences of bradycardia (5%), agitation (4%), and jitteriness (9%) have also been observed.

Geriatric Use: The effect of age on induction dose requirements for propofol was assessed in an open study involving 211 unpremedicated patients with approximately 30 patients in each decade between the ages of 16 and 80. The average dose to induce anesthesia was calculated for patients up to 54 years of age and for patients 55 years of age or older. The average dose to induce anesthesia in patients up to 54 years of age was 1.99 mg/kg and in patients above 54 it was 1.66 mg/kg. Subsequent clinical studies have demonstrated lower dosing requirements for subjects greater than 60 years of age.

A lower induction dose and a slower maintenance rate of administration of DIPRIVAN Injectable Emulsion should be used in elderly patients. In this group of patients, rapid (single or repeated) bolus administration should not be used in order to minimize undesirable cardiorespiratory depression including hypotension, apnea, airway obstruction, and/or oxygen desaturation. All dosing should be titrated according to patient condition and response. (See DOSAGE AND ADMINISTRATION—Elderly, debilitated, or ASA III/IV patients and CLINICAL PHARMACOLOGY—Geriatrics.)

ADVERSE REACTIONS

General

Adverse event information is derived from controlled clinical trials and worldwide marketing experience. In the description below, rates of the more common events represent US/Canadian clinical study results. Less frequent events are also derived from publications and marketing experience in over 8 million patients; there are insufficient data to support an accurate estimate of their incidence rates. These studies were conducted using a variety of premedicants, varying lengths of surgical/diagnostic procedures, and various other anesthetic/sedative agents. Most adverse events were mild and transient.

Anesthesia and MAC Sedation in Adults

The following estimates of adverse events for DIPRIVAN Injectable Emulsion include data from clinical trials in general anesthesia/MAC sedation (N=2889 adult patients). The adverse events listed below as probably causally related are those events in which the actual incidence rate in patients treated with DIPRIVAN Injectable Emulsion was greater

Incidence greater than 1%—Probably Causally Related

	Anesthesia/MAC Sedation	ICU Sedation
Cardiovascular:	Bradycardia Arrhythmia [Peds: 1.2%] Tachycardia Nodal [Peds: 1.6%] Hypotension* [Peds: 17%] (see also CLINICAL PHARMACOLOGY) [Hypertension Peds: 8%]	Bradycardia Decreased Cardiac Output Hypotension 26%
Central Nervous System:	Movement* [Peds: 17%]	
Injection Site:	Burning/Stinging or Pain, 17.6% [Peds: 10%]	
Metabolic/Nutritional:		Hyperlipemia*
Respiratory:	Apnea (see also CLINICAL PHARMACOLOGY)	Respiratory Acidosis During Weaning*
Skin and Appendages:	Rash [Peds: 5%] Pruritus [Peds: 2%]	

Events without an * or % had an incidence of 1%–3%
* Incidence of events 3% to 10%

Incidence less than 1%—Probably Causally Related

	Anesthesia/MAC Sedation	ICU Sedation
Body as a Whole:	Anaphylaxis/Anaphylactoid Reaction, Perinatal Disorder [Tachycardia], [Bigeminy], [Bradycardia] [Premature Ventricular Contractions], [Hemorrhage], [ECG Abnormal], [Arrhythmia Atrial], [Fever], [Extremities Pain], [Anticholinergic Syndrome]	
Cardiovascular:	Premature Atrial Contractions, Syncope	
Central Nervous System:	Hypertonia/Dystonia, Paresthesia	Agitation
Digestive:	[Hypersalivation], [Nausea]	
Hemic/Lymphatic:	[Leukocytosis]	
Injection Site:	[Phlebitis], [Pruritus]	
Metabolic:	[Hypomagnesemia]	
Musculoskeletal:	Myalgia	
Nervous:	[Dizziness], [Agitation], [Chills], [Somnolence], [Delirium]	
Respiratory:	Wheezing, [Cough], [Laryngospasm], [Hypoxia]	Decreased Lung Function
Skin and Appendages:	Flushing, Pruritus	
Special Senses:	Amblyopia [Vision Abnormal]	
Urogenital:	Cloudy Urine	Green Urine

Incidence less than 1%—Causal Relationship Unknown

	Anesthesia/MAC Sedation	ICU Sedation
Body as a Whole:	Asthenia, Awareness, Chest Pain, Extremities Pain, Fever, Increased Drug Effect, Neck Rigidity/Stiffness, Trunk Pain	Fever, Sepsis, Trunk Pain, Whole Body Weakness
Cardiovascular:	Arrhythmia, Atrial Fibrillation, Atrioventricular Heart Block, Bigeminy, Bleeding, Bundle Branch Block, Cardiac Arrest, ECG Abnormal, Edema, Extrasystole, Heart Block, Hypertension, Myocardial Infarction, Myocardial Ischemia, Premature Ventricular Contractions, ST Segment Depression, Supraventricular Tachycardia, Tachycardia, Ventricular Fibrillation	Arrhythmia, Atrial Fibrillation, Bigeminy, Cardiac Arrest, Extrasystole, Right Heart Failure, Ventricular Tachycardia
Central Nervous System:	Abnormal Dreams, Agitation, Amorous Behavior, Anxiety, Bucking/Jerking/Thrashing, Chills/Shivering, Clonic/Myoclonic Movement, Combativeness, Confusion, Delirium, Depression, Dizziness, Emotional Lability, Euphoria, Fatigue, Hallucinations, Headache, Hypotonia, Hysteria, Insomnia, Moaning, Neuropathy, Opisthotonos, Rigidity, Seizures, Somnolence, Tremor, Twitching	Chills/Shivering, Intracranial Hypertension, Seizures, Somnolence, Thinking Abnormal
Digestive:	Cramping, Diarrhea, Dry Mouth, Enlarged Parotid, Nausea, Swallowing, Vomiting	Ileus, Liver Function Abnormal
Hematologic/Lymphatic:	Coagulation Disorder, Leukocytosis	
Injection Site:	Hives/Itching, Phlebitis, Redness/Discoloration	
Metabolic/Nutritional:	Hyperkalemia, Hyperlipemia	BUN Increased, Creatinine Increased, Dehydration, Hyperglycemia, Metabolic Acidosis, Osmolality Increased
Respiratory:	Bronchospasm, Burning in Throat, Cough, Dyspnea, Hiccough, Hyperventilation, Hypoventilation, Hypoxia, Laryngospasm, Pharyngitis, Sneezing, Tachypnea, Upper Airway Obstruction	Hypoxia
Skin and Appendages:	Conjunctival Hyperemia, Diaphoresis, Urticaria	Rash
Special Senses:	Diplopia, Ear Pain, Eye Pain, Nystagmus, Taste Perversion, Tinnitus	
Urogenital:	Oliguria, Urine Retention	Kidney Failure

than the comparator incidence rate in these trials. Therefore, incidence rates for anesthesia and MAC sedation in adults generally represent estimates of the percentage of clinical trial patients which appeared to have probable causal relationship.

The adverse experience profile from reports of 150 patients in the MAC sedation clinical trials is similar to the profile established with DIPRIVAN Injectable Emulsion during anesthesia (see below). During MAC sedation clinical trials, significant respiratory events included cough, upper airway obstruction, apnea, hypoventilation, and dyspnea.

Anesthesia In Pediatric Patients

Generally the adverse experience profile from reports of 506 DIPRIVAN Injectable Emulsion pediatric patients from 6 days through 16 years of age in the US/Canadian anesthesia clinical trials is similar to the profile established with DIPRIVAN Injectable Emulsion during anesthesia in adults (see Pediatric percentages [Peds %] below). Although not reported as an adverse event in clinical trials, apnea is frequently observed in pediatric patients.

ICU Sedation In Adults

The following estimates of adverse events include data from clinical trials in ICU sedation (N=159 adult patients). Probably related incidence rates for ICU sedation were determined by individual case report form review. Probable causality was based upon an apparent dose response relationship and/or positive responses to rechallenge. In many instances the presence of concomitant disease and concomitant therapy made the causal relationship unknown. Therefore, incidence rates for ICU sedation generally represent estimates of the percentage of clinical trial patients which appeared to have a probable causal relationship.

[See table at top of previous page]

DRUG ABUSE AND DEPENDENCE

Rare cases of self-administration of DIPRIVAN Injectable Emulsion by health care professionals have been reported, including some fatalities. DIPRIVAN Injectable Emulsion should be managed to prevent the risk of diversion, including restriction of access and accounting procedures as appropriate to the clinical setting.

OVERDOSAGE

If overdosage occurs, DIPRIVAN Injectable Emulsion administration should be discontinued immediately. Overdosage is likely to cause cardiorespiratory depression. Respiratory depression should be treated by artificial ventilation with oxygen. Cardiovascular depression may require repositioning of the patient by raising the patient's legs, increasing the flow rate of intravenous fluids, and administering pressor agents and/or anticholinergic agents.

DOSAGE AND ADMINISTRATION

Dosage and rate of administration should be individualized and titrated to the desired effect, according to clinically relevant factors including preinduction and concomitant medications, age, ASA physical classification, and level of debilitation of the patient.

The following is abbreviated dosage and administration information which is only intended as a general guide in the use of DIPRIVAN Injectable Emulsion. Prior to administering DIPRIVAN Injectable Emulsion, it is imperative that the physician review and be completely familiar with the specific dosage and administration information detailed in the CLINICAL PHARMACOLOGY—Individualization of Dosage section.

In the elderly, debilitated, or ASA III/IV patients, rapid bolus doses should not be the method of administration. (See WARNINGS.)

Intensive Care Unit Sedation:

STRICT ASEPTIC TECHNIQUE MUST ALWAYS BE MAINTAINED DURING HANDLING. DIPRIVAN INJECTABLE EMULSION IS A SINGLE-USE PARENTERAL PRODUCT WHICH CONTAINS 0.005% DISODIUM EDETATE TO RETARD THE RATE OF GROWTH OF MICROORGANISMS IN THE EVENT OF ACCIDENTAL EXTRINSIC CONTAMINATION. HOWEVER, DIPRIVAN INJECTABLE EMULSION CAN STILL SUPPORT THE GROWTH OF MICROORGANISMS AS IT IS NOT AN ANTIMICROBIALLY PRESERVED PRODUCT UNDER USP STANDARDS. ACCORDINGLY, STRICT ASEPTIC TECHNIQUE MUST STILL BE ADHERED TO. DO NOT USE IF CONTAMINATION IS SUSPECTED. (See DOSAGE AND ADMINISTRATION, Handling Procedures.)

DIPRIVAN Injectable Emulsion should be individualized according to the patient's condition and response, blood lipid profile, and vital signs. (See PRECAUTIONS—ICU Sedation.) For intubated, mechanically ventilated adult patients, Intensive Care Unit (ICU) sedation should be initiated slowly with a continuous infusion in order to titrate to desired clinical effect and minimize hypotension. When indicated, initiation of sedation should begin at 5 μg/kg/min (0.3 mg/kg/h). The infusion rate should be increased by increments of 5 to 10 μg/kg/min (0.3 to 0.6 mg/kg/h) until the desired level of sedation is achieved. A minimum period of 5 minutes between adjustments should be allowed for onset of peak drug effect. Most adult patients require maintenance rates of 5 to 50 μg/kg/min (0.3 to 3 mg/kg/h) or higher. Dosages of DIPRIVAN Injectable Emulsion should be reduced in patients who have received large dosages of narcotics. Conversely, the DIPRIVAN Injectable Emulsion dosage requirement may be reduced by adequate management of pain with analgesic agents. As with other sedative medications, there is interpatient variability in dosage requirements, and these requirements may change with time. (See dosage guide.) **EVALUATION OF LEVEL OF SEDATION AND ASSESSMENT OF CNS FUNCTION SHOULD BE CARRIED OUT DAILY THROUGHOUT MAINTENANCE TO DETERMINE THE MINIMUM DOSE OF DIPRIVAN INJECTABLE EMULSION REQUIRED FOR SEDATION (SEE CLINICAL TRIALS, ICU SEDATION).** Bolus administration of 10 or 20 mg should only be used to rapidly increase depth of sedation in patients where hypotension is not likely to occur. Patients with compromised myocardial function, intravascular volume depletion, or abnormally low vascular tone (e.g., sepsis) may be more susceptible to hypotension. (See PRECAUTIONS.)

EDTA is a strong chelator of trace metals—including zinc. Although with DIPRIVAN Injectable Emulsion there are no reports of decreased zinc levels or zinc deficiency-related adverse events, DIPRIVAN Injectable Emulsion should not be infused for longer than 5 days without providing a drug holiday to safely replace estimated or measured urine zinc losses.

At high doses (2–3 grams per day), EDTA has been reported, on rare occasions, to be toxic to the renal tubules. Studies to-date, in patients with normal or impaired renal function have not shown any alteration in renal function with DIPRIVAN Injectable Emulsion containing 0.005% disodium edetate. In patients at risk for renal impairment, urinalysis and urine sediment should be checked before initiation of sedation and then be monitored on alternate days during sedation.

SUMMARY OF DOSAGE GUIDELINES—

Dosages and rates of administration in the following table should be individualized and titrated to clinical response. Safety and dosing requirements for induction of anesthesia in pediatric patients have only been established for children 3 years of age or older. Safety and dosing requirements for the maintenance of anesthesia have only been established for children 2 months of age and older. For complete dosage information, see CLINICAL PHARMACOLOGY— Individualization of Dosage.

[See table above]

INDICATION	DOSAGE AND ADMINISTRATION
Induction of General Anesthesia	**Healthy Adults Less Than 55 Years of Age:** 40 mg every 10 seconds until induction onset (2 to 2.5 mg/kg). **Elderly, Debilitated, or ASA III/IV Patients:** 20 mg every 10 seconds until induction onset (1 to 1.5 mg/kg). **Cardiac Anesthesia:**20 mg every 10 seconds until induction onset (0.5 to 1.5 mg/kg). **Neurosurgical Patients:** 20 mg every 10 seconds until induction onset (1 to 2 mg/kg). **Pediatric Patients—healthy, from 3 years to 16 years of age:** 2.5 to 3.5 mg/kg administered over 20–30 seconds. (See PRECAUTIONS—Pediatric Use: and CLINICAL PHARMACOLOGY—Pediatric patients)
Maintenance of General Anesthesia:	**Infusion** **Healthy Adults Less Than 55 Years of Age:** 100 to 200 μg/kg/min (6 to 12 mg/kg/h). **Elderly, Debilitated, ASA III/IV Patients:** 50 to 100 μg/kg/min (3 to 6 mg/kg/h). **Cardiac Anesthesia:**Most patients require: Primary DIPRIVAN Injectable Emulsion with Secondary Opioid—100–150 μg/kg/min Low-dose DIPRIVAN Injectable Emulsion with Primary Opioid—50–100 μg/kg/min (See CLINICAL PHARMACOLOGY, Table 5) **Neurosurgical Patients:** 100 to 200 μg/kg/min (6 to 12 mg/kg/h). **Pediatric Patients—healthy, from 2 months of age to 16 years of age:** 125 to 300 μg/kg/min (7.5 to 18 mg/kg/h) Following the first half hour of maintenance, if clinical signs of light anesthesia are not present, the infusion rate should be decreased. (See PRECAUTIONS—Pediatric Use: and CLINICAL PHARMACOLOGY—Pediatric patients)
Maintenance of General Anesthesia:	**Intermittent Bolus** **Healthy Adults Less Than 55 Years of Age:** Increments of 20 to 50 mg as needed.
Initiation of MAC Sedation	**Healthy Adults Less Than 55 Years of Age:** Slow infusion or slow injection techniques are recommended to avoid apnea or hypotension. Most patients require an infusion of 100 to 150 μg/kg/min (6 to 9 mg/kg/h) for 3 to 5 minutes or a slow injection of 0.5 mg/kg over 3 to 5 minutes followed immediately by a maintenance infusion. **Elderly, Debilitated, Neurosurgical, or ASA III/IV Patients:** Most patients require dosages similar to healthy adults. Rapid boluses are to be avoided. (See WARNINGS.)
Maintenance of MAC Sedation	**Healthy Adults Less Than 55 Years of Age:** A variable rate infusion technique is preferable over an intermittent bolus technique. Most patients require an infusion of 25 to 75 μg/kg/min (1.5 to 4.5 mg/kg/h) or incremental bolus doses of 10 mg or 20 mg. **In Elderly, Debilitated, Neurosurgical, or ASA III/IV Patients:** Most patients require 80% of the usual adult dose. A rapid (single or repeated) bolus dose should not be used. (See WARNINGS.)
Initiation and Maintenance of ICU Sedation in Intubated, Mechanically Ventilated	**Adult Patients**—Because of the residual effects of previous anesthetic or sedative agents, in most patients the initial infusion should be 5 μg/kg/min (0.3 mg/kg/h) for at least 5 minutes. Subsequent increments of 5 to 10 μg/kg/min (0.3 to 0.6 mg/kg/h) over 5 to 10 minutes may be used until desired clinical effect is achieved. Maintenance rates of 5 to 50 μg/kg/min (0.3 to 3 mg/kg/h) or higher may be required. **Evaluation of clinical effect and assessment of CNS function should be carried out daily throughout maintenance to determine the minimum dose of DIPRIVAN Injectable Emulsion required for sedation.** **The tubing and any unused portions of DIPRIVAN Injectable Emulsion should be discarded after 12 hours because DIPRIVAN Injectable Emulsion contains no preservatives and is capable of supporting growth of microorganisms. (See WARNINGS, and DOSAGE AND ADMINISTRATION.)**

Compatibility and Stability: DIPRIVAN Injectable Emulsion should not be mixed with other therapeutic agents prior to administration.

Dilution Prior to Administration: DIPRIVAN Injectable Emulsion is provided as a ready to use formulation. However, should dilution be necessary, it should only be diluted with 5% Dextrose Injection, USP, and it should not be diluted to a concentration less than 2 mg/mL because it is an emulsion. In diluted form it has been shown to be more stable when in contact with glass than with plastic (95% potency after 2 hours of running infusion in plastic).

Administration with Other Fluids: Compatibility of DIPRIVAN Injectable Emulsion with the coadministration of blood/serum/plasma has not been established. (See WARNINGS.) When administered using a y-type infusion set, DIPRIVAN Injectable Emulsion has been shown to be compatible with the following intravenous fluids.

— 5% Dextrose Injection, USP
— Lactated Ringers Injection, USP
— Lactated Ringers and 5% Dextrose Injection
— 5% Dextrose and 0.45% Sodium Chloride Injection, USP
— 5% Dextrose and 0.2% Sodium Chloride Injection, USP

Assembly Instructions for Pre-Filled Syringe

1. Remove the Luer connector from packaging.
2. Remove glass syringe barrel from tray and check for cracks or leaks. Shake. Remove the plastic cover. Apply-

Continued on next page

Diprivan—Cont.

ing moderate pressure, disinfect the surface of the rubber stopper using the alcohol swab provided in the package prior to attachment of the Luer connector.

3. Pull off needle cover from Luer connector. The bevel of the needle spike is slightly bent (c-tip) to prevent potential coring.

4. Stand the syringe barrel vertically on a hard surface and push Luer connector on to syringe barrel so needle penetrates rubber seal and connector slides over the aluminum seal until firmly seated. (Fig. 1)

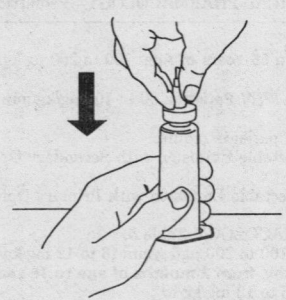

5. Add plunger rod by screwing clockwise. CAUTION: the rod must be fully screwed on, otherwise it may detach which could result in siphoning of the syringe contents. (Fig. 2)

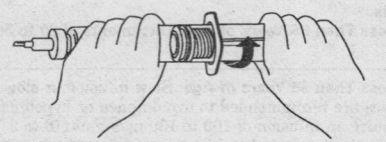

6. Unscrew Luer cover and remove excess nitrogen gas from the syringe (a small nitrogen gas bubble may remain). Assemble administration line and connect syringe.

Handling Procedures
General

Parenteral drug products should be inspected visually for particulate matter and discoloration prior to administration whenever solution and container permit.

Clinical experience with the use of in-line filters and DIPRIVAN Injectable Emulsion during anesthesia or ICU/MAC sedation is limited. DIPRIVAN Injectable Emulsion should only be administered through a filter with a pore size of 5 μm or greater unless it has been demonstrated that the filter does not restrict the flow of DIPRIVAN Injectable Emulsion and/or cause the breakdown of the emulsion. Filters should be used with caution and where clinically appropriate. Continuous monitoring is necessary due to the potential for restricted flow and/or breakdown of the emulsion. Do not use if there is evidence of separation of the phases of the emulsion.

Rare cases of self-administration of DIPRIVAN Injectable Emulsion by health care professionals have been reported, including some fatalities (See DRUG ABUSE AND DEPENDENCE).

STRICT ASEPTIC TECHNIQUE MUST ALWAYS BE MAINTAINED DURING HANDLING. DIPRIVAN INJECTABLE EMULSION IS A SINGLE-USE PARENTERAL PRODUCT WHICH CONTAINS 0.005% DISODIUM EDETATE TO RETARD THE RATE OF GROWTH OF MICROORGANISMS IN THE EVENT OF ACCIDENTAL EXTRINSIC CONTAMINATION. HOWEVER, DIPRIVAN INJECTABLE EMULSION CAN STILL SUPPORT THE GROWTH OF MICROORGANISMS AS IT IS NOT AN ANTIMICROBIALLY PRESERVED PRODUCT UNDER USP STANDARDS. ACCORDINGLY, STRICT ASEPTIC TECHNIQUE MUST STILL BE ADHERED TO. DO NOT USE IF CONTAMINATION IS SUSPECTED. DISCARD UNUSED PORTIONS AS DIRECTED WITHIN THE REQUIRED TIME LIMITS (SEE DOSAGE AND ADMINISTRATION, HANDLING PROCEDURES). THERE HAVE BEEN REPORTS IN WHICH FAILURE TO USE ASEPTIC TECHNIQUE WHEN HANDLING DIPRIVAN INJECTABLE EMULSION WAS ASSOCIATED WITH MICROBIAL CONTAMINATION OF THE PRODUCT AND WITH FEVER, INFECTION/SEPSIS, OTHER LIFE-THREATENING ILLNESS, AND/OR DEATH.

Guidelines for Aseptic Technique for General Anesthesia/MAC Sedation

DIPRIVAN Injectable Emulsion should be prepared for use just prior to initiation of each individual anesthetic/sedative procedure. The vial/pre-filled syringe rubber stopper should be disinfected using 70% isopropyl alcohol. DIPRIVAN Injectable Emulsion should be drawn into sterile syringes immediately after vials are opened. When withdrawing DIPRIVAN Injectable Emulsion from vials, a sterile vent spike should be used. The syringe(s) should be labeled with appropriate information including the date and time the vial was opened. Administration should commence promptly and be completed within 6 hours after the vials or pre-filled syringes have been opened.

DIPRIVAN Injectable Emulsion should be prepared for single-patient use only. Any unused portions of DIPRIVAN Injectable Emulsion, reservoirs, dedicated administration tubing and/or solutions containing DIPRIVAN Injectable Emulsion must be discarded at the end of the anesthetic

procedure or at 6 hours, whichever occurs sooner. The IV line should be flushed every 6 hours and at the end of the anesthetic procedure to remove residual DIPRIVAN Injectable Emulsion.

Guidelines for Aseptic Technique for ICU Sedation

DIPRIVAN Injectable Emulsion should be prepared for single-patient use only. When DIPRIVAN Injectable Emulsion is administered directly from the vial/pre-filled syringe, strict aseptic techniques must be followed. The vial/pre-filled syringe rubber stopper should be disinfected using 70% isopropyl alcohol. A sterile vent spike and sterile tubing must be used for administration of DIPRIVAN Injectable Emulsion. As with other lipid emulsions, the number of IV line manipulations should be minimized. Administration should commence promptly and must be completed within 12 hours after the vial has been spiked. The tubing and any unused portions of DIPRIVAN Injectable Emulsion must be discarded after 12 hours.

If DIPRIVAN Injectable Emulsion is transferred to a syringe or other container prior to administration, the handling procedures for General anesthesia/MAC sedation should be followed, and the product should be discarded and administration lines changed after 6 hours.

HOW SUPPLIED

DIPRIVAN Injectable Emulsion is available in ready to use 20 mL infusion vials, 50 mL infusion vials, 100 mL infusion vials, and 50 mL pre-filled syringes containing 10 mg/mL of propofol.

20 mL infusion vials (NDC 0310-0300-22)
50 mL infusion vials (NDC 0310-0300-50)
100 mL infusion vials (NDC 0310-0300-11)
50 mL pre-filled syringes (NDC 0310-300-54)

Propofol undergoes oxidative degradation, in the presence of oxygen, and is therefore packaged under nitrogen to eliminate this degradation path. Store between 4–22°C (40–72°F). Do not freeze. Shake well before use.

All trademarks are the property of the AstraZeneca group
© AstraZeneca 2001
Manufactured for:
AstraZeneca Pharmaceuticals LP
Wilmington, DE 19850
By: AstraZeneca S.p.A.
Caponago, Italy
Made in Italy
64180-02
AstraZeneca
Rev 2/01

ELAVIL® ℞
(AMITRIPTYLINE HCl)
Tablets and Injection

Prescribing information for this product, which appears on pages 626–628 of the 2001 PDR, has been revised. Please write "See Supplement A" next to the product heading.
Under the CONTRAINDICATIONS section, the following appears as a new 3rd paragraph:
"ELAVIL should not be given concurrently with Cisapride due to the potential for increased QT interval and increased risk for arrhythmia."

NOLVADEX® ℞
[nol ′va-dex]
tamoxifen citrate

Prescribing information for this product, which appears on pages 633–639 of the 2001 PDR, has been completely revised as follows. Please write "See Supplement A" next to the product heading.

DESCRIPTION

NOLVADEX® (tamoxifen citrate) Tablets, a nonsteroidal antiestrogen, are for oral administration. NOLVADEX Tablets are available as:

10 mg Tablets. Each tablet contains 15.2 mg of tamoxifen citrate which is equivalent to 10 mg of tamoxifen.

20 mg Tablets. Each tablet contains 30.4 mg of tamoxifen citrate which is equivalent to 20 mg of tamoxifen.

Inactive Ingredients: carboxymethylcellulose calcium, magnesium stearate, mannitol and starch.

Chemically, NOLVADEX is the trans-isomer of a triphenylethylene derivative. The chemical name is (Z)2-[4-(1,2-diphenyl-1-butenyl) phenoxy]-N, N-dimethylethanamine 2-hydroxy-1,2,3-propanetricarboxylate (1:1). The structural and empirical formulas are:

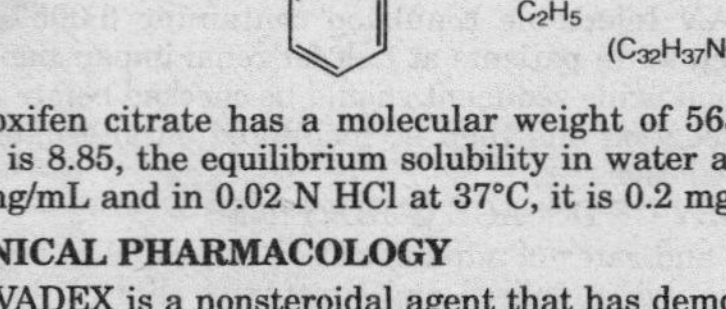

$$(CH_3)_2N(CH_2)_2O \cdots \quad C=C \quad \cdot C_6H_8O_7 \\ C_2H_5 \\ (C_{32}H_{37}NO_8)$$

Tamoxifen citrate has a molecular weight of 563.62, the pKa′ is 8.85, the equilibrium solubility in water at 37°C is 0.5 mg/mL and in 0.02 N HCl at 37°C, it is 0.2 mg/mL.

CLINICAL PHARMACOLOGY

NOLVADEX is a nonsteroidal agent that has demonstrated potent antiestrogenic properties in animal test systems. The antiestrogenic effects may be related to its ability to compete with estrogen for binding sites in target tissues such as

breast. Tamoxifen inhibits the induction of rat mammary carcinoma induced by dimethylbenzanthracene (DMBA) and causes the regression of already established DMBA-induced tumors. In this rat model, tamoxifen appears to exert its antitumor effects by binding the estrogen receptors. In cytosols derived from human breast adenocarcinomas, tamoxifen competes with estradiol for estrogen receptor protein.

Tamoxifen is extensively metabolized after oral administration. Studies in women receiving 20 mg of ^{14}C tamoxifen have shown that approximately 65% of the administered dose is excreted from the body over a period of 2 weeks with fecal excretion the primary route of elimination. The drug is excreted mainly as polar conjugates, with unchanged drug and unconjugated metabolites accounting for less than 30% of the total fecal radioactivity.

N-desmethyl tamoxifen is the major metabolite found in patients' plasma. The biological activity of N-desmethyl tamoxifen appears to be similar to that of tamoxifen. 4-Hydroxytamoxifen and a side chain primary alcohol derivative of tamoxifen have been identified as minor metabolites in plasma.

Following a single oral dose of 20 mg tamoxifen, an average peak plasma concentration of 40 ng/mL (range 35 to 45 ng/mL) occurred approximately 5 hours after dosing. The decline in plasma concentrations of tamoxifen is biphasic with a terminal elimination half-life of about 5 to 7 days. The average peak plasma concentration of N-desmethyl tamoxifen is 15 ng/mL (range 10 to 20 ng/mL). Chronic administration of 10 mg tamoxifen given twice daily for 3 months to patients results in average steady-state plasma concentrations of 120 ng/mL (range 67–183 ng/mL) for tamoxifen and 336 ng/mL (range 148–654 ng/mL) for N-desmethyl tamoxifen. The average steady-state plasma concentrations of tamoxifen and N-desmethyl tamoxifen after administration of 20 mg tamoxifen once daily for 3 months are 122 ng/mL (range 71–183 ng/mL) and 353 ng/mL (range 152–706 ng/mL), respectively. After initiation of therapy, steady-state concentrations for tamoxifen are achieved in about 4 weeks and steady-state concentrations for N-desmethyl tamoxifen are achieved in about 8 weeks, suggesting a half-life of approximately 14 days for this metabolite.

In a 3-month crossover steady-state bioavailability study with NOLVADEX 10 mg twice a day vs. NOLVADEX 20 mg given once daily, NOLVADEX 20 mg taken once daily had similar bioavailability to NOLVADEX 10 mg taken twice a day.

Clinical Studies—Metastatic Breast Cancer
Premenopausal Women (NOLVADEX vs. Ablation)—Three prospective, randomized studies (Ingle, Pritchard, Buchanan) compared NOLVADEX to ovarian ablation (oophorectomy or ovarian irradiation) in premenopausal women with advanced breast cancer. Although the objective response rate, time to treatment failure, and survival were similar with both treatments, the limited patient accrual prevented a demonstration of equivalence. In an overview analysis of survival data from the 3 studies, the hazard ratio for death (NOLVADEX/ovarian ablation) was 1.00 with two-sided 95% confidence intervals of 0.73 to 1.37. Elevated serum and plasma estrogens have been observed in premenopausal women receiving NOLVADEX, but the data from the randomized studies do not suggest an adverse effect of this increase. A limited number of premenopausal patients with disease progression during NOLVADEX therapy responded to subsequent ovarian ablation.

Male Breast Cancer—Published results from 122 patients (119 evaluable) and case reports in 16 patients (13 evaluable) treated with NOLVADEX have shown that NOLVADEX is effective for the palliative treatment of male breast cancer. Sixty-six of these 132 evaluable patients responded to NOLVADEX which constitutes a 50% objective response rate.

Clinical Studies—Adjuvant Breast Cancer
Overview—The Early Breast Cancer Trialists' Collaborative Group (EBCTCG) conducted worldwide overviews of systemic adjuvant therapy for early breast cancer in 1985, 1990, and again in 1995. In 1998, 10-year outcome data were reported for 36,689 women in 55 randomized trials of adjuvant NOLVADEX using doses of 20–40 mg/day for 1-5+ years. Twenty-five percent of patients received 1 year or less of trial treatment, 52% received 2 years, and 23% received about 5 years. Forty-eight percent of tumors were estrogen receptor (ER) positive (> 10 fmol/mg), 21% were ER poor (< 10 fmol/l), and 31% were ER unknown. Among 29,441 patients with ER positive or unknown breast cancer, 58% were entered into trials comparing NOLVADEX to no adjuvant therapy and 42% were entered into trials comparing NOLVADEX in combination with chemotherapy vs. the same chemotherapy alone. Among these patients, 54% had node positive disease and 46% had node negative disease.

Among women with ER positive or unknown breast cancer and positive nodes who received about 5 years of treatment, overall survival at 10 years was 61.4% for NOLVADEX vs. 50.5% for control (logrank 2p < 0.00001). The recurrence-free rate at 10 years was 59.7% for NOLVADEX vs. 44.5% for control (logrank 2p < 0.00001). Among women with ER positive or unknown breast cancer and negative nodes who received about 5 years of treatment, overall survival at 10 years was 78.9% for NOLVADEX vs. 73.3% for control (logrank 2p < 0.00001). The recurrence-free rate at 10 years was 79.2% for NOLVADEX versus 64.3% for control (logrank 2p < 0.00001).

The effect of the scheduled duration of tamoxifen may be described as follows. In women with ER positive or unknown breast cancer receiving 1 year or less, 2 years or about 5 years of NOLVADEX, the proportional reductions in mortality were 12%, 17% and 26%, respectively (trend significant at 2p < 0.003). The corresponding reductions in breast cancer recurrence were 21%, 29% and 47% (trend significant at 2p < 0.00001).

Benefit is less clear for women with ER poor breast cancer in whom the proportional reduction in recurrence was 10% (2p=0.007) for all durations taken together, or 9% (2p=0.02) if contralateral breast cancers are excluded. The corresponding reduction in mortality was 6% (NS). The effects of about 5 years of NOLVADEX on recurrence and mortality were similar regardless of age and concurrent chemotherapy. There was no indication that doses greater than 20 mg per day were more effective.

Node Positive—Individual Studies—Two studies (Hubay and NSABP B-09) demonstrated an improved disease-free survival following radical or modified radical mastectomy in postmenopausal women or women 50 years of age or older with surgically curable breast cancer with positive axillary nodes when NOLVADEX was added to adjuvant cytotoxic chemotherapy. In the Hubay study, NOLVADEX was added to "low-dose" CMF (cyclophosphamide, methotrexate and fluorouracil). In the NSABP B-09 study, NOLVADEX was added to melphalan [L-phenylalanine mustard (P)] and fluorouracil (F).

In the Hubay study, patients with a positive (more than 3 fmol) estrogen receptor were more likely to benefit. In the NSABP B-09 study in women age 50–59 years, only women with both estrogen and progesterone receptor levels 10 fmol or greater clearly benefited, while there was a nonstatistically significant trend toward adverse effect in women with both estrogen and progesterone receptor levels less than 10 fmol. In women age 60–70 years, there was a trend toward a beneficial effect of NOLVADEX without any clear relationship to estrogen or progesterone receptor status.

Three prospective studies (ECOG-1178, Toronto, NATO) using NOLVADEX adjuvantly as a single agent demonstrated an improved disease-free survival following total mastectomy and axillary dissection for postmenopausal women with positive axillary nodes compared to placebo/no treatment controls. The NATO study also demonstrated an overall survival benefit.

Node Negative—Individual Studies—NSABP B-14, a prospective, double-blind, randomized study, compared NOLVADEX to placebo in women with axillary node-negative, estrogen-receptor positive (≥10 fmol/mg cytosol protein) breast cancer (as adjuvant therapy, following total mastectomy and axillary dissection, or segmental resection, axillary dissection, and breast radiation). After five years of treatment, there was a significant improvement in disease-free survival in women receiving NOLVADEX. This benefit was apparent both in women under age 50 and in women at or beyond age 50.

One additional randomized study (NATO) demonstrated improved disease-free survival for NOLVADEX compared to no adjuvant therapy following total mastectomy and axillary dissection in postmenopausal women with axillary node-negative breast cancer. In this study, the benefits of NOLVADEX appeared to be independent of estrogen receptor status.

Duration of Therapy—In the EBCTCG 1995 overview, the reduction in recurrence and mortality was greater in those studies that used tamoxifen for about 5 years than in those that used tamoxifen for a shorter period of therapy.

In the NSABP B-14 trial, in which patients were randomized to NOLVADEX 20 mg/day for 5 years vs. placebo and were disease-free at the end of this 5-year period were offered rerandomization to an additional 5 years of NOLVADEX or placebo. With 4 years of follow-up after this rerandomization, 92% of the women that received 5 years of NOLVADEX were alive and disease-free, compared to 86% of the women scheduled to receive 10 years of NOLVADEX (p=0.003). Overall survivals were 96% and 94%, respectively (p=0.08). Results of the B-14 study suggest that continuation of therapy beyond 5 years does not provide additional benefit.

A Scottish trial of 5 years of tamoxifen vs. indefinite treatment found a disease-free survival of 70% in the five-year group and 61% in the indefinite group, with 6.2 years median follow-up (HR=1.27, 95% CI 0.87–1.85).

In a large randomized trial conducted by the Swedish Breast Cancer Cooperative Group of adjuvant NOLVADEX 40 mg/day for 2 or 5 years, overall survival at 10 years was estimated to be 80% in the patients in the 5-year tamoxifen group, compared with 74% among corresponding patients in the 2-year treatment group (p=0.03). Disease-free survival at 10 years was 73% in the 5-year group and 67% in the 2-year group (p=0.009). Compared with 2 years of tamoxifen treatment, 5 years of treatment resulted in a slightly greater reduction in the incidence of contralateral breast cancer at 10 years, but this difference was not statistically significant.

Contralateral Breast Cancer—The incidence of contralateral breast cancer is reduced in breast cancer patients (premenopausal and postmenopausal) receiving NOLVADEX compared to placebo. Data on contralateral breast cancer are available from 32,422 out of 36,689 patients in the 1995 overview analysis of the Early Breast Cancer Trialists Collaborative Group (EBCTCG). In clinical trials with NOLVADEX of 1 year or less, 2 years, and about 5 years duration, the proportional reductions in the incidence rate of contralateral breast cancer among women receiving NOLVADEX were 13% (NS), 26% (2p = 0.004) and 47% (2p < 0.00001), with a significant trend favoring longer tamoxifen duration (2p = 0.008). The proportional reductions in the incidence of con-

tralateral breast cancer were independent of age and ER status of the primary tumor. Treatment with about 5 years of NOLVADEX reduced the annual incidence rate of contralateral breast cancer from 7.6 per 1,000 patients in the control group compared with 3.9 per 1,000 patients in the tamoxifen group.

In a large randomized trial in Sweden (the Stockholm Trial) of adjuvant NOLVADEX 40 mg/day for 2–5 years, the incidence of second primary breast tumors was reduced 40% (p<0.01) on tamoxifen compared to control. In the NSABP B-14 trial in which patients were randomized to NOLVADEX 20 mg/day for 5 years vs. placebo, the incidence of second primary breast cancers was also significantly re-

duced (p<0.01). In NSABP B-14, the annual rate of contralateral breast cancer was 8.0 per 1000 patients in the placebo group compared with 5.0 per 1,000 patients in the tamoxifen group, at 10 years after first randomization.

Clinical Studies—Ductal Carcinoma in Situ: NSABP B-24, a double-blind, randomized trial included women with ductal carcinoma in situ (DCIS). This trial compared the addition of NOLVADEX or placebo to treatment with lumpectomy and radiation therapy for women with DCIS. The primary objective was to determine whether 5 years of NOLVADEX therapy (20 mg/day) would reduce the incidence of invasive

Continued on next page

Table 1—Major Outcomes of the NSABP B-24 Trial

Type of Event	Lumpectomy, radiotherapy and placebo		Lumpectomy, radiotherapy and NOLVADEX		RR	95% CI Limits
	No. of events	Rate per 1000 women per year	No. of events	Rate per 1000 women per year		
Invasive Breast Cancer (Primary Endpoint)	74	16.73	44	9.60	0.57	0.39 to 0.84
- ipsilateral	47	10.61	27	5.90	0.56	0.33 to 0.91
- contralateral	25	5.64	17	3.71	0.66	0.33 to 1.27
- Side undetermined	2		0			
DCIS (Secondary Endpoints)	56	12.66	41	8.95	0.71	0.46 to 1.08
- ipsilateral	46	10.40	38	8.29	0.88	0.51 to 1.25
- contralateral	10	2.26	3	0.65	0.29	0.05 to 1.13
- all breast cancer events	129	29.16	84	18.34	0.63	0.47 to 0.83
- all ipsilateral events	96	21.70	65	14.19	0.65	0.47 to 0.91
- all contralateral events	37	8.36	20	4.37	0.52	0.29 to 0.92
- Deaths	32		28			
- Endometrial Cancer	2	0.45	7	1.53	3.39	0.64 to 33.42
- Second primary malignancies (other than endometrial cancer)	30		29			
- Stroke	2		7			
- Thromboembolic events (DVT, PE)	5		15			

Table 2. Demographic Characteristics of Women in the NSABP P-1 Trial

Characteristic	Placebo		Tamoxifen	
	#	%	#	%
Age (yrs.)				
35–39	184	3	158	2
40–49	2,394	36	2,411	37
50–59	2,011	31	2,019	31
60–69	1,588	24	1,563	24
≥70	393	6	393	6
Age at first live birth (yrs.)				
Nulliparous	1,202	18	1,205	18
12–19	915	14	946	15
20–24	2,448	37	2,449	37
25–29	1,399	21	1,367	21
≥30	606	9	577	9
Race				
White	6,333	96	6,323	96
Black	109	2	103	2
Other	128	2	118	2
Age at menarche				
≥14	1,243	19	1,170	18
12–13	3,610	55	3,610	55
≤11	1,717	26	1,764	27
# of first degree relatives with breast cancer				
0	1,584	24	1,525	23
1	3,714	57	3,744	57
2+	1,272	19	1,275	20
Prior Hysterectomy				
No	4,173	63.5	4,018	62.4
Yes	2,397	36.5	2,464	37.7
# of previous breast biopsies				
0	2,935	45	2,923	45
1	1,833	28	1,850	28
≥2	1,802	27	1,771	27
History of atypical hyperplasia in the breast				
No	5,958	91	5,969	91
Yes	612	9	575	9
History of LCIS at entry				
No	6,165	94	6,135	94
Yes	405	6	409	6
5-year predicted breast cancer risk (%)				
≤2.00	1,646	25	1,626	25
2.01–3.00	2,028	31	2,057	31
3.01–5.00	1,787	27	1,707	26
≥5.01	1,109	17	1,162	18
Total	6,570	100.0	6,544	100.0

Nolvadex—Cont.

breast cancer in the ipsilateral (the same) or contralateral (the opposite) breast.
In this trial 1,804 women were randomized to receive either NOLVADEX or placebo for 5 years: 902 women were randomized to NOLVADEX 10 mg tablets twice a day and 902 women were randomized to placebo. As of December 31, 1998, follow-up data were available for 1,798 women and the median duration of follow-up was 74 months.
The NOLVADEX and placebo groups were well balanced for baseline demographic and prognostic factors. Over 80% of the tumors were less than or equal to 1 cm in their maximum dimension, were not palpable, and were detected by mammography alone. Over 60% of the study population was postmenopausal. In 16% of patients, the margin of the resected specimen was reported as being positive after surgery. Approximately half of the tumors were reported to contain comedo necrosis.
For the primary endpoint, the incidence of invasive breast cancer was reduced by 43% among women assigned to NOLVADEX (44 cases—NOLVADEX, 74 cases—placebo; p=0.004; relative risk (RR)=0.57, 95% CI: 0.39–0.84). No data are available regarding the ER status of the invasive cancers. The stage distribution of the invasive cancers at diagnosis was similar to that reported annually in the SEER data base.
Results are shown in Table 1. For each endpoint the following results are presented: the number of events and rate per 1,000 women per year for the placebo and NOLVADEX groups; and the relative risk (RR) and its associated 95% confidence interval (CI) between NOLVADEX and placebo. Relative risks less than 1.0 indicate a benefit of NOLVADEX therapy. The limits of the confidence intervals can be used to assess the statistical significance of the benefits of NOLVADEX therapy. If the upper limit of the CI is less than 1.0, then a statistically significant benefit exists.
[See table 1 at top of previous page]
Survival was similar in the placebo and NOLVADEX groups. At 5 years from study entry, survival was 97% for both groups.

Clinical Studies—Reduction in Breast Cancer Incidence in High Risk Women

The Breast Cancer Prevention Trial (BCPT, NSABP P-1) was a double-blind, randomized, placebo-controlled trial with a primary objective to determine whether 5 years of NOLVADEX therapy (20 mg/day) would reduce the incidence of invasive breast cancer in women at high risk for the disease (See **INDICATIONS AND USAGE**). Secondary objectives included an evaluation of the incidence of ischemic heart disease; the effects on the incidence of bone fractures; and other events that might be associated with the use of NOLVADEX, including: endometrial cancer, pulmonary embolus, deep vein thrombosis, stroke, and cataract formation and surgery (See **WARNINGS**).
The Gail Model was used to calculate predicted breast cancer risk for women who were less than 60 years of age and did not have lobular carcinoma in situ (LCIS). The following risk factors were used: age; number of first-degree female relatives with breast cancer; previous breast biopsies; presence or absence of atypical hyperplasia; nulliparity; age at first live birth; and age at menarche. A 5-year predicted risk of breast cancer of ≥ 1.67% was required for entry into the trial.
In this trial, 13,388 women of at least 35 years of age were randomized to receive either NOLVADEX or placebo for five years. The median duration of treatment was 3.5 years. As of January 31, 1998, follow-up data is available for 13,114 women. Twenty-seven percent of women randomized to placebo (1,782) and 24% of women randomized to NOLVADEX (1,596) completed 5 years of therapy. The demographic characteristics of women on the trial with follow-up data are shown in Table 2.
[See table 2 on previous page]
Results are shown in Table 3. After a median follow-up of 4.2 years, the incidence of invasive breast cancer was reduced by 44% among women assigned to NOLVADEX (86 cases-NOLVADEX, 156 cases-placebo; p<0.00001; relative risk (RR)=0.56, 95% CI: 0.43–0.72). A reduction in the incidence of breast cancer was seen in each prospectively specified age group (≤ 49, 50-59, ≥ 60), in women with or without LCIS, and in each of the absolute risk levels specified in Table 3. A non-significant decrease in the incidence of ductal carcinoma in situ (DCIS) was seen (23-NOLVADEX, 35-placebo; RR=0.66; 95% CI: 0.39–1.11).
There was no statistically significant difference in the number of myocardial infarctions, severe angina, or acute ischemic cardiac events between the two groups (61-NOLVADEX, 59-placebo; RR=1.04, 95% CI: 0.73–1.49).
No overall difference in mortality (53 deaths in NOLVADEX group vs. 65 deaths in placebo group) was present. No difference in breast cancer-related mortality was observed (4 deaths in NOLVADEX group vs. 5 deaths in placebo group).
Although there was a non-significant reduction in the number of hip fractures (9 on NOLVADEX, 20 on placebo) in the NOLVADEX group, the number of wrist fractures was similar in the two treatment groups (69 on NOLVADEX, 74 on placebo). No information regarding bone mineral density or other markers of osteoporosis is available.
The risks of NOLVADEX therapy include endometrial cancer, DVT, PE, stroke, cataract formation and cataract surgery (See Table 3). In the NSABP P-1 trial, 33 cases of endometrial cancer were observed in the NOLVADEX group vs. 14 in the placebo group (RR=2.48, 95% CI: 1.27–4.92). Deep vein thrombosis was observed in 30 women receiving NOLVADEX vs. 19 in women receiving placebo (RR=1.59, 95% CI: 0.86–2.98). Eighteen cases of pulmonary embolism were observed in the NOLVADEX group vs. 6 in the placebo group (RR=3.01, 95% CI: 1.15–9.27). There were 34 strokes on the NOLVADEX arm and 24 on the placebo arm (RR=1.42; 95% CI: 0.82–2.51). Cataract formation in women without cataracts at baseline was observed in 540 women taking NOLVADEX vs. 483 women receiving placebo (RR=1.13, 95% CI: 1.00–1.28). Cataract surgery (with or without cataracts at baseline) was performed in 201 women taking NOLVADEX vs. 129 women receiving placebo (RR=1.51, 95% CI: 1.21–1.89) (See **WARNINGS**).
Table 3 summarizes the major outcomes of the NSABP P-1 trial. For each endpoint, the following results are presented: the number of events and rate per 1000 women per year for the placebo and NOLVADEX groups; and the relative risk (RR) and its associated 95% confidence interval (CI) between NOLVADEX and placebo. Relative risks less than 1.0 indicate a benefit of NOLVADEX therapy. The limits of the confidence intervals can be used to assess the statistical significance of the benefits or risks of NOLVADEX therapy. If the upper limit of the CI is less than 1.0, then a statistically significant benefit exists.
For most participants, multiple risk factors would have been required for eligibility. This table considers risk factors individually, regardless of other co-existing risk factors, for women who developed breast cancer. The 5-year predicted absolute breast cancer risk accounts for multiple risk factors in an individual and should provide the best estimate of individual benefit (See **INDICATIONS AND USAGE**).
[See table 3 at left]

Table 3: Major Outcomes of the NSABP P-1 Trial

TYPE OF EVENT	# OF EVENTS PLACEBO	# OF EVENTS NOLVADEX	RATE/1000 WOMEN/YEAR PLACEBO	RATE/1000 WOMEN/YEAR NOLVADEX	RR	95% CI LIMITS
Invasive Breast Cancer	156	86	6.49	3.58	0.56	0.43–0.72
Age ≤49	59	38	6.34	4.11	0.65	0.43–0.98
Age 50–59	46	25	6.31	3.53	0.56	0.35–0.91
Age ≥60	51	23	7.17	3.22	0.45	0.27–0.74
Risk Factors for Breast Cancer						
History, LCIS						
No	140	78	6.23	3.51	0.56	0.43–0.74
Yes	16	8	12.73	6.33	0.50	0.21–1.17
History, Atypical Hyperplasia						
No	138	84	6.37	3.89	0.61	0.47–0.80
Yes	18	2	8.69	1.05	0.12	0.03–0.52
No. First Degree Relatives						
0	32	17	5.97	3.26	0.55	0.30–0.98
1	80	45	5.81	3.31	0.57	0.40–0.82
2	35	18	8.92	4.67	0.52	0.30–0.92
≥3	9	6	13.33	7.58	0.57	0.20–1.59
5-Year Predicted Breast Cancer Risk (as calculated by the Gail Model)						
≤2.00%	31	13	5.36	2.26	0.42	0.22–0.81
2.01–3.00%	39	28	5.25	3.83	0.73	0.45–1.18
3.01–5.00%	36	26	5.37	4.06	0.76	0.46–1.26
≥5.00%	50	19	13.15	4.71	0.36	0.21–0.61
DCIS	35	23	1.47	0.97	0.66	0.39–1.11
Fractures (protocol-specified sites)	92[1]	76[1]	3.87	3.20	0.61	0.83–1.12
Hip	20	9	0.84	0.38	0.45	0.18–1.04
Wrist[2]	74	69	3.11	2.91	0.93	0.67–1.29
Total Ischemic Events	59	61	2.47	2.57	1.04	0.71–1.51
Myocardial Infarction	27	27	1.13	1.13	1.00	0.57–1.78
Fatal	8	7	0.33	0.29	0.88	0.27–2.77
Nonfatal	19	20	0.79	0.84	1.06	0.54–2.09
Angina[3]	12	12	0.50	0.50	1.00	0.41–2.44
Acute Ischemic Syndrome[4]	20	22	0.84	0.92	1.11	0.58–2.13
Invasive Endometrial Cancer (among women without a hysterectomy)	14	33	0.92	2.29	2.48	1.27–4.92
Stroke[5]	24	34	1.00	1.43	1.42	0.82–2.51
Transient Ischemic Attack	21	18	0.88	0.75	0.86	0.43–1.70
Pulmonary Emboli[6]	6	18	0.25	0.75	3.01	1.15–9.27
Deep-Vein Thrombosis[7]	19	30	0.79	1.26	1.59	0.86–2.98
Cataracts Developing on Study[8]	483	540	22.51	25.41	1.13	1.00–1.28
Underwent Cataract Surgery[8]	63	101	31.83	4.57	1.62	1.18–2.22
Underwent Cataract Surgery[9]	129	201	5.44	8.56	1.58	1.26–1.97

[1]Two women had hip and wrist fractures
[2]Includes Colles' and other lower radius fractures
[3]Requiring angioplasty or CABG
[4]New Q-wave on ECG; no angina or elevation of serum enzymes; or angina requiring hospitalization without surgery
[5]Seven cases were fatal; three in the placebo group and four in the NOLVADEX group
[6]Three cases in the NOLVADEX group were fatal
[7]All but three cases in each group required hospitalization
[8]Based on women without cataracts at baseline (6,230-Placebo, 6,199-NOLVADEX)
[9]All women (6,707-Placebo, 6,681-NOLVADEX)

Table 4 describes the characteristics of the breast cancers in the NSABP P-1 trial and includes tumor size, nodal status, ER status. NOLVADEX decreased the incidence of small estrogen receptor positive tumors, but did not alter the incidence of estrogen receptor negative tumors or larger tumors.

Table 4: Characteristics of Breast Cancer in NSABP P-1 Trial

Staging Parameter	Placebo N=156	Tamoxifen N=86	Total N=242
Tumor size:			
T1	117	60	177
T2	28	20	48
T3	7	3	10
T4	1	2	3
Unknown	3	1	4
Nodal status:			
Negative	103	56	159
1–3 positive nodes	29	14	43
≥ 4 positive nodes	10	12	22
Unknown	14	4	18
Stage:			
I	88	47	135
II: node negative	15	9	24
II: node positive	33	22	55
III	6	4	10
IV	2[1]	1	3
Unknown	12	3	15
Estrogen receptor:			
Positive	115	38	153
Negative	27	36	63
Unknown	14	12	26

[1] One participant presented with a suspicious bone scan but did not have documented metastases. She subsequently died of metastatic breast cancer.

Interim results from 2 trials in addition to the NSABP P-1 trial examining the effects of tamoxifen in reducing breast cancer incidence have been reported.
The first was the Italian Tamoxifen Prevention trial. In this trial women between the ages of 35 and 70, who had had a total hysterectomy, were randomized to receive 20 mg tamoxifen or matching placebo for 5 years. The primary endpoints were occurrence of, and death from, invasive breast cancer. Women without any specific risk factors for breast cancer were to be entered. Between 1992 and 1997, 5408 women were randomized. Hormone Replacement Therapy (HRT) was used in 14% of participants. The trial closed in 1997 due to the large number of dropouts during the first year of treatment (26%). After 46 months of follow-up there were 22 breast cancers in women on placebo and 19 in women on tamoxifen. Although no decrease in breast cancer incidence was observed, there was a trend for a reduction in breast cancer among women receiving protocol therapy for at least 1 year (19-placebo, 11-tamoxifen). The small numbers of participants along with the low level

of risk in this otherwise healthy group precluded an adequate assessment of the effect of tamoxifen in reducing the incidence of breast cancer.

The second trial, the Royal Marsden Trial (RMT) was reported as an interim analysis. The RMT was begun in 1986 as a feasibility study of whether larger scale trials could be mounted. The trial was subsequently extended to a pilot trial to accrue additional participants to further assess the safety of tamoxifen. Twenty-four hundred and seventy-one women were entered between 1986 and 1996; they were selected on the basis of a family history of breast cancer. HRT was used in 40% of participants. In this trial, with a 70-month median follow-up, 34 and 36 breast cancers (8 noninvasive, 4 on each arm) were observed among women on tamoxifen and placebo, respectively. Patients in this trial were younger than those in the NSABP P-1 trial and may have been more likely to develop ER (-) tumors, which are unlikely to be reduced in number by tamoxifen therapy. Although women were selected on the basis of family history and were thought to have a high risk of breast cancer, few events occurred, reducing the statistical power of the study. These factors are potential reasons why the RMT may not have provided an adequate assessment of the effectiveness of tamoxifen in reducing the incidence of breast cancer.

In these trials, an increased number of cases of deep vein thrombosis, pulmonary embolus, stroke, and endometrial cancer were observed on the tamoxifen arm compared to the placebo arm. The frequency of events was consistent with the safety data observed in the NSABP P-1 trial.

INDICATIONS AND USAGE

Metastatic Breast Cancer: NOLVADEX is effective in the treatment of metastatic breast cancer in women and men. In premenopausal women with metastatic breast cancer, NOLVADEX is an alternative to oophorectomy or ovarian irradiation. Available evidence indicates that patients whose tumors are estrogen receptor positive are more likely to benefit from NOLVADEX therapy.

Adjuvant Treatment of Breast Cancer: NOLVADEX is indicated for the treatment of node-positive breast cancer in postmenopausal women following total mastectomy or segmental mastectomy, axillary dissection, and breast irradiation. In some NOLVADEX adjuvant studies, most of the benefit to date has been in the subgroup with four or more positive axillary nodes.

NOLVADEX is indicated for the treatment of axillary node-negative breast cancer in women following total mastectomy or segmental mastectomy, axillary dissection, and breast irradiation.

The estrogen and progesterone receptor values may help to predict whether adjuvant NOLVADEX therapy is likely to be beneficial.

NOLVADEX reduces the occurrence of contralateral breast cancer in patients receiving adjuvant NOLVADEX therapy for breast cancer.

Ductal Carcinoma in Situ (DCIS): In women with DCIS, following breast surgery and radiation, NOLVADEX is indicated to reduce the risk of invasive breast cancer. The decision regarding therapy with NOLVADEX for the reduction in breast cancer incidence should be based upon an individual assessment of the benefits and risks of NOLVADEX therapy. Current data from clinical trials support five years of adjuvant NOLVADEX therapy for patients with breast cancer.

Reduction in Breast Cancer Incidence in High Risk Women: NOLVADEX is indicated to reduce the incidence of breast cancer in women at high risk for breast cancer. This effect was shown in a study of 5 years planned duration with a median follow-up of 4.2 years. Twenty-five percent of the participants received drug for 5 years. The longer-term effects are not known. In this study, there was no impact of tamoxifen on overall or breast cancer-related mortality.

NOLVADEX is indicated only for high-risk women. "High risk" is defined as women at least 35 years of age with a 5-year predicted risk of breast cancer ≥ 1.67%, as calculated by the Gail Model.

Examples of combinations of factors predicting a 5-year risk ≥ 1.67% are:

Age 35 or older and any of the following combination of factors:
- One first degree relative with a history of breast cancer, 2 or more benign biopsies, and a history of a breast biopsy showing atypical hyperplasia; or
- At least 2 first degree relatives with a history of breast cancer, and a personal history of at least one breast biopsy; or
- LCIS

Age 40 or older and any of the following combination of factors:
- One first degree relative with a history of breast cancer, 2 or more benign biopsies, age at first live birth 25 or older, and age at menarche 11 or younger; or
- At least 2 first degree relatives with a history of breast cancer, and age at first live birth 19 or younger; or
- One first degree relative with a history of breast cancer, and a personal history of a breast biopsy showing atypical hyperplasia.

Age 45 or older and any of the following combination of factors:
- At least 2 first degree relatives with a history of breast cancer and age at first live birth 24 or younger; or
- One first degree relative with a history of breast cancer with a personal history of a benign breast biopsy, age at menarche 11 or less and age at first live birth 20 or more.

Age 50 or older and any of the following combination of factors:
- At least 2 first degree relatives with a history of breast cancer; or
- History of one breast biopsy showing atypical hyperplasia, and age at first live birth 30 or older and age at menarche 11 or less; or
- History of at least two breast biopsies with a history of atypical hyperplasia, and age at first live birth 30 or more.

Age 55 or older and any of the following combination of factors:
- One first degree relative with a history of breast cancer with a personal history of a benign breast biopsy, and age at menarche 11 or less; or
- History of at least 2 breast biopsies with a history of atypical hyperplasia, and age at first live birth 20 or older.

Age 60 or older and:
- 5-year predicted risk of breast cancer • 1.67%, as calculated by the Gail Model.

For women whose risk factors are not described in the above examples, the Gail Model is necessary to estimate absolute breast cancer risk. Health Care Professionals can obtain a Gail Model Risk Assessment Tool by dialing 1-800-544-2007.

There are no data available regarding the effect of NOLVADEX on breast cancer incidence in women with inherited mutations (BRCA1, BRCA2).

After an assessment of the risk of developing breast cancer, the decision regarding therapy with NOLVADEX for the reduction in breast cancer incidence should be based upon an individual assessment of the benefits and risks of NOLVADEX therapy. In the NSABP P-1 trial, NOLVADEX treatment lowered the risk of developing breast cancer during the follow-up period of the trial, but did not eliminate breast cancer risk (See Table 3 in **CLINICAL PHARMACOLOGY**).

CONTRAINDICATIONS

NOLVADEX is contraindicated in patients with known hypersensitivity to the drug or any of its ingredients.

Reduction in Breast Cancer Incidence in High Risk Women and Women with DCIS: NOLVADEX is contraindicated in women who require concomitant coumarin-type anticoagulant therapy or in women with a history of deep vein thrombosis or pulmonary embolus.

WARNINGS

Effects in Metastatic Breast Cancer Patients: As with other additive hormonal therapy (estrogens and androgens), hypercalcemia has been reported in some breast cancer patients with bone metastases within a few weeks of starting treatment with NOLVADEX. If hypercalcemia does occur, appropriate measures should be taken and, if severe, NOLVADEX should be discontinued.

Effects on the Uterus-Endometrial Cancer: As with other additive hormonal therapy (estrogens), an increased incidence of endometrial cancer has been reported in association with NOLVADEX treatment. The underlying mechanism is unknown, but may be related to the estrogen-like effect of NOLVADEX. Any patients receiving or having previously received NOLVADEX who report abnormal vaginal bleeding should be promptly evaluated. Patients receiving or having previously received NOLVADEX should have routine gynecological care and they should promptly inform their physician if they experience any abnormal gynecological symptoms, eg, menstrual irregularities, abnormal vaginal bleeding, changes in vaginal discharge, or pelvic pain or pressure.

In a large randomized trial in Sweden of adjuvant NOLVADEX 40 mg/day for 2–5 years, an increased incidence of uterine cancer was noted. Twenty-three of 1,372 patients randomized to receive NOLVADEX vs. 4 of 1,357 patients randomized to the observation group developed cancer of the uterus [RR = 5.6 (1.9–16.2), p<.001]. One of the patients with cancer of the uterus who was randomized to receive NOLVADEX never took the drug. After approximately 6.8 years of follow-up in the NSABP B-14 trial, 15 of 1,419 women randomized to receive NOLVADEX 20 mg/day for 5 years developed uterine cancer and 2 of the 1,424 women randomized to receive placebo, who subsequently were treated with NOLVADEX, also developed uterine cancer. Most of the uterine cancers were diagnosed at an early stage, but deaths from uterine cancer have been reported.

In the NSABP P-1 trial, among participants randomized to NOLVADEX there was a statistically significant increase in the incidence of endometrial cancer (33 cases of invasive endometrial cancer, compared to 14 cases among participants randomized to placebo (RR=2.48, 95% CI: 1.27–4.92). This increase was primarily observed among women at least 50 years of age at the time of randomization (26 cases of invasive endometrial cancer, compared to 6 cases among participants randomized to placebo (RR=4.50, 95% CI: 1.78–13.16). Among women ≤ 49 years of age at the time of randomization there were 7 cases of invasive endometrial cancer, compared to 8 cases among participants randomized to placebo (RR=0.94, 95% CI: 0.28–2.89). If age at the time of diagnosis is considered, there were 4 cases of endometrial cancer among participants ≤ 49 randomized to NOLVADEX compared to 2 among participants randomized to placebo (RR=2.21, 95% CI: 0.4–12.0). For women ≥ 50 at the time of diagnosis, there were 29 cases among participants randomized to NOLVADEX compared to 12 among women on placebo (RR=2.5, 95% CI: 1.3–4.9). The risk ratios were similar in the two groups, although fewer events occurred in younger women. Most (29 of 33 cases in the NOLVADEX group) endometrial cancers were diagnosed in symptomatic women, although 5 of 33 cases in the NOLVADEX group occurred in asymptomatic women. Among women receiving NOLVADEX the events appeared between 1 and 61 months (average=32 months) from the start of treatment.

Among participants receiving NOLVADEX, there were 33 cases of FIGO stage I [20 IA, 12 IB, and 1 IC] endometrial cancer. Among participants receiving placebo, there were 13 FIGO stage I cases [8 IA and 5 IB]. There was a single FIGO Stage IV endometrial cancer in a participant receiving placebo (See Table 3 in **CLINICAL PHARMACOLOGY**). The distribution of FIGO stage was similar between participants receiving NOLVADEX and placebo. Five women receiving NOLVADEX and 1 receiving placebo with FIGO Stage IB disease received postoperative radiation therapy in addition to surgery.

Endometrial sampling did not alter the endometrial cancer detection rate compared to women who did not undergo endometrial sampling (0.6% with sampling, 0.5% without sampling) for women with an intact uterus. There are no data to suggest that routine endometrial sampling in asymptomatic women taking NOLVADEX to reduce the incidence of breast cancer would be beneficial.

Non-Malignant Effects on the Uterus: An increased incidence of endometrial changes including hyperplasia and polyps have been reported in association with NOLVADEX treatment. The incidence and pattern of this increase suggest that the underlying mechanism is related to the estrogenic properties of NOLVADEX.

There have been a few reports of endometriosis and uterine fibroids in women receiving NOLVADEX. The underlying mechanism may be due to the partial estrogenic effect of NOLVADEX. Ovarian cysts have also been observed in a small number of premenopausal patients with advanced breast cancer who have been treated with NOLVADEX.

Thromboembolic Effects of NOLVADEX: As with other additive hormonal therapy (estrogen), there is evidence of an increased incidence of thromboembolic events, including deep vein thrombosis and pulmonary embolism, during NOLVADEX therapy. When NOLVADEX is coadminstered with chemotherapy, there may be a further increase in the incidence of thromboembolic effects. For treatment of breast cancer, the risks and benefits of NOLVADEX should be carefully considered in women with a history of thromboembolic events.

Data from the NSABP P-1 trial show that participants receiving NOLVADEX without a history of pulmonary emboli (PE) had a statistically significant increase in pulmonary emboli (18-NOLVADEX, 6-placebo, RR=3.01, 95% CI: 1.15–9.27). Three of the pulmonary emboli, all in the NOLVADEX arm, were fatal. Eighty-seven percent of the cases of pulmonary embolism occurred in women at least 50 years of age at randomization. Among women receiving NOLVADEX, the events appeared between 2 and 60 months (average=27 months) from the start of treatment.

In this same population, a non-statistically significant increase in deep vein thrombosis (DVT) was seen in the NOLVADEX group (30-NOLVADEX, 19-placebo; RR=1.59, 95% CI: 0.86–2.98). The same increase in relative risk was seen in women ≤ 49 and in women ≥ 50, although fewer events occurred in younger women. Women with thromboembolic events were at risk for a second related event (7 out of 25 women on placebo, 5 out of 48 women on NOLVADEX) and were at risk for complications of the event and its treatment (0/25 on placebo, 4/48 on NOLVADEX). Among women receiving NOLVADEX, deep vein thrombosis events occurred between 2 and 57 months (average=19 months) from the start of treatment.

There was a non-statistically significant increase in stroke among patients randomized to NOLVADEX (24-Placebo; 34-NOLVADEX; RR=1.42; 95% CI: 0.82–2.51). Six of the 24 strokes in the placebo group were considered hemorrhagic in origin and 10 of the 34 strokes in the NOLVADEX group were categorized as hemorrhagic. Seventeen of the 34 strokes in the NOLVADEX group were considered occlusive and 7 were considered to be of unknown etiology. Fourteen of the 24 strokes on the placebo arm were reported to be occlusive and 4 of unknown etiology. Among these strokes 3 strokes in the placebo group and 4 strokes in the NOLVADEX group were fatal. Eighty-eight percent of the strokes occurred in women at least 50 years of age at the time of randomization. Among women receiving NOLVADEX, the events occurred between 1 and 63 months (average=30 months) from the start of treatment.

Effects on the liver: Liver cancer: In the Swedish trial using adjuvant NOLVADEX 40 mg/day for 2–5 years, 3 cases of liver cancer have been reported in the NOLVADEX-treated group vs. 1 case in the observation group (See **PRECAUTIONS—Carcinogenesis**). In other clinical trials evaluating NOLVADEX, no cases of liver cancer have been reported to date.

One case of liver cancer was reported in NSABP P-1 in a participant randomized to NOLVADEX.

Effects on the liver: Non-malignant effects: NOLVADEX has been associated with changes in liver enzyme levels, and on rare occasions, a spectrum of more severe liver abnormalities including fatty liver, cholestasis, hepatitis and hepatic necrosis. A few of these serious cases included fatalities. In most reported cases the relationship to NOLVADEX is uncertain. However, some positive rechallenges and dechallenges have been reported.

In the NSABP P-1 trial, few grade 3–4 changes in liver function (SGOT, SGPT, bilirubin, alkaline phosphatase) were observed (10 on placebo and 6 on NOLVADEX). Serum lipids were not systematically collected.

Continued on next page

Nolvadex—Cont.

Other cancers: A number of second primary tumors, occurring at sites other than the endometrium, have been reported following the treatment of breast cancer with NOLVADEX in clinical trials. Data from the NSABP B-14 and P-1 studies show no increase in other (non-uterine) cancers among patients receiving NOLVADEX. Whether an increased risk for other (non-uterine) cancers is associated with NOLVADEX is still uncertain and continues to be evaluated.

Effects on the Eye: Ocular disturbances, including corneal changes, decrement in color vision perception, retinal vein thrombosis, and retinopathy have been reported in patients receiving NOLVADEX. An increased incidence of cataracts and the need for cataract surgery have been reported in patients receiving NOLVADEX.

In the NSABP P-1 trial, an increased risk of borderline significance of developing cataracts among those women without cataracts at baseline (540-NOLVADEX; 483-placebo; RR=1.13, 95% CI: 1.00–1.28) was observed. Among these same women, NOLVADEX was associated with an increased risk of having cataract surgery (101-NOLVADEX; 63-placebo; RR=1.62, 95% CI: 1.17–2.25) (See Table 3 in CLINICAL PHARMACOLOGY). Among all women on the trial (with or without cataracts at baseline), NOLVADEX was associated with an increased risk of having cataract surgery (201-NOLVADEX; 129-placebo; RR=1.51, 95% CI: 1.21–1.89). Eye examinations were not required during the study. No other conclusions regarding non-cataract ophthalmic events can be made.

Pregnancy Category D: NOLVADEX may cause fetal harm when administered to a pregnant woman. Women should be advised not to become pregnant while taking NOLVADEX and should use barrier or nonhormonal contraceptive measures if sexually active. Effects on reproductive functions are expected from the antiestrogenic properties of the drug. In reproductive studies in rats at dose levels equal to or below the human dose, nonteratogenic developmental skeletal changes were seen and were found reversible. In addition, in fertility studies in rats and in teratology studies in rabbits using doses at or below those used in humans, a lower incidence of embryo implantation and a higher incidence of fetal death or retarded in utero growth were observed, with slower learning behavior in some rat pups when compared to historical controls. Several pregnant marmosets were dosed during organogenesis or in the last half of pregnancy. No deformations were seen and, although the dose was high enough to terminate pregnancy in some animals, those that did maintain pregnancy showed no evidence of teratogenic malformations.

In rodent models of fetal reproductive tract development, tamoxifen (at doses 0.3 to 2.4-fold the human maximum recommended dose on a mg/m² basis) caused changes in both sexes that are similar to those caused by estradiol, ethynylestradiol and diethylstilbestrol. Although the clinical relevance of these changes is unknown, some of these changes, especially vaginal adenosis, are similar to those seen in young women who were exposed to diethylstilbestrol in utero and who have a 1 in 1000 risk of developing clear-cell adenocarcinoma of the vagina or cervix. To date, in utero exposure to tamoxifen has not been shown to cause vaginal adenosis, or clear-cell adenocarcinoma of the vagina or cervix, in young women. However, only a small number of young women have been exposed to tamoxifen in utero, and a smaller number have been followed long enough (to age 15–20) to determine whether vaginal or cervical neoplasia could occur as a result of this exposure.

There are no adequate and well controlled trials of tamoxifen in pregnant women. There have been a small number of reports of vaginal bleeding, spontaneous abortions, birth defects, and fetal deaths in pregnant women. If this drug is used during pregnancy, or the patient becomes pregnant while taking this drug, or within approximately two months after discontinuing therapy, the patient should be apprised of the potential risks to the fetus including the potential long-term risk of a DES-like syndrome.

Reduction in Breast Cancer Incidence in High Risk Women—Pregnancy Category D: For sexually active women of child-bearing potential, NOLVADEX therapy should be initiated during menstruation. In women with menstrual irregularity, a negative B-HCG immediately prior to the initiation of therapy is sufficient (See PRECAUTIONS—Information for Patients—Reduction in Breast Cancer Incidence in High Risk Women).

PRECAUTIONS

General: Decreases in platelet counts, usually to 50,000–100,000/mm³, infrequently lower, have been occasionally reported in patients taking NOLVADEX for breast cancer. In patients with significant thrombocytopenia, rare hemorrhagic episodes have occurred, but it is uncertain if these episodes are due to NOLVADEX therapy. Leukopenia has been observed, sometimes in association with anemia and/or thrombocytopenia. There have been rare reports of neutropenia and pancytopenia in patients receiving NOLVADEX; this can sometimes be severe.

In the NSABP P-1 trial, 6 women on NOLVADEX and 2 on placebo experienced grade 3–4 drops in platelet counts (≤50,000/mm³).

Information for Patients:

Reduction in Invasive Breast Cancer and DCIS in Women with DCIS: Women with DCIS treated with lumpectomy and radiation therapy who are considering NOLVADEX to reduce the incidence of a second breast cancer event should assess the risks and benefits of therapy, since treatment with

NOLVADEX decreased the incidence of invasive breast cancer, but has not been shown to affect survival (See Table 1 in CLINICAL PHARMACOLOGY.

Reduction in Breast Cancer Incidence in High Risk Women: Women who are at high risk for breast cancer can consider taking NOLVADEX therapy to reduce the incidence of breast cancer. Whether the benefits of treatment are considered to outweigh the risks depends on a woman's personal health history and on how she weighs the benefits and risks. NOLVADEX therapy to reduce the incidence of breast cancer may therefore not be appropriate for all women at high risk for breast cancer. Women who are considering NOLVADEX therapy should consult their health care professional for an assessment of the potential benefits and risks prior to starting therapy for reduction in breast cancer incidence (See Table 3 in CLINICAL PHARMACOLOGY). Women should understand that NOLVADEX reduces the incidence of breast cancer, but may not eliminate risk. NOLVADEX decreased the incidence of small estrogen receptor positive tumors, but did not alter the incidence of estrogen receptor negative tumors or larger tumors. In women with breast cancer who are at high risk of developing a second breast cancer, treatment with about 5 years of NOLVADEX reduced the annual incidence rate of a second breast cancer by approximately 50%. Women who are pregnant or who plan to become pregnant should not take NOLVADEX to reduce her risk of breast cancer. Effective nonhormonal contraception must be used by all premenopausal women taking NOLVADEX if they are sexually active. For sexually active women of child-bearing potential, NOLVADEX therapy should be initiated during menstruation. In women with menstrual irregularity, a negative B-HCG immediately prior to the initiation of therapy is sufficient (See WARNINGS—Pregnancy Category D).

Two European trials of tamoxifen to reduce the risk of breast cancer were conducted and showed no difference in the number of breast cancer cases between the tamoxifen and placebo arms. These studies had trial designs that differed from that of NSABP P-1, were smaller than NSABP P-1, and enrolled women at a lower risk for breast cancer than those in P-1.

Monitoring During NOLVADEX Therapy: Women taking or having previously taken NOLVADEX should be instructed to seek prompt medical attention for new breast lumps, vaginal bleeding, gynecologic symptoms (menstrual irregularities, changes in vaginal discharge, or pelvic pain or pressure), symptoms of leg swelling or tenderness, unexplained shortness of breath, or changes in vision. Women should inform all care providers, regardless of the reason for evaluation, that they take NOLVADEX.

Women taking NOLVADEX to reduce the incidence of breast cancer should have a breast examination, a mammogram, and a gynecologic examination prior to the initiation of therapy. These studies should be repeated at regular intervals while on therapy, in keeping with good medical practice. Women taking NOLVADEX as adjuvant breast cancer therapy should follow the same monitoring procedures as for women taking NOLVADEX for the reduction in the incidence of breast cancer. Women taking NOLVADEX as treatment for metastatic breast cancer should review this monitoring plan with their care provider and select the appropriate modalities and schedule of evaluation.

Laboratory Tests: Periodic complete blood counts, including platelet counts, and periodic liver function tests should be obtained.

Drug Interactions: When NOLVADEX is used in combination with coumarin-type anticoagulants, a significant increase in anticoagulant effect may occur. Where such coadministration exists, careful monitoring of the patient's prothrombin time is recommended.

In the NSABP P-1 trial, women who required coumarin-type anticoagulants for any reason were ineligible for participation in the trial (See CONTRAINDICATIONS).

There is an increased risk of thromboembolic events occurring when cytotoxic agents are used in combination with NOLVADEX.

Tamoxifen, N-desmethyl tamoxifen and 4-Hydroxytamoxifen have been found to be potent inhibitors of hepatic cytochrome p-450 mixed function oxidases. The effect of tamoxifen on metabolism and excretion of other antineoplastic drugs, such as cyclophosphamide and other drugs that require mixed function oxidases for activation, is not known.

One patient receiving NOLVADEX with concomitant phenobarbital exhibited a steady-state serum level of tamoxifen lower than that observed for other patients (ie, 26 ng/mL vs. mean value of 122 ng/mL). However, the clinical significance of this finding is not known.

Concomitant bromocriptine therapy has been shown to elevate serum tamoxifen and N-desmethyl tamoxifen.

Drug/Laboratory Testing Interactions: During postmarketing surveillance, T₄ elevations were reported for a few postmenopausal patients which may be explained by increases in thyroid-binding globulin. These elevations were not accompanied by clinical hyperthyroidism.

Variations in the karyopyknotic index on vaginal smears and various degrees of estrogen effect on Pap smears have been infrequently seen in postmenopausal patients given NOLVADEX.

In the postmarketing experience with NOLVADEX, infrequent cases of hyperlipidemias have been reported. Periodic monitoring of plasma triglycerides and cholesterol may be indicated in patients with pre-existing hyperlipidemias (See ADVERSE REACTIONS—Postmarketing experience section).

Carcinogenesis: A conventional carcinogenesis study in rats (doses of 5, 20, and 35 mg/kg/day for up to 2 years) revealed hepatocellular carcinoma at all doses, and the incidence of these tumors was significantly greater among rats given 20 or 35 mg/kg/day (69%) than those given 5 mg/kg/day (14%). The incidence of these tumors in rats given 5 mg/kg/day (29.5 mg/m²) was significantly greater than in controls.

In addition, preliminary data from 2 independent reports of 6-month studies in rats reveal liver tumors which in one study are classified as malignant (See WARNINGS).

Endocrine changes in immature and mature mice were investigated in a 13-month study. Granulosa cell ovarian tumors and interstitial cell testicular tumors were found in mice receiving NOLVADEX, but not in the controls.

Mutagenesis: Although no genotoxic potential was found in a conventional battery of in vivo and in vitro tests with pro- and eukaryotic test systems with drug metabolizing systems present, increased levels of DNA adducts have been found in the livers of rats exposed to tamoxifen. Tamoxifen also has been found to increase levels of micronucleus formation in vitro in human lymphoblastoid cell line (MCL-5). Based on these findings, tamoxifen is genotoxic in rodent and human MCL-5 cells.

Impairment of Fertility: Fertility in female rats was decreased following administration of 0.04 mg/kg for two weeks prior to mating through day 7 of pregnancy. There was a decreased number of implantations, and all fetuses were found dead.

Following administration to rats of 0.16 mg/kg from days 7–17 of pregnancy, there were increased numbers of fetal deaths. Administration of 0.125 mg/kg to rabbits during days 6–18 of pregnancy resulted in abortion or premature delivery. Fetal deaths occurred at higher doses. There were no teratogenic changes in either rat or rabbit segment II studies. Several pregnant marmosets were dosed with 10 mg/kg/day either during organogenesis or in the last half of pregnancy. No deformations were seen, and although the dose was high enough to terminate pregnancy in some animals, those that did maintain pregnancy showed no evidence of teratogenic malformations. Rats given 0.16 mg/kg from day 17 of pregnancy to 1 day before weaning demonstrated increased numbers of dead pups at parturition. It was reported that some rat pups showed slower learning behavior, but this did not achieve statistical significance in one study, and in another study where significance was reported, this was obtained by comparing dosed animals with controls of another study.

The recommended daily human dose of 20–40 mg corresponds to 0.4–0.8 mg/kg for an average 50 kg woman.

Pregnancy Category D: See WARNINGS.

Nursing Mothers: It is not known whether this drug is excreted in human milk. Because many drugs are excreted in human milk and because of the potential for serious adverse reactions in nursing infants from NOLVADEX, a decision should be made whether to discontinue nursing or to discontinue the drug, taking into account the importance of the drug to the mother.

Pediatric Use: The safety and efficacy of NOLVADEX in pediatric patients have not been established.

Geriatric Use: In the NSABP P-1 trial, the percentage of women at least 65 years of age was 16%. Women at least 70 years of age accounted for 6% of the participants. A reduction in breast cancer incidence was seen among participants in each of the subsets: A total of 28 and 10 invasive breast cancers were seen among participants 65 and older in the placebo and NOLVADEX groups, respectively. Across all other outcomes, the results in this subset reflect the results observed in the subset of women at least 50 years of age. No overall differences in tolerability were observed between older and younger patients (See CLINICAL PHARMACOLOGY—Clinical Studies—Reduction in Breast Cancer Incidence in High Risk Women section).

ADVERSE REACTIONS

Adverse reactions to NOLVADEX are relatively mild and rarely severe enough to require discontinuation of treatment in breast cancer patients.

Continued clinical studies have resulted in further information which better indicates the incidence of adverse reactions with NOLVADEX as compared to placebo.

Metastatic Breast Cancer: Increased bone and tumor pain and, also, local disease flare have occurred, which are sometimes associated with a good tumor response. Patients with increased bone pain may require additional analgesics. Patients with soft tissue disease may have sudden increases in the size of preexisting lesions, sometimes associated with marked erythema within and surrounding the lesions and/or the development of new lesions. When they occur, the bone pain or disease flare are seen shortly after starting NOLVADEX and generally subside rapidly.

In patients treated with NOLVADEX for metastatic breast cancer, the most frequent adverse reaction to NOLVADEX is hot flashes.

Other adverse reactions which are seen infrequently are hypercalcemia, peripheral edema, distaste for food, pruritus vulvae, depression, dizziness, light-headedness, headache, hair thinning and/or partial hair loss, and vaginal dryness.

Premenopausal Women: The following table summarizes the incidence of adverse reactions reported at a frequency of 2% or greater from clinical trials (Ingle, Pritchard, Buchanan) which compared NOLVADEX therapy to ovarian ablation in premenopausal patients with metastatic breast cancer.

Adverse Reactions*	NOLVADEX All Effects % of Women n=104	OVARIAN ABLATION All Effects % of Women n=100
Flush	33	46
Amenorrhea	16	69
Altered Menses	13	5
Oligomenorrhea	9	1
Bone Pain	6	6
Menstrual Disorder	6	4
Nausea	5	4
Cough/Coughing	4	1
Edema	4	1
Fatigue	4	1
Musculoskeletal Pain	3	0
Pain	3	4
Ovarian Cyst(s)	3	2
Depression	2	2
Abdominal Cramps	1	2
Anorexia	1	2

*Some women had more than one adverse reaction.

Male Breast Cancer: NOLVADEX is well tolerated in males with breast cancer. Reports from the literature and case reports suggest that the safety profile of NOLVADEX in males is similar to that seen in women. Loss of libido and impotence have resulted in discontinuation of tamoxifen therapy in male patients. Also, in oligospermic males treated with tamoxifen, LH, FSH, testosterone and estrogen levels were elevated. No significant clinical changes were reported.

Adjuvant Breast Cancer: In the NSABP B-14 study, women with axillary node-negative breast cancer were randomized to 5 years of NOLVADEX 20 mg/day or placebo following primary surgery. The reported adverse effects are tabulated below (mean follow-up of approximately 6.8 years) showing adverse events more common on NOLVADEX than on placebo. The incidence of hot flashes (64% vs. 48%), vaginal discharge (30% vs. 15%), and irregular menses (25% vs. 19%) were higher with NOLVADEX compared with placebo. All other adverse effects occurred with similar frequency in the 2 treatment groups, with the exception of thrombotic events; a higher incidence was seen in NOLVADEX-treated patients (through 5 years, 1.7% vs. 0.4%). Two of the patients treated with NOLVADEX who had thrombotic events died.

NSABP B-14 Study

Adverse Effect	% of Women NOLVADEX (n=1422)	Placebo (n=1437)
Hot Flashes	64	48
Fluid Retention	32	30
Vaginal Discharge	30	15
Nausea	26	24
Irregular Menses	25	19
Weight Loss (>5%)	23	18
Skin Changes	19	15
Increased SGOT	5	3
Increased Bilirubin	2	1
Increased Creatinine	2	1
Thrombocytopenia*	2	1
Thrombotic Events		
Deep Vein Thrombosis	0.8	0.2
Pulmonary Embolism	0.5	0.2
Superficial Phlebitis	0.4	0.0

*Defined as a platelet count of <100,000/mm^3

In the Eastern Cooperative Oncology Group (ECOG) adjuvant breast cancer trial, NOLVADEX or placebo was administered for 2 years to women following mastectomy. When compared to placebo, NOLVADEX showed a significantly higher incidence of hot flashes (19% vs. 8% for placebo). The incidence of all other adverse reactions was similar in the 2 treatment groups with the exception of thrombocytopenia where the incidence for NOLVADEX was 10% vs. 3% for placebo, an observation of borderline statistical significance.

In other adjuvant studies, Toronto and NOLVADEX Adjuvant Trial Organization (NATO), women received either NOLVADEX or no therapy. In the Toronto study, hot flashes were observed in 29% of patients for NOLVADEX vs. 1% in the untreated group. In the NATO trial, hot flashes and vaginal bleeding were reported in 2.8% and 2.0% of women, respectively, for NOLVADEX vs. 0.2% for each in the untreated group.

Ductal Carcinoma in Situ (DCIS): The type and frequency of adverse events in the NSABP B-24 trial were consistent with those observed in the other adjuvant trials conducted with NOLVADEX.

Reduction in Breast Cancer Incidence in High Risk Women: In the NSABP P-1 Trial, there was an increase in five serious adverse effects in the NOLVADEX group: endometrial cancer (33 cases in the NOLVADEX group vs. 14 in the placebo group); pulmonary embolism (18 cases in the NOLVADEX group vs. 6 in the placebo group); deep vein thrombosis (30 cases in the NOLVADEX group vs. 19 in the placebo group); stroke (34 cases in the NOLVADEX group vs. 24 in the placebo group); cataract formation (540 cases in the NOLVADEX group vs. 483 in the placebo group) and cataract surgery (101 cases in the NOLVADEX group vs. 63 in the placebo group) (See **WARNINGS** and Table 3 in **CLINICAL PHARMACOLOGY**).

The following table presents the adverse events observed in NSABP P-1 by treatment arm. Only adverse events more common on NOLVADEX than placebo are shown.

NSABP P-1 Trial: All Adverse Events

	% of Women NOLVADEX N=6681	PLACEBO N=6707
Self Reported Symptoms	N=6441[1]	N=6469[1]
Hot Flashes	80	68
Vaginal Discharges	55	35
Vaginal Bleeding	23	22
Laboratory Abnormalities	N=6520[2]	N=6535[2]
Platelets decreased	0.7	0.3
Adverse Effects	N=6492[3]	N=6484[3]
Other Toxicities		
Mood	11.6	10.8
Infection/Sepsis	6.0	5.1
Constipation	4.4	3.2
Alopecia	5.2	4.4
Skin	5.6	4.7
Allergy	2.5	2.1

[1]Number with Quality of Life Questionnaires
[2]Number with Treatment Follow-up Forms
[3]Number with Adverse Drug Reaction Forms

In the NSABP P-1 trial, 15.0% and 9.7% of participants receiving NOLVADEX and placebo therapy, respectively, withdrew from the trial for medical reasons. The following are the medical reasons for withdrawing from NOLVADEX and placebo therapy, respectively: Hot flashes (3.1% vs. 1.5%) and Vaginal Discharge (0.5% vs. 0.1%).

In the NSABP P-1 trial, 8.7% and 9.6% of participants receiving NOLVADEX and placebo therapy, respectively, withdrew for non-medical reasons.

On the NSABP P-1 trial, hot flashes of any severity occurred in 68% of women on placebo and in 80% of women on NOLVADEX. Severe hot flashes occurred in 28% of women on placebo and 45% of women on NOLVADEX. Vaginal discharge occurred in 35% and 55% of women on placebo and NOLVADEX respectively; and was severe in 4.5% and 12.3% respectively. There was no difference in the incidence of vaginal bleeding between treatment arms.

Postmarketing experience: Less frequently reported adverse reactions are vaginal bleeding, vaginal discharge, menstrual irregularities, skin rash and headaches. Usually these have not been of sufficient severity to require dosage reduction or discontinuation of treatment. Very rare reports of erythema multiforme, Stevens-Johnson syndrome, bullous pemphigoid and rare reports of hypersensitivity reactions including angioedema have been reported with NOLVADEX therapy. Rarely, elevation of serum triglyceride levels, in some cases with pancreatitis, may be associated with the use of NOLVADEX (see **PRECAUTIONS—Drug/Laboratory Testing Interactions** section).

OVERDOSAGE

Signs observed at the highest doses following studies to determine LD$_{50}$ in animals were respiratory difficulties and convulsions.

Acute overdosage in humans has not been reported. In a study of advanced metastatic cancer patients which specifically determined the maximum tolerated dose of NOLVADEX in evaluating the use of very high doses to reverse multidrug resistance, acute neurotoxicity manifested by tremor, hyperreflexia, unsteady gait and dizziness were noted. These symptoms occurred within 3–5 days of beginning NOLVADEX and cleared within 2–5 days after stopping therapy. No permanent neurologic toxicity was noted. One patient experienced a seizure several days after NOLVADEX was discontinued and neurotoxic symptoms had resolved. The causal relationship of the seizure to NOLVADEX therapy is unknown. Doses given in these patients were all greater than 400 mg/m^2 loading dose, followed by maintenance doses of 150 mg/m^2 of NOLVADEX given twice a day.

In the same study, prolongation of the QT interval on the electrocardiogram was noted when patients were given doses higher than 250 mg/m^2 loading dose, followed by maintenance doses of 80 mg/m^2 of NOLVADEX given twice a day. For a woman with a body surface area of 1.5 m^2 the minimal loading dose and maintenance doses given at which neurological symptoms and QT changes occurred were at least 6 fold higher in respect to the maximum recommended dose.

No specific treatment for overdosage is known; treatment must be symptomatic.

DOSAGE AND ADMINISTRATION

For patients with breast cancer, the recommended daily dose is 20–40 mg. Dosages greater than 20 mg per day should be given in divided doses (morning and evening).

In three single agent adjuvant studies in women, one 10 mg NOLVADEX tablet was administered two (ECOG and NATO) or three (Toronto) times a day for two years. In the NSABP B-14 adjuvant study in women with node-negative breast cancer, one 10 mg NOLVADEX tablet was given twice a day for at least 5 years. Results of the B-14 study suggest that continuation of therapy beyond five years does not provide additional benefit (see **CLINICAL PHARMACOLOGY**). In the EBCTCG 1995 overview, the reduction in recur-

rence and mortality was greater in those studies that used tamoxifen for about 5 years than in those that used tamoxifen for a shorter period of therapy. There was no indication that doses greater than 20 mg per day were more effective. Current data from clinical trials support 5 years of adjuvant NOLVADEX therapy for patients with breast cancer.

Ductal Carcinoma in Situ (DCIS): The recommended dose is NOLVADEX 20 mg daily for 5 years.

Reduction in Breast Cancer Incidence in High Risk Women: The recommended dose is NOLVADEX 20 mg daily for 5 years. There are no data to support the use of NOLVADEX other than for 5 years (See **CLINICAL PHARMACOLOGY—Clinical Studies—Reduction in Breast Cancer Incidence in High Risk Women**).

HOW SUPPLIED

10 mg Tablets containing tamoxifen as the citrate in an amount equivalent to 10 mg of tamoxifen (round, biconvex, uncoated, white tablet identified with NOLVADEX 600 debossed on one side and a cameo debossed on the other side) are supplied in bottles of 60 tablets, 180 tablets and 2500 tablets. NDC 0310-0600.

20 mg Tablets containing tamoxifen as the citrate in an amount equivalent to 20 mg of tamoxifen (round, biconvex, uncoated, white tablet identified with NOLVADEX 604 debossed on one side and a cameo debossed on the other side) are supplied in bottles of 30 tablets, 90 tablets and 1250 tablets. NDC 0310-0604.

Store at controlled room temperature, 20–25°C (68–77°F) [see USP]. Dispense in a well-closed, light-resistant container.

Patient Information about
NOLVADEX® (tamoxifen citrate) Tablets
for Breast Cancer Treatment and Reduction in the Incidence of Breast Cancer
Brand Name: **NOLVADEX®** (Nol 'va dex)
Generic Name: Tamoxifen (ta-MOX-i-fen)

Please read this information carefully before you begin taking NOLVADEX. It is important to read this information each time your prescription is filled or refilled in case new information is available. This summary does not tell you everything about NOLVADEX. Your health care professional is the best source of information about this medicine. You should talk with him or her before you begin taking NOLVADEX and at regular checkups. In addition, the professional package insert contains more detailed information on NOLVADEX.

What are the most important things I should know about NOLVADEX?

NOLVADEX has been shown to help women with advanced breast cancer and in clinical trials of over 30,000 women with early breast cancer it has been shown to reduce the risk of recurrence. Also in a trial of 13,000 women at high risk of breast cancer, NOLVADEX reduced the risk of developing the disease.

Like all medicines, NOLVADEX has some side effects. Most are mild and relate to its hormonal mode of action. NOLVADEX can, however, also increase the risk of some serious and potentially life-threatening conditions, including, uterine cancer, blood clots, and stroke. It can also increase the risk of getting cataracts or of needing cataract surgery. If you experience symptoms of any of these, tell your doctor immediately (see **"What should I avoid or do while taking NOLVADEX?"**). You and your doctor must carefully discuss your personal medical conditions, history, and preferences to decide whether the good NOLVADEX may do for you outweighs its potential risks. If you and your doctor decide that NOLVADEX therapy is right for you, you should look for symptoms indicating you might be experiencing one of the known risks of NOLVADEX.

What is NOLVADEX?

• NOLVADEX is a prescription medicine used to reduce the risk of getting breast cancer in women who have a high risk of getting breast cancer.

This effect was shown in the Breast Cancer Prevention Trial (BCPT, NSABP P-1), a large study where over 13,000 women at high risk for breast cancer were to take NOLVADEX or placebo (a pill without tamoxifen) for 5 years. High risk women were those who were at least 35 years old and had a combination of risks that made their chances of developing breast cancer greater than 1.67% in the next five years. The risk factors included early age at first menstrual period, late age at first pregnancy, no pregnancies, close family members with breast cancer (mother, sister, or daughter), history of previous breast biopsies, or high-risk changes in the breast seen on a biopsy. Twenty-five percent of the women in the study completed 5 years of treatment, and most women in this study have been followed for about 4 years. The study showed that NOLVADEX reduced the chance of getting breast cancer by 44%. The longer-term effects of NOLVADEX on reducing the chance of getting breast cancer are not known.

We do not know whether taking NOLVADEX for 5 years only delays the appearance of cancer, or actually decreases the number of tumors that will ever develop since long-term studies have not been completed.

Some women in this study also experienced serious side effects of NOLVADEX. They are described in detail in the section, **What are the possible side effects of NOLVADEX?**. Some of these women experienced complications related to the treatment of these side effects.

The following table of the major results from the study is intended to be an aid in weighing the potential benefit of a reduction in risk of breast cancer against the potential risk of serious side effects of NOLVADEX.

Continued on next page

Nolvadex—Cont.

	Cases per year out of 1000 women taking NOLVADEX	Cases per year out of 1000 women taking Placebo
Breast Cancer	3.6	6.5
Endometrial Cancer*	2.3	0.9
Blood clot in the lungs	0.8	0.3
Blood clot in the veins	1.3	0.8
Stroke	1.4	1.0
Cataracts	25.4	22.5
Cataract surgery	46.6	31.4

*In women with a uterus.

Two European trials of NOLVADEX in women with a high risk of breast cancer were also conducted. They showed no difference in the number of breast cancer cases between the women who took tamoxifen and those who got placebo. These studies had trial designs that differed from that of NSABP P-1, were smaller than P-1, and enrolled women at a lower risk for breast cancer than those in the P-1 trial.

• NOLVADEX is used to treat advanced breast cancer in women and men.

Three studies compared NOLVADEX to surgery or radiation to the ovaries in premenopausal women with advanced breast cancer and found that NOLVADEX was similar to surgery or radiation in causing tumor shrinkage.

Published studies have demonstrated that NOLVADEX is effective for the treatment of advanced breast cancer in men.

• In women with DCIS, following breast surgery and radiation, NOLVADEX is indicated to reduce the risk of invasive breast cancer. The decision regarding therapy with NOLVADEX for the reduction in breast cancer incidence should be based upon an individual assessment of the benefits and risks of NOLVADEX therapy.

A trial evaluated the addition of NOLVADEX to lumpectomy and radiation therapy in women with DCIS. The primary objective was to determine whether 5 years of NOLVADEX therapy would reduce the incidence of invasive breast cancer in the ipsilateral (the same) or contralateral (the opposite) breast. The incidence of invasive breast cancer was reduced by 43% among women treated with NOLVADEX.

• NOLVADEX is used to reduce the recurrence of breast cancer in women who have had surgery and/or radiation therapy to treat early breast cancer. NOLVADEX is also used in women with breast cancer who are at risk of developing a second breast cancer in the opposite breast.

The Early Breast Cancer Trialists Collaborative Group reviewed the 10-year results of studies of NOLVADEX for early breast cancer. Treatment with NOLVADEX for about 5 years reduced the risk of recurrence of breast cancer and improved overall survival. Treatment with about 5 years of NOLVADEX also reduced the chance of getting a second breast cancer in the opposite breast by approximately 50%, a result similar to that seen in the NSABP P-1 study.

• NOLVADEX is a tablet available in two dosage strengths: 10 mg tablets and 20 mg tablets. The active ingredient in each tablet is tamoxifen citrate.

How does NOLVADEX work?

NOLVADEX belongs to a group of medicines called antiestrogens. Antiestrogens work by blocking the effects of the hormone estrogen in the body. Estrogen may cause the growth of some types of breast tumors. NOLVADEX may block the growth of tumors that respond to estrogen.

Who should not take NOLVADEX?

• You should not take NOLVADEX to reduce the risk of getting breast cancer if you have ever had blood clots or if you develop blood clots that require medical treatment. However, if you are taking NOLVADEX for treatment of early or advanced breast cancer, the benefits of NOLVADEX may outweigh the risks associated with developing new blood clots. Your health care professional can assist you in deciding whether NOLVADEX is right for you.

• You should not take NOLVADEX if you are taking medicines to thin your blood (anticoagulants) like warfarin (Coumadin®*).

• You should not take NOLVADEX if you plan to become pregnant while taking NOLVADEX or during the two months after you stop taking it because NOLVADEX may harm your unborn child. You should see your doctor immediately and stop taking NOLVADEX if you become pregnant while taking the drug. Please talk with your doctor about birth control recommendations. If you are capable of becoming pregnant, you should start NOLVADEX during a menstrual period or if you have irregular periods have a negative pregnancy test before beginning to take NOLVADEX.

• You should not take NOLVADEX if you are breast-feeding.

• You should not take NOLVADEX if you have ever had an allergic reaction to NOLVADEX or tamoxifen citrate (the chemical name) or any of its ingredients.

• NOLVADEX is not known to reduce the risk of breast cancer in women with changes in breast cancer genes (BRCA1 or BRCA2).

• You should not take NOLVADEX to decrease the chance of getting breast cancer if you are less than age 35 because NOLVADEX has not been tested in younger women.

• You should not take NOLVADEX to reduce the risk of breast cancer unless you are at high risk of getting breast cancer. Certain conditions put women at high risk and it is possible to calculate this risk for any woman. Breast cancer risk assessment tools to help calculate your risk of breast cancer have been developed and are available to your health care professional. You should discuss your risks with your health care professional.

• Children should not take NOLVADEX because treatment for them has not been sufficiently studied.

How should I take NOLVADEX?

• Follow your doctor's instructions about when and how to take NOLVADEX. Read the label on the container. If you are unsure or have questions, ask your doctor or pharmacist.

• You will take NOLVADEX differently, depending on your diagnosis.

• For treatment of breast cancer in adult women and men, the usual dose is 20–40 mg a day. Take the tablets once or twice a day depending on the tablet strength prescribed. If your doctor has prescribed a different dose, do not change it unless he or she tells you to do so. For women with early breast cancer, NOLVADEX should be taken for 5 years. For women with advanced cancer, NOLVADEX should be taken until your doctor feels it is no longer indicated.

• For reduction of the risk of breast cancer, the usual dose is 20 mg a day, for five years.

• Take your medicine each day. You may find it easier to remember to take your medicine if you take it at the same time each day. If you forget to take a dose, take it as soon as you remember and then take the next dose as usual.

• Swallow the tablets whole with a drink of water.

• You can take NOLVADEX with or without food.

• Do not stop taking your tablets unless your doctor tells you to do so.

Are there other important factors to consider before taking NOLVADEX?

• Tell your doctor if you have ever had blood clots that required medical treatment.

• Because NOLVADEX may affect how other medicines work, always tell your doctor if you are taking any other prescription or non-prescription (over-the-counter) medications, particularly if you are taking warfarin to thin your blood.

• You should not become pregnant when taking NOLVADEX or during the two months after you stop taking it as NOLVADEX may harm your unborn child. Please contact your doctor for birth control recommendations. You should see your doctor immediately if you think you may have become pregnant after starting to take NOLVADEX.

What should I avoid or do while taking NOLVADEX?

• You should contact your doctor immediately if you notice any of the following symptoms. Some of these symptoms may suggest that you are experiencing a rare but serious side effect associated with NOLVADEX (see "What are the possible side effects of NOLVADEX?").

— new breast lumps
— vaginal bleeding
— changes in your menstrual cycle
— changes in vaginal discharge
— pelvic pain or pressure
— swelling or tenderness in your calf
— unexplained breathlessness (shortness of breath)
— sudden chest pain
— coughing up blood
— changes in your vision

If you see a health care professional who is new to you (an emergency room doctor, another doctor in the practice), tell him or her that you take NOLVADEX.

• Because NOLVADEX may affect how other medicines work, always tell your doctor if you are taking any other prescription or non-prescription (over-the-counter) medicines. Be sure to tell your doctor if you are taking warfarin (coumadin) to thin your blood.

• You should not become pregnant when taking NOLVADEX or during the two months after you stop taking it because NOLVADEX may harm your unborn child. You should see your doctor immediately if you think you may have become pregnant after starting to take NOLVADEX. Please talk with your doctor about birth control recommendations. If you are taking NOLVADEX to reduce your risk of getting breast cancer, and you are sexually active, NOLVADEX should be started during your menstrual period. If you have irregular periods, you should have a negative pregnancy test before you start NOLVADEX.

• If you are taking NOLVADEX to reduce your risk of getting breast cancer, you should know that NOLVADEX does not prevent all breast cancers. While you are taking NOLVADEX and in keeping with your doctor's recommendation, you should have annual gynecological check-ups which should include breast exams and mammograms. If breast cancer occurs, there is no guarantee that it will be detected at an early stage. This is why it is important to continue with regular check-ups.

What are the possible side effects of NOLVADEX?

Like many medicines, NOLVADEX causes side effects in most patients. The majority of the side effects seen with NOLVADEX have been mild and do not usually cause breast cancer patients to stop taking the medication. In women with breast cancer, withdrawal from NOLVADEX therapy is about 5%. Approximately 15% of women who took NOLVADEX to reduce the chance of getting breast cancer stopped treatment because of side effects.

The most common side effects reported with NOLVADEX are: hot flashes; vaginal discharge or bleeding; and menstrual irregularities (these side effects may be mild or may be a sign of a more serious side effect). Women may experience hair loss, skin rashes (itching or peeling skin) or headaches; however, hair loss is uncommon and is usually mild. A rare but serious side effect of NOLVADEX is a blood clot in the veins. Blood clots stop the flow of blood and can cause serious medical problems, disability, or death. Women who take NOLVADEX are at increased risk for developing blood clots in the lungs and legs. Some women may develop more than one blood clot, even if NOLVADEX is stopped. Women may also have complications from treating the clot, such as bleeding from thinning the blood too much. Symptoms of a blood clot in the lungs may include sudden chest pain, shortness of breath or coughing up blood. Symptoms of a blood clot in the legs are pain or swelling in the calves. A blood clot in the legs may move to the lungs. If you experience any of these symptoms of a blood clot, contact your doctor immediately.

NOLVADEX increases the chance of having a stroke, which can cause serious medical problems, disability, or death. If you experience any symptoms of stroke, such as weakness, difficulty walking or talking, or numbness, contact your doctor immediately.

NOLVADEX increases the chance of changes occurring in the lining of your uterus (endometrium), which can be serious and could include cancer of the uterus. If you have not had a hysterectomy (removal of the uterus), it is important for you to contact your doctor immediately if you experience any unusual vaginal discharge, vaginal bleeding, or menstrual irregularities; or pain or pressure in the pelvis (lower stomach). These may be caused by changes to the lining of your uterus (endometrium). It is important to bring them to your doctor's attention without delay as they can occasionally indicate the start of something more serious, and could include cancer of the uterus or other changes to the uterus. NOLVADEX may cause cataracts or changes to parts of the eye known as the cornea or retina. NOLVADEX can increase the chance of needing cataract surgery, and can cause blood clots in the veins of the eye. NOLVADEX can result in difficulty in distinguishing different colors. If you experience any changes in your vision, tell your doctor immediately.

Rare side effects, which may be serious, include certain liver problems such as jaundice (which may be seen as yellowing of the whites of the eyes) or hypertriglyceridemia (increased levels of fats in the blood) sometimes with pancreatitis (pain or tenderness in the upper abdomen). Stop taking NOLVADEX and contact your doctor immediately if you develop angioedema (swelling of the face, lips, tongue and/or throat).

If you are a woman receiving NOLVADEX for treatment of advanced breast cancer, and you experience excessive nausea, vomiting or thirst, tell your doctor immediately. This may mean that there are changes in the amount of calcium in your blood (hypercalcemia). Your doctor will evaluate this.

In patients with breast cancer, a temporary increase in the size of the tumor may occur and sometimes results in muscle aches/bone pain and skin redness. This condition may occur shortly after starting NOLVADEX and may be associated with a good response to treatment.

Many of these side effects happen only rarely. However, you should contact your doctor if you think you have any of these or any other problems with your NOLVADEX. Some side effects of NOLVADEX may become apparent soon after starting the drug, but others may first appear at any time during therapy.

This summary does not include all possible side effects with NOLVADEX. It is important to talk to your health care professional about possible side effects. If you want to read more, ask your doctor or pharmacist to give you the professional labeling.

How should I store NOLVADEX?

NOLVADEX Tablets should be stored at room temperature (68–77°F). Keep in a well-closed, light-resistant container. Keep out of the reach of children.

Do not take your tablets after the expiration date on the container. Be sure that any discarded tablets are out of the reach of children.

This leaflet provides you with a summary of information about NOLVADEX. Medicines are sometimes prescribed for uses other than those listed. NOLVADEX has been prescribed specifically for you by your doctor. Do not give your medicine to anyone else, even if they have a similar condition, because it may harm them.

If you have any questions or concerns, contact your doctor or pharmacist. Your pharmacist also has a longer leaflet about NOLVADEX written for health care professionals that you can ask to read. For more information about NOLVADEX or breast cancer, call 1-800-34 LIFE 4.

*Coumadin® is a registered trademark of DuPont Pharmaceuticals.

AstraZeneca Pharmaceuticals LP
Wilmington, Delaware 19850-5437
Rev Y 06/00 SIC 64143-01/NL
Printed in USA © 2000 AstraZeneca

SEROQUEL® ℞
[serō-quĕl]
(quetiapine fumarate)
Tablets

Prescribing information for this product, which appears on pages 639–643 of the 2001 PDR, has been revised. Please write "See Supplement A" next to the product heading.
The HOW SUPPLIED section was revised to add the 300 mg tablet strength.

SULAR® ℞
(nisoldipine)
Extended Release Tablets
For Oral Use

Prescribing information for this product, which appears on pages 645–647 of the 2001 PDR, has been completely revised as follows. Please write "See Supplement A" next to the product heading.

PROFESSIONAL INFORMATION

DESCRIPTION

SULAR® (nisoldipine) is an extended release tablet dosage form of the dihydropyridine calcium channel blocker nisoldipine. Nisoldipine is 3,5-pyridinedicarboxylic acid, 1,4-dihydro-2,6-dimethyl-4-(2-nitrophenyl)-, methyl 2-methylpropyl ester, $C_{20}H_{24}N_2O_6$, and has the structural formula:

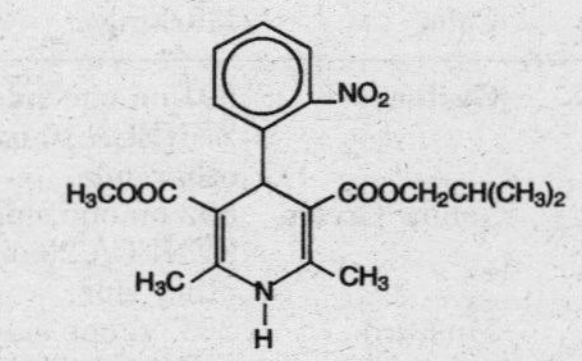

Nisoldipine is a yellow crystalline substance, practically insoluble in water but soluble in ethanol. It has a molecular weight of 388.4. SULAR tablets consist of an external coat and an internal core. Both coat and core contain nisoldipine, the coat as a slow release formulation and the core as a fast release formulation. SULAR tablets contain either 10, 20, 30 or 40 mg of nisoldipine for once-a-day oral administration.
Inert ingredients in the formulation are: hydroxypropylcellulose, lactose, corn starch, crospovidone, microcrystalline cellulose, sodium lauryl sulfate, povidone and magnesium stearate. The inert ingredients in the film coating are: hydroxypropylmethylcellulose, polyethylene glycol, ferric oxide, and titanium dioxide.

CLINICAL PHARMACOLOGY

Mechanism of Action
Nisoldipine is a member of the dihydropyridine class of calcium channel antagonists (calcium ion antagonists or slow channel blockers) that inhibit the transmembrane influx of calcium into vascular smooth muscle and cardiac muscle. It reversibly competes with other dihydropyridines for binding to the calcium channel. Because the contractile process of vascular smooth muscle is dependent upon the movement of extracellular calcium into the muscle through specific ion channels, inhibition of the calcium channel results in dilation of the arterioles. *In vitro* studies show that the effects of nisoldipine on contractile processes are selective, with greater potency on vascular smooth muscle than on cardiac muscle. Although, like other dihydropyridine calcium channel blockers, nisoldipine has negative inotropic effects *in vitro*, studies conducted in intact anesthetized animals have shown that the vasodilating effect occurs at doses lower than those that affect cardiac contractility.
The effect of nisoldipine on blood pressure is principally a consequence of a dose-related decrease of peripheral vascular resistance. While nisoldipine, like other dihydropyridines, exhibits a mild diuretic effect, most of the antihypertensive activity is attributed to its effect on peripheral vascular resistance.

Pharmacokinetics and Metabolism
Nisoldipine pharmacokinetics are independent of the dose in the range of 20 to 60 mg, with plasma concentrations proportional to dose. Nisoldipine accumulation, during multiple dosing, is predictable from a single dose.
Nisoldipine is relatively well absorbed into the systemic circulation with 87% of the radiolabeled drug recovered in urine and feces. The absolute bioavailability of nisoldipine is about 5%. Nisoldipine's low bioavailability is due, in part, to pre-systemic metabolism in the gut wall, and this metabolism decreases from the proximal to the distal parts of the intestine. Food with a high fat content has a pronounced effect on the release of nisoldipine from the coat-core formulation and results in a significant increase in peak concentration (C_{max}) by up to 300%. Total exposure, however, is decreased about 25%, presumably because more of the drug is released proximally. This effect appears to be specific for nisoldipine in the controlled release formulation, as a less pronounced food effect was seen with the immediate release tablet. Concomitant intake of a high fat meal with SULAR should be avoided.
Maximal plasma concentrations of nisoldipine are reached 6 to 12 hours after dosing. The terminal elimination half-life (reflecting post absorption clearance of nisoldipine) ranges from 7 to 12 hours. C_{max} and AUC increase by factors of approximately 1.3 and 1.5, respectively, from first dose to steady state. After oral administration, the concentration of (+) nisoldipine, the active enantiomer, is about 6 times higher than the (−) inactive enantiomer. The plasma protein binding of nisoldipine is very high, with less than 1% unbound over the plasma concentration range of 100 ng/mL to 10 mcg/mL.
Nisoldipine is highly metabolized; 5 major urinary metabolites have been identified. Although 60–80% of an oral dose undergoes urinary excretion, only traces of unchanged nisoldipine are found in urine. The major biotransformation pathway appears to be the hydroxylation of the isobutyl ester. A hydroxylated derivative of the side chain, present in plasma at concentrations approximately equal to the parent compound, appears to be the only active metabolite, and has about 10% of the activity of the parent compound. Cytochrome P_{450} enzymes are believed to play a major role in the metabolism of nisoldipine. The particular isoenzyme system responsible for its metabolism has not been identified, but other dihydropyridines are metabolized by cytochrome P_{450} IIIA4. Nisoldipine should not be administered with grapefruit juice as this has been shown, in a study of 12 subjects, to interfere with nisoldipine metabolism, resulting in a mean increase in C_{max} of about 3-fold (ranging up to about 7-fold) and AUC of almost 2-fold (ranging up to about 5-fold). A similar phenomenon has been seen with several other dihydropyridine calcium channel blockers.

Special Populations
Renal Dysfunction: Because renal elimination is not an important pathway, bioavailability and pharmacokinetics of SULAR were not significantly different in patients with various degrees of renal impairment. Dosing adjustments in patients with mild to moderate renal impairment are not necessary.
Geriatric: Elderly patients have been found to have 2 to 3 fold higher plasma concentrations (C_{max} and AUC) than young subjects. This should be reflected in more cautious dosing (See DOSAGE AND ADMINISTRATION).
Hepatic Insufficiency: In patients with liver cirrhosis given 10 mg SULAR, plasma concentrations of the parent compound were 4 to 5 times higher than those in healthy young subjects. Lower starting and maintenance doses should be used in cirrhotic patients (See DOSAGE AND ADMINISTRATION).
Gender and Race: The effect of gender or race on the pharmacokinetics of nisoldipine has not been investigated.
Disease States: Hypertension does not significantly alter the pharmacokinetics of nisoldipine.

Pharmacodynamics
Hemodynamic Effects
Administration of a single dose of nisoldipine leads to decreased systemic vascular resistance and blood pressure with a transient increase in heart rate. The change in heart rate is greater with immediate release nisoldipine preparations. The effect on blood pressure is directly related to the initial degree of elevation above normal. Chronic administration of nisoldipine results in a sustained decrease in vascular resistance and small increases in stroke index and left ventricular ejection fraction. A study of the immediate release formulation showed no effect of nisoldipine on the renin-angiotensin-aldosterone system or on plasma norepinephrine concentration in normals. Changes in blood pressure in hypertensive patients given SULAR were dose related over the range of 10–60 mg/day.
Nisoldipine does not appear to have significant negative inotropic activity in intact animals or humans, and did not lead to worsening of clinical heart failure in three small studies of patients with asymptomatic and symptomatic left ventricular dysfunction. There is little information, however, in patients with severe congestive heart failure, and all calcium channel blockers should be used with caution in any patient with heart failure.
Electrophysiologic Effects
Nisoldipine has no clinically important chronotropic effects. Except for mild shortening of sinus cycle, SA conduction time and AH intervals, single oral doses up to 20 mg of immediate release nisoldipine did not significantly change other conduction parameters. Similar electrophysiologic effects were seen with single iv doses, which could be blunted in patients pre-treated with beta-blockers. Dose and plasma level related flattening or inversion of T-waves have been observed in a few small studies. Such reports were concentrated in patients receiving rapidly increased high doses in one study; the phenomenon has not been a cause of safety concern in large clinical trials.

Clinical Studies in Hypertension
The antihypertensive efficacy of SULAR was studied in 5 double-blind, placebo-controlled, randomized studies, in which over 600 patients were treated with SULAR as monotherapy and about 300 with placebo; 4 of the five studies compared 2 or 3 fixed doses while the fifth allowed titration from 10–40 mg. Once daily administration of SULAR produced sustained reductions in systolic and diastolic blood pressures over the 24 hour dosing interval in both supine and standing positions. The mean placebo-subtracted reductions in supine systolic and diastolic blood pressure at trough, 24 hours post-dose, in these studies, are shown below. Changes in standing blood pressure were similar:

MEAN SUPINE THROUGH SYSTOLIC AND DIASTOLIC BLOOD PRESSURE CHANGES (mm Hg)

SULAR Dose (mg/day)	10 mg	20 mg	30 mg	40 mg	60 mg	10–40 mg titrated
Systolic	8	11	11	14	15	15
Diastolic	3	5	7	7	10	8

In patients receiving atenolol, supine blood pressure reductions with SULAR at 20, 40 and 60 mg once daily were 12/6, 19/8 and 22/10 mm Hg, respectively. The sustained antihypertensive effect of SULAR was demonstrated by 24 hour blood pressure monitoring and examination of peak and trough effects. The trough/peak ratios ranged from 70 to 100% for diastolic and systolic blood pressure. The mean change in heart rate in these studies was less than one beat per minute. In 4 of the 5 studies, patients received initial doses of 20–30 mg SULAR without incident (excessive effects on blood pressure or heart rate). The fifth study started patients on lower doses of SULAR.
Patient race and gender did not influence the blood pressure lowering effect of SULAR. Despite the higher plasma concentration of nisoldipine in the elderly, there was no consistent difference in their blood pressure response except that the 10 mg dose was somewhat more effective than in non-elderly patients. No postural effect on blood pressure was apparent and there was no evidence of tolerance to the antihypertensive effect of SULAR in patients treated for up to one year.

INDICATIONS AND USAGE

SULAR is indicated for the treatment of hypertension. It may be used alone or in combination with other antihypertensive agents.

CONTRAINDICATIONS

SULAR is contraindicated in patients with known hypersensitivity to dihydropyridine calcium channel blockers.

WARNINGS

Increased angina and/or myocardial infarction in patients with coronary artery disease: Rarely, patients, particularly those with severe obstructive coronary artery disease, have developed increased frequency, duration and/or severity of angina, or acute myocardial infarction on starting calcium channel blocker therapy or at the time of dosage increase. The mechanism of this effect has not been established. In controlled studies of SULAR in patients with angina this was seen about 1.5% of the time in patients given nisoldipine, compared with 0.9% in patients given placebo.

PRECAUTIONS

General
Hypotension: Because nisoldipine, like other vasodilators, decreases peripheral vascular resistance, careful monitoring of blood pressure during the initial administration and titration of SULAR is recommended. Close observation is especially important for patients already taking medications that are known to lower blood pressure. Although in most patients the hypotensive effect of SULAR is modest and well tolerated, occasional patients have had excessive and poorly tolerated hypotension. These responses have usually occurred during initial titration or at the time of subsequent upward dosage adjustment.
Congestive Heart Failure: Although acute hemodynamic studies of nisoldipine in patients with NYHA Class II-IV heart failure have not demonstrated negative inotropic effects, safety of SULAR in patients with heart failure has not been established. Caution therefore should be exercised when using SULAR in patients with heart failure or compromised ventricular function, particularly in combination with a beta-blocker.
Patients with Hepatic Impairment: Because nisoldipine is extensively metabolized by the liver and, in patients with cirrhosis, it reaches blood concentrations about 5 times those in normals, SULAR should be administered cautiously in patients with severe hepatic dysfunction (See DOSAGE AND ADMINISTRATION).
Information for Patients: SULAR is an extended release tablet and should be swallowed whole. Tablets should not be chewed, divided or crushed. SULAR should not be administered with a high fat meal. Grapefruit juice, which has been shown to increase significantly the bioavailability of nisoldipine and other dihydropyridine type calcium channel blockers, should not be taken with SULAR.
Laboratory Tests: SULAR is not known to interfere with the interpretation of laboratory tests.
Drug Interactions: A 30 to 45% increase in AUC and C_{max} of nisoldipine was observed with concomitant administration of cimetidine 400 mg twice daily. Ranitidine 150 mg twice daily did not interact significantly with nisoldipine (AUC was decreased by 15–20%). No pharmacodynamic effects of either histamine H_2 receptor antagonist were observed.
Coadministration of phenytoin with 40 mg SULAR tablets in epileptic patients lowered the nisoldipine plasma concentrations to undetectable levels. Coadministration of SULAR with phenytoin or any known CYP3A4 inducer should be avoided and alternative antihypertensive therapy should be considered.
Pharmacokinetic interactions between nisoldipine and beta-blockers (atenolol, propranolol) were variable and not signif-

Continued on next page

Sular—Cont.

icant. Propranolol attenuated the heart rate increase following administration of immediate release nisoldipine. The blood pressure effect of SULAR tended to be greater in patients on atenolol than in patients on no other antihypertensive therapy.
Quinidine at 648 mg bid decreased the bioavailability (AUC) of nisoldipine by 26%, but not the peak concentration. The immediate release, but not the coat-core formulation of nisoldipine increased plasma quinidine concentrations by about 20%. This interaction was not accompanied by ECG changes and its clinical significance is not known.
No significant interactions were found between nisoldipine and warfarin or digoxin.
Carcinogenesis, Mutagenesis, Impairment of Fertility: Dietary administration of nisoldipine to male and female rats for up to 24 months (mean doses up to 82 and 111 mg/kg/day, 16 and 19 times the maximum recommended human dose [MRHD] on a mg/m² basis, respectively) and female mice for up to 21 months (mean doses of up to 217 mg/kg/day, 20 times the MRHD on a mg/m² basis) revealed no evidence of tumorigenic effect of nisoldipine. In male mice receiving a mean dose of 163 mg nisoldipine/kg/day (16 times the MRHD of 60 mg/day on a mg/m² basis), an increased frequency of stomach papilloma, but still within the historical range, was observed. No evidence of stomach neoplasia was observed at lower doses (up to 58 mg/kg/day). Nisoldipine was negative when tested in a battery of genotoxicity assays including the Ames test and the CHO/HGRPT assay for mutagenicity and the *in vivo* mouse micronucleus test and *in vitro* CHO cell test for clastogenicity.
When administered to male and female rats at doses of up to 30 mg/kg/day (about 5 times the MRHD on a mg/m² basis) nisoldipine had no effect on fertility.
Pregnancy Category C: Nisoldipine was neither teratogenic nor fetotoxic at doses that were not maternally toxic. Nisoldipine was fetotoxic but not teratogenic in rats and rabbits at doses resulting in maternal toxicity (reduced maternal body weight gain). In pregnant rats, increased fetal resorption (post-implantation loss) was observed at 100 mg/kg/day and decreased fetal weight was observed at both 30 and 100 mg/kg/day. These doses are, respectively, about 5 and 16 times the MRHD when compared on a mg/m² basis. In pregnant rabbits, decreased fetal and placental weights were observed at a dose of 30 mg/kg/day, about 10 times the MRHD when compared on a mg/m² basis. In a study in which pregnant monkeys (both treated and control) had high rates of abortion and mortality, the only surviving fetus from a group exposed to a maternal dose of 100 mg nisoldipine/kg/day (about 30 times the MRHD when compared on a mg/m² basis) presented with forelimb and vertebral abnormalities not previously seen in control monkeys of the same strain. There are no adequate and well controlled studies in pregnant women. SULAR should be used in pregnancy only if the potential benefit justifies the potential risk to the fetus.
Nursing Mothers: It is not known whether nisoldipine is excreted in human milk. Because many drugs are excreted in human milk, a decision should be made to discontinue nursing, or to discontinue SULAR, taking into account the importance of the drug to the mother.
Pediatric Use: Safety and effectiveness in pediatric patients have not been established.
Geriatric Use: Clinical studies of nisoldipine did not include sufficient numbers of subjects aged 65 and over to determine whether they respond differently from younger subjects. Other reported clinical experience has not identified differences in responses between the elderly and younger patients. Patients over 65 are expected to develop higher plasma concentrations of nisoldipine. In general, dose selection for an elderly patient should be cautious, usually starting at the low end of the dosing range, reflecting the greater frequency of decreased hepatic, renal or cardiac function, and of concomitant disease or other drug therapy.

ADVERSE EXPERIENCES

More than 6000 patients world-wide have received nisoldipine in clinical trials for the treatment of hypertension, either as the immediate release or the SULAR extended release formulation. Of about 1,500 patients who received SULAR in hypertension studies, about 55% were exposed for at least 2 months and about one third were exposed for over 6 months, the great majority at doses of 20 to 60 mg daily.
SULAR is generally well-tolerated. In the U.S. clinical trials of SULAR in hypertension, 10.9% of the 921 SULAR patients discontinued treatment due to adverse events compared with 2.9% of 280 placebo patients. The frequency of discontinuations due to adverse experiences was related to dose, with a 5.4% discontinuation rate at 10 mg daily and a 10.9% discontinuation rate at 60 mg daily.
The most frequently occurring adverse experiences with SULAR are those related to its vasodilator properties; these are generally mild and only occasionally lead to patient withdrawal from treatment. The table below, from U.S. placebo-controlled parallel dose response trials of SULAR using doses from 10–60 mg once daily in patients with hypertension, lists all of the adverse events, regardless of the causal relationship to SULAR, for which the overall incidence on SULAR was both >1% and greater with SULAR than with placebo.

Adverse Event	Nisoldipine (%) (n=663)	Placebo (%) (n=280)
Peripheral Edema	22	10
Headache	22	15
Dizziness	5	4
Pharyngitis	5	4
Vasodilation	4	2
Sinusitis	3	2
Palpitation	3	1
Chest Pain	2	1
Nausea	2	1
Rash	2	1

Only peripheral edema and possibly dizziness appear to be dose related.

Adverse Event	Placebo	SULAR 10 mg	20 mg	30 mg	40 mg	60 mg
(Rates in %)	N=280	N=30	N=170	N=105	N=139	N=137
Peripheral Edema	10	7	15	20	27	29
Dizziness	4	7	3	3	4	10

The common adverse events occurred at about the same rate in men as in women, and at a similar rate in patients over age 65 as in those under that age, except that headache was much less common in older patients. Except for peripheral edema and vasodilation, which were more common in whites, adverse event rates were similar in blacks and whites.
The following adverse events occurred in ≤1 % of all patients treated for hypertension in U.S. and foreign clinical trials, or with unspecified incidence in other studies. Although a causal relationship of SULAR to these events cannot be established, they are listed to alert the physician to a possible relationship with SULAR treatment.
Body As A Whole: cellulitis, chills, facial edema, fever, flu syndrome, malaise
Cardiovascular: atrial fibrillation, cerebrovascular accident, congestive heart failure, first degree AV block, hypertension, hypotension, jugular venous distension, migraine, myocardial infarction, postural hypotension, ventricular extrasystoles, supraventricular tachycardia, syncope, systolic ejection murmur, T wave abnormalities on ECG (flattening, inversion, nonspecific changes), venous insufficiency
Digestive: abnormal liver function tests, anorexia, colitis, diarrhea, dry mouth, dyspepsia, dysphagia, flatulence, gastritis, gastrointestinal hemorrhage, gingival hyperplasia, glossitis, hepatomegaly, increased appetite, melena, mouth ulceration
Endocrine: diabetes mellitus, thyroiditis
Hemic and Lymphatic: anemia, ecchymoses, leukopenia, petechiae
Metabolic and Nutritional: gout, hypokalemia, increased serum creatine kinase, increased nonprotein nitrogen, weight gain, weight loss
Musculoskeletal: arthralgia, arthritis, leg cramps, myalgia, myasthenia, myositis, tenosynovitis
Nervous: abnormal dreams, abnormal thinking and confusion, amnesia, anxiety, ataxia, cerebral ischemia, decreased libido, depression, hypesthesia, hypertonia, insomnia, nervousness, paresthesia, somnolence, tremor, vertigo
Respiratory: asthma, dyspnea, end inspiratory wheeze and fine rales, epistaxis, increased cough, laryngitis, pharyngitis, pleural effusion, rhinitis, sinusitis
Skin and Appendages: acne, alopecia, dry skin, exfoliative dermatitis, fungal dermatitis, herpes simplex, herpes zoster, maculopapular rash, pruritus, pustular rash, skin discoloration, skin ulcer, sweating, urticaria
Special Senses: abnormal vision, amblyopia, blepharitis, conjunctivitis, ear pain, glaucoma, itchy eyes, keratoconjunctivitis, otitis media, retinal detachment, tinnitus, watery eyes, taste disturbance, temporary unilateral loss of vision, vitreous floater, watery eyes
Urogenital: dysuria, hematuria, impotence, nocturia, urinary frequency, increased BUN and serum creatinine, vaginal hemorrhage, vaginitis.
The following postmarketing event has been reported very rarely in patients receiving SULAR: systemic hypersensitivity reaction which may include one or more of the following; angioedema, shortness of breath, tachycardia, chest tightness, hypotension, and rash. A definite causal relationship with SULAR has not been established. An unusual event observed with immediate release nisoldipine but not observed with SULAR was one case of photosensitivity. Gynecomastia has been associated with the use of calcium channel blockers.

OVERDOSAGE

There is no experience with nisoldipine overdosage. Generally, overdosage with other dihydropyridines leading to pronounced hypotension calls for active cardiovascular support including monitoring of cardiovascular and respiratory function, elevation of extremities, judicious use of calcium infusion, pressor agents and fluids. Clearance of nisoldipine would be expected to be slowed in patients with impaired liver function. Since nisoldipine is highly protein bound, dialysis is not likely to be of any benefit; however, plasmapheresis may be beneficial.

DOSAGE AND ADMINISTRATION

The dosage of SULAR must be adjusted to each patient's needs. Therapy usually should be initiated with 20 mg orally once daily, then increased by 10 mg per week or longer intervals, to attain adequate control of blood pressure. Usual maintenance dosage is 20 to 40 mg once daily. Blood pressure response increases over the 10–60 mg daily dose range but adverse event rates also increase. Doses beyond 60 mg once daily are not recommended. SULAR has been used safely with diuretics, ACE inhibitors, and beta-blocking agents.
Patients over age 65, or patients with impaired liver function are expected to develop higher plasma concentrations of nisoldipine. Their blood pressure should be monitored closely during any dosage adjustment. A starting dose not exceeding 10 mg daily is recommended in these patient groups.
SULAR tablets should be administered orally once daily. Administration with a high fat meal can lead to excessive peak drug concentration and should be avoided. Grapefruit products should be avoided before and after dosing. SULAR is an extended release dosage form and tablets should be swallowed whole, not bitten, divided or crushed.

HOW SUPPLIED

SULAR extended release tablets are supplied as 10 mg, 20 mg, 30 mg, and 40 mg round film coated tablets. The different strengths can be identified as follows:

Strength	Color	Markings
10 mg	Oyster	891 on one side and ZENECA 10 on the other side.
20 mg	Yellow Cream	892 on one side and ZENECA 20 on the other side.
30 mg	Mustard	893 on one side and ZENECA 30 on the other side.
40 mg	Burnt Orange	894 on one side and ZENECA 40 on the other side.

SULAR Tablets are supplied in:

	Strength	NDC Code
Bottles of 100	10 mg	0310-0891-10
	20 mg	0310-0892-10
	30 mg	0310-0893-10
	40 mg	0310-0894-10
Unit Dose Packages of 100	10 mg	0310-0891-39
	20 mg	0310-0892-39
	30 mg	0310-0893-39

Protect from light and moisture. Store at controlled room temperature, 20–25°C (68–77°F) [see USP]. Dispense in tight, light-resistant containers.
SULAR® is a trademark of Bayer AG, used under license by Zeneca Inc.
ZENECA
Manufactured for:
Zeneca Pharmaceuticals
A Business Unit of Zeneca Inc.
Wilmington, Delaware 19850-5437
By: Bayer AG, Leverkusen, Germany
Made in Germany
64131-03 Rev 01/01

TENORMIN® Tablets ℞
TENORMIN® I.V. Injection
[*ten-or 'min*]
(atenolol)

Prescribing information for this product, which appears on pages 649–652 of the 2001 PDR, has been revised. Please write "See Supplement A" next to the product heading.
Under the HOW SUPPLIED section, the Hospital Unit Dose package sizes have been deleted.

ZOMIG® ℞
[*zō-mĭg*]
(zolmitriptan)
Tablets

ZOMIG-ZMT™ ℞
(zolmitriptan)
Orally Disintegrating Tablets

Prescribing information for this product, which appears on pages 665–668 of the 2001 PDR, has been completely revised as follows. Please write "See Supplement A" next to the product heading.

DESCRIPTION

ZOMIG® (zolmitriptan) Tablets contain zolmitriptan, which is a selective 5-hydroxytryptamine $_{1B/1D}$ (5-$HT_{1B/1D}$) receptor agonist. Zolmitriptan is chemically designated as (S)-4-

[[3-[2-(dimethylamino)ethyl]-1H-indol-5-yl]methyl]-2-oxazolidinone and has the following chemical structure:

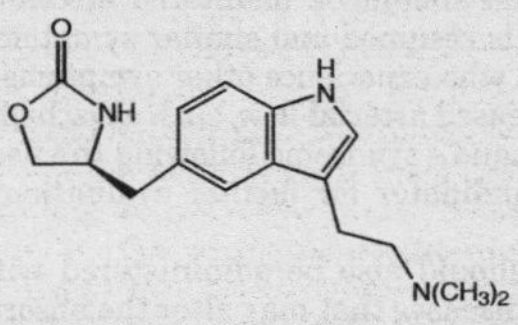

The empirical formula is $C_{16}H_{21}N_3O_2$, representing a molecular weight of 287.36. Zolmitriptan is a white to almost white powder that is readily soluble in water. ZOMIG Tablets are available as 2.5 mg (yellow) and 5 mg (pink) film coated tablets for oral administration. The film coated tablets contain anhydrous lactose NF, microcrystalline cellulose NF, sodium starch glycolate NF, magnesium stearate NF, hydroxypropyl methylcellulose USP, titanium dioxide USP, polyethylene glycol 400 NF, yellow iron oxide NF (2.5 mg tablet), red iron oxide NF (5 mg tablet), and polyethylene glycol 8000 NF.

ZOMIG-ZMT™ Orally Disintegrating Tablets are available as 2.5 mg white uncoated tablets for oral administration. The orally disintegrating tablets contain mannitol USP, microcrystalline cellulose NF, crospovidone NF, aspartame NF, sodium bicarbonate USP, citric acid anhydrous USP, colloidal silicon dioxide NF, magnesium stearate NF and orange flavor SN 027512.

CLINICAL PHARMACOLOGY

Mechanism of Action: Zolmitriptan binds with high affinity to human recombinant 5-HT_{1D} and 5-HT_{1B} receptors. Zolmitriptan exhibits modest affinity for 5-HT_{1A} receptors, but has no significant affinity (as measured by radioligand binding assays) or pharmacological activity at 5-HT_2, 5-HT_3, 5-HT_4, alpha$_1$-, alpha$_2$-, or beta$_1$- adrenergic; H_1, H_2, histaminic; muscarinic; dopamine$_1$, or dopamine$_2$ receptors. The N-desmethyl metabolite also has high affinity for 5-$HT_{1B/1D}$ and modest affinity for 5-HT_{1A} receptors.

Current theories proposed to explain the etiology of migraine headache suggest that symptoms are due to local cranial vasodilatation and/or to the release of sensory neuropeptides (vasoactive intestinal peptide, substance P and calcitonin gene-related peptide) through nerve endings in the trigeminal system. The therapeutic activity of zolmitriptan for the treatment of migraine headache can most likely be attributed to the agonist effects at the 5-$HT_{1B/1D}$ receptors on intracranial blood vessels (including the arterio-venous anastomoses) and sensory nerves of the trigeminal system which result in cranial vessel constriction and inhibition of pro-inflammatory neuropeptide release.

Clinical Pharmacokinetics and Bioavailability:

Absorption: Zolmitriptan is well absorbed after oral administration for both the conventional tablets and the orally disintegrating tablets. Zolmitriptan displays linear kinetics over the dose range of 2.5 to 50 mg.

The AUC and C_{max} of zolmitriptan are similar following administration of ZOMIG Tablets and ZOMIG-ZMT Orally Disintegrating Tablets, but the T_{max} is somewhat later with ZOMIG-ZMT, with a median T_{max} of 3 hours for the orally disintegrating tablet compared with 1.5 hours for the conventional tablet. The AUC, C_{max}, and T_{max} for the active N-desmethyl metabolite are similar for the two formulations.

During a moderate to severe migraine attack, mean AUC_{0-4} and C_{max} for zolmitriptan, dosed as a conventional tablet, were decreased by 40% and 25%, respectively, and mean T_{max} was delayed by one-half hour compared to the same patients during a migraine free period.

Food has no significant effect on the bioavailability of zolmitriptan. No accumulation occurred on multiple dosing.

Distribution: Mean absolute bioavailability is approximately 40%. The mean apparent volume of distribution is 7.0 L/kg. Plasma protein binding of zolmitriptan is 25% over the concentration range of 10–1000 ng/mL.

Metabolism: Zolmitriptan is converted to an active N-desmethyl metabolite such that the metabolite concentrations are about two thirds that of zolmitriptan. Because the 5-$HT_{1B/1D}$ potency of the metabolite is 2 to 6 times that of the parent, the metabolite may contribute a substantial portion of the overall effect after zolmitriptan administration.

Elimination: Total radioactivity recovered in urine and feces was 65% and 30% of the administered dose, respectively. About 8% of the dose was recovered in the urine as unchanged zolmitriptan. Indole acetic acid metabolite accounted for 31% of the dose, followed by N-oxide (7%) and N-desmethyl (4%) metabolites. The indole acetic acid and N-oxide metabolites are inactive.

Mean total plasma clearance is 31.5 mL/min/kg, of which one-sixth is renal clearance. The renal clearance is greater than the glomerular filtration rate suggesting renal tubular secretion.

Special Populations

Age: Zolmitriptan pharmacokinetics in healthy elderly non-migraineur volunteers (age 65–76 yrs) were similar to those in younger non-migraineur volunteers (age 18–39 yrs).

Gender: Mean plasma concentrations of zolmitriptan were up to 1.5-fold higher in females than males.

Renal Impairment: Clearance of zolmitriptan was reduced by 25% in patients with severe renal impairment (Clcr $\geq 5 \leq 25$ mL/min) compared to the normal group (Clcr $> = 70$ mL/min); no significant change in clearance was observed in the moderately renally impaired group (Clcr $\geq 26 \leq 50$ mL/min).

Hepatic Impairment: In severely hepatically impaired patients, the mean C_{max}, T_{max}, and $AUC_{0-\infty}$ of zolmitriptan were increased 1.5, 2 (2 vs 4 hr), and 3-fold, respectively, compared to normals. Seven out of 27 patients experienced 20 to 80 mm Hg elevations in systolic and/or diastolic blood pressure after a 10 mg dose. Zolmitriptan should be administered with caution in subjects with liver disease, generally using doses less than 2.5 mg (see WARNINGS and PRECAUTIONS).

Hypertensive Patients: No differences in the pharmacokinetics of zolmitriptan or its effects on blood pressure were seen in mild to moderate hypertensive volunteers compared to normotensive controls.

Race: Retrospective analysis of pharmacokinetic data between Japanese and Caucasians revealed no significant differences.

Drug Interactions: All drug interaction studies were performed in healthy volunteers using a single 10 mg dose of zolmitriptan and a single dose of the other drug except where otherwise noted.

Fluoxetine: The pharmacokinetics of zolmitriptan, as well as its effect on blood pressure, were unaffected by 4 weeks of pretreatment with oral fluoxetine (20 mg/day).

MAO Inhibitors: Following one week of administration of 150 mg bid moclobemide, a specific MAO-A inhibitor, there was an increase of about 25% in both C_{max} and AUC for zolmitriptan and a 3-fold increase in the C_{max} and AUC of the active N-desmethyl metabolite of zolmitriptan (see CONTRAINDICATIONS and PRECAUTIONS).

Selegiline, a selective MAO-B inhibitor, at a dose of 10 mg/day for 1 week, had no effect on the pharmacokinetics of zolmitriptan and its metabolite.

Propranolol: C_{max} and AUC of zolmitriptan increased 1.5-fold after one week of dosing with propranolol (160 mg/day). C_{max} and AUC of the N-desmethyl metabolite were reduced by 30% and 15%, respectively. There were no interactive effects on blood pressure or pulse rate following administration of propranolol with zolmitriptan.

Acetaminophen: A single 1 g dose of acetaminophen does not alter the pharmacokinetics of zolmitriptan and its N-desmethyl metabolite. However, zolmitriptan delayed the T_{max} of acetaminophen by one hour.

Metoclopramide: A single 10 mg dose of metoclopramide had no effect on the pharmacokinetics of zolmitriptan or its metabolites.

Oral Contraceptives: Retrospective analysis of pharmacokinetic data across studies indicated that mean plasma concentrations of zolmitriptan were generally higher in females taking oral contraceptives compared to those not taking oral contraceptives. Mean C_{max} and AUC of zolmitriptan were found to be higher by 30% and 50%, respectively, and T_{max} was delayed by one-half hour in females taking oral contraceptives. The effect of zolmitriptan on the pharmacokinetics of oral contraceptives has not been studied.

Cimetidine: Following the administration of cimetidine, the half-life and AUC of a 5 mg dose of zolmitriptan and its active metabolite were approximately doubled (see PRECAUTIONS).

Clinical Studies: The efficacy of ZOMIG Tablets in the acute treatment of migraine headaches was demonstrated in five randomized, double-blind, placebo controlled studies, of which 2 utilized the 1 mg dose, 2 utilized the 2.5 mg dose and 4 utilized the 5 mg dose; all studies used the marketed formulation. In study 1, patients treated their headaches in a clinic setting. In the other studies, patients treated their headaches as outpatients. In study 4, patients who had previously used sumatriptan were excluded, whereas in the other studies no such exclusion was applied. Patients enrolled in these 5 studies were predominantly female (82%) and Caucasian (97%) with a mean age of 40 years (range 12–65). Patients were instructed to treat a moderate to severe headache. Headache response, defined as a reduction in headache severity from moderate or severe pain to mild or no pain, was assessed at 1, 2, and, in most studies, 4 hours after dosing. Associated symptoms such as nausea, photophobia and phonophobia were also assessed. Maintenance of response was assessed for up to 24 hours postdose. A second dose of ZOMIG Tablets or other medication was allowed 2 to 24 hours after the initial treatment for persistent and recurrent headache. The frequency and time to use of these additional treatments were also recorded. In all studies, the effect of zolmitriptan was compared to placebo in the treatment of a single migraine attack.

In all five studies, the percentage of patients achieving headache response 2 hours after treatment was significantly greater among patients receiving ZOMIG Tablets at all doses (except for the 1 mg dose in the smallest study) compared to those who received placebo. In the two studies that evaluated the 1 mg dose, there was a statistically significant greater percentage of patients with headache response at 2 hours in the higher dose groups (2.5 and/or 5 mg) compared to the 1 mg dose group. There were no statistically significant differences between the 2.5 and 5 mg dose groups (or of doses up to 20 mg) for the primary end point of headache response at 2 hours in any study. The results of these controlled clinical studies are summarized in Table 1.

Comparisons of drug performance based upon results obtained in different clinical trials are never reliable. Because studies are conducted at different times, with different samples of patients, by different investigators, employing different criteria and/or different interpretations of the same criteria, under different conditions (dose, dosing regimen, etc.), quantitative estimates of treatment response and the timing of response may be expected to vary considerably from study to study.

Table 1: Percentage of Patients with Headache Response (Mild or no Headache) 2 Hours Following Treatment (n=number of patients randomized).

	Placebo	ZOMIG 1.0 mg	ZOMIG 2.5 mg	ZOMIG 5 mg
Study 1[a]	16% (n=19)	27% (n=22)	NA	60%*# (n=20)
Study 2	19% (n=88)	NA	NA	66%* (n=179)
Study 3	34% (n=121)	50%* (n=140)	65%*# (n=260)	67%*# (n=245)
Study 4[b]	44% (n=55)	NA	NA	59%* (n=491)
Study 5	36% (n=92)	NA NA	62%* (n=178)	NA

*p<0.05 in comparison with placebo.
#p<0.05 in comparison with 1 mg.
[a] This was the only study in which patients treated the headache in a clinic setting.
[b] This was the only study where patients were excluded who had previously used sumatriptan.
NA—not applicable

The estimated probability of achieving an initial headache response by 4 hours following treatment is depicted in Figure 1.

Figure 1: Estimated Probability Of Acheiving Initial Headache Response Within 4 Hours*

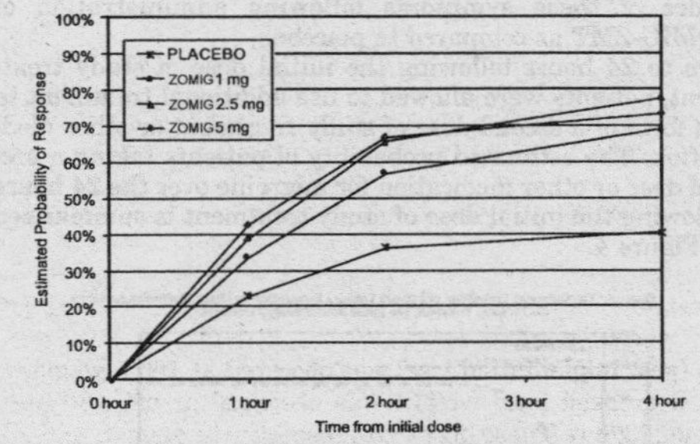

*Figure 1 shows the Kaplan-Meier plot of the probability over time of obtaining headache response (no or mild pain) following treatment with zolmitriptan. The averages displayed are based on pooled data from 3 placebo controlled, outpatient trials providing evidence of efficacy (Trials 2, 3 and 5). Patients not achieving headache response or taking additional treatment prior to 4 hours were censored at 4 hours.

For patients with migraine associated photophobia, phonophobia, and nausea at baseline, there was a decreased incidence of these symptoms following administration of ZOMIG as compared to placebo.

Two to 24 hours following the initial dose of study treatment, patients were allowed to use additional treatment for pain relief in the form of a second dose of study treatment or other medication. The estimated probability of patients taking a second dose or other medication for migraine over the 24 hours following the initial dose of study treatment is summarized in Figure 2.

Figure 2: The Estimated Probability Of Patients Taking A Second Dose Or Other Medication For Migraines Over The 24 Hours Following The Initial Dose Of Study Treatment*

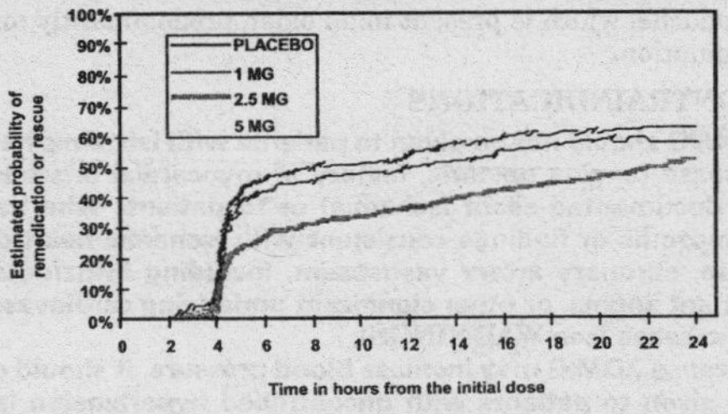

*This Kaplan-Meier plot is based on data obtained in 3 placebo controlled clinical trials (Study 2, 3 and 5). Patients not using additional treatments were censored at 24 hours. The plot includes both patients who had headache response at 2 hours and those who had no response to the initial dose. It should be noted that the protocols did not allow remedication within 2 hours postdose.

The efficacy of ZOMIG was unaffected by presence of aura; duration of headache prior to treatment; relationship to menses; gender, age or weight of the patient; pretreatment nausea or concomitant use of common migraine prophylactic drugs.

ZOMIG-ZMT Orally Disintegrating Tablets

The efficacy of ZOMIG-ZMT 2.5 mg was demonstrated in a randomized, placebo-controlled trial that was similar in design to the trials of ZOMIG Tablets. Patients were instructed to treat a moderate to severe headache. Of the 471 patients treated in the study, 87% were female and 97% were Caucasian, with a mean age of 41 years (range 18–62). At 2 hours post-dosing response rates in patients treated with ZOMIG-ZMT 2.5 mg was 63% compared to 22% in the

Continued on next page

Zomig—Cont.

placebo group. The difference was statistically significant. The estimated probability of achieving an initial headache response by 2 hours following treatment with ZOMIG-ZMT Tablets is depicted in Figure 3.

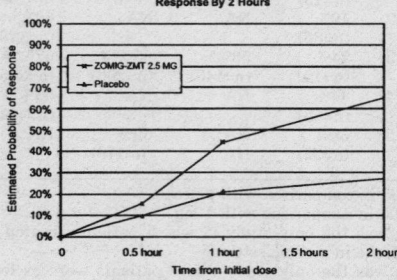

Figure 3: Estimated Probability Of Achieving Initial Headache Response By 2 Hours

Figure 3 shows the Kaplan-Meier plot of the probability over time of obtaining headache response (no or mild pain) following treatment with ZOMIG-ZMT Tablets or placebo. Patients taking additional treatment or not achieving headache response prior to 2 hours were censored at 2 hours. For patients with migraine-associated photophobia, phonophobia and nausea at baseline, there was a decreased incidence of these symptoms following administration of ZOMIG-ZMT as compared to placebo.

Two to 24 hours following the initial dose of study treatment, patients were allowed to use additional treatment in the form of a second dose of study treatment or other medication. The estimated probability of patients taking a second dose or other medication for migraine over the 24 hours following the initial dose of study treatment is summarized in Figure 4.

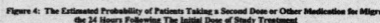
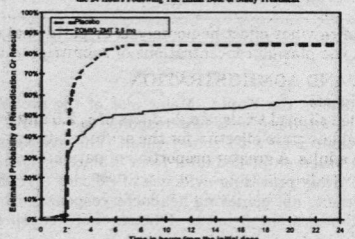

Figure 4: The Estimated Probability of Patients Taking a Second Dose or Other Medication for Migraine the 24 Hours Following The Initial Dose of Study Treatment

In this Kaplan-Meier plot, patients not using additional treatments were censored at 24 hours. The plot includes both patients who had headache response at 2 hours and those who had no response to the initial dose. Remedication was allowed 2 hours post-dose, and unlike the conventional tablet, remedication prior to 4 hours was not discouraged.

INDICATIONS AND USAGE: ZOMIG is indicated for the acute treatment of migraine with or without aura in adults.

ZOMIG is not intended for the prophylactic therapy of migraine or for use in the management of hemiplegic or basilar migraine (see CONTRAINDICATIONS). Safety and effectiveness of ZOMIG have not been established for cluster headache, which is present in an older, predominantly male population.

CONTRAINDICATIONS

ZOMIG should not be given to patients with ischemic heart disease (angina pectoris, history of myocardial infarction, or documented silent ischemia) or to patients who have symptoms or findings consistent with ischemic heart disease, coronary artery vasospasm, including Prinzmetal's variant angina, or other significant underlying cardiovascular disease (see WARNINGS).

Because ZOMIG may increase blood pressure, it should not be given to patients with uncontrolled hypertension (see WARNINGS).

ZOMIG should not be used within 24 hours of treatment with another 5-HT₁ agonist, or an ergotamine-containing or ergot-type medication like dihydroergotamine or methysergide.

ZOMIG should not be administered to patients with hemiplegic or basilar migraine.

Concurrent administration of MAO-A inhibitors or use of zolmitriptan within 2 weeks of discontinuation of MAO-A inhibitor therapy is contraindicated (see CLINICAL PHARMACOLOGY: Drug Interactions and PRECAUTIONS: Drug Interactions).

ZOMIG is contraindicated in patients who are hypersensitive to zolmitriptan or any of its inactive ingredients.

WARNINGS

ZOMIG should only be used where a clear diagnosis of migraine has been established.

Risk of Myocardial Ischemia and/or Infarction and Other Adverse Cardiac Events: ZOMIG should not be given to patients with documented ischemic or vasospastic coronary artery disease (see CONTRAINDICATIONS). It is strongly recommended that zolmitriptan not be given to patients in whom unrecognized coronary artery disease

(CAD) is predicted by the presence of risk factors (e.g., hypertension, hypercholesterolemia, smoker, obesity, diabetes, strong family history of CAD, female with surgical or physiological menopause, or male over 40 years of age) unless a cardiovascular evaluation provides satisfactory clinical evidence that the patient is reasonably free of coronary artery and ischemic myocardial disease or other significant underlying cardiovascular disease. The sensitivity of cardiac diagnostic procedures to detect cardiovascular disease or predisposition to coronary artery vasospasm is modest, at best. If, during the cardiovascular evaluation, the patient's medical history, electrocardiographic or other investigations reveal findings indicative of, or consistent with, coronary artery vasospasm or myocardial ischemia, zolmitriptan should not be administered (see CONTRAINDICATIONS). For patients with risk factors predictive of CAD, who are determined to have a satisfactory cardiovascular evaluation, it is strongly recommended that administration of the first dose of zolmitriptan take place in the setting of a physician's office or similar medically staffed and equipped facility unless the patient has previously received zolmitriptan. Because cardiac ischemia can occur in the absence of clinical symptoms, consideration should be given to obtaining on the first occasion of use an electrocardiogram (ECG) during the interval immediately following ZOMIG, in these patients with risk factors.

It is recommended that patients who are intermittent long-term users of ZOMIG and who have or acquire risk factors predictive of CAD, as described above, undergo periodic interval cardiovascular evaluation as they continue to use ZOMIG.

The systematic approach described above is intended to reduce the likelihood that patients with unrecognized cardiovascular disease will be inadvertently exposed to zolmitriptan.

Cardiac Events and Fatalities: Serious adverse cardiac events, including acute myocardial infarction, have been reported within a few hours following administration of zolmitriptan. Life-threatening disturbances of cardiac rhythm, and death have been reported within a few hours following the administration of other 5-HT₁ agonists. Considering the extent of use of 5-HT₁ agonists in patients with migraine, the incidence of these events is extremely low.

ZOMIG can cause coronary vasospasm; at least one of these events occurred in a patient with no cardiac disease history and with documented absence of coronary artery disease. Because of the close proximity of the events to ZOMIG use, a causal relationship cannot be excluded. In the cases where there has been known underlying coronary artery disease, the relationship is uncertain.

Patients with symptomatic Wolff-Parkinson-White syndrome or arrhythmias associated with other cardiac accessory conduction pathway disorders should not receive ZOMIG.

Premarketing experience with zolmitriptan: Among the more than 2,500 patients with migraine who participated in premarketing controlled clinical trials of ZOMIG Tablets, no deaths or serious cardiac events were reported.

Postmarketing experience with zolmitriptan: Serious cardiovascular events have been reported in association with the use of ZOMIG. The uncontrolled nature of postmarketing surveillance, however, makes it impossible to determine definitively the proportion of the reported cases that were actually caused by zolmitriptan or to reliably assess causation in individual cases.

Cerebrovascular Events and Fatalities with 5-HT₁ agonists: Cerebral hemorrhage, subarachnoid hemorrhage, stroke, and other cerebrovascular events have been reported in patients treated with 5-HT₁ agonists; and some have resulted in fatalities. In a number of cases, it appears possible that the cerebrovascular events were primary, the agonist having been administered in the incorrect belief that the symptoms experienced were a consequence of migraine, when they were not. It should be noted that patients with migraine may be at increased risk of certain cerebrovascular events (e.g., stroke, hemorrhage, transient ischemic attack).

Other Vasospasm-Related Events: 5-HT₁ agonists may cause vasospastic reactions other than coronary artery vasospasm. Both peripheral vascular ischemia and colonic ischemia with abdominal pain and bloody diarrhea have been reported with 5-HT₁ agonists.

Increase in Blood Pressure: Significant elevations in systemic blood pressure have been reported on rare occasions in patients with and without a history of hypertension treated with 5-HT₁ agonists. Zolmitriptan is contraindicated in patients with uncontrolled hypertension. In volunteers, an increase of 1 and 5 mm Hg in the systolic and diastolic blood pressure, respectively, was seen at 5 mg. In the headache trials, vital signs were measured only in the small inpatient study and no effect on blood pressure was seen. In a study of patients with moderate to severe liver disease, 7 of 27 experienced 20 to 80 mm Hg elevations in systolic and/or diastolic blood pressure after a dose of 10 mg of zolmitriptan (see CONTRAINDICATIONS).

An 18% increase in mean pulmonary artery pressure was seen following dosing with another 5-HT₁ agonist in a study evaluating subjects undergoing cardiac catheterization.

PRECAUTIONS

General: As with other 5-HT₁B/1D agonists, sensations of tightness, pain, pressure, and heaviness have been reported after treatment with ZOMIG Tablets in the precordium, throat, neck and jaw. Because zolmitriptan may cause coronary artery vasospasm, patients who experience signs or symptoms suggestive of angina following dosing should be

evaluated for the presence of CAD or a predisposition to Prinzmetal's variant angina before receiving additional doses of medication, and should be monitored electrocardiographically if dosing is resumed and similar symptoms recur. Similarly, patients who experience other symptoms or signs suggestive of decreased arterial flow, such as ischemic bowel syndrome or Raynaud's syndrome following the use of any 5-HT₁ agonist are candidates for further evaluation (see WARNINGS).

Zolmitriptan should also be administered with caution to patients with diseases that may alter the absorption, metabolism, or excretion of drugs, such as impaired hepatic function (see CLINICAL PHARMACOLOGY).

For a given attack, if a patient does not respond to the first dose of zolmitriptan, the diagnosis of migraine headache should be reconsidered before administration of a second dose.

Binding to Melanin-Containing Tissues: When pigmented rats were given a single oral dose of 10 mg/kg of radiolabeled zolmitriptan, the radioactivity in the eye after 7 days, the latest time point examined, was still 75% of the value measured after 4 hours. This suggests that zolmitriptan and/or its metabolites may bind to the melanin of the eye. Because there could be accumulation in melanin rich tissues over time, this raises the possibility that zolmitriptan could cause toxicity in these tissues after extended use. However, no effects on the retina related to treatment with zolmitriptan were noted in any of the toxicity studies. Although no systematic monitoring of ophthalmologic function was undertaken in clinical trials, and no specific recommendations for ophthalmologic monitoring are offered, prescribers should be aware of the possibility of long-term ophthalmologic effects.

Phenylketonurics: Phenylketonuric patients should be informed that ZOMIG-ZMT Tablets contain phenylalanine (a component of aspartame). Each 2.5 mg orally disintegrating tablet contains 2.81 mg phenylalanine.

Information for Patients: See PATIENT INFORMATION at the end of this labeling for the text of the separate leaflet provided for patients.

ZOMIG-ZMT Orally Disintegrating Tablets

The orally disintegrating tablet is packaged in a blister. Patients should be instructed not to remove the tablet from the blister until just prior to dosing. The blister pack should then be peeled open, and the orally disintegrating tablet placed on the tongue, where it will dissolve and be swallowed with the saliva.

Laboratory Tests: No monitoring of specific laboratory tests is recommended.

Drug Interactions: Ergot-containing drugs have been reported to cause prolonged vasospastic reactions. Because there is a theoretical basis that these effects may be additive, use of ergotamine-containing or ergot-type medications (like dihydroergotamine or methysergide) and zolmitriptan within 24 hours of each other should be avoided (see CONTRAINDICATIONS).

MAO-A inhibitors increase the systemic exposure of zolmitriptan. Therefore, the use of zolmitriptan in patients receiving MAO-A inhibitors is contraindicated (see CLINICAL PHARMACOLOGY and CONTRAINDICATIONS).

Concomitant use of other 5-HT₁B/1D agonists within 24 hours of ZOMIG treatment is not recommended (see CONTRAINDICATIONS).

Following administration of cimetidine, the half-life and AUC of zolmitriptan and its active metabolites were approximately doubled (see CLINICAL PHARMACOLOGY).

Selective serotonin reuptake inhibitors (SSRIs) (e.g., fluoxetine, fluvoxamine, paroxetine, sertraline) have been reported, rarely, to cause weakness, hyperreflexia, and incoordination when coadministered with 5-HT₁ agonists. If concomitant treatment with zolmitriptan and an SSRI is clinically warranted, appropriate observation of the patient is advised.

Drug/Laboratory Test Interactions: Zolmitriptan is not known to interfere with commonly employed clinical laboratory tests.

Carcinogenesis, Mutagenesis, Impairment of Fertility: Carcinogenesis: Carcinogenicity studies by oral gavage were carried out in mice and rats at doses up to 400 mg/kg/day. Mice were dosed for 85 weeks (males) and 92 weeks (females). The exposure (plasma AUC of parent drug) at the highest dose level was approximately 800 times that seen in humans after a single 10 mg dose (the maximum recommended total daily dose). There was no effect of zolmitriptan on tumor incidence. Control, low dose and middle dose rats were dosed for 104–105 weeks; the high dose group was sacrificed after 101 weeks (males) and 86 weeks (females) due to excess mortality. Aside from an increase in the incidence of thyroid follicular cell hyperplasia and thyroid follicular cell adenomas seen in male rats receiving 400 mg/kg/day, an exposure approximately 3000 times that seen in humans after dosing with 10 mg, no tumors were noted.

Mutagenesis: Zolmitriptan was mutagenic in an Ames test, in 2 of 5 strains of S. typhimurium tested, in the presence of, but not in the absence of, metabolic activation. It was not mutagenic in an *in vitro* mammalian gene cell mutation (CHO/HGPRT) assay. Zolmitriptan was clastogenic in an *in vitro* human lymphocyte assay both in the absence of and the presence of metabolic activation; it was not clastogenic in an *in vivo* mouse micronucleus assay. It was also not genotoxic in an unscheduled DNA synthesis study.

Impairment of Fertility: Studies of male and female rats administered zolmitriptan prior to and during mating and up to implantation have shown no impairment of fertility at doses up to 400 mg/kg/day. Exposure at this dose was approximately 3000 times exposure at the maximum recommended human dose of 10 mg/day.

Pregnancy: Pregnancy Category C: There are no adequate and well controlled studies in pregnant women; therefore, zolmitriptan should be used during pregnancy only if the potential benefit justifies the potential risk to the fetus. In reproductive toxicity studies in rats and rabbits, oral administration of zolmitriptan to pregnant animals was associated with embryolethality and fetal abnormalities. When pregnant rats were administered oral zolmitriptan during the period of organogenesis at doses of 100, 400 and 1200 mg/kg/day, there was a dose-related increase in embryolethality which became statistically significant at the high dose. The maternal plasma exposures at these doses were approximately 280, 1100 and 5000 times the exposure in humans receiving the maximum recommended total daily dose of 10 mg. The high dose was maternally toxic, as evidenced by a decreased maternal body weight gain during gestation. In a similar study in rabbits, embryolethality was increased at the maternally toxic doses of 10 and 30 mg/kg/day (maternal plasma exposures equivalent to 11 and 42 times exposure in humans receiving the maximum recommended total daily dose of 10 mg), and increased incidences of fetal malformations (fused sternebrae, rib anomalies) and variations (major blood vessel variations, irregular ossification pattern of ribs) were observed at 30 mg/kg/day. Three mg/kg/day was a no effect dose (equivalent to human exposure at a dose of 10 mg). When female rats were given zolmitriptan during gestation, parturition, and lactation, an increased incidence of hydronephrosis was found in the offspring at the maternally toxic dose of 400 mg/kg/day (1100 times human exposure).

Nursing Mothers: It is not known whether zolmitriptan is excreted in human milk. Because many drugs are excreted in human milk, caution should be exercised when zolmitriptan is administered to a nursing woman. Lactating rats dosed with zolmitriptan had milk levels equivalent to maternal plasma levels at 1 hour and 4 times higher than plasma levels at 4 hours.

Pediatric Use: Safety and effectiveness of ZOMIG in pediatric patients have not been established therefore, ZOMIG is not recommended for use in patients under 18 years of age. Postmarketing experience with other triptans includes a limited number of reports that describe pediatric patients who have experienced clinically serious adverse events that are similar in nature to those reported rarely in adults.

Use in the Elderly: Although the pharmacokinetic disposition of the drug in the elderly is similar to that seen in younger adults, there is no information about the safety and effectiveness of zolmitriptan in this population because patients over age 65 were excluded from the controlled clinical trials. (see CLINICAL PHARMACOLOGY: Special Populations)

ADVERSE REACTIONS

Serious cardiac events, including myocardial infarction, have occurred following the use of ZOMIG Tablets. These events are extremely rare and most have been reported in patients with risk factors predictive of CAD. Events reported, in association with drugs of this class, have included coronary artery vasospasm, transient myocardial ischemia, myocardial infarction, ventricular tachycardia, and ventricular fibrillation (see CONTRAINDICATIONS, WARNINGS, and PRECAUTIONS).

Incidence in Controlled Clinical Trials: Among 2,633 patients treated with ZOMIG Tablets in the active and placebo controlled trials, no patients withdrew for reasons related to adverse events, but as patients treated a single headache in these trials, the opportunity for discontinuation was limited. In a long-term, open label study where patients were allowed to treat multiple migraine attacks for up to 1 year, 8% (167 out of 2,058) withdrew from the trial because of adverse experience. The most common events were paresthesia, asthenia, nausea, dizziness, pain, chest or neck tightness or heaviness, somnolence, and warm sensation.

Table 2 lists the adverse events that occurred in ≥ 2% of the 2,074 patients in any one of the ZOMIG 1 mg, ZOMIG 2.5 mg or ZOMIG 5 mg Tablets dose groups of the controlled clinical trials. Only events that were more frequent in a ZOMIG Tablets group compared to the placebo groups are included. The events cited reflect experience gained under closely monitored conditions of clinical trials in a highly selected patient population. In actual clinical practice or in other clinical trials, these frequency estimates may not apply, as the conditions of use, reporting behavior, and the kinds of patients treated may differ.

Several of the adverse events appear dose related, notably paresthesia, sensation of heaviness or tightness in chest, neck, jaw, and throat, dizziness, somnolence, and possibly asthenia and nausea.

[See table above]

Table 2: Adverse Experience Incidence in Five Placebo-Controlled Migraine Clinical Trials: Events Reported By ≥ 2% Patients Treated With ZOMIG Tablets

Adverse Event Type	Placebo (n=401)	ZOMIG 1 mg (n=163)	ZOMIG 2.5 mg (n=498)	ZOMIG 5 mg (n=1012)
ATYPICAL SENSATIONS	**6%**	**12%**	**12%**	**18%**
Hypesthesia	1%	1%	1%	2%
Paresthesia (all types)	2%	5%	7%	9%
Sensation warm/cold	4%	6%	5%	7%
PAIN AND PRESSURE SENSATIONS	**7%**	**13%**	**14%**	**22%**
Chest—pain/tightness/pressure and/or heaviness	1%	2%	3%	4%
Neck/throat/jaw—pain/tightness/pressure	3%	4%	7%	10%
Heaviness other than chest or neck	1%	1%	2%	5%
Pain—location specified	1%	2%	2%	3%
Other—Pressure/tightness/heaviness	0%	2%	2%	2%
DIGESTIVE	**8%**	**11%**	**16%**	**14%**
Dry mouth	2%	5%	3%	3%
Dyspepsia	1%	3%	2%	1%
Dysphagia	0%	0%	0%	2%
Nausea	4%	4%	9%	6%
NEUROLOGICAL	**10%**	**11%**	**17%**	**21%**
Dizziness	4%	6%	8%	10%
Somnolence	3%	5%	6%	8%
Vertigo	0%	0%	0%	2%
OTHER				
Asthenia	3%	5%	3%	9%
Palpitations	1%	0%	<1%	2%
Myalgia	<1%	1%	1%	2%
Myasthenia	<1%	0%	1%	2%
Sweating	1%	0%	2%	3%

ZOMIG is generally well tolerated. Across all doses, most adverse reactions were mild and transient and did not lead to long-lasting effects. The incidence of adverse events in controlled clinical trials was not affected by gender, weight, or age of the patients; use of prophylactic medications; or presence of aura. There were insufficient data to assess the impact of race on the incidence of adverse events.

Other Events: In the paragraphs that follow, the frequencies of less commonly reported adverse clinical events are presented. Because the reports include events observed in open and uncontrolled studies, the role of ZOMIG in their causation cannot be reliably determined. Furthermore, variability associated with adverse event reporting, the terminology used to describe adverse events, etc., limit the value of the quantitative frequency estimates provided. Event frequencies are calculated as the number of patients who used ZOMIG Tablets (n=4,027) and reported an event divided by the total number of patients exposed to ZOMIG Tablets. All reported events are included except those already listed in the previous table, those too general to be informative, and those not reasonably associated with the use of the drug. Events are further classified within body system categories and enumerated in order of decreasing frequency using the following definitions: infrequent adverse events are those occurring in 1/100 to 1/1,000 patients and rare adverse events are those occurring in fewer than 1/1,000 patients.

Atypical sensations: Infrequent was hyperesthesia.

General: Infrequent were allergy reaction, chills, facial edema, fever, malaise and photosensitivity.

Cardiovascular: Infrequent were arrhythmias, hypertension and syncope. Rare were bradycardia, extrasystoles, postural hypotension, QT prolongation, tachycardia and thrombophlebitis.

Digestive: Infrequent were increased appetite, tongue edema, esophagitis, gastroenteritis, liver function abnormality and thirst. Rare were anorexia, constipation, gastritis, hematemesis, pancreatitis, melena, and ulcer.

Hemic: Infrequent was ecchymosis. Rare were cyanosis, thrombocytopenia, eosinophilia and leukopenia.

Metabolic: Infrequent was edema. Rare were hyperglycemia and alkaline phosphatase increased.

Musculoskeletal: Infrequent were back pain, leg cramps and tenosynovitis. Rare were arthritis, asthenia, tetany and twitching.

Neurological: Infrequent were agitation, anxiety, depression, emotional lability and insomnia. Rare were akathesia, amnesia, apathy, ataxia, dystonia, euphoria, hallucinations, cerebral ischemia, hyperkinesia, hypotonia, hypertonia and irritability.

Respiratory: Infrequent were bronchitis, bronchospasm, epistaxis, hiccup, laryngitis, and yawn. Rare were apnea and voice alteration.

Skin: Infrequent were pruritus, rash and urticaria.

Special Senses: Infrequent were dry eye, eye pain, hyperacusis, ear pain, parosmia, and tinnitus. Rare were diplopia and lacrimation.

Urogenital: Infrequent were hematuria, cystitis, polyuria, urinary frequency, urinary urgency. Rare were miscarriage and dysmenorrhea.

The adverse experiences profile seen with ZOMIG-ZMT Tablets was similar to that seen with ZOMIG Tablets.

Postmarketing Experience: The following section enumerates potentially important adverse events that have occurred in clinical practice and which have been reported spontaneously to various surveillance systems. The events enumerated represent reports arising from both domestic and nondomestic use of zolmitriptan. The events enumerated include all except those already listed in the ADVERSE REACTIONS section above or those too general to be informative. Because the reports cite events reported spontaneously from worldwide postmarketing experience, frequency of events and the role of zolmitriptan in their causation cannot be reliably determined.

Cardiovascular: Coronary artery vasospasm; transient myocardial ischemia, angina pectoris, and myocardial infarction.

DRUG ABUSE AND DEPENDENCE

The abuse potential of ZOMIG has not been assessed in clinical trials.

OVERDOSAGE

There is no experience with clinical overdose. Volunteers receiving single 50 mg oral doses of zolmitriptan commonly experienced sedation.

The elimination half-life of ZOMIG is 3 hours (see CLINICAL PHARMACOLOGY), and therefore monitoring of patients after overdose with ZOMIG should continue for at least 15 hours or while symptoms or signs persist.

There is no specific antidote to zolmitriptan. In cases of severe intoxication, intensive care procedures are recommended, including establishing and maintaining a patent airway, ensuring adequate oxygenation and ventilation, and monitoring and support of the cardiovascular system.

It is unknown what effect hemodialysis or peritoneal dialysis has on the plasma concentrations of zolmitriptan.

DOSAGE AND ADMINISTRATION

ZOMIG Tablets

In controlled clinical trials, single doses of 1, 2.5 and 5 mg of ZOMIG Tablets were effective for the acute treatment of migraines in adults. A greater proportion of patients had headache response following a 2.5 or 5 mg dose than following a 1 mg dose (see Table 1). In the only direct comparison of 2.5 and 5 mg, there was little added benefit from the larger dose but side effects are generally increased at 5 mg (see Table 2). Patients should, therefore, be started on 2.5 mg or lower. A dose lower than 2.5 mg can be achieved by manually breaking the scored 2.5 mg tablet in half.

If the headache returns, the dose may be repeated after 2 hours, not to exceed 10 mg within a 24-hour period. Controlled trials have not adequately established the effectiveness of a second dose if the initial dose is ineffective.

The safety of treating an average of more than three headaches in a 30-day period has not been established.

ZOMIG-ZMT Orally Disintegrating Tablets

In a controlled clinical trial, a single dose of 2.5 mg of ZOMIG-ZMT Tablets was effective for the acute treatment of migraines in adults.

If the headache returns, the dose may be repeated after 2 hours, not to exceed 10 mg within a 24-hour period. Controlled trials have not adequately established the effectiveness of a second dose if the initial dose is ineffective.

The safety of treating an average of more than three headaches in a 30-day period has not been established.

Administration with liquid is not necessary. The orally disintegrating tablet is packaged in a blister. Patients should be instructed not to remove the tablet from the blister until just prior to dosing. The blister pack should then be peeled open, and the orally disintegrating tablet placed on the tongue, where it will dissolve and be swallowed with the saliva. It is not recommended to break the orally disintegrating tablet.

Hepatic Impairment: Patients with moderate to severe hepatic impairment have decreased clearance of zolmitriptan and significant elevation in blood pressure was observed in some patients. Use of a low dose with blood pressure monitoring is recommended (see CLINICAL PHARMACOLOGY AND WARNINGS).

HOW SUPPLIED

2.5 mg Tablets—Yellow, biconvex, round, film-coated, scored tablets containing 2.5 mg of zolmitriptan identified with "ZOMIG" and "2.5" debossed on one side are supplied in cartons containing a blister pack of 6 tablets. (NDC 0310-0210-20).

2.5 mg Orally Disintegrating Tablets—White, flat faced, uncoated, bevelled tablet containing 2.5 mg of zolmitriptan identified with a debossed "Z" on one side are supplied in cartons containing a blister pack of 6 tablets. (NDC 0310-0209-20).

5 mg Tablets—Pink, biconvex, film-coated tablets containing 5 mg of zolmitriptan identified with "ZOMIG" and "5" debossed on one side are supplied in cartons containing a blister pack of 3 tablets. (NDC 0310-0211-25).

Continued on next page

Zomig—Cont.

Store both ZOMIG Tablets and ZOMIG-ZMT Tablets at controlled room temperature, 20–25°C (68–77°F) [see USP]. Protect from light and moisture.

PATIENT INFORMATION

The following wording is contained in a separate leaflet provided for patients.

ZOMIG®
(zolmitriptan) Tablets
ZOMIG-ZMT™
(zolmitriptan)
Orally Disintegrating Tablets
Patient Information about
ZOMIG (Zo-mig)
for Migraines

Generic Name: zolmitriptan (zol-mi-trip-tan)

Information for the Consumer on ZOMIG (zolmitriptan) Tablets: Please read this leaflet carefully before you administer ZOMIG Tablets. This provides a summary of the information available on your medicine. Please do not throw away this leaflet until you have finished your medicine. You may need to read this leaflet again. This leaflet does not contain all the information on ZOMIG Tablets. For further information or advice, ask your doctor or pharmacist.

Information About Your Medicine: The name of your medicine is ZOMIG Tablets. It can be obtained only by prescription from your doctor. The decision to use ZOMIG Tablets is one that you and your doctor should make jointly, taking into account your individual preferences and medical circumstances. If you have risk factors for heart disease (such as high blood pressure, high cholesterol, obesity, diabetes, smoking, strong family history of heart disease, or you are postmenopausal or a male over the age of 40), you should tell your doctor, who should evaluate you for heart disease in order to determine if ZOMIG Tablets are appropriate for you.

1. The Purpose of Your Medicine: ZOMIG Tablets are intended to relieve your migraine, but not to prevent or reduce the number of attacks you experience. Use ZOMIG Tablets only to treat an actual migraine attack.

2. Important Questions to Consider Before Using ZOMIG Tablets: If the answer to any of the following questions is **YES** or if you do not know the answer, then you must discuss it with your doctor before you use ZOMIG Tablets.

- Do you have any chest pain, heart disease, shortness of breath, or irregular heartbeats? Have you had a heart attack?
- Do you have risk factors for heart disease (such as high blood pressure, high cholesterol, obesity, diabetes, smoking, strong family history of heart disease, or you are postmenopausal or a male over the age of 40)?
- Do you have high blood pressure?
- Are you pregnant? Do you think you might be pregnant? Are you trying to become pregnant? Are you not using adequate contraception? Are you breast feeding an infant?
- If you are taking ZOMIG-ZMT™, are you sensitive to phenylalanine (a component of the artificial sweetener aspartame)?
- Have you ever had to stop taking this or any other medication because of an allergy or other problems?
- Are you taking any other migraine medications, including 5-HT_1 agonist or migraine medications containing ergotamine, dihydroergotamine, or methysergide?
- Are you taking any medication for depression (monoamine oxidase inhibitors or selective serotonin reuptake inhibitors [SSRIs])?
- Have you had, or do you have, any disease of the liver or kidney?
- Have you had, or do you have, epilepsy or seizures?
- Is this headache different from your usual migraine attacks?

Remember, if you answered **YES** to any of the above questions, then you must discuss it with your doctor.

3. The Use of ZOMIG Tablets During Pregnancy: Do not use ZOMIG Tablets if you are pregnant, think you might be pregnant, are trying to become pregnant, or are not using adequate contraception, unless you have discussed this with your doctor.

4. How to Use ZOMIG Tablets: Adults should be started on a 2.5 mg dose or lower administered by mouth. A dose lower than 2.5 mg can be achieved by manually breaking the conventional film-coated, scored 2.5 mg tablet in half. It is not recommended to break the ZOMIG-ZMT Tablet. If your headache comes back after your initial dose, a second dose may be administered anytime after 2 hours of administering the dose. For any attack where you have no response to the first dose, do not take a second dose without first consulting with your doctor. Do not administer more than a total of 10 mg of ZOMIG Tablets in any 24-hour period. Discard any unused tablets or its portion that have been removed from the blister packaging.

ZOMIG-ZMT Orally Disintegrating Tablets

The blister pack should be peeled open and the orally disintegrating tablet placed on the tongue, where it will dissolve and be swallowed with the saliva.

5. Side Effects to Watch For:

- Some patients experience pain or tightness in the chest or throat when using ZOMIG Tablets. If this happens to you, then discuss it with your doctor before using any more ZOMIG Tablets. If the chest pain is severe or does not go away, call your doctor immediately.
- Shortness of breath; wheeziness; heart throbbing; swelling of eyelids, face, or lips; or a skin rash, skin lumps, or hives happens rarely. If it happens to you, then tell your doctor immediately. Do not take any more ZOMIG Tablets unless your doctor tells you to do so.
- Some people may have feelings of tingling, heat, heaviness or pressure after treatment with ZOMIG Tablets. A few people may feel drowsy, dizzy, tired, or sick. Tell your doctor immediately if you have symptoms that you do not understand.

6. What to Do if an Overdose is Taken: If you have taken more medication than you have been told, contact either your doctor, hospital emergency department, or nearest poison control center immediately. This medicine was prescribed for your particular condition and should not be used by others or for any other condition.

7. Storing Your Medicine: Keep your medicine in a safe place where children cannot reach it. It may be harmful to children. Store your medication away from heat, light, moisture and at a controlled room temperature. If your medication has expired (the expiration date is printed on the treatment pack), throw it away as instructed. If your doctor decides to stop your treatment, do not keep any leftover medicine unless your doctor tells you to. Throw away your medicine as instructed. Be sure that discarded tablets are out of the reach of children.

All trademarks are the property of the AstraZeneca group
© AstraZeneca 2001

ZOMIG®
(zolmitriptan)
Tablets
Manufactured for:
AstraZeneca Pharmaceuticals LP
Wilmington, DE 19850
By: IPR Pharmaceuticals, Inc.
Carolina, PR 00984
ZOMIG-ZMT™
(zolmitriptan)
Orally Disintegrating Tablets
Manufactured for:
AstraZeneca Pharmaceuticals LP
Wilmington, Delaware 19850
By: CIMA Labs, Inc.
Eden Prairie, MN 55344
201653
Rev 02/01 AstraZeneca

Aventis Pharmaceuticals

300 SOMERSET CORPORATE BOULEVARD
BRIDGEWATER, NJ 08807-2854

Direct Inquiries to:
Customer Service
300 Somerset Boulevard
Bridgewater, NJ 08807-2854
(800) 207-8049

For Medical Information Contact:
Generally:
Medical Informatics
300 Somerset Boulevard
Bridgewater, NJ 08807-2854
(800) 633-1610

For information on the following products which are not described, contact the Customer Information Center at (800) 552-3656:

Bentyl® (dicyclomine hydrochloride USP) Capsules, Tablets, Injection, Syrup
Cantil® (mepenzolate bromide USP) Tablets
Cardizem® SR (diltiazem hydrochloride) Capsules
Cardizem® (diltiazem hydrochloride) Tablets
Cephulac® (lactulose solution)
Chronulac® (lactulose solution)
DDAVP® Rhinal Tube 2.5 mL (desmopressin acetate)
Hiprex® (methenamine hippurate)
Lasix® (furosemide) Tablets
Novafed® A (pseudoephedrine hydrochloride and chlorpheniramine maleate) Extended-Release Capsules
Tenuate® (diethylpropion hydrochloride USP) Tablets/Dospan

ALLEGRA® ℞

[ə- 'lĕgra]
(fexofenadine hydrochloride)
Capsules and Tablets

Prescribing information for this product, which appears on pages 673–675 of the 2001 PDR, has been completely revised as follows. Please write "See Supplement A" next to the product heading.

Prescribing Information as of November 2000

DESCRIPTION

Fexofenadine hydrochloride, the active ingredient of ALLEGRA, is a histamine H_1-receptor antagonist with the chemical name (±)-4-[1 hydroxy-4-[4-(hydroxydiphenyl methyl)-1-piperidinyl]-butyl]-α, α-dimethyl benzeneacetic acid hydrochloride. It has the following chemical structure

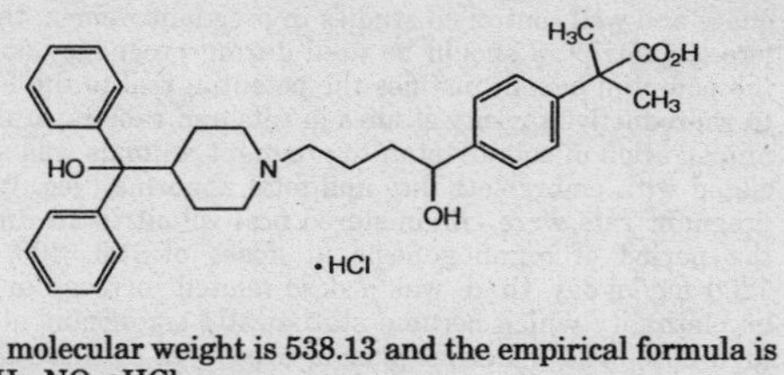

The molecular weight is 538.13 and the empirical formula is $C_{32}H_{39}NO_4 \cdot HCl$.

Fexofenadine hydrochloride is a white to off-white crystalline powder. It is freely soluble in methanol and ethanol, slightly soluble in chloroform and water, and insoluble in hexane. Fexofenadine hydrochloride is a racemate and exists as a zwitterion in aqueous media at physiological pH.

ALLEGRA is formulated as a capsule or tablet for oral administration. Each capsule contains 60 mg fexofenadine hydrochloride and the following excipients: croscarmellose sodium, gelatin, lactose, microcrystalline cellulose, and pregelatinized starch. The printed capsule shell is made from gelatin, iron oxide, silicon dioxide, sodium lauryl sulfate, titanium dioxide, and other ingredients.

Each tablet contains 30, 60, or 180 mg fexofenadine hydrochloride (depending on the dosage strength) and the following excipients: croscarmellose sodium, magnesium stearate, microcrystalline cellulose, and pregelatinized starch. The aqueous tablet film coating is made from hydroxypropyl methylcellulose, iron oxide blends, polyethylene glycol, povidone, silicone dioxide, and titanium dioxide.

CLINICAL PHARMACOLOGY

Mechanism of Action

Fexofenadine hydrochloride is an antihistamine with selective peripheral H_1-receptor antagonist activity. Both enantiomers of fexofenadine hydrochloride displayed approximately equipotent antihistaminic effects. Fexofenadine inhibited histamine release from peritoneal mast cells in rats. In laboratory animals, no anticholinergic, $alpha_1$-adrenergic or beta-adrenergic-receptor blocking effects were observed. No sedative or other central nervous system effects were observed. Radiolabeled tissue distribution studies in rats indicated that fexofenadine does not cross the blood-brain barrier.

Pharmacokinetics

Absorption:

Fexofenadine hydrochloride was rapidly absorbed following oral administration of a single dose of two 60 mg capsules to healthy male volunteers with a mean time to maximum plasma concentration occurring at 2.6 hours post-dose. After administration of a single 60 mg capsule to healthy subjects, the mean maximum plasma concentration was 131 ng/mL. Following single dose oral administrations of either the 60 and 180 mg tablet to healthy, adult male volunteers, mean maximum plasma concentrations were 142 and 494 ng/mL, respectively. The tablet formulations are bioequivalent to the capsule when administered at equal doses. Fexofenadine hydrochloride pharmacokinetics are linear for oral doses up to a total daily dose of 240 mg (120 mg twice daily).

Distribution:

Fexofenadine hydrochloride is 60% to 70% bound to plasma proteins, primarily albumin and α_1-acid glycoprotein.

Elimination:

The mean elimination half-life of fexofenadine was 14.4 hours following administration of 60 mg, twice daily, in normal volunteers.

Human mass balance studies documented a recovery of approximately 80% and 11% of the [^{14}C] fexofenadine hydrochloride dose in the feces and urine, respectively. Because the absolute bioavailability of fexofenadine hydrochloride has not been established, it is unknown if the fecal component represents unabsorbed drug or the result of biliary excretion.

Metabolism:

Approximately 5% of the total oral dose was metabolized.

Special Populations:

Special population pharmacokinetics (for geriatric subjects, renal and hepatic impairment), obtained after a single dose of 80 mg fexofenadine hydrochloride, were compared to those for normal subjects from a separate study of similar design. While subject weights were relatively uniform between studies, these adult special population patients were substantially older than the healthy, young volunteers. Thus, an age effect may be confounding the pharmacokinetic differences observed in some of the special populations.

Seasonal allergic rhinitis (SAR) and chronic idiopathic urticaria (CIU) patients. The pharmacokinetics of fexofenadine hydrochloride in seasonal allergic rhinitis and chronic idiopathic urticaria patients were similar to those in healthy subjects.

Geriatric Subjects. In older subjects (≥65 years old), peak plasma levels of fexofenadine were 99% greater than those observed in normal volunteers (<65 years old). Mean elimination half-lives were similar to those observed in normal volunteers.

Pediatric Patients. Cross study comparisons indicated that fexofenadine hydrochloride area under the curve (AUC) following oral administration of a 60 mg dose to 7–12 year old pediatric allergic rhinitis patients was 56% greater compared to healthy adult subjects given the same dose. Plasma exposure in pediatric patients given 30 mg fexofenadine hydrochloride is comparable to adults given 60 mg.

Renal Impairment. In patients with mild to moderate (creatinine clearance 41–80 mL/min) and severe (creatinine clearance 11–40 mL/min) renal impairment, peak plasma levels of fexofenadine were 87% and 111% greater, respectively, and mean elimination half-lives were 59% and 72% longer, respectively, than observed in normal volunteers. Peak plasma levels in patients on dialysis (creatinine clearance ≤10 mL/min) were 82% greater and half-life was 31% longer than observed in normal volunteers. Based on increases in bioavailability and half-life, a dose of 60 mg once daily is recommended as the starting dose in patients with decreased renal function. (See DOSAGE AND ADMINISTRATION).

Hepatic Impairment. The pharmacokinetics of fexofenadine hydrochloride in patients with hepatic disease did not differ substantially from that observed in healthy patients.

Effect of Gender. Across several trials, no clinically significant gender-related differences were observed in the pharmacokinetics of fexofenadine hydrochloride.

Pharmacodynamics

Wheal and Flare. Human histamine skin wheal and flare studies following single and twice daily doses of 20 and 40 mg fexofenadine hydrochloride demonstrated that the drug exhibits an antihistamine effect by 1 hour, achieves maximum effect at 2 to 3 hours, and an effect is still seen at 12 hours. There was no evidence of tolerance to these effects after 28 days of dosing.

Histamine skin wheal and flare studies in 7 to 12 year old patients showed that following a single dose of 30 or 60 mg, antihistamine effect was observed at 1 hour and reached a maximum by 3 hours. Greater than 49% inhibition of wheal area, and 74% inhibition of flare area were maintained for 8 hours following the 30 and 60 mg dose.

Effects on QT_c. In dogs (30 mg/kg/orally twice a day), and in rabbits (10 mg/kg, infused intravenously over 1 hour) fexofenadine hydrochloride did not prolong QT_c. In dogs the plasma fexofenadine concentration was approximately 9 times the therapeutic plasma concentrations in adults receiving the maximum recommended daily oral dose. In rabbits, the plasma fexofenadine concentration was approximately 20 times the therapeutic plasma concentration in adults receiving the maximum recommended daily oral dose. No effect was observed on calcium channel current, delayed potassium channel current, or action potential duration in guinea pig myocytes, sodium current in rat neonatal myocytes, or on several delayed rectifier potassium channels cloned from human heart at concentrations up to 1×10^{-5} M of fexofenadine hydrochloride.

No statistically significant increase in mean QT_c interval compared to placebo was observed in 714 seasonal allergic rhinitis patients given fexofenadine hydrochloride capsules in doses of 60 to 240 mg twice daily for two weeks. Pediatric patients from two placebo controlled trials (n=855) treated with up to 60 mg fexofenadine hydrochloride twice daily demonstrated no significant treatment or dose-related increases in QT_c. In addition, no statistically significant increase in mean QT_c interval compared to placebo was observed in 40 healthy volunteers given fexofenadine hydrochloride as an oral solution at doses up to 400 mg twice daily for 6 days, or in 231 healthy volunteers given fexofenadine hydrochloride 240 mg once daily for 1 year.

Clinical Studies

Seasonal Allergic Rhinitis:

Adults. In three, 2-week, multicenter, randomized, double-blind, placebo-controlled trials in patients 12 to 68 years of age with seasonal allergic rhinitis (n=1634), fexofenadine hydrochloride 60 mg twice daily significantly reduced total symptom scores (the sum of the individual scores for sneezing, rhinorrhea, itchy nose/palate/throat, itchy/watery/red eyes) compared to placebo. Statistically significant reductions in symptom scores were observed following the first 60 mg dose, with the effect maintained throughout the 12-hour interval. In these studies, there was no additional reduction in total symptom scores with higher doses of fexofenadine hydrochloride up to 240 mg twice daily.

In one 2-week, multicenter, randomized, double-blind clinical trial in patients 12 to 65 years of age with seasonal allergic rhinitis (n=863), fexofenadine hydrochloride 180 mg once daily significantly reduced total symptom scores (the sum of the individual scores for sneezing, rhinorrhea, itchy nose/palate/throat, itchy/watery/red eyes) compared to placebo. Although the number of patients in some of the subgroups was small, there were no significant differences in the effect of fexofenadine hydrochloride across subgroups of patients defined by gender, age, and race. Onset of action for reduction in total symptom scores, excluding nasal congestion, was observed at 60 minutes compared to placebo following a single 60 mg fexofenadine hydrochloride dose administered to patients with seasonal allergic rhinitis who were exposed to ragweed pollen in an environmental exposure unit. In one clinical trial conducted with ALLEGRA 60 mg capsules, and in one clinical trial conducted with ALLEGRA-D extended release tablets, onset of action was seen within 1 to 3 hours.

Pediatrics. Two 2-week multicenter, randomized, placebo-controlled, double-blind trials in 877 pediatric patients 6 to 11 years of age with seasonal allergic rhinitis were conducted at doses of 15, 30, and 60 mg twice daily. In one of these two studies, conducted in 411 pediatric patients, all three doses of fexofenadine hydrochloride significantly reduced total symptom scores (the sum of the individual scores for sneezing, rhinorrhea, itchy nose/palate/throat, itchy/watery/red eyes) compared to placebo, however a dose response relationship was not seen. The 60 mg twice daily dose did not provide any additional benefit over the 30 mg twice daily dose. Furthermore, exposure in pediatric patients given 30 mg fexofenadine hydrochloride is comparable to adults given 60 mg (see CLINICAL PHARMACOLOGY).

Chronic Idiopathic Urticaria:

Two 4-week multicenter, randomized, double-blind, placebo-controlled clinical trials compared four different doses of fexofenadine hydrochloride tablet (20, 60, 120, and 240 mg twice daily) to placebo in patients aged 12 to 70 years with chronic idiopathic urticaria (n=726). Efficacy was demonstrated by a significant reduction in mean pruritus scores (MPS), mean number of wheals (MNW), and mean total symptom scores (MTSS, the sum of the MPS and MNW score). Although all four doses were significantly superior to placebo, symptom reduction was greater and efficacy was maintained over the entire 4-week treatment period with fexofenadine hydrochloride doses of ≥60 mg twice daily. However, no additional benefit of the 120 or 240 mg fexofenadine hydrochloride twice daily dose was seen over the 60 mg twice daily dose in reducing symptom scores. There were no significant differences in the effect of fexofenadine hydrochloride across subgroups of patients defined by gender, age, weight, and race.

INDICATIONS AND USAGE

Seasonal Allergic Rhinitis

ALLEGRA is indicated for the relief of symptoms associated with seasonal allergic rhinitis in adults and children 6 years of age and older. Symptoms treated effectively were sneezing, rhinorrhea, itchy nose/palate/throat, itchy/watery/red eyes.

Chronic Idiopathic Urticaria

ALLEGRA is indicated for treatment of uncomplicated skin manifestations of chronic idiopathic urticaria in adults and children 6 years of age and older. It significantly reduces pruritus and the number of wheals.

CONTRAINDICATIONS

ALLEGRA is contraindicated in patients with known hypersensitivity to any of its ingredients.

PRECAUTIONS

Drug Interaction with Erythromycin and Ketoconazole

Fexofenadine hydrochloride has been shown to exhibit minimal (ca. 5%) metabolism. However, co-administration of fexofenadine hydrochloride with ketoconazole and erythromycin led to increased plasma levels of fexofenadine hydrochloride. Fexofenadine hydrochloride had no effect on the pharmacokinetics of erythromycin and ketoconazole. In two separate studies, fexofenadine hydrochloride 120 mg twice daily (two times the recommended twice daily dose) was co-administered with erythromycin 500 mg every 8 hours or ketoconazole 400 mg once daily under steady-state conditions to normal, healthy volunteers (n=24, each study). No differences in adverse events or QT_c interval were observed when patients were administered fexofenadine hydrochloride alone or in combination with erythromycin or ketoconazole. The findings of these studies are summarized in the following table:

[See table above]

Effects on steady-state fexofenadine hydrochloride pharmacokinetics after 7 days of co-administration with fexofenadine hydrochloride 120 mg every 12 hours (two times the recommended twice daily dose) in normal volunteers (n=24)

Concomitant Drug	C_{maxSS} *(Peak plasma concentration)*	$AUC_{SS(0-12h)}$ *(Extent of systemic exposure)*
Erythromycin (500 mg every 8 hrs)	+82%	+109%
Ketoconazole (400 mg once daily)	+135%	+164%

The changes in plasma levels were within the range of plasma levels achieved in adequate and well-controlled clinical trials.

The mechanism of these interactions has been evaluated in *in vitro, in situ,* and *in vivo* animal models. These studies indicate that ketoconazole or erythromycin co-administration enhances fexofenadine gastrointestinal absorption. *In vivo* animal studies also suggest that in addition to increasing absorption, ketoconazole decreases fexofenadine hydrochloride gastrointestinal secretion, while erythromycin may also decrease biliary excretion.

Drug Interactions with Antacids

Administration of 120 mg of fexofenadine hydrochloride (2 × 60 mg capsule) within 15 minutes of an aluminum and magnesium containing antacid (Maalox®) decreased fexofenadine AUC by 41% and C_{max} by 43%. ALLEGRA should not be taken closely in time with aluminum and magnesium containing antacids.

Carcinogenesis, Mutagenesis, Impairment of Fertility

The carcinogenic potential and reproductive toxicity of fexofenadine hydrochloride were assessed using terfenadine studies with adequate fexofenadine hydrochloride exposure (based on plasma area-under-the-concentration vs. time [AUC] values). No evidence of carcinogenicity was observed in an 18-month study in mice and in a 24-month study in rats at oral doses up to 150 mg/kg of terfenadine (which led to fexofenadine exposures that were respectively approximately 3 and 5 times the exposure from the maximum recommended daily oral dose of fexofenadine hydrochloride in adults and children).

In *in vitro* (Bacterial Reverse Mutation, CHO/HGPRT Forward Mutation, and Rat Lymphocyte Chromosomal Aberration assays) and *in vivo* (Mouse Bone Marrow Micronucleus assay) tests, fexofenadine hydrochloride revealed no evidence of mutagenicity.

In rat fertility studies, dose-related reductions in implants and increases in postimplantation losses were observed at an oral dose of 150 mg/kg of terfenadine (which led to fexofenadine hydrochloride exposures that were approximately 3 times the exposure of the maximum recommended daily oral dose of fexofenadine hydrochloride in adults).

Pregnancy

Teratogenic Effects: Category C. There was no evidence of teratogenicity in rats or rabbits at oral doses of terfenadine up to 300 mg/kg (which led to fexofenadine exposures that were approximately 4 and 31 times, respectively, the exposure from the maximum recommended daily oral dose of fexofenadine in adults).

There are no adequate and well controlled studies in pregnant women. Fexofenadine should be used during pregnancy only if the potential benefit justifies the potential risk to the fetus.

Nonteratogenic Effects. Dose-related decreases in pup weight gain and survival were observed in rats exposed to an oral dose of 150 mg/kg of terfenadine (approximately 3 times the maximum recommended daily oral dose of fexofenadine hydrochloride in adults based on comparison of fexofenadine hydrochloride AUCs).

Nursing Mothers

There are no adequate and well-controlled studies in women during lactation. Because many drugs are excreted in human milk, caution should be exercised when fexofenadine hydrochloride is administered to a nursing woman.

Pediatric Use

The recommended dose in patients 6 to 11 years of age is based on cross-study comparison of the pharmacokinetics of ALLEGRA in adults and pediatric patients and on the safety profile of fexofenadine hydrochloride in both adult and pediatric patients at doses equal to or higher than the recommended doses.

The safety of ALLEGRA tablets at a dose of 30 mg twice daily has been demonstrated in 438 pediatric patients 6 to 11 years of age in two placebo-controlled 2-week seasonal allergic rhinitis trials. The safety of ALLEGRA for the treatment of chronic idiopathic urticaria in patients 6 to 11 years of age is based on cross-study comparison of the pharmacokinetics of ALLEGRA in adult and pediatric patients and on the safety profile of fexofenadine in both adult and pediatric patients at doses equal to or higher than the recommended dose.

The effectiveness of ALLEGRA for the treatment of seasonal allergic rhinitis in patients 6 to 11 years of age was demonstrated in one trial (n=411) in which ALLEGRA tablets 30 mg twice daily significantly reduced total symptom scores compared to placebo, along with extrapolation of demonstrated efficacy in patients ages 12 years and above, and the pharmacokinetic comparisons in adults and children. The effectiveness of ALLEGRA for the treatment of chronic idiopathic urticaria in patients 6 to 11 years of age is based on an extrapolation of the demonstrated efficacy of ALLEGRA in adults with this condition and the likelihood that the disease course, pathophysiology and the drug's effect are substantially similar in children to that of adult patients.

The safety and effectiveness of ALLEGRA in pediatric patients under 6 years of age have not been established.

Geriatric Use

Clinical studies of ALLEGRA tablets and capsules did not include sufficient numbers of subjects aged 65 years and over to determine whether this population responds differently from younger patients. Other reported clinical experience has not identified differences in responses between the geriatric and younger patients. This drug is known to be substantially excreted by the kidney, and the risk of toxic reactions to this drug may be greater in patients with impaired renal function. Because elderly patients are more likely to have decreased renal function, care should be taken in dose selection, and may be useful to monitor renal function. (See CLINICAL PHARMACOLOGY).

ADVERSE REACTIONS

Seasonal Allergic Rhinitis

Adults. In placebo-controlled seasonal allergic rhinitis clinical trials in patients 12 years of age and older, which included 2461 patients receiving fexofenadine hydrochloride capsules at doses of 20 mg to 240 mg twice daily, adverse events were similar in fexofenadine hydrochloride and placebo-treated patients. All adverse events that were reported by greater than 1% of patients who received the recommended daily dose of fexofenadine hydrochloride (60 mg capsules twice daily), and that were more common with fexofenadine hydrochloride than placebo, are listed in Table 1.

In a placebo-controlled clinical study in the United States, which included 570 patients aged 12 years and older receiving fexofenadine hydrochloride tablets at doses of 120 or 180 mg once daily, adverse events were similar in

Continued on next page

Allegra—Cont.

fexofenadine hydrochloride and placebo-treated patients. Table 1 also lists adverse experiences that were reported by greater than 2% of patients treated with fexofenadine hydrochloride tablets at doses of 180 mg once daily and that were more common with fexofenadine hydrochloride than placebo.

The incidence of adverse events, including drowsiness, was not dose-related and was similar across subgroups defined by age, gender, and race.

[See table 1 above]

The frequency and magnitude of laboratory abnormalities were similar in fexofenadine hydrochloride and placebo-treated patients.

Pediatric. Table 2 lists adverse experiences in patients aged 6 to 11 years of age which were reported by greater than 2% of patients treated with fexofenadine hydrochloride tablets at a dose of 30 mg twice daily in placebo-controlled seasonal allergic rhinitis studies in the United States and Canada that were more common with fexofenadine hydrochloride than placebo.

[See table 2 above]

Chronic Idiopathic Urticaria

Adverse events reported by patients 12 years of age and older in placebo-controlled chronic idiopathic urticaria studies were similar to those reported in placebo-controlled seasonal allergic rhinitis studies. In placebo-controlled chronic idiopathic urticaria clinical trials, which included 726 patients 12 years of age and older receiving fexofenadine hydrochloride tablets at doses of 20 to 240 mg twice daily, adverse events were similar in fexofenadine hydrochloride and placebo-treated patients. Table 3 lists adverse experiences in patients aged 12 years and older which were reported by greater than 2% of patients treated with fexofenadine hydrochloride 60 mg tablets twice daily in controlled clinical studies in the United States and Canada and that were more common with fexofenadine hydrochloride than placebo. The safety of fexofenadine hydrochloride in the treatment of chronic idiopathic urticaria in pediatric patients 6 to 11 years of age is based on the safety profile of fexofenadine hydrochloride in adults and adolescent patients at doses equal to or higher than the recommended dose (see Pediatric Use).

[See table 3 above]

Events that have been reported during controlled clinical trials involving seasonal allergic rhinitis and chronic idiopathic urticaria patients with incidences less than 1% and similar to placebo and have been rarely reported during postmarketing surveillance include: insomnia, nervousness, and sleep disorders or paroniria. In rare cases, rash, urticaria, pruritus and hypersensitivity reactions with manifestations such as angioedema, chest tightness, dyspnea, flushing and systemic anaphylaxis have been reported.

OVERDOSAGE

Reports of fexofenadine hydrochloride overdose have been infrequent and contain limited information. However, dizziness, drowsiness, and dry mouth have been reported. Single doses of fexofenadine hydrochloride up to 800 mg (six normal volunteers at this dose level), and doses up to 690 mg twice daily for 1 month (three normal volunteers at this dose level) or 240 mg once daily for 1 year (234 normal volunteers at this dose level) were administered without the development of clinically significant adverse events as compared to placebo.

In the event of overdose, consider standard measures to remove any unabsorbed drug. Symptomatic and supportive treatment is recommended.

Hemodialysis did not effectively remove fexofenadine hydrochloride from blood (1.7% removed) following terfenadine administration.

No deaths occurred at oral doses of fexofenadine hydrochloride up to 5000 mg/kg in mice (110 times the maximum recommended daily oral dose in adults and 200 times the maximum recommended daily oral dose in children based on mg/m^2) and up to 5000 mg/kg in rats (230 times the maximum recommended daily oral dose in adults and 400 times the maximum recommended daily oral dose in children based on mg/m^2). Additionally, no clinical signs of toxicity or gross pathological findings were observed. In dogs, no evidence of toxicity was observed at oral doses up to 2000 mg/kg (300 times the maximum recommended daily oral dose in adults and 530 times the maximum recommended daily oral dose in children based on mg/m^2).

DOSAGE AND ADMINISTRATION

Seasonal Allergic Rhinitis

Adults and Children 12 Years and Older. The recommended dose of ALLEGRA is 60 mg twice daily, or 180 mg once daily. A dose of 60 mg once daily is recommended as the starting dose in patients with decreased renal function (see CLINICAL PHARMACOLOGY).

Children 6 to 11 Years. The recommended dose of ALLEGRA is 30 mg twice daily. A dose of 30 mg once daily is recommended as the starting dose in pediatric patients with decreased renal function (see CLINICAL PHARMACOLOGY).

Chronic Idiopathic Urticaria

Adults and Children 12 Years and Older. The recommended dose of ALLEGRA is 60 mg twice daily. A dose of 60 mg once daily is recommended as the starting dose in patients with decreased renal function (see CLINICAL PHARMACOLOGY).

Children 6 to 11 Years. The recommended dose of ALLEGRA is 30 mg twice daily. A dose of 30 mg once daily is recom-

mended as the starting dose in pediatric patients with decreased renal function (see CLINICAL PHARMACOLOGY).

HOW SUPPLIED

ALLEGRA 60 mg capsules are available in: high-density polyethylene (HDPE) bottles of 60 (NDC 0088-1102-41); HDPE bottles of 100 (NDC 0088-1102-47); HDPE bottles of 500 (NDC 0088-1102-55); and aluminum-foil blister packs of 100 (NDC 0088-1102-49).

ALLEGRA capsules have a white opaque cap and a pink opaque body. The capsules are imprinted in black ink, with "ALLEGRA" on the cap and "60 mg" on the body.

ALLEGRA 30 mg tablets are available in: high-density polyethylene (HDPE) bottles of 100 (NDC 0088-1106-47) with a polypropylene screw cap containing a pulp/wax liner with heat-sealed foil inner seal and HDPE bottles of 500 (NDC 0088-1106-55) with a polypropylene screw cap containing a pulp/wax liner with heat-sealed foil inner seal.

ALLEGRA 60 mg tablets are available in: HDPE bottles of 100 (NDC 0088-1107-47) with a polypropylene screw cap containing a pulp/wax liner with heat-sealed foil inner seal; HDPE bottles of 500 (NDC 0088-1107-55) with a polypropylene screw cap containing a pulp/wax liner with heat-sealed foil inner seal; and aluminum foil-backed clear blister packs of 100 (NDC 0088-1107-49).

ALLEGRA 180 mg tablets are available in: HDPE bottles of 100 (NDC 0088-1109-47) with a polypropylene screw cap containing a pulp/wax liner with heat-sealed foil inner seal; and HDPE bottles of 500 (NDC 0088-1109-55) with a polypropylene screw cap containing a pulp/wax liner with heat-sealed foil inner seal.

ALLEGRA tablets are coated with a peach colored film coating. Tablets have the following unique identifiers: 30 mg tablets have 03 on one side and either 0088 or scripted E on the other; 60 mg tablets have 06 on one side and either 0088 or scripted E on the other; and 180 mg tablets have 018 on one side and either 0088 or scripted E on the other.

Store ALLEGRA capsules and tablets at controlled room temperature 20–25°C (68–77°F). (See USP Controlled Room Temperature.) Foil-backed blister packs containing ALLEGRA capsules and all tablet packaging should be protected from excessive moisture.

Prescribing Information as of November 2000
Aventis Pharmaceuticals Inc.
Kansas City, MO 64137 USA
US Patents 4,254,129; 5,375,693; 5,578,610
www.allegra.com

allp1100p

Table 1

Adverse experiences in patients ages 12 years and older reported in placebo-controlled seasonal allergic rhinitis clinical trials in the United States

Twice daily dosing with fexofenadine capsules at rates of greater than 1%

Adverse experience	Fexofenadine 60 mg Twice Daily (n=679)	Placebo Twice Daily (n=671)
Viral Infection (cold, flu)	2.5%	1.5%
Nausea	1.6%	1.5%
Dysmenorrhea	1.5%	0.3%
Drowsiness	1.3%	0.9%
Dyspepsia	1.3%	0.6%
Fatigue	1.3%	0.9%

Once daily dosing with fexofenadine hydrochloride tablets at rates of greater than 2%

Adverse experience	Fexofenadine 180 mg once daily (n=283)	Placebo (n=293)
Headache	10.6%	7.5%
Upper Respiratory Tract Infection	3.2%	3.1%
Back Pain	2.8%	1.4%

Table 2

Adverse experiences reported in placebo-controlled seasonal allergic rhinitis studies in pediatric patients ages 6 to 11 in the United States and Canada at rates of greater than 2%

Adverse experience	Fexofenadine 30 mg twice daily (n=209)	Placebo (n=229)
Headache	7.2%	6.6%
Accidental Injury	2.9%	1.3%
Coughing	3.8%	1.3%
Fever	2.4%	0.9%
Pain	2.4%	0.4%
Otitis Media	2.4%	0.0%
Upper Respiratory Tract Infection	4.3%	1.7%

Table 3

Adverse experiences reported in patients 12 years and older in placebo-controlled chronic idiopathic urticaria studies in the United States and Canada at rates of greater than 2%

Adverse experience	Fexofenadine 60 mg twice daily (n=186)	Placebo (n=178)
Back Pain	2.2%	1.1%
Sinusitis	2.2%	1.1%
Dizziness	2.2%	0.6%
Drowsiness	2.2%	0.0%

ALLEGRA-D® ℞

[ə-'lĕgra-D]

(fexofenadine HCl 60 mg and pseudoephedrine HCl 120 mg) Extended-Release Tablets

Prescribing information for this product, which appears on pages 675–678 of the 2001 PDR, has been completely revised as follows. Please write "See Supplement A" next to the product heading.

Prescribing Information as of November 2000

DESCRIPTION

ALLEGRA-D® (fexofenadine hydrochloride and pseudoephedrine hydrochloride) Extended-Release Tablets for oral administration contain 60 mg fexofenadine hydrochloride for immediate-release and 120 mg pseudoephedrine hydrochloride for extended-release. Tablets also contain as excipients: microcrystalline cellulose, pregelatinized starch, croscarmellose sodium, magnesium stearate, carnauba wax, stearic acid, silicon dioxide, hydroxypropyl methylcellulose and polyethylene glycol.

Fexofenadine hydrochloride, one of the active ingredients of ALLEGRA-D, is a histamine H$_1$-receptor antagonist with the chemical name ($\pm$)-4-[1-hydroxy-4-[4-(hydroxydiphenylmethyl)-1-piperidinyl]-butyl]-α, α-dimethyl benzeneacetic acid hydrochloride and the following chemical structure:

• HCl

The molecular weight is 538.13 and the empirical formula is C$_{32}$H$_{39}$NO$_4$•HCl. Fexofenadine hydrochloride is a white to off-white crystalline powder. It is freely soluble in methanol and ethanol, slightly soluble in chloroform and water, and insoluble in hexane. Fexofenadine hydrochloride is a racemate and exists as a zwitterion in aqueous media at physiological pH.

Pseudoephedrine hydrochloride, the other active ingredient of ALLEGRA-D, is an adrenergic (vasoconstrictor) agent with the chemical name [S-(R*,R*)]-α-[1-(methylamino) ethyl]-benzenemethanol hydrochloride and the following chemical structure:

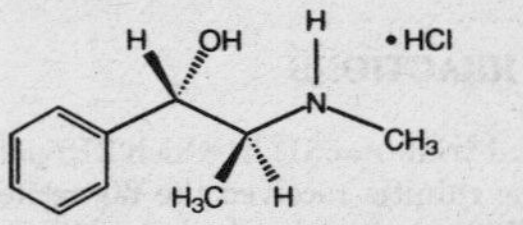

The molecular weight is 201.70. The molecular formula is $C_{10}H_{15}NO \bullet HCl$. Pseudoephedrine hydrochloride occurs as fine, white to off-white crystals or powder, having a faint characteristic odor. It is very soluble in water, freely soluble in alcohol, and sparingly soluble in chloroform.

CLINICAL PHARMACOLOGY

Mechanism of Action

Fexofenadine hydrochloride, the major active metabolite of terfenadine, is an antihistamine with selective peripheral H_1-receptor antagonist activity. Fexofenadine hydrochloride inhibited antigen-induced bronchospasm in sensitized guinea pigs and histamine release from peritoneal mast cells in rats. In laboratory animals, no anticholinergic or alpha$_1$-adrenergic-receptor blocking effects were observed. Moreover, no sedative or other central nervous system effects were observed. Radiolabeled tissue distribution studies in rats indicated that fexofenadine does not cross the blood-brain barrier.

Pseudoephedrine hydrochloride is an orally active sympathomimetic amine and exerts a decongestant action on the nasal mucosa. Pseudoephedrine hydrochloride is recognized as an effective agent for the relief of nasal congestion due to allergic rhinitis. Pseudoephedrine produces peripheral effects similar to those of ephedrine and central effects similar to, but less intense than, amphetamines. It has the potential for excitatory side effects. At the recommended oral dose, it has little or no pressor effect in normotensive adults.

Pharmacokinetics

The pharmacokinetics of fexofenadine hydrochloride and pseudoephedrine hydrochloride when administered separately have been well characterized. Fexofenadine pharmacokinetics were linear for oral doses of fexofenadine hydrochloride up to 120 mg twice daily. The mean elimination half-life of fexofenadine was 14.4 hours following administration of 60 mg fexofenadine hydrochloride, twice daily, to steady-state in normal volunteers. Human mass balance studies documented a recovery of approximately 80% and 11% of the [^{14}C] fexofenadine hydrochloride dose in the feces and urine, respectively. Approximately 5% of the total dose was metabolized. Because the absolute bioavailability of fexofenadine hydrochloride has not been established, it is unknown if the fecal component is unabsorbed drug or the result of biliary excretion. The pharmacokinetics of fexofenadine hydrochloride in seasonal allergic rhinitis patients were similar to those in healthy subjects. Peak fexofenadine plasma concentrations were similar between adolescent (12–16 years of age) and adult patients. Fexofenadine is 60% to 70% bound to plasma proteins, primarily albumin and α_1-acid glycoprotein.

Pseudoephedrine has been shown to have a mean elimination half-life of 4–6 hours which is dependent on urine pH. The elimination half-life is decreased at urine pH lower than 6 and may be increased at urine pH higher than 8.

The bioavailability of fexofenadine hydrochloride and pseudoephedrine hydrochloride from ALLEGRA-D Extended-Release Tablets is similar to that achieved with separate administration of the components. Coadministration of fexofenadine and pseudoephedrine does not significantly affect the bioavailability of either component.

Fexofenadine hydrochloride was rapidly absorbed following single-dose administration of the 60 mg fexofenadine hydrochloride/120 mg pseudoephedrine hydrochloride tablet with median time to mean maximum fexofenadine plasma concentration of 191 ng/mL occurring 2 hours postdose. Pseudoephedrine hydrochloride produced a mean single-dose pseudoephedrine peak plasma concentration of 206 ng/mL which occurred 6 hours postdose. Following multiple dosing to steady-state, a fexofenadine peak concentration of 255 ng/mL was observed 2 hours postdose. Following multiple dosing to steady-state, a pseudoephedrine peak concentration of 411 ng/mL was observed 5 hours postdose. Coadministration of ALLEGRA-D with a high-fat meal decreased fexofenadine plasma concentrations C_{max} (−46%) and AUC (−42%). Time to maximum concentration (T_{max}) was delayed by 50%. The rate or extent of pseudoephedrine absorption was not affected by food. It is recommended that the administration of ALLEGRA-D with food should be avoided. (See DOSAGE AND ADMINISTRATION).

Special Populations

Special population pharmacokinetics (for renal and hepatic impairment and age), obtained after a single dose of 80 mg fexofenadine hydrochloride, were compared to those from normal subjects in a separate study of similar design. While subject weights were relatively uniform between studies, these special population patients were substantially older than the healthy, young volunteers. Thus, an age effect may be confounding the pharmacokinetic differences observed in some of the special populations.

Effect of Age. In older subjects (≥65 years old), peak plasma levels of fexofenadine were 99% greater than those observed in younger subjects (<65 years old). Mean elimination half-lives were similar to those observed in younger subjects.

Renally Impaired. In patients with mild (creatinine clearance 41–80 mL/min) to severe (creatinine clearance 11–40 mL/min) renal impairment, peak plasma levels of fexofenadine were 87% and 111% greater, respectively, and mean elimination half-lives were 59% and 72% longer, respectively, than observed in normal volunteers. Peak plasma levels in patients on dialysis (creatinine clearance ≤10 mL/min) were 82% greater and half-life was 31% longer than observed in normal volunteers.

About 55–75% of an administered dose of pseudoephedrine hydrochloride is excreted unchanged in the urine; the remainder is apparently metabolized in the liver. Therefore, pseudoephedrine may accumulate in patients with renal insufficiency.

Based on increases in bioavailability and half-life of fexofenadine hydrochloride and pseudoephedrine hydrochloride, a dose of one tablet once daily is recommended as the starting dose in patients with decreased renal function (See DOSAGE AND ADMINISTRATION).

Hepatically Impaired. The pharmacokinetics of fexofenadine hydrochloride in patients with hepatic disease did not differ substantially from that observed in healthy subjects. The effect on pseudoephedrine pharmacokinetics is unknown.

Effect of Gender. Across several trials, no clinically significant gender-related differences were observed in the pharmacokinetics of fexofenadine hydrochloride.

Pharmacodynamics

Wheal and Flare. Human histamine skin wheal and flare studies following single and twice daily doses of 20 mg and 40 mg fexofenadine hydrochloride demonstrated that the drug exhibits an antihistamine effect by 1 hour, achieves maximum effect at 2–3 hours, and an effect is still seen at 12 hours. There was no evidence of tolerance to these effects after 28 days of dosing. The clinical significance of these observations is not known.

Effects on QT_c. In dogs, (10 mg/kg/day, orally for 5 days) and rabbits (10 mg/kg, intravenously over one hour) fexofenadine hydrochloride did not prolong QT_c at plasma concentrations that were at least 28 and 63 times, respectively, the therapeutic plasma concentrations in man (based on a 60 mg twice daily fexofenadine hydrochloride dose). No effect was observed on calcium channel current, delayed K^+ channel current, or action potential duration in guinea pig myocytes, Na^+ current in rat neonatal myocytes, or on the delayed rectifier K^+ channel cloned from human heart at concentrations up to 1×10^{-5} M of fexofenadine. This concentration was at least 32 times the therapeutic plasma concentration in man (based on a 60 mg twice daily fexofenadine hydrochloride dose).

No statistically significant increase in mean QT_c interval compared to placebo was observed in 714 seasonal allergic rhinitis patients given fexofenadine hydrochloride capsules in doses of 60 mg to 240 mg twice daily for two weeks or in 40 healthy volunteers given fexofenadine hydrochloride as an oral solution at doses up to 400 mg twice daily for 6 days. A one year study designed to evaluate safety and tolerability of 240 mg of fexofenadine hydrochloride (n=240) compared to placebo (n=237) in healthy subjects, did not reveal a statistically significant increase in the mean QT_c interval for the fexofenadine hydrochloride treated group when evaluated pretreatment and after 1, 2, 3, 6, 9, and 12 months of treatment.

Administration of the 60 mg fexofenadine hydrochloride/120 mg pseudoephedrine hydrochloride combination tablet for approximately 2 weeks to 213 patients with seasonal allergic rhinitis demonstrated no statistically significant increase in the mean QT_c interval compared to fexofenadine hydrochloride administered alone (60 mg twice daily, n=215), or compared to pseudoephedrine hydrochloride (120 mg twice daily, n=215) administered alone.

Clinical Studies

In a 2-week, multicenter, randomized, double-blind, active-controlled trial in patients 12–65 years of age with seasonal allergic rhinitis due to ragweed allergy (n=651), the 60 mg fexofenadine hydrochloride/120 mg pseudoephedrine hydrochloride combination tablet administered twice daily significantly reduced the intensity of sneezing, rhinorrhea, itchy nose/palate/throat, itchy/watery/red eyes, and nasal congestion.

In three, 2-week, multicenter, randomized, double-blind, placebo-controlled trials in patients 12–68 years of age with seasonal allergic rhinitis (n=1634), fexofenadine hydrochloride 60 mg twice daily significantly reduced total symptom scores (the sum of the individual scores for sneezing, rhinorrhea, itchy nose/palate/throat, itchy/watery/red eyes) compared to placebo. Statistically significant reductions in symptom scores were observed following the first 60 mg dose, with the effect maintained throughout the 12-hour interval. In general, there was no additional reduction in total symptom scores with higher doses of fexofenadine hydrochloride up to 240 mg twice daily. Although the number of subjects in some of the subgroups was small, there were no significant differences in the effect of fexofenadine hydrochloride across subgroups of patients defined by gender, age, and race. Onset of action for reduction in total symptom scores, excluding nasal congestion, was observed at 60 minutes compared to placebo following a single 60 mg fexofenadine hydrochloride dose administered to patients with seasonal allergic rhinitis who were exposed to ragweed pollen in an environmental exposure unit.

INDICATIONS AND USAGE

ALLEGRA-D is indicated for the relief of symptoms associated with seasonal allergic rhinitis in adults and children 12 years of age and older. Symptoms treated effectively include sneezing, rhinorrhea, itchy nose/palate/ and/or throat, itchy/watery/red eyes, and nasal congestion.

ALLEGRA-D should be administered when both the antihistaminic properties of fexofenadine hydrochloride and the nasal decongestant properties of pseudoephedrine hydrochloride are desired (see CLINICAL PHARMACOLOGY).

CONTRAINDICATIONS

ALLEGRA-D is contraindicated in patients with known hypersensitivity to any of its ingredients.

Due to its pseudoephedrine component, ALLEGRA-D is contraindicated in patients with narrow-angle glaucoma or urinary retention, and in patients receiving monoamine oxidase (MAO) inhibitor therapy or within fourteen (14) days of stopping such treatment (see Drug Interactions section). It is also contraindicated in patients with severe hypertension, or severe coronary artery disease, and in those who have shown hypersensitivity or idiosyncrasy to its components, to adrenergic agents, or to other drugs of similar chemical structures. Manifestations of patient idiosyncrasy to adrenergic agents include: insomnia, dizziness, weakness, tremor, or arrhythmias.

WARNINGS

Sympathomimetic amines should be used judiciously and sparingly in patients with hypertension, diabetes mellitus, ischemic heart disease, increased intraocular pressure, hyperthyroidism, renal impairment, or prostatic hypertrophy (see CONTRAINDICATIONS). Sympathomimetic amines may produce central nervous system stimulation with convulsions or cardiovascular collapse with accompanying hypotension.

PRECAUTIONS

General

Due to its pseudoephedrine component, ALLEGRA-D should be used with caution in patients with hypertension, diabetes mellitus, ischemic heart disease, increased intraocular pressure, hyperthyroidism, renal impairment, or prostatic hypertrophy (see WARNINGS and CONTRAINDICATIONS). Patients with decreased renal function should be given a lower initial dose (one tablet per day) because they have reduced elimination of fexofenadine and pseudoephedrine (See CLINICAL PHARMACOLOGY and DOSAGE AND ADMINISTRATION).

Information for Patients

Patients taking ALLEGRA-D tablets should receive the following information: ALLEGRA-D tablets are prescribed for the relief of symptoms of seasonal allergic rhinitis. Patients should be instructed to take ALLEGRA-D tablets only as prescribed. **Do not exceed the recommended dose.** If nervousness, dizziness, or sleeplessness occur, discontinue use and consult the doctor. Patients should also be advised against the concurrent use of ALLEGRA-D tablets with over-the-counter antihistamines and decongestants.

The product should not be used by patients who are hypersensitive to it or to any of its ingredients. Due to its pseudoephedrine component, this product should not be used by patients with narrow-angle glaucoma, urinary retention, or by patients receiving a monoamine oxidase (MAO) inhibitor or within 14 days of stopping use of MAO inhibitor. It also should not be used by patients with severe hypertension or severe coronary artery disease.

Patients should be told that this product should be used in pregnancy or lactation only if the potential benefit justifies the potential risk to the fetus or nursing infant. Patients should be cautioned not to break or chew the tablet. Patients should be directed to swallow the tablet whole. Patients should be instructed not to take the tablet with food. Patients should also be instructed to store the medication in a tightly closed container in a cool, dry place, away from children.

Drug Interactions

Fexofenadine hydrochloride and pseudoephedrine hydrochloride do not influence the pharmacokinetics of each other when administered concomitantly.

Fexofenadine has been shown to exhibit minimal (ca. 5%) metabolism. However, co-administration of fexofenadine with ketoconazole and erythromycin led to increased plasma levels of fexofenadine. Fexofenadine had no effect on the pharmacokinetics of erythromycin and ketoconazole. In two separate studies, fexofenadine HCl 120 mg BID (twice the recommended dose) was co-administered with erythromycin 500 mg every 8 hours or ketoconazole 400 mg once daily under steady-state conditions to normal, healthy volunteers (n=24, each study). No differences in adverse events or QT_c interval were observed when subjects were administered fexofenadine HCl alone or in combination with erythromycin or ketoconazole. The findings of these studies are summarized in the following table:

Effects on Steady-State Fexofenadine Pharmacokinetics After 7 Days of Co-Administration with Fexofenadine Hydrochloride 120 mg Every 12 Hours (twice recommended dose) in Normal Volunteers (n=24)

Concomitant Drug	$C_{max,SS}$ (Peak plasma concentration)	AUC_{SS} (0–12h) (Extent of systemic exposure)
Erythromycin (500 mg every 8 hrs)	+82%	+109%
Ketoconazole (400 mg once daily)	+135%	+164%

Continued on next page

Allegra-D—Cont.

The changes in plasma levels were within the range of plasma levels achieved in adequate and well-controlled clinical trials.
The mechanism of these interactions has been evaluated in in vitro, in situ and in vivo animal models. These studies indicate that ketoconazole or erythromycin co-administration enhances fexofenadine gastrointestinal absorption. In vivo animal studies also suggest that in addition to enhancing absorption, ketoconazole decreases fexofenadine gastrointestinal secretion, while erythromycin may also decrease biliary excretion.
ALLEGRA-D tablets (pseudoephedrine component) are contraindicated in patients taking monoamine oxidase inhibitors and for 14 days after stopping use of an MAO inhibitor. Concomitant use with antihypertensive drugs which interfere with sympathetic activity (eg, methyldopa, mecamylamine, and reserpine) may reduce their antihypertensive effects. Increased ectopic pacemaker activity can occur when pseudoephedrine is used concomitantly with digitalis.
Care should be taken in the administration of ALLEGRA-D concomitantly with other sympathomimetic amines because combined effects on the cardiovascular system may be harmful to the patient (see WARNINGS).

Carcinogenesis, Mutagenesis, Impairment of Fertility
There are no animal or in vitro studies on the combination product fexofenadine hydrochloride and pseudoephedrine hydrochloride to evaluate carcinogenesis, mutagenesis, or impairment of fertility.
The carcinogenic potential and reproductive toxicity of fexofenadine hydrochloride were assessed using terfenadine studies with adequate fexofenadine exposure (area-under-the plasma concentration versus time curve [AUC]). No evidence of carcinogenicity was observed when mice and rats were given daily oral doses up to 150 mg/kg of terfenadine for 18 and 24 months, respectively. In both species, 150 mg/kg of terfenadine produced AUC values of fexofenadine that were approximately 3 times the human AUC at the maximum recommended daily oral dose in adults.
Two-year feeding studies in rats and mice conducted under the auspices of the National Toxicology Program (NTP) demonstrated no evidence of carcinogenic potential with ephedrine sulfate, a structurally related drug with pharmacological properties similar to pseudoephedrine, at doses up to 10 and 27 mg/kg, respectively (approximately 1/3 and 1/2, respectively, the maximum recommended daily oral dose of pseudoephedrine hydrochloride in adults on a mg/m^2 basis).
In in-vitro (Bacterial Reverse Mutation, CHO/HGPRT Forward Mutation, and Rat Lymphocyte Chromosomal Aberration assays) and in vivo (Mouse Bone Marrow Micronucleus assay) tests, fexofenadine hydrochloride revealed no evidence of mutagenicity.
Reproduction and fertility studies with terfenadine in rats produced no effect on male or female fertility at oral doses up to 300 mg/kg/day. However, reduced implants and post implantation losses were reported at 300 mg/kg. A reduction in implants was also observed at an oral dose of 150 mg/kg/day. Oral doses of 150 and 300 mg/kg of terfenadine produced AUC values of fexofenadine that were approximately 3 and 4 times, respectively, the human AUC at the maximum recommended daily oral dose in adults.

Pregnancy
Teratogenic Effects: Category C. Terfenadine alone was not teratogenic in rats and rabbits at oral doses up to 300 mg/kg; 300 mg/kg of terfenadine produced fexofenadine AUC values that were approximately 4 and 30 times, respectively, the human AUC at the maximum recommended daily oral dose in adults.
The combination of terfenadine and pseudoephedrine hydrochloride in a ratio of 1:2 by weight was studied in rats and rabbits. In rats, an oral combination dose of 150/300 mg/kg produced reduced fetal weight and delayed ossification with a finding of wavy ribs. The dose of 150 mg/kg of terfenadine in rats produced an AUC value of fexofenadine that was approximately 3 times the human AUC at the maximum recommended daily oral dose in adults. The dose of 300 mg/kg of pseudoephedrine hydrochloride in rats was approximately 10 times the maximum recommended daily oral dose in adults on a mg/m^2 basis. In rabbits, an oral combination dose of 100/200 mg/kg produced decreased fetal weight. By extrapolation, the AUC of fexofenadine for 100 mg/kg orally of terfenadine was approximately 10 times the human AUC at the maximum recommended daily oral dose in adults. The dose of 200 mg/kg of pseudoephedrine hydrochloride was approximately 15 times the maximum recommended daily oral dose in adults on a mg/m^2 basis. There are no adequate and well-controlled studies in pregnant women. ALLEGRA-D should be used during pregnancy only if the potential benefit justifies the potential risk to the fetus.
Nonteratogenic Effects. Dose-related decreases in pup weight gain and survival were observed in rats exposed to an oral dose of 150 mg/kg of terfenadine; this dose produced an AUC of fexofenadine that was approximately 3 times the human AUC at the maximum recommended daily oral dose in adults.

Nursing Mothers
It is not known if fexofenadine is excreted in human milk. Because many drugs are excreted in human milk, caution should be used when fexofenadine hydrochloride is administered to a nursing woman. Pseudoephedrine hydrochloride administered alone distributes into breast milk of lactating human females. Pseudoephedrine concentrations in milk are consistently higher than those in plasma. The total amount of drug in milk as judged by AUC is 2 to 3 times greater than the plasma AUC. The fraction of a pseudoephedrine dose excreted in milk is estimated to be 0.4% to 0.7%. A decision should be made whether to discontinue nursing or to discontinue the drug, taking into account the importance of the drug to the mother. Caution should be exercised when ALLEGRA-D is administered to nursing women.

Pediatric Use
Safety and effectiveness of ALLEGRA-D in pediatric patients under the age of 12 years have not been established.

Geriatric Use
Clinical studies of ALLEGRA-D did not include sufficient numbers of patients aged 65 and older to determine whether they respond differently from younger patients. Other reported clinical experience has not identified differences in responses between the elderly and younger patients, although the elderly are more likely to have adverse reactions to sympathomimetic amines. In general, dose selection for an elderly patient should be cautious, usually starting at the low end of the dosing range, reflecting the greater frequency of decreased hepatic, renal, or cardiac function, and of concomitant disease or other drug therapy.
The pseudoephedrine component of ALLEGRA-D is known to be substantially excreted by the kidney, and the risk of toxic reactions to this drug may be greater in patients with impaired renal function. Because elderly patients are more likely to have decreased renal function, care should be taken in dose selection, and it may be useful to monitor renal function.

ADVERSE REACTIONS

ALLEGRA-D
In one clinical trial (n=651) in which 215 patients with seasonal allergic rhinitis received the 60 mg fexofenadine hydrochloride/120 mg pseudoephedrine hydrochloride combination tablet twice daily for up to 2 weeks, adverse events were similar to those reported either in patients receiving fexofenadine hydrochloride 60 mg alone (n=218 patients) or in patients receiving pseudoephedrine hydrochloride 120 mg alone (n=218). A placebo group was not included in this study.
The percent of patients who withdrew prematurely because of adverse events was 3.7% for the fexofenadine hydrochloride/pseudoephedrine hydrochloride combination group, 0.5% for the fexofenadine hydrochloride group, and 4.1% for the pseudoephedrine hydrochloride group. All adverse events that were reported by greater than 1% of patients who received the recommended daily dose of the fexofenadine hydrochloride/pseudoephedrine hydrochloride combination are listed in the following table.
[See table below]

Adverse Experiences Reported in One Active-Controlled Seasonal Allergic Rhinitis Clinical Trial at Rates of Greater than 1%

Adverse Experience	60 mg Fexofenadine Hydrochloride/120 mg Pseudoephedrine Hydrochloride Combination Tablet Twice Daily (n=215)	Fexofenadine Hydrochloride 60 mg Twice Daily (n=218)	Pseudoephedrine Hydrochloride 120 mg Twice Daily (n=218)
Headache	13.0%	11.5%	17.4%
Insomnia	12.6%	3.2%	13.3%
Nausea	7.4%	0.5%	5.0%
Dry Mouth	2.8%	0.5%	5.5%
Dyspepsia	2.8%	0.5%	0.9%
Throat Irritation	2.3%	1.8%	0.5%
Dizziness	1.9%	0.0%	3.2%
Agitation	1.9%	0.0%	1.4%
Back Pain	1.9%	0.5%	0.5%
Palpitation	1.9%	0.0%	0.9%
Nervousness	1.4%	0.5%	1.8%
Anxiety	1.4%	0.0%	1.4%
Upper Respiratory Infection	1.4%	0.9%	0.9%
Abdominal Pain	1.4%	0.5%	0.5%

Many of the adverse events occurring in the fexofenadine hydrochloride/pseudoephedrine hydrochloride combination group were adverse events also reported predominately in the pseudoephedrine hydrochloride group, such as insomnia, headache, nausea, dry mouth, dizziness, agitation, nervousness, anxiety, and palpitation.

Fexofenadine Hydrochloride
In placebo-controlled clinical trials, which included 2461 patients receiving fexofenadine hydrochloride at doses of 20 mg to 240 mg twice daily, adverse events were similar in fexofenadine hydrochloride and placebo-treated patients. The incidence of adverse events, including drowsiness, was not dose related and was similar across subgroups defined by age, gender, and race. The percent of patients who withdrew prematurely because of adverse events was 2.2% with fexofenadine hydrochloride vs 3.3% with placebo.
Events that have been reported during controlled clinical trials involving seasonal allergic rhinitis and chronic idiopathic urticaria patients with incidences less than 1% and similar to placebo and have been rarely reported during postmarketing surveillance include: insomnia, nervousness, and sleep disorders or paroniria. In rare cases, rash, urticaria, pruritus and hypersensitivity reactions with manifestations such as angioedema, chest tightness, dyspnea, flushing and systemic anaphylaxis have been reported.

Pseudoephedrine Hydrochloride
Pseudoephedrine hydrochloride may cause mild CNS stimulation in hypersensitive patients. Nervousness, excitability, restlessness, dizziness, weakness, or insomnia may occur. Headache, drowsiness, tachycardia, palpitation, pressor activity, and cardiac arrhythmias have been reported. Sympathomimetic drugs have also been associated with other untoward effects such as fear, anxiety, tenseness, tremor, hallucinations, seizures, pallor, respiratory difficulty, dysuria, and cardiovascular collapse.

OVERDOSAGE

Most reports of fexofenadine hydrochloride overdose contain limited information. However, dizziness, drowsiness, and dry mouth have been reported. For the pseudoephedrine hydrochloride component of ALLEGRA-D, information on acute overdose is limited to the marketing history of pseudoephedrine hydrochloride. Single doses of fexofenadine hydrochloride up to 800 mg (6 normal volunteers at this dose level), and doses up to 690 mg twice daily for one month (3 normal volunteers at this dose level), were administered without the development of clinically significant adverse events.
In large doses, sympathomimetics may give rise to giddiness, headache, nausea, vomiting, sweating, thirst, tachycardia, precordial pain, palpitations, difficulty in micturition, muscular weakness and tenseness, anxiety, restlessness, and insomnia. Many patients can present a toxic psychosis with delusions and hallucinations. Some may develop cardiac arrhythmias, circulatory collapse, convulsions, coma, and respiratory failure.
In the event of overdose, consider standard measures to remove any unabsorbed drug. Symptomatic and supportive treatment is recommended. Hemodialysis did not effectively remove fexofenadine from blood (up to 1.7% removed) following terfenadine administration.
The effect of hemodialysis on the removal of pseudoephedrine is unknown.
No deaths occurred in mature mice and rats at oral doses of fexofenadine hydrochloride up to 5000 mg/kg (approximately 170 and 340 times, respectively, the maximum recommended daily oral dose in adults on a mg/m^2 basis.) The median oral lethal dose in newborn rats was 438 mg/kg (approximately 30 times the maximum recommended daily oral dose in adults on a mg/m^2 basis). In dogs, no evidence of toxicity was observed at oral doses up to 2000 mg/kg (approximately 450 times the maximum recommended human daily oral dose in adults on a mg/m^2 basis). The oral median

lethal dose of pseudoephedrine hydrochloride in rats was 1674 mg/kg (approximately 55 times the maximum recommended daily oral dose in adults on a mg/m² basis).

DOSAGE AND ADMINISTRATION

The recommended dose of ALLEGRA-D is one tablet twice daily for adults and children 12 years of age and older. It is recommended that the administration of ALLEGRA-D with food should be avoided. A dose of one tablet once daily is recommended as the starting dose in patients with decreased renal function. (See CLINICAL PHARMACOLOGY and PRECAUTIONS.)

HOW SUPPLIED

ALLEGRA-D (fexofenadine hydrochloride and pseudoephedrine hydrochloride) Extended-Release Tablets are available in: high-density polyethylene (HDPE) bottles of 60 (NDC 0088-1090-41) with a polypropylene child-resistant cap containing a pulp/wax liner with heat-sealed foil inner seal; HDPE bottles of 100 (NDC 0088-1090-47) with a polypropylene screw cap containing a pulp/wax liner with heat-sealed foil inner seal; HDPE bottles of 500 (NDC 0088-1090-55) with a polypropylene screw cap containing a pulp/wax liner with heat-sealed foil inner seal; and aluminum foil-backed clear blister packs of 100 (NDC 0088-1090-49).

ALLEGRA-D is a two-layer tablet, one white layer and one tan layer with a clear film coating on the tablet. The tablets are engraved with "Allegra-D" on the white layer.

Store ALLEGRA-D Extended-Release Tablets at 20–25°C (68–77°F). (See USP Controlled Room Temperature.)

Prescribing Information as of November 2000

Aventis Pharmaceuticals Inc.
Kansas City, MO 64137 USA
US Patents 4,254,129; 5,375,693; 5,578,610.
www.allegra.com
alldp1100p

LANTUS® ℞

[*lăn' tus*]

(insulin glargine [rDNA origin] injection)

Prescribing information for this product, which appears on pages 709–713 of the 2001 PDR, has been completely revised as follows. Please write "See Supplement A" next to the product heading.

Prescribing Information as of February 2001

LANTUS® must not be diluted or mixed with any other insulin or solution.

DESCRIPTION

LANTUS® (insulin glargine [rDNA origin] injection) is a sterile solution of insulin glargine for use as an injection. Insulin glargine is a recombinant human insulin analog that is a long-acting (up to 24-hour duration of action), parenteral blood-glucose-lowering agent. (See CLINICAL PHARMACOLOGY). LANTUS is produced by recombinant DNA technology utilizing a non-pathogenic laboratory strain of *Escherichia coli* (K12) as the production organism. Insulin glargine differs from human insulin in that the amino acid asparagine at position A21 is replaced by glycine and two arginines are added to the C-terminus of the B-chain. Chemically, it is 21^{A}-Gly-30^{B}a-L-Arg-30^{B}b-L-Arg-human insulin and has the empirical formula $C_{267}H_{404}N_{72}O_{78}S_6$ and a molecular weight of 6063. It has the following structural formula:

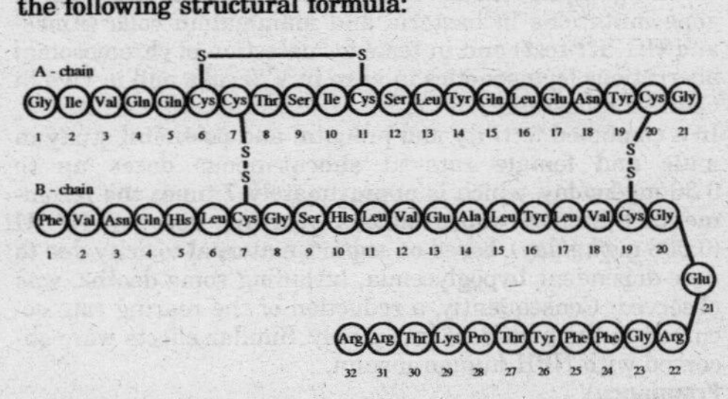

LANTUS consists of insulin glargine dissolved in a clear aqueous fluid. Each milliliter of LANTUS (insulin glargine injection) contains 100 IU (3.6378 mg) insulin glargine, 30 mcg zinc, 2.7 mg m-cresol, 20 mg glycerol 85%, and water for injection. The pH is adjusted by addition of aqueous solutions of hydrochloric acid and sodium hydroxide. LANTUS has a pH of approximately 4.

CLINICAL PHARMACOLOGY

Mechanism of Action

The primary activity of insulin, including insulin glargine, is regulation of glucose metabolism. Insulin and its analogs lower blood glucose levels by stimulating peripheral glucose uptake, especially by skeletal muscle and fat, and by inhibiting hepatic glucose production. Insulin inhibits lipolysis in the adipocyte, inhibits proteolysis, and enhances protein synthesis.

Pharmacodynamics

Insulin glargine is a human insulin analog that has been designed to have low aqueous solubility at neutral pH. At pH 4, as in the LANTUS injection solution, it is completely soluble. After injection into the subcutaneous tissue, the acidic solution is neutralized, leading to formation of microprecipitates from which small amounts of insulin glargine are slowly released, resulting in a relatively constant concentration/time profile over 24 hours with no pronounced peak. This profile allows once-daily dosing as a patient's basal insulin.

In clinical studies, the glucose-lowering effect on a molar basis (i.e., when given at the same doses) of intravenous insulin glargine is approximately the same as human insulin. In euglycemic clamp studies in healthy subjects or in patients with type 1 diabetes, the onset of action of subcutaneous insulin glargine was slower than NPH human insulin. The effect profile of insulin glargine was relatively constant with no pronounced peak and the duration of its effect was prolonged compared to NPH human insulin. *Figure 1* shows results from a study in patients with type 1 diabetes conducted for a maximum of 24 hours after the injection. The median time between injection and the end of pharmacological effect was 14.5 hours (range: 9.5 to 19.3 hours) for NPH human insulin, and 24 hours (range: 10.8 to >24.0 hours) (24 hours was the end of the observation period) for insulin glargine.

Figure 1. Activity Profile in Patients with Type 1 Diabetes†

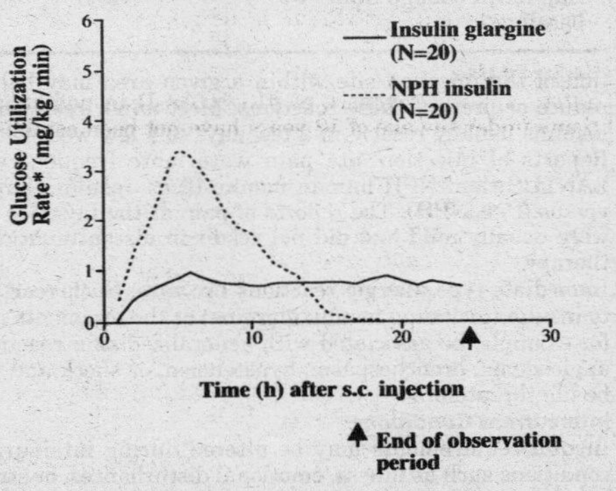

* Determined as amount of glucose infused to maintain constant plasma glucose levels (hourly mean values); indicative of insulin activity.

† Between-patient variability (CV, coefficient of variation); insulin glargine, 84% and NPH, 78%.

The longer duration of action (up to 24 hours) of LANTUS is directly related to its slower rate of absorption and supports once-daily subcutaneous administration. The time course of action of insulins, including LANTUS, may vary between individuals and/or within the same individual.

Pharmacokinetics

Absorption and Bioavailability. After subcutaneous injection of insulin glargine in healthy subjects and in patients with diabetes, the insulin serum concentrations indicated a slower, more prolonged absorption and a relatively constant concentration/time profile over 24 hours with no pronounced peak in comparison to NPH human insulin. Serum insulin concentrations were thus consistent with the time profile of the pharmacodynamic activity of insulin glargine.

After subcutaneous injection of 0.3 IU/kg insulin glargine in patients with type 1 diabetes, a relatively constant concentration/time profile has been demonstrated. The duration of action after abdominal, deltoid, or thigh subcutaneous administration was similar.

Metabolism. A metabolism study in humans indicates that insulin glargine is partly metabolized at the carboxyl terminus of the B chain in the subcutaneous depot to form two active metabolites with in vitro activity similar to that of insulin, M1 (21^{A}-Gly-insulin) and M2 (21^{A}-Gly-des-30^{B}-Thr-insulin). Unchanged drug and these degradation products are also present in the circulation.

Special Populations

Age, Race, and Gender. Information on the effect of age, race, and gender on the pharmacokinetics of LANTUS is not available. However, in controlled clinical trials in adults (n=3890) and a controlled clinical trial in pediatric patients (n=349), subgroup analyses based on age, race, and gender did not show differences in safety and efficacy between insulin glargine and NPH human insulin.

Smoking. The effect of smoking on the pharmacokinetics/pharmacodynamics of LANTUS has not been studied.

Pregnancy. The effect of pregnancy on the pharmacokinetics and pharmacodynamics of LANTUS has not been studied. (See PRECAUTIONS, Pregnancy)

Obesity. In controlled clinical trials, which included patients with Body Mass Index (BMI) up to and including 49.6 kg/m², subgroup analyses based on BMI did not show any differences in safety and efficacy between insulin glargine and NPH human insulin.

Renal Impairment. The effect of renal impairment on the pharmacokinetics of LANTUS has not been studied. However, some studies with human insulin have shown increased circulating levels of insulin in patients with renal failure. Careful glucose monitoring and dose adjustments of insulin, including LANTUS, may be necessary in patients with renal dysfunction. (See PRECAUTIONS, Renal Impairment)

Hepatic Impairment. The effect of hepatic impairment on the pharmacokinetics of LANTUS has not been studied. However, some studies with human insulin have shown increased circulating levels of insulin in patients with liver failure. Careful glucose monitoring and dose adjustments of insulin, including LANTUS, may be necessary in patients with hepatic dysfunction. (See PRECAUTIONS, Hepatic Impairment)

CLINICAL STUDIES

The safety and effectiveness of insulin glargine given once-daily at bedtime was compared to that of once-daily and twice-daily NPH human insulin in open-label, randomized, active-control, parallel studies of 2327 adult patients and 349 pediatric patients with type 1 diabetes mellitus and 1563 adult patients with type 2 diabetes mellitus (see Tables 1–3). In general, LANTUS achieved a level of glycemic control similar to NPH human insulin as measured by glycated hemoglobin (GHb). The overall rate of hypoglycemia did not differ between patients with diabetes treated with LANTUS compared with NPH human insulin.

Type 1 Diabetes—Adult (see Table 1). In two large, randomized, controlled clinical studies (Studies A and B), patients with type 1 diabetes (Study A; n=585, Study B; n=534) were randomized to basal-bolus treatment with LANTUS once daily or to NPH human insulin once or twice daily and treated for 28 weeks. Regular human insulin was administered before each meal. LANTUS was administered at bedtime. NPH human insulin was administered once daily at bedtime or in the morning and at bedtime when used twice daily. In one large, randomized, controlled clinical study (Study C), patients with type 1 diabetes (n=619) were treated for 16 weeks with a basal-bolus insulin regimen where insulin lispro was used before each meal. LANTUS was administered once daily at bedtime and NPH human insulin was administered once or twice daily. In these studies, LANTUS and NPH human insulin had a similar effect on glycohemoglobin with a similar overall rate of hypoglycemia.

[See table 1 above]

Table 1: Type 1 Diabetes Mellitus—Adult

	Study A		Study B		Study C	
Treatment duration	28 weeks		28 weeks		16 weeks	
Treatment in combination with	Regular insulin		Regular insulin		Insulin lispro	
	LANTUS	NPH	LANTUS	NPH	LANTUS	NPH
Number of subjects treated	292	293	264	270	310	309
GHb						
Endstudy mean	8.13	8.07	7.55	7.49	7.53	7.60
Adj. mean change from baseline	+0.21	+0.10	−0.16	−0.21	−0.07	−0.08
LANTUS—NPH	+0.11		+0.05		+0.01	
95% CI for Treatment difference	(−0.03; +0.24)		(−0.08; +0.19)		(−0.11; +0.13)	
Basal insulin dose						
Endstudy mean	19.2	22.8	24.8	31.3	23.9	29.2
Mean change from baseline	−1.7	−0.3	−4.1	+1.8	−4.5	+0.9
Total insulin dose						
Endstudy mean	46.7	51.7	50.3	54.8	47.4	50.7
Mean change from baseline	−1.1	−0.1	+0.3	+3.7	−2.9	+0.3
Fasting blood glucose (mg/dL)						
Endstudy mean	146.3	150.8	147.8	154.4	144.4	161.3
Adj. mean change from baseline	−21.1	−16.0	−20.2	−16.9	−29.3	−11.9

Type 1 Diabetes—Pediatric (see Table 2). In a randomized, controlled clinical study (Study D), pediatric patients (age range 6 to 15 years) with type 1 diabetes (n=349) were treated for 28 weeks with a basal-bolus insulin regimen where regular human insulin was used before each meal. LANTUS was administered once daily at bedtime and NPH human insulin was administered once or twice daily. Similar effects on glycohemoglobin and the incidence of hypoglycemia were observed in both treatment groups.

[See table 2 at top of next page]

Type 2 Diabetes—Adult (see Table 3). In a large, randomized, controlled clinical study (Study E) (n=570), LANTUS was evaluated for 52 weeks as part of a regimen of combination therapy with insulin and oral antidiabetic agents (a sulfonylurea, metformin, acarbose, or combinations of these drugs). LANTUS administered once daily at bedtime was as effective as NPH human insulin administered once daily at bedtime in reducing glycohemoglobin and fasting glucose. There was a low rate of hypoglycemia that was similar in LANTUS and NPH human insulin treated patients. In a large, randomized, controlled clinical study (Study F), in patients with type 2 diabetes not using oral antidiabetic agents (n=518), a basal-bolus regimen of LANTUS once daily at bedtime or NPH human insulin administered once or twice

Continued on next page

Lantus—Cont.

daily was evaluated for 28 weeks. Regular human insulin was used before meals as needed. LANTUS had similar effectiveness as either once- or twice-daily NPH human insulin in reducing glycohemoglobin and fasting glucose with a similar incidence of hypoglycemia.
[See table 3 to the right]

Table 2: Type 1 Diabetes Mellitus—Pediatric

	Study D LANTUS	Study D NPH
Treatment duration	28 weeks	
Treatment in combination with	Regular insulin	
Number of subjects treated	174	175
GHb		
Endstudy mean	8.91	9.18
Adj. mean change from baseline	+0.28	+0.27
LANTUS—NPH	+0.01	
95% CI for Treatment difference	(−0.24; +0.26)	
Basal insulin dose		
Endstudy mean	18.2	21.1
Mean change from baseline	−1.3	+2.4
Total insulin dose		
Endstudy mean	45.0	46.0
Mean change from baseline	+1.9	+3.4
Fasting blood glucose (mg/dL)		
Endstudy mean	171.9	182.7
Adj. mean change from baseline	−23.2	−12.2

Table 3: Type 2 Diabetes Mellitus—Adult

	Study E LANTUS	Study E NPH	Study F LANTUS	Study F NPH
Treatment duration	52 weeks		28 weeks	
Treatment in combination with	Oral agents		Regular insulin	
Number of subjects treated	289	281	259	259
GHb				
Endstudy mean	8.51	8.47	8.14	7.96
Adj. mean change from baseline	−0.46	−0.38	−0.41	−0.59
LANTUS—NPH	−0.08		+0.17	
95% CI for Treatment difference	(−0.28; +0.12)		(−0.00; +0.35)	
Basal insulin dose				
Endstudy mean	25.9	23.6	42.9	52.5
Mean change from baseline	+11.5	+9.0	−1.2	+7.0
Total insulin dose				
Endstudy mean	25.9	23.6	74.3	80.0
Mean change from baseline	+11.5	+9.0	+10.0	+13.1
Fasting blood glucose (mg/dL)				
Endstudy mean	126.9	129.4	141.5	144.5
Adj. mean change from baseline	−49.0	−46.3	−23.8	−21.6

INDICATIONS AND USAGE

LANTUS is indicated for once-daily subcutaneous administration at bedtime in the treatment of adult and pediatric patients with type 1 diabetes mellitus or adult patients with type 2 diabetes mellitus who require basal (long-acting) insulin for the control of hyperglycemia.

CONTRAINDICATIONS

LANTUS is contraindicated in patients hypersensitive to insulin glargine or the excipients.

WARNINGS

Hypoglycemia is the most common adverse effect of insulin, including LANTUS. As with all insulins, the timing of hypoglycemia may differ among various insulin formulations. Glucose monitoring is recommended for all patients with diabetes.

Any change of insulin should be made cautiously and only under medical supervision. Changes in insulin strength, manufacturer, type (e.g., regular, NPH, or insulin analogs), species (animal, human), or method of manufacture (recombinant DNA versus animal-source insulin) may result in the need for a change in dosage. Concomitant oral antidiabetic treatment may need to be adjusted.

PRECAUTIONS

General

LANTUS is not intended for intravenous administration. The prolonged duration of activity of insulin glargine is dependent on injection into subcutaneous tissue. Intravenous administration of the usual subcutaneous dose could result in severe hypoglycemia.

LANTUS must not be diluted or mixed with any other insulin or solution. If LANTUS is diluted or mixed, the solution may become cloudy, and the pharmacokinetic/pharmacodynamic profile (e.g., onset of action, time to peak effect) of LANTUS and/or the mixed insulin may be altered in an unpredictable manner. When LANTUS and regular human insulin were mixed immediately before injection in dogs, a delayed onset of action and time to maximum effect for regular human insulin was observed. The total bioavailability of the mixture was also slightly decreased compared to separate injections of LANTUS and regular human insulin. The relevance of these observations in dogs to humans is not known.

As with all insulin preparations, the time course of LANTUS action may vary in different individuals or at different times in the same individual and the rate of absorption is dependent on blood supply, temperature, and physical activity.

Insulin may cause sodium retention and edema, particularly if previously poor metabolic control is improved by intensified insulin therapy.

Hypoglycemia

As with all insulin preparations, hypoglycemic reactions may be associated with the administration of LANTUS. Hypoglycemia is the most common adverse effect of insulins. Early warning symptoms of hypoglycemia may be different or less pronounced under certain conditions, such as long duration of diabetes, diabetic nerve disease, use of medications such as beta-blockers, or intensified diabetes control. (See PRECAUTIONS, Drug Interactions). Such situations may result in severe hypoglycemia (and, possibly, loss of consciousness) prior to patient's awareness of hypoglycemia.

The time of occurrence of hypoglycemia depends on the action profile of the insulins used and may, therefore, change when the treatment regimen is changed. Patients being switched from twice daily NPH insulin to once-daily LANTUS should have their LANTUS dose reduced by 20% from the previous total daily NPH dose to reduce the risk of hypoglycemia. (See DOSAGE AND ADMINISTRATION, Changeover to LANTUS)

The prolonged effect of subcutaneous LANTUS may delay recovery from hypoglycemia.

In a clinical study, symptoms of hypoglycemia or counterregulatory hormone responses were similar after intravenous insulin glargine and regular human insulin both in healthy subjects and patients with type 1 diabetes.

Renal Impairment

Although studies have not been performed in patients with diabetes and renal impairment, LANTUS requirements may be diminished because of reduced insulin metabolism, similar to observations found with other insulins. (See CLINICAL PHARMACOLOGY, Special Populations)

Hepatic Impairment

Although studies have not been performed in patients with diabetes and hepatic impairment, LANTUS requirements may be diminished due to reduced capacity for gluconeogenesis and reduced insulin metabolism, similar to observations found with other insulins. (See CLINICAL PHARMACOLOGY, Special Populations)

Injection Site and Allergic Reactions

As with any insulin therapy, lipodystrophy may occur at the injection site and delay insulin absorption. Other injection site reactions with insulin therapy include redness, pain, itching, hives, swelling, and inflammation. Continuous rotation of the injection site within a given area may help to reduce or prevent these reactions. Most minor reactions to insulins usually resolve in a few days to a few weeks.

Reports of injection site pain were more frequent with LANTUS than NPH human insulin (2.7% insulin glargine versus 0.7% NPH). The reports of pain at the injection site were usually mild and did not result in discontinuation of therapy.

Immediate-type allergic reactions are rare. Such reactions to insulin (including insulin glargine) or the excipients may, for example, be associated with generalized skin reactions, angioedema, bronchospasm, hypotension, or shock and may be life threatening.

Intercurrent Conditions

Insulin requirements may be altered during intercurrent conditions such as illness, emotional disturbances, or stress.

Information for Patients

LANTUS must only be used if the solution is clear and colorless with no particles visible. (See DOSAGE AND ADMINISTRATION, Preparation and Handling) **Patients must be advised that LANTUS must not be diluted or mixed with any other insulin or solution.** (See PRECAUTIONS, General)

Patients should be instructed on self-management procedures including glucose monitoring, proper injection technique, and hypoglycemia and hyperglycemia management. Patients must be instructed on handling of special situations such as intercurrent conditions (illness, stress, or emotional disturbances), an inadequate or skipped insulin dose, inadvertent administration of an increased insulin dose, inadequate food intake, or skipped meals. Refer patients to the LANTUS Information for the Patient circular for additional information.

As with all patients who have diabetes, the ability to concentrate and/or react may be impaired as a result of hypoglycemia or hyperglycemia.

Patients with diabetes should be advised to inform their doctor if they are pregnant or are contemplating pregnancy.

Drug Interactions

A number of substances affect glucose metabolism and may require insulin dose adjustment and particularly close monitoring.

The following are examples of substances that may increase the blood-glucose-lowering effect and susceptibility to hypoglycemia: oral antidiabetic products, ACE inhibitors, disopyramide, fibrates, fluoxetine, MAO inhibitors, propoxyphene, salicylates, somatostatin analog (e.g., octreotide), sulfonamide antibiotics.

The following are examples of substances that may reduce the blood-glucose-lowering effect of insulin: corticosteroids, danazol, diuretics, sympathomimetic agents (e.g., epinephrine, albuterol, terbutaline), isoniazid, phenothiazine derivatives, somatropin, thyroid hormones, estrogens, progestogens (e.g., in oral contraceptives).

Beta-blockers, clonidine, lithium salts, and alcohol may either potentiate or weaken the blood-glucose-lowering effect of insulin. Pentamidine may cause hypoglycemia, which may sometimes be followed by hyperglycemia. In addition, under the influence of sympatholytic medicinal products such as beta-blockers, clonidine, guanethidine, and reserpine, the signs of hypoglycemia may be reduced or absent.

Carcinogenesis, Mutagenesis, Impairment of Fertility

In mice and rats, standard two-year carcinogenicity studies with insulin glargine were performed at doses up to 0.455 mg/kg, which is for the rat approximately 10 times and for the mouse approximately 5 times the recommended human subcutaneous starting dose of 10 IU (0.008 mg/kg/day), based on mg/m^2. The findings in female mice were not conclusive due to excessive mortality in all dose groups during the study. Histiocytomas were found at injection sites in male rats (statistically significant) and male mice (not statistically significant) in acid vehicle containing groups. These tumors were not found in female animals, in saline control, or insulin comparator groups using a different vehicle. The relevance of these findings to humans is unknown.

Insulin glargine was not mutagenic in tests for detection of gene mutations in bacteria and mammalian cells (Ames- and HGPRT-test) and in tests for detection of chromosomal aberrations (cytogenetics in vitro in V79 cells and in vivo in Chinese hamsters).

In a combined fertility and prenatal and postnatal study in male and female rats at subcutaneous doses up to 0.36 mg/kg/day, which is approximately 7 times the recommended human subcutaneous starting dose of 10 IU (0.008 mg/kg/day), based on mg/m^2, maternal toxicity due to dose-dependent hypoglycemia, including some deaths, was observed. Consequently, a reduction of the rearing rate occurred in the high-dose group only. Similar effects were observed with NPH human insulin.

Pregnancy

Teratogenic Effects: Pregnancy Category C. Subcutaneous reproduction and teratology studies have been performed with insulin glargine and regular human insulin in rats and Himalayan rabbits. The drug was given to female rats before mating, during mating, and throughout pregnancy at doses up to 0.36 mg/kg/day, which is approximately 7 times the recommended human subcutaneous starting dose of 10 IU (0.008 mg/kg/day), based on mg/m^2. In rabbits, doses of 0.072 mg/kg/day, which is approximately 2 times the recommended human subcutaneous starting dose of 10 IU (0.008 mg/kg/day), based on mg/m^2, were administered during organogenesis. The effects of insulin glargine did not generally differ from those observed with regular human insulin in rats or rabbits. However, in rabbits, five fetuses from two litters of the high-dose group exhibited dilation of the cerebral ventricles. Fertility and early embryonic development appeared normal.

There are no well-controlled clinical studies of the use of insulin glargine in pregnant women. It is essential for patients with diabetes or a history of gestational diabetes to maintain good metabolic control before conception and throughout pregnancy. Insulin requirements may decrease during the first trimester, generally increase during the second and third trimesters, and rapidly decline after delivery.

Careful monitoring of glucose control is essential in such patients. Because animal reproduction studies are not always predictive of human response, this drug should be used during pregnancy only if clearly needed.

Nursing Mothers

It is unknown whether insulin glargine is excreted in significant amounts in human milk. Many drugs, including human insulin, are excreted in human milk. For this reason, caution should be exercised when LANTUS is administered to a nursing woman. Lactating women may require adjustments in insulin dose and diet.

Pediatric Use

Safety and effectiveness of LANTUS have been established in the age group 6 to 15 years with type 1 diabetes.

Geriatric Use

In controlled clinical studies comparing insulin glargine to NPH human insulin, 593 of 3890 patients with type 1 and type 2 diabetes were 65 years and older. The only difference in safety or effectiveness in this subpopulation compared to the entire study population was an expected higher incidence of cardiovascular events in both insulin glargine and NPH human insulin-treated patients.

In elderly patients with diabetes, the initial dosing, dose increments, and maintenance dosage should be conservative to avoid hypoglycemic reactions. Hypoglycemia may be difficult to recognize in the elderly. (See PRECAUTIONS, Hypoglycemia)

ADVERSE REACTIONS

The adverse events commonly associated with LANTUS include the following:

Body as a whole: allergic reactions (See PRECAUTIONS)

Skin and appendages: injection site reaction, lipodystrophy, pruritus, rash (See PRECAUTIONS)

Other: hypoglycemia (See WARNINGS and PRECAUTIONS)

In clinical studies in adult patients, there was a higher incidence of treatment-emergent injection site pain in LANTUS-treated patients (2.7%) compared to NPH insulin-treated patients (0.7%). The reports of pain at the injection site were usually mild and did not result in discontinuation of therapy. Other treatment-emergent injection site reactions occurred at similar incidences with both insulin glargine and NPH human insulin.

Retinopathy was evaluated in the clinical studies by means of retinal adverse events reported and fundus photography. The numbers of retinal adverse events reported for LANTUS and NPH treatment groups were similar for patients with type 1 and type 2 diabetes. Progression of retinopathy was investigated by fundus photography using a grading protocol derived from the Early Treatment Diabetic Retinopathy Study (ETDRS). In one clinical study involving patients with type 2 diabetes, a difference in the number of subjects with ≥3-step progression in ETDRS scale over a 6-month period was noted by fundus photography (7.5% in LANTUS group versus 2.7% in NPH treated group). The overall relevance of this isolated finding cannot be determined due to the small number of patients involved, the short follow-up period, and the fact that this finding was not observed in other clinical studies.

OVERDOSAGE

An excess of insulin relative to food intake, energy expenditure, or both may lead to severe and sometimes long-term and life-threatening hypoglycemia. Mild episodes of hypoglycemia can usually be treated with oral carbohydrates. Adjustments in drug dosage, meal patterns, or exercise may be needed.

More severe episodes with coma, seizure, or neurologic impairment may be treated with intramuscular/subcutaneous glucagon or concentrated intravenous glucose. After apparent clinical recovery from hypoglycemia, continued observation and additional carbohydrate intake may be necessary to avoid reoccurrence of hypoglycemia.

DOSAGE AND ADMINISTRATION

LANTUS is a recombinant human insulin analog. Its potency is approximately the same as human insulin. It exhibits a relatively constant glucose-lowering profile over 24 hours that permits once-daily dosing.

LANTUS should be administered subcutaneously once a day at bedtime. LANTUS is not intended for intravenous administration. (See PRECAUTIONS). Intravenous administration of the usual subcutaneous dose could result in severe hypoglycemia. The desired blood glucose levels as well as the doses and timing of antidiabetic medications must be determined individually. Blood glucose monitoring is recommended for all patients with diabetes. The prolonged duration of activity of LANTUS is dependent on injection into subcutaneous space.

As with all insulins, injection sites within an injection area (abdomen, thigh or deltoid) must be rotated from one injection to the next.

In clinical studies, there was no relevant difference in insulin glargine absorption after abdominal, deltoid, or thigh subcutaneous administration. As for all insulins, the rate of absorption, and consequently the onset and duration of action, may be affected by exercise and other variables.

LANTUS is not the insulin of choice for the treatment of diabetic ketoacidosis. Intravenous short-acting insulin is the preferred treatment.

Pediatric Use

LANTUS can be safely administrated to pediatric patients ≥6 years of age. Administration to pediatric patients <6 years has not been studied. Based on the results of a study in pediatric patients, the dose recommendation for changeover to LANTUS is the same as described for adults in DOSAGE AND ADMINISTRATION, Changeover to LANTUS.

Initiation of LANTUS Therapy

In a clinical study with insulin naïve patients with type 2 diabetes already treated with oral antidiabetic drugs, LANTUS was started at an average dose of 10 IU once daily, and subsequently adjusted according to the patient's need to a total daily dose ranging from 2 to 100 IU.

Changeover to LANTUS

If changing from a treatment regimen with an intermediate- or long-acting insulin to a regimen with LANTUS, the amount and timing of short-acting insulin or fast-acting insulin analog or the dose of any oral antidiabetic drug may need to be adjusted. In clinical studies, when patients were transferred from once-daily NPH human insulin or ultralente human insulin to once-daily LANTUS, the initial dose was usually not changed. However, when patients were transferred from twice-daily NPH human insulin to LANTUS once daily at bedtime, to reduce the risk of hypoglycemia, the initial dose (IU) was usually reduced by approximately 20% (compared to total daily IU of NPH human insulin) within the first week of treatment and then adjusted based on patient response. (See PRECAUTIONS, Hypoglycemia)

A program of close metabolic monitoring under medical supervision is recommended during transfer and in the initial weeks thereafter. The amount and timing of short-acting insulin or fast-acting insulin analog may need to be adjusted. This is particularly true for patients with acquired antibodies to human insulin needing high-insulin doses and occurs with all insulin analogs. Dose adjustment of LANTUS and other insulins or oral antidiabetic drugs may be required; for example, if the patient's weight or lifestyle changes or other circumstances arise that increase susceptibility to hypoglycemia or hyperglycemia. (See PRECAUTIONS, Hypoglycemia)

The dose may also have to be adjusted during intercurrent illness. (See PRECAUTIONS, Intercurrent Conditions)

Preparation and Handling

Parenteral drug products should be inspected visually prior to administration whenever the solution and the container permit. LANTUS must only be used if the solution is clear and colorless with no particles visible.

The syringes must not contain any other medicinal product or residue.

Mixing and diluting. LANTUS must not be diluted or mixed with any other insulin or solution. (See PRECAUTIONS, General)

Cartridge version only: If the OptiPen™ One Insulin Delivery Device malfunctions, LANTUS may be drawn from the cartridge into a U 100 syringe and injected.

HOW SUPPLIED

LANTUS 100 units per mL (U 100) is available in the following package sizes:

10 mL vials (NDC 0088-2220-33)

3 mL cartridges*, package of 5 (NDC 0088-2220-52)

*Cartridges are for use only in the OptiPen™ One Insulin Delivery Device

Storage

Unopened LANTUS vials and cartridges should be stored in a refrigerator, 36°F–46°F (2°C–8°C). LANTUS should not be stored in the freezer and it should not be allowed to freeze. If refrigeration is not possible, the 10 mL vial or cartridge of LANTUS in use can be kept unrefrigerated for up to 28 days away from direct heat and light, as long as the temperature is not greater than 86°F (30°C). Unrefrigerated 10 mL vials and cartridges must be used within the 28-day period or they must be discarded.

Once the cartridge is placed in an OptiPen One, it should not be put in the refrigerator.

Prescribing Information as of February 2001

Manufactured by:
Aventis Pharma Deutschland GmbH
D-65926 Frankfurt am Main
Germany

Manufactured for:
Aventis Pharmaceuticals Inc.
Kansas City, MO 64137 USA
US Patents 5,656,722, 5,370,629, and 5,509,905
Made in Germany
www.aventispharma-us.com

LANTUS®

(insulin glargine [Recombinant DNA origin] injection)

Patient Information for the LANTUS Vial

This leaflet tells you about LANTUS (LAN-tus) and about how to use LANTUS in a vial. At the end of the leaflet is a list of vocabulary words you may find useful. Read this information carefully before you use LANTUS. Read the information you get when you refill your LANTUS prescriptions because there may be new information. This leaflet does not take the place of complete discussions with your health care professional. If you have questions about LANTUS or about diabetes, talk with your health care professional.

What is the most important information I should know about LANTUS?

[See figure at top of next column]

Do not dilute or mix LANTUS with any other insulin or solution. It will not work as intended, and you may lose blood sugar control, which could be serious.

What is LANTUS?

LANTUS is a long-acting synthetic (man-made) human insulin to treat diabetes. You need a prescription to get

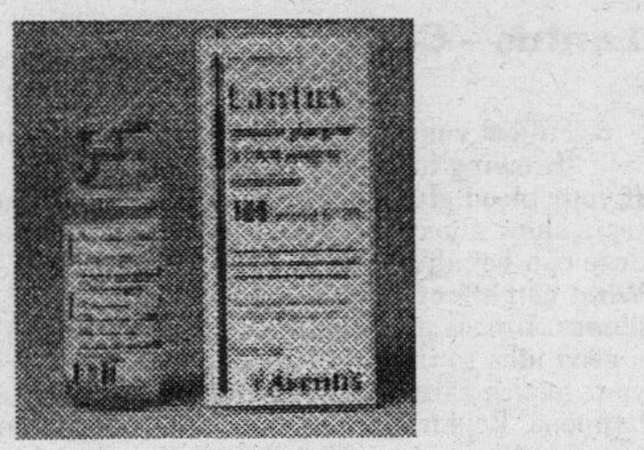

LANTUS. Always be sure the pharmacy gives you the right insulin. The carton and vial should look like the ones in this picture.

Diabetes is a disease caused when the body cannot produce or use insulin. Insulin is a hormone produced by the pancreas. Your body needs insulin to turn glucose (sugar) from food into energy. If your body does not make enough insulin, you need another source of insulin so you will not have too much sugar in your blood. That is why you must take insulin injections.

LANTUS is similar to the insulin made by your body. It is used once a day to lower blood glucose. Like other insulins, you take LANTUS by injecting it in the fatty layer under the skin (subcutaneously). The dose your health care professional prescribes helps keep the glucose level in your blood close to normal.

You will be able to tell if LANTUS is working by testing your blood and/or urine for glucose.

LANTUS contains active and inactive ingredients. The active ingredient is insulin. It is dissolved in a colorless sterile (germ-free) fluid. The concentration is 100 units/mL (U-100). Inactive ingredients are zinc, glycerol, m-cresol, and water for injection.

Insulin injections play an important role in keeping your diabetes in control. But the way you live—your diet, careful monitoring of your glucose levels, exercise, and planned physical activity—all work with your insulin to help you control your diabetes.

Who should not take LANTUS?

You should not take LANTUS if you are allergic to insulin or any of the inactive ingredients in LANTUS.

How should I take LANTUS?

Inject LANTUS under your skin once a day at bedtime. You do not need to shake the vial before use. You should look at the medicine in the vial. If the medicine is cloudy or has particles in it, throw the vial away and get a new one.

What sort of syringe should I use?

Always use a syringe that is marked for U-100 insulin preparations. If you use the wrong syringe, you may get the wrong dose and develop a blood glucose level that is too low or too high.

Use disposable syringes and needles only once. Throw them away properly. Use a new needle and syringe every time you dose. Never share needles and syringes.

How do I draw the insulin into the syringe?

Do not dilute or mix LANTUS with any other insulin or solution. The syringe must not contain any other medicine or residue.

Follow these steps:

1. Wash your hands.
2. Check the insulin to make sure it is clear and colorless. Do not use it if it is cloudy or if you see particles.
3. If you are using a new vial, remove the protective cap. Do not remove the stopper.
4. Wipe the top of the vial with an alcohol swab.
5. Draw air into the syringe equal to your insulin dose. Put the needle through the rubber top of the vial and push the plunger to inject the air into the vial.
6. Leave the syringe in the vial and turn both upside down. Hold the syringe and vial firmly in one hand.
7. Make sure the tip of the needle is in the insulin. With your free hand, pull the plunger to withdraw the correct dose into the syringe.
8. Before you take the needle out of the vial, check the syringe for air bubbles. If bubbles are in the medicine, hold the syringe straight up and tap the side of the syringe until the bubbles float to the top. Push the bubbles out with the plunger and draw insulin back in until you have the correct dose.
9. Remove the needle from the vial. Do not let the needle touch anything. You are now ready to inject.

How do I inject LANTUS?

Do not mix or dilute LANTUS with any other insulin or solution or LANTUS will not work as intended, and you may lose blood sugar control, which could be serious. You do not have to shake the vial before use.

Follow these steps:

1. Decide on an injection area—either upper arm, thigh, or abdomen. Injection sites within an injection area must be different from one injection to the next.
2. Use alcohol to clean the skin where you are going to inject.
3. Pinch the skin and hold it. Stick the needle in the way your doctor, nurse, or diabetes educator showed you.
4. Slowly push in the plunger of the syringe all the way, making sure you have injected all the insulin. Leave the needle in the skin for several seconds.
5. Pull the needle straight out and gently press on the spot where you injected yourself for several seconds. Do not rub the area.

Continued on next page

Lantus—Cont.

6. Follow your health care professional's instructions for throwing away the needle and syringe.

If your blood glucose reading is high or low, or if your urine tests show glucose, tell your health care professional so the dose can be adjusted.

What can affect how much insulin I need?

Illness. Illness may change how much insulin you need. It is a good idea to think ahead and make a "sick day" plan with your health care professional so you will be ready when this happens. Be sure to test your blood and urine often and call your health care professional if you are sick.

Pregnancy and nursing. If you are pregnant or nursing, or if you plan to get pregnant, talk with your health care professional before you take LANTUS. Your diabetes may be harder to control when you are pregnant. It is important for you to monitor your glucose closer than usual during this time.

Medicines. Other medicines can change the way insulin works. Therefore, tell your health care professional about all other medicines you are taking. Your insulin dosage may need to be changed by your health care professional. Do not change your medicine doses yourself.

For example, your body may need more insulin if you take birth control, thyroid, decongestant, or diet pills. Your body may need less insulin if you are taking antidepressants, antidiabetic pills, or ACE inhibitors (used to lower blood pressure and for certain heart conditions).

Exercise. Exercise may change the way your body uses insulin. Be sure to check with your health care professional before you start an exercise program.

Travel. If you travel across time zones, talk with your health care professional about how to time your injections. When you travel, wear your medical alert identification. Take extra insulin and supplies with you.

What if I want to drink alcohol?

Before you drink alcohol, talk to your health care professional about its effect on diabetes.

What are the possible side effects of insulins?

1. **Allergic reactions:**

In rare cases, a patient may be allergic to an insulin product. Severe insulin allergies may be life-threatening. If you think you are having an allergic reaction, get medical help right away. Signs of insulin allergy are:

- a rash all over your body
- shortness of breath
- wheezing (trouble breathing)
- a fast pulse
- sweating
- low blood pressure

2. **Hypoglycemia:**

Hypoglycemia is often called an "insulin reaction" or "low blood sugar." It may occur when you do not have enough glucose in your blood. Common causes of hypoglycemia are illness, emotional or physical stress, too much insulin, too little food or missed meals, and too much exercise.

Some of the symptoms of hypoglycemia are:

- sudden cold sweat
- feeling shaky or nervous
- feeling very tired
- feeling sick to your stomach
- feeling dizzy
- blurry vision
- headache
- confusion
- personality changes

Early warning signs of hypoglycemia may be different or less noticeable in some people. That is why it is important to check your glucose as you have been advised by your doctor. If you have hypoglycemia, your body needs sugar. That is why you should carry sugar, candy mints, or glucose tablets with you. Learn to recognize the signs and eat or drink something that has some sugar in it.

Hypoglycemia can be very dangerous. Severe hypoglycemia can cause confusion, seizures, and loss of consciousness. Someone with hypoglycemia who cannot take sugar by mouth needs medical help fast. Without immediate medical help, serious reactions or even death could occur.

You will have mild hypoglycemia once in a while when a meal is delayed, if you get sick, or if you are late with your insulin injection. But if hypoglycemia happens often or is severe, tell your health care professional about it. Also, if you have trouble recognizing the symptoms of hypoglycemia, talk with your health care professional.

3. **Hyperglycemia:**

Hyperglycemia occurs when you have too much glucose in your blood. Usually, it means there is not enough insulin to break down the food you eat into energy your body can use. Hyperglycemia can be caused by a fever, an infection, stress, eating more than you should, taking less insulin than prescribed, or it can be part of the natural progression of diabetes. Routine testing of your blood or urine will let you know if you have hyperglycemia. If your tests are often high, tell your health care professional so your dose of medicine can be changed.

If your glucose is often high, you can develop a very serious condition called diabetic ketoacidosis. Ketoacidosis can be life-threatening. If your blood tests show high amounts of glucose or your urine tests show high amounts of glucose or acetone, or if you have signs of ketoacidosis, you need to get medical help quickly. Do not use LANTUS to treat diabetic ketoacidosis. Signs of ketoacidosis are:

- sleepiness
- flushed (red) face
- thirst
- loss of appetite
- fruity odor on your breath

Signs of severe ketoacidosis are:

- heavy breathing
- fast pulse

4. **Possible reactions on the skin at the injection site:**

Injecting insulin can cause the following reactions on the skin at the injection site:

- a little depression in the skin (lipoatrophy)
- skin thickening (lipohypertrophy)
- red, swelling, itchy skin (injection site reaction)

An injection site reaction should clear up in a few days or a few weeks. If it does not go away and it continues to occur, tell your health care professional.

You can reduce the chance of getting lipoatrophy and lipohypertrophy if you change the injection site each time. Tell your health care professional if you have these problems. You may need to learn to inject your insulin a different way.

How should I store LANTUS?

Store new LANTUS vials in the refrigerator (not the freezer) between 36°F–46°F (2°C–8°C). Do not freeze LANTUS. If a vial freezes, throw it away.

Once a vial is opened, you can keep it in the refrigerator or as cool as possible (below 86°F [30°C]). The 10 mL vial is good for 28 days. Keep LANTUS out of direct heat and light. For example, do not leave it in your car on a summer day.

VOCABULARY

Glucose—A form of sugar that the body uses for fuel. It is made when food is broken down in the digestive system. Blood carries glucose to the cells.

Hypoglycemia—Also called insulin reaction. It means that glucose levels in the blood are too low.

Hyperglycemia—Too much glucose in the blood. Usually testing, not symptoms, reveals a too-high level.

Insulin—A hormone that helps the cells in your body use glucose.

LANTUS—A long-acting insulin similar to insulin made by your body. It is used once a day at bedtime to lower blood glucose.

Lipoatrophy (LIP-o-AT-troe-fee)—Loss of fat under the skin. Can be caused by repeated insulin injections in the same place.

Lipohypertrophy (LIP-o-hi-PER-troe-fee)—A lump under the skin caused by an overgrowth of fat cells. Can be caused by repeated insulin injections in the same place.

Ketoacidosis (kee-toe-as-ih-DOE-sis)—A dangerous condition caused when the body does not have enough insulin.

Pancreas (PAN-kree-as)—A gland near the stomach that produces insulin.

Subcutaneous (sub-ku-TAE-nee-us)—The fatty layer under the skin.

ADDITIONAL INFORMATION

DIABETES FORECAST is a national magazine designed especially for patients with diabetes and their families and is available by subscription from the American Diabetes Association, National Service Center, 1701 N. Beauregard Street, Alexandria, Virginia 22311, 1-800-DIABETES (1-800-342-2383).

Another publication, **DIABETES COUNTDOWN**, is available from the Juvenile Diabetes Foundation International (JDF), 120 Wall Street, 19th Floor, New York, New York 10005, 1-800-JDF-CURE (1-800-533-2873). You may also visit the JDF website at www.jdf.org.

To get more information about diabetes, check with your doctor or diabetes educator. To get more information about LANTUS, ask your health care professional or call 1-800-552-3656.

February 2001

Package insert circular number: 50056938

Aventis Pharmaceuticals Inc.

Kansas City, MO 64137 USA

©2001

lanvp0201p

LOVENOX® ℞

(enoxaparin sodium)

Injection

Prescribing Information as of January 2000

Prescribing information for this product, which appears on pages 713–717 of the 2001 PDR, has been completely revised as follows. Please write "See Supplement A" next to the product heading.

SPINAL / EPIDURAL HEMATOMAS

When neuraxial anesthesia (epidural/spinal anesthesia) or spinal puncture is employed, patients anticoagulated or scheduled to be anticoagulated with low molecular weight heparins or heparinoids for prevention of thromboembolic complications are at risk of developing an epidural or spinal hematoma which can result in long-term or permanent paralysis.

The risk of these events is increased by the use of indwelling epidural catheters for administration of analgesia or by the concomitant use of drugs affecting hemostasis such as non steroidal anti-inflammatory drugs (NSAIDs), platelet inhibitors, or other anticoagulants. The risk also appears to be increased by traumatic or repeated epidural or spinal puncture.

Patients should be frequently monitored for signs and symptoms of neurological impairment. If neurologic compromise is noted, urgent treatment is necessary. The physician should consider the potential benefit versus risk before neuraxial intervention in patients anticoagulated or to be anticoagulated for thromboprophylaxis (see also **WARNINGS, Hemorrhage,** and **PRECAUTIONS, Drug Interactions**).

DESCRIPTION

Lovenox Injection is a sterile solution containing enoxaparin sodium, a low molecular weight heparin. It is available in: prefilled syringes (30 and 40 mg), graduated prefilled syringes (60, 80, and 100 mg), and ampules (30 mg). Each dosage unit contains 10 mg enoxaparin sodium per 0.1 mL Water for Injection. The solution is preservative-free and intended for use only as a single-dose injection. (See **DOSAGE AND ADMINISTRATION** and **HOW SUPPLIED** for dosage unit descriptions.) The pH of the injection is 5.5 to 7.5, with an approximate anti-Factor Xa activity per dosage unit of 1000 IU per every 10 mg of enoxaparin sodium (with reference to the W.H.O. First International Low Molecular Weight Heparin Reference Standard). Nitrogen is used in the headspace to inhibit oxidation.

Enoxaparin is obtained by alkaline degradation of heparin benzyl ester derived from porcine intestinal mucosa. Its structure is characterized by a 2-O-sulfo-4-enepyranosuronic acid group at the non-reducing end and a 2-N,6-O-disulfo-D-glucosamine at the reducing end of the chain. The substance is the sodium salt. The average molecular weight is about 4500 daltons. The molecular weight distribution is:

<2000 daltons	≤20%
2000 to 8000 daltons	≥68%
>8000 daltons	≤15%

STRUCTURAL FORMULA

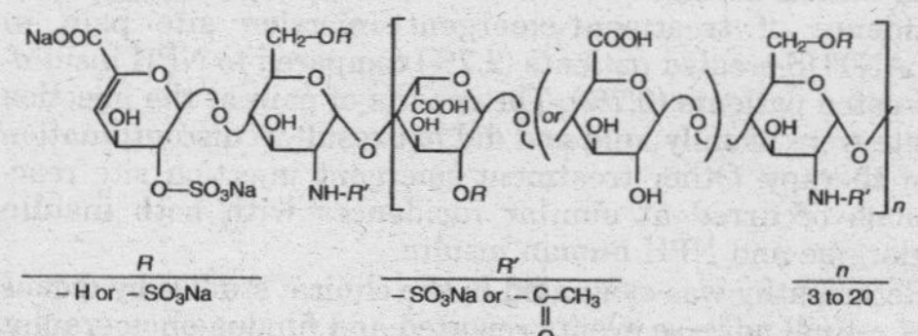

CLINICAL PHARMACOLOGY

Enoxaparin is a low molecular weight heparin which has antithrombotic properties. In humans, enoxaparin given at a dose of 1.5 mg/kg subcutaneously (SC) is characterized by a higher ratio of anti-Factor Xa to anti-Factor IIa activity (mean±SD, 14.0±3.1) (based on areas under anti-Factor activity versus time curves) compared to the ratios observed for heparin (mean±SD, 1.220±0.13). Increases of up to 1.8 times the control values were seen in the thrombin time (TT) and the activated partial thromboplastin time (aPTT). Enoxaparin at a 1 mg/kg dose, administered SC every 12 hours to patients in a large clinical trial resulted in aPTT values of 45 seconds or less in the majority of patients (n = 1607).

Pharmacodynamics: Maximum anti-Factor Xa and anti-thrombin (anti-Factor IIa) activities occur 3 to 5 hours after SC injection of enoxaparin. Mean peak anti-Factor Xa activity was 0.16 IU/mL (1.58 µg/mL) and 0.38 IU/mL (3.83 µg/mL) after the 20 mg and the 40 mg clinically tested SC doses, respectively. Mean (n = 46) peak anti-Factor Xa activity was 1.1 IU/mL at steady state in patients with unstable angina receiving 1.0 mg/kg SC every 12 hours for 14 days. Mean absolute bioavailability of enoxaparin, given SC, based on anti-Factor Xa activity is 92% in healthy volunteers. The volume of distribution of anti-Factor Xa activity is about 6 L. Following intravenous (i.v.) dosing, the total body clearance of enoxaparin is 26 mL/min. After i.v. dosing of enoxaparin labeled with the gamma-emitter, ^{99m}Tc, 40% of radioactivity and 8 to 20% of anti-Factor Xa activity were recovered in urine in 24 hours. Elimination half-life based on anti-Factor Xa activity was 4.5 hours after SC administration. Following a 40 mg SC once a day dose, significant anti-Factor Xa activity persists in plasma for about 12 hours.

Following SC dosing, the apparent clearance (CL/F) of enoxaparin is approximately 15 mL/min. Apparent clearance and A_{max} derived from anti-Factor Xa values following single SC dosing (40 mg and 60 mg) were slightly higher in males than in females. The source of the gender difference in these parameters has not been conclusively identified, however, body weight may be a contributing factor.

Apparent clearance and A_{max} derived from anti-Factor Xa values following single and multiple SC dosing in elderly subjects were close to those observed in young subjects. Following once a day SC dosing of 40 mg enoxaparin, the Day 10 mean area under anti-Factor Xa activity versus time curve (AUC) was approximately 15% greater than the mean Day 1 AUC value. In subjects with moderate renal impairment (creatinine clearance 30 to 80 mL/min), anti-Factor Xa CL/F values were similar to those in healthy subjects. However, mean CL/F values of subjects with severe renal impairment (creatinine clearance <30 mL/min), were approximately 30% lower than the mean CL/F value of control group subjects. (See **PRECAUTIONS.**)

CLINICAL TRIALS

Hip or Knee Replacement Surgery: Lovenox Injection has been shown to prevent post-operative deep vein thrombosis (DVT) following hip or knee replacement surgery.

In a double-blind study, Lovenox Injection 30 mg every 12 hours SC was compared to placebo in patients with hip replacement. After hemostasis was established, treatment was initiated 12 to 24 hours after surgery and was continued for 10 to 14 days after surgery. The data are provided below.

Efficacy of Lovenox Injection in Hip Replacement Surgery

	Dosing Regimen	
Indication	Lovenox 30 mg q12h SC n (%)	Placebo q12h SC n (%)
All Treated Hip Replacement Patients	50 (100)	50 (100)
Treatment Failures Total DVT (%)	5 (10)[1]	23 (46)
Proximal DVT (%)	1 (2)[2]	11 (22)

[1]p value versus placebo = 0.0002
[2]p value versus placebo = 0.0134

A double-blind, multicenter study compared three dosing regimens of Lovenox Injection in patients with hip replacement. Treatment was initiated within two days after surgery and was continued for 7 to 11 days after surgery. The data are provided below.

Efficacy of Lovenox Injection in Hip Replacement Surgery

	Lovenox Dosing Regimen		
Indication	10 mg q.d. SC n (%)	30 mg q12h SC n (%)	40 mg q.d. SC n (%)
All Treated Hip Replacement Patients	161 (100)	208 (100)	199 (100)
Treatment Failures Total DVT (%)	40 (25)	22 (11)[1]	27 (14)
Proximal DVT (%)	17 (11)	8 (4)[2]	9 (5)

[1]p value versus Lovenox 10 mg once a day = 0.0008
[2]p value versus Lovenox 10 mg once a day = 0.0168

There was no significant difference between the 30 mg every 12 hours and 40 mg once a day regimens.
Extended Prophylaxis in Hip Replacement Surgery: In a study of extended prophylaxis for patients undergoing hip replacement surgery, patients were treated, while hospitalized, with enoxaparin 40 mg SC, initiated up to 12 hours prior to surgery for the prevention of post-operative deep vein thrombosis. At the end of the peri-operative period, all patients underwent bilateral venography. In a double-blind design, those patients with no venous thromboembolic disease were randomized to a post-discharge regimen of either enoxaparin 40 mg (n = 90) once a day SC or to placebo (n = 89) for 3 weeks. In this population of patients, the incidence of deep vein thrombosis during extended prophylaxis was significantly lower for enoxaparin compared to placebo. The data are provided below.

Efficacy of Lovenox Injection with Extended Prophylaxis Following Hip Replacement Surgery

	Post Discharge Dosing Regimen	
Indication (Post-Discharge)	Lovenox 40 mg q.d. SC n (%)	Placebo q.d. SC n (%)
All Treated Extended Prophylaxis Patients	90 (100)	89 (100)
Treatment Failures Total DVT (%)	6 (7)[1] (95% CI: 3 to 14)	18 (20) (95% CI: 12 to 30)
Proximal DVT (%)	5 (6)[2] (95% CI: 2 to 13)	7 (8) (95% CI: 3 to 16)

[1]p value versus placebo = 0.008
[2]p value versus placebo = 0.537

In a second study, patients undergoing hip replacement surgery were treated, while hospitalized, with enoxaparin 40 mg SC, initiated up to 12 hours prior to surgery. All patients were examined for clinical signs and symptoms of venous thromboembolic disease. In a double-blind design, patients without clinical signs and symptoms of venous thromboembolic disease were randomized to a post-discharge regimen of either enoxaparin 40 mg (n = 131) once a day SC or to placebo (n = 131) for 3 weeks. Similar to the first study the incidence of deep vein thrombosis during extended prophylaxis was significantly lower for enoxaparin compared to placebo, with a statistically significant difference in both total DVT (enoxaparin 21 [16%] versus placebo 45 [34%]; p = 0.001) and proximal DVT (enoxaparin 8 [6%] versus placebo 28 [21%]; p = <0.001).
In a double-blind study, Lovenox Injection 30 mg every 12 hours SC was compared to placebo in 99 patients under-

going knee replacement surgery. After hemostasis was established, treatment was initiated 12 to 24 hours after surgery and was continued up to 15 days after surgery. The incidence of proximal and total deep vein thrombosis after surgery was significantly lower for enoxaparin compared to placebo. The data are provided below.

Efficacy of Lovenox Injection in Knee Replacement Surgery

	Dosing Regimen	
Indication	Lovenox 30 mg q12h SC n (%)	Placebo q12h SC n (%)
All Treated Knee Replacements Patients	47 (100)	52 (100)
Treatment Failures Total DVT (%)	5 (11)[1] (95% CI: 1 to 21)	32 (62) (95% CI: 47 to 76)
Proximal DVT (%)	0 (0)[2] (95% Upper CL: 5)	7 (13) (95% CI: 3 to 24)

[1]p value versus placebo = 0.001
CI = Confidence Interval
[2]p value versus placebo = 0.013
CL = Confidence Limit

Additionally, in an open-label, parallel group, randomized clinical study, Lovenox Injection 30 mg every 12 hours SC in patients undergoing elective knee replacement surgery was compared to heparin 5000 U every 8 hours SC. Treatment was initiated after surgery and continued up to 14 days. The incidence of deep vein thrombosis was significantly lower for enoxaparin compared to heparin.

Efficacy of Lovenox Injection in Abdominal Surgery Patients with Cancer

	Dosing Regimen	
Indication	Lovenox 40 mg q.d. SC n (%)	Heparin 5000 U q8h SC n (%)
All Treated Abdominal Surgery Patients	555 (100)	560 (100)
Treatment Failures Total VTE[1] (%)	56 (10.1) (95% CI[2]: 8 to 13)	63 (11.3) (95% CI: 9 to 14)
DVT Only (%)	54 (9.7) (95% CI: 7 to 12)	61 (10.9) (95% CI: 8 to 13)

[1]VTE=Venous thromboembolic events which included DVT, PE, and death considered to be thromboembolic in origin.
[2]CI=Confidence Interval

Efficacy of Lovenox Injection in Colorectal Surgery

	Dosing Regimen	
Indication	Lovenox 40 mg q.d. SC n (%)	Heparin 5000 U q8h SC n (%)
All Treated Colorectal Surgery Patients	673 (100)	674 (100)
Treatment Failures Total VTE[1] (%)	48 (7.1) (95% CI[2]: 5 to 9)	45 (6.7) (95% CI: 5 to 9)
DVT Only (%)	47 (7.0) (95% CI: 5 to 9)	44 (6.5) (95% CI: 5 to 8)

[1]VTE=Venous thromboembolic events which included DVT, PE, and death considered to be thromboembolic in origin.
[2]CI=Confidence Interval

Efficacy of Lovenox Injection in Treatment of Deep Vein Thrombosis and Pulmonary Embolism

	Dosing Regimen[1]		
Indication	Lovenox 1.5 mg/kg q.d. SC n (%)	Lovenox 1.0 mg/kg q12h SC n (%)	Heparin aPTT Adjusted i.v. Therapy n (%)
All Treated DVT Patients with and without PE	298 (100)	312 (100)	290 (100)
Patient Outcome Total VTE[2] (%)	13 (4.4)[3]	9 (2.9)[3]	12 (4.1)
DVT Only (%)	11 (3.7)	7 (2.2)	8 (2.8)
Proximal DVT (%)	9 (3.0)	6 (1.9)	7 (2.4)
PE (%)	2 (0.7)	2 (0.6)	4 (1.4)

[1] All patients were also treated with warfarin sodium commencing within 72 hours of Lovenox or standard heparin therapy.
[2] VTE = venous thromboembolic event (deep vein thrombosis [DVT] and/or pulmonary embolism [PE]).
[3] The 95% Confidence Intervals for the treatment differences for total VTE were:
Lovenox once a day versus heparin (−3.0 to 3.5)
Lovenox every 12 hours versus heparin (−4.2 to 1.7).

Abdominal Surgery: In a double-blind, parallel group study of 1115 patients undergoing elective cancer surgery of the gastrointestinal, urological, or gynecological tract, Lovenox Injection 40 mg SC, administered once a day, beginning 2 hours prior to surgery and continuing for a maximum of 12 days after surgery, was comparable to heparin 5000 U every 8 hours SC in preventing deep vein thrombosis (DVT). The data are provided below.
[See first table above]
In a second double-blind, parallel group study, Lovenox Injection 40 mg SC once a day was compared to heparin 5000 U every 8 hours SC in 1347 patients undergoing colorectal surgery (one-third with cancer). Treatment was initiated approximately 2 hours prior to surgery and continued for approximately 7 to 10 days after surgery. The data are provided below.
[See second table above]
Treatment of Deep Vein Thrombosis and Pulmonary Embolism: In a multicenter, parallel group study, 900 patients with acute lower extremity deep vein thrombosis (DVT) with or without pulmonary embolism (PE) were randomized to an inpatient (hospital) treatment of either (i) Lovenox Injection 1.5 mg/kg once a day SC, (ii) Lovenox Injection 1.0 mg/kg every 12 hours SC, or (iii) heparin i.v. bolus (5000 IU) followed by a continuous infusion (administered to achieve an aPTT of 55 to 85 seconds). All patients also received warfarin sodium (dose adjusted according to PT to achieve an International Normalization Ratio [INR] of 2.0 to 3.0), commencing within 72 hours of initiation of Lovenox Injection or standard heparin therapy, and continuing for 90 days. Lovenox Injection or standard heparin therapy was administered for a minimum of 5 days and until the targeted warfarin sodium INR was achieved. Both Lovenox Injection regimens were equivalent to standard heparin therapy in the prevention of recurrent venous thromboembolism (DVT and/or PE).

Continued on next page

Lovenox—Cont.

[See third table at top of previous page]
Similarly, in a multicenter, open-label, parallel group study, 501 patients with acute proximal deep vein thrombosis were randomized to enoxaparin or heparin. Patients who could not receive outpatient therapy were excluded from entering the study. Eligible patients could be treated in the hospital, but ONLY enoxaparin patients were permitted to go home on therapy (72%). Patients were randomized to either Lovenox Injection 1 mg/kg every 12 hours SC or heparin i.v. bolus (5000 IU) followed by a continuous infusion administered to achieve an aPTT of 60 to 85 seconds (in-patient treatment). All patients also received warfarin sodium as described in the previous study. Lovenox Injection or standard heparin therapy was administered for a minimum of 5 days. Lovenox Injection was equivalent to standard heparin therapy in the prevention of recurrent venous thromboembolism.

[See first table at right]

Unstable Angina and Non-Q-Wave Myocardial Infarction: In a multicenter, double-blind, parallel group study, 3171 patients who recently experienced unstable angina or non-Q-wave myocardial infarction were randomized to either Lovenox Injection 1 mg/kg every 12 hours SC or heparin i.v. bolus (5000 U) followed by a continuous infusion (adjusted to achieve an aPTT of 55 to 85 seconds). **All** patients were also treated with aspirin 100 to 325 mg per day. Treatment was initiated within 24 hours of the event and continued until clinical stabilization, revascularization procedures, or hospital discharge, with a maximal duration of 8 days of therapy. The combined incidence of the triple endpoint of death, myocardial infarction, or recurrent angina was lower for Lovenox Injection compared with heparin therapy at 14 days after initiation of treatment. The lower incidence of the triple endpoint was sustained up to 30 days after initiation of treatment. These results were observed in an analysis of both all-randomized and all-treated patients.

Urgent revascularization procedures were performed less frequently in the Lovenox Injection group as compared to the heparin group, 6.3% compared to 8.2% at 30 days (p = 0.047).

[See second table at right]

The combined incidence of death or myocardial infarction at all time points was lower for Lovenox Injection compared to standard heparin therapy, but did not achieve statistical significance. The data are provided below.

[See third table at right]

INDICATIONS AND USAGE

- Lovenox Injection is indicated for the prevention of deep vein thrombosis, which may lead to pulmonary embolism:
  - in patients undergoing hip replacement surgery, during and following hospitalization;
  - in patients undergoing knee replacement surgery;
  - in patients undergoing abdominal surgery who are at risk for thromboembolic complications. Patients at risk include patients who are over 40 years of age, obese, undergoing surgery under general anesthesia lasting longer than 30 minutes or who have additional risk factors such as malignancy or a history of deep vein thrombosis or pulmonary embolism.
- Lovenox Injection is indicated for:
  - the **inpatient treatment** of acute deep vein thrombosis **with and without pulmonary embolism**, when administered in conjunction with warfarin sodium;
  - the **outpatient treatment** of acute deep vein thrombosis **without pulmonary embolism** when administered in conjunction with warfarin sodium.
- Lovenox Injection is indicated for the prevention of ischemic complications of unstable angina and non-Q-wave myocardial infarction, when concurrently administered with aspirin.

See **DOSAGE AND ADMINISTRATION: Adult Dosage** for appropriate dosage regimens.

CONTRAINDICATIONS

Lovenox Injection is contraindicated in patients with active major bleeding, in patients with thrombocytopenia associated with a positive *in vitro* test for anti-platelet antibody in the presence of enoxaparin sodium, or in patients with hypersensitivity to enoxaparin sodium.

Patients with known hypersensitivity to heparin or pork products should not be treated with Lovenox Injection.

WARNINGS

Lovenox Injection is not intended for intramuscular administration.

Lovenox Injection cannot be used interchangeably (unit for unit) with heparin or other low molecular weight heparins as they differ in manufacturing process, molecular weight distribution, anti-Xa and anti-IIa activities, units, and dosage. Each of these medicines has its own instructions for use.

Lovenox Injection should be used with extreme caution in patients with a history of heparin-induced thrombocytopenia.

Hemorrhage: Lovenox Injection, like other anticoagulants, should be used with extreme caution in conditions with increased risk of hemorrhage, such as bacterial endocarditis, congenital or acquired bleeding disorders, active ulcerative and angiodysplastic gastrointestinal disease, hemorrhagic

Efficacy of Lovenox Injection in Treatment of Deep Vein Thrombosis

Indication	Dosing Regimen[1]	
	Lovenox 1.0 mg/kg q12h SC n (%)	Heparin aPTT Adjusted i.v. Therapy n (%)
All Treated DVT Patients	247 (100)	254 (100)
Patient Outcome Total VTE[2] (%)	13 (5.3)[3]	17 (6.7)
DVT Only (%)	11 (4.5)	14 (5.5)
Proximal DVT (%)	10 (4.0)	12 (4.7)
PE (%)	2 (0.8)	3 (1.2)

[1] All patients were also treated with warfarin sodium commencing on the evening of the second day of Lovenox or standard heparin therapy.
[2] VTE=venous thromboembolic event (deep vein thrombosis [DVT] and/or pulmonary embolism [PE]).
[3] The 95% Confidence Intervals for the treatment difference for total VTE was: Lovenox versus heparin (−5.6 to 2.7).

Efficacy of Lovenox Injection in Unstable Angina and Non-Q-Wave Myocardial Infarction (Combined Endpoint of Death, Myocardial Infarction, or Recurrent Angina)

Indication	Dosing Regimen[1]		Reduction (%)	p Value
	Lovenox 1 mg/kg q12h SC n (%)	Heparin aPTT Adjusted i.v. Therapy n (%)		
All Randomized Unstable Angina and Non-Q-Wave MI Patients	1607 (100)	1564 (100)		
Timepoint[2]				
48 Hours	99 (6.2)	115 (7.4)	1.2	0.178
14 Days	266 (16.6)	309 (19.8)	3.2	0.019
30 Days	318 (19.8)	364 (23.3)	3.5	0.016

[1] All patients were also treated with aspirin 100 to 325 mg per day.
[2] Evaluation timepoints are after initiation of treatment. Therapy continued for up to 8 days (median duration of 2.6 days).

Efficacy of Lovenox Injection in Unstable Angina and Non-Q-Wave Myocardial Infarction (Combined Endpoint of Death or Myocardial Infarction)

Indication	Dosing Regimen[1]		Reduction (%)	p Value
	Lovenox 1 mg/kg q 12h SC n (%)	Heparin aPTT Adjusted i.v. Therapy n (%)		
All Randomized Unstable Angina and Non-Q-Wave MI Patients	1607 (100)	1564 (100)		
Timepoint[2]				
48 Hours	18 (1.1)	21 (1.3)	0.2	0.119
14 Days	79 (4.9)	96 (6.1)	1.2	0.132
30 Days	99 (6.2)	121 (7.7)	1.5	0.081

[1] All patients were also treated with aspirin 100 to 325 mg per day.
[2] Evaluation timepoints are after initiation of treatment. Therapy continued for up to 8 days (median duration of 2.6 days).

stroke, or shortly after brain, spinal, or ophthalmological surgery, or in patients treated concomitantly with platelet inhibitors.

Cases of epidural or spinal hematomas have been reported with the associated use of enoxaparin and spinal/epidural anesthesia or spinal puncture resulting in long-term or permanent paralysis. The risk of these events is higher with the use of post-operative indwelling epidural catheters or by the concomitant use of additional drugs affecting hemostasis such as NSAIDs (see boxed WARNING; ADVERSE REACTIONS, Ongoing Safety Surveillance; and PRECAUTIONS, Drug Interactions).

Major hemorrhages including retroperitoneal and intracranial bleeding have been reported. Some of these cases have been fatal. Bleeding can occur at any site during therapy with enoxaparin. An unexplained fall in hematocrit or blood pressure should lead to a search for a bleeding site.

Thrombocytopenia: Thrombocytopenia can occur with the administration of Lovenox Injection.

Moderate thrombocytopenia (platelet counts between 100,000/mm³ and 50,000/mm³) occurred at a rate of 1.3% in patients given Lovenox Injection, 1.2% in patients given heparin, and 0.6% in patients given placebo in clinical trials.

Platelet counts less than 50,000/mm³ occurred at a rate of 0.1% in patients given Lovenox Injection, in 0.2% of patients given heparin, and 0% of patients given placebo in the same trials.

Thrombocytopenia of any degree should be monitored closely. If the platelet count falls below 100,000/mm³, enoxaparin should be discontinued. Rare cases of thrombocytopenia with thrombosis have also been observed in clinical practice. Some of these cases were complicated by organ infarction or limb ischemia.

PRECAUTIONS

General: Lovenox Injection should not be mixed with other injections or infusions.

Lovenox Injection should be used with care in patients with a bleeding diathesis, uncontrolled arterial hypertension or a history of recent gastrointestinal ulceration, diabetic retinopathy, and hemorrhage. Elderly patients and patients with renal insufficiency may show delayed elimination of enoxaparin. Enoxaparin should be used with care in these patients. Adjustment of enoxaparin sodium dose may be considered for low weight (<45 kg) patients and/or for patients with severe renal impairment (creatinine clearance <30mL/min).

If thromboembolic events occur despite enoxaparin prophylaxis, appropriate therapy should be initiated.

Laboratory Tests: Periodic complete blood counts, including platelet count, and stool occult blood tests are recommended during the course of treatment with Lovenox Injection. When administered at recommended prophylaxis doses, routine coagulation tests such as Prothrombin Time (PT) and Activated Partial Thromboplastin Time (aPTT) are relatively insensitive measures of Lovenox Injection activity and, therefore, unsuitable for monitoring. Anti-Factor Xa may be used to monitor the anticoagulant effect of Lovenox Injection in patients with significant renal impairment. If during Lovenox Injection therapy abnormal coagulation parameters or bleeding should occur, anti-Factor Xa levels may be used to monitor the anticoagulant effects of Lovenox Injection (see CLINICAL PHARMACOLOGY: Pharmacodynamics).

Drug Interactions: Unless really needed, agents which may enhance the risk of hemorrhage should be discontinued prior to initiation of Lovenox Injection therapy. These agents include medications such as: anticoagulants, platelet inhibitors including acetylsalicylic acid, salicylates, NSAIDs (including ketorolac tromethamine), dipyridamole, or sulfinpyrazone. If co-administration is essential, conduct close clinical and laboratory monitoring (see **PRECAUTIONS: Laboratory Tests**). **Carcinogenesis, Mutagenesis, Impairment of Fertility:** No long-term studies in animals have been performed to evaluate the carcinogenic potential of enoxaparin. Enoxaparin was not mutagenic in *in vitro* tests, including the Ames test, mouse lymphoma cell forward mutation test, and human lymphocyte chromosomal aberration test, and the *in vivo* rat bone marrow chromosomal aberration test. Enoxaparin was found to have no effect on fertility or reproductive performance of male and female rats at SC doses up to 20 mg/kg/day or 141 mg/m²/day. The maximum human dose in clinical trials was 2.0 mg/kg/day or 78 mg/m²/day (for an average body weight of 70 kg, height of 170 cm, and body surface area of 1.8 m²).

Pregnancy: *Teratogenic Effects:* Pregnancy Category B: Teratology studies have been conducted in pregnant rats and rabbits at SC doses of enoxaparin up to 30 mg/kg/day or 211 mg/m²/day and 410 mg/m²/day, respectively. There was no evidence of teratogenic effects or fetotoxicity due to enoxaparin. There are, however, no adequate and well-controlled studies in pregnant women. Because animal reproduction studies are not always predictive of human response, this drug should be used during pregnancy only if clearly needed. *Non-teratogenic Effects:* There have been a few spontaneous post-marketing reports of fetal death when pregnant women received enoxaparin. Causality of the cases has not been determined. In one case, placental hemorrhage and detachment were found in association with the fetal death. If enoxaparin is used during pregnancy, or if the patient becomes pregnant while taking this drug, the patient should be apprised of the potential hazard to the fetus.

Nursing Mothers: It is not known whether this drug is excreted in human milk. Because many drugs are excreted in human milk, caution should be exercised when enoxaparin is administered to nursing women.

Pediatric Use: Safety and effectiveness of enoxaparin in pediatric patients have not been established.

ADVERSE REACTIONS

Hemorrhage: The incidence of major hemorrhagic complications during Lovenox Injection treatment has been low. The following rates of major bleeding events have been reported during clinical trials.

[See first table at right]

NOTE: At no time point were the 40 mg once a day pre-operative and the 30 mg every 12 hours post-operative hip replacement surgery prophylactic regimens compared in clinical trials.

Injection site hematomas during the extended prophylaxis period after hip replacement surgery occurred in 9% of the enoxaparin patients versus 1.8% of the placebo patients.

Major Bleeding Episodes in Abdominal and Colorectal Surgery[1]

Indications	Dosing Regimen	
	Lovenox 40 mg q.d. SC	Heparin 5000 U q8h SC
Abdominal Surgery	n = 555 23 (4%)	n = 560 16 (3%)
Colorectal Surgery	n = 673 28 (4%)	n = 674 21 (3%)

[1] Bleeding complications were considered major: (1) if the hemorrhage caused a significant clinical event, or (2) if accompanied by a hemoglobin decrease ≥2g/dL or transfusion of 2 or more units of blood products. Retroperitoneal, intraocular, and intracranial hemorrhages were always considered major.

Major Bleeding Episodes in Deep Vein Thrombosis and Pulmonary Embolism Treatment[1]

Indication	Dosing Regimen[2]		
	Lovenox 1.5 mg/kg q.d. SC	Lovenox 1.0 mg/kg q12h SC	Heparin aPTT Adjusted i.v. Therapy
Deep Vein Thrombosis and Pulmonary Embolism Treatment	n = 298 5 (2%)	n = 559 9 (2%)	n = 554 9 (2%)

[1] Bleeding complications were considered major: (1) if the hemorrhage caused a significant clinical event, or (2) if accompanied by a hemoglobin decrease ≥2g/dL or transfusion of 2 or more units of blood products. Retroperitoneal, intraocular, and intracranial hemorrhages were always considered major.

[2] All patients also received warfarin sodium (dose-adjusted according to PT to achieve an INR of 2.0 to 3.0) commencing within 72 hours of Lovenox or standard heparin therapy and continuing for up to 90 days.

Major Bleeding Episodes in Hip or Knee Replacement Surgery[1]

Indications	Dosing Regimen		
	Lovenox 40 mg q.d. SC	Lovenox 30 mg q12h SC	Heparin 15,000 U/24h SC
Hip Replacement Surgery Without Extended Prophylaxis[2]		n = 786 31 (4%)	n = 541 32 (6%)
Hip Replacement Surgery With Extended Prophylaxis Peri-operative Period[3]	n = 288 4 (2%)		
Extended Prophylaxis Period[4]	n = 221 0 (0%)		
Knee Replacement Surgery Without Extended Prophylaxis[2]		n = 294 3 (1%)	n = 225 3 (1%)

[1] Bleeding complications were considered major: (1) if the hemorrhage caused a significant clinical event, or (2) if accompanied by a hemoglobin decrease ≥2g/dL or transfusion of 2 or more units of blood products. Retroperitoneal and intracranial hemorrhages were always considered major. In the knee replacement surgery trials, intraocular hemorrhages were also considered major hemorrhages.

[2] Lovenox 30 mg every 12 hours SC initiated 12 to 24 hours after surgery and continued for up to 14 days after surgery.

[3] Lovenox 40 mg SC once a day initiated up to 12 hours prior to surgery and continued for up to 7 days after surgery.

[4] Lovenox 40 mg SC once a day for up to 21 days after discharge.

Adverse Events Occurring at ≥2% Incidence in Lovenox Injection Treated Patients[1] Undergoing Hip or Knee Replacement Surgery

Adverse Event	Lovenox 40 mg q.d. SC				Lovenox 30 mg q12h SC		Heparin 15,000 U/24h SC		Placebo q12h SC	
	Peri-operative Period n = 288[2]		Extended Prophylaxis Period n = 131[3]		n = 1080		n = 766		n = 115	
	Severe	Total	Severe	Total	Severe	Total	Severe	Total	Severe	Total
Fever	0%	8%	0%	0%	<1%	5%	<1%	4%	0%	3%
Hemorrhage	<1%	13%	0%	5%	<1%	4%	1%	4%	0%	3%
Nausea					<1%	3%	<1%	2%	0%	2%
Anemia	0%	16%	0%	<2%	<1%	23%	2%	5%	<1%	7%
Edema					<1%	2%	<1%	2%	0%	2%
Peripheral edema	0%	6%	0%	0%	<1%	3%	<1%	4%	0%	3%

[1] Excluding unrelated adverse events.

[2] Data represents Lovenox 40 mg SC once a day initiated up to 12 hours prior to surgery in 288 hip replacement surgery patients who received enoxaparin perioperatively in an unblinded fashion in one clinical trial.

[3] Data represents Lovenox 40 mg SC once a day given in a blinded fashion as extended prophylaxis at the end of the peri-operative period in 131 of the original 288 hip replacement surgery patients for up to 21 days in one clinical trial.

Adverse Events Occurring at ≥2% Incidence in Lovenox Injection Treated Patients[1] Undergoing Treatment for Deep Vein Thrombosis and Pulmonary Embolism

Adverse Event	Dosing Regimen					
	Lovenox 1.5 mg/kg q.d. SC n = 298		Lovenox 1.0 mg/kg q12h SC n = 559		Heparin aPTT Adjusted i.v. Therapy n = 544	
	Severe	Total	Severe	Total	Severe	Total
Injection Site Hemorrhage	0%	5%	0%	3%	<1%	<1%
Injection Site Pain	0%	2%	0%	2%	0%	0%
Hematuria	0%	2%	0%	<1%	<1%	2%

[1] Excluding unrelated adverse events.

Major Bleeding Episodes in Unstable Angina and Non-Q-Wave Myocardial Infarction

Indication	Dosing Regimen	
	Lovenox[1] 1 mg/kg q12h SC	Heparin[1] aPTT Adjusted i.v. Therapy
Unstable Angina and Non-Q-Wave MI[2,3]	n = 1578 17 (1%)	n = 1529 18 (1%)

[1] The rates represent major bleeding on study medication up to 12 hours after dose.

[2] Aspirin therapy was administered concurrently (100 to 325 mg per day).

[3] Bleeding complications were considered major: (1) if the hemorrhage caused a significant clinical event, or (2) if accompanied by a hemoglobin decrease by ≥3g/dL or transfusion of 2 or more units of blood products. Intraocular, retroperitoneal, and intracranial hemorrhages were always considered major.

Thrombocytopenia: see **WARNINGS: Thrombocytopenia.**
Elevations of Serum Aminotransferases: Asymptomatic increases in aspartate (AST [SGOT]) and alanine (ALT [SGPT]) aminotransferase levels greater than three times the upper limit of normal of the laboratory reference range have been reported in up to 6.1% and 5.9% of patients, respectively, during treatment with Lovenox Injection. Similar significant increases in aminotransferase levels have also been observed in patients and healthy volunteers treated with heparin and other low molecular weight heparins. Such elevations are fully reversible and are rarely associated with increases in bilirubin.

Since aminotransferase determinations are important in the differential diagnosis of myocardial infarction, liver disease, and pulmonary emboli, elevations that might be caused by drugs like Lovenox Injection should be interpreted with caution.

Local Reactions: Mild local irritation, pain, hematoma, ecchymosis, and erythema may follow SC injection of Lovenox Injection.

Other: Other adverse effects that were thought to be possibly or probably related to treatment with Lovenox Injection, heparin, or placebo in clinical trials with patients undergoing hip or knee replacement surgery, abdominal or colorectal surgery, or treatment for DVT and that occurred at a rate of at least 2% in the enoxaparin group, are provided below.

[See second table above]

Continued on next page

Lovenox—Cont.

Adverse Events Occurring at ≥2% Incidence in Lovenox Injection Treated Patients[1] Undergoing Abdominal or Colorectal Surgery

	Dosing Regimen			
	Lovenox 40 mg q.d. SC n = 1228		Heparin 5000 U q8h SC n = 1234	
Adverse Event	Severe	Total	Severe	Total
Hemorrhage	<1%	7%	<1%	6%
Anemia	<1%	3%	<1%	3%
Ecchymosis	0%	3%	0%	3%

[1] Excluding unrelated adverse events.

[See 3rd table at top of previous page]

Adverse Events in Lovenox Injection Treated Patients With Unstable Angina or Non-Q-Wave Myocardial Infarction: Non-hemorrhagic clinical events reported to be related to enoxaparin therapy occurred at an incidence of ≤1%.

Non-major hemorrhagic episodes, primarily injection site ecchymoses and hematomas, were more frequently reported in patients treated with SC enoxaparin than in patients treated with i.v. heparin.

Serious adverse events with Lovenox Injection or heparin in a clinical trial in patients with unstable angina or non-Q-wave myocardial infarction that occurred at a rate of at least 0.5% in the enoxaparin group, are provided below (irrespective of relationship to drug therapy).

Serious Adverse Events Occurring at ≥0.5% Incidence in Lovenox Injection Treated Patients With Unstable Angina or Non-Q-Wave Myocardial Infarction

	Dosing Regimen	
Adverse Event	Lovenox 1 mg/kg q12 h SC n = 1578 n (%)	Heparin aPTT Adjusted i.v. Therapy n = 1529 n (%)
Atrial fibrillation	11 (0.70)	3 (0.20)
Heart failure	15 (0.95)	11 (0.72)
Lung edema	11 (0.70)	11 (0.72)
Pneumonia	13 (0.82)	9 (0.59)

Ongoing Safety Surveillance: Since 1993, there have been more than 68 reports of epidural or spinal hematoma formation with concurrent use of enoxaparin and spinal/epidural anesthesia or spinal puncture. The majority of patients had a post-operative indwelling epidural catheter placed for analgesia or received additional drugs affecting hemostasis such as NSAIDs. Many of the epidural or spinal hematomas caused neurologic injury, including long-term or permanent paralysis. Because these events were reported voluntarily from a population of unknown size, estimates of frequency cannot be made.

Other reports include: local reactions at the injection site (*i.e.*, skin necrosis, nodules, inflammation, oozing), systemic allergic reactions (*i.e.*, pruritus, urticaria, anaphylactoid reactions), vesiculobullous rash, purpura, thrombocytosis, and thrombocytopenia with thrombosis (see **WARNINGS, Thrombocytopenia**). Very rare cases of hyperlipidemia have been reported, with one case of hyperlipidemia, with marked hypertriglyceridemia, reported in a diabetic pregnant woman; causality has not been determined.

OVERDOSAGE

Symptoms/Treatment: Accidental overdosage following administration of Lovenox Injection may lead to hemorrhagic complications. Injected Lovenox Injection may be largely neutralized by the slow i.v. injection of protamine sulfate (1% solution). The dose of protamine sulfate should be equal to the dose of Lovenox Injection injected: 1 mg protamine sulfate should be administered to neutralize 1 mg Lovenox Injection. A second infusion of 0.5 mg protamine sulfate per 1 mg of Lovenox Injection may be administered if the aPTT measured 2 to 4 hours after the first infusion remains prolonged. However, even with higher doses of protamine, the aPTT may remain more prolonged than under normal conditions found following administration of heparin. In all cases, the anti-Factor Xa activity is never completely neutralized (maximum about 60%). Particular care should be taken to avoid overdosage with protamine sulfate. Administration of protamine sulfate can cause severe hypotensive and anaphylactoid reactions. Because fatal reactions, often resembling anaphylaxis, have been reported with protamine sulfate, it should be given only when resuscitation techniques and treatment of anaphylactic shock are readily available. For additional information consult the labeling of Protamine Sulfate Injection, USP, products.

A single SC dose of 46.4 mg/kg enoxaparin was lethal to rats. The symptoms of acute toxicity were ataxia, decreased motility, dyspnea, cyanosis, and coma.

DOSAGE AND ADMINISTRATION

All patients should be evaluated for a bleeding disorder before administration of Lovenox Injection, unless the medication is needed urgently. Since coagulation parameters are unsuitable for monitoring Lovenox Injection activity, routine monitoring of coagulation parameters is not required (see **PRECAUTIONS, Laboratory Tests**).

Adult Dosage: *Hip or Knee Replacement Surgery:* In patients undergoing hip or knee replacement surgery, the recommended dose of Lovenox Injection is **30 mg every 12 hours** administered by SC injection. Provided that hemostasis has been established, the initial dose should be given 12 to 24 hours after surgery. Up to 14 days administration (average duration 7 to 10 days) of Lovenox Injection 30 mg every 12 hours has been well tolerated in controlled clinical trials. For hip replacement surgery, a dose of **40 mg once a day** SC, given initially 12 (±3) hours prior to surgery, may be considered. Following the initial phase of thromboprophylaxis in hip replacement surgery patients (Lovenox Injection 30 mg every 12 hours or 40 mg once a day), continued prophylaxis with Lovenox Injection 40 mg once a day administered by SC injection for 3 weeks is recommended.

Abdominal Surgery: In patients undergoing abdominal surgery who are at risk for thromboembolic complications, the recommended dose of Lovenox Injection is **40 mg once a day** administered by SC injection with the initial dose given 2 hours prior to surgery. The usual duration of administration is 7 to 10 days; up to 12 days administration has been well tolerated in clinical trials.

Treatment of Deep Vein Thrombosis and Pulmonary Embolism: In **outpatient treatment**, patients with acute deep vein thrombosis without pulmonary embolism who can be treated at home, the recommended dose of Lovenox Injection is **1.0 mg/kg every 12 hours** administered SC. In **inpatient (hospital) treatment**, patients with acute deep vein thrombosis with pulmonary embolism or patients with acute deep vein thrombosis without pulmonary embolism (who are not candidates for outpatient treatment), the recommended dose of Lovenox Injection is **1.0 mg/kg every 12 hours** administered SC or **1.5 mg/kg once a day** administered SC at the same time every day. In both outpatient and inpatient (hospital) treatments, warfarin sodium therapy should be initiated when appropriate (usually within 72 hours of Lovenox Injection). Lovenox Injection should be continued for a minimum of 5 days and until a therapeutic oral anticoagulant effect has been achieved (International Normalization Ratio 2.0 to 3.0). The average duration of administration is 7 days; up to 17 days Lovenox Injection administration has been well tolerated in controlled clinical trials.

Unstable Angina and Non-Q-Wave Myocardial Infarction: In patients with unstable angina or non-Q-wave myocardial infarction, the recommended dose of Lovenox Injection is **1 mg/kg** administered SC **every 12 hours** in conjunction with oral aspirin therapy (100 to 325 mg once daily). Treatment with Lovenox Injection should be prescribed for a minimum of 2 days and continued until clinical stabilization. The usual duration of treatment is 2 to 8 days. To minimize the risk of bleeding following vascular instrumentation during the treatment of unstable angina, adhere precisely to the intervals recommended between Lovenox Injection doses. The vascular access sheath for instrumentation should remain in place for 6 to 8 hours following a dose of Lovenox Injection. The next scheduled dose should be given no sooner than 6 to 8 hours after sheath removal. The site of the procedure should be observed for signs of bleeding or hematoma formation.

Administration: Enoxaparin injection is a clear, colorless to pale yellow sterile solution, and as with other parenteral drug products, should be inspected visually for particulate matter and discoloration prior to administration.

When using Lovenox Injection ampules, to assure withdrawal of the appropriate volume of drug, the use of a tuberculin syringe or equivalent is recommended.

Lovenox Injection is administered by SC injection. It must not be administered by intramuscular injection. Lovenox Injection is intended for use under the guidance of a physician. Patients may self-inject only if their physician determines that it is appropriate and with medical follow-up, as necessary. Proper training in subcutaneous injection technique (with or without the assistance of an injection device) should be provided.

Subcutaneous Injection Technique: Patients should be lying down and Lovenox Injection administered by deep SC injection. To avoid the loss of drug when using the 30 and 40 mg prefilled syringes, do not expel the air bubble from the syringe before the injection. Administration should be alternated between the left and right anterolateral and left and right posterolateral abdominal wall. The whole length of the needle should be introduced into a skin fold held between the thumb and forefinger; the skin fold should be held throughout the injection. To minimize bruising, do not rub the injection site after completion of the injection. An automatic injector, Lovenox EasyInjector™, is available for patients to administer Lovenox Injection packaged in 30 mg and 40 mg prefilled syringes. Please see directions accompanying the Lovenox EasyInjector™ automatic injection device.

HOW SUPPLIED

Lovenox (enoxaparin sodium) Injection is available in:

[See table below]

Store at Controlled Room Temperature, 15–25°C (59–77°F) [see USP].

Keep out of the reach of children.

Lovenox Injection prefilled and graduated prefilled syringes manufactured in France.

Lovenox Injection ampules manufactured in England.

AVENTIS PHARMACEUTICALS PRODUCTS INC.

COLLEGEVILLE, PA 19426

Rev. 1/00A

Dosage Unit	Strength[1]	Package size (per carton)	Anti-Xa Activity[2]	NDC # 0075-
Ampules	30 mg/0.3 mL	10 ampules	3000 IU	0624-03
Prefilled Syringes[3]	30 mg/0.3 mL	10 syringes	3000 IU	0624-30
	40 mg/0.4 mL	10 syringes	4000 IU	0620-40
Graduated Prefilled Syringes[3]	60 mg/0.6 mL	10 syringes	6000 IU	0621-60
	80 mg/0.8 mL	10 syringes	8000 IU	0622-80
	100 mg/1.0 mL	10 syringes	10 000 IU	0623-00

[1] Strength represents the number of milligrams of enoxaparin sodium in Water for Injection. Lovenox ampules and prefilled syringes contain 10 mg enoxaparin sodium per 0.1 mL Water for Injection.

[2] Approximate anti-Factor Xa activity based on reference to the W.H.O. First International Low Molecular Weight Heparin Reference Standard.

[3] Each Lovenox syringe is affixed with a 27 gauge x 1/2 inch needle.

NILANDRON® ℞
(nilutamide)
Tablets

Prescribing information for this product, which appears on pages 720–722 of the 2001 PDR, has been completely revised as follows. Please write "See Supplement A" next to the product heading.

Prescribing Information as of October 2000

DESCRIPTION

NILANDRON® tablets contain nilutamide, a nonsteroidal, orally active antiandrogen having the chemical name 5,5-dimethyl-3-[4-nitro-3-(trifluoromethyl)phenyl]-2,4-imidazolidinedione with the following structural formula:

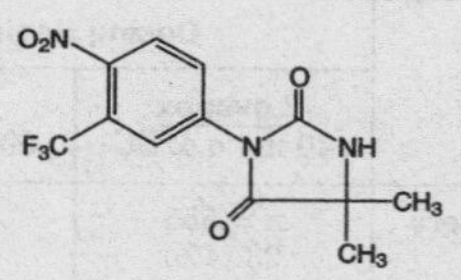

Nilutamide is a microcrystalline, white to practically white powder with a molecular weight of 317.25. Its molecular formula is $C_{12}H_{10}F_3N_3O_4$.

It is freely soluble in ethyl acetate, acetone, chloroform, ethyl alcohol, dichloromethane, and methanol. It is slightly soluble in water [< 0.1% W/V at 25°C (77°F)]. It melts between 153°C and 156°C (307.4°F and 312.8°F).

Each NILANDRON tablet contains 50 mg or 150 mg of nilutamide. Other ingredients in NILANDRON tablets are corn starch, lactose, povidone, docusate sodium, magnesium stearate, and talc.

CLINICAL PHARMACOLOGY

Mechanism of Action

Prostate cancer is known to be androgen sensitive and responds to androgen ablation. In animal studies, nilutamide has demonstrated antiandrogenic activity without other hormonal (estrogen, progesterone, mineralocorticoid, and glucocorticoid) effects. In vitro, nilutamide blocks the effects of testosterone at the androgen receptor level. In vivo, nilutamide interacts with the androgen receptor and prevents the normal androgenic response.

Pharmacokinetics

Absorption: Analysis of blood, urine, and feces samples following a single oral 150-mg dose of [^{14}C]-nilutamide in patients with metastatic prostate cancer showed that the drug is rapidly and completely absorbed and that it yields high and persistent plasma concentrations. In a two-way crossover bioavailability study between a single NILANDRON 150 mg tablet and three NILANDRON 50 mg tablets, it was found that the two treatments were bioequivalent.

Distribution: After absorption of the drug, there is a detectable distribution phase. There is moderate binding of the drug to plasma proteins and low binding to erythrocytes. The binding is nonsaturable except in the case of alpha-1-glycoprotein, which makes a minor contribution to the total concentration of proteins in the plasma. The results of binding studies do not indicate any effects that would cause nonlinear pharmacokinetics.

Metabolism: The results of a human metabolism study using ^{14}C-radiolabelled tablets show that nilutamide is extensively metabolized and less than 2% of the drug is excreted unchanged in urine after 5 days. Five metabolites have been isolated from human urine. Two metabolites display an asymmetric center, due to oxidation of a methyl group, resulting in the formation of D- and L-isomers. One of the metabolites was shown, in vitro, to possess 25 to 50% of the pharmacological activity of the parent drug, and the D-isomer of the active metabolite showed equal or greater potency compared to the L-isomer. However, the pharmacokinetics and the pharmacodynamics of the metabolites have not been fully investigated.

Elimination: The majority (62%) of orally administered [^{14}C]-nilutamide is eliminated in the urine during the first 120 hours after a single 150-mg dose. Fecal elimination is negligible, ranging from 1.4% to 7% of the dose after 4 to 5 days. Excretion of radioactivity in urine likely continues beyond 5 days. The mean elimination half-life of nilutamide determined in studies in which subjects received a single dose of 100–300 mg ranged from 38.0 to 59.1 hours with most values between 41 and 49 hours. The elimination of at least one metabolite is generally longer than that of unchanged nilutamide (59–126 hours). During multiple dosing of 3×50 mg twice a day, steady state was reached within 2 to 4 weeks for most patients, and mean steady state AUC_{0-12} was 110% higher than the $AUC_{0-\infty}$ obtained from the first dose of 3×50 mg. These data and in vitro metabolism data suggest that, upon multiple dosing, metabolic enzyme inhibition may occur for this drug.

Clinical Studies
Nilutamide through its antiandrogenic activity can complement surgical castration, which suppresses only testicular androgens. The effects of the combined therapy were studied in patients with previously untreated metastatic prostate cancer.

In a double-blind, randomized, multicenter study that enrolled 457 patients (225 treated with orchiectomy and NILANDRON, 232 treated with orchiectomy and placebo), the NILANDRON group showed a statistically significant benefit in time to progression and time to death. The results are summarized below.

	NILANDRON	PLACEBO
Median Survival (months)	27.3	23.6
Progression-Free Survival (months)	21.1	14.9
Complete or Partial Regression	41%	24%
Improvement in Bone Pain	54%	37%

INDICATIONS AND USAGE
Metastatic Prostate Cancer
NILANDRON tablets are indicated for use in combination with surgical castration for the treatment of metastatic prostate cancer (Stage D_2).
For maximum benefit, NILANDRON treatment must begin on the same day as or on the day after surgical castration.

CONTRAINDICATIONS
NILANDRON tablets are contraindicated:
- in patients with severe hepatic impairment (baseline hepatic enzymes should be evaluated prior to treatment)
- in patients with severe respiratory insufficiency
- in patients with hypersensitivity to nilutamide or any component of this preparation.

WARNINGS

Interstitial Pneumonitis
Interstitial pneumonitis has been reported in 2% of patients in controlled clinical trials in patients exposed to nilutamide. A small study in Japanese subjects showed that 8 of 47 patients (17%) developed interstitial pneumonitis. Reports of interstitial changes including pulmonary fibrosis that led to hospitalization and death have been reported rarely post-marketing. Symptoms included exertional dyspnea, cough, chest pain, and fever. X-rays showed interstitial or alveolo-interstitial changes, and pulmonary function tests revealed a restrictive pattern with decreased DLco. Most cases occurred within the first 3 months of treatment with NILANDRON, and most reversed with discontinuation of therapy.
A routine chest X-ray should be performed prior to initiating treatment with NILANDRON. Baseline pulmonary function tests may be considered. Patients should be instructed to report any new or worsening shortness of breath that they experience while on NILANDRON. If symptoms occur, NILANDRON should be immediately discontinued until it can be determined if the symptoms are drug related.

Hepatitis
Rare cases of death or hospitalization due to severe liver injury have been reported post-marketing in association with

the use of NILANDRON. Hepatotoxicity in these reports generally occurred within the first 3 to 4 months of treatment. Hepatitis or marked increases in liver enzymes leading to drug discontinuation occurred in 1% of NILANDRON patients in controlled clinical trials.
Serum transaminase levels should be measured prior to starting treatment with NILANDRON, at regular intervals for the first 4 months of treatment, and periodically thereafter. Liver function tests should also be obtained at the first sign or symptom suggestive of liver dysfunction, e.g. nausea, vomiting, abdominal pain, fatigue, anorexia, "flu-like" symptoms, dark urine, jaundice, or right upper quadrant tenderness. If at any time, a patient has jaundice, or their ALT rises above 2 times the upper limit of normal, NILANDRON should be immediately discontinued with close followup of liver function tests until resolution.

Use in Women
NILANDRON has no indication for women, and should not be used in this population, particularly for non-serious or non-life threatening conditions.

Other
Foreign postmarketing surveillance has revealed isolated cases of aplastic anemia in which a causal relationship with NILANDRON could not be ascertained.

PRECAUTIONS
Information for Patients
Patients should be informed that NILANDRON tablets should be started on the day of, or on the day after, surgical castration. They should also be informed that they should not interrupt their dosing of NILANDRON or stop taking this medication without consulting their physician.
Because of the possibility of interstitial pneumonitis, patients should also be told to report immediately any dyspnea or aggravation of pre-existing dyspnea.
Because of the possibility of hepatitis, patients should be told to consult with their physician should nausea, vomiting, abdominal pain, or jaundice occur.
Because of the possibility of an intolerance to alcohol (facial flushes, malaise, hypotension) following ingestion of NILANDRON, it is recommended that intake of alcoholic beverages be avoided by patients who experience this reaction. This effect has been reported in about 5% of patients treated with NILANDRON.
In clinical trials, 13% to 57% of patients receiving NILANDRON reported a delay in adaptation to dark, ranging from seconds to a few minutes, when passing from a lighted area to a dark area. This effect sometimes does not abate as drug treatment is continued. Patients who experience this effect should be cautioned about driving at night or through tunnels. This effect can be alleviated by the wearing of tinted glasses.

Drug Interactions
In vitro, nilutamide has been shown to inhibit the activity of liver cytochrome P-450 isoenzymes and, therefore, may reduce the metabolism of compounds requiring these systems. Consequently, drugs with a low therapeutic margin, such as vitamin K antagonists, phenytoin, and theophylline, could have a delayed elimination and increases in their serum half-life leading to a toxic level. The dosage of these drugs or others with a similar metabolism may need to be modified if they are administered concomitantly with nilutamide. For example, when vitamin K antagonists are administered concomitantly with nilutamide, prothrombin time should be carefully monitored and, if necessary, the dosage of vitamin K antagonists should be reduced.

Carcinogenesis, Mutagenesis, Impairment of Fertility
Administration of nilutamide to rats for 18 months at doses of 0, 5, 15, or 45 mg/kg/day produced benign Leydig cell tumors in 35% of the high-dose male rats (AUC exposures in high-dose rats were approximately 1–2 times human AUC exposures with therapeutic doses). The increased incidence of Leydig cell tumors is secondary to elevated luteinizing hormone (LH) concentrations resulting from loss of feedback inhibition at the pituitary. Elevated LH and testosterone concentrations are not observed in castrated men receiving NILANDRON. Nilutamide had no effect on the incidence, size, or time of onset of any spontaneous tumor in rats.
Nilutamide displayed no mutagenic effects in a variety of in vitro and in vivo tests (Ames test, mouse micronucleus test, and two chromosomal aberration tests).
In reproduction studies in rats, nilutamide had no effect on the reproductive function of males and females, and no lethal, teratogenic, or growth-suppressive effects on fetuses were found. The maximal dose at which nilutamide did not affect reproductive function in either sex or have an effect on fetuses was estimated to be 45 mg/kg orally (AUC exposures in rats approximately 1–2 times human therapeutic AUC exposures).

Pregnancy
Pregnancy Category C; Animal reproduction studies have not been conducted with nilutamide. It is also not known whether nilutamide can cause fetal harm when administered to a pregnant woman or can affect reproductive capacity. Nilutamide should be given to a pregnant woman only if clearly needed.

Pediatric Use
Safety and effectiveness in pediatric patients have not been determined.

Animal Pharmacology and Toxicology
Administration of NILANDRON to beagle dogs resulted in drug-related deaths at dose levels that produce AUC exposures in dogs much lower than the AUC exposures of men receiving the therapeutic doses of 150 and 300 mg/day. Nilutamide-induced toxicity in dogs was cumulative with

progressively lower doses producing death when given for longer durations. Nilutamide given to dogs at 60 mg/kg/day (1–2 times human AUC exposure) for 1 month produced 100% mortality. Administration of 20 and 30 mg/kg/day nilutamide (1/2–1 times human AUC exposure) for 6 months resulted in 20% and 70% mortality in treated dogs. Administration to dogs of 3, 6, and 12 mg/kg/day nilutamide (1/10–1/2 human AUC exposure) for 1 year resulted in 8%, 33%, and 50% mortality, respectively. **A "no-effect level" for nilutamide-induced mortality in dogs was not identified.** Pathology data from the one-year oral toxicity study suggest that the deaths in dogs were secondary to liver toxicity. Marked-to-massive hepatocellular swelling and vacuolization were observed in affected dogs. Liver toxicity in dogs was not consistently associated with elevations of liver enzymes. Administration of nilutamide to rats at a dose level of 45 mg/kg/day (AUC exposure in rats 1–2 times human therapeutic AUC exposures) for 18 months increased the incidence of lung pathology (granulomatous inflammation and chronic alveolitis).
The hepatic and pulmonary adverse effects observed in nilutamide-treated animals and men are similar to effects observed with another nitroaromatic compound, nitrofurantoin. Nilutamide and nitrofurantoin are both metabolized in vitro to nitroanion free-radicals by microsomal NADPH-cytochrome P450 reductase in the lungs and liver of rats and humans.

ADVERSE REACTIONS
The following adverse experiences were reported during a multicenter clinical trial comparing NILANDRON + surgical castration versus placebo + surgical castration. The most frequently reported (greater than 5%) adverse experiences during treatment with NILANDRON tablets in combination with surgical castration are listed below. For comparison, adverse experiences seen with surgical castration and placebo are also listed.

Adverse Experience	NILANDRON + surgical castration (N=225) % All	Placebo + surgical castration (N=232) % All
Cardiovascular System		
Hypertension	5.3	2.6
Digestive System		
Nausea	9.8	6.0
Constipation	7.1	3.9
Endocrine System		
Hot flushes	28.4	22.4
Metabolic and Nutritional System		
Increased AST	8.0	3.9
Increased ALT	7.6	4.3
Nervous System		
Dizziness	7.1	3.4
Respiratory System		
Dyspnea	6.2	7.3
Special Senses		
Impaired adaptation to dark	12.9	1.3
Abnormal vision	6.7	1.7
Urogenital System		
Urinary tract infection	8.0	9.1

The overall incidence of adverse experiences was 86% (194/225) for the NILANDRON group and 81% (188/232) for the placebo group. The following adverse experiences were reported during a multicenter clinical trial comparing NILANDRON + leuprolide versus placebo + leuprolide. The most frequently reported (greater than 5%) adverse experiences during treatment with NILANDRON tablets in combination with leuprolide are listed below. For comparison, adverse experiences seen with leuprolide and placebo are also listed.

Adverse Experience	NILANDRON + leuprolide (N=209) % All	Placebo + leuprolide (N=202) % All
Body as a Whole		
Pain	26.8	27.7
Headache	13.9	10.4
Asthenia	19.1	20.8
Back pain	11.5	16.8
Abdominal pain	10.0	5.4
Chest pain	7.2	4.5
Flu syndrome	7.2	3.0
Fever	5.3	6.4
Cardiovascular System		
Hypertension	9.1	9.9
Digestive System		
Nausea	23.9	8.4
Constipation	19.6	16.8
Anorexia	11.0	6.4
Dyspepsia	6.7	4.5
Vomiting	5.7	4.0

Continued on next page

Nilandron—Cont.

Endocrine System		
Hot flushes	66.5	59.4
Impotence	11.0	12.9
Libido decreased	11.0	4.5
Hemic and Lymphatic System		
Anemia	7.2	6.4
Metabolic and Nutritional System		
Increased AST	12.9	13.9
Peripheral edema	12.4	17.3
Increased ALT	9.1	8.9
Musculoskeletal System		
Bone Pain	6.2	5.0
Nervous System		
Insomnia	16.3	15.8
Dizziness	10.0	11.4
Depression	8.6	7.4
Hypesthesia	5.3	2.0
Respiratory System		
Dyspnea	10.5	7.4
Upper respiratory infection	8.1	10.9
Pneumonia	5.3	3.5
Skin and Appendages		
Sweating	6.2	3.0
Body hair loss	5.7	0.5
Dry skin	5.3	2.5
Rash	5.3	4.0
Special Senses		
Impaired adaptation to dark	56.9	5.4
Chromatopsia	8.6	0.0
Impaired adaptation to light	7.7	1.0
Abnormal vision	6.2	4.5
Urogenital System		
Testicular atrophy	16.3	12.4
Gynecomastia	10.5	11.9
Urinary tract infection	8.6	21.3
Hematuria	8.1	7.9
Urinary tract disorder	7.2	10.4
Nocturia	6.7	6.4

The overall incidence of adverse experiences is 99.5% (208/209) for the NILANDRON group and 98.5% (199/202) for the placebo group. Some frequently occurring adverse experiences, for example hot flushes, impotence, and decreased libido, are known to be associated with low serum androgen levels and known to occur with medical or surgical castration alone. Notable was the higher incidence of visual disturbances (variously described as impaired adaptation to darkness, abnormal vision, and colored vision), which led to treatment discontinuation in 1% to 2% of patients.

Interstitial pneumonitis occurred in one (<1%) patient receiving NILANDRON in combination with surgical castration and in seven patients (3%) receiving NILANDRON in combination with leuprolide and one patient receiving placebo in combination with leuprolide. Overall, it has been reported in 2% of patients receiving NILANDRON. This included a report of interstitial pneumonitis in 8 of 47 patients (17%) in a small study performed in Japan.

In addition, the following adverse experiences were reported in 2 to 5% of patients treated with NILANDRON in combination with leuprolide or orchiectomy.

Body as a Whole: Malaise (2%).

Cardiovascular System: Angina (2%), heart failure (3%), syncope (2%).

Digestive System: Diarrhea (2%), gastrointestinal disorder (2%), gastrointestinal hemorrhage (2%), melena (2%).

Metabolic and Nutritional System: Alcohol intolerance (5%), edema (2%), weight loss (2%).

Musculoskeletal System: Arthritis (2%).

Nervous System: Dry mouth (2%), nervousness (2%), paresthesia (3%).

Respiratory System: Cough increased (2%), interstitial lung disease (2%), lung disorder (4%), rhinitis (2%).

Skin and Appendages: Pruritus (2%).

Special Senses: Cataract (2%), photophobia (2%).

Laboratory Values: Haptoglobin increased (2%), leukopenia (3%), alkaline phosphatase increased (3%), BUN increased (2%), creatinine increased (2%), hyperglycemia (4%).

OVERDOSAGE

One case of massive overdosage has been published. A 79-year-old man attempted suicide by ingesting 13 g of nilutamide (i.e., 43 times the maximum recommended dose). Despite immediate gastric lavage and oral administration of activated charcoal, plasma nilutamide levels peaked at 6 times the normal range 2 hours after ingestion. There were no clinical signs or symptoms or changes in parameters such as transaminases or chest X-ray. Maintenance treatment (150 mg/day) was resumed 30 days later.

In repeated-dose tolerance studies, doses of 600 mg/day and 900 mg/day were administered to 9 and 4 patients, respectively. The ingestion of these doses was associated with gastrointestinal disorders, including nausea and vomiting, malaise, headache, and dizziness. In addition, a transient elevation in hepatic enzyme levels was noted in one patient.

Since nilutamide is protein bound, dialysis may not be useful as treatment for overdose. As in the management of overdosage with any drug, it should be borne in mind that multiple agents may have been taken. If vomiting does not occur spontaneously, it should be induced if the patient is alert. General supportive care, including frequent monitoring of the vital signs and close observation of the patient, is indicated.

DOSAGE AND ADMINISTRATION

The recommended dosage is 300 mg once a day for 30 days, followed thereafter by 150 mg once a day. NILANDRON tablets can be taken with or without food.

HOW SUPPLIED

NILANDRON (nilutamide) 50 mg tablets are supplied in boxes of 90 tablets. Each box contains 6 child-resistant, PVC, aluminum foil-backed blisters of 15 tablets (NDC 0088-1110-35). Each white, biconvex, cylindrical (7 mm in diameter) tablet has a triangular logo on one side and an internal reference number (168) on the other.

NILANDRON 150 mg tablets are supplied in boxes of 30 tablets. Each box contains 6 child-resistant, PVC, aluminum foil-backed blisters of 5 tablets (NDC 0088-1111-14). Each white, biconvex, cylindrical (10 mm in diameter) tablet has a triangular logo on one side and an internal reference number (168D) on the other.

Store at 25°C (77°F); excursions permitted between 15–30°C (59–86°F) [see USP Controlled Room Temperature]. Protect from light.

Prescribing information as of October 2000
Manufactured by Usiphar, 60200 Compiegne, France for:
Aventis Pharmaceuticals Inc.
Kansas City, MO 64137
Made in France
www.aventispharma-us.com
nilp1000p

Bayer Corporation

Pharmaceutical Division
400 MORGAN LANE
WEST HAVEN, CT 06516

For Medical Information Contact:
Director, Medical Services
(800) 468-0894
(203) 812-2000

CIPRO® ℞
(ciprofloxacin hydrochloride)
TABLETS

CIPRO® ℞
(ciprofloxacin)
5% and 10% ORAL SUSPENSION

Prescribing information for this product, which appears on pages 847-852 of the 2001 PDR, has been completely revised as follows. Please write "See Supplement A" next to the product heading.

DESCRIPTION

CIPRO® (ciprofloxacin hydrochloride) Tablets and CIPRO® (ciprofloxacin) Oral Suspension are synthetic broad spectrum antimicrobial agents for oral administration. Ciprofloxacin hydrochloride, USP, a fluoroquinolone, is the monohydrochloride monohydrate salt of 1-cyclopropyl-6-fluoro-1, 4-dihydro-4-oxo-7-(1-piperazinyl)-3-quinolinecarboxylic acid. It is a faintly yellowish to light yellow crystalline substance with a molecular weight of 385.8. Its empirical formula is $C_{17}H_{18}FN_3O_3 \cdot HCl \cdot H_2O$ and its chemical structure is as follows:

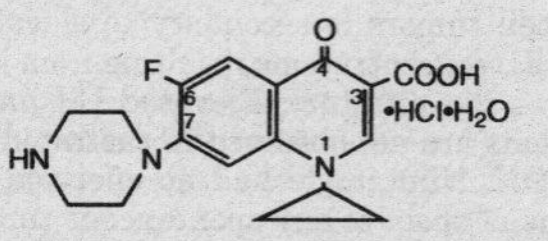

Ciprofloxacin is 1-cyclopropyl-6-fluoro-1, 4-dihydro-4-oxo-7-(1-piperazinyl)-3-quinolinecarboxylic acid. Its empirical formula is $C_{17}H_{18}FN_3O_3$ and its molecular weight is 331.4. It is a faintly yellowish to light yellow crystalline substance and its chemical structure is as follows:

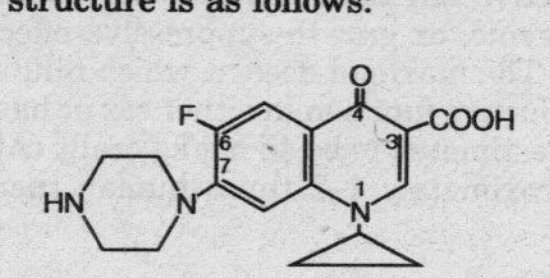

Ciprofloxacin differs from other quinolones in that it has a fluorine atom at the 6-position, a piperazine moiety at the 7-position, and a cyclopropyl ring at the 1-position.

CIPRO® film-coated tablets are available in 100-mg, 250-mg, 500-mg and 750-mg (ciprofloxacin equivalent) strengths. The inactive ingredients are starch, microcrystalline cellulose, silicon dioxide, crospovidone, magnesium stearate, hydroxypropyl methylcellulose, titanium dioxide, polyethylene glycol and water.

Ciprofloxacin Oral Suspension is available in 5% (5 g ciprofloxacin in 100 mL) and 10% (10 g ciprofloxacin in 100 mL) strengths. Ciprofloxacin Oral Suspension is a white to slightly yellowish suspension with strawberry flavor which may contain yellow-orange droplets. It is composed of ciprofloxacin microcapsules and diluent which are mixed prior to dispensing (See instructions for USE/HANDLING). The components of the suspension have the following compositions:

Microcapsules—ciprofloxacin, polyvinylpyrrolidone, methacrylic acid copolymer, hydroxypropyl methylcellulose, magnesium stearate, and Polysorbate 20.

Diluent—medium-chain triglycerides, sucrose, lecithin, water, and strawberry flavor.

CLINICAL PHARMACOLOGY

Ciprofloxacin given as an oral tablet is rapidly and well absorbed from the gastrointestinal tract after oral administration. The absolute bioavailability is approximately 70% with no substantial loss by first pass metabolism. Ciprofloxacin maximum serum concentrations and area under the curve are shown in the chart for the 250-mg to 1000-mg dose range.

Dose (mg)	Maximum Serum Concentration (µg/mL)	Area Under Curve (AUC) (µg • hr/mL)
250	1.2	4.8
500	2.4	11.6
750	4.3	20.2
1000	5.4	30.8

Maximum serum concentrations are attained 1 to 2 hours after oral dosing. Mean concentrations 12 hours after dosing with 250, 500, or 750-mg are 0.1, 0.2, and 0.4 µg/mL, respectively. The serum elimination half-life in subjects with normal renal function is approximately 4 hours. Serum concentrations increase proportionately with doses up to 1000-mg.

A 500-mg oral dose given every 12 hours has been shown to produce an area under the serum concentration time curve (AUC) equivalent to that produced by an intravenous infusion of 400 mg ciprofloxacin given over 60 minutes every 12 hours. A 750-mg oral dose given every 12 hours has been shown to produce an AUC at steady-state equivalent to that produced by an intravenous infusion of 400 mg over 60 minutes every 8 hours. A 750-mg oral dose results in a C_{max} similar to that observed with a 400-mg I.V. dose. A 250-mg oral dose given every 12 hours produces an AUC equivalent to that produced by an infusion of 200 mg ciprofloxacin given every 12 hours.

[See table below]

The serum elimination half-life in subjects with normal renal function is approximately 4 hours. Approximately 40 to 50% of an orally administered dose is excreted in the urine as unchanged drug. After a 250-mg oral dose, urine concentrations of ciprofloxacin usually exceed 200 µg/mL during the first two hours and are approximately 30 µg/mL at 8 to 12 hours after dosing. The urinary excretion of ciprofloxacin is virtually complete within 24 hours after dosing. The renal clearance of ciprofloxacin, which is approximately 300 mL/minute, exceeds the normal glomerular filtration rate of 120 mL/minute. Thus, active tubular secretion would seem to play a significant role in its elimination. Co-administration of probenecid with ciprofloxacin results in about a 50% reduction in the ciprofloxacin renal clearance and a 50% increase in its concentration in the systemic circulation. Although bile concentrations of ciprofloxacin are several fold higher than serum concentrations after oral dosing, only a small amount of the dose administered is recovered from the bile as unchanged drug. An additional 1 to 2% of the dose is recovered from the bile in the form of metabolites. Approximately 20 to 35% of an oral dose is recovered from the feces within 5 days after dosing. This may arise from either biliary clearance or transintestinal elimination. Four metabolites have been identified in human urine which together account for approximately 15% of an oral dose. The metabolites have antimicrobial activity, but are less active than unchanged ciprofloxacin.

With oral administration, a 500-mg dose, given as 10 mL of the 5% CIPRO® Suspension (containing 250-mg ciprofloxacin/5mL) is bioequivalent to the 500-mg tablet. A 10 mL volume of the 5% CIPRO® Suspension (containing 250-mg ciprofloxacin/5mL) is bioequivalent to a 5 mL volume of the 10% CIPRO® Suspension (containing 500-mg ciprofloxacin/5mL).

When CIPRO® Tablet is given concomitantly with food, there is a delay in the absorption of the drug, resulting in peak concentrations that occur closer to 2 hours after dosing rather than 1 hour whereas there is no delay observed when

Steady-state Pharmacokinetic Parameter Following Multiple Oral and I.V. Doses

Parameters	500 mg q12h, P.O.	400 mg q12h, I.V.	750 mg q12h, P.O.	400 mg q8h, I.V.
AUC (µg•hr/mL)	13.7[a]	12.7[a]	31.6[b]	32.9[c]
C_{max} (µg/mL)	2.97	4.56	3.59	4.07

[a] AUC_{0-12h}
[b] AUC 24h=$AUC_{0-12h} \times 2$
[c] AUC 24h=$AUC_{0-8h} \times 3$

CIPRO® Suspension is given with food. The overall absorption of CIPRO® Tablet or CIPRO® Suspension, however, is not substantially affected. The pharmacokinetics of ciprofloxacin given as the suspension are also not affected by food. Concurrent administration of antacids containing magnesium hydroxide or aluminum hydroxide may reduce the bioavailability of ciprofloxacin by as much as 90%. (See **PRECAUTIONS.**)

The serum concentrations of ciprofloxacin and metronidazole were not altered when these two drugs were given concomitantly.

Concomitant administration of ciprofloxacin with theophylline decreases the clearance of theophylline resulting in elevated serum theophylline levels and increased risk of a patient developing CNS or other adverse reactions. Ciprofloxacin also decreases caffeine clearance and inhibits the formation of paraxanthine after caffeine administration. (See **PRECAUTIONS.**)

Pharmacokinetic studies of the oral (single dose) and intravenous (single and multiple dose) forms of ciprofloxacin indicate that plasma concentrations of ciprofloxacin are higher in elderly subjects (>65 years) as compared to young adults. Although the C_{max} is increased 16-40%, the increase in mean AUC is approximately 30%, and can be at least partially attributed to decreased renal clearance in the elderly. Elimination half-life is only slightly (~20%) prolonged in the elderly. These differences are not considered clinically significant. (See **PRECAUTIONS: Geriatric Use.**)

In patients with reduced renal function, the half-life of ciprofloxacin is slightly prolonged. Dosage adjustments may be required. (See **DOSAGE AND ADMINISTRATION.**)

In preliminary studies in patients with stable chronic liver cirrhosis, no significant changes in ciprofloxacin pharmacokinetics have been observed. The kinetics of ciprofloxacin in patients with acute hepatic insufficiency, however, have not been fully elucidated.

The binding of ciprofloxacin to serum proteins is 20 to 40% which is not likely to be high enough to cause significant protein binding interactions with other drugs.

After oral administration, ciprofloxacin is widely distributed throughout the body. Tissue concentrations often exceed serum concentrations in both men and women, particularly in genital tissue including the prostate. Ciprofloxacin is present in active form in the saliva, nasal and bronchial secretions, mucosa of the sinuses, sputum, skin blister fluid, lymph, peritoneal fluid, bile, and prostatic secretions. Ciprofloxacin has also been detected in lung, skin, fat, muscle, cartilage, and bone. The drug diffuses into the cerebrospinal fluid (CSF); however, CSF concentrations are generally less than 10% of peak serum concentrations. Low levels of the drug have been detected in the aqueous and vitreous humors of the eye.

Microbiology: Ciprofloxacin has *in vitro* activity against a wide range of gram-negative and gram-positive organisms. The bactericidal action of ciprofloxacin results from interference with the enzyme DNA gyrase which is needed for the synthesis of bacterial DNA. Ciprofloxacin does not cross-react with other antimicrobial agents such as beta-lactams or aminoglycosides; therefore, organisms resistant to these drugs may be susceptible to ciprofloxacin. *In vitro* studies have shown that additive activity often results when ciprofloxacin is combined with other antimicrobial agents such as beta-lactams, aminoglycosides, clindamycin, or metronidazole. Synergy has been reported particularly with the combination of ciprofloxacin and a beta-lactam; antagonism is observed only rarely.

Ciprofloxacin has been shown to be active against most strains of the following microorganisms, both *in vitro* and in clinical infections as described in the **INDICATIONS AND USAGE** section of the package insert for CIPRO® (ciprofloxacin hydrochloride) Tablets and CIPRO® (ciprofloxacin) 5% and 10% Oral Suspension.

Aerobic gram-positive microorganisms
Enterococcus faecalis
  (Many strains are only moderately susceptible.)
Staphylococcus aureus (methicillin susceptible)
Staphylococcus epidermidis
Staphylococcus saprophyticus
Streptococcus pneumoniae
Streptococcus pyogenes
Aerobic gram-negative microorganisms
Campylobacter jejuni
Citrobacter diversus
Citrobacter freundii
Enterobacter cloacae
Escherichia coli
Haemophilus influenzae
Haemophilus parainfluenzae
Klebsiella pneumoniae
Moraxella catarrhalis
Morganella morganii
Neisseria gonorrhoeae
Proteus mirabilis
Proteus vulgaris
Providencia rettgeri
Providencia stuartii
Pseudomonas aeruginosa
Salmonella typhi
Serratia marcescens
Shigella boydii
Shigella dysenteriae
Shigella flexneri
Shigella sonnei
Ciprofloxacin has been shown to be active against most strains of the following microorganisms, both *in vitro* and in

clinical infections as described in the **INDICATIONS AND USAGE** section of the package insert for CIPRO® I.V. (ciprofloxacin for intravenous infusion).
Aerobic gram-positive microorganisms
Enterococcus faecalis
  (Many strains are only moderately susceptible.)
Staphylococcus aureus (methicillin susceptible)
Staphylococcus epidermidis
Staphylococcus saprophyticus
Streptococcus pneumoniae
Streptococcus pyogenes
Aerobic gram-negative microorganisms
Citrobacter diversus
Citrobacter freundii
Enterobacter cloacae
Escherichia coli
Haemophilus influenzae
Haemophilus parainfluenzae
Klebsiella pneumoniae
Morganella morganii
Proteus mirabilis
Proteus vulgaris
Providencia rettgeri
Providencia stuartii
Pseudomonas aeruginosa
Serratia marcescens
Ciprofloxacin has been shown to be active against *Bacillus anthracis* both *in vitro* and by use of serum levels as a surrogate marker (see **INDICATIONS AND USAGE** and **INHALATIONAL ANTHRAX—ADDITIONAL INFORMATION**).

The following *in vitro* data are available, **but their clinical significance is unknown.**

Ciprofloxacin exhibits *in vitro* minimum inhibitory concentrations (MICs) of 1 μg/mL or less against most (≥90%) strains of the following microorganisms; however, the safety and effectiveness of ciprofloxacin in treating clinical infections due to these microorganisms have not been established in adequate and well-controlled clinical trials.

Aerobic gram-positive microorganisms
Staphylococcus haemolyticus
Staphylococcus hominis
Aerobic gram-negative microorganisms
Acinetobacter lwoffi
Aeromonas hydrophila
Edwardsiella tarda
Enterobacter aerogenes
Klebsiella oxytoca
Legionella pneumophila
Pasteurella multocida
Salmonella enteritidis
Vibrio cholerae
Vibrio parahaemolyticus
Vibrio vulnificus
Yersinia enterocolitica
Most strains of *Burkholderia cepacia* and some strains of *Stenotrophomonas maltophilia* are resistant to ciprofloxacin as are most anaerobic bacteria, including *Bacteroides fragilis* and *Clostridium difficile*.

Ciprofloxacin is slightly less active when tested at acidic pH. The inoculum size has little effect when tested *in vitro*. The minimal bactericidal concentration (MBC) generally does not exceed the minimal inhibitory concentration (MIC) by more than a factor of 2. Resistance to ciprofloxacin *in vitro* develops slowly (multiple-step mutation).

Susceptibility Tests
Dilution Techniques: Quantitative methods are used to determine antimicrobial minimum inhibitory concentrations (MICs). These MICs provide estimates of the susceptibility of bacteria to antimicrobial compounds. The MICs should be determined using a standardized procedure. Standardized procedures are based on a dilution method[1] (broth or agar) or equivalent with standardized inoculum concentrations and standardized concentrations of ciprofloxacin powder. The MIC values should be interpreted according to the following criteria:

For testing aerobic microorganisms other than *Haemophilus influenzae, Haemophilus parainfluenzae,* and *Neisseria gonorrhoeae*[a]:

MIC (μg/mL)	Interpretation
≤1	Susceptible (S)
2	Intermediate (I)
≥4	Resistant (R)

[a] These interpretive standards are applicable only to broth microdilution susceptibility tests with streptococci using cation-adjusted Mueller-Hinton broth with 2-5% lysed horse blood.

For testing *Haemophilus influenzae* and *Haemophilus parainfluenzae*[b]:

MIC (μg/mL)	Interpretation
≤1	Susceptible (S)

[b]This interpretive standard is applicable only to broth microdilution susceptibility tests with *Haemophilus influenzae* and *Haemophilus parainfluenzae* using *Haemophilus* Test Medium[1].

The current absence of data on resistant strains precludes defining any results other than "Susceptible". Strains yield-

ing MIC results suggestive of a "nonsusceptible" category should be submitted to a reference laboratory for further testing.

For testing *Neisseria gonorrhoeae*[c]:

MIC (μg/mL)	Interpretation
≤0.06	Susceptible (S)

[c] This interpretive standard is applicable only to agar dilution test with GC agar base and 1% defined growth supplement.

The current absence of data on resistant strains precludes defining any results other than "Susceptible". Strains yielding MIC results suggestive of a "nonsusceptible" category should be submitted to a reference laboratory for further testing.

A report of "Susceptible" indicates that the pathogen is likely to be inhibited if the antimicrobial compound in the blood reaches the concentrations usually achievable. A report of "Intermediate" indicates that the result should be considered equivocal, and, if the microorganism is not fully susceptible to alternative, clinically feasible drugs, the test should be repeated. This category implies possible clinical applicability in body sites where the drug is physiologically concentrated or in situations where high dosage of drug can be used. This category also provides a buffer zone which prevents small uncontrolled technical factors from causing major discrepancies in interpretation. A report of "Resistant" indicates that the pathogen is not likely to be inhibited if the antimicrobial compound in the blood reaches the concentrations usually achievable; other therapy should be selected. Standardized susceptibility test procedures require the use of laboratory control microorganisms to control the technical aspects of the laboratory procedures. Standard ciprofloxacin powder should provide the following MIC values:

Organism		MIC (μg/mL)
E. faecalis	ATCC 29212	0.25 – 2.0
E. coli	ATCC 25922	0.004 – 0.015
H. influenzae[a]	ATCC 49247	0.004 – 0.03
N. gonorrhoeae[b]	ATCC 49226	0.001 – 0.008
P. aeruginosa	ATCC 27853	0.25 – 1.0
S. aureus	ATCC 29213	0.12 – 0.5

[a] This quality control range is applicable to only *H. influenzae* ATCC 49247 tested by a broth microdilution procedure using *Haemophilus* Test Medium (HTM)[1].
[b] This quality control range is applicable to only *N. gonorrhoeae* ATCC 49226 tested by an agar dilution procedure using GC agar base and 1% defined growth supplement.

Diffusion Techniques: Quantitative methods that require measurement of zone diameters also provide reproducible estimates of the susceptibility of bacteria to antimicrobial compounds. One such standardized procedure[2] requires the use of standardized inoculum concentrations. This procedure uses paper disks impregnated with 5-μg ciprofloxacin to test the susceptibility of microorganisms to ciprofloxacin.

Reports from the laboratory providing results of the standard single-disk susceptibility test with a 5-μg ciprofloxacin disk should be interpreted according to the following criteria:

For testing aerobic microorganisms other than *Haemophilus influenzae, Haemophilus parainfluenzae,* and *Neisseria gonorrhoeae*[a]:

Zone Diameter (mm)	Interpretation
≥21	Susceptible (S)
16–20	Intermediate (I)
≤15	Resistant (R)

[a] These zone diameter standards are applicable only to tests performed for streptococci using Mueller-Hinton agar supplemented with 5% sheep blood incubated in 5% CO_2.

For testing *Haemophilus influenzae* and *Haemophilus parainfluenzae*[b]:

Zone Diameter (mm)	Interpretation
≥21	Susceptible (S)

[b]This zone diameter standard is applicable only to tests with *Haemophilus influenzae* and *Haemophilus parainfluenzae* using *Haemophilus* Test Medium (HTM)[2].

The current absence of data on resistant strains precludes defining any results other than "Susceptible". Strains yielding zone diameter results suggestive of a "nonsusceptible" category should be submitted to a reference laboratory for further testing.

For testing *Neisseria gonorrhoeae*[c]:

Zone Diameter (mm)	Interpretation
≥36	Susceptible (S)

[c]This zone diameter standard is applicable only to disk diffusion tests with GC agar base and 1% defined growth supplement.

The current absence of data on resistant strains precludes defining any results other than "Susceptible". Strains yield-

Continued on next page

Cipro—Cont.

ing zone diameter results suggestive of a "nonsusceptible" category should be submitted to a reference laboratory for further testing.

Interpretation should be as stated above for results using dilution techniques. Interpretation involves correlation of the diameter obtained in the disk test with the MIC for ciprofloxacin.

As with standardized dilution techniques, diffusion methods require the use of laboratory control microorganisms that are used to control the technical aspects of the laboratory procedures. For the diffusion technique, the 5-µg ciprofloxacin disk should provide the following zone diameters in these laboratory test quality control strains:

Organism		Zone Diameter (mm)
E. coli	ATCC 25922	30 – 40
H. influenzae[a]	ATCC 49247	34 – 42
N. gonorrhoeae[b]	ATCC 49226	48 – 58
P. aeruginosa	ATCC 27853	25 – 33
S. aureus	ATCC 25923	22 – 30

[a] These quality control limits are applicable to only H. influenzae ATCC 49247 testing using Haemophilus Test Medium (HTM)[2].
[b] These quality control limits are applicable only to tests conducted with N. gonorrhoeae ATCC 49226 performed by disk diffusion using GC agar base and 1% defined growth supplement.

INDICATIONS AND USAGE

CIPRO® is indicated for the treatment of infections caused by susceptible strains of the designated microorganisms in the conditions listed below. Please see DOSAGE AND ADMINISTRATION for specific recommendations.

Acute Sinusitis caused by Haemophilus infuenzae, Streptococcus pneumoniae, or Moraxella catarrhalis.

Lower Respiratory Tract Infections caused by Escherichia coli, Klebsiella pneumoniae, Enterobacter cloacae, Proteus mirabilis, Pseudomonas aeruginosa, Haemophilus influenzae, Haemophilus parainfluenzae, or Streptococcus pneumoniae. Also, Moraxella catarrhalis for the treatment of acute exacerbations of chronic bronchitis.

NOTE: Although effective in clinical trials, ciprofloxacin is not a drug of first choice in the treatment of presumed or confirmed penumonia secondary to Streptococcos pneumoniae.

Urinary Tract Infections caused by Escherichia coli, Klebsiella pneumoniae, Enterobacter cloacae, Serratia marcescens, Proteus mirabilis, Providencia rettgeri, Morganella morganii, Citrobacter diversus, Citrobacter freundii, Pseudomonas aeruginosa, Staphylococcus epidermidis, Staphylococcus saprophyticus, or Enterococcus faecalis.

Acute Uncomplicatd Cystitis in females caused by Escherichia coli or Staphylococcus saprophyticus. (See DOSAGE AND ADMINISTRATION.)

Chronic Bacterial Prostatitis caused by Escherichia coli or Proteus mirabilis.

Complicated Intra-Abdominal Infections (used in combination with metronidazole) caused by Escherichia coli, Pseudomonas aeruginosa, Proteus mirabilis, Klebsiella pneumoniae, or Bacteroides fragilis. (See DOSAGE AND ADMINISTRATION.)

Skin and Skin Structure Infections caused by Escherichia coli, Klebsiella pneumoniae, Enterobacter cloacae, Proteus mirabilis, Proteus vulgaris, Providencia stuartii, Morganella morganii, Citrobacter freundii, Pseudomonas aeruginosa, Staphylococcus aureus (methicillin susceptible), Staphylococcus epidermidis, or Streptococcus pyogenes.

Bone and Joint Infections caused by Enterobacter cloacae, Serratia marcescens, or Pseudomonas aeruginosa.

Infectious Diarrhea caused by Escherichia coli (enterotoxigenic strains), Campylobacter jejuni, Shigella boydii*, Shigella dysenteriae, Shigella flexneri or Shigella sonnei* when antibacterial therapy is indicated.

Typhoid Fever (Enteric Fever) caused by Salmonella typhi.
NOTE: The efficacy of ciprofloxacin in the eradication of the chronic typhoid carrier state has not been demonstrated.

Uncomplicated cervical and urethral gonorrhea due to Neisseria gonorrhoeae.

Inhalational anthrax (post-exposure): To reduce the incidence or progression of disease following exposure to aerosolized Bacillus anthracis.

Ciprofloxacin serum conentrations achieved in humans serve as a surrogate endpoint reasonably likely to predict clinical benefit and provide the basis for this indication.[4] (See also INHALATIONAL ANTHRAX—ADDITIONAL INFORMATION).

*Although treatment of infections due to this organism in this organ system demonstrated a clinically significant outcome, efficacy was studied in fewer than 10 patients.

If anaerobic organisms are suspected of contributing to the infection, appropriate therapy should be administered.

Appropriate culture and susceptibility tests should be performed before treatment in order to isolate and identify organisms causing infection and to determine their susceptibility to ciprofloxacin. Therapy with CIPRO® may be initiated before results of these tests are known; once results become available appropriate therapy should be continued.

As with other drugs, some strains of Pseudomonas aeruginosa may develop resistance fairly rapidly during treatment with ciprofloxacin. Culture and susceptibility testing per-

formed periodically during therapy will provide information not only on the therapeutic effect of the antimicrobial agent but also on the possible emergence of bacterial resistance.

CONTRAINDICATIONS

CIPRO® (ciprofloxacin hydrochloride) is contraindicated in persons with a history of hypersensitivity to ciprofloxacin or any member of the quinolone class of antimicrobial agents.

WARNINGS

THE SAFETY AND EFFECTIVENESS OF CIPROFLOXACIN IN PEDIATRIC PATIENTS AND ADOLESCENTS (LESS THAN 18 YEARS OF AGE),—EXCEPT FOR USE IN INHALATIONAL ANTHRAX (POST-EXPOSURE), PREGNANT WOMEN, AND LACTATING WOMEN HAVE NOT BEEN ESTABLISHED. (See PRECAUTIONS: Pediatric Use, Pregnancy, and Nursing Mothers subsections.) The oral administration of ciprofloxacin caused lameness in immature dogs. Histopathological examination of the weight-bearing joints of these dogs revealed permanent lesions of the cartilage. Related quinolone-class drugs also produce erosions of cartilage of weight-bearing joints and other signs of arthropathy in immature animals of various species. (See ANIMAL PHARMACOLOGY.)

Convulsions, increased intracranial pressure, and toxic psychosis have been reported in patients receiving quinolones, including ciprofloxacin. Ciprofloxacin may also cause central nervous system (CNS) events including: dizziness, confusion, tremors, hallucinations, depression, and, rarely, suicidal thoughts or acts. These reactions may occur following the first dose. If these reactions occur in patients receiving ciprofloxacin, the drug should be discontinued and appropriate measures instituted. As with all quinolones, ciprofloxacin should be used with caution in patients with known or suspected CNS disorders that may predispose to seizures or lower the seizure threshold (e.g. severe cerebral arteriosclerosis, epilepsy), or in the presence of other risk factors that may predispose to seizures or lower the seizure threshold (e.g. certain drug therapy, renal dysfunction). (See PRECAUTIONS: General, Information for Patients, Drug Interactions and ADVERSE REACTIONS.)

SERIOUS AND FATAL REACTIONS HAVE BEEN REPORTED IN PATIENTS RECEIVING CONCURRENT ADMINISTRATION OF CIPROFLOXACIN AND THEOPHYLLINE. These reactions have included cardiac arrest, seizure, status epilepticus, and respiratory failure. Although similar serious adverse effects have been reported in patients receiving theophylline alone, the possibility that these reactions may be potentiated by ciprofloxacin cannot be eliminated. If concomitant use cannot be avoided, serum levels of theophylline should be monitored and dosage adjustments made as appropriate.

Serious and occasionally fatal hypersensitivity (anaphylactic) reactions, some following the first dose, have been reported in patients receiving quinolone therapy. Some reactions were accompanied by cardiovascular collapse, loss of consciousness, tingling, pharyngeal or facial edema, dyspnea, urticaria, and itching. Only a few patients had a history of hypersensitivity reactions. Serious anaphylactic reactions require immediate emergency treatment with epinephrine. Oxygen, intravenous steroids, and airway management, including intubation, should be administered as indicated.

Severe hypersensitivity reactions characterized by rash, fever, eosinophilia, jaundice, and hepatic necrosis with fatal outcome have also been rarely reported in patients receiving ciprofloxacin along with other drugs. The possibility that these reactions were related to ciprofloxacin cannot be excluded. Ciprofloxacin should be discontinued at the first appearance of a skin rash or any other sign of hypersensitivity.

Pseudomembranous colitis has been reported with nearly all antibacterial agents, including ciprofloxacin, and may range in severity from mild to life-threatening. Therefore, it is important to consider this diagnosis in patients who present with diarrhea subsequent to the administration of antibacterial agents.

Treatment with antibacterial agents alters the normal flora of the colon and may permit overgrowth of clostridia. Studies indicate that a toxin produced by Clostridium difficile is one primary cause of "antibiotic-associated colitis."

After the diagnosis of pseudomembranous colitis has been established, therapeutic measures should be initiated. Mild cases of pseudomembranous colitis usually respond to drug discontinuation alone. In moderate to severe cases, consideration should be given to management with fluids and electrolytes, protein supplementation, and treatment with an antibacterial drug clinically effective against C. difficile colitis.

Achilles and other tendon ruptures that required surgical repair or resulted in prolonged disability have been reported with ciprofloxacin and other quinolones. Ciprofloxacin should be discontinued if the patient experiences pain, inflammation, or rupture of a tendon.

Ciprofloxacin has not been shown to be effective in the treatment of syphilis. Antimicrobial agents used in high dose for short periods of time to treat gonorrhea may mask or delay the symptoms of incubating syphilis. All patients with gonorrhea should have a serologic test for syphilis at the time of diagnosis. Patients treated with ciprofloxacin should have a follow-up serologic test for syphilis after three months.

PRECAUTIONS

General: Crystals of ciprofloxacin have been observed rarely in the urine of human subjects but more frequently in the urine of laboratory animals, which is usually alkaline. (See ANIMAL PHARMACOLOGY.) Crystalluria related to ciprofloxacin has been reported only rarely in humans because human urine is usually acidic. Alkalinity of the urine should be avoided in patients receiving ciprofloxacin. Pa-

tients should be well hydrated to prevent the formation of highly concentrated urine.

Quinolones, including ciprofloxacin, may also cause central nervous system (CNS) events, including: nervousness, agitation, insomnia, anxiety, nightmares or paranoia. (See WARNINGS, Information for Patients, and Drug Interactions.)

Alteration of the dosage regimen is necessary for patients with impairment of renal function. (See DOSAGE AND ADMINISTRATION.)

Moderate to severe phototoxicity manifested as an exaggerated sunburn reaction has been observed in patients who are exposed to direct sunlight while receiving some members of the quinolone class of drugs. Excessive sunlight should be avoided. Therapy should be discontinued if phototoxicity occurs.

As with any potent drug, periodic assessment of organ system functions, including renal, hepatic, and hematopoietic function, is advisable during prolonged therapy.

Information for Patients:
Patients should be advised:
- that ciprofloxacin may be taken with or without meals and to drink fluids liberally. As with other quinolones, concurrent administration of ciprofloxacin with magnesium/aluminum antacids, or sucralfate, Videx® (didanosine) chewable/buffered tablets or pediatric powder, or with other products containing calcium, iron or zinc should be avoided. These products may be taken two hours after or six hours before ciprofloxacin. Ciprofloxacin should not be taken concurrently with milk or yogurt alone, since absorption of ciprofloxacin may be significantly reduced. Dietary calcium as part of a meal, however, does not significantly affect ciprofloxacin absorption.
- that ciprofloxacin may be associated with hypersensitivity reactions, even following a single dose, and to discontinue the drug at the first sign of a skin rash or other allergic reaction.
- to avoid excessive sunlight or artificial ultraviolet light while receiving ciprofloxacin and to discontinue therapy if phototoxicity occurs.
- to discontinue treatment; rest and refrain from exercise; and inform their physician if they experience pain, inflammation, or rupture of a tendon.
- that ciprofloxacin may cause dizziness and lightheadedness; therefore, patients should know how they react to this drug before they operate an automobile or machinery or engage in activities requiring mental alertness or coordination.
- that ciprofloxacin may increase the effects of theophylline and caffeine. There is a possibility of caffeine accumulation when products containing caffeine are consumed while taking quinolones.
- that convulsions have been reported in patients taking quinolones, including ciprofloxacin, and to notify their physician before taking the drug if there is a history of this condition.

Drug Interactions: As with some other quinolones, concurrent administration of ciprofloxacin with theophylline may lead to elevated serum concentrations of theophylline and prolongation of its elimination half-life. This may result in increased risk of theophylline-related adverse reactions. (See WARNINGS.) If concomitant use cannot be avoided, serum levels of theophylline should be monitored and dosage adjustments made as appropriate.

Some quinolones, including ciprofloxacin, have also been shown to interfere with the metabolism of caffeine. This may lead to reduced clearance of caffeine and a prolongation of its serum half-life.

Concurrent administration of a quinolone, including ciprofloxacin, with multivalent cation-containing products such as magnesium/aluminum antacids, sucralfate, Videx® (didanosine) chewable/buffered tablets or pediatric powder, or products containing calcium, iron, or zinc may substantially decrease its absorption, resulting in serum and urine levels considerably lower than desired. (See DOSAGE AND ADMINISTRATION for current administration of these agents with ciprofloxacin.)

Histamine H_2-receptor antagonists appear to have no significant effect on the bioavailability of ciprofloxacin.

Altered serum levels of phenytoin (increased and decreased) have been reported in patients receiving concomitant ciprofloxacin.

The concomitant administration of ciprofloxacin with the sulfonylurea glyburide has, on rare occasions, resulted in severe hypoglycemia.

Some quinolones, including ciprofloxacin, have been associated with transient elevations in serum creatinine in patients receiving cyclosporine concomitantly.

Quinolones have been reported to enhance the effects of the oral anticoagulant warfarin or its derivatives. When these products are administered concomitantly, prothrombin time or other suitable coagulation tests should be closely monitored.

Probenecid interferes with renal tubular secretion of ciprofloxacin and produces an increase in the level of ciprofloxacin in the serum. This should be considered if patients are receiving both drugs concomitantly.

As with other broad spectrum antimicrobial agents, prolonged use of ciprofloxacin may result in overgrowth of nonsusceptible organisms. Repeated evaluation of the patient's condition and microbial susceptibility testing is essential. If superinfection occurs during therapy, appropriate measures should be taken.

Carcinogenesis, Mutagenesis, Impairment of Fertility: Eight in vitro mutagenicity tests have been conducted with ciprofloxacin, and the test results are listed below:

Salmonella/Microsome Test (Negative)
E. coli DNA Repair Assay (Negative)
Mouse Lymphoma Cell Forward Mutation Assay (Positive)
Chinese Hamster V_{79} Cell HGPRT Test (Negative)

Syrian Hamster Embryo Cell Transformation Assay (Negative)

Saccharomyces cerevisiae Point Mutation Assay (Negative)

Saccharomyces cerevisiae Mitotic Crossover and Gene Conversion Assay (Negative)

Rat Hepatocyte DNA Repair Assay (Positive)

Thus, 2 of the 8 tests were positive, but results of the following 3 *in vivo* test systems gave negative results:

Rat Hepatocyte DNA Repair Assay

Micronucleus Test (Mice)

Dominant Lethal Test (Mice)

Long-term carcinogenicity studies in mice and rats have been completed. After daily oral doses of 750 mg/kg (mice) and 250 mg/kg (rats) were administered for up to 2 years, there was no evidence that ciprofloxacin had any carcinogenic or tumorigenic effects in these species.

Results from photo co-carcinogenicity testing indicate that ciprofloxacin does not reduce the time to appearance of UV-induced skin tumors as compared to vehicle control. Hairless (Skh-1) mice were exposed to UVA light for 3.5 hours five times every two weeks for up to 78 weeks while concurrently being administered ciprofloxacin. The time to development of the first skin tumors was 50 weeks in mice treated concomitantly with UVA and ciprofloxacin (mouse dose approximately equal to maximum recommended human dose based upon mg/m^2), as opposed to 34 weeks when animals were treated with both UVA and vehicle. The times to development of skin tumors ranged from 16–32 weeks in mice treated concomitantly with UVA and other quinolones.[3]

In this model, mice treated with ciprofloxacin alone did not develop skin or systemic tumors. There are no data from similar models using pigmented mice and/or fully haired mice. The clinical significance of these findings to humans is unknown.

Fertility studies performed in rats at oral doses of ciprofloxacin up to 100 mg/kg (0.8 times the highest recommended human dose of 1200 mg based upon body surface area) revealed no evidence of impairment.

Pregnancy: Teratogenic Effects. Pregnancy Category C: Reproduction studies have been performed in rats and mice using oral doses up to 100 mg/kg (0.6 and 0.3 times the maximum daily human dose based upon body surface area, respectively) and have revealed no evidence of harm to the fetus due to ciprofloxacin. In rabbits, ciprofloxacin (30 and 100 mg/kg orally) produced gastrointestinal disturbances resulting in maternal weight loss and an increased incidence of abortion, but no teratogenicity was observed at either dose. After intravenous administration of doses up to 20 mg/kg, no maternal toxicity was produced in the rabbit, and no embryotoxicity or teratogenicity was observed. There are, however, no adequate and well-controlled studies in pregnant women. Ciprofloxacin should be used during pregnancy only if the potential benefit justifies the potential risk to the fetus. (See **WARNINGS.**)

Nursing Mothers: Ciprofloxacin is excreted in human milk. Because of the potential for serious adverse reactions in infants nursing from mothers taking ciprofloxacin, a decision should be made whether to discontinue nursing or to discontinue the drug, taking into account the importance of the drug to the mother.

Pediatric Use: Safety and effectiveness in pediatric patients and adolescents less than 18 years of age have not been established, except for use in inhalational anthrax (post-exposure). Ciprofloxacin causes arthropathy in juvenile animals. (See **WARNINGS.**)

For the indication of inhalational anthrax (post-exposure), the risk-benefit assessment indicates that administration of ciprofloxacin to pediatric patients is appropriate. For information regarding pediatric dosing in inhalational anthrax (post-exposure), see **DOSAGE AND ADMINISTRATION** and **INHALATIONAL ANTHRAX—ADDITIONAL INFORMATION.**

Short-term safety data from a single trial in pediatric cystic fibrosis patients are available. In a randomized, double-blind clinical trial for the treatment of acute pulmonary exacerbations in cystic fibrosis patients (ages 5–17 years), 67 patients received ciprofloxacin I.V. 10 mg/kg/dose q8h for one week followed by ciprofloxacin tablets 20 mg/kg/dose q12h to complete 10–21 days treatment and 62 patients received the combination of ceftazidime I.V. 50 mg/kg/dose q8h and tobramycin I.V. 3 mg/kg/dose q8h for a total of 10–21 days. Patients less than 5 years of age were not studied. Safety monitoring in the study included periodic range of motion examinations and gait assessments by treatment-blinded examiners. Patients were followed for an average of 23 days after completing treatment (range 0–93 days). This study was not designed to determine long term effects and the safety of repeated exposure to ciprofloxacin.

In the study, injection site reactions were more common in the ciprofloxacin group (24%) than in the comparison group (8%). Other adverse events were similar in nature and frequency between treatment arms. Musculoskeletal adverse events were reported in 22% of the patients in the ciprofloxacin group and 21% in the comparison group. Decreased range of motion was reported in 12% of the subjects in the ciprofloxacin group and 16% in the comparison group. Arthralgia was reported in 10% of the patients in the ciprofloxacin group and 11% in the comparison group. One of sixty-seven patients developed arthritis of the knee nine days after a ten day course of treatment with ciprofloxacin. Clinical symptoms resolved, but an MRI showed knee effusion without other abnormalities eight months after treatment. However, the relationship of this event to the patient's course of ciprofloxacin can not be definitively determined, particularly since patients with cystic fibrosis may develop arthralgias/arthritis as part of their underlying disease process.

Hepatic	—	Elevations of ALT (SGPT) (1.9%), AST (SGOT) (1.7%), alkaline phosphatase (0.8%), LDH (0.4%), serum bilirubin (0.3%).
Hematologic	—	Eosinophilia (0.6%), leukopenia (0.4%), decreased blood platelets (0.1%), elevated blood platelets (0.1%), pancytopenia (0.1%).
Renal	—	Elevations of serum creatinine (1.1%), BUN (0.9%), CRYSTALLURIA, CYLINDRURIA, AND HEMATURIA HAVE BEEN REPORTED.

Geriatric Use: In a retrospective analysis of 23 multiple-dose controlled clinical trials of ciprofloxacin encompassing over 3500 ciprofloxacin treated patients, 25% of patients were greater than or equal to 65 years of age and 10% were greater than or equal to 75 years of age. No overall differences in safety or effectiveness were observed between these subjects and younger subjects, and other reported clinical experience has not identified differences in responses between the elderly and younger patients, but greater sensitivity of some older individuals on any drug therapy cannot be ruled out. Ciprofloxacin is known to be substantially excreted by the kidney, and the risk of adverse reactions may be greater in patients with impaired renal function. No alteration of dosage is necessary for patients greater than 65 years of age with normal renal function. However, since some older individuals experience reduced renal function by virtue of their advanced age, care should be taken in dose selection for elderly patients, and renal function monitoring may be useful in these patients. (See **CLINICAL PHARMACOLOGY** and **DOSAGE AND ADMINISTRATION.**)

ADVERSE REACTIONS

During clinical investigation with the tablet, 2,799 patients received 2,868 courses of the drug. Adverse events that were considered likely to be drug related occurred in 7.3% of patients treated, possibly related in 9.2% (total of 16.5% thought to be possibly or probably related to drug therapy), and remotely related in 3.0%. Ciprofloxacin was discontinued because of an adverse event in 3.5% of patients treated, primarily involving the gastrointestinal system (1.5%), skin (0.6%), and central nervous system (0.4%).

The most frequently reported events, drug related or not, were nausea (5.2%), diarrhea (2.3%), vomiting (2.0%), abdominal pain/discomfort (1.7%), headache (1.2%), restlessness (1.1%), and rash (1.1%).

Additional events that occurred in less than 1% of ciprofloxacin patients are listed below.

CARDIOVASCULAR: palpitation, atrial flutter, ventricular ectopy, syncope, hypertension, angina pectoris, myocardial infarction cardiopulmonary arrest, cerebral thrombosis

CENTRAL NERVOUS SYSTEM: dizziness, lightheadedness, insomnia, nightmares, hallucinations, manic reaction, irritability, tremor, ataxia, convulsive seizures, lethargy, drowsiness, weakness, malaise, anorexia, phobia, depersonalization, depression, paresthesia (See above.) (See **PRECAUTIONS.**)

GASTROINTESTINAL: painful oral mucosa, oral candidiasis, dysphagia, intestinal perforation, gastrointestinal bleeding (See above.) Cholestatic jaundice has been reported.

MUSCULOSKELETAL: arthralgia or back pain, joint stiffness, achiness, neck or chest pain, flare up of gout

RENAL/UROGENITAL: interstitial nephritis, nephritis, renal failure, polyuria, urinary retention, urethral bleeding, vaginitis, acidosis

RESPIRATORY: dyspnea, epistaxis, laryngeal or pulmonary edema, hiccough, hemoptysis, bronchospasm, pulmonary embolism

SKIN/HYPERSENSITIVITY: pruritus, urticaria, photosensitivity, flushing, fever, chills, angioedema, edema of the face, neck, lips, conjunctivae or hands, cutaneous candidiasis, hyperpigmentation, erythema nodosum (See above.)

Allergic reactions ranging from urticaria to anaphylactic reactions have been reported. (See **WARNINGS.**)

SPECIAL SENSES: blurred vision, disturbed vision (change in color perception, overbrightness of lights), decreased visual acuity, diplopia, eye pain, tinnitus, hearing loss, bad taste

Most of the adverse events reported were described as only mild or moderate in severity, abated soon after the drug was discontinued, and required no treatment.

In several instances nausea, vomiting, tremor, irritability, or palpitation were judged by investigators to be related to elevated serum levels of theophylline possibly as a result of drug interaction with ciprofloxacin.

In domestic clinical trials involving 214 patients receiving a single 250-mg oral dose, approximately 5% of patients reported adverse experiences without reference to drug relationship. The most common adverse experiences were vaginitis (2%), headache (1%), and vaginal pruritus (1%). Additional reactions, occurring in 0.3%–1% of patients, were abdominal discomfort, lymphadenopathy, foot pain, dizziness, and breast pain. Less than 20% of these patients had laboratory values obtained, and these results were generally consistent with the pattern noted for multi-dose therapy.

In randomized, double-blind controlled clinical trials comparing ciprofloxacin tablets (500 mg BID) to cefuroxime axetil (250 mg–500 mg BID) and to clarithromycin (500 mg BID) in patients with respiratory tract infections, ciprofloxacin demonstrated a CNS adverse event profile comparable to the control drugs.

Post-Marketing Adverse Events: Additional adverse events, regardless of relationship to drug, reported from worldwide marketing experience with quinolones, including ciprofloxacin, are:

BODY AS A WHOLE: change in serum phenytoin

CARDIOVASCULAR: postural hypotension, vasculitis

CENTRAL NERVOUS SYSTEM: agitation, confusion, delirium, dysphasia, myoclonus, nystagmus, toxic psychosis

GASTROINTESTINAL: constipation, dyspepsia, flatulence, hepatic necrosis, jaundice, pancreatitis, pseudomembranous colitis (The onset of pseudomembranous colitis symptoms may occur during or after antimicrobial treatment.)

HEMIC/LYMPHATIC: agranulocytosis, hemolytic anemia, methemoglobinemia, prolongation of prothrombin time

METABOLIC/NUTRITIONAL: elevation of serum triglycerides, cholesterol, blood glucose, serum potassium

MUSCULOSKELETAL: myalgia, possible exacerbation of myasthenia gravis, tendinitis/tendon rupture

RENAL/UROGENITAL: albuminuria, candiduria, renal calculi, vaginal candidiasis

SKIN/HYPERSENSITIVITY: anaphylactic reactions, erythema multiforme/Stevens-Johnson syndrome, exfoliative dermatitis, toxic epidermal necrolysis

SPECIAL SENSES: anosmia, taste loss (See **PRECAUTIONS.**)

Adverse Laboratory Changes: Changes in laboratory parameters listed as adverse events without regard to drug relationship are listed below:

[See table above]

Other changes occurring in less than 0.1% of courses were: elevation of serum gammaglutamyl transferase, elevation of serum amylase, reduction in blood glucose, elevated uric acid, decrease in hemoglobin, anemia, bleeding diathesis, increase in blood monocytes, leukocytosis.

OVERDOSAGE

In the event of acute overdosage, the stomach should be emptied by inducing vomiting or by gastric lavage. The patient should be carefully observed and given supportive treatment. Adequate hydration must be maintained. Only a small amount of ciprofloxacin (<10%) is removed from the body after hemodialysis or peritoneal dialysis.

In mice, rats, rabbits and dogs, significant toxicity including tonic/clonic convulsions was observed at intravenous doses of ciprofloxacin between 125 and 300 mg/kg.

Single doses of ciprofloxacin were relatively non-toxic via the oral route of administration in mice, rats, and dogs. No deaths occurred within a 14-day post treatment observation period at the highest oral doses tested; up to 5000 mg/kg in either rodent species, or up to 2500 mg/kg in the dog. Clinical signs observed included hypoactivity and cyanosis in both rodent species and severe vomiting in dogs. In rabbits, significant mortality was seen at doses of ciprofloxacin > 2500 mg/kg. Mortality was delayed in these animals, occurring 10–14 days after dosing.

DOSAGE AND ADMINISTRATION

The recommended adult dosage for acute sinusitis is 500-mg every 12 hours.

Lower respiratory tract infections may be treated with 500-mg every 12 hours. For more severe or complicated infections, a dosage of 750-mg may be given every 12 hours.

Severe/complicated urinary tract infections or urinary tract infections caused by organisms not highly susceptible to ciprofloxacin may be treated with 500-mg every 12 hours.

For other mild/moderate urinary infections, the usual adult dosage is 250-mg every 12 hours.

In acute uncomplicated cystitis in females, the usual dosage is 100-mg or 250-mg every 12 hours. For acute uncomplicated cystitis in females, 3 days of treatment is recommended while 7 to 14 days is suggested for other mild/moderate, severe or complicated urinary tract infections.

The recommended adult dosage for chronic bacterial prostatitis is 500-mg every 12 hours.

The recommended adult dosage for oral sequential therapy of complicated intra-abdominal infections is 500-mg every 12 hours. (To provide appropriate anaerobic activity, metronidazole should be given according to product labeling.) (See CIPRO® I.V. package insert.)

Skin and skin structure infections and bone and joint infections may be treated with 500-mg every 12 hours. For more severe or complicated infections, a dosage of 750-mg may be given every 12 hours.

The recommended adult dosage for infectious diarrhea or typhoid fever is 500-mg every 12 hours. For the treatment of uncomplicated urethral and cervical gonococcal infections, a single 250-mg dose is recommended.

See Instructions To The Pharmacist for Use/Handling of CIPRO® Oral Suspension.

[See first table at top of next page]

One teaspoonful (5 mL) of 5% ciprofloxacin oral suspension = 250-mg of ciprofloxacin.

One teaspoonful (5 mL) of 10% ciprofloxacin oral suspension = 500-mg of ciprofloxacin.

See Instructions for USE/HANDLING.

Continued on next page

Cipro—Cont.

Dosage	Volume (mL) of Oral Suspension	
	5%	10%
250-mg	5 mL	2.5 mL
500-mg	10 mL	5 mL
750-mg	15 mL	7.5 mL

CIPRO (ciprofloxacin) 5% and 10% Oral Suspension should not be administered through feeding tubes due to its physical characteristics.

Complicated Intra-Abdominal Infections: Sequential therapy [parenteral to oral—400-mg CIPRO® I.V. q 12 h (plus I.V. metronidazole) → 500-mg CIPRO® Tablets q 12 h (plus oral metronidazole)] can be instituted at the discretion of the physician.

The determination of dosage for any particular patient must take into consideration the severity and nature of the infection, the susceptibility of the causative organism, the integrity of the patient's host-defense mechanisms, and the status of renal function and hepatic function.

The duration of treatment depends upon the severity of infection. Generally ciprofloxacin should be continued for at least 2 days after the signs and symptoms of infection have disappeared. The usual duration is 7 to 14 days; however, for severe and complicated infections more prolonged therapy may be required. Bone and joint infections may require treatment for 4 to 6 weeks longer. Chronic Bacterial Prostatitis should be treated for 28 days. Infectious diarrhea may be treated for 5–7 days. Typhoid fever should be treated for 10 days.

Ciprofloxacin should be administered at least 2 hours before or 6 hours after magnesium/aluminum antacids, or sucralfate, Videx® (didanosine) chewable/buffered tablets or pediatric powder for oral solution, or other products containing calcium, iron or zinc.

Impaired Renal Function: Ciprofloxacin is eliminated primarily by renal excretion; however, the drug is also metabolized and partially cleared through the biliary system of the liver and through the intestine. These alternate pathways of drug elimination appear to compensate for the reduced renal excretion in patients with renal impairment. Nonetheless, some modification of dosage is recommended, particularly for patients with severe renal dysfunction. The following table provides dosage guidelines for use in patients with renal impairment; however, monitoring of serum drug levels provides the most reliable basis for dosage adjustment:

RECOMMENDED STARTING AND MAINTENANCE DOSES FOR PATIENTS WITH IMPAIRED RENAL FUNCTION

Creatinine Clearance (mL/min)	Dose
>50	See Usual Dosage.
30–50	250–500 mg q 12 h
5–29	250–500 mg q 18 h
Patients on hemodialysis or Peritoneal dialysis	250–500 mg q 24 h (after dialysis)

When only the serum creatinine concentration is known, the following formula may be used to estimate creatinine clearance.

[See second table above]

The serum creatinine should represent a steady state of renal function.

In patients with severe infections and severe renal impairment, a unit dose of 750-mg may be administered at the intervals noted above; however, patients should be carefully monitored and the serum ciprofloxacin concentration should be measured periodically. Peak concentrations (1–2 hours after dosing) should generally range from 2 to 4 µg/mL.

For patients with changing renal function or for patients with renal impairment and hepatic insufficiency, measurement of serum concentrations of ciprofloxacin will provide additional guidance for adjusting dosage.

HOW SUPPLIED

CIPRO® (ciprofloxacin hydrochloride) Tablets are available as round, slightly yellowish film-coded tablets containing 100-mg or 250-mg ciprofloxacin. The 100-mg tablet is coded with the word "CIPRO" on one side and "100" on the reverse side. The 250-mg tablet is coded with the word "CIPRO" on one side and "250" on the reverse side. CIPRO® is also available as capsule shaped, slightly yellowish film-coated tablets containing 500-mg or 750-mg ciprofloxacin. The 500-mg tablet is coded with the word "CIPRO" on one side and "500" on the reverse side. The 750-mg tablet is coded with the word "CIPRO" on one side and "750" on the reverse side. CIPRO® 250-mg, 500-mg, and 750-mg are available in bottles of 50, 100, and Unit Dose packages of 100. The 100-mg strength, is available only as CIPRO® Cystitis pack containing 6 tablets for use only in female patients with acute uncomplicated cystitis.

[See third table above]

Store below 30°C (86°F).

CIPRO® Oral Suspension is supplied in 5% (5g ciprofloxacin in 100 mL) and 10% (10g ciprofloxacin in 100 mL) strengths. The drug product is composed of two components (microcapsules and diluent) which are mixed prior to dispensing. See Instructions To The Pharmacist For Use/ Handling.

[See fourth table above]

Microcapsules and diluent should be stored below 25°C (77°F) and protected from freezing.

Reconstituted product may be stored below 30°C (86°F). Protect from freezing. A teaspoon is provided for the patient.

DOSAGE GUIDELINES

Infection	Type or Severity	Unit Dose	Frequency	Usual Durations†
Acute Sinusitis	Mild/Moderate	500-mg	q 12 h	10 Days
Lower Respiratory Tract	Mild/Moderate	500-mg	q 12 h	7 to 14 Days
	Severe/Complicated	750-mg	q 12 h	7 to 14 Days
Urinary Tract	Acute Uncomplicated	100-mg or 250-mg	q 12 h	3 Days
	Mild/Moderate	250-mg	q 12 h	7 to 14 Days
	Severe/Complicated	500-mg	q 12 h	7 to 14 Days
Chronic Bacterial Prostatitis	Mild/Moderate	500-mg	q 12 h	28 Days
Intra-Abdominal*	Complicated	500-mg	q 12 h	7 to 14 Days
Skin and Skin Structure	Mild/Moderate	500-mg	q 12 h	7 to 14 Days
	Severe/Complicated	750-mg	q 12 h	7 to 14 Days
Bone and Joint	Mild/Moderate	500-mg	q 12 h	≥4 to 6 weeks
	Severe/Complicated	750-mg	q 12 h	≥4 to 6 weeks
Infectious Diarrhea	Mild/Moderate/Severe	500-mg	q 12 h	5 to 7 Days
Typhoid Fever	Mild/Moderate	500-mg	q 12 h	10 Days
Urethral and Cervical Gonococcal Infections	Uncomplicated	250-mg	single dose	single dose
Inhalational anthrax (post-exposure)**	Adult	500-mg	q 12 h	60 Days
	Pediatric	15 mg/kg per dose, not to exceed 500-mg per dose	q 12 h	60 Days

* used in conjunction with metronidazole

† Generally ciprofloxacin should be continued for at least 2 days after the signs and symptoms of infection have disappeared, except for inhalational anthrax (post-exposure).

** Drug administration should begin as soon as possible after suspected or confirmed exposure. This indication is based on a surrogate endpoint, ciprofloxacin serum concentrations achieved in humans, reasonably likely to predict clinical benefit.[4] For a discussion of ciprofloxacin serum concentrations in various human populations, see **INHALATIONAL ANTHRAX—ADDITIONAL INFORMATION.**

Men: Creatinine clearance (mL/min) = $\dfrac{\text{Weight (kg)} \times (140 - \text{age})}{72 \times \text{serum creatinine (mg/dL)}}$

Women: 0.85 × the value calculated for men.

	Strength	NDC Code	Tablet Identification	
Bottles of 50:	750-mg	NDC 0026-8514-50	CIPRO	750
Bottles of 100:	250-mg	NDC 0026-8512-51	CIPRO	250
	500-mg	NDC 0026-8513-51	CIPRO	500
Unit Dose Package of 100:	250-mg	NDC 0026-8512-48	CIPRO	250
	500-mg	NDC 0026-8513-48	CIPRO	500
	750-mg	NDC 0026-8514-48	CIPRO	750
Cystitis: Package of 6:	100-mg	NDC 0026-8511-06	CIPRO	100

Total volume after reconstitution	Ciprofloxacin contents after reconstitution	Ciprofloxacin contents per bottle	NDC Code
100 mL	250 mg/5 mL	5,000 mg	0026-8551-36
100 mL	500 mg/5 mL	10,000 mg	0026-8553-36

ANIMAL PHARMACOLOGY

Ciprofloxacin and other quinolones have been shown to cause arthropathy in immature animals of most species tested. (See **WARNINGS.**) Damage of weight bearing joints was observed in juvenile dogs and rats. In young beagles, 100 mg/kg ciprofloxacin, given daily for 4 weeks, caused degenerative articular changes of the knee joint. At 30 mg/kg, the effect on the joint was minimal. In a subsequent study in beagles, removal of weight bearing from the joint reduced the lesions but did not totally prevent them.

Crystalluria, sometimes associated with secondary nephropathy, occurs in laboratory animals dosed with ciprofloxacin. This is primarily related to the reduced solubility of ciprofloxacin under alkaline conditions, which predominate in the urine of test animals; in man, crystalluria is rare since human urine is typically acidic. In rhesus monkeys, crystalluria without nephropathy has been noted after single oral doses as low as 5 mg/kg. After 6 months of intravenous dosing at 10 mg/kg/day, no nephropathological changes were noted; however, nephropathy was observed after dosing at 20 mg/kg/day for the same duration.

In dogs, ciprofloxacin at 3 and 10 mg/kg by rapid IV injection (15 sec.) produces pronounced hypotensive effects. These effects are considered to be related to histamine release, since they are partially antagonized by pyrilamine, an antihistamine. In rhesus monkeys, rapid IV injection also produces hypotension but the effect in this species is inconsistent and less pronounced.

In mice, concomitant administration of nonsteroidal anti-inflammatory drugs such as phenylbutazone and indomethacin with quinolones has been reported to enhance the CNS stimulatory effect of quinolones.

Ocular toxicity seen with some related drugs has not been observed in ciprofloxacin-treated animals.

CLINICAL STUDIES

Acute Sinusitis Studies

Ciprofloxacin tablets (500-mg BID) were evaluated for the treatment of acute sinusitis in two randomized, double-blind, controlled clinical trials conducted in the United States. Study 1 compared ciprofloxacin with cefuroxime axetil (250-mg BID) and enrolled 501 patients (400 of which were valid for the primary efficacy analysis). Study 2 compared ciprofloxacin with clarithromycin (500-mg BID) and enrolled 560 patients (418 of whom were valid for the primary efficacy analysis). The primary test of cure endpoint was a follow-up visit performed approximately 30 days after the completion of treatment with study medication. Clinical response data from these studies is summarized below:

Drug Regimen	Clinical Response Resolution at 30 Day Follow-up n (%)
STUDY 1	
CIPRO 500-mg BID × 10 days	152/197 (77)
Cefuroxime Axetil 250-mg BID × 10 days	145/203 (71)
STUDY 2	
CIPRO 500-mg BID × 10 days	168/212 (79)
Clarithromycin 500-mg BID × 14 days	169/206 (82)

In ciprofloxacin-treated patients enrolled in controlled and uncontrolled acute sinusitis studies, all of which included antral puncture, bacteriological eradication/presumed eradication was documented at the 30 day follow-up visit in 44 of

Drug Regimen	Clinical Response Resolution n (%)	Bacteriological Response By Organism (Eradication Rate)	
		E. coli n (%)	S. saprophyticus n (%)
STUDY 1			
CIPRO 100-mg BID × 3 days	82/94 (87)	64/70 (91)	8/8 (100)
CIPRO 250-mg BID × 7 days	81/86 (94)	67/69 (97)	4/4 (100)
STUDY 2			
CIPRO 100-mg BID × 3 days	134/141 (95)	117/123 (95)	8/8 (100)
Control (3 days)	128/133 (96)	103/105 (98)	10/10 (100)

50 (88%) *H. influenzae*, 17 of 21 (80.9%) *M. catarrhalis*, and 42 of 51 (82.3%) *S. pneumoniae*. Patients infected with *S. pneumoniae* strains whose baseline susceptibilities were intermediate or resistant to ciprofloxacin had a lower success rate than patients infected with susceptible strains.

Uncomplicated Cystitis Studies

Efficacy: Two U.S. double-blind, controlled clinical studies of acute uncomplicated cystitis in women compared ciprofloxacin 100-mg BID for 3 days to ciprofloxacin 250-mg BID for 7 days or control drug. In these two studies, using strict evaluability criteria and microbiologic and clinical response criteria at the 5–9 day post-therapy follow-up, the following clinical resolution and bacterial eradication rates were obtained:

[See table above]

INHALATIONAL ANTHRAX – ADDITIONAL INFORMATION

The mean serum concentrations of ciprofloxacin associated with a statistically significant improvement in survival in the rhesus monkey model of inhalational anthrax are reached or exceeded in adult and pediatric patients receiving oral and intravenous regimens. (See **DOSAGE AND ADMINISTRATION**.) Ciprofloxacin pharmacokinetics have been evaluated in various human populations. The mean peak serum concentration achieved at steady-state in human adults receiving 500 mg orally every 12 hours is 2.97 µg/mL, and 4.56 µg/mL following 400 mg intravenously every 12 hours. The mean trough serum concentration at steady-state for both of these regimens is 0.2 µg/mL. In a study of 10 pediatric patients between 6 and 16 years of age, the mean peak plasma concentration achieved is 8.3 µg/mL and trough concentrations range from 0.09 to 0.26 µg/mL, following two 30-minute intravenous infusions of 10 mg/kg administered 12 hours apart. After the second intravenous infusion patients switched to 15 mg/kg orally every 12 hours achieve a mean peak concentration of 3.6 µg/mL, after the initial oral dose. Long-term safety data, including effects on cartilage, following the administration of ciprofloxacin to pediatric patients are limited. (For additional information, see **PRECAUTIONS: Pediatric Use.**) Ciprofloxacin serum concentrations achieved in humans serve as a surrogate endpoint reasonably likely to predict clinical benefit and provide the basis for this indication.[4]

A placebo-controlled animal study in rhesus monkeys exposed to an inhaled mean dose of 11 LD_{50} ($\sim$5.5 × 10⁵) spores (range 5–30 LD_{50}) of *B. anthracis* was conducted. The minimal inhibitory concentration (MIC) of ciprofloxacin for the anthrax strain used in this study was 0.08 µg/mL. In the animals studied, mean serum concentrations of ciprofloxacin achieved at expected T_{max} (1 hour post-dose) following oral dosing to steady-state ranged from 0.98 to 1.69 µg/mL. Mean steady-state trough concentrations at 12 hours post-dose ranged from 0.12 to 0.19 µg/mL.[5] Mortality due to anthrax for animals that received a 30-day regimen of oral ciprofloxacin beginning 24 hours post-exposure was significantly lower (1/9), compared to the placebo group (9/10) [p=0.001]. The one ciprofloxacin-treated animal that died of anthrax did so following the 30-day drug administration period.[6]

Instructions To The Pharmacist For Use/Handling Of CIPRO® Oral Suspension:

Preparation of the suspension:

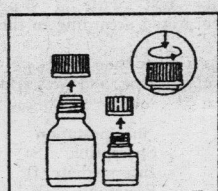

1. The small bottle contains the microcapsules, the large bottle contains the diluent.

2. Open both bottles. Child-proof cap: Press down according to instructions on the cap while turning to the left.

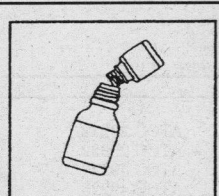

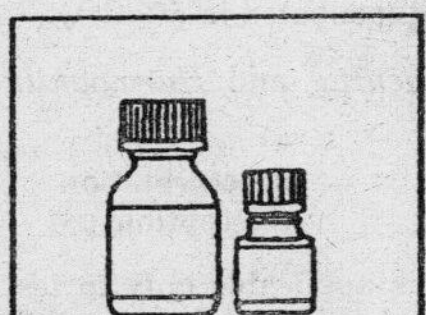

3. Pour the microcapsules completely into the large bottle of diluent. **Do not add water to the suspension.**

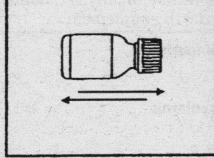

4. Remove the top layer of the diluent bottle label (to reveal the CIPRO® Oral Suspension label).

5. Close the large bottle completely according to the directions on the cap and shake vigorously for about 15 seconds. The suspension is ready for use.

Instructions To The Patient For Taking CIPRO® Oral Suspension:

Shake vigorously each time before use for approximately 15 seconds.

Swallow the prescribed amount of suspension. Do not chew the microcapsules. Reclose the bottle completely after use according to the instructions on the cap. Shake vigorously each time before use for approximately 15 seconds. The product can be used for 14 days when stored in a refrigerator or at room temperature (below 86°F). After treatment has been completed, any remaining suspension should not be reused.

REFERENCES

1. National Committee for Clinical Laboratory Standards, Methods for Dilution Antimicrobial Susceptibility Tests for Bacteria That Grow Aerobically-Fifth Edition. Approved Standard NCCLS Document M7-A5, Vol. 20, No. 2, NCCLS, Wayne, PA, January, 2000. **2.** National Committee for Clinical Laboratory Standards, Performance Standards for Antimicrobial Disk Susceptibility Tests-Seventh Edition. Approved Standard NCCLS Document M2-A7, Vol. 20, No. 1, NCCLS, Wayne, PA, January, 2000. **3.** Report presented at the FDA's Anti-Infective Drug and Dermatological Drug Product's Advisory Committee meeting, March 31, 1993, Silver Spring, MD. Report available from FDA, CDER, Advisors and Consultants Staff, HFD-21, 1901 Chapman Avenue, Room 200, Rockville, MD 20852, USA. **4.** 21 CFR 314.510 (Subpart H—Accelerated Approval of New Drugs for Life-Threatening Illnesses) **5.** Kelly DJ, et al. Serum concentrations of penicillin, doxycycline, and ciprofloxacin during prolonged therapy in rhesus monkeys. J Infect Dis 1992; 166: 1184–7. **6.** Friedlander AM, et al. Postexposure prophylaxis against experimental inhalational anthrax. J Infect Dis 1993; 167: 1239–42.

Bayer Corporation
Pharmaceutical Division
400 Morgan Lane
West Haven, CT 06516 USA
℞ Only
PZ500174   10/00   Bay o 9867   5202-2-A-U.S.-11
© 2000 Bayer Corporation   10007
CIPRO® (ciprofloxacin) 5% and 10% ORAL SUSPENSION
Made in Italy
Printed in U.S.A.

CIPRO® I.V.   ℞

(ciprofloxacin)

For Intravenous Infusion

Prescribing Information for this product, which appears on pages 852–856 of the 2001 PDR, has been completely revised as follows. Please write "See Supplement A" alongside product heading.

DESCRIPTION

CIPRO® I.V. (ciprofloxacin) is a synthetic broad-spectrum antimicrobial agent for intravenous (I.V.) administration. Ciprofloxacin, a fluoroquinolone, is 1-cyclopropyl-6-fluoro-1, 4-dihydro-4-oxo-7-(1-piperazinyl) -3- quinolinecarboxylic

acid. Its empirical formula is $C_{17}H_{18}FN_3O_3$ and its chemical structure is:

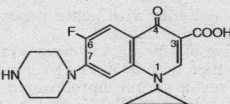

Ciprofloxacin is a faint to light yellow crystalline powder with a molecular weight of 331.4. It is soluble in dilute (0.1N) hydrochloric acid and is practically insoluble in water and ethanol. Ciprofloxacin differs from other quinolones in that it has a fluorine atom at the 6-position, a piperazine moiety at the 7-position, and a cyclopropyl ring at the 1-position. CIPRO® I.V. solutions are available as sterile 1.0% aqueous concentrates, which are intended for dilution prior to administration, and as 0.2% ready-for-use infusion solutions in 5% Dextrose Injection. All formulas contain lactic acid as a solubilizing agent and hydrochloric acid for pH adjustment. The pH range for the 1.0% aqueous concentrates in vials is 3.3 to 3.9. The pH range for the 0.2% ready-for-use infusion solutions is 3.5 to 4.6.

The plastic container is fabricated from a specially formulated polyvinyl chloride. Solutions in contact with the plastic container can leach out certain of its chemical components in very small amounts within the expiration period, e.g., di(2-ethylhexyl) phthalate (DEHP), up to 5 parts per million. The suitability of the plastic has been confirmed in tests in animals according to USP biological tests for plastic containers as well as by tissue culture toxicity studies.

CLINICAL PHARMACOLOGY

Following 60-minute intravenous infusions of 200 mg and 400 mg ciprofloxacin to normal volunteers, the mean maximum serum concentrations achieved were 2.1 and 4.6 µg/mL, respectively; the concentrations at 12 hours were 0.1 and 0.2 µg/mL, respectively.

[See first table at top of next page]

The pharmacokinetics of ciprofloxacin are linear over the dose range of 200 to 400 mg administered intravenously. The serum elimination half-life is approximately 5–6 hours and the total clearance is around 35 L/hr. Comparison of the pharmacokinetic parameters following the 1st and 5th I.V. dose on a q 12 h regimen indicates no evidence of drug accumulation.

The absolute bioavailability of oral ciprofloxacin is within a range of 70–80% with no substantial loss by first pass metabolism. An intravenous infusion of 400 mg ciprofloxacin given over 60 minutes every 12 hours has been shown to produce an area under the serum concentration time curve (AUC) equivalent to that produced by a 500-mg oral dose given every 12 hours. An intravenous infusion of 400 mg ciprofloxacin given over 60 minutes every 8 hours has been shown to produce an AUC at steady-state equivalent to that produced by a 750-mg oral dose given every 12 hours. A 400-mg I.V. dose results in a C_{max} similar to that observed with a 750-mg oral dose. An infusion of 200 mg ciprofloxacin given every 12 hours produces an AUC equivalent to that produced by a 250-mg oral dose given every 12 hours.

[See second table at top of next page]

After intravenous administration, approximately 50% to 70% of the dose is excreted in the urine as unchanged drug. Following a 200-mg I.V. dose, concentrations in the urine exceed 200 µg/mL 0–2 hours after dosing and are generally greater than 15 µg/mL 8–12 hours after dosing. Following a 400-mg I.V. dose, urine concentrations generally exceed 400 µg/mL 0–2 hours after dosing and are usually greater than 30 µg/mL 8–12 hours after dosing. The renal clearance is approximately 22 L/hr. The urinary excretion of ciprofloxacin is virtually complete by 24 hours after dosing. The serum concentrations of ciprofloxacin and metronidazole were not altered when these two drugs were given concomitantly.

Co-administration of probenecid with ciprofloxacin results in about 50% reduction in the ciprofloxacin renal clearance and a 50% increase in its concentration in the systemic circulation. Although bile concentrations of ciprofloxacin are severalfold higher than serum concentrations after intravenous dosing, only a small amount of the administered dose (<1%) is recovered from the bile as unchanged drug. Approximately 15% of an I.V. dose is recovered from the feces within 5 days after dosing.

After I.V. administration, three metabolites of ciprofloxacin have been identified in human urine which together account for approximately 10% of the intravenous dose.

Pharmacokinetic studies of the oral (single dose) and intravenous (single and multiple dose) forms of ciprofloxacin indicate that plasma concentrations of ciprofloxacin are higher in elderly subjects (>65 years) as compared to young adults. Although the C_{max} is increased 16–40%, the increase in mean AUC is approximately 30%, and can be at least partially attributed to decreased renal clearance in the elderly. Elimination half-life is only slightly ($\sim$20%) prolonged in the elderly. These differences are not considered clinically significant. (See **PRECAUTIONS: Geriatric Use.**)

In patients with reduced renal function, the half-life of ciprofloxacin is slightly prolonged and dosage adjustments may be required. (See **DOSAGE AND ADMINISTRATION.**)

In preliminary studies in patients with stable chronic liver cirrhosis, no significant changes in ciprofloxacin pharmaco-

Continued on next page

Cipro I.V.—Cont.

kinetics have been observed. However, the kinetics of ciprofloxacin in patients with acute hepatic insufficiency have not been fully elucidated.

Following infusion of 400 mg I.V. ciprofloxacin every eight hours in combination with 50 mg/kg I.V. piperacillin sodium every 4 hours, mean serum ciprofloxacin concentrations were 3.02 µg/mL ½ hour and 1.18 µg/mL between 6–8 hours after the end of infusion.

The binding of ciprofloxacin to serum proteins is 20 to 40%. After intravenous administration, ciprofloxacin is present in saliva, nasal and bronchial secretions, sputum, skin blister fluid, lymph, peritoneal fluid, bile, and prostatic secretions. It has also been detected in the lung, skin, fat, muscle, cartilage, and bone. Although the drug diffuses into cerebrospinal (CSF), CSF concentrations are generally less than 10% of peak serum concentrations. Levels of the drug in the aqueous and vitreous chambers of the eye are lower than in serum.

Microbiology: Ciprofloxacin has in vitro activity against a wide range of gram-negative and gram-positive microorganisms. The bactericidal action of ciprofloxacin results from interference with the enzyme DNA gyrase which is needed for the synthesis of bacterial DNA.

Ciprofloxacin has been shown to be active against most strains of the following microorganisms, both in vitro and in clinical infections as described in the **INDICATIONS AND USAGE** section of the package insert for CIPRO® I.V. (ciprofloxacin for intravenous infusion).

Aerobic gram-positive microorganisms
Enterococcus faecalis
   (Many strains are only moderately susceptible.)
Staphylococcus aureus
   (methicillin susceptible)
Staphylococcus epidermidis
Staphylococcus saprophyticus
Streptococcus pneumoniae
Streptococcus pyogenes
Aerobic gram-negative microorganisms
Citrobacter diversus
Citrobacter freundii
Enterobacter cloacae
Escherichia coli
Haemophilus influenzae
Haemophilus parainfluenzae
Klebsiella pneumoniae
Moraxella catarrhalis
Morganella morganii
Proteus mirabilis
Proteus vulgaris
Providencia rettgeri
Providencia stuartii
Pseudomonas aeruginosa
Serratia marcescens

Ciprofloxacin has been shown to be active against most strains of the following microorganisms, both in vitro and in clinical infections as described in the **INDICATIONS AND USAGE** section of the package insert for CIPRO® (ciprofloxacin hydrochloride) Tablets.

Aerobic gram-positive microorganisms
Enterococcus faecalis
   (Many strains are only moderately susceptible.)
Staphylococcus aureus
   (methicillin susceptible)
Staphylococcus epidermidis
Staphylococcus saprophyticus
Streptococcus pneumoniae
Streptococcus pyogenes
Aerobic gram-negative microorganisms
Campylobacter jejuni
Citrobacter diversus
Citrobacter freundii
Enterobacter cloacae
Escherichia coli
Haemophilus influenzae
Haemophilus parainfluenzae
Klebsiella pneumoniae
Moraxella catarrhalis
Morganella morganii
Neisseria gonorrhoeae
Proteus mirabilis
Proteus vulgaris
Providencia rettgeri
Providencia stuartii
Pseudomonas aeruginosa
Salmonella typhi
Serratia marcescens
Shigella boydii
Shigella dysenteriae
Shigella flexneri
Shigella sonnei

Ciprofloxacin has been shown to be active against *Bacillus anthracis* both in vitro and by use of serum levels as a surrogate marker (see **INDICATIONS AND USAGE** and **INHALATIONAL ANTHRAX—ADDITIONAL INFORMATION**).

The following in vitro data are available, **but their clinical significance is unknown.**

Ciprofloxacin exhibits in vitro minimum inhibitory concentrations (MICs) of 1 µg/mL or less against most ($\geq$90%) strains of the following microorganisms; however, the safety and effectiveness of ciprofloxacin in treating clinical infections due to these microorganisms have not been established in adequate and well-controlled clinical trials.

Steady-state Ciprofloxacin Serum Concentrations (µg/mL) After 60-minute I.V. Infusions q 12 h.

Dose	Time after starting the infusion					
	30 min	1 hr	3 hr	6 hr	8 hr	12 hr
200 mg	1.7	2.1	0.6	0.3	0.2	0.1
400 mg	3.7	4.6	1.3	0.7	0.5	0.2

Steady-state Pharmacokinetic Parameter Following Multiple Oral and I.V. Doses

Parameters	500 mg q12h, P.O.	400 mg q12h, I.V.	750 mg q12h, P.O.	400 mg q8h, I.V.
AUC (µg•hr/mL)	13.7[a]	12.7[a]	31.6[b]	32.9[c]
C_{max} (µg/mL)	2.97	4.56	3.59	4.07

[a] AUC_{0-12h}
[b] $AUC\ 24h = AUC_{0-12h} \times 2$
[c] $AUC\ 24h = AUC_{0-8h} \times 3$

Organism		MIC (µg/mL)
E. faecalis	ATCC 29212	0.25 –2.0
E. coli	ATCC 25922	0.004–0.015
H. influenzae[a]	ATCC 49247	0.004–0.03
N. gonorrhoeae[b]	ATCC 49226	0.001–0.008
P. aeruginosa	ATCC 27853	0.25 –1.0
S. aureus	ATCC 29213	0.12 –0.5

[a] This quality control range is applicable to only *H. influenzae* ATCC 49247 tested by a broth microdilution procedure using *Haemophilus* Test Medium (HTM)[1].

[b] This quality control range is applicable to only *N. gonorrhoeae* ATCC 49226 tested by an agar dilution procedure using GC agar base and 1% defined growth supplement.

Aerobic gram-positive microorganisms
Staphylococcus haemolyticus
Staphylococcus hominis
Aerobic gram-negative microorganisms
Acinetobacter lwoffi
Aeromonas hydrophila
Edwardsiella tarda
Enterobacter aerogenes
Klebsiella oxytoca
Legionella pneumophila
Pasteurella multocida
Salmonella enteritidis
Vibrio cholerae
Vibrio parahaemolyticus
Vibrio vulnificus
Yersinia enterocolitica

Most strains of *Burkholderia cepacia* and some strains of *Stenotrophomonas maltophilia* are resistant to ciprofloxacin as are most anaerobic bacteria, including *Bacteroides fragilis* and *Clostridium difficile*.

Ciprofloxacin is slightly less active when tested at acidic pH. The inoculum size has little effect when tested in vitro. The minimum bactericidal concentration (MBC) generally does not exceed the minimum inhibitory concentration (MIC) by more than a factor of 2. Resistance to ciprofloxacin in vitro usually develops slowly (multiple-step mutation).

Ciprofloxacin does not cross-react with other antimicrobial agents such as beta-lactams or aminoglycosides; therefore, organisms resistant to these drugs may be susceptible to ciprofloxacin.

In vitro studies have shown that additive activity often results when ciprofloxacin is combined with other antimicrobial agents such as beta-lactams, aminoglycosides, clindamycin, or metronidazole. Synergy has been reported particularly with the combination of ciprofloxacin and beta-lactam; antagonism is observed only rarely.

Susceptibility Tests

Dilution Techniques: Quantitative methods are used to determine antimicrobial minimum inhibitory concentrations (MICs). These MICs provide estimates of the susceptibility of bacteria to antimicrobial compounds. The MICs should be determined using a standardized procedure. Standardized procedures are based on a dilution method[1] (broth or agar) or equivalent with standardized inoculum concentrations and standardized concentrations of ciprofloxacin powder. The MIC values should be interpreted according to the following criteria:

For testing aerobic microorganisms other than *Haemophilus influenzae*, *Haemophilus parainfluenzae*, and *Neisseria gonorrhoeae*[a]:

MIC (µg/mL)	Interpretation
≤ 1	Susceptible (S)
2	Intermediate (I)
≥ 4	Resistant (R)

[a] These interpretive standards are applicable only to broth microdilution susceptibility tests with streptococci using cation-adjusted Mueller-Hinton broth with 2–5% lysed horse blood.

For testing *Haemophilus influenzae* and *Haemophilus parainfluenzae*[b]:

MIC (µg/mL)	Interpretation
≤ 1	Susceptible (S)

[b] This interpretive standard is applicable only to broth microdilution susceptibility tests with *Haemophilus influenzae* and *Haemophilus parainfluenzae* using *Haemophilus* Test Medium[1].

The current absence of data on resistant strains precludes defining any results other than "Susceptible". Strains yielding MIC results suggestive of a "nonsusceptible" category should be submitted to a reference laboratory for further testing.

For testing *Neisseria gonorrhoeae*[c]:

MIC (µg/mL)	Interpretation
≤ 0.06	Susceptible (S)

[c] This interpretive standard is applicable only to agar dilution test with GC agar base and 1% defined growth supplement.

The current absence of data on resistant strains precludes defining any results other than "Susceptible". Strains yielding MIC results suggestive of a "nonsusceptible" category should be submitted to a reference laboratory for further testing.

A report of "Susceptible" indicates that the pathogen is likely to be inhibited if the antimicrobial compound in the blood reaches the concentrations usually achievable. A report of "Intermediate" indicates that the result should be considered equivocal, and, if the microorganism is not fully susceptible to alternative, clinically feasible drugs, the test should be repeated. This category implies possible clinical applicability in body sites where the drug is physiologically concentrated or in situations where high dosage of drug can be used. This category also provides a buffer zone which prevents small uncontrolled technical factors from causing major discrepancies in interpretation. A report of "Resistant" indicates that the pathogen is not likely to be inhibited if the antimicrobial compound in the blood reaches the concentrations usually achievable; other therapy should be selected. Standardized susceptibility test procedures require the use of laboratory control microorganisms to control the technical aspects of the laboratory procedures. Standard ciprofloxacin powder should provide the following MIC values:

[See third table above]

Diffusion Techniques: Quantitative methods that require measurement of zone diameters also provide reproducible estimates of the susceptibility of bacteria to antimicrobial compounds. One such standardized procedure[2] requires the use of standardized inoculum concentrations. This procedure uses paper disks impregnated with 5-µg ciprofloxacin to test the susceptibility of microorganisms to ciprofloxacin.

Reports from the laboratory providing results of the standard single-disk susceptibility test with a 5-µg ciprofloxacin disk should be interpreted according to the following criteria:

For testing aerobic microorganisms other than *Haemophilus influenzae*, *Haemophilus parainfluenzae*, and *Neisseria gonorrhoeae*[a]:

Zone Diameter (mm)	Interpretation
≥ 21	Susceptible (S)
16–20	Intermediate (I)
≤ 15	Resistant (R)

[a] These zone diameter standards are applicable only to tests performed for streptococci using Mueller-Hinton agar supplemented with 5% sheep blood incubated in 5% CO_2.

For testing *Haemophilus influenzae* and *Haemophilus parainfluenzae*[b]:

Zone Diameter (mm)	Interpretation
≥ 21	Susceptible (S)

[b] This zone diameter standard is applicable only to tests with *Haemophilus influenzae* and *Haemophilus parainfluenzae* using *Haemophilus* Test Medium (HTM)[2].

The current absence of data on resistant strains precludes defining any results other than "Susceptible". Strains yielding zone diameter results suggestive of a "nonsusceptible" category should be submitted to a reference laboratory for further testing.
For testing *Neisseria gonorrhoeae*[c]:

Zone Diameter (mm)	Interpretation
≥36	Susceptible (S)

[c] This zone diameter standard is applicable only to disk diffusion tests with GC agar base and 1% defined growth supplement.

The current absence of data on resistant strains precludes defining any results other than "Susceptible". Strains yielding zone diameter results suggestive of a "nonsusceptible" category should be submitted to a reference laboratory for further testing.
Interpretation should be as stated above for results using dilution techniques. Interpretation involves correlation of the diameter obtained in the disk test with the MIC for ciprofloxacin.
As with standardized dilution techniques, diffusion methods require the use of laboratory control microorganisms that are used to control the technical aspects of the laboratory procedures. For the diffusion technique, the 5-μg ciprofloxacin disk should provide the following zone diameters in these laboratory test quality control strains:
[See first table above]

INDICATIONS AND USAGE

CIPRO® I.V. is indicated for the treatment of infections caused by susceptible strains of the designated microorganisms in the conditions listed below when the intravenous administration offers a route of administration advantageous to the patient. Please see **DOSAGE AND ADMINISTRATION** for specific recommendations.

Urinary Tract Infections caused by *Escherichia coli* (including cases with secondary bacteremia), *Klebsiella pneumoniae* subspecies *pneumoniae, Enterobacter cloacae, Serratia marcescens, Proteus mirabilis, Providencia rettgeri, Morganella morganii, Citrobacter diversus, Citrobacter freundii, Pseudomonas aeruginosa, Staphylococcus epidermidis, Staphylococcus saprophyticus*, or *Enterococcus faecalis*.

Lower Respiratory Infections caused by *Escherichia coli, Klebsiella pneumoniae* subspecies *pneumoniae, Enterobacter cloacae, Proteus mirabilis, Pseudomonas aeruginosa, Haemophilus influenzae, Haemophilus parainfluenzae*, or *Streptococcus pneumoniae*.

NOTE: Although effective in clinical trials, ciprofloxacin is not a drug of first choice in the treatment of presumed or confirmed pneumonia secondary to *Streptococcus pneumoniae*.

Nosocomial Pneumonia caused by *Haemophilus influenzae* or *Klebsiella pneumoniae*.

Skin and Skin Structure Infections caused by *Escherichia coli, Klebsiella pneumoniae* subspecies *pneumoniae, Enterobacter cloacae, Proteus mirabilis, Proteus vulgaris, Providencia stuartii, Morganella morganii, Citrobacter freundii, Pseudomonas aeruginosa, Staphylococcus aureus* (methicillin susceptible), *Staphylococcus epidermidis*, or *Streptococcus pyogenes*.

Bone and Joint Infections caused by *Enterobacter cloacae, Serratia marcescens*, or *Pseudomonas aeruginosa*.

Complicated Intra-Abdominal Infections (used in conjunction with metronidazole) caused by *Escherichia coli, Pseudomonas aeruginosa, Proteus mirabilis, Klebsiella pneumonia*, or *Bacteroides fragilis*. (See **DOSAGE AND ADMINISTRATION**.)

Acute Sinusitis caused by *Haemophilus influenzae, Streptococcus pneumoniae*, or *Moraxella catarrhalis*.

Chronic Bacterial Prostatitis caused by *Escherichia coli* or *Proteus mirabilis*.

Empirical Therapy for Febrile Neutropenic Patients in combination with piperacillin sodium. (See **DOSAGE AND ADMINISTRATION** and **CLINICAL STUDIES**.)

Inhalational anthrax (post-exposure): To reduce the incidence or progression of disease following exposure to aerosolized *Bacillus anthracis*.

Ciprofloxacin serum concentrations achieved in humans serve as a surrogate endpoint reasonably likely to predict clinical benefit and provide the basis for this indication.[4] (See also, **INHALATIONAL ANTHRAX—ADDITIONAL INFORMATION**).

If anaerobic organisms are suspected of contributing to the infection, appropriate therapy should be administered.

Appropriate culture and susceptibility tests should be performed before treatment in order to isolate and identify organisms causing infection and to determine their susceptibility to ciprofloxacin. Therapy with CIPRO® I.V. may be initiated before results of these tests are known; once results become available, appropriate therapy should be continued.

As with other drugs, some strains of *Pseudomonas aeruginosa* may develop resistance fairly rapidly during treatment with ciprofloxacin. Culture and susceptibility testing performed periodically during therapy will provide information not only on the therapeutic effect of the antimicrobial agent but also on the possible emergence of bacterial resistance.

CLINICAL STUDIES

EMPIRICAL THERAPY IN FEBRILE NEUTROPENIC PATIENTS

The safety and efficacy of ciprofloxacin, 400 mg I.V. q 8h, in combination with piperacillin sodium 50 mg/kg I.V. q 4h, for the empirical therapy of febrile neutropenic patients were studied in one large pivotal multicenter, randomized trial and were compared to those of tobramycin, 2 mg/kg I.V. q 8h, in combination with piperacillin sodium, 50 mg/kg I.V. q 4h.

Organism		Zone Diameter (mm)
E. coli	ATCC 25922	30–40
H. influenzae[a]	ATCC 49247	34–42
N. gonorrhoeae[b]	ATCC 49226	48–58
P. aeruginosa	ATCC 27853	25–33
S. aureus	ATCC 25923	22–30

[a] These quality control limits are applicable to only *H. influenzae* ATCC 49247 testing using *Haemophilus* Test Medium (HTM)[2].
[b] These quality control limits are applicable only to tests conducted with *N. gonorrhoeae* ATCC 49226 performed by disk diffusion using GC agar base and 1% defined growth supplement.

Total	Ciprofloxacin/Piperacillin N = 233		Tobramycin/Piperacillin N = 237	
Median Age (years)	47.0	(range 19–84)	50.0	(range 18–81)
Male	114	(48.9%)	117	(49.4%)
Female	119	(51.1%)	120	(50.6%)
Leukemia/Bone Marrow Transplant	165	(70.8%)	158	(66.7%)
Solid Tumor/Lymphoma	68	(29.2%)	79	(33.3%)
Medial Duration of Neutropenia (days)	15.0	(range 1–61)	14.0	(range 1–89)

Outcomes	Ciprofloxacin/Piperacillin N = 233 Success (%)		Tobramycin/Piperacillin N = 237 Success (%)	
Clinical Resolution of Initial Febrile Episode with No Modifications of Empirical Regimen*	63	(27.0%)	52	(21.9%)
Clinical Resolution of Initial Febrile Episode Including Patients with Modifications of Empirical Regimen	187	(80.3%)	185	(78.1%)
Overall Survival	224	(96.1%)	223	(94.1%)

* To be evaluated as a clinical resolution, patients had to have: (1) resolution of fever; (2) microbiological eradication of infection (if an infection was microbiologically documented); (3) resolution of signs/symptoms of infection; and (4) no modification of empirical antibiotic regimen.

The demographics of the evaluable patients were as follows:
[See second table above]
Clinical response rates observed in this study were as follows:
[See third table above]

CONTRAINDICATIONS

CIPRO® I.V. (ciprofloxacin) is contraindicated in persons with a history of hypersensitivity to ciprofloxacin or any member of the quinolone class of antimicrobial agents.

WARNINGS

THE SAFETY AND EFFECTIVENESS OF CIPROFLOXACIN IN PEDIATRIC PATIENTS AND ADOLESCENTS (LESS THAN 18 YEARS OF AGE),—EXCEPT FOR USE IN INHALATIONAL ANTHRAX (POST-EXPOSURE), PREGNANT WOMEN, AND LACTATING WOMEN HAVE NOT BEEN ESTABLISHED. (See **PRECAUTIONS: Pediatric Use, Pregnancy,** and **Nursing Mothers** subsections.) Ciprofloxacin causes lameness in immature dogs. Histopathological examination of the weight-bearing joints of these dogs revealed permanent lesions of the cartilage. Related quinolone-class drugs also produce erosions of cartilage of weight-bearing joints and other signs of arthropathy in immature animals of various species. (See **ANIMAL PHARMACOLOGY**.)

Convulsions, increased intracranial pressure, and toxic psychosis have been reported in patients receiving quinolones, including ciprofloxacin. Ciprofloxacin may also cause central nervous system (CNS) events including: dizziness, confusion, tremors, hallucinations, depression, and rarely, suicidal thoughts or acts. These reactions may occur following the first dose. If these reactions occur in patients receiving ciprofloxacin, the drug should be discontinued and appropriate measures instituted. As with all quinolones, ciprofloxacin should be used with caution in patients with known or suspected CNS disorders that may predispose to seizures or lower the seizure threshold (e.g. severe cerebral arteriosclerosis, epilepsy), or in the presence of other risk factors that may predispose to seizures or lower the seizure threshold (e.g. certain drug therapy, renal dysfunction). (See **PRECAUTIONS: General: Information for Patients, Drug Interactions** and **ADVERSE REACTIONS**.)

SERIOUS AND FATAL REACTIONS HAVE BEEN REPORTED IN PATIENTS RECEIVING CONCURRENT ADMINISTRATION OF INTRAVENOUS CIPROFLOXACIN AND THEOPHYLLINE. These reactions have included cardiac arrest, seizure, status epilepticus, and respiratory failure. Although similar serious adverse events have been reported in patients receiving theophylline alone, the possibility that these reactions may be potentiated by ciprofloxacin cannot be eliminated. If concomitant use cannot be avoided, serum levels of theophylline should be monitored and dosage adjustments made as appropriate.

Serious and occasionally fatal hypersensitivity (anaphylactic) reactions, some following the first dose, have been reported in patients receiving quinolone therapy. Some reactions were accompanied by cardiovascular collapse, loss of consciousness, tingling, pharyngeal or facial edema, dyspnea, urticaria, and itching. Only a few patients had a history of hypersensitivity reactions. Serious anaphylactic reactions require immediate emergency treatment with epinephrine and other resuscitation measures, including oxygen, intravenous oxygen, intravenous fluids, intravenous antihistamines, corticosteroids, pressor amines, and airway management, as clinically indicated.

Severe hypersensitivity reactions characterized by rash, fever, eosinophilia, jaundice, and hepatic necrosis with fatal outcome have also been reported extremely rarely in patients receiving ciprofloxacin along with other drugs. The possibility that these reactions were related to ciprofloxacin cannot be excluded. Ciprofloxacin should be discontinued at the first appearance of a skin rash or any other sign of hypersensitivity.

Pseudomembranous colitis has been reported with nearly all antibacterial agents, including ciprofloxacin, and may range in severity from mild to life-threatening. Therefore, it is important to consider this diagnosis in patients who present with diarrhea subsequent to the administration of antibacterial agents.

Treatment with antibacterial agents alters the normal flora of the colon and may permit overgrowth of clostridia. Studies indicate that a toxin produced by *Clostridium difficile* is one primary cause of "antibiotic-associated colitis".

After the diagnosis of pseudomembranous colitis has been established, therapeutic measures should be initiated. Mild cases of pseudomembranous colitis usually respond to drug discontinuation alone. In moderate to severe cases, consideration should be given to management with fluids and electrolytes, protein supplementation and treatment with an antibacterial drug clinically effective against *C. difficile* colitis.

Achilles and other tendon ruptures that required surgical repair or resulted in prolonged disability have been reported with ciprofloxacin and other quinolones. Ciprofloxacin should be discontinued if the patient experiences pain, inflammation, or rupture of a tendon.

PRECAUTIONS

General: INTRAVENOUS CIPROFLOXACIN SHOULD BE ADMINISTERED BY SLOW INFUSION OVER A PERIOD OF 60 MINUTES. Local I.V. site reactions have been reported with the intravenous administration of ciprofloxacin. These reactions are more frequent if infusion time is 30 minutes or less or if small veins of the hand are used. (See **ADVERSE REACTIONS**.)

Quinolones, including ciprofloxacin, may also cause central nervous system (CNS) events, including nervousness, agitation, insomnia, anxiety, nightmares or paranoia. (See **WARNINGS, Information for Patients,** and **Drug Interactions**.)

Crystals of ciprofloxacin have been observed rarely in the urine of human subjects but more frequently in the urine of laboratory animals, which is usually alkaline. (See **ANI-**

Continued on next page

Cipro I.V.—Cont.

MAL PHARMACOLOGY.) Crystalluria related to ciprofloxacin has been reported only rarely in humans because human urine is usually acidic. Alkalinity of the urine should be avoided in patients receiving ciprofloxacin. Patients should be well hydrated to prevent the formation of highly concentrated urine.

Alteration of the dosage regimen is necessary for patients with impairment of renal function. (See **DOSAGE AND ADMINISTRATION**.)

Moderate to severe phototoxicity manifested as an exaggerated sunburn reaction has been observed in some patients who were exposed to direct sunlight while receiving some members of the quinolone class of drugs. Excessive sunlight should be avoided.

As with any potent drug, periodic assessment of organ system functions, including renal, hepatic, and hematopoietic, is advisable during prolonged therapy.

Information For Patients: Patients should be advised that ciprofloxacin may be associated with hypersensitivity reactions, even following a single dose, and to discontinue the drug at the first sign of a skin rash or other allergic reaction. Ciprofloxacin may cause dizziness and lightheadedness; therefore, patients should know how they react to this drug before they operate an automobile or machinery or engage in activities requiring mental alertness or coordination.

Patients should be advised that ciprofloxacin may increase the effects of theophylline and caffeine. There is a possibility of caffeine accumulation when products containing caffeine are consumed while taking ciprofloxacin.

Patients should be advised to discontinue treatment; rest and refrain from exercise; and inform their physician if they experience pain, inflammation, or rupture of a tendon.

Patients should be advised that convulsions have been reported in patients taking quinolones, including ciprofloxacin, and to notify their physician before taking the drug if there is a history of this condition.

Drug Interactions: As with some other quinolones, concurrent administration of ciprofloxacin with theophylline may lead to elevated serum concentrations of theophylline and prolongation of its elimination half-life. This may result in increased risk of theophylline-related adverse reactions. (See **WARNINGS**.) If concomitant use cannot be avoided, serum levels of theophylline should be monitored and dosage adjustments made as appropriate.

Some quinolones, including ciprofloxacin, have also been shown to interfere with the metabolism of caffeine. This may lead to reduced clearance of caffeine and prolongation of its serum half-life.

Some quinolones, including ciprofloxacin, have been associated with transient elevations in serum creatinine in patients receiving cyclosporine concomitantly.

Altered serum levels of phenytoin (increased and decreased) have been reported in patients receiving concomitant ciprofloxacin.

The concomitant administration of ciprofloxacin with the sulfonylurea has, in some patients, resulted in severe hypoglycemia. Fatalities have been reported.

Quinolones have been reported to enhance the effects of the oral anticoagulant warfarin or its derivatives. When these products are administered concomitantly, prothrombin time or other suitable coagulation tests should be closely monitored.

Probenecid interferes with renal tubular secretion of ciprofloxacin and produces an increase in the level of ciprofloxacin in the serum. This should be considered if patients are receiving both drugs concomitantly.

As with other broad-spectrum antimicrobial agents, prolonged use of ciprofloxacin may result in overgrowth of non-susceptible organisms. Repeated evaluation of the patient's condition and microbial susceptibility testing are essential. If superinfection occurs during therapy, appropriate measures should be taken.

Carcinogenesis, Mutagenesis, Impairment of Fertility: Eight *in vitro* mutagenicity tests have been conducted with ciprofloxacin. Test results are listed below:

Salmonella/Microsome Test (Negative)
E. coli DNA Repair Assay (Negative)
Mouse Lymphoma Cell Forward Mutation Assay (Positive)
Chinese Hamster V$_{79}$ Cell HGPRT Test (Negative)
Syrian Hamster Embryo Cell Transformation Assay (Negative)
Saccharomyces cerevisiae Point Mutation Assay (Negative)
Saccharomyces cerevisiae Mitotic Crossover and Gene Conversion Assay (Negative)
Rat Hepatocyte DNA Repair Assay (Positive)

Thus, two of the eight tests were positive, but results of the following three *in vivo* test systems gave negative results:

Rat Hepatocyte DNA Repair Assay
Micronucleus Test (Mice)
Dominant Lethal Test (Mice)

Long-term carcinogenicity studies in mice and rats have been completed. After daily oral doses of 750 mg/kg (mice) and 250 mg/kg (rats) were administered for up to 2 years, there was no evidence that ciprofloxacin had any carcinogenic or tumorigenic effects in these species.

Results from photo co-carcinogenicity testing indicate that ciprofloxacin dose not reduce the time to appearance of UV-induced skin tumors as compared to vehicle control. Hairless (Skh-1) mice were exposed to UVA light for 3.5 hours five times every two weeks for up to 78 weeks while concur-

rently being administered ciprofloxacin. The time to development of the first skin tumors was 50 weeks in mice treated concomitantly with UVA and ciprofloxacin (mouse dose approximately equal to maximum recommended human dose based upon mg/m^2), as opposed to 34 weeks when animals were treated with both UVA and vehicle. The times to development of skin tumors ranged from 16–32 weeks in mice treated concomitantly with UVA and other quinolones.[3]

In this model, mice treated with ciprofloxacin alone did not develop skin or systemic tumors. There are no data from similar models using pigmented mice and/or fully haired mice. The clinical significance of these findings to humans in unknown.

Fertility studies performed in rats at oral doses of ciprofloxacin up to 100 mg/kg (0.8 times the highest recommended human dose of 1200 mg based upon body surface area) revealed no evidence of impairment.

Pregnancy: Teratogenic Effects. Pregnancy Category C: Reproduction studies have been performed in rats and mice using oral doses of up to 100 mg/kg (0.8 and 0.4 times the maximum daily human dose based upon body surface area, respectively) and I.V. doses of up to 30 mg/kg (0.24 and 0.12 times the maximum daily human dose based upon body surface area, respectively) and have revealed no evidence of harm to the fetus due to ciprofloxacin. In rabbits, ciprofloxacin (30 and 100 mg/kg orally) produced gastrointestinal disturbances resulting in maternal weight loss and an increased incidence of abortion, but no teratogenicity was observed at either dose. After intravenous administration of doses up to 20 mg/kg, no maternal toxicity was produced in the rabbit, and no embryotoxicity or teratogenicity was observed. There are, however, no adequate and well-controlled studies in pregnant women. Ciprofloxacin should be used during pregnancy only if the potential benefit justifies the potential risk to the fetus. (See **WARNINGS**.)

Nursing Mothers: Ciprofloxacin is excreted in human milk. Because of the potential for serious adverse reactions in infants nursing from mothers taking ciprofloxacin, a decision should be made whether to discontinue nursing or to discontinue the drug, taking into account the importance of the drug to the mother.

Pediatric Use: Safety and effectiveness in pediatric patients and adolescents less than 18 years of age have not been established, except for use in inhalational anthrax (post-exposure). Ciprofloxacin causes arthropathy in juvenile animals. (See **WARNINGS**.)

For the indication of inhalational anthrax (post-exposure), the risk-benefit assessment indicates that administration of ciprofloxacin to pediatric patients is appropriate. For information regarding pediatric dosing in inhalational anthrax (post-exposure), see **DOSAGE AND ADMINISTRATION** and **INHALATIONAL ANTHRAX—ADDITIONAL INFORMATION**.

Short-term safety data from a single trial in pediatric cystic fibrosis patients are available. In a randomized, double-blind clinical trial for the treatment of acute pulmonary exacerbations in cystic fibrosis patients (ages 5–17 years), 67 patients received ciprofloxacin I.V. 10 mg/kg/dose q8h for one week followed by ciprofloxacin tablets 20 mg/kg/dose q12h to complete 10–21 days treatment and 62 patients received the combination of ceftazidime I.V. 50 mg/kg/dose q8h and tobramycin I.V. 3 mg/kg/dose q8h for a total of 10–21 days. Patients less than 5 years of age were not studied. Safety monitoring in the study included periodic range of motion examinations and gait assessments by treatment-blinded examiners. Patients were followed for an average of 23 days after completing treatment (range 0–93 days). This study was not designed to determine long term effects and the safety of repeated exposure to ciprofloxacin.

In the study, injection site reactions were more common in the ciprofloxacin group (24%) than in the comparison group (8%). Other adverse events were similar in nature and frequency between treatment arms. Musculoskeletal adverse events were reported in 22% of the patients in the ciprofloxacin group and 21% in the comparison group. Decreased range of motion was reported in 12% of the subjects in the ciprofloxacin group and 16% in the comparison group. Arthralgia was reported in 10% of the patients in the ciprofloxacin group and 11% in the comparison group. One of sixty-seven patients developed arthritis of the knee nine days after a ten day course of treatment with ciprofloxacin. Clinical symptoms resolved, but an MRI showed knee effusion without other abnormalities eight months after treatment. However, the relationship of this event to the patient's course of ciprofloxacin can not be definitively determined, particularly since patients with cystic fibrosis may develop arthralgias/arthritis as part of their underlying disease process.

Geriatric Use: In a retrospective analysis of 23 multiple-dose controlled clinical trials of ciprofloxacin encompassing over 3500 ciprofloxacin treated patients, 25% of patients were greater than or equal to 65 years of age and 10% were greater than or equal to 75 years of age. No overall differences in safety or effectiveness were observed between these subjects and younger subjects, and other reported clinical experience has not identified differences in responses between the elderly and younger patients, but greater sensitivity of some older individuals on any drug therapy cannot be ruled out. Ciprofloxacin is known to be substantially excreted by the kidney, and the risk of adverse reactions may be greater in patients with impaired renal function. No alteration of dosage is necessary for patients greater than 65 years of age with normal renal function. However, since some older individuals experience reduced renal function by virtue of their

advanced age, care should be taken in dose selection for elderly patients, and renal function monitoring may be useful in these patients. (See **CLINICAL PHARMACOLOGY** and **DOSAGE AND ADMINISTRATION**.)

ADVERSE REACTIONS

The most frequently reported events, without regard to drug relationship, among patients treated with intravenous ciprofloxacin were nausea, diarrhea, central nervous system disturbance, local I.V. site reactions, abnormalities of liver associated enzymes (hepatic enzymes), and eosinophilia. Headache, restlessness, and rash were also noted in greater than 1% of patients treated with the most common doses of ciprofloxacin.

Local I.V. site reactions have been reported with the intravenous administration of ciprofloxacin. These reactions are more frequent if the infusion time is 30 minutes or less. These may appear as local skin reactions which resolve rapidly upon completion of the infusion. Subsequent intravenous administration is not contraindicated unless the reactions recur or worsen.

Additional events, without regard to drug relationship or route of administration, that occurred in 1% or less of ciprofloxacin patients are listed below:

CARDIOVASCULAR: cardiovascular collapse, cardiopulmonary arrest, myocardial infarction, arrhythmia, tachycardia, palpitation, cerebral thrombosis, syncope, cardiac murmur, hypertension, hypotension, angina pectoris

CENTRAL NERVOUS SYSTEM: convulsive seizures, paranoia, toxic psychosis, depression, dysphasia, phobia, depersonalization, manic reaction, unresponsiveness, ataxia, confusion, hallucinations, dizziness, lightheadedness, paresthesia, anxiety, tremor, insomnia, nightmares, weakness, drowsiness, irritability, malaise, lethargy

GASTROINTESTINAL: ileus, jaundice, gastrointestinal bleeding, C. difficile associated diarrhea, pseudomembranous colitis, pancreatitis, hepatic necrosis, intestinal perforation, dyspepsia, epigastric or abdominal pain, vomiting, constipation, oral ulceration, oral candidiasis, mouth dryness, anorexia, dysphagia, flatulence

I.V. INFUSION SITE: thrombophlebitis, burning, pain, pruritus, paresthesia, erythema, swelling

MUSCULOSKELETAL: arthralgia, jaw, arm or back pain, joint stiffness, neck and chest pain, achiness, flare up of gout

RENAL/UROGENITAL: renal failure, interstitial nephritis, hemorrhagic cystitis, renal calculi, frequent urination, acidosis, urethral bleeding, polyuria, urinary retention, gynecomastia, candiduria, vaginitis. Crystalluria, cylindruria, hematuria, and albuminuria have also been reported.

RESPIRATORY: respiratory arrest, pulmonary embolism, dyspnea, pulmonary edema, respiratory distress, pleural effusion, hemoptysis, epistaxis, hiccough

SKIN/HYPERSENSITIVITY: anaphylactic reactions, erythema multiforme/Stevens-Johnson syndrome, exfoliative dermatitis, toxic epidermal necrolysis, vasculitis, angioedema, edema of the lips, face, neck, conjunctivae, hands or lower extremities, purpura, fever, chills, flushing, pruritus, urticaria, cutaneous candidiasis, vesicles, increased perspiration, hyperpigmentation, erythema nodosum, photosensitivity (See **WARNINGS**.)

SPECIAL SENSES: decreased visual acuity, blurred vision, disturbed vision (flashing lights, change in color perception, overbrightness of lights, diplopia), eye pain, anosmia, hearing loss, tinnitus, nystagmus, a bad taste

Also reported were agranulocytosis, prolongation of prothrombin time, and possible exacerbation of myasthenia gravis.

Many of these events were described as only mild or moderate in severity, abated soon after the drug was discontinued, and required no treatment.

In several instances, nausea, vomiting, tremor, irritability, or palpitation were judged by investigators to be related to elevated serum levels of theophylline possibly as a result of drug interaction with ciprofloxacin.

In randomized, double-blind controlled clinical trials comparing ciprofloxacin (I.V. and I.V. P.O sequential) with intravenous beta-lactam control antibiotics, the CNS adverse event profile of ciprofloxacin was comparable to that of the control drugs.

Post-Marketing Adverse Events: Additional adverse events, regardless of relationship to drug, reported from worldwide marketing experience with quinolones, including ciprofloxacin, are:

BODY AS A WHOLE: change in serum phenytoin
CARDIOVASCULAR: postural hypotension, vasculitis
CENTRAL NERVOUS SYSTEM: agitation, delirium, myoclonus, toxic psychosis
HEMIC/LYMPHATIC: hemolytic anemia, methemoglobinemia
METABOLIC/NUTRITIONAL: elevation of serum triglycerides, cholesterol, blood glucose, serum potassium
MUSCULOSKELTAL: myalgia, tendinitis/tendon rupture
RENAL/UROGENITAL: vaginal candidiasis
(See **PRECAUTIONS**.)

Adverse Laboratory Changes: The most frequently reported changes in laboratory parameters with intravenous ciprofloxacin therapy, without regard to drug relationship are listed below:

Hepatic—   elevations of AST (SGOT), ALT (SGPT), alkaline phosphatase, LDH, and serum bilirubin;

Hematologic— elevated eosinophil and platelet counts, decresed platelet counts, hemoglobin and/or hematocrit;

Renal— elevations of serum creatinine, BUN, and uric acid;

Other— elevations of serum creatinine, phosphokinase, serum theophylline (in patients receiving theophylline concomitantly), blood glucose, and triglycerides.

Other changes occurring infrequently were: decreased leukocyte count, elevated atypical lymphocyte count, immature WBCs, elevated serum calcium, elevation of serum gamma-glutamyl transpeptidase (γ GT), decreased BUN, decreased uric acid, decreased total serum protein, decreased serum albumin, decreased serum potassium, elevated serum potassium, elevated serum cholesterol.

Other changes occurring rarely during administration of ciprofloxacin were: elevation of serum amylase, decrease of blood glucose, pancytopenia, leukocytosis, elevated sedimentation rate, change in serum phenytoin, decreased prothrombin time, hemolytic anemia, and bleeding diathesis.

OVERDOSAGE

In the event of acute overdosage, the patient should be carefully observed and given supportive treatment. Adequate hydration must be maintained. Only a small amount of ciprofloxacin (<10%) is removed from the body after hemodialysis or peritoneal dialysis.

In mice, rats, rabbits and dogs, significant toxicity including tonic/clonic convulsions was observed at intravenous doses of ciprofloxacin between 125 and 300 mg/kg.

DOSAGE AND ADMINISTRATION

The recommended adult dosage for urinary tract infections of mild to moderate severity is 200 mg I.V. every 12 hours. For severe or complicated urinary tract infections, the recommended dosage is 400 mg I.V. every 12 hours.

The recommended adult dosage for lower respiratory tract infections, skin and skin structure infections, and bone and joint infections of mild to moderate severity is 400 mg I.V. every 12 hours.

For severe/complicated infections of the lower respiratory tract, skin and skin structure, and bone and joint, the recommended adult dosage is 400 mg I.V. every 8 hours.

The recommended adult dosage for mild, moderate, and severe nosocomial pneumonia is 400 mg I.V. every 8 hours.

Complicated Intra-Abdominal Infections: Sequential therapy [parenteral to oral—400 mg CIPRO® I.V. q 12 h (plus I.V. metronidazole) → 500 mg CIPRO® I.V. Tablets q 12 h (plus oral metronidazole)] can be instituted at the discretion of the physician. Metronidazole should be given according to product labeling to provide appropriate anaerobic coverage.

The recommended dosage for mild to moderate Acute Sinusitis and Chronic Bacterial Prostatitis is 400 mg I.V. every 12 hours.

The recommended adult dosage for empirical therapy of febrile neutropenic patients is 400 mg I.V. every 8 hours in combination with piperacillin sodium 50 mg/kg I.V. q 4 hours, not to exceed 24 g/day (300 mg/kg/day), for 7–14 days.

The determination of dosage for any particular patient must take into consideration the severity and nature of the infection, the susceptibility of the causative microorganism, the integrity of the patient's host-defense mechanisms and the status of renal and hepatic function.

[See first table above]

CIPRO® I.V. should be administered by intravenous infusion over a period of 60 minutes.

Parenteral drug products should be inspected visually for particulate matter and discoloration prior to administration.

Ciprofloxacin hydrochloride (CIPRO® Tablets) for oral administration are available. Parenteral therapy may be changed to oral CIPRO® Tablets when the condition warrants, at the discretion of the physician. For complete dosage and administration information, see CIPRO® Tablets package insert.

Impaired Renal Function: The following table provides dosage guidelines for use in patients with renal impairment; however, monitoring of serum drug levels provides the most reliable basis for dosage adjustment.

[See second table above]

When only the serum creatinine concentration is known, the following formula may be used to estimate creatinine clearance:

[See third table above]

The serum creatinine should represent a steady state of renal function.

For patients with changing renal function or for patients with renal impairment and hepatic insufficiency, measurement of serum concentrations of ciprofloxacin will provide additional guidance for adjusting dosage.

INTRAVENOUS ADMINISTRATION

CIPRO® I.V. should be administered by intravenous infusion over a period of 60 minutes. Slow infusion of a dilute solution into a large vein will minimize patient discomfort and reduce the risk of venous irritation.

Vials (Injection Concentrate): THIS PREPARATION MUST BE DILUTED BEFORE USE. The intravenous dose should be prepared by aseptically withdrawing the concentrate from the vial of CIPRO® I.V. This should be diluted with a suitable intravenous solution to a final concentration of 1–2 mg/mL. (See **COMPATIBILITY AND STABILITY**.) The resulting solution should be infused over a period of 60 minutes by direct infusion or through a Y-type intravenous infusion set which may already be in place.

If this method or the "piggyback" method of administration is used, it is advisable to discontinue temporarily the administration of any other solutions during the infusion of CIPRO® I.V.

Flexible Containers: CIPRO® I.V. is also available as a 0.2% premixed solution in 5% dextrose in flexible containers of 100 mL or 200 mL. The solutions in flexible containers may be infused as described above.

COMPATIBILITY AND STABILITY

Ciprofloxacin injection 1% (10 mg/mL), when diluted with the following intravenous solutions to concentrations of 0.5 to 2.0 mg/mL, is stable for up to 14 days at refrigerated or room temperature storage.

0.9% Sodium Chloride Injection, USP
5% Dextrose Injection, USP
Sterile Water for Injection
10% Dextrose for Injection
5% Dextrose and 0.225% Sodium Chloride for Injection
5% Dextrose and 0.45% Sodium Chloride for Injection
Lactated Ringer's for Injection

If CIPRO® I.V. is to be given concomitantly with another drug, each drug should be given separately in accordance with the recommended dosage and route of administration for each drug.

HOW SUPPLIED

CIPRO® I.V. (ciprofloxacin) is available as a clear, colorless to slightly yellowish solution. CIPRO® I.V. is available in 200 mg and 400 mg strengths. The concentrate is supplied in vials while the premixed solution is supplied in flexible containers as follows:

VIAL:	SIZE	STRENGTH	NDC NUMBER
	20 mL	200 mg, 1%	0026-8562-20
	40 mL	400 mg, 1%	0026-8564-64

FLEXIBLE CONTAINER: manufactured for Bayer Corporation by Abbott Laboratories, North Chicago, IL 60064.

[See fourth table above]

FLEXIBLE CONTAINER: manufactured for Bayer Corporation by Baxter Healthcare Corporation, Deerfield, IL 60015.

[See fifth table above]

STORAGE

Vial: Store between 5–30°C (41–86°F).

Flexible Container: Store between 5–25°C (41–77°F).

Protect from light, avoid excessive heat, protect from freezing.

CIPRO® I.V. (ciprofloxacin) is also available in a 120 mL Pharmacy Bulk Package.

Ciprofloxacin is also available as CIPRO® (ciprofloxacin HCl) Tablets 100, 250, 500, and 750 mg and CIPRO® (ciprofloxacin) 5% and 10% Oral Suspension.

ANIMAL PHARMACOLOGY

Ciprofloxacin and other quinolones have been shown to cause arthropathy in immature animals of most species tested. (See **WARNINGS**.) Damage of weight-bearing joints was observed in juvenile dogs and rats. In young beagles, 100 mg/kg ciprofloxacin given daily for 4 weeks caused degenerative articular changes of the knee joint. At 30 mg/kg, the effect on the joint was minimal. In a subsequent study in beagles, removal of weight-bearing from the joint reduced the lesions but did not totally prevent them.

Crystalluria, sometimes associated with secondary nephropathy, occurs in laboratory animals dosed with ciprofloxacin. This is primarily related to the reduced solubility of ciprofloxacin under alkaline conditions, which predominate in the urine of test animals; in man, crystalluria is rare since human urine is typically acidic. In rhesus monkeys, crystalluria without nephropathy has been noted after in-

Continued on next page

DOSAGE GUIDELINES
Intravenous

Infection†	Type or Severity	Unit Dose	Frequency	Daily Dose
Urinary tract	Mild/Moderate	200 mg	q 12h	400 mg
	Severe/Complicated	400 mg	q 12h	800 mg
Lower Respiratory Tract	Mild/Moderate	400 mg	q 12h	800 mg
	Severe/Complicated	400 mg	q 8h	1200 mg
Nosocomial Pneumonia	Mild/Moderate/Severe	400 mg	q 8h	1200 mg
Skin and Skin Structure	Mild/Moderate	400 mg	q 12h	800 mg
	Severe/Complicated	400 mg	q 8h	1200 mg
Bone and Joint	Mild/Moderate	400 mg	q 12h	800 mg
	Severe/Complicated	400 mg	q 8h	1200 mg
Intra-Abdominal*	Complicated	400 mg	q 12h	800 mg
Acute Sinusitis	Mild/Moderate	400 mg	q 12h	800 mg
Chronic Bacterial Prostatitis	Mild/Moderate	400 mg	q 12h	800 mg
Empirical Therapy in Febrile Neutropenic Patients	Severe Ciprofloxacin	400 mg	q 8h	1200 mg
	+ Piperacillin	50 mg/kg	q 4h	Not to exceed 24 g/day
Inhalational anthrax (post-exposure)**	Adult	400 mg	q 12h	800 mg
	Pediatric	10 mg/kg per dose, not to exceed 400 mg per dose	q 12h	Not to exceed 800 mg

* used in conjunction with metronidazole. (See product labeling for prescribing information.)
† DUE TO THE DESIGNATED PATHOGENS (See **INDICATIONS AND USAGE**.)
Drug administration should begin as soon as possible after suspected or confirmed exposure. This indication is based on a surrogate endpoint, ciprofloxacin serum concentrations achieved in humans. For a discussion of ciprofloxacin serum concentrations in various human populations, see **INHALATIONAL ANTHRAX—ADDITIONAL INFORMATION. Total duration of ciprofloxacin administration (IV or oral) for inhalational anthrax (post-exposure) is 60 days.

RECOMMENDED STARTING AND MAINTENANCE DOSES FOR PATIENTS WITH IMPAIRED RENAL FUNCTION

Creatinine Clearance (mL/min)	Dosage
> 30	See usual dosage.
5 – 29	200 – 400 mg q 18–24 hr

Men: Creatinine clearance (mL/min) = $\dfrac{\text{Weight (kg)} \times (140 - \text{age})}{72 \times \text{serum creatinine (mg/dL)}}$

Women: 0.85 × the value calculated for men.

SIZE	STRENGTH	NDC NUMBER
100 mL 5% dextrose	200 mg, 0.2%	0026-8552-36
200 mL 5% dextrose	400 mg, 0.2%	0026-8554-63

SIZE	STRENGTH	NDC NUMBER
100 mL 5% dextrose	200 mg, 0.2%	0026-8527-36
200 mL 5% dextrose	400 mg, 0.2%	0026-8527-63

Cipro I.V.—Cont.

travenous doses as low as 5 mg/kg. After 6 months of intravenous dosing at 10 mg/kg/day, no nephropathological changes were noted; however, nephropathy was observed after dosing at 20 mg/kg/day for the same duration.
In dogs, ciprofloxacin administered at 3 and 10 mg/kg by rapid intravenous injection (15 sec.) produces pronounced hypotensive effects. These effects are considered to be related to histamine release because they are partially antagonized by pyrilamine, an antihistamine. In rhesus monkeys, rapid intravenous injection also produces hypotension, but the effect in this species is inconsistent and less pronounced.
In mice, concomitant administration of nonsteroidal anti-inflammatory drugs, such as phenylbutazone and indomethacin, with quinolones has been reported to enhance the CNS stimulatory effect of quinolones.
Ocular toxicity, seen with some related drugs, has not been observed in ciprofloxacin-treated animals.

INHALATIONAL ANTHRAX—ADDITIONAL INFORMATION

The mean serum concentrations of ciprofloxacin associated with a statistically significant improvement in survival in the rhesus monkey model of inhalational anthrax are reached or exceeded in adult and pediatric patients receiving oral and intravenous regimens. (See **DOSAGE AND ADMINISTRATION.**) Ciprofloxacin pharmacokinetics have been evaluated in various human populations. The mean peak serum concentration achieved at steady-state in human adults receiving 500 mg orally every 12 hours is 2.97 μg/mL, and 4.56 μg/mL following 400 mg intravenously every 12 hours. The mean trough serum concentration at steady-state for both of these regimens is 0.2 μg/mL. In a study of 10 pediatric patients between 6 and 16 years of age, the mean peak plasma concentration achieved is 8.3 μg/mL and trough concentrations range from 0.09 to 0.26 μg/mL, following two 30-minute intravenous infusions of 10 mg/kg administered 12 hours apart. After the second intravenous infusion patients switched to 15 mg/kg orally every 12 hours achieve a mean peak concentration of 3.6 μg/mL after the initial oral dose. Long-term safety data, including effects on cartilage, following the administration of ciprofloxacin to pediatric patients are limited. (For additional information, see **PRECAUTIONS, Pediatric Use.**) Ciprofloxacin serum concentrations achieved in humans serve as a surrogate endpoint reasonably likely to predict clinical benefit and provide the basis for this indication.[4]
A placebo-controlled animal study in rhesus monkeys exposed to an inhaled mean dose of 11 LD_{50} (~5.5 × 10^5) spores (range 5–30 LD_{50}) of *B. anthracis* was conducted. The minimal inhibitory concentration (MIC) of ciprofloxacin for the anthrax strain used in this study was 0.08 μg/mL. In the animals studied, mean serum concentrations of ciprofloxacin achieved at expected T_{max} (1 hour post-dose) following oral dosing to steady-state ranged form 0.98 to 1.69 μg/mL.[5] Mean steady-state trough concentrations at 12 hours post-dose ranged from 0.12 to 0.19 μg/mL.[5] Mortality due to anthrax for animals that received a 30-day regimen of oral ciprofloxacin beginning 24 hours post-exposure was significantly lower (1/9), compared to the placebo group (9/10) [p=0.001]. The one ciprofloxacin-treated animal that died of anthrax did so following the 30-day administration period.[6]

REFERENCES

1. National Committee for Clinical Laboratory Standards, Methods for Dilution Antimicrobial Susceptibility Tests for Bacteria That Grow Aerobically—Fifth Edition. Approved Standard NCCLS Document M7–A5, Vol. 20, No.2, NCCLS, Wayne, PA, January, 2000. **2.** National Committee for Clinical Laboratory Standards, Performance Standards for Antimicrobial Disk Susceptibility Tests—Seventh Edition. Approved Standard NCCLS Document M2–A7, Vol. 20, No. 1, NCCLS, Wayne, PA, January, 2000. **3.** Report presented at the FDA's Anti-Infective Drug and Dermatological Drug Product's Advisory Committee meeting, March 31, 1993, Silver Spring, MD. Report available from FDA, CDER, Advisors and Consultants Staff, HFD-21, 1901 Chapman Avenue, Room 200, Rockville, MD 20852, USA. **4.** 21 CFR 314.510 (Subpart H—Accelerated Approval of New Drugs for Life-Threatening Illnesses). **5.** Kelly DJ, et al. Serum concentrations of penicillin, doxycycline, and ciprofloxacin during prolonged therapy in rhesus monkeys. J Infect Dis 1992; 166: 1184–7. **6.** Friedlander AM, et. al. Postexposure prophylaxis against experimental inhalational anthrax. J Infect Dis 1993; 167: 1239–42.

Manufactured for:
Bayer Corporation
Pharmaceutical Division
400 Morgan Lane
West Haven, CT 06516 USA
Rx Only
PZ500175 11/00 BAY q 3939 5202-4-A-U.S.-8

58-6307 Printed in U.S.A.

CIPRO® I.V. ℞
(ciprofloxacin)
For Intravenous Infusion

Prescribing Information for this product, which appears on pages 856–860 of the 2001 PDR, has been completely revised as follows. Please write "See Supplement A" alongside product heading.

PHARMACY BULK PACKAGE—NOT FOR DIRECT INFUSION

DESCRIPTION

The pharmacy bulk package is a single-entry container of a sterile preparation for parenteral use that contains many single doses. It contains ciprofloxacin as a 1% aqueous solution concentrate. The contents are intended for use in a pharmacy admixture program and are restricted to the preparation of admixtures for intravenous infusion.
CIPRO® I.V. (ciprofloxacin) is a synthetic broad-spectrum antimicrobial agent for intravenous (I.V.) administration. Ciprofloxacin, a fluoroquinolone, is 1-cyclopropyl-6-fluoro-1, 4-dihydro-4-oxo-7-(1-piperazinyl)-3-quino-linecarboxylic acid. Its empirical formula is $C_{17}H_{18}FN_3O_3$ and its chemical structure is:

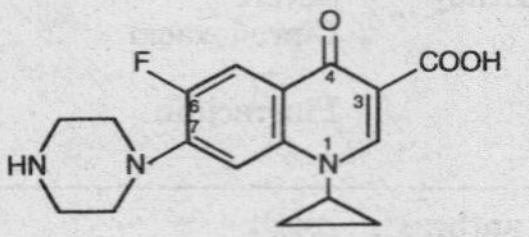

Ciprofloxacin is a faint to light yellow crystalline powder with a molecular weight of 331.4. It is soluble in dilute (0.1N) hydrochloric acid and is practically insoluble in water and ethanol. Ciprofloxacin differs from other quinolones in that it has a fluorine atom at the 6-position, a piperazine moiety at the 7-position, and a cyclopropyl ring at the 1-position. CIPRO® I.V. solutions are available as sterile 1.0% aqueous concentrate, which is intended for dilution prior to administration. Ciprofloxacin solution contains lactic acid as a solubilizing agent and hydrochloric acid for pH adjustment. The pH range for the 1.0% aqueous concentrate is 3.3 to 3.9.

CLINICAL PHARMACOLOGY

Following 60-minute intravenous infusions of 200 mg and 400 mg ciprofloxacin to normal volunteers, the mean maximum serum concentrations achieved were 2.1 and 4.6 μg/mL, respectively; the concentrations at 12 hours were 0.1 and 0.2 μg/mL, respectively.
[See first table below]
The pharmacokinetics of ciprofloxacin are linear over the dose range of 200 to 400 mg administered intravenously. The serum elimination half-life is approximately 5–6 hours and the total clearance is around 35 L/hr. Comparison of the pharmacokinetic parameters following the 1st and 5th I.V. dose on a q 12 h regimen indicates no evidence of drug accumulation.
The absolute bioavailability of oral ciprofloxacin is within a range of 70–80% with no substantial loss by first pass metabolism. An intravenous infusion of 400 mg ciprofloxacin given over 60 minutes every 12 hours has been shown to produce an area under the serum concentration time curve (AUC) equivalent to that produced by a 500-mg oral dose given every 12 hours. An intravenous infusion of 400 mg ciprofloxacin given over 60 minutes every 8 hours has been shown to produce an AUC at steady-state equivalent to that produced by a 750-mg oral dose given every 12 hours. A 400-mg I.V. dose results in a C_{max} similar to that observed with a 750-mg oral dose. An infusion of 200 mg ciprofloxacin given every 12 hours produces an AUC equivalent to that produced by a 250-mg oral dose given every 12 hours.
[See second table below]
After intravenous administration, approximately 50% to 70% of the dose is excreted in the urine as unchanged drug. Following a 200-mg I.V. dose, concentrations in the urine usually exceed 200 μg/mL 0–2 hours after dosing and are generally greater than 15 μg/mL 8–12 hours after dosing. Following a 400-mg I.V. dose, urine concentrations generally exceed 400 μg/mL 0–2 hours after dosing and are usually greater than 30 μg/mL 8–12 hours after dosing. The renal clearance is approximately 22 L/hr. The urinary excretion of ciprofloxacin is virtually complete by 24 hours after dosing.
The serum concentrations of ciprofloxacin and metronidazole were not altered when these two drugs were given concomitantly.
Co-administration of probenecid with ciprofloxacin results in about a 50% reduction in the ciprofloxacin renal clearance and a 50% increase in its concentration in the systemic circulation. Although bile concentrations of ciprofloxacin are severalfold higher than serum concentrations after intravenous dosing, only a small amount of the administered dose (<1%) is recovered from the bile as unchanged drug. Approximately 15% of an I.V. dose is recovered from the feces within 5 days after dosing.
After I.V. administration, three metabolites of ciprofloxacin have been identified in human urine which together account for approximately 10% of the intravenous dose.
Pharmacokinetic studies of the oral (single dose) and intravenous (single and multiple dose) forms of ciprofloxacin indicate that plasma concentrations of ciprofloxacin are higher in elderly subjects (>65 years) as compared to young adults. Although the C_{max} is increased 16–40%, the increase in mean AUC is approximately 30%, and can be at least partially attributed to decreased renal clearance in the elderly. Elimination half-life is only slightly (~20%) prolonged in the elderly. These differences are not considered clinically significant. (See **PRECAUTIONS: Geriatric Use.**)
In patients with reduced renal function, the half-life of ciprofloxacin is slightly prolonged and dosage adjustments may be required. (See **DOSAGE AND ADMINISTRATION.**)
In preliminary studies in patients with stable chronic liver cirrhosis, no significant changes in ciprofloxacin pharmacokinetics have been observed. However, the kinetics of ciprofloxacin in patients with acute hepatic insufficiency have not been fully elucidated.
Following infusion of 400 mg I.V. ciprofloxacin every eight hours in combination with 50 mg/kg I.V. piperacillin sodium every 4 hours, mean serum ciprofloxacin concentrations were 3.02 μg/mL 1/2 hour and 1.18 μg/mL between 6–8 hours after the end of infusion.
The binding of ciprofloxacin to serum proteins is 20 to 40%.
After intravenous administration, ciprofloxacin is present in saliva, nasal and bronchial secretions, sputum, skin blister fluid, lymph, peritoneal fluid, bile, and prostatic secretions. It has also been detected in the lung, skin, fat, muscle, cartilage, and bone. Although the drug diffuses into cerebrospinal fluid (CSF), CSF concentrations are generally less than 10% of peak serum concentrations. Levels of the drug in the aqueous and vitreous chambers of the eye are lower than in serum.
Microbiology: Ciprofloxacin has *in vitro* activity against a wide range of gram-negative and gram-positive microorganisms. The bactericidal action of ciprofloxacin results from interference with the enzyme DNA gyrase which is needed for the synthesis of bacterial DNA.
Ciprofloxacin has been shown to be active against most strains of the following microorganisms, both *in vitro* and in clinical infections as described in the **INDICATIONS AND USAGE** section of the package insert for CIPRO® I.V. (ciprofloxacin for intravenous infusion).

Aerobic gram-positive microorganisms
Enterococcus faecalis
(Many strains are only moderately susceptible.)
Staphylococcus aureus
(methicillin susceptible)
Staphylococcus epidermidis
Staphylococcus saprophyticus
Streptococcus pneumoniae
Streptococcus pyogenes

Aerobic gram-negative microorganisms
Citrobacter diversus
Citrobacter freundii
Enterobacter cloacae
Escherichia coli
Haemophilus influenzae
Haemophilus parainfluenzae
Klebsiella pneumoniae
Moraxella catarrhalis
Morganella morganii
Proteus mirabilis
Proteus vulgaris
Providencia rettgeri
Providencia stuartii
Pseudomonas aeruginosa

Steady-state Ciprofloxacin Serum Concentrations (μg/mL) After 60-minute I.V. Infusions q 12 h.

	Time after starting the infusion						
Dose	**30 min**	**1 hr**	**3 hr**	**6 hr**	**8 hr**	**12 hr**
200 mg	1.7	2.1	0.6	0.3	0.2	0.1
400 mg	3.7	4.6	1.3	0.7	0.5	0.2

Steady-state Pharmacokinetic Parameter Following Multiple Oral and I.V. Doses

Parameters	500 mg q12h, P.O.	400 mg q12h, I.V.	750 mg q12h, P.O.	400 mg q8h, I.V.
AUC (μg•hr/mL)	13.7[a]	12.7[a]	31.6[b]	32.9[c]
C_{max} (μg/mL)	2.97	4.56	3.59	4.07

[a] $AUC_{0\text{-}12h}$
[b] AUC 24h=$AUC_{0\text{-}12h}$ × 2
[c] AUC 24h=$AUC_{0\text{-}8h}$ × 3

Serratia marcescens

Ciprofloxacin has been shown to be active against most strains of the following microorganisms, both *in vitro* and in clinical infections as described in the **INDICATIONS AND USAGE** section of the package insert for CIPRO® (ciprofloxacin hydrochloride) Tablets.

Aerobic gram-positive microorganisms

Enterococcus faecalis
(Many strains are only moderately susceptible.)
Staphylococcus aureus
(methicillin susceptible)
Staphylococcus epidermidis
Staphylococcus saprophyticus
Streptococcus pneumoniae
Streptococcus pyogenes

Aerobic gram-negative microorganisms

Campylobacter jejuni
Citrobacter diversus
Citrobacter freundii
Enterobacter cloacae
Escherichia coli
Haemophilus influenzae
Haemophilus parainfluenzae
Klebsiella pneumoniae
Moraxella catarrhalis
Morganella morganii
Neisseria gonorrhoeae
Proteus mirabilis
Proteus vulgaris
Providencia rettgeri
Providencia stuartii
Pseudomonas aeruginosa
Salmonella typhi
Serratia marcescens
Shigella boydii
Shigella dysenteriae
Shigella flexneri
Shigella sonnei

Ciprofloxacin has been shown to be active against *Bacillus anthracis* both *in vitro* and by use of serum levels as a surrogate marker (see **INDICATIONS AND USAGE** and **INHALATIONAL ANTHRAX—ADDITIONAL INFORMATION**).

The following *in vitro* data are available, **but their clinical significance is unknown.**

Ciprofloxacin exhibits *in vitro* minimum inhibitory concentrations (MICs) of 1 µg/mL or less against most (≥90%) strains of the following microorganisms; however, the safety and effectiveness of ciprofloxacin in treating clinical infections due to these microorganisms have not been established in adequate and well-controlled clinical trials.

Aerobic gram-positive microorganisms

Staphylococcus haemolyticus
Staphylococcus hominis

Aerobic gram-negative microorganisms

Acinetobacter Iwoffi
Aeromonas hydrophila
Edwardsiella tarda
Enterobacter aerogenes
Klebsiella oxytoca
Legionella pneumophila
Pasteurella multocida
Salmonella enteritidis
Vibrio cholerae
Vibrio parahaemolyticus
Vibrio vulnificus
Yersinia enterocolitica

Most strains of *Burkholderia cepacia* and some strains of *Stenotrophomonas maltophilia* are resistant to ciprofloxacin as are most anaerobic bacteria, including *Bacteroides fragilis* and *Clostridium difficile*.

Ciprofloxacin is slightly less active when tested at acidic pH. The inoculum size has little effect when tested *in vitro*. The minimum bactericidal concentration (MBC) generally does not exceed the minimum inhibitory concentration (MIC) by more than a factor of 2. Resistance to ciprofloxacin *in vitro* usually develops slowly (multiple-step mutation).

Ciprofloxacin does not cross-react with other antimicrobial agents such as beta-lactams or aminoglycosides; therefore, organisms resistant to these drugs may be susceptible to ciprofloxacin.

In vitro studies have shown that additive activity often results when ciprofloxacin is combined with other antimicrobial agents such as beta-lactams, aminoglycosides, clindamycin, or metronidazole. Synergy has been reported particularly with the combination of ciprofloxacin and a beta-lactam; antagonism is observed only rarely.

Susceptibility Tests

Dilution Techniques: Quantitative methods are used to determine antimicrobial minimum inhibitory concentrations (MICs). These MICs provide estimates of the susceptibility of bacteria to antimicrobial compounds. The MICs should be determined using a standardized procedure. Standardized procedures are based on a dilution method[1] (broth and agar) or equivalent with standardized inoculum concentrations and standardized concentrations of ciprofloxacin powder. The MIC values should be interpreted according to the following criteria:

For testing aerobic microorganisms other than *Haemophilus influenzae, Haemophilus parainfluenzae,* and *Neisseria gonorrhoeae*[a]:

MIC (µg/mL)	Interpretation
≤1	Susceptible (S)
2	Intermediate (I)
≥4	Resistant (R)

[a] These interpretive standards are applicable only to broth microdilution susceptibility tests with streptococci using cation-adjusted Mueller-Hinton broth with 2–5% lysed horse blood.

For testing *Haemophilus influenzae,* and *Haemophilus parainfluenzae*[b]:

MIC (µg/mL)	Interpretation
≤1	Susceptible (S)

[b] This interpretive standard is applicable only to broth microdilution susceptibility tests with *Haemophilus influenzae* and *Haemophilus parainfluenzae* using *Haemophilus* Test Medium[1].

The current absence of data on resistant strains precludes defining any results other than "Susceptible". Strains yielding MIC results suggestive of a "nonsusceptible" category should be submitted to a reference laboratory for further testing.

For testing *Neisseria gonorrhoeae*[c]:

MIC (µg/mL)	Interpretation
≤0.06	Susceptible (S)

[c] This interpretive standard is applicable only to agar dilution test with GC agar base and 1% defined growth supplement.

The current absence of data on resistant strains precludes defining any results other than "Susceptible". Strains yielding MIC results suggestive of a "nonsusceptible" category should be submitted to a reference laboratory for further testing.

A report of "Susceptible" indicates that the pathogen is likely to be inhibited if the antimicrobial compound in the blood reaches the concentrations usually achievable. A report of "Intermediate" indicates that the result should be considered equivocal, and, if the microorganism is not fully susceptible to alternative, clinically feasible drugs, the test should be repeated. This category implies possible clinical applicability in body sites where the drug is physiologically concentrated or in situations where high dosage of drug can be used. This category also provides a buffer zone which prevents small uncontrolled technical factors from causing major discrepancies in interpretation. A report of "Resistant" indicates that the pathogen is not likely to be inhibited if the antimicrobial compound in the blood reaches the concentrations usually achievable; other therapy should be selected.

Standardized susceptibility test procedures require the use of laboratory control microorganisms to control the technical aspects of the laboratory procedures. Standard ciprofloxacin powder should provide the following MIC values:

Organism		MIC (µg/mL)
E. faecalis	ATCC 29212	0.25 – 2.0
E. coli	ATCC 25922	0.004 – 0.015
H. influenzae[a]	ATCC 49247	0.004 – 0.03
N. gonorrhoeae[b]	ATCC 49226	0.001 – 0.008
P. aeruginosa	ATCC 27853	0.25 – 1.0
S. aureus	ATCC 29213	0.12 – 0.5

[a] This quality control range is applicable to only *H. influenzae* ATCC 49247 tested by a broth microdilution procedure using *Haemophilus* Test Medium (HTM)[1].

[b] This quality control range is applicable to only *N. gonorrhoeae* ATCC 49226 tested by an agar dilution procedure using GC agar base and 1% defined growth supplement.

Diffusion Techniques: Quantitative methods that require measurement of zone diameters also provide reproducible estimates of the susceptibility of bacteria to antimicrobial compounds. One such standardized procedure[2] requires the use of standardized inoculum concentrations. This procedure uses paper disks impregnated with 5-µg ciprofloxacin to test the susceptibility of microorganisms to ciprofloxacin.

Reports from the laboratory providing results of the standard single-disk susceptibility test with a 5-µg ciprofloxacin disk should be interpreted according to the following criteria:

For testing aerobic microorganisms other than *Haemophilus influenzae, Haemophilus parainfluenzae,* and *Neisseria gonorrhoeae*[a]:

Zone Diameter (mm)	Interpretation
≥21	Susceptible (S)
16–20	Intermediate (I)
≤15	Resistant (R)

[a] These zone diameter standards are applicable only to tests performed for streptococci using Mueller-Hinton agar supplemented with 5% sheep blood incubated in 5% CO_2.

For testing *Haemophilus influenzae* and *Haemophilus parainfluenzae*[b]:

Zone Diameter (mm)	Interpretation
≥21	Susceptible (S)

[b] This zone diameter standard is applicable only to tests with *Haemophilus influenzae* and *Haemophilus parainfluenzae* using *Haemophilus* Test Medium (HTM)[2].

The current absence of data on resistant strains precludes defining any results other than "Susceptible". Strains yielding zone diameter results suggestive of a "nonsusceptible" category should be submitted to a reference laboratory for further testing.

For testing *Neisseria gonorrhoeae*[c]:

Zone Diameter (mm)	Interpretation
≥36	Susceptible (S)

[c] This zone diameter standard is applicable only to disk diffusion tests with GC agar base and 1% defined growth supplement.

The current absence of data on resistant strains precludes defining any results other than "Susceptible". Strains yielding zone diameter results suggestive of a "nonsusceptible" category should be submitted to a reference laboratory for further testing.

Interpretation should be as stated above for results using dilution techniques. Interpretation involves correlation of the diameter obtained in the disk test with the MIC for ciprofloxacin.

As with standardized dilution techniques, diffusion methods require the use of laboratory control microorganisms that are used to control the technical aspects of the laboratory procedures. For the diffusion technique, the 5-µg ciprofloxacin disk should provide the following zone diameters in these laboratory test quality control strains:

Organism		Zone Diameter (mm)
E. coli	ATCC 25922	30–40
H. influenzae[a]	ATCC 49247	34–42
N. gonorrhoeae[b]	ATCC 49226	48–58
P. aeruginosa	ATCC 27853	25–33
S. aureus	ATCC 25923	22–30

[a] These quality control limits are applicable to only *H. influenzae* ATCC 49247 testing using *Haemophilus* Test Medium (HTM)[2].

[b] These quality control limits are applicable only to tests conducted with *N. gonorrhoeae* ATCC 49226 performed by disk diffusion using GC agar base and 1% defined growth supplement.

INDICATIONS AND USAGE

CIPRO® I.V. is indicated for the treatment of infections caused by susceptible strains of the designated microorganisms in the conditions listed below when the intravenous administration offers a route of administration advantageous to the patient. Please see **DOSAGE AND ADMINISTRATION** for specific recommendations.

Urinary Tract Infections caused by *Escherichia coli* (including cases with secondary bacteremia), *Klebsiella pneumoniae* subspecies *pneumoniae, Enterobacter cloacae, Serratia marcescens, Proteus mirabilis, Providencia rettgeri, Morganella morganii, Citrobacter diversus, Citrobacter freundii, Pseudomonas aeruginosa, Staphylococcus epidermidis, Staphylococcus saprophyticus,* or *Enterococcus faecalis*.

Lower Respiratory Infections caused by *Escherichia coli, Klebsiella pneumoniae* subspecies *pneumoniae, Enterobacter cloacae, Proteus mirabilis, Pseudomonas aeruginosa, Haemophilus influenzae, Haemophilus parainfluenzae,* or *Streptococcus pneumoniae*.

NOTE: Although effective in clinical trials, ciprofloxacin is not a drug of first choice in the treatment of presumed or confirmed pneumonia secondary to *Streptococcus pneumoniae*.

Nosocomial Pneumonia caused by *Haemophilus influenzae* or *Klebsiella pneumoniae*.

Skin and Skin Structure Infections caused by *Escherichia coli, Klebsiella pneumoniae* subspecies *pneumoniae, Enterobacter cloacae, Proteus mirabilis, Proteus vulgaris, Providencia stuartii, Morganella morganii, Citrobacter freundii, Pseudomonas aeruginosa, Staphylococcus aureus* (methicillin susceptible), *Staphylococcus epidermidis,* or *Streptococcus pyogenes*.

Bone and Joint Infections caused by *Enterobacter cloacae, Serratia marcescens,* or *Pseudomonas aeruginosa*.

Complicated Intra-Abdominal Infections (used in conjunction with metronidazole) caused by *Escherichia coli, Pseudomonas aeruginosa, Proteus mirabilis, Klebsiella pneumoniae,* or *Bacteroides fragilis*. (See **DOSAGE AND ADMINISTRATION.**)

Acute Sinusitis caused by *Haemophilus influenzae, Streptococcus pneumoniae,* or *Moraxella catarrhalis*.

Chronic Bacterial Prostatitis caused by *Escherichia coli* or *Proteus mirabilis*.

Empirical Therapy for Febrile Neutropenic Patients in combination with piperacillin sodium. (See **DOSAGE AND ADMINISTRATION** and **CLINICAL STUDIES.**)

Inhalational anthrax (post-exposure): To reduce the incidence or progression of disease following exposure to aerosolized *Bacillus anthracis*.

Ciprofloxacin serum concentrations achieved in humans serve as a surrogate endpoint reasonably likely to predict

Continued on next page

Cipro I.V. Bulk—Cont.

clinical benefit and provide the basis for this indication.[4] (See also, **INHALATIONAL ANTHRAX—ADDITIONAL INFORMATION**).

If anaerobic organisms are suspected of contributing to the infection, appropriate therapy should be administered.

Appropriate culture and susceptibility tests should be performed before treatment in order to isolate and identify organisms causing infection and to determine their susceptibility to ciprofloxacin. Therapy with CIPRO® I.V. may be initiated before results of these tests are known; once results become available, appropriate therapy should be continued.

As with other drugs, some strains of *Pseudomonas aeruginosa* may develop resistance fairly rapidly during treatment with ciprofloxacin. Culture and susceptibility testing performed periodically during therapy will provide information not only on the therapeutic effect of the antimicrobial agent but also on the possible emergence of bacterial resistance.

CLINICAL STUDIES

EMPIRICAL THERAPY IN FEBRILE NEUTROPENIC PATIENTS
The safety and efficacy of ciprofloxacin, 400 mg I.V. q 8h, in combination with piperacillin sodium, 50 mg/kg I.V. q 4h, for the empirical therapy of febrile neutropenic patients were studied in one large pivotal multicenter, randomized trial and were compared to those of tobramycin, 2 mg/kg I.V. q 8h, in combination with piperacillin sodium, 50 mg/kg I.V. q 4h.

The demographics of the evaluable patients were as follows: [See first table above]

Clinical response rates observed in this study were as follows:
[See second table above]

CONTRAINDICATIONS

CIPRO® I.V. (ciprofloxacin) is contraindicated in persons with a history of hypersensitivity to ciprofloxacin or any member of the quinolone class of antimicrobial agents.

WARNINGS

THE SAFETY AND EFFECTIVENESS OF CIPROFLOXACIN IN PEDIATRIC PATIENTS AND ADOLESCENTS (LESS THAN 18 YEARS OF AGE),—EXCEPT FOR USE IN INHALATIONAL ANTHRAX (POST-EXPOSURE), PREGNANT WOMEN, AND LACTATING WOMEN HAVE NOT BEEN ESTABLISHED. (See **PRECAUTIONS: Pediatric Use, Pregnancy,** and **Nursing Mothers** subsections.) Ciprofloxacin causes lameness in immature dogs. Histopathological examination of the weight-bearing joints of these dogs revealed permanent lesions of the cartilage. Related quinolone-class drugs also produce erosions of cartilage of weight-bearing joints and other signs of arthropathy in immature animals of various species. (See **ANIMAL PHARMACOLOGY**.)

Convulsions, increased intracranial pressure, and toxic psychosis have been reported in patients receiving quinolones, including ciprofloxacin. Ciprofloxacin may also cause central nervous system (CNS) events including: dizziness, confusion, tremors, hallucinations, depression, and, rarely, suicidal thoughts or acts. These reactions may occur following the first dose. If these reactions occur in patients receiving ciprofloxacin, the drug should be discontinued and appropriate measures instituted. As with all quinolones, ciprofloxacin should be used with caution in patients with known or suspected CNS disorders that may predispose to seizures or lower the seizure threshold (e.g. severe cerebral arteriosclerosis, epilepsy), or in the presence of other risk factors that may predispose to seizures or lower the seizure threshold (e.g. certain drug therapy, renal dysfunction). (See **PRECAUTIONS: General, Information for Patients, Drug Interactions** and **ADVERSE REACTIONS**.)

SERIOUS AND FATAL REACTIONS HAVE BEEN REPORTED IN PATIENTS RECEIVING CONCURRENT ADMINISTRATION OF INTRAVENOUS CIPROFLOXACIN AND THEOPHYLLINE. These reactions have included cardiac arrest, seizure, status epilepticus, and respiratory failure. Although similar serious adverse events have been reported in patients receiving theophylline alone, the possibility that these reactions may be potentiated by ciprofloxacin cannot be eliminated. If concomitant use cannot be avoided, serum levels of theophylline should be monitored and dosage adjustments made as appropriate.

Serious and occasionally fatal hypersensitivity (anaphylactic) reactions, some following the first dose, have been reported in patients receiving quinolone therapy. Some reactions were accompanied by cardiovascular collapse, loss of consciousness, tingling, pharyngeal or facial edema, dyspnea, urticaria, and itching. Only a few patients had a history of hypersensitivity reactions. Serious anaphylactic reactions require immediate emergency treatment with epinephrine and other resuscitation measures, including oxygen, intravenous fluids, intravenous antihistamines, corticosteroids, pressor amines, and airway management, as clinically indicated.

Severe hypersensitivity reactions characterized by rash, fever, eosinophilia, jaundice, and hepatic necrosis with fatal outcome have also been reported extremely rarely in patients receiving ciprofloxacin along with other drugs. The possibility that these reactions were related to ciprofloxacin cannot be excluded. Ciprofloxacin should be discontinued at the first appearance of a skin rash or any other sign of hypersensitivity.

Pseudomembranous colitis has been reported with nearly all antibacterial agents, including ciprofloxacin, and may

Total	Ciprofloxacin/Piperacillin N = 233	Tobramycin/Piperacillin N = 237
Median Age (years)	47.0 (range 19–84)	50.0 (range 18–81)
Male	114 (48.9%)	117 (49.4%)
Female	119 (51.1%)	120 (50.6%)
Leukemia/Bone Marrow Transplant	165 (70.8%)	158 (66.7%)
Solid Tumor/Lymphoma	68 (29.2%)	79 (33.3%)
Median Duration of Neutropenia (days)	15.0 (range 1–61)	14.0 (range 1–89)

Outcomes	Ciprofloxacin/Piperacillin N = 233 Success (%)	Tobramycin/Piperacillin N = 237 Success (%)
Clinical Resolution of Initial Febrile Episode with No Modifications of Empirical Regimen*	63 (27.0%)	52 (21.9%)
Clinical Resolution of Initial Febrile Episode Including Patients with Modifications of Empirical Regimen	187 (80.3%)	185 (78.1%)
Overall Survival	224 (96.1%)	223 (94.1%)

* To be evaluated as a clinical resolution, patients had to have: (1) resolution of fever; (2) microbiological eradication of infection (if an infection was microbiologically documented); (3) resolution of signs/symptoms of infection; and (4) no modification of empirical antibiotic regimen.

range in severity from mild to life-threatening. Therefore, it is important to consider this diagnosis in patients who present with diarrhea subsequent to the administration of antibacterial agents.

Treatment with antibacterial agents alters the normal flora of the colon and may permit overgrowth of clostridia. Studies indicate that a toxin produced by *Clostridium difficile* is one primary cause of "antibiotic-associated colitis".

After the diagnosis of pseudomembranous colitis has been established, therapeutic measures should be initiated. Mild cases of pseudomembranous colitis usually respond to drug discontinuation alone. In moderate to severe cases, consideration should be given to management with fluids and electrolytes, protein supplementation and treatment with an antibacterial drug clinically effective against *C. difficile* colitis.

Achilles and other tendon ruptures that required surgical repair or resulted in prolonged disability have been reported with ciprofloxacin and other quinolones. Ciprofloxacin should be discontinued if the patient experiences pain, inflammation, or rupture of a tendon.

PRECAUTIONS

General: INTRAVENOUS CIPROFLOXACIN SHOULD BE ADMINISTERED BY SLOW INFUSION OVER A PERIOD OF 60 MINUTES. Local I.V. site reactions have been reported with the intravenous administration of ciprofloxacin. These reactions are more frequent if infusion time is 30 minutes or less or if small veins of the hand are used. (See **ADVERSE REACTIONS**.)

Quinolones, including ciprofloxacin, may also cause central nervous system (CNS) events, including nervousness, agitation, insomnia, anxiety, nightmares or paranoia. (See **WARNINGS, Information for Patients,** and **Drug Interactions**.)

Crystals of ciprofloxacin have been observed rarely in the urine of human subjects but more frequently in the urine of laboratory animals, which is usually alkaline. (See **ANIMAL PHARMACOLOGY**.) Crystalluria related to ciprofloxacin has been reported only rarely in humans because human urine is usually acidic. Alkalinity of the urine should be avoided in patients receiving ciprofloxacin. Patients should be well hydrated to prevent the formation of highly concentrated urine.

Alteration of the dosage regimen is necessary for patients with impairment of renal function. (See **DOSAGE AND ADMINISTRATION**.)

Moderate to severe phototoxicity manifested as an exaggerated sunburn reaction has been observed in some patients who were exposed to direct sunlight while receiving some members of the quinolone class of drugs. Excessive sunlight should be avoided.

As with any potent drug, periodic assessment of organ system functions, including renal, hepatic, and hematopoietic, is advisable during prolonged therapy.

Information For Patients: Patients should be advised that ciprofloxacin may be associated with hypersensitivity reactions, even following a single dose, and to discontinue the drug at the first sign of a skin rash or other allergic reaction. Ciprofloxacin may cause dizziness and lightheadedness; therefore, patients should know how they react to this drug before they operate an automobile or machinery or engage in activities requiring mental alertness or coordination.

Patients should be advised that ciprofloxacin may increase the effects of theophylline and caffeine. There is a possibility of caffeine accumulation when products containing caffeine are consumed while taking ciprofloxacin.

Patients should be advised to discontinue treatment; rest and refrain from exercise; and inform their physician if they experience pain, inflammation, or rupture of a tendon.

Patients should be advised that convulsions have been reported in patients taking quinolones, including ciprofloxacin, and to notify their physician before taking the drug if there is a history of this condition.

Drug Interactions: As with some other quinolones, concurrent administration of ciprofloxacin with theophylline may lead to elevated serum concentrations of theophylline and prolongation of its elimination half-life. This may result in increased risk of theophylline-related adverse reactions. (See **WARNINGS**.) If concomitant use cannot be avoided, serum levels of theophylline should be monitored and dosage adjustments made as appropriate.

Some quinolones, including ciprofloxacin, have also been shown to interfere with the metabolism of caffeine. This may lead to reduced clearance of caffeine and prolongation of its serum half-life.

Some quinolones, including ciprofloxacin, have been associated with transient elevations in serum creatinine in patients receiving cyclosporine concomitantly.

Altered serum levels of phenytoin (increased and decreased) have been reported in patients receiving concomitant ciprofloxacin.

The concomitant administration of ciprofloxacin with the sulfonylurea glyburide has, in some patients, resulted in severe hypoglycemia. Fatalities have been reported.

Quinolones have been reported to enhance the effects of the oral anticoagulant warfarin or its derivatives. When these products are administered concomitantly, prothrombin time or other suitable coagulation tests should be closely monitored.

Probenecid interferes with renal tubular secretion of ciprofloxacin and produces an increase in the level of ciprofloxacin in the serum. This should be considered if patients are receiving both drugs concomitantly.

As with other broad-spectrum antimicrobial agents, prolonged use of ciprofloxacin may result in overgrowth of nonsusceptible organisms. Repeated evaluation of the patient's condition and microbial susceptibility testing is essential. If superinfection occurs during therapy, appropriate measures should be taken.

Carcinogenesis, Mutagenesis, Impairment of Fertility: Eight *in vitro* mutagenicity tests have been conducted with ciprofloxacin. Test results are listed below:

Salmonella/Microsome Test (Negative)
E. coli DNA Repair Assay (Negative)
Mouse Lymphoma Cell Forward Mutation Assay (Positive)
Chinese Hamster V_{79} Cell HGPRT Test (Negative)
Syrian Hamster Embryo Cell Transformation Assay (Negative)
Saccharomyces cerevisiae Point Mutation Assay (Negative)
Saccharomyces cerevisiae Mitotic Crossover and Gene Conversion Assay (Negative)
Rat Hepatocyte DNA Repair Assay (Positive)

Thus, two of the eight tests were positive, but results of the following three *in vivo* test systems gave negative results:

Rat Hepatocyte DNA Repair Assay
Micronucleus Test (Mice)
Dominant Lethal Test (Mice)

Long-term carcinogenicity studies in mice and rats have been completed. After daily oral doses of 750 mg/kg (mice) and 250 mg/kg (rats) were administered for up to 2 years, there was no evidence that ciprofloxacin had any carcinogenic or tumorigenic effects in these species.

Results from photo co-carcinogenicity testing indicate that ciprofloxacin does not reduce the time to appearance of UV-induced skin tumors as compared to vehicle control. Hairless (Skh-1) mice were exposed to UVA light for 3.5 hours five times every two weeks for up to 78 weeks while concurrently being administered ciprofloxacin. The time to development of the first skin tumors was 50 weeks in mice treated concomitantly with UVA and ciprofloxacin (mouse dose approximately equal to maximum recommended human dose based upon mg/m^2), as opposed to 34 weeks when animals were treated with both UVA and vehicle. The times to development of skin tumors ranged from 16–32 weeks in mice treated concomitantly with UVA and other quinolones.[3]

In this model, mice treated with ciprofloxacin alone did not develop skin or systemic tumors. There are no data from similar models using pigmented mice and/or fully haired mice. The clinical significance of these findings to humans is unknown.
Fertility studies performed in rats at oral doses of ciprofloxacin up to 100 mg/kg (0.8 times the highest recommended human dose of 1200 mg based upon body surface area) revealed no evidence of impairment.
Pregnancy: Teratogenic Effects. Pregnancy Category C: Reproduction studies have been performed in rats and mice using oral doses of up to 100 mg/kg (0.8 and 0.4 times the maximum daily human dose based upon body surface area, respectively) and I.V. doses of up to 30 mg/kg (0.24 and 0.12 times the maximum daily human dose based upon body surface area, respectively) and have revealed no evidence of harm to the fetus due to ciprofloxacin. In rabbits, ciprofloxacin (30 and 100 mg/kg orally) produced gastrointestinal disturbances resulting in maternal weight loss and an increased incidence of abortion, but no teratogenicity was observed at either dose. After intravenous administration of doses up to 20 mg/kg, no maternal toxicity was produced in the rabbit, and no embryotoxicity or teratogenicity was observed. There are, however, no adequate and well-controlled studies in pregnant women. Ciprofloxacin should be used during pregnancy only if the potential benefit justifies the potential risk to the fetus. (See **WARNINGS**.)
Nursing Mothers: Ciprofloxacin is excreted in human milk. Because of the potential for serious adverse reactions in infants nursing from mothers taking ciprofloxacin, a decision should be made whether to discontinue nursing or to discontinue the drug, taking into account the importance of the drug to the mother.
Pediatric Use: Safety and effectiveness in pediatric patients and adolescents less than 18 years of age have not been established, except for use in inhalational anthrax (post-exposure). Ciprofloxacin causes arthropathy in juvenile animals. (See **WARNINGS**.)
For the indication of inhalational anthrax (post-exposure), the risk-benefit assessment indicates that administration of ciprofloxacin to pediatric patients is appropriate. For information regarding pediatric dosing in inhalational anthrax (post-exposure), see **DOSAGE AND ADMINISTRATION** and **INHALATIONAL ANTHRAX—ADDITIONAL INFORMATION**.
Short-term safety data from a single trial in pediatric cystic fibrosis patients are available. In a randomized, double-blind clinical trial for the treatment of acute pulmonary exacerbations in cystic fibrosis patients (ages 5–17 years), 67 patients received ciprofloxacin I.V. 10 mg/kg/dose q8h for one week followed by ciprofloxacin tablets 20 mg/kg/dose q12h to complete 10–21 days treatment and 62 patients received the combination of ceftazidime I.V. 50 mg/kg/dose q8h and tobramycin I.V. 3 mg/kg/dose q8h for a total of 10–21 days. Patients less than 5 years of age were not studied. Safety monitoring in the study included periodic range of motion examinations and gait assessments by treatment-blinded examiners. Patients were followed for an average of 23 days after completing treatment (range 0–93 days). This study was not designed to determine long term effects and the safety of repeated exposure to ciprofloxacin.
In the study, injection site reactions were more common in the ciprofloxacin group (24%) than in the comparison group (8%). Other adverse events were similar in nature and frequency between treatment arms. Musculoskeletal adverse events were reported in 22% of the patients in the ciprofloxacin group and 21% in the comparison group. Decreased range of motion was reported in 12% of the subjects in the ciprofloxacin group and 16% in the comparison group. Arthralgia was reported in 10% of the patients in the ciprofloxacin group and 11% in the comparison group. One of sixty-seven patients developed arthritis of the knee nine days after a ten day course of treatment with ciprofloxacin. Clinical symptoms resolved, but an MRI showed knee effusion without other abnormalities eight months after treatment. However, the relationship of this event to the patient's course of ciprofloxacin can not be definitively determined, particularly since patients with cystic fibrosis may develop arthralgias/arthritis as part of their underlying disease process.
Geriatric Use: In a retrospective analysis of 23 multiple-dose controlled clinical trials of ciprofloxacin encompassing over 3500 ciprofloxacin treated patients, 25% of patients were greater than or equal to 65 years of age and 10% were greater than or equal to 75 years of age. No overall differences in safety or effectiveness were observed between these subjects and younger subjects, and other reported clinical experience has not identified differences in responses between the elderly and younger patients, but greater sensitivity of some older individuals on any drug therapy cannot be ruled out. Ciprofloxacin is known to be substantially excreted by the kidney, and the risk of adverse reactions may be greater in patients with impaired renal function. No alteration of dosage is necessary for patients greater than 65 years of age with normal renal function. However, since some older individuals experience reduced renal function by virtue of their advanced age, care should be taken in dose selection for elderly patients, and renal function monitoring may be useful in these patients. (See **CLINICAL PHARMACOLOGY** and **DOSAGE AND ADMINISTRATION**.)

ADVERSE REACTIONS

The most frequently reported events, without regard to drug relationship, among patients treated with intravenous ciprofloxacin were nausea, diarrhea, central nervous system disturbance, local I.V. site reactions, abnormalities of liver associated enzymes (hepatic enzymes), and eosinophilia. Headache, restlessness, and rash were also noted in greater than 1% of patients treated with the most common doses of ciprofloxacin.
Local I.V. site reactions have been reported with the intravenous administration of ciprofloxacin. These reactions are more frequent if the infusion time is 30 minutes or less. These may appear as local skin reactions which resolve rapidly upon completion of the infusion. Subsequent intravenous administration is not contraindicated unless the reactions recur or worsen.
Additional events, without regard to drug relationship or route of administration, that occurred in 1% or less of ciprofloxacin patients are listed below:
CARDIOVASCULAR: cardiovascular collapse, cardiopulmonary arrest, myocardial infarction, arrhythmia, tachycardia, palpitation, cerebral thrombosis, syncope, cardiac murmur, hypertension, hypotension, angina pectoris
CENTRAL NERVOUS SYSTEM: convulsive seizures, paranoia, toxic psychosis, depression, dysphasia, phobia, depersonalization, manic reaction, unresponsiveness, ataxia, confusion, hallucinations, dizziness, lightheadedness, paresthesia, anxiety, tremor, insomnia, nightmares, weakness, drowsiness, irritability, malaise, lethargy
GASTROINTESTINAL: ileus, jaundice, gastrointestinal bleeding, *C. difficile* associated diarrhea, pseudomembranous colitis, pancreatitis, hepatic necrosis, intestinal perforation, dyspepsia, epigastric or abdominal pain, vomiting, constipation, oral ulceration, oral candidiasis, mouth dryness, anorexia, dysphagia, flatulence
I.V. INFUSION SITE: thrombophlebitis, burning, pain, pruritus, paresthesia, erythema, swelling
MUSCULOSKELETAL: arthralgia, jaw, arm or back pain, joint stiffness, neck and chest pain, achiness, flare up of gout
RENAL/UROGENITAL: renal failure, interstitial nephritis, hemorrhagic cystitis, renal calculi, frequent urination, acidosis, urethral bleeding, polyuria, urinary retention, gynecomastia, candiduria, vaginitis. Crystalluria, cylindruria, hematuria, and albuminuria have also been reported.
RESPIRATORY: respiratory arrest, pulmonary embolism, dyspnea, pulmonary edema, respiratory distress, pleural effusion, hemoptysis, epistaxis, hiccough
SKIN/HYPERSENSITIVITY: anaphylactic reactions, erythema multiforme/Stevens-Johnson syndrome, exfoliative dermatitis, toxic epidermal necrolysis, vasculitis, angioedema, edema of the lips, face, neck, conjunctivae, hands or lower extremities, purpura, fever, chills, flushing, pruritus, urticaria, cutaneous candidiasis, vesicles, increased perspiration, hyperpigmentation, erythema nodosum, photosensitivity (See **WARNINGS**.)
SPECIAL SENSES: decreased visual acuity, blurred vision, disturbed vision (flashing lights, change in color perception, overbrightness of lights, diplopia), eye pain, anosmia, hearing loss, tinnitus, nystagmus, a bad taste
Also reported were agranulocytosis, prolongation of prothrombin time, and possible exacerbation of myasthenia gravis.
Many of these events were described as only mild or moderate in severity, abated soon after the drug was discontinued, and required no treatment.
In several instances, nausea, vomiting, tremor, irritability, or palpitation were judged by investigators to be related to elevated serum levels of theophylline possibly as a result of drug interaction with ciprofloxacin.
In randomized, double-blind controlled clinical trials comparing ciprofloxacin (I.V. and I.V. P.O. sequential) with intravenous beta-lactam control antibiotics, the CNS adverse event profile of ciprofloxacin was comparable to that of the control drugs.
Post-Marketing Adverse Events: Additional adverse events, regardless of relationship to drug, reported from worldwide marketing experience with quinolones, including ciprofloxacin, are:
BODY AS A WHOLE: change in serum phenytoin
CARDIOVASCULAR: postural hypotension, vasculitis
CENTRAL NERVOUS SYSTEM: agitation, delirium, myoclonus, toxic psychosis
HEMIC/LYMPHATIC: hemolytic anemia, methemoglobinemia
METABOLIC/NUTRITIONAL: elevation of serum triglycerides, cholesterol, blood glucose, serum potassium
MUSCULOSKELETAL: myalgia, tendinitis/tendon rupture
RENAL/UROGENITAL: vaginal candidiasis
(See **PRECAUTIONS**.)
Adverse Laboratory Changes: The most frequently reported changes in laboratory parameters with intravenous ciprofloxacin therapy, without regard to drug relationship are listed below:
[See first table above]

Hepatic	—	elevations of AST (SGOT), ALT (SGPT), alkaline phosphatase, LDH, and serum bilirubin;
Hematologic	—	elevated eosinophil and platelet counts, decreased platelet counts, hemoglobin and/or hematocrit;
Renal	—	elevations of serum creatinine, BUN, and uric acid;
Other	—	elevations of serum creatinine, phosphokinase, serum theophylline (in patients receiving theophylline concomitantly), blood glucose, and triglycerides.

Other changes occurring infrequently were: decreased leukocyte count, elevated atypical lymphocyte count, immature WBCs, elevated serum calcium, elevation of serum gamma-glutamyl transpeptidase (γ GT), decreased BUN, decreased uric acid, decreased total serum protein, decreased serum albumin, decreased serum potassium, elevated serum potassium, elevated serum cholesterol.
Other changes occurring rarely during administration of ciprofloxacin were: elevation of serum amylase, decrease of blood glucose, pancytopenia, leukocytosis, elevated sedi-

DOSAGE GUIDELINES
Intravenous

Infection†	Type or Severity	Unit Dose	Frequency	Daily Dose
Urinary tract	Mild/Moderate Severe/Complicated	200 mg 400 mg	q 12h q 12h	400 mg 800 mg
Lower Respiratory Tract	Mild/Moderate Severe/Complicated	400 mg 400 mg	q 12h q 8h	800 mg 1200 mg
Nosocomial Pneumonia	Mild/Moderate/Severe	400 mg	q 8h	1200 mg
Skin and Skin Structure	Mild/Moderate Severe/Complicated	400 mg 400 mg	q 12h q 8h	800 mg 1200 mg
Bone and Joint	Mild/Moderate Severe/Complicated	400 mg 400 mg	q 12h q 8h	800 mg 1200 mg
Intra-Abdominal*	Complicated	400 mg	q 12h	800 mg
Acute Sinusitis	Mild/Moderate	400 mg	q 12h	800 mg
Chronic Bacterial Prostatitis	Mild/Moderate	400 mg	q 12h	800 mg
Empirical Therapy in Febrile Neutropenic Patients	Severe Ciprofloxacin + Piperacillin	400 mg 50 mg/kg	q 8h q 4h	1200 mg Not to exceed 24 g/day
Inhalational anthrax (post-exposure)**	Adult	400 mg	q 12h	800 mg
	Pediatric	10 mg/kg per dose, not to exceed 400 mg per dose	q 12h	Not to exceed 800 mg

* used in conjunction with metronidazole. (See product labeling for prescribing information.)
† DUE TO THE DESIGNATED PATHOGENS (See **INDICATIONS AND USAGE**.)
** Drug administration should begin as soon as possible after suspected or confirmed exposure. This indication is based on a surrogate endpoint, ciprofloxacin serum concentrations achieved in humans. For a discussion of ciprofloxacin serum concentrations in various human populations, see **INHALATIONAL ANTHRAX—ADDITIONAL INFORMATION**. Total duration of ciprofloxacin administration (IV or oral) for inhalational anthrax (post-exposure) is 60 days.

Continued on next page

Cipro I.V. Bulk—Cont.

mentation rate, change in serum phenytoin, decreased prothrombin time, hemolytic anemia, and bleeding diathesis.

OVERDOSAGE

In the event of acute overdosage, the patient should be carefully observed and given supportive treatment. Adequate hydration must be maintained. Only a small amount of ciprofloxacin (<10%) is removed from the body after hemodialysis or peritoneal dialysis.

In mice, rats, rabbits and dogs, significant toxicity including tonic/clonic convulsions was observed at intravenous doses of ciprofloxacin between 125 and 300 mg/kg.

DOSAGE AND ADMINISTRATION

The recommended adult dosage for urinary tract infections of mild to moderate severity is 200 mg I.V. every 12 hours. For severe or complicated urinary tract infections, the recommended dosage is 400 mg I.V. every 12 hours.

The recommended adult dosage for lower respiratory tract infections, skin and skin structure infections, and bone and joint infections of mild to moderate severity is 400 mg I.V. every 12 hours.

For severe/complicated infections of the lower respiratory tract, skin and skin structure, and bone and joint, the recommended adult dosage is 400 mg I.V. every 8 hours.

The recommended adult dosage for mild, moderate, and severe nosocomial pneumonia is 400 mg I.V. every 8 hours.

Complicated Intra-Abdominal Infections: Sequential therapy [parenteral to oral - 400 mg CIPRO® I.V. q 12 h (plus I.V. metronidazole) → 500 mg CIPRO® Tablets q 12 h (plus oral metronidazole)] can be instituted at the discretion of the physician. Metronidazole should be given according to product labeling to provide appropriate anaerobic coverage.

The recommended dosage for mild to moderate Acute Sinusitis and Chronic Bacterial Prostatitis is 400 mg I.V. every 12 hours.

The recommended adult dosage for empirical therapy of febrile neutropenic patients is 400 mg I.V. every 8 hours in combination with piperacillin sodium 50 mg/kg I.V. q 4 hours, not to exceed 24 g/day (300 mg/kg/day), for 7–14 days.

The determination of dosage for any particular patient must take into consideration the severity and nature of the infection, the susceptibility of the causative microorganism, the integrity of the patient's host-defense mechanisms and the status of renal and hepatic function.

[See second table at top of previous page]

After dilution CIPRO® I.V. should be administered by intravenous infusion over a period of 60 minutes.

Parenteral drug products should be inspected visually for particulate matter and discoloration prior to administration.

Ciprofloxacin hydrochloride (CIPRO® Tablets) for oral administration are available. Parenteral therapy may be changed to oral CIPRO® Tablets when the condition warrants, at the discretion of the physician. For complete dosage and administration information, see CIPRO® Tablets package insert.

Impaired Renal Function: The following table provides dosage guidelines for use in patients with renal impairment; however, monitoring of serum drug levels provides the most reliable basis for dosage adjustment.

RECOMMENDED STARTING AND MAINTENANCE DOSES FOR PATIENTS WITH IMPAIRED RENAL FUNCTION

Creatinine Clearance (mL/min)	Dosage
> 30	See usual dosage.
5–29	200 - 400 mg q 18–24 hr

When only the serum creatinine concentration is known, the following formula may be used to estimate creatinine clearance:

[See first table above]

The serum creatinine should represent a steady state of renal function.

For patients with changing renal function or for patients with renal impairment and hepatic insufficiency, measurement of serum concentrations of ciprofloxacin will provide additional guidance for adjusting dosage.

INTRAVENOUS ADMINISTRATION

After dilution, CIPRO® I.V. should be administered by intravenous infusion over a period of 60 minutes. Slow infusion of a dilute solution into a large vein will minimize patient discomfort and reduce the risk of venous irritation.

PHARMACY BULK PACKAGE: The pharmacy bulk package is a single-entry container of a sterile preparation for parenteral use that contains many single doses. It contains ciprofloxacin as a 1% aqueous solution concentrate. The contents are intended for use in a pharmacy admixture program and are restricted to the preparation of admixture for intravenous infusion. **THE CLOSURE SHALL BE PENETRATED ONLY ONE TIME** with a suitable sterile transfer set or dispensing device which allows measured dispensing of the contents.

The pharmacy bulk package is to be used only in a suitable work area such as laminar flow hood or an equivalent clean air or compounding area. **THIS PREPARATION MUST BE DILUTED BEFORE USE.** The intravenous dose should be prepared by aseptically withdrawing the CIPRO® I.V. concentrate from the pharmacy bulk package and diluting the appropriate volume with a suitable intravenous solution to a final concentration of 0.5–2 mg/mL. (See **COMPATIBILITY AND STABILITY**.) The resulting solution should be infused over a period of 60 minutes by direct infusion or through a

$$\text{Men: Creatinine clearance (mL/min)} = \frac{\text{Weight (kg)} \times (140 - \text{age})}{72 \times \text{serum creatinine (mg/dL)}}$$

Women: 0.85 × the value calculated for men.

CONTAINER	SIZE	STRENGTH	NDC NUMBER
Pharmacy Bulk Package:	120 mL	1200-mg, 1%	0026-8566-65

CIPRO® I.V. (ciprofloxacin) is also available as follows:

VIAL:	SIZE	STRENGTH	NDC NUMBER
	20 mL	200 mg, 1%	0026-8562-20
	40 mL	400 mg, 1%	0026-8564-64

FLEXIBLE CONTAINER: manufactured for Bayer Corporation by Abbott Laboratories, North Chicago, IL 60064.

	SIZE	STRENGTH	NDC NUMBER
	100 mL 5% dextrose	200 mg, 0.2%	0026-8552-36
	200 mL 5% dextrose	400 mg, 0.2%	0026-8554-63

FLEXIBLE CONTAINER: manufactured for Bayer Corporation by Baxter Healthcare Corporation, Deerfield, IL 60015.

	SIZE	STRENGTH	NDC NUMBER
	100 mL 5% dextrose	200 mg, 0.2%	0026-8527-36
	200 mL 5% dextrose	400 mg, 0.2%	0026-8527-63

Y-type intravenous set which may already be in place. If this method or the "piggyback" method of administration is used, it is advisable to discontinue the administration of any other intravenous solutions during the infusion of CIPRO® I.V.

COMPATIBILITY AND STABILITY

Ciprofloxacin injection 1% (10 mg/mL), when diluted with the following intravenous solutions to concentrations of 0.5 to 2.0 mg/mL, is stable for up to 14 days at refrigerated or room temperature storage.

0.9% Sodium Chloride Injection, USP
5% Dextrose Injection, USP
Sterile Water for Injection
10% Dextrose for Injection
5% Dextrose and 0.225% Sodium Chloride for Injection
5% Dextrose and 0.45% Sodium Chloride for Injection
Lactated Ringer's for Injection

If CIPRO® I.V. is to be given concomitantly with another drug, each drug should be given separately in accordance with the recommended dosage and route of administration for each drug.

HOW SUPPLIED

CIPRO® I.V. (ciprofloxacin) is available as a clear, colorless to slightly yellowish solution supplied in the pharmacy bulk package as follows:

[See second table above]

Ciprofloxacin is also available as CIPRO® (ciprofloxacin HCl) Tablets 100, 250, 500, and 750 mg and CIPRO® (ciprofloxacin) 5% and 10% Oral Suspension.

STORAGE

Store between 5–30°C (41–86°F).
Protect from light, avoid excessive heat, protect from freezing.

ANIMAL PHARMACOLOGY

Ciprofloxacin and other quinolones have been shown to cause arthropathy in immature animals of most species tested. (See **WARNINGS**.) Damage of weight-bearing joints was observed in juvenile dogs and rats. In young beagles, 100 mg/kg ciprofloxacin given daily for 4 weeks caused degenerative articular changes of the knee joint. At 30 mg/kg, the effect on the joint was minimal. In a subsequent study in beagles, removal of weight-bearing from the joint reduced the lesions but did not totally prevent them.

Crystalluria, sometimes associated with secondary nephropathy, occurs in laboratory animals dosed with ciprofloxacin. This is primarily related to the reduced solubility of ciprofloxacin under alkaline conditions, which predominate in the urine of test animals; in man, crystalluria is rare since human urine is typically acidic. In rhesus monkeys, crystalluria without nephropathy has been noted after intravenous doses as low as 5 mg/kg. After 6 months of intravenous dosing at 10 mg/kg/day, no nephropathological changes were noted; however, nephropathy was observed after dosing at 20 mg/kg/day for the same duration.

In dogs, ciprofloxacin administered at 3 and 10 mg/kg by rapid intravenous injection (15 sec.) produces pronounced hypotensive effects. These effects are considered to be related to histamine release because they are partially antagonized by pyrilamine, an antihistamine. In rhesus monkeys, rapid intravenous injection also produces hypotension, but the effect in this species is inconsistent and less pronounced. In mice, concomitant administration of nonsteroidal anti-inflammatory drugs, such as phenylbutazone and indomethacin, with quinolones has been reported to enhance the CNS stimulatory effect of quinolones.

Ocular toxicity, seen with some related drugs, has not been observed in ciprofloxacin-treated animals.

INHALATIONAL ANTHRAX—ADDITIONAL INFORMATION

The mean serum concentrations of ciprofloxacin associated with a statistically significant improvement in survival in the rhesus monkey model of inhalational anthrax are reached or exceeded in adult and pediatric patients receiving oral and intravenous regimens. (See **DOSAGE AND ADMINISTRATION**.) Ciprofloxacin pharmacokinetics have been evaluated in various human populations. The mean peak serum concentration achieved at steady-state in human adults receiving 500 mg orally every 12 hours is 2.97 µg/mL, and 4.56 µg/mL following 400 mg intravenously every 12 hours. The mean trough serum concentration at steady-state for both of these regimens is 0.2 µg/mL. In a study of 10 pediatric patients between 6 and 16 years of age, the mean peak plasma concentration achieved is 8.3 µg/mL

and trough concentrations range from 0.09 to 0.26 µg/mL, following two 30-minute intravenous infusions of 10 mg/kg administered 12 hours apart. After the second intravenous infusion patients switched to 15 mg/kg orally every 12 hours achieve a mean peak concentration of 3.6 µg/mL after the initial oral dose. Long-term safety data, including effects on cartilage, following the administration of ciprofloxacin to pediatric patients are limited. For additional information, see **PRECAUTIONS, Pediatric Use**.) Ciprofloxacin serum concentrations achieved in humans serve as a surrogate endpoint reasonably likely to predict clinical benefit and provide the basis for this indication.[4]

A placebo-controlled animal study in rhesus monkeys exposed to an inhaled mean dose of 11 LD_{50} (~5.5 × 10⁵) spores (range 5–30 LD_{50}) of B. anthracis was conducted. The minimal inhibitory concentration (MIC) of ciprofloxacin for the anthrax strain used in this study was 0.08 µg/mL. In the animals studied, mean serum concentrations of ciprofloxacin achieved at expected T_{max} (1 hour post-dose) following oral dosing to steady-state ranged from 0.98 to 1.69 µg/mL. Mean steady-state trough concentrations at 12 hours post-dose ranged from 0.12 to 0.19 µg/mL.[5] Mortality due to anthrax for animals that received a 30-day regimen of oral ciprofloxacin beginning 24 hours post-exposure was significantly lower (1/9), compared to the placebo group (9/10) [p=0.001]. The one ciprofloxacin-treated animal that died of anthrax did so following the 30-day drug administration period.[6]

REFERENCES

1. National Committee for Clinical Laboratory Standards, Methods for Dilution Antimicrobial Susceptibility Tests for Bacteria That Grow Aerobically-Fifth Edition. Approved Standard NCCLS Document M7-A5, Vol. 20, No. 2, NCCLS, Wayne, PA, January, 2000. 2. National Committee for Clinical Laboratory Standards, Performance Standards for Antimicrobial Disk Susceptibility Tests-Seventh Edition. Approved Standard NCCLS Document M2-A7, Vol. 20, No. 1, NCCLS, Wayne, PA, January, 2000. 3. Report presented at the FDA's Anti-Infective Drug and Dermatological Drug Product's Advisory Committee meeting, March 31, 1993, Silver Spring, MD. Report available from FDA, CDER, Advisors and Consultants Staff, HFD-21, 1901 Chapman Avenue, Room 200, Rockville, MD 20852, USA. 4. 21 CFR 314.510 (Subpart H – Accelerated Approval of New Drugs for Life-Threatening Illnesses). 5. Kelly DJ, et al. Serum concentrations of penicillin, doxycycline, and ciprofloxacin during prolonged therapy in rhesus monkeys. J Infect Dis 1992; 166: 1184–7. 6. Friedlander AM, et al. Postexposure prophylaxis against experimental inhalational anthrax. J Infect Dis 1993; 167: 1239–42.

Manufactured for:
Bayer Corporation
Pharmaceutical Division
400 Morgan Lane
West Haven, CT 06516 USA
℞ Only
PZ500176   11/00   BAY q 3939   5202-4-A-U.S.-7
©2000 Bayer Corporation   10046
Printed in U.S.A.

To keep your **PDR** up to date throughout the year, note these revisions on the corresponding pages of the annual volume. Simply write **"See Supplement A"** next to the product heading.

Boehringer Ingelheim Pharmaceuticals, Inc.

A subsidiary of Boehringer Ingelheim Corporation
900 RIDGEBURY ROAD
POST OFFICE BOX 368
RIDGEFIELD, CT 06877-0368

For Medical Information Contact:
1-800-542-6257
or email:
druginfo@rdg.boehringer-ingelheim.com

VIRAMUNE® ℞
[*vī'ră-mūne*]
(nevirapine) 200 mg Tablets
VIRAMUNE® ℞
(nevirapine) Oral Suspension 50 mg/5ml
Rx only

Prescribing information for this product, which appears on pages 2838–2842 of the 2001 PDR, has been completely revised as follows. Please write "See Supplement A" alongside product heading.

WARNING
Severe, life-threatening, and in some cases fatal hepatotoxicity, including fulminant and cholestatic hepatitis, hepatic necrosis and hepatic failure, has been reported in patients treated with VIRAMUNE®. In some cases, patients presented with non-specific prodromal signs or symptoms of hepatitis and progressed to hepatic failure. Some events occurred after short-term exposure to VIRAMUNE. Patients with signs or symptoms of hepatitis must seek medical evaluation immediately and should be advised to discontinue VIRAMUNE. (See WARNINGS)
Severe, life-threatening skin reactions, including fatal cases, have occurred in patients treated with VIRAMUNE. These have included cases of Stevens-Johnson syndrome, toxic epidermal necrolysis, and hypersensitivity reactions characterized by rash, constitutional findings, and organ dysfunction. Patients developing signs or symptoms of severe skin reactions or hypersensitivity reactions must discontinue VIRAMUNE as soon as possible. (See WARNINGS)
The first 12 weeks of therapy with VIRAMUNE are a critical period during which it is essential that patients be monitored intensively to detect potentially life-threatening hepatotoxicity or skin reactions. VIRAMUNE should not be restarted following severe hepatic, skin or hypersensitivity reactions. In addition, the 14-day lead-in period with VIRAMUNE 200 mg daily dosing must be strictly followed. (See WARNINGS)
Resistant virus emerges rapidly and uniformly when VIRAMUNE is administered as monotherapy. Therefore, VIRAMUNE should always be administered in combination with other antiretroviral agents.

DESCRIPTION

VIRAMUNE is the brand name for nevirapine (NVP), a non-nucleoside reverse transcriptase inhibitor with activity against Human Immunodeficiency Virus Type 1 (HIV-1). Nevirapine is structurally a member of the dipyridodiazepinone chemical class of compounds.
VIRAMUNE Tablets are for oral administration. Each tablet contains 200 mg of nevirapine and the inactive ingredients microcrystalline cellulose, lactose monohydrate, povidone, sodium starch glycolate, colloidal silicon dioxide and magnesium stearate.
VIRAMUNE Oral Suspension is for oral administration. Each 5 mL of VIRAMUNE® suspension contains 50 mg of nevirapine (as nevirapine hemihydrate). The suspension also contains the following excipients: carbomer 934P, methylparaben, propylparaben, sorbitol, sucrose, polysorbate 80, sodium hydroxide and water.
The chemical name of nevirapine is 11-cyclopropyl-5,11-dihydro-4-methyl-6H-dipyrido [3,2-b:2',3'-][1,4] diazepin-6-one. Nevirapine is a white to off-white crystalline powder with the molecular weight of 266.3 and the molecular formula $C_{15}H_{14}N_4O$. Nevirapine has the following structural formula:

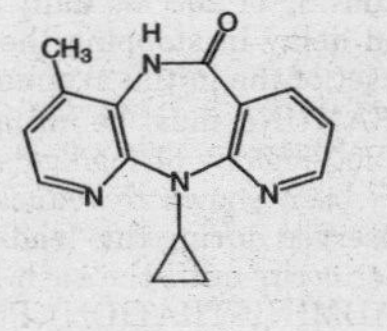

MICROBIOLOGY

Mechanism of Action:
Nevirapine is a non-nucleoside reverse transcriptase inhibitor (NNRTI) of HIV-1. Nevirapine binds directly to reverse transcriptase (RT) and blocks the RNA-dependent and DNA-dependent DNA polymerase activities by causing a disruption of the enzyme's catalytic site. The activity of nevirapine does not compete with template or nucleoside triphosphates. HIV-2 RT and eukaryotic DNA polymerases (such as human DNA polymerases α, β, γ, or δ) are not inhibited by nevirapine.
In Vitro HIV Susceptibility:
The relationship between *in vitro* susceptibility of HIV-1 to nevirapine and the inhibition of HIV-1 replication in humans has not been established. The *in vitro* antiviral activity of nevirapine was measured in peripheral blood mononuclear cells, monocyte derived macrophages, and lymphoblastoid cell lines. IC_{50} values (50% inhibitory concentration) ranged from 10-100 nM against laboratory and clinical isolates of HIV-1. In cell culture, nevirapine demonstrated additive to synergistic activity against HIV in drug combination regimens with zidovudine (ZDV), didanosine (ddI), stavudine (d4T), lamivudine (3TC), saquinavir, and indinavir.
Resistance:
HIV isolates with reduced susceptibility (100-250-fold) to nevirapine emerge *in vitro*. Genotypic analysis showed mutations in the HIV RT gene at amino acid positions 181 and/or 106 depending upon the virus strain and cell line employed. Time to emergence of nevirapine resistance *in vitro* was not altered when selection included nevirapine in combination with several other NNRTIs.
Phenotypic and genotypic changes in HIV-1 isolates from patients treated with either nevirapine (n=24) or nevirapine and ZDV (n=14) were monitored in Phase I/II trials over 1 to ≥12 weeks. After 1 week of nevirapine monotherapy, isolates from 3/3 patients had decreased susceptibility to nevirapine *in vitro*; one or more of the RT mutations at amino acid positions 103, 106, 108, 181, 188 and 190 were detected in some patients as early as 2 weeks after therapy initiation. By week eight of nevirapine monotherapy, 100% of the patients tested (n=24) had HIV isolates with a >100-fold decrease in susceptibility to nevirapine *in vitro* compared to baseline, and had one or more of the nevirapine-associated RT resistance mutations; 19 of 24 patients (80%) had isolates with a position 181 mutation regardless of dose. Nevirapine+ZDV combination therapy did not alter the emergence rate of nevirapine-resistant virus or the magnitude of nevirapine resistance *in vitro*; however, a different RT mutation pattern, predominantly distributed amongst amino acid positions 103, 106, 188, and 190, was observed. In patients (6 of 14) whose baseline isolates possessed a wild type RT gene, nevirapine+ZDV combination therapy did not appear to delay emergence of ZDV-resistant RT mutations. The clinical relevance of phenotypic and genotypic changes associated with nevirapine therapy has not been established.
Cross-resistance:
Rapid emergence of HIV strains which are cross-resistant to NNRTIs has been observed *in vitro*. Data on cross-resistance between the NNRTI nevirapine and nucleoside analogue RT inhibitors are very limited. In four patients, ZDV-resistant isolates tested *in vitro* retained susceptibility to nevirapine and in six patients, nevirapine-resistant isolates were susceptible to ZDV and ddI. Cross-resistance between nevirapine and HIV protease inhibitors is unlikely because the enzyme targets involved are different.

ANIMAL PHARMACOLOGY

Animal studies have shown that nevirapine is widely distributed to nearly all tissues and readily crosses the blood-brain barrier.

CLINICAL PHARMACOLOGY

Pharmacokinetics in Adults:
Absorption and Bioavailability: Nevirapine is readily absorbed (>90%) after oral administration in healthy volunteers and in adults with HIV-1 infection. Absolute bioavailability in 12 healthy adults following single-dose administration was 93 ± 9% (mean ± SD) for a 50 mg tablet and 91 ± 8% for an oral solution. Peak plasma nevirapine concentrations of 2 ± 0.4 µg/mL (7.5 µM) were attained by 4 hours following a single 200 mg dose. Following multiple doses, nevirapine peak concentrations appear to increase linearly in the dose range of 200 to 400 mg/day. Steady state trough nevirapine concentrations of 4.5 ± 1.9 µg/mL (17 ± 7 µM), (n = 242) were attained at 400 mg/day. Nevirapine tablets and suspension have been shown to be comparably bioavailable and interchangeable at doses up to 200 mg. When VIRAMUNE (200 mg) was administered to 24 healthy adults (12 female, 12 male), with either a high fat breakfast (857 kcal, 50 g fat, 53% of calories from fat) or antacid (Maalox® 30 mL), the extent of nevirapine absorption (AUC) was comparable to that observed under fasting conditions. In a separate study in HIV-1 infected patients (n=6), nevirapine steady-state systemic exposure ($AUC_τ$) was not significantly altered by ddI, which is formulated with an alkaline buffering agent. VIRAMUNE may be administered with or without food, antacid or ddI.
Distribution: Nevirapine is highly lipophilic and is essentially nonionized at physiologic pH. Following intravenous administration to healthy adults, the apparent volume of distribution (Vdss) of nevirapine was 1.21 ± 0.09 L/kg, suggesting that nevirapine is widely distributed in humans. Nevirapine readily crosses the placenta and is found in breast milk. (See PRECAUTIONS, *Nursing Mothers*) Nevirapine is about 60% bound to plasma proteins in the plasma concentration range of 1-10 µg/mL. Nevirapine concentrations in human cerebrospinal fluid (n=6) were 45% (± 5%) of the concentrations in plasma; this ratio is approximately equal to the fraction not bound to plasma protein.
Metabolism/Elimination: *In vivo* studies in humans and *in vitro* studies with human liver microsomes have shown that nevirapine is extensively biotransformed via cytochrome P450 (oxidative) metabolism to several hydroxylated metabolites. *In vitro* studies with human liver microsomes suggest that oxidative metabolism of nevirapine is mediated primarily by cytochrome P450 isozymes from the CYP3A family, although other isozymes may have a secondary role. In a mass balance/excretion study in eight healthy male volunteers dosed to steady state with nevirapine 200 mg given twice daily followed by a single 50 mg dose of ^{14}C-nevirapine, approximately 91.4 ± 10.5% of the radiolabeled dose was recovered, with urine (81.3 ± 11.1%) representing the primary route of excretion compared to feces (10.1 ± 1.5%). Greater than 80% of the radioactivity in urine was made up of glucuronide conjugates of hydroxylated metabolites. Thus cytochrome P450 metabolism, glucuronide conjugation, and urinary excretion of glucuronidated metabolites represent the primary route of nevirapine biotransformation and elimination in humans. Only a small fraction (<5%) of the radioactivity in urine (representing <3% of the total dose) was made up of parent compound; therefore, renal excretion plays a minor role in elimination of the parent compound.
Nevirapine has been shown to be an inducer of hepatic cytochrome P450 metabolic enzymes. The pharmacokinetics of autoinduction are characterized by an approximately 1.5 to 2 fold increase in the apparent oral clearance of nevirapine as treatment continues from a single dose to two-to-four weeks of dosing with 200-400 mg/day. Autoinduction also results in a corresponding decrease in the terminal phase half-life of nevirapine in plasma from approximately 45 hours (single dose) to approximately 25-30 hours following multiple dosing with 200-400 mg/day.
Pharmacokinetics in Special Populations:
Renal/Hepatic Dysfunction: The pharmacokinetics of nevirapine have not been evaluated in patients with either renal or hepatic dysfunction.
Gender: In one Phase I study in healthy volunteers (15 females, 15 males), the weight-adjusted apparent volume of distribution (Vdss/F) of nevirapine was higher in the female subjects (1.54 L/kg) compared to the males (1.38 L/kg), suggesting that nevirapine was distributed more extensively in the female subjects. However, this difference was offset by a slightly shorter terminal-phase half-life in the females resulting in no significant gender difference in nevirapine oral clearance or plasma concentrations following either single- or multiple-dose administration(s).
Race: An evaluation of nevirapine plasma concentrations (pooled data from several clinical trials) from HIV-1-infected patients (27 Black, 24 Hispanic, 189 Caucasian) revealed no marked difference in nevirapine steady-state trough concentrations (median C_{minss} = 4.7 µg/mL Black, 3.8 µg/mL Hispanic, 4.3 µg/mL Caucasian) with long-term nevirapine treatment at 400 mg/day. However, the pharmacokinetics of nevirapine have not been evaluated specifically for the effects of ethnicity.
Geriatric Patients: Nevirapine pharmacokinetics in HIV-1 infected adults do not appear to change with age (range 18–68 years); however, nevirapine has not been extensively evaluated in patients beyond the age of 55 years.
Pediatric Patients: See PRECAUTIONS, *Pediatric Use*.
Drug Interactions: *Nucleoside Analogues:* No dosage adjustments are required when VIRAMUNE is taken in combination with ZDV, ddI, or zalcitabine (ddC). Results from studies in HIV-1 infected patients who were administered VIRAMUNE with different combinations of ddI or ddC, on a background of ZDV therapy, indicated that no clinically significant pharmacokinetic interactions occurred when the nucleoside analogues were administered in combination with VIRAMUNE.
Protease Inhibitors: In the following three studies, VIRAMUNE was given 200 mg once daily for two weeks followed by 200 mg twice daily for 28 days:
Ritonavir: No dosage adjustments are required when VIRAMUNE is taken in combination with ritonavir. Results from a 49-day study in HIV-infected patients (n=14) administered VIRAMUNE and ritonavir (600 mg b.i.d. [using a gradual dose escalation regimen]) indicated that their coadministration did not affect ritonavir AUC or C_{max}. Comparison of nevirapine pharmacokinetics from this study to historical data suggested that coadministration did not affect the pharmacokinetics of nevirapine.
Indinavir: Results from a 36-day study in HIV-infected patients (n=19) administered VIRAMUNE and indinavir (800 mg q8h) indicated that their coadministration led to a 28% mean decrease (95% CI -39, -16) in indinavir AUC and an 11% mean decrease (95% CI -49, +59) in indinavir C_{max}. The clinical significance of this interaction is not known. Comparison of nevirapine pharmacokinetics from this study to historical data suggested that coadministration did not affect the pharmacokinetics of nevirapine.
Saquinavir: Results from a 42-day study in HIV-infected patients (n=23) administered VIRAMUNE and saquinavir (hard gelatin capsules, 600 mg t.i.d.) indicated that their coadministration led to a 24% mean decrease (95% CI -42, -1) in saquinavir AUC and a 28% mean decrease (95% CI -47, -1) in saquinavir C_{max}. The clinical significance of this interaction is not known. Coadministration did not affect the pharmacokinetics of nevirapine.
In vitro: Studies using human liver microsomes indicated that the formation of nevirapine hydroxylated metabolites was not affected by the presence of dapsone, rifabutin,

Continued on next page

Viramune—Cont.

rifampin, and trimethoprim/sulfamethoxazole. Ketoconazole significantly inhibited the formation of nevirapine hydroxylated metabolites.

In vivo: ketoconazole: VIRAMUNE and ketoconazole should not be administered concomitantly. Ketoconazole AUC and C_{max} decreased by a median 63% (95% CI -95, +33) and 40% (95% CI -52, +11), respectively, in HIV-infected patients (n=22) who were given VIRAMUNE 200 mg once daily for two weeks followed by 200 mg twice daily for two weeks along with ketoconazole 400 mg daily. (See PRECAUTIONS, *Drug Interactions*) Comparison of the pharmacokinetics from this study to historical data suggested that coadministration with ketoconazole may result in a 15-30% increase in nevirapine plasma concentrations. The clinical significance of this observation is not known.

Monitoring of nevirapine plasma concentrations in patients who received long-term VIRAMUNE treatment indicate that steady-state nevirapine trough plasma concentrations were elevated in patients who received cimetidine (+21%, n=11) and macrolides (+12%, n=24), known inhibitors of CYP3A.

Steady-state nevirapine trough concentrations were reduced in patients who received rifabutin (-16%, n=19) and rifampin (-37%, n=3), known inducers of CYP3A. Nevirapine is an inducer of CYP3A, with maximal induction occurring within 2–4 weeks of initiating multiple-dose therapy. Other compounds that are substrates of CYP3A may have decreased plasma concentrations when co-administered with VIRAMUNE. Therefore, careful monitoring of the therapeutic effectiveness of CYP3A-metabolized drugs is recommended when taken in combination with VIRAMUNE. (See PRECAUTIONS, *Drug Interactions*, for recommendations regarding rifampin, rifabutin, oral contraceptives and methadone)

INDICATIONS AND USAGE

VIRAMUNE (nevirapine) is indicated for use in combination with other antiretroviral agents for the treatment of HIV-1 infection. This indication is based on analyses of changes in surrogate endpoints. At present, there are no results from controlled clinical trials evaluating the effect of VIRAMUNE in combination with other antiretroviral agents on the clinical progression of HIV-1 infection, such as the incidence of opportunistic infections or survival.

Resistant virus emerges rapidly and uniformly when VIRAMUNE is administered as monotherapy. Therefore, VIRAMUNE should always be administered in combination with at least one additional antiretroviral agent.

Description of Clinical Studies:

Patients with a prior history of nucleoside therapy:

ACTG 241 compared treatment with VIRAMUNE+ZDV+ddI versus ZDV+ddI in 398 HIV-1 infected patients (median age 38 years, 74% Caucasian, 80% male) with CD4+ cell counts ≤350 cells/mm^3 (mean 153 cells/mm^3) and a mean baseline plasma HIV-1 RNA concentration of 4.59 $\log_{10}$ copies/mL (38,905 copies/mL), who had received at least 6 months of nucleoside therapy prior to enrollment (median 115 weeks). Treatment doses were VIRAMUNE, 200 mg daily for two weeks, followed by 200 mg twice daily, or placebo; ZDV, 200 mg three times daily; ddI, 200 mg twice daily. Mean changes in CD4+ cell counts are shown in Figure 1. For 198 patients in the virology sub-study, mean HIV-1 RNA concentration changes from baseline are shown in Figure 2.

Figure 1: Mean Change From Baseline for CD4+ Cell Count (absolute number of CD4+ cells/mm^3), Trial ACTG 241

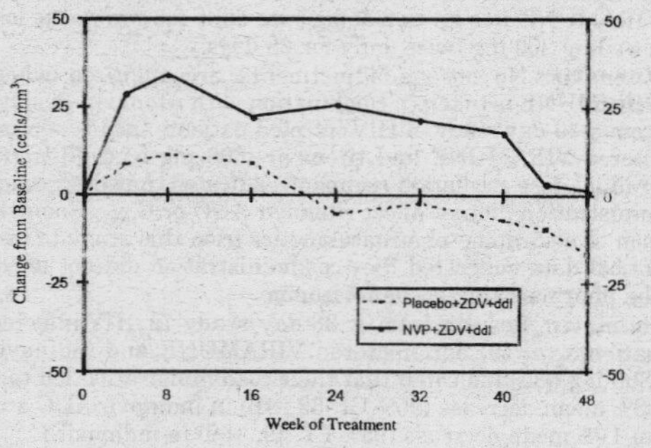

Number of patients with CD4+ cell counts at each timepoint

	Baseline	Week 16	Week 32	40-48 Weeks
NVP+ZDV+ddI	196	177	157	161
Placebo+ZDV+ddI	196	176	160	167

[See figure at top of next column]

Trial BI 1037 compared treatment with VIRAMUNE+ZDV versus ZDV in 60 HIV-1-infected patients (median age 33 years, 70% Caucasian, 93% male) with CD4+ cell counts between 200 and 500 cells/mm^3 (mean 373 cells/mm^3) and a mean baseline plasma HIV-1 RNA concentration of 4.24 $\log_{10}$ copies/mL (17,378 copies/mL), who had received between 3 and 24 months of prior ZDV therapy (median 35 weeks). Treatment doses were VIRAMUNE 200 mg daily for 2 weeks, followed by 200 mg twice daily, or placebo; ZDV, 500-600 mg/day. Mean changes in CD4+ cell counts are shown in Figure 3. Mean HIV-1 RNA concentration changes from baseline are shown in Figure 4.

Figure 2: Mean Change From Baseline in HIV-1 RNA* Concentrations ($\log_{10}$ copies/mL), Virology Sub-study of Trial ACTG 241

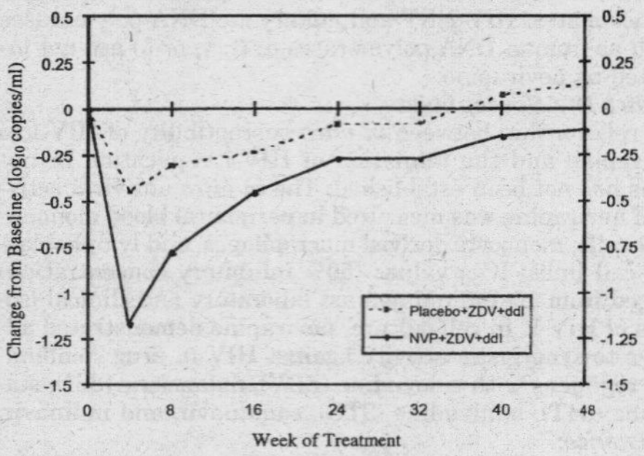

Number of patients with HIV-1 RNA data at each timepoint

	Baseline	Week 16	Week 32	40-48 Weeks
NVP+ZDV+ddI	95	84	75	74
Placebo+ZDV+ddI	93	82	75	75

* the clinical significance of changes in serum viral RNA measurements during treatment with VIRAMUNE has not been established

Figure 3: Mean Change From Baseline for/CD4+ Cell Count (absolute number of CD4+ cells/mm^3), Trial BI 1037

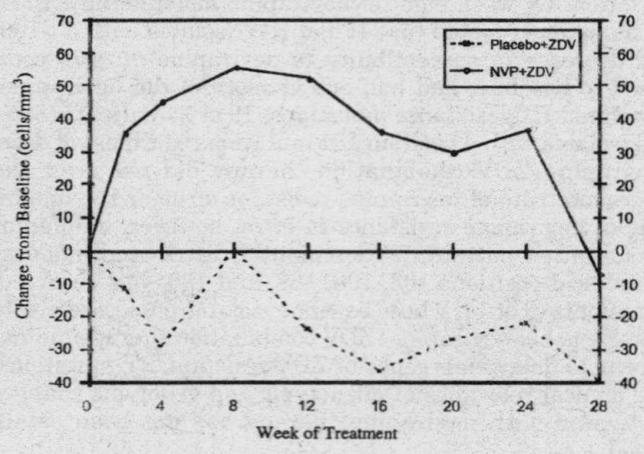

Number of patients with CD4+ cell counts at each timepoint

	Baseline	Week 8	Week 16	20-28 Weeks
NVP+ZDV	30	28	26	26
Placebo+ZDV	30	30	28	29

Figure 4: Mean Change From Baseline in HIV-1 RNA Concentrations ($\log_{10}$ copies/mL), Trial BI 1037

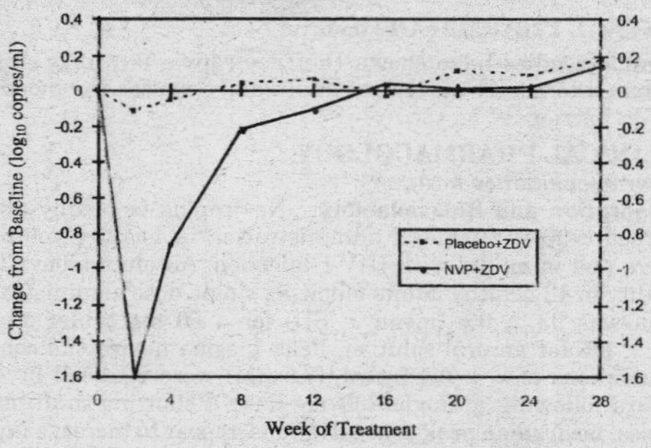

Number of patients with HIV-1 RNA data at each timepoint

	Baseline	Week 8	Week 16	20-28 Weeks
NVP+ZDV	30	27	26	26
Placebo+ZDV	30	29	23	29

Patients without a history of prior antiretroviral therapy:

BI Trial 1046 compared treatment with VIRAMUNE+ZDV+ddI versus VIRAMUNE+ZDV versus ZDV+ddI in 151 HIV-1-infected patients (median age 36 years, 94% Caucasian, 93% male) with CD4+ cell counts of 200–600 cells/mm^3 (mean 376 cells/mm^3) and a mean baseline plasma HIV-1 RNA concentration of 4.41 $\log_{10}$ copies/mL (25,704 copies/mL). Treatment doses were VIRAMUNE, 200 mg daily for two weeks, followed by 200 mg twice daily, or placebo; ZDV, 200 mg three times daily; ddI, 125 or 200 mg twice daily. Changes in CD4+ cell counts at 24 weeks: mean levels of CD4+ cell counts in those randomized to VIRAMUNE+ZDV+ddI and ZDV+ddI remained significantly above baseline; however there was no significant difference between these arms. Changes in HIV-1 viral RNA at 24 weeks: there was no significant difference as measured by mean changes in plasma viral RNA between those randomized to VIRAMUNE+ZDV+ddI and ZDV+ddI. However, the proportion of patients whose HIV-1 RNA decreased below the limit of detection (400 copies/mL) was significantly greater for the VIRAMUNE+ZDV+ddI group (27/36 or 75%), when compared to the ZDV+ddI group (18/39 or 46%) or the VIRAMINE+ZDV group (0/28 or 0%); the clinical significance of this finding is unknown.

CONTRAINDICATIONS

VIRAMUNE is contraindicated in patients with clinically significant hypersensitivity to any of the components contained in the tablet or the oral suspension.

WARNINGS

General:

The first 12 weeks of therapy with VIRAMUNE are a critical period during which intensive monitoring of patients is required to detect potentially life-threatening hepatic events and skin reactions. The optimal frequency of monitoring during this time period has not been established. Some experts recommend clinical and laboratory monitoring more often than once per month, and in particular, would include monitoring of liver function tests at baseline, prior to dose escalation and at two weeks post dose escalation. After the initial 12-week period, frequent clinical and laboratory monitoring should continue throughout VIRAMUNE treatment. In addition, the 14-day lead-in period with VIRAMUNE 200-mg daily dosing has been demonstrated to reduce the frequency of rash.

Hepatic Events:

Severe, life-threatening, and in some cases fatal hepatotoxicity, including fulminant and cholestatic hepatitis, hepatic necrosis and hepatic failure, have been reported in patients treated with VIRAMUNE. Serious hepatic events occur most frequently during the first 12 weeks of VIRAMUNE therapy, and have been reported to occur as early as within the first few weeks of therapy. However, approximately one third of cases have been reported to occur after the critical 12-week period. In some cases, patients presented with non-specific, prodromal signs or symptoms of fatigue, malaise, anorexia, nausea, jaundice, liver tenderness or hepatomegaly, with or without initially abnormal serum transaminase levels. These events progressed to hepatic failure with transaminase elevation, with or without hyperbilirubinemia, prolonged partial thromboplastin time, or eosinophilia. Rash and fever accompanied some of these hepatic events. Patients with signs or symptoms of hepatitis must immediately seek medical evaluation, have liver function tests performed, and be advised to discontinue VIRAMUNE as soon as possible.

In addition, serious hepatotoxicity (including liver failure requiring transplantation in one instance) has been reported in HIV-uninfected individuals receiving multiple doses of VIRAMUNE in the setting of post-exposure prophylaxis, an unapproved use.

Increased AST or ALT levels and/or history of hepatitis B and C infection prior to the start of antiretroviral therapy are associated with a greater risk of hepatic adverse events. **Intensive clinical and laboratory monitoring, including liver function tests, is essential at baseline and during the first 12 weeks of treatment. (See WARNINGS, *General*) Monitoring should continue at frequent intervals thereafter, depending on the patient's clinical status. Liver function tests should be performed if a patient experiences signs or symptoms suggestive of hepatitis and/or hypersensitivity reaction. Physicians and patients should be vigilant for the appearance of signs or symptoms of hepatitis, such as fatigue, malaise, anorexia, nausea, jaundice, bilirubinuria, acholic stools, liver tenderness or hepatomegaly. The diagnosis of hepatotoxicity should be considered in this setting, even if liver function tests are initially normal or alternative diagnoses are possible. (See PRECAUTIONS, *Information for Patients*; ADVERSE REACTIONS; DOSAGE AND ADMINISTRATION)**

If clinical hepatitis occurs, VIRAMUNE should be permanently discontinued and not restarted after recovery.

Skin Reactions:

Severe, life-threatening skin reactions, including fatal cases, have been reported with VIRAMUNE treatment. These have included cases of Stevens-Johnson syndrome, toxic epidermal necrolysis, and hypersensitivity reactions characterized by rash, constitutional findings, and organ dysfunction. Patients developing signs or symptoms of severe skin reactions or hypersensitivity reactions (including, but not limited to, severe rash or rash accompanied by fever, general malaise, fatigue, muscle or joint aches, blisters, oral lesions, conjunctivitis, facial edema, and/or hepatitis, eosinophilia, granulocytopenia, lymphadenopathy, and renal dysfunction) must permanently discontinue VIRAMUNE and seek medical evaluation immediately. (See PRECAUTIONS, *Information for Patients*; ADVERSE REACTIONS) VIRAMUNE should not be restarted following severe skin rash or hypersensitivity reaction. Some of the risk factors for developing serious cutaneous reactions include failure to follow the initial dosing of 200 mg daily during the 14-day lead-in period and delay in stopping the nevirapine treatment after the onset of the initial symptoms.

Therapy with VIRAMUNE must be initiated with a 14-day lead-in period of 200 mg/day (4 mg/kg/day in pediatric patients), which has been shown to reduce the frequency of rash. If rash is observed during this lead-in period, dose escalation should not occur until the rash has resolved. (See DOSAGE AND ADMINISTRATION) Patients should be monitored closely if isolated rash of any severity occurs.

In a clinical trial, concomitant prednisone use (40 mg/day for the first 14 days of VIRAMUNE® administration) was associated with an increase in incidence and severity of rash during the first 6 weeks of VIRAMUNE therapy. Therefore, use of prednisone to prevent VIRAMUNE-associated rash is not recommended.

St. John's Wort:
Concomitant use of St. John's wort (hypericum perforatum) or St. John's wort containing products and VIRAMUNE is not recommended. Coadministration of Non-Nucleoside Reverse Transcriptase Inhibitors (NNRTIs), including VIRAMUNE, with St. John's wort is expected to substantially decrease NNRTI concentrations and may result in sub-optimal levels of VIRAMUNE and lead to loss of virologic response and possible resistance to VIRAMUNE or to the class of NNRTIs.

PRECAUTIONS
General:
Nevirapine is extensively metabolized by the liver and nevirapine metabolites are extensively eliminated by the kidney. However, the pharmacokinetics of nevirapine have not been evaluated in patients with either hepatic or renal dysfunction. Therefore, VIRAMUNE should be used with caution in these patient populations.

The duration of clinical benefit from antiretroviral therapy may be limited. Patients receiving VIRAMUNE or any other antiretroviral therapy may continue to develop opportunistic infections and other complications of HIV infection, and therefore should remain under close clinical observation by physicians experienced in the treatment of patients with associated HIV diseases.

When administering VIRAMUNE as part of an antiretroviral regimen, the complete product information for each therapeutic component should be consulted before initiation of treatment.

Drug Interactions:
The induction of CYP3A by nevirapine may result in lower plasma concentrations of other concomitantly administered drugs that are extensively metabolized by CYP3A. (See CLINICAL PHARMACOLOGY) Thus, if a patient has been stabilized on a dosage regimen for a drug metabolized by CYP3A, and begins treatment with VIRAMUNE, dose adjustments may be necessary.

Rifampin/Rifabutin: There are insufficient data to assess whether dose adjustments are necessary when nevirapine and rifampin or rifabutin are coadministered. Therefore, these drugs should only be used in combination if clearly indicated and with careful monitoring.

Ketoconazole: VIRAMUNE and ketoconazole should not be administered concomitantly. Coadministration of nevirapine and ketoconazole resulted in a significant reduction in ketoconazole plasma concentrations. (See CLINICAL PHARMACOLOGY, Drug Interactions)

Oral Contraceptives: There are no clinical data on the effects of nevirapine on the pharmacokinetics of oral contraceptives. Nevirapine may decrease plasma concentrations of oral contraceptives (also other hormonal contraceptives); therefore, these drugs should not be administered concomitantly with VIRAMUNE.

Methadone: Based on the known metabolism of methadone, nevirapine may decrease plasma concentrations of methadone by increasing its hepatic metabolism. Narcotic withdrawal syndrome has been reported in patients treated with VIRAMUNE and methadone concomitantly. Methadone-maintained patients beginning nevirapine therapy should be monitored for evidence of withdrawal and methadone dose should be adjusted accordingly.

Information for Patients:
Patients should be informed of the possibility of severe liver disease or skin reactions associated with VIRAMUNE that may result in death. Patients developing signs or symptoms of liver disease or skin reactions should be instructed to seek medical attention immediately, including performance of laboratory monitoring. Symptoms of liver disease include fatigue, malaise, anorexia, nausea, jaundice, acholic stools, liver tenderness or hepatomegaly. Symptoms of severe skin or hypersensitivity reactions include rash accompanied by fever, general malaise, fatigue, muscle or joint aches, blisters, oral lesions, conjunctivitis, facial edema and/or hepatitis.

Severe liver disease occurs most frequently during the first 12 weeks of therapy. Intensive clinical and laboratory monitoring, including liver function tests, is essential during this period. Approximately one third of severe liver disease occurs after 12 weeks, therefore monitoring should continue at frequent intervals thereafter, depending on the patient's clinical status. Patients with signs and symptoms of hepatitis should seek medical evaluation immediately. If VIRAMUNE is discontinued due to hepatitis it should not be restarted. Patients should be advised that history of hepatitis B or C infection and/or increased liver function tests prior to the start of antiretroviral therapy are associated with a greater risk of hepatic events with VIRAMUNE.

The majority of rashes associated with VIRAMUNE occur within the first 6 weeks of initiation of therapy. Patients should be instructed that if any rash occurs during the two-week lead-in period, the VIRAMUNE dose should not be escalated until the rash resolves. Any patient experiencing severe rash or hypersensitivity reactions should discontinue VIRAMUNE and consult a physician. VIRAMUNE should not be restarted following severe skin rash or hypersensitivity reaction.

Oral contraceptives and other hormonal methods of birth control should not be used as a method of contraception in women taking VIRAMUNE. (See PRECAUTIONS, Drug Interactions)

Patients should be informed that VIRAMUNE therapy has not been shown to reduce the risk of transmission of HIV-1 to others through sexual contact or blood contamination. The long term effects of VIRAMUNE are unknown at this time.

VIRAMUNE is not a cure for HIV-1 infection; patients may continue to experience illnesses associated with advanced HIV-1 infection, including opportunistic infections. Treatment with VIRAMUNE has not been shown to reduce the incidence or frequency of such illnesses; patients should be advised to remain under the care of a physician when using VIRAMUNE.

Patients should be informed to take VIRAMUNE every day as prescribed. Patients should not alter the dose without consulting their doctor. If a dose is missed, patients should take the next dose as soon as possible. However, if a dose is skipped, the patient should not double the next dose. Patients should be advised to report to their doctor the use of any other medications. Based on the known metabolism of methadone, nevirapine may decrease plasma concentrations of methadone by increasing its hepatic metabolism. Narcotic withdrawal syndrome has been reported in patients treated with VIRAMUNE and methadone concomitantly. Methadone-maintained patients beginning nevirapine therapy should be monitored for evidence of withdrawal and methadone dose should be adjusted accordingly.

VIRAMUNE may interact with some drugs, therefore, patients should be advised to report to their doctor the use of any other prescription, non-prescription medication or herbal products, particularly St. John's wort.

The Patient Package Insert provides written information for the patient, and should be dispensed with each new prescription and refill.

Carcinogenesis, Mutagenesis, Impairment of Fertility:
Long-term carcinogenicity studies of nevirapine in animals are currently in progress. In genetic toxicology assays, nevirapine showed no evidence of mutagenic or clastogenic activity in a battery of in vitro and in vivo assays including microbial assays for gene mutation (Ames: Salmonella strains and E. coli), mammalian cell gene mutation assays (CHO/HGPRT), cytogenetic assays using a Chinese hamster ovary cell line and a mouse bone marrow micronucleus assay following oral administration. In reproductive toxicology studies, evidence of impaired fertility was seen in female rats at doses providing systemic exposure, based on AUC, approximately equivalent to that provided with the recommended clinical dose of VIRAMUNE.

Pregnancy: Pregnancy Category C:
No observable teratogenicity was detected in reproductive studies performed in pregnant rats and rabbits. In rats, a significant decrease in fetal body weight occurred at doses providing systemic exposure approximately 50% higher, based on AUC, than that seen at the recommended human clinical dose.

The maternal and developmental no-observable-effect level dosages in rats and rabbits produced systemic exposures approximately equivalent to or approximately 50% higher, respectively, than those seen at the recommended daily human dose, based on AUC. There are no adequate and well-controlled studies in pregnant women. VIRAMUNE should be used during pregnancy only if the potential benefit justifies the potential risk to the fetus.

Antiretroviral Pregnancy Registry:
To monitor maternal-fetal outcomes of pregnant women exposed to VIRAMUNE, an Antiretroviral Pregnancy Registry has been established. Physicians are encouraged to register patients by calling (800) 258-4263.

Nursing Mothers:
Preliminary results from an ongoing pharmacokinetic study (ACTG 250) of 10 HIV-1-infected pregnant women who were administered a single oral dose of 100 or 200 mg VIRAMUNE at a median of 5.8 hours before delivery, indicate that nevirapine readily crosses the placenta and is found in breast milk.

Consistent with the recommendation by the U.S. Public Health Service Centers for Disease Control and Prevention that HIV-infected mothers not breast-feed their infants to avoid risking postnatal transmission of HIV, mothers should discontinue nursing if they are receiving VIRAMUNE.

Pediatric Use:
The pharmacokinetics of nevirapine have been studied in two open-label studies in children with HIV-1 infection. In one study (BI 853; ACTG 165), nine HIV-1-infected children ranging in age from 9 months to 14 years were administered a single dose (7.5 mg, 30 mg, or 120 mg per m², n=3 per dose) of nevirapine suspension after an overnight fast. The mean nevirapine apparent clearance adjusted for body weight was greater in children compared to adults.

In a multiple dose study (BI 882; ACTG 180), nevirapine suspension or tablets (240 or 400 mg/m²/day) were administered as monotherapy or in combination with ZDV or ZDV+ddI to 37 HIV-1-infected pediatric patients with the following demographics: male (54%), racial minority groups (73%), median age of 11 months (range: 2 months-15 years). The majority of these patients received 120 mg/m²/day of nevirapine for approximately 4 weeks followed by 120 mg/ m²/b.i.d. (patients > 9 years of age) or 200 mg/m²/b.i.d. (patients ≤ 9 years of age). Nevirapine apparent clearance adjusted for body weight reached maximum values by age 1 to 2 years and then decreased with increasing age. Nevirapine apparent clearance adjusted for body weight was at least two-fold greater in children younger than 8 years compared to adults. The relationship between nevirapine clearance with long term drug administration and age is shown in Figure 5. The pediatric dosing regimens were selected in order to achieve steady-state plasma concentrations in pediatric patients that approximate those in adults. (See DOSAGE AND ADMINISTRATION, Pediatric Patients)

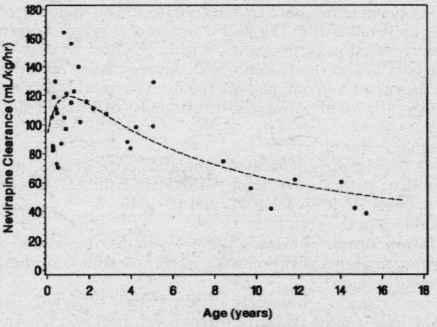

Figure 5: Nevirapine Apparent Clearance (mL/kg/hr) in Pediatric Patients

Evaluation of the pharmacokinetics of nevirapine in neonates is ongoing.

Safety was assessed in trial BI 882 in which patients were followed for a mean duration of 33.9 months (range: 6.8 months to 5.3 years, including long-term follow-up in 29 of these patients in trial BI 892). The most frequently reported adverse events related to VIRAMUNE in pediatric patients were similar to those observed in adults, with the exception of granulocytopenia which was more commonly observed in children. Serious adverse events were assessed in ACTG 245, a double-blind, placebo controlled trial of VIRAMUNE (n = 305) in which pediatric patients received combination treatment with VIRAMUNE. In this trial two patients were reported to experience Stevens-Johnson syndrome or Stevens-Johnson/toxic epidermal necrolysis transition syndrome. Cases of allergic reaction, including one case of anaphylaxis, were also reported. The evaluation of the antiviral activity of VIRAMUNE in pediatric patients is ongoing.

Table 1 summarizes the marked laboratory abnormalities occurring in pediatric patients in Trial BI 882 and in follow-up Trial BI 892.

Table 1: Number of Pediatric Patients (%) with Marked Laboratory Abnormalities in Trials BI 882 and BI 892 Combined.

	No. (%) of Patients n=37
Hematology	
Decreased Hg (<8.0 g/dL)	7 (19)
Decreased platelets (<50,000/mm³)	4 (11)
Decreased neutrophils (<750/mm³)	14 (38)
Increased MCV (>100 F/L)	13 (35)
Blood Chemistry	
Increased ALT (>250 U/L)	4 (11)
Increased AST (>250 U/L)	5 (14)
Increased GGT (>450 U/L)	4 (11)
Increased total bilirubin (>2.5 mg/dL)	1 (3)
Increased alkaline phosphatase (>2x ULN)	19 (51)
Increased amylase (>2x ULN)	6 (16)

ADVERSE REACTIONS
Adults:
The safety of VIRAMUNE has been assessed in 2861 patients in clinical trials. The experience from clinical trials and clinical practice has shown that the most serious adverse reactions are clinical hepatitis/hepatic failure, Stevens-Johnson syndrome, toxic epidermal necrolysis, and hypersensitivity reactions. Clinical hepatitis/hepatic failure may be isolated or associated with signs of hypersensitivity including, but not limited to, severe rash or rash accompanied by fever, general malaise, fatigue, muscle or joint aches, blisters, oral lesions, conjunctivitis, facial edema, and/or hepatitis, eosinophilia, granulocytopenia, and renal dysfunction.

Cases of hepatitis, severe and life-threatening hepatotoxicity, and fatal fulminant hepatitis, have been reported in patients treated with VIRAMUNE. The first 12 weeks of treatment is a critical period, but such events may also occur later. In clinical trials, the risk of hepatitis is approximately 1%. Increased AST or ALT levels and/or history of hepatitis B or C infection prior to the start of antiretroviral therapy are associated with a greater risk of hepatic adverse events. (See WARNINGS)

The most common clinical toxicity of VIRAMUNE is rash, with VIRAMUNE-attributable rash occurring in 16% of patients in combination regimens in Phase II/III controlled studies. Thirty-five percent of patients treated with VIRAMUNE experienced rash compared with 19% of patients treated in control groups of either ZDV+ddI or ZDV alone (Table 2). Severe or life-threatening rash occurred in

Continued on next page

Viramune—Cont.

6.6% of VIRAMUNE-treated patients compared with 1.3% of patients treated in the control groups.

Rashes are usually mild to moderate, maculopapular erythematous cutaneous eruptions, with or without pruritus, located on the trunk, face and extremities. The majority of rashes occurred within the first 6 weeks of therapy. Severe rashes occurred most frequently within the first 28 days of treatment; 25% of the patients with severe rashes required hospitalization; and one patient required surgical intervention. Overall, 7% of patients discontinued VIRAMUNE due to rash.

[See table 2 above]

Table 3 lists treatment-related clinical adverse events that occurred in patients receiving VIRAMUNE in ACTG 241 and in Trials BI 1037, BI 1011, and BI 1046.

[See table 3 to the right]

Laboratory Abnormalities: Table 4 summarizes marked laboratory abnormalities occurring in four controlled studies.

[See table 4 below]

Because clinical hepatitis has been reported in VIRAMUNE-treated patients, intensive clinical and laboratory monitoring, including liver function tests, is essential at baseline and during the first 12 weeks of treatment. Monitoring should continue at frequent intervals thereafter, depending on the patient's clinical status. (See WARNINGS) Asymptomatic elevations in GGT levels are more frequent in VIRAMUNE recipients than in controls. Asymptomatic elevations in GGT, without elevations in other liver function tests, are not a contraindication to continue VIRAMUNE therapy.

Post Marketing Surveillance: In addition to the adverse events identified during clinical trials, the following events have been reported with the use of VIRAMUNE in clinical practice

Body as a Whole: drug withdrawal (see PRECAUTIONS: Drug Interactions)

Liver and Biliary: jaundice, fulminant and cholestatic hepatitis, hepatic necrosis, hepatic failure

Hematology: eosinophilia

Skin and Appendages: allergic reactions including anaphylaxis, angioedema, bullous eruptions, and urticaria have all been reported. In addition, hypersensitivity reactions with rash associated with constitutional findings such as fever, blistering, oral lesions, conjunctivitis, facial edema, muscle or joint aches, general malaise or significant hepatic abnormalities (See WARNINGS) plus one or more of the following: hepatitis, eosinophilia, granulocytopenia and/or renal dysfunction have been reported with the use of VIRAMUNE.

Pediatric Patients:

The most frequently reported adverse events related to VIRAMUNE in pediatric patients were similar to those observed in adults, with the exception of granulocytopenia which was more commonly observed in children. (See PRECAUTIONS: Pediatric Use) The safety profile of VIRAMUNE in neonates has not been established.

OVERDOSAGE

There is no known antidote for VIRAMUNE overdosage. Cases of VIRAMUNE overdose at doses ranging from 800 to 1800 mg per day for up to 15 days have been reported. Patients have experienced events including edema, erythema nodosum, fatigue, fever, headache, insomnia, nausea, pulmonary infiltrates, rash, vertigo, vomiting and weight decrease. All events subsided following discontinuation of VIRAMUNE.

DOSAGE AND ADMINISTRATION

Adults:

The recommended dose for VIRAMUNE is one 200 mg tablet daily for the first 14 days (this lead-in period should be used because it has been found to lessen the frequency of rash), followed by one 200 mg tablet twice daily, in combination with antiretroviral agents. For concomitantly administered antiretroviral therapy, the manufacturer's recommended dosage and monitoring should be followed.

Pediatric Patients:

The recommended oral dose of VIRAMUNE for pediatric patients 2 months up to 8 years of age is 4 mg/kg once daily for the first 14 days followed by 7 mg/kg twice daily thereafter. For patients 8 years and older the recommended dose is 4 mg/kg once daily for two weeks followed by 4 mg/kg twice daily thereafter. The total daily dose should not exceed 400 mg for any patient.

VIRAMUNE suspension should be shaken gently prior to administration. It is important to administer the entire measured dose of suspension by using an oral dosing syringe or dosing cup. An oral dosing syringe is recommended, particularly for volumes of 5 mL or less. If a dosing cup is used, it should be thoroughly rinsed with water and the rinse should also be administered to the patient.

Monitoring of Patients:

Intensive clinical and laboratory monitoring, including liver function tests, is essential at baseline and during the first 12 weeks of treatment with VIRAMUNE. The optimal frequency of monitoring during this period has not been established. Some experts recommend clinical and laboratory monitoring more often than once per month, and in particular, would include monitoring of liver function tests at baseline, prior to dose escalation and at two weeks post dose escalation. After the initial 12-week period, frequent clinical and laboratory monitoring should continue throughout VIRAMUNE treatment. (See WARNINGS)

Table 2: Percentage of Patients with Rashes in Adult Controlled Trials[a]

	ACTG 241[b]		BI 1037		BI 1011[c]		BI 1046			COMBINED DATA	
	NVP+ZDV+ddl	ZDV+ddl	NVP+ZDV	ZDV	NVP+ZDV	ZDV	NVP+ZDV	NVP+ZDV+ddl	ZDV+ddl	NVP	Control
n	197	201	30	30	25	24	47	51	53	350	308
Rash events of all Grades and all causality	39.6%	23.9%	26.7%	6.7%	32.0%	4.2%	31.9%	29.4%	13.2%	35.4%	18.8%
Grade 3 or 4 rash events; all causality	8.1%	1.5%	3.3%	0%	8.0%	0%	4.3%	3.9%	1.9%	6.6%	1.3%

a At recommended dose of one 200 mg tablet daily for the first 14 days followed by one 200 mg tablet twice daily
b Trial ACTG 241 was designed to report Grade 3/4 (severe or life-threatening) events; except for several pre-specified events including rash for which all grades are reported
c Trial BI 1011 was an open-label comparison of NVP added to ZDV versus ZDV alone in patients with ≥ 6 months prior antiretroviral therapy

Table 3: Comparative Incidence of Selected Drug-Related Events in Adult Controlled Trials

	ACTG 241 Grade 3/4 Events		Trials BI 1037 and BI 1011[a] All Severities		Trial BI 1046 All Severities			COMBINED DATA	
	NVP+ZDV+ddl	ZDV+ddl	NVP+ZDV	ZDV Alone	NVP+ZDV	NVP+ZDV+ddl	ZDV+ddl	NVP	Control
Number of patients	197	201	55	30	47	51	53	350	284
Overall incidence of related adverse events	31%	23%	42%	33%	87%	71%	57%	46%	30%
Rash	8	2	20	3	24	24	6	14	2
Nausea	4	3	9	3	43	41	30	15	8
Headache	2	2	11	0	23	12	11	8	3
Abnormal LFT	5	3	2	3	17	10	4	7	3
Fatigue	1	0	10	0	19	16	23	7	4
Fever	3	1	11	3	6	4	6	5	2
Vomiting	2	1	4	0	15	6	8	5	2
Myalgia	1	0	2	3	13	8	8	4	1
Somnolence	0	0	6	0	4	8	8	3	1
Abdominal pain	1	1	2	0	13	2	2	3	1
Arthralgia	0	0	2	0	4	6	0	2	0
Hepatitis	1	0	4	0	2	0	0	1	0
Paraesthesia	1	0	2	0	2	2	0	1	0
Ulcerative Stomatitis	0	0	4	0	2	0	0	1	0
Diarrhea	2	2	0	0	11	12	13	4	4
Peripheral Neuropathy	0	2	0	0	0	0	0	0	1

a Total does not include patients who received ZDV alone in open label trial BI 1011.

Table 4: Percentage of Adult Patients with Marked Laboratory Abnormalities

	Data combined for controlled trials ACTG 241, BI 1037, BI 1011 & BI 1046	
	VIRAMUNE n=350	Control n=308
Hematology		
Decreased Hg (<8.0 g/dL)	1.1%	1.6%
Decreased platelets (<50,000/mm³)	0.9	0.6
Decreased neutrophils (<750/mm³)	9.1	9.4
Blood Chemistry		
Increased ALT (>250 U/L)	5.1	3.9
Increased AST (>250 U/L)	3.4	2.3
Increased GGT (>450 U/L)	3.1	1.3
Increased total bilirubin (>2.5 mg/dL)	0.6	1.6

Dosage Adjustment:

VIRAMUNE should be discontinued if patients experience severe rash or a rash accompanied by constitutional findings. (See WARNINGS) Patients experiencing rash during the 14-day lead-in period of 200 mg/day (4 mg/kg/day in pediatric patients) should not have their VIRAMUNE dose increased until the rash has resolved. (See PRECAUTIONS, Information for Patients)

If clinical hepatitis occurs, VIRAMUNE should be permanently discontinued and not restarted after recovery.

Patients who interrupt VIRAMUNE dosing for more than 7 days should restart the recommended dosing, using one 200 mg tablet daily (4 mg/kg/day in pediatric patients) for the first 14 days (lead-in) followed by one 200 mg tablet twice daily (4 or 7 mg/kg twice daily, according to age, for pediatric patients).

No data are available to recommend a dosage of VIRAMUNE in patients with hepatic dysfunction, renal insufficiency, or undergoing dialysis.

HOW SUPPLIED

VIRAMUNE (nevirapine) Tablets, 200 mg, are white, oval, biconvex tablets, 9.3 mm × 19.1 mm. One side is embossed with "54 193", with a single bisect separating the "54" and "193". The opposite side has a single bisect.

VIRAMUNE Tablets are supplied in bottles of 100 (NDC 0597-0046-01), bottles of 60 (NDC 0597-0046-60), and individually blister-sealed unit-dose cartons of 100 tablets as 10 × 10 cards (NDC 0597-0046-61).

VIRAMUNE (nevirapine) Oral Suspension, is a white to off-white preserved suspension containing 50 mg nevirapine (as nevirapine hemihydrate) in each 5 mL. VIRAMUNE suspension is supplied in plastic bottles with child-resistant closures containing 240 mL of suspension (NDC 0597-0047-24). VIRAMUNE Tablets and Oral Suspension should be stored at 15°C–30°C (59°F–86°F).

Revise 11/02/00   4077435//03
4077435/US/3

Boehringer Ingelheim Pharmaceuticals, Inc.
Ridgefield, CT 06877 USA

Centocor, Inc.
**200 GREAT VALLEY PARKWAY
MALVERN, PA 19355**

Direct General Inquiries to:
Ph: (610) 651-6000
    (888) 874-3083
Fax: (610) 651-6100

Medical Emergency Contact:
Ph: 1-800-457-6399
For Medical Information/Adverse Experience Reporting Contact:
Medical Information & Product Surveillance
Ph: (800) 457-6399
Fax: 610-889-4410

REMICADE®
**Infliximab recombinant
for IV Injection**

Prescribing Information for this product, which appears on pages 1085–1088 of the 2001 PDR, has been completely revised as follows. Please write "See Supplement A" next to the product heading.

DESCRIPTION:

REMICADE® (infliximab) is a chimeric IgG1k monoclonal antibody with an approximate molecular weight of 149,100 daltons. It is composed of human constant and murine variable regions. Infliximab binds specifically to human tumor necrosis factor alpha (TNFα) with an association constant of 10^{10} M^{-1}. Infliximab is produced by a recombinant cell line cultured by continuous perfusion and is purified by a series of steps that includes measures to inactivate and remove viruses.

REMICADE is supplied as a sterile, white, lyophilized powder for intravenous infusion. Following reconstitution with 10 mL of Sterile Water for Injection, USP, the resulting pH is approximately 7.2. Each single-use vial contains 100 mg infliximab, 500 mg sucrose, 0.5 mg polysorbate 80, 2.2 mg monobasic sodium phosphate, monohydrate, and 6.1 mg dibasic sodium phosphate, dihydrate. No preservatives are present.

CLINICAL PHARMACOLOGY:
General

Infliximab neutralizes the biological activity of TNFα by binding with high affinity to the soluble and transmembrane forms of TNFα and inhibits binding of TNFα with its receptors.[1–4] Infliximab does not neutralize TNFβ (lymphotoxin α), a related cytokine that utilizes the same receptors as TNFα. Biological activities attributed to TNFα include: induction of pro-inflammatory cytokines such as interleukins (IL) 1 and 6, enhancement of leukocyte migration by increasing endothelial layer permeability and expression of adhesion molecules by endothelial cells and leukocytes, activation of neutrophil and eosinophil functional activity, induction of acute phase reactants and other liver proteins, as well as tissue degrading enzymes produced by synoviocytes and/or chondrocytes. Cells expressing transmembrane TNFα bound by infliximab can be lysed *in vitro* by complement or effector cells.[2] Infliximab inhibits the functional activity of TNFα in a wide variety of *in vitro* bioassays utilizing human fibroblasts, endothelial cells, neutrophils,[3] B and T lymphocytes and epithelial cells. Anti-TNFα antibodies reduce disease activity in the cotton-top tamarin colitis model, and decrease synovitis and joint erosions in a murine model of collagen-induced arthritis. Infliximab prevents disease in transgenic mice that develop polyarthritis as a result of constitutive expression of human TNFα, and, when administered after disease onset, allows eroded joints to heal.

Pharmacodynamics

Elevated concentrations of TNFα have been found in the joints of rheumatoid arthritis patients[5] and the stools of Crohn's disease patients[6] and correlate with elevated disease activity. In rheumatoid arthritis, treatment with REMICADE reduced infiltration of inflammatory cells into inflamed areas of the joint as well as expression of molecules mediating cellular adhesion [E-selectin, intercellular adhesion molecule-1 (ICAM-1) and vascular cell adhesion mole-

cule-1 (VCAM-1)], chemoattraction [IL-8 and monocyte chemotactic protein (MCP-1)] and tissue degradation [matrix metalloproteinase (MMP) 1 and 3].[4] In Crohn's disease, treatment with REMICADE reduced infiltration of inflammatory cells and TNFα production in inflamed areas of the intestine, and reduced the proportion of mononuclear cells from the lamina propria able to express TNFα and interferon.[4] After treatment with REMICADE, patients with rheumatoid arthritis or Crohn's disease exhibited decreased levels of serum IL-6 and C-reactive protein (CRP) compared to baseline. Peripheral blood lymphocytes from REMICADE-treated patients showed no significant decrease in number or in proliferative responses to *in vitro* mitogenic stimulation when compared to cells from untreated patients.

Pharmacokinetics

Single intravenous infusions of 3 mg/kg to 20 mg/kg showed a predictable and linear relationship between the dose administered and the maximum serum concentration and area under the concentration-time curve. The volume of distribution at steady state was independent of dose and indicated that infliximab was distributed primarily within the vascular compartment. Median pharmacokinetic results for doses of 3 mg/kg to 10 mg/kg in rheumatoid arthritis and 5 mg/kg in Crohn's disease indicate that the terminal half-life of infliximab is 8.0 to 9.5 days.

Following an initial dose of REMICADE, repeated infusions at 2 and 6 weeks in fistulizing Crohn's disease and rheumatoid arthritis patients resulted in predictable concentration-time profiles following each treatment. No systemic accumulation of infliximab occurred upon continued repeated treatment with 3 mg/kg or 10 mg/kg at 4- or 8-week intervals in rheumatoid arthritis patients or patients with moderate or severe Crohn's disease retreated with 4 infusions of 10 mg/kg REMICADE at 8-week intervals. The proportion of patients with rheumatoid arthritis who had undetectable infliximab concentrations at 8 weeks following an infusion was approximately 25% for those receiving 3 mg/kg every 8 weeks, 15% for patients administered 3 mg/kg every 4 weeks, and 0% for patients receiving 10 mg/kg every 4 or 8 weeks. No major differences in clearance or volume of distribution were observed in patient subgroups defined by age or weight. It is not known if there are differences in clearance or volume of distribution between gender subgroups or in patients with marked impairment of hepatic or renal function.

CLINICAL STUDIES:
Rheumatoid Arthritis

The safety and efficacy of REMICADE when given in conjunction with methotrexate (MTX) were assessed in a multicenter, randomized, double-blind, placebo-controlled study of 428 patients with active rheumatoid arthritis despite treatment with MTX (the Anti-TNF Trial in Rheumatoid Arthritis with Concomitant Therapy or ATTRACT). Patients enrolled had a median age of 54 years, median disease duration of 8.4 years, median swollen and tender joint count of 20 and 31 respectively, and were on a median dose of 15 mg/wk of MTX. Patients received either placebo + MTX or one of 4 doses/schedules of REMICADE + MTX: 3 mg/kg or 10 mg/kg of REMICADE by intravenous infusion (IV) at weeks 0, 2 and 6 followed by additional infusions every 4 or 8 weeks in combination with MTX. Concurrent use of stable doses of folic acid, oral corticosteroids (≤10 mg/day) and/or nonsteroidal anti-inflammatory drugs was also permitted.

Clinical Response

All doses/schedules of REMICADE + MTX resulted in improvement in signs and symptoms as measured by the American College of Rheumatology response criteria (ACR 20)[7] through 54 weeks (Figure 1).

TABLE 1
COMPONENTS OF ACR 20

Parameter (medians)	Placebo + MTX		3 mg/kg q 8 wks REMICADE + MTX	
	Baseline	Week 54	Baseline	Week 54
No. of Tender Joints	24	16	32	10
No. of Swollen Joints	19	13	19	9
Pain[a]	6.7	6.1	7.0	4.8
Physician's Global Assessment[a]	6.5	5.2	6.1	2.6
Patient's Global Assessment[a]	6.2	6.2	6.6	4.5
Disability Index (HAQ)[b]	1.8	1.5	1.8	1.5
CRP (mg/dL)	3.0	2.3	3.1	0.8

[a] Visual Analog Scale (0=best, 10=worst)
[b] Health Assessment Questionnaire, measurement of 8 categories: dressing and grooming, arising, eating, walking, hygiene, reach, grip, and activities(0=best, 3=worst)[8]

TABLE 2
PERCENTAGE OF PATIENTS WHO ACHIEVED AN ACR RESPONSE AT WEEKS 30 AND 54
REMICADE + MTX

Response	Placebo + MTX (n=88)	3 mg/kg* q 8 wks (n=86)	3 mg/kg* q 4 wks (n=86)	10 mg/kg* q 8 wks (n=87)	10 mg/kg* q 4 wks (n=81)
ACR 50					
Week 30	5%	27%	29%	31%	26%
Week 54	9%	21%	34%	40%	38%
ACR 70					
Week 30	0%	8%	11%	18%	11%
Week 54	2%	11%	18%	26%	19%

* $p < 0.05$ for each outcome compared to placebo

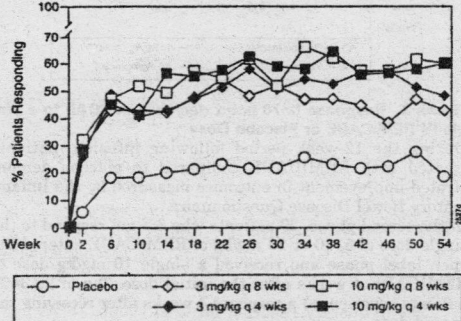

| Week | 0 2 6 10 14 18 22 26 30 34 38 42 46 50 54 |

—O— Placebo   —◇— 3 mg/kg q 8 wks   —□— 10 mg/kg q 8 wks
—◆— 3 mg/kg q 4 wks   —■— 10 mg/kg q 4 wks
All groups received concomitant MTX.

Figure 1 Percentage of Patients who Achieved an ACR 20
Compared to placebo + MTX, all doses/schedules of REMICADE + MTX consistently resulted in greater effects on each component of the ACR 20, except for the HAQ, where only the 3 higher doses/schedules showed improvements in HAQ. Results from patients receiving 3 mg/kg q 8 weeks are shown in Table 1. Responses to the higher doses or more frequent administrations were similarly distributed.

[See first table above]

All doses/schedules of REMICADE + MTX resulted in a higher number of patients experiencing ACR 50 and ACR 70 compared to placebo + MTX (Table 2).

[See second table above]

Health outcome measures were assessed by the SF-36 questionnaire. The eight subscales of the SF-36 were combined into two summary scales, the physical component summary (PCS) and the mental component summary (MCS).[9] At week 54, patients treated with 3 mg/kg or 10 mg/kg of REMICADE every 8 or 4 weeks showed significantly more improvement in the PCS compared to the placebo group, and no change in the MCS.

Radiographic Response

Structural damage in both hands and feet was assessed radiographically at week 54 by the change from baseline in the van der Heijde-modified Sharp score, a composite score of structural damage that measures the number and size of joint erosions and the degree of joint space narrowing in hands/wrists and feet.[10] Approximately 80% of patients had paired x-ray data. Results are shown in Table 3.

[See table at top of next page]

Data on use of REMICADE without concurrent MTX are limited (see *Precautions, Immunogenicity*).[11,12]

Active Crohn's Disease

The safety and efficacy of REMICADE were assessed in a randomized, double-blind, placebo-controlled dose ranging study of 108 patients with moderate to severe active Crohn's disease[13] [Crohn's Disease Activity Index (CDAI) ≥220 and ≤400]. All patients had experienced an inadequate response to prior conventional therapies, including corticosteroids (60% of patients), 5-aminosalicylates (5-ASA) (60%) and/or 6-mercaptopurine/azathioprine (6-MP/AZA) (37%). Concurrent use of stable dose regimens of corticosteroids, 5-ASA, 6-MP and/or AZA was permitted and 92% of patients continued to receive at least one of these medications.

Continued on next page

Remicade—Cont.

The study was divided into three phases. In the first phase, patients were randomized to receive a single IV dose of placebo, 5, 10 or 20 mg/kg of REMICADE. The primary endpoint was the proportion of patients who experienced a clinical response, defined as a decrease in CDAI by ≥70 points from baseline at the 4-week evaluation and without an increase in Crohn's disease medications or surgery for Crohn's disease. Patients who responded at week 4 were followed to week 12. Secondary endpoints included the proportion of patients who were in clinical remission at week 4 (CDAI <150), and clinical response over time.

At week four, 4 of 25 (16%) of the placebo patients achieved a clinical response vs. 22 of 27 (82%) of the patients receiving 5 mg/kg REMICADE ($p < 0.001$, two-sided, Fisher's Exact test). One of 25 (4%) placebo patients and 13 of 27 (48%) patients receiving 5 mg/kg REMICADE achieved a CDAI <150 at week 4. The maximum response to any dose of REMICADE was observed within 2 to 4 weeks. The proportion of patients responding gradually diminished over the 12 weeks of the evaluation period. There was no evidence of a dose response; doses higher than 5 mg/kg did not result in a greater proportion of responders. Results are shown in Figure 3.

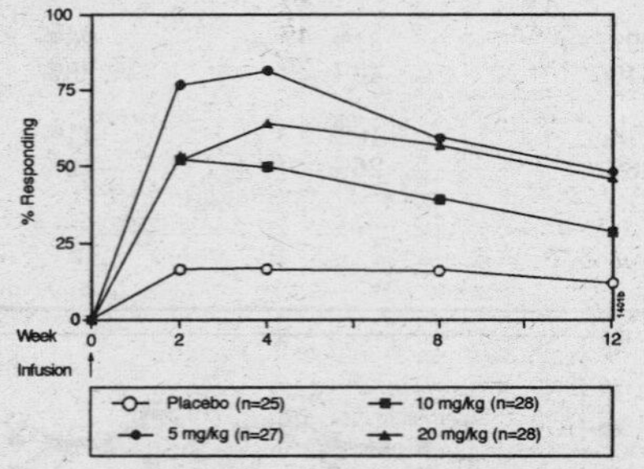

Figure 3 Response (≥70 point decrease in CDAI) to a Single IV REMICADE or Placebo Dose

During the 12-week period following infusion, patients treated with REMICADE compared to placebo demonstrated improvement in outcomes measured by the Inflammatory Bowel Disease Questionnaire.

In the second phase, 29 patients who did not respond to the single dose of 5, 10 or 20 mg/kg of REMICADE entered the open label phase and received a single 10 mg/kg dose of REMICADE 4 weeks after the initial dose. Ten of 29(34%) patients experienced a response 4 weeks after receiving the second dose.

Patients who remained in clinical response at week 8 during the first or second phase were eligible for the retreatment phase. Seventy-three patients were re-randomized at week 12 to receive 4 infusions of placebo or 10 mg/kg REMICADE at 8-week intervals (weeks 12, 20, 28, 36) and were followed to week 48. In the limited data set available, no significant differences were observed between the REMICADE and placebo re-treated groups.

Fistulizing Crohn's Disease

The safety and efficacy of REMICADE were assessed in a randomized, double-blind, placebo-controlled study of 94 patients with fistulizing Crohn's disease with fistula(s) that were of at least 3 months duration.[14] Concurrent use of stable doses of corticosteroids, 5-ASA, antibiotics, MTX, 6-MP and/or AZA was permitted, and 83% of patients continued to receive at least one of these medications. Fifty-two (55%) had multiple cutaneously draining fistulas, 90% of patients had fistula(s) in the perianal area and 10% had abdominal fistula(s).

Patients received 3 doses of placebo, 5 or 10 mg/kg REMICADE at weeks 0, 2 and 6 and were followed up to 26 weeks. The primary endpoint was the proportion of patients who experienced a clinical response, defined as ≥50% reduction from baseline in the number of fistula(s) draining upon gentle compression, on at least two consecutive visits, without an increase in medication or surgery for Crohn's disease. Eight of 31 (26%) patients in the placebo arm achieved a clinical response vs. 21 of the 31 (68%) patients in the 5 mg/kg REMICADE arm ($p = 0.002$, two-sided, Fisher's Exact test). Eighteen of 32 (56%) patients in the 10 mg/kg arm achieved a clinical response.

The median time to onset of response in the REMICADE-treated group was 2 weeks. The median duration of response was 12 weeks; after 22 weeks there was no difference between either dose of REMICADE and placebo in the proportion of patients in response (Figure 4). New fistula(s) developed in approximately 15% of both REMICADE- and placebo-treated patients.

[See figure at top of next column]

Figure 4 Response [fistula(s) closure] with Three Doses of REMICADE or Placebo

Seven of 60 (12%) evaluable REMICADE-treated patients, compared to 1 of 31 (3.5%) placebo-treated patients, developed an abscess in the area of fistulas between 8 and 16 weeks after the last infusion of REMICADE. Six of the REMICADE patients who developed an abscess had experienced a clinical response (see *ADVERSE REACTIONS, Infections*).

Dose regimens other than dosing at weeks 0, 2 and 6 have not been studied. Studies have not been done to assess the effects of REMICADE on healing of the internal fistular canal, on closure of non-cutaneously draining fistulas (e.g., entero-entero), or on cutaneously draining fistulas in locations other than perianal and periabdominal.

TABLE 3
RADIOGRAPHIC CHANGE FROM BASELINE TO WEEK 54

Median (10, 90 percentiles) Week 54	Placebo + MTX (N=64)	REMICADE + MTX 3 mg/kg q 8 wks (N=71)	3 mg/kg q 4 wks (N=71)	10 mg/kg q 8 wks (N=77)	10 mg/kg q 4 wks (N=66)	p-value*
Total Score						
Baseline	55 (14, 188)	57 (15, 187)	45 (8, 162)	56 (6, 143)	43 (7, 178)	
Change from baseline	4.0 (−1.0, 19.0)	0.5 (−3.0, 5.5)	0.1 (−5.2, 9.0)	0.5 (−4.8, 5.0)	−0.5 (−5.7, 4.0)	p<0.001
Erosion Score						
Baseline	25 (8, 110)	29 (9, 100)	22 (3, 91)	22 (3, 80)	26 (4, 104)	
Change from baseline	2.0 (−1.0, 9.7)	0.0 (−3.0 4.3)	−0.3 (−3.1, 2.5)	0.5 (−3.0, 2.5)	−0.5 (−2.7, 2.5)	p<0.001
JSN Score						
Baseline	26 (3, 88)	29 (4, 80)	20 (3, 83)	24 (1, 79)	25 (3, 77)	
Change from baseline	1.5 (−0.8, 8.0)	0.0 (−2.5, 4.5)	0.0 (−3.4, 5.0)	0.0 (−3.0, 2.5)	0.0 (−3.0, 3.5)	p<0.001

* For comparisons of each dose against placebo

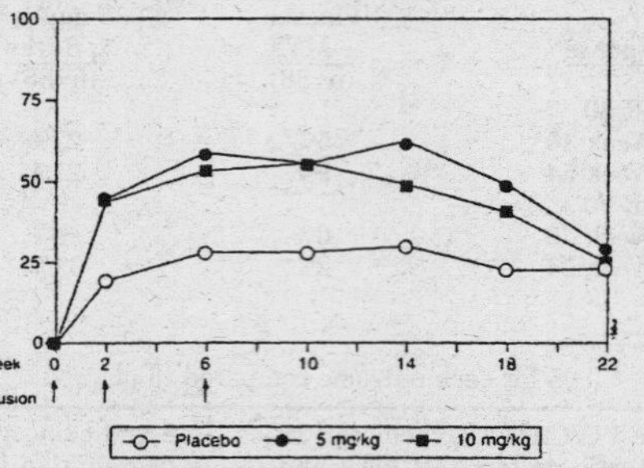

INDICATIONS AND USAGE:

Rheumatoid Arthritis

REMICADE, in combination with methotrexate, is indicated for reducing signs and symptoms and inhibiting the progression of structural damage in patients with moderately to severely active rheumatoid arthritis who have had an inadequate response to methotrexate.

Crohn's Disease

REMICADE is indicated for the reduction in signs and symptoms of Crohn's disease in patients with moderately to severely active Crohn's disease who have had an inadequate response to conventional therapy.

The safety and efficacy of therapy continued beyond a single dose have not been established (see *DOSAGE AND ADMINISTRATION*).

REMICADE is indicated for the reduction in the number of draining enterocutaneous fistulas in patients with fistulizing Crohn's disease.

The safety and efficacy of therapy continued beyond three doses have not been established (see *DOSAGE AND ADMINSTRATION*).

CONTRAINDICATIONS:

REMICADE should not be administered to patients with known hypersensitivity to any murine proteins or other component of the product.

WARNINGS:

RISK OF INFECTIONS

SERIOUS INFECTIONS, INCLUDING SEPSIS AND DISSEMINATED TUBERCULOSIS, HAVE BEEN REPORTED IN PATIENTS RECEIVING TNF-BLOCKING AGENTS, INCLUDING REMICADE. SOME OF THESE INFECTIONS HAVE BEEN FATAL. MANY OF THE SERIOUS INFECTIONS IN PATIENTS TREATED WITH REMICADE HAVE OCCURRED IN PATIENTS ON CONCOMITANT IMMUNOSUPPRESSIVE THERAPY THAT, IN ADDITION TO THEIR CROHN'S DISEASE OR RHEUMATOID ARTHRITIS, COULD PREDISPOSE THEM TO INFECTIONS.

CAUTION SHOULD BE EXERCISED WHEN CONSIDERING THE USE OF REMICADE IN PATIENTS WITH A CHRONIC INFECTION OR A HISTORY OF RECURRENT INFECTION. REMICADE SHOULD NOT BE GIVEN TO PATIENTS WITH A CLINICALLY IMPORTANT, ACTIVE INFECTION. PATIENTS SHOULD BE MONITORED FOR SIGNS AND SYMPTOMS OF INFECTION WHILE ON OR AFTER TREATMENT WITH REMICADE. NEW INFECTIONS SHOULD BE CLOSELY MONITORED. IF A PATIENT DEVELOPS A SERIOUS INFECTION INCLUDING SEPSIS, REMICADE THERAPY SHOULD BE DISCONTINUED (see *ADVERSE REACTIONS, Infections*). PATIENTS SHOULD BE EVALUATED FOR THE RISK OF TUBERCULOSIS, INCLUDING LATENT TUBERCULOSIS.[15] TREATMENT FOR TUBERCULOSIS SHOULD BE INITIATED PRIOR TO TREATMENT WITH REMICADE.

Hypersensitivity

REMICADE has been associated with hypersensitivity reactions that vary in their time of onset. Most hypersensitivity reactions, which include urticaria, dyspnea, and/or hypotension, have occurred during or within 2 hours of infliximab infusion. However, in some cases, serum sickness-like reactions have been observed in Crohn's disease patients 3 to 12 days after REMICADE therapy was reinstituted following an extended period without REMICADE treatment. Symptoms associated with these reactions include fever, rash, headache, sore throat, myalgias, polyarthralgias, hand and facial edema and/or dysphagia. These reactions were associated with marked increase in antibodies to infliximab, loss of detectable serum concentrations of REMICADE, and possible loss of drug efficacy. REMICADE should be discontinued for severe reactions. Medications for the treatment of hypersensitivity reactions (e.g., acetaminophen, antihistamines, corticosteroids and/or epinephrine) should be available for immediate use in the event of a reaction (see *ADVERSE REACTIONS, Infusion-related Reactions*).

Neurologic Events

Infliximab and other agents that inhibit TNF have been associated in rare cases with exacerbation of clinical symptoms and/or radiographic evidence of de-myelinating disease. Prescribers should exercise caution in considering the use of REMICADE in patients with pre-existing or recent onset of central nervous system de-myelinating disorders.

PRECAUTIONS

Autoimmunity

Treatment with REMICADE may result in the formation of autoantibodies and, rarely, in the development of a lupus-like syndrome. If a patient develops symptoms suggestive of a lupus-like syndrome following treatment with REMICADE, treatment should be discontinued (see *ADVERSE REACTIONS, Autoantibodies/Lupus-like Syndrome*).

Malignancy

Patients with long duration of Crohn's disease or rheumatoid arthritis and chronic exposure to immunosuppressant therapies are more prone to develop lymphomas (see *ADVERSE REACTIONS, Malignancies/Lymphoproliferative Disease*). The impact of treatment with REMICADE on these phenomena is unknown.

Immunogenicity

Treatment with REMICADE can be associated with the development of antibodies to infliximab. One hundred thirty-four of the 199 Crohn's disease patients treated with REMICADE were evaluated for the development of infliximab-specific antibodies; 18 (13%) were antibody-positive (the majority at low titer, <1:20). Patients who were antibody-positive were more likely to experience an infusion reaction (see *ADVERSE REACTIONS, Infusion-related Reactions*). Antibody development was lower among rheumatoid arthritis and Crohn's disease patients receiving immunosuppressant therapies such as 6-MP, AZA or MTX. With repeated dosing of REMICADE, serum concentrations of infliximab were higher in rheumatoid arthritis patients who received concomitant MTX. There are limited data available on the development of antibodies to infliximab in patients receiving long-term treatment with REMICADE. Because immunogenicity analyses are product-specific, comparison of antibody rates to those from other products is not appropriate.

Vaccinations

No data are available on the response to vaccination or on the secondary transmission of infection by live vaccines in patients receiving anti-TNF therapy. It is recommended that live vaccines not be given concurrently.

Drug Interactions

Specific drug interaction studies, including interactions with MTX, have not been conducted. The majority of patients in rheumatoid arthritis or Crohn's disease clinical studies received one or more concomitant medications. In rheumatoid arthritis, concomitant medications besides MTX were nonsteroidal anti-inflammatory agents, folic acid, corticosteroids and/or narcotics. Concomitant Crohn's disease medications were antibiotics, antivirals, corticosteroids, 6-MP/AZA and aminosalicylates. Patients with Crohn's disease who received immunosuppressants tended to experience fewer infusion reactions compared to patients on no immunosuppressants (see *PRECAUTIONS, Immunogenicity* and *ADVERSE REACTIONS, Infusion-related Reactions*).

Carcinogenesis, Mutagenesis and Impairment of Fertility

Long-term studies in animals have not been performed to evaluate the carcinogenic potential. No clastogenic or mutagenic effects of infliximab were observed in the *in vivo* mouse micronucleus test or the *Salmonella-Escherichia coli* (Ames) assay, respectively. Chromosomal aberrations were not observed in an assay performed using human lymphocytes. Tumorigenicity studies in mice deficient in TNFα demonstrated no increase in tumors when challenged with known tumor initiators and/or promoters. It is not known

Table 4
ADVERSE EVENTS IN RHEUMATOID ARTHRITIS AND CROHN'S DISEASE STUDIES

	RHEUMATOID ARTHRITIS		CROHN'S DISEASE	
	Placebo (n=133)	REMICADE (n=555)	Placebo (n=56)	REMICADE (n=199)
Avg. weeks of follow-up	35.9	41.2	14.7	27.0
Respiratory				
Upper respiratory infection	17%	26%	9%	16%
Coughing	7%	13%	0%	5%
Sinusitis	4%	13%	2%	5%
Pharyngitis	6%	11%	5%	9%
Rhinitis	7%	9%	4%	6%
Bronchitis	5%	6%	2%	7%
Gastrointestinal				
Nausea	18%	17%	4%	17%
Diarrhea	14%	13%	2%	3%
Abdominal Pain	8%	10%	4%	12%
Vomiting	10%	7%	0%	9%
Dyspepsia	5%	6%	0%	5%
Other				
Headache	14%	22%	21%	23%
Rash	5%	12%	5%	6%
Dizziness	10%	10%	9%	8%
Urinary tract infection	7%	8%	4%	3%
Fatigue	5%	8%	5%	11%
Fever	6%	8%	7%	10%
Pain	8%	8%	5%	9%
Back pain	3%	6%	4%	5%
Pruritus	0%	6%	2%	5%
Arthralgia	2%	6%	2%	5%
Chest pain	5%	5%	5%	6%

whether infliximab can impair fertility in humans. No impairment of fertility was observed in a fertility and general reproduction toxicity study conducted in mice using an analogous antibody that selectively inhibits the functional activity of mouse TNFα.

Pregnancy Category B

Since infliximab does not cross-react with TNFα in species other than humans and chimpanzees, animal reproduction studies have not been conducted with REMICADE. No evidence of maternal toxicity, embryotoxicity or teratogenicity was observed in a developmental toxicity study conducted in mice using an analogous antibody that selectively inhibits the functional activity of mouse TNFα. Doses of 10 to 15 mg/kg in pharmacodynamic animal models with the anti-TNF analogous antibody produced maximal pharmacologic effectiveness. Doses up to 40 mg/kg were shown to produce no adverse effects in animal reproduction studies. It is not known whether REMICADE can cause fetal harm when administered to a pregnant woman or can affect reproduction capacity. REMICADE should be given to a pregnant woman only if clearly needed.

Nursing Mothers

It is not known whether infliximab is excreted in human milk or absorbed systemically after ingestion. Because many drugs and immunoglobulins are excreted in human milk, and because of the potential for adverse reactions in nursing infants from REMICADE, a decision should be made whether to discontinue nursing or to discontinue the drug, taking into account the importance of the drug to the mother.

Pediatric Use

Safety and effectiveness of REMICADE in patients with juvenile rheumatoid arthritis and in pediatric patients with Crohn's disease have not been established.

Geriatric Use

In the ATTRACT study, no overall differences were observed in effectiveness or safety in 72 patients aged 65 or older compared to younger patients. In Crohn's disease studies, there were insufficient numbers of patients aged 65 and over to determine whether they respond differently from patients aged 18 to 65. Because there is a higher incidence of infections in the elderly population in general, caution should be used in treating the elderly (see *ADVERSE REACTIONS, Infections*).

ADVERSE REACTIONS:

A total of 771 patients were treated with REMICADE in clinical studies. In both rheumatoid arthritis and Crohn's disease studies, approximately 6% of patients discontinued REMICADE because of adverse experiences. The most common reasons for discontinuation of treatment were dyspnea, urticaria and headache. Adverse events have been reported in a higher proportion of patients receiving the 10 mg/kg dose than the 3 mg/kg dose.

Infusion-related Reactions

Acute infusion reactions

An infusion reaction was defined as any adverse event occurring during the infusion or within 1 to 2 hours after the infusion. Nineteen percent of REMICADE-treated patients in all clinical studies experienced an infusion reaction compared to 8% of placebo-treated patients. Among the 4797 REMICADE infusions, 3% were accompanied by nonspecific symptoms such as fever or chills, 1% were accompanied by cardiopulmonary reactions (primarily chest pain, hypotension, hypertension or dyspnea), <1% were accompanied by pruritus, urticaria, or the combined symptoms of pruritus/urticaria and cardiopulmonary reactions. Serious infusion reactions including anaphylaxis were infrequent. Less than 2% of patients discontinued REMICADE because of infusion reactions, and all patients recovered with treatment and/or discontinuation of infusion. REMICADE infusions beyond the initial infusion in rheumatoid arthritis patients were not associated with a higher incidence of reactions.

Patients with Crohn's disease who became positive for antibodies to infliximab were more likely to develop infusion reactions than were those who were negative (36% vs. 11% respectively). Use of concomitant immunosuppressant agents appeared to reduce the frequency of antibodies to infliximab and infusion reactions (see *PRECAUTIONS, Immunogenicity and Drug Interactions*).

Reactions following readministration

In a clinical study of forty patients with Crohn's disease retreated with infliximab following a 2 to 4 year period without infliximab treatment, 10 patients experienced adverse events manifesting 3 to 12 days following infusion of which 6 were considered serious. Signs and symptoms included myalgia and/or arthralgia with fever and/or rash, with some patients also experiencing pruritus, facial, hand or lip edema, dysphagia, urticaria, sore throat, and headache. Patients experiencing these adverse events had not experienced infusion-related adverse events associated with their initial infliximab therapy. Of the 40 patients enrolled, these adverse events occurred in 9 of 23 (39%) who had received liquid formulation which is no longer in use and 1 of 17 (6%) who received lyophilized formulation. The clinical data are not adequate to determine if occurrence of these reactions is due to differences in formulation. Patients' signs and symptoms improved substantially or resolved with treatment in all cases. There are insufficient data on the incidence of these events after drug-free intervals of less than 2 years. However, these events have been observed infrequently in clinical studies and post-marketing surveillance at intervals of less than 1 year.

Infections

In REMICADE clinical studies, treated infections were reported in 32% of REMICADE-treated patients (average of 37 weeks of follow-up) and in 22% of placebo-treated patients (average of 29 weeks of follow-up). The infections most frequently reported were upper respiratory tract infections (including sinusitis, pharyngitis, and bronchitis) and urinary tract infections. No increased risk of serious infections or sepsis were observed with REMICADE compared to placebo in the ATTRACT study. Among REMICADE-treated patients, these serious infections included pneumonia, cellulitis and sepsis. In the ATTRACT study, one patient died with miliary tuberculosis and one died with disseminated coccidioidomycosis. Other cases of tuberculosis, including disseminated tuberculosis, also have been reported post-marketing. Although the relationship to REMICADE is unknown, most of the cases of tuberculosis occurred within the first two months after initiation of therapy with infliximab and may reflect recrudesence of latent disease (see *WARNINGS, RISK OF INFECTIONS*). Twelve percent of patients with fistulizing Crohn's disease developed a new abscess 8 to 16 weeks after the last infusion of REMICADE (see *CLINICAL STUDIES, Fistulizing Crohn's Disease*).

Autoantibodies/Lupus-like Syndrome

In the ATTRACT rheumatoid arthritis study through week 54, 49% of REMICADE-treated patients developed antinuclear antibodies (ANA) between screening and last evaluation, compared to 21% of placebo-treated patients. Anti-dsDNA antibodies developed in approximately 10% of REMICADE-treated patients, compared to none of the placebo-treated patients. No association was seen between REMICADE dose/schedule and development of ANA or anti-dsDNA.

Of Crohn's disease patients treated with REMICADE who were evaluated for antinuclear antibodies (ANA), 34% developed ANA between screening and last evaluation. Anti-dsDNA antibodies developed in approximately 9% of Crohn's disease patients treated with REMICADE. The development of anti-dsDNA antibodies was not related to either the dose or duration of REMICADE treatment. However, baseline therapy with an immunosuppressant in Crohn's disease patients was associated with reduced development of anti-dsDNA antibodies (3% compared to 21% in patients not receiving any immunosuppressant). Crohn's disease patients were approximately 2 times more likely to develop anti-dsDNA antibodies if they were ANA-positive at study entry. In clinical studies, three patients developed clinical symptoms consistent with a lupus-like syndrome, two with rheumatoid arthritis and one with Crohn's disease. All three patients improved following discontinuation of therapy and appropriate medical treatment. No cases of lupus-like reactions have been observed in up to three years of long-term follow-up (see *PRECAUTIONS, Autoimmunity*).

Malignancies/Lymphoproliferative Disease

In completed clinical studies of REMICADE for up to 54 weeks, 7 of 771 patients developed 8 new or recurrent malignancies. These were non-Hodgkins B-cell lymphoma, breast cancer, melanoma, squamous, rectal adenocarcinoma and basal cell carcinoma. There are insufficient data to determine whether REMICADE contributed to the development of these malignancies. The observed rates and incidences were similar to those expected for the populations studied[16,17] (see *PRECAUTIONS, Malignancy*).

Other Adverse Reactions

Adverse events occurring at a frequency of at least 5% in all patients treated with REMICADE are shown in Table 4. Patients with Crohn's disease who were treated with REMICADE were more likely than patients with rheumatoid arthritis to experience adverse events associated with gastrointestinal symptoms.

[See table above]

Serious adverse events (all occurred at frequencies <2%) by body system in all patients treated with REMICADE are as follows:

Body as a whole: abdominal hernia, asthenia, chest pain, diaphragmatic hernia, edema, fall, pain

Blood: splenic infarction, splenomegaly

Cardiovascular: hypertension, hypotension, syncope

Central & Peripheral Nervous: encephalopathy, dizziness, headache, spinal stenosis, upper motor neuron lesion

Autoimmunity: lupus erythematosus syndrome, worsening rheumatoid arthritis, rheumatoid nodules

Ear and Hearing: ceruminosis

Eye and Vision: endophthalmitis

Gastrointestinal: abdominal pain, appendicitis, Crohn's disease, diarrhea, gastric ulcer, gastrointestinal hemorrhage, intestinal obstruction, intestinal perforation, intestinal stenosis, nausea, pancreatitis, peritonitis, proctalgia, vomiting

Heart Rate and Rhythm: arrhythmia, atrioventricular block, bradycardia, cardiac arrest, palpitation, tachycardia

Liver and Biliary: biliary pain, cholecystitis, cholelithiasis, hepatitis cholestatic

Metabolic and Nutritional: dehydration, pancreatic insufficiency, weight decrease

Musculoskeletal: arthralgia, arthritis, back pain, bone fracture, hemarthrosis, intervertebral disk herniation, joint cyst, joint degeneration, myalgia, osteoarthritis, osteoporosis, spondylolisthesis, symphyseolysis, tendon disorder, tendon injury

Myo-, Endo-, Pericardial and Coronary Valve: angina pectoris, cardiac failure, myocardial ischemia

Neoplasms: basal cell, breast, lymphoma, melanoma, rectal adenocarcinoma, skin

Platelet, Bleeding and Clotting: thrombocytopenia

Psychiatric: anxiety, confusion, delirium, depression, somnolence, suicide attempt

Red Blood Cell: anemia

Reproductive: endometriosis

Resistance Mechanism: abscess, bacterial infection, cellulitis, fever, fungal infection, herpes zoster, infection, inflammation, sepsis

Respiratory: adult respiratory distress syndrome, bronchitis, coughing, dyspnea, pleural effusion, pleurisy, pneumonia, pneumothorax, pulmonary edema, pulmonary infiltration, respiratory insufficiency, upper respiratory tract infection

Skin and Appendages: furunculosis, increased sweating, injection site inflammation, rash, ulceration

Urinary: azotemia, dysuria, hydronephrosis, kidney infarction, pyelonephritis, renal calculus, renal failure, ureteral obstruction

Vascular (Extracardiac): brain infarction, peripheral ischemia, pulmonary embolism, thrombophlebitis deep

White cell and Reticuloendothelial: leukopenia, lymphadenopathy, lymphangitis

A greater proportion of patients enrolled into the ATTRACT study who received REMICADE plus MTX experienced mild, transient elevations (<2 times the upper limit of normal) in AST or ALT (35% and 32% respectively) compared to patients treated with placebo with MTX (24% each). Six (1.8%) patients treated with REMICADE and MTX experienced more prolonged elevations in their ALT.

OVERDOSAGE:

Single doses up to 20 mg/kg have been administered without any direct toxic effect. In case of overdosage, it is recommended that the patient be monitored for any signs or symptoms of adverse reactions or effects and appropriate symptomatic treatment instituted immediately.

DOSAGE AND ADMINISTRATION:

Rheumatoid Arthritis

The recommended dose of REMICADE is 3mg/kg given as an intravenous infusion followed with additional similar doses at 2 and 6 weeks after the first infusion then every 8 weeks thereafter. REMICADE should be given in combi-

Continued on next page

Remicade—Cont.

nation with methotrexate. For patients who have an incomplete response, consideration may be given to adjusting the dose up to 10 mg/kg or treating as often as every 4 weeks.

Crohn's Disease

The recommended dose of REMICADE is 5 mg/kg given as a single intravenous infusion for treatment of moderately to severely active Crohn's disease. In patients with fistulizing disease, an initial 5 mg/kg dose should be followed with additional 5 mg/kg doses at 2 and 6 weeks after the first infusion.

There are insufficient safety and efficacy data for the use of REMICADE in Crohn's disease beyond the recommended duration (see *WARNINGS, Hypersensitivity; ADVERSE REACTIONS, Infusion-related Reactions;* and *INDICATIONS AND USAGE*).

Preparation and administration instructions: Use aseptic technique.

REMICADE vials do not contain antibacterial preservatives. Therefore, the vials after reconstitution should be used immediately, not re-entered or stored. The diluent to be used for reconstitution is 10 mL of Sterile Water for Injection, USP. The total dose of the reconstituted product must be further diluted to 250 mL with 0.9% Sodium Chloride Injection, USP. The infusion concentration should range between 0.4 mg/mL and 4 mg/mL. The REMICADE infusion should begin within 3 hours of preparation.

1. Calculate the dose and the number of REMICADE vials needed. Each REMICADE vial contains 100 mg of infliximab. Calculate the total volume of reconstituted REMICADE solution required.
2. Reconstitute each REMICADE vial with 10 mL of Sterile Water for Injection, USP, using a syringe equipped with a 21-gauge or smaller needle. Remove the flip-top from the vial and wipe the top with an alcohol swab. Insert the syringe needle into the vial through the center of the rubber stopper and direct the stream of Sterile Water for Injection, USP, to the glass wall of the vial. Do not use the vial if the vacuum is not present. Gently swirl the solution by rotating the vial to dissolve the lyophilized powder. Avoid prolonged or vigorous agitation. DO NOT SHAKE. Foaming of the solution on reconstitution is not unusual. Allow the reconstituted solution to stand for 5 minutes. The solution should be colorless to light yellow and opalescent, and the solution may develop a few translucent particles as infliximab is a protein. Do not use if opaque particles, discoloration, or other foreign particles are present.
3. Dilute the total volume of the reconstituted REMICADE solution dose to 250 mL with 0.9% Sodium Chloride Injection, USP, by withdrawing a volume of 0.9% Sodium Chloride Injection, USP, equal to the volume of reconstituted REMICADE from the 0.9% Sodium Chloride Injection, USP, 250 mL bottle or bag. Slowly add the total volume of reconstituted REMICADE solution to the 250 mL infusion bottle or bag. Gently mix.
4. The infusion solution must be administered over a period of not less than 2 hours and must use an infusion set with an in-line, sterile, non-pyrogenic, low-protein-binding filter (pore size of 1.2-μm or less). Any unused portion of the infusion solution should not be stored for reuse.
5. No physical biochemical compatibility studies have been conducted to evaluate the co-administration of REMICADE with other agents. REMICADE should not be infused concomitantly in the same intravenous line with other agents.
6. Parenteral drug products should be inspected visually for particulate matter and discoloration prior to administration, whenever solution and container permit. If visibly opaque particles, discoloration or other foreign particulates are observed, the solution should not be used.

Storage

Store the lyophilized product under refrigeration at 2°C to 8°C (36°F to 46°F). Do not freeze. Do not use beyond the expiration date. This product contains no preservative.

HOW SUPPLIED:

REMICADE lyophilized concentrate for IV injection is supplied in individually-boxed single-use vials in the following strength:

NDC 57894-030-01 100 mg infliximab in a 20-mL vial

REFERENCES:

1. Knight DM, Trinh H, Le J, et al. Construction and initial characterization of a mouse-human chimeric anti-TNF antibody. Molec *Immunol* 1993;30:1443–1453.
2. Scallon BJ, Moore MA, Trinh H, et al. Chimeric anti-TNFα monoclonal antibody cA2 binds recombinant transmembrane TNFα and activates immune effector functions. *Cytokine* 1995;7:251–259.
3. Siegel SA, Shealy DJ, Nakada MT, et al. The mouse/human chimeric monoclonal antibody cA2 neutralizes TNF *in vitro* and protects transgenic mice from cachexia and TNF lethality *in vivo. Cytokine* 1995;7:15–25.
4. Data on file.
5. Chu CQ, Field M, Feldmann M, et al. Localization of tumor necrosis factor α in synovial tissues and at the cartilage-pannus junction in patients with rheumatoid arthritis. *Arthritis and Rheum* 1991;34:1125–1132.
6. Braegger CP, Nicholls S, Murch SH, et al. Tumour necrosis factor alpha in stool as a marker of intestinal inflammation. *Lancet* 1992;339:89–91.
7. Felson DT, Anderson JJ, Boers M, et al. American College of Rheumatology preliminary definition of improvement in rheumatoid arthritis. *Arthritis Rheum* 1995;38(6):727–735.
8. Fries JF, Spitz PW, Young DY. The dimensions of health outcomes: the health assessment questionnaire, disability and pain scales. *J Rheumatol* 1982;9(5):789–793.
9. Ware JE Jr, Sherbourne CD. The MOS 36-item short-form health survey (SF-36). I. Conceptual framework and item selection. *Med Care* 1992;30(6):473–483.
10. Van der Heijde DM, van Leeuwen MA, van Riel PL, et al. Biannual radiographic assessments of hands and feet in a three-year prospective followup of patients with early rheumatoid arthritis. *Arthritis Rheum* 1992;35(1):26–34.
11. Maini RN, Breedveld FC, Kalden JR, et al. Therapeutic efficacy of multiple intravenous infusions of anti-tumor necrosis factor α monoclonal antibody combined with low-dose weekly methotrexate in rheumatoid arthritis. *Arthritis Rheum* 1998;41(9);1552–1563.
12. Elliott MJ, Maini RN, Feldmann M, et al. Randomised double-blind comparison of chimeric monoclonal antibody to tumour necrosis factor alpha (cA2) vs. placebo in rheumatoid arthritis. Lancet 1994;344(8930):1105-1110.
13. Targan SR, Hanauer SR, van Deventer SJH, et al. A short-term study of chimeric monoclonal antibody cA2 to tumor necrosis factor α for Crohn's disease. *N Engl J Med* 1997;337(15):1029–1035.
14. Present DH, Rutgeerts P, Targan S, et al. Infliximab for the treatment of fistulas in patients with Crohn's disease. N Engl J Med 1999;340:1398–1405.
15. American Thoracic Society, Centers for Disease Control and Prevention. Targeted tuberculin testing and treatment of latent tuberculosis infection. *Am J Respir Crit Care Med* 2000;161:S221–S247.
16. Greenstein AJ, Mullin GE, Strauchen JA, et al. Lymphoma in inflammatory bowel disease. *Cancer* 1992;69:1119–1121.
17. Jones M, Symmons D, Finn J, et al. Does exposure to immunosuppressive therapy increase the 10 year malignancy and mortality risks in rheumatoid arthritis? A matched cohort study. *Br J Rheum* 1996;35:738–745.

© Centocor, Inc. 2000 License #1242
Malvern, PA 19355, USA Revised 1 December 2000
1-800-457-6399 IN00160

DuPont Pharma
WILMINGTON, DE 19880

DUPONT PHARMA
Chestnut Run Plaza, Hickory Run
P.O. Box 80723
Wilmington, DE 19880-0723
(302) 992-5000
www.dupontpharma.com

Address all product-related inquiries to:
Medical Affairs Department

For Product Information/Adverse Drug Experience Reporting, call
Product Information
(302) 992-4240 or 1-800-474-2762

COUMADIN® TABLETS ℞
(Warfarin Sodium Tablets, USP) Crystalline
Anticoagulant

COUMADIN® FOR INJECTION ℞
(Warfarin Sodium for Injection, USP)
Rx only

Prescribing information for this product, which appears on pages 1137-1141 of the 2001 PDR, has been completely revised as follows. Please write "See Supplement A" next to the product heading.

DESCRIPTION

COUMADIN (crystalline warfarin sodium), is an anticoagulant which acts by inhibiting vitamin K-dependent coagulation factors. Chemically, it is 3-(α-acetonylbenzyl)-4-hydroxycoumarin and is a racemic mixture of the R- and S-enantiomers. Crystalline warfarin sodium is an isopropanol clathrate. The crystallization of warfarin sodium virtually eliminates trace impurities present in amorphous warfarin. Its empirical formula is $C_{19}H_{15}NaO_4$ and its structural formula may be represented by the following:

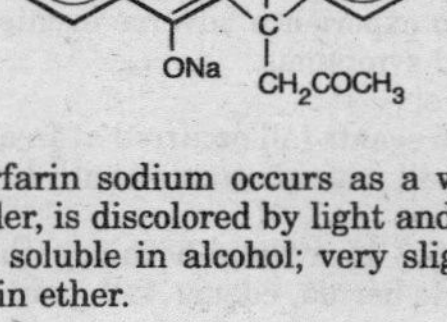

Crystalline warfarin sodium occurs as a white, odorless, crystalline powder, is discolored by light and is very soluble in water; freely soluble in alcohol; very slightly soluble in chloroform and in ether.

COUMADIN Tablets for oral use also contain:

All strengths:	Lactose, starch and magnesium stearate
1 mg:	D&C Red No. 6 Barium Lake
2 mg:	FD&C Blue No. 2 Aluminum Lake and FD&C Red No. 40 Aluminum Lake
2-1/2 mg:	D&C Yellow No. 10 Aluminum Lake and FD&C Blue No. 1 Aluminum Lake
3 mg:	FD&C Yellow No. 6 Aluminum Lake, FD&C Blue No. 2 Aluminum Lake and FD&C Red No. 40 Aluminum Lake
4 mg:	FD&C Blue No. 1 Aluminum Lake
5 mg:	FD&C Yellow No. 6 Aluminum Lake
6 mg:	FD&C Yellow No. 6 Aluminum Lake and FD&C Blue No. 1 Aluminum Lake
7-1/2 mg:	D&C Yellow No. 10 Aluminum Lake and FD&C Yellow No. 6 Aluminum Lake
10 mg:	Dye Free

COUMADIN for Injection is supplied as a sterile, lyophilized powder, which, after reconstitution with 2.7 mL sterile Water for Injection, contains:

Warfarin Sodium	2 mg/mL
Sodium Phosphate, Dibasic, Heptahydrate	4.98 mg/mL
Sodium Phosphate, Monobasic, Monohydrate	0.194 mg/mL
Sodium Chloride	0.1 mg/mL
Mannitol	38.0 mg/mL
Sodium Hydroxide, as needed for pH adjustment to	8.1 to 8.3

CLINICAL PHARMACOLOGY

COUMADIN and other coumarin anticoagulants act by inhibiting the synthesis of vitamin K dependent clotting factors, which include Factors II, VII, IX and X, and the anticoagulant proteins C and S. Half-lives of these clotting factors are as follows: Factor II — 60 hours, VII — 4–6 hours, IX — 24 hours, and X — 48–72 hours. The half-lives of proteins C and S are approximately 8 hours and 30 hours, respectively. The resultant *in vivo* effect is a sequential depression of Factors VII, IX, X and II activities. Vitamin K is an essential cofactor for the post ribosomal synthesis of the vitamin K dependent clotting factors. The vitamin promotes the biosynthesis of γ-carboxyglutamic acid residues in the proteins which are essential for biological activity. Warfarin is thought to interfere with clotting factor synthesis by inhibition of the regeneration of vitamin K_1 epoxide. The degree of depression is dependent upon the dosage administered. Therapeutic doses of warfarin decrease the total amount of the active form of each vitamin K dependent clotting factor made by the liver by approximately 30% to 50%. An anticoagulation effect generally occurs within 24 hours after drug administration. However, peak anticoagulant effect may be delayed 72 to 96 hours. The duration of action of a single dose of racemic warfarin is 2 to 5 days. The effects of COUMADIN may become more pronounced as effects of daily maintenance doses overlap. Anticoagulants have no direct effect on an established thrombus, nor do they reverse ischemic tissue damage. However, once a thrombus has occurred, the goal of anticoagulant treatment is to prevent further extension of the formed clot and prevent secondary thromboembolic complications which may result in serious and possibly fatal sequelae.

Pharmacokinetics: COUMADIN is a racemic mixture of the R- and S-enantiomers. The S-enantiomer exhibits 2–5 times more anticoagulant activity than the R-enantiomer in humans, but generally has a more rapid clearance.

Absorption: COUMADIN is essentially completely absorbed after oral administration with peak concentration generally attained within the first 4 hours.

Distribution: There are no differences in the apparent volumes of distribution after intravenous and oral administration of single doses of warfarin solution. Warfarin distributes into a relatively small apparent volume of distribution of about 0.14 liter/kg. A distribution phase lasting 6 to 12 hours is distinguishable after rapid intravenous or oral administration of an aqueous solution. Using a one compartment model, and assuming complete bioavailability, estimates of the volumes of distribution of R- and S-warfarin are similar to each other and to that of the racemate. Concentrations in fetal plasma approach the maternal values, but warfarin has not been found in human milk (see WARNINGS—Lactation). Approximately 99% of the drug is bound to plasma proteins.

Metabolism: The elimination of warfarin is almost entirely by metabolism. COUMADIN is stereoselectively metabolized by hepatic microsomal enzymes (cytochrome P-450) to inactive hydroxylated metabolites (predominant route) and by reductases to reduced metabolites (warfarin alcohols). The warfarin alcohols have minimal anticoagulant activity. The metabolites are principally excreted into the urine; and to a lesser extent into the bile. The metabolites of warfarin that have been identified include dehydrowarfarin, two diastereoisomer alcohols, 4'-, 6-, 7-, 8- and 10-hydroxywarfarin. The Cytochrome P-450 isozymes involved in the metabolism of warfarin include 2C9, 2C19, 2C8, 2C18, 1A2, and 3A4. 2C9 is likely to be the principal form of human liver P-450 which modulates the *in vivo* anticoagulant activity of warfarin.

Excretion: The terminal half-life of warfarin after a single dose is approximately one week; however, the effective half-life ranges from 20 to 60 hours, with a mean of about 40 hours. The clearance of R-warfarin is generally half that of S-warfarin; thus as the volumes of distribution are similar, the half-life of R-warfarin is longer than that of S-warfarin. The half-life of R-warfarin ranges from 37 to 89 hours, while that of S-warfarin ranges from 21 to 43 hours. Studies with radiolabeled drug have demonstrated that up to 92% of the orally administered dose is recovered in urine. Very little warfarin is excreted unchanged in urine. Urinary excretion is in the form of metabolites.

Elderly: Patients 60 years or older appear to exhibit greater than expected PT/INR response to the anticoagulant effects of warfarin. The cause of the increased sensitivity to the anticoagulant effects of warfarin in this age group is unknown. This increased anticoagulant effect from warfarin may be due to a combination of pharmacokinetic and pharmacodynamic factors. Racemic warfarin clearance may be unchanged or reduced with increasing age. Limited information suggests there is no difference in the clearance of S-warfarin in the elderly versus young subjects. However, there may be a slight decrease in the clearance of R-warfarin in the elderly as compared to the young. Therefore, as patient age increases, a lower dose of warfarin is usually required to produce a therapeutic level of anticoagulation.

Asians: Asian patients may require lower initiation and maintenance doses of warfarin. One non-controlled study conducted in 151 Chinese outpatients reported a mean daily warfarin requirement of 3.3±1.4 mg to achieve an INR of 2 to 2.5. These patients were stabilized on warfarin for various indications. Patient age was the most important determinant of warfarin requirement in Chinese patients with a progressively lower warfarin requirement with increasing age.

Renal Dysfunction: Renal clearance is considered to be a minor determinant of anticoagulant response to warfarin. No dosage adjustment is necessary for patients with renal failure.

Hepatic Dysfunction: Hepatic dysfunction can potentiate the response to warfarin through impaired synthesis of clotting factors and decreased metabolism of warfarin.

The administration of COUMADIN via the intravenous (IV) route should provide the patient with the same concentration of an equal oral dose, but maximum plasma concentration will be reached earlier. However, the full anticoagulant effect of a dose of warfarin may not be achieved until 72–96 hours after dosing, indicating that the administration of IV COUMADIN should not provide any increased biological effect or earlier onset of action.

Clinical Trials

Atrial Fibrillation (AF): In five prospective randomized controlled clinical trials involving 3711 patients with non-rheumatic AF, warfarin significantly reduced the risk of systemic thromboembolism including stroke (See Table 1). The risk reduction ranged from 60% to 86% in all except one trial (CAFA: 45%) which stopped early due to published positive results from two of these trials. The incidence of major bleeding in these trials ranged from 0.6 to 2.7% (See Table 1). Meta-analysis findings of these studies revealed that the effects of warfarin in reducing thromboembolic events including stroke were similar at either moderately high INR (2.0–4.5) or low INR (1.4–3.0). There was a significant reduction in minor bleeds at the low INR. Similar data from clinical studies in valvular atrial fibrillation patients are not available.

[See table 1 above]

TABLE 1
CLINICAL STUDIES OF WARFARIN IN NON-RHEUMATIC AF PATIENTS*

Study	N Warfarin-Treated Patients	N Control Patients	PT Ratio	INR	Thromboembolism % Risk Reduction	Thromboembolism *p*-value	% Major Bleeding Warfarin-Treated Patients	% Major Bleeding Control Patients
AFASAK	335	336	1.5–2.0	2.8–4.2	60	0.027	0.6	0.0
SPAF	210	211	1.3–1.8	2.0–4.5	67	0.01	1.9	1.9
BAATAF	212	208	1.2–1.5	1.5–2.7	86	<0.05	0.9	0.5
CAFA	187	191	1.3–1.6	2.0–3.0	45	0.25	2.7	0.5
SPINAF	260	265	1.2–1.5	1.4–2.8	79	0.001	2.3	1.5

* All study results of warfarin vs. control are based on intention-to-treat analysis and include ischemic stroke and systemic thromboembolism, excluding hemorrhage and transient ischemic attacks.

Myocardial Infarction: WARIS (The Warfarin Re-Infarction Study) was a double-blind, randomized study of 1214 patients 2 to 4 weeks post-infarction treated with warfarin to a target INR of 2.8 to 4.8. [But note that a lower INR was achieved and increased bleeding was associated with INR's above 4.0; (see DOSAGE AND ADMINISTRATION)]. The primary endpoint was a combination of total mortality and recurrent infarction. A secondary endpoint of cerebrovascular events was assessed. Mean follow-up of the patients was 37 months. The results for each endpoint separately, including an analysis of vascular death, are provided in the following table:

[See table 2 above]

TABLE 2

Event	Warfarin (N=607)	Placebo (N=607)	RR (95%CI)	% Risk Reduction (p-value)
Total Patient Years of Follow-up	2018	1944		
Total Mortality	94 (4.7/100 py)	123 (6.3/100 py)	0.76 (0.60, 0.97)	24 (p=0.030)
Vascular Death	82 (4.1/100 py)	105 (5.4/100 py)	0.78 (0.60, 1.02)	22 (p=0.068)
Recurrent MI	82 (4.1/100 py)	124 (6.4/100 py)	0.66 (0.51, 0.85)	34 (p=0.001)
Cerebrovascular Event	20 (1.0/100 py)	44 (2.3/100 py)	0.46 (0.28, 0.75)	54 (p=0.002)

RR=Relative risk; Risk reduction=(I - RR); CI=Confidence interval; MI=Myocardial infarction; py=patient years

Mechanical and Bioprosthetic Heart Valves: In a prospective, randomized, open label, positive-controlled study (Mok et al, 1985) in 254 patients, the thromboembolic-free interval was found to be significantly greater in patients with mechanical prosthetic heart valves treated with warfarin alone compared with dipyridamole-aspirin (p<0.005) and pentoxifylline-aspirin (p<0.05) treated patients. Rates of thromboembolic events in these groups were 2.2, 8.6, and 7.9/100 patient years, respectively. Major bleeding rates were 2.5, 0.0, and 0.9/100 patient years, respectively.

In a prospective, open label, clinical trial (Saour et al, 1990) comparing moderate (INR 2.65) vs. high intensity (INR 9.0) warfarin therapies in 258 patients with mechanical prosthetic heart valves, thromboembolism occurred with similar frequency in the two groups (4.0 and 3.7 events/100 patient years, respectively). Major bleeding was more common in the high intensity group (2.1 events/100 patient years) vs. 0.95 events/100 patient years in the moderate intensity group.

In a randomized trial (Turpie et al, 1988) in 210 patients comparing two intensities of warfarin therapy (INR 2.0–2.25 vs. INR 2.5–4.0) for a three-month period following tissue heart valve replacement, thromboembolism occurred with similar frequency in the two groups (major embolic events 2.0% vs. 1.9%, respectively and minor embolic events 10.8% vs. 10.2%, respectively). Major bleeding complications were more frequent with the higher intensity (major hemorrhages 4.6%) vs. none in the lower intensity.

INDICATIONS AND USAGE

COUMADIN is indicated for the prophylaxis and/or treatment of venous thrombosis and its extension, and pulmonary embolism.

COUMADIN is indicated for the prophylaxis and/or treatment of the thromboembolic complications associated with atrial fibrillation and/or cardiac valve replacement.

COUMADIN is indicated to reduce the risk of death, recurrent myocardial infarction, and thromboembolic events such as stroke or systemic embolization after myocardial infarction.

CONTRAINDICATIONS

Anticoagulation is contraindicated in any localized or general physical condition or personal circumstance in which the hazard of hemorrhage might be greater than the potential clinical benefits of anticoagulation, such as:

Pregnancy: COUMADIN is contraindicated in women who are or may become pregnant because the drug passes through the placental barrier and may cause fatal hemorrhage to the fetus *in utero*. Furthermore, there have been reports of birth malformations in children born to mothers who have been treated with warfarin during pregnancy.

Embryopathy characterized by nasal hypoplasia with or without stippled epiphyses (chondrodysplasia punctata) has been reported in pregnant women exposed to warfarin during the first trimester. Central nervous system abnormalities also have been reported, including dorsal midline dysplasia characterized by agenesis of the corpus callosum, Dandy-Walker malformation, and midline cerebellar atrophy. Ventral midline dysplasia, characterized by optic atrophy, and eye abnormalities have been observed. Mental retardation, blindness, and other central nervous system abnormalities have been reported in association with second and third trimester exposure. Although rare, teratogenic reports following *in utero* exposure to warfarin include urinary tract anomalies such as single kidney, asplenia, anencephaly, spina bifida, cranial nerve palsy, hydrocephalus, cardiac defects and congenital heart disease, polydactyly, deformities of toes, diaphragmatic hernia, corneal leukoma, cleft palate, cleft lip, schizencephaly, and microcephaly.

Spontaneous abortion and still birth are known to occur and a higher risk of fetal mortality is associated with the use of warfarin. Low birth weight and growth retardation have also been reported.

Women of childbearing potential who are candidates for anticoagulant therapy should be carefully evaluated and the indications critically reviewed with the patient. If the patient becomes pregnant while taking this drug, she should be apprised of the potential risks to the fetus, and the possibility of termination of the pregnancy should be discussed in light of those risks.

Hemorrhagic tendencies or blood dyscrasias.

Recent or contemplated surgery of: (1) central nervous system; (2) eye; (3) traumatic surgery resulting in large open surfaces.

Bleeding tendencies associated with active ulceration or overt bleeding of: (1) gastrointestinal, genitourinary or respiratory tracts; (2) cerebrovascular hemorrhage; (3) aneurysms-cerebral, dissecting aorta; (4) pericarditis and pericardial effusions; (5) bacterial endocarditis.

Threatened abortion, eclampsia and preeclampsia.

Inadequate laboratory facilities.

Unsupervised patients with senility, alcoholism, or psychosis or other lack of patient cooperation.

Spinal puncture and other diagnostic or therapeutic procedures with potential for uncontrollable bleeding.

Miscellaneous: major regional, lumbar block anesthesia, malignant hypertension and known hypersensitivity to warfarin or to any other components of this product.

WARNINGS

The most serious risks associated with anticoagulant therapy with warfarin sodium are hemorrhage in any tissue or organ and, less frequently (<0.1%), necrosis and/or gangrene of skin and other tissues. The risk of hemorrhage is related to the level of intensity and the duration of anticoagulant therapy. Hemorrhage and necrosis have in some cases been reported to result in death or permanent disability. Necrosis appears to be associated with local thrombosis and usually appears within a few days of the start of anticoagulant therapy. In severe cases of necrosis, treatment through debridement or amputation of the affected tissue, limb, breast or penis has been reported. Careful diagnosis is required to determine whether necrosis is caused by an underlying disease. Warfarin therapy should be discontinued when warfarin is suspected to be the cause of developing necrosis and heparin therapy may be considered for anticoagulation. Although various treatments have been attempted, no treatment for necrosis has been considered uniformly effective. See below for information on predisposing conditions. These and other risks associated with anticoagulant therapy must be weighed against the risk of thrombosis or embolization in untreated cases.

It cannot be emphasized too strongly that treatment of each patient is a highly individualized matter. COUMADIN (Warfarin Sodium), a narrow therapeutic range (index) drug, may be affected by factors such as other drugs and dietary Vitamin K. Dosage should be controlled by periodic determinations of prothrombin time (PT)/International Normalized Ratio (INR) or other suitable coagulation tests. Determinations of whole blood clotting and bleeding times are not effective measures for control of therapy. Heparin prolongs the one-stage PT. When heparin and COUMADIN are administered concomitantly, refer below to CONVERSION FROM HEPARIN THERAPY for recommendations.

Caution should be observed when COUMADIN is administered in any situation or in the presence of any predisposing condition where added risk of hemorrhage, necrosis, and/or gangrene is present.

Anticoagulation therapy with COUMADIN may enhance the release of atheromatous plaque emboli, thereby increasing the risk of complications from systemic cholesterol microembolization, including the "purple toes syndrome." Discontinuation of COUMADIN therapy is recommended when such phenomena are observed.

Systemic atheroemboli and cholesterol microemboli can present with a variety of signs and symptoms including purple toes syndrome, livedo reticularis, rash, gangrene, abrupt and intense pain in the leg, foot, or toes, foot ulcers, myalgia, penile gangrene, abdominal pain, flank or back pain, hematuria, renal insufficiency, hypertension, cerebral ischemia, spinal cord infarction, pancreatitis, symptoms simulating polyarteritis, or any other sequelae of vascular compromise due to embolic occlusion. The most commonly involved visceral organs are the kidneys followed by the pancreas, spleen, and liver. Some cases have progressed to necrosis or death.

Purple toes syndrome is a complication of oral anticoagulation characterized by a dark, purplish or mottled color of the toes, usually occurring between 3–10 weeks, or later, after the initiation of therapy with warfarin or related compounds. Major features of this syndrome include purple color of plantar surfaces and sides of the toes that blanches on moderate pressure and fades with elevation of the legs; pain and tenderness of the toes; waxing and waning of the color over time. While the purple toes syndrome is reported to be reversible, some cases progress to gangrene or necrosis which may require debridement of the affected area, or may lead to amputation.

Heparin-induced thrombocytopenia: COUMADIN should be used with caution in patients with heparin-induced thrombocytopenia and deep venous thrombosis. Cases of venous limb ischemia, necrosis, and gangrene have occurred in patients with heparin-induced thrombocytopenia and deep venous thrombosis when heparin treatment was discontin-

Continued on next page

Coumadin—Cont.

ued and warfarin therapy was started or continued. In some patients sequelae have included amputation of the involved area and/or death (Warkentin et al, 1997).

A severe elevation (>50 seconds) in activated partial thromboplastin time (aPTT) with a PT/INR in the desired range has been identified as an indication of increased risk of postoperative hemorrhage.

The decision to administer anticoagulants in the following conditions must be based upon clinical judgment in which the risks of anticoagulant therapy are weighed against the benefits:

Lactation: Based on very limited published data, warfarin has not been detected in the breast milk of mothers treated with warfarin. The same limited published data reports that breast-fed infants, whose mothers were treated with warfarin, had neither detectable warfarin in their plasma, nor clinically significant changes in coagulation tests. Although warfarin was not detected in the plasma of the breast-fed infants, the possibility of an anticoagulant effect by warfarin cannot be excluded. It is prudent to perform coagulation tests on infants at risk for bleeding tendencies before advising women taking warfarin to breast-feed. Effects in premature infants have not been evaluated.

Severe to moderate hepatic or renal insufficiency.
Infectious diseases or disturbances of intestinal flora: sprue, antibiotic therapy.
Trauma which may result in internal bleeding.
Surgery or trauma resulting in large exposed raw surfaces.
Indwelling catheters.

Severe to moderate hypertension.
Known or suspected deficiency in protein C mediated anticoagulant response: Hereditary or acquired deficiencies of protein C or its cofactor, protein S, have been associated with tissue necrosis following warfarin administration. Not all patients with these conditions develop necrosis, and tissue necrosis occurs in patients without these deficiencies. Inherited resistance to activated protein C has been described in many patients with venous thromboembolic disorders but has not yet been evaluated as a risk factor for tissue necrosis. The risk associated with these conditions, both for recurrent thrombosis and for adverse reactions, is difficult to evaluate since it does not appear to be the same for everyone. Decisions about testing and therapy must be made on an individual basis. It has been reported that concomitant anticoagulation therapy with heparin for 5 to 7 days during initiation of therapy with COUMADIN may minimize the incidence of tissue necrosis. Warfarin therapy should be discontinued when warfarin is suspected to be the cause of developing necrosis and heparin therapy may be considered for anticoagulation.
Miscellaneous: polycythemia vera, vasculitis, and severe diabetes.

Minor and severe allergic/hypersensitivity reactions and anaphylactic reactions have been reported.

In patients with acquired or inherited warfarin resistance, decreased therapeutic responses to COUMADIN have been reported. Exaggerated therapeutic responses have been reported in other patients.

Patients with congestive heart failure may exhibit greater than expected PT/INR response to COUMADIN, thereby requiring more frequent laboratory monitoring, and reduced doses of COUMADIN.

Concomitant use of anticoagulants with streptokinase or urokinase is not recommended and may be hazardous. (Please note recommendations accompanying these preparations.)

PRECAUTIONS

Periodic determination of PT/INR or other suitable coagulation test is essential.

Numerous factors, alone or in combination, including travel, changes in diet, environment, physical state and medication, including botanicals, may influence response of the patient to anticoagulants. It is generally good practice to monitor the patient's response with additional PT/INR determinations in the period immediately after discharge from the hospital, and whenever other medications, including botanicals, are initiated, discontinued or taken irregularly. The following factors are listed for reference; however, other factors may also affect the anticoagulant response.

Drugs may interact with COUMADIN through pharmacodynamic or pharmacokinetic mechanisms. Pharmacodynamic mechanisms for drug interactions with COUMADIN are synergism (impaired hemostasis, reduced clotting factor synthesis), competitive antagonism (vitamin K), and altered physiologic control loop for vitamin K metabolism (hereditary resistance). Pharmacokinetic mechanisms for drug interactions with COUMADIN are mainly enzyme induction, enzyme inhibition, and reduced plasma protein binding. It is important to note that some drugs may interact by more than one mechanism.

The following factors, alone or in combination, may be responsible for INCREASED PT/INR response:
[See table to the left]
The following factors, alone or in combination, may be responsible for DECREASED PT/INR response:

ENDOGENOUS FACTORS:

blood dyscrasias - see CONTRAINDICATIONS	diarrhea	hyperthyroidism
cancer	elevated temperature	poor nutritional state
collagen vascular disease	hepatic disorders	steatorrhea
congestive heart failure	infectious hepatitis	vitamin K deficiency
	jaundice	

EXOGENOUS FACTORS:
Potential drug interactions with COUMADIN are listed below by drug class and by specific drugs.

Classes of Drugs

5-lipoxygenase Inhibitor	Antiplatelet Drugs/Effects	Leukotriene Receptor Antagonist
Adrenergic Stimulants, Central	Antithyroid Drugs†	Monoamine Oxidase Inhibitors
Alcohol Abuse Reduction Preparations	Beta-Adrenergic Blockers	Narcotics, prolonged
Analgesics	Cholelitholytic Agents	Nonsteroidal Anti-Inflammatory Agents
Anesthetics, Inhalation	Diabetes Agents, Oral	Psychostimulants
Antiandrogen	Diuretics†	Pyrazolones
Antiarrhythmics†	Fungal Medications, Systemic†	Salicylates
Antibiotics†	Gastric Acidity and Peptic Ulcer Agents†	Selective Serotonin Reuptake Inhibitors
Aminoglycosides (oral)	Gastrointestinal Prokinetic Agents	Steroids, Adrenocortical†
Cephalosporins, parenteral	Ulcerative Colitis Agents	Steroids, Anabolic (17-Alkyl Testosterone Derivatives)
Macrolides	Gout Treatment Agents	Thrombolytics
Miscellaneous	Hemorrheologic Agents	Thyroid Drugs
Penicillins, intravenous, high dose	Hepatotoxic Drugs	Tuberculosis Agents†
Quinolones (fluoroquinolones)	Hyperglycemic Agents	Uricosuric Agents
Sulfonamides, long acting	Hypertensive Emergency Agents	Vaccines
Tetracyclines	Hypnotics†	Vitamins†
Anticoagulants	Hypolipidemics†	
Anticonvulsants†	Bile Acid-Binding Resins†	
Antidepressants†	Fibric Acid Derivatives	
Antimalarial Agents	HMG-CoA Reductase Inhibitors†	
Antineoplastics†		
Antiparasitic/Antimicrobials		

Specific Drugs Reported

acetaminophen	fluconazole	paroxetine
alcohol†	fluorouracil	penicillin G, intravenous
allopurinol	fluoxetine	pentoxifylline
aminosalicylic acid	flutamide	phenylbutazone
amiodarone HCl	fluvastatin	phenytoin†
aspirin	fluvoxamine	piperacillin
azithromycin	gemfibrozil	piroxicam
capecitabine	glucagon	prednisone†
cefamandole	halothane	propafenone
cefazolin	heparin	propoxyphene
cefoperazone	ibuprofen	propranolol
cefotetan	ifosfamide	propylthiouracil†
cefoxitin	indomethacin	quinidine
ceftriaxone	influenza virus vaccine	quinine
celecoxib	itraconazole	ranitidine†
cerivastatin	ketoprofen	rofecoxib
chenodiol	ketorolac	sertraline
chloramphenicol	levamisole	simvastatin
chloral hydrate†	levofloxacin	stanozolol
chlorpropamide	levothyroxine	streptokinase
cholestyramine†	liothyronine	sulfamethizole
cimetidine	lovastatin	sulfamethoxazole
ciprofloxacin	mefenamic acid	sulfinpyrazone
cisapride	methimazole†	sulfisoxazole
clarithromycin	methyldopa	sulindac
clofibrate	methylphenidate	tamoxifen
COUMADIN overdose	methylsalicylate ointment (topical)	tetracycline
cyclophosphamide†	metronidazole	thyroid
danazol	miconazole	ticarcillin
dextran	moricizine hydrochloride†	ticlopidine
dextrothyroxine	nalidixic acid	tissue plasminogen activator (t-PA)
diazoxide	naproxen	tolbutamide
diclofenac	neomycin	tramadol
dicumarol	norfloxacin	trimethoprim/sulfamethoxazole
diflunisal	ofloxacin	urokinase
disulfiram	olsalazine	valproate
doxycycline	omeprazole	vitamin E
erythromycin	oxaprozin	zafirlukast
ethacrynic acid	oxymetholone	zileuton
fenofibrate		
fenoprofen		

also: other medications affecting blood elements which may modify hemostasis
   dietary deficiencies
   prolonged hot weather
   unreliable PT/INR determinations
†Increased and decreased PT/INR responses have been reported.

ENDOGENOUS FACTORS:

edema	hypothyroidism
hereditary coumarin resistance	nephrotic syndrome
hyperlipemia	

EXOGENOUS FACTORS:
Potential drug interactions with COUMADIN (Warfarin Sodium) are listed below by drug class and by specific drugs.
[See first table at top of next page]
Because a patient may be exposed to a combination of the above factors, the net effect of COUMADIN on PT/INR response may be unpredictable. More frequent PT/INR monitoring is therefore advisable. Medications of unknown interaction with coumarins are best regarded with caution. When these medications are started or stopped, more frequent PT/INR monitoring is advisable.

It has been reported that concomitant administration of warfarin and ticlopidine may be associated with cholestatic hepatitis.

Botanical (Herbal) Medicines: Caution should be exercised when botanical medicines (botanicals) are taken concomitantly with COUMADIN. Few adequate, well-controlled studies exist evaluating the potential for metabolic and/or pharmacologic interactions between botanicals and COUMADIN. Due to a lack of manufacturing standardization with botanical medicinal preparations, the amount of active ingredients may vary. This could further confound the ability to assess potential interactions and effects on anticoagulation. It is good practice to monitor the patient's response with additional PT/INR determinations when initiating or discontinuing botanicals.

Specific botanicals reported to affect COUMADIN therapy include the following:

• Bromelains, danshen, dong quai (*Angelica sinensis*), garlic, and Ginkgo biloba are associated most often with an INCREASE in the effects of COUMADIN.

Classes of Drugs

Adrenal Corticol Steroid Inhibitors	Antipsychotic Medications	Hypolipidemics†
Antacids	Antithyroid Drugs†	Bile Acid-Binding Resins†
Antianxiety Agents	Barbiturates	HMG-CoA Reductase
Antiarrhythmics†	Diuretics†	Inhibitors†
Antibiotics†	Enteral Nutritional Supplements	Immunosuppressives
Anticonvulsants†	Fungal Medications, Systemic†	Oral Contraceptives, Estrogen
Antidepressants†	Gastric Acidity and Peptic	Containing
Antihistamines	Ulcer Agents†	Selective Estrogen Receptor
Antineoplastics†	Hypnotics†	Modulators
		Steroids, Adrenocortical†
		Tuberculosis Agents†
		Vitamins†

Specific Drugs Reported

alcohol†	COUMADIN underdosage	phenobarbital
aminoglutethimide	cyclophosphamide†	phenytoin†
amobarbital	dicloxacillin	prednisone†
atorvastatin	ethchlorvynol	primidone
azathioprine	glutethimide	propylthiouracil†
butabarbital	griseofulvin	raloxifene
butalbital	haloperidol	ranitidine†
carbamazepine	meprobamate	rifampin
chloral hydrate†	6-mercaptopurine	secobarbital
chlordiazepoxide	methimazole†	spironolactone
chlorthalidone	moricizine hydrochloride†	sucralfate
cholestyramine†	nafcillin	trazodone
clozapine	paraldehyde	vitamin C (high dose)
corticotropin	pentobarbital	vitamin K
cortisone		

also: diet high in vitamin K
      unreliable PT/INR determinations
†Increased and decreased PT/INR responses have been reported.

Botanicals that contain coumarins with potential anticoagulant effects:

Alfalfa	Celery	Parsley
Angelica (Dong Quai)	Chamomile (German and	Passion Flower
Aniseed	Roman)	Prickly Ash (Northern)
Arnica	Dandelion[3]	Quassia
Asa Foetida	Fenugreek	Red Clover
Bogbean[1]	Horse Chestnut	Sweet Clover
Boldo	Horseradish	Sweet Woodruff
Buchu	Licorice[3]	Tonka Beans
Capsicum[2]	Meadowsweet[1]	Wild Carrot
Cassia[3]	Nettle	Wild Lettuce

Miscellaneous botanicals with anticoagulant properties:

Bladder Wrack (*Fucus*)	Pau d'arco	

Botanicals that contain salicylate and/or have antiplatelet properties:

Agrimony[4]	Dandelion[3]	Meadowsweet[1]
Aloe Gel	Feverfew	Onion[5]
Aspen	Garlic[5]	Policosanol
Black Cohosh	German Sarsaparilla	Poplar
Black Haw	Ginger	Senega
Bogbean[1]	Ginkgo Biloba	Tamarind
Cassia[3]	Ginseng (*Panax*)[5]	Willow
Clove	Licorice[3]	Wintergreen

Botanicals with fibrinolytic properties:

Bromelains	Garlic[5]	Inositol Nicotinate
Capsicum[2]	Ginseng (*Panax*)[5]	Onion[5]

Botanicals with coagulant properties:

Agrimony[4]	Mistletoe	
Goldenseal	Yarrow	

[1]Contains coumarins and salicylate.
[2]Contains coumarins and has fibrinolytic properties.
[3]Contains coumarins and has antiplatelet properties.
[4]Contains salicylate and has coagulant properties.
[5]Has antiplatelet and fibrinolytic properties.

- Coenzyme Q[10] (ubidecarenone) and St. John's wort are associated most often with a DECREASE in the effects of COUMADIN.

Some botanicals may cause bleeding events when taken alone (e.g., garlic and Ginkgo biloba) and may have anticoagulant, antiplatelet, and/or fibrinolytic properties. These effects would be expected to be additive to the anticoagulant effects of COUMADIN. Conversely, other botanicals may have coagulant properties when taken alone or may decrease the effects of COUMADIN.

Some botanicals that may affect coagulation are listed below for reference; however, this list should not be considered all-inclusive. Many botanicals have several common names and scientific names. The most widely recognized common botanical names are listed.
[See second table above]

Effect on Other Drugs: Coumarins may also affect the action of other drugs. Hypoglycemic agents (chlorpropamide and tolbutamide) and anticonvulsants (phenytoin and phenobarbital) may accumulate in the body as a result of interference with either their metabolism or excretion.

Special Risk Patients: COUMADIN is a narrow therapeutic range (index) drug, and caution should be observed when warfarin sodium is administered to certain patients such as

the elderly or debilitated or when administered in any situation or physical condition where added risk of hemorrhage is present.

Intramuscular (I.M.) injections of concomitant medications should be confined to the upper extremities which permits easy access for manual compression, inspections for bleeding and use of pressure bandages.

Caution should be observed when COUMADIN (or warfarin) is administered concomitantly with nonsteroidal anti-inflammatory drugs (NSAIDs), including aspirin, to be certain that no change in anticoagulation dosage is required. In addition to specific drug interactions that might affect PT/INR, NSAIDs, including aspirin, can inhibit platelet aggregation, and can cause gastrointestinal bleeding, peptic ulceration and/or perforation.

Acquired or inherited warfarin resistance should be suspected if large daily doses of COUMADIN are required to maintain a patient's PT/INR within a normal therapeutic range.

Information for Patients: The objective of anticoagulant therapy is to decrease the clotting ability of the blood so that thrombosis is prevented, while avoiding spontaneous bleeding. Effective therapeutic levels with minimal complications are in part dependent upon cooperative and well-instructed

patients who communicate effectively with their physician. Patients should be advised: Strict adherence to prescribed dosage schedule is necessary. Do not take or discontinue any other medication, including salicylates (e.g., aspirin and topical analgesics), other over-the-counter medications, and botanical (herbal) products (e.g., bromelains, coenzyme Q[10], danshen, dong quai, garlic, Ginkgo biloba, and St. John's wort) except on advice of the physician. Avoid alcohol consumption. Do not take COUMADIN during pregnancy and do not become pregnant while taking it (see CONTRAINDICATIONS). Avoid any activity or sport that may result in traumatic injury. Prothrombin time tests and regular visits to physician or clinic are needed to monitor therapy. Carry identification stating that COUMADIN is being taken. If the prescribed dose of COUMADIN is forgotten, notify the physician immediately. Take the dose as soon as possible on the same day but do not take a double dose of COUMADIN the next day to make up for missed doses. The amount of vitamin K in food may affect therapy with COUMADIN. Eat a normal, balanced diet maintaining a consistent amount of vitamin K. Avoid drastic changes in dietary habits, such as eating large amounts of green leafy vegetables. Contact physician to report any illness, such as diarrhea, infection or fever. Notify physician immediately if any unusual bleeding or symptoms occur. Signs and symptoms of bleeding include: pain, swelling or discomfort, prolonged bleeding from cuts, increased menstrual flow or vaginal bleeding, nosebleeds, bleeding of gums from brushing, unusual bleeding or bruising, red or dark brown urine, red or tar black stools, headache, dizziness, or weakness. If therapy with COUMADIN is discontinued, patients should be cautioned that the anticoagulant effects of COUMADIN may persist for about 2 to 5 days. **Patients should be informed that all warfarin sodium, USP, products represent the same medication, and should not be taken concomitantly, as overdosage may result.**

Carcinogenesis, Mutagenesis, Impairment of Fertility: Carcinogenicity and mutagenicity studies have not been performed with COUMADIN. The reproductive effects of COUMADIN have not been evaluated.

Use in Pregnancy: Pregnancy Category X—See CONTRAINDICATIONS.

Pediatric Use: Safety and effectiveness in pediatric patients below the age of 18 have not been established, in randomized, controlled clinical trials. However, the use of COUMADIN in pediatric patients is well-documented for the prevention and treatment of thromboembolic events. Difficulty achieving and maintaining therapeutic PT/INR ranges in the pediatric patient has been reported. More frequent PT/INR determinations are recommended because of possible changing warfarin requirements.

Geriatric Use: Patients 60 years or older appear to exhibit greater than expected PT/INR response to the anticoagulant effects of warfarin (see CLINICAL PHARMACOLOGY). COUMADIN is contraindicated in any unsupervised patient with senility. Caution should be observed with administration of warfarin sodium to elderly patients in any situation or physical condition where added risk of hemorrhage is present. Low initiation and maintenance doses of COUMADIN are recommended for elderly patients (see DOSAGE AND ADMINISTRATION).

ADVERSE REACTIONS

Potential adverse reactions to COUMADIN may include:

- Fatal or nonfatal hemorrhage from any tissue or organ. This is a consequence of the anticoagulant effect. The signs, symptoms, and severity will vary according to the location and degree or extent of the bleeding. Hemorrhagic complications may present as paralysis; paresthesia; headache, chest, abdomen, joint, muscle or other pain; dizziness; shortness of breath, difficult breathing or swallowing; unexplained swelling; weakness; hypotension; or unexplained shock. Therefore, the possibility of hemorrhage should be considered in evaluating the condition of any anticoagulated patient with complaints which do not indicate an obvious diagnosis. Bleeding during anticoagulant therapy does not always correlate with PT/INR. (See OVERDOSAGE—Treatment.)
- Bleeding which occurs when the PT/INR is within the therapeutic range warrants diagnostic investigation since it may unmask a previously unsuspected lesion, e.g., tumor, ulcer, etc.
- Necrosis of skin and other tissues. (See WARNINGS.)
- Adverse reactions reported infrequently include: hypersensitivity/allergic reactions, systemic cholesterol microembolization, purple toes syndrome, hepatitis, cholestatic hepatic injury, jaundice, elevated liver enzymes, vasculitis, edema, fever, rash, dermatitis, including bullous eruptions, urticaria, abdominal pain including cramping, flatulence/bloating, fatigue, lethargy, malaise, asthenia, nausea, vomiting, diarrhea, pain, headache, dizziness, taste perversion, pruritus, alopecia, cold intolerance, and paresthesia including feeling cold and chills.

Rare events of tracheal or tracheobronchial calcification have been reported in association with long-term warfarin therapy. The clinical significance of this event is unknown. Priapism has been associated with anticoagulant administration, however, a causal relationship has not been established.

OVERDOSAGE

Signs and Symptoms: Suspected or overt abnormal bleeding (e.g., appearance of blood in stools or urine, hematuria, excessive menstrual bleeding, melena, petechiae, excessive bruising or persistent oozing from superficial injuries) are early manifestations of anticoagulation beyond a safe and satisfactory level.

Continued on next page

Coumadin—Cont.

Treatment: Excessive anticoagulation, with or without bleeding, may be controlled by discontinuing COUMADIN therapy and if necessary, by administration of oral or parenteral vitamin K_1. (Please see recommendations accompanying vitamin K_1 preparations prior to use.)

Such use of vitamin K_1 reduces response to subsequent COUMADIN therapy. Patients may return to a pretreatment thrombotic status following the rapid reversal of a prolonged PT/INR. Resumption of COUMADIN administration reverses the effect of vitamin K, and a therapeutic PT/INR can again be obtained by careful dosage adjustment. If rapid anticoagulation is indicated, heparin may be preferable for initial therapy.

If minor bleeding progresses to major bleeding, give 5 to 25 mg (rarely up to 50 mg) parenteral vitamin K_1. In emergency situations of severe hemorrhage, clotting factors can be returned to normal by administering 200 to 500 mL of fresh whole blood or fresh frozen plasma, or by giving commercial Factor IX complex.

A risk of hepatitis and other viral diseases is associated with the use of these blood products; Factor IX complex is also associated with an increased risk of thrombosis. Therefore, these preparations should be used only in exceptional or life-threatening bleeding episodes secondary to COUMADIN (Warfarin Sodium) overdosage.

Purified Factor IX preparations should not be used because they cannot increase the levels of prothrombin, Factor VII and Factor X which are also depressed along with the levels of Factor IX as a result of COUMADIN treatment. Packed red blood cells may also be given if significant blood loss has occurred. Infusions of blood or plasma should be monitored carefully to avoid precipitating pulmonary edema in elderly patients or patients with heart disease.

DOSAGE AND ADMINISTRATION

The dosage and administration of COUMADIN must be individualized for each patient according to the particular patient's PT/INR response to the drug. The dosage should be adjusted based upon the patient's PT/INR. (See LABORATORY CONTROL below for full discussion on INR.)

Venous Thromboembolism (including pulmonary embolism): Available clinical evidence indicates that an INR of 2.0–3.0 is sufficient for prophylaxis and treatment of venous thromboembolism and minimizes the risk of hemorrhage associated with higher INRs. In patients with risk factors for recurrent venous thromboembolism including venous insufficiency, inherited thrombophilia, idiopathic venous thromboembolism, and a history of thrombotic events, consideration should be given to longer term therapy (Schulman et al, 1995 and Schulman et al, 1997).

Atrial Fibrillation: Five recent clinical trials evaluated the effects of warfarin in patients with non-valvular atrial fibrillation (AF). Meta-analysis findings of these studies revealed that the effects of warfarin in reducing thromboembolic events including stroke were similar at either moderately high INR (2.0–4.5) or low INR (1.4–3.0). There was a significant reduction in minor bleeds at the low INR. Similar data from clinical studies in valvular atrial fibrillation patients are not available. The trials in non-valvular atrial fibrillation support the American College of Chest Physicians' (ACCP) recommendation that an INR of 2.0–3.0 be used for long term warfarin therapy in appropriate AF patients.

Post-Myocardial Infarction: In post-myocardial infarction patients, COUMADIN therapy should be initiated early (2–4 weeks post-infarction) and dosage should be adjusted to maintain an INR of 2.5–3.5 long-term. The recommendation is based on the results of the WARIS study in which treatment was initiated 2 to 4 weeks after the infarction. In patients thought to be at an increased risk of bleeding complications or on aspirin therapy, maintenance of COUMADIN therapy at the lower end of this INR range is recommended.

Mechanical and Bioprosthetic Heart Valves: In patients with mechanical heart valve(s), long term prophylaxis with warfarin to an INR of 2.5–3.5 is recommended. In patients with bioprosthetic heart valve(s), based on limited data, the American College of Chest Physicians recommends warfarin therapy to an INR of 2.0–3.0 for 12 weeks after valve insertion. In patients with additional risk factors such as atrial fibrillation or prior thromboembolism, consideration should be given for longer term therapy.

Recurrent Systemic Embolism: In cases where the risk of thromboembolism is great, such as in patients with recurrent systemic embolism, a higher INR may be required.

An INR of greater than 4.0 appears to provide no additional therapeutic benefit in most patients and is associated with a higher risk of bleeding.

Initial Dosage: The dosing of COUMADIN must be individualized according to patient's sensitivity to the drug as indicated by the PT/INR. Use of a large loading dose may increase the incidence of hemorrhagic and other complications, does not offer more rapid protection against thrombi formation, and is not recommended. Lower initiation and maintenance doses are recommended for elderly and/or debilitated patients and patients with potential to exhibit greater than expected PT/INR response to COUMADIN (see PRECAUTIONS). Based on limited data, Asian patients may also require lower initiation and maintenance doses of COUMADIN (see CLINICAL PHARMACOLOGY). It is recommended that COUMADIN therapy be initiated with a dose of 2 to 5 mg per day with dosage adjustments based on the results of PT/INR determinations.

TABLE 3
Relationship Between INR and PT Ratios For Thromboplastins With Different ISI Values (Sensitivities)

	PT RATIOS				
	ISI 1.0	ISI 1.4	ISI 1.8	ISI 2.3	ISI 2.8
INR = 2.0–3.0	2.0–3.0	1.6–2.2	1.5–1.8	1.4–1.6	1.3–1.5
INR = 2.5–3.5	2.5–3.5	1.9–2.4	1.7–2.0	1.5–1.7	1.4–1.6

	100's	1000's	Hospital Unit-Dose Blister Package of 100
1 mg pink	NDC 0056-0169-70	NDC 0056-0169-90	NDC 0056-0169-75
2 mg lavender	NDC 0056-0170-70	NDC 0056-0170-90	NDC 0056-0170-75
2-1/2 mg green	NDC 0056-0176-70	NDC 0056-0176-90	NDC 0056-0176-75
3 mg tan	NDC 0056-0188-70	NDC 0056-0188-90	NDC 0056-0188-75
4 mg blue	NDC 0056-0168-70	NDC 0056-0168-90	NDC 0056-0168-75
5 mg peach	NDC 0056-0172-70	NDC 0056-0172-90	NDC 0056-0172-75
6 mg teal	NDC 0056-0189-70	NDC 0056-0189-90	NDC 0056-0189-75
7-1/2 mg yellow	NDC 0056-0173-70		NDC 0056-0173-75
10 mg white (Dye Free)	NDC 0056-0174-70		NDC 0056-0174-75

Maintenance: Most patients are satisfactorily maintained at a dose of 2 to 10 mg daily. Flexibility of dosage is provided by breaking scored tablets in half. The individual dose and interval should be gauged by the patient's prothrombin response.

Duration of Therapy: The duration of therapy in each patient should be individualized. In general, anticoagulant therapy should be continued until the danger of thrombosis and embolism has passed.

Missed Dose: The anticoagulant effect of COUMADIN persists beyond 24 hours. If the patient forgets to take the prescribed dose of COUMADIN at the scheduled time, the dose should be taken as soon as possible on the same day. The patient should not take the missed dose by doubling the daily dose to make up for missed doses, but should refer back to his or her physician.

Intravenous Route of Administration: COUMADIN for Injection provides an alternate administration route for patients who cannot receive oral drugs. The IV dosages would be the same as those that would be used orally if the patient could take the drug by the oral route. COUMADIN for Injection should be administered as a slow bolus injection over 1 to 2 minutes into a peripheral vein. It is not recommended for intramuscular administration. The vial should be reconstituted with 2.7 mL of sterile Water for Injection and inspected for particulate matter and discoloration immediately prior to use. Do not use if either particulate matter and/or discoloration is noted. After reconstitution, COUMADIN for Injection is chemically and physically stable for 4 hours at room temperature. It does not contain any antimicrobial preservative and, thus, care must be taken to assure the sterility of the prepared solution. The vial is not recommended for multiple use and unused solution should be discarded.

LABORATORY CONTROL The PT reflects the depression of vitamin K dependent Factors VII, X and II. There are several modifications of the one-stage PT and the physician should become familiar with the specific method used in his laboratory. The degree of anticoagulation indicated by any range of PTs may be altered by the type of thromboplastin used; the appropriate therapeutic range must be based on the experience of each laboratory. The PT should be determined daily after the administration of the initial dose until PT/INR results stabilize in the therapeutic range. Intervals between subsequent PT/INR determinations should be based upon the physician's judgment of the patient's reliability and response to COUMADIN in order to maintain the individual within the therapeutic range. Acceptable intervals for PT/INR determinations are normally within the range of one to four weeks after a stable dosage has been determined. To ensure adequate control, it is recommended that additional PT tests are done when other warfarin products are interchanged with warfarin sodium tablets, USP, as well as whenever other medications are initiated, discontinued, or taken irregularly (see PRECAUTIONS).

Different thromboplastin reagents vary substantially in their sensitivity to sodium warfarin-induced effects on PT. To define the appropriate therapeutic regimen it is important to be familiar with the sensitivity of the thromboplastin reagent used in the laboratory and its relationship to the International Reference Preparation (IRP), a sensitive thromboplastin reagent prepared from human brain.

A system of standardizing the PT in oral anticoagulant control was introduced by the World Health Organization in 1983. It is based upon the determination of an International Normalized Ratio (INR) which provides a common basis for communication of PT results and interpretations of therapeutic ranges. The INR system of reporting is based on a logarithmic relationship between the PT ratios of the test and reference preparation. The INR is the PT ratio that would be obtained if the International Reference Preparation (IRP), which has an ISI of 1.0, were used to perform the test. Early clinical studies of oral anticoagulants, which formed the basis for recommended therapeutic ranges of 1.5 to 2.5 times control mean normal PT, used sensitive human brain thromboplastin. When using the less sensitive rabbit brain thromboplastins commonly employed in PT assays today, adjustments must be made to the targeted PT range that reflect this decrease in sensitivity.

The INR can be calculated as: INR = $(\text{observed PT ratio})^{ISI}$ where the ISI (International Sensitivity Index) is the correction factor in the equation that relates the PT ratio of the local reagent to the reference preparation and is a measure of the sensitivity of a given thromboplastin to reduction of vitamin K-dependent coagulation factors; the lower the ISI, the more "sensitive" the reagent and the closer the derived INR will be to the observed PT ratio.[1]

The proceedings and recommendations of the 1992 National Conference on Antithrombotic Therapy[2–4] review and evaluate issues related to oral anticoagulant therapy and the sensitivity of thromboplastin reagents and provide additional guidelines for defining the appropriate therapeutic regimen.

The conversion of the INR to PT ratios for the less-intense (INR 2.0–3.0) and more intense (INR 2.5–3.5) therapeutic range recommended by the ACCP for thromboplastins over a range of ISI values is shown in Table 3.[5]

[See table above]

TREATMENT DURING DENTISTRY AND SURGERY The management of patients who undergo dental and surgical procedures requires close liaison between attending physicians, surgeons and dentists. PT/INR determination is recommended just prior to any dental or surgical procedure. In patients undergoing minimal invasive procedures who must be anticoagulated prior to, during, or immediately following these procedures, adjusting the dosage of COUMADIN to maintain the PT/INR at the low end of the therapeutic range may safely allow for continued anticoagulation. The operative site should be sufficiently limited and accessible to permit the effective use of local procedures for hemostasis. Under these conditions, dental and minor surgical procedures may be performed without undue risk of hemorrhage. Some dental or surgical procedures may necessitate the interruption of COUMADIN therapy. When discontinuing COUMADIN even for a short period of time, the benefits and risks should be strongly considered.

CONVERSION FROM HEPARIN THERAPY Since the anticoagulant effect of COUMADIN is delayed, heparin is preferred initially for rapid anticoagulation. Conversion to COUMADIN may begin concomitantly with heparin therapy or may be delayed 3 to 6 days. To ensure continuous anticoagulation, it is advisable to continue full dose heparin therapy and that COUMADIN therapy be overlapped with heparin for 4 to 5 days, until COUMADIN has produced the desired therapeutic response as determined by PT/INR. When COUMADIN has produced the desired PT/INR or prothrombin activity, heparin may be discontinued.

COUMADIN may increase the aPTT test, even in the absence of heparin. During initial therapy with COUMADIN, the interference with heparin anticoagulation is of minimal clinical significance.

As heparin may affect the PT/INR, patients receiving both heparin and COUMADIN should have blood for PT/INR determination drawn at least:

- 5 hours after the last IV bolus dose of heparin, or
- 4 hours after cessation of a continuous IV infusion of heparin, or
- 24 hours after the last subcutaneous heparin injection.

HOW SUPPLIED

Tablets: For oral use, single scored with one face imprinted numerically with 1, 2, 2-1/2, 3, 4, 5, 6, 7-1/2 or 10 superimposed and inscribed with "COUMADIN" and with the opposite face inscribed with "DuPont." COUMADIN is available in bottles and Hospital Unit-Dose Blister Packages with potencies and colors as follows:

[See table above]

Protect from light. Store at controlled room temperature (59°–86°F, 15°–30°C). Dispense in a tight, light-resistant container as defined in the USP.

Hospital Unit-Dose Blister Packages are to be stored in carton until contents have been used.

Injection: Available for intravenous use only. Not recommended for intramuscular administration. Reconstitute with 2.7 mL of sterile Water for Injection to yield 2 mg/mL. Net contents 5.4 mg lyophilized powder. Maximum yield 2.5 mL.

5 mg vial (box of 6) NDC 0590-0324-35

Protect from light. Keep vial in box until used. Store at controlled room temperature (59°–86°F, 15°–30°C).
After reconstitution, store at controlled room temperature (59°–86°F, 15°–30°C) and use within 4 hours. Do not refrigerate. Discard any unused solution.

REFERENCES
1. Poller, L.: Laboratory Control of Anticoagulant Therapy. Seminars in Thrombosis and Hemostasis, Vol. 12, No. 1, pp. 13–19, 1986.
2. Hirsh, J.: Is the Dose of Warfarin Prescribed by American Physicians Unnecessarily High? Arch Int Med, Vol. 147, pp. 769–771, 1987.
3. Cook, D.J., Guyatt, H.G., Laupacis, A., Sackett, D.L.: Rules of Evidence and Clinical Recommendations on the Use of Antithrombotic Agents. Chest ACCP Consensus Conference on Antithrombotic Therapy. Chest, Vol. 102(Suppl), pp. 305S–311S, 1992.
4. Hirsh, J., Dalen, J., Deykin, D., Poller, L.: Oral Anticoagulants Mechanism of Action, Clinical Effectiveness, and Optimal Therapeutic Range. Chest ACCP Consensus Conference on Antithrombotic Therapy. Chest, Vol. 102(Suppl), pp. 312S–326S, 1992.
5. Hirsh, J., M.D., F.C.C.P.: Hamilton Civic Hospitals Research Center, Hamilton, Ontario, Personal Communication.

Distributed by:
DuPont Pharma
Wilmington, Delaware 19880
COUMADIN® and the color and configuration of COUMADIN tablets are trademarks of DuPont Pharmaceuticals Company. Any unlicensed use of these trademarks is expressly prohibited under the U.S. Trademark Act.
Printed in U.S.A.   Copyright © DuPont Pharma 2001
6550-00/January, 2001

ESI Lederle Inc.
P.O. BOX 41502
PHILADELPHIA, PA 19101

Direct Inquiries to:
Professional Service
(610) 688-4400

For Emergency Medical Information Contact:
Day: (800) 934–5556 8:30 AM to 4:30 PM
       (Eastern Standard Time), Weekdays only
Night: (610) 688-4400 (Emergencies only; non-emergencies should wait until the next day)
For Medical/Pharmacy Inquiries on Marketed Products Call:
(800) 934–5556 8:30 AM to 4:30 PM
(Eastern Standard Time), Weekdays only

AYGESTIN®   ℞
[ā-jĕs′tĭn]
(norethindrone acetate tablets, USP)

Prescribing information for this product, which appears on pages 1218–1219 of the 2001 PDR, has been revised as follows. Please write "See Supplement A" next to the product heading.
Item 6 under the heading GENERAL PRECAUTIONS in the **PRECAUTIONS** section should be deleted and replaced with the following:
6. Data suggest that progestin therapy may have adverse effects on lipid and carbohydrate metabolism. The choice of progestin, its dose, and its regimen may be important in minimizing these adverse effects, but these issues will require further study before they are clarified. Women with hyperlipidemias and/or diabetes should be monitored closely during progestin therapy.
Item 7, which starts "7. A decrease in glucose tolerance...," under the heading GENERAL PRECAUTIONS in the **PRECAUTIONS** section should be deleted and items 8 and 9 of this section should be renumbered 7 and 8, respectively.

In the PDR annual,
the **Brand and Generic Name Index**
(PINK section)
alphabetizes drugs under both
brand and generic names.

Glaxo Wellcome Inc.
FIVE MOORE DRIVE
RESEARCH TRIANGLE PARK, NC 27709

For Medical Information for Healthcare Professionals Contact:
1-888-825-5249

In Emergencies:
Medical Information: 1-800-334-0089

For Consumer inquiries Contact:
1-888-825-5249

ACLOVATE®   ℞
[a′klō-vāt″]
(alclometasone dipropionate cream)
Cream, 0.05%

ACLOVATE®   ℞
(alclometasone dipropionate ointment)
Ointment, 0.05%
For Dermatologic Use Only—
Not for Ophthalmic Use.

Prescribing information for this product, which appears on page(s) 1335–1336 of the 2001 PDR, has been revised as follows. Please write "See Supplement A" next to the product heading.
The following subsection was added to the **PRECAUTIONS** *section.*
Geriatric Use: A limited number of patients at or above 65 years of age have been treated with ACLOVATE Cream and Ointment in US clinical trials. The number of patients is too small to permit separate analysis of efficacy and safety. No adverse events were reported with ACLOVATE Ointment in geriatric patients, and the single adverse reaction reported with ACLOVATE Cream in this population was similar to those reactions reported by younger patients. Based on available data, no adjustment of dosage of ACLOVATE Cream and Ointment in geriatric patients is warranted.
The following subsection was added to the **DOSAGE AND ADMINISTRATION** *section.*
Geriatric Use: In studies where geriatric patients (65 years of age or older, see PRECAUTIONS) have been treated with ACLOVATE Cream or Ointment, safety did not differ from that in younger patients; therefore, no dosage adjustment is recommended.
Manufactured for Glaxo Wellcome Inc.
Research Triangle Park, NC 27709
by Schering Corporation, Kenilworth, NJ 07033
July 2000/RL-846

AGENERASE®   ℞
[ă-jĭn′ə-rās]
(amprenavir)
Capsules

Prescribing information for this product, which appears on page(s) 1336–1341 of the 2001 PDR, has been revised. Please write "See Supplement A" next to the product heading.
The following ingredient information was updated in the **DESCRIPTION** *section.*
Each 150-mg capsule contains the inactive ingredients TPGS, PEG 400 740 mg, and propylene glycol 57 mg.
Each 150-mg AGENERASE Capsule contains 109 IU vitamin E in the form of TPGS. The total amount of vitamin E in the recommended daily adult dose of AGENERASE is 1744 IU.
The following sentence was added to the beginning of the **WARNINGS** *section.*
ALERT: Find out about medicines that should not be taken with AGENERASE.
The following paragraph was added to the **WARNINGS** *section.*
Concomitant use of AGENERASE and St. John's wort (hypericum perforatum) or products containing St. John's wort is not recommended. Coadministration of protease inhibitors, including AGENERASE, with St. John's wort is expected to substantially decrease protease inhibitor concentrations and may result in suboptimal levels of amprenavir and lead to loss of virologic response and possible resistance to AGENERASE or to the class of protease inhibitors.
The following paragraphs were revised in the **PRECAUTIONS: Information for Patients** *subsection.*
A statement to patients and health care providers is included on the product's bottle label: **ALERT: Find out about medicines that should NOT be taken with AGENERASE.** A Patient Package Insert (PPI) for AGENERASE Capsules is available for patient information.
AGENERASE may interact with some drugs; therefore, patients should be advised to report to their doctor the use of any other prescription, nonprescription medication, or herbal products, particularly St. John's wort.
References to **pravastatin** *were deleted from the* **PRECAUTIONS: Drug Interactions** *subsection.*
In the **ADVERSE REACTIONS** *section, the following row was added to the* **Other Potentially Significant Drug Interactions** *section of* **Table 7: Drug Interactions with AGENERASE.**

Other: St. John's wort	May decrease amprenavir concentrations.

The following paragraph was added to the beginning of the **PATIENT INFORMATION** *section.*
ALERT: Find out about medicines that should not be taken with AGENERASE. Please also read the section "MEDICINES YOU SHOULD NOT TAKE WITH AGENERASE."
The Heading **"MEDICINES YOU SHOULD NOT TAKE WITH AGENERASE"** *was added and a paragraph underneath it was revised to:*
- Taking AGENERASE with St. John's Wort (hypericum perforatum, a nonprescription herbal product) or products containing St. John's Wort is not recommended. Talk with your doctor if you are taking or are planning to take St. John's Wort because St. John's Wort may reduce the effect of AGENERASE.
The heading **"Medicines That Require Dose Adjustments or Special Attention From Your Doctor"** *was added and a paragraph underneath it was revised to:*
- It is not recommended that you take AGENERASE with the cholesterol-lowering drugs MEVACOR® (lovastatin) or ZOCOR® (simvastatin) because of the possible drug interactions. There is also an increased risk of drug interactions between AGENERASE and LIPITOR® (atorvastatin), and BAYCOL® (cerivastatin). Talk to your doctor if you are taking or are planning to take these or other drugs for lowering cholesterol.
AGENERASE is a registered trademark of the Glaxo Wellcome group of companies.
*The brands listed are trademarks of their respective owners and are not trademarks of the Glaxo Wellcome group of companies. The makers of these brands are not affiliated with and do not endorse Glaxo Wellcome or its products.
AGENERASE Capsules are manufactured by
R.P. Scherer, Beinheim, France
for Glaxo Wellcome Inc., Research Triangle Park, NC 27709
Licensed from Vertex Pharmaceuticals Incorporated
Cambridge, MA 02139
US Patent Nos. 5,585,397; 5,723,490; and 5,646,180
©Copyright 1999, 2000, 2001, Glaxo Wellcome Inc. All rights reserved.
January 2001/RL-899

AGENERASE®   ℞
[ă-jĭn′ə-rās]
(amprenavir)
Oral Solution

Prescribing information for this product, which appears on pages 1341–1346 of the 2001 PDR, has been revised. Please write "See Supplement A" next to the product heading.
The following ingredient information was updated in the **DESCRIPTION** *section.*
Each mL of AGENERASE Oral Solution contains 46 IU vitamin E in the form of TPGS.
The following sentence was added to the beginning of the **WARNINGS** *section.*
ALERT: Find out about medicines that should not be taken with AGENERASE.
The following paragraph was added to the **WARNINGS** *section.*
Concomitant use of AGENERASE and St. John's wort (hypericum perforatum) or products containing St. John's wort is not recommended. Coadministration of protease inhibitors, including AGENERASE, with St. John's wort is expected to substantially decrease protease inhibitor concentrations and may result in suboptimal levels of amprenavir and lead to loss of virologic response and possible resistance to AGENERASE or to the class of protease inhibitors.
The following paragraphs were revised in the **PRECAUTIONS: Information for Patients** *subsection.*
A statement to patients and health care providers is included on the product's bottle label: **ALERT: Find out about medicines that should NOT be taken with AGENERASE.** A Patient Package Insert (PPI) for AGENERASE Oral Solution is available for patient information.
AGENERASE may interact with some drugs; therefore, patients should be advised to report to their doctor the use of any other prescription, nonprescription medication, or herbal products, particularly St. John's wort.
References to **pravastatin** *were deleted from the* **PRECAUTIONS: Drug Interactions** *subsection.*
In the **ADVERSE REACTIONS** *section, the following row was added to the* **Other Potentially Significant Drug Interactions** *section of* **Table 7: Drug Interactions with AGENERASE.**

Other: St. John's wort	May decrease amprenavir concentrations.

The following paragraph was added to the beginning of the **PATIENT INFORMATION** *section.*
ALERT: Find out about medicines that should not be taken with AGENERASE. Please also read the section "MEDICINES YOU SHOULD NOT TAKE WITH AGENERASE."
The heading **"MEDICINES YOU SHOULD NOT TAKE WITH AGENERASE"** *was added and a paragraph underneath it was revised to:*

Continued on next page

Agenerase Oral Solution—Cont.

• Taking AGENERASE with St. John's Wort (hypericum perforatum, a nonprescription herbal product) or products containing St. John's Wort is not recommended. Talk with your doctor if you are taking or are planning to take St. John's Wort because St. John's Wort may reduce the effect of AGENERASE.

The heading "Medicines That Require Dose Adjustments or Special Attention From Your Doctor" was added and a paragraph underneath it was revised to:

• It is not recommended that you take AGENERASE with the cholesterol-lowering drugs MEVACOR® (lovastatin) or ZOCOR® (simvastatin) because of the possible drug interactions. There is also an increased risk of drug interactions between AGENERASE and LIPITOR® (atorvastatin), and BAYCOL® (cerivastatin). Talk to your doctor if you are taking or are planning to take these or other drugs for lowering cholesterol.

AGENERASE is a registered trademark of the Glaxo Wellcome group of companies.

*The brands listed are trademarks of their respective owners and are not trademarks of the Glaxo Wellcome group of companies. The makers of these brands are not affiliated with and do not endorse Glaxo Wellcome or its products.
Glaxo Wellcome Inc., Research Triangle Park, NC 27709
Licensed from Vertex Pharmaceuticals Incorporated
Cambridge, MA 02139
US Patent Nos. 5,585,397; 5,723,490; and 5,646,180
©Copyright 1999, 2000, 2001, Glaxo Wellcome Inc. All rights reserved.
January 2001/RL-900

ALKERAN®
[ăl-kur 'ăn]
(melphalan)
2-mg Scored Tablets

Prescribing information for this product, which appears on pages 1348–1349 of the 2001 PDR, has been revised. Please write "See Supplement A" next to the product heading.
The following sentence was revised in the Pregnancy: Pregnancy Category D subsection.

Melphalan was embryolethal and teratogenic in rats following oral (6 to 18 mg/m² per day for 10 days) and intraperitoneal (18 mg/m²) administration.
Manufactured by Catalytica Pharmaceuticals, Inc.
Greenville, NC 27834
for Glaxo Wellcome Inc., Research Triangle Park, NC 27709
©Copyright 1996, Glaxo Wellcome Inc. All rights reserved.
August 1999/RL-746

CEFTIN® Tablets
[sef 'tin]
(cefuroxime axetil tablets)
CEFTIN® for Oral Suspension
(cefuroxime axetil powder for oral suspension)

Prescribing information for this product, which appears on pages 1358–1362 of the 2001 PDR, has been revised. Please write "See Supplement A" next to the product heading.
The following packs were deleted from the HOW SUPPLIED section.

20 Tablets/Bottle	NDC 0173-0395-00
Unit Dose Packs of 100 Tablets	NDC 0173-0395-02
50-mL Suspension	NDC 0173-0406-01

Glaxo Wellcome Inc., Research Triangle Park, NC 27709
US Patent Nos. 4,562,181; 4,865,851; and 4,897,270
©Copyright 1996, 2000, Glaxo Wellcome Inc. All rights reserved.
August 2000/RL-842

COMBIVIR® Tablets
[kom 'bə-vir]
(lamivudine/zidovudine tablets)

Prescribing information for this product, which appears on pages 1365–1368 of the 2001 PDR, has been revised. Please write "See Supplement A" next to the product heading.
The following ingredient information was updated in the DESCRIPTION section.

Each film-coated tablet contains 150 mg of lamivudine, 300 mg of zidovudine, and the inactive ingredients colloidal silicon dioxide, hydroxypropyl methylcellulose, magnesium stearate, microcrystalline cellulose, polyethylene glycol, polysorbate 80, sodium starch glycolate, and titanium dioxide.
The following subsection was deleted from CLINICAL PHARMACOLOGY.
Geriatric Patients: Lamivudine and zidovudine pharmacokinetics have not been studied in patients over 65 years of age.
The following subsection was added to PRECAUTIONS.
Geriatric Use: Clinical studies of COMBIVIR did not include sufficient numbers of subjects aged 65 and over to determine whether they respond differently from younger subjects. In general, dose selection for an elderly patient should be cautious, reflecting the greater frequency of decreased hepatic, renal, or cardiac function, and of concomitant disease or other drug therapy. COMBIVIR is not recommended for

patients with impaired renal function (i.e., creatinine clearance ≤50 mL/min; see PRECAUTIONS: Patients with Impaired Renal Function and DOSAGE AND ADMINISTRATION).
Glaxo Wellcome Inc., Research Triangle Park, NC 27709
Lamivudine is manufactured under agreement from BioChem Pharma Inc.
Laval, Quebec, Canada
US Patent Nos. 5,047,407; 4,818,538; 4,828,838; 4,724,232; 4,833,130; 4,837,208; 5,859,021; and 5,905,082
October 2000/RL-874

CUTIVATE®
[kyoot' ə-vāt]
(fluticasone propionate cream)
Cream, 0.05%

For Dermatologic Use Only—
Not for Ophthalmic Use.

Prescribing information for this product, which appears on pages 1368–1370 of the 2001 PDR, has been revised. Please write "See Supplement A" next to the product heading.
The following subsection was added to the PRECAUTIONS section.
Geriatric Use: A limited number of patients above 65 years of age (n = 133) have been treated with CUTIVATE Cream in US and non-US clinical trials. While the number of patients is too small to permit separate analysis of efficacy and safety, the adverse reactions reported in this population were similar to those reported by younger patients. Based on available data, no adjustment of dosage of CUTIVATE in geriatric patients is warranted.
The following subsection was added to DOSAGE AND ADMINISTRATION section.
Geriatric Use: In studies where geriatric patients (65 years of age or older, see PRECAUTIONS) have been treated with CUTIVATE Cream, safety did not differ from that in younger patients; therefore, no dosage adjustment is recommended.
Glaxo Wellcome Inc., Research Triangle Park, NC 27709
August 1999/RL-865

CUTIVATE®
[kyoot' ə-vāt ']
(fluticasone propionate ointment)
Ointment, 0.005%

For Dermatologic Use Only—
Not for Ophthalmic Use.

Prescribing information for this product, which appears on pages 1370–1371 of the 2001 PDR, has been revised. Please write "See Supplement A" next to the product heading.
The following subsection was added to the PRECAUTIONS section.
Geriatric Use: A limited number of patients above 65 years of age (n = 214) have been treated with CUTIVATE Ointment in US and non-US clinical trials. While the number of patients is too small to permit separate analysis of efficacy and safety, the adverse reactions reported in this population were similar to those reported by younger patients. Based on available data, no adjustment of dosage of CUTIVATE in geriatric patients is warranted.
The following subsection was added to DOSAGE AND ADMINISTRATION section.
Geriatric Use: In studies where geriatric patients (65 years of age or older, see PRECAUTIONS) have been treated with CUTIVATE Ointment, safety did not differ from that in younger patients; therefore, no dosage adjustment is recommended.
Glaxo Wellcome Inc., Research Triangle Park, NC 27709
August 1999/RL-866

DIGIBIND®
[dij ' ə-bīnd]
DIGOXIN IMMUNE FAB (OVINE)

Prescribing information for this product, which appears on pages 1372–1373 of the 2001 PDR, has been revised. Please write "See Supplement A" next to the product heading.
Added the following subsection to PRECAUTIONS:
Geriatric Use: Of the 150 subjects in an open-label study of DIGIBIND, 42% were 65 and over, while 21% were 75 and over. In a post-marketing surveillance study that enrolled 717 adults, 84% were 60 and over, and 60% were 70 and over. No overall differences in safety or effectiveness were observed between these subjects and younger subjects, and other reported clinical experience has not identified differences in responses between the elderly and younger patients, but greater sensitivity of some older individuals cannot be ruled out.
The kidney excretes the Fab fragment-digoxin complex, and the risk of digoxin release with recurrence of toxicity is potentially increased when excretion of the complex is slowed by renal failure. However, recurrence of toxicity was reported for only 2.8% of patients in the surveillance study and the only factor associated with recurrence of toxicity was inadequacy of initial dose—not renal function. Calculation of dose is the same for patients of all ages and for patients with normal and impaired renal function. Because el-

derly patients are more likely to have decreased renal function, it may be useful to monitor renal function and to observe for possible recurrence of toxicity.
THE WELLCOME FOUNDATION LTD., Beckenham, Kent, England BR3 3BS
U.S. License No. 129
Distributed by: Glaxo Wellcome Inc., Research Triangle Park, NC 27709
February 2001/RL-906

EPIVIR® Tablets
[ep' ə-vir]
(lamivudine tablets)
EPIVIR® Oral Solution
(lamivudine oral solution)

Prescribing information for this product, which appears on pages 1374–1377 of the 2001 PDR, has been completely revised as follows. Please write "See Supplement A" next to the product heading.

> WARNING: LACTIC ACIDOSIS AND SEVERE HEPATOMEGALY WITH STEATOSIS, INCLUDING FATAL CASES, HAVE BEEN REPORTED WITH THE USE OF NUCLEOSIDE ANALOGUES ALONE OR IN COMBINATION, INCLUDING LAMIVUDINE AND OTHER ANTIRETROVIRALS (SEE WARNINGS).
> EPIVIR TABLETS AND ORAL SOLUTION (USED TO TREAT HIV INFECTION) CONTAIN A HIGHER DOSE OF THE ACTIVE INGREDIENT (LAMIVUDINE) THAN EPIVIR-HBV® TABLETS AND ORAL SOLUTION (USED TO TREAT CHRONIC HEPATITIS B). PATIENTS WITH HIV INFECTION SHOULD RECEIVE ONLY DOSING FORMS APPROPRIATE FOR TREATMENT OF HIV (SEE WARNINGS AND PRECAUTIONS).

DESCRIPTION
EPIVIR (also known as 3TC) is a brand name for lamivudine, a synthetic nucleoside analogue with activity against human immunodeficiency virus-1 (HIV-1) and hepatitis B virus (HBV). The chemical name of lamivudine is (2R,cis)-4-amino-1-(2-hydroxymethyl-1,3-oxathiolan-5-yl)-(1H)-pyrimidin-2-one. Lamivudine is the (-)enantiomer of a dideoxy analogue of cytidine. Lamivudine has also been referred to as (-)2′,3′-dideoxy, 3′-thiacytidine. It has a molecular formula of $C_8H_{11}N_3O_3S$ and a molecular weight of 229.3. Lamivudine is a white to off-white crystalline solid with a solubility of approximately 70 mg/mL in water at 20°C.
EPIVIR Tablets are for oral administration. Each tablet contains 150 mg of lamivudine and the inactive ingredients magnesium stearate, microcrystalline cellulose, and sodium starch glycolate. Opadry YS-1-7706-G White is the coloring agent in the tablet coating.
EPIVIR Oral Solution is for oral administration. One milliliter (1 mL) of EPIVIR Oral Solution contains 10 mg of lamivudine (10 mg/mL) in an aqueous solution and the inactive ingredients artificial strawberry and banana flavors, citric acid (anhydrous), methylparaben, propylene glycol, propylparaben, sodium citrate (dihydrate), and sucrose.

MICROBIOLOGY
Mechanism of Action: Lamivudine is a synthetic nucleoside analogue. Intracellularly, lamivudine is phosphorylated to its active 5′-triphosphate metabolite, lamivudine triphosphate (L-TP). The principal mode of action of L-TP is inhibition of reverse transcriptase (RT) via DNA chain termination after incorporation of the nucleoside analogue. L-TP is a weak inhibitor of mammalian DNA polymerases α and β, and mitochondrial DNA polymerase.
Antiviral Activity In Vitro: The relationship between in vitro susceptibility of HIV to lamivudine and the inhibition of HIV replication in humans has not been established. In vitro activity of lamivudine against HIV-1 was assessed in a number of cell lines (including monocytes and fresh human peripheral blood lymphocytes) using standard susceptibility assays. IC_{50} values (50% inhibitory concentrations) were in the range of 2 nM to 15 μM. Lamivudine had anti–HIV-1 activity in all acute virus-cell infections tested. In HIV-1–infected MT-4 cells, lamivudine in combination with zidovudine had synergistic antiretroviral activity. Synergistic activity of lamivudine/zidovudine was also shown in a variable-ratio study. Please see the EPIVIR-HBV package insert for information regarding activity of lamivudine in studies using in vitro model systems such as transfected cells for study of HBV replication.
Drug Resistance: Lamivudine-resistant isolates of HIV-1 have been selected in vitro. The resistant isolates showed reduced susceptibility to lamivudine and genotypic analysis showed that the resistance was due to specific substitution mutations in the HIV-1 reverse transcriptase at codon 184 from methionine to either isoleucine or valine. HIV-1 strains resistant to both lamivudine and zidovudine have been isolated.
Susceptibility of clinical isolates to lamivudine and zidovudine was monitored in controlled clinical trials. In patients receiving lamivudine monotherapy or combination therapy with lamivudine plus zidovudine, HIV-1 isolates from most patients became phenotypically and genotypically resistant to lamivudine within 12 weeks. In some patients harboring zidovudine-resistant virus, phenotypic sensitivity to zidovudine by 12 weeks of treatment was restored. Combination therapy with lamivudine plus zidovudine delayed the emergence of mutations conferring resistance to zidovudine.
Mutations in the HBV polymerase YMDD motif have been associated with reduced susceptibility of HBV to lamivudine

in vitro. In studies of non-HIV-infected patients with chronic hepatitis B, HBV isolates with YMDD mutations were detected in some patients who received lamivudine daily for 6 months or more, and were associated with evidence of diminished treatment response; similar HBV mutants have been reported in HIV-infected patients who received lamivudine-containing antiretroviral regimens in the presence of concurrent infection with hepatitis B virus (see PRECAUTIONS).

Cross-Resistance: Cross-resistance among certain reverse transcriptase inhibitors has been observed. Cross-resistance between lamivudine and zidovudine has not been reported. In some patients treated with lamivudine alone or in combination with zidovudine, isolates have emerged with a mutation at codon 184 which confers resistance to lamivudine. In the presence of the 184 mutation, cross-resistance to didanosine and zalcitabine has been seen in some patients; the clinical significance is unknown. In some patients treated with zidovudine plus didanosine or zalcitabine, isolates resistant to multiple reverse transcriptase inhibitors, including lamivudine, have emerged.

CLINICAL PHARMACOLOGY

Pharmacokinetics in Adults: The pharmacokinetic properties of lamivudine have been studied in asymptomatic, HIV-infected adult patients after administration of single intravenous (IV) doses ranging from 0.25 to 8 mg/kg, as well as single and multiple (twice-daily regimen) oral doses ranging from 0.25 to 10 mg/kg.

The pharmacokinetic properties of lamivudine have also been studied as single and multiple oral doses ranging from 5 mg to 600 mg per day administered to HBV-infected patients.

Absorption and Bioavailability: Lamivudine was rapidly absorbed after oral administration in HIV-infected patients. Absolute bioavailability in 12 adult patients was 86% ± 16% (mean ± SD) for the tablet and 87% ± 13% for the oral solution. After oral administration of 2 mg/kg twice a day to 9 adults with HIV, the peak serum lamivudine concentration (C_{max}) was 1.5 ± 0.5 µg/mL (mean ± SD). The area under the plasma concentration versus time curve (AUC) and C_{max} increased in proportion to oral dose over the range from 0.25 to 10 mg/kg.

An investigational 25-mg dosage form of lamivudine was administered orally to 12 asymptomatic, HIV-infected patients on 2 occasions, once in the fasted state and once with food (1099 kcal; 75 grams fat, 34 grams protein, 72 grams carbohydrate). Absorption of lamivudine was slower in the fed state (T_{max}: 3.2 ± 1.3 hours) compared with the fasted state (T_{max}: 0.9 ± 0.3 hours); C_{max} in the fed state was 40% ± 23% (mean ± SD) lower than in the fasted state. There was no significant difference in systemic exposure (AUC∞) in the fed and fasted states; therefore, EPIVIR Tablets and Oral Solution may be administered with or without food.

The accumulation ratio of lamivudine in HIV-positive asymptomatic adults with normal renal function was 1.50 following 15 days of oral administration of 2 mg/kg b.i.d.

Distribution: The apparent volume of distribution after IV administration of lamivudine to 20 patients was 1.3 ± 0.4 L/kg, suggesting that lamivudine distributes into extravascular spaces. Volume of distribution was independent of dose and did not correlate with body weight.

Binding of lamivudine to human plasma proteins is low (<36%). *In vitro* studies showed that, over the concentration range of 0.1 to 100 µg/mL, the amount of lamivudine associated with erythrocytes ranged from 53% to 57% and was independent of concentration.

Metabolism: Metabolism of lamivudine is a minor route of elimination. In man, the only known metabolite of lamivudine is the trans-sulfoxide metabolite. Within 12 hours after a single oral dose of lamivudine in 6 HIV-infected adults, 5.2% ± 1.4% (mean ± SD) of the dose was excreted as the trans-sulfoxide metabolite in the urine. Serum concentrations of this metabolite have not been determined.

Elimination: The majority of lamivudine is eliminated unchanged in urine. In 9 healthy subjects given a single 300-mg oral dose of lamivudine, renal clearance was 199.7 ± 56.9 mL/min (mean ± SD). In 20 HIV-infected patients given a single IV dose, renal clearance was 280.4 ± 75.2 mL/min (mean ± SD), representing 71% ± 16% (mean ± SD) of total clearance of lamivudine.

In most single-dose studies in HIV-infected patients, HBV-infected patients, or healthy subjects with serum sampling for 24 hours after dosing, the observed mean elimination half-life ($t_{½}$) ranged from 5 to 7 hours. In HIV-infected patients, total clearance was 398.5 ± 69.1 mL/min (mean ± SD). Oral clearance and elimination half-life were independent of dose and body weight over an oral dosing range from 0.25 to 10 mg/kg.

Special Populations: *Adults with Impaired Renal Function:* The pharmacokinetic properties of lamivudine have been determined in a small group of HIV-infected adults with impaired renal function (Table 1).

[See table 1 above]

Exposure (AUC∞), C_{max}, and half-life increased with diminishing renal function (as expressed by creatinine clearance). Apparent total oral clearance (Cl/F) of lamivudine decreased as creatinine clearance decreased. T_{max} was not significantly affected by renal function. Based on these observations, it is recommended that the dosage of lamivudine be modified in patients with renal impairment (see DOSAGE AND ADMINISTRATION).

Based on a study in otherwise healthy subjects with impaired renal function, hemodialysis increased lamivudine

Table 1: Pharmacokinetic Parameters (Mean ± SD) After a Single 300-mg Oral Dose of Lamivudine in 3 Groups of Adults With Varying Degrees of Renal Function

Parameter	Creatinine Clearance Criterion (Number of Subjects) >60 mL/min (n = 6)	10-30 mL/min (n = 4)	<10 mL/min (n = 6)
Creatinine clearance (mL/min)	111 ± 14	28 ± 8	6 ± 2
C_{max} (µg/mL)	2.6 ± 0.5	3.6 ± 0.8	5.8 ± 1.2
AUC∞ (µg•h/mL)	11.0 ± 1.7	48.0 ± 19	157 ± 74
Cl/F (mL/min)	464 ± 76	114 ± 34	36 ± 11

Table 2: Number of Patients (%) With At Least One HIV Disease Progression Event or Death

Endpoint	Current Therapy (n = 460)	EPIVIR plus Current Therapy (n = 896)	EPIVIR plus a NNRTI* plus Current Therapy (n = 460)
HIV progression or death	90 (19.6%)	86 (9.6%)	41 (8.9%)
Death	27 (5.9%)	23 (2.6%)	14 (3.0%)

*An investigational non-nucleoside reverse transcriptase inhibitor not approved in the United States.

clearance from a mean of 64 to 88 mL/min; however, the length of time of hemodialysis (4 hours) was insufficient to significantly alter mean lamivudine exposure after a single-dose administration. Therefore, it is recommended, following correction of dose for creatinine clearance, that no additional dose modification be made after routine hemodialysis. It is not known whether lamivudine can be removed by peritoneal dialysis or continuous (24-hour) hemodialysis.

The effects of renal impairment on lamivudine pharmacokinetics in pediatric patients are not known.

Adults with Impaired Hepatic Function: The pharmacokinetic properties of lamivudine have been determined in adults with impaired hepatic function. Pharmacokinetic parameters were not altered by diminishing hepatic function; therefore, no dose adjustment for lamivudine is required for patients with impaired hepatic function. Safety and efficacy of lamivudine have not been established in the presence of decompensated liver disease.

Pediatric Patients: For pharmacokinetic properties of lamivudine in pediatric patients, see PRECAUTIONS: Pediatric Use.

Geriatric Patients: Lamivudine pharmacokinetics have not been specifically studied in patients over 65 years of age.

Gender: There are no significant gender differences in lamivudine pharmacokinetics.

Race: There are no significant racial differences in lamivudine pharmacokinetics.

Drug Interactions: No clinically significant alterations in lamivudine or zidovudine pharmacokinetics were observed in 12 asymptomatic HIV-infected adult patients given a single dose of zidovudine (200 mg) in combination with multiple doses of lamivudine (300 mg q 12 h).

Lamivudine and trimethoprim/sulfamethoxazole (TMP/SMX) were coadministered to 14 HIV-positive patients in a single-center, open-label, randomized, crossover study. Each patient received treatment with a single 300-mg dose of lamivudine and TMP 160 mg/SMX 800 mg once a day for 5 days with concomitant administration of lamivudine 300 mg with the fifth dose in a crossover design.

Coadministration of TMP/SMX with lamivudine resulted in an increase of 44% ± 23% (mean ± SD) in lamivudine AUC∞, a decrease of 29% ±13% in lamivudine oral clearance, and a decrease of 30% ± 36% in lamivudine renal clearance. The pharmacokinetic properties of TMP and SMX were not altered by coadministration with lamivudine.

There was no significant pharmacokinetic interaction between lamivudine and interferon alfa in a study of 19 healthy male subjects.

INDICATIONS AND USAGE

EPIVIR in combination with other antiretroviral agents is indicated for the treatment of HIV infection (see Description of Clinical Studies).

Description of Clinical Studies: *Clinical Endpoint Study in Adults:* B3007 (CAESAR) was a multicenter, double-blind, placebo-controlled study comparing continued current therapy [zidovudine alone (62% of patients) or zidovudine with didanosine or zalcitabine (38% of patients)] to the addition of EPIVIR or EPIVIR plus an investigational non-nucleoside reverse transcriptase inhibitor, randomized 1:2:1. A total of 1816 HIV-infected adults with 25 to 250 CD4 cells/mm^3 (median = 122 cells/mm^3) at baseline were enrolled: median age was 36 years, 87% were male, 84% were nucleoside-experienced, and 16% were therapy-naive. The median duration on study was 12 months. Results are summarized in Table 2.

[See table 2 above]

Clinical Endpoint Study in Pediatric Patients: ACTG300 was a multicenter, randomized, double-blind study that provided for comparison of EPIVIR plus RETROVIR® (zidovudine) to didanosine monotherapy. A total of 471 symptomatic, HIV-infected therapy-naive (≤56 days of antiretroviral therapy) pediatric patients were enrolled in these 2 treatment arms. The median age was 2.7 years (range 6 weeks to 14 years), 58% were female, and 86% were non-Caucasian. The mean baseline CD4 cell count was 868 cells/mm^3 (mean: 1060 cells/mm^3 and range: 0 to 4650 cells/mm^3 for patients ≤5 years of age; mean 419 cells/mm^3 and range: 0 to 1555 cells/mm^3 for patients >5 years of age) and the mean baseline plasma HIV RNA was 5.0 $\log_{10}$ copies/mL. The median duration on study was 10.1 months for the patients receiving EPIVIR plus RETROVIR and 9.2 months for patients receiving didanosine monotherapy. Results are summarized in Table 3.

[See table 3 at bottom of next page]

Surrogate Endpoint Studies: Therapy-Naive Adults: A3001 was a randomized, double-blind study comparing EPIVIR 150 mg b.i.d. plus RETROVIR 200 mg t.i.d.; EPIVIR 300 mg b.i.d. plus RETROVIR; EPIVIR 300 mg b.i.d.; and RETROVIR. Three hundred sixty-six adults enrolled: male (87%), Caucasian (61%), median age of 34 years, asymptomatic HIV infection (80%), baseline CD4 cell counts of 200 to 500 cells/mm^3 (median = 352 cells/mm^3), and mean baseline plasma HIV RNA of 4.47 ($\log_{10}$ copies/mL). B3001 was a randomized, double-blind study comparing EPIVIR 300 mg b.i.d. plus RETROVIR 200 mg t.i.d. versus RETROVIR. One hundred twenty-nine adults enrolled: male (74%), Caucasian (82%), median age of 33 years, asymptomatic HIV infection (64%), and baseline CD4 cell counts of 100 to 400 cells/mm^3 (median = 260 cells/mm^3). Mean changes in CD4 cell count and HIV RNA through 24 weeks of treatment for study A3001 are summarized in Figures 1 and 2, respectively. Mean change in CD4 cell count through 24 weeks of treatment for study B3001 is summarized in Figure 3.

Figure 1: Mean Absolute CD4 Cell Count Change (cells/mm^3) From Baseline in Study A3001

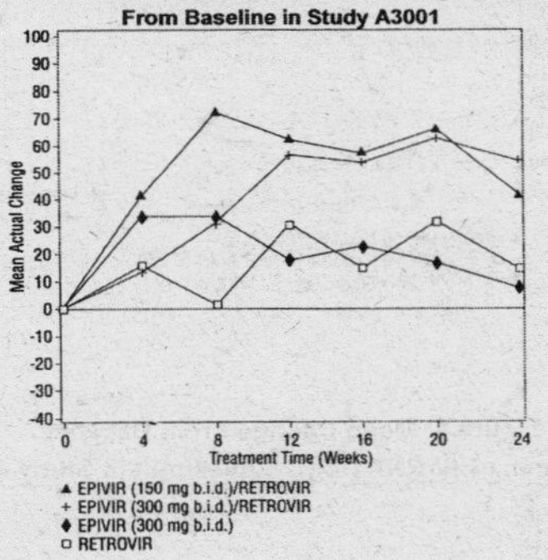

Figure 2: Mean Change From Baseline in Plasma HIV RNA ($\log_{10}$ copies/mL) in Study A3001

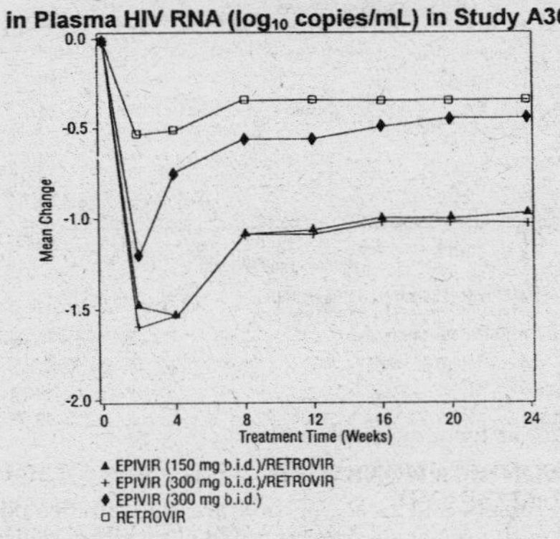

[See figure at top of next column]

Therapy-Experienced Adults (≥24 Weeks of Prior Zidovudine Therapy): A3002 was a randomized, double-blind study comparing EPIVIR 150 mg b.i.d. plus RETROVIR 200 mg t.i.d.; EPIVIR 300 mg b.i.d. plus RETROVIR; and RETROVIR plus zalcitabine 0.75 mg t.i.d. Two hundred fifty-

Continued on next page

Epivir—Cont.

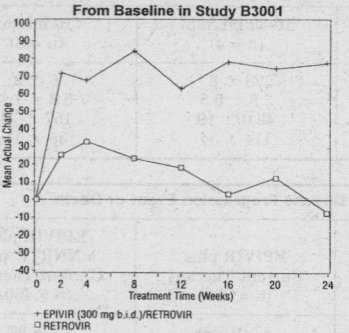

Figure 3: Mean Absolute CD4 Cell Count Change (cells/mm³)
From Baseline in Study B3001

+ EPIVIR (300 mg b.i.d.)/RETROVIR
□ RETROVIR

four adults enrolled: male (83%), Caucasian (63%), median age of 37 years, asymptomatic HIV infection (58%), median duration of prior zidovudine use of 24 months, baseline CD4 cell counts of 100 to 300 cells/mm³ (median = 211 cells/mm³), and mean baseline plasma HIV RNA of 4.60 ($\log_{10}$ copies/mL). B3002 was a randomized, double-blind study comparing EPIVIR 150 mg b.i.d. plus RETROVIR, EPIVIR 300 mg b.i.d. plus RETROVIR, and RETROVIR. Two hundred twenty-three adults enrolled: male (83%), Caucasian (96%), median age of 36 years, asymptomatic HIV infection (53%), median duration of prior zidovudine use of 23 months, and baseline CD4 cell counts of 100 to 400 cells/mm³ (median = 241 cells/mm³). Mean changes in CD4 cell count and HIV RNA through 24 weeks of treatment in study A3002 are summarized in Figures 4 and 5, respectively. Mean change in CD4 cell count through 24 weeks of treatment for study B3002 is summarized in Figure 6.

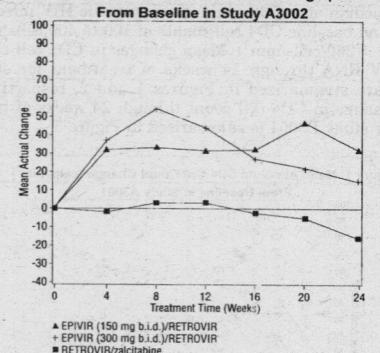

Figure 4: Mean Absolute CD4 Cell Count Change (cells/mm³)
From Baseline in Study A3002

▲ EPIVIR (150 mg b.i.d.)/RETROVIR
+ EPIVIR (300 mg b.i.d.)/RETROVIR
■ RETROVIR/zalcitabine

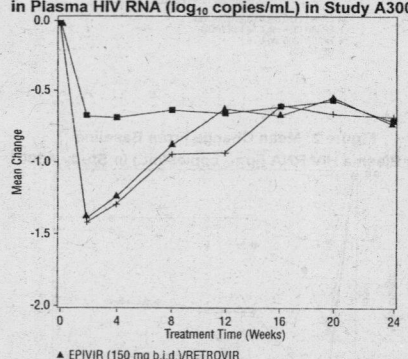

Figure 5: Mean Change From Baseline
in Plasma HIV RNA ($\log_{10}$ copies/mL) in Study A3002

▲ EPIVIR (150 mg b.i.d.)/RETROVIR
+ EPIVIR (300 mg b.i.d.)/RETROVIR
■ RETROVIR/zalcitabine

[See figure at top of next column]

CONTRAINDICATIONS

EPIVIR Tablets and Oral Solution are contraindicated in patients with previously demonstrated clinically significant hypersensitivity to any of the components of the products.

WARNINGS

In pediatric patients with a history of prior antiretroviral nucleoside exposure, a history of pancreatitis, or other significant risk factors for the development of pancreatitis, EPIVIR should be used with caution. Treatment with EPIVIR should be stopped immediately if clinical signs, symptoms, or laboratory abnormalities suggestive of pancreatitis occur (see ADVERSE REACTIONS).

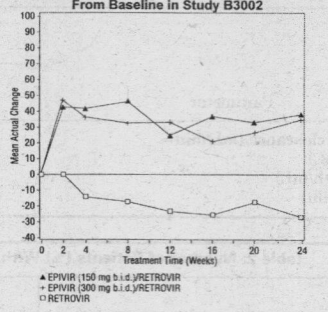

Figure 6: Mean Absolute CD4 Cell Count Change (cells/mm³)
From Baseline in Study B3002

▲ EPIVIR (150 mg b.i.d.)/RETROVIR
+ EPIVIR (300 mg b.i.d.)/RETROVIR
□ RETROVIR

Lactic Acidosis/Severe Hepatomegaly with Steatosis: Lactic acidosis and severe hepatomegaly with steatosis, including fatal cases, have been reported with the use of nucleoside analogues alone or in combination, including lamivudine and other antiretrovirals. A majority of these cases have been in women. Obesity and prolonged nucleoside exposure may be risk factors. Particular caution should be exercised when administering EPIVIR to any patient with known risk factors for liver disease; however, cases have also been reported in patients with no known risk factors. Treatment with EPIVIR should be suspended in any patient who develops clinical or laboratory findings suggestive of lactic acidosis or pronounced hepatotoxicity (which may include hepatomegaly and steatosis even in the absence of marked transaminase elevations).

Important Differences Among Lamivudine-Containing Products: EPIVIR Tablets and Oral Solution contain a higher dose of the same active ingredient (lamivudine) than in EPIVIR-HBV Tablets and Oral Solution. EPIVIR-HBV was developed for patients with chronic hepatitis B. The formulation and dosage of lamivudine in EPIVIR-HBV are not appropriate for patients dually infected with HIV and HBV. Lamivudine has not been adequately studied for treatment of chronic hepatitis B in patients dually infected with HIV and HBV. If treatment with EPIVIR-HBV is prescribed for chronic hepatitis B for a patient with unrecognized or untreated HIV infection, rapid emergence of HIV resistance is likely to result because of the subtherapeutic dose and the inappropriateness of monotherapy HIV treatment. If a decision is made to administer lamivudine to patients dually infected with HIV and HBV, EPIVIR Tablets, EPIVIR Oral Solution, or COMBIVIR® (lamivudine/zidovudine) Tablets should be used as part of an appropriate combination regimen. COMBIVIR (a fixed-dose combination tablet of lamivu-

dine and zidovudine) should not be administered concomitantly with either EPIVIR, EPIVIR-HBV, or RETROVIR.

Posttreatment Exacerbations of Hepatitis: In clinical trials in non-HIV-infected patients treated with lamivudine for chronic hepatitis B, clinical and laboratory evidence of exacerbations of hepatitis have occurred after discontinuation of lamivudine. These exacerbations have been detected primarily by serum ALT elevations in addition to re-emergence of HBV DNA. Although most events appear to have been self-limited, fatalities have been reported in some cases. Similar events have been reported from post-marketing experience after changes from lamivudine-containing HIV treatment regimens to non-lamivudine-containing regimens in patients infected with both HIV and HBV. The causal relationship to discontinuation of lamivudine treatment is unknown. Patients should be closely monitored with both clinical and laboratory followup for at least several months after stopping treatment. There is insufficient evidence to determine whether re-initiation of lamivudine alters the course of posttreatment exacerbations of hepatitis.

PRECAUTIONS

Patients with Impaired Renal Function: Reduction of the dosage of EPIVIR is recommended for patients with impaired renal function (see CLINICAL PHARMACOLOGY and DOSAGE AND ADMINISTRATION).

Patients with HIV and Hepatitis B Virus Coinfection: Safety and efficacy of lamivudine have not been established for treatment of chronic hepatitis B in patients dually infected with HIV and HBV. In non-HIV-infected patients treated with lamivudine for chronic hepatitis B, emergence of lamivudine-resistant HBV has been detected and has been associated with diminished treatment response (see EPIVIR-HBV package insert for additional information). Emergence of hepatitis B virus variants associated with resistance to lamivudine has also been reported in HIV-infected patients who have received lamivudine-containing antiretroviral regimens in the presence of concurrent infection with hepatitis B virus.

Information for Patients: EPIVIR is not a cure for HIV infection and patients may continue to experience illnesses associated with HIV infection, including opportunistic infections. Patients should remain under the care of a physician when using EPIVIR. Patients should be advised that the use of EPIVIR has not been shown to reduce the risk of transmission of HIV to others through sexual contact or blood contamination.

Patients should be advised that EPIVIR Tablets and Oral Solution contain a higher dose of the same active ingredient (lamivudine) as EPIVIR-HBV Tablets and Oral Solution. If a decision is made to include lamivudine in the HIV treatment regimen of a patient dually infected with HIV and HBV, the formulation and dosage of lamivudine in EPIVIR (not EPIVIR-HBV) should be used.

Table 3: Number of Patients (%) Reaching a Primary Clinical Endpoint (Disease Progression or Death)

Endpoint	EPIVIR plus RETROVIR (n = 236)	Didanosine (n = 235)
HIV disease progression or death (total)	15 (6.4%)	37 (15.7%)
Physical growth failure	7 (3.0%)	6 (2.6%)
Central nervous system deterioration	4 (1.7%)	12 (5.1%)
CDC Clinical Category C	2 (0.8%)	8 (3.4%)
Death	2 (0.8%)	11 (4.7%)

Table 4: Selected Clinical Adverse Events (≥5% Frequency) in Four Controlled Clinical Trials (A3001, A3002, B3001, B3002)

Adverse Event	EPIVIR 150 mg b.i.d. plus RETROVIR (n = 251)	RETROVIR (n = 230)
Body as a whole		
Headache	35%	27%
Malaise & fatigue	27%	23%
Fever or chills	10%	12%
Digestive		
Nausea	33%	29%
Diarrhea	18%	22%
Nausea & vomiting	13%	12%
Anorexia and/or decreased appetite	10%	7%
Abdominal pain	9%	11%
Abdominal cramps	6%	3%
Dyspepsia	5%	5%
Nervous system		
Neuropathy	12%	10%
Insomnia & other sleep disorders	11%	7%
Dizziness	10%	4%
Depressive disorders	9%	4%
Respiratory		
Nasal signs & symptoms	20%	11%
Cough	18%	13%
Skin		
Skin rashes	9%	6%
Musculoskeletal		
Musculoskeletal pain	12%	10%
Myalgia	8%	6%
Arthralgia	5%	5%

Patients should be advised that the long-term effects of EPIVIR are unknown at this time.

EPIVIR Tablets and Oral Solution are for oral ingestion only.

Patients should be advised of the importance of taking EPIVIR exactly as it is prescribed.

Parents or guardians should be advised to monitor pediatric patients for signs and symptoms of pancreatitis.

Drug Interaction: TMP 160 mg/SMX 800 mg once daily has been shown to increase lamivudine exposure (AUC). The effect of higher doses of TMP/SMX on lamivudine pharmacokinetics has not been investigated (see CLINICAL PHARMACOLOGY).

Carcinogenesis, Mutagenesis, and Impairment of Fertility: Long-term carcinogenicity studies with lamivudine in mice and rats showed no evidence of carcinogenic potential at exposures up to 10 times (mice) and 58 times (rats) those observed in humans at the recommended therapeutic dose for HIV infection. Lamivudine was not active in a microbial mutagenicity screen or an *in vitro* cell transformation assay, but showed weak *in vitro* mutagenic activity in a cytogenetic assay using cultured human lymphocytes and in the mouse lymphoma assay. However, lamivudine showed no evidence of *in vivo* genotoxic activity in the rat at oral doses of up to 2000 mg/kg producing plasma levels of 35 to 45 times those in humans at the recommended dose for HIV infection. In a study of reproductive performance, lamivudine administered to rats at doses up to 4000 mg/kg per day, producing plasma levels 47 to 70 times those in humans, revealed no evidence of impaired fertility and no effect on the survival, growth, and development to weaning of the offspring.

Pregnancy: Pregnancy Category C. Reproduction studies have been performed in rats and rabbits at orally administered doses up to 4000 mg/kg per day and 1000 mg/kg per day respectively, producing plasma levels up to approximately 35 times that for the adult HIV dose. No evidence of teratogenicity due to lamivudine was observed. Evidence of early embryolethality was seen in the rabbit at exposure levels similar to those observed in humans, but there was no indication of this effect in the rat at exposure levels up to 35 times that in humans. Studies in pregnant rats and rabbits showed that lamivudine is transferred to the fetus through the placenta. There are no adequate and well-controlled studies in pregnant women. Because animal reproductive toxicity studies are not always predictive of human response, lamivudine should be used during pregnancy only if the potential benefits outweigh the risks.

Antiretroviral Pregnancy Registry: To monitor maternal-fetal outcomes of pregnant women exposed to lamivudine, a Pregnancy Registry has been established. Physicians are encouraged to register patients by calling 1-800-258-4263.

Nursing Mothers: The Centers for Disease Control and Prevention recommend that HIV-infected mothers not breastfeed their infants to avoid risking postnatal transmission of HIV infection. A study in which lactating rats were administered 45 mg/kg of lamivudine showed that lamivudine concentrations in milk were slightly greater than those in plasma. Although it is not known if lamivudine is excreted in human milk, there is the potential for adverse effects from lamivudine in nursing infants. **Mothers should be instructed not to breastfeed if they are receiving lamivudine.**

Pediatric Use: *HIV:* The safety and effectiveness of EPIVIR in combination with other antiretroviral agents have been established in pediatric patients 3 months of age and older.

In Study A2002, pharmacokinetic properties of lamivudine were assessed in a subset of 57 HIV-infected pediatric patients (age range: 4.8 months to 16 years, weight range: 5 to 66 kg) after oral and IV administration of 1, 2, 4, 8, 12, and 20 mg/kg per day. In the 9 infants and children (range: 5 months to 12 years of age) receiving oral solution 4 mg/kg twice daily (the usual recommended pediatric dose), absolute bioavailability was 66% ± 26% (mean ± SD), which was less than the 86% ± 16% (mean ± SD) observed in adults. The mechanism for the diminished absolute bioavailability of lamivudine in infants and children is unknown.

Systemic clearance decreased with increasing age in pediatric patients, as shown in Figure 7.

Figure 7: Systemic Clearance (L/hr*kg) of Lamivudine in Relation to Age

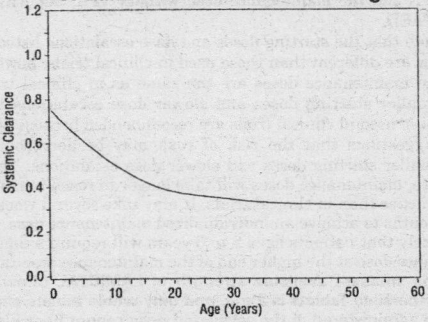

After oral administration of lamivudine 4 mg/kg twice daily to 11 pediatric patients ranging from 4 months to 14 years of age, C_{max} was 1.1 ± 0.6 µg/mL and half-life was 2.0 ± 0.6 hours. (In adults with similar blood sampling, the half-life was 3.7 ± 1 hours.) Total exposure to lamivudine,

Table 5: Frequencies of Selected Laboratory Abnormalities in Adults in Four 24-Week Surrogate Endpoint Studies (A3001, A3002, B3001, B3002) and a Clinical Endpoint Study (B3007)

Test (Abnormal Level)	24-Week Surrogate Endpoint Studies		Clinical Endpoint Study*	
	EPIVIR plus RETROVIR	RETROVIR	EPIVIR plus Current Therapy	Placebo plus Current Therapy†
Neutropenia (ANC<750/mm³)	7.2%	5.4%	15%	13%
Anemia (Hgb<8.0 g/dL)	2.9%	1.8%	2.2%	3.4%
Thrombocytopenia (platelets<50,000/mm³)	0.4%	1.3%	2.8%	3.8%
ALT (>5.0 × ULN)	3.7%	3.6%	3.8%	1.9%
AST (>5.0 × ULN)	1.7%	1.8%	4.0%	2.1%
Bilirubin (>2.5 × ULN)	0.8%	0.4%	ND	ND
Amylase (>2.0 × ULN)	4.2%	1.5%	2.2%	1.1%

* The median duration on study was 12 months.
† Current therapy was either zidovudine, zidovudine plus didanosine, or zidovudine plus zalcitabine.
ULN = Upper limit of normal.
ANC = Absolute neutrophil count.
ND = Not done.

Table 6: Selected Clinical Adverse Events and Physical Findings (≥5% Frequency) in Pediatric Patients in Study ACTG300

Adverse Event	EPIVIR plus RETROVIR (n = 236)	Didanosine (n = 235)
Body as a whole		
Fever	25%	32%
Digestive		
Hepatomegaly	11%	11%
Nausea & vomiting	8%	7%
Diarrhea	8%	6%
Stomatitis	6%	12%
Splenomegaly	5%	8%
Respiratory		
Cough	15%	18%
Abnormal breath sounds/wheezing	7%	9%
Ear, Nose and Throat		
Signs or symptoms of ears*	7%	6%
Nasal discharge or congestion	8%	11%
Other		
Skin rashes	12%	14%
Lymphadenopathy	9%	11%

*Includes pain, discharge, erythema, or swelling of an ear.

Table 7: Frequencies of Selected Laboratory Abnormalities in Pediatric Patients in Study ACTG300

Test (Abnormal Level)	EPIVIR plus RETROVIR	Didanosine
Neutropenia (ANC<400/mm³)	8%	3%
Anemia (Hgb<7.0 g/dL)	4%	2%
Thrombocytopenia (platelets<50,000/mm³)	1%	3%
ALT (>10 × ULN)	1%	3%
AST (>10 × ULN)	2%	4%
Lipase (>2.5 × ULN)	3%	3%
Total Amylase (>2.5 × ULN)	3%	3%

ULN = Upper limit of normal.
ANC = Absolute neutrophil count.

as reflected by mean AUC values, was comparable between pediatric patients receiving an 8-mg/kg-per-day dose and adults receiving a 4-mg/kg-per-day dose.

Distribution of lamivudine into cerebrospinal fluid (CSF) was assessed in 38 pediatric patients after multiple oral dosing with lamivudine. CSF samples were collected between 2 and 4 hours postdose. At the dose of 8 mg/kg per day, CSF lamivudine concentrations in 8 patients ranged from 5.6% to 30.9% (mean ± SD of 14.2% ± 7.9%) of the concentration in a simultaneous serum sample, with CSF lamivudine concentrations ranging from 0.04 to 0.3 µg/mL. The effect of renal impairment on lamivudine pharmacokinetics in pediatric patients is not known.

The safety and pharmacokinetic properties of EPIVIR in combination with other antiretroviral agents have not been established in pediatric patients less than 3 months of age. See INDICATIONS AND USAGE: Description of Clinical Studies, CLINICAL PHARMACOLOGY, WARNINGS, ADVERSE REACTIONS, and DOSAGE AND ADMINISTRATION.

HBV: See the complete prescribing information for EPIVIR-HBV Tablets and Oral Solution for additional information on the pharmacokinetics of lamivudine in HBV-infected children.

ADVERSE REACTIONS
Clinical Trials in HIV: *Adults:* Selected clinical adverse events with a ≥5% frequency during therapy with EPIVIR 150 mg b.i.d. plus RETROVIR 200 mg t.i.d. compared with zidovudine are listed in Table 4.
[See table at bottom of previous page]
Pancreatitis was observed in 3 of the 656 adult patients (<0.5%) who received EPIVIR in controlled clinical trials.

Selected laboratory abnormalities observed during therapy are summarized in Table 5.
[See table 5 above]
Pediatric Patients: Selected clinical adverse events and physical findings with a ≥5% frequency during therapy with EPIVIR 4 mg/kg twice daily plus RETROVIR 160 mg/m² 3 times daily compared with didanosine in therapy-naive (≤56 days of antiretroviral therapy) pediatric patients are listed in Table 6.
[See table 6 above]
Selected laboratory abnormalities experienced by therapy-naive (≤56 days of antiretroviral therapy) pediatric patients are listed in Table 7.
[See table 7 above]
Pancreatitis, which has been fatal in some cases, has been observed in antiretroviral nucleoside-experienced pediatric patients receiving EPIVIR alone or in combination with other antiretroviral agents. In an open-label dose-escalation study (A2002), 14 patients (14%) developed pancreatitis while receiving monotherapy with EPIVIR. Three of these patients died of complications of pancreatitis. In a second open-label study (A2005), 12 patients (18%) developed pancreatitis. In Study ACTG300, pancreatitis was not observed in 236 patients randomized to EPIVIR plus RETROVIR.
Pancreatitis was observed in 1 patient in this study who received open-label EPIVIR in combination with RETROVIR and ritonavir following discontinuation of didanosine monotherapy.
Paresthesias and peripheral neuropathies were reported in 15 patients (15%) in Study A2002, 6 patients (9%) in Study A2005, and 2 patients (<1%) in Study ACTG300.

Continued on next page

Epivir—Cont.

Lamivudine in Patients with Chronic Hepatitis B: Clinical trials in chronic hepatitis B used a lower dose of lamivudine (100 mg daily) than the dose used to treat HIV. The most frequent adverse events with lamivudine versus placebo were ear, nose, and throat infections (25% versus 21%); malaise and fatigue (24% versus 28%); and headache (21% versus 21%), respectively. The most frequent laboratory abnormalities reported with lamivudine were elevated ALT, elevated serum lipase, elevated CPK, and posttreatment elevations of liver function tests. Emergence of HBV viral mutants during lamivudine treatment, associated with reduced drug susceptibility and diminished treatment response, was also reported (also see WARNINGS and PRECAUTIONS). Please see the complete prescribing information for EPIVIR-HBV Tablets and Oral Solution for more information.
Observed During Clinical Practice: In addition to adverse events reported from clinical trials, the following events have been identified during post-approval use of lamivudine. Because they are reported voluntarily from a population of unknown size, estimates of frequency cannot be made. These events have been chosen for inclusion due to a combination of their seriousness, frequency of reporting, or potential causal connection to lamivudine.
Digestive: Stomatitis.
Endocrine and Metabolic: Hyperglycemia.
General: Weakness.
Hemic and Lymphatic: Anemia, lymphadenopathy, splenomegaly.
Hepatic and Pancreatic: Lactic acidosis and hepatic steatosis, pancreatitis, posttreatment exacerbation of hepatitis B (see WARNINGS and PRECAUTIONS).
Hypersensitivity: Anaphylaxis, urticaria.
Musculoskeletal: Muscle weakness, CPK elevation, rhabdomyolysis.
Nervous: Paresthesia, peripheral neuropathy.
Respiratory: Abnormal breath sounds/wheezing.
Skin: Alopecia, rash, pruritus.

OVERDOSAGE

There is no known antidote for EPIVIR. One case of an adult ingesting 6 g of EPIVIR was reported; there were no clinical signs or symptoms noted and hematologic tests remained normal. Two cases of pediatric overdose were reported in ACTG300. One case was a single dose of 7 mg/kg of EPIVIR; the second case involved use of 5 mg/kg of EPIVIR twice daily for 30 days. There were no clinical signs or symptoms noted in either case. It is not known whether lamivudine can be removed by peritoneal dialysis or hemodialysis.

DOSAGE AND ADMINISTRATION

Adults: The recommended oral dose of EPIVIR for adults is 150 mg twice daily, administered in combination with other antiretroviral agents. If lamivudine is administered to a patient dually infected with HIV and HBV, the dosage indicated for HIV therapy should be used as part of an appropriate combination regimen (see WARNINGS).
Pediatric Patients: The recommended oral dose of EPIVIR for HIV-infected pediatric patients 3 months up to 16 years of age is 4 mg/kg twice daily (up to a maximum of 150 mg twice a day), administered in combination with other antiretroviral agents.
Dose Adjustment: It is recommended that doses of EPIVIR be adjusted in accordance with renal function (see Table 8). (See CLINICAL PHARMACOLOGY section.)

Table 8: Adjustment of Dosage of EPIVIR in Adults and Adolescents in Accordance With Creatinine Clearance

Creatinine Clearance (mL/min)	Recommended Dosage of EPIVIR
≥50	150 mg twice daily
30-49	150 mg once daily
15-29	150 mg first dose, then 100 mg once daily
5-14	150 mg first dose, then 50 mg once daily
<5	50 mg first dose, then 25 mg once daily

Insufficient data are available to recommend a dosage of EPIVIR in patients undergoing dialysis. Although there are insufficient data to recommend a specific dose adjustment of EPIVIR in pediatric patients with renal impairment, a reduction in the dose and/or an increase in the dosing interval should be considered.

HOW SUPPLIED

EPIVIR Tablets, 150 mg, are white, modified diamond-shaped, film-coated tablets imprinted with "150" on one side and "GX CJ7" on the reverse side. They are available in bottles of 60 tablets (NDC 0173-0470-01) with child-resistant closures.
Store in tightly closed bottles at 25°C (77°F) (see USP Controlled Room Temperature).
EPIVIR Oral Solution, a clear, colorless to pale yellow, strawberry-banana flavored liquid, contains 10 mg of lamivudine in each 1 mL in plastic bottles of 240 mL (NDC 0173-0471-00) with child-resistant closures. This product does not require reconstitution.
Store in tightly closed bottles at 25°C (77°F) (see USP Controlled Room Temperature).
Glaxo Wellcome Inc., Research Triangle Park, NC 27709
Manufactured under agreement from **BioChem Pharma Inc.** 275 Armand Frappier Blvd., Laval, Quebec, Canada H7V 4A7
EPIVIR® Oral Solution Manufactured in England
US Patent No. 5,047,407

January 2001/RL-901

FLOLAN® ℞
[*flō 'lan*]
(epoprostenol sodium)
for Injection

Prescribing information for this product, which appears on pages 1384–1388 of the 2001 PDR, has been revised. Please write "See Supplement A" next to the product heading.
The following paragraph was revised in the **PRECAUTIONS: Drug Interactions** *subsection.*
In a pharmacokinetic substudy in patients with congestive heart failure receiving furosemide or digoxin in whom FLOLAN therapy was initiated, apparent oral clearance values for furosemide (n = 23) and digoxin (n = 30) were decreased by 13% and 15%, respectively, on the second day of therapy and had returned to baseline values by day 87. The change in furosemide clearance value is not likely to be clinically significant. However patients on digoxin may show elevations of digoxin concentrations after initiation of FLOLAN therapy, which may be clinically significant in patients prone to digoxin toxicity.
The following paragraph was revised in the **ADVERSE REACTIONS: Adverse Events During Chronic Administration for PH/SSD** *subsection.*
Although the relationship to FLOLAN administration has not been established, pulmonary embolism has been reported in several patients taking FLOLAN and there have been reports of hepatic failure.
The following paragraph was revised in the **ADVERSE REACTIONS: Observed During Clinical Practice** *subsection.*
Blood and Lymphatic: anemia, hypersplenism, pancytopenia, splenomegaly.
The following paragraph was revised in the **OVERDOSAGE** *section.*
One patient with secondary pulmonary hypertension accidentally received 50 mL of an unspecified concentration of FLOLAN. The patient vomited and became unconscious with an initially unrecordable blood pressure. FLOLAN was discontinued and the patient regained consciousness within seconds. In clinical practice, fatal occurrences of hypoxemia, hypotension, and respiratory arrest have been reported following overdosage of FLOLAN.
Glaxo Wellcome Inc., Research Triangle Park, NC 27709
US Patent Nos. 4,539,333 and 4,883,812 (Use Patent)

Sterile Diluent for FLOLAN manufactured by
Catalytica Pharmaceuticals, Inc., Greenville, NC 27834
for Glaxo Wellcome Inc., Research Triangle Park, NC 27709
October 2000/RL-877

FLONASE® ℞
[*flō' nāz*]
(fluticasone propionate)
Nasal Spray, 50 mcg

For Intranasal Use Only.
SHAKE GENTLY BEFORE USE.

Prescribing information for this product, which appears on pages 1388–1390 of the 2001 PDR, has been revised. Please write "See Supplement A" next to the product heading.
The following sentence was added to the **CLINICAL PHARMACOLOGY: Metabolism** *subsection.*
Since fluticasone propionate is a substrate of cytochrome P450 3A4, caution should be exercised when cytochrome P450 3A4 inhibitors (e.g., ritonavir, ketoconazole) are coadministered with fluticasone propionate as this could result in increased plasma concentrations of fluticasone propionate.
Glaxo Wellcome Inc., Research Triangle Park, NC 27709

U.S. Patent 4,335,121
October 2000/RL-868

IMITREX® ℞
[*ĭm '-ĭ-trĕx* "]
(sumatriptan succinate)
Tablets

Prescribing information for this product, which appears on pages 1407–1412 of the 2001 PDR, has been revised. Please write "See Supplement A" next to the product heading.
The following sentence in the **DESCRIPTION** *section was revised to include information on the new 100-mg tablet.*
Each IMITREX Tablet for oral administration contains 35, 70, or 140 mg of sumatriptan succinate equivalent to 25, 50, or 100 mg of sumatriptan, respectively.
The following two paragraphs in the **HOW SUPPLIED** *section were revised to include information on the new 100-mg tablet.*
HOW SUPPLIED: IMITREX Tablets, 25, 50, and 100 mg of sumatriptan (base) as the succinate. IMITREX Tablets, 100 mg, are light pink, capsule-shaped, film-coated tablets embossed with "Imitrex" on one side and "100" on the other in blister packs of 9 tablets (NDC 0173-0450-03).
The patent numbers statement was revised as shown below.
Glaxo Wellcome Inc., Research Triangle Park, NC 27709
US Patent Nos. 4,816,470; 5,037,845; 5,863,559; and 6,020,001

September 2000/RL-859

LAMICTAL® ℞
[*la-mik' tal*]
(lamotrigine)
Tablets

LAMICTAL® ℞
(lamotrigine)
Chewable Dispersible Tablets

Prescribing information for this product, which appears on pages 1412–1418 of the 2001 PDR, has been revised. Please write "See Supplement A" next to the product heading.
The following paragraph in the **DESCRIPTION** *section was revised to add information on the new 2-mg strength of LAMICTAL® (lamotrigine) Chewable Dispersible Tablets:*
LAMICTAL Chewable Dispersible Tablets are supplied for oral administration. The tablets contain 2 mg (white), 5 mg (white), or 25 mg (white) of lamotrigine and the following inactive ingredients: blackcurrant flavor, calcium carbonate, low-substituted hydroxypropylcellulose, magnesium aluminum silicate, magnesium stearate, povidone, saccharin sodium, and sodium starch glycolate.
The following paragraph was deleted from the **WARNINGS** *section:*
Special Dosing Considerations for Pediatric Patients: The lowest available strength of LAMICTAL Chewable Dispersible Tablets is 5 mg, and only whole tablets should be administered. Since the dosing of LAMICTAL in pediatric patients is based on body weight and the lowest tablet strength is 5 mg, some low-weight pediatric patients should not receive LAMICTAL. Specifically, pediatric patients who weigh less than 17 kg (37 lb) should not receive LAMICTAL because therapy cannot be initiated using the dosing guidelines and the currently available tablet strengths (see DOSAGE AND ADMINISTRATION).
The following **DOSAGE AND ADMINISTRATION** *subsections were revised to:*
Adjunctive Therapy with LAMICTAL: This section provides specific dosing recommendations for patients 2 to 12 years of age and patients greater than 12 years of age. Within each of these age-groups, specific dosing recommendations are provided depending upon whether or not the patient is receiving VPA (Tables 8 and 9 for patients 2 to 12 years of age, Tables 10 and 11 for patients greater than 12 years of age). In addition, the section provides a discussion of dosing for those patients receiving concomitant AEDs that have not been systematically evaluated in combination with LAMICTAL.
For dosing guidelines for LAMICTAL below, enzyme-inducing antiepileptic drugs (EIAEDs) include phenytoin, carbamazepine, phenobarbital, and primidone.
Patients 2 to 12 Years of Age: Recommended dosing guidelines for LAMICTAL added to an antiepileptic drug (AED) regimen containing VPA are summarized in Table 8. Recommended dosing guidelines for LAMICTAL added to EIAEDs are summarized in Table 9.
LAMICTAL Added to AEDs Other Than EIAEDs and VPA: The effect of AEDs other than EIAEDs and VPA on the metabolism of LAMICTAL is not currently known. Therefore, no specific dosing guidelines can be provided in that situation. Conservative starting doses and dose escalations (as with concomitant VPA) would be prudent; maintenance dosing would be expected to fall between the maintenance dose with VPA and the maintenance dose without VPA, but with an EIAED.
Note that the starting doses and dose escalations listed below are different than those used in clinical trials; however, the maintenance doses are the same as in clinical trials. Smaller starting doses and slower dose escalations than those used in clinical trials are recommended because of the suggestions that the risk of rash may be decreased by smaller starting doses and slower dose escalations. Therefore, maintenance doses will take longer to reach in clinical practice than in clinical trials. It may take several weeks to months to achieve an individualized maintenance dose. It is likely that patients aged 2 to 6 years will require a maintenance dose at the higher end of the maintenance dose range.
The smallest available strength of LAMICTAL Chewable Dispersible Tablets is 2 mg, and only whole tablets should be administered. If the calculated dose cannot be achieved using whole tablets, the dose should be rounded down to the nearest whole tablet (see HOW SUPPLIED and PATIENT INFORMATION for a description of the LAMICTAL Chewable Dispersible Tablet available sizes).
[See table 8 at top of next page]
[See table 9 at top of next page]

Table 8: LAMICTAL Added to an AED Regimen Containing VPA in Patients 2 to 12 Years of Age

Weeks 1 and 2	0.15 mg/kg/day in one or two divided doses, rounded down to the nearest whole tablet. Only whole tablets should be used for dosing.
Weeks 3 and 4	0.3 mg/kg/day in one or two divided doses, rounded down to the nearest whole tablet.

Weight based dosing can be achieved by using the following guide:

If the patient's weight is		Give this daily dose, using the most appropriate combination of Lamictal 2 mg and 5 mg tablets	
Greater than	And less than	Weeks 1 and 2	Weeks 3 and 4
6.7 kg	14 kg	2 mg every *other* day	2 mg every day
14.1 kg	27 kg	2 mg every day	4 mg every day
27.1 kg	34 kg	4 mg every day	8 mg every day
34.1 kg	40 kg	5 mg every day	10 mg every day

Usual maintenance dose: 1 to 5 mg/kg/day (maximum 200 mg/day in one or two divided doses). To achieve the usual maintenance dose, subsequent doses should be increased every 1 to 2 weeks as follows: calculate 0.3 mg/kg/day, round this amount down to the nearest whole tablet, and add this amount to the previously administered daily dose.

Table 9: LAMICTAL Added to EIAEDs (Without VPA) in Patients 2 to 12 Years of Age

Weeks 1 and 2	0.6 mg/kg/day in two divided doses, rounded down to the nearest whole tablet.
Weeks 3 and 4	1.2 mg/kg/day in two divided doses, rounded down to the nearest whole tablet.

Usual maintenance dose: 5 to 15 mg/kg/day (maximum 400 mg/day in two divided doses). To achieve the usual maintenance dose, subsequent doses should be increased every 1 to 2 weeks as follows: calculate 1.2 mg/kg/day, round this amount down to the nearest whole tablet, and add this amount to the previously administered daily dose.

Table 10: LAMICTAL Added to an AED Regimen Containing VPA in Patients Over 12 Years of Age

Weeks 1 and 2	25 mg every *other* day
Weeks 3 and 4	25 mg every day

Usual maintenance dose: 100 to 400 mg/day (1 or 2 divided doses). To achieve maintenance, doses may be increased by 25 to 50 mg/day every 1 to 2 weeks. The usual maintenance dose in patients adding LAMICTAL to VPA alone ranges from 100 to 200 mg/day.

Table 11: LAMICTAL Added to EIAEDs (Without VPA) in Patients Over 12 Years of Age

Weeks 1 and 2	50 mg/day
Weeks 3 and 4	100 mg/day in two divided doses

Usual maintenance dose: 300 to 500 mg/day (in two divided doses). To achieve maintenance, doses may be increased by 100 mg/day every 1 to 2 weeks.

Patients Over 12 Years of Age: Recommended dosing guidelines for LAMICTAL added to VPA are summarized in Table 10. Recommended dosing guidelines for LAMICTAL added to EIAEDs are summarized in Table 11.
LAMICTAL Added to AEDs Other Than EIAEDs and VPA: The effect of AEDs other than EIAEDs and VPA on the metabolism of LAMICTAL is not currently known. Therefore, no specific dosing guidelines can be provided in that situation. Conservative starting doses and dose escalations (as with concomitant VPA) would be prudent; maintenance dosing would be expected to fall between the maintenance dose with VPA and the maintenance dose without VPA, but with an EIAED.
[See table 10 above]
[See table 11 above]
Conversion From a Single EIAED to Monotherapy With LAMICTAL in Patients ≥16 Years of Age: The goal of the transition regimen is to effect the conversion to monotherapy with LAMICTAL under conditions that ensure adequate seizure control while mitigating the risk of serious rash associated with the rapid titration of LAMICTAL. The conversion regimen involves two steps. In the first, LAMICTAL is titrated to the targeted dose while maintaining the dose of the EIAED at a fixed level; in the second step, the EIAED is gradually withdrawn over a period of 4 weeks.
The recommended maintenance dose of LAMICTAL as monotherapy is 500 mg/day given in two divided doses. LAMICTAL should be added to an EIAED to achieve a dose of 500 mg/day according to the guidelines in Table 11 above. The regimen for the withdrawal of the concomitant EIAED is based on experience gained in the controlled monotherapy clinical trial. In that trial, the concomitant EIAED was withdrawn by 20% decrements each week over a 4-week period.
Because of an increased risk of rash, the recommended initial dose and subsequent dose escalations of LAMICTAL should not be exceeded (see BOX WARNING).
Usual Maintenance Dose: The usual maintenance doses identified in the tables above are derived from dosing regimens employed in the placebo-controlled adjunctive studies in which the efficacy of LAMICTAL was established. In pa-

tients receiving multidrug regimens employing EIAEDs **without VPA**, maintenance doses of adjunctive LAMICTAL as high as 700 mg/day have been used. In patients receiving **VPA alone**, maintenance doses of adjunctive LAMICTAL as high as 200 mg/day have been used. The advantage of using doses above those recommended in the tables above has not been established in controlled trials.
The **HOW SUPPLIED** *section was revised to:*
HOW SUPPLIED: LAMICTAL Tablets, 25 mg, white, scored, shield-shaped tablets debossed with "LAMICTAL" and "25", bottles of 100 (NDC 0173-0633-02).
Store at 25°C (77°F); excursions permitted to 15–30°C (59–86°F) [see USP Controlled Room Temperature] in a dry place.
LAMICTAL Tablets, 100 mg, peach, scored, shield-shaped tablets debossed with "LAMICTAL" and "100", bottles of 100 (NDC 0173-0642-55).
LAMICTAL Tablets, 150 mg, cream, scored, shield-shaped tablets debossed with "LAMICTAL" and "150", bottles of 60 (NDC 0173-0643-60).
LAMICTAL Tablets, 200 mg, blue, scored, shield-shaped tablets debossed with "LAMICTAL" and "200", bottles of 60 (NDC 0173-0644-60).
Store at 25°C (77°F); excursions permitted to 15–30°C (59–86°F) [see USP Controlled Room Temperature] in a dry place and protect from light.
LAMICTAL Chewable Dispersible Tablets, 2 mg, white to off-white, round tablets debossed with "LTG" over "2", bottles of 30 (NDC 0173-0699-00). ORDER DIRECTLY FROM GLAXO WELLCOME, INC. 1-800-334-4153.
LAMICTAL Chewable Dispersible Tablets, 5 mg, white to off-white, caplet-shaped tablets debossed with "GX CL2", bottles of 100 (NDC 0173-0526-00).
LAMICTAL Chewable Dispersible Tablets, 25 mg, white, super elliptical-shaped tablets debossed with "GX CL5", bottles of 100 (NDC 0173-0527-00).
Store at 25°C (77°F); excursions permitted to 15–30°C (59–86°F) [see USP Controlled Room Temperature] in a dry place.

The beginning of the **PATIENT INFORMATION** *section was revised to:*

Information for the Patient
LAMICTAL® (lamotrigine) Tablets

 25 mg, white imprinted with LAMICTAL 25	 100 mg, peach imprinted with LAMICTAL 100
 150 mg, cream imprinted with LAMICTAL 150	 200 mg, blue imprinted with LAMICTAL 200

LAMICTAL® (lamotrigine)
Chewable Dispersible Tablets

 2 mg, white imprinted with LTG 2	 5 mg, white imprinted with GX CL2

 25 mg, white imprinted with GX CL5

NOTE: The pictures above show actual tablet shape and size and the wording describes the color and printing that is on each strength of LAMICTAL Tablets and Chewable Dispersible Tablets. Before taking your medicine, it is important to compare the tablets you receive from your doctor or pharmacist with these pictures to make sure you have received the correct medicine.
Glaxo Wellcome Inc., Research Triangle Park, NC 27709
US Patent No. 4,602,017 and 5,698,226
©Copyright 1998, 1999, 2000, Glaxo Wellcome Inc. All rights reserved.
September 2000/RL-860

LANOXIN®   Ŗ
[lă-nŏx'ĭn"]
(digoxin)
Injection
500 mcg (0.5 mg) in 2 mL (250 mcg [0.25 mg] per mL)

Prescribing information for this product, which appears on pages 1425–1429 of the 2001 PDR, has been revised as follows. Please write "See Supplement A" next to the product heading.
The following sentence was revised in the **DESCRIPTION** *section.*
LANOXIN Injection is a sterile solution of digoxin for intravenous or intramuscular injection.
Manufactured by Catalytica Pharmaceuticals, Inc., Greenville, NC 27834
for Glaxo Wellcome Inc., Research Triangle Park, NC 27709
©Copyright 1996, 1998, 2000, Glaxo Wellcome Inc. All rights reserved.
July 2000/RL-829

LANOXIN®   Ŗ
[lă-nŏx'ĭn"]
(digoxin)
Injection Pediatric
100 mcg (0.1 mg) in 1 mL

Prescribing information for this product, which appears on pages 1429–1432 of the 2001 PDR, has been revised as follows. Please write "See Supplement A" next to the product heading.
The following sentence was revised in the **DESCRIPTION** *section.*
LANOXIN Injection Pediatric is a sterile solution of digoxin for intravenous or intramuscular injection.
Manufactured by Catalytica Pharmaceuticals, Inc. Greenville, NC 27834

Continued on next page

Lanoxin Pediatric—Cont.

for Glaxo Wellcome Inc., Research Triangle Park, NC 27709
©Copyright 1996, 1998, 2000, Glaxo Wellcome Inc. All rights
reserved.
July 2000/RL-830

MALARONE™ ℞
[*mal' ə-rōn*]
(atovaquone and proguanil hydrochloride)
Tablets
MALARONE™ ℞
(atovaquone and proguanil hydrochloride)
Pediatric Tablets

Prescribing information for this product, which appears on
pages 1439–1442 of the 2001 PDR, has been revised as fol-
lows. Please write "See Supplement A" next to the product
heading.

DESCRIPTION
MALARONE (atovaquone and proguanil hydrochloride) is a
fixed-dose combination of the antimalarial agents atovaquone and proguanil hydrochloride. The chemical name of
atovaquone is *trans*-2-[4-(4-chlorophenyl)cyclohexyl]-3-hy-
droxy-1,4-naphthalenedione. Atovaquone is a yellow crystalline solid that is practically insoluble in water. It has a molecular weight of 366.84 and the molecular formula
$C_{22}H_{19}ClO_3$. The compound has the following structural formula:

The chemical name of proguanil hydrochloride is 1-(4-chlo-
rophenyl)-5-isopropyl-biguanide hydrochloride. Proguanil
hydrochloride is a white crystalline solid that is sparingly
soluble in water. It has a molecular weight of 290.22 and the
molecular formula $C_{11}H_{16}ClN_5$•HCl. The compound has the
following structural formula:

MALARONE Tablets and MALARONE Pediatric Tablets
are for oral administration. Each MALARONE Tablet contains 250 mg of atovaquone and 100 mg of proguanil hydrochloride and each MALARONE Pediatric Tablet contains
62.5 mg of atovaquone and 25 mg of proguanil hydrochloride. The inactive ingredients in both tablets are low-substituted hydroxypropyl cellulose, magnesium stearate, microcrystalline cellulose, poloxamer 188, povidone K30, and sodium starch glycolate. The tablet coating contains red iron
oxide, polyethylene glycol 400, hydroxypropyl methylcellulose, polyethylene glycol 8000, and titanium dioxide.

CLINICAL PHARMACOLOGY
Microbiology:
Mechanism of Action: The constituents of MALARONE,
atovaquone and proguanil hydrochloride, interfere with 2 different pathways involved in the biosynthesis of pyrimidines
required for nucleic acid replication. Atovaquone is a selective inhibitor of parasite mitochondrial electron transport.
Proguanil hydrochloride primarily exerts its effect by means
of the metabolite cycloguanil, a dihydrofolate reductase inhibitor. Inhibition of dihydrofolate reductase in the malaria
parasite disrupts deoxythymidylate synthesis.
Activity In Vitro and In Vivo: Atovaquone and cycloguanil
(an active metabolite of proguanil) are active against the
erythrocytic and exoerythrocytic stages of *Plasmodium* spp.
Enhanced efficacy of the combination compared to either
atovaquone or proguanil hydrochloride alone was demonstrated in clinical studies in both immune and nonimmune
patients (see CLINICAL STUDIES).
Drug Resistance: Strains of *P. falciparum* with decreased
susceptibility to atovaquone or proguanil/cycloguanil alone
can be selected in vitro or in vivo. The combination of atovaquone and proguanil hydrochloride may not be effective for
treatment of recrudescent malaria that develops after prior
therapy with the combination.
Pharmacokinetics:
Absorption: Atovaquone is a highly lipophilic compound
with low aqueous solubility. The bioavailability of atovaquone shows considerable inter-individual variability.
Dietary fat taken with atovaquone increases the rate and
extent of absorption, increasing AUC 2 to 3 times and C_{max}
5 times over fasting. The absolute bioavailability of the tablet formulation of atovaquone when taken with food is 23%.
MALARONE Tablets should be taken with food or a milky
drink.
Proguanil hydrochloride is extensively absorbed regardless
of food intake.

Table 1: Adverse Experiences in Clinical Trials of MALARONE for Prophylaxis of Malaria

| Adverse Event | Percent of Subjects With Adverse Experiences (Percent of Subjects With Adverse Experiences Attributable to Therapy) | | | | |
| | Adults | | | Children and Adolescents | |
	Placebo (n = 206)	MALARONE* (n = 206)	MALARONE† (n = 381)	Placebo (n = 140)	MALARONE (n = 125)
Headache	27 (7)	22 (3)	17 (5)	21 (14)	19 (14)
Fever	13 (1)	5 (0)	3 (0)	11 (<1)	6 (0)
Myalgia	11 (0)	12 (0)	7 (0)	0 (0)	0 (0)
Abdominal pain	10 (5)	9 (4)	6 (3)	29 (29)	33 (31)
Cough	8 (<1)	6 (<1)	4 (1)	9 (0)	9 (0)
Diarrhea	8 (3)	6 (2)	4 (1)	3 (1)	2 (0)
Upper respiratory infection	7 (0)	8 (0)	5 (0)	0 (0)	<1 (0)
Dyspepsia	5 (4)	3 (2)	2 (1)	0 (0)	0 (0)
Back Pain	4 (0)	4 (0)	4 (0)	0 (0)	0 (0)
Gastritis	3 (2)	3 (3)	2 (2)	0 (0)	0 (0)
Vomiting	2 (<1)	1 (<1)	<1 (<1)	6 (6)	7 (7)
Flu syndrome	1 (0)	2 (0)	0 (0)	6 (6)	9 (9)
Any adverse event	65 (32)	54 (17)	49 (17)	62 (41)	60 (42)

*Subjects receiving the recommended dose of atovaquone and proguanil hydrochloride in placebo-controlled trials.
†Subjects receiving the recommended dose of atovaquone and proguanil hydrochloride in any trial.

Distribution: Atovaquone is highly protein bound (>99%)
over the concentration range of 1 to 90 mcg/mL. The apparent volume of distribution of atovaquone after oral administration is approximately 3.5 L/kg.
Proguanil is 75% protein bound. The apparent volume of
distribution is approximately 42 L/kg.
In human plasma, the binding of atovaquone and proguanil
was unaffected by the presence of the other.
Metabolism: In a study where ^{14}C-labelled atovaquone was
administered to healthy volunteers, greater than 94% of the
dose was recovered as unchanged atovaquone in the feces
over 21 days. There was little or no excretion of atovaquone
in the urine (less than 0.6%). There is indirect evidence that
atovaquone may undergo limited metabolism; however, a
specific metabolite has not been identified. Between 40% to
60% of proguanil is excreted by the kidneys. Proguanil is metabolized to cycloguanil (primarily via CYP2C19) and 4-chlo-
rophenylbiguanide. The main routes of elimination are hepatic biotransformation and renal excretion.
Elimination: The elimination half-life of atovaquone is
about 2 to 3 days in adult patients.
The mean oral clearance of atovaquone is approximately
0.04 L/h per kg.
The mean oral clearance of proguanil is 3.22 L/h per kg. The
elimination half-life of proguanil is 12 to 21 hours in both
adult patients and pediatric patients, but may be longer in
individuals who are slow metabolizers.
Special Populations:
Pediatrics: The pharmacokinetics of proguanil and cycloguanil are similar in adult patients and pediatric patients.
However, the elimination half-life of atovaquone is shorter in
pediatric patients (1 to 2 days) than in adult patients (2 to 3
days).
Geriatrics: No studies have been carried out in geriatric patients to assess the pharmacokinetics in this patient population. Since geriatric patients may have reduced renal function, caution should be taken when treating geriatric patients with MALARONE (see Special Populations: Renal
Impairment and PRECAUTIONS).
Hepatic Impairment: The pharmacokinetics of
MALARONE have not been studied in patients with hepatic
impairment. The effect of hepatic dysfunction on the conversion of proguanil to cycloguanil is unknown.
Renal Impairment: In patients with mild to moderate renal
impairment, oral clearance and/or AUC data for atovaquone,
proguanil, and cycloguanil are within the range of values observed in patients with normal renal function. In patients
with severe renal impairment (creatinine clearance
<30 mL/min), atovaquone C_{max} and AUC are reduced but the
elimination half-lives for proguanil and cycloguanil are prolonged, with corresponding increases in AUC, resulting in
the potential of drug accumulation with repeated dosing (see
CONTRAINDICATIONS).
Drug Interactions: There are no pharmacokinetic interactions between atovaquone and proguanil at the recommended dose.
Concomitant treatment with **tetracycline** has been associated with approximately a 40% reduction in plasma concentrations of atovaquone.
Concomitant treatment with **metoclopramide** has also been
associated with decreased bioavailability of atovaquone.
Concomitant administration of **rifampin** or **rifabutin** is
known to reduce atovaquone levels by approximately 50%
and 34%, respectively (see PRECAUTIONS: Drug Interactions). The mechanisms of these interactions are unknown.
Atovaquone is highly protein bound (>99%) but does not displace other highly protein-bound drugs in vitro, indicating

significant drug interactions arising from displacement are
unlikely (see PRECAUTIONS: Drug Interactions). Proguanil is metabolized primarily by CYP2C19. Potential
pharmacokinetic interactions with other substrates or inhibitors of this pathway are unknown.

INDICATIONS AND USAGE
Prevention of Malaria: MALARONE is indicated for the
prophylaxis of *P. falciparum* malaria, including in areas
where chloroquine resistance has been reported (see CLINI-
CAL STUDIES).
Treatment of Malaria: MALARONE is indicated for the
treatment of acute, uncomplicated *P. falciparum* malaria.
MALARONE has been shown to be effective in regions where
the drugs chloroquine, halofantrine, mefloquine, and amodi-
aquine may have unacceptable failure rates, presumably due
to drug resistance.

CONTRAINDICATIONS
MALARONE is contraindicated in individuals with known
hypersensitivity to atovaquone proguanil hydrochloride or
any component of the formulation. During clinical trials,
one case of anaphylaxis following treatment with atova-
quone/proguanil was observed.
MALARONE is contraindicated for prophylaxis of *P. falciparum* malaria in patients with severe renal impairment
(creatinine clearance <30 mL/min) (see CLINICAL PHAR-
MACOLOGY: Special Populations: Renal Impairment).

PRECAUTIONS
General: MALARONE has not been evaluated for the treatment of cerebral malaria or other severe manifestations of
complicated malaria, including hyperparasitemia, pulmonary edema, or renal failure. Patients with severe malaria
are not candidates for oral therapy.
Absorption of atovaquone may be reduced in patients with
diarrhea or vomiting. If MALARONE is used in patients
who are vomiting (see DOSAGE AND ADMINISTRATION),
parasitemia should be closely monitored and the use of an
antiemetic considered. Vomiting occurred in up to 19% of pediatric patients given treatment doses of MALARONE. In
the controlled clinical trials of MALARONE, 15.3% of adults
who were treated with atovaquone/proguanil received an
antiemetic drug during that part of the trial when they received atovaquone/proguanil. Of these patients, 98.3% were
successfully treated. In patients with severe or persistent
diarrhea or vomiting, alternative antimalarial therapy may
be required.
Parasite relapse occurred commonly when *P. vivax* malaria
was treated with MALARONE alone.
In the event of recrudescent *P. falciparum* infections after
treatment with MALARONE or failure of chemoprophylaxis
with MALARONE, patients should be treated with a different blood schizonticide.
In patients with severe renal impairment (creatinine clearance <30 mL/min), alternatives to MALARONE should be
recommended for treatment of acute *P. falciparum* malaria
whenever possible (see CONTRAINDICATIONS and CLIN-
ICAL PHARMACOLOGY: Special Populations: Renal Impairment). The concomitant administration of MALARONE
and any other medication containing proguanil hydrochloride should be avoided.
Information for Patients: Patients should be instructed:
• to take MALARONE tablets at the same time each day
  with food or a milky drink.
• to take a repeat dose of MALARONE if vomiting occurs
  within 1 hour after dosing.

- to consult a healthcare professional regarding alternative forms of prophylaxis if prophylaxis with MALARONE is prematurely discontinued for any reason.
- that protective clothing, insect repellents, and bednets are important components of malaria prophylaxis.
- that no chemoprophylactic regimen is 100% effective; therefore, patients should seek medical attention for any febrile illness that occurs during or after return from a malaria-endemic area and inform their healthcare professional that they may have been exposed to malaria.
- that falciparum malaria carries a higher risk of death and serious complications in pregnant women than in the general population. Pregnant women anticipating travel to malarious areas should discuss the risks and benefits of such travel with their physicians (see Pregnancy section).

Drug Interactions: Concomitant treatment with **tetracycline** has been associated with approximately a 40% reduction in plasma concentrations of atovaquone. Parasitemia should be closely monitored in patients receiving tetracycline. While antiemetics may be indicated for patients receiving MALARONE, **metoclopramide** may reduce the bioavailability of atovaquone and should be used only if other antiemetics are not available.

Concomitant administration of **rifampin or rifabutin** is known to reduce atovaquone levels by approximately 50% and 34%, respectively. The concomitant administration of MALARONE and rifampin or rifabutin is not recommended. Atovaquone is highly protein bound (>99%) but does not displace other highly protein-bound drugs in vitro, indicating significant drug interactions arising from displacement are unlikely.

Potential interactions between proguanil or cycloguanil and other drugs that are CYP2C19 substrates or inhibitors are unknown.

Carcinogenesis, Mutagenesis, Impairment of Fertility:
Atovaquone: Carcinogenicity studies in rats were negative; 24-month studies in mice showed treatment-related increases in incidence of hepatocellular adenoma and hepatocellular carcinoma at all doses tested which ranged from approximately 5 to 8 times the average steady-state plasma concentrations in humans during prophylaxis of malaria. Atovaquone alone was negative with or without metabolic activation in the Ames *Salmonella* mutagenicity assay, the Mouse Lymphoma mutagenesis assay, and the Cultured Human Lymphocyte cytogenetic assay. No evidence of genotoxicity was observed in the in vivo Mouse Micronucleus assay.
Proguanil: Carcinogenicity studies with proguanil have not been completed. Proguanil was not genotoxic in in vitro or in vivo studies.

Proguanil alone was negative with or without metabolic activation in the Ames *Salmonella* mutagenicity assay and the Mouse Lymphoma mutagenesis assay. No evidence of genotoxicity was observed in the in vivo Mouse Micronucleus assay.

Genotoxicity studies have not been performed with atovaquone in combination with proguanil. Effects of MALARONE on male and female reproductive performance are unknown.

Pregnancy: Pregnancy Category C. Falciparum malaria carries a higher risk of morbidity and mortality in pregnant women than in the general population. Maternal death and fetal loss are both known complications of falciparum malaria in pregnancy. In pregnant women who must travel to malaria-endemic areas, personal protection against mosquito bites should always be employed (see Information for Patients) in addition to antimalarials.

Atovaquone was not teratogenic and did not cause reproductive toxicity in rats at maternal plasma concentrations up to 5 to 6.5 times the estimated human exposure during treatment of malaria. Following single-dose administration of ^{14}C-labeled atovaquone to pregnant rats, concentrations of radiolabel in rat fetuses were 18% (mid-gestation) and 60% (late gestation) of concurrent maternal plasma concentrations. In rabbits, atovaquone caused maternal toxicity at plasma concentrations that were approximately 0.6 to 1.3 times the estimated human exposure during treatment of malaria. Adverse fetal effects in rabbits, including decreased fetal body lengths and increased early resorptions and postimplantation losses, were observed only in the presence of maternal toxicity. Concentrations of atovaquone in rabbit fetuses averaged 30% of the concurrent maternal plasma concentrations.

The combination of atovaquone and proguanil hydrochloride was not teratogenic in rats at plasma concentrations up to 1.7 and 0.10 times, respectively, the estimated human exposure during treatment of malaria. In rabbits, the combination of atovaquone and proguanil hydrochloride was not teratogenic or embryotoxic to rabbit fetuses at plasma concentrations up to 0.34 and 0.82 times, respectively, the estimated human exposure during treatment of malaria.

While there are no adequate and well-controlled studies of atovaquone and/or proguanil hydrochloride in pregnant women, MALARONE may be used if the potential benefit justifies the potential risk to the fetus. The proguanil component of MALARONE acts by inhibiting the parasitic dihydrofolate reductase (see CLINICAL PHARMACOLOGY: Microbiology: Mechanism of Action). However, there are no clinical data indicating that folate supplementation diminishes drug efficacy, and for women of childbearing age receiving folate supplements to prevent neural tube birth defects, such supplements may be continued while taking MALARONE.

Nursing Mothers: It is not known whether atovaquone is excreted into human milk. In a rat study, atovaquone concen-

trations in the milk were 30% of the concurrent atovaquone concentrations in the maternal plasma.
Proguanil is excreted into human milk in small quantities. Caution should be exercised when MALARONE is administered to a nursing woman.
Pediatric Use: Safety and effectiveness for the treatment and prophylaxis of malaria in pediatric patients who weigh less than 11 kg have not been established.
Geriatric Use: Clinical studies of MALARONE did not include sufficient numbers of subjects aged 65 and over to determine whether they respond differently from younger subjects. In general, dose selection for an elderly patient should be cautious, reflecting the greater frequency of decreased hepatic, renal, or cardiac function, and of concomitant disease or other drug therapy (see CLINICAL PHARMACOLOGY: Special Populations: Geriatrics).

ADVERSE REACTIONS
Because MALARONE contains atovaquone and proguanil hydrochloride, the type and severity of adverse reactions associated with each of the compounds may be expected. The higher treatment doses of MALARONE were less well tolerated than the lower prophylactic doses.
Among adults who received MALARONE for treatment of malaria, attributable adverse experiences that occurred in ≥5% of patients were abdominal pain (17%), nausea (12%), vomiting (12%), headache (10%), diarrhea (8%), asthenia (8%), anorexia (5%), and dizziness (5%). Treatment was discontinued prematurely due to an adverse experience in 4 of 436 adults treated with MALARONE.
Among pediatric patients who received MALARONE for the treatment of malaria, attributable adverse experiences that occurred in ≥5% of patients were vomiting (10%) and pruritus (6%). Vomiting occurred in 43 of 319 (13%) pediatric patients who did not have symptomatic malaria but were given treatment doses of MALARONE for 3 days in a clinical trial. The design of this clinical trial required that any patient who vomited be withdrawn from the trial. Among pediatric patients with symptomatic malaria treated with MALARONE, treatment was discontinued prematurely due to an adverse experience in 1 of 116 (0.9%).

Abnormalities in laboratory tests reported in clinical trials were limited to elevations of transaminases in malaria patients being treated with MALARONE. The frequency of these abnormalities varied substantially across studies of treatment and were not observed in the randomized portions of the prophylaxis trials.
In one phase III trial of malaria treatment in Thai adults, early elevations of ALT and AST were observed to occur more frequently in patients treated with MALARONE compared to patients treated with an active control drug. Rates for patients who had normal baseline levels of these clinical laboratory parameters were: Day 7: ALT 26.7% vs. 15.6%; AST 16.9% vs. 8.6%. By day 14 of this 28-day study, the frequency of transaminase elevations equalized across the two groups.
In this and other studies in which transaminase elevations occurred, they were noted to persist for up to 4 weeks following treatment with MALARONE for malaria. None were associated with untoward clinical events.
Among subjects who received MALARONE for prophylaxis of malaria, adverse experiences occurred in similar proportions of subjects receiving MALARONE or placebo (Table 1). The most commonly reported adverse experiences possibly attributable to MALARONE or placebo were headache and abdominal pain. Prophylaxis with MALARONE was discontinued prematurely due to a treatment-related adverse experience in 3 of 381 adults and 0 of 125 pediatric patients. [See table 1 at top of previous page]

OVERDOSAGE
There have been no reports of overdosage from the administration of MALARONE.
There is no known antidote for atovaquone, and it is currently unknown if atovaquone is dialyzable. The median lethal dose is higher than the maximum oral dose tested in mice and rats (1825 mg/kg per day). Overdoses up to 31,500 mg of atovaquone have been reported. In one such patient who also took an unspecified dose of dapsone, methemoglobinemia occurred. Rash has also been reported after overdose.

Continued on next page

Table 2: Dosage for Prevention of Malaria in Pediatric Patients

Weight (kg)	Atovaquone/Proguanil HCl Total Daily Dose	Dosage Regimen
11–20	62.5 mg/25 mg	1 MALARONE Pediatric Tablet daily
21–30	125 mg/50 mg	2 MALARONE Pediatric Tablets as a single dose daily
31–40	187.5 mg/75 mg	3 MALARONE Pediatric Tablets as a single dose daily
>40	250 mg/100 mg	1 MALARONE Tablet (adult strength) as a single dose daily

Table 3: Dosage for Treatment of Acute Malaria in Pediatric Patients

Weight (kg)	Atovaquone/Proguanil HCl Total Daily Dose	Dosage Regimen
11–20	250 mg/100 mg	1 MALARONE Tablet (adult strength) daily for 3 consecutive days
21–30	500 mg/200 mg	2 MALARONE Tablets (adult strength) as a single dose daily for 3 consecutive days
31–40	750 mg/300 mg	3 MALARONE Tablets (adult strength) as a single dose daily for 3 consecutive days
>40	1 g/400 mg	4 MALARONE Tablets (adult strength) as a single dose daily for 3 consecutive days

Table 4: Parasitological Response in Clinical Trials of MALARONE for Treatment of *P. falciparum* Malaria

Study Site	MALARONE*		Comparator		
	Evaluable Patients (n)	% Sensitive Response**	Drug(s)	Evaluable Patients (n)	% Sensitive Response**
Brazil	74	98.6%	Quinine and tetracycline	76	100.0%
Thailand	79	100.0%	Mefloquine	79	86.1%
France†	21	100.0%	Halofantrine	18	100.0%
Kenya†‡	81	93.8%	Halofantrine	83	90.4%
Zambia	80	100.0%	Pyrimethamine/ sulfadoxine (P/S)	80	98.8%
Gabon†	63	98.4%	Amodiaquine	63	81.0%
Philippines	54	100.0%	Chloroquine (Cq) Cq and P/S	23 32	30.4% 87.5%
Peru	19	100.0%	Chloroquine P/S	13 7	7.7% 100.0%

*MALARONE = 1000 mg atovaquone and 400 mg proguanil hydrochloride (or equivalent based on body weight for patients weighing ≤40 kg) once daily for 3 days.
**Elimination of parasitemia with no recurrent parasitemia during follow-up for 28 days.
†Patients hospitalized only for acute care. Follow-up conducted in outpatients.
‡Study in pediatric patients 3 to 12 years of age.

Malarone—Cont.

Overdoses of proguanil hydrochloride as large as 1500 mg have been followed by complete recovery, and doses as high as 700 mg twice daily have been taken for over 2 weeks without serious toxicity. Adverse events occasionally associated with proguanil hydrochloride doses of 100 to 200 mg/day, such as epigastric discomfort and vomiting, would be likely to occur with overdose. There are also reports of reversible hair loss and scaling of the skin on the palms and/or soles, reversible aphthous ulceration, and hematologic side effects.

DOSAGE AND ADMINISTRATION

The daily dose should be taken at the same time each day with food or a milky drink. In the event of vomiting within 1 hour after dosing, a repeat dose should be taken.

Prevention of Malaria: Prophylactic treatment with MALARONE should be started 1 or 2 days before entering a malaria-endemic area and continued daily during the stay and for 7 days after return.

Adults: One MALARONE Tablet (adult strength = 250 mg atovaquone/100 mg proguanil hydrochloride) per day.

Pediatric Patients: The dosage for prevention of malaria in pediatric patients is based upon body weight (Table 2).

[See table 2 at top of previous page]

Treatment of Acute Malaria:

Adults: Four MALARONE Tablets (adult strength; total daily dose 1 g atovaquone/400 mg proguanil hydrochloride) as a single dose daily for 3 consecutive days.

Pediatric Patients: The dosage for treatment of acute malaria in pediatric patients is based upon body weight (Table 3).

[See table 3 at top of previous page]

Patients with Renal Impairment: MALARONE should not be used for malaria prophylaxis in patients with severe renal impairment (creatinine clearance <30 mL/min), and alternatives to MALARONE should be recommended for treatment of acute *P. falciparum* malaria whenever possible (see CONTRAINDICATIONS, PRECAUTIONS: General, and CLINICAL PHARMACOLOGY: Special Populations). No dosage adjustments are needed in patients with mild to moderate renal impairment.

HOW SUPPLIED

MALARONE Tablets, containing 250 mg atovaquone and 100 mg proguanil hydrochloride, are pink, film-coated, round, biconvex tablets engraved with "GX CM3" on one side.

Bottle of 100 tablets with child-resistant closure (NDC 0173-0675-01).

MALARONE Pediatric Tablets, containing 62.5 mg atovaquone and 25 mg proguanil hydrochloride, are pink, film-coated, round, biconvex tablets engraved with "GX CG7" on one side.

Bottle of 100 tablets with child-resistant closure (NDC 0173-0676-01).

Store at 25°C (77°F); excursions permitted to 15° to 30°C (59° to 86°F) (see USP Controlled Room Temperature).

ANIMAL TOXICOLOGY

Fibrovascular proliferation in the right atrium, pyelonephritis, bone marrow hypocellularity, lymphoid atrophy, and gastritis/enteritis were observed in dogs treated with proguanil hydrochloride for 6 months at a dose of 12 mg/kg per day (approximately 3.9 times the recommended daily human dose for malaria prophylaxis on a mg/m^2 basis). Bile duct hyperplasia, gall bladder mucosal atrophy, and interstitial pneumonia were observed in dogs treated with proguanil hydrochloride for 6 months at a dose of 4 mg/kg per day (approximately 1.3 times the recommended daily human dose for malaria prophylaxis on a mg/m^2 basis). Mucosal hyperplasia of the cecum and renal tubular basophilia were observed in rats treated with proguanil hydrochloride for 6 months at a dose of 20 mg/kg per day (approximately 1.6 times the recommended daily human dose for malaria prophylaxis on a mg/m^2 basis). Adverse heart, lung, liver, and gall bladder effects observed in dogs and kidney effects observed in rats were not shown to be reversible.

CLINICAL STUDIES

Treatment of Acute Malarial Infections: In 3 phase II clinical trials, atovaquone alone, proguanil hydrochloride alone, and the combination of atovaquone and proguanil hydrochloride were evaluated for the treatment of acute, uncomplicated malaria caused by *P. falciparum*. Among 156 evaluable patients, the parasitological cure rate was 59/89 (66%) with atovaquone alone, 1/17 (6%) with proguanil hydrochloride alone, and 50/50 (100%) with the combination of atovaquone and proguanil hydrochloride.

MALARONE was evaluated for treatment of acute, uncomplicated malaria caused by *P. falciparum* in 8 phase III controlled clinical trials. Among 471 evaluable patients treated with the equivalent of 4 MALARONE Tablets once daily for 3 days, 464 had a sensitive response (elimination of parasitemia with no recurrent parasitemia during follow-up for 28 days) (see Table 4). Seven patients had a response of R1 resistance (elimination of parasitemia but with recurrent parasitemia between 7 and 28 days after starting treatment). In these trials, the response to treatment with MALARONE was similar to treatment with the comparator drug in 4 trials, and better than the response to treatment with the comparator drug in the other 4 trials.

The overall efficacy in 521 evaluable patients was 98.7% (see Table 4).

[See table 4 at top of previous page]

Eighteen of 521 (3.5%) evaluable patients with acute falciparum malaria presented with a pretreatment serum creatinine greater than 2.0 mg/dL (range 2.1 to 4.3 mg/dL). All were successfully treated with MALARONE and 17 of 18 (94.4%) had normal serum creatinine levels by day 7.

Data from a phase II trial of atovaquone conducted in Zambia suggested that approximately 40% of the study population in this country were HIV-infected patients. The enrollment criteria were similar for the phase III trial of MALARONE conducted in Zambia and the results are presented in Table 4. Efficacy rates for MALARONE in this study population were high and comparable to other populations studied.

The efficacy of MALARONE in the treatment of the erythrocytic phase of nonfalciparum malaria was assessed in a small number of patients. Of the 23 patients in Thailand infected with *P. vivax* and treated with atovaquone/proguanil hydrochloride 1000 mg/400 mg daily for 3 days, parasitemia cleared in 21 (91.3%) at 7 days. Parasite relapse occurred commonly when *P. vivax* malaria was treated with MALARONE alone. Seven patients in Gabon with malaria due to *P. ovale* or *P. malariae* were treated with atovaquone/proguanil hydrochloride 1000 mg/400 mg daily for 3 days. All 6 evaluable patients (3 with *P. malariae*, 2 with *P. ovale*, and 1 with mixed *P. falciparum* and *P. ovale*) were cured at 28 days. Relapsing malarias including *P. vivax* and *P. ovale* require additional treatment to prevent relapse.

Prevention of Malaria: MALARONE was evaluated for prophylaxis of malaria in 4 clinical trials in malaria-endemic areas.

Three placebo-controlled studies of 10 to 12 weeks' duration were conducted among residents of malaria-endemic areas in Kenya, Zambia, and Gabon. Of a total of 669 randomized patients (including 264 pediatric patients 5 to 16 years of age), 103 were withdrawn for reasons other than falciparum malaria or drug-related adverse events. (Fifty-five percent of these were lost to follow-up and 45% were withdrawn for protocol violations.) The results are listed in Table 5.

Table 5: Prevention of Parasitemia in Controlled Clinical Trials of MALARONE for Prophylaxis of *P. falciparum* Malaria

	MALARONE	Placebo
Total number of patients randomized	326	341
Failed to complete study	57	44
Developed parasitemia (*P. falciparum*)	2	92

In a 10-week study in 175 South African subjects who moved into malaria-endemic areas and were given prophylaxis with 1 MALARONE Tablet daily, parasitemia developed in 1 subject who missed several doses of medication. Since no placebo control was included, the incidence of malaria in this study was not known. In a malaria challenge study conducted in healthy US volunteers, atovaquone alone prevented malaria in 6/6 individuals, whereas 4/4 placebo-treated volunteers developed malaria. Although these data suggest that MALARONE prophylaxis is effective in both malaria-immune and nonimmune subjects, differences in the response rates may occur.

Causal Prophylaxis: In separate studies with small numbers of volunteers, atovaquone and proguanil hydrochloride were independently shown to have causal prophylactic activity directed against liver-stage parasites of *P. falciparum*. Six patients given a single dose of atovaquone 250 mg 24 hours prior to malaria challenge were protected from developing malaria, whereas all 4 placebo-treated patients developed malaria.

During the 4 weeks following cessation of prophylaxis in clinical trial participants who remained in malaria-endemic areas and were available for evaluation, malaria developed in 24/211 (11.4%) subjects who took placebo and 9/328 (2.7%) who took MALARONE. While new infections could not be distinguished from recrudescent infections, all but 1 of the infections in patients treated with MALARONE occurred more than 15 days after stopping therapy, probably representing new infections. The single case occurring on day 8 following cessation of therapy with MALARONE probably represents a failure of prophylaxis with MALARONE.

The possibility that delayed cases of *P. falciparum* malaria may occur some time after stopping prophylaxis with MALARONE cannot be ruled out. Hence, returning travelers developing febrile illnesses should be investigated for malaria.

Glaxo Wellcome Inc., Research Triangle Park, NC 27709

US Patent Nos. 5,053,432 and 5,998,449

©Copyright 2000, Glaxo Wellcome Inc. All rights reserved.

November 2000/RL-881

NAVELBINE® ℞

[*na 'vəl-bēn*]

(vinorelbine tartrate)

Injection

Prescribing information for this product, which appears on pages 1448–1451 of the 2001 PDR, has been revised as follows. Please write "See Supplement A" next to the product heading.

The following paragraph was revised in the **WARNINGS** *section.*

Reported cases of interstitial pulmonary changes and ARDS, most of which were fatal, occurred in patients treated with single-agent NAVELBINE. The mean time to onset of these symptoms after vinorelbine administration was 1 week (range 3 to 8 days). Patients with alterations in their baseline pulmonary symptoms or with new onset of dyspnea, cough, hypoxia, or other symptoms should be evaluated promptly.

The following paragraph was revised in the **ADVERSE REACTIONS: Observed During Clinical Practice** *subsection.*

Gastrointestinal: Dysphagia, mucositis, and pancreatitis have been reported.

Manufactured by Pierre Fabre Medicament Production, 64320 Idron, FRANCE

for Glaxo Wellcome Inc., Research Triangle Park, NC 27709

Under license of Pierre Fabre Médicament - Centre National de la Recherche Scientifique-France

US Patent No. 4,307,100

©Copyright 1996, 2000, Glaxo Wellcome Inc. All rights reserved.

October 2000/RL-872

OXISTAT® ℞

[*öx 'ē-stat"*]

(oxiconazole nitrate cream)

Cream, 1%*

OXISTAT®

(oxiconazole nitrate lotion)

Lotion, 1%*

***Potency expressed as oxiconazole**

FOR TOPICAL DERMATOLOGIC USE ONLY—NOT FOR OPHTHALMIC OR INTRAVAGINAL USE

Prescribing information for this product, which appears on pages 1451–1452 of the 2001 PDR, has been revised as follows. Please write "See Supplement A" next to the product heading.

Added the following subsection to the **PRECAUTIONS** *section.*

Geriatric Use: A limited number of patients at or above 65 years of age (n = 508) have been treated with OXISTAT Cream in US and non-US clinical trials, and a limited number (n = 43) have been treated with OXISTAT Lotion in US clinical trials. The number of patients is too small to permit separate analysis of efficacy and safety. No adverse events were reported with OXISTAT Lotion in geriatric patients, and the adverse reactions reported with OXISTAT Cream in this population were similar to those reported by younger patients. Based on available data, no adjustment of dosage of OXISTAT Cream and Lotion in geriatric patients is warranted.

Added the following subsection to the **DOSAGE AND ADMINISTRATION** *section.*

Geriatric Use: In studies where geriatric patients (65 years of age or older, see PRECAUTIONS) have been treated with OXISTAT Cream or Lotion, safety did not differ from that in younger patients; therefore, no dosage adjustment is recommended.

Glaxo Wellcome Inc., Research Triangle Park, NC 27709

July 2000/RL-847

RETROVIR® ℞

[*re 'trō-vir*]

(zidovudine)

IV Infusion

For Intravenous Infusion Only

Prescribing information for this product, which appears on pages 1460–1464 of the 2001 PDR, has been revised as follows. Please write "See Supplement A" next to the product heading.

The **CLINICAL PHARMACOLOGY: Pharmacokinetics: Nursing Mothers** *subsection was revised to:*

The Centers for Disease Control and Prevention recommend that HIV-infected mothers not breastfeed their infants to avoid risking postnatal transmission of HIV. After administration of a single dose of 200 mg zidovudine to 13 HIV-infected women, the mean concentration of zidovudine was similar in human milk and serum (see PRECAUTIONS: Nursing Mothers).

The **PRECAUTIONS: Nursing Mothers** *subsection was revised to:*

The Centers for Disease Control and Prevention recommended that HIV-infected women not breastfeed their infants to avoid risking postnatal transmission of HIV. Zidovudine is excreted in human milk (see CLINICAL PHARMACOLOGY: Pharmacokinetics: Nursing Mothers). Because of both the potential for HIV transmission and the potential for serious adverse reactions in nursing infants, **mothers should be instructed not to breastfeed if they are receiving RETROVIR** (see Pediatric Use and INDICATIONS AND USAGE: Maternal-Fetal HIV Transmission).

The **PRECAUTIONS: Pediatric Use** *subsection was revised to:*

Pediatric Use: RETROVIR has been studied in HIV-infected pediatric patients over 3 months of age who have HIV-related symptoms or who are asymptomatic with abnormal laboratory values indicating significant HIV-related immunosuppression (see ADVERSE REACTIONS, DOSAGE AND ADMINISTRATION, INDICATIONS AND USAGE: Description of Clinical Studies, and CLINICAL PHARMACOLOGY: Pharmacokinetics).

Manufactured by Catalytica Pharmaceuticals, Inc.
Greenville, NC 27834
for Glaxo Wellcome Inc., Research Triangle Park, NC 27709
©Copyright 1996, 2000, Glaxo Wellcome Inc. All rights reserved.
September 2000/RL-863

SEREVENT®   ℞
[*ser' a-vent*]
(salmeterol xinafoate)
Inhalation Aerosol

Bronchodilator Aerosol
For Oral Inhalation Only

Prescribing information for this product, which appears on pages 1464–1468 of the 2001 PDR has been revised. Please write "See Supplement A" next to the product heading.
The **CLINICAL PHARMACOLOGY: Pharmacokinetics** *subsection was revised to the following.*

Pharmacokinetics: Salmeterol xinafoate, an ionic salt, dissociates in solution so that the salmeterol and 1-hydroxy-2-naphthoic acid (xinafoate) moieties are absorbed, distributed, metabolized, and excreted independently. Salmeterol acts locally in the lung; therefore, plasma levels do not predict therapeutic effect.

Absorption: Because of the small therapeutic dose, systemic levels of salmeterol are low or undetectable after inhalation of recommended doses (42 mcg of salmeterol inhalation aerosol twice daily). Following chronic administration of an inhaled dose of 42 mcg twice daily, salmeterol was detected in plasma within 5 to 10 minutes in 6 asthmatic patients; plasma concentrations were very low, with peak concentrations of 150 pg/mL and no accumulation with repeated doses. Larger inhaled doses gave approximately proportionally increased blood levels. In these patients, a second peak concentration of 115 pg/mL occurred at about 45 minutes, probably due to absorption of the swallowed portion of the dose (most of the dose delivered by a metered-dose inhaler is swallowed).

Distribution: Binding of salmeterol to human plasma proteins averages 96% in vitro over the concentration range of 8 to 7722 ng of salmeterol base per milliliter, much higher than those achieved following therapeutic doses of salmeterol.

Metabolism: Salmeterol base is extensively metabolized by hydroxylation, with subsequent elimination predominantly in the feces. No significant amount of unchanged salmeterol base was detected in either urine or feces.

Excretion: In 2 healthy subjects who received 1 mg of radiolabeled salmeterol (as salmeterol xinafoate) orally, approximately 25% and 60% of the radiolabeled salmeterol was eliminated in urine and feces, respectively, over a period of 7 days. The terminal elimination half-life was about 5.5 hours (1 volunteer only).

The xinafoate moiety has no apparent pharmacologic activity. The xinafoate moiety is highly protein bound (>99%) and has a long elimination half-life of 11 days.

Special Populations: The pharmacokinetics of salmeterol base has not been studied in elderly patients or in patients with hepatic or renal impairment. Since salmeterol is predominantly cleared by hepatic metabolism, liver function impairment may lead to accumulation of salmeterol in plasma. Therefore, patients with hepatic disease should be closely monitored.

The first two paragraphs of the **CLINICAL PHARMACOLOGY: Pharmacodynamics** *subsection were revised to the following.*

Pharmacodynamics: Inhaled salmeterol, like other beta-adrenergic agonist drugs, can in some patients produce dose-related cardiovascular effects and effects on blood glucose and/or serum potassium (see PRECAUTIONS). The cardiovascular effects (heart rate, blood pressure) associated with salmeterol occur with similar frequency, and are of similar type and severity, as those noted following albuterol administration. The effects of rising doses of salmeterol and standard inhaled doses of albuterol were studied in volunteers and in patients with asthma. Salmeterol doses up to 84 mcg administered as inhalation aerosol resulted in heart rate increases of 3 to 16 beats/min, about the same as albuterol dosed at 180 mcg by inhalation aerosol (4 to 10 beats/min). In 2 double-blind asthma studies, patients receiving either 42 mcg of salmeterol inhalation aerosol twice daily (n = 81) or 180 mcg of albuterol inhalation aerosol 4 times daily (n = 80) underwent continuous electrocardiographic monitoring during four 24-hour periods; no clinically significant dysrhythmias were noted. Continuous electrocardiographic monitoring was also performed in 2 double-blind studies in COPD patients (see ADVERSE REACTIONS).

The following subsection was added to **CLINICAL TRIALS.**

Effects in Patients With Asthma on Concomitant Inhaled Corticosteroids: In 4 clinical trials in adult and adolescent patients with asthma (n = 1922), the effect of adding salmeterol to inhaled corticosteroid therapy was evaluated. The studies utilized the inhalation aerosol formulation of salmeterol xinafoate for a treatment period of 6 months. They compared the addition of salmeterol therapy to an increase (at least doubling) of the inhaled corticosteroid dose.

Two randomized, double-blind, parallel group clinical trials (n = 997) enrolled patients (ages 18–82 years) with persistent asthma who were previously maintained but not adequately controlled on inhaled corticosteroid therapy. During the 2-week run-in period, all patients were switched to beclomethasone dipropionate 168 mcg twice daily. Patients still not adequately controlled were randomized to either the addition of salmeterol inhalation aerosol 42 mcg twice daily or an increase of beclomethasone dipropionate to 336 mcg twice daily. As compared to the doubled dose of beclomethasone dipropionate, the addition of salmeterol resulted in statistically significantly greater improvements in pulmonary function and asthma symptoms, and statistically significantly greater reduction in supplemental albuterol use. The percent of patients who experienced asthma exacerbations overall was not different between groups (i.e., 16.2% in the salmeterol group versus 17.9% in the higher dose beclomethasone dipropionate group).

Two randomized, double-blind, parallel group clinical trials (n = 925) enrolled patients (ages 12–78 years) with persistent asthma who were previously maintained but not adequately controlled on prior therapy. During the 2- to 4-week run-in period, all patients were switched to fluticasone propionate 88 mcg twice daily. Patients still not adequately controlled were randomized to either the addition of salmeterol inhalation aerosol 42 mcg twice daily or an increase of fluticasone propionate to 220 mcg twice daily. As compared to the increased (2.5 times) dose of fluticasone propionate, the addition of salmeterol resulted in statistically significantly greater improvements in pulmonary function and asthma symptoms, and statistically significantly greater reduction in supplemental albuterol use. Fewer patients receiving salmeterol experienced asthma exacerbations than those receiving the higher dose of fluticasone propionate (8.8% versus 13.8%).

The following paragraph was revised in the **INDICATIONS AND USAGE: Asthma** *subsection.*

SEREVENT Inhalation Aerosol may be used alone or in combination with inhaled or systemic corticosteroid therapy.
The following paragraph was revised in the **WARNINGS** *section.*

4. Do Not Use SEREVENT Inhalation Aerosol as a Substitute for Oral or Inhaled Corticosteroids: The use of beta-adrenergic agonist bronchodilators alone may not be adequate to control asthma in many patients. Early consideration should be given to adding anti-inflammatory agents, e.g., corticosteroids. There are no data demonstrating that SEREVENT Inhalation Aerosol has a clinical anti-inflammatory effect and could be expected to take the place of corticosteroids. Patients who already require oral or inhaled corticosteroids for treatment of asthma should be continued on this type of treatment even if they feel better as a result of initiating SEREVENT Inhalation Aerosol. Any change in corticosteroid dosage should be made ONLY after clinical evaluation (see PRECAUTIONS: Information for Patients).
The following paragraphs were revised in the **ADVERSE REACTIONS: Asthma** *subsection.*

Data from small dose-response studies show an apparent dose relationship for tremor, nervousness, and palpitations. In clinical trials evaluating concurrent therapy of salmeterol with inhaled corticosteroids, adverse events were consistent with those previously reported for salmeterol, or might otherwise be expected with the use of inhaled corticosteroids.

Glaxo Wellcome Inc., Research Triangle Park, NC 27709
US Patent Nos. 4,992,474; 5,225,445; and 5,380,922
©Copyright 1994, 1998, 2000, Glaxo Wellcome Inc. All rights reserved.
July 2000/RL-851

SEREVENT® DISKUS®   ℞
[*sĕr' ə-vent dĭsk' us*]
(salmeterol xinafoate inhalation powder)

For Oral Inhalation Only

Prescribing information for this product, which appears on pages 1468–1471 of the 2001 PDR, has been revised. Please write "See Supplement A" next to the product heading.
The **CLINICAL PHARMACOLOGY: Pharmacokinetics** *subsection was revised to the following.*

Pharmacokinetics: Salmeterol xinafoate, an ionic salt, dissociates in solution so that the salmeterol and 1-hydroxy-2-naphthoic acid (xinafoate) moieties are absorbed, distributed, metabolized, and excreted independently. Salmeterol acts locally in the lung; therefore, plasma levels do not predict therapeutic effect.

Absorption: Because of the small therapeutic dose, systemic levels of salmeterol are low or undetectable after inhalation of recommended doses (50 mcg of salmeterol inhalation powder twice daily). Following chronic administration of an inhaled dose of 50 mcg of salmeterol inhalation powder twice daily, salmeterol was detected in plasma within 5 to 45 minutes in 7 asthmatic patients; plasma concentrations were very low, with mean peak concentrations of 167 pg/mL at 20 minutes and no accumulation with repeated doses.

Distribution: Binding of salmeterol to human plasma proteins averages 96% in vitro over the concentration range of 8 to 7722 ng of salmeterol base per milliliter, much higher than those achieved following therapeutic doses of salmeterol.

Metabolism: Salmeterol base is extensively metabolized by hydroxylation, with subsequent elimination predominantly in the feces. No significant amount of unchanged salmeterol base was detected in either urine or feces.

Excretion: In 2 healthy subjects who received 1 mg of radiolabeled salmeterol (as salmeterol xinafoate) orally, approximately 25% and 60% of the radiolabeled salmeterol was eliminated in urine and feces, respectively, over a period of 7 days. The terminal elimination half-life was about 5.5 hours (1 volunteer only).

The xinafoate moiety has no apparent pharmacologic activity. The xinafoate moiety is highly protein bound (>99%) and has a long elimination half-life of 11 days.

Special Populations: The pharmacokinetics of salmeterol base has not been studied in elderly patients or in patients with hepatic or renal impairment. Since salmeterol is predominantly cleared by hepatic metabolism, liver function impairment may lead to accumulation of salmeterol in plasma. Therefore, patients with hepatic disease should be closely monitored.

The first paragraph of the **CLINICAL PHARMACOLOGY: Pharmacodynamics** *subsection was revised to the following.*
Inhaled salmeterol, like other beta-adrenergic agonist drugs, can in some patients produce dose-related cardiovascular effects and effects on blood glucose and/or serum potassium (see PRECAUTIONS). The cardiovascular effects (heart rate, blood pressure) associated with salmeterol inhalation aerosol occur with similar frequency, and are of similar type and severity, as those noted following albuterol administration.

The following subsection was added to **CLINICAL TRIALS.**

Effects in Patients With Asthma on Concomitant Inhaled Corticosteroids: In 4 clinical trials in adult and adolescent patients with asthma (n = 1922), the effect of adding salmeterol to inhaled corticosteroid therapy was evaluated. The studies utilized the inhalation aerosol formulation of salmeterol xinafoate for a treatment period of 6 months. They compared the addition of salmeterol therapy to an increase (at least doubling) of the inhaled corticosteroid dose.

Two randomized, double-blind, controlled, parallel group clinical trials (n = 997) enrolled patients (ages 18–82 years) with persistent asthma who were previously maintained but not adequately controlled on inhaled corticosteroid therapy. During the 2-week run-in period all patients were switched to beclomethasone dipropionate 168 mcg twice daily. Patients still not adequately controlled were randomized to either the addition of salmeterol inhalation aerosol 42 mcg twice daily or an increase of beclomethasone dipropionate to 336 mcg twice daily. As compared to the doubled dose of beclomethasone dipropionate, the addition of salmeterol resulted in statistically significantly greater improvements in pulmonary function and asthma symptoms, and statistically significantly greater reduction in supplemental albuterol use. The percent of patients who experienced asthma exacerbations overall was not different between groups (i.e., 16.2% in the salmeterol group versus 17.9% in the higher dose beclomethasone dipropionate group).

Two randomized, double-blind, parallel group clinical trials (n = 925) enrolled patients (ages 12–78 years) with persistent asthma who were previously maintained but not adequately controlled on prior therapy. During the 2- to 4-week run-in period, all patients were switched to fluticasone propionate 88 mcg twice daily. Patients still not adequately controlled were randomized to either the addition of salmeterol inhalation aerosol 42 mcg twice daily or an increase of fluticasone propionate to 220 mcg twice daily. As compared to the increased (2.5 times) dose of fluticasone propionate, the addition of salmeterol resulted in statistically significantly greater improvements in pulmonary function and asthma symptoms, and statistically significantly greater reduction in supplemental albuterol use. Fewer patients receiving salmeterol experienced asthma exacerbations than those receiving the higher dose of fluticasone propionate (8.8% versus 13.8%)

The following paragraph was revised in the **INDICATIONS AND USAGE** *section.*
SEREVENT DISKUS may be used alone or in combination with inhaled or systemic corticosteroid therapy.
The following paragraph was revised in the **WARNINGS** *section.*

4. Do Not Use SEREVENT DISKUS as a Substitute for Oral or Inhaled Corticosteroids: The use of beta-adrenergic agonist bronchodilators alone may not be adequate to control asthma in many patients. Early consideration should be given to adding anti-inflammatory agents, e.g., corticosteroids. There are no data demonstrating that SEREVENT DISKUS has a clinical anti-inflammatory effect and could be expected to take the place of corticosteroids. Patients who already require oral or inhaled corticosteroids for treatment of asthma should be continued on a suitable dose to maintain clinical stability even if they feel better as a result of initiating SEREVENT DISKUS. Any change in corticosteroid dosage should be made ONLY after clinical evaluation (see PRECAUTIONS: Information for Patients).
The following paragraph was added to the **ADVERSE REACTIONS** *section.*
In clinical trials evaluating concurrent therapy of salmeterol with inhaled corticosteroids, adverse events were consistent with those previously reported for salmeterol, or might otherwise be expected with the used of inhaled corticosteroids.

Continued on next page

Serevent Diskus—Cont.

Glaxo Wellcome Inc., Research Triangle Park, NC 27709
US Patent Nos. 4,992,474; 5,225,445; 5,126,375; 5,860,419; 5,873,360; 5,590,645; and Des. 342,994
©Copyright 1997, 2000, Glaxo Wellcome Inc. All rights reserved.
July 2000/RL-852

TEMOVATE® ℞
[tim 'ō-vāt]
(clobetasol propionate cream)
Cream, 0.05%

TEMOVATE® ℞
(clobetasol propionate ointment)
Ointment, 0.05%

For Dermatologic Use Only—
Not for Ophthalmic Use.
FOR TOPICAL DERMATOLOGIC USE ONLY—
NOT FOR OPHTHALMIC, ORAL, OR INTRAVAGINAL USE

Prescribing information for this product, which appears on pages 1473–1474 of the 2001 PDR, has been revised as follows. Please "See Supplement A" next to the product heading.

"Children" was changed to "pediatric patients" in the following sentence in **INDICATIONS AND USAGE**. Use in pediatric patients under 12 years of age is not recommended.

The following paragraph was revised in the **PRECAUTIONS: Carcinogenesis, Mutagenesis, Impairment of Fertility** *subsection.*

Studies in the rat following subcutaneous administration at dosage levels up to 50 mcg/kg per day revealed that the females exhibited an increase in the number of resorbed embryos and a decrease in the number of living fetuses at the highest dose.

The following paragraphs were revised in the **PRECAUTIONS: Pregnancy** *subsection.*

Teratogenicity studies in mice using the subcutaneous route resulted in fetotoxicity at the highest dose tested (1 mg/kg) and teratogenicity at all dose levels tested down to 0.03 mg/kg. These doses are approximately 1.4 and 0.04 times, respectively, the human topical dose of TEMOVATE Cream and Ointment. Abnormalities seen included cleft palate and skeletal abnormalities.

In rabbits, clobetasol propionate was teratogenic at doses of 3 and 10 mcg/kg. These doses are approximately 0.02 and 0.05 times, respectively, the human topical dose of TEMOVATE Cream and Ointment. Abnormalities seen included cleft palate, cranioschisis, and other skeletal abnormalities.

The first two sentences of the **PRECAUTIONS: Pediatric Use** *subsection were revised to:*

Safety and effectiveness of TEMOVATE Cream and Ointment in pediatric patients have not been established. Use in pediatric patients under 12 years of age is not recommended.

The following subsection was added to **PRECAUTIONS**.

Geriatric Use: A limited number of patients at or above 65 years of age have been treated with TEMOVATE Cream (n = 231) and with TEMOVATE Ointment (n = 101) in US and non-US clinical trials. While the number of patients is too small to permit separate analysis of efficacy and safety, the adverse reactions reported in this population were similar to those reported by younger patients. Based on available data, no adjustment of dosage of TEMOVATE Cream and Ointment in geriatric patients is warranted.

The first sentence of the **DOSAGE AND ADMINISTRATION** *section was revised to:*

Apply a thin layer of TEMOVATE Cream or Ointment to the affected skin areas twice daily and rub in gently and completely (see INDICATIONS AND USAGE).

The following subsection was added to **DOSAGE AND ADMINISTRATION**.

Geriatric Use: In studies where geriatric patients (65 years of age or older, see PRECAUTIONS) have been treated with TEMOVATE Cream or Ointment, safety did not differ from that in younger patients; therefore, no dosage adjustment is recommended.

Glaxo Wellcome Inc., Research Triangle Park, NC 27709
July 2000/RL-848

TEMOVATE® ℞
[tim 'ō-vāt]
(clobetasol propionate gel)
Gel, 0.05%

FOR TOPICAL DERMATOLOGIC USE ONLY—
NOT FOR OPHTHALMIC, ORAL, OR INTRAVAGINAL USE

Prescribing information for this product, which appears on page 1474 of the 2001 PDR, has been revised as follows. Please write "See Supplement A" next to the product heading.

"Children" was changed to "pediatric patients" in the following sentence in **INDICATIONS AND USAGE**.

Use in pediatric patients under 12 years of age is not recommended.

The following sentence was revised in the **PRECAUTIONS: General** *subsection.*

Patients applying a topical steroid to a large surface area or to areas under occlusion should be evaluated periodically for evidence of HPA axis suppression.

In the following sentence, "children" was changed to "pediatric patients".

Pediatric patients may be more susceptible to systemic toxicity from equivalent doses due to their larger skin surface to body mass ratios (see PRECAUTIONS: Pediatric Use).

The following paragraph was revised in the **PRECAUTIONS: Carcinogenesis, Mutagenesis, Impairment of Fertility** *subsection.*

Studies in the rat following subcutaneous administration at dosage levels up to 50 mcg/kg per day revealed that the females exhibited an increase in the number of resorbed embryos and a decrease in the number of living fetuses at the highest dose.

The following paragraphs were revised in the **PRECAUTIONS: Pregnancy** *subsection.*

Clobetasol propionate has not been tested for teratogenicity when applied topically; however, it is absorbed percutaneously, and when administered subcutaneously it was a significant teratogen in both the rabbit and mouse. Clobetasol propionate has greater teratogenic potential than steroids that are less potent.

Teratogenicity studies in mice using the subcutaneous route resulted in fetotoxicity at the highest dose tested (1 mg/kg) and teratogenicity at all dose levels tested down to 0.03 mg/kg. These doses are approximately 1.4 and 0.04 times, respectively, the human topical dose of TEMOVATE Gel. Abnormalities seen included cleft palate and skeletal abnormalities.

In rabbits, clobetasol propionate was teratogenic at doses of 3 and 10 mcg/kg. These doses are approximately 0.02 and 0.05 times, respectively, the human topical dose of TEMOVATE Gel. Abnormalities seen included cleft palate, cranioschisis, and other skeletal abnormalities.

The following sentence was revised in the **PRECAUTIONS: Pediatric Use** *subsection.*

They are therefore also at greater risk of adrenal insufficiency after withdrawal of treatment and of Cushing's syndrome while on treatment.

The following subsection was added to **PRECAUTIONS.**

Geriatric Use: A limited number of patients at or above 65 years of age (n = 37) have been treated with TEMOVATE Gel in US clinical trials. The number of patients is too small to permit separate analysis of efficacy and safety, and no adverse events were reported in geriatric patients. Based on available data, no adjustment of dosage of TEMOVATE Gel in geriatric patients is warranted.

The following subsection was added to **DOSAGE AND ADMINISTRATION**.

Geriatric Use: In studies where geriatric patients (65 years of age or older, see PRECAUTIONS) have been treated with TEMOVATE Gel, safety did not differ from that in younger patients; therefore, no dosage adjustment is recommended.

Glaxo Wellcome Inc., Research Triangle Park, NC 27709
July 2000/RL-849

TEMOVATE® ℞
[tim 'ō-vāt]
(clobetasol propionate scalp application)
Scalp Application, 0.05%

For Dermatologic Use Only—
Not for Ophthalmic Use.
FOR TOPICAL DERMATOLOGIC USE ONLY—
NOT FOR OPHTHALMIC, ORAL, OR INTRAVAGINAL USE

Prescribing information for this product, which appears on pages 1474–1475 of the 2001 PDR, has been revised as follows. Please write "See Supplement A" next to the product heading.

"Children" was changed to "pediatric patients" in the following sentence in the **INDICATIONS AND USAGE** *section.*

This product is not recommended for use in pediatric patients under 12 years of age.

"Children" was changed to "pediatric patients" in the following sentence in the **PRECAUTIONS: General** *subsection.*

Pediatric patients may absorb proportionally larger amounts of topical corticosteroids and thus be more susceptible to systemic toxicity (see PRECAUTIONS: Pediatric Use).

The following subsections were revised in the **PRECAUTIONS** *section.*

Carcinogenesis, Mutagenesis, Impairment of Fertility: Long-term animal studies have not been performed to evaluate the carcinogenic potential of clobetasol propionate.

Studies in the rat following subcutaneous administration at dosage levels up to 50 mcg/kg per day revealed that the females exhibited an increase in the number of resorbed embryos and a decrease in the number of living fetuses at the highest dose.

Clobetasol propionate was nonmutagenic in 3 different test systems: the Ames test, the *Saccharomyces cerevisiae* gene conversion assay, and the *E. coli* B WP2 fluctuation test.

Pregnancy: *Teratogenic Effects:* Pregnancy Category C. Corticosteroids have been shown to be teratogenic in laboratory animals when administered systemically at relatively low dosage levels. Some corticosteroids have been shown to be teratogenic after dermal application to laboratory animals.

Clobetasol propionate has not been tested for teratogenicity when applied topically; however, it is absorbed percutaneously, and when administered subcutaneously it was a significant teratogen in both the rabbit and mouse. Clobetasol propionate has greater teratogenic potential than steroids that are less potent.

Teratogenicity studies in mice using the subcutaneous route resulted in fetotoxicity at the highest dose tested (1 mg/kg) and teratogenicity at all dose levels tested down to 0.03 mg/kg. These doses are approximately 1.4 and 0.04 times, respectively, the human topical dose of TEMOVATE Scalp Application. Abnormalities seen included cleft palate and skeletal abnormalities.

In rabbits, clobetasol propionate was teratogenic at doses of 3 and 10 mcg/kg. These doses are approximately 0.02 and 0.05 times, respectively, the human topical dose of TEMOVATE Scalp Application. Abnormalities seen included cleft palate, cranioschisis, and other skeletal abnormalities.

There are no adequate and well-controlled studies of the teratogenic potential of clobetasol propionate in pregnant women. TEMOVATE Scalp Application should be used during pregnancy only if the potential benefit justifies the potential risk to the fetus.

Nursing Mothers: Systemically administered corticosteroids appear in human milk and could suppress growth, interfere with endogenous corticosteroid production, or cause other untoward effects. It is not known whether topical administration of corticosteroids could result in sufficient systemic absorption to produce detectable quantities in human milk. Because many drugs are excreted in human milk, caution should be exercised when TEMOVATE Scalp Application is administered to a nursing woman.

Pediatric Use: Use of TEMOVATE Scalp Application in pediatric patients under 12 years of age is not recommended.

Pediatric patients may demonstrate greater susceptibility to topical corticosteroid-induced HPA axis suppression and Cushing's syndrome than mature patients because of a larger skin surface area to body weight ratio.

HPA axis suppression, Cushing's syndrome, linear growth retardation, delayed weight gain, and intracranial hypertension have been reported in children receiving topical corticosteroids. Manifestations of adrenal suppression in children include low plasma cortisol levels and an absence of response to ACTH stimulation. Manifestations of intracranial hypertension include bulging fontanelles, headaches, and bilateral papilledema.

The following subsection was added to the **PRECAUTIONS** *section.*

Geriatric Use: A limited number of patients at or above 65 years of age (n = 65) have been treated with TEMOVATE Scalp Application in US and non-US clinical trials. While the number of patients is too small to permit separate analysis of efficacy and safety, the adverse reactions reported in this population were similar to those reported by younger patients. Based on available data, no adjustment of dosage of TEMOVATE Scalp Application in geriatric patients is warranted.

The following subsection was added to the **DOSAGE AND ADMINISTRATION** *section.*

Geriatric Use: In studies where geriatric patients (65 years of age or older, see PRECAUTIONS) have been treated with TEMOVATE Scalp Application, safety did not differ from that in younger patients; therefore, no dosage adjustment is recommended.

Glaxo Wellcome Inc., Research Triangle Park, NC 27709
August 2000/RL-845

TEMOVATE E® ℞
[tim 'ō-vāt "]
(clobetasol propionate emollient cream)
Emollient, 0.05%
FOR TOPICAL DERMATOLOGIC USE ONLY—NOT FOR OPHTHALMIC, ORAL, OR INTRAVAGINAL USE

Prescribing information for this product, which appears on pages 1475–1476 of the 2001 PDR, has been revised. Please write "See Supplement A" next to the product heading.

"Children" was changed to "pediatric patients" in the following sentence in **INDICATIONS AND USAGE**: Use in pediatric patients under 12 years of age is not recommended.

The following paragraph was revised in the **PRECAUTIONS: Carcinogenesis, Mutagenesis, Impairment of Fertility** *subsection.*

Studies in the rat following subcutaneous administration at dosage levels up to 50 mcg/kg per day revealed that the females exhibited an increase in the number of resorbed embryos and a decrease in the number of living fetuses at the highest dose.

The following paragraphs were revised in the **PRECAUTIONS: Pregnancy** *subsection.*

Clobetasol propionate has not been tested for teratogenicity when applied topically; however, it is absorbed percutaneously, and when administered subcutaneously it was a significant teratogen in both the rabbit and mouse. Clobetasol propionate has greater teratogenic potential than steroids that are less potent.

Teratogenicity studies in mice using the subcutaneous route resulted in fetotoxicity at the highest dose tested (1 mg/kg) and teratogenicity at all dose levels tested down to 0.03 mg/kg. These doses are approximately 1.4 and 0.04 times, respectively, the human topical dose of TEMOVATE E Emollient. Abnormalities seen included cleft palate and skeletal abnormalities.

In rabbits, clobetasol propionate was teratogenic at doses of 3 and 10 mcg/kg. These doses are approximately 0.02 and 0.05 times, respectively, the human topical dose of TEMOVATE E Emollient. Abnormalities seen included cleft palate, cranioschisis, and other skeletal abnormalities.

The first two sentences of the **PRECAUTIONS: Pediatric Use** *subsection were revised to:*

Safety and effectiveness of TEMOVATE E Emollient in pediatric patients have not been established. Use in pediatric patients under 12 years of age is not recommended.

The following subsection was added to **PRECAUTIONS**:

Geriatric Use: A limited number of patients at or above 65 years of age (n = 34) have been treated with TEMOVATE E Emollient in US clinical trials. While the number of patients is too small to permit separate analysis of efficacy and safety, the single adverse reaction reported in this population was similar to those reactions reported by younger patients. Based on available data, no adjustment of dosage of TEMOVATE E Emollient in geriatric patients is warranted.

The **OVERDOSAGE** *section was revised to:*

Topically applied TEMOVATE E Emollient can be absorbed in sufficient amounts to produce systemic effects (see PRECAUTIONS).

The following sentence was deleted from the second paragraph of the **DOSAGE AND ADMINISTRATION** *section:*

Use in children under 12 years of age is not recommended.

The following sentence was revised in the third paragraph:

As with other highly active corticosteroids, therapy should be discontinued when control has been achieved. If no improvement is seen within 2 weeks, reassessment of diagnosis may be necessary.

The following subsection was added to **DOSAGE AND ADMINISTRATION**:

Geriatric Use: In studies where geriatric patients (65 years of age or older, see PRECAUTIONS) have been treated with TEMOVATE E Emollient, safety did not differ from that in younger patients; therefore, no dosage adjustment is recommended.

Glaxo Wellcome Inc., Research Triangle Park, NC 27709
July 2000/RL-850

VALTREX® ℞

[val'trĕx]
(valacyclovir hydrochloride)
Caplets

Prescribing information for this product, which appears on pages 1476–1478 of the 2001 PDR, has been revised. Please write "See Supplement A" next to the product heading.

The **PRECAUTIONS: Geriatric Use** *subsection has been revised to:*

Geriatric Use: Of the total number of subjects in clinical studies of VALTREX, 861 were 65 and over, and 344 were 75 and over. Other clinical experience has identified a greater number of reports and increased severity of CNS adverse events in elderly patients as compared to younger patients (see ADVERSE REACTIONS: Observed During Clinical Practice). Dose selection for an elderly patient should be cautious, reflecting the greater frequency of decreased renal function. This drug is known to be substantially excreted by the kidney, and the risk of toxic reactions to this drug may be greater in patients with impaired renal function. Because elderly patients are more likely to have reduced renal function, care should be taken in dose selection, and it may be useful to monitor renal function (see CLINICAL PHARMACOLOGY and DOSAGE AND ADMINISTRATION: Table 4).

The following two listings were revised in the **ADVERSE REACTIONS: Observed During Clinical Practice** *subsection:*

CNS Symptoms: Aggressive behavior; agitation; coma; confusion; decreased consciousness, encephalopathy; mania, and psychosis, including auditory and visual hallucinations (see PRECAUTIONS).

Eye: Visual abnormalties.

Manufactured by Catalytica Pharmaceuticals, Inc.
Greenville, NC 27834
for Glaxo Wellcome Inc., Research Triangle Park, NC 27709
US Patent Nos. 4,567,182; 4,957,924; 5,879,706; and 6,107,302
©Copyright 1996, 1999, 2000, Glaxo Wellcome Inc. All rights reserved.
October 2000/RL-871

ZIAGEN® ℞

[zī' ə-jin]
(abacavir sulfate)
Tablets

ZIAGEN® ℞

(abacavir sulfate)
Oral Solution

Prescribing information for this product, which appears on pages 1497–1500 of the 2001 PDR, has been completely revised as follows. Please write "See Supplement A" next to the product heading.

WARNING: FATAL HYPERSENSITIVITY REACTIONS HAVE BEEN ASSOCIATED WITH THERAPY WITH ZIAGEN. PATIENTS DEVELOPING SIGNS OR SYMPTOMS OF HYPERSENSITIVITY (WHICH INCLUDE FEVER; SKIN RASH; FATIGUE; GASTROINTESTINAL SYMPTOMS SUCH AS NAUSEA, VOMITING, DIARRHEA, OR ABDOMINAL PAIN; AND RESPIRATORY SYMPTOMS SUCH AS PHARYNGITIS, DYSPNEA, OR COUGH) SHOULD DISCONTINUE ZIAGEN AS SOON AS A HYPERSENSITIVITY REACTION IS SUSPECTED. TO AVOID A DELAY IN DIAGNOSIS AND MINIMIZE THE RISK OF A LIFE-THREATENING HYPERSENSITIVITY REACTION, ZIAGEN SHOULD BE PERMANENTLY DISCONTINUED IF HYPERSENSITIVITY CAN NOT BE RULED OUT, EVEN WHEN OTHER DIAGNOSES ARE POSSIBLE (E.G., ACUTE ONSET RESPIRATORY DISEASES, GASTROENTERITIS, OR REACTIONS TO OTHER MEDICATIONS).

ZIAGEN SHOULD NOT BE RESTARTED FOLLOWING A HYPERSENSITIVITY REACTION BECAUSE MORE SEVERE SYMPTOMS WILL RECUR WITHIN HOURS AND MAY INCLUDE LIFE-THREATENING HYPOTENSION AND DEATH.

SEVERE OR FATAL HYPERSENSITIVITY REACTIONS CAN OCCUR WITHIN HOURS AFTER REINTRODUCTION OF ZIAGEN IN PATIENTS WHO HAVE NO IDENTIFIED HISTORY OR UNRECOGNIZED SYMPTOMS OF HYPERSENSITIVITY TO ABACAVIR THERAPY (see WARNINGS, PRECAUTIONS: Information for Patients, and ADVERSE REACTIONS).

LACTIC ACIDOSIS AND SEVERE HEPATOMEGALY WITH STEATOSIS, INCLUDING FATAL CASES, HAVE BEEN REPORTED WITH THE USE OF NUCLEOSIDE ANALOGUES ALONE OR IN COMBINATION, INCLUDING ZIAGEN AND OTHER ANTIRETROVIRALS (SEE WARNINGS).

DESCRIPTION

ZIAGEN is the brand name for abacavir sulfate, a synthetic carbocyclic nucleoside analogue with inhibitory activity against HIV. The chemical name of abacavir sulfate is (1*S*,*cis*)-4-[2-amino-6-(cyclopropylamino)-9*H*-purin-9-yl]-2-cyclopentene-1-methanol sulfate (salt) (2:1). Abacavir sulfate is the enantiomer with *1S, 4R* absolute configuration on the cyclopentene ring. It has a molecular formula of $(C_{14}H_{18}N_6O)_2 \bullet H_2SO_4$ and a molecular weight of 670.76 daltons.

Abacavir sulfate is a white to off-white solid with a solubility of approximately 77 mg/mL in distilled water at 25°C. It has an octanol/water (pH 7.1 to 7.3) partition coefficient (log *P*) of approximately 1.20 at 25°C.

ZIAGEN Tablets are for oral administration. Each tablet contains abacavir sulfate equivalent to 300 mg of abacavir and the inactive ingredients colloidal silicon dioxide, magnesium stearate, microcrystalline cellulose, and sodium starch glycolate. The tablets are coated with a film that is made of hydroxypropyl methylcellulose, polysorbate 80, synthetic yellow iron oxide, titanium dioxide, and triacetin.

ZIAGEN Oral Solution is for oral administration. One milliliter (1 mL) of ZIAGEN Oral Solution contains abacavir sulfate equivalent to 20 mg of abacavir (20 mg/mL) in an aqueous solution and the inactive ingredients artificial strawberry and banana flavors, citric acid (anhydrous), methylparaben and propylparaben (added as preservatives), propylene glycol, saccharin sodium, sodium citrate (dihydrate), and sorbitol solution.

In vivo, abacavir sulfate dissociates to its free base, abacavir. In this insert, all dosages for ZIAGEN are expressed in terms of abacavir.

MICROBIOLOGY

Mechanism of Action: Abacavir is a carbocyclic synthetic nucleoside analogue. Intracellularly, abacavir is converted by cellular enzymes to the active metabolite carbovir triphosphate. Carbovir triphosphate is an analogue of deoxyguanosine-5′-triphosphate (dGTP). Carbovir triphosphate inhibits the activity of HIV-1 reverse transcriptase (RT) both by competing with the natural substrate dGTP and by its incorporation into viral DNA. The lack of a 3′-OH group in the incorporated nucleoside analogue prevents the formation of the 5′ to 3′ phosphodiester linkage essential for DNA chain elongation, and therefore, the viral DNA growth is terminated.

Antiviral Activity *In Vitro*: The *in vitro* anti-HIV-1 activity of abacavir was evaluated against a T-cell tropic laboratory strain HIV-1 IIIB in lymphoblastic cell lines, a monocyte/macrophage tropic laboratory strain HIV-1 BaL in primary monocytes/macrophages, and clinical isolates in peripheral blood mononuclear cells. The concentration of drug necessary to inhibit viral replication by 50 percent (IC_{50}) ranged from 3.7 to 5.8 μM against HIV-1 IIIB, and was 0.26 ± 0.18 μM (1 μM = 0.28 mcg/mL) against 8 clinical isolates. The IC_{50} of abacavir against HIV-1 BaL varied from 0.07 to 1.0 μM. Abacavir had synergistic activity in combination with amprenavir, nevirapine, and zidovudine, and additive activity in combination with didanosine, lamivudine, stavudine, and zalcitabine *in vitro.* These drug combinations have not been adequately studied in humans. The relationship between *in vitro* susceptibility of HIV to abacavir and the inhibition of HIV replication in humans has not been established.

Drug Resistance: HIV-1 isolates with reduced sensitivity to abacavir have been selected *in vitro* and were also obtained from patients treated with abacavir. Genetic analysis of isolates from abacavir-treated patients showed point mutations in the reverse transcriptase gene that resulted in amino acid substitutions at positions K65R, L74V, Y115F, and M184V. Phenotypic analysis of HIV-1 isolates that harbored abacavir-associated mutations from 17 patients after 12 weeks of abacavir monotherapy exhibited a 3-fold decrease in susceptibility to abacavir *in vitro.*

Genetic analysis of HIV-1 isolates from 21 previously antiretroviral therapy-naive patients with confirmed virologic failure (plasma HIV-1 RNA ≥400 copies/mL) after 16 to 48 weeks of abacavir/lamivudine/zidovudine therapy showed that 16/21 isolates had abacavir/lamivudine-associated mutation M184V, either alone (11/21), or in combination with Y115F (1/21) or zidovudine-associated (4/21) mutations at the last time point. Phenotypic data available on isolates from 10 patients showed that 7 of the 10 isolates had 25- to 86-fold decreases in susceptibility to lamivudine *in vitro.* Likewise, isolates from 2 of these 7 patients had 7- to 10-fold decreases in susceptibility to abacavir *in vitro.* The clinical relevance of genotypic and phenotypic changes associated with abacavir therapy has not been established, but is currently under evaluation.

Cross-Resistance: Recombinant laboratory strains of HIV-1 (HXB2) containing multiple reverse transcriptase mutations conferring abacavir resistance exhibited cross-resistance to lamivudine, didanosine, and zalcitabine *in vitro.* For clinical information in treatment-experienced patients, see INDICATIONS AND USAGE: Description of Clinical Studies and PRECAUTIONS.

CLINICAL PHARMACOLOGY

Pharmacokinetics in Adults: The pharmacokinetic properties of abacavir have been studied in asymptomatic, HIV-infected adult patients after administration of a single intravenous (IV) dose of 150 mg and after single and multiple oral doses. The pharmacokinetic properties of abacavir were independent of dose over the range of 300 to 1200 mg/day.

Absorption and Bioavailability: Abacavir was rapidly and extensively absorbed after oral administration. The geometric mean absolute bioavailability of the tablet was 83%. After oral administration of 300 mg twice daily in 20 patients, the steady-state peak serum abacavir concentration (C_{max}) was 3.0 ± 0.89 mcg/mL (mean ± SD) and $AUC_{(0-12\ h)}$ was 6.02 ± 1.73 mcg•h/mL. Bioavailability of abacavir tablets was assessed in the fasting and fed states. There was no significant difference in systemic exposure (AUC∞) in the fed and fasting states; therefore, ZIAGEN Tablets may be administered with or without food. Systemic exposure to abacavir was comparable after administration of ZIAGEN Oral Solution and ZIAGEN Tablets. Therefore, these products may be used interchangeably.

Distribution: The apparent volume of distribution after IV administration of abacavir was 0.86 ± 0.15 L/kg, suggesting that abacavir distributes into extravascular space. In 3 subjects, the CSF $AUC_{(0-6\ h)}$ to plasma abacavir $AUC_{(0-6\ h)}$ ratio ranged from 27% to 33%.

Binding of abacavir to human plasma proteins is approximately 50%. Binding of abacavir to plasma proteins was independent of concentration. Total blood and plasma drug-related radioactivity concentrations are identical, demonstrating that abacavir readily distributes into erythrocytes.

Metabolism: In humans, abacavir is not significantly metabolized by cytochrome P450 enzymes. The primary routes of elimination of abacavir are metabolism by alcohol dehydrogenase (to form the 5′-carboxylic acid) and glucuronyl transferase (to form the 5′-glucuronide). The metabolites do not have antiviral activity. *In vitro* experiments reveal that abacavir does not inhibit human CYP3A4, CYP2D6, or CYP2C9 activity at clinically relevant concentrations.

Elimination: Elimination of abacavir was quantified in a mass balance study following administration of a 600-mg dose of ^{14}C-abacavir: 99% of the radioactivity was recovered, 1.2% was excreted in the urine as abacavir, 30% as the 5′-carboxylic acid metabolite, 36% as the 5′-glucuronide metabolite, and 15% as unidentified minor metabolites in the urine. Fecal elimination accounted for 16% of the dose.

In single-dose studies, the observed elimination half-life ($t_{1/2}$) was 1.54 ± 0.63 hours. After intravenous administration, total clearance was 0.80 ± 0.24 L/hr per kg (mean ± SD).

Special Populations: *Adults With Impaired Renal Function:* The pharmacokinetic properties of ZIAGEN have not been determined in patients with impaired renal function. Renal excretion of unchanged abacavir is a minor route of elimination in humans.

Pediatric Patients: The pharmacokinetics of abacavir have been studied after either single or repeat doses of ZIAGEN in 68 pediatric patients. Following multiple-dose administration of ZIAGEN 8 mg/kg twice daily, steady-state $AUC_{(0-12\ h)}$ and C_{max} were 9.8 ± 4.56 mcg•h/mL and 3.71 ± 1.36 mcg/mL (mean ± SD), respectively (see PRECAUTIONS: Pediatric Use).

Geriatric Patients: The pharmacokinetics of ZIAGEN have not been studied in patients over 65 years of age.

Gender: The pharmacokinetics of ZIAGEN with respect to gender have not been determined.

Race: The pharmacokinetics of ZIAGEN with respect to race have not been determined.

Drug Interactions: In human liver microsomes, abacavir did not inhibit cytochrome P450 isoforms (2C9, 2D6, 3A4). Based on these data, it is unlikely that clinically significant drug interactions will occur between abacavir and drugs metabolized through these pathways.

Due to their common metabolic pathways via glucuronyl transferase with zidovudine, 15 HIV-infected patients were enrolled in a crossover study evaluating single doses of abacavir (600 mg), lamivudine (150 mg), and zidovudine (300 mg) alone or in combination. Analysis showed no clinically relevant changes in the pharmacokinetics of abacavir with the addition of lamivudine or zidovudine or the combination of lamivudine and zidovudine. Lamivudine exposure (AUC decreased 15%) and zidovudine exposure (AUC increased 10%) did not show clinically relevant changes with concurrent abacavir.

Continued on next page

Ziagen—Cont.

Due to their common metabolic pathways via alcohol dehydrogenase, the pharmacokinetic interaction between abacavir and ethanol was studied in 24 HIV-infected male patients. Each patient received the following treatments on separate occasions: a single 600-mg dose of abacavir, 0.7 g/kg ethanol (equivalent to 5 alcoholic drinks), and abacavir 600 mg plus 0.7 g/kg ethanol. Coadministration of ethanol and abacavir resulted in a 41% increase in abacavir $AUC\infty$ and a 26% increase in abacavir $t_{1/2}$. In males, abacavir had no effect on the pharmacokinetic properties of ethanol, so no clinically significant interaction is expected in men. This interaction has not been studied in females.

Methadone: In a study of 11 HIV-infected subjects receiving methadone-maintenance therapy (40 mg and 90 mg daily), with 600 mg of ZIAGEN twice daily (twice the current recommended dose), oral methadone clearance increased 22% (90% CI 6% to 42%). This alteration will not result in a methadone dose modification in the majority of patients; however, an increased methadone dose may be required in a small number of patients.

INDICATIONS AND USAGE

ZIAGEN Tablets and Oral Solution, in combination with other antiretroviral agents, are indicated for the treatment of HIV-1 infection. This indication is based on 2 controlled trials of 16 and 48 weeks' duration that evaluated suppression of HIV RNA and changes in CD4 cell count. At present, there are no results from controlled trials evaluating the effect of ZIAGEN on clinical progression of HIV (see Description of Clinical Studies).

Description of Clinical Studies: *Therapy-Naive Adults:* CNAAB3003 is a multicenter, double-blind, placebo-controlled study in which 173 HIV-infected, therapy-naive adults were randomized to receive either ZIAGEN (300 mg twice daily), lamivudine (150 mg twice daily), and zidovudine (300 mg twice daily) or lamivudine (150 mg twice daily) and zidovudine (300 mg twice daily). The duration of double-blind treatment was 16 weeks. Study participants were: male (76%), Caucasian (54%), African-American (28%), and Hispanic (16%). The median age was 34 years, the median pretreatment CD4 cell count was 450 cells/mm^3, and median plasma HIV-1 RNA was 4.5 $\log_{10}$ copies/mL. Proportions of patients with plasma HIV-1 RNA <400 copies/mL (using Roche Amplicor HIV-1 MONITOR® Test) through 16 weeks of treatment are summarized in Figure 1.

Figure 1: Proportions of Patients with HIV-1 RNA <400 copies/mL in Study CNAAB3003[1]

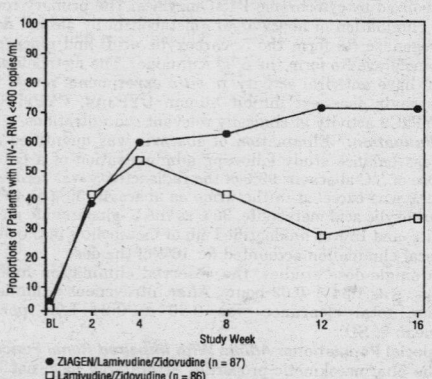

- ● ZIAGEN/Lamivudine/Zidovudine (n = 87)
- □ Lamivudine/Zidovudine (n = 86)

[1]Missing data were considered as HIV-1 RNA ≥400 copies/mL.

After 16 weeks of therapy, the median CD4 increases from baseline were 47 cells/mm^3 in the group receiving ZIAGEN and 112 cells/mm^3 in the placebo group.

CNAAB3005 was a multicenter, double-blind, controlled study in which 562 HIV-infected, therapy-naive adults with a pre-entry plasma HIV-1 RNA >10,000 copies/mL were randomized to receive either ZIAGEN (300 mg twice daily) plus COMBIVIR (lamivudine 150 mg/zidovudine 300 mg twice daily), or indinavir (800 mg 3 times a day) plus COMBIVIR twice daily. Study participants were male (87%), Caucasian (73%), African-American (15%), and Hispanic (9%). At baseline the median age was 36 years, the median pretreatment CD4 cell count was 360 cells/mm^3, and median plasma HIV-1 RNA was 4.8 $\log_{10}$ copies/mL. Proportions of patients with plasma HIV-1 RNA <400 cop-

ies/mL (using Roche Amplicor HIV-1 MONITOR Test) through 48 weeks of treatment are summarized in Figure 2.

Figure 2: Proportions of Patients with HIV-1 RNA <400 copies/mL in Study CNAAB3005[1]

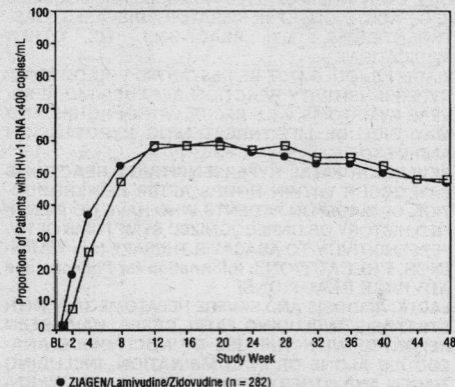

- ● ZIAGEN/Lamivudine/Zidovudine (n = 282)
- □ Indinavir/Lamivudine/Zidovudine (n = 280)

[1]Discontinuations of randomized therapy or missing data were considered as HIV-1 RNA ≥400 copies/mL.

Through week 48, an overall mean increase in CD4 cells of about 150 cells/mm^3 was observed in both treatment arms. [See table below]

Therapy-Experienced Pediatric Patients: CNAA3006 is a randomized, double-blind study comparing ZIAGEN 8 mg/kg twice daily, lamivudine 4 mg/kg twice daily, and zidovudine 180 mg/m^2 twice daily versus lamivudine 4 mg/kg twice daily and zidovudine 180 mg/m^2 twice daily. Two hundred and five pediatric patients were enrolled: female (56%), Caucasian (17%), African-American (50%), Hispanic (30%), median age of 5.4 years, baseline CD4 cell percent >15% (median = 27%), and median baseline plasma HIV-1 RNA of 4.6 $\log_{10}$ copies/mL. Eighty percent and 55% of patients had prior therapy with zidovudine and lamivudine, respectively, most often in combination. The median duration of prior nucleoside analogue therapy was 2 years. Proportions of patients with plasma HIV-1 RNA levels ≤10,000 and <400 copies/mL, respectively, through 24 weeks of treatment are summarized in Figure 3.

Figure 3: Proportions of Patients with Plasma HIV-1 RNA ≤10,000 copies/mL or <400 copies/mL Through Week 24 In Study CNAA3006[1,2]

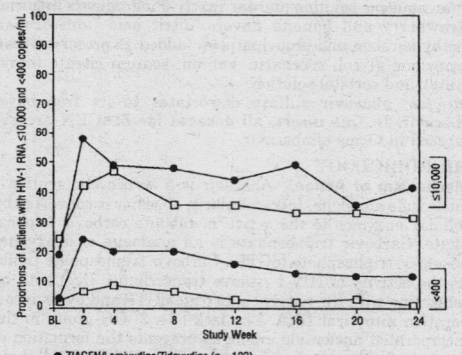

- ● ZIAGEN/Lamivudine/Zidovudine (n = 102)
- □ Lamivudine/Zidovudine (n = 103)

[1]Missing data were considered as above the HIV-1 RNA threshold.
[2]No significant difference was observed at 24 weeks for the ≤10,000 copies/mL threshold.

After 16 weeks of therapy, the median CD4 increases from baseline were 69 cells/mm^3 in the group receiving ZIAGEN and 9 cells/mm^3 in the control group.

CONTRAINDICATIONS

Abacavir sulfate has been associated with fatal hypersensitivity reactions. ZIAGEN SHOULD NOT BE RESTARTED FOLLOWING A HYPERSENSITIVITY REACTION TO ABACAVIR (see WARNINGS, PRECAUTIONS, and ADVERSE REACTIONS).

ZIAGEN Tablets and Oral Solution are contraindicated in patients with previously demonstrated hypersensitivity to any of the components of the products (see WARNINGS).

WARNINGS

Hypersensitivity Reaction: Fatal hypersensitivity reactions have been associated with therapy with ZIAGEN. Patients developing signs or symptoms of hypersensitivity (which include fever; skin rash; fatigue; gastrointestinal symptoms such as nausea, vomiting, diarrhea, or abdominal pain; and respiratory symptoms such as pharyngitis, dyspnea, or cough) should discontinue ZIAGEN as soon as a hypersensitivity reaction is first suspected, and should seek medical evaluation immediately. To avoid a delay in diagnosis and minimize the risk of a life-threatening hypersensitivity reaction, ZIAGEN should be permanently discontinued if hypersensitivity can not be ruled out, even when other diagnoses are possible (e.g., acute onset respiratory diseases, gastroenteritis, or reactions to other medications).

ZIAGEN SHOULD NOT be restarted following a hypersensitivity reaction because more severe symptoms will recur within hours and may include life-threatening hypotension and death. Severe or fatal hypersensitivity reactions can occur within hours after reintroduction of ZIAGEN in patients who have no identified history or unrecognized symptoms of hypersensitivity to abacavir therapy.

When therapy with ZIAGEN has been discontinued for reasons other than symptoms of a hypersensitivity reaction, and if reinitiation of therapy is under consideration, the reason for discontinuation should be evaluated to ensure that the patient did not have symptoms of a hypersensitivity reaction. If hypersensitivity can not be ruled out, abacavir should **NOT** be reintroduced. If symptoms consistent with hypersensitivity are not identified, reintroduction can be undertaken with continued monitoring for symptoms of a hypersensitivity reaction. Patients should be made aware that a hypersensitivity reaction can occur with reintroduction of abacavir, and that abacavir reintroduction should be undertaken only if medical care can be readily accessed by the patient or others (see ADVERSE REACTIONS).

In clinical trials, hypersensitivity reactions have been reported in approximately 5% of adult and pediatric patients receiving abacavir. Symptoms usually appear within the first 6 weeks of treatment with ZIAGEN although these reactions may occur at any time during therapy (see PRECAUTIONS: Information for Patients and ADVERSE REACTIONS).

Abacavir Hypersensitivity Reaction Registry: To facilitate reporting of hypersensitivity reactions and collection of information on each case, an Abacavir Hypersensitivity Registry has been established. Physicians should register patients by calling 1-800-270-0425.

Lactic Acidosis/Severe Hepatomegaly with Steatosis: Lactic acidosis and severe hepatomegaly with steatosis, including fatal cases, have been reported with the use of nucleoside analogues alone or in combination, including abacavir and other antiretrovirals. A majority of these cases have been in women. Obesity and prolonged nucleoside exposure may be risk factors. Particular caution should be exercised when administering ZIAGEN to any patient with known risk factors for liver disease; however, cases have also been reported in patients with no known risk factors. Treatment with ZIAGEN should be suspended in any patient who develops clinical or laboratory findings suggestive of lactic acidosis or pronounced hepatotoxicity (which may include hepatomegaly and steatosis even in the absence of marked transaminase elevations).

PRECAUTIONS

General: Abacavir should always be used in combination with other antiretroviral agents. Abacavir should not be added as a single agent when antiretroviral regimens are changed due to loss of virologic response.

Therapy-Experienced Patients: In clinical trials, patients with prolonged prior nucleoside reverse transcriptase inhibitor (NRTI) exposure or who had HIV-1 isolates that contained multiple mutations conferring resistance to NRTIs had limited response to abacavir. The potential for cross-resistance between abacavir and other NRTIs should be considered when choosing new therapeutic regimens in therapy-experienced patients (see MICROBIOLOGY: Cross-Resistance).

Information for Patients: Patients should be advised that a Medication Guide and Warning Card summarizing the symptoms of abacavir hypersensitivity reactions should be dispensed by the pharmacist with each new prescription and refill of ZIAGEN. The complete text of the Medication Guide is reprinted at the end of this document. Patients should be instructed to carry the Warning Card with them. Patients should be advised of the possibility of a hypersensitivity reaction to ZIAGEN that may result in death. Patients developing signs or symptoms of hypersensitivity (which include fever; skin rash; fatigue; gastrointestinal symptoms such as nausea, vomiting, diarrhea, or abdominal pain; and respiratory symptoms such as sore throat, shortness of breath, or cough) should discontinue treatment with ZIAGEN and seek medical evaluation immediately. **ZIAGEN SHOULD NOT be restarted following a hypersensitivity reaction because more severe symptoms will recur within hours and may include life-threatening hypotension and death.** Patients who have interrupted ZIAGEN for reasons other than symptoms of hypersensitivity (for example, those who have an interruption in drug supply) should be made aware that a severe or fatal hypersensitivity reaction can occur with reintroduction of abacavir. Patients should be instructed not to reintroduce abacavir without medical consultation and that reintroduction of abacavir should be undertaken only if medical care can be readily accessed by the patient or others (see ADVERSE REACTIONS and WARNINGS).

Table 1: Outcomes of Randomized Treatment Through Week 48 (CNAAB3005)

Outcome	ZIAGEN/Lamivudine/ Zidovudine (n = 282)	Indinavir/ Lamivudine/Zidovudine (n = 280)
HIV RNA <400 copies/mL	46%	47%
HIV RNA ≥400 copies/mL*	29%	28%
CDC Class C event	2%	<1%
Discontinued due to adverse reactions	9%	11%
Discontinued due to other reasons†	6%	6%
Randomized but never initiated treatment	7%	5%

*Includes viral rebound and failure to achieve confirmed <400 copies/mL by Week 48.
† Includes consent withdrawn, lost to follow up, protocol violations, those with missing data, and other.

ZIAGEN is not a cure for HIV infection and patients may continue to experience illnesses associated with HIV infection, including opportunistic infections. Patients should remain under the care of a physician when using ZIAGEN. Patients should be advised that the use of ZIAGEN has not been shown to reduce the risk of transmission of HIV to others through sexual contact or blood contamination.

Patients should be advised that the long-term effects of ZIAGEN are unknown at this time.

ZIAGEN Tablets and Oral Solution are for oral ingestion only.

Patients should be advised of the importance of taking ZIAGEN exactly as it is prescribed.

Drug Interactions: Pharmacokinetic properties of abacavir were not altered by the addition of either lamivudine or zidovudine or the combination of lamivudine and zidovudine. No clinically significant changes to lamivudine or zidovudine pharmacokinetics were observed following concomitant administration of abacavir.

Abacavir has no effect on the pharmacokinetic properties of ethanol. Ethanol decreases the elimination of abacavir causing an increase in overall exposure (see CLINICAL PHARMACOLOGY: Drug Interactions). The addition of methadone has no clinically significant effect on the pharmacokinetic properties of abacavir. In a study of 11 HIV-infected subjects receiving methadone-maintenance therapy (40 mg and 90 mg daily), with 600 mg of ZIAGEN twice daily (twice the current recommended dose), oral methadone clearance increased 22% (90% CI 6% to 42%) This alteration will not result in a methadone dose modification in the majority of patients; however, an increased methadone dose may be required in a small number of patients.

Carcinogenesis, Mutagenesis, and Impairment of Fertility: Abacavir induced chromosomal aberrations both in the presence and absence of metabolic activation in an *in vitro* cytogenetic study in human lymphocytes. Abacavir was mutagenic in absence of metabolic activation, although it was not mutagenic in the presence of metabolic activation in an L5178Y mouse lymphoma assay. At systemic exposures approximately 9 times higher than that in humans at the therapeutic dose, abacavir was clastogenic in males and not clastogenic in females in an *in vivo* mouse bone marrow micronucleus assay.

Abacavir was not mutagenic in bacterial mutagenicity assays in the presence and absence of metabolic activation. Abacavir had no adverse effects on the mating performance or fertility of male and female rats at doses of up to 500 mg/kg per day, a dose expected to produce exposures approximately 8-fold higher than that in humans at the therapeutic dose based on body surface area comparisons.

Pregnancy: Pregnancy Category C. Studies in pregnant rats showed that abacavir is transferred to the fetus through the placenta. Developmental toxicity (depressed fetal body weight and reduced crown-rump length) and increased incidences of fetal anasarca and skeletal malformations were observed when rats were treated with abacavir at doses of 1000 mg/kg during organogenesis. This dose produced 35 times the human exposure, based on AUC. In a fertility study, evidence of toxicity to the developing embryo and fetuses (increased resorptions, decreased fetal body weights) occurred only at 500 mg/kg per day. The offspring of female rats treated with abacavir at 500 mg/kg per day (beginning at embryo implantation and ending at weaning) showed increased incidence of stillbirth and lower body weights throughout life. In the rabbit, there was no evidence of drug-related developmental toxicity and no increases in fetal malformations at doses up to 700 mg/kg (8.5 times the human exposure at the recommended dose, based on AUC).

There are no adequate and well-controlled studies in pregnant women. ZIAGEN should be used during pregnancy only if the potential benefits outweigh the risk.

Antiretroviral Pregnancy Registry: To monitor maternal-fetal outcomes of pregnant women exposed to ZIAGEN, an Antiretroviral Pregnancy Registry has been established. Physicians are encouraged to register patients by calling 1-800-258-4263.

Nursing Mothers: The Centers for Disease Control and Prevention recommend that HIV-infected mothers not breastfeed their infants to avoid risking postnatal transmission of HIV infection. Although it is not known if abacavir is excreted in human milk, abacavir is secreted into the milk of lactating rats. Because of both the potential for HIV transmission and the potential for serious adverse reactions in nursing infants, **mothers should be instructed not to breastfeed if they are receiving ZIAGEN.**

Pediatric Use: The safety and effectiveness of ZIAGEN have been established in pediatric patients aged 3 months to 13 years. Use of ZIAGEN in these age groups is supported by pharmacokinetic studies and evidence from adequate and well-controlled studies of ZIAGEN in adults and pediatric patients (see CLINICAL PHARMACOLOGY: Pharmacokinetics: Special Populations: Pediatric Patients; INDICATIONS AND USAGE: Description of Clinical Studies; WARNINGS; ADVERSE REACTIONS; and DOSAGE AND ADMINISTRATION).

Geriatric Use: Clinical studies of ZIAGEN did not include sufficient numbers of patients aged 65 and over to determine whether they respond differently from younger patients. In general, dose selection for an elderly patient should be cautious, reflecting the greater frequency of decreased hepatic, renal, or cardiac function, and of concomitant disease or other drug therapy.

ADVERSE REACTIONS

Hypersensitivity Reaction: Fatal hypersensitivity reactions have been associated with therapy with ZIAGEN.

Table 2: Selected Clinical Adverse Events Grades 1–4 (≥5% Frequency) in Therapy-Naive Adults (CNAAB3003) Through 16 Weeks of Treatment

Adverse Event	ZIAGEN/Lamivudine/ Zidovudine (n = 83)	Lamivudine/Zidovudine (n = 81)
Nausea	47%	41%
Nausea and vomiting	16%	11%
Diarrhea	12%	11%
Loss of appetite/anorexia	11%	10%
Insomnia and other sleep disorders	7%	5%

Table 3: Selected Clinical Adverse Events Grades 1–4 (≥5% Frequency) in Therapy-Naive Adults (CNAAB3005) Through 48 Weeks of Treatment

Adverse Event	ZIAGEN/Lamivudine/Zidovudine (n = 262)	Indinavir/Lamivudine/Zidovudine (n = 264)
Nausea	60%	61%
Nausea and vomiting	30%	27%
Diarrhea	26%	27%
Loss of appetite/anorexia	15%	11%
Insomnia and other sleep disorders	13%	12%
Fever and/or chills	20%	13%
Headache	28%	25%
Malaise and/or fatigue	44%	41%

Table 4: Selected Clinical Adverse Events Grades 1–4 (≥5% Frequency) in Therapy-Experienced Pediatric Patients (CNAA3006) Through 16 Weeks of Treatment

Adverse Event	ZIAGEN/Lamivudine/ Zidovudine (n = 102)	Lamivudine/Zidovudine (n = 103)
Nausea and vomiting	38%	18%
Fever	19%	12%
Headache	16%	12%
Diarrhea	16%	15%
Skin rashes	11%	8%
Loss of appetite/anorexia	9%	2%

Therapy with ZIAGEN SHOULD NOT be restarted following a hypersensitivity reaction because more severe symptoms will recur within hours and may include life-threatening hypotension and death. Patients developing signs or symptoms of hypersensitivity should discontinue treatment as soon as a hypersensitivity reaction is first suspected, and should seek medical evaluation immediately. To avoid a delay in diagnosis and minimize the risk of a life-threatening hypersensitivity reaction, ZIAGEN should be permanently discontinued if hypersensitivity can not be ruled out, even when other diagnoses are possible (e.g., acute onset respiratory diseases, gastroenteritis, or reactions to other medications).

Severe or fatal hypersensitivity reactions can occur within hours after reintroduction of ZIAGEN in patients who have no identified history or unrecognized symptoms of hypersensitivity to abacavir therapy (see WARNINGS and PRECAUTIONS: Information for Patients).

When therapy with ZIAGEN has been discontinued for reasons other than symptoms of a hypersensitivity reaction, and if reinitiation of therapy is under consideration, the reason for discontinuation should be evaluated to ensure that the patient did not have symptoms of a hypersensitivity reaction. If hypersensitivity can not be ruled out, abacavir should **NOT** be reintroduced. If symptoms consistent with hypersensitivity are not identified, reintroduction can be undertaken with continued monitoring for symptoms of hypersensitivity reaction. Patients should be made aware that a hypersensitivity reaction can occur with reintroduction of abacavir, and that abacavir reintroduction should be undertaken only if medical care can be readily accessed by the patient or others (see WARNINGS).

In clinical studies, approximately 5% of adult and pediatric patients receiving ZIAGEN developed a hypersensitivity reaction. This reaction is characterized by the appearance of symptoms indicating multi-organ/body system involvement. Symptoms usually appear within the first 6 weeks of treatment with ZIAGEN, although these reactions may occur at any time during therapy. Frequently observed signs and symptoms include fever; skin rash; fatigue; and gastrointestinal symptoms such as nausea, vomiting, diarrhea, or abdominal pain. Other signs and symptoms include malaise, lethargy, myalgia, myolysis, arthralgia, edema, pharyngitis, cough, dyspnea, headache, and paresthesia. Some patients who experienced a hypersensitivity reaction were initially thought to have acute onset or worsening respiratory disease. The diagnosis of hypersensitivity reaction should be carefully considered for patients presenting with symptoms of acute onset respiratory diseases, even if alternative respiratory diagnoses (pneumonia, bronchitis, pharyngitis, or flu-like illness) are possible.

Physical findings include lymphadenopathy, mucous membrane lesions (conjunctivitis and mouth ulcerations), and rash. The rash usually appears maculopapular or urticarial but may be variable in appearance. Hypersensitivity reactions have occurred without rash.

Laboratory abnormalities include elevated liver function tests, increased creatinine phosphokinase or creatinine, and lymphopenia. Anaphylaxis, liver failure, renal failure, hypotension, and death have occurred in association with hypersensitivity reactions. Symptoms worsen with continued therapy but often resolve upon discontinuation of ZIAGEN.

Risk factors that may predict the occurrence or severity of hypersensitivity to abacavir have not been identified.

Therapy-Naive Adults: Selected clinical adverse events with a ≥5% frequency during therapy with ZIAGEN 300 mg twice daily, lamivudine 150 mg twice daily, and zidovudine 300 mg twice daily compared with lamivudine 150 mg twice daily and zidovudine 300 mg twice daily from CNAAB3003 are listed in Table 2.

[See table 2 above]

Selected clinical adverse events with a ≥5% frequency during therapy with ZIAGEN 300 mg twice daily, lamivudine 150 mg twice daily, and zidovudine 300 mg twice daily compared with indinavir 800 mg 3 times daily, lamivudine 150 mg twice daily, and zidovudine 300 mg twice daily from CNAAB3005 are listed in Table 3.

[See table 3 above]

Five subjects in the abacavir arm of study CNAAB3005 experienced worsening of pre-existing depression compared to none in the indinavir arm. The background rates of pre-existing depression were similar in the 2 treatment arms.

Pediatric Patients: Selected clinical adverse events with a ≥5% frequency during therapy with ZIAGEN 8 mg/kg twice daily, lamivudine 4 mg/kg twice daily, and zidovudine 180 mg/m² twice daily compared with lamivudine 4 mg/kg twice daily and zidovudine 180 mg/m² twice daily from CNAA3006 are listed in Table 4.

[See table 4 above]

Laboratory Abnormalities: Laboratory abnormalities (anemia, neutropenia, liver function test abnormalities, and CPK elevations) were observed with similar frequencies in the 2 treatment groups in studies CNAAB3003 and CNAA3006. Mild elevations of blood glucose were more frequent in subjects receiving abacavir. In study CNAAB3003, triglyceride elevations (all grades) were more common on the abacavir arm (25%) than on the placebo arm (11%). In study CNAAB3005, hyperglycemia and disorders of lipid metabolism occurred with similar frequency in the abacavir and indinavir treatment arms.

Other Adverse Events: In addition to adverse events in Tables 2, 3, and 4, other adverse events observed in the expanded access program were pancreatitis and increased GGT.

OVERDOSAGE

There is no known antidote for ZIAGEN. It is not known whether abacavir can be removed by peritoneal dialysis or hemodialysis.

DOSAGE AND ADMINISTRATION

A Medication Guide and Warning Card that provide information about recognition of hypersensitivity reactions should be dispensed with each new prescription and refill.

To facilitate reporting of hypersensitivity reactions and collection of information on each case, an Abacavir Hypersensitivity Registry has been established. Physicians should register patients by calling 1-800-270-0425.

ZIAGEN may be taken with or without food.

Adults: The recommended oral dose of ZIAGEN for adults is 300 mg twice daily in combination with other antiretroviral agents.

Continued on next page

Ziagen—Cont.

Adolescents and Pediatric Patients: The recommended oral dose of ZIAGEN for adolescents and pediatric patients 3 months to up to 16 years of age is 8 mg/kg twice daily (up to a maximum of 300 mg twice daily) in combination with other antiretroviral agents.

Dose Adjustment in Hepatic Impairment: Insufficient data are available to recommend a dosage of ZIAGEN in patients with hepatic impairment.

HOW SUPPLIED

ZIAGEN is available as tablets and oral solution.
ZIAGEN Tablets: Each tablet contains abacavir sulfate equivalent to 300 mg abacavir. The tablets are yellow, biconvex, capsule-shaped, film-coated, and imprinted with "GX 623" on one side with no marking on the reverse side. They are packaged as follows:
Bottles of 60 tablets (NDC 0173-0661-01).
Unit dose blister packs of 60 tablets (NDC 0173-0661-00).
Each pack contains 6 blister cards of 10 tablets each.
Store at controlled room temperature of 20° to 25°C (68° to 77°F) (see USP).
ZIAGEN Oral Solution: It is a clear to opalescent, yellowish, strawberry-banana-flavored liquid. Each mL of the solution contains abacavir sulfate equivalent to 20 mg of abacavir. It is packaged in plastic bottles as follows:
Bottles of 240 mL (NDC 0173-0664-00) with child-resistant closure. This product does not require reconstitution.
Store at controlled room temperature of 20° to 25°C (68° to 77°F) (see USP). DO NOT FREEZE. May be refrigerated.
Glaxo Wellcome Inc., Research Triangle Park, NC 27709
US Patent Nos. 5,034,394 and 5,089,500
©Copyright 1998, 2000, Glaxo Wellcome Inc. All rights reserved.
December 2000/RL-882

MEDICATION GUIDE

ZIAGEN® (z-EYE-uh-jen) (abacavir sulfate) Tablets and Oral Solution
Generic name: abacavir (uh-BACK-ah-veer) sulfate tablets and oral solution
Read the Medication Guide you get each time you fill your prescription for Ziagen. There may be new information since you filled your last prescription

---

What is the most important information I should know about Ziagen?
About 1 in 20 patients (5%) who take Ziagen will have **a serious allergic reaction (hypersensitivity reaction) that may cause death if the drug is not stopped right away.**
You may be having this reaction if:

(1) you get a skin rash, or
(2) you get 1 or more symptoms from at least 2 of the following groups:
• **Fever**
• **Nausea, vomiting, diarrhea, abdominal (stomach area) pain**
• **Extreme tiredness, achiness, generally ill feeling**
• **Sore throat, shortness of breath, cough**
If you think you may be having a reaction, **STOP taking Ziagen and call your doctor right away.**

If you stop treatment with Ziagen because of this serious reaction, **NEVER take Ziagen (abacavir) again.** If you take Ziagen again after you have had this serious reaction, **you could die within hours.**
Some patients who have stopped taking Ziagen (abacavir) and who have then started taking Ziagen (abacavir) again have had serious or life-threatening allergic (hypersensitivity) reactions. If you must stop treatment with Ziagen for reasons other than symptoms of hypersensitivity, do not begin taking it again without talking to your health care provider. If your health care provider decides that you may begin taking Ziagen again, you should do so only in a setting with other people to get access to a doctor if needed.
A written list of these symptoms is on the Warning Card your pharmacist gives you. Carry this Warning Card with you.
Ziagen can have other serious side effects. Be sure to read the section below titled "What are the possible side effects of Ziagen?"

What is Ziagen?
Ziagen is a medication used to treat HIV infection. Ziagen is taken by mouth as a tablet or a strawberry-banana-flavored liquid. Ziagen is a medicine called a nucleoside analogue reverse transcriptase inhibitor (NRTI). Ziagen is only proven to work when taken in combination with other anti-HIV medications. When used in combination with these other medications, Ziagen helps lower the amount of HIV found in your blood. This helps to keep your immune system as healthy as possible so that it can help fight infection.
Ziagen does not cure HIV infection or AIDS. Ziagen has not been studied long enough to know if it will help you live longer or have fewer of the medical problems that are associated with HIV infection or AIDS. Therefore, you must see your health care provider regularly.
Who should not take Ziagen?
Do not take Ziagen if you have ever had a serious allergic reaction (a hypersensitivity reaction) to abacavir (as Ziagen or Trizivir™ [abacavir, lamivudine, and zidovudine] Tablets). If you have had such a reaction, return all of your unused Ziagen to your doctor or pharmacist.

How should I take Ziagen?
To help make sure that your anti-HIV therapy is as effective as possible, take your Ziagen exactly as your doctor prescribes it. Do not skip any doses.
The usual dosage for adults (at least 16 years of age) is one 300-mg tablet twice a day. You can take Ziagen with food or on an empty stomach.
Adolescents and children 3 months and older can also take Ziagen. Your doctor will tell you if the oral solution or tablet is best for your child. Also, your child's doctor will decide the right dose based on your child's weight and age. Ziagen has not been studied in children under 3 months of age.
If you miss a dose of Ziagen, take the missed dose right away. Then, take the next dose at the usual scheduled time. Do not let your Ziagen run out. The amount of virus in your blood may increase if your anti-HIV drugs are stopped, even for a short time. Also, the virus in your body may become harder to treat.
What should I avoid while taking Ziagen?
Practice safe sex while using Ziagen. Do not use or share dirty needles. Ziagen does not reduce the risk of passing HIV to others through sexual contact or blood contamination.
Talk to your doctor if you are pregnant or if you become pregnant while taking Ziagen. Ziagen has not been studied in pregnant women. It is not known whether Ziagen will harm the unborn child.
Mothers with HIV should not breastfeed their babies because HIV is passed to the baby through breast milk. Also Ziagen can be passed to babies in breast milk and could cause the child to have side effects.
What are the possible side effects of Ziagen?
Life-threatening allergic reaction. Ziagen has caused some people to have a life-threatening reaction (hypersensitivity reaction) that can cause death. How to recognize a possible reaction, and what to do are discussed in "What is the most important information I should know about Ziagen?" at the beginning of this Medication Guide.
Lactic Acidosis and severe liver problems. Ziagen can cause a serious condition called lactic acidosis and, in some cases, this condition can cause death. Nausea and tiredness that don't get better may be symptoms of lactic acidosis. Women are more likely than men to get this rare but serious side effect.
Ziagen can cause other side effects. In studies, the most common side effects with Ziagen were nausea, vomiting, malaise or fatigue, headache, diarrhea, and loss of appetite. Most of these side effects did not cause people to stop taking Ziagen.
This listing of side effects is not complete. Your doctor or pharmacist can discuss with you a more complete list of side effects with Ziagen.
Ask a health care professional about any concerns about Ziagen. If you want more information, ask your doctor or pharmacist for the labeling for Ziagen that was written for health care professionals.
Do not use Ziagen for a condition for which it was not prescribed. Do not given Ziagen to other persons.
Glaxo Wellcome Inc., Research Triangle Park, NC 27709
December 2000/MG-012
This Medication Guide has been approved by the US Food and Drug Administration.

ZOFRAN® ℞
[zō' fran]
(ondansetron hydrochloride)
Injection
ZOFRAN® ℞
(ondansetron hydrochloride)
Injection Premixed

Prescribing information for this product, which appears on pages 1503–1507 of the 2001 PDR, has been revised. Please write "See Supplement A" next to the product heading.
The **CLINICAL PHARMACOLOGY: Pharmacokinetics** *subsection was revised to the following:*
Pharmacokinetics: Ondansetron is extensively metabolized in humans, with approximately 5% of a radiolabeled dose recovered as the parent compound from the urine. The primary metabolic pathway is hydroxylation on the indole ring followed by glucuronide or sulfate conjugation.
Although some nonconjugated metabolites have pharmacologic activity, these are not found in plasma at concentrations likely to significantly contribute to the biological activity of ondansetron.
In vitro metabolism studies have shown that ondansetron is a substrate for human hepatic cytochrome P-450 enzymes, including CYP1A2, CYP2D6, and CYP3A4. In terms of overall ondansetron turnover, CYP3A4 played the predominant role. Because of the multiplicity of metabolic enzymes capable of metabolizing ondansetron, it is likely that inhibition or loss of one enzyme (e.g., CYP2D6 genetic deficiency) will

be compensated by others and may result in little change in overall rates of ondansetron elimination. Ondansetron elimination may be affected by cytochrome P-450 inducers. In a pharmacokinetic study of 16 epileptic patients maintained chronically on carbamazepine or phenytoin, reduction in AUC, C_{max} and $T_{1/2}$ of ondansetron was observed. This resulted in a significant increase in clearance. However, on the basis of available data, no dosage adjustment is recommended (see PRECAUTIONS: Drug Interactions).
In normal volunteers, the following mean pharmacokinetic data have been determined following a single 0.15-mg/kg I.V. dose.
[See table below]
A reduction in clearance and increase in elimination half-life are seen in patients over 75 years of age. In clinical trials with cancer patients, safety and efficacy were similar in patients over 65 years of age and those under 65 years of age; there was an insufficient number of patients over 75 years of age to permit conclusions in that age-group. No dosage adjustment is recommended in the elderly.
In patients with mild-to-moderate hepatic impairment, clearance is reduced twofold and mean half-life is increased to 11.6 hours compared to 5.7 hours in normals. In patients with severe hepatic impairment (Child-Pugh score[1] of 10 or greater), clearance is reduced twofold to threefold and apparent volume of distribution is increased with a resultant increase in half-life to 20 hours. In patients with severe hepatic impairment, a total daily dose of 8 mg should not be exceeded.
Due to the very small contribution (5%) of renal clearance to the overall clearance, renal impairment was not expected to significantly influence the total clearance of ondansetron. However, ondansetron mean plasma clearance was reduced by about 41% in patients with severe renal impairment (creatinine clearance <30 mL/min). This reduction in clearance is variable and was not consistent with an increase in half-life. No reduction in dose or dosing frequency in these patients is warranted.
In adult cancer patients, the mean elimination half-life was 4.0 hours, and there was no difference in the multidose pharmacokinetics over a 4-day period. In a study of 21 pediatric cancer patients (aged 4 to 18 years) who received three I.V. doses of 0.15 mg/kg of ondansetron at 4-hour intervals, patients older than 15 years of age exhibited ondansetron pharmacokinetic parameters similar to those of adults. Patients aged 4 to 12 years generally showed higher clearance and somewhat larger volume of distribution than adults. Most pediatric patients younger than 15 years of age with cancer had a shorter (2.4 hours) ondansetron plasma half-life than patients older than 15 years of age. It is not known whether these differences in ondansetron plasma half-life may result in differences in efficacy between adults and some young pediatric patients (see CLINICAL TRIALS: Pediatric Studies).
In a study of 21 pediatric patients (aged 3 to 12 years) who were undergoing surgery requiring anesthesia for a duration of 45 minutes to 2 hours, a single I.V. dose of ondansetron, 2 mg (3 to 7 years) or 4 mg (8 to 12 years), was administered immediately prior to anesthesia induction. Mean weight-normalized clearance and volume of distribution values in these pediatric surgical patients were similar to those previously reported for young adults. Mean terminal half-life was slightly reduced in pediatric patients (range, 2.5 to 3 hours) in comparison with adults (range, 3 to 3.5 hours).
In normal volunteers (19 to 39 years old, n = 23), the peak plasma concentration was 264 ng/mL following a single 32-mg dose administered as a 15-minute I.V. infusion. The mean elimination half-life was 4.1 hours. Systemic exposure to 32 mg of ondansetron was not proportional to dose as measured by comparing dose-normalized AUC values to an 8-mg dose. This is consistent with a small decrease in systemic clearance with increasing plasma concentrations.
A study was performed in normal volunteers (n = 56) to evaluate the pharmacokinetics of a single 4-mg dose administered as a 5-minute infusion compared to a single intramuscular injection. Systemic exposure as measured by mean AUC was equivalent, with values of 156 [95% CI 136, 180] and 161 [95% CI 137, 190] ng•h/mL for I.V. and I.M. groups, respectively. Mean peak plasma concentrations were 42.9 [95% CI 33.8, 54.4] ng/mL at 10 minutes after I.V. infusion and 31.9 [95% CI 26.3, 38.6] ng/mL at 41 minutes after I.M. injection. The mean elimination half-life was not affected by route of administration.
Plasma protein binding of ondansetron as measured in vitro was 70% to 76%, with binding constant over the pharmacologic concentration range (10 to 500 ng/mL). Circulating drug also distributes into erythrocytes.
A positive lymphoblast transformation test to ondansetron has been reported, which suggests immunologic sensitivity to ondansetron.
The second paragraph of the **PRECAUTIONS: Drug Interactions** *subsection was revised to the following:*

Table 1: Pharmacokinetics in Normal Volunteers

Age-group	n	Peak Plasma Concentration (ng/mL)	Mean Elimination Half-life (h)	Plasma Clearance (L/h/kg)
19–40	11	102	3.5	0.381
61–74	12	106	4.7	0.319
≥75	11	170	5.5	0.262

In a cross-over study in 76 pediatric patients, I.V. ondansetron did not increase blood levels of high-dose methotrexate.

The **DOSAGE AND ADMINISTRATION: Dosage Adjustment for Patients With Impaired Hepatic Function** *subsection was revised to the following:*

In patients with severe hepatic impairment (Child-Pugh[1] score of 10 or greater), a single maximal daily dose of 8 mg to be infused over 15 minutes beginning 30 minutes before the start of the emetogenic chemotherapy is recommended. There is no experience beyond first-day administration of ondansetron.

Glaxo Wellcome Inc., Research Triangle Park, NC 27709
ZOFRAN® Injection Premixed:
Manufactured for Glaxo Wellcome Inc.
Research Triangle Park, NC 27709
by Abbott Laboratories, North Chicago, IL 60064
US Patent Nos. 4,695,578; 4,753,789; and 5,578,628
©Copyright 1996, 1998, 1999, 2000, Glaxo Wellcome Inc. All rights reserved.
December 2000/RL-887

ZOFRAN® ℞
[*zō' fran*]
(ondansetron hydrochloride)
Tablets

ZOFRAN ODT® ℞
(ondansetron)
Orally Disintegrating Tablets

ZOFRAN® ℞
(ondansetron hydrochloride)
Oral Solution

Prescribing information for this product which appears on pages 1507–1510 of the 2001 PDR, has been completely revised as follows. Please write "See Supplement A" next to the product heading.

DESCRIPTION

The active ingredient in ZOFRAN Tablets and ZOFRAN Oral Solution is ondansetron hydrochloride (HCl) as the dihydrate, the racemic form of ondansetron and a selective blocking agent of the serotonin 5-HT_3 receptor type. Chemically it is (±) 1, 2, 3, 9-tetrahydro-9-methyl-3-[(2-methyl-1H-imidazol-1-yl)methyl]-4H-carbazol-4-one, monohydrochloride, dihydrate.

The empirical formula is $C_{18}H_{19}N_3O{\bullet}HCl{\bullet}2H_2O$, representing a molecular weight of 365.9.

Ondansetron HCl dihydrate is a white to off-white powder that is soluble in water and normal saline.

The active ingredient in ZOFRAN ODT Orally Distintegrating Tablets is ondansetron base, the racemic form of ondansetron, and a selective blocking agent of the serotonin 5-HT_3 receptor type. Chemically it is (±) 1, 2, 3, 9-tetrahydro-9-methyl-3-[(2-methyl-1H-imidazol-1-yl)methyl]-4H-carbazol-4-one.

The empirical formula is $C_{18}H_{19}N_3O$ representing a molecular weight of 293.4.

Each 4-mg ZOFRAN Tablet for oral administration contains ondansetron HCl dihydrate equivalent to 4 mg of ondansetron. Each 8-mg ZOFRAN Tablet for oral administration contains ondansetron HCl dihydrate equivalent to 8 mg of ondansetron. Each 24-mg ZOFRAN Tablet for oral administration contains ondansetron HCl dihydrate equivalent to 24 mg of ondansetron. Each tablet also contains the inactive ingredients lactose, microcrystalline cellulose, pregelatinized starch, hydroxypropyl methylcellulose, magnesium stearate, titanium dioxide, triacetin, iron oxide yellow (8-mg tablet only), and iron oxide red (24-mg tablet only).

Each 4-mg ZOFRAN ODT Orally Disintegrating Tablet for oral administration contains 4 mg ondansetron base. Each 8-mg ZOFRAN ODT Orally Disintegrating Tablet for oral administration contains 8 mg ondansetron base. Each ZOFRAN ODT Tablet also contains the inactive ingredients aspartame, gelatin, mannitol, methylparaben sodium, propylparaben sodium, and strawberry flavor. ZOFRAN ODT Tablets are a freeze-dried, orally administered formulation of ondansetron which rapidly disintegrates on the tongue and does not require water to aid dissolution or swallowing.

Each 5 mL of ZOFRAN Oral Solution contains 5 mg of ondansetron HCl dihydrate equivalent to 4 mg of ondansetron. ZOFRAN Oral Solution contains the inactive ingredients citric acid anhydrous, purified water, sodium benzoate, sodium citrate, sorbitol, and strawberry flavor.

CLINICAL PHARMACOLOGY

Pharmacodynamics: Ondansetron is a selective 5-HT_3 receptor antagonist. While its mechanism of action has not been fully characterized, ondansetron is not a dopamine-receptor antagonist. Serotonin receptors of the 5-HT_3 type are present both peripherally on vagal nerve terminals and centrally in the chemoreceptor trigger zone of the area postrema. It is not certain whether ondansetron's antiemetic action is mediated centrally, peripherally, or in both sites. However, cytotoxic chemotherapy appears to be associated with release of serotonin from the enterochromaffin cells of the small intestine. In humans, urinary 5-HIAA (5-hydroxyindoleacetic acid) excretion increases after cisplatin administration in parallel with the onset of emesis. The released serotonin may stimulate the vagal afferents through the 5-HT_3 receptors and initiate the vomiting reflex.

In animals, the emetic response to cisplatin can be prevented by pretreatment with an inhibitor of serotonin synthesis, bilateral abdominal vagotomy and greater splanchnic nerve section, or pretreatment with a serotonin 5-HT_3 receptor antagonist.

In normal volunteers, single intravenous doses of 0.15 mg/kg of ondansetron had no effect on esophageal motility, gastric motility, lower esophageal sphincter pressure, or small intestinal transit time. Multiday administration of ondansetron has been shown to slow colonic transit in normal volunteers. Ondansetron has no effect on plasma prolactin concentrations.

Ondansetron does not alter the respiratory depressant effects produced by alfentanil or the degree of neuromuscular blockade produced by atracurium. Interactions with general or local anesthetics have not been studied.

Pharmacokinetics: Ondansetron is extensively metabolized in humans, with approximately 5% of a radiolabeled dose recovered from the urine as the parent compound. The primary metabolic pathway is hydroxylation on the indole ring followed by subsequent glucuronide or sulfate conjugation. Although some nonconjugated metabolites have pharmacologic activity, these are not found in plasma at concentrations likely to significantly contribute to the biological activity of ondansetron.

In vitro metabolism studies have shown that ondansetron is a substrate for human hepatic cytochrome P-450 enzymes, including CYP1A2, CYP2D6, and CYP3A4. In terms of overall ondansetron turnover, CYP3A4 played the predominant role. Because of the multiplicity of metabolic enzymes capable of metabolizing ondansetron, it is likely that inhibition or loss of one enzyme (e.g., CYP2D6 genetic deficiency) will be compensated by others and may result in little change in overall rates of ondansetron elimination. Ondansetron elimination may be affected by cytochrome P-450 inducers. In a pharmacokinetic study of 16 epileptic patients maintained chronically on carbamazepine or phenytoin, reduction in AUC, C_{max} and $T_{½}$ of ondansetron was observed. This resulted in a significant increase in clearance. However, on the basis of available data, no dosage adjustment is recommended (see PRECAUTIONS: Drug Interactions).

Ondansetron is well absorbed from the gastrointestinal tract and undergoes some first-pass metabolism. Mean bioavailability in healthy subjects, following administration of a single 8-mg tablet, is approximately 56%. Ondansetron systemic exposure does not increase proportionately to dose. AUC from a 16-mg tablet was 24% greater than predicted from an 8-mg tablet dose. This may reflect some reduction of first-pass metabolism at higher oral doses. Bioavailability is also slightly enhanced by the presence of food but unaffected by antacids. Gender differences were shown in the disposition of ondansetron given as a single dose. The extent and rate of ondansetron's absorption is greater in women than men. Slower clearance in women, a smaller apparent volume of distribution (adjusted for weight), and higher absolute bioavailability resulted in higher plasma ondansetron levels. These higher plasma levels may in part be explained by differences in body weight between men and women. It is not known whether these gender-related differences were clinically important. More detailed pharmacokinetic information is contained in Tables 1 and 2 taken from two studies.

[See table 1 above]

[See table 2 above]

Table 1: Pharmacokinetics in Normal Volunteers: Single 8-mg ZOFRAN Tablet Dose

Age-group (years)	Mean Weight (kg)	n	Peak Plasma Concentration (ng/mL)	Time of Peak Plasma Concentration (h)	Mean Elimination Half-life (h)	Systemic Plasma Clearance L/h/kg	Absolute Bioavailability
18–40 M	69.0	6	26.2	2.0	3.1	0.403	0.483
F	62.7	5	42.7	1.7	3.5	0.354	0.663
61–74 M	77.5	6	24.1	2.1	4.1	0.384	0.585
F	60.2	6	52.4	1.9	4.9	0.255	0.643
≥75 M	78.0	5	37.0	2.2	4.5	0.277	0.619
F	67.6	6	46.1	2.1	6.2	0.249	0.747

Table 2: Pharmacokinetics in Normal Volunteers: Single 24-mg ZOFRAN Tablet Dose

Age-group (years)	Mean Weight (kg)	n	Peak Plasma Concentration (ng/mL)	Time of Peak Plasma Concentration (h)	Mean Elimination Half-life (h)
18–43 M	84.1	8	125.8	1.9	4.7
F	71.8	8	194.4	1.6	5.8

A reduction in clearance and increase in elimination half-life are seen in patients over 75 years of age. In clinical trials with cancer patients, safety and efficacy was similar in patients over 65 years of age and those under 65 years of age; there was an insufficient number of patients over 75 years of age to permit conclusions in that age-group. No dosage adjustment is recommended in the elderly.

In patients with mild-to-moderate hepatic impairment, clearance is reduced twofold and mean half-life is increased to 11.6 hours compared to 5.7 hours in normals. In patients with severe hepatic impairment (Child-Pugh[1] score of 10 or greater), clearance is reduced twofold to threefold and apparent volume of distribution is increased with a resultant increase in half-life to 20 hours. In patients with severe hepatic impairment, a total daily dose of 8 mg should not be exceeded.

Due to the very small contribution (5%) of renal clearance to the overall clearance, renal impairment was not expected to significantly influence the total clearance of ondansetron. However, ondansetron oral mean plasma clearance was reduced by about 50% in patients with severe renal impairment (creatinine clearance <30 mL/min). This reduction in clearance is variable and was not consistent with an increase in half-life. No reduction in dose or dosing frequency in these patients is warranted.

Plasma protein binding of ondansetron as measured in vitro was 70% to 76% over the concentration range of 10 to 500 ng/mL. Circulating drug also distributes into erythrocytes.

Four- and 8-mg doses of either ZOFRAN Oral Solution or ZOFRAN ODT Orally Disintegrating Tablets are bioequivalent to corresponding doses of ZOFRAN Tablets and may be used interchangeably. One 24-mg ZOFRAN Tablet is bioequivalent to and interchangeable with three 8-mg ZOFRAN Tablets.

CLINICAL TRIALS

Chemotherapy-Induced Nausea and Vomiting: ***Highly Emetogenic Chemotherapy:*** In two randomized, double-blind, monotherapy trials, a single 24-mg ZOFRAN Tablet was superior to a relevant historical placebo control in the prevention of nausea and vomiting associated with highly emetogenic cancer chemotherapy, including cisplatin ≥50 mg/m². Steroid administration was excluded from these clinical trials. More than 90% of patients receiving a cisplatin dose ≥50 mg/m² in the historical placebo comparator experienced vomiting in the absence of antiemetic therapy.

The first trial compared oral doses of ondansetron 24 mg once a day, 8 mg twice a day, and 32 mg once a day in 357 adult cancer patients receiving chemotherapy regimens con-

Table 3: Emetic Episodes: Treatment Response

	Ondansetron 8-mg b.i.d. ZOFRAN Tablets*	Placebo	*P* Value
Number of patients	33	34	
Treatment response			
0 Emetic episodes	20 (61%)	2 (6%)	<0.001
1–2 Emetic episodes	6 (18%)	8 (24%)	
More than 2 emetic episodes/withdrawn	7 (21%)	24 (71%)	<0.001
Median number of emetic episodes	0.0	Undefined†	
Median time to first emetic episode (h)	Undefined‡	6.5	

*The first dose was administered 30 minutes before the start of emetogenic chemotherapy, with a subsequent dose 8 hours after the first dose. An 8-mg ZOFRAN Tablet was administered twice a day for 2 days after completion of chemotherapy.
† Median undefined since at least 50% of the patients were withdrawn or had more than two emetic episodes.
‡ Median undefined since at least 50% of patients did not have any emetic episodes.

Continued on next page

Zofran—Cont.

taining cisplatin ≥50 mg/m^2. A total of 66% of patients in the ondansetron 24 mg once a day group, 55% in the ondansetron 8 mg twice a day group, and 55% in the ondansetron 32 mg once a day group completed the 24-hour study period with zero emetic episodes and no rescue antiemetic medications, the primary endpoint of efficacy. Each of the three treatment groups was shown to be statistically significantly superior to a historical placebo control.

In the same trial, 56% of patients receiving oral ondansetron 24 mg once a day experienced no nausea during the 24-hour study period, compared with 36% of patients in the oral ondansetron 8 mg twice a day group (p = 0.001) and 50% in the oral ondansetron 32 mg once a day group.

In a second trial, efficacy of the oral ondansetron 24 mg once a day regimen in the prevention of nausea and vomiting associated with highly emetogenic cancer chemotherapy, including cisplatin ≥50 mg/m^2, was confirmed.

Moderately Emetogenic Chemotherapy: In one double-blind US study in 67 patients, ZOFRAN Tablets 8 mg administered twice a day were significantly more effective than placebo in preventing vomiting induced by cyclophosphamide-based chemotherapy containing doxorubicin. Treatment response is based on the total number of emetic episodes over the 3-day study period. The results of this study are summarized in Table 3:

[See table 3 at top of previous page]

In one double-blind US study in 336 patients, ZOFRAN Tablets 8 mg administered twice a day were as effective as ZOFRAN Tablets 8 mg administered three times a day in preventing nausea and vomiting induced by cyclophosphamide-based chemotherapy containing either methotrexate or doxorubicin. Treatment response is based on the total number of emetic episodes over the 3-day study period. The results of this study are summarized in Table 4:

[See table 4 above]

Table 4: Emetic Episodes: Treatment Response

	Ondansetron	
	8-mg b.i.d. ZOFRAN Tablets*	8-mg t.i.d. ZOFRAN Tablets†
Number of patients	165	171
Treatment response		
0 Emetic episodes	101 (61%)	99 (58%)
1–2 Emetic episodes	16 (10%)	17 (10%)
More than 2 emetic episodes/withdrawn	48 (29%)	55 (32%)
Median number of emetic episodes	0.0	0.0
Median time to first emetic episode (h)	Undefined‡	Undefined‡
Median nausea scores (0–100)§	6	6

*The first dose was administered 30 minutes before the start of emetogenic chemotherapy, with a subsequent dose 8 hours after the first dose. An 8-mg ZOFRAN Tablet was administered twice a day for 2 days after completion of chemotherapy.

† The first dose was administered 30 minutes before the start of emetogenic chemotherapy, with subsequent doses 4 and 8 hours after the first dose. An 8-mg ZOFRAN Tablet was administered three times a day for 2 days after completion of chemotherapy.

‡ Median undefined since at least 50% of patients did not have any emetic episodes.

§ Visual analog scale assessment: 0 = no nausea, 100 = nausea as bad as it can be.

Re-treatment: In uncontrolled trials, 148 patients receiving cyclophosphamide-based chemotherapy were re-treated with ZOFRAN Tablets 8 mg t.i.d. of oral ondansetron during subsequent chemotherapy for a total of 396 re-treatment courses. No emetic episodes occurred in 314 (79%) of the re-treatment courses, and only one to two emetic episodes occurred in 43 (11%) of the re-treatment courses.

Pediatric Studies: Three open-label, uncontrolled, foreign trials have been performed with 182 pediatric patients 4 to 18 years old with cancer who were given a variety of cisplatin or noncisplatin regimens. In these foreign trials, the initial dose of ZOFRAN® (ondansetron HCl) Injection ranged from 0.04 to 0.87 mg/kg for a total dose of 2.16 to 12 mg. This was followed by the administration of ZOFRAN Tablets ranging from 4 to 24 mg daily for 3 days. In these studies, 58% of the 170 evaluable patients had a complete response (no emetic episodes) on day 1. Two studies showed the response rates for patients less than 12 years of age who received ZOFRAN Tablets 4 mg three times a day to be similar to those in patients 12 to 18 years of age who received ZOFRAN Tablets 8 mg three times daily. Thus, prevention of emesis in these pediatric patients was essentially the same as for patients older than 18 years of age. Overall, ZOFRAN Tablets were well tolerated in these pediatric patients.

Radiation-Induced Nausea and Vomiting: *Total Body Irradiation:* In a randomized, double-blind study in 20 patients, ZOFRAN Tablets (8 mg given 1.5 hours before each fraction of radiotherapy for 4 days) were significantly more effective than placebo in preventing vomiting induced by total body irradiation. Total body irradiation consisted of 11 fractions (120 cGy per fraction) over 4 days for a total of 1320 cGy. Patients received three fractions for 3 days, then two fractions on day 4.

Single High-Dose Fraction Radiotherapy: Ondansetron was significantly more effective than metoclopramide with respect to complete control of emesis (0 emetic episodes) in a double-blind trial in 105 patients receiving single high-dose radiotherapy (800 to 1000 cGy) over an anterior or posterior field size of ≥80 cm^2 to the abdomen. Patients received the first dose of ZOFRAN Tablets (8 mg) or metoclopramide (10 mg) 1 to 2 hours before radiotherapy. If radiotherapy was given in the morning, two additional doses of study treatment were given (one tablet late afternoon and one tablet before bedtime). If radiotherapy was given in the afternoon, patients took only one further tablet that day before bedtime. Patients continued the oral medication on a t.i.d. basis for 3 days.

Daily Fractionated Radiotherapy: Ondansetron was significantly more effective than prochlorperazine with respect to complete control of emesis (0 emetic episodes) in a double-blind trial in 135 patients receiving a 1- to 4-week course of fractionated radiotherapy (180 cGY doses) over a field size of ≥100 cm^2 to the abdomen. Patients received the first dose of ZOFRAN Tablets (8 mg) or prochlorperazine (10 mg) 1 to 2 hours before the patient received the first daily radiotherapy fraction, with two subsequent doses on a t.i.d. basis. Patients continued the oral medication on a t.i.d. basis on each day of radiotherapy.

Postoperative Nausea and Vomiting: Surgical patients who received ondansetron 1 hour before the induction of general balanced anesthesia (barbiturate: thiopental, methohexital, or thiamylal; opioid: alfentanil, sufentanil, morphine, or fentanyl; nitrous oxide; neuromuscular blockade: succinylcholine/curare or gallamine and/or vecuronium, pancuronium, or atracurium; and supplemental isoflurane or enflurane) were evaluated in two double-blind studies (one US study, one foreign) involving 865 patients. ZOFRAN Tablets (16 mg) were significantly more effective than placebo in preventing postoperative nausea and vomiting.

The study populations in all trials thus far consisted of women undergoing inpatient surgical procedures. No studies have been performed in males. No controlled clinical study comparing ZOFRAN Tablets to ZOFRAN Injection has been performed.

Table 5: Principal Adverse Events in US Trials: Single Day Therapy With 24-mg ZOFRAN Tablets (Highly Emetogenic Chemotherapy)

Event	Ondansetron 24 mg q.d. n = 300	Ondansetron 8 mg b.i.d. n = 124	Ondansetron 32 mg q.d. n = 117
Headache	33 (11%)	16 (13%)	17 (15%)
Diarrhea	13 (4%)	9 (7%)	3 (3%)

INDICATIONS AND USAGE

1. Prevention of nausea and vomiting associated with highly emetogenic cancer chemotherapy, including cisplatin ≥50 mg/m^2.
2. Prevention of nausea and vomiting associated with initial and repeat courses of moderately emetogenic cancer chemotherapy.
3. Prevention of nausea and vomiting associated with radiotherapy in patients receiving either total body irradiation, single high-dose fraction to the abdomen, or daily fractions to the abdomen.
4. Prevention of postoperative nausea and/or vomiting. As with other antiemetics, routine prophylaxis is not recommended for patients in whom there is little expectation that nausea and/or vomiting will occur postoperatively. In patients where nausea and/or vomiting must be avoided postoperatively, ZOFRAN Tablets, ZOFRAN ODT Orally Disintegrating Tablets, and ZOFRAN Oral Solution are recommended even where the incidence of postoperative nausea and/or vomiting is low.

CONTRAINDICATIONS

ZOFRAN Tablets, ZOFRAN ODT Orally Disintegrating Tablets, and ZOFRAN Oral Solution are contraindicated for patients known to have hypersensitivity to the drug.

WARNINGS

Hypersensitivity reactions have been reported in patients who have exhibited hypersensitivity to other selective 5-HT_3 receptor antagonists.

PRECAUTIONS

Ondansetron is not a drug that stimulates gastric or intestinal peristalsis. It should not be used instead of nasogastric suction. The use of ondansetron in patients following abdominal surgery or in patients with chemotherapy-induced nausea and vomiting may mask a progressive ileus and/or gastric distension.

Information for Patients: *Phenylketonurics:* Phenylketonuric patients should be informed that ZOFRAN ODT Orally Disintegrating Tablets contain phenylalanine (a component of aspartame). Each 4-mg and 8-mg orally disintegrating tablet contains <0.03 mg phenylalanine.

Patients should be instructed not to remove ZOFRAN ODT Tablets from the blister until just prior to dosing. The tablet should not be pushed through the foil. With dry hands, the blister backing should be peeled completely off the blister. The tablet should be gently removed and immediately placed on the tongue to dissolve and be swallowed with the saliva. Peelable illustrated stickers are affixed to the product carton that can be provided with the prescription to ensure proper use and handling of the product.

Drug Interactions: Ondansetron does not itself appear to induce or inhibit the cytochrome P-450 drug-metabolizing enzyme system of the liver. Because ondansetron is metabolized by hepatic cytochrome P-450 drug-metabolizing enzymes, inducers or inhibitors of these enzymes may change the clearance and, hence, the half-life of ondansetron. On the basis of available data, no dosage adjustment is recommended for patients on these drugs. Tumor response to chemotherapy in the P 388 mouse leukemia model is not affected by ondansetron. In humans, carmustine, etoposide, and cisplatin do not affect the pharmacokinetics of ondansetron. In a crossover study in 76 pediatric patients, I.V. ondansetron did not increase blood levels of high-dose methotrexate.

Use in Surgical Patients: The coadministration of ondansetron had no effect on the pharmacokinetics and pharmacodynamics of temazepam.

Carcinogenesis, Mutagenesis, Impairment of Fertility: Carcinogenic effects were not seen in 2-year studies in rats and mice with oral ondansetron doses up to 10 and 30 mg/kg per day, respectively. Ondansetron was not mutagenic in standard tests for mutagenicity. Oral administration of ondansetron up to 15 mg/kg per day did not affect fertility or general reproductive performance of male and female rats.

Pregnancy: *Teratogenic Effects:* Pregnancy Category B. Reproduction studies have been performed in pregnant rats and rabbits at daily oral doses up to 15 and 30 mg/kg per day, respectively, and have revealed no evidence of impaired fertility or harm to the fetus due to ondansetron. There are, however, no adequate and well-controlled studies in pregnant women. Because animal reproduction studies are not always predictive of human response, this drug should be used during pregnancy only if clearly needed.

Nursing Mothers: Ondansetron is excreted in the breast milk of rats. It is not known whether ondansetron is excreted in human milk. Because many drugs are excreted in human milk, caution should be exercised when ondansetron is administered to a nursing woman.

Pediatric Use: Little information is available about dosage in pediatric patients 4 years of age or younger (see CLINICAL PHARMACOLOGY and DOSAGE AND ADMINISTRATION sections for use in pediatric patients 4 to 18 years of age).

Geriatric Use: Of the total number of subjects enrolled in cancer chemotherapy-induced and postoperative nausea and vomiting in US- and foreign-controlled clinical trials, for which there were subgroup analyses, 938 were 65 years of age and over. No overall differences in safety or effectiveness were observed between these subjects and younger subjects, and other reported clinical experience has not identified differences in responses between the elderly and younger patients, but greater sensitivity of some older individuals cannot be ruled out. Dosage adjustment is not needed in patients over the age of 65 (see CLINICAL PHARMACOLOGY).

ADVERSE REACTIONS

The following have been reported as adverse events in clinical trials of patients treated with ondansetron, the active ingredient of ZOFRAN. A causal relationship to therapy with ZOFRAN has been unclear in many cases.

Chemotherapy-Induced Nausea and Vomiting: The adverse events in Table 5 have been reported in ≥5% of adult patients receiving a single 24-mg ZOFRAN Tablet in two trials. These patients were receiving concurrent highly emetogenic cisplatin-based chemotherapy regimens (cisplatin dose ≥50 mg/m^2).

[See table 5 above]

The adverse events in Table 6 have been reported in ≥5% of adults receiving either 8 mg of ZOFRAN Tablets two or three times a day for 3 days or placebo in four trials. These patients were receiving concurrent moderately emetogenic chemotherapy, primarily cyclophosphamide-based regimens.

[See table 6 at top of next page]

Central Nervous System: There have been rare reports consistent with, but not diagnostic of, extrapyramidal reactions in patients receiving ondansetron.

Hepatic: In 723 patients receiving cyclophosphamide-based chemotherapy in US clinical trials, AST and/or ALT values have been reported to exceed twice the upper limit of normal

Table 6: Principal Adverse Events in US Trials: 3 Days of Therapy With 8 mg ZOFRAN Tablets (Moderately Emetogenic Chemotherapy)

Event	Ondansetron 8 mg b.i.d. n = 242	Ondansetron 8 mg t.i.d. n = 415	Placebo n = 262
Headache	58 (24%)	113 (27%)	34 (13%)
Malaise/fatigue	32 (13%)	37 (9%)	6 (2%)
Constipation	22 (9%)	26 (6%)	1 (<1%)
Diarrhea	15 (6%)	16 (4%)	10 (4%)
Dizziness	13 (5%)	18 (4%)	12 (5%)

Table 7: Frequency of Adverse Events From Controlled Studies With ZOFRAN Tablets (Postoperative Nausea and Vomiting)

Adverse Event	Ondansetron 16 mg (n = 550)	Placebo (n = 531)
Wound problem	152 (28%)	162 (31%)
Drowsiness/sedation	112 (20%)	122 (23%)
Headache	49 (9%)	27 (5%)
Hypoxia	49 (9%)	35 (7%)
Pyrexia	45 (8%)	34 (6%)
Dizziness	36 (7%)	34 (6%)
Gynecological disorder	36 (7%)	33 (6%)
Anxiety/agitation	33 (6%)	29 (5%)
Bradycardia	32 (6%)	30 (6%)
Shiver(s)	28 (5%)	30 (6%)
Urinary retention	28 (5%)	18 (3%)
Hypotension	27 (5%)	32 (6%)
Pruritus	27 (5%)	20 (4%)

in approximately 1% to 2% of patients receiving ZOFRAN Tablets. The increases were transient and did not appear to be related to dose or duration of therapy. On repeat exposure, similar transient elevations in transaminase values occurred in some courses, but symptomatic hepatic disease did not occur. The role of cancer chemotherapy in these biochemical changes cannot be clearly determined.

There have been reports of liver failure and death in patients with cancer receiving concurrent medications including potentially hepatotoxic cytotoxic chemotherapy and antibiotics. The etiology of the liver failure is unclear.

Integumentary: Rash has occurred in approximately 1% of patients receiving ondansetron.

Other: Rare cases of anaphylaxis, bronchospasm, tachycardia, angina (chest pain), hypokalemia, electrocardiographic alterations, vascular occlusive events, and grand mal seizures have been reported. Except for bronchospasm and anaphylaxis, the relationship to ZOFRAN was unclear.

Radiation-Induced Nausea and Vomiting: The adverse events reported in patients receiving ZOFRAN Tablets and concurrent radiotherapy were similar to those reported in patients receiving ZOFRAN Tablets and concurrent chemotherapy. The most frequently reported adverse events were headache, constipation, and diarrhea.

Postoperative Nausea and Vomiting: The adverse events in Table 7 have been reported in ≥5% of patients receiving ZOFRAN Tablets at a dosage of 16 mg orally in clinical trials. With the exception of headache, rates of these events were not significantly different in the ondansetron and placebo groups. These patients were receiving multiple concomitant perioperative and postoperative medications.
[See table 7 above]
Preliminary observations in a small number of subjects suggest a higher incidence of headache when ZOFRAN ODT Orally Disintegrating Tablets are taken with water, when compared to without water.

Observed During Clinical Practice: In addition to adverse events reported from clinical trials, the following events have been identified during post-approval use of oral formulations of ZOFRAN. Because they are reported voluntarily from a population of unknown size, estimates of frequency cannot be made. The events have been chosen for inclusion due to a combination of their seriousness, frequency of reporting, or potential causal connection to ZOFRAN.

General: Flushing. Rare cases of hypersensitivity reactions, sometimes severe (e.g., anaphylaxis/anaphylactoid reactions, angioedema, bronchospasm, shortness of breath, hypotension, laryngeal edema, stridor) have also been reported. Laryngospasm, shock, and cardiopulmonary arrest have occurred during allergic reactions in patients receiving injectable ondansetron.

Hepatobiliary: Liver enzyme abnormalities

Lower Respiratory: Hiccups

Neurology: Oculogyric crisis, appearing alone, as well as with other dystonic reactions

Skin: Urticaria

DRUG ABUSE AND DEPENDENCE

Animal studies have shown that ondansetron is not discriminated as a benzodiazepine nor does it substitute for benzodiazepines in direct addiction studies.

OVERDOSAGE

There is no specific antidote for ondansetron overdose. Patients should be managed with appropriate supportive therapy. Individual intravenous doses as large as 150 mg and total daily intravenous doses as large as 252 mg have been

inadvertently administered without significant adverse events. These doses are more than 10 times the recommended daily dose.

In addition to the adverse events listed above, the following events have been described in the setting of ondansetron overdose: "Sudden blindness" (amaurosis) of 2 to 3 minutes' duration plus severe constipation occurred in one patient that was administered 72 mg of ondansetron intravenously as a single dose. Hypotension (and faintness) occurred in a patient that took 48 mg of ZOFRAN Tablets. Following infusion of 32 mg over only a 4-minute period, a vasovagal episode with transient second-degree heart block was observed. In all instances, the events resolved completely.

DOSAGE AND ADMINISTRATION

Instructions for Use/Handling ZOFRAN ODT Orally Disintegrating Tablets: Do not attempt to push ZOFRAN ODT Tablets through the foil backing. With dry hands, PEEL BACK the foil backing of one blister and GENTLY remove the tablet. IMMEDIATELY place the ZOFRAN ODT Tablet on top of the tongue where it will dissolve in seconds, then swallow with saliva. Administration with liquid is not necessary.

Prevention of Nausea and Vomiting Associated With Highly Emetogenic Cancer Chemotherapy: The recommended adult oral dosage of ZOFRAN is a single 24-mg tablet administered 30 minutes before the start of single-day highly emetogenic chemotherapy, including cisplatin ≥50 mg/m². Multiday, single-dose administration of ZOFRAN 24-mg Tablets has not been studied.

Pediatric Use: There is no experience with the use of 24-mg ZOFRAN Tablets in pediatric patients.

Geriatric Use: The dosage recommendation is the same as for the general population.

Prevention of Nausea and Vomiting Associated With Moderately Emetogenic Cancer Chemotherapy: The recommended adult oral dosage is one 8-mg ZOFRAN Tablet or one 8-mg ZOFRAN ODT Tablet or 10 mL (2 teaspoonfuls equivalent to 8 mg of ondansetron) of ZOFRAN Oral Solution given twice a day. The first dose should be administered 30 minutes before the start of emetogenic chemotherapy, with a subsequent dose 8 hours after the first dose. One 8-mg ZOFRAN Tablet or one 8-mg ZOFRAN ODT Tablet or 10 mL (2 teaspoonfuls equivalent to 8 mg of ondansetron) of ZOFRAN Oral Solution should be administered twice a day (every 12 hours) for 1 to 2 days after completion of chemotherapy.

Pediatric Use: For pediatric patients 12 years of age and older, the dosage is the same as for adults. For pediatric patients 4 through 11 years of age, the dosage is one 4-mg ZOFRAN Tablet or one 4-mg ZOFRAN ODT Tablet or 5 mL (1 teaspoonful equivalent to 4 mg of ondansetron) of ZOFRAN Oral Solution given three times a day. The first dose should be administered 30 minutes before the start of emetogenic chemotherapy, with subsequent doses 4 and 8 hours after the first dose. One 4-mg ZOFRAN Tablet or one 4-mg ZOFRAN ODT Tablet or 5 mL (1 teaspoonful equivalent to 4 mg of ondansetron) of ZOFRAN Oral Solution should be administered three times a day (every 8 hours) for 1 to 2 days after completion of chemotherapy.

Geriatric Use: The dosage is the same as for the general population.

Prevention of Nausea and Vomiting Associated With Radiotherapy, Either Total Body Irradiation, or Single High-Dose Fraction or Daily Fractions to the Abdomen: The recommended oral dosage is one 8-mg ZOFRAN Tablet or one 8-mg ZOFRAN ODT Tablet or 10 mL (2 teaspoonfuls equiv-

alent to 8 mg of ondansetron) of ZOFRAN Oral Solution given three times a day.

For total body irradiation, one 8-mg ZOFRAN Tablet or one 8-mg ZOFRAN ODT Tablet or 10 mL (2 teaspoonfuls equivalent to 8 mg of ondansetron) of ZOFRAN Oral Solution should be administered 1 to 2 hours before each fraction of radiotherapy administered each day.

For single high-dose fraction radiotherapy to the abdomen, one 8-mg ZOFRAN Tablet or one 8-mg ZOFRAN ODT Tablet or 10 mL (2 teaspoonfuls equivalent to 8 mg of ondansetron) of ZOFRAN Oral Solution should be administered 1 to 2 hours before radiotherapy, with subsequent doses every 8 hours after the first dose for 1 to 2 days after completion of radiotherapy.

For daily fractionated radiotherapy to the abdomen, one 8-mg ZOFRAN Tablet or one 8-mg ZOFRAN ODT Tablet or 10 mL (2 teaspoonfuls equivalent to 8 mg of ondansetron) of ZOFRAN Oral Solution should be administered 1 to 2 hours before radiotherapy, with subsequent doses every 8 hours after the first dose for each day radiotherapy is given.

Pediatric Use: There is no experience with the use of ZOFRAN Tablets, ZOFRAN ODT Tablets, or ZOFRAN Oral Solution in the prevention of radiation-induced nausea and vomiting in pediatric patients.

Geriatric Use: The dosage recommendation is the same as for the general population.

Postoperative Nausea and Vomiting: The recommended dosage is 16 mg given as two 8-mg ZOFRAN Tablets or two 8-mg ZOFRAN ODT Tablets or 20 mL (4 teaspoonfuls equivalent to 16 mg of ondansetron) of ZOFRAN Oral Solution 1 hour before induction of anesthesia.

Pediatric Use: There is no experience with the use of ZOFRAN Tablets, ZOFRAN ODT Tablets, or ZOFRAN Oral Solution in the prevention of postoperative nausea and vomiting in pediatric patients.

Geriatric Use: The dosage is the same as for the general population.

Dosage Adjustment for Patients With Impaired Renal Function: The dosage recommendation is the same as for the general population. There is no experience beyond first-day administration of ondansetron.

Dosage Adjustment for Patients With Impaired Hepatic Function: In patients with severe hepatic impairment (Child-Pugh[1] score of 10 or greater), clearance is reduced and apparent volume of distribution is increased with a resultant increase in plasma half-life. In such patients, a total daily dose of 8 mg should not be exceeded.

HOW SUPPLIED

ZOFRAN Tablets, 4 mg (ondansetron HCl dihydrate equivalent to 4 mg of ondansetron), are white, oval, film-coated tablets engraved with "Zofran" on one side and "4" on the other in daily unit dose packs of 3 tablets (NDC 0173-0446-04), bottles of 30 tablets (NDC 0173-0446-00), and unit dose packs of 100 tablets (NDC 0173-0446-02).

ZOFRAN Tablets, 8 mg (ondansetron HCl dihydrate equivalent to 8 mg of ondansetron), are yellow, oval, film-coated tablets engraved with "Zofran" on one side and "8" on the other in daily unit dose packs of 3 tablets (NDC 0173-0447-04), bottles of 30 tablets (NDC 0173-0447-00), and unit dose packs of 100 tablets (NDC 0173-0447-02).

Store between 2° and 30°C (36° and 86°F). Protect from light. Store blisters and bottles in cartons.

ZOFRAN Tablets, 24 mg (ondansetron HCl dihydrate equivalent to 24 mg of ondansetron), are pink, oval, film-coated tablets engraved with "GX CF7" on one side and "24" on the other in daily unit dose packs of 1 tablet (NDC 0173-0680-00).

Store between 2° and 30°C (36° and 86°F).

ZOFRAN ODT Orally Disintegrating Tablets, 4 mg (as 4 mg ondansetron base) are white, round and plano-convex tablets debossed with a "Z4" on one side in unit dose packs of 30 tablets (NDC 0173-0569-00).

ZOFRAN ODT Orally Disintegrating Tablets, 8 mg (as 8 mg ondansetron base) are white, round and plano-convex tablets debossed with a "Z8" on one side in unit dose packs of 10 tablets (NDC 0173-0570-04) and 30 tablets (NDC 0173-0570-00).

Store between 2° and 30°C (36° and 86°F).

ZOFRAN Oral Solution, a clear, colorless to light yellow liquid with a characteristic strawberry odor, contains 5 mg of ondansetron HCl dihydrate equivalent to 4 mg of ondansetron per 5 mL in amber glass bottles of 50 mL with child-resistant closures (NDC 0173-0489-00).

Store upright between 15° and 30°C (59° and 86°F). Protect from light. Store bottles upright in cartons.

REFERENCE
1. Pugh RNH, Murray-Lyon IM, Dawson JL, Pietroni MC, Williams R. Transection of the oesophagus for bleeding oesophageal varices. *Brit J Surg.* 1973;60:646–649.

ZOFRAN Tablets and Oral Solution:
Glaxo Wellcome Inc., Research Triangle Park, NC 27709

ZOFRAN ODT Orally Disintegrating Tablets:
Manufactured for Glaxo Wellcome Inc., Research Triangle Park, NC 27709

by Scherer DDS, Blagrove, Swindon, Wiltshire, UK SN5 8RU

US Patent Nos. 4,695,578; 4,753,789; 5,344,658; 5,578,628; 5,854,270; 5,955,488; and 6,063,802

December 2000/RL-888

Continued on next page

ZOVIRAX® ℞
[zō vī' rax]
(acyclovir)
Capsules

ZOVIRAX® ℞
(acyclovir)
Tablets

ZOVIRAX® ℞
(acyclovir)
Suspension

Prescribing information for this product, which appears on pages 1510–1512 of the 2001 PDR, has been revised. Please write "See Supplement A" next to the product heading.
The **PRECAUTIONS: Pregnancy** *subsection was revised to the following:*
Pregnancy: Teratogenic Effects: Pregnancy Category B. Acyclovir was not teratogenic in the mouse (450 mg/kg per day, PO), rabbit (50 mg/kg per day, SC and IV), or rat (50 mg/kg per day, SC). These exposures resulted in plasma levels 9 and 18, 16 and 106, and 11 and 22 times, respectively, human levels.
There are no adequate and well-controlled studies in pregnant women. A prospective epidemiologic registry of acyclovir use during pregnancy was established in 1984 and completed in April 1999. There were 749 pregnancies followed in women exposed to systemic acyclovir during the first trimester of pregnancy resulting in 756 outcomes. The occurrence rate of birth defects approximates that found in the general population. However, the small size of the registry is insufficient to evaluate the risk for less common defects or to permit reliable or definitive conclusions regarding the safety of acyclovir in pregnant women and their developing fetuses. Acyclovir should be used during pregnancy only if the potential benefit justifies the potential risk to the fetus.
The following listings were revised in the **PRECAUTIONS: Observed During Clinical Practice** *subsection:*
General: Anaphylaxis, angioedema, fever, headache, pain, peripheral edema.
Nervous: Aggressive behavior, agitation, ataxia, coma, confusion, decreased consciousness, delirium, dizziness, encephalopathy, hallucinations, paresthesia, psychosis, seizure, somnolence, tremors. These symptoms may be marked, particularly in older adults or in patients with renal impairment (see PRECAUTIONS).
Hemic and Lymphatic: Anemia, leukopenia, lymphadenopathy, thrombocytopenia.
Hepatobiliary Tract and Pancreas: Elevated liver function tests, hepatitis, hyperbilirubinemia, jaundice.
The following sentence was revised in the **OVERDOSAGE** *section:*
Adverse events that have been reported in association with overdosage include agitation, coma, convulsions, and lethargy.
Glaxo Wellcome Inc., Research Triangle Park, NC 27709
©Copyright 1996, 2000, 2001, Glaxo Wellcome Inc. All rights reserved.
January 2001/RL-902

ZYBAN® ℞
[zī' ban]
(bupropion hydrochloride)
Sustained-Release Tablets

Prescribing information for this product, which appears on pages 1515–1519 of the 2001 PDR, has been revised. Please write "See Supplement A" next to the product heading.
The **CLINICAL PHARMACOLOGY: Population Subgroups: *Hepatic*** *subsection was revised to the following:*
The effect of hepatic impairment on the pharmacokinetics of bupropion was characterized in two single-dose studies, one in patients with alcoholic liver disease and one in patients with mild to severe cirrhosis. The first study showed that the half-life of hydroxybupropion was significantly longer in 8 patients with alcoholic liver disease than in 8 healthy volunteers (32±14 hours versus 21±5 hours, respectively). Although not statistically significant, the AUCs for bupropion and hydroxybupropion were more variable and tended to be greater (by 53% to 57%) in patients with alcoholic liver disease. The differences in half-life for bupropion and the other metabolites in the two patient groups were minimal.
The second study showed that there were no statistically significant differences in the pharmacokinetics of bupropion and its active metabolites in 9 patients with mild to moderate hepatic cirrhosis compared to 8 healthy volunteers. There was, however, more variability observed in some of the pharmacokinetic parameters for bupropion (AUC, C_{max}, and T_{max}) and its active metabolites ($t_{½}$) in patients with mild to moderate hepatic cirrhosis. In addition, in patients with severe hepatic cirrhosis, the bupropion C_{max} and AUC were substantially increased (mean difference: by approximately 70% and 3-fold, respectively) and more variable when compared to values in healthy volunteers; the mean bupropion half-life was also longer (by approximately 40%). For the metabolites, the mean C_{max} was lower (by approximately 30% to 70%), the mean AUC tended to be higher (by approximately 30% to 50%), the median T_{max} was later (by approximately 20 hours), and the mean half-lives were longer (by approximately 2- to 4-fold) in patients with severe hepatic cirrhosis than in healthy volunteers (see WARNINGS, PRECAUTIONS, and DOSAGE AND ADMINISTRATION).
The following sentence was revised in the **WARNINGS** *section:*
- **Patient factors: Predisposing factors that may increase the risk of seizure with bupropion use include history of head trauma or prior seizure, central nervous system (CNS) tumor, the presence of severe hepatic cirrhosis, and concomitant medications that lower seizure threshold.**

The following subsection was added to the **WARNINGS** *section:*
Hepatic Impairment: ZYBAN should be used with extreme caution in patients with severe hepatic cirrhosis. In these patients a reduced frequency of dosing is required, as peak bupropion levels are substantially increased and accumulation is likely to occur in such patients to a greater extent than usual. The dose should not exceed 150 mg every other day in these patients (see CLINICAL PHARMACOLOGY, PRECAUTIONS, and DOSAGE AND ADMINISTRATION).
The following subsection was added to the **PRECAUTIONS** *section:*
Hepatic Impairment: ZYBAN should be used with extreme caution in patients with severe hepatic cirrhosis. In these patients, a reduced frequency of dosing is required. ZYBAN should be used with caution in patients with hepatic impairment (including mild to moderate hepatic cirrhosis) and reduced frequency of dosing should be considered in patients with mild to moderate hepatic cirrhosis.
All patients with hepatic impairment should be closely monitored for possible adverse effects that could indicate high drug and metabolite levels (see CLINICAL PHARMACOLOGY, WARNINGS, and DOSAGE AND ADMINISTRATION).
The following subsection was revised in the **PRECAUTIONS** *section:*
Renal Impairment: No studies have been conducted in patients with renal impairment. Bupropion is extensively metabolized in the liver to active metabolites, which are further metabolized and excreted by the kidneys. ZYBAN should be used with caution in patients with renal impairment and a reduced frequency of dosing should be considered as bupropion and its metabolites may accumulate in such patients to a greater extent than usual. The patient should be closely monitored for possible adverse effects that could indicate high drug or metabolite levels.
The following paragraph was revised in the **PRECAUTIONS: Geriatric Use** *subsection:*
Bupropion is extensively metabolized in the liver to active metabolites, which are further metabolized and excreted by the kidneys. The risk of toxic reaction to this drug may be greater in patients with impaired renal function. Because elderly patients are more likely to have decreased renal function, care should be taken in dose selection, and it may be useful to monitor renal function (see PRECAUTIONS: Renal Impairment and DOSAGE AND ADMINISTRATION).
The following subsections were added to **DOSAGE AND ADMINISTRATION:**
Dosage Adjustment for Patients with Impaired Hepatic Function: ZYBAN should be used with extreme caution in patients with severe hepatic cirrhosis. The dose should not exceed 150 mg every other day in these patients. ZYBAN should be used with caution in patients with hepatic impairment (including mild to moderate hepatic cirrhosis) and a reduced frequency of dosing should be considered in patients with mild to moderate hepatic cirrhosis (see CLINICAL PHARMACOLOGY, WARNINGS, and PRECAUTIONS).
Dosage Adjustment for Patients with Impaired Renal Function: ZYBAN should be used with caution in patients with renal impairment and a reduced frequency of dosing should be considered (see CLINICAL PHARMACOLOGY and PRECAUTIONS).
The following was added to the **PATIENT INFORMATION** *section:*
4. Are there any concerns for patients with liver or kidney disease?
If you have liver or kidney disease, tell your doctor before taking ZYBAN. Depending on the severity of your condition, your doctor may need to adjust your dosage.
Manufactured by Catalytica Pharmaceuticals, Inc.
Greenville, NC 27834
for Glaxo Wellcome Inc., Research Triangle Park, NC 27709
US Patent Nos. 5,358,970; 5,427,798; 5,731,000; and 5,763,493
©Copyright 1997, 1998, 1999, 2000, Glaxo Wellcome Inc. All rights reserved.
May 2000/RL-813

To keep your **PDR** up to date throughout the year, note these revisions on the corresponding pages of the annual volume. Simply write **"See Supplement A"** next to the product heading.

Knoll Laboratories

A Division of
Knoll Pharmaceutical Company
3000 CONTINENTAL DRIVE NORTH
MOUNT OLIVE, NJ 07828-1234

Direct Inquiries to:
BASF Group
Customer Information Center:
General Information (800) 240-3820

Customer Operations: Orders, Credits/Returns, Wholesaler and Hospital Inquiries, Deductions, New Accounts (800) 526-0710

For Medical Information Contact:
(800) 526-0221

AKINETON® TABLETS AND AMPULES ℞
[ā-kĭn 'ĕ-ton]
biperiden hydrochloride and biperiden lactate

Prescribing information for this product, which appears on pages 1617–1618 of the 2001 PDR, has been revised. Please write "See Supplement A" next to the product heading.
Under © the following must be changed
©2000 Knoll Pharmaceutical Company.
AKINETON is a registered trademark of Knoll AG.
Manufactured for:
PAR PHARMACEUTICAL, INC.
Spring Valley, New York 10977
Manufactured by:
Knoll Laboratories
A Division of
Knoll Pharmaceutical Company
Mount Olive, New Jersey 07828
Issued: 08/00 0900002-3

DILAUDID® CII ℞
[dī "law 'dĭd]
hydromorphone hydrochloride
Rx only

Prescribing information for this product, which appears on pages 1618–1619 of the 2001 PDR, has been revised. Please write "See Supplement A" next to the product heading.

PRECAUTIONS
Special Risk Patients: DILAUDID should be used with caution in elderly or debilitated patients and those with impaired renal or hepatic function, hypothyroidism, Addison's disease, prostatic hypertrophy or urethral stricture. As with any narcotic analgesic agent, the usual precautions should be observed and the possibility of respiratory depression should be kept in mind.
Cough Reflex: DILAUDID suppresses the cough reflex; as with all narcotics, caution should be exercised when DILAUDID is used postoperatively and in patients with pulmonary disease.
Usage in Ambulatory Patients: Narcotics may impair the mental and/or physical abilities required for the performance of potentially hazardous tasks such as driving a car or operating machinery; patients should be cautioned accordingly.
Drug Interactions: Patients receiving other narcotic analgesics, general anesthetics, phenothiazines, tranquilizers, sedative hypnotics, tricyclic antidepressants or other CNS depressants (including alcohol) concomitantly with DILAUDID may exhibit an additive CNS depression. When such combined therapy is contemplated, the dose of one or both agents should be reduced.
Parenteral Administration: The parenteral form of DILAUDID may be given intravenously, but the injection should be given very slowly. Rapid intravenous injection of narcotic analgesics increases the possibility of side effects such as hypotension and respiratory depression.
Reports of mild to severe seizures and myoclonus have been reported in severely compromised patients, administered high doses of parenteral hydromorphone, for cancer and severe pain. Opioid administration at very high doses is associated with seizures and myoclonus in a variety of diseases where pain control is the primary focus.
Pregnancy: Pregnancy Category C. DILAUDID has been shown to be teratogenic in hamsters when given in doses 600 times the human dose. There are no adequate and well-controlled studies in pregnant women. DILAUDID should be used during pregnancy only if the potential benefit justifies the potential risk to the fetus.
Nonteratogenic effects: Babies born to mothers who have been taking opioids regularly prior to delivery will be physically dependent. The withdrawal signs include irritability and excessive crying, tremors, hyperactive reflexes, increased respiratory rate, increased stools, sneezing, yawning, vomiting, and fever. The intensity of the syndrome does not always correlate with the duration of maternal opioid use or dose. There is no consensus on the best method of managing withdrawal. Chlorpromazine 0.7 to 1.0 mg/kg q6h, phenobarbital 2 mg/kg q6h, and paregoric 2 to 4 drops/kg q4h, have been used to treat withdrawal symptoms in infants. The duration of therapy is 4 to 28 days, with the dosages decreased as tolerated.
Labor and Delivery: As with all narcotics, administration of DILAUDID to the mother shortly before delivery may re-

sult in some degree of respiratory depression in the newborn, especially if higher doses are used.

Nursing Mothers: It is not known whether this drug is excreted in human milk. Because many drugs are excreted in human milk and because of the potential for serious adverse reactions in nursing infants from DILAUDID, a decision should be made whether to discontinue nursing or to discontinue the drug, taking into account the importance of the drug to the mother.

Pediatric Use: Safety and effectiveness in children have not been established.

Geriatric Use: Clinical studies of DILAUDID did not include sufficient numbers of subjects aged 65 and over to determine whether they respond differently from younger subjects. Other reported clinical experience has not identified differences in responses between the elderly and younger patients. In general, dose selection for an elderly patient should be cautious, usually starting at the low end of the dosing range, reflecting the greater frequency of decreased hepatic, renal, or cardiac function, and of concomitant disease or other drug therapy.

Revised: December 1999   0900105-3

Knoll Pharmaceutical Company
3000 CONTINENTAL DRIVE NORTH
MOUNT OLIVE, NJ 07828

BASF Group

Direct Inquiries to:
BASF Group
Customer Information Center:
General Information (800) 240-3820

Customer Operations: Orders, Credits/Returns,
Wholesaler and Hospital Inquiries,
Deductions, New Accounts (800) 526-0710

For Medical Information Contact:
(800) 526-0221

TARKA®   ℞
(Trandolapril/Verapamil
Hydrochloride ER Tablets)

Prescribing information for this product, which appears on pages 1644–1648 of the 2001 PDR, has been revised. Please write "See Supplement A" next to the product heading.
Under HOW SUPPLIED

HOW SUPPLIED

TARKA 2/180 mg tablets are supplied as pink, oval, film-coated tablets containing 2 mg trandolapril in an immediate release form and 180 mg verapamil hydrochloride in a sustained release form. The tablet is embossed with the Knoll triangle and 182 on one side and plain on the other side.
NDC 0048-5921-80 — bottles of 100

TARKA 1/240 mg tablets are supplied as white, oval, film-coated tablets containing 1 mg trandolapril in an immediate release form and 240 mg verapamil hydrochloride in a sustained release form. The tablet is embossed with the Knoll triangle and 241 on one side and plain on the other side.
NDC 0048-5912-40 — bottles of 100

TARKA 2/240 mg tablets are supplied as gold, oval, film-coated tablets containing 2 mg trandolapril in an immediate release form and 240 mg verapamil hydrochloride in a sustained release form. The tablet is embossed with the Knoll triangle and 242 on one side and plain on the other side.
NDC 0048-5922-40 — bottles of 100

TARKA 4/240 mg tablets are supplied as reddish-brown, oval, film-coated tablets containing 4 mg trandolapril in an immediate release form and 240 mg verapamil hydrochloride in a sustained release form. The tablet is embossed with the Knoll triangle and 244 on one side and plain on the other side.
NDC 0048-5942-40 — bottles of 100

Dispense in well-closed container with safety closure.
Storage: Store at 15°–25°C (59°–77°F) see USP.
Revised August 2000   0900055-4

To keep your **PDR** up to date
throughout the year, note these revisions
on the corresponding pages of the annual
volume. Simply write **"See Supplement A"**
next to the product heading.

LEDERLE PHARMACEUTICAL
Division American Cyanamid Company
Pearl River, NY 10965
US Gov't. License No. 17

For Medical Information Contact:
MARKETED ONCOLOGY PRODUCTS:
Immunex Corporation
Professional Services Department
51 University Street
Seattle, WA 98101
(800) IMMUNEX

OTHER MARKETED DRUG PRODUCTS:
Lederle Pharmaceutical/Wyeth-Ayerst Pharmaceuticals
Medical Affairs Department
P.O. Box 8299
Philadelphia, PA 19101
Day: (800) 934-5556
8:30 AM to 4:30 PM
(Eastern Standard Time),
Weekdays only
Night: (610) 688-4400 (Emergencies only; non-emergencies should wait until the next day)

MARKETED VACCINES AND TINE TESTS:
Lederle Pharmaceutical/Wyeth-Ayerst Pharmaceuticals
Medical Affairs Department
P.O. Box 8299
Philadelphia, PA 19101
Day: (800) 934-5556
8:30 AM to 4:30 PM
(Eastern Standard Time),
Weekdays only
Night: (610) 688-4400 (Emergencies only; non-emergencies should wait until the next day)

SUPRAX®   ℞
[*sū 'präcks*]
Cefixime
Oral

Prescribing information for this product, which appears on pages 1680–1682 of the 2001 PDR, has been revised as follows. Please write "See Supplement A" next to the product heading.

The following sentence should be added after the first paragraph, which is set in boldface type, of the **WARNINGS** section:

Anaphylactoid reactions have been reported with the use of cefixime.

The following paragraph should be added to the end of the **Drug Interactions** section under **PRECAUTIONS**, just after the paragraph following the subheading "*Carbamazepine*":

Warfarin and Anticoagulants: Increased prothrombin time, with or without clinical bleeding, has been reported when cefixime is administered concomitantly.

The word "Anaphylaxis" should be added after the subheading "*Hypersensitivity Reactions*" in the **ADVERSE REACTIONS** section, and the words "angioedema, and facial edema" should be added after the word "pruritis" in this section.

The words "hepatitis, jaundice" should be added to the end of the list of adverse reactions following the subheading "*Hepatic*" in the **ADVERSE REACTIONS** section.

The words "acute renal failure" should be added to the end of the list of adverse reactions following the subheading "*Renal*" in the **ADVERSE REACTIONS** section.

The word "seizures" should be added to the list of adverse reactions following the subheading "*Central Nervous System*" in the **ADVERSE REACTIONS** section.

The following subheading and adverse reaction should be added after the list of reactions following the subheading "*Central Nervous System*" in the **ADVERSE REACTIONS** section:

Abnormal Laboratory Tests: Hyperbilirubinemia

The words "toxic epidermal necrolysis" should be added after the word "candidiasis" in the list of adverse reactions that follows the subheading "*Other*" in the **ADVERSE REACTIONS** section.

In the **ADVERSE REACTIONS** section, the list of adverse reactions that follows the subheading "*Adverse reactions:*" under the paragraph that explains the adverse reactions associated with cephalosporin-class antibiotics should be deleted and replaced with the following:

Adverse reactions: Allergic reactions, superinfection, renal dysfunction, toxic nephropathy, hepatic dysfunction including cholestasis, aplastic anemia, hemolytic anemia, hemorrhage, and colitis.

In the list of adverse reactions following the heading "*Abnormal Laboratory Tests*" the words "elevated bilirubin" should be deleted.

The manufacturing information should be deleted and replaced with the following:

Marketed by:
LEDERLE PHARMACEUTICAL
Division of American Cyanamid
Pearl River, NY 10965

Ligand Pharmaceuticals Incorporated
10275 SCIENCE CENTER DRIVE
SAN DIEGO, CA 92121

Direct Inquiries to:
(858) 550-7500
Customer Service
(877) 454-4263
Medical Information
(800) 964-5836
Reimbursement Support
(877) 654-4263

TARGRETIN®   ℞
[*tahr-greh' tan*]
(bexarotene)
Capsules, 75 mg
Rx only.

Prescribing information for this product, which appears on pages 3487–3490 of the 2001 PDR, has been completely revised as follows. Please write "See Supplement A" next to the product heading.

> Targretin® capsules are a member of the retinoid class of drugs that is associated with birth defects in humans. Targretin® capsules also caused birth defects when administered orally to pregnant rats. Targretin® capsules must not be administered to a pregnant woman. See CONTRAINDICATIONS.

DESCRIPTION

Targretin® (bexarotene) is a member of a subclass of retinoids that selectively activate retinoid X receptors (RXRs). These retinoid receptors have biologic activity distinct from that of retinoic acid receptors (RARs). Each soft gelatin capsule for oral administration contains 75 mg of bexarotene. The chemical name is 4-[1-(5,6,7,8-tetrahydro-3,5,5,8,8-pentamethyl-2-naphthalenyl) ethenyl] benzoic acid, and the structural formula is as follows:

Bexarotene is an off-white to white powder with a molecular weight of 348.48 and a molecular formula of $C_{24}H_{28}O_2$. It is insoluble in water and slightly soluble in vegetable oils and ethanol, USP.

Each Targretin® (bexarotene) capsule also contains the following inactive ingredients: polyethylene glycol 400, NF, polysorbate 20, NF, povidone, USP, and butylated hydroxyanisole, NF. The capsule shell contains gelatin, NF, sorbitol special-glycerin blend, and titanium dioxide, USP.

CLINICAL PHARMACOLOGY
Mechanism of Action

Bexarotene selectively binds and activates retinoid X receptor subtypes (RXRα, RXRβ, RXRγ). RXRs can form heterodimers with various receptor partners such as retinoic acid receptors (RARs), vitamin D receptor, thyroid receptor, and peroxisome proliferator activator receptors (PPARs). Once activated, these receptors function as transcription factors that regulate the expression of genes that control cellular differentiation and proliferation. Bexarotene inhibits the growth *in vitro* of some tumor cell lines of hematopoietic and squamous cell origin. It also induces tumor regression *in vivo* in some animal models. The exact mechanism of action of bexarotene in the treatment of cutaneous T-cell lymphoma (CTCL) is unknown.

Pharmacokinetics
General

After oral administration of Targretin® capsules, bexarotene is absorbed with a T_{max} of about two hours. Terminal half-life of bexarotene is about seven hours. Studies in patients with advanced malignancies show approximate single dose linearity within the therapeutic range and low accumulation with multiple doses. Plasma bexarotene AUC and C_{max} values resulting from a 75 to 300 mg dose were 35% and 48% higher, respectively, after a fat-containing meal than after a glucose solution (see **PRECAUTIONS: Drug-Food Interaction** and **DOSAGE AND ADMINISTRATION**). Bexarotene is highly bound (>99%) to plasma proteins. The plasma proteins to which bexarotene binds have not been elucidated, and the ability of bexarotene to displace drugs bound to plasma proteins and the ability of drugs to displace bexarotene binding have not been studied (see **PRECAUTIONS: Protein Binding**). The uptake of bexarotene by organs or tissues has not been evaluated.

Metabolism

Four bexarotene metabolites have been identified in plasma: 6- and 7-hydroxy-bexarotene and 6- and 7-oxo-bexarotene. *In vitro* studies suggest that cytochrome P450 3A4 is the major cytochrome P450 responsible for formation of the oxidative metabolites and that the oxidative metabolites may be glucuronidated. The oxidative metabolites are active in *in vitro* assays of retinoid receptor activation, but the relative contribution of the parent and any metabolites to the efficacy and safety of Targretin® capsules is unknown.

Continued on next page

Targretin—Cont.

Elimination
The renal elimination of bexarotene and its metabolites was examined in patients with Type 2 diabetes mellitus. Neither bexarotene nor its metabolites were excreted in urine in appreciable amounts. Bexarotene is thought to be eliminated primarily through the hepatobiliary system.

Special Populations
Elderly: Bexarotene C_{max} and AUC were similar in advanced cancer patients <60 years old and in patients >60 years old, including a subset of patients >70 years old.
Pediatric: Studies to evaluate bexarotene pharmacokinetics in the pediatric population have not been conducted (see PRECAUTIONS: *Pediatric Use*).
Gender: The pharmacokinetics of bexarotene were similar in male and female patients with advanced cancer.
Ethnic Origin: The effect of ethnic origin on bexarotene pharmacokinetics is unknown.
Renal Insufficiency: No formal studies have been conducted with Targretin® capsules in patients with renal insufficiency. Urinary elimination of bexarotene and its known metabolites is a minor excretory pathway (<1% of administered dose), but because renal insufficiency can result in significant protein binding changes, pharmacokinetics may be altered in patients with renal insufficiency (see PRECAUTIONS: *Renal Insufficiency*).
Hepatic Insufficiency: No specific studies have been conducted with Targretin® capsules in patients with hepatic insufficiency. Because less than 1% of the dose is excreted in the urine unchanged and there is *in vitro* evidence of extensive hepatic contribution to bexarotene elimination, hepatic impairment would be expected to lead to greatly decreased clearance (see WARNINGS: *Hepatic insufficiency*).

Drug-Drug Interactions
No specific studies to evaluate drug interactions with bexarotene have been conducted. Bexarotene oxidative metabolites appear to be formed by cytochrome P450 3A4.
Because bexarotene is metabolized by cytochrome P450 3A4, ketoconazole, itraconazole, erythromycin, gemfibrozil, grapefruit juice, and other inhibitors of cytochrome P450 3A4 would be expected to lead to an increase in plasma bexarotene concentrations. Furthermore, rifampin, phenytoin, phenobarbital and other inducers of cytochrome P450 3A4 may cause a reduction in plasma bexarotene concentrations. Concomitant administration of Targretin® capsules and gemfibrozil resulted in substantial increases in plasma concentrations of bexarotene, probably at least partially related to cytochrome P450 3A4 inhibition by gemfibrozil. Under similar conditions, bexarotene concentrations were not affected by concomitant atorvastatin administration. Concomitant administration of gemfibrozil with Targretin® capsules is not recommended (see PRECAUTIONS: *Drug-Drug Interactions*).
Concomitant administration of Targretin® capsules and tamoxifen in women with breast cancer who were progressing on tamoxifen resulted in a modest decrease in plasma concentrations of tamoxifen, possibly through an induction of cytochrome P450 3A4. Based on this known interaction, bexarotene may theoretically increase the rate of metabolism and reduce plasma concentrations of other substrates metabolized by cytochrome P450 3A4, including hormonal contraceptives (see CONTRAINDICATIONS: *Pregnancy: Category X* and PRECAUTIONS: *Drug-Drug Interactions*).

Clinical Studies
Targretin® capsules were evaluated in 152 patients with advanced and early stage cutaneous T-cell lymphoma (CTCL) in two multicenter, open-label, historically-controlled clinical studies conducted in the U.S., Canada, Europe, and Australia.
The advanced disease patients had disease refractory to at least one prior systemic therapy (median of two, range one to six prior systemic therapies) and had been treated with a median of five (range 1 to 11) prior systemic, irradiation, and/or topical therapies. Early disease patients were intolerant to, had disease that was refractory to, or had reached a response plateau of six months on, at least two prior therapies. The patients entered had been treated with a median of 3.5 (range 2 to 12) therapies (systemic, irradiation, and/or topical).
The two clinical studies enrolled a total of 152 patients, 102 of whom had disease refractory to at least one prior systemic therapy, 90 with advanced disease and 12 with early disease. This is the patient population for whom Targretin® capsules are indicated.
Patients were initially treated with a starting dose of 650 mg/m²/day with a subsequent reduction of starting dose to 500 mg/m²/day. Neither of these starting doses was tolerated, and the starting dose was then reduced to 300 mg/m²/day. If, however, a patient on 300 mg/m²/day of Targretin® capsules showed no response after eight or more weeks of therapy, the dose could be increased to 400 mg/m²/day.
Tumor response was assessed in both studies by observation of up to five baseline-defined index lesions using a Composite Assessment of Index Lesion Disease Severity (CA). This endpoint was based on a summation of the grades, for all index lesions, of erythema, scaling, plaque elevation, hypopigmentation or hyperpigmentation, and area of involvement. Also considered in response assessment was the presence or absence of cutaneous tumors and extracutaneous disease manifestations.
All tumor responses required confirmation over at least two assessments separated by at least four weeks. A partial response was defined as an improvement of at least 50% in the index lesions without worsening, or development of new cutaneous tumors or non-cutaneous manifestations. A complete clinical response required complete disappearance of all manifestations of disease, but did not require confirmation by biopsy.
At the initial dose of 300 mg/m²/day, 1/62 (1.6%) of patients had a complete clinical tumor response and 19/62 (30%) of patients had a partial tumor response. The rate of relapse (25% increase in CA or worsening of other aspects of disease) in the 20 patients who had a tumor response was 6/20 (30%) over a median duration of observation of 21 weeks, and the median duration of tumor response had not been reached. Responses were seen as early as 4 weeks and new responses continued to be seen at later visits.

INDICATIONS AND USAGE
Targretin® (bexarotene) capsules are indicated for the treatment of cutaneous manifestations of cutaneous T-cell lymphoma in patients who are refractory to at least one prior systemic therapy.

CONTRAINDICATIONS
Targretin® capsules are contraindicated in patients with a known hypersensitivity to bexarotene or other components of the product.

Pregnancy: Category X
Targretin® (bexarotene) capsules may cause fetal harm when administered to a pregnant woman. Targretin® capsules must not be given to a pregnant woman or a woman who intends to become pregnant. If a woman becomes pregnant while taking Targretin® capsules, Targretin® capsules must be stopped immediately and the woman given appropriate counseling.
Bexarotene caused malformations when administered orally to pregnant rats during days 7–17 of gestation. Developmental abnormalities included incomplete ossification at 4 mg/kg/day and cleft palate, depressed eye bulge/microphthalmia, and small ears at 16 mg/kg/day. The plasma AUC of bexarotene in rats at 4 mg/kg/day is approximately one third the AUC in humans at the recommended daily dose. At doses greater than 10 mg/kg/day, bexarotene caused developmental mortality. The no effect dose for fetal effects in rats was 1 mg/kg/day (producing an AUC approximately one sixth of the AUC at the recommended human daily dose).
Women of child-bearing potential should be advised to avoid becoming pregnant when Targretin® capsules are used. The possibility that a woman of child-bearing potential is pregnant at the time therapy is instituted should be considered. A negative pregnancy test (e.g., serum beta-human chorionic gonadotropin, beta-HCG) with a sensitivity of at least 50 mIU/L should be obtained within one week prior to Targretin® capsules therapy, and the pregnancy test must be repeated at monthly intervals while the patient remains on Targretin® capsules. Effective contraception must be used for one month prior to the initiation of therapy, during therapy and for at least one month following discontinuation of therapy; it is recommended that two reliable forms of contraception be used simultaneously unless abstinence is the chosen method. Bexarotene can potentially induce metabolic enzymes and thereby theoretically reduce the plasma concentrations of hormonal contraceptives (see CLINICAL PHARMACOLOGY: *Drug-Drug Interactions* and PRECAUTIONS: *Drug-Drug Interactions*). Thus, if treatment with Targretin® capsules is intended in a woman with child-bearing potential, it is strongly recommended that one of the two reliable forms of contraception should be non-hormonal. Male patients with sexual partners who are pregnant, possibly pregnant, or who could become pregnant must use condoms during sexual intercourse while taking Targretin® capsules and for at least one month after the last dose of drug. Targretin® capsules therapy should be initiated on the second or third day of a normal menstrual period. No more than a one month supply of Targretin® capsules should be given to the patient so that the results of pregnancy testing can be assessed and counseling regarding avoidance of pregnancy and birth defects can be reinforced.

WARNINGS
Lipid abnormalities: Targretin® capsules induce major lipid abnormalities in most patients. These must be monitored and treated during long-term therapy. About 70% of patients with CTCL who received an initial dose of ≥300 mg/m²/day of Targretin® capsules had fasting triglyceride levels greater than 2.5 times the upper limit of normal. About 55% had values over 800 mg/dL with a median of about 1200 mg/dL in those patients. Cholesterol elevations above 300 mg/dL occurred in approximately 60% and 75% of patients with CTCL who received an initial dose of 300 mg/m²/day or greater than 300 mg/m²/day, respectively. Decreases in high density lipoprotein (HDL) cholesterol to less than 25 mg/dL were seen in about 55% and 90% of patients receiving an initial dose of 300 mg/m²/day or greater than 300 mg/m²/day, respectively, of Targretin® capsules. The effects on triglycerides, HDL cholesterol, and total cholesterol were reversible with cessation of therapy, and could generally be mitigated by dose reduction or concomitant antilipemic therapy.
Fasting blood lipid determinations should be performed before Targretin® capsules therapy is initiated and weekly until the lipid response to Targretin® capsules is established, which usually occurs within two to four weeks, and at eight week intervals thereafter. Fasting triglycerides should be normal or normalized with appropriate intervention prior to initiating Targretin® capsules therapy. Attempts should be made to maintain triglyceride levels below 400 mg/dL to reduce the risk of clinical sequelae (see WARNINGS: *Pancreatitis*). If fasting triglycerides are elevated or become elevated during treatment, antilipemic therapy should be instituted, and if necessary, the dose of Targretin® capsules reduced or suspended. In the 300 mg/m²/day initial dose group, 60% of patients were given lipid lowering drugs. Atorvastatin was used in 48% (73/152) of patients with CTCL. Because of a potential drug-drug interaction (see PRECAUTIONS: *Drug-Drug Interactions*), gemfibrozil is not recommended for use with Targretin® capsules.
Pancreatitis: Acute pancreatitis has been reported in four patients with CTCL and in six patients with non-CTCL cancers treated with Targretin® capsules; the cases were associated with marked elevations of fasting serum triglycerides, the lowest being 770 mg/dL in one patient. One patient with advanced non-CTCL cancer died of pancreatitis. Patients with CTCL who have risk factors for pancreatitis (e.g., prior pancreatitis, uncontrolled hyperlipidemia, excessive alcohol consumption, uncontrolled diabetes mellitus, biliary tract disease, and medications known to increase triglyceride levels or to be associated with pancreatic toxicity) should generally not be treated with Targretin® capsules (see WARNINGS: *Lipids abnormalities* and PRECAUTIONS: *Laboratory Tests*).
Liver function test abnormalities: For patients with CTCL receiving an initial dose of 300 mg/m²/day of Targretin® capsules, elevations in liver function tests (LFTs) have been observed in 5% (SGOT/AST), 2% (SGPT/ALT), and 0% (bilirubin). In contrast, with an initial dose greater than 300 mg/m²/day of Targretin® capsules, the incidence of LFT elevations was higher at 7% (SGOT/AST), 9% (SGPT/ALT), and 6% (bilirubin). Two patients developed cholestasis, including one patient who died of liver failure. In clinical trials, elevation of LFTs resolved within one month in 80% of patients following a decrease in dose or discontinuation of therapy. Baseline LFTs should be obtained, and LFTs should be carefully monitored after one, two and four weeks of treatment initiation, and if stable, at least every eight weeks thereafter during treatment. Consideration should be given to a suspension or discontinuation of Targretin® capsules if test results reach greater than three times the upper limit of normal values for SGOT/AST, SGPT/ALT, or bilirubin.
Hepatic insufficiency: No specific studies have been conducted with Targretin® capsules in patients with hepatic insufficiency. Because less than 1% of the dose is excreted in the urine unchanged and there is *in vitro* evidence of extensive hepatic contribution to bexarotene elimination, hepatic impairment would be expected to lead to greatly decreased clearance. Targretin® capsules should be used only with great caution in this population.
Thyroid axis alterations: Targretin® capsules induce biochemical evidence of or clinical hypothyroidism in about half of all patients treated, causing a reversible reduction in thyroid hormone (total thyroxine [total T4]) and thyroid-stimulating hormone (TSH) levels. The incidence of decreases in TSH and total T4 were about 60% and 45%, respectively, in patients with CTCL receiving an initial dose of 300 mg/m²/day. Hypothyroidism was reported as an adverse event in 29% of patients. Treatment with thyroid hormone supplements should be considered in patients with laboratory evidence of hypothyroidism. In the 300 mg/m²/day initial dose group, 37% of patients were treated with thyroid hormone replacement. Baseline thyroid function tests should be obtained and patients monitored during treatment.
Leukopenia: A total of 18% of patients with CTCL receiving an initial dose of 300 mg/m²/day of Targretin® capsules had reversible leukopenia in the range of 1000 to <3000 WBC/mm³. Patients receiving an initial dose greater than 300 mg/m²/day of Targretin® capsules had an incidence of leukopenia of 43%. No patient with CTCL treated with Targretin® capsules developed leukopenia of less than 1000 WBC/mm³. The time to onset of leukopenia was generally four to eight weeks. The leukopenia observed in most patients was explained by neutropenia. In the 300 mg/m²/day initial dose group, the incidence of NCI Grade 3 and Grade 4 neutropenia, respectively, was 12% and 4%. The leukopenia and neutropenia experienced during Targretin® capsules therapy resolved after dose reduction or discontinuation of treatment, on average within 30 days in 93% of the patients with CTCL and 82% of patients with non-CTCL cancers. Leukopenia and neutropenia were rarely associated with severe sequelae or serious adverse events. Determination of WBC with differential should be obtained at baseline and periodically during treatment.
Cataracts: Posterior subcapsular cataracts were observed in preclinical toxicity studies in rats and dogs administered bexarotene daily for 6 months. In 15 of 79 patients who had serial slit lamp examinations, new cataracts or worsening of previous cataracts were found. Because of the high prevalence and rate of cataract formation in older patient populations, the relationship of Targretin® capsules and cataracts cannot be determined in the absence of an appropriate control group. Patients treated with Targretin® capsules who experience visual difficulties should have an appropriate ophthalmologic evaluation.

PRECAUTIONS
Pregnancy: Category X. See CONTRAINDICATIONS.
General: Targretin® capsules should be used with caution in patients with a known hypersensitivity to retinoids. Clinical instances of cross-reactivity have not been noted.
Vitamin A Supplementation: In clinical studies, patients were advised to limit vitamin A intake to

≤15,000 IU/day. Because of the relationship of bexarotene to vitamin A, patients should be advised to limit vitamin A supplements to avoid potential additive toxic effects.

Patients with Diabetes Mellitus: Caution should be used when administering Targretin® capsules in patients using insulin, agents enhancing insulin secretion (e.g., sulfonylureas), or insulin-sensitizers (e.g., troglitazone). Based on the mechanism of action, Targretin® capsules could enhance the action of these agents, resulting in hypoglycemia. Hypoglycemia has not been associated with the use of Targretin® capsules as monotherapy.

Photosensitivity: Retinoids as a class have been associated with photosensitivity. *In vitro* assays indicate that bexarotene is a potential photosensitizing agent. Mild phototoxicity manifested as sunburn and skin sensitivity to sunlight was observed in patients who were exposed to direct sunlight while receiving Targretin® capsules. Patients should be advised to minimize exposure to sunlight and artificial ultraviolet light while receiving Targretin® capsules.

Laboratory Tests

Blood lipid determinations should be performed before Targretin® capsules are given. Fasting triglycerides should be normal or normalized with appropriate intervention prior to therapy. Hyperlipidemia usually occurs within the initial two to four weeks. Therefore, weekly lipid determinations are recommended during this interval. Subsequently, in patients not hyperlipidemic, determinations can be performed less frequently (see **WARNINGS:** *Lipid abnormalities*).

A white blood cell count with differential should be obtained at baseline and periodically during treatment. Baseline liver function tests should be obtained and should be carefully monitored after one, two and four weeks of treatment initiation, and if stable, periodically thereafter during treatment. Baseline thyroid function tests should be obtained and then monitored during treatment as indicated (see **WARNINGS:** *Leukopenia, Liver function test abnormalities, and Thyroid axis alterations*).

Drug-Food Interaction

In all clinical trials, patients were instructed to take Targretin® capsules with or immediately following a meal. In one clinical study, plasma bexarotene AUC and C_{max} values were substantially higher following a fat-containing meal versus those following the administration of a glucose solution. Because safety and efficacy data are based upon administration with food, it is recommended that Targretin® capsules be administered with food (see **CLINICAL PHARMACOLOGY:** *Pharmacokinetics* and **DOSAGE AND ADMINISTRATION**).

Drug-Drug Interactions

No formal studies to evaluate drug interactions with bexarotene have been conducted. Bexarotene oxidative metabolites appear to be formed by cytochrome P450 3A4. On the basis of the metabolism of bexarotene by cytochrome P450 3A4, ketoconazole, itraconazole, erythromycin, gemfibrozil, grapefruit juice, and other inhibitors of cytochrome P450 3A4 would be expected to lead to an increase in plasma bexarotene concentrations. Furthermore, rifampin, phenytoin, phenobarbital, and other inducers of cytochrome P450 3A4 may cause a reduction in plasma bexarotene concentrations.

Concomitant administration of Targretin® capsules and gemfibrozil resulted in substantial increases in plasma concentrations of bexarotene, probably at least partially related to cytochrome P450 3A4 inhibition by gemfibrozil. Under similar conditions, bexarotene concentrations were not affected by concomitant atorvastatin administration. Concomitant administration of gemfibrozil with Targretin® capsules is not recommended.

Concomitant administration of Targretin® capsules and tamoxifen in women with breast cancer who were progressing on tamoxifen resulted in a modest decrease in plasma concentrations of tamoxifen, possibly through an induction of cytochrome P450 3A4. Based on this known interaction, bexarotene may theoretically increase the rate of metabolism and reduce plasma concentrations of other substrates metabolized by cytochrome P450 3A4, including hormonal contraceptives (see **CLINICAL PHARMACOLOGY:** *Drug-Drug Interactions* and **CONTRAINDICATIONS:** *Pregnancy:* Category X). Thus, if treatment with Targretin® capsules is intended in a woman with child-bearing potential, it is strongly recommended that two reliable forms of contraception be used concurrently, one of which should be non-hormonal.

Renal Insufficiency

No formal studies have been conducted with Targretin® capsules in patients with renal insufficiency. Urinary elimination of bexarotene and its known metabolites is a minor excretory pathway for bexarotene (<1% of administered dose), but because renal insufficiency can result in significant protein binding changes, and bexarotene is >99% protein bound, pharmacokinetics may be altered in patients with renal insufficiency.

Protein Binding

Bexarotene is highly bound (>99%) to plasma proteins. The plasma proteins to which bexarotene binds have not been elucidated, and the ability of bexarotene to displace drugs bound to plasma proteins and the ability of drugs to displace bexarotene binding have not been studied.

Drug/Laboratory Test Interactions

CA125 assay values in patients with ovarian cancer may be increased by Targretin® capsule therapy.

Carcinogenesis, Mutagenesis, Impairment of Fertility

Long-term studies in animals to assess the carcinogenic potential of bexarotene have not been conducted. Bexarotene is not mutagenic to bacteria (Ames assay) or mammalian cells (mouse lymphoma assay). Bexarotene was not clastogenic *in vivo* (micronucleus test in mice). No formal fertility studies were conducted with bexarotene. Bexarotene caused testicular degeneration when oral doses of 1.5 mg/kg/day were given to dogs for 91 days (producing an AUC of approximately one fifth the AUC at the recommended human daily dose).

Use in Nursing Mothers

It is not known whether bexarotene is excreted in human milk. Because many drugs are excreted in human milk and because of the potential for serious adverse reactions in nursing infants from bexarotene, a decision should be made whether to discontinue nursing or to discontinue the drug, taking into account the importance of the drug to the mother.

Pediatric Use

Safety and effectiveness in pediatric patients have not been established.

Geriatric Use

Of the total patients with CTCL in clinical studies of Targretin® capsules, 64% were 60 years or older, while 33% were 70 years or older. No overall differences in safety were observed between patients 70 years or older and younger patients, but greater sensitivity of some older individuals to Targretin® capsules cannot be ruled out. Responses to Targretin® capsules were observed across all age group decades, without preference for any individual age group decade.

Continued on next page

Table 1. Adverse Events with Incidence ≥10% in CTCL Trials

Body System Adverse Event[1,2]	Initial Assigned Dose Group (mg/m²/day)	
	300 N=84 N (%)	>300 N=53 N (%)
METABOLIC AND NUTRITIONAL DISORDERS		
Hyperlipemia	66 (78.6)	42 (79.2)
Hypercholesteremia	27 (32.1)	33 (62.3)
Lactic dehydrogenase increased	6 (7.1)	7 (13.2)
BODY AS A WHOLE		
Headache	25 (29.8)	22 (41.5)
Asthenia	17 (20.2)	24 (45.3)
Infection	11 (13.1)	12 (22.6)
Abdominal pain	9 (10.7)	2 (3.8)
Chills	8 (9.5)	7 (13.2)
Fever	4 (4.8)	9 (17.0)
Flu syndrome	3 (3.6)	7 (13.2)
Back pain	2 (2.4)	6 (11.3)
Infection bacterial	1 (1.2)	7 (13.2)
ENDOCRINE		
Hypothyroidism	24 (28.6)	28 (52.8)
SKIN AND APPENDAGES		
Rash	14 (16.7)	12 (22.6)
Dry skin	9 (10.7)	5 (9.4)
Exfoliative dermatitis	8 (9.5)	15 (28.3)
Alopecia	3 (3.6)	6 (11.3)
HEMIC AND LYMPHATIC SYSTEM		
Leukopenia	14 (16.7)	25 (47.2)
Anemia	5 (6.0)	13 (24.5)
Hypochromic anemia	3 (3.6)	7 (13.2)
DIGESTIVE SYSTEM		
Nausea	13 (15.5)	4 (7.5)
Diarrhea	6 (7.1)	22 (41.5)
Vomiting	3 (3.6)	7 (13.2)
Anorexia	2 (2.4)	12 (22.6)
CARDIOVASCULAR SYSTEM		
Peripheral edema	11 (13.1)	6 (11.3)
NERVOUS SYSTEM		
Insomnia	4 (4.8)	6 (11.3)

[1] Preferred English term coded according to Ligand-modified COSTART 5 Dictionary.
[2] Patients are counted at most once in each AE category.

Table 2. Incidence of Moderately Severe and Severe Adverse Events Reported in at Least Two Patients (CTCL Trials)

Body System Adverse Event[1,2]	Initial Assigned Dose Group (mg/m²/day)			
	300 (N=84)		>300 (N=53)	
	Mod Sev N (%)	Severe N (%)	Mod Sev N (%)	Severe N (%)
BODY AS A WHOLE				
Asthenia	1 (1.2)	0 (0.0)	11 (20.8)	0 (0.0)
Headache	3 (3.6)	0 (0.0)	5 (9.4)	1 (1.9)
Infection bacterial	1 (1.2)	0 (0.0)	0 (0.0)	2 (3.8)
CARDIOVASCULAR SYS.				
Peripheral edema	2 (2.4)	1 (1.2)	0 (0.0)	0 (0.0)
DIGESTIVE SYSTEM				
Anorexia	0 (0.0)	0 (0.0)	3 (5.7)	0 (0.0)
Diarrhea	1 (1.2)	1 (1.2)	2 (3.8)	1 (1.9)
Pancreatitis	1 (1.2)	0 (0.0)	3 (5.7)	0 (0.0)
Vomiting	0 (0.0)	0 (0.0)	2 (3.8)	0 (0.0)
ENDOCRINE				
Hypothyroidism	1 (1.2)	1 (1.2)	2 (3.8)	0 (0.0)
HEM. & LYMPH. SYS.				
Leukopenia	3 (3.6)	0 (0.0)	6 (11.3)	1 (1.9)
META. AND NUTR. DIS.				
Bilirubinemia	0 (0.0)	1 (1.2)	2 (3.8)	0 (0.0)
Hypercholesteremia	2 (2.4)	0 (0.0)	5 (9.4)	0 (0.0)
Hyperlipemia	16 (19.0)	6 (7.1)	17 (32.1)	5 (9.4)
SGOT/AST increased	0 (0.0)	0 (0.0)	2 (3.8)	0 (0.0)
SGPT/ALT increased	0 (0.0)	0 (0.0)	2 (3.8)	0 (0.0)
RESPIRATORY SYSTEM				
Pneumonia	0 (0.0)	0 (0.0)	2 (3.8)	2 (3.8)
SKIN AND APPENDAGES				
Exfoliative dermatitis	0 (0.0)	1 (1.2)	3 (5.7)	1 (1.9)
Rash	1 (1.2)	2 (2.4)	1 (1.9)	0 (0.0)

[1] Preferred English term coded according to Ligand-modified COSTART 5 Dictionary.
[2] Patients are counted at most once in each AE category. Patients are classified by the highest severity within each row.

Targretin—Cont.

ADVERSE REACTIONS

The safety of Targretin® capsules has been evaluated in clinical studies of 152 patients with CTCL who received Targretin® capsules for up to 97 weeks and in 352 patients in other studies. The mean duration of therapy for the 152 patients with CTCL was 166 days. The most common adverse events reported with an incidence of at least 10% in patients with CTCL treated at an initial dose of 300 mg/m²/day of Targretin® capsules are shown in Table 1. The events at least possibly related to treatment are lipid abnormalities (elevated triglycerides, elevated total and LDL cholesterol and decreased HDL cholesterol), hypothyroidism, headache, asthenia, rash, leukopenia, anemia, nausea, infection, peripheral edema, abdominal pain, and dry skin. Most adverse events occurred at a higher incidence in patients treated at starting doses of greater than 300 mg/m²/day (see Table 1).

[See table 1 at top of previous page]

Adverse events leading to dose reduction or study drug discontinuation in at least two patients were hyperlipemia, neutropenia/leukopenia, diarrhea, fatigue/lethargy, hypothyroidism, headache, liver function test abnormalities, rash, pancreatitis, nausea, anemia, allergic reaction, muscle spasm, pneumonia, and confusion.

The moderately severe (NCI Grade 3) and severe (NCI Grade 4) adverse events reported in two or more patients with CTCL treated at an initial dose of 300 mg/m²/day of Targretin® capsules (see Table 2) were hypertriglyceridemia, pruritus, headache, peripheral edema, leukopenia, rash, and hypercholesteremia. Most of these moderately severe or severe adverse events occurred at a higher rate in patients treated at starting doses of greater than 300 mg/m²/day than in patients treated at a starting dose of 300 mg/m²/day.

[See middle table at top of previous page]

As shown in Table 3, in patients with CTCL receiving an initial dose of 300 mg/m²/day, the incidence of NCI Grade 3 or 4 elevations in triglycerides and total cholesterol was 28% and 25%, respectively. In contrast, in patients with CTCL receiving greater than 300 mg/m²/day, the incidence of NCI Grade 3 or 4 elevated triglycerides and total cholesterol was 45% and 45%, respectively. Other Grade 3 and 4 laboratory abnormalities are shown in Table 3.

[See table 3 below]

In addition to the 152 patients enrolled in the two CTCL studies, 352 patients received Targretin® capsules as monotherapy for various advanced malignancies at doses from 5 mg/m²/day to 1000 mg/m²/day. The common adverse events (incidence greater than 10%) were similar to those seen in patients with CTCL.

In the 504 patients (CTCL and non-CTCL) who received Targretin® capsules as monotherapy, drug-related serious adverse events that were fatal, in one patient each, were acute pancreatitis, subdural hematoma, and liver failure.

In the patients with CTCL receiving an initial dose of 300 mg/m²/day of Targretin® capsules, adverse events reported at an incidence of less than 10% and not included in Tables 1–3 or discussed in other parts of labeling and possibly related to treatment were as follows:

Body as a Whole: chills, cellulitis, chest pain, sepsis, and monilia.

Cardiovascular: hemorrhage, hypertension, angina pectoris, right heart failure, syncope, and tachycardia.

Digestive: constipation, dry mouth, flatulence, colitis, dyspepsia, cheilitis, gastroenteritis, gingivitis, liver failure, and melena.

Hemic and Lymphatic: eosinophilia, thrombocythemia, coagulation time increased, lymphocytosis, and thrombocytopenia.

Metabolic and Nutritional: LDH increased, creatinine increased, hypoproteinemia, hyperglycemia, weight decreased, weight increased, and amylase increased.

Musculoskeletal: arthralgia, myalgia, bone pain, myasthenia, and arthrosis.

Nervous: depression, agitation, ataxia, cerebrovascular accident, confusion, dizziness, hyperesthesia, hypesthesia, and neuropathy.

Respiratory: pharyngitis, rhinitis, dyspnea, pleural effusion, bronchitis, cough increased, lung edema, hemoptysis, and hypoxia.

Skin and Appendages: skin ulcer, acne, alopecia, skin nodule, macular papular rash, pustular rash, serous drainage, and vesicular bullous rash.

Special Senses: dry eyes, conjunctivitis, ear pain, blepharitis, corneal lesion, keratitis, otitis externa, and visual field defect.

Urogenital: albuminuria, hematuria, urinary incontinence, urinary tract infection, urinary urgency, dysuria, kidney function abnormal, and breast pain.

OVERDOSAGE

Doses up to 1000 mg/m²/day of Targretin® capsules have been administered in short-term studies in patients with advanced cancer without acute toxic effects. Single doses of 1500 mg/kg and 720 mg/kg were tolerated without significant toxicity in rats and dogs, respectively. These doses are approximately 30 and 50 times, respectively, the recommended human dose on a mg/m² basis.

No clinical experience with an overdose of Targretin® capsules has been reported. Any overdose with Targretin® capsules should be treated with supportive care for the signs and symptoms exhibited by the patient.

DOSAGE AND ADMINISTRATION

The recommended initial dose of Targretin® capsules is 300 mg/m²/day. (See Table 4.) Targretin® capsules should be taken as a single oral daily dose with a meal. See CONTRAINDICATIONS: *Pregnancy: Category X* section for precautions to prevent pregnancy and birth defects in women of child-bearing potential.

Table 4. Targretin® Capsule Initial Dose Calculation According to Body Surface Area

Initial Dose Level (300 mg/m²/day)		Number of 75 mg Targretin® Capsules
Body Surface Area (m²)	Total Daily Dose (mg/day)	
0.88 – 1.12	300	4
1.13 – 1.37	375	5
1.38 – 1.62	450	6
1.63 – 1.87	525	7
1.88 – 2.12	600	8
2.13 – 2.37	675	9
2.38 – 2.62	750	10

Dose Modification Guidelines: The 300 mg/m²/day dose level of Targretin® capsules may be adjusted to 200 mg/m²/day then to 100 mg/m²/day, or temporarily suspended, if necessitated by toxicity. When toxicity is controlled, doses may be carefully readjusted upward. If there is no tumor response after eight weeks of treatment and if the initial dose of 300 mg/m²/day is well tolerated, the dose may be escalated to 400 mg/m²/day with careful monitoring.

Duration of Therapy: In clinical trials in CTCL, Targretin® capsules were administered for up to 97 weeks. Targretin® capsules should be continued as long as the patient is deriving benefit.

HOW SUPPLIED

Targretin® capsules are supplied as 75 mg off-white, oblong soft gelatin capsules, imprinted with "Targretin", in high density polyethylene bottles with child-resistant closures.

Bottles of 100 capsules .... NDC 64365-502-01

Store at 2°–25°C (36°–77°F). Avoid exposing to high temperatures and humidity after the bottle is opened. Protect from light.

Manufactured for: Ligand Pharmaceuticals Incorporated
San Diego, CA 92121

by: R.P. Scherer
St. Petersburg, FL 33716

Ligand Part #3000207 (Rev. 0101)
Anderson Part #5422101-02

Merck & Co., Inc.
WEST POINT, PA 19486

For Medical Information Contact:

Generally:
Product and service information:
Call the Merck National Service Center, 8:00 AM to 7:00 PM (ET), Monday through Friday:
(800) NSC-MERCK
(800) 672-6372
FAX: (800) MERCK-68
FAX: (800) 637-2568

Adverse Drug Experiences:
Call the Merck National Service Center, 8:00 AM to 7:00 PM (ET), Monday through Friday:
(800) NSC-MERCK
(800) 672-6372

In Emergencies:
24-hour emergency information for healthcare professionals:
(800) NSC-MERCK
(800) 672-6372

Sales and Ordering:
For product orders and direct account inquiries only, call the Order Management Center,
8:00 AM to 7:00 PM (ET), Monday through Friday:
(800) MERCK RX
(800) 637-2579

AGGRASTAT® ℞
(tirofiban hydrochloride injection premixed)
AGGRASTAT® ℞
(tirofiban hydrochloride injection)

Prescribing information for this product, which appears on pages 1868–1872 of the 2001 PDR, has been revised as follows. Please write "See Supplement A" alongside product heading.

In the **DESCRIPTION** section, in the last paragraph, replace the first sentence with the following:
AGGRASTAT Injection is a sterile concentrated solution for intravenous infusion after dilution and is supplied in a 25 mL or a 50 mL vial.

In the **WARNINGS** section, in the first paragraph, add the following sentence at the end:
Fatal bleedings have been reported (see ADVERSE REACTIONS).

Also in the **WARNINGS** section, in the second paragraph, after "<150,000/mm³" add ", in patients with hemorrhagic retinopathy, and in chronic hemodialysis patients."

In the **PRECAUTIONS** section, under *Bleeding Precautions*, replace the *Laboratory Monitoring* subsection with the following:

Laboratory Monitoring: Platelet counts, and hemoglobin and hematocrit should be monitored prior to treatment, within 6 hours following the loading infusion, and at least daily thereafter during therapy with AGGRASTAT (or more frequently if there is evidence of significant decline). In patients who have previously received GP IIb/IIIa receptor antagonists, consideration should be given to earlier monitoring of platelet count. If the patient experiences a platelet decrease to <90,000/mm³, additional platelet counts should be performed to exclude pseudothrombocytopenia. If thrombocytopenia is confirmed, AGGRASTAT and heparin should be discontinued and the condition appropriately monitored and treated.

In addition, the activated partial thromboplastin time (APTT) should be determined before treatment and the anticoagulant effects of heparin should be carefully monitored by repeated determinations of APTT and the dose should be adjusted accordingly (see also DOSAGE AND ADMINISTRATION). Potentially life-threatening bleeding may occur especially when heparin is administered with other products affecting hemostasis, such as GP IIb/IIIa receptor an-

---

Table 3. Treatment-Emergent Abnormal Laboratory Values in CTCL Trials

Analyte	Initial Assigned Dose (mg/m²/day)			
	300 N=83[1]		>300 N=53[1]	
	Grade 3[2] (%)	Grade 4[2] (%)	Grade 3 (%)	Grade 4 (%)
Triglycerides[3]	21.3	6.7	31.8	13.6
Total Cholesterol[3]	18.7	6.7	15.9	29.5
Alkaline Phosphatase	1.2	0.0	0.0	1.9
Hyperglycemia	1.2	0.0	5.7	0.0
Hypocalcemia	1.2	0.0	0.0	0.0
Hyponatremia	1.2	0.0	9.4	0.0
SGPT/ALT	1.2	0.0	1.9	1.9
Hyperkalemia	0.0	0.0	1.9	0.0
Hypernatremia	0.0	1.2	0.0	0.0
SGOT/AST	0.0	0.0	1.9	1.9
Total Bilirubin	0.0	0.0	0.0	1.9
ANC	12.0	3.6	18.9	7.5
ALC	7.2	0.0	15.1	0.0
WBC	3.6	0.0	11.3	0.0
Hemoglobin	0.0	0.0	1.9	0.0

[1] Number of patients with at least one analyte value post-baseline.

[2] Adapted from NCI Common Toxicity Criteria, Grade 3 and 4, Version 2.0. Patients are considered to have had a Grade 3 or 4 value if either of the following occurred: a) Value becomes Grade 3 or 4 during the study; b) Value is abnormal at or baseline and worsens to Grade 3 or 4 on study, including all values beyond study drug discontinuation, as defined in data handling conventions.

[3] The denominator used to calculate the incidence rates for fasting Total Cholesterol and Triglycerides were N=75 for the 300 mg/m²/day initial dose group and N=44 for the >300 mg/m²/day initial dose group.

tagonists. To monitor unfractionated heparin, APTT should be monitored 6 hours after the start of the heparin infusion; heparin should be adjusted to maintain APTT at approximately 2 times control.

In the **ADVERSE REACTIONS** section, replace the *Allergic Reactions/Readministration* subsection with the following:

Although no patients in the clinical trial database developed anaphylaxis and/or hives requiring discontinuation of the infusion of tirofiban, anaphylaxis has been reported in post-marketing experience (see also *Post-Marketing Experience, Hypersensitivity*). No information is available regarding the development of antibodies to tirofiban.

Also in the **ADVERSE REACTIONS** section, under *Laboratory Findings*, add the following sentence at the end of the second paragraph:

Platelet decreases have been observed in patients with no prior history of thrombocytopenia upon readministration of GP IIb/IIIa receptor antagonists.

Also in the **ADVERSE REACTIONS** section, replace the *Post-Marketing Experience* subsection with the following:

The following additional adverse reactions have been reported in post-marketing experience:

Bleeding: Intracranial bleeding, retroperitoneal bleeding, hemopericardium and pulmonary (alveolar) hemorrhage. Fatal bleedings have been reported rarely; *Body as a Whole*: Acute and/or severe decreases in platelet counts which may be associated with chills, low-grade fever, or bleeding complications (see *Laboratory Findings* above); *Hypersensitivity*: Severe allergic reactions including anaphylactic reactions. The reported cases have occurred during the first day of tirofiban infusion, during initial treatment, and during readministration of tirofiban. Some cases have been associated with severe thrombocytopenia (platelet counts ($<10{,}000/mm^3$).

In the **DOSAGE AND ADMINISTRATION** section, under *Directions for Use*, replace the first paragraph with the following:

Prior to use, AGGRASTAT Injection (250 mcg/mL) must be diluted to the same strength as AGGRASTAT Injection Premixed (50 mcg/mL). This may be achieved, for example, using one of the following three methods:

1. If using a 500 mL bag of sterile 0.9% sodium chloride or 5% dextrose in water, withdraw and discard 100 mL from the bag and replace this volume with 100 mL of AGGRASTAT Injection (from four 25 mL vials or two 50 mL vials) **OR**
2. If using a 250 mL bag of sterile 0.9% sodium chloride or 5% dextrose in water, withdraw and discard 50 mL from the bag and replace this volume with 50 mL of AGGRASTAT Injection (from two 25 mL vials or one 50 mL vial), **OR**
3. If using a 100 mL bag of sterile 0.9% sodium chloride or 5% dextrose in water, add the contents of a 25 mL vial to the bag.

Mix well prior to administration.

Also in the **DOSAGE AND ADMINISTRATION** section, under *Recommended Dosage*, add the following paragraph between the first paragraph and the table:

AGGRASTAT Injection must first be diluted to the same strength as AGGRASTAT Injection Premixed, as noted under *Directions for Use*.

In the **HOW SUPPLIED** section, replace No. 3713 with the following:

No. 3713 — AGGRASTAT Injection 6.25 mg per 25 mL (250 mcg per mL) and 12.5 mg per 50 mL (250 mcg per mL) are non-preserved, clear, colorless concentrated sterile solutions for intravenous infusion after dilution and are supplied as follows:

NDC 0006-3713-25, 25 mL vials.
NDC 0006-3713-50, 50 mL vials.

Revisions based on 9123308, issued December 2000.

ARAMINE® Injection ℞
(metaraminol bitartrate)

Prescribing information for this product, which appears on page 1882 of the 2001 PDR, has been revised as follows. Please write "See Supplement A" alongside product heading.

In the **HOW SUPPLIED** section, delete "(6505-00-753-9601 10 mL vial)" and replace the *Storage* subsection with the following:

Storage

Store at 25°C (77°F); excursions permitted to 15–30°C (59–86°F) [see USP Controlled Room Temperature]. Store container in carton until contents have been used. Protect from light. Protect from freezing.

Revisions based on 9050625, issued August 1999.

COMVAX® ℞
[Haemophilus b conjugate (meningococcal protein conjugate) and hepatitis B (recombinant) vaccine]

Prescribing information for this product, which appears on pages 1893–1895 of the 2001 PDR, has been revised as follows. Please write "See Supplement A" alongside product heading.

In the **ADVERSE REACTIONS** section, replace the *Post-Marketing Experience* subsection with the following:

Post-Marketing Experience

As with any vaccine, there is the possibility that broad use of COMVAX could reveal adverse experiences not observed in clinical trials. The following additional adverse reactions have been reported with use of the marketed vaccine.

Hypersensitivity

Anaphylaxis, angioedema, urticaria, erythema multiforme

Hematologic

Thrombocytopenia

Also in the **ADVERSE REACTIONS** section, under *Potential Adverse Effects*, under *RECOMBIVAX HB*, replace the *Hypersensitivity* subsection with the following:

Symptoms of hypersensitivity including reports of rash, pruritus, edema, arthralgia, dyspnea, hypotension, and ecchymoses

Also in the **ADVERSE REACTIONS** section, under *Potential Adverse Effects*, under *RECOMBIVAX HB*, in the *Hematologic* subsection, delete "; thrombocytopenia".

Revisions based on 9024703, issued May 2000.

COSMEGEN® for Injection ℞
(Dactinomycin for Injection)
(Actinomycin D)

Prescribing Information for this product, which appears on pages 1898–1900 of the 2001 PDR, has been revised as follows. Please write "See Supplement A" alongside product heading.

At the beginning, replace the boxed **WARNING** and **DOSAGE** text with the following:

> **WARNING**
> COSMEGEN* (Dactinomycin for Injection) should be administered only under the supervision of a physician who is experienced in the use of cancer chemotherapeutic agents.
> This drug is **HIGHLY TOXIC** and both powder and solution must be handled and administered with care. Inhalation of dust or vapors and contact with skin or mucous membranes, especially those of the eyes, must be avoided. Due to the toxic properties of dactinomycin (e.g., corrosivity, carcinogenicity, mutagenicity, teratogenicity), special handling procedures should be reviewed prior to handling and followed diligently. Dactinomycin is extremely corrosive to soft tissue. If extravasation occurs during intravenous use, severe damage to soft tissues will occur. In at least one instance, this has led to contracture of the arms.

In the **CLINICAL PHARMACOLOGY** section, under *Action*, in the second paragraph, in the second sentence, after "their use in the", delete "palliative". Also in this paragraph, add the following as the last sentence:

Dactinomycin is believed to produce its cytotoxic effects by binding DNA and inhibiting RNA synthesis.

Add a new **CLINICAL STUDIES** section after the **CLINICAL PHARMACOLOGY** section.

CLINICAL STUDIES

A wide variety of single agent and combination chemotherapy regimens with COSMEGEN have been studied. Because chemotherapeutic regimens are constantly changing, the decision to employ COSMEGEN should be directly supervised by physicians familiar with current oncologic practices and new advances in therapy.

Wilms' Tumor

The neoplasm responding most frequently to COSMEGEN is Wilms' tumor. Data from the National Wilms' Tumor Studies (NWTS-1, NWTS-2, NWTS-3 and NWTS-4) support the use of COSMEGEN in Wilms' tumor. The NWTS-3 evaluated results in 1,439 patients randomized to various regimens incorporating COSMEGEN (see table below).

[See first table at top of next page]

It should be noted that the complete results from NWTS-4 have not yet been published. Changes in NWTS-4 and NWTS-5 have consisted of alterations in duration as well as dose intensity of COSMEGEN. As a consequence, appropriate consultation with physicians experienced in the management of Wilms' tumor should be sought.

Childhood Rhabdomyosarcoma

The Third Intergroup Rhabdomyosarcoma Study (IRS-III) studied 1,062 previously untreated pediatric patients and young adults (≤21 years of age) and compared outcomes amongst a number of treatment regimens. COSMEGEN was included in all arms as a standard component of the treatment regimen; thus, comparative data are not available from this study. Nevertheless, it does provide information on treatment outcomes in a large group of closely studied patients. For treatment purposes, patients were stratified according to clinical group, histologic subtype, and site of disease. Patients in most strata were randomized, but clinical group I patients with favorable histology were not randomized and treated according to a single regimen.

[See second table at top of next page]

Metastatic Nonseminomatous Testicular Cancer

Combinations of vinblastine, cyclophosphamide, COSMEGEN, bleomycin and cisplatin (VAB-6 regimen) have been employed in the treatment of metastatic nonseminomatous testicular cancer. In a retrospective analysis of 142 evaluable patients with primary advanced stage II or clinical stage III testicular cancer 112 (79%) achieved a complete response (CR) after treatment with VAB-6 alone or in combination with surgery. Relapses were uncommon (12%) and 117 of 166 patients (71%) were categorized as alive without evidence of disease during the four years covered by the study.

Ewing's Sarcoma

COSMEGEN in conjunction with vincristine, doxorubicin, cyclophosphamide and radiotherapy has been used in the management of both metastatic and non-metastatic Ewing's sarcoma. Of 120 previously untreated patients with non-metastatic disease treated with COSMEGEN as part of maintenance therapy in the United Kingdom Children's Cancer Study Group Ewing's Tumor Study (ET-1), 49 (41%) were free of disease at 5 years and 53 (44%) were alive at 5 years. Outcomes in regional and metastatic disease for previously untreated patients administered COSMEGEN resulted in 31 of 44 patients (70%) achieving a CR after a median time on study of 83 weeks. Eight of 44 (18%) patients achieved a partial response (PR) and the remaining 5 (11%) demonstrated no response to the regimen.

Gestational Trophoblastic Neoplasia

Single agent COSMEGEN has been used in the management of nonmetastatic gestational trophoblastic neoplasia. In a series of 31 patients with nonmetastatic disease, complete and sustained remissions were achieved with COSMEGEN alone in 94% of treated patients. Alternating combination regimens incorporating COSMEGEN in conjunction with etoposide, methotrexate, vincristine and cyclophosphamide (EMA-CO regimen) have also been used in the treatment of poor prognosis gestational trophoblastic neoplasia. Administration of EMA-CO to 148 women with poor prognosis gestational trophoblastic neoplasia resulted in 110 (80%) complete and 25 (18%) partial responses after a mean follow-up of 50.4 months. Overall survival during the study period was 85% and relapses were uncommon (5.4%). Meticulous monitoring of beta-hCG (human chorionic gonadotropin) must be incorporated into the treatment regimen.

Regional Perfusion in Locally Recurrent and Locoregional Solid Malignancies

COSMEGEN, as a component of regional perfusion, has been administered as palliative treatment and as an adjunct to tumor resection in the management of locally recurrent and locoregional sarcomas, carcinomas and adenocarcinomas.

Replace the **INDICATIONS AND USAGE** section with the following:

INDICATIONS AND USAGE

COSMEGEN, as part of a combination chemotherapy and/or multi-modality treatment regimen, is indicated for the treatment of Wilms' tumor, childhood rhabdomyosarcoma, Ewing's sarcoma and metastatic, nonseminomatous testicular cancer.

COSMEGEN is indicated as a single agent, or as part of a combination chemotherapy regimen, for the treatment of gestational trophoblastic neoplasia.

COSMEGEN, as a component of regional perfusion, is indicated for the palliative and/or adjunctive treatment of locally recurrent or locoregional solid malignancies.

Replace the **CONTRAINDICATIONS** section with the following:

CONTRAINDICATIONS

COSMEGEN should not be given at or about the time of infection with chickenpox or herpes zoster because of the risk of severe generalized disease which may result in death.

Add the following as a new **WARNINGS** section after the **CONTRAINDICATIONS** section:

WARNINGS

Reports indicate an increased incidence of second primary tumors (including leukemia) following treatment with radiation and antineoplastic agents, such as COSMEGEN. Multi-modal therapy creates the need for careful, long-term observation of cancer survivors.

Pregnancy Category D

COSMEGEN may cause fetal harm when administered to a pregnant woman. COSMEGEN has been shown to cause malformations and embryotoxicity in rat, rabbit, and hamster when given in doses of 50–100 mcg/kg (approximately 0.5–2 times the maximum recommended daily human dose on a body surface area basis). If this drug is used during pregnancy, or if the patient becomes pregnant while receiving this drug, the patient should be apprised of the potential hazard to the fetus. Women of childbearing potential must be warned to avoid becoming pregnant.

After the **WARNINGS** section, replace the remainder of the Prescribing Information with the following:

PRECAUTIONS

General

This drug is **HIGHLY TOXIC** and both powder and solution must be handled and administered with care (see boxed warning and HOW SUPPLIED, *Special Handling*). Since COSMEGEN is extremely corrosive to soft tissues, it is intended for intravenous use. Inhalation of dust or vapors and contact with skin or mucous membranes, especially those of the eyes, must be avoided. Appropriate protective equipment should be worn when handling COSMEGEN. Should accidental eye contact occur, copious irrigation for at least 15 minutes with water, normal saline or a balanced salt

Continued on next page

Information on the Merck & Co. products listed on these pages is from the full prescribing information in use April 1, 2001.

Cosmegen—Cont.

ophthalmic irrigating solution should be instituted immediately, followed by prompt ophthalmologic consultation. Should accidental skin contact occur, the affected part must be irrigated immediately with copious amounts of water for at least 15 minutes while removing contaminated clothing and shoes. Medical attention should be sought immediately. Contaminated clothing should be destroyed and shoes cleaned thoroughly before reuse (see HOW SUPPLIED, *Special Handling*).

As with all antineoplastic agents, COSMEGEN is a toxic drug and very careful and frequent observation of the patient for adverse reactions is necessary. These reactions may involve any tissue of the body, most commonly the hematopoietic system resulting in myelosuppression. The possibility of an anaphylactoid reaction should be borne in mind.

It is extremely important to observe the patient daily for toxic side effects when combination chemotherapy is employed, since a full course of therapy occasionally is not tolerated. If stomatitis, diarrhea, or severe hematopoietic depression appear during therapy, these drugs should be discontinued until the patient has recovered.

COSMEGEN (Dactinomycin for Injection) and Radiation Therapy
An increased incidence of gastrointestinal toxicity and marrow suppression has been reported with combined therapy incorporating COSMEGEN and radiation. Moreover, the normal skin, as well as the buccal and pharyngeal mucosa, may show early erythema. A smaller than usual radiation dose administered in combination with COSMEGEN causes erythema and vesiculation, which progress more rapidly through the stages of tanning and desquamation. Healing may occur in four to six weeks rather than two to three months. Erythema from previous radiation therapy may be reactivated by COSMEGEN alone, even when radiotherapy was administered many months earlier, and especially when the interval between the two forms of therapy is brief. This potentiation of radiation effect represents a special problem when the radiotherapy involves the mucous membrane. When irradiation is directed toward the nasopharynx, the combination may produce severe oropharyngeal mucositis. *Severe reactions may ensue if high doses of both COSMEGEN and radiation therapy are used or if the patient is particularly sensitive to such combined therapy.*

Particular caution is necessary when administering COSMEGEN within two months of irradiation for the treatment of right-sided Wilms' tumor, since hepatomegaly and elevated AST levels have been noted.

In general, COSMEGEN should not be concomitantly administered with radiotherapy in the treatment of Wilms' tumor unless the benefit outweighs the risk.

COSMEGEN (Dactinomycin for Injection) and Regional Perfusion Therapy
Complications of the perfusion technique are related mainly to the amount of drug that escapes into the systemic circulation and may consist of hematopoietic depression, absorption of toxic products from massive destruction of neoplastic tissue, increased susceptibility to infection, impaired wound healing, and superficial ulceration of the gastric mucosa. Other side effects may include edema of the extremity involved, damage to soft tissues of the perfused area, and (potentially) venous thrombosis.

Laboratory Tests
Many abnormalities of renal, hepatic, and bone marrow function have been reported in patients with neoplastic diseases receiving COSMEGEN. Renal, hepatic, and bone marrow functions should be assessed frequently.

Drug/Laboratory Test Interactions
Dactinomycin may interfere with bioassay procedures for the determination of antibacterial drug levels.

Carcinogenesis, Mutagenesis, Impairment of Fertility
Reports indicate an increased incidence of second primary tumors (including leukemia) following treatment with radiation and antineoplastic agents, such as COSMEGEN. Multi-modal therapy creates the need for careful, long-term observation of cancer survivors.

The International Agency on Research on Cancer has judged that dactinomycin is a positive carcinogen in animals. Local sarcomas were produced in mice and rats after repeated subcutaneous or intraperitoneal injection. Mesenchymal tumors occurred in male F344 rats given intraperitoneal injections of 50 mcg/kg, 2 to 5 times per week for 18 weeks. The first tumor appeared at 23 weeks.

Dactinomycin has been shown to be mutagenic in a number of test systems *in vitro* and *in vivo* including human fibroblasts and leukocytes, and HeLa cells. DNA damage and cytogenetic effects have been demonstrated in the mouse and the rat.

Adequate fertility studies have not been reported, although, reports suggest an increased incidence of infertility following treatment with other antineoplastic agents.

Pregnancy
Pregnancy Category D
(See WARNINGS.)

Nursing Mothers
It is not known whether this drug is excreted in human milk. Because many drugs are excreted in human milk and because of the potential for serious adverse reactions in nursing infants from COSMEGEN, a decision should be made as to discontinuation of nursing and/or drug, taking into account the important of the drug to the mother.

The Third National Wilms' Tumor Study

Stage	Regimen	4-Year Relapse Free Survival (%)	4-Year Overall Survival (%)
I (favorable histology)	L	89.0	95.6
	EE	91.8	97.4
II (favorable histology)	DD	87.9	93.6
	DD2	86.9	89.6
	K	87.4	91.1
	K2	90.1	94.9
III (favorable histology)	DD1	82.0	90.9
	DD2	85.9	86.7
	K1	71.4	85.2
	K2	76.8	85.1
IV (favorable histology)	DD-RT	71.9	78.4
	J	77.9	86.6
I-III (unfavorable histology)	DD-RT	67.1	68.3
	J	62.4	68.4
IV (unfavorable histology)	DD-RT	58.3	58.3
	J	52.9	52.3

L = COSMEGEN and vincristine (10 weeks)
EE = COSMEGEN and vincristine (26 weeks)
DD = COSMEGEN, doxorubicin, and vincristine (65 weeks)
DD1 = COSMEGEN, doxorubicin, and vincristine (65 weeks) preceded by radiation therapy (1000 rads)
DD2 = COSMEGEN, doxorubicin, and vincristine (65 weeks) preceded by radiation therapy (2000 rads)
DD-RT = COSMEGEN, doxorubicin, and vincristine (65 weeks) preceded by radiation therapy (dose according to age)
K = COSMEGEN and vincristine (65 weeks)
K1 = COSMEGEN and vincristine (65 weeks) preceded by radiation therapy (1000 rads)
K2 = COSMEGEN and vincristine (65 weeks) preceded by radiation therapy (2000 rads)
J = COSMEGEN, doxorubicin, cyclophosphamide, and vincristine (65 weeks)

The Third Intergroup Rhabdomyosarcoma Study

Group	Number of Arms	Chemotherapy Regimen	5-Year Progression Free Survival (%) (mean±SEM)	5-Year Overall Survival (%) (mean±SEM)
I (favorable histology)	1 (non-randomized)	cyclic sequential VA (1 year)	83±3	93±2
II (favorable histology, excluding orbit, head and paratesticular sites)	2 (randomized)	VA, doxorubicin and RT (1 year)	77±6	89±5
		VA and RT (1 year)	56±10	54±13
III (excluding special pelvic, orbit, scalp, parotid, oral cavity, larynx, oropharynx and cheek)	3 (randomized)	pulsed VAC and RT (2 years)	70±6	70±6
		pulsed VADRC-VAC, CDDP and RT (2 years)	62±5	63±5
		pulsed VADRC-VAC, CDDP, VP-16 and RT (2 years)	56±4	64±5
IV (all)	3 (randomized)	pulsed VAC and RT (2 years)	27±8	27±6
		pulsed VADRC-VAC, CDDP and RT (2 years)	27±8	31±6
		pulsed VADRC-VAC, CDDP, VP-16 and RT (2 years)	30±6	29±7

VA = vincristine/COSMEGEN
VADRC = vincristine/doxorubicin/cyclophosphamide
VAC = vincristine/COSMEGEN/cyclophosphamide
CDDP = cisplatin
VP-16 = etoposide
RT = radiation therapy

Pediatric Use
The greater frequency of toxic effects of COSMEGEN in infants suggest that this drug should be administered to infants only over the age of 6 to 12 months.

ADVERSE REACTIONS

Toxic effects (excepting nausea and vomiting) usually do not become apparent until two to four days after a course of therapy is stopped, and may not peak until one to two weeks have elapsed. Deaths have been reported. However, adverse reactions are usually reversible on discontinuance of therapy. They include the following:
Miscellaneous: malaise, fatigue, lethargy, fever, myalgia, proctitis, hypocalcemia, growth retardation, infection.
Oral: cheilitis, dysphagia, esophagitis, ulcerative stomatitis, pharyngitis.
Lung: pneumonitis.
Gastrointestinal: anorexia, nausea, vomiting, abdominal pain, diarrhea, gastrointestinal ulceration, liver toxicity including ascites, hepatomegaly, hepatic veno-occlusive disease, hepatitis, and liver function test abnormalities. Nausea and vomiting, which occur early during the first few hours after administration, may be alleviated by the administration of anti-emetics.
Hematologic: anemia, even to the point of aplastic anemia, agranulocytosis, leukopenia, thrombocytopenia, pancytopenia, reticulocytopenia. Platelet and white cell counts should be performed *frequently* to detect severe hematopoietic depression. If either count markedly decreases, the drug should be withheld to allow marrow recovery. This often takes up to three weeks.
Dermatologic: alopecia, skin eruptions, acne, flare-up of erythema or increased pigmentation of previously irradiated skin.

Soft tissues: Dactinomycin is extremely corrosive. If extravasation occurs during intravenous use, severe damage to soft tissues will occur. In at least one instance, this has led to contracture of the arms. Epidermolysis, erythema, and edema, at times severe, have been reported with regional limb perfusion.
Laboratory Tests
Many abnormalities of renal, hepatic, and bone marrow function have been reported in patients with neoplastic diseases receiving COSMEGEN. Renal, hepatic, and bone marrow functions should be assessed frequently.

OVERDOSAGE

Dactinomycin was lethal to mice and rats at intravenous doses of 700 and 500 mcg/kg, respectively (approximately 3.8 and 5.4 times the maximum recommended daily human dose on a body surface area basis, respectively).

DOSAGE AND ADMINISTRATION

Toxic reactions due to COSMEGEN are frequent and may be severe (see ADVERSE REACTIONS), thus limiting in many instances the amount that may be administered. However, the severity of toxicity varies markedly and is only partly dependent on the dose employed.
Intravenous Use
The dosage of COSMEGEN varies depending on the tolerance of the patient, the size and location of the neoplasm, and the use of other forms of therapy. It may be necessary to decrease the usual dosages suggested below when additional chemotherapy or radiation therapy is used concomitantly or has been used previously.
The dosage for COSMEGEN is calculated in micrograms (mcg). The dose intensity per 2-week cycle for adults or children should not exceed 15 mcg/kg/day or

400–600 mcg/m²/day intravenously for five days. Calculation of the dosage for obese or edematous patients should be performed on the basis of surface area in an effort to more closely relate dosage to lean body mass.

A wide variety of single agent and combination chemotherapy regimens with COSMEGEN may be employed. Because chemotherapeutic regimens are constantly changing, dosing and administration should be performed under the direct supervision of physicians familiar with current oncologic practices and new advances in therapy. The following suggested regimens are based upon a review of current literature concerning therapy with COSMEGEN and are on a per cycle basis.

Wilms' Tumor, Childhood Rhabdomyosarcoma and Ewing's Sarcoma

Regimens of 15 mcg/kg intravenously daily for five days administered in various combinations and schedules with other chemotherapeutic agents have been utilized in the treatment of Wilms' tumor, rhabdomyosarcoma and Ewing's sarcoma.

Metastatic Nonseminomatous Testicular Cancer

1000 mcg/m² intravenously on Day 1 as part of a combination regimen with cyclophosphamide, bleomycin, vinblastine, and cisplatin.

Gestational Trophoblastic Neoplasia

12 mcg/kg intravenously daily for five days as a single agent.

500 mcg intravenously on Days 1 and 2 as part of a combination regimen with etoposide, methotrexate, folinic acid, vincristine, cyclophosphamide and cisplatin.

Regional Perfusion in Locally Recurrent and Locoregional Solid Malignancies

The dosage schedules and the technique itself vary from one investigator to another; the published literature, therefore, should be consulted for details. In general, the following doses are suggested:

50 mcg (0.05 mg) per kilogram of body weight for lower extremity or pelvis.

35 mcg (0.035 mg) per kilogram of body weight for upper extremity.

It may be advisable to use lower doses in obese patients, or when previous chemotherapy or radiation therapy has been employed.

Preparation of Solution for Intravenous Administration

This drug is **HIGHLY TOXIC** and both powder and solution must be handled and administered with care (see boxed warning and HOW SUPPLIED, *Special Handling*). Since COSMEGEN is extremely corrosive to soft tissues, it is intended for intravenous use. Inhalation of dust or vapors and contact with skin or mucous membranes, especially those of the eyes, must be avoided. Appropriate protective equipment should be worn when handling COSMEGEN. Should accidental eye contact occur, copious irrigation for at least 15 minutes with water, normal saline or a balanced salt ophthalmic irrigating solution should be instituted immediately, followed by prompt ophthalmologic consultation. Should accidental skin contact occur, the affected part must be irrigated immediately with copious amounts of water for at least 15 minutes while removing contaminated clothing and shoes. Medical attention should be sought immediately. Contaminated clothing should be destroyed and shoes cleaned thoroughly before reuse. (See HOW SUPPLIED, *Special Handling*.)

Reconstitute COSMEGEN by adding 1.1 mL of **Sterile Water for Injection (without preservative)** using aseptic precautions. The resulting solution of COSMEGEN will contain approximately 500 mcg (0.5 mg) per mL.

Parenteral drug products should be inspected visually for particulate matter and discoloration prior to administration, whenever solution and container permit. When reconstituted, COSMEGEN is a clear, gold-colored solution.

Once reconstituted, the solution of COSMEGEN can be added to infusion solutions of Dextrose Injection 5 percent or Sodium Chloride Injection either directly or to the tubing of a running intravenous infusion.

Although reconstituted COSMEGEN is chemically stable, the product does not contain a preservative and accidental microbial contamination might result. Any unused portion should be discarded. Use of water containing preservatives (benzyl alcohol or parabens) to reconstitute COSMEGEN for Injection, results in the formation of a precipitate.

Partial removal of COSMEGEN from intravenous solutions by cellulose ester membrane filters used in some intravenous in-line filters has been reported.

Since dactinomycin is extremely corrosive to soft tissue, precautions for materials of this nature should be observed.

If the drug is given directly into the vein without the use of an infusion, the "two-needle technique" should be used. Reconstitute and withdraw the calculated dose from the vial with one sterile needle. Use another sterile needle for direct injection into the vein.

Discard any unused portion of the COSMEGEN solution.

Management of Extravasation

Care in the administration of COSMEGEN will reduce the chance of perivenous infiltration (see boxed warning and ADVERSE REACTIONS). It may also decrease the chance of local reactions such as urticaria and erythematous streaking. On intravenous administration of COSMEGEN, extravasation may occur with or without an accompanying burning or stinging sensation, even if blood returns well on aspiration of the infusion needle. If any signs or symptoms of extravasation have occurred, the injection or infusion should be immediately terminated and restarted in another vein. If extravasation is suspected, intermittent application of ice to the site for 15 minutes q.i.d. for 3 days may be use-

ful. The benefit of local administration of drugs has not been clearly established. Because of the progressive nature of extravasation reactions, close observation and plastic surgery consultation is recommended. Blistering, ulceration and/or persistent pain are indications for wide excision surgery, followed by split-thickness skin grafting.

HOW SUPPLIED

No. 3298 — COSMEGEN for Injection is a lyophilized powder. In the dry form the compound is an amorphous yellow to orange powder. The solution is clear and gold-colored. COSMEGEN for Injection is supplied as follows:

NDC 0006-3298-22 in vials containing 0.5 mg (500 micrograms) of dactinomycin and 20.0 mg of mannitol.

Storage

Store at 25°C (77°F); excursions permitted to 15–30°C (59–86°F) [see USP Controlled Room Temperature]. Protect from light and humidity.

Special Handling

Animal studies have shown dactinomycin to be corrosive to skin, irritating to the eyes and mucous membranes of the respiratory tract and highly toxic by the oral route. It has also been shown to be carcinogenic, mutagenic, embryotoxic and teratogenic. Due to the drug's toxic properties, appropriate precautions including the use of appropriate safety equipment are recommended for the preparation of COSMEGEN for parenteral administration. Inhalation of dust or vapors and contact with skin or mucous membranes, especially those of the eyes, must be avoided. The National Institutes of Health presently recommends that the preparation of injectable antineoplastic drugs should be performed in a Class II laminar flow biological safety cabinet. Personnel preparing drugs of this class should wear chemical resistant, impervious gloves, safety goggles, outer garments and shoe covers. Additional body garments should be used based upon the task being performed (e.g., sleevelets, apron, gauntlets, disposable suits) to avoid exposed skin surfaces and inhalation of vapors and dust. Appropriate techniques should be used to remove potentially contaminated clothing.

Several other guidelines for proper handling and disposal of antineoplastic drugs have been published and should be considered.

Accidental Contact Measures

Should accidental eye contact occur, copious irrigation for at least 15 minutes with water, normal saline or a balanced salt ophthalmic irrigating solution should be instituted immediately, followed by prompt ophthalmologic consultation. Should accidental skin contact occur, the affected part must be irrigated immediately with copious amounts of water for at least 15 minutes while removing contaminated clothing and shoes. Medical attention should be sought immediately. Contaminated clothing should be destroyed and shoes cleaned thoroughly before reuse (see PRECAUTIONS, *General* and DOSAGE AND ADMINISTRATION, *Preparation of Solution for Intravenous Administration*).

Revisions based on 9000831, issued July 2000.

COSOPT® Sterile Ophthalmic Solution ℞
(dorzolamide hydrochloride-timolol maleate ophthalmic solution)

Prescribing information for this product, which appears on pages 1900–1902 of the 2001 PDR, has been revised as follows. Please write "See Supplement A" alongside product heading.

In the **HOW SUPPLIED** section, in the second paragraph, after "OCUMETER®*", add "PLUS container,".

Also in the **HOW SUPPLIED** section, the NDC items should read as follows:

NDC 0006-3628-35, 5 mL.
NDC 0006-3628-36, 10 mL.

After the **HOW SUPPLIED** section, add the **INSTRUCTIONS FOR USE** section.

INSTRUCTIONS FOR USE

Please follow these instructions carefully when using COSOPT*. Use COSOPT as prescribed by your doctor.

1. If you use other topically applied ophthalmic medications, they should be administered at least 10 minutes before or after COSOPT.
2. Wash hands before each use.

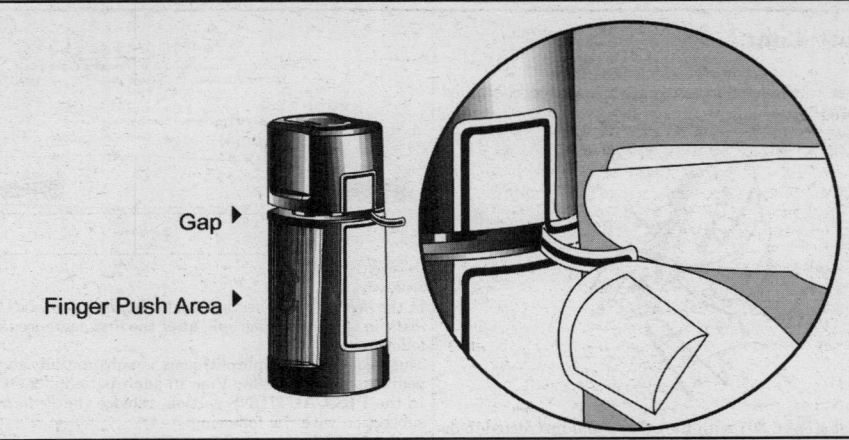

Gap ▶
Finger Push Area ▶

3. Before using the medication, be sure the Safety Strip on the front of the bottle is unbroken. A gap between the bottle and the cap is normal for an unopened bottle.

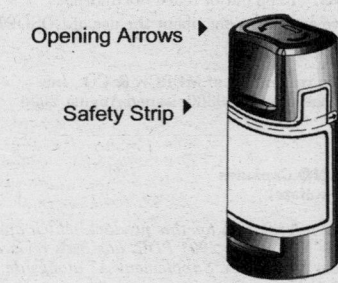

Opening Arrows ▶
Safety Strip ▶

4. Tear off the Safety Strip to break the seal. [See figure above]
5. To open the bottle, unscrew the cap by turning as indicated by the arrows.

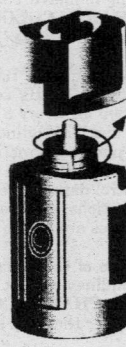

6. Tilt your head back and pull your lower eyelid down slightly to form a pocket between your eyelid and your eye.

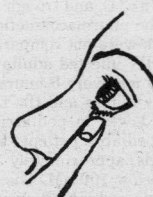

7. Invert the bottle, grasping it with the thumb or index finger over the Finger Push Area as shown. Press lightly until a single drop is dispensed into the eye as directed by your doctor.
DO NOT TOUCH YOUR EYE OR EYELID WITH THE DROPPER TIP.
Ophthalmic medications, if handled improperly, can become contaminated by common bacteria known to cause eye infections. Serious damage to the eye and subsequent loss of vision may result from using contaminated ophthalmic medications. If you think your medication may be contaminated, or if you develop an eye infection,

Continued on next page

Cosopt—Cont.

contact your doctor immediately concerning continued use of this bottle.

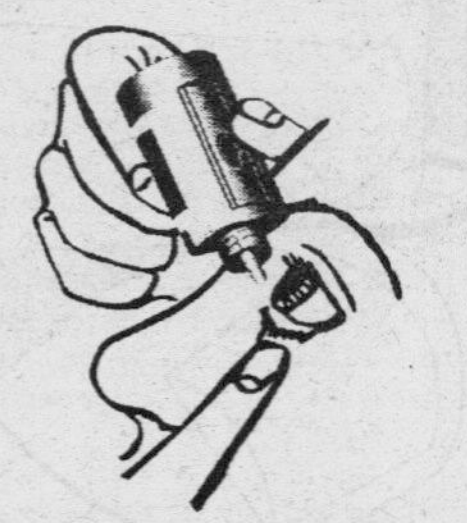

8. Repeat steps 6 & 7 with the other eye if instructed to do so by your doctor.
9. Replace the cap by turning until it is firmly touching the bottle.
10. The dispenser tip is designed to provide a pre-measured drop; therefore, do NOT enlarge the hole of the dispenser.

WARNING: Keep out of reach of children.

If you have any questions about the use of COSOPT, please consult your doctor.

*Registered trademark of MERCK & CO., Inc.
Revisions based on 9359300, issued August 2000.

CRIXIVAN® Capsules ℞
(indinavir sulfate)

Prescribing information for this product, which appears on pages 1904–1909 of the 2001 PDR, has been revised as follows. Please write "See Supplement A" alongside product heading.

In the **DESCRIPTION** section, in the first paragraph, replace the second sentence with the following:
CRIXIVAN Capsules are formulated as a sulfate salt and are available for oral administration in strengths of 100, 200, 333, and 400 mg of indinavir (corresponding to 125, 250, 416.3, and 500 mg indinavir sulfate, respectively).
In the **CLINICAL PHARMACOLOGY** section, under *Special Populations*, replace the *Gender* subsection with the following:
Gender: The effect of gender on the pharmacokinetics of indinavir was evaluated in 10 HIV seropositive women who received CRIXIVAN 800 mg every 8 hours with zidovudine 200 mg every 8 hours and lamivudine 150 mg twice a day for one week. Indinavir pharmacokinetic parameters in these women were compared in those in HIV seropositive men (pooled historical control data). Differences in indinavir exposure, peak concentrations, and trough concentrations between males and females are shown in Table 1 below:
[See table below]
The clinical significance of these gender differences in the pharmacokinetics of indinavir is not known.
Also in the **CLINICAL PHARMACOLOGY** section, under *Special Populations*, after the *Race* subsection, add the following subsection:
Pediatric: The optimal dosing regimen for use of indinavir in pediatric patients has not been established. In HIV-infected pediatric patients (age 4–5 years), a dosage regimen of indinavir capsules, 500 mg/m^2 every 8 hours, produced AUC_{0-8hr} of 38,742 ± 24,098 nM•hour (n=34), C_{max} of 17,181 ± 9809 nM (n=34), and trough concentrations of 134 ± 91 nM (n=28). The pharmacokinetic profiles of indinavir in pediatric patients were not comparable to profiles previously observed in HIV-infected adults receiving the recommended dose of 800 mg every 8 hours. The AUC and C_{max} values were slightly higher and the trough concentrations were considerably lower in pediatric patients. Approximately 50% of the pediatric patients had trough values below 100 nM; whereas, approximately 10% of adult patients had trough levels below 100 nM. The relationship between specific trough values and inhibition of HIV replication has not been established.
Also in the **CLINICAL PHARMACOLOGY** section, under *Drugs That Should Not Be Coadministered With CRIXIVAN*, add "(See WARNINGS.)" after the last sentence.
In the **INDICATIONS AND USAGE** section, under *Description of Studies,* in the second paragraph, replace the fifth sentence with the following:
The mean baseline HIV RNA was 4.95 $\log_{10}$ copies/mL (89,035 copies/mL).
Also in the **INDICATIONS AND USAGE** section, replace Figure 1 with the following:
[See figure at top of next column]

Table 1

PK Parameter	% change in PK parameter for females relative to males	90% Confidence Interval
AUC_{0-8h} (nM•hr)	↓13%	(↓32%, ↑12%)
C_{max} (nM)	↓13%	(↓32%, ↑10%)
C_{8h} (nM)	↓22%	(↓47%, ↑15%)

↓ Indicates a decrease in the PK parameter; ↑ indicates an increase in the PK parameter.

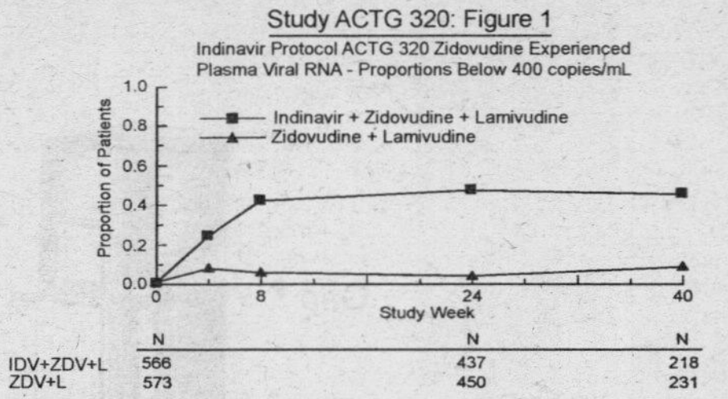
Study ACTG 320: Figure 1
Indinavir Protocol ACTG 320 Zidovudine Experienced
Plasma Viral RNA - Proportions Below 400 copies/mL
Proportion of Patients
1.0
0.8
0.6
0.4
0.2
0.0
Indinavir + Zidovudine + Lamivudine
Zidovudine + Lamivudine
0
8
24
40
Study Week
N N N
IDV+ZDV+L 566 437 218
ZDV+L 573 450 231

In the **WARNINGS** section, under *Nephrolithiasis / Urolithiasis,* in the first paragraph, after the first sentence, add the following:
The frequency of nephrolithiasis is substantially higher in pediatric patients (29%) than in adult patients (9.3%).
In the **PRECAUTIONS** section, replace the *Pediatric Use* subsection with the following:
Pediatric Use
The optimal dosing regimen for use of indinavir in pediatric patients has not been established. A dose of 500 mg/m^2 every eight hours has been studied in uncontrolled studies of 70 children, 3 to 18 years of age. The pharmacokinetic profiles of indinavir at this dose were not comparable to profiles previously observed in adults receiving the recommended dose (see CLINICAL PHARMACOLOGY, *Pediatric*). Although viral suppression was observed in some of the 32 children who were followed on this regimen through 24 weeks, a substantially higher rate of nephrolithiasis was reported when compared to adult historical data (see WARNINGS, *Nephrolithiasis / Urolithiasis*). Physicians considering the use of indinavir in pediatric patients without other protease inhibitor options should be aware of the limited data available in this population and the increased risk of nephrolithiasis.
In the **ADVERSE REACTIONS** section, rename the first subsection "*Clinical Trials in Adults*", and in Table 4, under "Study 028", under the "CRIXIVAN plus Zidovudine" column, within the "Asthenia/fatigue" row, replace "14.2" with "4.2".
In the **DOSAGE AND ADMINISTRATION** section, replace the first paragraph with the following:
The recommended dosage of CRIXIVAN is 800 mg (usually **two** 400-mg capsules) orally every 8 hours.
Also in the **DOSAGE AND ADMINISTRATION** section, in the third paragraph, replace "the patient" with "adults".
In the **HOW SUPPLIED** section, below "CRIXIVAN Capsules are supplied as follows:", set the following:
No. 3755–100 mg capsules: semi-translucent white capsules coded **"CRIXIVAN™ 100 mg"** in green. Available as:
NDC 0006-0570-62 unit of use bottles of 180 (with desiccant).
Also in the **HOW SUPPLIED** section, under "No. 3758", under the first **NDC** item, add the following:
NDC 0006-0573-40 unit-of-use bottles of 120 (with desiccant)
Revisions based on 7979819, issued November 2000.
In the Patient Information, under **How does CRIXIVAN work?**, delete the last paragraph.
Under **How should I take CRIXIVAN?**, in item 6, replace the first sentence with the following:
It is critical to drink plenty of fluids while taking CRIXIVAN. Adults should drink at least six 8-ounce glasses of liquids (preferably water) throughout the day, every day. Your health care provider will give you further instructions on the amount of fluid that you should drink.
Under **What are the possible side effects of CRIXIVAN?**, in the second paragraph, replace the third sentence with the following:
Drinking at least six 8-ounce glasses of liquids (preferably water) each day should help reduce the chances of forming a kidney stone (see **How should I take CRIXIVAN?**).
Revisions based on 9024513, issued October 2000.

ELSPAR® ℞
(asparaginase)

Prescribing information for this product, which appears on pages 1927–1929 of the 2001 PDR, has been revised as follows. Please write "See Supplement A" alongside product heading.

In the boxed **WARNINGS** at the beginning of the Prescribing Information, replace the second paragraph with the following:
Special handling procedures should be followed (see DOSAGE AND ADMINISTRATION, *Special Handling*).
Also in the boxed **WARNINGS**, delete the third paragraph, which begins "The following data...".
In the **PRECAUTIONS** section, under *General,* replace the first paragraph with the following:
This drug may have toxic properties and must be handled and administered with care. ELSPAR may be irritating to eyes, skin, and the upper respiratory tract. Inhalation of dust or aerosols and contact with skin or mucous membranes, especially those of the eyes, must be avoided. (See DOSAGE AND ADMINISTRATION, *Special Handling*.)
In the **DOSAGE AND ADMINISTRATION** section, replace the first paragraph with the following:
This drug may have toxic properties and must be handled and administered with care. Special handling procedures should be reviewed prior to handling and followed diligently during reconstitution and administration. Inhalation of dust or aerosols and contact with skin or mucous membranes, especially those of the eyes, must be avoided. (See DOSAGE AND ADMINISTRATION, *Special Handling*.)
Replace the heading **"DIRECTIONS FOR RECONSTITUTION"** with *"Directions for Reconstitution"* (this will now be a subsection under the **DOSAGE AND ADMINISTRATION** section), and replace the first paragraph currently under **DIRECTIONS FOR RECONSTITUTION** with the following:
This drug may have toxic properties and must be handled and administered with care. Inhalation of dust or aerosols and contact with skin or mucous membranes, especially those of the eyes, must be avoided. Appropriate protective equipment should be worn when handling ELSPAR. (See *Special Handling*.)
In the first paragraph of *Special Handling*, currently under **DIRECTIONS FOR RECONSTITUTION**, in the sentence beginning "Due to the drug's..." add "potential" after "drug's", and in the sentence beginning "Inhalation of dust..." replace "vapors" with "aerosols".
Revisions based on 7407114, issued August 2000.

FLEXERIL* Tablets ℞
(cyclobenzaprine HCl)

This product is marketed by ALZA Pharmaceuticals, a division of ALZA Corporation. Please refer to ALZA Pharmaceuticals for prescribing information.

*Registered trademark of ALZA Corporation.

FOSAMAX® ℞
(ALENDRONATE SODIUM TABLETS)

Prescribing information for this product, which appears on pages 1930–1936 of the 2001 PDR, has been completely revised as follows. Please write "See Supplement A" alongside product heading.

DESCRIPTION
FOSAMAX* (alendronate sodium) is a bisphosphonate that acts as a specific inhibitor of osteoclast-mediated bone resorption. Bisphosphonates are synthetic analogs of pyrophosphate that bind to the hydroxyapatite found in bone.
Alendronate sodium is chemically described as (4-amino-1-hydroxybutylidene) bisphosphonic acid monosodium salt trihydrate.
The empirical formula of alendronate sodium is $C_4H_{12}NNaO_7P_2 \cdot 3H_2O$ and its formula weight is 325.12. The structural formula is:

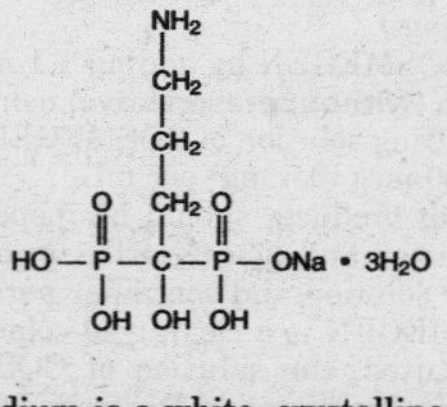
NH2
CH2
CH2
O CH2 O
HO—P—C—P—ONa • 3H2O
OH OH OH

Alendronate sodium is a white, crystalline, nonhygroscopic powder. It is soluble in water, very slightly soluble in alcohol, and practically insoluble in chloroform.
Tablets FOSAMAX for oral administration contain 6.53, 13.05, 45.68, 52.21 or 91.37 mg of alendronate monosodium salt trihydrate, which is the molar equivalent of 5, 10, 35, 40 and 70 mg, respectively, of free acid, and the following inactive ingredients: microcrystalline cellulose, anhydrous lactose, croscarmellose sodium, and magnesium stearate. Tablets FOSAMAX 10 mg also contain carnauba wax.

*Registered trademark of MERCK & CO., Inc.

CLINICAL PHARMACOLOGY
Mechanism of Action
Animal studies have indicated the following mode of action. At the cellular level, alendronate shows preferential localization to sites of bone resorption, specifically under osteoclasts. The osteoclasts adhere normally to the bone surface but lack the ruffled border that is indicative of active resorption of active resorption. Alendronate does not interfere with osteoclast recruitment or attachment, but it does inhibit osteoclast activity. Studies in mice on the localization of radioactive [^{3}H]alendronate in bone showed about 10-fold higher uptake on osteoclast surfaces than on osteoblast surfaces. Bones examined 6 and 49 days after [^{3}H]alendronate administration in rats and mice, respectively, showed that normal bone was formed on top of the alendronate, which was incorporated inside the matrix. While incorporated in bone matrix, alendronate is not pharmacologically active. Thus, alendronate must be continuously administered to suppress osteoclasts on newly formed resorption surfaces. Histomorphometry in baboons and rats showed that alendronate treatment reduces bone turnover (i.e., the number of

sites at which bone is remodeled). In addition, bone formation exceeds bone resorption at these remodeling sites, leading to progressive gains in bone mass.

Pharmacokinetics

Absorption

Relative to an intravenous (IV) reference dose, the mean oral bioavailability of alendronate in women was 0.64% for doses ranging from 5 to 70 mg when administered after an overnight fast and two hours before a standardized breakfast. Oral bioavailability of the 10 mg tablet in men (0.59%) was similar to that in women when administered after an overnight fast and 2 hours before breakfast.

A study examining the effect of timing of a meal on the bioavailability of alendronate was performed in 49 postmenopausal women. Bioavailability was decreased (by approximately 40%) when 10 mg alendronate was administered either 0.5 or 1 hour before a standardized breakfast, when compared to dosing 2 hours before eating. In studies of treatment and prevention of osteoporosis, alendronate was effective when administered at least 30 minutes before breakfast.

Bioavailability was negligible whether alendronate was administered with or up to two hours after a standardized breakfast. Concomitant administration of alendronate with coffee or orange juice reduced bioavailability by approximately 60%.

Distribution

Preclinical studies (in male rats) show that alendronate transiently distributes to soft tissues following 1 mg/kg IV administration but is then rapidly redistributed to bone or excreted in the urine. The mean steady-state volume of distribution, exclusive of bone, is at least 28 L in humans. Concentrations of drug in plasma following therapeutic oral doses are too low (less than 5 ng/mL) for analytical detection. Protein binding in human plasma is approximately 78%.

Metabolism

There is no evidence that alendronate is metabolized in animals or humans.

Excretion

Following a single IV dose of [^{14}C]alendronate, approximately 50% of the radioactivity was excreted in the urine within 72 hours and little or no radioactivity was recovered in the feces. Following a single 10 mg IV dose, the renal clearance of alendronate was 71 mL/min (64, 78; 90% confidence interval [CI]), and systemic clearance did not exceed 200 mL/min. Plasma concentrations fell by more than 95% within 6 hours following IV administration. The terminal half-life in humans is estimated to exceed 10 years, probably reflecting release of alendronate from the skeleton. Based on the above, it is estimated that after 10 years of oral treatment with FOSAMAX (10 mg daily) the amount of alendronate released daily from the skeleton is approximately 25% of that absorbed from the gastrointestinal tract.

Special Populations

Pediatric: Alendronate pharmacokinetics have not been investigated in patients <18 years of age.

Gender: Bioavailability and the fraction of an IV dose excreted in urine were similar in men and women.

Geriatric: Bioavailability and disposition (urinary excretion) were similar in elderly and younger patients. No dosage adjustment is necessary (see DOSAGE AND ADMINISTRATION).

Race: Pharmacokinetic differences due to race have not been studied.

Renal Insufficiency: Preclinical studies show that, in rats with kidney failure, increasing amounts of drug are present in plasma, kidney, spleen, and tibia. In healthy controls, drug that is not deposited in bone is rapidly excreted in the urine. No evidence of saturation of bone uptake was found after 3 weeks dosing with cumulative IV doses of 35 mg/kg in young male rats. Although no clinical information is available, it is likely that, as in animals, elimination of alendronate via the kidney will be reduced in patients with impaired renal function. Therefore, somewhat greater accumulation of alendronate in bone might be expected in patients with impaired renal function.

No dosage adjustment is necessary for patients with mild-to-moderate renal insufficiency (creatinine clearance 35 to 60 mL/min). **FOSAMAX is not recommended for patients with more severe renal insufficiency (creatinine clearance <35 mL/min) due to lack of experience with alendronate in renal failure.**

Hepatic Insufficiency: As there is evidence that alendronate is not metabolized or excreted in the bile, no studies were conducted in patients with hepatic insufficiency. No dosage adjustment is necessary.

Drug Interactions (also see PRECAUTIONS, *Drug Interactions*)

Intravenous ranitidine was shown to double the bioavailability of oral alendronate. The clinical significance of this increased bioavailability and whether similar increases will occur in patients given oral H$_2$-antagonists is unknown.

In healthy subjects, oral prednisone (20 mg three times daily for five days) did not produce a clinically meaningful change in the oral bioavailability of alendronate (a mean increase ranging from 20 to 44%).

Products containing calcium and other multivalent cations are likely to interfere with absorption of alendronate.

Pharmacodynamics

Alendronate is a bisphosphonate that binds to bone hydroxyapatite and specifically inhibits the activity of osteoclasts, the bone-resorbing cells. Alendronate reduces bone resorption with no direct effect on bone formation, although

the latter process is ultimately reduced because bone resorption and formation are coupled during bone turnover.

Osteoporosis in postmenopausal women

Osteoporosis is characterized by low bone mass that leads to an increased risk of fracture. The diagnosis can be confirmed by the finding of low bone mass, evidence of fracture on x-ray, a history of osteoporotic fracture, or height loss or kyphosis, indicative of vertebral (spinal) fracture. Osteoporosis occurs in both males and females but is most common among women following the menopause, when bone turnover increases and the rate of bone resorption exceeds that of bone formation. These changes result in progressive bone loss and lead to osteoporosis in a significant proportion of women over age 50. Fractures, usually of the spine, hip, and wrist, are the common consequences. From age 50 to age 90, the risk of hip fracture in white women increases 50-fold and the risk of vertebral fracture 15- to 30-fold. It is estimated that approximately 40% of 50-year-old women will sustain one or more osteoporosis-related fractures of the spine, hip, or wrist during their remaining lifetimes. Hip fractures, in particular, are associated with substantial morbidity, disability, and mortality.

Daily oral doses of alendronate (5, 20, and 40 mg for six weeks) in postmenopausal women produced biochemical changes indicative of dose-dependent inhibition of bone resorption, including decreases in urinary calcium and urinary markers of bone collagen degradation (such as deoxypyridinoline and cross-linked N-telopeptides of type I collagen). These biochemical changes tended to return toward baseline values as early as 3 weeks following the discontinuation of therapy with alendronate and did not differ from placebo after 7 months.

Long-term treatment of osteoporosis with FOSAMAX 10 mg/day (for up to five years) reduced urinary excretion of markers of bone resorption, deoxypyridinoline and cross-linked N-telopeptides of type I collagen, by approximately 50% and 70%, respectively, to reach levels similar to those seen in healthy premenopausal women. Similar decreases were seen in patients in osteoporosis prevention studies who received FOSAMAX 5 mg/day. The decrease in the rate of bone resorption indicated by these markers was evident as early as one month and at three to six months reached a plateau that was maintained for the entire duration of treatment with FOSAMAX. In osteoporosis treatment studies FOSAMAX 10 mg/day decreased the markers of bone formation, osteocalcin and bone specific alkaline phosphatase by approximately 50%, and total serum alkaline phosphatase, by approximately 25 to 30% to reach a plateau after 6 to 12 months. In osteoporosis prevention studies FOSAMAX 5 mg/day decreased osteocalcin and total serum alkaline phosphatase by approximately 40% and 15%, respectively. Similar reductions in the rate of bone turnover were observed in postmenopausal women during one-year studies with once weekly FOSAMAX 70 mg for the treatment of osteoporosis and once weekly FOSAMAX 35 mg for the prevention of osteoporosis. These data indicate that the rate of bone turnover reached a new steady-state, despite the progressive increase in the total amount of alendronate deposited within bone.

As a result of inhibition of bone resorption, asymptomatic reductions in serum calcium and phosphate concentrations were also observed following treatment with FOSAMAX. In the long-term studies, reductions from baseline in serum calcium (approximately 2%) and phosphate (approximately 4 to 6%) were evident the first month after the initiation of FOSAMAX 10 mg. No further decreases in serum calcium were observed for the five-year duration of treatment, however, serum phosphate returned toward prestudy levels during years three through five. Similar reductions were observed with FOSAMAX 5 mg/day. In one-year studies with once weekly FOSAMAX 35 and 70 mg, similar reductions were observed at 6 and 12 months. The reduction in serum phosphate may reflect not only the positive bone mineral balance due to FOSAMAX but also a decrease in renal phosphate reabsorption.

Osteoporosis in men

Treatment of men with osteoporosis with FOSAMAX 10 mg/day for two years reduced urinary excretion of cross-linked N-telopeptides of type I collagen by approximately 60% and bone-specific alkaline phosphatase by approximately 40%.

Glucocorticoid-induced Osteoporosis

Sustained use of glucocorticoids is commonly associated with development of osteoporosis and resulting fractures (especially vertebral, hip, and rib). It occurs both in males and females of all ages. Osteoporosis occurs as a result of inhibited bone formation and increased bone resorption resulting in net bone loss. Alendronate decreases bone resorption without directly inhibiting bone formation.

In clinical studies of up to two years' duration, FOSAMAX 5 and 10 mg/day reduced cross-linked N-telopeptides of type I collagen (a marker of bone resorption) by approximately 60% and reduced bone-specific alkaline phosphatase and total serum alkaline phosphatase (markers of bone formation) by approximately 15 to 30% and 8 to 18%, respectively. As a result of inhibition of bone resorption, FOSAMAX 5 and 10 mg/day induced asymptomatic decreases in serum calcium (approximately 1 to 2%) and serum phosphate (approximately 1 to 8%).

Paget's disease of bone

Paget's disease of bone is a chronic, focal skeletal disorder characterized by greatly increased and disorderly bone remodeling. Excessive osteoclastic bone resorption is followed by osteoblastic new bone formation, leading to the replacement of the normal bone architecture by disorganized, enlarged, and weakened bone structure.

Clinical manifestations of Paget's disease range from no symptoms to severe morbidity due to bone pain, bone deformity, pathological fractures, and neurological and other complications. Serum alkaline phosphatase, the most frequently used biochemical index of disease activity, provides an objective measure of disease severity and response to therapy.

FOSAMAX decreases the rate of bone resorption directly, which leads to an indirect decrease in bone formation. In clinical trials, FOSAMAX 40 mg once daily for six months produced significant decreases in serum alkaline phosphatase as well as in urinary markers of bone collagen degradation. As a result of the inhibition of bone resorption, FOSAMAX induced generally mild, transient, and asymptomatic decreases in serum calcium and phosphate.

Clinical Studies

Treatment of osteoporosis

Postmenopausal women

Effect of bone mineral density

The efficacy of FOSAMAX 10 mg once daily in postmenopausal women, 44 to 84 years of age, with osteoporosis (lumbar spine bone mineral density [BMD] of at least 2 standard deviations below the premenopausal mean) was demonstrated in four double-blind, placebo-controlled clinical studies of two or three years' duration. These included two three-year, multicenter studies of virtually identical design, one performed in the United States (U.S.) and the other in 15 different countries (Multinational), which enrolled 478 and 516 patients, respectively. The following graph shows the mean increases in BMD of the lumbar spine, femoral neck, and trochanter in patients receiving FOSAMAX 10 mg/day relative to placebo-treated patients at three years for each of these studies.

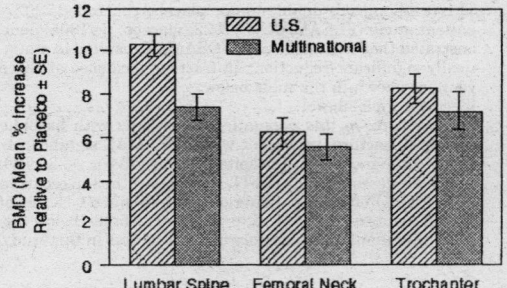

Osteoporosis Treatment Studies in Postmenopausal Women

Increase in BMD
FOSAMAX 10 mg/day at Three Years

At three years significant increases in BMD, relative both to baseline and placebo, were seen at each measurement site in each study in patients who received FOSAMAX 10 mg/day. Total body BMD also increased significantly in each study, suggesting that the increases in bone mass of the spine and hip did not occur at the expense of other skeletal sites. Increases in BMD were evident as early as three months and continued throughout the three years of treatment. (See figures below for lumbar spine results.) In the two-year extension of these studies, treatment of 147 patients with FOSAMAX 10 mg/day resulted in continued increases in BMD at the lumbar spine and trochanter (absolute additional increases between years 3 and 5: lumbar spine, 0.94%; trochanter, 0.88%). BMD at the femoral neck, forearm and total body were maintained. FOSAMAX was similarly effective regardless of age, race, baseline rate of bone turnover, and baseline BMD in the range studied (at least 2 standard deviations below the premenopausal mean). Thus, overall FOSAMAX reverses the loss of bone mineral density, a central factor in the progression of osteoporosis.

[See figure at top of next page]

In patients with postmenopausal osteoporosis treated with FOSAMAX 10 mg/day for one or two years, the effects of treatment withdrawal were assessed. Following discontinuation, there were no further increases in bone mass and the rates of bone loss were similar to those of the placebo groups. These data indicate that continued treatment with FOSAMAX is required to maintain the effect of the drug.

The therapeutic equivalence of once weekly FOSAMAX 70 mg (n=519) and FOSAMAX 10 mg daily (n=370) was demonstrated in a one-year, double-blind, multicenter study of postmenopausal women with osteoporosis. In the primary analysis of completers, the mean increases from baseline in lumbar spine BMD at one year were 5.1% (4.8, 5.4%; 95% CI) in the 70-mg once-weekly group (n=440) and 5.4% (5.0, 5.8%; 95% CI) in the 10-mg daily group (n=330). The two treatment groups were also similar with regard to BMD in-

Continued on next page

Information on the Merck & Co. products listed on these pages is from the full prescribing information in use April 1, 2001.

Fosamax—Cont.

creases at other skeletal sites. The results of the intention-to-treat analysis were consistent with the primary analysis of completers.

Effect on fracture incidence

Data on the effects of FOSAMAX on fracture incidence are derived from three clinical studies: 1) U.S. and Multinational combined: a study of patients with a BMD T-score at or below minus 2.5 with or without a prior vertebral fracture, 2) Three-Year Study of the Fracture Intervention Trial (FIT): a study of patients with at least one baseline vertebral fracture, and 3) Four-Year Study of FIT: a study of patients with low bone mass but without a baseline vertebral fracture.

To assess the effects of FOSAMAX on the incidence of vertebral fractures (detected by digitized radiography; approximately one third of these were clinically symptomatic), the U.S. and Multinational studies were combined in an analysis that compared placebo to the pooled dosage groups of FOSAMAX (5 or 10 mg for three years or 20 mg for two years followed by 5 mg for one year). There was a statistically significant reduction in the proportion of patients treated with FOSAMAX experiencing one or more new vertebral fractures relative to those treated with placebo (3.2% vs. 6.2%; a 48% relative risk reduction). A reduction in the total number of new vertebral fractures (4.2 vs. 11.3 per 100 patients) was also observed. In the pooled analysis, patients who received FOSAMAX had a loss in stature that was statistically significantly less than was observed in those who received placebo (−3.0 mm vs. −4.6 mm).

The Fracture Intervention Trial (FIT) consisted of two studies in postmenopausal women: the Three-Year Study of patients who had at least one baseline radiographic vertebral fracture and the Four-Year Study of patients with low bone mass but without a baseline vertebral fracture. In both studies of FIT, 96% of randomized patients completed the studies (i.e. had a closeout visit at the scheduled end of the study); approximately 80% of patients were still taking study medication upon completion.

Fracture Intervention Trial: Three-Year Study (patients with at least one baseline radiographic vertebral fracture)

This randomized, double-blind, placebo-controlled, 2027-patient study (FOSAMAX, n=1022; placebo, n=1005) demonstrated that treatment with FOSAMAX resulted in statistically significant reductions in fracture incidence at three years as shown in the table below.

[See first table above]

Furthermore, in this population of patients with baseline vertebral fracture, treatment with FOSAMAX significantly reduced the incidence of hospitalizations (25.0% vs. 30.7%). In the Three-Year Study of FIT, fractures of the hip occurred in 22 (2.2%) of 1005 patients on placebo and 11 (1.1%) of 1022 patients on FOSAMAX, p=0.047. The figure below displays the cumulative incidence of hip fractures in this study.

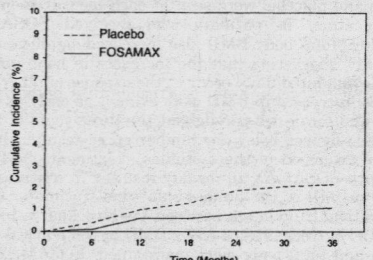

Cumulative Incidence of Hip Fractures in the Three-Year Study of FIT
(patients with radiographic vertebral fracture at baseline)

Fracture Intervention Trial: Four-Year Study (patients with low bone mass but without a baseline radiographic vertebral fracture)

This randomized, double-blind, placebo-controlled, 4432-patient study (FOSAMAX, n=2214; placebo, n=2218) further investigated the reduction in fracture incidence due to FOSAMAX. The intent of the study was to recruit women with osteoporosis, defined as a baseline femoral neck BMD at least two standard deviations below the mean for young adult women. However, due to subsequent revisions to the normative values for femoral neck BMD, 31% of patients were found not to meet this entry criterion and thus this study included both osteoporotic and non-osteoporotic women. The results are shown in the table below for the patients with osteoporosis.

[See second table above]

Fracture results across studies

In the Three-Year Study of FIT, FOSAMAX reduced the percentage of women experiencing at least one new radiographic vertebral fracture from 15.0% to 7.9% (47% relative risk reduction, p<0.001); in the Four-Year Study of FIT, the percentage was reduced from 3.8% to 2.1% (44% relative risk reduction, p=0.001); and in the combined U.S./Multinational studies, from 6.2% to 3.2% (48% relative risk reduction, p=0.034).

FOSAMAX reduced the percentage of women experiencing multiple (two or more) new vertebral fractures from 4.2% to 0.6% (87% relative risk reduction, p<0.001) in the combined U.S./Multinational studies and from 4.9% to 0.5%

(90% relative risk reduction, p<0.001) in the Three-Year Study of FIT. In the Four-Year Study of FIT, FOSAMAX reduced the percentage of osteoporotic women experiencing multiple vertebral fractures from 0.6% to 0.1% (78% relative risk reduction, p=0.035).

Thus, FOSAMAX reduced the incidence of radiographic vertebral fractures in osteoporotic women whether or not they had a previous radiographic vertebral fracture.

FOSAMAX, over a three- or four-year period, was associated with statistically significant reductions in loss of height vs. placebo in patients with and without baseline radiographic vertebral fracture. At the end of the FIT studies the between-treatment group differences were 3.2 mm in the Three-Year Study and 1.3 mm in the Four-Year Study.

Bone histology

Bone histology in 270 postmenopausal patients with osteoporosis treated with FOSAMAX at doses ranging from 1 to 20 mg/day for one, two, or three years revealed normal mineralization and structure, as well as the expected decrease in bone turnover relative to placebo. These data, together with the normal bone histology and increased bone strength observed in rats and baboons exposed to long-term alendronate treatment, support the conclusion that bone formed during therapy with FOSAMAX is of normal quality.

Men

The efficacy of FOSAMAX 10 mg once daily in men with osteoporosis was demonstrated in a two-year, double-blind, placebo-controlled, multicenter study, which enrolled a total

of 241 men between the ages of 31 and 87 (mean, 63). All patients in the trial had either: 1) a BMD T-score ≤−2 at the femoral neck and ≤−1 at the lumbar spine, or 2) a baseline osteoporotic fracture and a BMD T-score ≤−1 at the femoral neck. At two years, the mean increases relative to placebo in BMD in men receiving FOSAMAX 10 mg/day were significant at the following sites: lumbar spine, 5.3%; femoral neck, 2.6%; trochanter, 3.1%; and total body, 1.6%. BMD responses were similar regardless of age (≥65 years vs. <65 years), gonadal function (baseline testosterone <9 ng/dl vs. ≥ 9 ng/dl), or baseline BMD (femoral neck and lumbar spine T-score ≤−2.5 vs. >−2.5). Treatment with FOSAMAX also reduced height loss (FOSAMAX, −0.6 mm vs. placebo, −2.4 mm).

Prevention of osteoporosis in postmenopausal women

Prevention of bone loss was demonstrated in two double-blind, placebo-controlled studies of postmenopausal women 40–60 years of age. One thousand six hundred nine patients (FOSAMAX 5 mg/day; n=498) who were at least six months postmenopausal were entered into a two-year study without regard to their baseline BMD. In the other study, 447 patients (FOSAMAX 5 mg/day; n=88), who were between six months and three years postmenopause, were treated for up to three years. In the placebo-treated patients BMD losses of approximately 1% per year were seen at the spine, hip (femoral neck and trochanter) and total body. In contrast, FOSAMAX 5 mg/day prevented bone loss in the majority of patients and induced significant increases in

---

Osteoporosis Treatment Studies in Postmenopausal Women

Time Course of Effect of FOSAMAX 10 mg/day Versus Placebo: Lumbar Spine BMD Percent Change From Baseline

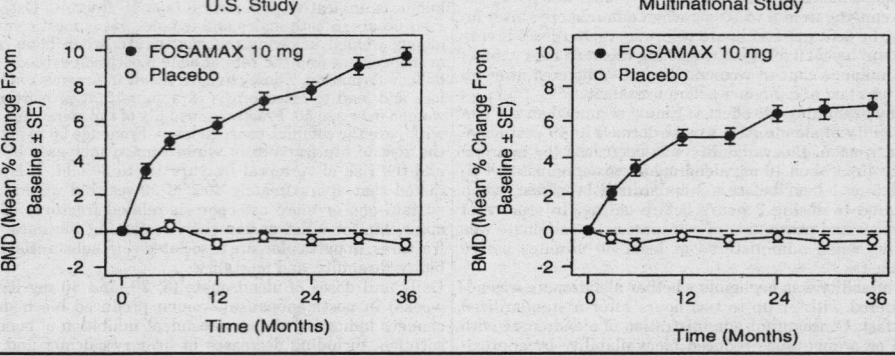

Effect of FOSAMAX on Fracture Incidence in the Three-Year Study of FIT
(patients with vertebral fracture at baseline)

	Percent of Patients		Absolute Reduction in Fracture Incidence	Relative Reduction in Fracture Risk %
	FOSAMAX (n=1022)	Placebo (n=1005)		
Patients with:				
Vertebral fractures (diagnosed by X-ray)[†]				
≥1 new vertebral fracture	7.9	15.0	7.1	47***
≥2 new vertebral fractures	0.5	4.9	4.4	90***
Clinical (symptomatic) fractures				
Any clinical (symptomatic) fracture	13.8	18.1	4.3	26‡
≥1 clinical (symptomatic) vertebral fracture	2.3	5.0	2.7	54**
Hip fracture	1.1	2.2	1.1	51*
Wrist (forearm) fracture	2.2	4.1	1.9	48*

[†]Number evaluable for vertebral fractures: FOSAMAX, n=984; placebo, n=966
*p<0.05, **p<0.01, ***p<0.001, ‡p=0.007

Effect of FOSAMAX on Fracture Incidence in Osteoporotic[†] Patients in the Four-Year Study of FIT
(patients without vertebral fracture at baseline)

	Percent of Patients		Absolute Reduction in Fracture Incidence	Relative Reduction in Fracture Risk %
	FOSAMAX (n=1545)	Placebo (n=1521)		
Patients with:				
Vertebral fractures (diagnosed by X-ray)[††]				
≥1 new vertebral fracture	2.5	4.8	2.3	48***
≥2 new vertebral fractures	0.1	0.6	0.5	78*
Clinical (symptomatic) fractures				
Any clinical (symptomatic) fracture	12.9	16.2	3.3	22**
≥1 clinical (symptomatic) vertebral fracture	1.0	1.6	0.6	41 (NS)[†††]
Hip fracture	1.0	1.4	0.4	29 (NS)[†††]
Wrist (forearm) fracture	3.9	3.8	−0.1	NS[†††]

[†]Baseline femoral neck BMD at least 2 SD below the mean for young adult women
[††]Number evaluable for vertebral fractures: FOSAMAX, n=1426; placebo, n=1428
[†††]Not significant. This study was not powered to detect differences at these sites.
*p=0.035, **p=0.01, ***p<0.001

mean bone mass at each of these sites (see figures below). In addition, FOSAMAX 5 mg/day reduced the rate of bone loss at the forearm by approximately half relative to placebo. FOSAMAX 5 mg/day was similarly effective in this population regardless of age, time since menopause, race and baseline rate of bone turnover.

[See figure at right]

The therapeutic equivalence of once weekly FOSAMAX 35 mg (n=362) and FOSAMAX 5 mg daily (n=361) was demonstrated in a one-year, double-blind, multicenter study of postmenopausal women without osteoporosis. In the primary analysis of completers, the mean increases from baseline in lumbar spine BMD at one year were 2.9% (2.6, 3.2%; 95% CI) in the 35-mg once-weekly group (n=307) and 3.2% (2.9, 3.5%; 95% CI) in the 5-mg daily group (n=298). The two treatment groups were also similar with regard to BMD increases at other skeletal sites. The results of the intention-to-treat analysis were consistent with the primary analysis of completers.

Bone histology
Bone histology was normal in the 28 patients biopsied at the end of three years who received FOSAMAX at doses of up to 10 mg/day.

Concomitant use with estrogen/hormone replacement therapy (HRT)
The effects on BMD of treatment with FOSAMAX 10 mg once daily and conjugated estrogen (0.625 mg/day) either alone or in combination were assessed in a two-year, double-blind, placebo-controlled study of hysterectomized postmenopausal osteoporotic women (n=425). At two years, the increases in lumbar spine BMD from baseline were significantly greater with the combination (8.3%) than with either estrogen or FOSAMAX alone (both 6.0%).
The effects on BMD when FOSAMAX was added to stable doses (for at least one year) of HRT (estrogen ± progestin) were assessed in a one-year, double-blind, placebo-controlled study in postmenopausal osteoporotic women (n=428). The addition of FOSAMAX 10 mg once daily to HRT produced, at one year, significantly greater increases in lumbar spine BMD (3.7%) than HRT alone (1.1%).
In these studies, significant increases or favorable trends in BMD for combined therapy compared with HRT alone were seen at the total hip, femoral neck, and trochanter. No significant effect was seen for total body BMD.
Histomorphometric studies of transiliac biopsies in 92 subjects showed normal bone architecture. Compared to placebo there was a 98% suppression of bone turnover (as assessed by mineralizing surface) after 18 months of combined treatment with FOSAMAX and HRT, 94% on FOSAMAX alone, and 78% on HRT alone. The long-term effects of combined FOSAMAX and HRT on fracture occurrence and fracture healing have not been studied.

Glucocorticoid-induced osteoporosis
The efficacy of FOSAMAX 5 and 10 mg once daily in men and women receiving glucocorticoids (at least 7.5 mg/day of prednisone or equivalent) was demonstrated in two, one-year, double-blind, randomized, placebo-controlled, multicenter studies of virtually identical design, one performed in the United States and the other in 15 different countries (Multinational [which also included FOSAMAX 2.5 mg/day]). These studies enrolled 232 and 328 patients, respectively, between the ages of 17 and 83 with a variety of glucocorticoid-requiring diseases. Patients received supplemental calcium and vitamin D. The following figure shows the mean increases relative to placebo in BMD of the lumbar spine, femoral neck, and trochanter in patients receiving FOSAMAX 5 mg/day for each study.

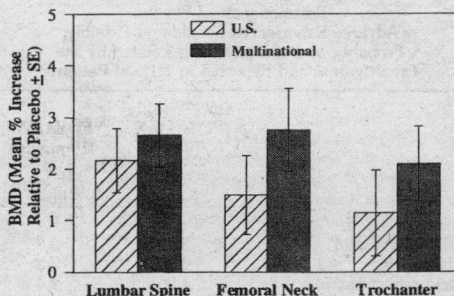

Studies in Glucocorticoid - Treated Patients
Increase in BMD
FOSAMAX 5 mg/day at One Year

After one year, significant increases relative to placebo in BMD were seen in the combined studies at each of these sites in patients who received FOSAMAX 5 mg/day. In the placebo-treated patients, a significant decrease in BMD occurred at the femoral neck (−1.2%), and smaller decreases were seen at the lumbar spine and trochanter. Total body BMD was maintained with FOSAMAX 5 mg/day. The increases in BMD with FOSAMAX 10 mg/day were similar to those with FOSAMAX 5 mg/day in all patients except for postmenopausal women not receiving estrogen therapy. In these women, the increases (relative to placebo) with FOSAMAX 10 mg/day were greater than those with FOSAMAX 5 mg/day at the lumbar spine (4.1% vs. 1.6%) and trochanter (2.8% vs. 1.7%), but not at other sites. FOSAMAX was effective regardless of dose or duration of glucocorticoid use. In addition, FOSAMAX was similarly effective regardless of age (<65 vs. ≥65 years), race (Cauca-

sian vs. other races), gender, underlying disease, baseline BMD, baseline bone turnover, and use with a variety of common medications.
Bone histology was normal in the 49 patients biopsied at the end of one year who received FOSAMAX at doses of up to 10 mg/day.
Of the original 560 patients in these studies, 208 patients who remained on at least 7.5 mg/day of prednisone or equivalent continued into a one-year double-blind extension. After two years of treatment, spine BMD increased by 3.7% and 5.0% relative to placebo with FOSAMAX 5 and 10 mg/day, respectively. Significant increases in BMD (relative to placebo) were also observed at the femoral neck, trochanter, and total body.
After one year, 2.3% of patients treated with FOSAMAX 5 or 10 mg/day (pooled) vs. 3.7% of those treated with placebo experienced a new vertebral fracture (not significant). However, in the population studied for two years, treatment with FOSAMAX (pooled dosage groups: 5 or 10 mg for two years or 2.5 mg for one year followed by 10 mg for one year) significantly reduced the incidence of patients with a new vertebral fracture (FOSAMAX 0.7% vs. placebo 6.8%).

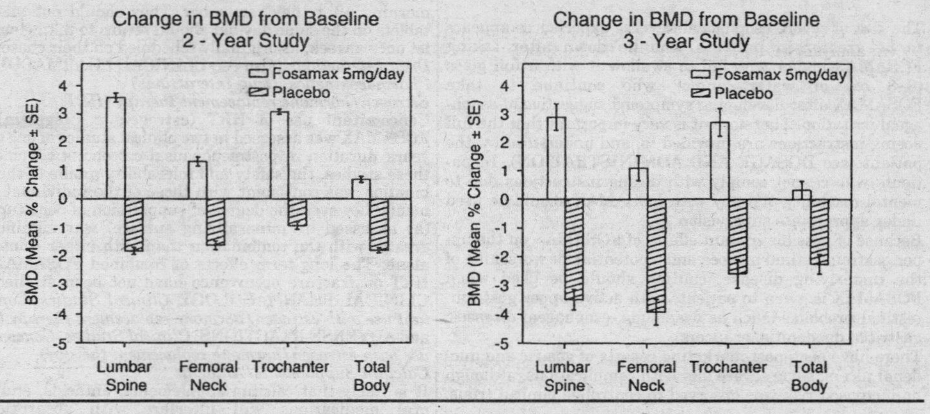

Paget's disease of bone
The efficacy of FOSAMAX 40 mg once daily for six months was demonstrated in two double-blind clinical studies of male and female patients with moderate to severe Paget's disease (alkaline phosphatase at least twice the upper limit of normal): a placebo-controlled multinational study and a U.S. comparative study with etidronate disodium 400 mg/day. The following figure shows the mean percent changes from baseline in serum alkaline phosphatase for up to six months of randomized treatment.

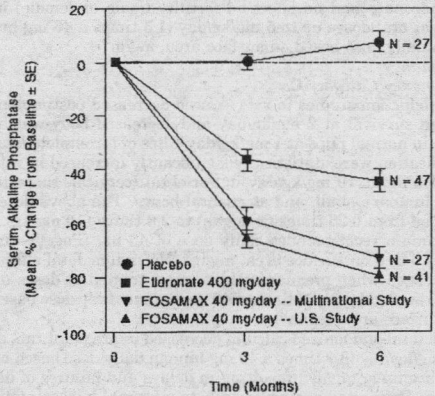

Studies in Paget's Disease of Bone
Effect on Serum Alkaline Phosphatase of FOSAMAX 40 mg/day Versus Placebo or Etidronate 400 mg/day

At six months the suppression in alkaline phosphatase in patients treated with FOSAMAX was significantly greater than that achieved with etidronate and contrasted with the complete lack of response in placebo-treated patients. Response (defined as either normalization of serum alkaline phosphatase or decrease from baseline ≥60%) occurred in approximately 85% of patients treated with FOSAMAX in the combined studies vs. 30% in the etidronate group and 0% in the placebo group. FOSAMAX was similarly effective irrespective of age, gender, race, prior use of other bisphosphonates, or baseline alkaline phosphatase within the range studied (at least twice the upper limit of normal).
Bone histology was evaluated in 33 patients with Paget's disease treated with FOSAMAX 40 mg/day for 6 months. As in patients treated for osteoporosis (see *Clinical Studies, Treatment of osteoporosis in postmenopausal women, Bone histology*), FOSAMAX did not impair mineralization, and the expected decrease in the rate of bone turnover was observed. Normal lamellar bone was produced during treatment with FOSAMAX, even where preexisting bone was wo-

ven and disorganized. Overall, bone histology data support the conclusion that bone formed during treatment with FOSAMAX is of normal quality.

ANIMAL PHARMACOLOGY
The relative inhibitory activities on bone resorption and mineralization of alendronate and etidronate were compared in the Schenk assay, which is based on histological examination of the epiphyses of growing rats. In this assay, the lowest dose of alendronate that interfered with bone mineralization (leading to osteomalacia) was 6000-fold the antiresorptive dose. The corresponding ratio for etidronate was one to one. These data suggest that alendronate administered in therapeutic doses is highly unlikely to induce osteomalacia.

INDICATIONS AND USAGE
FOSAMAX is indicated for:
- Treatment and prevention of osteoporosis in postmenopausal women
  - For the treatment of osteoporosis, FOSAMAX increases bone mass and reduces the incidence of fractures, including those of the hip and spine (vertebral compression fractures). Osteoporosis may be confirmed by the finding of low bone mass (for example, at least 2 standard deviations below the premenopausal mean) or by the presence or history of osteoporotic fracture. (See CLINICAL PHARMACOLOGY, *Pharmacodynamics*.)
  - For the prevention of osteoporosis, FOSAMAX may be considered in postmenopausal women who are at risk of developing osteoporosis and for whom the desired clinical outcome is to maintain bone mass and to reduce the risk of future fracture.
  Bone loss is particularly rapid in postmenopausal women younger than age 60. Risk factors often associated with the development of postmenopausal osteoporosis include early menopause; moderately low bone mass (for example, at least 1 standard deviation below the mean for healthy young adult women); thin body build; Caucasian or Asian race; and family history of osteoporosis. The presence of such risk factors may be important when considering the use of FOSAMAX for prevention of osteoporosis.
- Treatment to increase bone mass in men with osteoporosis
- Treatment of glucocorticoid-induced osteoporosis in men and women receiving glucocorticoids in a daily dosage equivalent to 7.5 mg or greater of prednisone and who have low bone mineral density (see PRECAUTIONS, *Glucocorticoid-induced osteoporosis*). Patients treated with glucocorticoids should receive adequate amounts of calcium and vitamin D.
- Treatment of Paget's disease of bone in men and women
  - Treatment is indicated in patients with Paget's disease of bone having alkaline phosphatase at least two times the upper limit of normal, or those who are symptomatic, or those at risk for future complications from their disease.

CONTRAINDICATIONS
- Abnormalities of the esophagus which delay esophageal emptying such as stricture or achalasia
- Inability to stand or sit upright for at least 30 minutes
- Hypersensitivity to any component of this product
- Hypocalcemia (see PRECAUTIONS, *General*)

WARNINGS
FOSAMAX, like other bisphosphonates, may cause local irritation of the upper gastrointestinal mucosa.
Esophageal adverse experiences, such as esophagitis, esophageal ulcers and esophageal erosions, occasionally with bleeding and rarely followed by esophageal stricture, have been reported in patients receiving treatment with FOSAMAX. In some cases these have been severe and required hospitalization. Physicians should therefore be alert to any signs or symptoms signaling a possible esophageal reaction and patients should be instructed to discontinue FOSAMAX and seek medical attention if they develop dysphagia, odynophagia, retrosternal pain or new or worsening heartburn.

Continued on next page

Information on the Merck & Co. products listed on these pages is from the full prescribing information in use April 1, 2001.

Osteoporosis Prevention Studies in Postmenopausal Women

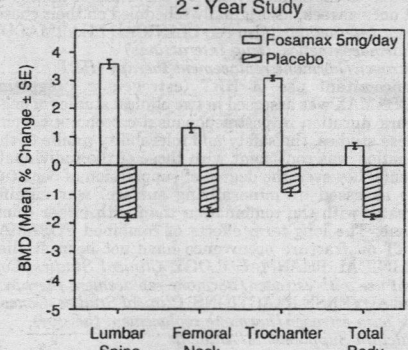

Change in BMD from Baseline
2 - Year Study

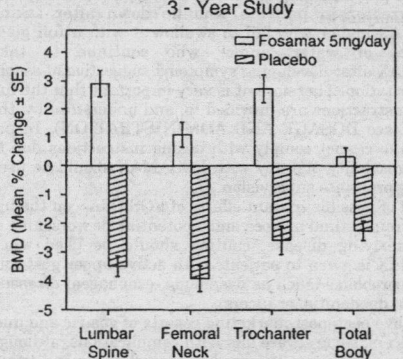

Change in BMD from Baseline
3 - Year Study

Fosamax—Cont.

The risk of severe esophageal adverse experiences appears to be greater in patients who lie down after taking FOSAMAX and/or who fail to swallow it with a full glass (6–8 oz) of water, and/or who continue to take FOSAMAX after developing symptoms suggestive of esophageal irritation. Therefore, it is very important that the full dosing instructions are provided to, and understood by, the patient (see DOSAGE AND ADMINISTRATION). In patients who cannot comply with dosing instructions due to mental disability, therapy with FOSAMAX should be used under appropriate supervision.

Because of possible irritant effects of FOSAMAX on the upper gastrointestinal mucosa and a potential for worsening of the underlying disease, caution should be used when FOSAMAX is given to patients with active upper gastrointestinal problems (such as dysphagia, esophageal diseases, gastritis, duodenitis, or ulcers).

There have been post-marketing reports of gastric and duodenal ulcers, some severe and with complications, although no increased risk was observed in controlled clinical trials.

PRECAUTIONS

General

Causes of osteoporosis other than estrogen deficiency, aging, and glucocorticoid use should be considered.

Hypocalcemia must be corrected before initiating therapy with FOSAMAX (see CONTRAINDICATIONS). Other disturbances of mineral metabolism (such as vitamin D deficiency) should also be effectively treated. Presumably due to the effects of FOSAMAX on increasing bone mineral, small asymptomatic decreases in serum calcium and phosphate may occur, especially in patients with Paget's disease, in whom the pretreatment rate of bone turnover may be greatly elevated and in patients receiving glucocorticoids, in whom calcium absorption may be decreased.

Ensuring adequate calcium and vitamin D intake is especially important in patients with Paget's disease of bone and in patients receiving glucocorticoids.

Renal insufficiency

FOSAMAX is not recommended for patients with renal insufficiency (creatinine clearance <35 mL/min). (See DOSAGE AND ADMINISTRATION.)

Glucocorticoid-induced osteoporosis

The risk versus benefit of FOSAMAX for treatment at daily dosages of glucocorticoids less than 7.5 mg of prednisone or equivalent has not been established (see INDICATIONS AND USAGE). Before initiating treatment, the hormonal status of both men and women should be ascertained and appropriate replacement considered.

A bone mineral density measurement should be made at the initiation of therapy and repeated after 6 to 12 months of combined FOSAMAX and glucocorticoid treatment.

The efficacy of FOSAMAX for the treatment of glucocorticoid-induced osteoporosis has been shown in patients with a median bone mineral density which was 1.2 standard deviations below the mean for healthy young adults.

The efficacy of FOSAMAX has been established in studies of two years' duration. The greatest increase in bone mineral density occurred in the first year with maintenance or smaller gains during the second year. Efficacy of FOSAMAX beyond two years has not been studied.

The efficacy of FOSAMAX in respect to fracture prevention has been demonstrated for vertebral fractures. However, this finding was based on very few fractures that occurred primarily in postmenopausal women. The efficacy for prevention of non-vertebral fractures has not been demonstrated.

Information for Patients

General

Physicians should instruct their patients to read the patient package insert before starting therapy with FOSAMAX and to reread it each time the prescription is renewed.

Patients should be instructed to take supplemental calcium and vitamin D, if daily dietary intake is inadequate. Weight-bearing exercise should be considered along with the modification of certain behavioral factors, such as cigarette smoking and/or excessive alcohol consumption, if these factors exist.

Dosing Instructions

Patients should be instructed that the expected benefits of FOSAMAX may only be obtained when each tablet is swallowed with plain water the first thing upon arising for the day at least 30 minutes before the first food, beverage, or medication of the day. Even dosing with orange juice or coffee has been shown to markedly reduce the absorption of FOSAMAX (see CLINICAL PHARMACOLOGY, *Pharmacokinetics, Absorption*).

To facilitate delivery to the stomach and thus reduce the potential for esophageal irritation patients should be instructed to swallow FOSAMAX with a full glass of water (6–8 oz) and not to lie down for at least 30 minutes and until after their first food of the day. Patients should not chew or suck on the tablet because of a potential for oropharyngeal ulceration. Patients should be specifically instructed not to take FOSAMAX at bedtime or before arising for the day. Patients should be informed that failure to follow these instructions may increase their risk of esophageal problems. Patients should be instructed that if they develop symptoms of esophageal disease (such as difficulty or pain upon swallowing, retrosternal pain or new or worsening heartburn) they should stop taking FOSAMAX and consult their physician.

Patients should be instructed that if they miss a dose of once weekly FOSAMAX, they should take one tablet on the morning after they remember. They should not take two tablets on the same day but should return to taking one tablet once a week, as originally scheduled on their chosen day.

Drug Interactions (also see CLINICAL PHARMACOLOGY, *Pharmacokinetics, Drug Interactions*)

Estrogen/hormone replacement therapy (HRT)

Concomitant use of HRT (estrogen ± progestin) and FOSAMAX was assessed in two clinical studies of one or two years' duration in postmenopausal osteoporotic women. In these studies, the safety and tolerability profile of the combination was consistent with those of the individual treatments; however, the degree of suppression of bone turnover (as assessed by mineralizing surface) was significantly greater with the combination than with either component alone. The long-term effects of combined FOSAMAX and HRT on fracture occurrence have not been studied (see CLINICAL PHARMACOLOGY, *Clinical Studies, Concomitant use with estrogen/hormone replacement therapy (HRT)* and ADVERSE REACTIONS, *Clinical Studies, Concomitant use with estrogen/hormone replacement therapy*).

Calcium Supplements/Antacids

It is likely that calcium supplements, antacids, and some oral medications will interfere with absorption of FOSAMAX. Therefore, patients must wait at least one-half hour after taking FOSAMAX before taking any other oral medications.

Aspirin

In clinical studies, the incidence of upper gastrointestinal adverse events was increased in patients receiving concomitant therapy with daily doses of FOSAMAX greater than 10 mg and aspirin-containing products.

Nonsteroidal Anti-inflammatory Drugs (NSAIDs)

FOSAMAX may be administered to patients taking NSAIDs. In a 3-year, controlled, clinical study (n=2027) during which a majority of patients received concomitant NSAIDs, the incidence of upper gastrointestinal adverse events was similar in patients taking FOSAMAX 5 or 10 mg/day compared to those taking placebo. However, since NSAID use is associated with gastrointestinal irritation, caution should be used during concomitant use with FOSAMAX.

Carcinogenesis, Mutagenesis, Impairment of Fertility

Harderian gland (a retro-orbital gland not present in humans) adenomas were increased in high-dose female mice (p=0.003) in a 92-week oral carcinogenicity study at doses of alendronate of 1, 3, and 10 mg/kg/day (males) or 1, 2, and 5 mg/kg/day (females). These doses are equivalent to 0.12 to 1.2 times a maximum recommended daily dose of 40 mg (Paget's disease) based on surface area, mg/m^2. The relevance of this finding to humans is unknown.

Parafollicular cell (thyroid) adenomas were increased in high-dose male rats (p=0.003) in a 2-year oral carcinogenicity study at doses of 1 and 3.75 mg/kg body weight. These doses are equivalent to 0.26 and 1 times a 40 mg human daily dose based on surface area, mg/m^2. The relevance of this finding to humans is unknown.

Alendronate was not genotoxic in the *in vitro* microbial mutagenesis assay with and without metabolic activation, in an *in vitro* mammalian cell mutagenesis assay, in an *in vitro* alkaline elution assay in rat hepatocytes, and in an *in vivo* chromosomal aberration assay in mice. In an *in vitro* chromosomal aberration assay in Chinese hamster ovary cells, however, alendronate gave equivocal results.

Alendronate had no effect on fertility (male or female) in rats at oral doses up to 5 mg/kg/day (1.3 times a 40 mg human daily dose based on surface area, mg/m^2).

Pregnancy

Pregnancy Category C:

Reproduction studies in rats showed decreased postimplantation survival at 2 mg/kg/day and decreased body weight gain in normal pups at 1 mg/kg/day. Sites of incomplete fetal ossification were statistically significantly increased in rats beginning at 10 mg/kg/day in vertebral (cervical, thoracic, and lumbar), skull, and sternebral bones. The above doses ranged from 0.26 times (1 mg/kg) to 2.6 times (10 mg/kg) a maximum recommended daily dose of 40 mg (Paget's disease) based on surface area, mg/m^2. No similar fetal effects were seen when pregnant rabbits were treated at doses up to 35 mg/kg/day (10.3 times a 40 mg human daily dose based on surface area, mg/m^2).

Both total and ionized calcium decreased in pregnant rats at 15 mg/kg/day (3.9 times a 40 mg human daily dose based on surface area, mg/m^2) resulting in delays and failures of delivery. Protracted parturition due to maternal hypocalcemia occurred in rats at doses as low as 0.5 mg/kg/day (0.13 times a 40 mg human daily dose based on surface area, mg/m^2) when rats were treated from before mating through gestation. Maternotoxicity (late pregnancy deaths) occurred in the female rats treated with 15 mg/kg/day for varying periods of time ranging from treatment only during pre-mating to treatment only during early, middle, or late gestation; these deaths were lessened but not eliminated by cessation of treatment. Calcium supplementation either in the drinking water or by minipump could not ameliorate the hypocalcemia or prevent maternal and neonatal deaths due to delays in delivery; calcium supplementation IV prevented maternal, but not fetal deaths.

There are no studies in pregnant women. FOSAMAX should be used during pregnancy only if the potential benefit justifies the potential risk to the mother and fetus.

Nursing Mothers

It is not known whether alendronate is excreted in human milk. Because many drugs are excreted in human milk, caution should be exercised when FOSAMAX is administered to nursing women.

Pediatric Use

Safety and effectiveness in pediatric patients have not been established.

Use in the Elderly

Of the patients receiving FOSAMAX in the United States and Multinational osteoporosis treatment studies in women, the osteoporosis study in men, glucocorticoid-induced osteoporosis studies, and Paget's disease studies (see CLINICAL PHARMACOLOGY, *Clinical Studies*), 45%, 50%, 37%, and 70%, respectively, were 65 years of age or over. No overall differences in efficacy or safety were observed between these patients and younger patients but greater sensitivity of some older individuals cannot be ruled out.

ADVERSE REACTIONS

Clinical Studies

In clinical studies of up to five years in duration adverse experiences associated with FOSAMAX usually were mild, and generally did not require discontinuation of therapy.

FOSAMAX has been evaluated for safety in approximately 8000 postmenopausal women in clinical studies.

Treatment of osteoporosis

Postmenopausal women

In two identically designed, three-year, placebo-controlled, double-blind, multicenter studies (United States and Multinational; n=994), discontinuation of therapy due to any clinical adverse experience occurred in 4.1% of 196 patients treated with FOSAMAX 10 mg/day and 6.0% of 397 patients treated with placebo. In the Fracture Intervention Trial (n=6459), discontinuation of therapy due to any clinical adverse experience occurred in 9.1% of 3236 patients treated with FOSAMAX 5 mg/day for 2 years and 10 mg/day for either one or two additional years and 10.1% of 3223 patients treated with placebo. Discontinuations due to upper gastrointestinal adverse experiences were: FOSAMAX, 3.2%; placebo, 2.7%. In these study populations, 49–54% had a history of gastrointestinal disorders at baseline and 54–89% used nonsteroidal anti-inflammatory drugs or aspirin at some time during the studies. Adverse experiences from these studies considered by the investigators as possibly, probably, or definitely drug related in ≥1% of patients treated with either FOSAMAX or placebo are presented in the following table.

[See first table at top of next page]

Rarely, rash and erythema have occurred.

One patient treated with FOSAMAX (10 mg/day), who had a history of peptic ulcer disease and gastrectomy and who was taking concomitant aspirin developed an anastomotic ulcer with mild hemorrhage, which was considered drug related. Aspirin and FOSAMAX were discontinued and the patient recovered.

The adverse experience profile was similar for the 401 patients treated with either 5 or 20 mg doses of FOSAMAX in the United States and Multinational studies.

The adverse experience profile for the 296 patients who received continued treatment with either 5 or 10 mg doses of FOSAMAX in the two-year extension of these studies (treatment years 4 and 5) was similar to that observed during the three-year placebo-controlled period. During the extension period, of the 151 patients treated with FOSAMAX 10 mg/day, the proportion of patients who discontinued therapy due to any clinical adverse experience was similar to that during the first three years of the study.

In a one-year, double-blind multicenter study, the overall safety and tolerability profiles of once weekly FOSAMAX 70 mg and FOSAMAX 10 mg daily were similar. The adverse experiences considered by the investigators as possibly, probably, or definitely drug related in ≥1% of patients in either treatment group are presented in the following table.

Osteoporosis Treatment Studies in Postmenopausal Women
Adverse Experiences Considered Possibly, Probably, or Definitely Drug Related by the Investigators and Reported in ≥1% of Patients

	Once Weekly FOSAMAX 70 mg % (n = 519)	FOSAMAX 10 mg/day % (n = 370)
Gastrointestinal		
abdominal pain	3.7	3.0
dyspepsia	2.7	2.2
acid regurgitation	1.9	2.4
nausea	1.9	2.4
abdominal distension	1.0	1.4
constipation	0.8	1.6
flatulence	0.4	1.6
gastritis	0.2	1.1
gastric ulcer	0.0	1.1
Musculoskeletal		
musculoskeletal (bone, muscle, joint) pain	2.9	3.2
muscle cramp	0.2	1.1

Men

In a two-year, placebo-controlled, double-blind, multicenter study, discontinuation of therapy due to any clinical adverse experience occurred in 2.7% of men treated with FOSAMAX 10 mg/day and 10.5% of men treated with placebo. The adverse experiences considered by the investigators as possibly, probably, or definitely drug related in ≥2% of patients treated with either FOSAMAX 10 mg/day or placebo are presented in the following table.

Osteoporosis Study in Men
Adverse Experiences Considered Possibly, Probably, or Definitely Drug Related by the Investigators and Reported in ≥2% of Patients

	FOSAMAX 10 mg/day % (n = 146)	Placebo % (n = 95)
Gastrointestinal		
acid regurgitation	4.1	3.2
flatulence	4.1	1.1
dyspepsia	3.4	0.0
abdominal pain	2.1	1.1
nausea	2.1	0.0

Prevention of osteoporosis in postmenopausal women
The safety of FOSAMAX 5 mg/day in postmenopausal women 40–60 years of age has been evaluated in three double-blind, placebo-controlled studies involving over 1,400 patients randomized to receive FOSAMAX for either two or three years. In these studies the overall safety profiles of FOSAMAX 5 mg/day and placebo were similar. Discontinuation of therapy due to any clinical adverse experience occurred in 7.5% of 642 patients treated with FOSAMAX 5 mg/day and 5.7% of 648 patients treated with placebo.
In a one-year, double-blind multicenter study, the overall safety and tolerability profiles of once weekly FOSAMAX 35 mg and FOSAMAX 5 mg daily were similar.
The adverse experiences from these studies considered by the investigators as possibly, probably, or definitely drug related in ≥1% of patients treated with either once weekly FOSAMAX 35 mg, FOSAMAX 5 mg/day or placebo are presented in the following table.
[See second table to right]
Concomitant use with estrogen/hormone replacement therapy
In two studies (of one and two years' duration) of postmenopausal osteoporotic women (total: n=853), the safety and tolerability profile of combined treatment with FOSAMAX 10 mg once daily and estrogen ± progestin (n=354) was consistent with those of the individual treatments.
Treatment of glucocorticoid-induced osteoporosis
In two, one-year, placebo-controlled, double-blind, multicenter studies in patients receiving glucocorticoid treatment, the overall safety and tolerability profiles of FOSAMAX 5 and 10 mg/day were generally similar to that of placebo. The adverse experiences considered by the investigators as possibly, probably, or definitely drug related in ≥1% of patients treated with either FOSAMAX 5 or 10 mg/day or placebo are presented in the following table.
[See third table to right]
The overall safety and tolerability profile in the glucocorticoid-induced osteoporosis population that continued therapy for the second year of the studies (FOSAMAX: n=147) was consistent with that observed in the first year.
Paget's disease of bone
In clinical studies (osteoporosis and Paget's disease), adverse experiences reported in 175 patients taking FOSAMAX 40 mg/day for 3–12 months were similar to those in postmenopausal women treated with FOSAMAX 10 mg/day. However, there was an apparent increased incidence of upper gastrointestinal adverse experiences in patients taking FOSAMAX 40 mg/day (17.7% FOSAMAX vs. 10.2% placebo). One case of esophagitis and two cases of gastritis resulted in discontinuation of treatment.
Additionally, musculoskeletal (bone, muscle or joint) pain, which has been described in patients with Paget's disease treated with other bisphosphonates, was considered by the investigators as possibly, probably, or definitely drug related in approximately 6% of patients treated with FOSAMAX 40 mg/day versus approximately 1% of patients treated with placebo, but rarely resulted in discontinuation of therapy. Discontinuation of therapy due to any clinical adverse experience occurred in 6.4% of patients with Paget's disease treated with FOSAMAX 40 mg/day and 2.4% of patients treated with placebo.
Laboratory Test Findings
In double-blind, multicenter, controlled studies, asymptomatic, mild, and transient decreases in serum calcium and phosphate were observed in approximately 18% and 10%, respectively, of patients taking FOSAMAX versus approximately 12% and 3% of those taking placebo. However, the incidences of decreases in serum calcium to <8.0 mg/dL (2.0 mM) and serum phosphate to ≤2.0 mg/dL (0.65 mM) were similar in both treatment groups.
Post-Marketing Experience
The following adverse reactions have been reported in postmarketing use:
Body as a Whole: hypersensitivity reactions including urticaria and rarely angioedema.
Gastrointestinal: esophagitis, esophageal erosions, esophageal ulcers, rarely esophageal stricture, and oropharyngeal ulceration. Gastric or duodenal ulcers, some severe and with complications have also been reported (see WARNINGS, PRECAUTIONS, *Information for Patients*, and DOSAGE AND ADMINISTRATION).
Skin: rash (occasionally with photosensitivity).
Special Senses: rarely uveitis.

Osteoporosis Treatment Studies in Postmenopausal Women
Adverse Experiences Considered Possibly, Probably, or Definitely Drug Related by the Investigators and Reported in ≥1% of Patients

	United States/Multinational Studies		Fracture Intervention Trial	
	FOSAMAX* % (n = 196)	Placebo % (n = 397)	FOSAMAX** % (n = 3236)	Placebo % (n = 3223)
Gastrointestinal				
abdominal pain	6.6	4.8	1.5	1.5
nausea	3.6	4.0	1.1	1.5
dyspepsia	3.6	3.5	1.1	1.2
constipation	3.1	1.8	0.0	0.2
diarrhea	3.1	1.8	0.6	0.3
flatulence	2.6	0.5	0.2	0.3
acid regurgitation	2.0	4.3	1.1	0.9
esophageal ulcer	1.5	0.0	0.1	0.1
vomiting	1.0	1.5	0.2	0.3
dysphagia	1.0	0.0	0.1	0.1
abdominal distention	1.0	0.8	0.0	0.0
gastritis	0.5	1.3	0.6	0.7
Musculoskeletal				
musculoskeletal (bone, muscle or joint) pain	4.1	2.5	0.4	0.3
muscle cramp	0.0	1.0	0.2	0.1
Nervous System/Psychiatric				
headache	2.6	1.5	0.2	0.2
dizziness	0.0	1.0	0.0	0.1
Special Senses				
taste perversion	0.5	1.0	0.1	0.0

*10 mg/day for three years
**5 mg/day for 2 years and 10 mg/day for either 1 or 2 additional years

Osteoporosis Prevention Studies in Postmenopausal Women
Adverse Experiences Considered Possibly, Probably, or Definitely Drug Related by the Investigators and Reported in ≥1% of Patients

	Two/Three-Year Studies		One-Year Study	
	FOSAMAX 5 mg/day % (n = 642)	Placebo % (n = 648)	FOSAMAX 5 mg/day % (n = 361)	Once Weekly FOSAMAX 35 mg % (n = 362)
Gastrointestinal				
dyspepsia	1.9	1.4	2.2	1.7
abdominal pain	1.7	3.4	4.2	2.2
acid regurgitation	1.4	2.5	4.2	4.7
nausea	1.4	1.4	2.5	1.4
diarrhea	1.1	1.7	1.1	0.6
constipation	0.9	0.5	1.7	0.3
abdominal distention	0.2	0.3	1.4	1.1
Musculoskeletal				
musculoskeletal (bone, muscle or joint) pain	0.8	0.9	1.9	2.2

One-Year Studies in Glucocorticoid-Treated Patients
Adverse Experiences Considered Possibly, Probably, or Definitely Drug Related by the Investigators and Reported in ≥1% of Patients

	FOSAMAX 10 mg/day % (n = 157)	FOSAMAX 5 mg/day % (n = 161)	Placebo % (n = 159)
Gastrointestinal			
abdominal pain	3.2	1.9	0.0
acid regurgitation	2.5	1.9	1.3
constipation	1.3	0.6	0.0
melena	1.3	0.0	0.0
nausea	0.6	1.2	0.6
diarrhea	0.0	0.0	1.3
Nervous System/Psychiatric			
headache	0.6	0.0	1.3

OVERDOSAGE

Significant lethality after single oral doses was seen in female rats and mice at 552 mg/kg (3256 mg/m^2) and 966 mg/kg (2898 mg/m^2), respectively. In males, these values were slightly higher, 626 and 1280 mg/kg, respectively. There was no lethality in dogs at oral doses up to 200 mg/kg (4000 mg/m^2).
No specific information is available on the treatment of overdosage with FOSAMAX. Hypocalcemia, hypophosphatemia, and upper gastrointestinal adverse events, such as upset stomach, heartburn, esophagitis, gastritis, or ulcer, may result from oral overdosage. Milk or antacids should be given to bind alendronate. Due to the risk of esophageal irritation, vomiting should not be induced and the patient should remain fully upright.
Dialysis would not be beneficial.

DOSAGE AND ADMINISTRATION

FOSAMAX must be taken *at least* one-half hour before the first food, beverage, or medication of the day with plain water only (see PRECAUTIONS, *Information for Patients*). Other beverages (including mineral water), food, and some medications are likely to reduce the absorption of FOSAMAX (see PRECAUTIONS, *Drug Interactions*). Waiting less than 30 minutes, or taking FOSAMAX with food, beverages (other than plain water) or other medications will lessen the effect of FOSAMAX by decreasing its absorption into the body.
To facilitate delivery to the stomach and thus reduce the potential for esophageal irritation, FOSAMAX should only be swallowed upon arising for the day with a full glass of water (6–8 oz) and patients should not lie down for at least 30 minutes and until after their first food of the day. FOSAMAX should not be taken at bedtime or before arising for the day. Failure to follow these instructions may increase the risk of esophageal adverse experiences (see WARNINGS, PRECAUTIONS, *Information for Patients*).
Patients should receive supplemental calcium and vitamin D, if dietary intake is inadequate (see PRECAUTIONS, *General*).
No dosage adjustment is necessary for the elderly or for patients with mild-to-moderate renal insufficiency (creatinine

Continued on next page

Information on the Merck & Co. products listed on these pages is from the full prescribing information in use April 1, 2001.

Fosamax—Cont.

clearance 35 to 60 mL/min). FOSAMAX is not recommended for patients with more severe renal insufficiency (creatinine clearance <35 mL/min) due to lack of experience.

Treatment of osteoporosis in postmenopausal women (see INDICATIONS AND USAGE)

The recommended dosage is:
- one 70 mg tablet once weekly

or
- one 10 mg tablet once daily

Treatment to increase bone mass in men with osteoporosis

The recommended dosage is one 10 mg tablet once daily.

Prevention of osteoporosis in postmenopausal women (see INDICATIONS AND USAGE)

The recommended dosage is:
- one 35 mg tablet once weekly

or
- one 5 mg tablet once daily

The safety of treatment and prevention of osteoporosis with FOSAMAX has been studied for up to 7 years.

Treatment of glucocorticoid-induced osteoporosis in men and women

The recommended dosage is one 5 mg tablet once daily, except for postmenopausal women not receiving estrogen, for whom the recommended dosage is one 10 mg tablet once daily.

Paget's disease of bone in men and women

The recommended treatment regimen is 40 mg once a day for six months.

Retreatment of Paget's disease

In clinical studies in which patients were followed every six months, relapses during the 12 months following therapy occurred in 9% (3 out of 32) of patients who responded to treatment with FOSAMAX. Specific retreatment data are not available, although responses to FOSAMAX were similar in patients who had received prior bisphosphonate therapy and those who had not. Retreatment with FOSAMAX may be considered, following a six-month post-treatment evaluation period in patients who have relapsed, based on increases in serum alkaline phosphatase, which should be measured periodically. Retreatment may also be considered in those who failed to normalize their serum alkaline phosphatase.

HOW SUPPLIED

No. 3759—Tablets FOSAMAX, 5 mg, are white, round, uncoated tablets with an outline of a bone image on one side and code MRK 925 on the other. They are supplied as follows:

NDC 0006-0925-31 unit-of-use bottles of 30.
NDC 0006-0925-58 unit-of-use bottles of 100.

No. 3797—Tablets FOSAMAX, 10 mg, are white, oval, wax-polished tablets with code MRK on one side and 936 on the other. They are supplied as follows:

NDC 0006-0936-31 unit-of-use bottles of 30
NDC 0006-0936-58 unit-of-use bottles of 100
NDC 0006-0936-28 unit dose packages of 100
NDC 0006-0936-82 bottles of 1,000
NDC 0006-0936-72 carton of 25 UNIBLISTER™ cards of 31 tablets each.

No. 3813—Tablets FOSAMAX, 35 mg, are white, oval, uncoated tablets with code 77 on one side and a bone image on the other. They are supplied as follows:

NDC 0006-0077-44 unit-of-use blister package of 4
NDC 0006-0077-21 unit dose packages of 20.

No. 3592—Tablets FOSAMAX, 40 mg, are white, triangular-shaped, uncoated tablets with code MRK 212 on one side and FOSAMAX on the other. They are supplied as follows:
NDC 0006-0212-31 unit-of-use bottles of 30.

No. 3814—Tablets FOSAMAX, 70 mg, are white, oval, uncoated tablets with code 31 on one side and an outline of a bone image on the other. They are supplied as follows:

NDC 0006-0031-44 unit-of-use blister package of 4
NDC 0006-0031-21 unit dose packages of 20.

Storage

Store in a well-closed container at room temperature, 15–30°C (59–86°F).

7957017   Issued October 2000
COPYRIGHT ©MERCK & CO., Inc., 1995, 1997, 2000
All rights reserved.

Patient Information about

FOSAMAX® (FOSS-ah-max) for Osteoporosis

Generic name: alendronate sodium (a-LEN-dro-nate)

Please read this information before you start taking FOSAMAX*. Also, read the leaflet each time you renew your prescription, just in case anything has changed. Remember, this leaflet does not take the place of careful discussions with your doctor. You and your doctor should discuss FOSAMAX when you start taking your medication and at regular checkups.

* Registered trademark of MERCK & CO., Inc.

How should I take FOSAMAX?

These are the important things you must do to help make sure you will benefit from FOSAMAX:

1. **After getting up for the day and before taking your first food, beverage, or other medication, swallow your FOSAMAX tablet with a full glass (6–8 oz) of** <u>plain water</u> **only.**

   Not mineral water
   Not coffee or tea
   Not juice

   Do not chew or suck on a tablet of FOSAMAX.

2. **After swallowing your FOSAMAX tablet do not lie down—stay fully upright (sitting, standing or walking) for at least 30 minutes** <u>and</u> **do not lie down until after your first food of the day.** This will help the FOSAMAX tablet reach your stomach quickly and help reduce the potential for irritation of your esophagus (the tube that connects your mouth with your stomach).

3. **After swallowing your FOSAMAX tablet, wait at least 30 minutes before taking your first food, beverage, or other medication of the day,** including antacids, calcium supplements and vitamins. FOSAMAX is effective only if taken when your stomach is empty.

4. **Do not take FOSAMAX at bedtime or before getting up for the day.**

5. **If you have difficulty or pain upon swallowing, chest pain, or new or worsening heartburn, stop taking FOSAMAX and call your doctor.**

6. Take one FOSAMAX tablet once a day, every day.

7. It is important that you continue taking FOSAMAX for as long as your doctor prescribes it. FOSAMAX can treat your osteoporosis or help you from getting osteoporosis only if you continue to take it.

8. If you miss a dose do not take it later in the day. Continue your usual schedule of 1 tablet once a day the next morning.

What is FOSAMAX?

FOSAMAX is for:

- **The treatment or prevention of osteoporosis (thinning of bone) in women after menopause. It reduces the chance of having a hip or spinal fracture.**
- **Treatment to increase bone mass in men with osteoporosis.**
- **The treatment of osteoporosis in both men and women receiving corticosteroid medications (for example, prednisone).**

You will find more information about osteoporosis at the end of this leaflet.

How does FOSAMAX work?

FOSAMAX works by:
- Reducing the activity of the cells that cause bone loss
- Decreasing the faster rate of bone loss that occurs after menopause or with use of corticosteroid medications
- Increasing the amount of bone in most patients

These effects are seen as soon as three months after therapy with FOSAMAX has begun. These effects continue as long as you keep taking FOSAMAX. The density of bone is maintained or increased and the bone is less likely to fracture.

Who should not take FOSAMAX?

Patients with:
- Certain disorders of the esophagus (the tube that connects your mouth with your stomach)
- Inability to stand or sit upright for at least 30 minutes
- Low levels of calcium in their blood
- Severe kidney disease
- Allergy to FOSAMAX

Patients who are:
- Pregnant or Nursing
  If you are pregnant or nursing, you should not be taking FOSAMAX. Talk to your doctor.

What other medical problems should I discuss with my doctor?

Talk to your doctor about any:
- Problems with swallowing
- Stomach or digestive problems
- Other medical problems you have or have had in the past

What are the possible side effects of FOSAMAX?

Some patients may develop severe digestive reactions including irritation, inflammation or ulceration (occasionally with bleeding) of the esophagus (the tube that connects your mouth with your stomach). These reactions can cause chest pain, heartburn or difficulty or pain upon swallowing. This may occur especially if patients do not drink a full glass of water with FOSAMAX and/or if they lie down in less than 30 minutes or before their first food of the day. Esophageal reactions may worsen if patients continue to take FOSAMAX after developing symptoms suggesting irritation of the esophagus.

Like all prescription drugs, FOSAMAX may cause side effects. Side effects usually have been mild. They generally have not caused patients to stop taking FOSAMAX. Some patients treated with FOSAMAX experienced abdominal (stomach) pain. This is the most commonly reported side effect. Less frequently reported side effects are:

Nausea, heartburn, irritation or pain of the esophagus (the tube that connects your mouth with your stomach), vomiting, difficulty swallowing, a full or bloated feeling in the stomach, constipation, diarrhea, black and/or bloody stools, stomach or other peptic ulcers (some severe), and gas.

Bone, muscle or joint pain, headache, or an altered sense of taste were also experienced by some patients. Rarely, a rash (occasionally made worse by sunlight) or eye pain have occurred. Allergic reactions such as hives or, rarely, swelling of the face, lips, tongue and/or throat which may cause difficulty in breathing or swallowing have also been reported. Mouth ulcers have occurred when the tablet was chewed or dissolved in the mouth.

Anytime you have a medical problem you think may be related to FOSAMAX, talk to your doctor.

What should I know about osteoporosis?

Normally your bones are being rebuilt all the time. First, old bone is removed (resorbed). Then a similar amount of new bone is formed. This balanced process keeps your skeleton healthy and strong.

Osteoporosis is a thinning and weakening of the bones. It is common in women after menopause and may also occur in men. It may also be caused by certain medications called corticosteroids in both men and women. At the start osteoporosis usually has no symptoms, but it can result in fractures (broken bones). Fractures usually cause pain. Fractures of the bones of the spine may not be painful, but over time they cause height loss. Eventually the spine becomes curved and the body becomes bent over. Fractures may happen during normal, everyday activity, such as lifting, or from minor injury that would normally not cause bone to break. Fractures most often occur at the hip, spine, or wrist. This can lead to pain, severe disability, or loss of mobility.

Osteoporosis in men and in postmenopausal women

Osteoporosis often occurs in women several years after the menopause, which happens when the ovaries stop producing the female hormone, estrogen, or are removed (which may occur, for example, at the time of a hysterectomy). Osteoporosis can also occur in men due to several causes, including aging and/or a low level of the male hormone, testosterone. In all instances, bone is removed faster than it is formed, so bone loss occurs and bones become weaker. Therefore, maintaining bone mass is important to keep your bones healthy.

Osteoporosis in men and women caused by corticosteroids

Corticosteroids can cause bone to be removed faster than it is formed, so bone loss occurs and bones become weaker. Therefore, maintaining bone mass is important to keep your bones healthy. It is important to take your corticosteroid medication as recommended by your doctor.

How can osteoporosis be treated or prevented?

- **Medication.**
  Your doctor has prescribed FOSAMAX. FOSAMAX acts specifically on your bones. FOSAMAX is not a hormone and does not have the benefits and risks of estrogen (hormone replacement therapy used in postmenopausal women) elsewhere in your body.

- **Lifestyle changes.**
  In addition to FOSAMAX, your doctor may recommend one or more of the following lifestyle changes:
  - **Stop smoking.** Smoking appears to increase the risk of osteoporosis.
  - **Reduce the use of alcohol.** Too much alcohol appears to increase the risk of osteoporosis and injuries that may cause fractures.
  - **Exercise regularly.** Like muscles, bones need exercise to stay strong and healthy. Exercise must be safe to prevent injuries including fractures. You should consult your doctor before you begin any exercise program.
  - **Eat a balanced diet.** Adequate dietary calcium is important. Your doctor can advise you whether you need to change your diet or take any dietary supplements such as calcium or vitamin D.

This medication was prescribed for your particular condition. Do not use it for another condition or give the drug to others. Keep FOSAMAX and all medicines out of the reach of children. If you suspect that more than the prescribed dose of this medicine has been taken, drink a full glass of milk and contact your local poison control center or emergency room immediately. Do not induce vomiting. Do not lie down.

This leaflet provides a summary of information about FOSAMAX. If you have any questions or concerns about either FOSAMAX or osteoporosis, talk to your doctor. In addition, talk to your pharmacist or other health care provider.

7969410   Issued October 2000
COPYRIGHT © MERCK & CO., Inc., 1995, 1997, 2000
All rights reserved.

Patient Information about

Once Weekly FOSAMAX® (FOSS-ah-max) for Osteoporosis

Generic name: alendronate sodium (a-LEN-dro-nate)

Please read this information before you start taking once weekly FOSAMAX*. Also, read the leaflet each time you renew your prescription, just in case anything has changed. Remember, this leaflet does not take the place of careful discussions with your doctor. You and your doctor should discuss FOSAMAX when you start taking your medication and at regular checkups.

*Registered trademark of MERCK & CO., Inc.

How should I take once weekly FOSAMAX?

These are the important things you must do to help make sure you will benefit from FOSAMAX:

1. **Choose the day of the week that best fits your schedule. Every week, take one FOSAMAX tablet on your chosen day.**

2. **After getting up for the day and before taking your first food, beverage, or other medication, swallow your FOSAMAX tablet with a full glass (6–8 oz) of** <u>plain water</u> **only.**

   Not mineral water
   Not coffee or tea
   Not juice

   Do not chew or suck on a tablet of FOSAMAX.

3. **After swallowing your FOSAMAX tablet do not lie down—stay fully upright (sitting, standing or walking) for at least 30 minutes** <u>and</u> **do not lie down until after your first food of the day.** This will help the FOSAMAX tablet reach your stomach quickly and help reduce the potential for irritation of your esophagus (the tube that connects your mouth with your stomach).

4. **After swallowing your FOSAMAX tablet, wait at least 30 minutes before taking your first food, beverage, or other medication of the day,** including antacids, calcium supplements and vitamins. FOSAMAX is effective only if taken when your stomach is empty.

5. **Do not take FOSAMAX at bedtime or before getting up for the day.**

6. **If you have difficulty or pain upon swallowing, chest pain, or new or worsening heartburn, stop taking FOSAMAX and call your doctor.**
7. If you miss a dose, take only one FOSAMAX tablet on the morning after you remember. *Do not take two tablets on the same day.* Return to taking one tablet once a week, as originally scheduled on your chosen day.
8. It is important that you continue taking FOSAMAX for as long as your doctor prescribes it. FOSAMAX can treat your osteoporosis or help you from getting osteoporosis only if you continue to take it.

What is FOSAMAX?

FOSAMAX is for the treatment or prevention of osteoporosis (thinning of bone) in women after menopause. It reduces the chance of having a hip or spinal fracture.

You will find more information about osteoporosis at the end of this leaflet.

How does FOSAMAX work?

FOSAMAX works by:

- Reducing the activity of the cells that cause bone loss
- Decreasing the faster rate of bone loss that occurs after menopause
- Increasing the amount of bone in most patients

These effects are seen as soon as three months after therapy with FOSAMAX has begun. These effects continue as long as you keep taking FOSAMAX. The density of bone is maintained or increased and the bone is less likely to fracture.

Who should not take FOSAMAX?

Patients with:

- Certain disorders of the esophagus (the tube that connects your mouth with your stomach)
- Inability to stand or sit upright for at least 30 minutes
- Low levels of calcium in their blood
- Severe kidney disease
- Allergy to FOSAMAX

Patients who are:

- Pregnant or Nursing
  If you are pregnant or nursing, you should not be taking FOSAMAX. Talk to your doctor.

What other medical problems should I discuss with my doctor?

Talk to your doctor about any:

- Problems with swallowing
- Stomach or digestive problems
- Other medical problems you have or have had in the past

What are the possible side effects of FOSAMAX?

Some patients may develop severe digestive reactions including irritation, inflammation or ulceration (occasionally with bleeding) of the esophagus (the tube that connects your mouth with your stomach). These reactions can cause chest pain, heartburn or difficulty or pain upon swallowing. This may occur especially if patients do not drink a full glass of water with FOSAMAX and/or if they lie down in less than 30 minutes or before their first food of the day. Esophageal reactions may worsen if patients continue to take FOSAMAX after developing symptoms suggesting irritation of the esophagus.

Like all prescription drugs, FOSAMAX may cause side effects. Side effects usually have been mild. They generally have not caused patients to stop taking FOSAMAX. Some patients treated with FOSAMAX experienced abdominal (stomach) pain. This is the most commonly reported side effect. Less frequently reported side effects are:

Nausea, heartburn, irritation or pain of the esophagus (the tube that connects your mouth with your stomach), vomiting, difficulty swallowing, a full or bloated feeling in the stomach, constipation, diarrhea, black and/or bloody stools, stomach or other peptic ulcers (some severe), and gas.

Bone, muscle or joint pain, headache, or an altered sense of taste were also experienced by some patients. Rarely, a rash (occasionally made worse by sunlight) or eye pain have occurred. Allergic reactions such as hives or, rarely, swelling of the face, lips, tongue and/or throat which may cause difficulty in breathing or swallowing have also been reported. Mouth ulcers have occurred when the tablet was chewed or dissolved in the mouth.

Anytime you have a medical problem you think may be related to FOSAMAX, talk to your doctor.

What should I know about osteoporosis?

Normally your bones are being rebuilt all the time. First, old bone is removed (resorbed). Then a similar amount of new bone is formed. This balanced process keeps your skeleton healthy and strong.

Osteoporosis is a thinning and weakening of the bones. Osteoporosis often occurs in women several years after the menopause, which happens when the ovaries stop producing the female hormone, estrogen, or are removed (which may occur, for example, at the time of a hysterectomy). After menopause, bone is removed faster than it is formed, so bone loss occurs and bones become weaker. Therefore, maintaining bone mass is important to keep your bones healthy. At the start osteoporosis usually has no symptoms, but it can result in fractures (broken bones). Fractures usually cause pain. Fractures of the bones of the spine may not be painful, but over time they cause height loss. Eventually the spine becomes curved and the body becomes bent over. Fractures may happen during normal, everyday activity, such as lifting, or from minor injury that would normally not cause bone to break. Fractures most often occur at the hip, spine, or wrist. This can lead to pain, severe disability, or loss of mobility.

How can osteoporosis in postmenopausal women be treated or prevented?

- **Medication.**
  Your doctor has prescribed FOSAMAX. FOSAMAX acts specifically on your bones. FOSAMAX is not a hormone and does not have the benefits and risks of estrogen (hormone replacement therapy) elsewhere in your body.
- **Lifestyle changes.**
  In addition to FOSAMAX, your doctor may recommend one or more of the following lifestyle changes:
  - **Stop smoking.** Smoking appears to increase the risk of osteoporosis.
  - **Reduce the use of alcohol.** Too much alcohol appears to increase the risk of osteoporosis and injuries that may cause fractures.
  - **Exercise regularly.** Like muscles, bones need exercise to stay strong and healthy. Exercise must be safe to prevent injuries including fractures. You should consult your doctor before you begin any exercise program.
  - **Eat a balanced diet.** Adequate dietary calcium is important. Your doctor can advise you whether you need to change your diet or take any dietary supplements such as calcium or vitamin D.

This medication was prescribed for your particular condition. Do not use it for another condition or give the drug to others. Keep FOSAMAX and all medicines out of the reach of children. If you suspect that more than the prescribed dose of this medicine has been taken, drink a full glass of milk and contact your local poison control center or emergency room immediately. Do not induce vomiting. Do not lie down.

This leaflet provides a summary of information about FOSAMAX. If you have any questions or concerns about either FOSAMAX or osteoporosis, talk to your doctor. In addition, talk to your pharmacist or other health care provider.

9364100 Issued October 2000

COPYRIGHT © MERCK & CO., Inc., 2000
All rights reserved.

MAXALT® Tablets
(rizatriptan benzoate)

MAXALT-MLT® Orally Disintegrating Tablets
(rizatriptan benzoate)

Prescribing information for this product, which appears on pages 1956–1960 of the 2001 PDR, has been revised as follows. Please write "See Supplement A" alongside product heading.

In the product heading, after MAXALT-MLT, change the ™ trademark symbol to the ® registered trademark symbol.

In the **CLINICAL PHARMACOLOGY** section, under *Clinical Studies,* at the end, add the following paragraph:

In a single study in adolescents (n=291), there were no statistically significant differences between treatment groups. The headache response rates at 2 hours were 66% and 56% for MAXALT 5 mg Tablets and placebo, respectively.

In the **PRECAUTIONS** section, under *Pediatric Use*, add the following at the end:

The efficacy of MAXALT Tablets (5 mg) in patients aged 12 to 17 years was not established in a randomized placebo-controlled trial of 291 adolescent migraineurs (see *Clinical Studies*). Adverse events observed were similar in nature to those reported in clinical trials in adults. Postmarketing experience with other triptans includes a limited number of reports that describe pediatric patients who have experienced clinically serious adverse events that are similar in nature to those reported rarely in adults. The long-term safety of rizatriptan in pediatric patients has not been studied.

In the **ADVERSE REACTIONS** section, under *Post-Marketing Experience,* replace the last paragraph with the following:

The following adverse reactions have also been reported:
Skin and Skin Appendage: Toxic epidermal necrolysis.
Special Senses: Dysgeusia.

Revisions based on 9122107, issued July 2000.

In the Patient Information, in the product heading, after MAXALT-MLT, replace "™" with "®".

Under **What are the possible side effects of MAXALT?**, in the fourth paragraph, after "side effects", add "reported in studies or general use". In the **Skin** subsection, after "hives," add "severe sloughing of the skin,". In the **Special Senses** subsection, at the end, add "bad taste." After the **Miscellaneous** subsection, delete the sentence "In addition, bad taste has occurred."

Revisions based on 9122202, issued July 2000.

MEVACOR® Tablets ℞
(lovastatin)

Prescribing information for this product, which appears on pages 1968–1971 of the 2001 PDR, has been revised as follows. Please write "See Supplement A" alongside product heading.

In the **CLINICAL PHARMACOLOGY** section, under *Pharmacokinetics*, add the following paragraph at the end:

Lovastatin is a substrate for cytochrome P450 isoform 3A4 (CYP3A4) (see PRECAUTONS, *Drug Interactions.*) Grapefruit juice contains one or more components that inhibit CYP3A4 and can increase the plasma concentrations of drugs metabolized by CYP3A4. In one study**, 10 subjects consumed 200 mL of double-strength grapefruit juice (one can of frozen concentrate diluted with one rather than 3 cans of water) three times daily for 2 days and an additional 200 mL double-strength grapefruit juice together with and 30 and 90 minutes following a single dose of 80 mg lovastatin on the third day. This regimen of grapefruit juice resulted in a mean increase in the serum concentration of lovastatin and its β-hydroxyacid metabolite (as measured by the area under the concentration-time curve) of 15-fold and 5-fold, respectively [as measured using a chemical assay—high performance liquid chromatography]. In a second study, 15 subjects consumed one 8 oz glass of single-strength grapefruit juice (one can of frozen concentrate diluted with 3 cans of water) with breakfast for 3 consecutive days and a single dose of 40 mg lovastatin in the evening of the third day. This regimen of grapefruit juice resulted in a mean increase in the plasma concentration (as measured by the area under the concentration-time curve) of active and total HMG-CoA reductase inhibitory activity [using an enzyme inhibition assay both before (for active inhibitors) and after (for total inhibitors) base hydrolysis] of 1.34-fold and 1.36-fold, respectively, and of lovastatin and its β-hydroxyacid metabolite [measured using a chemical assay—liquid chromatography/tandem mass spectrometry—different from that used in the first** study] of 1.94-fold and 1.57-fold, respectively. The effect of amounts of grapefruit juice between those used in these two studies of lovastatin pharmacokinetics has not been studied.

**Kantola, T, et al., Clin Pharmacol Ther 1998; 63(4):397–402.

In the **WARNINGS** section, under *Myopathy caused by drug interactions*, replace the second paragraph with the following:

In addition, the risk of myopathy may be increased by high levels of HMG-CoA reductase inhibitory activity in plasma. Lovastatin is metabolized by the cytochrome P450 isoform 3A4 (CYP3A4). Potent inhibitors of this metabolic pathway can raise the plasma levels of HMG-CoA reductase inhibitory activity and may increase the risk of myopathy. These include cyclosporine; the azole antifungals, itraconazole and ketoconazole; the macrolide antibiotics, erythromycin and clarithromycin; HIV protease inhibitors; the antidepressant nefazodone; and large quantities of grapefruit juice (> 1 quart daily) (see below; CLINICAL PHARMACOLOGY, *Pharmacokinetics*; PRECAUTIONS, *Drug Interactions*; and DOSAGE AND ADMINISTRATION).

Although the data are insufficient for lovastatin, the risk of myopathy appears to be increased when verapamil, but not other calcium channel blockers, is used concomitantly with a closely related HMG-CoA reductase inhibitor (see PRECAUTIONS, *Drug Interactions*).

Also in the **WARNINGS** section, under *Reducing the risk of myopathy*, replace the last paragraph with the following:

In patients taking concomitant cyclosporine, fibrates or niacin, the dose of lovastatin should generally not exceed 20 mg/day (see DOSAGE AND ADMINISTRATION and DOSAGE AND ADMINISTRATION, *Concomitant Lipid-Lowering Therapy*), as the risk of myopathy increases substantially at higher doses. Concomitant use of lovastatin with itraconazole, ketoconazole, erythromycin, clarithromycin, HIV protease inhibitors, nefazodone, or large quantities of grapefruit juice (> 1 quart daily) is not recommended. If no alternative to a short course of treatment with itraconazole, ketoconazole, erythromycin, or clarithromycin is available, a brief suspension of lovastatin therapy during such treatment can be considered as there are no known adverse consequences to brief interruptions of long-term cholesterol-lowering therapy.

In the **PRECAUTIONS** section, under *Drug Interactions*, replace the first paragraph with the following:

Gemfibrozil and other fibrates, lipid-lowering doses (≥ 1 g/day) of niacin (nicotinic acid): These drugs increase the risk of myopathy when given concomitantly with lovastatin, probably because they can produce myopathy when given alone (see WARNINGS, *Skeletal Muscle*). There is no evidence to suggest that these agents affect the pharmacokinetics of lovastatin.

CYP3A4 Interactions: Lovastatin has no CYP3A4 inhibitory activity; therefore, it is not expected to affect the plasma concentrations of other drugs metabolized by CYP3A4. However, lovastatin itself is a substrate for CYP3A4. Potent inhibitors of CYP3A4 may increase the risk of myopathy by increasing the plasma concentration of HMG-CoA reductase inhibitory activity during lovastatin therapy. These inhibitors include cyclosporine, itraconazole, ketoconazole, erythromycin, clarithromycin, HIV protease inhibitors, nefazodone, and large quantities of grapefruit juice (> 1 quart daily) (see CLINICAL PHARMACOLOGY, *Pharmacokinetics* and WARNINGS, *Skeletal Muscle*).

Grapefruit juice contains one or more components that inhibit CYP3A4 and can increase the plasma concentrations of drugs metabolized by CYP3A4. Large quantities of grapefruit juice (> 1 quart daily) significantly increase the serum concentrations of lovastatin and its β-hydroxyacid metabo-

Continued on next page

Information on the Merck & Co. products listed on these pages is from the full prescribing information in use April 1, 2001.

Mevacor—Cont.

lite during lovastatin therapy and should be avoided (see CLINICAL PHARMACOLOGY, *Pharmacokinetics* and WARNINGS, *Skeletal Muscle*).

Although the data are insufficient for lovastatin, the risk of myopathy appears to be increased when verapamil, but not other calcium channel blockers, is used concomitantly with a closely related HMG-CoA reductase inhibitor (see WARNINGS, *Skeletal Muscle*).

Also in the **PRECAUTIONS** section, under *Drug Interactions*, delete the third paragraph that begins "Antipyrine: Lovastatin . . .".

In the **ADVERSE REACTIONS** section, under *Hypersensitivity Reactions*, after "polymyalgia rheumatica," add "dermatomyositis,".

In the **DOSAGE AND ADMINISTRATION** section, under *Concomitant Lipid-Lowering Therapy*, replace the last sentence with the following:

However, if MEVACOR is used in combination with fibrates or niacin, the dose of MEVACOR should generally not exceed 20 mg/day (see WARNINGS, *Skeletal Muscle* and PRECAUTIONS, *Drug Interactions*).

Revisions based on 7825349, issued September 2000.

PEPCID® Tablets   ℞
(famotidine)
PEPCID® for Oral Suspension   ℞
(famotidine)
PEPCID RPD® Orally Disintegrating Tablets   ℞
(famotidine)

Prescribing information for this product, which appears on pages 1988–1990 of the 2001 PDR, has been revised as follows. Please write "See Supplement A" alongside product heading.

In the **PRECAUTIONS** section, replace the entire *Use in Elderly Patients* subsection with the following:
Geriatric Use
Of the 4,966 subjects in clinical studies who were treated with famotidine, 488 subjects (9.8%) were 65 and older, and 88 subjects (1.7%) were greater than 75 years of age. No overall differences in safety or effectiveness were observed between these subjects and younger subjects, and other reported clinical experience has not identified differences in responses between the elderly and younger patients, but greater sensitivity of some older individuals cannot be ruled out.

No dosage adjustment is required based on age (see CLINICAL PHARMACOLOGY IN ADULTS, *Pharmacokinetics*). This drug is known to be substantially excreted by the kidney, and the risk of toxic reactions to this drug may be greater in patients with impaired renal function. Because elderly patients are more likely to have decreased renal function, care should be taken in dose selection, and it may be useful to monitor renal function. Dosage adjustment in the case of severe renal impairment is necessary (see PRECAUTIONS, *Patients with Severe Renal Insufficiency* and DOSAGE AND ADMINISTRATION, *Dosage Adjustment for Patients with Severe Renal Insufficiency*).

In the **HOW SUPPLIED** section, replace the *Storage* subsection with the following:
Storage
Store PEPCID Tablets and PEPCID RPD Orally Disintegrating Tablets at 25°C (77°F); excursions permitted to 15–30°C (59–86°F) [see USP Controlled Room Temperature].
Store PEPCID for Oral Suspension dry powder and suspension at 25°C (77°F); excursions permitted to 15–30°C (59–86°F) [see USP Controlled Room Temperature]. Suspension: Protect from freezing. Discard unused suspension after 30 days.
Revisions based on 7825034, issued May 2000.

PEPCID® Injection Premixed   ℞
(famotidine)
PEPCID® Injection   ℞
(famotidine)

Prescribing information for this product, which appears on pages 1990–1993 of the 2001 PDR, has been revised as follows. Please write "See Supplement A" alongside product heading.

In the **PRECAUTIONS** section, replace the entire *Use in Elderly Patients* subsection with the following:
Geriatric Use
Of the 4,966 subjects in clinical studies who were treated with famotidine, 488 subjects (9.8%) were 65 and older, and 88 subjects (1.7%) were greater than 75 years of age. No overall differences in safety or effectiveness were observed between these subjects and younger subjects, and other reported clinical experience has not identified differences in responses between the elderly and younger patients, but greater sensitivity of some older individuals cannot be ruled out.

No dosage adjustment is required based on age (see CLINICAL PHARMACOLOGY IN ADULTS, *Pharmacokinetics*). This drug is known to be substantially excreted by the kidney, and the risk of toxic reactions to this drug may be greater in patients with impaired renal function. Because elderly patients are more likely to have decreased renal

function, care should be taken in dose selection, and it may be useful to monitor renal function. Dosage adjustment in the case of severe renal impairment is necessary (see PRECAUTIONS, *Patients with Severe Renal Insufficiency* and DOSAGE AND ADMINISTRATION, *Dosage Adjustment for Patients with Severe Renal Insufficiency*).
Revision based on 9042509, issued May 2000.

SINGULAIR® Tablets and Chewable Tablets   ℞
(montelukast sodium)

The Prescribing information for this product, which appears on pages 2018–2022 of the 2001 PDR, has been revised as follows. Please write "See Supplement A" alongside product heading.

In the **ADVERSE REACTIONS** section, under *Post-Marketing Experience*, in the first paragraph, after "dyspepsia" add ", diarrhea, and myalgia including muscle cramps." Revision based on 9088808, issued August 2000.

In the Patient Information, under **What are the possible side effects of SINGULAIR?**, in the paragraph beginning "Less common side effects...", at the end of the bulleted list, add the following:

• muscle aches and muscle cramps
Revision based on 9094208, issued August 2000.

TRUSOPT® Sterile Ophthalmic Solution 2%
(dorzolamide hydrochloride ophthalmic solution)

Prescribing information for this product, which appears on pages 2033–2035 of the 2001 PDR, has been revised as follows. Please write "See Supplement A" alongside product heading.

In the **PRECAUTIONS** section, under *General,* add the following paragraph at the end:
Choroidal detachment has been reported with administration of aqueous suppressant therapy (e.g., dorzolamide) after filtration procedures.

In the **ADVERSE REACTIONS** section, under *Clinical practice:*, in the last sentence, after "transient myopia," add "choroidal detachment following filtration surgery,".

In the **HOW SUPPLIED** section, in the second paragraph, after "OCUMETER®*" add "PLUS container,".

Also in the **HOW SUPPLIED** section, replace the NDC codes with the following:
NDC 0006-3519-35, 5 mL
NDC 0006-3519-36, 10 mL.

After the **HOW SUPPLIED** section, add the **INSTRUCTIONS FOR USE** section.

INSTRUCTIONS FOR USE

Please follow these instructions carefully when using TRUSOPT*. Use TRUSOPT as prescribed by your doctor.
1. If you use other topically applied ophthalmic medications, they should be administered at least 10 minutes before or after TRUSOPT.
2. Wash hands before each use.
3. Before using the medication, be sure the Safety Strip on the front of the bottle is unbroken. A gap between the bottle and the cap is normal for an unopened bottle.

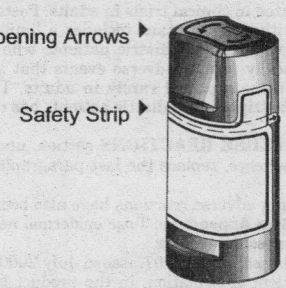

Opening Arrows ▶

Safety Strip ▶

4. Tear off the Safety Strip to break the seal. [See figure below]

5. To open the bottle, unscrew the cap by turning as indicated by the arrows.

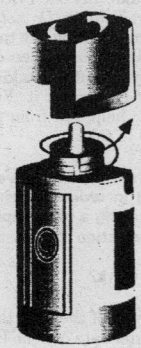

6. Tilt your head back and pull your lower eyelid down slightly to form a pocket between your eyelid and your eye.

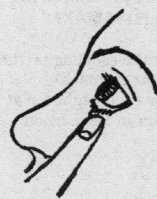

7. Invert the bottle, grasping it with the thumb or index finger over the Finger Push Area as shown. Press lightly until a single drop is dispensed into the eye as directed by your doctor.
DO NOT TOUCH YOUR EYE OR EYELID WITH THE DROPPER TIP.
Ophthalmic medications, if handled improperly, can become contaminated by common bacteria known to cause eye infections. Serious damage to the eye and subsequent loss of vision may result from using contaminated ophthalmic medications. If you think your medication may be contaminated, or if you develop an eye infection, contact your doctor immediately concerning continued use of this bottle.

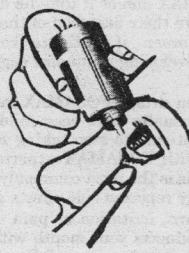

8. Repeat steps 6 & 7 with the other eye if instructed to do so by your doctor.
9. Replace the cap by turning until it is firmly touching the bottle.
10. The dispenser tip is designed to provide a pre-measured drop; therefore, do NOT enlarge the hole of the dispenser.

WARNING: Keep out of reach of children.

If you have any questions about the use of TRUSOPT, please consult your doctor.

---

*Registered trademark of MERCK & CO., Inc.
Revisions based on 9368201, issued January 2001.

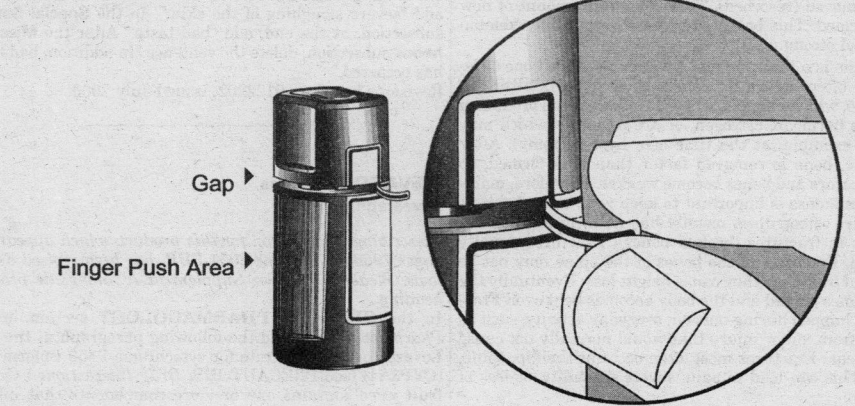

Gap ▶

Finger Push Area ▶

VIOXX® ℞
(rofecoxib tablets and oral suspension)

Prescribing information for this product, which appears on pages 2049–2053 of the 2001 PDR, has been revised as follows. Please write "See Supplement A" alongside product heading.

In the **PRECAUTIONS** section, under *Drug Interactions,* in the *Lithium* subsection, after the first sentence, add the following:

In post-marketing experience there have been reports of increases in plasma lithium levels.

In the **ADVERSE REACTIONS** section, in the *Gastrointestinal* subsection, after "gastrointestinal bleeding," add "*hepatitis,*" and after "intestinal obstruction," add *"jaundice,"*. In the *Hemic and lymphatic* subsection, before "lymphoma," add *"agranulocytosis, leukopenia,"* and after "lymphoma" add *", thrombocytopenia."* In the *Psychiatric* subsection, before *"hallucinations."* add *"confusion,"*. Below the *Psychiatric* subsection, add the following new subsection:

Skin and Skin Appendages: severe skin reactions, including Stevens-Johnson syndrome.

Revisions based on 9183806, issued July 2000.

In the Patient Information, under **Can I take VIOXX with other medicines?**, after the last bullet, add the following:

• lithium (a medicine used to treat a certain type of depression.)

Under **What are the possible side effects of VIOXX?**, at the end of the second bulleted paragraph, add "Severe skin reactions have also been reported." In the fourth bulleted paragraph, replace the first sentence with the following:

Severe liver problems, including hepatitis and jaundice, occur rarely in patients taking NSAIDs, including VIOXX.

Also under **What are the possible side effects of VIOXX?**, replace the paragraph after the bullets with the following:

In addition, the following side effects have been reported: confusion, hair loss, hallucinations, low blood cell counts, unusual headache with stiff neck (aseptic meningitis).

Revisions based on 9183902, issued July 2000.

VIVACTIL* Tablets ℞
(protriptyline HCl)

This product is marketed by Odyssey Pharmaceuticals, a subsidiary of Sidmak Labs. Please refer to Odyssey Pharmaceuticals for prescribing information.

*Registered trademark of Sidmak Labs.

ZOCOR® Tablets ℞
(simvastatin)

Prescribing information for this product, which appears on pages 2054–2058 of the 2001 PDR, has been revised as follows. Please write "See Supplement A" alongside product heading.

In the **CLINICAL PHARMACOLOGY** section, under *Pharmacokinetics,* add the following paragraphs at the end:

In a study of 12 healthy volunteers, simvastatin at the 80-mg dose had no effect on the metabolism of the probe cytochrome P450 isoform 3A4 (CYP3A4) substrates midazolam and erythromycin. This indicates that simvastatin is not an inhibitor of CYP3A4, and, therefore, is not expected to affect the plasma levels of other drugs metabolized by CYP3A4.

Simvastatin is a substrate for CYP3A4 (see PRECAUTIONS, *Drug Interactions*). Grapefruit juice contains one or more components that inhibit CYP3A4 and can increase the plasma concentrations of drugs metabolized by CYP3A4. In one study**, 10 subjects consumed 200 mL of double-strength grapefruit juice (one can of frozen concentrate diluted with one rather than 3 cans of water) three times daily for 2 days and an additional 200 mL double-strength grapefruit juice together with and 30 and 90 minutes following a single dose of 60 mg simvastatin on the third day. This regimen of grapefruit juice resulted in mean increases in the concentration (as measured by the area under the concentration-time curve) of active and total HMG-CoA reductase inhibitory activity [measured using a radioenzyme inhibition assay both before (for active inhibitors) and after (for total inhibitors) base hydrolysis] of 2.4-fold and 3.6-fold, respectively, and of simvastatin and its β-hydroxyacid metabolite [measured using a chemical assay—liquid chromatography/tandem mass spectrometry of 16-fold and 7-fold, respectively. In a second study, 16 subjects consumed one 8 oz glass of single-strength grapefruit juice (one can of frozen concentrate diluted with 3 cans of water) with breakfast for 3 consecutive days and a single dose of 20 mg simvastatin in the evening of the third day. This regimen of grapefruit juice resulted in a mean increase in the plasma concentration (as measured by the area under the concentration-time curve) of active and total HMG-CoA reductase inhibitory activity [using a validated enzyme inhibition assay different from that used in the first** study, both before (for active inhibitors) and after simvastatin and its β-hydroxyacid metabolite [measured using a chemical assay—liquid chromatography/tandem mass spectrometry] of 1.88-fold and 1.31-fold, respectively. The effect of amounts of grapefruit juice between those used in these two studies on simvastatin pharmacokinetics has not been studied.

** Lilja JJ, Kivisto KT, Neuvonen PJ, Clin Pharmacol Ther 1998;64(5):477–83.

In the **WARNINGS** section, under *Myopathy caused by drug interactions,* replace the second paragraph with the following two paragraphs:

In addition, the risk of myopathy may be increased by high levels of HMG-CoA reductase inhibitory activity in plasma. Simvastatin is metabolized by the cytochrome P450 isoform 3A4 (CYP3A4). Potent inhibitors of this metabolic pathway can raise the plasma levels of HMG-CoA reductase inhibitory activity and may increase the risk of myopathy. These include cyclosporine; the azole antifungals, itraconazole and ketoconazole; the macrolide antibiotics, erythromycin and clarithromycin; HIV protease inhibitors; the antidepressant nefazodone; and large quantities of grapefruit juice (> 1 quart daily) (see below; CLINICAL PHARMACOLOGY, *Pharmacokinetics;* PRECAUTIONS, *Drug Interactions;* and DOSAGE AND ADMINISTRATION, *Dosage in Patients taking Cyclosporine*).

The risk of myopathy appears to be increased by concomitant administration of verapamil, but not by other calcium channel blockers (see PRECAUTIONS, *Drug Interactions*). Because concomitant use of calcium channel blockers with simvastatin in clinical trials was substantial and far greater than with any of the interacting drugs listed above, it is possible to calculate incidence: 4 of 635 patients taking verapamil concomitantly with simvastatin in clinical trials experienced myopathy (0.63%). By comparison, in the same trials myopathy occurred in 2 of 2,343 patients taking diltiazem with simvastatin (0.085%) and 1 of 1,046 (0.096%) taking amlodipine. In patients taking simvastatin with none of these three calcium channel blockers, the incidence of myopathy was 13 of 21,224 patients (0.061%).

Also in the **WARNINGS** section, under *Reducing the risk of myopathy,* replace the fifth paragraph with the following:

In patients taking concomitant cyclosporine, fibrates or niacin, the dose of simvastatin should generally not exceed 10 mg/day (see DOSAGE AND ADMINISTRATION, *Dosage in Patients taking Cyclosporine* and *Concomitant Lipid-Lowering Therapy*), as the risk of myopathy increases substantially at higher doses. Concomitant use of simvastatin with itraconazole, ketoconazole, erythromycin, clarithromycin, HIV protease inhibitors, nefazodone, or large quantities of grapefruit juice (>1 quart daily) is not recommended. If no alternative to a short course of treatment with itraconazole, ketoconazole, erythromycin, or clarithromycin is available, a brief suspension of simvastatin therapy during such treatment can be considered as there are no known adverse consequences to brief interruptions of long-term cholesterol-lowering therapy.

In the **PRECAUTIONS** section, under *Drug Interactions,* replace the first two paragraphs with the following four paragraphs:

Gemfibrozil and other fibrates, lipid-lowering doses (≥1g/day) of niacin (nicotinic acid): These drugs increase the risk of myopathy when given concomitantly with simvastatin, probably because they can produce myopathy when given alone (see WARNINGS, *Skeletal Muscle*). There is no evidence to suggest that these agents affect the pharmacokinetics of simvastatin.

CYP3A4 Interactions: Simvastatin has no CYP3A4 inhibitory activity; therefore, it is not expected to affect the plasma concentrations of other drugs metabolized by CYP3A4 (see CLINICAL PHARMACOLOGY, *Pharmacokinetics*). However, simvastatin itself is a substrate for CYP3A4. Potent inhibitors of CYP3A4 may increase the risk of myopathy by increasing the plasma concentration of HMG-CoA reductase inhibitory activity during simvastatin therapy. These inhibitors include cyclosporine, itraconazole, ketoconazole, erythromycin, clarithromycin, HIV protease inhibitors, nefazodone, and large quantities of grapefruit juice (>1 quart daily) (see CLINICAL PHARMACOLOGY, *Pharmacokinetics* and WARNINGS, *Skeletal Muscle*).

Grapefruit juice contains one or more components that inhibit CYP3A4 and can increase the plasma concentrations of drugs metabolized by CYP3A4. Large quantities of grapefruit juice (>1 quart daily) significantly increase the serum concentrations of simvastatin and its β-hydroxyacid metabolite during simvastatin therapy and should be avoided; the serum concentration of HMG-CoA reductase inhibitory activity is increased to a lesser extent (see CLINICAL PHARMACOLOGY, *Pharmacokinetics* and WARNINGS, *Skeletal Muscle.*

The risk of myopathy appears to be increased by concomitant administration of verapamil, but not by other calcium channel blockers (see WARNINGS, *Skeletal Muscle*).

In the **ADVERSE REACTIONS** section, under *Hypersensitivity Reactions,* after "rheumatica," add "dermatomyositis,".

In the **DOSAGE AND ADMINISTRATION** section, replace the paragraph under *Concomitant Lipid-Lowering Therapy* with the following:

ZOCOR is effective alone or when used concomitantly with bile-acid sequestrants. Use of ZOCOR with fibrates or niacin should generally be avoided. However, if ZOCOR is used in combination with fibrates or niacin, the dose of ZOCOR should generally not exceed 10 mg/day (see WARNINGS, *Skeletal Muscle* and PRECAUTIONS, *Drug Interactions*.)

Revisions based on 7825439, issued September 2000.

Novartis Pharmaceuticals Corporation

NOVARTIS PHARMACEUTICALS CORPORATION
59 Route 10
East Hanover, NJ 07936
(for branded products)

GENEVA PHARMACEUTICALS, INC.
A NOVARTIS COMPANY
2655 West Midway Boulevard
PO Box 446
Broomfield, CO 80038-0446
(for branded generic product listing refer to Geneva Pharmaceuticals, Inc.)

For Information Contact (*branded products*):
Customer Response Department
(888) NOW-NOVARTIS [888-669-6682]
Global Internet Address:
http: //www.novartis.com

For Information Contact (*branded generic products*):
Customer Support Department
(800) 525-8747
(303) 466-2400
FAX: (303) 438-4600

EXELON® ℞
[*ĕx ' ə-lŏn*]
(rivastigmine tartrate)
Capsules
Rx only

Prescribing information for this product, which appears on page(s) 2171–2174 of the 2001 PDR, has been completely revised as follows. Please write "See Supplement A" next to the product heading.

DESCRIPTION

Exelon® (rivastigmine tartrate) is a reversible cholinesterase inhibitor and is known chemically as (S)-N-Ethyl-N-methyl-3-[1-(dimethylamino)ethyl]-phenyl carbamate hydrogen-(2R,3R)-tartrate. Rivastigmine tartrate is commonly referred to in the pharmacological literature as SDZ ENA 713 or ENA 713. It has an empirical formula of $C_{14}H_{22}N_2O_2 \bullet C_4H_6O_6$ (hydrogen tartrate salt – hta salt) and a molecular weight of 400.43 (hta salt). Rivastigmine tartrate is a white to off-white, fine crystalline powder that is very soluble in water, soluble in ethanol and acetonitrile, slightly soluble in n-octanol and very slightly soluble in ethyl acetate. The distribution coefficient at 37°C in n-octanol/phosphate buffer solution pH 7 is 3.0.

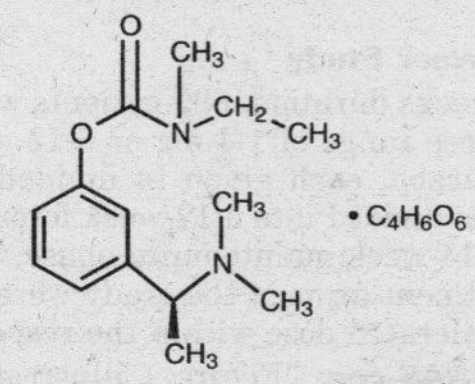

Exelon is supplied as capsules containing rivastigmine tartrate, equivalent to 1.5, 3, 4.5 and 6 mg of rivastigmine base for oral administration. Inactive ingredients are hydroxypropyl methylcellulose, magnesium stearate, microcrystalline cellulose, and silicon dioxide. Each hard-gelatin capsule contains gelatin, titanium dioxide and red and/or yellow iron oxides.

CLINICAL PHARMACOLOGY

Mechanism of Action

Pathological changes in Dementia of the Alzheimer type involve cholinergic neuronal pathways that project from the basal forebrain to the cerebral cortex and hippocampus. These pathways are thought to be intricately involved in memory, attention, learning, and other cognitive processes. While the precise mechanism of rivastigmine's action is unknown, it is postulated to exert its therapeutic effect by enhancing cholinergic function. This is accomplished by increasing the concentration of acetylcholine through reversible inhibition of its hydrolysis by cholinesterase. If this proposed mechanism is correct, Exelon's effect may lessen as the disease process advances and fewer cholinergic neurons remain functionally intact. There is no evidence that rivastigmine alters the course of the underlying dementing process. After a 6-mg dose of rivastigmine, anticholinesterase activity is present in CSF for about 10 hours, with a maximum inhibition of about 60% five hours after dosing.

Clinical Trial Data

The effectiveness of Exelon® (rivastigmine tartrate) as a treatment for Alzheimer's Disease is demonstrated by the results of two randomized, double-blind, placebo-controlled clinical investigations in patients with Alzheimer's Disease [diagnosed by NINCDS-ADRDA and DSM-IV criteria, Mini-Mental State Examination (MMSE) ≥10 and ≤26, and the Global Deterioration Scale (GDS)]. The mean age of patients participating in Exelon trials was 73 years with a range of 41-95. Approximately 59% of patients were women and 41% were men. The racial distribution was Caucasian 87%, Black 4% and Other races 9%.

Continued on next page

Exelon Capsules—Cont.

Study Outcome Measures: In each study, the effectiveness of Exelon was evaluated using a dual outcome assessment strategy.

The ability of Exelon to improve cognitive performance was assessed with the cognitive subscale of the Alzheimer's Disease Assessment Scale (ADAS-cog), a multi item instrument that has been extensively validated in longitudinal cohorts of Alzheimer's Disease patients. The ADAS-cog examines selected aspects of cognitive performance including elements of memory, orientation, attention, reasoning, language and praxis. The ADAS-cog scoring range is from 0 to 70, with higher scores indicating greater cognitive impairment. Elderly normal adults may score as low as 0 or 1, but it is not unusual for non-demented adults to score slightly higher.

The patients recruited as participants in each study had mean scores on ADAS-cog of approximately 23 units, with a range from 1 to 61. Experience gained in longitudinal studies of ambulatory patients with mild to moderate Alzheimer's Disease suggest that they gain 6-12 units a year on the ADAS-cog. Lesser degrees of change, however, are seen in patients with very mild or very advanced disease because the ADAS-cog is not uniformly sensitive to change over the course of the disease. The annualized rate of decline in the placebo patients participating in Exelon trials was approximately 3-8 units per year.

The ability of Exelon to produce an overall clinical effect was assessed using a Clinician's Interview Based Impression of Change that required the use of caregiver information, the CIBIC-Plus. The CIBIC-Plus is not a single instrument and is not a standardized instrument like the ADAS-cog. Clinical trials for investigational drugs have used a variety of CIBIC formats, each different in terms of depth and structure. As such, results from a CIBIC-Plus reflect clinical experience from the trial or trials in which it was used and can not be compared directly with the results of CIBIC-Plus evaluations from other clinical trials. The CIBIC-Plus used in the Exelon trials was a structured instrument based on a comprehensive evaluation at baseline and subsequent time-points of three domains: patient cognition, behavior and functioning, including assessment of activities of daily living. It represents the assessment of a skilled clinician using validated scales based on his/her observation at interviews conducted separately with the patient and the caregiver familiar with the behavior of the patient over the interval rated. The CIBIC-Plus is scored as a seven point categorical rating, ranging from a score of 1, indicating "markedly improved," to a score of 4, indicating "no change" to a score of 7, indicating "marked worsening." The CIBIC-Plus has not been systematically compared directly to assessments not using information from caregivers (CIBIC) or other global methods.

U.S. Twenty-Six-Week Study

In a study of 26 weeks duration, 699 patients were randomized to either a dose range of 1-4 mg or 6-12 mg of Exelon per day or to placebo, each given in divided doses. The 26-week study was divided into a 12-week forced dose titration phase and a 14-week maintenance phase. The patients in the active treatment arms of the study were maintained at their highest tolerated dose within the respective range.

Effects on the ADAS-cog: Figure 1 illustrates the time course for the change from baseline in ADAS-cog scores for all three dose groups over the 26 weeks of the study. At 26 weeks of treatment, the mean differences in the ADAS-cog change scores for the Exelon-treated patients compared to the patients on placebo were 1.9 and 4.9 units for the 1-4 mg and 6-12 mg treatments, respectively. Both treatments were statistically significantly superior to placebo and the 6-12 mg/day range was significantly superior to the 1-4 mg/day range.

Figure 1: Time-course of the Change from Baseline in ADAS-cog Score for Patients Completing 26 Weeks of Treatment

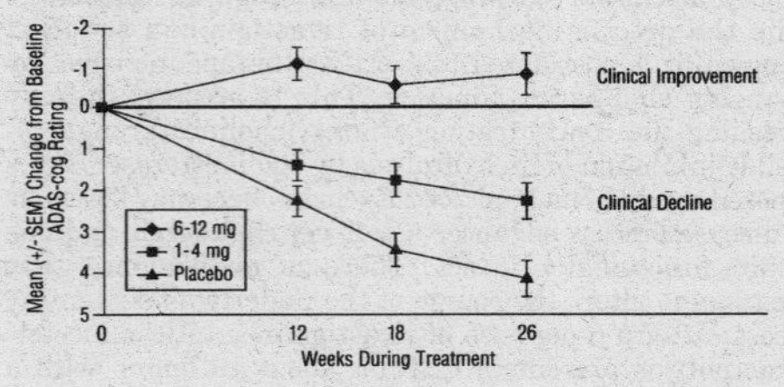
Mean (+/- SEM) Change from Baseline ADAS-cog Rating
Clinical Improvement
Clinical Decline
6-12 mg
1-4 mg
Placebo
Weeks During Treatment

Figure 2 illustrates the cumulative percentages of patients from each of the three treatment groups who had attained at least the measure of improvement in ADAS-cog score shown on the X axis. Three change scores, (7-point and 4-point reductions from baseline or no change in score) have been identified for illustrative purposes, and the percent of patients in each group achieving that result is shown in the inset table.

The curves demonstrate that both patients assigned to Exelon and placebo have a wide range of responses, but that the Exelon groups are more likely to show the greater improvements. A curve for an effective treatment would be shifted to the left of the curve for placebo, while an ineffective or deleterious treatment would be superimposed upon, or shifted to the right of the curve for placebo, respectively.

Figure 2: Cumulative Percentage of Patients Completing 26 Weeks of Double-blind Treatment with Specified Changes from Baseline ADAS-cog Scores. The Percentages of Randomized Patients who Completed the Study were: Placebo 84%, 1-4 mg 85%, and 6-12 mg 65%.

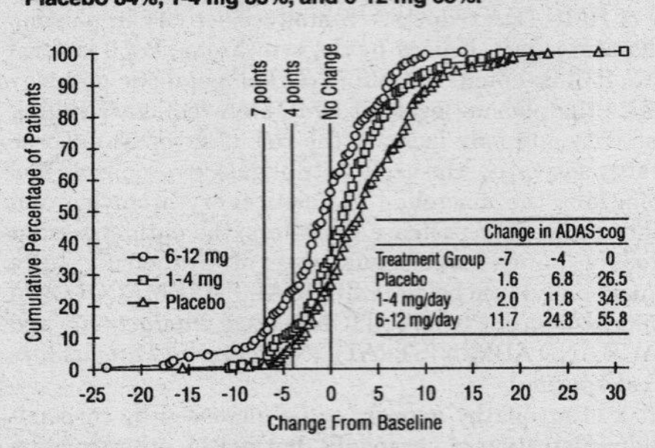
Cumulative Percentage of Patients
7 points
4 points
No Change
6-12 mg
1-4 mg
Placebo
Change in ADAS-cog
Treatment Group -7 -4 0
Placebo 1.6 6.8 26.5
1-4 mg/day 2.0 11.8 34.5
6-12 mg/day 11.7 24.8 55.8
Change From Baseline

Effects on the CIBIC-Plus: Figure 3 is a histogram of the frequency distribution of CIBIC-Plus scores attained by patients assigned to each of the three treatment groups who completed 26 weeks of treatment. The mean Exelon-placebo differences for these groups of patients in the mean rating of change from baseline were 0.32 units and 0.35 units for 1-4 mg and 6-12 mg of Exelon, respectively. The mean ratings for the 6-12 mg/day and 1-4 mg/day groups were statistically significantly superior to placebo. The differences between the 6-12 mg/day and the 1-4 mg/day groups were statistically significant.

Figure 3: Frequency Distribution of CIBIC-Plus Scores at Week 26

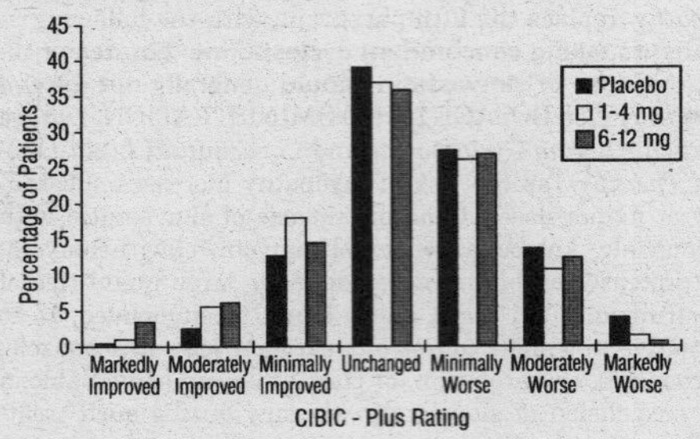
Percentage of Patients
Placebo
1-4 mg
6-12 mg
Markedly Improved
Moderately Improved
Minimally Improved
Unchanged
Minimally Worse
Moderately Worse
Markedly Worse
CIBIC - Plus Rating

Global Twenty-Six-Week Study

In a second study of 26 weeks duration, 725 patients were randomized to either a dose range of 1-4 mg or 6-12 mg of Exelon per day or to placebo, each given in divided doses. The 26-week study was divided into a 12-week forced dose titration phase and a 14-week maintenance phase. The patients in the active treatment arms of the study were maintained at their highest tolerated dose within the respective range.

Effects on the ADAS-cog: Figure 4 illustrates the time course for the change from baseline in ADAS-cog scores for all three dose groups over the 26 weeks of the study. At 26 weeks of treatment, the mean differences in the ADAS-cog change scores for the Exelon-treated patients compared to the patients on placebo were 0.2 and 2.6 units for the 1-4 mg and 6-12 mg treatments, respectively. The 6-12 mg/day group was statistically significantly superior to placebo, as well as to the 1-4 mg/day group. The difference between the 1-4 mg/day group and placebo was not statistically significant.

Figure 4: Time-course of the Change from Baseline in ADAS-cog Score for Patients Completing 26 Weeks of Treatment

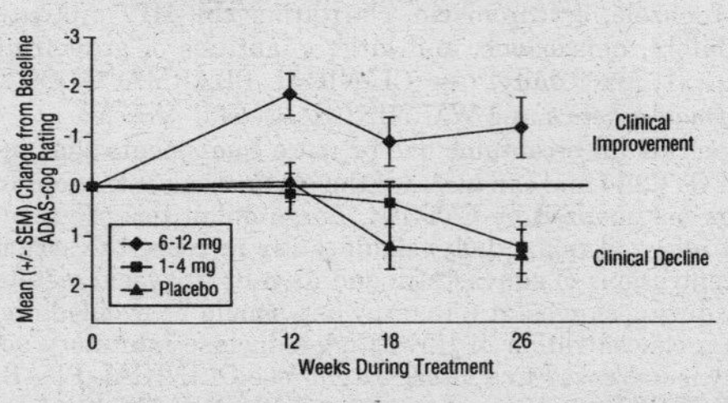
Mean (+/- SEM) Change from Baseline ADAS-cog Rating
Clinical Improvement
Clinical Decline
6-12 mg
1-4 mg
Placebo
Weeks During Treatment

Figure 5 illustrates the cumulative percentages of patients from each of the three treatment groups who had attained at least the measure of improvement in ADAS-cog score shown on the X axis. Similar to the U.S. 26-week study, the curves demonstrate that both patients assigned to Exelon and placebo have a wide range of responses, but that the 6-12 mg/day Exelongroup is more likely to show the greater improvements.

[See figure at top of next column]

Effects on the CIBIC-Plus: Figure 6 is a histogram of the frequency distribution of CIBIC-Plus scores attained by patients assigned to each of the three treatment groups who completed 26 weeks of treatment. The mean Exelon-placebo differences for these groups of patients for the mean rating of change from baseline were 0.14 units and 0.41 units for 1-4 mg and 6-12 mg of Exelon, respectively. The mean ratings for the 6-12 mg/day group was statistically significantly superior to placebo. The comparison of the mean ratings for the 1-4 mg/day group and placebo group was not statistically significant.

Figure 5: Cumulative Percentage of Patients Completing 26 Weeks of Double-blind Treatment with Specified Changes from Baseline ADAS-cog Scores. The Percentages of Randomized Patients who Completed the Study were: Placebo 87%, 1-4 mg 86%, and 6-12 mg 67%.

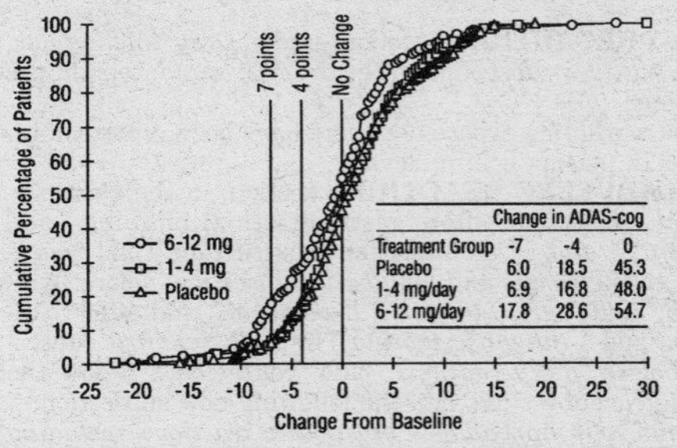
Cumulative Percentage of Patients
7 points
4 points
No Change
6-12 mg
1-4 mg
Placebo
Change in ADAS-cog
Treatment Group -7 -4 0
Placebo 6.0 18.5 45.3
1-4 mg/day 6.9 16.8 48.0
6-12 mg/day 17.8 28.6 54.7
Change From Baseline

Figure 6: Frequency Distribution of CIBIC-Plus Scores at Week 26

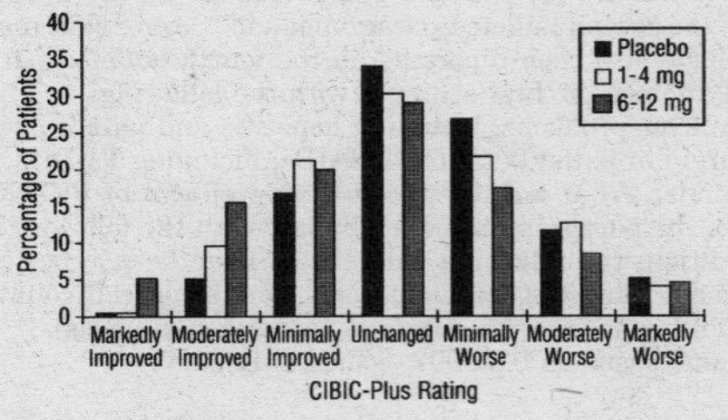
Percentage of Patients
Placebo
1-4 mg
6-12 mg
Markedly Improved
Moderately Improved
Minimally Improved
Unchanged
Minimally Worse
Moderately Worse
Markedly Worse
CIBIC-Plus Rating

U.S. Fixed Dose Study

In a study of 26 weeks' duration, 702 patients were randomized to doses of 3, 6, or 9 mg/day of Exelon or to placebo, each given in divided doses. The fixed-dose study design, which included a 12-week forced titration phase and a 14-week maintenance phase, led to a high dropout rate in the 9 mg/day group because of poor tolerability. At 26 weeks of treatment, significant differences were observed for the ADAS-cog mean change from baseline for the 9 mg/day and 6 mg/day groups, compared to placebo. No significant differences were observed between any of the Exelon dose groups and placebo for the analysis of the CIBIC-Plus mean rating of change. Although no significant differences were observed between Exelon treatment groups, there was a trend toward numerical superiority with higher doses.

Age, Gender and Race: Patient's age, gender, or race did not predict clinical outcome to Exelon treatment.

Pharmacokinetics

Rivastigmine is well absorbed with absolute bioavailability of about 40% (3-mg dose). It shows linear pharmacokinetics up to 3 mg BID but is non-linear at higher doses. Doubling the dose from 3 to 6 mg BID results in a 3-fold increase in AUC. The elimination half-life is about 1.5 hours, with most elimination as metabolites via the urine.

Absorption: Rivastigmine is rapidly and completely absorbed. Peak plasma concentrations are reached in approximately 1 hour. Absolute bioavailability after a 3-mg dose is about 36%. Administration of Exelon with food delays absorption (t_{max}) by 90 min, lowers C_{max} by approximately 30% and increases AUC by approximately 30%.

Distribution: Rivastigmine is widely distributed throughout the body with a volume of distribution in the range of 1.8-2.7 L/kg. Rivastigmine penetrates the blood brain barrier, reaching CSF peak concentrations in 1.4-2.6 hours. Mean AUC_{1-12hr} ratio of CSF/plasma averaged 40 ± 0.5% following 1-6 mg BID doses.

Rivastigmine is about 40% bound to plasma proteins at concentrations of 1-400 ng/mL, which cover the therapeutic concentration range. Rivastigmine distributes equally between blood and plasma with a blood-to-plasma partition ratio of 0.9 at concentrations ranging from 1-400 ng/mL.

Metabolism: Rivastigmine is rapidly and extensively metabolized, primarily via cholinesterase-mediated hydrolysis to the decarbamylated metabolite. Based on evidence from *in vitro* and animal studies the major cytochrome P450 isozymes are minimally involved in rivastigmine metabolism. Consistent with these observations is the finding that no drug interactions related to cytochrome P450 have been observed in humans (see Drug-Drug Interactions).

Elimination: The major pathway of elimination is via the kidneys. Following administration of ^{14}C-rivastigmine to 6 healthy volunteers total recovery of radioactivity over 120 hours was 97% in urine and 0.4% in feces. No parent drug was detected in urine. The sulfate conjugate of the decarbamylated metabolite is the major component excreted in urine and represents 40% of the dose. Mean oral clearance of rivastigmine is 1.8 ± 0.6 L/min after 6 mg BID.

Special Populations

Hepatic Disease: Following a single 3-mg dose, mean oral clearance of rivastigmine was 60% lower in hepatically impaired patients (n=10, biopsy proven) than in healthy subjects (n=10). After multiple 6 mg BID oral dosing, the mean clearance of rivastigmine was 65% lower in mild (n=7, Child-Pugh score 5-6) and moderate (n=3, Child-Pugh score 7-9) hepatically impaired patients (biopsy proven, liver cirrhosis) than in healthy subjects (n=10). Dosage adjustment is not necessary in hepatically impaired patients as the dose of drug is individually titrated to tolerability.

Renal Disease: Following a single 3-mg dose, mean oral clearance of rivastigmine is 64% lower in moderately impaired renal patients (n=8, GFR=10-50 mL/min) than in healthy subjects (n=10, GFR≥60 mL/min); Cl/F=1.7 L/min (cv=45%) and 4.8 L/min (cv=80%), respectively. In severely impaired renal patients (n=8, GFR<10 mL/min), mean oral clearance of rivastigmine is 43% higher than in healthy subjects (n=10, GFR≥60 mL/min); Cl/F=6.9 L/min and 4.8 L/min, respectively. For unexplained reasons, the severely impaired renal patients had a higher clearance of rivastigmine than moderately impaired patients. However, dosage adjustment may not be necessary in renally impaired patients as the dose of the drug is individually titrated to tolerability.

Age: Following a single 2.5 mg oral dose to elderly volunteers (>60 years of age, n=24) and younger volunteers (n=24), mean oral clearance of rivastigmine was 30% lower in elderly (7 L/min) than in younger subjects (10 L/min).

Gender and Race: No specific pharmacokinetic study was conducted to investigate the effect of gender and race on the disposition of Exelon, but a population pharmacokinetic analysis indicates that gender (n=277 males and 348 females) and race (n=575 White, 34 Black, 4 Asian, and 12 Other) did not affect the clearance of Exelon.

Nicotine Use: Population PK analysis showed that nicotine use increases the oral clearance of rivastigmine by 23% (n=75 Smokers and 549 Nonsmokers).

Drug-Drug Interactions

Effect of Exelon on the Metabolism of Other Drugs: Rivastigmine is primarily metabolized through hydrolysis by esterases. Minimal metabolism occurs via the major cytochrome P450 isoenzymes. Based on *in vitro* studies, no pharmacokinetic drug interactions with drugs metabolized by the following isoenzyme systems are expected: CYP1A2, CYP2D6, CYP3A4/5, CYP2E1, CYP2C9, CYP2C8, or CYP2C19.

No pharmacokinetic interaction was observed between rivastigmine and digoxin, warfarin, diazepam, or fluoxetine in studies in healthy volunteers. The elevation of prothrombin time induced by warfarin is not affected by administration of Exelon.

Effect of Other Drugs on the Metabolism of Exelon: Drugs that induce or inhibit CYP450 metabolism are not expected to alter the metabolism of rivastigmine. Single dose pharmacokinetic studies demonstrated that the metabolism of rivastigmine is not significantly affected by concurrent administration of digoxin, warfarin, diazepam, or fluoxetine. Population PK analysis with a database of 625 patients showed that the pharmacokinetics of rivastigmine were not influenced by commonly prescribed medications such as antacids (n=77), antihypertensives (n=72), β-blockers (n=42), calcium channel blockers (n=75), antidiabetics (n=21), nonsteroidal anti-inflammatory drugs (n=79), estrogens (n=70), salicylate analgesics (n=177), antianginals (n=35), and antihistamines (n=15). In addition, in clinical trials, no increased risk of clinically relevant untoward effects was observed in patients treated concomitantly with Exelon and these agents.

INDICATIONS AND USAGE

Exelon® (rivastigmine tartrate) is indicated for the treatment of mild to moderate dementia of the Alzheimer's type.

CONTRAINDICATIONS

Exelon® (rivastigmine tartrate) is contraindicated in patients with known hypersensitivity to rivastigmine, other carbamate derivatives or other components of the formulation (see DESCRIPTION).

WARNINGS

Gastrointestinal Adverse Reactions

Exelon® (rivastigmine tartrate) use is associated with significant gastrointestinal adverse reactions, including nausea and vomiting, anorexia, and weight loss. For this reason, patients should always be started at a dose of 1.5 mg BID and titrated to their maintenance dose. If treatment is interrupted for longer than several days, treatment should be reinitiated with the lowest daily dose (see DOSAGE AND ADMINISTRATION) to reduce the possibility of severe vomiting and its potentially serious sequelae (e.g., there has been one post-marketing report of severe vomiting with esophageal rupture following inappropriate reinitiation of treatment with a 4.5-mg dose after 8 weeks of treatment interruption).

Nausea and Vomiting: **In the controlled clinical trials, 47% of the patients treated with an Exelon dose in the therapeutic range of 6-12 mg/day (n=1189) developed nausea (compared with 12% in placebo). A total of 31% of Exelon-treated patients developed at least one episode of vomiting (compared with 6% for placebo). The rate of vomiting was higher during the titration phase (24% vs. 3% for placebo) than in the maintenance phase (14% vs. 3% for placebo). The rates were higher in women than men. Five percent of patients discontinued for vomiting, compared to less than 1% for patients on placebo. Vomiting was severe in 2% of Exelon-treated patients and was rated as mild or moderate each in 14% of patients. The rate of nausea was higher during the titration phase (43% vs. 9% for placebo) than in the maintenance phase (17% vs. 4% for placebo).**

Weight Loss: **In the controlled trials, approximately 26% of women on high doses of Exelon (greater than 9 mg/day) had weight loss of equal to or greater than 7% of their baseline weight compared to 6% in the placebo-treated patients. About 18% of the males in the high dose group experienced a similar degree of weight loss compared to 4% in placebo-treated patients. It is not clear how much of the weight loss was associated with anorexia, nausea, vomiting, and the diarrhea associated with the drug.**

Table 1. Most Frequent Adverse Events Leading to Withdrawal from Clinical Trials during Titration and Maintenance in Patients Receiving 6-12 mg/day Exelon® Using a Forced Dose Titration

Study Phase	Titration		Maintenance		Overall	
	Placebo (n=868)	Exelon ≥6-12 mg/day (n=1189)	Placebo (n=788)	Exelon ≥6-12 mg/day (n=987)	Placebo (n=868)	Exelon ≥6-12 mg/day (n=1189)
Event/% Discontinuing						
Nausea	<1	8	<1	1	1	8
Vomiting	<1	4	<1	1	<1	5
Anorexia	0	2	<1	1	<1	3
Dizziness	<1	2	<1	1	<1	2

Anorexia: In the controlled clinical trials, of the patients treated with an Exelon dose of 6-12 mg/day, 17% developed anorexia compared to 3% of the placebo patients. Neither the time course or the severity of the anorexia is known.

Peptic Ulcers/Gastrointestinal Bleeding: Because of their pharmacological action, cholinesterase inhibitors may be expected to increase gastric acid secretion due to increased cholinergic activity. Therefore, patients should be monitored closely for symptoms of active or occult gastrointestinal bleeding, especially those at increased risk for developing ulcers, e.g., those with a history of ulcer disease or those receiving concurrent nonsteroidal anti-inflammatory drugs (NSAIDS). Clinical studies of Exelon have shown no significant increase, relative to placebo, in the incidence of either peptic ulcer disease or gastrointestinal bleeding.

Anesthesia

Exelon as a cholinesterase inhibitor, is likely to exaggerate succinylcholine-type muscle relaxation during anesthesia.

Cardiovascular Conditions

Drugs that increase cholinergic activity may have vagotonic effects on heart rate (e.g., bradycardia). The potential for this action may be particularly important to patients with "sick sinus syndrome" or other supraventricular cardiac conduction conditions. In clinical trials, Exelon was not associated with any increased incidence of cardiovascular adverse events, heart rate or blood pressure changes, or ECG abnormalities. Syncopal episodes have been reported in 3% of patients receiving 6-12 mg/day of Exelon, compared to 2% of placebo patients.

Genitourinary

Although this was not observed in clinical trials of Exelon, drugs that increase cholinergic activity may cause urinary obstruction.

Neurological Conditions

Seizures: Drugs that increase cholinergic activity are believed to have some potential for causing seizures. However, seizure activity also may be a manifestation of Alzheimer's Disease.

Pulmonary Conditions

Like other drugs that increase cholinergic activity, Exelon should be used with care in patients with a history of asthma or obstructive pulmonary disease.

PRECAUTIONS

Information for Patients and Caregivers

Caregivers should be advised of the high incidence of nausea and vomiting associated with the use of the drug along with the possibility of anorexia and weight loss. Caregivers should be encouraged to monitor for these adverse events and inform the physician if they occur. It is critical to inform caregivers that if therapy has been interrupted for more than several days, the next dose should not be administered until they have discussed this with the physician.

Drug-Drug Interactions

Effect of Exelon® (rivastigmine tartrate) on the Metabolism of Other Drugs: Rivastigmine is primarily metabolized through hydrolysis by esterases. Minimal metabolism occurs via the major cytochrome P450 isoenzymes. Based on *in vitro* studies, no pharmacokinetic drug interactions with drugs metabolized by the following isoenzyme systems are expected: CYP1A2, CYP2D6, CYP3A4/5, CYP2E1, CYP2C9, CYP2C8, or CYP2C19.

No pharmacokinetic interaction was observed between rivastigmine and digoxin, warfarin, diazepam, or fluoxetine in studies in healthy volunteers. The elevation of prothrombin time induced by warfarin is not affected by administration of Exelon.

Effect of Other Drugs on the Metabolism of Exelon: Drugs that induce or inhibit CYP450 metabolism are not expected to alter the metabolism of rivastigmine. Single dose pharmacokinetic studies demonstrated that the metabolism of rivastigmine is not significantly affected by concurrent administration of digoxin, warfarin, diazepam, or fluoxetine. Population PK analysis with a database of 625 patients showed that the pharmacokinetics of rivastigmine were not influenced by commonly prescribed medications such as antacids (n=77), antihypertensives (n=72), β-blockers (n=42), calcium channel blockers (n=75), antidiabetics (n=21), nonsteroidal anti-inflammatory drugs (n=79), estrogens (n=70), salicylate analgesics (n=177), antianginals (n=35), and antihistamines (n=15).

Use with Anticholinergics: Because of their mechanism of action, cholinesterase inhibitors have the potential to interfere with the activity of anticholinergic medications.

Use with Cholinomimetics and Other Cholinesterase Inhibitors: A synergistic effect may be expected when cholinesterase inhibitors are given concurrently with succinylcholine, similar neuromuscular blocking agents or cholinergic agonists such as bethanechol.

Carcinogenesis, Mutagenesis, Impairment of Fertility

In carcinogenicity studies conducted at dose levels up to 1.1 mg-base/kg/day in rats and 1.6 mg-base/kg/day in mice, rivastigmine was not carcinogenic. These dose levels are approximately 0.9 times and 0.7 times the maximum recommended human daily dose of 12 mg/day on a mg/m^2 basis.

Rivastigmine was clastogenic in two *in vitro* assays in the presence, but not the absence, of metabolic activation. It caused structural chromosomal aberrations in V79 Chinese hamster lung cells and both structural and numerical (polyploidy) chromosomal aberrations in human peripheral blood lymphocytes. Rivastigmine was not genotoxic in three *in vitro* assays: the Ames test, the unscheduled DNA synthesis (UDS) test in rat hepatocytes (a test for induction of DNA repair synthesis), and the HGPRT test in V79 Chinese hamster cells. Rivastigmine was not clastogenic in the *in vivo* mouse micronucleus test.

Rivastigmine had no effect on fertility or reproductive performance in the rat at dose levels up to 1.1 mg-base/kg/day. This dose is approximately 0.9 times the maximum recommended human daily dose of 12 mg/day on a mg/m^2 basis.

Pregnancy

Pregnancy Category B: Reproduction studies conducted in pregnant rats at doses up to 2.3 mg-base/kg/day (approximately 2 times the maximum recommended human dose on a mg/m^2 basis) and in pregnant rabbits at doses up to 2.3 mg-base/kg/day (approximately 4 times the maximum recommended human dose on a mg/m^2 basis) revealed no evidence of teratogenicity. Studies in rats showed slightly decreased fetal/pup weights, usually at doses causing some maternal toxicity; decreased weights were seen at doses which were several fold lower than the maximum recommended human dose on a mg/m^2 basis. There are no adequate or well-controlled studies in pregnant women. Because animal reproduction studies are not always predictive of human response, Exelon should be used during pregnancy only if the potential benefit justifies the potential risk to the fetus.

Nursing Mothers

It is not known whether rivastigmine is excreted in human breast milk. Exelon has no indication for use in nursing mothers.

Pediatric Use

There are no adequate and well-controlled trials documenting the safety and efficacy of Exelon in any illness occurring in children.

ADVERSE REACTIONS

Adverse Events Leading to Discontinuation

The rate of discontinuation due to adverse events in controlled clinical trials of Exelon® (rivastigmine tartrate) was 15% for patients receiving 6-12 mg/day compared to 5% for patients on placebo during forced weekly dose titration. While on a maintenance dose, the rates were 6% for patients on Exelon compared to 4% for those on placebo.

The most common adverse events leading to discontinuation, defined as those occurring in at least 2% of patients and at twice the incidence seen in placebo patients, are shown in Table 1.

[See table above]

Most Frequent Adverse Clinical Events Seen in Association with the Use of Exelon

The most common adverse events, defined as those occurring at a frequency of at least 5% and twice the placebo rate, are largely predicted by Exelon's cholinergic effects. These include nausea, vomiting, anorexia, dyspepsia, and asthenia.

Gastrointestinal Adverse Reactions

Exelon use is associated with significant nausea, vomiting, and weight loss (see WARNINGS).

Adverse Events Reported in Controlled Trials

Table 2 lists treatment emergent signs and symptoms that were reported in at least 2% of patients in placebo-controlled trials and for which the rate of occurrence was greater for patients treated with Exelon doses of 6-12 mg/day than for those treated with placebo. The prescriber should be aware that these figures cannot be used to predict the frequency of adverse events in the course of usual medical practice when patient characteristics and other factors may differ from those prevailing during clinical studies. Similarly, the cited frequencies cannot be directly compared with figures obtained from other clinical investigations involving different treatments, uses, or investigators. An inspection of these frequencies, however, does provide the prescriber with one basis by which to estimate the relative contribution of drug and non-drug factors to the adverse event incidences in the population studied.

In general, adverse reactions were less frequent later in the course of treatment.

Continued on next page

Exelon Capsules—Cont.

No systematic effect of race or age could be determined on the incidence of adverse events in the controlled studies. Nausea, vomiting and weight loss were more frequent in women than men.

Table 2. Adverse Events Reported in Controlled Clinical Trials in at Least 2% of Patients Receiving Exelon® (6-12 mg/day) and at a Higher Frequency than Placebo-treated Patients

Body System/Adverse Event	Placebo (n=868)	Exelon (6-12 mg/day) (n=1189)
Percent of Patients with any Adverse Event	79	92
Autonomic Nervous System		
Sweating increased	1	4
Syncope	2	3
Body as a Whole		
Accidental Trauma	9	10
Fatigue	5	9
Asthenia	2	6
Malaise	2	5
Influenza-like Symptoms	2	3
Weight Decrease	<1	3
Cardiovascular Disorders, General		
Hypertension	2	3
Central and Peripheral Nervous System		
Dizziness	11	21
Headache	12	17
Somnolence	3	5
Tremor	1	4
Gastrointestinal System		
Nausea	12	47
Vomiting	6	31
Diarrhea	11	19
Anorexia	3	17
Abdominal Pain	6	13
Dyspepsia	4	9
Constipation	4	5
Flatulence	2	4
Eructation	1	2
Psychiatric Disorders		
Insomnia	7	9
Confusion	7	8
Depression	4	6
Anxiety	3	5
Hallucination	3	4
Aggressive Reaction	2	3
Resistance Mechanism Disorders		
Urinary Tract Infection	6	7
Respiratory System		
Rhinitis	3	4

Other adverse events observed at a rate of 2% or more on Exelon 6-12 mg/day but at a greater or equal rate on placebo were chest pain, peripheral edema, vertigo, back pain, arthralgia, pain, bone fracture, agitation, nervousness, delusion, paranoid reaction, upper respiratory tract infections, infection (general), coughing, pharyngitis, bronchitis, rash (general), urinary incontinence.

Other Adverse Events Observed During Clinical Trials

Exelon has been administered to over 5297 individuals during clinical trials worldwide. Of these, 4326 patients have been treated for at least 3 months, 3407 patients have been treated for at least 6 months, 2150 patients have been treated for 1 year, 1250 have been treated for 2 years, and 168 have been treated for over 3 years. With regard to exposure to the highest dose, 2809 patients were exposed to doses of 10-12 mg, 2615 patients treated for 3 months, 2328 patients treated for 6 months, 1378 patients treated for 1 year, 917 patients treated for 2 years, and 129 treated for over 3 years.

Treatment emergent signs and symptoms that occurred during 8 controlled clinical trials and 9 open-label trials in North America, Western Europe, Australia, South Africa, and Japan were recorded as adverse events by the clinical investigators using terminology of their own choosing. To provide an overall estimate of the proportion of individuals having similar types of events, the events were grouped into a smaller number of standardized categories using a modified WHO dictionary, and event frequencies were calculated across all studies. These categories are used in the listing below. The frequencies represent the proportion of 5297 patients from these trials who experienced that event while receiving Exelon. All adverse events occurring in at least 6 patients (approximately 0.1%) are included, except for those already listed elsewhere in labeling, WHO terms too general to be informative, relatively minor events, or events unlikely to be drug caused. Events are classified by body system and listed using the following definitions: frequent adverse events — those occurring in at least 1/100 patients; infrequent adverse events — those occurring in 1/100 to 1/1000 patients. These adverse events are not necessarily related to Exelon treatment and in most cases were observed at a similar frequency in placebo-treated patients in the controlled studies.

Autonomic Nervous System: *Infrequent:* Cold clammy skin, dry mouth, flushing, increased saliva.

Body as a Whole: *Frequent:* Accidental trauma, fever, edema, allergy, hot flushes, rigors. *Infrequent:* Edema periorbital or facial, hypothermia, edema, feeling cold, halitosis.

Cardiovascular System: *Frequent:* Hypotension, postural hypotension, cardiac failure.

Central and Peripheral Nervous System: *Frequent:* Abnormal gait, ataxia, paraesthesia, convulsions. *Infrequent:* Paresis, apraxia, aphasia, dysphonia, hyperkinesia, hyperreflexia, hypertonia, hypoesthesia, hypokinesia, migraine, neuralgia, nystagmus, peripheral neuropathy.

Endocrine System: *Infrequent:* Goitre, hypothyroidism.

Gastrointestinal System: *Frequent:* Fecal incontinence, gastritis. *Infrequent:* Dysphagia, esophagitis, gastric ulcer, gastritis, gastroesophageal reflux, GI hemorrhage, hernia, intestinal obstruction, melena, rectal hemorrhage, gastroenteritis, ulcerative stomatitis, duodenal ulcer, hematemesis, gingivitis, tenesmus, pancreatitis, colitis, glossitis.

Hearing and Vestibular Disorders: *Frequent:* Tinnitus.

Heart Rate and Rhythm Disorders: *Frequent:* Atrial fibrillation, bradycardia, palpitation. *Infrequent:* AV block, bundle branch block, sick sinus syndrome, cardiac arrest, supraventricular tachycardia, extrasystoles, tachycardia.

Liver and Biliary System Disorders: *Infrequent:* Abnormal hepatic function, cholecystitis.

Metabolic and Nutritional Disorders: *Frequent:* Dehydration, hypokalemia. *Infrequent:* Diabetes mellitus, gout, hypercholesterolemia, hyperlipemia, hypoglycemia, cachexia, thirst, hyperglycemia, hyponatremia.

Musculoskeletal Disorders: *Frequent:* Arthritis, leg cramps, myalgia. *Infrequent:* Cramps, hernia, muscle weakness.

Myo-, Endo-, Pericardial and Valve Disorders: *Frequent:* Angina pectoris, myocardial infarction.

Platelet, Bleeding, and Clotting Disorders: *Frequent:* Epistaxis. *Infrequent:* Hematoma, thrombocytopenia, purpura.

Psychiatric Disorders: *Frequent:* Paranoid reaction, confusion. *Infrequent:* Abnormal dreaming, amnesia, apathy, delirium, dementia, depersonalization, emotional lability, impaired concentration, decreased libido, personality disorder, suicide attempt, increased libido, neurosis, suicidal ideation, psychosis.

Red Blood Cell Disorders: *Frequent:* Anemia. *Infrequent:* Hypochromic anemia.

Reproductive Disorders (Female & Male): *Infrequent:* Breast pain, impotence, atrophic vaginitis.

Resistance Mechanism Disorders: *Infrequent:* Cellulitis, cystitis, herpes simplex, otitis media.

Respiratory System: *Infrequent:* Bronchospasm, laryngitis, apnea.

Skin and Appendages: *Frequent:* Rashes of various kinds (maculopapular, eczema, bullous, exfoliative, psoriaform, erythematous). *Infrequent:* Alopecia, skin ulceration, urticaria, dermatitis contact.

Special Senses: *Infrequent:* Perversion of taste, loss of taste.

Urinary System Disorders: *Frequent:* Hematuria. *Infrequent:* Albuminuria, oliguria, acute renal failure, dysuria, micturition urgency, nocturia, polyuria, renal calculus, urinary retention.

Vascular (extracardiac) Disorders: *Infrequent:* Hemorrhoids, peripheral ischemia, pulmonary embolism, thrombosis, thrombophlebitis deep, aneurysm, hemorrhage intracranial.

Vision Disorders: *Frequent:* Cataract. *Infrequent:* Conjunctival hemorrhage, blepharitis, diplopia, eye pain, glaucoma.

White Cell and Resistance Disorders: *Infrequent:* Lymphadenopathy, leukocytosis.

Post-Introduction Reports

Voluntary reports of adverse events temporally associated with Exelon that have been received since market introduction that are not listed above, and that may or may not be causally related to the drug include the following:

Skin and Appendages: Stevens-Johnson syndrome.

OVERDOSAGE

Because strategies for the management of overdose are continually evolving, it is advisable to contact a Poison Control Center to determine the latest recommendations for the management of an overdose of any drug.

As Exelon® (rivastigmine tartrate) has a short plasma half-life of about one hour and a moderate duration of acetylcholinesterase inhibition of 8-10 hours, it is recommended that in cases of asymptomatic overdoses, no further dose of Exelon should be administered for the next 24 hours.

As in any case of overdose, general supportive measures should be utilized. Overdosage with cholinesterase inhibitors can result in cholinergic crisis characterized by severe nausea, vomiting, salivation, sweating, bradycardia, hypotension, respiratory depression, collapse and convulsions. Increasing muscle weakness is a possibility and may result in death if respiratory muscles are involved. Atypical responses in blood pressure and heart rate have been reported with other drugs that increase cholinergic activity when co-administered with quaternary anticholinergics such as glycopyrrolate. Due to the short half-life of Exelon, dialysis (hemodialysis, peritoneal dialysis, or hemofiltration) would not be clinically indicated in the event of an overdose.

In overdoses accompanied by severe nausea and vomiting, the use of antiemetics should be considered. In a documented case of a 46 mg overdose with Exelon, the patient experienced vomiting, incontinence, hypertension, psychomotor retardation, and loss of consciousness. The patient fully recovered within 24 hours and conservative management was all that was required for treatment.

DOSAGE AND ADMINISTRATION

The dosage of Exelon® (rivastigmine tartrate) shown to be effective in controlled clinical trials is 6-12 mg/day, given as twice a day dosing (daily doses of 3 to 6 mg BID). There is evidence from the clinical trials that doses at the higher end of this range may be more beneficial.

The starting dose of Exelon is 1.5 mg twice a day (BID). If this dose is well tolerated, after a minimum of two weeks of treatment, the dose may be increased to 3 mg BID. Subsequent increases to 4.5 mg BID and 6 mg BID should be attempted after a minimum of 2 weeks at the previous dose. If adverse effects (e.g., nausea, vomiting, abdominal pain, loss of appetite) cause intolerance during treatment, the patient should be instructed to discontinue treatment for several doses and then restart at the same or next lower dose level. If treatment is interrupted for longer than several days, treatment should be reinitiated with the lowest daily dose and titrated as described above (see WARNINGS). The maximum dose is 6 mg BID (12 mg/day).

Exelon should be taken with meals in divided doses in the morning and evening.

HOW SUPPLIED

Exelon® (rivastigmine tartrate) capsules equivalent to 1.5 mg, 3 mg, 4.5 mg, or 6 mg of rivastigmine base are available as follows:

1.5 mg Capsule — yellow, "Exelon 1,5 mg" is printed in red on the body of the capsule.

Bottles of 60	NDC 0078-0323-44
Bottles of 500	NDC 0078-0323-08
Unit Dose (blister pack) Box of 100 (strips of 10)	NDC 0078-0323-06

3 mg Capsule — orange, "Exelon 3 mg" is printed in red on the body of the capsule.

Bottles of 60	NDC 0078-0324-44
Bottles of 500	NDC 0078-0324-08
Unit Dose (blister pack) Box of 100 (strips of 10)	NDC 0078-0324-06

4.5 mg Capsule — red, "Exelon 4,5 mg" is printed in white on the body of the capsule.

Bottles of 60	NDC 0078-0325-44
Bottles of 500	NDC 0078-0325-08
Unit Dose (blister pack) Box of 100 (strips of 10)	NDC 0078-0325-06

6 mg Capsule — orange and red, "Exelon 6 mg" is printed in red on the body of the capsule.

Bottles of 60	NDC 0078-0326-44
Bottles of 500	NDC 0078-0326-08
Unit Dose (blister pack) Box of 100 (strips of 10)	NDC 0078-0326-06

Store below 77°F (25°C) in a tight container.

T2000-74
REV: JANUARY 2001 Printed in U.S.A. 89007403
Manufactured by
Novartis Pharma AG
Basle, Switzerland
Manufactured for
Novartis Pharmaceuticals Corporation
East Hanover, New Jersey 07936

EXELON® ℞

[ĕx' ə-lŏn]

(rivastigmine tartrate)
Oral Solution
Rx only

Prescribing information for this product, which appears on pages 2174–2177 of the 2001 PDR, has been completely revised as follows. Please write "See Supplement A" next to the product heading.

DESCRIPTION

Exelon® (rivastigmine tartrate) is a reversible cholinesterase inhibitor and is known chemically as (S)-N-Ethyl-N-methyl-3-[1-(dimethylamino)ethyl]-phenyl carbamate hydrogen-(2R,3R)-tartrate. Rivastigmine tartrate is commonly referred to in the pharmacological literature as SDZ ENA 713 or ENA 713. It has an empirical formula of $C_{14}H_{22}N_2O_2 \bullet C_4H_6O_6$ (hydrogen tartrate salt – hta salt) and a molecular weight of 400.43 (hta salt). Rivastigmine tartrate is a white to off-white, fine crystalline powder that is very soluble in water, soluble in ethanol and acetonitrile, slightly soluble in n-octanol and very slightly soluble in ethyl acetate. The distribution coefficient at 37°C in n-octanol/phosphate buffer solution pH 7 is 3.0.

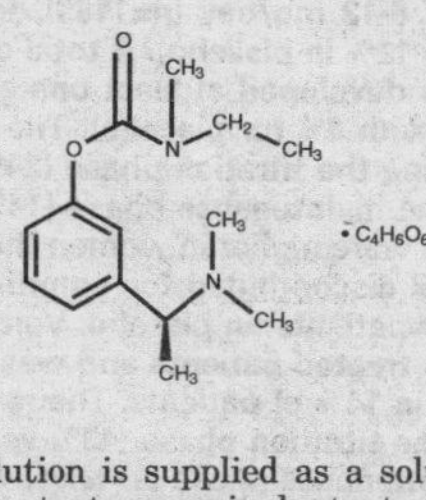

Exelon Oral Solution is supplied as a solution containing rivastigmine tartrate, equivalent to 2 mg/mL of rivastigmine base for oral administration. Inactive ingredients are citric acid, D&C yellow #10, purified water, sodium benzoate and sodium citrate.

CLINICAL PHARMACOLOGY

Mechanism of Action

Pathological changes in Dementia of the Alzheimer type involve cholinergic neuronal pathways that project from the basal forebrain to the cerebral cortex and hippocampus. These pathways are thought to be intricately involved in memory, attention, learning, and other cognitive processes. While the precise mechanism of rivastigmine's action is unknown, it is postulated to exert its therapeutic effect by enhancing cholinergic function. This is accomplished by increasing the concentration of acetylcholine through reversible inhibition of its hydrolysis by cholinesterase. If this proposed mechanism is correct, Exelon's effect may lessen as the disease process advances and fewer cholinergic neurons remain functionally intact. There is no evidence that rivastigmine alters the course of the underlying dementing process. After a 6-mg dose of rivastigmine, anticholinesterase activity is present in CSF for about 10 hours, with a maximum inhibition of about 60% five hours after dosing.

Clinical Trial Data

The effectiveness of Exelon® (rivastigmine tartrate) as a treatment for Alzheimer's Disease is demonstrated by the results of two randomized, double-blind, placebo-controlled clinical investigations in patients with Alzheimer's Disease [diagnosed by NINCDS-ADRDA and DSM-IV criteria, Mini-Mental State Examination (MMSE) ≥10 and ≤26, and the Global Deterioration Scale (GDS)]. The mean age of patients participating in Exelon trials was 73 years with a range of 41-95. Approximately 59% of patients were women and 41% were men. The racial distribution was Caucasian 87%, Black 4% and Other races 9%.

Study Outcome Measures: In each study, the effectiveness of Exelon was evaluated using a dual outcome assessment strategy.

The ability of Exelon to improve cognitive performance was assessed with the cognitive subscale of the Alzheimer's Disease Assessment Scale (ADAS-cog), a multi-item instrument that has been extensively validated in longitudinal cohorts of Alzheimer's Disease patients. The ADAS-cog examines selected aspects of cognitive performance including elements of memory, orientation, attention, reasoning, language and praxis. The ADAS-cog scoring range is from 0 to 70, with higher scores indicating greater cognitive impairment. Elderly normal adults may score as low as 0 or 1, but it is not unusual for non-demented adults to score slightly higher.

The patients recruited as participants in each study had mean scores on ADAS-cog of approximately 23 units, with a range from 1 to 61. Experience gained in longitudinal studies of ambulatory patients with mild to moderate Alzheimer's Disease suggest that they gain 6-12 units a year on the ADAS-cog. Lesser degrees of change, however, are seen in patients with very mild or very advanced disease because the ADAS-cog is not uniformly sensitive to change over the course of the disease. The annualized rate of decline in the placebo patients participating in Exelon trials was approximately 3-8 units per year.

The ability of Exelon to produce an overall clinical effect was assessed using a Clinician's Interview Based Impression of Change that required the use of caregiver information, the CIBIC-Plus. The CIBIC-Plus is not a single instrument and is not a standardized instrument like the ADAS-cog. Clinical trials for investigational drugs have used a variety of CIBIC formats, each different in terms of depth and structure. As such, results from a CIBIC-Plus reflect clinical experience from the trial or trials in which it was used and can not be compared directly with the results of CIBIC-Plus evaluations from other clinical trials. The CIBIC-Plus used in the Exelon trials was a structured instrument based on a comprehensive evaluation at baseline and subsequent timepoints of three domains: patient cognition, behavior and functioning, including assessment of activities of daily living. It represents the assessment of a skilled clinician using validated scales based on his/her observation at interviews conducted separately with the patient and the caregiver familiar with the behavior of the patient over the interval rated. The CIBIC-Plus is scored as a seven point categorical rating, ranging from a score of 1, indicating "markedly improved," to a score of 4, indicating "no change" to a score of 7, indicating "marked worsening." The CIBIC-Plus has not been systematically compared directly to assessments not using information from caregivers (CIBIC) or other global methods.

U.S. Twenty-Six-Week Study

In a study of 26 weeks duration, 699 patients were randomized to either a dose range of 1-4 mg or 6-12 mg of Exelon per day or to placebo, each given in divided doses. The 26-week study was divided into a 12-week forced dose titration phase and a 14-week maintenance phase. The patients in the active treatment arms of the study were maintained at their highest tolerated dose within the respective range.

Effects on the ADAS-cog: Figure 1 illustrates the time course for the change from baseline in ADAS-cog scores for all three dose groups over the 26 weeks of the study. At 26 weeks of treatment, the mean differences in the ADAS-cog change scores for the Exelon-treated patients compared to the patients on placebo were 1.9 and 4.9 units for the 1-4 mg and 6-12 mg treatments, respectively. Both treatments were statistically significantly superior to placebo and the

6-12 mg/day range was significantly superior to the 1-4 mg/day range.

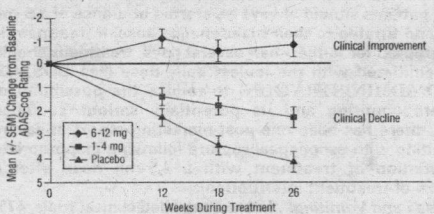

Figure 1: Time-course of the Change from Baseline in ADAS-cog Score for Patients Completing 26 Weeks of Treatment

Figure 2 illustrates the cumulative percentages of patients from each of the three treatment groups who had attained at least the measure of improvement in ADAS-cog score shown on the X axis. Three change scores, (7-point and 4-point reductions from baseline or no change in score) have been identified for illustrative purposes, and the percent of patients in each group achieving that result is shown in the inset table.

The curves demonstrate that both patients assigned to Exelon and placebo have a wide range of responses, but that the Exelon groups are more likely to show the greater improvements. A curve for an effective treatment would be shifted to the left of the curve for placebo, while an ineffective or deleterious treatment would be superimposed upon, or shifted to the right of the curve for placebo, respectively.

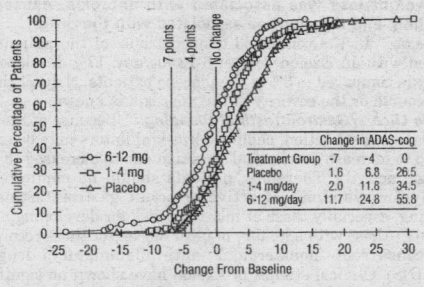

Figure 2: Cumulative Percentage of Patients Completing 26 Weeks of Double-blind Treatment with Specified Changes from Baseline ADAS-cog Scores. The Percentages of Randomized Patients who Completed the Study were: Placebo 84%, 1-4 mg 85%, and 6-12 mg 65%.

Treatment Group	Change in ADAS-cog -7	-4	0
Placebo	1.6	6.8	26.5
1-4 mg/day	2.0	11.8	34.5
6-12 mg/day	11.7	24.8	55.8

Effects on the CIBIC-Plus: Figure 3 is a histogram of the frequency distribution of CIBIC-Plus scores attained by patients assigned to each of the three treatment groups who completed 26 weeks of treatment. The mean Exelon-placebo differences for these groups of patients in the mean rating of change from baseline were 0.32 units and 0.35 units for 1-4 mg and 6-12 mg of Exelon, respectively. The mean ratings for the 6-12 mg/day and 1-4 mg/day groups were statistically significantly superior to placebo. The differences between the 6-12 mg/day and the 1-4 mg/day groups were statistically significant.

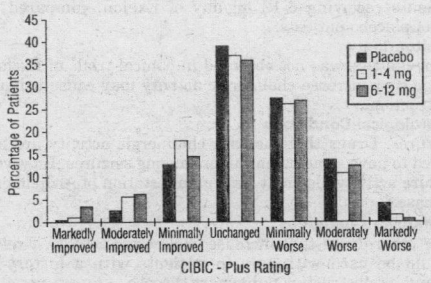

Figure 3: Frequency Distribution of CIBIC-Plus Scores at Week 26

Global Twenty-Six-Week Study

In a second study of 26 weeks duration, 725 patients were randomized to either a dose range of 1-4 mg or 6-12 mg of Exelon per day or to placebo, each given in divided doses. The 26-week study was divided into a 12-week forced dose titration phase and a 14-week maintenance phase. The patients in the active treatment arms of the study were maintained at their highest tolerated dose within the respective range.

Effects on the ADAS-cog: Figure 4 illustrates the time course for the change from baseline in ADAS-cog scores for all three dose groups over the 26 weeks of the study. At 26 weeks of treatment, the mean differences in the ADAS-cog change scores for the Exelon-treated patients compared to the patients on placebo were 0.2 and 2.6 units for the 1-4 mg and 6-12 mg treatments, respectively. The 6-12 mg/day group was statistically significantly superior to placebo, as well as to the 1-4 mg/day group. The difference between the 1-4 mg/day group and placebo was not statistically significant.

[See figure at top of next column]

Figure 5 illustrates the cumulative percentages of patients from each of the three treatment groups who had attained at least the measure of improvement in ADAS-cog score

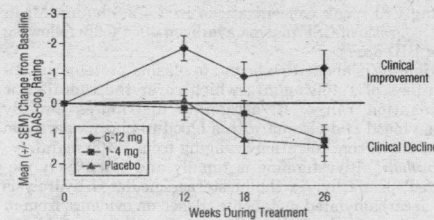

Figure 4: Time-course of the Change from Baseline in ADAS-cog Score for Patients Completing 26 Weeks of Treatment

shown on the X axis. Similar to the U.S. 26-week study, the curves demonstrate that both patients assigned to Exelon and placebo have a wide range of responses, but that the 6-12 mg/day Exelon group is more likely to show the greater improvements.

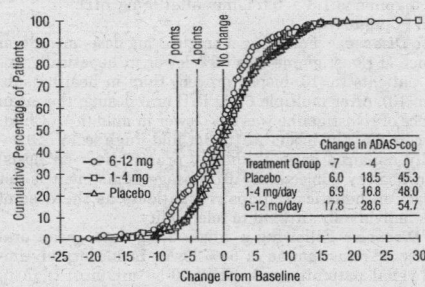

Figure 5: Cumulative Percentage of Patients Completing 26 Weeks of Double-blind Treatment with Specified Changes from Baseline ADAS-cog Scores. The Percentages of Randomized Patients who Completed the Study were: Placebo 87%, 1-4 mg 86%, and 6-12 mg 67%.

Treatment Group	Change in ADAS-cog -7	-4	0
Placebo	6.0	18.5	45.3
1-4 mg/day	6.9	16.8	48.0
6-12 mg/day	17.8	28.6	54.7

Effects on the CIBIC-Plus: Figure 6 is a histogram of the frequency distribution of CIBIC-Plus scores attained by patients assigned to each of the three treatment groups who completed 26 weeks of treatment. The mean Exelon-placebo differences for these groups of patients for the mean rating of change from baseline were 0.14 units and 0.41 units for 1-4 mg and 6-12 mg of Exelon, respectively. The mean ratings for the 6-12 mg/day group was statistically significantly superior to placebo. The comparison of the mean ratings for the 1-4 mg/day group and placebo group was not statistically significant.

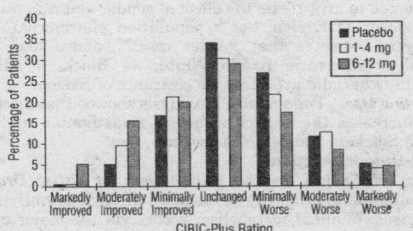

Figure 6: Frequency Distribution of CIBIC-Plus Scores at Week 26

U.S. Fixed Dose Study

In a study of 26 weeks' duration, 702 patients were randomized to doses of 3, 6, or 9 mg/day of Exelon or to placebo, each given in divided doses. The fixed-dose study design, which included a 12-week forced titration phase and a 14-week maintenance phase, led to a high dropout rate in the 9 mg/day group because of poor tolerability. At 26 weeks of treatment, significant differences were observed for the ADAS-cog mean change from baseline for the 9 mg/day and 6 mg/day groups, compared to placebo. No significant differences were observed between any of the Exelon dose groups and placebo for the analysis of the CIBIC-Plus mean rating of change. Although no significant differences were observed between Exelon treatment groups, there was a trend toward numerical superiority with higher doses.

Age, Gender and Race:
Patient's age, gender, or race did not predict clinical outcome to Exelon treatment.

Pharmacokinetics

Rivastigmine is well absorbed with absolute bioavailability of about 40% (3-mg dose). It shows linear pharmacokinetics up to 3 mg BID but is non-linear at higher doses. Doubling the dose from 3 to 6 mg BID results in a 3-fold increase in AUC. The elimination half-life is about 1.5 hours, with most elimination as metabolites via the urine.

Absorption: Rivastigmine is rapidly and completely absorbed. Peak plasma concentrations are reached in approximately 1 hour. Absolute bioavailability after a 3-mg dose is about 36%. Administration of Exelon with food delays absorption (t_{max}) by 90 min, lowers C_{max} by approximately 30% and increases AUC by approximately 30%.

Distribution: Rivastigmine is widely distributed throughout the body with a volume of distribution in the range of 1.8-2.7 L/kg. Rivastigmine penetrates the blood brain barrier,

Continued on next page

Exelon Oral Solution—Cont.

reaching CSF peak concentrations in 1.4-2.6 hours. Mean $AUC_{1\text{-}12hr}$ ratio of CSF/plasma averaged 40 ± 0.5% following 1-6 mg BID doses.

Rivastigmine is about 40% bound to plasma proteins at concentrations of 1-400 ng/mL, which cover the therapeutic concentration range. Rivastigmine distributes equally between blood and plasma with a blood-to-plasma partition ratio of 0.9 at concentrations ranging from 1-400 ng/mL.

Metabolism: Rivastigmine is rapidly and extensively metabolized, primarily via cholinesterase-mediated hydrolysis to the decarbamylated metabolite. Based on evidence from *in vitro* and animal studies the major cytochrome P450 isozymes are minimally involved in rivastigmine metabolism. Consistent with these observations is the finding that no drug interactions related to cytochrome P450 have been observed in humans (see Drug-Drug Interactions).

Elimination: The major pathway of elimination is via the kidneys. Following administration of ^{14}C-rivastigmine to 6 healthy volunteers total recovery of radioactivity over 120 hours was 97% in urine and 0.4% in feces. No parent drug was detected in urine. The sulfate conjugate of the decarbamylated metabolite is the major component excreted in urine and represents 40% of the dose. Mean oral clearance of rivastigmine is 1.8 ± 0.6 L/min after 6 mg BID.

Special Populations

Hepatic Disease: Following a single 3-mg dose, mean oral clearance of rivastigmine was 60% lower in hepatically impaired patients (n=10, biopsy proven) than in healthy subjects (n=10). After multiple 6 mg BID oral dosing, the mean clearance of rivastigmine was 65% lower in mild (n=7, Child-Pugh score 5-6) and moderate (n=3, Child-Pugh score 7-9) hepatically impaired patients (biopsy proven, liver cirrhosis) than in healthy subjects (n=10). Dosage adjustment is not necessary in hepatically impaired patients as the dose of drug is individually titrated to tolerability.

Renal Disease: Following a single 3-mg dose, mean oral clearance of rivastigmine is 64% lower in moderately impaired renal patients (n=8, GFR=10-50 mL/min) than in healthy subjects (n=10, GFR≥60 mL/min); Cl/F=1.7 L/min (cv=45%) and 4.8 L/min (cv=80%), respectively. In severely impaired renal patients (n=8, GFR<10 mL/min), mean oral clearance of rivastigmine is 43% higher than in healthy subjects (n=10, GFR≥60 mL/min); Cl/F=6.9 L/min and 4.8 L/min, respectively. For unexplained reasons, the severely impaired renal patients had a higher clearance of rivastigmine than moderately impaired patients. However, dosage adjustment may not be necessary in renally impaired patients as the dose of the drug is individually titrated to tolerability.

Age: Following a single 2.5 mg oral dose to elderly volunteers (>60 years of age, n=24) and younger volunteers (n=24), mean oral clearance of rivastigmine was 30% lower in elderly (7 L/min) than in younger subjects (10 L/min).

Gender and Race: No specific pharmacokinetic study was conducted to investigate the effect of gender and race on the disposition of Exelon, but a population pharmacokinetic analysis indicates that gender (n=277 males and 348 females) and race (n=575 White, 34 Black, 4 Asian, and 12 Other) did not affect the clearance of Exelon.

Nicotine Use: Population PK analysis showed that nicotine use increases the oral clearance of rivastigmine by 23% (n=75 Smokers and 549 Nonsmokers).

Drug-Drug Interactions

Effect of Exelon on the Metabolism of Other Drugs: Rivastigmine is primarily metabolized through hydrolysis by esterases. Minimal metabolism occurs via the major cytochrome P450 isoenzymes. Based on *in vitro* studies, no pharmacokinetic drug interactions with drugs metabolized by the following isoenzyme systems are expected: CYP1A2, CYP2D6, CYP3A4/5, CYP2E1, CYP2C9, CYP2C8, or CYP2C19.

No pharmacokinetic interaction was observed between rivastigmine and digoxin, warfarin, diazepam, or fluoxetine in studies in healthy volunteers. The elevation of prothrombin time induced by warfarin is not affected by administration of Exelon.

Effect of Other Drugs on the Metabolism of Exelon: Drugs that induce or inhibit CYP450 metabolism are not expected to alter the metabolism of rivastigmine. Single dose pharmacokinetic studies demonstrated that the metabolism of rivastigmine is not significantly affected by concurrent administration of digoxin, warfarin, diazepam, or fluoxetine. Population PK analysis with a database of 625 patients showed that the pharmacokinetics of rivastigmine were not influenced by commonly prescribed medications such as antacids (n=77), antihypertensives (n=72), β-blockers (n=42), calcium channel blockers (n=75), antidiabetics (n=21), nonsteroidal anti-inflammatory drugs (n=79), estrogens (n=70), salicylate analgesics (n=177), antianginals (n=35), and antihistamines (n=15). In addition, in clinical trials, no increased risk of clinically relevant untoward effects was observed in patients treated concomitantly with Exelon and these agents.

INDICATIONS AND USAGE

Exelon® (rivastigmine tartrate) is indicated for the treatment of mild to moderate dementia of the Alzheimer's type.

CONTRAINDICATIONS

Exelon® (rivastigmine tartrate) is contraindicated in patients with known hypersensitivity to rivastigmine, other carbamate derivatives or other components of the formulation (see DESCRIPTION).

WARNINGS

Gastrointestinal Adverse Reactions

Exelon® (rivastigmine tartrate) use is associated with significant gastrointestinal adverse reactions, including nausea and vomiting, anorexia, and weight loss. For this reason, patients should always be started at a dose of 1.5 mg BID and titrated to their maintenance dose. If treatment is interrupted for longer than several days, treatment should be reinitiated with the lowest daily dose (see DOSAGE AND ADMINISTRATION) to reduce the possibility of severe vomiting and its potentially serious sequelae (e.g., there has been one post-marketing report of severe vomiting with esophageal rupture following inappropriate reinitiation of treatment with a 4.5-mg dose after 8 weeks of treatment interruption).

Nausea and Vomiting: **In the controlled clinical trials, 47% of the patients treated with an Exelon dose in the therapeutic range of 6-12 mg/day (n=1189) developed nausea (compared with 12% in placebo). A total of 31% of Exelon-treated patients developed at least one episode of vomiting (compared with 6% for placebo). The rate of vomiting was higher during the titration phase (24% vs. 3% for placebo) than in the maintenance phase (14% vs. 3% for placebo). The rates were higher in women than men. Five percent of patients discontinued for vomiting, compared to less than 1% for patients on placebo. Vomiting was severe in 2% of Exelon-treated patients and was rated as mild or moderate each in 14% of patients. The rate of nausea was higher during the titration phase (43% vs. 9% for placebo) than in the maintenance phase (17% vs. 4% for placebo).**

Weight Loss: **In the controlled trials, approximately 26% of women on high doses of Exelon (greater than 9 mg/day) had weight loss of equal to or greater than 7% of their baseline weight compared to 6% in the placebo-treated patients. About 18% of the males in the high dose group experienced a similar degree of weight loss compared to 4% in placebo-treated patients. It is not clear how much of the weight loss was associated with anorexia, nausea, vomiting, and the diarrhea associated with the drug.**

Anorexia: In the controlled clinical trials, of the patients treated with an Exelon dose of 6-12 mg/day, 17% developed anorexia compared to 3% of the placebo patients. Neither the time course or the severity of the anorexia is known.

Peptic Ulcers/Gastrointestinal Bleeding: Because of their pharmacological action, cholinesterase inhibitors may be expected to increase gastric acid secretion due to increased cholinergic activity. Therefore, patients should be monitored closely for symptoms of active or occult gastrointestinal bleeding, especially those at increased risk for developing ulcers, e.g., those with a history of ulcer disease or those receiving concurrent nonsteroidal anti-inflammatory drugs (NSAIDS). Clinical studies of Exelon have shown no significant increase, relative to placebo, in the incidence of either peptic ulcer disease or gastrointestinal bleeding.

Anesthesia

Exelon as a cholinesterase inhibitor, is likely to exaggerate succinylcholine-type muscle relaxation during anesthesia.

Cardiovascular Conditions

Drugs that increase cholinergic activity may have vagotonic effects on heart rate (e.g., bradycardia). The potential for this action may be particularly important to patients with "sick sinus syndrome" or other supraventricular cardiac conduction conditions. In clinical trials, Exelon was not associated with any increased incidence of cardiovascular adverse events, heart rate or blood pressure changes, or ECG abnormalities. Syncopal episodes have been reported in 3% of patients receiving 6-12 mg/day of Exelon, compared to 2% of placebo patients.

Genitourinary

Although this was not observed in clinical trials of Exelon, drugs that increase cholinergic activity may cause urinary obstruction.

Neurological Conditions

Seizures: Drugs that increase cholinergic activity are believed to have some potential for causing seizures. However, seizure activity also may be a manifestation of Alzheimer's Disease.

Pulmonary Conditions

Like other drugs that increase cholinergic activity, Exelon should be used with care in patients with a history of asthma or obstructive pulmonary disease.

PRECAUTIONS

Information for Patients and Caregivers

Caregivers should be advised of the high incidence of nausea and vomiting associated with the use of the drug along with the possibility of anorexia and weight loss. Caregivers should be encouraged to monitor for these adverse events and inform the physician if they occur. It is critical to inform caregivers that if therapy has been interrupted for more than several days, the next dose should not be administered until they have discussed this with the physician.

Caregivers should be instructed in the correct procedure for administering Exelon® (rivastigmine tartrate) Oral Solution. In addition, they should be informed of the existence of an Instruction Sheet (included with the product) describing how the solution is to be administered. They should be urged to read this sheet prior to administering Exelon Oral Solution. Caregivers should direct questions about the administration of the solution to either their physician or pharmacist.

Drug-Drug Interactions

Effect of Exelon® on the Metabolism of Other Drugs: Rivastigmine is primarily metabolized through hydrolysis by esterases. Minimal metabolism occurs via the major cytochrome P450 isoenzymes. Based on *in vitro* studies, no pharmacokinetic drug interactions with drugs metabolized by the following isoenzyme systems are expected: CYP1A2, CYP2D6, CYP3A4/5, CYP2E1, CYP2C9, CYP2C8, or CYP2C19.

No pharmacokinetic interaction was observed between rivastigmine and digoxin, warfarin, diazepam, or fluoxetine in studies in healthy volunteers. The elevation of prothrombin time induced by warfarin is not affected by administration of Exelon.

Effect of Other Drugs on the Metabolism of Exelon: Drugs that induce or inhibit CYP450 metabolism are not expected to alter the metabolism of rivastigmine. Single dose pharmacokinetic studies demonstrated that the metabolism of rivastigmine is not significantly affected by concurrent administration of digoxin, warfarin, diazepam, or fluoxetine. Population PK analysis with a database of 625 patients showed that the pharmacokinetics of rivastigmine were not influenced by commonly prescribed medications such as antacids (n=77), antihypertensives (n=72), β-blockers (n=42), calcium channel blockers (n=75), antidiabetics (n=21), nonsteroidal anti-inflammatory drugs (n=79), estrogens (n=70), salicylate analgesics (n=177), antianginals (n=35), and antihistamines (n=15).

Use with Anticholinergics: Because of their mechanism of action, cholinesterase inhibitors have the potential to interfere with the activity of anticholinergic medications.

Use with Cholinomimetics and Other Cholinesterase Inhibitors: A synergistic effect may be expected when cholinesterase inhibitors are given concurrently with succinylcholine, similar neuromuscular blocking agents or cholinergic agonists such as bethanechol.

Carcinogenesis, Mutagenesis, Impairment of Fertility

In carcinogenicity studies conducted at dose levels up to 1.1 mg-base/kg/day in rats and 1.6 mg-base/kg/day in mice, rivastigmine was not carcinogenic. These dose levels are approximately 0.9 times and 0.7 times the maximum recommended human daily dose of 12 mg/day on a mg/m^2 basis.

Rivastigmine was clastogenic in two *in vitro* assays in the presence, but not the absence, of metabolic activation. It caused structural chromosomal aberrations in V79 Chinese hamster lung cells and both structural and numerical (polyploidy) chromosomal aberrations in human peripheral blood lymphocytes. Rivastigmine was not genotoxic in three *in vitro* assays: the Ames test, the unscheduled DNA synthesis (UDS) test in rat hepatocytes (a test for induction of DNA repair synthesis), and the HGPRT test in V79 Chinese hamster cells. Rivastigmine was not clastogenic in the *in vivo* mouse micronucleus test.

Rivastigmine had no effect on fertility or reproductive performance in the rat at dose levels up to 1.1 mg-base/kg/day. This dose is approximately 0.9 times the maximum recommended human daily dose of 12 mg/day on a mg/m^2 basis.

Pregnancy

Pregnancy Category B: Reproduction studies conducted in pregnant rats at doses up to 2.3 mg-base/kg/day (approximately 2 times the maximum recommended human dose on a mg/m^2 basis) and in pregnant rabbits at doses up to 2.3 mg-base/kg/day (approximately 4 times the maximum recommended human dose on a mg/m^2 basis) revealed no evidence of teratogenicity. Studies in rats showed slightly decreased fetal/pup weights, usually at doses causing some maternal toxicity; decreased weights were seen at doses which were several fold lower than the maximum recommended human dose on a mg/m^2 basis. There are no adequate or well-controlled studies in pregnant women. Because animal reproduction studies are not always predictive of human response, Exelon should be used during pregnancy only if the potential benefit justifies the potential risk to the fetus.

Nursing Mothers

It is not known whether rivastigmine is excreted in human breast milk. Exelon has no indication for use in nursing mothers.

Pediatric Use

There are no adequate and well-controlled trials documenting the safety and efficacy of Exelon in any illness occurring in children.

ADVERSE REACTIONS

Adverse Events Leading to Discontinuation

The rate of discontinuation due to adverse events in controlled clinical trials of Exelon® (rivastigmine tartrate) was 15% for patients receiving 6-12 mg/day compared to 5% for patients on placebo during forced weekly dose titration. While on a maintenance dose, the rates were 6% for patients on Exelon compared to 4% for those on placebo.

The most common adverse events leading to discontinuation, defined as those occurring in at least 2% of patients and at twice the incidence seen in placebo patients, are shown in Table 1.

[See table 1 at top of next page]

Most Frequent Adverse Clinical Events Seen in Association with the Use of Exelon

The most common adverse events, defined as those occurring at a frequency of at least 5% and twice the placebo rate, are largely predicted by Exelon's cholinergic effects. These include nausea, vomiting, anorexia, dyspepsia, and asthenia.

Gastrointestinal Adverse Reactions

Exelon use is associated with significant nausea, vomiting, and weight loss (see WARNINGS).

Adverse Events Reports in Controlled Trials

Table 2 lists treatment emergent signs and symptoms that were reported in at least 2% of patients in placebo-controlled trials and for which the rate of occurrence was greater for patients treated with Exelon doses of 6-12 mg/day than for those treated with placebo. The prescriber should be aware that these figures cannot be used to predict the frequency of adverse events in the course of usual medical practice when patient characteristics and other factors may differ from those prevailing during clinical studies. Similarly, the cited frequencies cannot be directly compared with figures obtained from other clinical investigations involving different treatments, uses, or investigators. An inspection of these frequencies, however, does provide the prescriber with one basis by which to estimate the relative contribution of drug and non-drug factors to the adverse event incidences in the population studied.

In general, adverse reactions were less frequent later in the course of treatment.

No systematic effect of race or age could be determined on the incidence of adverse events in the controlled studies. Nausea, vomiting and weight loss were more frequent in women than men.

[See table 2 to right]

Other adverse events observed at a rate of 2% or more on Exelon 6-12 mg/day but at a greater or equal rate on placebo were chest pain, peripheral edema, vertigo, back pain, arthralgia, pain, bone fracture, agitation, nervousness, delusion, paranoid reaction, upper respiratory tract infections, infection (general), coughing, pharyngitis, bronchitis, rash (general), urinary incontinence.

Other Adverse Events During Clinical Trials

Exelon has been administered to over 5297 individuals during clinical trials worldwide. Of these, 4326 patients have been treated for at least 3 months, 3407 patients have been treated for at least 6 months, 2150 patients have been treated for 1 year, 1250 have been treated for 2 years, and 168 have been treated for over 3 years. With regard to exposure to the highest dose, 2809 patients were exposed to doses of 10-12 mg, 2615 patients treated for 3 months, 2328 patients treated for 6 months, 1378 patients treated for 1 year, 917 patients treated for 2 years, and 129 treated for over 3 years.

Treatment emergent signs and symptoms that occurred during 8 controlled clinical trials and 9 open-label trials in North America, Western Europe, Australia, South Africa, and Japan were recorded as adverse events by the clinical investigators using terminology of their own choosing. To provide an overall estimate of the proportion of individuals having similar types of events, the events were grouped into a smaller number of standardized categories using a modified WHO dictionary, and event frequencies were calculated across all studies. These categories are used in the listing below. The frequencies represent the proportion of 5297 patients from these trials who experienced that event while receiving Exelon. All adverse events occurring in at least 6 patients (approximately 0.1%) are included, except for those already listed elsewhere in labeling, WHO terms too general to be informative, relatively minor events, or events unlikely to be drug caused. Events are classified by body system and listed using the following definitions: frequent adverse events – those occurring in at least 1/100 patients; infrequent adverse events – those occurring in 1/100 to 1/1000 patients. These adverse events are not necessarily related to Exelon treatment and in most cases were observed at a similar frequency in placebo-treated patients in the controlled studies.

Autonomic Nervous System: *Infrequent:* Cold clammy skin, dry mouth, flushing, increased saliva.
Body as a Whole: *Frequent:* Accidental trauma, fever, edema, allergy, hot flushes, rigors. *Infrequent:* Edema periorbital or facial, hypothermia, edema, feeling cold, halitosis.
Cardiovascular System: *Frequent:* Hypotension, postural hypotension, cardiac failure.
Central and Peripheral Nervous System: *Frequent:* Abnormal gait, ataxia, paraesthesia, convulsions. *Infrequent:* Paresis, apraxia, aphasia, dysphonia, hyperkinesia, hyperreflexia, hypertonia, hypoesthesia, hypokinesia, migraine, neuralgia, nystagmus, peripheral neuropathy.
Endocrine System: *Infrequent:* Goitre, hypothyroidism.
Gastrointestinal System: *Frequent:* Fecal incontinence, gastritis. *Infrequent:* Dysphagia, esophagitis, gastric ulcer, gastritis, gastroesophageal reflux, GI hemorrhage, hernia, intestinal obstruction, melena, rectal hemorrhage, gastroenteritis, ulcerative stomatitis, duodenal ulcer, hematemesis, gingivitis, tenesmus, pancreatitis, colitis, glossitis.
Hearing and Vestibular Disorders: *Frequent:* Tinnitus.
Heart Rate and Rhythm Disorders: *Frequent:* Atrial fibrillation, bradycardia, palpitation. *Infrequent:* AV block, bundle branch block, sick sinus syndrome, cardiac arrest, supraventricular tachycardia, extrasystoles, tachycardia.
Liver and Biliary System Disorders: *Infrequent:* Abnormal hepatic function, cholecystitis.
Metabolic and Nutritional Disorders: *Frequent:* Dehydration, hypokalemia. *Infrequent:* Diabetes mellitus, gout, hypercholesterolemia, hyperlipemia, hypoglycemia, cachexia, thirst, hyperglycemia, hyponatremia.
Musculoskeletal Disorders: *Frequent:* Arthritis, leg cramps, myalgia. *Infrequent:* Cramps, hernia, muscle weakness.
Myo-, Endo-, Pericardial and Valve Disorders: *Frequent:* Angina pectoris, myocardial infarction.
Platelet, Bleeding, and Clotting Disorders: *Frequent:* Epistaxis. *Infrequent:* Hematoma, thrombocytopenia, purpura.
Psychiatric Disorders: *Frequent:* Paranoid reaction, confusion. *Infrequent:* Abnormal dreaming, amnesia, apathy, delirium, dementia, depersonalization, emotional lability, impaired concentration, decreased libido, personality disorder,

suicide attempt, increased libido, neurosis, suicidal ideation, psychosis.
Red Blood Cell Disorders: *Frequent:* Anemia. *Infrequent:* Hypochromic anemia.
Reproductive Disorders (Female & Male): *Infrequent:* Breast pain, impotence, atrophic vaginitis.
Resistance Mechanism Disorders: *Infrequent:* Cellulitis, cystitis, herpes simplex, otitis media.
Respiratory System: *Infrequent:* Bronchospasm, laryngitis, apnea.
Skin and Appendages: *Frequent:* Rashes of various kinds (maculopapular, eczema, bullous, exfoliative, psoriaform, erythematous). *Infrequent:* Alopecia, skin ulceration, urticaria, dermatitis contact.
Special Senses: *Infrequent:* Perversion of taste, loss of taste.
Urinary System Disorders: *Frequent:* Hematuria. *Infrequent:* Albuminuria, oliguria, acute renal failure, dysuria, micturition urgency, nocturia, polyuria, renal calculus, urinary retention.
Vascular (extracardiac) Disorders: *Infrequent:* Hemorrhoids, peripheral ischemia, pulmonary embolism, thrombosis, thrombophlebitis deep, aneurysm, hemorrhage intracranial.
Vision Disorders: *Frequent:* Cataract. *Infrequent:* Conjunctival hemorrhage, blepharitis, diplopia, eye pain, glaucoma.
White Cell and Resistance Disorders: *Infrequent:* Lymphadenopathy, leukocytosis.

Post-Introduction Reports
Voluntary reports of adverse events temporally associated with Exelon that have been received since market introduction that are not listed above, and that may or may not be causally related to the drug include the following:
Skin and Appendages: Stevens-Johnson syndrome.

OVERDOSAGE
Because strategies for the management of overdose are continually evolving, it is advisable to contact a Poison Control Center to determine the latest recommendations for the management of an overdose of any drug.
As Exelon® (rivastigmine tartrate) has a short plasma half-life of about one hour and a moderate duration of acetylcho-

linesterase inhibition of 8-10 hours, it is recommended that in cases of asymptomatic overdoses, no further dose of Exelon should be administered for the next 24 hours.
As in any case of overdose, general supportive measures should be utilized. Overdosage with cholinesterase inhibitors can result in cholinergic crisis characterized by severe nausea, vomiting, salivation, sweating, bradycardia, hypotension, respiratory depression, collapse and convulsions. Increasing muscle weakness is a possibility and may result in death if respiratory muscles are involved. Atypical responses in blood pressure and heart rate have been reported with other drugs that increase cholinergic activity when co-administered with quaternary anticholinergics such as glycopyrrolate. Due to the short half-life of Exelon, dialysis (hemodialysis, peritoneal dialysis, or hemofiltration) would not be clinically indicated in the event of an overdose.
In overdoses accompanied by severe nausea and vomiting, the use of antiemetics should be considered. In a documented case of a 46 mg overdose with Exelon, the patient experienced vomiting, incontinence, hypertension, psychomotor retardation, and loss of consciousness. The patient fully recovered within 24 hours and conservative management was all that was required for treatment.

DOSAGE AND ADMINISTRATION
The dosage of Exelon® (rivastigmine tartrate) shown to be effective in controlled clinical trials is 6-12 mg/day, given as twice a day dosing (daily doses of 3 to 6 mg BID). There is evidence from the clinical trials that doses at the higher end of this range may be more beneficial.
The starting dose of Exelon is 1.5 mg twice a day (BID). If this dose is well tolerated, after a minimum of two weeks of treatment, the dose may be increased to 3 mg BID. Subsequent increases to 4.5 mg BID and 6 mg BID should be attempted after a minimum of 2 weeks at the previous dose. If adverse effects (e.g., nausea, vomiting, abdominal pain, loss of appetite) cause intolerance during treatment, the patient should be instructed to discontinue treatment for several doses and then restart at the same or next lower dose level. If treatment is interrupted for longer than several days,

Continued on next page

Table 1. Most Frequent Adverse Events Leading to Withdrawal from Clinical Trials during Titration and Maintenance in Patients Receiving 6-12 mg/day Exelon® Using a Forced Dose Titration

Study Phase	Titration		Maintenance		Overall	
	Placebo (n=868)	Exelon ≥6–12 mg/day (n=1189)	Placebo (n=788)	Exelon ≥6–12 mg/day (n=987)	Placebo (n=868)	Exelon ≥6–12 mg/day (n=1189)
Event/% Discontinuing						
Nausea	<1	8	<1	1	1	8
Vomiting	<1	4	<1	1	<1	5
Anorexia	0	2	<1	1	<1	3
Dizziness	<1	2	<1	1	<1	2

Table 2. Adverse Events Reported in Controlled Clinical Trials in at Least 2% of Patients Receiving Exelon® (6-12 mg/day) and at a Higher Frequency than Placebo-treated Patients

Body System/Adverse Event	Placebo (n=868)	Exelon (6-12 mg/day) (n=1189)
Percent of Patients with any Adverse Event	79	92
Autonomic Nervous System		
Sweating increased	1	4
Syncope	2	3
Body as a Whole		
Accidental Trauma	9	10
Fatigue	5	9
Asthenia	2	6
Malaise	2	5
Influenza-like Symptoms	2	3
Weight Decrease	<1	3
Cardiovascular Disorders, General		
Hypertension	2	3
Central and Peripheral Nervous System		
Dizziness	11	21
Headache	12	17
Somnolence	3	5
Tremor	1	4
Gastrointestinal System		
Nausea	12	47
Vomiting	6	31
Diarrhea	11	19
Anorexia	3	17
Abdominal Pain	6	13
Dyspepsia	4	9
Constipation	4	5
Flatulence	2	4
Eructation	1	2
Psychiatric Disorders		
Insomnia	7	9
Confusion	7	8
Depression	4	6
Anxiety	3	5
Hallucination	3	4
Aggressive Reaction	2	3
Resistance Mechanism Disorders		
Urinary Tract Infection	6	7
Respiratory System		
Rhinitis	3	4

Exelon Oral Solution—Cont.

treatment should be reinitiated with the lowest daily dose and titrated as described above (see WARNINGS). The maximum dose is 6 mg BID (12 mg/day).
Exelon should be taken with meals in divided doses in the morning and evening.
Recommendations for Administration: Caregivers should be instructed in the correct procedure for administering Exelon Oral Solution. In addition, they should be directed to the Instruction Sheet (included with the product) describing how the solution is to be administered. Caregivers should direct questions about the administration of the solution to either their physician or pharmacist (see PRECAUTIONS: Information for Patients and Caregivers).
Patients should be instructed to remove the oral dosing syringe provided in its protective case, and using the provided syringe, withdraw the prescribed amount of Exelon Oral Solution from the container. Each dose of Exelon Oral Solution may be swallowed directly from the syringe or first mixed with a small glass of water, cold fruit juice or soda. Patients should be instructed to stir and drink the mixture.
Exelon Oral Solution and Exelon Capsules may be interchanged at equal doses.

HOW SUPPLIED

Exelon® (rivastigmine tartrate Oral Solution is supplied as 120 mL of a clear, yellow solution (2 mg/mL base) in a 4 ounce USP Type III amber glass bottle with a child-resistant 28 mm cap, 0.5 mm foam liner, dip tube and self-aligning plug. The oral solution is packaged with a dispenser set which consists of an assembled oral dosing syringe that allows dispensing a maximum volume of 3 mL corresponding to a 6 mg dose, with a plastic tube container.
Bottles of 120 mL .... NDC 0078-0339-31
Store below 77°F (25°C) in an upright position and protect from freezing.
When Exelon Oral Solution is combined with cold fruit juice or soda, the mixture is stable at room temperature for up to 4 hours.

Exelon® *(rivastigmine tartrate)* Oral Solution Instructions for Use

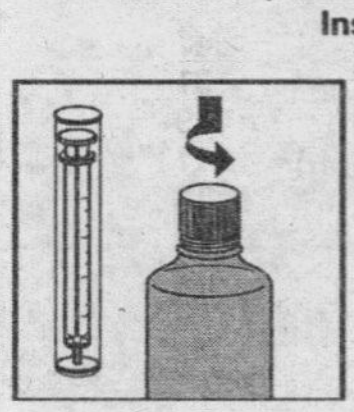

1. Remove oral dosing syringe from its protective case. Push down and twist child resistant closure to open bottle.

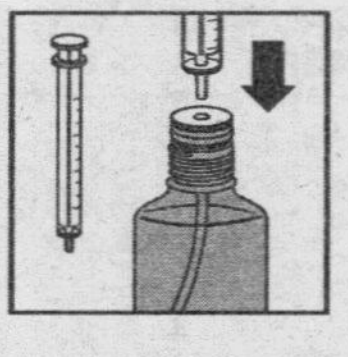

2. Insert tip of syringe into opening of white stopper.

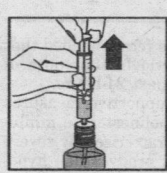

3. While holding the syringe, pull the plunger up to the level (see markings on side of syringe) that equals the dose prescribed by your doctor.

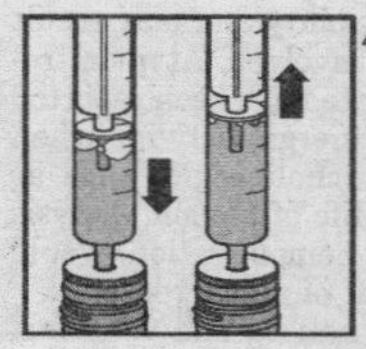

4. Before removing syringe containing prescribed dose from bottle, push out **large** bubbles by moving plunger up and down a few times. After the large bubbles are gone, pull the plunger again to the level that equals the dose prescribed by your doctor. Do not worry about a few tiny bubbles. This will not affect your dose in any away. Remove the syringe from the bottle.

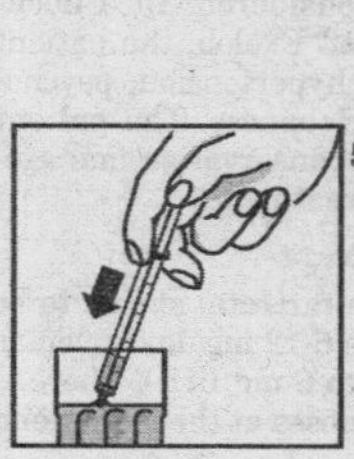

5. You may swallow Exelon Oral Solution directly from the syringe or mix with a small glass of water, cold fruit juice or soda. If mixing with water, juice or soda, be sure to stir completely and to drink the entire mixture. DO NOT MIX WITH OTHER LIQUIDS.

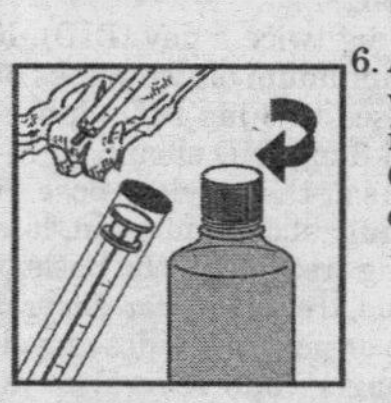

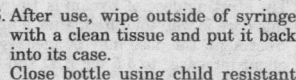

6. After use, wipe outside of syringe with a clean tissue and put it back into its case. Close bottle using child resistant closure.

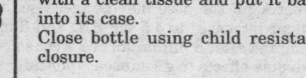

Store Exelon Oral Solution at room temperature (below 77° F) in an upright position. Do not place in freezer.

(86000501 4/00)
REV: JANUARY 2001 Printed in U.S.A. 89009402
4088-42
T2001-01

Manufactured by
Novartis Consumer Health, Incorporated
Lincoln, Nebraska 68517
Manufactured for
Novartis Pharmaceuticals Corporation
East Hanover, New Jersey 07936

FEMARA® ℞

[fĕm-ara]
(letrozole tablets)
2.5 mg Tablets
Rx only

Prescribing information for this product, which appears on pages 2177–2179 of the 2001 PDR, has been completely revised as follows. Please write "See Supplement A" next to the product heading.

DESCRIPTION

Femara® (letrozole tablets) for oral administration contains 2.5 mg of letrozole, a nonsteroidal aromatase inhibitor (inhibitor of estrogen synthesis). It is chemically described as 4,4′-(1H-1,2,4-Triazol-1-ylmethylene)dibenzonitrile, and its structural formula is

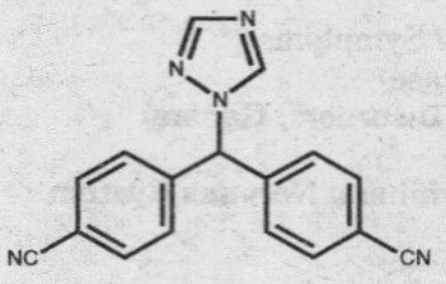

Letrozole is a white to yellowish crystalline powder, practically odorless, freely soluble in dichloromethane, slightly soluble in ethanol, and practically insoluble in water. It has a molecular weight of 285.31, empirical formula $C_{17}H_{11}N_5$, and a melting range of 184°C–185°C.
Femara® (letrozole tablets) is available as 2.5 mg tablets for oral administration.
Inactive Ingredients. Colloidal silicon dioxide, ferric oxide, hydroxypropyl methylcellulose, lactose monohydrate, magnesium stearate, maize starch, microcrystalline cellulose, polyethylene glycol, sodium starch glycolate, talc, and titanium dioxide.

CLINICAL PHARMACOLOGY

Mechanism of Action
The growth of some cancers of the breast is stimulated or maintained by estrogens. Treatment of breast cancer thought to be hormonally responsive (i.e., estrogen and/or progesterone receptor positive or receptor unknown) has included a variety of efforts to decrease estrogen levels (ovariectomy, adrenalectomy, hypophysectomy) or inhibit estrogen effects (antiestrogens and progestational agents). These interventions lead to decreased tumor mass or delayed progression of tumor growth in some women.
In postmenopausal women, estrogens are mainly derived from the action of the aromatase enzyme, which converts adrenal androgens (primarily androstenedione and testosterone) to estrone and estradiol. The suppression of estrogen biosynthesis in peripheral tissues and in the cancer tissue itself can therefore be achieved by specifically inhibiting the aromatase enzyme.
Letrozole is a nonsteroidal competitive inhibitor of the aromatase enzyme system; it inhibits the conversion of androgens to estrogens. In adult nontumor- and tumor-bearing female animals, letrozole is as effective as ovariectomy in reducing uterine weight, elevating serum LH, and causing the regression of estrogen-dependent tumors. In contrast to ovariectomy, treatment with letrozole does not lead to an increase in serum FSH. Letrozole selectively inhibits gonadal steroidogenesis but has no significant effect on adrenal mineralocorticoid or glucocorticoid synthesis.
Letrozole inhibits the aromatase enzyme by competitively binding to the heme of the cytochrome P450 subunit of the enzyme, resulting in a reduction of estrogen biosynthesis in all tissues. Treatment of women with letrozole significantly lowers serum estrone, estradiol and estrone sulfate and has not been shown to significantly affect adrenal corticosteroid synthesis, aldosterone synthesis, or synthesis of thyroid hormones.

Pharmacokinetics
Letrozole is rapidly and completely absorbed from the gastrointestinal tract and absorption is not affected by food. It is metabolized slowly to an inactive metabolite whose glucuronide conjugate is excreted renally, representing the major clearance pathway. About 90% of radiolabeled letrozole is recovered in urine. Letrozole's terminal elimination half-life is about 2 days and steady-state plasma concentration after daily 2.5 mg dosing is reached in 2-6 weeks. Plasma concentrations at steady-state are 1.5 to 2 times higher than predicted from the concentrations measured after a single dose, indicating a slight non-linearity in the pharmacokinetics of letrozole upon daily administration of 2.5 mg. These steady-state levels are maintained over extended periods, however, and continuous accumulation of letrozole does not occur. Letrozole is weakly protein bound and has a large volume of distribution (approximately 1.9 L/kg).

Metabolism and Excretion
Metabolism to a pharmacologically-inactive carbinol metabolite (4,4′-methanol-bisbenzonitrile) and renal excretion of the glucuronide conjugate of this metabolite is the major pathway of letrozole clearance. Of the radiolabel recovered in urine, at least 75% was the glucuronide of the carbinol metabolite, about 9% was two unidentified metabolites, and 6% was unchanged letrozole.
In human microsomes with specific CYP isozyme activity, CYP3A4 metabolized letrozole to the carbinol metabolite while CYP2A6 formed both this metabolite and its ketone analog. In human liver microsomes, letrozole strongly inhibited CYP2A6 and moderately inhibited CYP2C19.

Special Populations
Pediatric, Geriatric and Race
In the study populations (adults ranging in age from 35 to >80 years), no change in pharmacokinetic parameters was observed with increasing age. Differences in letrozole pharmacokinetics between adult and pediatric populations have not been studied. Differences in letrozole pharmacokinetics due to race have not been studied.
Renal Insufficiency
In a study of volunteers with varying renal function (24-hour creatinine clearance: 9-116 mL/min), no effect of renal function on the pharmacokinetics of single doses of 2.5 mg of Femara® (letrozole tablets) was found. In addition, in a study of 347 patients with advanced breast cancer, about half of whom received 2.5 mg Femara and half 0.5 mg Femara, renal impairment (calculated creatinine clearance: 20-50 mL/min) did not affect steady-state plasma letrozole concentration.
Hepatic Insufficiency
In a study of subjects with varying degrees of non-metastatic hepatic dysfunction (e.g., cirrhosis, Child-Pugh classification A and B), the mean AUC values of the volunteers with moderate hepatic impairment were 37% higher than in normal subjects, but still within the range seen in subjects without impaired function. Patients with severe hepatic impairment (Child-Pugh classification C) have not been studied (see DOSAGE AND ADMINISTRATION, Hepatic Impairment).
Drug/Drug Interactions
A pharmacokinetic interaction study with cimetidine showed no clinically significant effect on letrozole pharmacokinetics. An interaction study with warfarin showed no clinically significant effect of letrozole on warfarin pharmacokinetics.
There is no clinical experience to date on the use of Femara in combination with other anticancer agents.

Pharmacodynamics
In postmenopausal patients with advanced breast cancer, daily doses of 0.1 mg to 5 mg Femara suppress plasma concentrations of estradiol, estrone, and estrone sulfate by 75%-95% from baseline with maximal suppression achieved within two-three days. Suppression is dose-related, with doses of 0.5 mg and higher giving many values of estrone and estrone sulfate that were below the limit of detection in the assays. Estrogen suppression was maintained throughout treatment in all patients treated at 0.5 mg or higher.
Letrozole is highly specific in inhibiting aromatase activity. There is no impairment of adrenal steroidogenesis. No clinically-relevant changes were found in the plasma concentrations of cortisol, aldosterone, 11-deoxycortisol, 17-hydroxy-progesterone, ACTH or in plasma renin activity among postmenopausal patients treated with a daily dose of Femara 0.1 mg to 5 mg. The ACTH stimulation test performed after 6 and 12 weeks of treatment with daily doses of 0.1, 0.25, 0.5, 1, 2.5, and 5 mg did not indicate any attenuation of aldosterone or cortisol production. Glucocorticoid or mineralocorticoid supplementation is, therefore, not necessary.
No changes were noted in plasma concentrations of androgens (androstenedione and testosterone) among healthy postmenopausal women after 0.1, 0.5, and 2.5 mg single doses of Femara or in plasma concentrations of androstenedione among postmenopausal patients treated with daily doses of 0.1 mg to 5 mg. This indicates that the blockade of estrogen biosynthesis does not lead to accumulation of androgenic precursors. Plasma levels of LH and FSH were not affected by letrozole in patients, nor was thyroid function as evaluated by TSH levels, T3 uptake, and T4 levels.

Clinical Studies

First-Line Breast Cancer
A randomized, double-blinded, multinational trial compared Femara 2.5 mg with tamoxifen 20 mg in 907 postmenopausal patients with locally advanced (Stage IIIB or locoregional recurrence not amenable to treatment with surgery or radiation) or metastatic breast cancer. Time to progression (TTP) was the primary endpoint of the trial. Selected baseline characteristics for this study are shown in Table 1.

Table 1: Selected Study Population Demographics

Baseline Status	Femara® N = 453	tamoxifen N = 454
Stage of Disease		
IIIB	6%	7%
IV	93%	92%
Receptor Status		
ER and PR Positive	38%	41%
ER or PR Positive	26%	26%
Both unknown	34%	33%
ER^- or PR^-/other unknown	<1%	0

Previous Antiestrogen Therapy

Adjuvant	19%	18%
None	81%	82%

Dominant Site of Disease

Soft Tissue	25%	25%
Bone	32%	29%
Visceral	43%	46%

Femara was superior to tamoxifen in TTP and rate of objective tumor response (see Table 2). No differences were seen in duration of tumor response. Results from the prospectively defined secondary endpoint of time to treatment failure and clinical benefit were supportive of the results of the primary efficacy endpoint.

Table 2 summarizes the results of the trial, with a total median follow-up of approximately 18 months. (All analyses are unadjusted and use 2-sided p-values.)

[See table 2 to right]

Figure 1 shows the Kaplan-Meier curves for TTP.

Table 3 shows results in the subgroup and women who had received prior antiestrogen adjuvant therapy and Table 4 shows results by disease site.

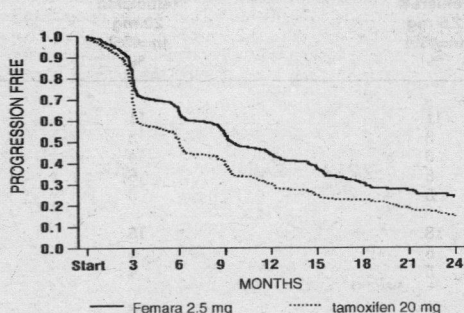

Figure 1
KAPLAN-MEIER ESTIMATES OF TIME TO PROGRESSION
(TAMOXIFEN STUDY)

— Femara 2.5 mg   .... tamoxifen 20 mg

[See table 3 above]
[See table 4 to right]

Second-Line Breast Cancer

Femara was initially studied at doses of 0.1 mg to 5.0 mg daily in six non-comparative Phase I/II trials in 181 postmenopausal estrogen/progesterone receptor positive or unknown advanced breast cancer patients previously treated with at least anti-estrogen therapy. Patients had received other hormonal therapies and also may have received cytotoxic therapy. Eight (20%) of forty patients treated with Femara 2.5 mg daily in Phase I/II trials achieved an objective tumor response (complete or partial response).

Two large randomized controlled multinational (predominantly European) trials were conducted in patients with advanced breast cancer who had progressed despite antiestrogen therapy. Patients were randomized to Femara 0.5 mg daily, Femara 2.5 mg daily, or a comparator (megestrol acetate 160 mg daily in one study; and aminoglutethimide 250 mg b.i.d. with corticosteroid supplementation in the other study). In each study over 60% of the patients had received therapeutic antiestrogens, and about one-fifth of these patients had had an objective response. The megestrol acetate controlled study was double-blind; the other study was open label. Selected baseline characteristics for each study are shown in Table 5.

[See table 5 to right]

Confirmed objective tumor response (complete response plus partial response) was the primary endpoint of the trials. Responses were measured according to the Union Internationale Contre le Cancer (UICC) criteria and verified by independent, blinded review. All responses were confirmed by a second evaluation 4-12 weeks after the documentation of the initial response.

Table 6 shows the results for the first trial, with a minimum follow-up of 15 months, that compared Femara 0.5 mg, Femara 2.5 mg, and megestrol acetate 160 mg daily. (All analyses are unadjusted.)

[see table 6 to right]

The Kaplan-Meier Curve for progression for the megestrol acetate study is shown in Figure 2.

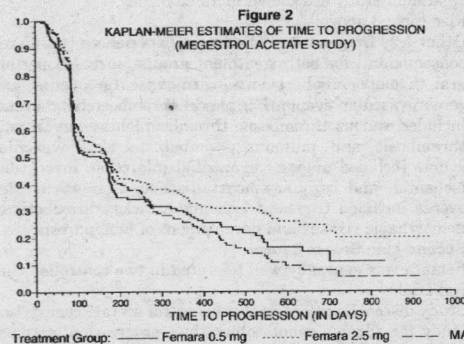

Figure 2
KAPLAN-MEIER ESTIMATES OF TIME TO PROGRESSION
(MEGESTROL ACETATE STUDY)

TIME TO PROGRESSION (IN DAYS)

Treatment Group: —— Femara 0.5 mg   .... Femara 2.5 mg   — — — MA

The results for the study comparing Femara to aminoglutethimide, with a minimum follow-up of nine months, are shown in Table 7. (Unadjusted analyses are used.)

Table 2: Results

	Femara® 2.5 mg N = 453	tamoxifen 20 mg N = 454	ratio (95% CI) p-value (2-sided)
Median Time to Progression	9.4 months	6.0 months	0.70 (0.60, 0.82)[1] p=0.0001
Objective Response Rate (CR + PR)	137 (30%)	92 (20%)	1.71 (1.26, 2.32)[2] p=0.0006
(CR)	34 (8%)	13 (3%)	2.75 (1.43, 5.29)[2] p=0.002

[1]Hazard ratio
[2]Odds ratio

Table 3: Efficacy in Patients Who Received Prior Antiestrogen Adjuvant Therapy

	Femara® 2.5 mg N = 84	tamoxifen 20 mg N = 83	p-value (2-sided)
Median Time to Progression	8.8 months	5.9 months	0.04[1]
Objective Response Rate (CR + PR)	29%	8%	0.002[2]

[1]Hazard ratio
[2]Odds ratio

Table 4: Efficacy by Disease Site

	Femara® 2.5 mg N = 453	tamoxifen 20 mg N = 454	p-value (2-sided)
Dominant Disease Site			
Soft Tissue:	N = 113	N = 116	
Median TTP	12.9 months	6.4 months	0.05[1]
Objective Response Rate	48%	35%	0.04[2]
Bone:	N = 146	N = 130	
Median TTP	9.7 months	6.2 months	0.01[1]
Objective Response Rate	22%	14%	0.08[2]
Visceral:	N = 194	N = 208	
Median TTP	8.2 months	4.7 months	0.001[1]
Objective Response Rate	26%	16%	0.02[2]

[1]Hazard ratio
[2]Odds ratio

Table 5: Selected Study Population Demographics

Parameter	megestrol acetate study	aminoglutethimide study
No. of Participants	552	557
Receptor Status		
ER/PR Positive	57%	56%
ER/PR Unknown	43%	44%
Previous Therapy		
Adjuvant Only	33%	38%
Therapeutic +/− Adj.	66%	62%
Sites of Disease		
Soft Tissue	56%	50%
Bone	50%	55%
Visceral	40%	44%

Table 6: Megestrol Acetate Study Results

	Femara® 0.5 mg N = 188	Femara® 2.5 mg N = 174	megestrol acetate N = 190
Objective Response (CR + PR)	22 (11.7%)	41 (23.6%)	31 (16.3%)
Median Duration of Response	552 days	(Not reached)	561 days
Median Time to Progression	154 days	170 days	168 days
Median Survival	633 days	730 days	659 days
Odds Ratio for Response	Femara 2.5: Femara 0.5 = 2.33 (95% CI: 1.32, 4.17); p=0.004*		Femara 2.5: megestrol = 1.58 (95% CI: 0.94, 2.66); p=0.08*
Relative Risk of Progression	Femara 2.5: Femara 0.5 = 0.81 (95% CI: 0.63, 1.03); p=0.09*		Femara 2.5: megestrol = 0.77 (95% CI: 0.60, 0.98); p=0.03*

*two-sided p-value

[See table 7 at top of next page]
The Kaplan-Meier Curve for progression for the aminoglutethimide study is shown in Figure 3.
[See figure 3 at top of next page]

INDICATIONS AND USAGE

Femara® (letrozole tablets) is indicated for first-line treatment of postmenopausal women with hormone receptor positive or hormone receptor unknown locally advanced or metastatic breast cancer. Femara is also indicated for the treatment of advanced breast cancer in postmenopausal women with disease progression following antiestrogen therapy.

CONTRAINDICATIONS

Femara® (letrozole tablets) is contraindicated in patients with known hypersensitivity to Femara or any of its excipients.

WARNINGS

Pregnancy

Letrozole may cause fetal harm when administered to pregnant women. Studies in rats at doses equal to or greater than 0.003 mg/kg (about 1/100 the daily maximum recommended human dose on a mg/m[2] basis) administered during

Continued on next page

Femara—Cont.

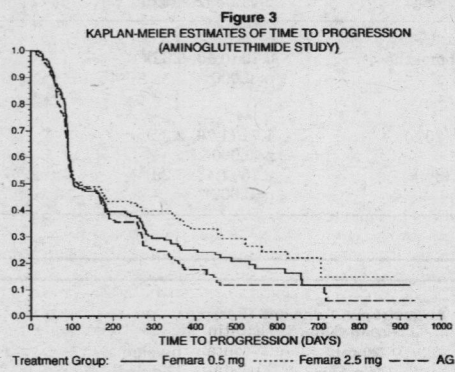

Figure 3
KAPLAN-MEIER ESTIMATES OF TIME TO PROGRESSION
(AMINOGLUTETHIMIDE STUDY)

TIME TO PROGRESSION (DAYS)

Treatment Group: —— Femara 0.5 mg ········ Femara 2.5 mg — — — AG

the period of organogenesis, have shown that letrozole is embryotoxic and fetotoxic, as indicated by intrauterine mortality, increased resorption, increased postimplantation loss, decreased numbers of live fetuses and fetal anomalies including absence and shortening of renal papilla, dilation of ureter, edema and incomplete ossification of frontal skull and metatarsals. Letrozole was teratogenic in rats. A 0.03 mg/kg dose (about 1/10 the daily maximum recommended human dose on a mg/m² basis) caused fetal domed head and cervical/centrum vertebral fusion.

Letrozole is embryotoxic at doses equal to or greater than 0.002 mg/kg and fetotoxic when administered to rabbits at 0.02 mg/kg (about 1/100,000 and 1/10,000 the daily maximum recommended human dose on a mg/m² basis, respectively). Fetal anomalies included incomplete ossification of the skull, sternebrae, and fore- and hindlegs.

There are no studies in pregnant women. Femara® (letrozole tablets) is indicated for post-menopausal women. If there is exposure to letrozole during pregnancy, the patient should be apprised of the potential hazard to the fetus and potential risk for loss of the pregnancy.

PRECAUTIONS
Laboratory Tests
No dose-related effect of Femara® (letrozole tablets) on any hematologic or clinical chemistry parameter was evident. Moderate decreases in lymphocyte counts, of uncertain clinical significance, were observed in some patients receiving Femara 2.5 mg. This depression was transient in about half of those affected. Two patients on Femara developed thrombocytopenia; relationship to the study drug was unclear. Patient withdrawal due to laboratory abnormalities, whether related to study treatment or not, was infrequent.

Increases in SGOT, SGPT, and gamma GT ≥5 times the upper limit of normal (ULN) and of bilirubin ≥1.5 times the ULN were most often associated with metastatic disease in the liver. About 3% of study participants receiving Femara had abnormalities in liver chemistries not associated with documented metastases; these abnormalities may have been related to study drug therapy. In the megestrol acetate comparative study about 8% of patients treated with megestrol acetate had abnormalities in liver chemistries that were not associated with documented liver metastases; in the aminoglutethimide study about 10% of aminoglutethimide-treated patients had abnormalities in liver chemistries not associated with hepatic metastases.

Drug Interactions
Clinical interaction studies with cimetidine and warfarin indicated that the coadministration of Femara with these drugs does not result in clinically-significant drug interactions. (See CLINICAL PHARMACOLOGY.)
There is no clinical experience to date on the use of Femara in combination with other anticancer agents.
Drug/Laboratory Test-Interactions
None observed.
Carcinogenesis, Mutagenesis, Impairment of Fertility
A conventional carcinogenesis study in mice at doses of 0.6 to 60 mg/kg/day (about one to 100 times the daily maximum recommended human dose on a mg/m² basis) administered by oral gavage for up to 2 years revealed a dose-related increase in the incidence of benign ovarian stromal tumors. The incidence of combined hepatocellular adenoma and carcinoma showed a significant trend in females when the high dose group was excluded due to low survival. In a separate study, plasma AUC_{0-12hr} levels in mice at 60 mg/kg/day were 55 times higher than the AUC_{0-24hr} level in breast cancer patients at the recommended dose. The carcinogenicity study in rats at oral doses of 0.1 to 10 mg/kg/day (about 0.4 to 40 times the daily maximum recommended human dose on a mg/m² basis) for up to 2 years also produced an increase in the incidence of benign ovarian stromal tumors at 10 mg/kg/day. Ovarian hyperplasia was observed in females at doses equal to or greater than 0.1 mg/kg/day. At 10 mg/kg/day, plasma AUC_{0-24hr} levels in rats were 80 times higher than the level in breast cancer patients at the recommended dose.

Letrozole was not mutagenic in in vitro tests (Ames and E.coli bacterial tests) but was observed to be a potential

clastogen in in vitro assays (CHO K1 and CCL 61 Chinese hamster ovary cells). Letrozole was not clastogenic in vivo (micronucleus test in rats).
Studies to investigate the effect of letrozole on fertility have not been conducted; however, repeated dosing caused sexual inactivity in females and atrophy of the reproductive tract in males and females at doses of 0.6, 0.1 and 0.03 mg/kg in mice, rats and dogs, respectively (about one, 0.4 and 0.4 the daily maximum recommended human dose on a mg/m² basis, respectively).
Pregnancy
Pregnancy Category D (see WARNINGS).
Nursing Mothers
It is not known if letrozole is excreted in human milk. Because many drugs are excreted in human milk, caution should be exercised when letrozole is administered to a nursing woman (see WARNINGS and PRECAUTIONS).
Pediatric Use
The safety and effectiveness in pediatric patients have not been established.
Geriatric Use
The median age of patients in the trial that compared Femara 2.5 mg daily to tamoxifen 20 mg daily as first-line therapy was 65 years. About 1/3 of the patients were ≥70 years old. Femara time to tumor progression and tumor response rate were better in patients ≥70 than in patients <70 years of age.
The mean age of patients in the two second-line randomized trials, that compared Femara (0.5 mg and 2.5 mg) to megestrol acetate and to aminoglutethimide, was 64 years. Thirty percent of patients were ≥70 years old. The proportion of patients responding to each dose of Femara was similar for women ≥70 years old and <70 years old.

ADVERSE REACTIONS
Femara® (letrozole tablets) was generally well tolerated across all studies as first-line and second-line treatment for

breast cancer and adverse reaction rates were similar in both settings.
First-Line Breast Cancer
A total of 455 patients was treated for a median time of exposure of 11 months. The incidence of adverse experiences was similar for Femara and tamoxifen. The most frequently reported adverse experiences were bone pain, hot flushes, back pain, nausea, arthralgia and dyspnea. Discontinuations for adverse experiences other than progression of tumor occurred in 10/455 (2%) of patients on Femara and in 15/455 (3%) of patients on tamoxifen.
Adverse events, regardless of relationship to study drug, that were reported in at least 5% of the patients treated with Femara 2.5 mg or tamoxifen 20 mg in the first-line treatment study are shown in Table 8.
[See table 8 above]
Other less frequent (≤2%) adverse experiences considered consequential for both treatment groups, included peripheral thromboembolic events, cardiovascular events, and cerebrovascular events. Peripheral thromboembolic events included venous thrombosis, thrombophlebitis, portal vein thrombosis and pulmonary embolism. Cardiovascular events included angina, myocardial infarction, myocardial ischemia, and coronary heart disease. Cerebrovascular events included transient ischemic attacks, thrombotic or hemorrhagic strokes and development of hemiparesis.
Second-Line Breast Cancer
Femara was generally well tolerated in two controlled clinical trials.
Study discontinuations in the megestrol acetate comparison study for adverse events other than progression of tumor occurred in 5/188 (2.7%) of patients on Femara 0.5 mg, in 4/174 (2.3%) of the patients on Femara 2.5 mg, and in 15/190 (7.9%) of patients on megestrol acetate. There were fewer thromboembolic events at both Femara doses than on

Table 7. Aminoglutethimide Study Results

	Femara® 0.5 N = 193	Femara® 2.5 N = 185	aminoglutethimide N = 179
Objective Response (CR + PR)	34 (17.6%)	34 (18.4%)	22 (12.3%)
Median Duration of Response	619 days	706 days	450 days
Median Time to Progression	103 days	123 days	112 days
Median Survival	636 days	792 days	592 days
Odds Ratio for Response	Femara 2.5: Femara 0.5 = 1.05 (95% Cl: 0.62, 1.79); p=0.85*		Femara 2.5: aminoglutethimide=1.61 (95% Cl: 0.90, 2.87); p=0.11*
Relative Risk of Progression	Femara 2.5: Femara 0.5 = 0.86 (95% Cl: 0.68, 1.11); p=0.25*		Femara 2.5: aminoglutethimide=0.74 (95% Cl: 0.57, 0.94); p=0.02*

*two-sided p-value

Table 8: Percentage (%) of Patients with Adverse Events

Adverse Experience	Femara® 2.5 mg (n=455) %	tamoxifen 20 mg (n=455) %
Body as a Whole		
Fatigue	11	11
Chest pain	8	8
Weight decreased	6	4
Pain-not otherwise specified	5	6
Weakness	5	3
Cardiovascular		
Hot flushes	18	15
Edema-lower limb	5	5
Hypertension	5	4
Digestive System		
Nausea	15	16
Constipation	9	9
Diarrhea	7	4
Vomiting	7	7
Appetite decreased	4	6
Pain-abdominal	4	5
Infections/Infestations		
Influenza	5	4
Musculoskeletal System		
Pain-bone	20	18
Pain-back	17	17
Arthralgia	14	13
Pain-limb	8	7
Nervous System		
Headache	8	7
Insomnia	6	4
Reproductive		
Breast Pain	5	6
Respiratory System		
Dyspnea	14	15
Coughing	11	10
Skin and Appendages		
Alopecia/hair thinning	5	4
Surgical/Medical Procedures		
Post-mastectomy lymphoedema	7	6

Table 9: Percentage (%) of Patients with Adverse Events

Adverse Experience	Pooled Femara® 2.5 mg (n=359) %	Pooled Femara® 0.5 mg (n=380) %	megestrol acetate 160 mg (n=189) %	aminoglutethimide 500 mg (n=178) %
Body as a Whole				
Fatigue	8	6	11	3
Chest pain	6	3	7	3
Peripheral edema[1]	5	5	8	3
Asthenia	4	5	4	5
Weight increase	2	2	9	3
Cardiovascular				
Hypertension	5	7	5	6
Digestive System				
Nausea	13	15	9	14
Vomiting	7	7	5	9
Constipation	6	7	9	7
Diarrhea	6	5	3	4
Pain-abdominal	6	5	9	8
Anorexia	5	3	5	5
Dyspepsia	3	4	6	5
Infections/Infestations				
Viral infection	6	5	6	3
Lab Abnormality				
Hypercholesterolemia	3	3	0	6
Musculoskeletal System				
Musculoskeletal[2]	21	22	30	14
Arthralgia	8	8	8	3
Nervous System				
Headache	9	12	9	7
Somnolence	3	2	2	9
Dizziness	3	5	7	3
Respiratory System				
Dyspnea	7	9	16	5
Coughing	6	5	7	5
Skin and Appendages				
Hot flushes	6	5	4	3
Rash[3]	5	4	3	12
Pruritus	1	2	5	3

[1] Includes peripheral edema, leg edema, dependent edema, edema
[2] Includes musculoskeletal pain, skeletal pain, back pain, arm pain, leg pain
[3] Includes rash, erythematous rash, maculopapular rash, psoriaform rash, vesicular rash

the megestrol acetate arm (2 of 362 patients or 0.6% vs. 9 of 190 patients or 4.7%). There was also less vaginal bleeding (1 of 362 patients or 0.3% vs. 6 of 190 patients or 3.2%) on letrozole than on megestrol acetate. In the aminoglutethimide comparison study, discontinuations for reasons other than progression occurred in 6/193 (3.1%) of patients on 0.5 mg Femara, 7/185 (3.8%) of patients on 2.5 mg Femara, and 7/178 (3.9%) of patients on aminoglutethimide.

Comparisons of the incidence of adverse events revealed no significant differences between the high and low dose Femara groups in either study. Most of the adverse events observed in all treatment groups were mild to moderate in severity and it was generally not possible to distinguish adverse reactions due to treatment from the consequences of the patient's metastatic breast cancer, the effects of estrogen deprivation, or intercurrent illness.

Adverse events, regardless of relationship to study drug, that were reported in at least 5% of the patients treated with Femara 0.5 mg, Femara 2.5 mg, megestrol acetate, or aminoglutethimide in the two controlled trials are shown in Table 9.
[See table above]

Other less frequent (<5%) adverse experiences considered consequential and reported in at least 3 patients treated with Femara, included hypercalcemia, fracture, depression, anxiety, pleural effusion, alopecia, increased sweating and vertigo.

OVERDOSAGE

Isolated cases of Femara® (letrozole tablets) overdose have been reported. In these instances, the highest single dose ingested was 62.5 mg or 25 tablets. While no serious adverse events were reported in these cases, because of the limited data available, no firm recommendations for treatment can be made. However, emesis could be induced if the patient is alert. In general, supportive care and frequent monitoring of vital signs are also appropriate. In single dose studies the highest dose used was 30 mg, which was well tolerated; in multiple dose trials, the largest dose of 10 mg was well tolerated.

Lethality was observed in mice and rats following single oral doses that were equal to or greater than 2000 mg/kg (about 4000 to 8000 times the daily maximum recommended human dose on a mg/m² basis); death was associated with reduced motor activity, ataxia and dyspnea. Lethality was observed in cats following single IV doses that were equal to or greater than 10 mg/kg (about 50 times the daily maximum recommended human dose on a mg/m² basis); death was preceded by depressed blood pressure and arrhythmias.

DOSAGE AND ADMINISTRATION

Adult and Elderly Patients

The recommended dose of Femara® (letrozole tablets) is one 2.5 mg tablet administered once a day, without regard to meals. Treatment with Femara should continue until tumor progression is evident. No dose adjustment is required for elderly patients. Patients treated with Femara do not require glucocorticoid or mineralocorticoid replacement therapy.

Renal Impairment

(See CLINICAL PHARMACOLOGY.) No dosage adjustment is required for patients with renal impairment if creatinine clearance is ≥10 mL/min.

Hepatic Impairment

(See CLINICAL PHARMACOLOGY.) Although letrozole blood concentrations were modestly increased in subjects with moderate hepatic impairment due to cirrhosis, no dosage adjustment is recommended for patients with mild-to-moderate hepatic impairment. Patients with severe impairment of liver function have not been studied. Because letrozole is eliminated almost exclusively by hepatic metabolism, patients with severe impairment of liver function should be dosed with caution.

HOW SUPPLIED

2.5 mg tablets — dark yellow, film-coated, round, slightly biconvex, with beveled edges (imprinted with the letters FV on one side and CG on the other side).
Packaged in HDPE bottles with a safety screw cap.
Bottles of 30 tablets .... NDC 0078-0249-15
Store at 25°C (77°F); excursions permitted to 15°C-30°C (59°F-86°F) [see USP Controlled Room Temperature].

T2001-03
REV: JANUARY 2001   Printed in U.S.A.   89010302
Manufactured by
Novartis Consumer Health Incorporated
Lincoln, Nebraska 68517
Manufactured for
Novartis Pharmaceuticals Corporation
East Hanover, New Jersey 07936

LESCOL®
(fluvastatin sodium)
Capsules

LESCOL® XL
(fluvastatin sodium)
Extended-Release Tablets

Rx only

Prescribing information for this product, which appears on pages 2181–2184 of the 2001 PDR, has been completely revised as follows. Please write "See Supplement A" next to the product heading.

Prescribing Information

DESCRIPTION

Lescol® (fluvastatin sodium), is a water-soluble cholesterol lowering agent which acts through the inhibition of 3-hydroxy-3-methylglutaryl-coenzyme A (HMG-CoA) reductase.

Fluvastatin sodium is $[R^*, S^*-(E)]-(\pm)-7-[3-(4-fluorophenyl)-1-(1-methylethyl)-1H-indol-2-yl]-3,5-dihydroxy-6-heptenoic$ acid, monosodium salt. The empirical formula of fluvastatin

sodium is $C_{24}H_{25}FNO_4 \cdot Na$, its molecular weight is 433.46 and its structural formula is:

$C_{24}H_{25}FNO_4 \cdot Na$ Mol. wt. 433.46

This molecular entity is the first entirely synthetic HMG-CoA reductase inhibitor, and is in part structurally distinct from the fungal derivatives of this therapeutic class.

Fluvastatin sodium is a white to pale yellow, hygroscopic powder soluble in water, ethanol and methanol. Lescol is supplied as capsules containing fluvastatin sodium, equivalent to 20 mg or 40 mg of fluvastatin, for oral administration. Lescol® XL (fluvastatin sodium) is supplied as extended-release tablets containing fluvastatin sodium, equivalent to 80 mg of fluvastatin, for oral administration.

Active Ingredient: fluvastatin sodium
Inactive Ingredients in capsules: gelatin, magnesium stearate, microcrystalline cellulose, pregelatinized starch (corn), red iron oxide, sodium lauryl sulfate, talc, titanium dioxide, yellow iron oxide, and other ingredients.
Capsules may also include: benzyl alcohol, black iron oxide, butylparaben, carboxymethylcellulose sodium, edetate calcium disodium, methylparaben, propylparaben, silicon dioxide and sodium propionate.
Inactive Ingredients in extended-release tablets: microcrystalline cellulose, hydroxypropyl cellulose, hydroxypropyl methyl cellulose, potassium bicarbonate, povidone, magnesium stearate, iron oxide yellow, titanium dioxide and polyethylene glycol 8000.

CLINICAL PHARMACOLOGY

A variety of clinical studies have demonstrated that elevated levels of total cholesterol (Total-C), low density lipoprotein cholesterol (LDL-C), triglycerides (TG) and apolipoprotein B (a membrane transport complex for LDL-C) promote human atherosclerosis. Similarly, decreased levels of HDL-cholesterol (HDL-C) and its transport complex, apolipoprotein A, are associated with the development of atherosclerosis. Epidemiologic investigations have established that cardiovascular morbidity and mortality vary directly with the level of Total-C and LDL-C and inversely with the level of HDL-C.

Like LDL, cholesterol-enriched triglyceride-rich lipoproteins, including VLDL, IDL and remnants, can also promote atherosclerosis. Elevated plasma triglycerides are frequently found in a triad with low HDL-C levels and small LDL particles, as well as in association with non-lipid metabolic risk factors for coronary heart disease. As such, total plasma TG has not consistently been shown to be an independent risk factor for CHD. Furthermore, the independent effect of raising HDL or lowering TG on the risk of coronary and cardiovascular morbidity and mortality has not been determined.

In patients with hypercholesterolemia and mixed dyslipidemia, treatment with Lescol® (fluvastatin sodium) or Lescol® XL (fluvastatin sodium) reduced Total-C, LDL-C, apolipoprotein B, and triglycerides while producing an increase in HDL-C. Increases in HDL-C are greater in patients with low HDL-C (<35 mg/dL). Neither agent had a consistent effect on either Lp(a) or fibrinogen. The effect of Lescol or Lescol XL induced changes in lipoprotein levels, including reduction of serum cholesterol, on cardiovascular morbidity or mortality has not been determined.

Mechanism of Action

Lescol is a competitive inhibitor of HMG-CoA reductase, which is responsible for the conversion of 3-hydroxy-3-methylglutaryl-coenzyme A (HMG-CoA) to mevalonate, a precursor of sterols, including cholesterol. The inhibition of cholesterol biosynthesis reduces the cholesterol in hepatic cells, which stimulates the synthesis of LDL receptors and thereby increases the uptake of LDL particles. The end result of these biochemical processes is a reduction of the plasma cholesterol concentration.

Pharmacokinetics/Metabolism

Oral Absorption

Fluvastatin is absorbed rapidly and completely following oral administration of the capsule, with peak concentrations reached in less than 1 hour. Following administration of a 10 mg dose, the absolute bioavailability is 24% (range 9%-50%). Administration with food reduces the rate but not the extent of absorption. At steady-state, administration of fluvastatin with the evening meal results in a two-fold decrease in C_{max} and more than two-fold increase in t_{max} as compared to administration 4 hours after the evening meal. No significant differences in extent of absorption or in the lipid-lowering effects were observed between the two administrations. After single or multiple doses above 20 mg, fluvastatin exhibits saturable first-pass metabolism resulting in higher-than-expected plasma fluvastatin concentrations.

Fluvastatin has two optical enantiomers, an active 3R,5S and an inactive 3S,5R form. In vivo studies showed that stereo-selective hepatic binding of the active form occurs during the first pass resulting in a difference in the peak levels of the two enantiomers, with the active to inactive

Continued on next page

Lescol—Cont.

peak concentration ratio being about 0.7. The approximate ratio of the active to inactive approaches unity after the peak is seen and thereafter the two enantiomers decline with the same half-life. After an intravenous administration, bypassing the first-pass metabolism, the ratios of the enantiomers in plasma were similar throughout the concentration-time profiles.

Fluvastatin administered as Lescol XL 80 mg tablets reaches peak concentration in approximately 3 hours under fasting conditions, after a low-fat meal, or 2.5 hours after a low-fat meal. The mean relative bioavailability of the XL tablet is approximately 29% (range: 9%-66%) compared to that of the Lescol immediate release capsule administered under fasting conditions. Administration of a high fat meal delayed the absorption (T_{max}: 6H) and increased the bioavailability of the XL tablet by approximately 50%. Once Lescol XL begins to be absorbed, fluvastatin concentrations rise rapidly. The maximum concentration seen after a high fat meal is much less than the peak concentration following a single dose or twice daily dose of the 40 mg Lescol capsule. Overall variability in the pharmacokinetics of Lescol XL is large (42%-64% CV for C_{max} and AUC), and especially so after a high fat meal (63%-89% for C_{max} and AUC). Intra-subject variability in the pharmacokinetics of Lescol XL under fasting conditions (about 25% for C_{max} and AUC) tends to be much smaller as compared to the overall variability. Multiple peaks in plasma fluvastatin concentrations have been observed after Lescol XL administration.

Distribution
Fluvastatin is 98% bound to plasma proteins. The mean volume of distribution (VD_{ss}) is estimated at 0.35 L/kg. The parent drug is targeted to the liver and no active metabolites are present systemically. At therapeutic concentrations, the protein binding of fluvastatin is not affected by warfarin, salicylic acid and glyburide.

Metabolism
Fluvastatin is metabolized in the liver, primarily via hydroxylation of the indole ring at the 5- and 6-positions. N-dealkylation and beta-oxidation of the side-chain also occurs. The hydroxy metabolites have some pharmacologic activity, but do not circulate in the blood. Both enantiomers of fluvastatin are metabolized in a similar manner.

In vitro studies demonstrated that fluvastatin undergoes oxidative metabolism, predominantly via 2C9 isozyme systems (75%). Other isozymes that contribute to fluvastatin metabolism are 2C8 (~5%) and 3A4 (~20%). *(See PRECAUTIONS: Drug Interactions Section)*.

Elimination
Fluvastatin is primarily (about 90%) eliminated in the feces as metabolites, with less than 2% present as unchanged drug. Urinary recovery is about 5%. After a radiolabeled dose of fluvastatin, the clearance was 0.8 L/h/kg. Following multiple oral doses of radiolabeled compound, there was no accumulation of fluvastatin; however, there was a 2.3 fold accumulation of total radioactivity.

Steady-state plasma concentrations show no evidence of accumulation of fluvastatin following immediate release capsule administration of up to 80 mg daily, as evidenced by a beta-elimination half-life of less than 3 hours. However, under conditions of maximum rate of absorption (i.e., fasting) systemic exposure to fluvastatin is increased 33% to 53% compared to a single 20 mg or 40 mg dose of the immediate release capsule. Accumulation following once daily administration of the 80 mg Lescol XL tablet has not been studied. Single-dose and steady-state pharmacokinetic parameters in 33 subjects with hypercholesterolemia for the capsules and single dose data in 24 healthy subjects for the extended-release tablets are summarized below:
[See table 1 above]

Special Populations
Renal Insufficiency: No significant (<6%) renal excretion of fluvastatin occurs in humans.

Hepatic Insufficiency: Fluvastatin is subject to saturable first-pass metabolism/sequestration by the liver and is eliminated primarily via the biliary route. Therefore, the potential exists for drug accumulation in patients with hepatic insufficiency. Caution should therefore be exercised when fluvastatin sodium is administered to patients with a history of liver disease or heavy alcohol ingestion *(see WARNINGS)*. Fluvastatin AUC and C_{max} values increased by about 2.5 fold in hepatic insufficiency patients. This result was attributed to the decreased presystemic metabolism due to hepatic dysfunction. The enantiomer ratios of the two isomers of fluvastatin in hepatic insufficiency patients were comparable to those observed in healthy subjects.

Age: Plasma levels of fluvastatin are not affected by age.

Gender: Women tend to have slightly higher (but statistically insignificant) fluvastatin concentrations than men for the immediate release capsule. This is most likely due to body weight differences, as adjusting for body weight decreases the magnitude of the differences seen. For Lescol XL, there are 67% and 77% increases in systemic availability for women over men under fasted and high fat meal conditions.

Pediatric: No data are available. Fluvastatin is not indicated for use in the pediatric population.

CLINICAL STUDIES
Hypercholesterolemia (heterozygous familial and non familial) and Mixed Dyslipidemia
In 12 placebo-controlled studies in patients with Type IIa or IIb hyperlipoproteinemia, Lescol® (fluvastatin sodium) alone was administered to 1621 patients in daily dose regimens of 20 mg, 40 mg, and 80 mg (40 mg twice daily) for at least 6 weeks duration. After 24 weeks of treatment, daily doses of 20 mg, 40 mg, and 80 mg (40 mg twice daily) resulted in median LDL-C reductions of 22% (n=747), 25% (n=748) and 36% (n=257), respectively. Lescol treatment produced dose-related reductions in Apo B and in triglycerides and increases in HDL-C. The median (25th, 75th percentile) percent changes from baseline in HDL-C after 12 weeks of treatment with Lescol at daily doses of 20 mg, 40 mg and 80 mg (40 mg twice daily) were +2 (-4,+10), +5 (-2,+12), and +4 (-3,+12), respectively. In a subgroup of patients with primary mixed dyslipidemia, defined as baseline TG levels ≥200 mg/dL, treatment with Lescol also produced significant decreases in Total-C, LDL-C, TG and Apo B and variable increases in HDL-C. The median (25th, 75th percentile) percent changes from baseline in HDL-C after 12 weeks of treatment with Lescol at daily doses of 20 mg, 40 mg and 80 mg (40 mg twice daily) in this population were +4 (-2,+12), +8 (+1,+15), and +4 (-3,+13), respectively.

In a long-term open-label free titration study, after 96 weeks LDL-C decreases of 25% (20 mg, n=68), 31% (40 mg, n=298) and 34% (80 mg, n=209) were seen. No consistent effect on Lp(a) was observed.

Lescol® XL (fluvastatin sodium) Extended-Release Tablets have been studied in five controlled studies of patients with Type IIa or IIb hyperlipoproteinemia. Lescol XL was administered to over 900 patients in trials from 4 to 26 weeks in duration. In the three largest of these studies, Lescol XL given as a single daily dose of 80 mg significantly reduced Total-C, LDL-C, TG and Apo B. Therapeutic response is well established within two weeks, and a maximum response is achieved within four weeks. After four weeks of therapy, the median decrease in LDL-C was 38% and at week 24 endpoint the median LDL-C decrease was 35%. Significant increases in HDL-C were also observed. The median (25th and 75th percentile) percent changes from baseline in HDL-C for Lescol XL were +7(+0,+15) after 24 weeks of treatment.
[See table 2 above]

In patients with primary mixed dyslipidemia (Fredrickson Type IIb) as defined by baseline plasma triglycerides levels ≥200 mg/dL, Lescol XL 80 mg produced a median reduction in triglycerides of 25%. In these patients, Lescol XL 80 mg produced median (25th and 75th percentile) percent change from baseline in HDL-C of +11(+3,+20). Significant decreases in Total-C, LDL-C, and Apo B were also achieved. In these studies, patients with triglycerides >400 mg/dL were excluded.

Atherosclerosis
In the Lipoprotein and Coronary Atherosclerosis Study (LCAS), the effect of Lescol therapy on coronary atherosclerosis was assessed by quantitative coronary angiography (QCA) in patients with coronary artery disease and mild to moderate hypercholesterolemia (baseline LDL-C range 115-190 mg/dL). In this randomized double-blind, placebo controlled trial, 429 patients were treated with conventional measures (Step 1 AHA Diet) and either Lescol 40 mg/day or placebo. In order to provide treatment to patients receiving placebo with LDL-C levels ≥160 mg/dL at baseline, adjunctive therapy with cholestyramine was added after week 12 to all patients in the study with baseline LDL-C values of ≥160 mg/dL. These baseline levels were present in 25% of the study population. Quantitative coronary angiograms were evaluated at baseline and 2.5 years in 340 (79%) angiographic evaluable patients.

Lescol significantly slowed the progression of coronary atherosclerosis. Compared to placebo, Lescol significantly slowed the progression of lesions as measured by within-patient per-lesion change in minimum lumen diameter (MLD), the primary endpoint (see Figure 1 below), percent diameter stenosis (Figure 2), and the formation of new lesions (13% of all fluvastatin patients versus 22% of all placebo patients). Additionally, a significant difference in favor of Lescol was found between all fluvastatin and all placebo patients in the distribution among the three categories of definite progression, definite regression, and mixed or no change. Beneficial angiographic results (change in MLD) were independent of patients' gender and consistent across a range of baseline LDL-C levels.

Table 1
Single-dose and steady-state pharmacokinetic parameters

	C_{max} (ng/mL) mean ± SD (range)	AUC (ng·h/mL) mean ± SD (range)	t_{max} (hr) mean ± SD (range)	CL/F (L/hr) mean ± SD (range)	$t_{1/2}$ (hr) mean ± SD (range)
Capsules					
20 mg single dose (n=17)	166±106 (48.9-517)	207±65 (111-88)	0.9±0.4 (0.5-2.0)	107±38.1 (69.5-181)	2.5±1.7 (0.5-6.6)
20 mg twice daily (n=17)	200±86 (71.8-366)	275±111 (91.6-467)	1.2±0.9 (0.5-4.0)	87.8±45 (42.8-218)	2.8±1.7 (0.9-6.0)
40 mg single dose (n=16)	273±189 (72.8-812)	456±259 (207-1221)	1.2±0.7 (0.75-3.0)	108±44.7 (32.8-193)	2.7±1.3 (0.8-5.9)
40 mg twice daily (n=16)	432±236 (119-990)	697±275 (359-1559)	1.2±0.6 (0.5-2.5)	64.2±21.1 (25.7-111)	2.7±1.3 (0.7-5.0)
Extended-Release Tablets 80 mg single dose (n=24)					
Fasting	126±53 (37-242)	579±341 (144-1760)	3.2±2.6 (1-12)		
Fed State-High Fat Meal	183±163 (21-733)	861±632 (199-3132)	6 (2-24)		

Table 2
Median Percent Change in Lipid Parameters from Baseline to Week 24 Endpoint
All Placebo-Controlled Studies (Lescol) and Active Controlled Trials (Lescol XL)

Dose	Total Chol. N	% Δ	TG N	% Δ	LDL N	% Δ	Apo B N	% Δ	HDL N	% Δ
All Patients										
Lescol 20 mg[1]	747	-17	747	-12	747	-22	114	-19	747	+3
Lescol 40 mg[1]	748	-19	748	-14	748	-25	125	-18	748	+4
Lescol 40 mg twice daily[1]	257	-27	257	-18	257	-36	232	-28	257	+6
Lescol XL 80 mg[2]	750	-25	750	-19	748	-35	745	-27	750	+7
Baseline TG ≥200 mg/dL										
Lescol 20 mg[1]	148	-16	148	-17	148	-22	23	-19	148	+6
Lescol 40 mg[1]	179	-18	179	-20	179	-24	47	-18	179	+7
Lescol 40 mg twice daily[1]	76	-27	76	-23	76	-35	69	-28	76	+9
Lescol XL 80 mg[2]	239	-25	239	-25	237	-33	235	-27	239	+11

[1] Data for Lescol from 12 placebo controlled trials
[2] Data for Lescol XL 80 mg tablet from three 24 week controlled trials

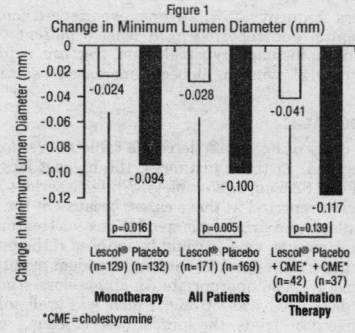

Figure 1
Change in Minimum Lumen Diameter (mm)

Monotherapy: Lescol® (n=129) -0.024, Placebo (n=132) -0.094, p=0.016
All Patients: Lescol® (n=171) -0.028, Placebo (n=169) -0.100, p=0.005
Combination Therapy: Lescol® + CME* (n=42) -0.041, Placebo + CME* (n=37) -0.117, p=0.139

*CME=cholestyramine

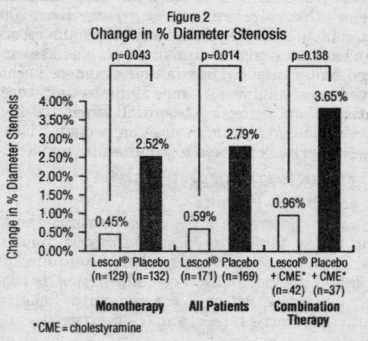

Figure 2
Change in % Diameter Stenosis

Monotherapy: Lescol® (n=129) 0.45%, Placebo (n=132) 2.52%, p=0.043
All Patients: Lescol® (n=171) 0.59%, Placebo (n=169) 2.79%, p=0.014
Combination Therapy: Lescol® + CME* (n=42) 0.96%, Placebo + CME* (n=37) 3.65%, p=0.138

*CME = cholestyramine

INDICATIONS AND USAGE

Therapy with lipid-altering agents should be a component of multiple risk factor intervention in those individuals at significantly increased risk for atherosclerosis vascular disease due to hypercholesterolemia.

Hypercholesterolemia (heterozygous familial and non familial) and Mixed Dyslipidemia

Lescol® (fluvastatin sodium) and Lescol® XL (fluvastatin sodium) are indicated as an adjunct to diet to reduce elevated total cholesterol (Total-C), LDL-C, TG and Apo B levels, and to increase HDL-C in patients with primary hypercholesterolemia and mixed dyslipidemia (Fredrickson Type IIa and IIb) whose response to dietary restriction of saturated fat and cholesterol and other non-pharmacological measures has not been adequate.

Atherosclerosis

Lescol and Lescol XL are also indicated to slow the progression of coronary atherosclerosis in patients with coronary heart disease as part of a treatment strategy to lower total and LDL cholesterol to target levels.

Therapy with lipid-altering agents should be considered only after secondary causes for hyperlipidemia such as poorly controlled diabetes mellitus, hypothyroidism, nephrotic syndrome, dysproteinemias, obstructive liver disease, other medication, or alcoholism, have been excluded. Prior to initiation of fluvastatin sodium, a lipid profile should be performed to measure Total-C, HDL-C and TG. For patients with TG <400 mg/dL (<4.5 mmol/L), LDL-C can be estimated using the following equation:

LDL-C = Total-C - HDL-C - 1/5 TG

For TG levels >400 mg/dL (>4.5 mmol/L), this equation is less accurate and LDL-C concentrations should be determined by ultracentrifugation. In many hypertriglyceridemic patients LDL-C may be low or normal despite elevated Total-C. In such cases, Lescol is not indicated.

Lipid determinations should be performed at intervals of no less than 4 weeks and dosage adjusted according to the patient's response to therapy.

The National Cholesterol Education Program (NCEP) Treatment Guidelines are summarized below:

[See table 3 above]

At the time of hospitalization for an acute coronary event, consideration can be given to initiating drug therapy at discharge if the LDL-C level is ≥130 mg/dL (NCEP-ATP II).

Since the goal of treatment is to lower LDL-C, the NCEP recommends that the LDL-C levels be used to initiate and assess treatment response. Only if LDL-C levels are not available, should the Total-C be used to monitor therapy.

[See table 4 above]

Neither Lescol nor Lescol XL have been studied in conditions where the major abnormality is elevation of chylomicrons, VLDL, or IDL (i.e., hyperlipoproteinemia Types I, III, IV, or V).

CONTRAINDICATIONS

Hypersensitivity to any component of this medication. Lescol® (fluvastatin sodium) and Lescol® XL (fluvastatin sodium) are contraindicated in patients with active liver disease or unexplained, persistent elevations in serum transaminases *(see WARNINGS)*.

Pregnancy and Lactation

Atherosclerosis is a chronic process and discontinuation of lipid-lowering drugs during pregnancy should have little impact on the outcome of long-term therapy of primary hypercholesterolemia. Cholesterol and other products of cholesterol biosynthesis are essential components for fetal development (including synthesis of steroids and cell membranes). Since HMG-CoA reductase inhibitors decrease cholesterol synthesis and possibly the synthesis of other biologically active substances derived from cholesterol, they may cause fetal harm when administered to pregnant women. Therefore, HMG-CoA reductase inhibitors are contraindicated during pregnancy and in nursing mothers. **Fluvastatin sodium should be administered to women of childbearing age only when such patients are highly unlikely to conceive and have been informed of the potential hazards.** If the patient becomes pregnant while taking this class of drug, therapy should be discontinued and the patient apprised of the potential hazard to the fetus.

WARNINGS

Liver Enzymes

Biochemical abnormalities of liver function have been associated with HMG-CoA reductase inhibitors and other lipid-lowering agents. Approximately 1.1% of patients treated with Lescol® (fluvastatin sodium) capsules in worldwide trials developed dose-related, persistent elevations of transaminase levels to more than 3 times the upper limit of normal. Fourteen of these patients (0.6%) were discontinued from therapy. In all clinical trials, a total of 33/2969 patients (1.1%) had persistent transaminase elevations with an average fluvastatin exposure of approximately 71.2 weeks; 19 of these patients (0.6%) were discontinued. The majority of patients with these abnormal biochemical findings were asymptomatic.

In a pooled analysis of all placebo-controlled studies in which Lescol capsules were used, persistent transaminase elevations (>3 times the upper limit of normal [ULN] on two consecutive weekly measurements) occurred in 0.2%, 1.5%, and 2.7% of patients treated with 20, 40, and 80 mg (titrated to 40 mg twice daily) Lescol capsules, respectively. Ninety-one percent of the cases of persistent liver function test abnormalities (20 of 22 patients) occurred within 12 weeks of therapy and in all patients with persistent liver function test abnormalities there was an abnormal liver function test present at baseline or by week 8.

Table 3
National Cholesterol Education Program (NCEP) Treatment Guidelines

Definite Atherosclerotic Disease*	Two or More Other Risk Factors**	LDL-Cholesterol mg/dL (mmol/L) Initiation Level	Goal
NO	NO	≥190 (≥4.9)	<160 (<4.1)
NO	YES	≥160 (≥4.1)	<130 (<3.4)
YES	YES or NO	≥130 (≥3.4)	≤100 (≤2.6)

*Coronary heart disease or peripheral vascular disease (including symptomatic carotid artery disease).

**Other risk factors for coronary heart disease (CHD) include: age (males: ≥45 years; females: ≥55 years or premature menopause without estrogen replacement therapy); family history of premature CHD; current cigarette smoking; hypertension; confirmed HDL-C <35 mg/dL (<0.91 mmol/L); and diabetes mellitus. Subtract one risk factor if HDL-C is ≥60 mg/dL (≥1.6 mmol/L).

Table 4
Classification of Hyperlipoproteinemias

Type	Lipoproteins Elevated	Lipid Elevations: Major	Minor
I (rare)	Chylomicrons	TG	↑ → C
IIa	LDL	C	–
IIb	LDL, VLDL	C	TG
III (rare)	IDL	C/TG	–
IV	VLDL	TG	↑ → C
V (rare)	Chylomicrons, VLDL	TG	↑ → C

C = cholesterol, TG = triglycerides, LDL = low density lipoprotein, VLDL = very low density lipoprotein, IDL = intermediate density lipoprotein

In the pooled analysis of the 24-week controlled trials, persistent transaminase elevation occurred in 1.9%, 1.8% and 4.9% of patients treated with Lescol® XL (fluvastatin sodium) 80 mg, Lescol 40 mg and Lescol 40 mg twice daily, respectively. In 13 of 16 patients treated with Lescol XL the abnormality occurred within 12 weeks of initiation of treatment with Lescol XL 80 mg.

It is recommended that liver function tests be performed before the initiation of therapy and at 12 weeks following initiation of treatment or elevation in dose. Patients who develop transaminase elevations or signs and symptoms of liver disease should be monitored to confirm the finding and should be followed thereafter with frequent liver function tests until the levels return to normal. Should an increase in AST or ALT of three times the upper limit of normal or greater persist (found on two consecutive occasions) withdrawal of fluvastatin sodium therapy is recommended.

Active liver disease or unexplained transaminase elevations are contraindications to the use of Lescol and Lescol XL *(see CONTRAINDICATIONS)*. Caution should be exercised when fluvastatin sodium is administered to patients with a history of liver disease or heavy alcohol ingestion *(see CLINICAL PHARMACOLOGY: Pharmacokinetics/Metabolism)*. Such patients should be closely monitored.

Skeletal Muscle

Rhabdomyolysis with renal dysfunction secondary to myoglobinuria has been reported with fluvastatin and with other drugs in this class. Myopathy, defined as muscle aching or muscle weakness in conjunction with increases in creatine phosphokinase (CPK) values to greater than 10 times the upper limit of normal, has been reported.

Myopathy should be considered in any patients with diffuse myalgias, muscle tenderness or weakness, and/or marked elevation of CPK. Patients should be advised to report promptly unexplained muscle pain, tenderness or weakness, particularly if accompanied by malaise or fever. Fluvastatin sodium therapy should be discontinued if markedly elevated CPK levels occur or myopathy is diagnosed or suspected. Fluvastatin sodium therapy should also be temporarily withheld in any patient experiencing an acute or serious condition predisposing to the development of renal failure secondary to rhabdomyolysis, e.g., sepsis; hypotension; major surgery; trauma; severe metabolic, endocrine, or electrolyte disorders; or uncontrolled epilepsy.

The risk of myopathy and or rhabdomyolysis during treatment with HMG-CoA reductase inhibitors has been reported to be increased if therapy with either cyclosporine, gemfibrozil, erythromycin, or niacin is administered concurrently. Myopathy was not observed in a clinical trial in 74 patients involving patients who were treated with fluvastatin sodium together with niacin.

Uncomplicated myalgia has been observed infrequently in patients treated with Lescol at rates indistinguishable from placebo.

The use of fibrates alone may occasionally be associated with myopathy. The combined use of HMG-CoA reductase inhibitors and fibrates should generally be avoided.

PRECAUTIONS

General

Before instituting therapy with Lescol® (fluvastatin sodium) or Lescol® XL (fluvastatin sodium), an attempt should be made to control hypercholesterolemia with appropriate diet, exercise, and weight reduction in obese patients, and to treat other underlying medical problems *(see INDICATIONS AND USAGE)*.

The HMG-CoA reductase inhibitors may cause elevation of creatine phosphokinase and transaminase levels *(see WARNINGS and ADVERSE REACTIONS)*. This should be considered in the differential diagnosis of chest pain in a patient on therapy with fluvastatin sodium.

Homozygous Familial Hypercholesterolemia

HMG-CoA reductase inhibitors are reported to be less effective in patients with rare homozygous familial hypercholesterolemia, possibly because these patients have few functional LDL receptors.

Information for Patients

Patients should be advised to report promptly unexplained muscle pain, tenderness or weakness, particularly if accompanied by malaise or fever.

Women should be informed that if they become pregnant while receiving Lescol or Lescol XL the drug should be discontinued immediately to avoid possible harmful effects on a developing fetus from a relative deficit of cholesterol and biological products derived from cholesterol. In addition, Lescol or Lescol XL should not be taken during nursing. *(See CONTRAINDICATIONS.)*

Drug Interactions

The below listed drug interaction information is derived from studies using immediate release fluvastatin. Similar studies have not been conducted using the Lescol XL tablet.

Immunosuppressive Drugs, Gemfibrozil, Niacin (Nicotinic Acid), Erythromycin *(See WARNINGS: Skeletal Muscle).*

In vitro data indicate that fluvastatin metabolism involves multiple Cytochrome P450 (CYP) isozymes. CYP2C9 isoenzyme is primarily involved in the metabolism of fluvastatin (~75%), while CYP2C8 and CYP3A4 isoenzymes are involved to a much less extent, i.e. ~5% and ~20%, respectively. If one pathway is inhibited in the elimination process of fluvastatin other pathways may compensate.

In vivo drug interaction studies with CYP3A4 inhibitors/substrates such as cyclosporine, erythromycin, and itraconazle result in minimal changes in the pharmacokinetics of fluvastatin, confirming less involvement of CYP3A4 isozyme. Concomitant administration of fluvastatin and phenytoin increased the levels of phenytoin and fluvastatin, suggesting predominant involvement of CYP2C9 in fluvastatin metabolism.

Niacin/Propranolol: Concomitant administration of immediate release fluvastatin sodium with niacin or propranolol has no effect on the bioavailability of fluvastatin sodium.

Cholestyramine: Administration of immediate release fluvastatin sodium concomitantly with, or up to 4 hours after cholestyramine, results in fluvastatin decreases of more than 50% for AUC and 50%-80% for C_{max}. However, administration of immediate release fluvastatin sodium 4 hours after cholestyramine resulted in a clinically significant additive effect compared with that achieved with either component drug.

Cyclosporine: Plasma cyclosporine levels remain unchanged when fluvastatin (20 mg daily) was administered concurrently in renal transplant recipients on stable cyclosporine regimens. Fluvastatin AUC increased 1.9 fold, and C_{max} increased 1.3 fold compared to historical controls.

Continued on next page

Lescol—Cont.

Digoxin: In a crossover study involving 18 patients chronically receiving digoxin, a single 40 mg dose of immediate release fluvastatin had no effect on digoxin AUC, but had an 11% increase in digoxin C_{max} and small increase in digoxin urinary clearance.

Erythromycin: Erythromycin (500 mg, single dose) did not affect steady-state plasma levels of fluvastatin (40 mg daily).

Itraconazole: Concomitant administration of fluvastatin (40 mg) and itraconazole (100 mg daily x 4 days) does not affect plasma itraconazole or fluvastatin levels.

Gemfibrozil: There is no change in either fluvastatin (20 mg twice daily) or gemfibrozil (600 mg twice daily) plasma levels when these drugs are co-administered.

Phenytoin: Single morning dose administration of phenytoin (300 mg extended release) increased mean steady-state fluvastatin (40 mg) C_{max} by 27% and AUC by 40% whereas fluvastatin increased the mean phenytoin C_{max} by 5% and AUC by 20%. Patients on phenytoin should continue to be monitored appropriately when fluvastatin therapy is initiated or when the fluvastatin dosage is changed.

Diclofenac: Concurrent administration of fluvastatin (40 mg) increased the mean C_{max} and AUC of diclofenac by 60% and 25% respectively.

Tolbutamide: In healthy volunteers, concurrent administration of either single or multiple daily doses of fluvastatin sodium (40 mg) with tolbutamide (1 g) did not affect the plasma levels of either drug to a clinically significant extent.

Glibenclamide (Glyburide): In glibenclamide-treated NIDDM patients (n=32), administration of fluvastatin (40 mg twice daily for 14 days) increased the mean C_{max}, AUC, and $t_{1/2}$ of glibenclamide approximately 50%, 69% and 121%, respectively. Glibenclamide (5-20 mg daily) increased the mean C_{max} and AUC of fluvastatin by 44% and 51%, respectively. In this study there were no changes in glucose, insulin and C-peptide levels. However, patients on concomitant therapy with glibenclamide (glyburide) and fluvastatin should continue to be monitored appropriately when their fluvastatin dose is increased to 40 mg twice daily.

Losartan: Concomitant administration of fluvastatin with losartan has no effect on the bioavailability of either losartan or its active metabolite.

Cimetidine/Ranitidine/Omeprazole: Concomitant administration of immediate release fluvastatin sodium with cimetidine, ranitidine and omeprazole results in a significant increase in the fluvastatin C_{max} (43%, 70% and 50%, respectively) and AUC (24%-33%), with an 18%-23% decrease in plasma clearance.

Rifampicin: Administration of immediate release fluvastatin sodium to subjects pretreated with rifampicin results in significant reduction in C_{max} (59%) and AUC (51%), with a large increase (95%) in plasma clearance.

Warfarin: In vitro protein binding studies demonstrated no interaction at therapeutic concentrations. Concomitant administration of a single dose of warfarin (30 mg) in young healthy males receiving immediate release fluvastatin sodium (40 mg/day × 8 days) resulted in no elevation of racemic warfarin concentration. There was also no effect on prothrombin complex activity when compared to concomitant administration of placebo and warfarin. However, bleeding and/or increased prothrombin times have been reported in patients taking coumarin anticoagulants concomitantly with other HMG-CoA reductase inhibitors. Therefore, patients receiving warfarin-type anticoagulants should have their prothrombin times closely monitored when fluvastatin sodium is initiated or the dosage of fluvastatin sodium is changed.

Endocrine Function

HMG-CoA reductase inhibitors interfere with cholesterol synthesis and lower circulating cholesterol levels and, as such, might theoretically blunt adrenal or gonadal steroid hormone production.

Fluvastatin exhibited no effect upon non-stimulated cortisol levels and demonstrated no effect upon thyroid metabolism as assessed by TSH. Small declines in total testosterone have been noted in treated groups, but no commensurate elevation in LH occurred, suggesting that the observation was not due to a direct effect upon testosterone production. No effect upon FSH in males was noted. Due to the limited number of premenopausal females studied to date, no conclusions regarding the effect of fluvastatin upon female sex hormones may be made.

Two clinical studies in patients receiving fluvastatin at doses up to 80 mg daily for periods of 24 to 28 weeks demonstrated no effect of treatment upon the adrenal response to ACTH stimulation. A clinical study evaluated the effect of fluvastatin at doses up to 80 mg daily for 28 weeks upon the gonadal response to HCG stimulation. Although the mean total testosterone response was significantly reduced (p<0.05) relative to baseline in the 80 mg group, it was not significant in comparison to the changes noted in groups receiving either 40 mg of fluvastatin or placebo.

Patients treated with fluvastatin sodium who develop clinical evidence of endocrine dysfunction should be evaluated appropriately. Caution should be exercised if an HMG-CoA reductase inhibitor or other agent used to lower cholesterol levels is administered to patients receiving other drugs (e.g., ketoconazole, spironolactone, or cimetidine) that may decrease the levels of endogenous steroid hormones.

CNS Toxicity

CNS effects, as evidenced by decreased activity, ataxia, loss of righting reflex, and ptosis were seen in the following animal studies: the 18-month mouse carcinogenicity study at 50 mg/kg/day, the 6-month dog study at 36 mg/kg/day, the 6-month hamster study at 40 mg/kg/day, and in acute, high-

dose studies in rats and hamsters (50 mg/kg), rabbits (300 mg/kg) and mice (1500 mg/kg). CNS toxicity in the acute high-dose studies was characterized (in mice) by conspicuous vacuolation in the ventral white columns of the spinal cord at a dose of 5000 mg/kg and (in rat) by edema with separation of myelinated fibers of the ventral spinal tracts and sciatic nerve at a dose of 1500 mg/kg. CNS toxicity, characterized by periaxonal vacuolation, was observed in the medulla of dogs that died after treatment for 5 weeks with 48 mg/kg/day; this finding was not observed in the remaining dogs when the dose level was lowered to 36 mg/kg/day. CNS vascular lesions, characterized by perivascular hemorrhages, edema, and mononuclear cell infiltration of perivascular spaces, have been observed in dogs treated with other members of this class. No CNS lesions have been observed after chronic treatment for up to 2 years with fluvastatin in the mouse (at doses up to 350 mg/kg/day), rat (up to 24 mg/kg/day), or dog (up to 16 mg/kg/day).

Prominent bilateral posterior Y suture lines in the ocular lens were seen in dogs after treatment with 1, 8, and 16 mg/kg/day for 2 years.

Carcinogenesis, Mutagenesis, Impairment of Fertility

A 2-year study was performed in rats at dose levels of 6, 9, and 18-24 (escalated after 1 year) mg/kg/day. These treatment levels represented plasma drug levels of approximately 9, 13, and 26-35 times the mean human plasma drug concentration after a 40 mg oral dose. A low incidence of forestomach squamous papillomas and 1 carcinoma of the forestomach at the 24 mg/kg/day dose level was considered to reflect the prolonged hyperplasia induced by direct contact exposure to fluvastatin sodium rather than to a systemic effect of the drug. In addition, an increased incidence of thyroid follicular cell adenomas and carcinomas was recorded for males treated with 18-24 mg/kg/day. The increased incidence of thyroid follicular cell neoplasm in male rats with fluvastatin sodium appears to be consistent with findings from other HMG-CoA reductase inhibitors. In contrast to other HMG-CoA reductase inhibitors, no hepatic adenomas or carcinomas were observed.

The carcinogenicity study conducted in mice at dose levels of 0.3, 15 and 30 mg/kg/day revealed, as in rats, a statistically significant increase in forestomach squamous cell papillomas in males and females at 30 mg/kg/day and in females at 15 mg/kg/day. These treatment levels represented plasma drug levels of approximately 0.05, 2, and 7 times the mean human plasma drug concentration after a 40 mg oral dose. No evidence of mutagenicity was observed in vitro, with or without rat-liver metabolic activation, in the following studies: microbial mutagen tests using mutant strains of *Salmonella typhimurium* or *Escherichia coli*; malignant transformation assay in BALB/3T3 cells; unscheduled DNA synthesis in rat primary hepatocytes; chromosomal aberrations in V79 Chinese Hamster cells; HGPRT V79 Chinese Hamster cells. In addition, there was no evidence of mutagenicity in vivo in either a rat or mouse micronucleus test.

In a study in rats at dose levels for females of 0.6, 2 and 6 mg/kg/day and at dose levels for males of 2, 10 and 20 mg/kg/day, fluvastatin sodium had no adverse effects on the fertility or reproductive performance.

Seminal vesicles and testes were small in hamsters treated for 3 months at 20 mg/kg/day (approximately three times the 40 milligram human daily dose based on surface area, mg/m²). There was tubular degeneration and aspermatogenesis in testes as well as vesiculitis of seminal vesicles. Vesiculitis of seminal vesicles and edema of the testes were also seen in rats treated for 2 years at 18 mg/kg/day (approximately 4 times the human C_{max} achieved with a 40 milligram daily dose).

Pregnancy

Pregnancy Category X

See CONTRAINDICATIONS.

Fluvastatin sodium produced delays in skeletal development in rats at doses of 12 mg/kg/day and in rabbits at doses of 10 mg/kg/day. Malaligned thoracic vertebrae were seen in rats at 36 mg/kg, a dose that produced maternal toxicity. These doses resulted in 2 times (rat at 12 mg/kg) or 5 times (rabbit at 10 mg/kg) the 40 mg human exposure based on mg/m² surface area. A study in which female rats were dosed during the third trimester at 12 and 24 mg/kg/day resulted in maternal mortality at or near term and postpartum. In addition, fetal and neonatal lethality were apparent. No effects on the dam or fetus occurred at 2 mg/kg/day. A second study at levels of 2, 6, 12 and 24 mg/kg/day confirmed the findings in the first study with neonatal mortality beginning at 6 mg/kg. A modified Segment III study was performed at dose levels of 12 or 24 mg/kg/day with or without the presence of concurrent supplementation with mevalonic acid, a product of HMG-CoA reductase which is essential for cholesterol biosynthesis. The concurrent administration of mevalonic acid completely prevented the maternal and neonatal mortality but did not prevent low body weights in pups at 24 mg/kg on days 0 and 7 postpartum. Therefore, the maternal and neonatal lethality observed with fluvastatin sodium reflect its exaggerated pharmacologic effect during pregnancy. There are no data with fluvastatin sodium in pregnant women. However, rare reports of congenital anomalies have been received following intrauterine exposure to other HMG-CoA reductase inhibitors. There has been one report of severe congenital bony deformity, tracheo-esophageal fistula, and anal atresia (VATER association) in a baby born to a woman who took another HMG-CoA reductase inhibitor with dextroamphetamine sulfate during the first trimester of pregnancy. **Lescol or Lescol XL should be administered to women of child-bearing potential only when such patients are highly unlikely to conceive and have been informed of the potential**

hazards. If a woman becomes pregnant while taking Lescol or Lescol XL, the drug should be discontinued and the patient advised again as to the potential hazards to the fetus.

Nursing Mothers

Based on preclinical data, drug is present in breast milk in a 2:1 ratio (milk:plasma). Because of the potential for serious adverse reactions in nursing infants, nursing women should not take Lescol or Lescol XL *(see CONTRAINDICATIONS).*

Pediatric Use

Safety and effectiveness in individuals less than 18 years old have not been established. Treatment in patients less than 18 years of age is not recommended at this time.

Geriatric Use

The effect of age on the pharmacokinetics of immediate release fluvastatin sodium was evaluated. Results indicate that for the general patient population plasma concentrations of fluvastatin sodium do not vary as a function of age. *(See also CLINICAL PHARMACOLOGY: Pharmacokinetics/Metabolism.)* Elderly patients (≥65 years of age) demonstrated a greater treatment response in respect to LDL-C, Total-C and LDL/HDL ratio than patients <65 years of age.

ADVERSE REACTIONS

In all clinical studies of Lescol® (fluvastatin sodium), 1.0% (32/2969) of fluvastatin-treated patients were discontinued due to adverse experiences attributed to study drug (mean exposure approximately 16 months ranging in duration from 1 to >36 months). This results in an exposure adjusted rate of 0.8% (32/4051) per patient year in fluvastatin patients in controlled studies compared to an incidence of 1.1% (4/355) in placebo patients. Adverse reactions have usually been of mild to moderate severity.

In controlled clinical studies, 3.9% (36/912) of patients treated with Lescol® XL (fluvastatin sodium) 80 mg discontinued due to adverse events (causality not determined).

Adverse experiences occurring in the Lescol and Lescol XL controlled studies with a frequency >2%, regardless of causality, include the following:

Table 5
Adverse experiences occurring in >2% patients in Lescol and Lescol XL controlled studies

Adverse Event	Lescol[1] (%) (N=2326)	Placebo[1] (%) (N=960)	Lescol XL[2] (%) (N=912)
Integumentary			
Rash	2.3	2.4	1.6
Musculoskeletal			
Back Pain	5.7	6.6	4.7
Myalgia	5.0	4.5	3.8
Arthralgia	4.0	4.1	1.3
Arthritis	2.1	2.0	1.3
Arthropathy	NA	NA	3.2
Respiratory			
Upper Respiratory Tract Infection	16.2	16.5	12.5
Pharyngitis	3.8	3.8	2.4
Rhinitis	4.7	4.9	1.5
Sinusitis	2.6	1.9	3.5
Coughing	2.4	2.9	1.9
Bronchitis	1.8	1.0	2.6
Gastrointestinal			
Dyspepsia	7.9	3.2	3.5
Diarrhea	4.9	4.2	3.3
Abdominal Pain	4.9	3.8	3.7
Nausea	3.2	2.0	2.5
Constipation	3.1	3.3	2.3
Flatulence	2.6	2.5	1.4
Misc. Tooth Disorder	2.1	1.7	1.4
Central Nervous System			
Dizziness	2.2	2.5	1.9
Psychiatric Disorders			
Insomnia	2.7	1.4	0.8
Genitourinary			
Urinary Tract Infection	1.6	1.1	2.7
Miscellaneous			
Headache	8.9	7.8	4.7
Influenza-Like Symptoms	5.1	5.7	7.1
Accidental Trauma	5.1	4.8	4.2
Fatigue	2.7	2.3	1.6
Allergy	2.3	2.2	1.0

[1] Controlled trials with Lescol Capsules (20 and 40 mg daily and 40 mg twice daily)
[2] Controlled trials with Lescol XL 80 mg Tablets

The following effects have been reported with drugs in this class. Not all the effects listed below have necessarily been associated with fluvastatin sodium therapy.

Skeletal: muscle cramps, myalgia, myopathy, rhabdomyolysis, arthralgias.

Neurological: dysfunction of certain cranial nerves (including alteration of taste, impairment of extra-ocular movement, facial paresis), tremor, dizziness, vertigo, memory loss, paresthesia, peripheral neuropathy, peripheral nerve palsy, psychic disturbances, anxiety, insomnia, depression.

Hypersensitivity Reactions: An apparent hypersensitivity syndrome has been reported rarely which has included one or more of the following features: anaphylaxis, angioedema, lupus erythematosus-like syndrome, polymyalgia rheumatica, vasculitis, purpura, thrombocytopenia, leukopenia, hemo-

lytic anemia, positive ANA, ESR increase, eosinophilia, arthritis, arthralgia, urticaria, asthenia, photosensitivity, fever, chills, flushing, malaise, dyspnea, toxic epidermal necrolysis, erythema multiforme, including Stevens-Johnson syndrome.
Gastrointestinal: pancreatitis, hepatitis, including chronic active hepatitis, cholestatic jaundice, fatty change in liver, and, rarely, cirrhosis, fulminant hepatic necrosis, and hepatoma; anorexia, vomiting.
Skin: alopecia, pruritus. A variety of skin changes (e.g., nodules, discoloration, dryness of skin/mucous membranes, changes to hair/nails) have been reported.
Reproductive: gynecomastia, loss of libido, erectile dysfunction.
Eye: progression of cataracts (lens opacities), ophthalmoplegia.
Laboratory Abnormalities: elevated transaminases, alkaline phosphatase, γ-glutamyl transpeptidase, and bilirubin; thyroid function abnormalities.

Concomitant Therapy
Fluvastatin sodium has been administered concurrently with cholestyramine and nicotinic acid. No adverse reactions unique to the combination or in addition to those previously reported for this class of drugs alone have been reported. Myopathy and rhabdomyolysis (with or without acute renal failure) have been reported when another HMG-CoA reductase inhibitor was used in combination with immunosuppressive drugs, gemfibrozil, erythromycin, or lipid-lowering doses of nicotinic acid. Concomitant therapy with HMG-CoA reductase inhibitors and these agents is generally not recommended. (See WARNINGS: Skeletal Muscle.)

OVERDOSAGE
The approximate oral LD_{50} is greater than 2 g/kg in mice and greater than 0.7 g/kg in rats.
The maximum single oral dose of Lescol® (fluvastatin sodium) capsules received by healthy volunteers was 80 mg. No clinically significant adverse experiences were seen at this dose. The maximum dose administered with an extended-release formulation was 640 mg for two weeks. This dose was not well tolerated and produced a variety of GI complaints and an increase in transaminase values (i.e., SGOT and SGPT).
There has been a single report of 2 children, one 2 years old and the other 3 years of age, either of whom may have possibly ingested fluvastatin sodium. The maximum amount of fluvastatin sodium that could have been ingested was 80 mg (4 × 20 mg capsules). Vomiting was induced by ipecac in both children and no capsules were noted in their emesis. Neither child experienced any adverse symptoms and both recovered from the incident without problems.
Should an accidental overdose occur, treat symptomatically and institute supportive measures as required. The dialyzability of fluvastatin sodium and of its metabolites in humans is not known at present.
Information about the treatment of overdose can often be obtained from a certified Regional Poison Control Center. Telephone numbers of certified Regional Poison Control Centers are listed in the Physicians' Desk Reference®.*

DOSAGE AND ADMINISTRATION
The patient should be placed on a standard cholesterol-lowering diet before receiving Lescol® (fluvastatin sodium) or Lescol® XL (fluvastatin sodium) and should continue on this diet during treatment with Lescol or Lescol XL. (See NCEP Treatment Guidelines for details on dietary therapy.) For patients requiring LDL-C reduction to a goal of ≥25%, the recommended starting dose is 40 mg as one capsule, 80 mg as one Lescol XL tablet administered as a single dose in the evening or 80 mg in divided doses of the 40 mg capsule given twice daily. For patients requiring LDL-C reduction to a goal of <25% a starting dose of 20 mg may be used. The recommended dosing range is 20-80 mg/day. Lescol or Lescol XL may be taken without regard to meals, since there are no apparent differences in the lipid-lowering effects of fluvastatin sodium administered with the evening meal or 4 hours after the evening meal. Since the maximal reductions in LDL-C of a given dose are seen within 4 weeks, periodic lipid determinations should be performed and dosage adjustment made according to the patient's response to therapy and established treatment guidelines. The therapeutic effect of Lescol or Lescol XL is maintained with prolonged administration.

Concomitant Therapy
Lipid-lowering effects on total cholesterol and LDL cholesterol are additive when immediate release Lescol is combined with a bile-acid binding resin or niacin. When administering a bile-acid resin (e.g., cholestyramine) and fluvastatin sodium, Lescol should be administered at bedtime, at least 2 hours following the resin to avoid a significant interaction due to drug binding to resin. (See also ADVERSE REACTIONS: Concomitant Therapy.)

Dosage in Patients with Renal Insufficiency
Since fluvastatin sodium is cleared hepatically with less than 6% of the administered dose excreted into the urine, dose adjustments for mild to moderate renal impairment are not necessary. Fluvastatin has not been studied at doses greater than 40 mg in patients with severe renal impairment; therefore caution should be exercised when treating such patients at higher doses.

HOW SUPPLIED
Lescol® (fluvastatin sodium) Capsules
20 mg
Brown and light brown imprinted twice with "⚕" and "20" on one half and "LESCOL" and the Lescol® (fluvastatin sodium) logo twice on the other half of the capsule.

Bottles of 30 capsules .... (NDC 0078-0176-15)
Bottles of 100 capsules .... (NDC 0078-0176-05)
40 mg
Brown and gold imprinted twice with "⚕" and "40" on one half and "LESCOL" and the Lescol® (fluvastatin sodium) logo twice on the other half of the capsule.
Bottles of 30 capsules .... (NDC 0078-0234-15)
Bottles of 100 capsules .... (NDC 0078-0234-05)
Lescol® XL (fluvastatin sodium) Extended-Release Tablets
80 mg
Yellow, round, slightly biconvex film-coated tablet with beveled edges debossed with "Lescol XL" on one side and "80" on the other.
Bottles of 30 tablets .... (NDC 0078-0354-15)
Bottle of 100 tablets .... (NDC 0078-0354-05)
Store and Dispense
Store at 25°C (77°F); excursions permitted to 15°C-30°C (59°F-86°F). [See USP Controlled Room Temperature]. Dispense in a tight container. Protect from light.

---

*Trademark of Medical Economics Company, Inc.
Distributed by:
Novartis Pharmaceuticals Corporation
East Hanover, New Jersey 07936

REV: JANUARY 2001   Printed in U.S.A.
©2001 Novartis

T2001-02
89011103

NEORAL® Soft Gelatin Capsules ℞
[nē ŏ 'ral]
(cyclosporine capsules, USP) MODIFIED
NEORAL® Oral Solution
(cyclosporine oral solution, USP) MODIFIED
Rx only

Prescribing information for this product, which appears on pages 2199–2206 of the 2001 PDR, has been completely revised as follows. Please write "See Supplement A" next to the product heading.

WARNING
Only physicians experienced in management of systemic immunosuppressive therapy for the indicated disease should prescribe Neoral®. At doses used in solid organ transplantation, only physicians experienced in immunosuppressive therapy and management of organ transplant recipients should prescribe Neoral®. Patients receiving the drug should be managed in facilities equipped and staffed with adequate laboratory and supportive medical resources. The physician responsible for maintenance therapy should have complete information requisite for the follow-up of the patient.
Neoral®, a systemic immunosuppressant, may increase the susceptibility to infection and the development of neoplasia. In kidney, liver, and heart transplant patients Neoral® may be administered with other immunosuppressive agents. Increased susceptibility to infection and the possible development of lymphoma and other neoplasms may result from the increase in the degree of immunosuppression in transplant patients.

Neoral® Soft Gelatin Capsules (cyclosporine capsules, USP) MODIFIED and Neoral® Oral Solution (cyclosporine oral solution, USP) MODIFIED have increased bioavailability in comparison to Sandimmune® Soft Gelatin Capsules (cyclosporine capsules, USP) and Sandimmune® Oral Solution (cyclosporine oral solution, USP). Neoral® and Sandimmune® are not bioequivalent and cannot be used interchangeably without physician supervision. For a given trough concentration, cyclosporine exposure will be greater with Neoral® than with Sandimmune®. If a patient who is receiving exceptionally high doses of Sandimmune® is converted to Neoral®, particular caution should be exercised. Cyclosporine blood concentrations should be monitored in transplant and rheumatoid arthritis patients taking Neoral® to avoid toxicity due to high concentrations. Dose adjustments should be made in transplant patients to minimize possible organ rejection due to low concentrations. Comparison of blood concentrations in the published literature with blood concentrations obtained using current assays must be done with detailed knowledge of the assay methods employed.

For Psoriasis Patients (See also Boxed WARNINGS above)
Psoriasis patients previously treated with PUVA and to a lesser extent, methotrexate or other immunosuppressive agents, UVB, coal tar, or radiation therapy, are at an increased risk of developing skin malignancies when taking Neoral®.
Cyclosporine, the active ingredient in Neoral®, in recommended dosages, can cause systemic hypertension and nephrotoxicity. The risk increases with increasing dose and duration of cyclosporine therapy. Renal dysfunction, including structural kidney damage, is a potential consequence of cylcosporine, and therefore, renal function must be monitored during therapy.

DESCRIPTION
Neoral® is an oral formulation of cyclosporine that immediately forms a microemulsion in an aqueous environment. Cyclosporine, the active principle in Neoral®, is a cyclic polypeptide immunosuppressant agent consisting of 11 amino acids. It is produced as a metabolite by the fungus species *Beauveria nivea*.
Chemically, cyclosporine is designated as $[R-[R^*,R^*-(E)]]$-cyclic-(L-alanyl-D-alanyl-N-methyl-L-leucyl-N-methyl-L-leucyl-N-methyl-L-valyl-3-hydroxy-N,4-dimethyl-L-2-amino-6-octenoyl-L-α-amino-butyryl-N-methylglycyl-N-methyl-L-leucyl-L-valyl-N-methyl-L-leucyl).
Neoral® Soft Gelatin Capsules (cyclosporine capsules, USP) MODIFIED are available in 25 mg and 100 mg strengths.
Each 25 mg capsule contains:
cyclosporine .... 25 mg
alcohol, USP dehydrated .... 11.9% v/v (9.5% wt/vol.)
Each 100 mg capsule contains:
cyclosporine .... 100 mg
alcohol, USP dehydrated .... 11.9% v/v (9.5% wt/vol.)
Inactive Ingredients: Corn oil-mono-di-triglycerides, polyoxyl 40 hydrogenated castor oil NF, DL-α-tocopherol USP, gelatin NF, glycerol, iron oxide black, propylene glycol USP, titanium dioxide USP, carmine, and other ingredients.
Neoral® Oral Solution (cyclosporine oral solution, USP) MODIFIED is available in 50 mL bottles.
Each mL contains:
cyclosporine .... 100 mg/mL
alcohol, USP dehydrated .... 11.9% v/v (9.5% wt/vol.)
Inactive Ingredients: Corn oil-mono-di-triglycerides, polyoxyl 40 hydrogenated castor oil NF, DL-α-tocopherol USP, propylene glycol USP.
The chemical structure of cyclosporine (also known as cyclosporin A) is:

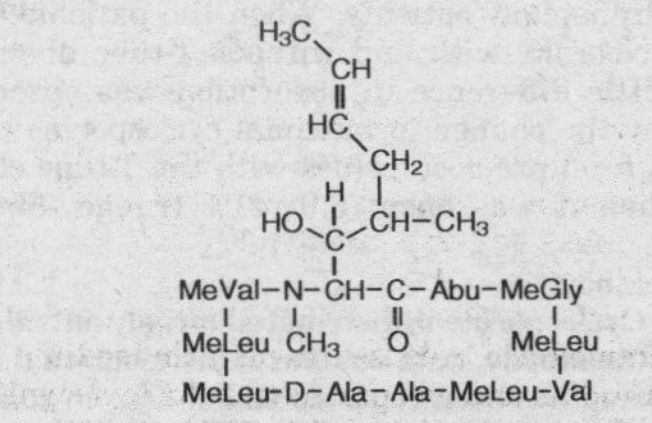

MeVal–N–CH–C–Abu–MeGly
MeLeu CH₃ O   MeLeu
MeLeu–D-Ala–Ala–MeLeu–Val
$C_{62}H_{111}N_{11}O_{12}$ Mol. Wt. 1202.63

CLINICAL PHARMACOLOGY
Cyclosporine is a potent immunosuppressive agent that in animals prolongs survival of allogeneic transplants involving skin, kidney, liver, heart, pancreas, bone marrow, small intestine, and lung. Cyclosporine has been demonstrated to suppress some humoral immunity and to a greater extent, cell-mediated immune reactions such as allograft rejection, delayed hypersensitivity, experimental allergic encephalomyelitis, Freund's adjuvant arthritis, and graft vs. host disease in many animal species for a variety of organs.
The effectiveness of cyclosporine results from specific and reversible inhibition of immunocompetent lymphocytes in the G_0- and G_1-phase of the cell cycle. T-lymphocytes are preferentially inhibited. The T-helper cell is the main target, although the T-suppressor cell may also be suppressed. Cyclosporine also inhibits lymphokine production and release including interleukin-2.
No effects on phagocytic function (changes in enzyme secretions, chemotactic migration of granulocytes, macrophage migration, carbon clearance *in vivo*) have been detected in animals. Cyclosporine does not cause bone marrow suppression in animal models or man.
Pharmacokinetics: The immunosuppressive activity of cyclosporine is primarily due to parent drug. Following oral administration, absorption of cyclosporine is incomplete. The extent of absorption of cyclosporine is dependent on the individual patient, the patient population, and the formulation. Elimination of cyclosporine is primarily biliary with only 6% of the dose (parent drug and metabolites) excreted in urine. The disposition of cyclosporine from blood is generally biphasic, with a terminal half-life of approximately 8.4 hours (range 5-18 hours). Following intravenous administration, the blood clearance of cyclosporine (assay: HPLC) is approximately 5-7 mL/min/kg in adult recipients of renal or liver allografts. Blood cyclosporine clearance appears to be slightly slower in cardiac transplant patients.
The Neoral® Soft Gelatin Capsules (cyclosporine capsules, USP) MODIFIED and Neoral® Oral Solution (cyclosporine oral solution, USP) MODIFIED are bioequivalent.
The relationship between administered dose and exposure (area under the concentration versus time curve, AUC) is linear within the therapeutic dose range. The intersubject variability (total, %CV) of cyclosporine exposure (AUC) when Neoral® or Sandimmune® is administered ranges from approximately 20% to 50% in renal transplant patients. This intersubject variability contributes to the need for individualization of the dosing regimen for optimal therapy *(see DOSAGE AND ADMINISTRATION)*. Intrasubject variability of AUC in renal transplant recipients (%CV) was 9%-21% for Neoral® and 19%-26% for Sandimmune®. In the same studies, intrasubject variability of trough concentrations (%CV) was 17%-30% for Neoral® and 16%-38% for Sandimmune®.
Absorption: Neoral® has increased bioavailability compared to Sandimmune®. The absolute bioavailability of

Continued on next page

Neoral—Cont.

cyclosporine administered as Sandimmune® is dependent on the patient population, estimated to be less than 10% in liver transplant patients and as great as 89% in some renal transplant patients. The absolute bioavailability of cyclosporine administered as Neoral® has not been determined in adults. In studies of renal transplant, rheumatoid arthritis and psoriasis patients, the mean cyclosporine AUC was approximately 20% to 50% greater and the peak blood cyclosporine concentration (C_{max}) was approximately 40% to 106% greater following administration of Neoral® compared to following administration of Sandimmune®. The dose normalized AUC in *de novo* liver transplant patients administered Neoral® 28 days after transplantation was 50% greater and C_{max} was 90% greater than in those patients administered Sandimmune®. AUC and C_{max} are also increased (Neoral® relative to Sandimmune®) in heart transplant patients, but data are very limited. Although the AUC and C_{max} values are higher on Neoral® relative to Sandimmune®, the pre-dose trough concentrations (dose-normalized) are similar for the two formulations.

Following oral administration of Neoral®, the time to peak blood cyclosporine concentrations (T_{max}) ranged from 1.5-2.0 hours. The administration of food with Neoral® decreases the cyclosporine AUC and C_{max}. A high fat meal (669 kcal, 45 grams fat) consumed within one-half hour before Neoral® administration decreased the AUC by 13% and C_{max} by 33%. The effects of a low fat meal (667 kcal, 15 grams fat) were similar.

The effect of T-tube diversion of bile on the absorption of cyclosporine from Neoral® was investigated in eleven *de novo* liver transplant patients. When the patients were administered Neoral® with and without T-tube diversion of bile, very little difference in absorption was observed, as measured by the change in maximal cyclosporine blood concentrations from pre-dose values with the T-tube closed relative to when it was open: 6.9±41% (range -55% to 68%).

[See first table above]

Distribution: Cyclosporine is distributed largely outside the blood volume. The steady state volume of distribution during intravenous dosing has been reported as 3-5 L/kg in solid organ transplant recipients. In blood, the distribution is concentration dependent. Approximately 33%-47% is in plasma, 4%-9% in lymphocytes, 5%-12% in granulocytes, and 41%-58% in erythrocytes. At high concentrations, the binding capacity of leukocytes and erythrocytes becomes saturated. In plasma, approximately 90% is bound to proteins, primarily lipoproteins. Cyclosporine is excreted in human milk. *(See PRECAUTIONS, Nursing Mothers)*

Metabolism: Cyclosporine is extensively metabolized by the cytochrome P-450 3A enzyme system in the liver, and to a lesser degree in the gastrointestinal tract, and the kidney. The metabolism of cyclosporine can be altered by the coadministration of a variety of agents. *(See PRECAUTIONS, Drug Interactions)* At least 25 metabolites have been identified from human bile, feces, blood, and urine. The biological activity of the metabolites and their contributions to toxicity are considerably less than those of the parent compound. The major metabolites (M1, M9, and M4N) result from oxidation at the 1-beta, 9-gamma, and 4-N-demethylated positions, respectively. At steady state following the oral administration of Sandimmune®, the mean AUCs for blood concentrations of M1, M9, and M4N are about 70%, 21%, and 7.5% of the AUC for blood cyclosporine concentrations, respectively. Based on blood concentration data from stable renal transplant patients (13 patients administered Neoral® and Sandimmune® in a crossover study), and bile concentration data from *de novo* liver transplant patients (4 administered Neoral®, 3 administered Sandimmune®), the percentage of dose present as M1, M9, and M4N metabolites is similar when either Neoral® or Sandimmune® is administered.

Excretion: Only 0.1% of a cyclosporine dose is excreted unchanged in the urine. Elimination is primarily biliary with only 6% of the dose (parent drug and metabolites) excreted in the urine. Neither dialysis nor renal failure alter cyclosporine clearance significantly.

Drug Interactions: *(See PRECAUTIONS, Drug Interactions)* When diclofenac or methotrexate was co-administered with cyclosporine in rheumatoid arthritis patients, the AUC of diclofenac and methotrexate, each was significantly increased. *(See PRECAUTIONS, Drug Interactions)* No clinically significant pharmacokinetic interactions occurred between cyclosporine and aspirin, ketoprofen, piroxicam, or indomethacin.

Special Populations: ***Pediatric Population:*** Pharmacokinetic data from pediatric patients administered Neoral® or Sandimmune® are very limited. In 15 renal transplant patients aged 3-16 years, cyclosporine whole blood clearance after IV administration of Sandimmune® was 10.6±3.7 mL/min/kg (assay: Cyclo-trac specific RIA). In a study of 7 renal transplant patients aged 2-16, the cyclosporine clearance ranged from 9.8-15.5 mL/min/kg. In 9 liver transplant patients aged 0.6-5.6 years, clearance was 9.3±5.4 mL/min/kg (assay: HPLC).

In the pediatric population, Neoral® also demonstrates an increased bioavailability as compared to Sandimmune®. In 7 liver *de novo* transplant patients aged 1.4-10 years, the absolute bioavailability of Neoral® was 43% (range 30%-68%) and for Sandimmune® in the same individuals absolute bioavailability was 28% (range 17%-42%).

[See second table above]

Pharmacokinetic Parameters (mean ± SD)

Patient Population	Dose/ day[1] (mg/d)	Dose/ weight (mg/kg/d)	AUC[2] (ng·hr/mL)	C_{max} (ng/mL)	Trough[3] (ng/mL)	CL/F (mL/min)	CL/F (mL/min/ kg)
De novo renal transplant[4] Week 4 (N=37)	597±174	7.95±2.81	8772±2089	1802±428	361±129	593±204	7.8±2.9
Stable renal transplant[4] (N=55)	344±122	4.10±1.58	6035±2194	1333±469	251±116	492±140	5.9±2.1
De novo liver transplant[5] Week 4 (N=18)	458±190	6.89±3.68	7187±2816	1555±740	268±101	577±309	8.6±5.7
De novo rheumatoid arthritis[6] (N=23)	182±55.6	2.37±0.36	2641±877	728±263	96.4±37.7	613±196	8.3±2.8
De novo psoriasis[6] Week 4 (N=18)	189±69.8	2.48±0.65	2324±1048	655±186	74.9±46.7	723±186	10.2±3.9

[1]Total daily dose was divided into two doses administered every 12 hours
[2]AUC was measured over one dosing interval
[3]Trough concentration was measured just prior to the morning Neoral® dose, approximately 12 hours after the previous dose
[4]Assay: TDx specific monoclonal fluorescence polarization immunoassay
[5]Assay: Cyclo-trac specific monoclonal radioimmunoassay
[6]Assay: INCSTAR specific monoclonal radioimmunoassay

Pediatric Pharmacokinetic Parameters (mean ± SD)

Patient Population	Dose/day (mg/d)	Dose/weight (mg/kg/d)	AUC[1] (ng·hr/mL)	C_{max} (ng/mL)	CL/F (mL/min)	CL/F (mL/min/kg)
Stable liver transplant[2]						
Age 2-8, Dosed TID (N=9)	101±25	5.95±1.32	2163±801	629±219	285±94	16.6±4.3
Age 8-15, Dosed BID (N=8)	188±55	4.96±2.09	4272±1462	975±281	378±80	10.2±4.0
Stable liver transplant[3]						
Age 3, Dosed BID (N=1)	120	8.33	5832	1050	171	11.9
Age 8-15, Dosed BID (N=5)	158±55	5.51±1.91	4452±2475	1013±635	328±121	11.0±1.9
Stable renal transplant[3]						
Age 7-15, Dosed BID (N=5)	328±83	7.37±4.11	6922±1988	1827±487	418±143	8.7±2.9

[1]AUC was measured over one dosing interval
[2]Assay: Cyclo-trac specific monoclonal radioimmunoassay
[3]Assay: TDx specific monoclonal fluorescence polarization immunoassay

Geriatric Population: Comparison of single dose data from both normal elderly volunteers (N=18, mean age 69 years) and elderly rheumatoid arthritis patients (N=16, mean age 68 years) to single dose data in young adult volunteers (N=16, mean age 26 years) showed no significant difference in the pharmacokinetic parameters.

CLINICAL TRIALS

Rheumatoid Arthritis: The effectiveness of Sandimmune® and Neoral® in the treatment of severe rheumatoid arthritis was evaluated in 5 clinical studies involving a total of 728 cyclosporine treated patients and 273 placebo treated patients.

A summary of the results is presented for the "responder" rates per treatment group, with a responder being defined as a patient having *completed* the trial with a 20% improvement in the tender and the swollen joint count and a 20% improvement in 2 of 4 of investigator global, patient global, disability, and erythrocyte sedimentation rates (ESR) for the Studies 651 and 652 and 3 of 5 of investigator global, patient global, disability, visual analog pain, and ESR for Studies 2008, 654 and 302.

Study 651 enrolled 264 patients with active rheumatoid arthritis with at least 20 involved joints, who had failed at least one major RA drug, using a 3:3:2 randomization to one of the following three groups: (1) cyclosporine dosed at 2.5-5 mg/kg/day, (2) methotrexate at 7.5-15 mg/week, or (3) placebo. Treatment duration was 24 weeks. The mean cyclosporine dose at the last visit was 3.1 mg/kg/day. See Graph below.

Study 652 enrolled 250 patients with active RA with >6 active painful or tender joints who had failed at least one major RA drug. Patients were randomized using a 3:3:2 randomization to 1 of 3 treatment arms: (1) 1.5-5 mg/kg/day of cyclosporine, (2) 2.5-5 mg/kg/day of cyclosporine, and (3) placebo. Treatment duration was 16 weeks. The mean cyclosporine dose for group 2 at the last visit was 2.92 mg/kg/day. See Graph below.

Study 2008 enrolled 144 patients with active RA and >6 active joints who had unsuccessful treatment courses of aspirin and gold or Penicillamine. Patients were randomized to 1 of 2 treatment groups (1) cyclosporine 2.5-5 mg/kg/day with adjustments after the first month to achieve a target trough level and (2) placebo. Treatment duration was 24 weeks. The mean cyclosporine dose at the last visit was 3.63 mg/kg/day. See Graph below.

Study 654 enrolled 148 patients who remained with active joint counts of 6 or more despite treatment with maximally tolerated methotrexate doses for at least three months. Patients continued to take their current dose of methotrexate and were randomized to receive, in addition, one of the following medications: (1) cyclosporine 2.5 mg/kg/day with dose increases of 0.5 mg/kg/day at weeks 2 and 4 if there was no evidence of toxicity and further increases of 0.5 mg/kg/day at weeks 8 and 16 if a <30% decrease in active joint count occurred without any significant toxicity; dose decreases could be made at any time for toxicity or (2) placebo. Treatment duration was 24 weeks. The mean cyclosporine dose at the last visit was 2.8 mg/kg/day (range: 1.3-4.1). See Graph below.

Study 302 enrolled 299 patients with severe active RA, 99% of whom were unresponsive or intolerant to at least one prior major RA drug. Patients were randomized to 1 of 2 treatment groups (1) Neoral® and (2) cyclosporine, both of which were started at 2.5 mg/kg/day and increased after 4 weeks for inefficacy in increments of 0.5 mg/kg/day to a maximum of 5 mg/kg/day and decreased at any time for toxicity. Treatment duration was 24 weeks. The mean cyclosporine dose at the last visit was 2.91 mg/kg/day (range: 0.72-5.17) for Neoral® and 3.27 mg/kg/day (range: 0.73-5.68) for cyclosporine. See Graph below.

[See figure at top of next page]

INDICATIONS AND USAGE

Kidney, Liver, and Heart Transplantation: Neoral® is indicated for the prophylaxis of organ rejection in kidney, liver, and heart allogeneic transplants. Neoral® has been used in combination with azathioprine and corticosteroids.

Rheumatoid Arthritis: Neoral® is indicated for the treatment of patients with severe active, rheumatoid arthritis where the disease has not adequately responded to methotrexate. Neoral® can be used in combination with methotrexate in rheumatoid arthritis patients who do not respond adequately to methotrexate alone.

Psoriasis: Neoral® is indicated for the treatment of *adult, nonimmunocompromised* patients with severe (i.e., extensive and/or disabling), recalcitrant, plaque psoriasis who have failed to respond to at least one systemic therapy (eg., PUVA, retinoids, or methotrexate) or in patients for whom other systemic therapies are contraindicated, or cannot be tolerated. While rebound rarely occurs, most patients will experience relapse with Neoral® as with other therapies upon cessation of treatment.

CONTRAINDICATIONS

General: Neoral® is contraindicated in patients with a hypersensitivity to cyclosporine or to any of the ingredients of the formulation.

Rheumatoid Arthritis: Rheumatoid arthritis patients with abnormal renal function, uncontrolled hypertension, or malignancies should not receive Neoral®.

Psoriasis: Psoriasis patients who are treated with Neoral® should not receive concomitant PUVA or UVB therapy, methotrexate or other immunosuppressive agents, coal tar or radiation therapy. Psoriasis patients with abnormal renal function, uncontrolled hypertension, or malignancies should not receive Neoral®.

WARNINGS: *(See also Boxed WARNING)* **All Patients:** Cyclosporine, the active ingredient of Neoral®, can cause nephrotoxicity and hepatotoxicity. The risk increases with increasing doses of cyclosporine. Renal dysfunction including structural kidney damage is a potential consequence of

Neoral® and therefore renal function must be monitored during therapy. **Care should be taken in using cyclosporine with nephrotoxic drugs.** ***(See PRECAUTIONS)***

Patients receiving Neoral® require frequent monitoring of serum creatinine. *(See Special Monitoring under DOSAGE AND ADMINISTRATION)* Elderly patients should be monitored with particular care, since decreases in renal function also occur with age. If patients are not properly monitored and doses are not properly adjusted, cyclosporine therapy can be associated with the occurrence of structural kidney damage and persistent renal dysfunction.

An increase in serum creatinine and BUN may occur during Neoral® therapy and reflect a reduction in the glomerular filtration rate. Impaired renal function at any time requires close monitoring, and frequent dosage adjustment may be indicated. The frequency and severity of serum creatinine elevations increase with dose and duration of cyclosporine therapy. These elevations are likely to become more pronounced without dose reduction or discontinuation.

Because Neoral® is not bioequivalent to Sandimmune®, conversion from Neoral® to Sandimmune® using a 1:1 ratio (mg/kg/day) may result in lower cyclosporine blood concentrations. Conversion from Neoral® to Sandimmune® should be made with increased monitoring to avoid the potential of underdosing.

Kidney, Liver, and Heart Transplant: Cyclosporine, the active ingredient of Neoral®, can cause nephrotoxicity and hepatotoxicity when used in high doses. It is not unusual for serum creatinine and BUN levels to be elevated during cyclosporine therapy. These elevations in renal transplant patients do not necessarily indicate rejection, and each patient must be fully evaluated before dosage adjustment is initiated.

Based on the historical Sandimmune® experience with oral solution, nephrotoxicity associated with cyclosporine had been noted in 25% of cases of renal transplantation, 38% of cases of cardiac transplantation, and 37% of cases of liver transplantation. Mild nephrotoxicity was generally noted 2-3 months after renal transplant and consisted of an arrest in the fall of the pre-operative elevations of BUN and creatinine at a range of 35-45 mg/dl and 2.0-2.5 mg/dl respectively. These elevations were often responsive to cyclosporine dosage reduction.

More overt nephrotoxicity was seen early after transplantation and was characterized by a rapidly rising BUN and creatinine. Since these events are similar to renal rejection episodes, care must be taken to differentiate between them. This form of nephrotoxicity is usually responsive to cyclosporine dosage reduction.

Although specific diagnostic criteria which reliably differentiate renal graft rejection from drug toxicity have not been found, a number of parameters have been significantly associated with one or the other. It should be noted however, that up to 20% of patients may have simultaneous nephrotoxicity and rejection.

[See table at right]

A form of a cyclosporine-associated nephropathy is characterized by serial deterioration in renal function and morphologic changes in the kidneys. From 5%-15% of transplant recipients who have received cyclosporine will fail to show a reduction in rising serum creatinine despite a decrease or discontinuation of cyclosporine therapy. Renal biopsies from these patients will demonstrate one or several of the following alterations: tubular vacuolization, tubular microcalcifications, peritubular capillary congestion, arteriolopathy, and a striped form of interstitial fibrosis with tubular atrophy. Though none of these morphologic changes is entirely specific, a diagnosis of cyclosporine-associated structural nephrotoxicity requires evidence of these findings.

When considering the development of cyclosporine-associated nephropathy, it is noteworthy that several authors have reported an association between the appearance of interstitial fibrosis and higher cumulative doses or persistently high circulating trough levels of cyclosporine. This is particularly true during the first 6 post-transplant months when the dosage tends to be highest and when, in kidney recipients, the organ appears to be most vulnerable to the toxic effects of cyclosporine. Among other contributing factors to the development of interstitial fibrosis in these patients are prolonged perfusion time, warm ischemia time, as well as episodes of acute toxicity, and acute and chronic rejection. The reversibility of interstitial fibrosis and its correlation to renal function have not yet been determined. Reversibility of arteriolopathy has been reported after stopping cyclosporine or lowering the dosage.

Impaired renal function at any time requires close monitoring, and frequent dosage adjustment may be indicated.

In the event of severe and unremitting rejection, when rescue therapy with pulse steroids and monoclonal antibodies fail to reverse the rejection episode, it may be preferable to switch to alternative immunosuppressive therapy rather than increase the Neoral® dose to excessive levels.

Occasionally patients have developed a syndrome of thrombocytopenia and microangiopathic hemolytic anemia which may result in graft failure. The vasculopathy can occur in the absence of rejection and is accompanied by avid platelet consumption within the graft as demonstrated by Indium 111 labeled platelet studies. Neither the pathogenesis nor the management of this syndrome is clear. Though resolution has occurred after reduction or discontinuation of cyclosporine and 1) administration of streptokinase and heparin or 2) plasmapheresis, this appears to depend upon early detection with Indium 111 labeled platelet scans. *(See ADVERSE REACTIONS)*

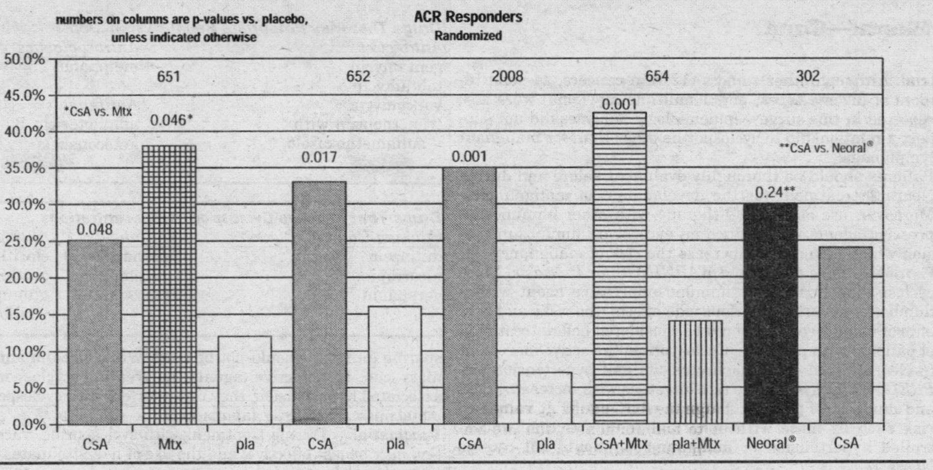
numbers on columns are p-values vs. placebo, unless indicated otherwise
ACR Responders
Randomized
50.0%
45.0%
40.0%
35.0%
30.0%
25.0%
20.0%
15.0%
10.0%
5.0%
0.0%
651
652
2008
654
302
*CsA vs. Mtx
0.046*
0.048
0.017
0.001
0.001
**CsA vs. Neoral®
0.24**
CsA
Mtx
pla
CsA
pla
CsA
pla
CsA+Mtx
pla+Mtx
Neoral®
CsA

Nephrotoxicity vs. Rejection

Parameter	Nephrotoxicity	Rejection
History	Donor > 50 years old or hypotensive Prolonged kidney preservation Prolonged anastomosis time Concomitant nephrotoxic drugs	Anti-donor immune response Retransplant patient
Clinical	Often > 6 weeks postop[b] Prolonged initial nonfunction (acute tubular necrosis)	Often < 4 weeks postop[b] Fever > 37.5°C Weight gain > 0.5 kg Graft swelling and tenderness Decrease in daily urine volume > 500 mL (or 50%)
Laboratory	CyA serum trough level > 200 ng/mL Gradual rise in Cr (< 0.15 mg/dl/day)[a] Cr plateau < 25% above baseline BUN/Cr ≥ 20	CyA serum trough level < 150 ng/mL Rapid rise in Cr (> 0.3 mg/dl/day)[a] Cr > 25% above baseline BUN/Cr < 20
Biopsy	Arteriolopathy (medial hypertrophy[a], hyalinosis, nodular deposits, intimal thickening, endothelial vacuolization, progressive scarring) Tubular atrophy, isometric vacuolization, isolated calcifications Minimal edema Mild focal infiltrates[c] Diffuse interstitial fibrosis, often striped form	Endovasculitis[c] (proliferation[a], intimal arteritis[b], necrosis, sclerosis) Tubulitis with RBC[b] and WBC[b] casts, some irregular vacuolization Interstitial edema[c] and hemorrhage[b] Diffuse moderate to severe mononuclear infiltrates[d] Glomerulitis (mononuclear cells)[c]
Aspiration Cytology	CyA deposits in tubular and endothelial cells Fine isometric vacuolization of tubular cells	Inflammatory infiltrate with mononuclear phagocytes, macrophages, lymphoblastoid cells, and activated T-cells These strongly express HLA-DR antigens
Urine Cytology	Tubular cells with vacuolization and granularization	Degenerative tubular cells, plasma cells, and lymphocyturia > 20% of sediment
Manometry	Intracapsular pressure < 40 mm Hg[b]	Intracapsular pressure > 40 mm Hg[b]
Ultrasonography	Unchanged graft cross sectional area	Increase in graft cross sectional area AP diameter ≥ Transverse diameter
Magnetic Resonance Imagery	Normal appearance	Loss of distinct corticomedullary junction, swelling image intensity of parachyma approaching that of psoas, loss of hilar fat
Radionuclide Scan	Normal or generally decreased perfusion Decrease in tubular function (^{131}I-hippuran) > decrease in perfusion (^{99m}Tc DTPA)	Patchy arterial flow Decrease in perfusion > decrease in tubular function Increased uptake of Indium 111 labeled platelets or Tc-99m in colloid
Therapy	Responds to decreased cyclosporine	Responds to increased steroids or antilymphocyte globulin

[a]$p < 0.05$, [b]$p < 0.01$, [c]$p < 0.001$, [d]$p < 0.0001$

Significant hyperkalemia (sometimes associated with hyperchloremic metabolic acidosis) and hyperuricemia have been seen occasionally in individual patients.

Hepatotoxicity associated with cyclosporine use had been noted in 4% of cases of renal transplantation, 7% of cases of cardiac transplantation, and 4% of cases of liver transplantation. This was usually noted during the first month of therapy when high doses of cyclosporine were used and consisted of elevations of hepatic enzymes and bilirubin. The chemistry elevations usually decreased with a reduction in dosage.

As in patients receiving other immunosuppressants, those patients receiving cyclosporine are at increased risk for development of lymphomas and other malignancies, particularly those of the skin. The increased risk appears related to the intensity and duration of immunosuppression rather than to the use of specific agents. Because of the danger of oversuppression of the immune system resulting in increased risk of infection or malignancy, a treatment regimen containing multiple immunosuppressants should be used with caution.

There have been reports of convulsions in adult and pediatric patients receiving cyclosporine, particularly in combination with high dose methylprednisolone.

Encephalopathy has been described both in post-marketing reports and in the literature. Manifestations include impaired consciousness, convulsions, visual disturbances (including blindness), loss of motor function, movement disorders and psychiatric disturbances. In many cases, changes in the white matter have been detected using imaging techniques and pathologic specimens. Predisposing factors such as hypertension, hypomagnesemia, hypocholesterolemia, high-dose corticosteroids, high cyclosporine blood concentrations, and graft-versus-host disease have been noted in many but not all of the reported cases. The changes in most cases have been reversible upon discontinuation of cyclosporine, and in some cases improvement was noted after reduction of dose. It appears that patients receiving liver transplant are more susceptible to encephalopathy than those receiving kidney transplant.

Care should be taken in using cyclosporine with nephrotoxic drugs. *(See PRECAUTIONS)*

Rheumatoid Arthritis: Cyclosporine nephropathy was detected in renal biopsies of 6 out of 60 (10%) rheumatoid arthritis patients after the average treatment duration of 19 months. Only one patient, out of these 6 patients, was treated with a dose ≤4 mg/kg/day. Serum creatinine improved in all but one patient after discontinuation of cyclosporine. The "maximal creatinine increase" appears to be a factor in predicting cyclosporine nephropathy.

There is a potential, as with other immunosuppressive agents, for an increase in the occurrence of malignant lymphomas with cyclosporine. It is not clear whether the risk with cyclosporine is greater than that in Rheumatoid Arthritis patients or in Rheumatoid Arthritis patients on cytotoxic treatment for this indication. Five cases of lymphoma were detected: four in a survey of approximately 2,300 patients treated with cyclosporine for rheumatoid arthritis, and another case of lymphoma was reported in a clinical

Continued on next page

Neoral—Cont.

trial. Although other tumors (12 skin cancers, 24 solid tumors of diverse types, and 1 multiple myeloma) were also reported in this survey, epidemiologic analyses did not support a relationship to cyclosporine other than for malignant lymphomas.

Patients should be thoroughly evaluated before and during Neoral® treatment for the development of malignancies. Moreover, use of Neoral® therapy with other immunosuppressive agents may induce an excessive immunosuppression which is known to increase the risk of malignancy.

Psoriasis: *(See also Boxed WARNINGS for Psoriasis)* Since cyclosporine is a potent immunosuppressive agent with a number of potentially serious side effects, the risks and benefits of using Neoral® should be considered before treatment of patients with psoriasis. Cyclosporine, the active ingredient in Neoral®, can cause nephrotoxicity and hypertension *(see PRECAUTIONS)* and the risk increases with increasing dose and duration of therapy. Patients who may be at increased risk such as those with abnormal renal function, uncontrolled hypertension or malignancies, should not receive Neoral®.

Renal dysfunction is a potential consequence of Neoral® therefore renal function must be monitored during therapy. Patients receiving Neoral® require frequent monitoring of serum creatinine. *(See Special Monitoring under DOSAGE AND ADMINISTRATION)* Elderly patients should be monitored with particular care, since decreases in renal function also occur with age. If patients are not properly monitored and doses are not properly adjusted, cyclosporine therapy can cause structural kidney damage and persistent renal dysfunction.

An increase in serum creatinine and BUN may occur during Neoral® therapy and reflects a reduction in the glomerular filtration rate.

Kidney biopsies from 86 psoriasis patients treated for a mean duration of 23 months with 1.2-7.6 mg/kg/day of cyclosporine showed evidence of cyclosporine nephropathy in 18/86 (21%) of the patients. The pathology consisted of renal tubular atrophy and interstitial fibrosis. On repeat biopsy of 13 of these patients maintained on various dosages of cyclosporine for a mean of 2 additional years, the number with cyclosporine induced nephropathy rose to 26/86 (30%). The majority of patients (19/26) were on a dose of ≥5.0 mg/kg/day (the highest recommended dose is 4 mg/kg/day). The patients were also on cyclosporine for greater than 15 months (18/26) and/or had a clinically significant increase in serum creatinine for greater than 1 month (21/26). Creatinine levels returned to normal range in 7 of 11 patients in whom cyclosporine therapy was discontinued.

There is an increased risk for the development of skin and lymphoproliferative malignancies in cyclosporine-treated psoriasis patients. The relative risk of malignancies is comparable to that observed in psoriasis patients treated with other immunosuppressive agents.

Tumors were reported in 32 (2.2%) of 1439 psoriasis patients treated with cyclosporine worldwide from clinical trials. Additional tumors have been reported in 7 patients in cyclosporine postmarketing experience. Skin malignancies were reported in 16 (1.1%) of these patients; all but 2 of them had previously received PUVA therapy. Methotrexate was received by 7 patients. UVB and coal tar had been used by 2 and 3 patients, respectively. Seven patients had either a history of previous skin cancer or a potentially predisposing lesion was present prior to cyclosporine exposure. Of the 16 patients with skin cancer, 11 patients had 18 squamous cell carcinomas and 7 patients had 10 basal cell carcinomas. There were two lymphoproliferative malignancies; one case of non-Hodgkin's lymphoma which required chemotherapy, and one case of mycosis fungoides which regressed spontaneously upon discontinuation of cyclosporine. There were four cases of benign lymphocytic infiltration: 3 regressed spontaneously upon discontinuation of cyclosporine, while the fourth regressed despite continuation of the drug. The remainder of the malignancies, 13 cases (0.9%), involved various organs.

Patients should not be treated concurrently with cyclosporine and PUVA or UVB, other radiation therapy, or other immunosuppressive agents, because of the possibility of excessive immunosuppression and the subsequent risk of malignancies. *(See CONTRAINDICATIONS)* Patients should also be warned to protect themselves appropriately when in the sun, and to avoid excessive sun exposure. Patients should be thoroughly evaluated before and during treatment for the presence of malignancies remembering that malignant lesions may be hidden by psoriatic plaques. Skin lesions not typical of psoriasis should be biopsied before starting treatment. Patients should be treated with Neoral® only after complete resolution of suspicious lesions, and only if there are no other treatment options. *(See Special Monitoring for Psoriasis Patients)*

PRECAUTIONS

General: ***Hypertension:*** Cyclosporine is the active ingredient of Neoral®. Hypertension is a common side effect of cyclosporine therapy which may persist. *(See ADVERSE REACTIONS and DOSAGE AND ADMINISTRATION for monitoring recommendations)* Mild or moderate hypertension is encountered more frequently than severe hypertension and the incidence decreases over time. In recipients of kidney, liver, and heart allografts treated with cyclosporine, antihypertensive therapy may be required. *(See Special Monitoring of Rheumatoid Arthritis and Psoriasis Patients)* However, since cyclosporine may cause hyperkalemia, potassium-sparing diuretics should not be used. While calcium antagonists can be effective agents in treating cyclosporine-associated hypertension, they can interfere with cyclosporine metabolism. *(See Drug Interactions)*

Drugs That May Potentiate Renal Dysfunction

Antibiotics	*Antineoplastics*	*Anti-inflammatory Drugs*	*Gastrointestinal Agents*
gentamycin	melphalan	azapropazon	cimetidine
tobramycin		diclofenac	ranitidine
vancomycin	*Antifungals*	naproxen	*Immunosuppressives*
trimethoprim with sulfamethoxazole	amphotericin B	sulindac	tacrolimus
	ketoconazole	colchicine	

Drugs That Increase Cyclosporine Concentrations

Calcium Channel Blockers	*Antifungals*	*Antibiotics*	*Glucocorticoids*	*Other Drugs*	
diltiazem	fluconazole	clarithromycin	methylprednisolone	allopurinol	danazol
nicardipine	itraconazole	erythromycin		bromocriptine	metoclopramide
verapamil	ketoconazole	quinupristin/ dalfopristin			colchicine
					amiodarone

Vaccination: During treatment with cyclosporine, vaccination may be less effective; and the use of live attenuated vaccines should be avoided.

Special Monitoring of Rheumatoid Arthritis Patients: Before initiating treatment, a careful physical examination, including blood pressure measurements (on at least two occasions) and two creatinine levels to estimate baseline should be performed. Blood pressure and serum creatinine should be evaluated every 2 weeks during the initial 3 months and then monthly if the patient is stable. It is advisable to monitor serum creatinine and blood pressure always after an increase of the dose of nonsteroidal anti-inflammatory drugs and after initiation of new nonsteroidal anti-inflammatory drug therapy during Neoral® treatment. If co-administered with methotrexate, CBC and liver function tests are recommended to be monitored monthly. *(See also PRECAUTIONS, General, Hypertension)*

In patients who are receiving cyclosporine, the dose of Neoral® should be decreased by 25%-50% if hypertension occurs. If hypertension persists, the dose of Neoral® should be further reduced or blood pressure should be controlled with antihypertensive agents. In most cases, blood pressure has returned to baseline when cyclosporine was discontinued.

In placebo-controlled trials of rheumatoid arthritis patients, systolic hypertension (defined as an occurrence of two systolic blood pressure readings >140 mmHg) and diastolic hypertension (defined as two diastolic blood pressure readings >90 mmHg) occurred in 33% and 19% of patients treated with cyclosporine, respectively. The corresponding placebo rates were 22% and 8%.

Special Monitoring for Psoriasis Patients: Before initiating treatment, a careful dermatological and physical examination, including blood pressure measurements (on at least two occasions) should be performed. Since Neoral® is an immunosuppressive agent, patients should be evaluated for the presence of occult infection on their first physical examination and for the presence of tumors initially, and throughout treatment with Neoral®. Skin lesions not typical for psoriasis should be biopsied before starting Neoral®. Patients with malignant or premalignant changes of the skin should be treated with Neoral® only after appropriate treatment of such lesions and if no other treatment option exists.

Baseline laboratories should include serum creatinine (on two occasions), BUN, CBC, serum magnesium, potassium, uric acid, and lipids.

The risk of cyclosporine nephropathy is reduced when the starting dose is low (2.5 mg/kg/day), the maximum dose does not exceed 4.0 mg/kg/day, serum creatinine is monitored regularly while cyclosporine is administered, and the dose of Neoral® is decreased when the rise in creatinine is greater than or equal to 25% above the patients pretreatment level. The increase in creatinine is generally reversible upon timely decrease of the dose of Neoral® or its discontinuation.

Serum creatinine and BUN should be evaluated every 2 weeks during the initial 3 months of therapy and then monthly if the patient is stable. If the serum creatinine is greater than or equal to 25% above the patient's pretreatment level, serum creatinine should be repeated within two weeks. If the change in serum creatinine remains greater than or equal to 25% above baseline, Neoral® should be reduced by 25%-50%. If at **any time** the serum creatinine increases by greater than or equal to 50% above pretreatment level, Neoral® should be reduced by 25%-50%. Neoral® should be discontinued if reversibility (within 25% of baseline) of serum creatinine is not achievable after two dosage modifications. It is advisable to monitor serum creatinine after an increase of the dose of nonsteroidal anti-inflammatory drug and after initiation of new nonsteroidal anti-inflammatory therapy during Neoral® treatment.

Blood pressure should be evaluated every 2 weeks during the initial 3 months of therapy and then monthly if the patient is stable, or more frequently when dosage adjustments are made. Patients without a history of previous hypertension before initiation of treatment with Neoral®, should have the drug reduced by 25%-50% if found to have sustained hypertension. If the patient continues to be hypertensive despite multiple reductions of Neoral®, then Neoral® should be discontinued. For patients with treated hypertension, before the initiation of Neoral® therapy, their medication should be adjusted to control hypertension while on Neoral®. Neoral® should be discontinued if a change in hypertension management is not effective or tolerable.

CBC, uric acid, potassium, lipids, and magnesium should also be monitored every 2 weeks for the first 3 months of therapy, and then monthly if the patient is stable or more frequently when dosage adjustments are made. Neoral® dosage should be reduced by 25%-50% for any abnormality of clinical concern.

In controlled trials of cyclosporine in psoriasis patients, cyclosporine blood concentrations did not correlate well with either improvement or with side effects such as renal dysfunction.

Information for Patients: Patients should be advised that any change of cyclosporine formulation should be made cautiously and only under physician supervision because it may result in the need for a change in dosage.

Patients should be informed of the necessity of repeated laboratory tests while they are receiving cyclosporine. Patients should be advised of the potential risks during pregnancy and informed of the increased risk of neoplasia. Patients should also be informed of the risk of hypertension and renal dysfunction.

Patients should be advised that during treatment with cyclosporine, vaccination may be less effective and the use of live attenuated vaccines should be avoided.

Patients should be given careful dosage instructions. Neoral® Oral Solution (cyclosporine oral solution, USP) MODIFIED should be diluted, preferably with orange or apple juice that is at room temperature. The combination of Neoral® Oral Solution (cyclosporine oral solution, USP) MODIFIED with milk can be unpalatable.

Patients should be advised to take Neoral® on a consistent schedule with regard to time of day and relation to meals. Grapefruit and grapefruit juice affect metabolism, increasing blood concentration of cyclosporine, thus should be avoided.

Laboratory Tests: In all patients treated with cyclosporine, renal and liver functions should be assessed repeatedly by measurement of serum creatinine, BUN, serum bilirubin, and liver enzymes. Serum lipids, magnesium, and potassium should also be monitored. Cyclosporine blood concentrations should be routinely monitored in transplant patients *(see DOSAGE AND ADMINISTRATION, Blood Concentration Monitoring in Transplant Patients)*, and periodically monitored in rheumatoid arthritis patients.

Drug Interactions: All of the individual drugs cited below are well substantiated to interact with cyclosporine. In addition, concomitant non-steroidal anti-inflammatory drugs, particularly in the setting of dehydration, may potentiate renal dysfunction.

[See first table above]

Drugs That Alter Cyclosporine Concentrations: Compounds that decrease cyclosporine absorption such as orlistat should be avoided. Cyclosporine is extensively metabolized cytochrome P-450 3A. Substances that inhibit this enzyme could decrease metabolism and increase cyclosporine concentrations. Substances that are inducers of cytochrome P-450 activity could increase metabolism and decrease cyclosporine concentrations. Monitoring of circulating cyclosporine concentrations and appropriate Neoral® dosage adjustment are essential when these drugs are used concomitantly. *(See Blood Concentration Monitoring)*

[See second table above]

The HIV protease inhibitors (e.g., indinavir, nelfinavir, ritonavir, and saquinavir) are known to inhibit cytochrome P-450 3A and thus could potentially increase the concentrations of cyclosporine, however no formal studies of the interaction are available. Care should be exercised when these drugs are administered concomitantly.

Grapefruit and grapefruit juice affect metabolism, increasing blood concentrations of cyclosporine, thus should be avoided.

Drugs/Dietary Supplements That Decrease Cyclosporine Concentrations

Antibiotics	*Anticonvulsants*	*Other Drugs/ Dietary Supplements*
nafcillin	carbamazepine	octreotide
rifampin	phenobarbital	ticlopidine
	phenytoin	orlistat
		St. John's Wort

There have been reports of a serious drug interaction between cyclosporine and the herbal dietary supplement, St. John's Wort. This interaction has been reported to produce a marked reduction in the blood concentrations of cyclosporine, resulting in subtherapeutic levels, rejection of transplanted organs, and graft loss.

Rifabutin is known to increase the metabolism of other drugs metabolized by the cytochrome P-450 system. The interaction between rifabutin and cyclosporine has not been studied. Care should be exercised when these two drugs are administered concomitantly.

Nonsteroidal Anti-inflammatory Drug (NSAID) Interactions: Clinical status and serum creatinine should be closely monitored when cyclosporine is used with nonsteroidal anti-inflammatory agents in rheumatoid arthritis patients. *(See WARNINGS)*

Pharmacodynamic interactions have been reported to occur between cyclosporine and both naproxen and sulindac, in that concomitant use is associated with additive decreases in renal function, as determined by ^{99m}Tc-diethylenetriaminepentaacetic acid (DTPA) and (*p*-aminohippuric acid) PAH clearances. Although concomitant administration of diclofenac does not affect blood levels of cyclosporine, it has been associated with approximate doubling of diclofenac blood levels and occasional reports of reversible decreases in renal function. Consequently, the dose of diclofenac should be in the lower end of the therapeutic range.

Methotrexate Interaction: Preliminary data indicate that when methotrexate and cyclosporine were co-administered to rheumatoid arthritis patients (N=20), methotrexate concentrations (AUCs) were increased approximately 30% and the concentrations (AUCs) of its metabolite, 7-hydroxy methotrexate, were decreased by approximately 80%. The clinical significance of this interaction is not known. Cyclosporine concentrations do not appear to have been altered (N=6).

Other Drug Interactions: Reduced clearance of prednisolone, digoxin, and lovastatin has been observed when these drugs are administered with cyclosporine. In addition, a decrease in the apparent volume of distribution of digoxin has been reported after cyclosporine administration. Severe digitalis toxicity has been seen within days of starting cyclosporine in several patients taking digoxin. Cyclosporine should not be used with potassium-sparing diuretics because hyperkalemia can occur.

During treatment with cyclosporine, vaccination may be less effective. The use of live vaccines should be avoided. Myositis has occurred with concomitant lovastatin, frequent gingival hyperplasia with nifedipine, and convulsions with high dose methylprednisolone.

Psoriasis patients receiving other immunosuppressive agents or radiation therapy (including PUVA and UVB) should not receive concurrent cyclosporine because of the possibility of excessive immunosuppression.

For additional information on Cyclosporine Drug Interactions please contact Novartis Medical Affairs Department at 888-NOW-NOVA [888-669-6682].

Carcinogenesis, Mutagenesis, and Impairment of Fertility: Carcinogenicity studies were carried out in male and female rats and mice. In the 78-week mouse study, evidence of a statistically significant trend was found for lymphocytic lymphomas in females, and the incidence of hepatocellular carcinomas in mid-dose males significantly exceeded the control value. In the 24-month rat study, pancreatic islet cell adenomas significantly exceeded the control rate in the low dose level. Doses used in the mouse and rat studies were 0.01 to 0.16 times the clinical maintenance dose (6 mg/kg). The hepatocellular carcinomas and pancreatic islet cell adenomas were not dose related. Published reports indicate that co-treatment of hairless mice with UV irradiation and cyclosporine or other immunosuppressive agents shorten the time to skin tumor formation compared to UV irradiation alone.

Cyclosporine was not mutagenic in appropriate test systems. Cyclosporine has not been found to be mutagenic/genotoxic in the Ames Test, the V79-HGPRT Test, the micronucleus test in mice and Chinese hamsters, the chromosome-aberration tests in Chinese hamster bone-marrow, the mouse dominant lethal assay, and the DNA-repair test in sperm from treated mice. A recent study analyzing sister chromatid exchange (SCE) induction by cyclosporine using human lymphocytes *in vitro* gave indication of a positive effect (i.e., induction of SCE), at high concentrations in this system.

No impairment in fertility was demonstrated in studies in male and female rats.

Widely distributed papillomatosis of the skin was observed after chronic treatment of dogs with cyclosporine at 9 times the human initial psoriasis treatment dose of 2.5 mg/kg, where doses are expressed on a body surface area basis. This papillomatosis showed a spontaneous regression upon discontinuation of cyclosporine.

An increased incidence of malignancy is a recognized complication of immunosuppression in recipients of organ transplants and patients with rheumatoid arthritis and psoriasis. The most common forms of neoplasms are non-Hodgkin's lymphoma and carcinomas of the skin. The risk of malignancies in cyclosporine recipients is higher than in the normal, healthy population but similar to that in patients receiving other immunosuppressive therapies. Reduction or discontinuance of immunosuppression may cause the lesions to regress.

In psoriasis patients on cyclosporine, development of malignancies, especially those of the skin has been reported. *(See WARNINGS)* Skin lesions not typical for psoriasis should be biopsied before starting cyclosporine treatment. Patients with malignant or premalignant changes of the skin should be treated with cyclosporine only after appropriate treatment of such lesions and if no other treatment option exists.

Pregnancy: *Pregnancy Category C.* Cyclosporine was not teratogenic in appropriate test systems. Only at dose levels toxic to dams, were adverse effects seen in reproduction studies in rats. Cyclosporine has been shown to be embryo- and fetotoxic in rats and rabbits following oral administration at maternally toxic doses. Fetal toxicity was noted in rats at 0.8 and rabbits at 5.4 times the transplant doses in humans of 6.0 mg/kg, where dose corrections are based on body surface area. Cyclosporine was embryo- and fetotoxic as indicated by increased pre- and postnatal mortality and reduced fetal weight together with related skeletal retardation.

There are no adequate and well-controlled studies in pregnant women. Neoral® should be used during pregnancy only if the potential benefit justifies the potential risk to the fetus.

The following data represent the reported outcomes of 116 pregnancies in women receiving cyclosporine during pregnancy, 90% of whom were transplant patients, and most of whom received cyclosporine throughout the entire gestational period. The only consistent patterns of abnormality were premature birth (gestational period of 28 to 36 weeks) and low birth weight for gestational age. Sixteen fetal losses occurred. Most of the pregnancies (85 of 100) were complicated by disorders; including, pre-eclampsia, eclampsia, premature labor, abruptio placentae, oligohydramnios, Rh incompatibility, and fetoplacental dysfunction. Pre-term delivery occurred in 47%. Seven malformations were reported in 5 viable infants and in 2 cases of fetal loss. Twenty-eight percent of the infants were small for gestational age. Neonatal complications occurred in 27%. Therefore, the risks and benefits of using Neoral® during pregnancy should be carefully weighed.

Because of the possible disruption of maternal-fetal interaction, the risk/benefit ratio of using Neoral® in psoriasis patients during pregnancy should carefully be weighed with serious consideration for discontinuation of Neoral®.

Nursing Mothers: Since cyclosporine is excreted in human milk, breast-feeding should be avoided.

Pediatric Use: Although no adequate and well-controlled studies have been completed in children, transplant recipients as young as one year of age have received Neoral® with no unusual adverse effects. The safety and efficacy of Neoral® treatment in children with juvenile rheumatoid arthritis or psoriasis below the age of 18 have not been established.

Geriatric Use: In rheumatoid arthritis clinical trials with cyclosporine, 17.5% of patients were age 65 or older. These patients were more likely to develop systolic hypertension on therapy, and more likely to show serum creatinine rises ≥50% above the baseline after 3-4 months of therapy.

ADVERSE REACTIONS

Kidney, Liver, and Heart Transplantation: The principal adverse reactions of cyclosporine therapy are renal dysfunction, tremor, hirsutism, hypertension, and gum hyperplasia.

Hypertension, which is usually mild to moderate, may occur in approximately 50% of patients following renal transplantation and in most cardiac transplant patients.

Glomerular capillary thrombosis has been found in patients treated with cyclosporine and may progress to graft failure. The pathologic changes resembled those seen in the hemolytic-uremic syndrome and included thrombosis of the renal microvasculature, with platelet-fibrin thrombi occluding glomerular capillaries and afferent arterioles, microangiopathic hemolytic anemia, thrombocytopenia, and decreased renal function. Similar findings have been observed when other immunosuppressives have been employed post-transplantation.

Hypomagnesemia has been reported in some, but not all, patients exhibiting convulsions while on cyclosporine therapy. Although magnesium-depletion studies in normal subjects suggest that hypomagnesemia is associated with neurologic disorders, multiple factors, including hypertension, high dose methylprednisolone, hypocholesterolemia, and nephrotoxicity associated with high plasma concentrations of cyclosporine appear to be related to the neurological manifestations of cyclosporine toxicity.

In controlled studies, the nature, severity, and incidence of the adverse events that were observed in 493 transplanted patients treated with Neoral® were comparable with those observed in 208 transplanted patients who received Sandimmune® in these same studies when the dosage of the two drugs was adjusted to achieve the same cyclosporine blood trough concentrations.

Based on the historical experience with Sandimmune®, the following reactions occurred in 3% or greater of 892 patients involved in clinical trials of kidney, heart, and liver transplants.

[See first table above]

		Randomized Kidney Patients		Cyclosporine Patients (Sandimmune®)		
Body System	**Adverse Reactions**	**Sandimmune® (N=227) %**	**Azathioprine (N=228) %**	**Kidney (N=705) %**	**Heart (N=112) %**	**Liver (N=75) %**
Genitourinary	Renal Dysfunction	32	6	25	38	37
Cardiovascular	Hyertension	26	18	13	53	27
	Cramps	4	<1	2	<1	0
Skin	Hirsutism	21	<1	21	28	45
	Acne	6	8	2	2	1
Central Nervous System	Tremor	12	0	21	31	55
	Convulsions	3	1	1	4	5
	Headache	2	<1	2	15	4
Gastrointestinal	Gum Hyperplasia	4	0	9	5	16
	Diarrhea	3	<1	3	4	8
	Nausea/Vomiting	2	<1	4	10	4
	Hepatotoxicity	<1	<1	4	7	4
	Abdominal Discomfort	<1	0	<1	7	0
Autonomic Nervous System	Paresthesia	3	0	1	2	1
	Flushing	<1	0	4	0	4
Hematopoietic	Leukopenia	2	19	<1	6	0
	Lymphoma	<1	0	1	6	1
Respiratory	Sinusitis	<1	0	4	3	7
Miscellaneous	Gynecomastia	<1	0	<1	4	3

Among 705 kidney transplant patients treated with cyclosporine oral solution (Sandimmune®) in clinical trials, the reason for treatment discontinuation was renal toxicity in 5.4%, infection in 0.9%, lack of efficacy in 1.4%, acute tubular necrosis in 1.0%, lymphoproliferative disorders in 0.3%, hypertension in 0.3%, and other reasons in 0.7% of the patients.

The following reactions occurred in 2% or less of Sandimmune®-treated patients: allergic reactions, anemia, anorexia, confusion, conjunctivitis, edema, fever, brittle fingernails, gastritis, hearing loss, hiccups, hyperglycemia, muscle pain, peptic ulcer, thrombocytopenia, tinnitus.

The following reactions occurred rarely: anxiety, chest pain, constipation, depression, hair breaking, hematuria, joint pain, lethargy, mouth sores, myocardial infarction, night sweats, pancreatitis, pruritus, swallowing difficulty, tingling, upper GI bleeding, visual disturbance, weakness, weight loss.

[See second table above]

Infectious Complications in Historical Randomized Studies in Renal Transplant Patients Using Sandimmune®

Complication	**Cyclosporine Treatment (N=227) % of Complications**	**Azathioprine with Steroids* (N=228) % of Complications**
Septicemia	5.3	4.8
Abscesses	4.4	5.3
Systemic Fungal Infection	2.2	3.9
Local Fungal Infection	7.5	9.6
Cytomegalovirus	4.8	12.3
Other Viral Infections	15.9	18.4
Urinary Tract Infections	21.1	20.2
Wound and Skin Infections	7.0	10.1
Pneumonia	6.2	9.2

*Some patients also received ALG.

Rheumatoid Arthritis: The principal adverse reactions associated with the use of cyclosporine in rheumatoid arthritis are renal dysfunction *(see WARNINGS)*, hypertension *(see PRECAUTIONS)*, headache, gastrointestinal disturbances, and hirsutism/hypertrichosis.

In rheumatoid arthritis patients treated in clinical trials within the recommended dose range, cyclosporine therapy was discontinued in 5.3% of the patients because of hypertension and in 7% of the patients because of increased creatinine. These changes are usually reversible with timely

Continued on next page

Neoral—Cont.

dose decrease or drug discontinuation. The frequency and severity of serum creatinine elevations increase with dose and duration of cyclosporine therapy. These elevations are likely to become more pronounced without dose reduction or discontinuation.

The following adverse events occurred in controlled clinical trials:

[See table to the right]

In addition, the following adverse events have been reported in 1% to <3% of the rheumatoid arthritis patients in the cyclosporine treatment group in controlled clinical trials.
Autonomic Nervous System: dry mouth, increased sweating;
Body as a Whole: allergy, asthenia, hot flushes, malaise, overdose, procedure NOS*, tumor NOS*, weight decrease, weight increase;
Cardiovascular: abnormal heart sounds, cardiac failure, myocardial infarction, peripheral ischemia;
Central and Peripheral Nervous System: hypoesthesia, neuropathy, vertigo;
Endocrine: goiter;
Gastrointestinal: constipation, dysphagia, enanthema, eructation, esophagitis, gastric ulcer, gastritis, gastroenteritis, gingival bleeding, glossitis, gingiva ulcer, salivary gland enlargement, tongue disorder, tooth disorder;
Infection: abscess, bacterial infection, cellulitis, folliculitis, fungal infection, herpes simplex, herpes zoster, renal abscess, moniliasis, tonsillitis, viral infection;
Hematologic: anemia, epistaxis, leukopenia, lymphadenopathy;
Liver and Biliary System: bilirubinemia;
Metabolic and Nutritional: diabetes mellitus, hyperkalemia, hyperuricemia, hypoglycemia;
Musculoskeletal System: arthralgia, bone fracture, bursitis, joint dislocation, myalgia, stiffness, synovial cyst, tendon disorder;
Neoplasms: breast fibroadenosis, carcinoma;
Psychiatric: anxiety, confusion, decreased libido, emotional lability, impaired concentration, increased libido, nervousness, paroniria, somnolence;
Reproductive (Female): breast pain, uterine hemorrhage;
Respiratory System: abnormal chest sounds, bronchospasm;
Skin and Appendages: abnormal pigmentation, angioedema, dermatitis, dry skin, eczema, nail disorder, pruritus, skin disorder, urticaria;
Special Senses: abnormal vision, cataract, conjunctivitis, deafness, eye pain, taste perversion, tinnitus, vestibular disorder;
Urinary System: abnormal urine, hematuria, increased BUN, micturition urgency, nocturia, polyuria, pyelonephritis, urinary incontinence.

---

*NOS = Not Otherwise Specified.
Psoriasis: The principal adverse reactions associated with the use of cyclosporine in patients with psoriasis are renal dysfunction, headache, hypertension, hypertriglyceridemia, hirsutism/hypertrichosis, paresthesia or hyperesthesia, influenza-like symptoms, nausea/vomiting, diarrhea, abdominal discomfort, lethargy, and musculoskeletal or joint pain. In psoriasis patients treated in US controlled clinical studies within the recommended dose range, cyclosporine therapy was discontinued in 1.0% of the patients because of hypertension and in 5.4% of the patients because of increased creatinine. In the majority of cases, these changes were reversible after dose reduction or discontinuation of cyclosporine.

There has been one reported death associated with the use of cyclosporine in psoriasis. A 27-year-old male developed renal deterioration and was continued on cyclosporine. He had progressive renal failure leading to death.

Frequency and severity of serum creatinine increases with dose and duration of cyclosporine therapy. These elevations are likely to become more pronounced and may result in irreversible renal damage without dose reduction or discontinuation.

[See table at bottom of next page]

The following events occurred in 1% to less than 3% of psoriasis patients treated with cyclosporine:

Body as a Whole: fever, flushes, hot flushes; *Cardiovascular:* chest pain; *Central and Peripheral Nervous System:* appetite increased, insomnia, dizziness, nervousness, vertigo; *Gastrointestinal:* abdominal distention, constipation, gingival bleeding; *Liver and Biliary System:* hyperbilirubinemia; *Neoplasms:* skin malignancies [squamous cell (0.9%) and basal cell (0.4%) carcinomas]; *Reticuloendothelial:* platelet, bleeding, and clotting disorders, red blood cell disorder; *Respiratory:* infection, viral and other infection; *Skin and Appendages:* acne, folliculitis, keratosis, pruritus, rash, dry skin; *Urinary System:* micturition frequency; *Vision:* abnormal vision.

Mild hypomagnesemia and hyperkalemia may occur but are asymptomatic. Increases in uric acid may occur and attacks of gout have been rarely reported. A minor and dose related hyperbilirubinemia has been observed in the absence of hepatocellular damage. Cyclosporine therapy may be associated with a modest increase of serum triglycerides or cholesterol. Elevations of triglycerides (>750 mg/dL) occur in about 15% of psoriasis patients; elevations of cholesterol (>300 mg/dL) are observed in less than 3% of psoriasis patients. Generally these laboratory abnormalities are reversible upon dose reduction or discontinuation of cyclosporine.

Neoral®/Sandimmune® Rheumatoid Arthritis
Percentage of Patients with Adverse Events ≥3% in any Cyclosporine Treated Group

Body System	Preferred term	Studies 651+652+2008 Sandimmune®† (N=269)	Study 302 Sandimmune® (N=155)	Study 654 Sandimmune® (N=74)	Study 654 Methotrexate & Placebo (N=73)	Study 302 Neoral® (N=143)	Studies 651+652+2008 Placebo (N=201)
Autonomic Nervous System Disorders							
	Flushing	2%	2%	3%	0%	5%	2%
Body As A Whole—General Disorders							
	Accidental Trauma	0%	1%	10%	4%	4%	0%
	Edema NOS*	5%	14%	12%	4%	10%	<1%
	Fatigue	6%	3%	8%	12%	3%	7%
	Fever	2%	3%	0%	0%	2%	4%
	Influenza-like symptoms	<1%	6%	1%	0%	3%	2%
	Pain	6%	9%	10%	15%	13%	4%
	Rigors	1%	1%	4%	0%	3%	1%
Cardiovascular Disorders							
	Arrhythmia	2%	5%	5%	6%	2%	1%
	Chest Pain	4%	5%	1%	1%	6%	1%
	Hypertension	8%	26%	16%	12%	25%	2%
Central and Peripheral Nervous System Disorders							
	Dizziness	8%	6%	7%	3%	8%	3%
	Headache	17%	23%	22%	11%	25%	9%
	Migraine	2%	3%	0%	0%	3%	1%
	Paresthesia	8%	7%	8%	4%	11%	1%
	Tremor	8%	7%	7%	3%	13%	4%
Gastrointestinal System Disorders							
	Abdominal Pain	15%	15%	15%	7%	15%	10%
	Anorexia	3%	3%	1%	0%	3%	3%
	Diarrhea	12%	12%	18%	15%	13%	8%
	Dyspepsia	12%	12%	10%	8%	8%	4%
	Flatulence	5%	5%	5%	4%	4%	1%
	Gastrointestinal Disorder NOS*	0%	2%	1%	4%	4%	0%
	Gingivitis	4%	3%	0%	0%	0%	1%
	Gum Hyperplasia	2%	4%	1%	3%	4%	1%
	Nausea	23%	14%	24%	15%	18%	14%
	Rectal Hemorrhage	0%	3%	0%	0%	1%	1%
	Stomatitis	7%	5%	16%	12%	6%	8%
	Vomiting	9%	8%	14%	7%	6%	5%
Hearing and Vestibular Disorders							
	Ear Disorder NOS*	0%	5%	0%	0%	1%	0%
Metabolic and Nutritional Disorders							
	Hypomagnesemia	0%	4%	0%	0%	6%	0%
Musculoskeletal System Disorders							
	Arthropathy	0%	5%	0%	1%	4%	0%
	Leg Cramps/Involuntary Muscle Contractions	2%	11%	11%	3%	12%	1%
Psychiatric Disorders							
	Depression	3%	6%	3%	1%	1%	2%
	Insomnia	4%	1%	1%	0%	3%	2%
Renal							
	Creatinine elevations ≥30%	43%	39%	55%	19%	48%	13%
	Creatinine elevations ≥50%	24%	18%	26%	8%	18%	3%
Reproductive Disorders, Female							
	Leukorrhea	1%	0%	4%	0%	1%	0%
	Menstrual Disorder	3%	2%	1%	0%	1%	1%
Respiratory System Disorders							
	Bronchitis	1%	3%	1%	0%	1%	3%
	Coughing	5%	3%	5%	7%	4%	4%
	Dyspnea	5%	1%	3%	3%	1%	2%
	Infection NOS*	9%	5%	0%	7%	3%	10%
	Pharyngitis	3%	5%	5%	6%	4%	4%
	Pneumonia	1%	0%	4%	0%	1%	1%
	Rhinitis	0%	3%	11%	10%	1%	0%
	Sinusitis	4%	4%	8%	4%	3%	3%
	Upper Respiratory Tract	0%	14%	23%	15%	13%	0%
Skin and Appendages Disorders							
	Alopecia	3%	0%	1%	1%	4%	4%
	Bullous Eruption	1%	0%	4%	1%	1%	1%
	Hypertrichosis	19%	17%	12%	0%	15%	3%
	Rash	7%	12%	10%	7%	8%	10%
	Skin Ulceration	1%	1%	3%	4%	0%	2%
Urinary System Disorders							
	Dysuria	0%	0%	11%	3%	1%	2%
	Micturition Frequency	2%	4%	3%	1%	2%	2%
	NPN, Increased	0%	19%	12%	0%	18%	0%
	Urinary Tract Infection	0%	3%	5%	4%	3%	0%
Vascular (Extracardiac) Disorders							
	Purpura	3%	4%	1%	1%	2%	0%

†Includes patients in 2.5 mg/kg/day dose group only. *NOS = Not Otherwise Specified.

OVERDOSAGE

There is a minimal experience with cyclosporine overdosage. Forced emesis can be of value up to 2 hours after administration of Neoral®. Transient hepatotoxicity and nephrotoxicity may occur which should resolve following drug withdrawal. General supportive measures and symptomatic treatment should be followed in all cases of overdosage. Cyclosporine is not dialyzable to any great extent, nor is it cleared well by charcoal hemoperfusion. The oral dosage at which half of experimental animals are estimated to die is 31 times, 39 times, and >54 times the human maintenance dose for transplant patients (6mg/kg; corrections based on body surface area) in mice, rats, and rabbits.

DOSAGE AND ADMINISTRATION

Neoral® Soft Gelatin Capsules (cyclosporine capsules, USP) MODIFIED and Neoral® Oral Solution (cyclosporine oral solution, USP) MODIFIED
Neoral® has increased bioavailability in comparison to Sandimmune®. Neoral® and Sandimmune® are not bioequivalent and cannot be used interchangeably without physician supervision.
The daily dose of Neoral® should always be given in two divided doses (BID). It is recommended that Neoral® be administered on a consistent schedule with regard to time of day and relation to meals. Grapefruit and grapefruit juice affect metabolism, increasing blood concentration of cyclosporine, thus should be avoided.

Newly Transplanted Patients: The initial oral dose of Neoral® can be given 4-12 hours prior to transplantation or be given postoperatively. The initial dose of Neoral® varies depending on the transplanted organ and the other immunosuppressive agents included in the immunosuppressive protocol. In newly transplanted patients, the initial oral dose of Neoral® is the same as the initial oral dose of Sandimmune®. Suggested initial doses are available from the results of a 1994 survey of the use of Sandimmune® in US transplant centers. The mean ± SD initial doses were 9±3 mg/kg/day for renal transplant patients (75 centers), 8±4 mg/kg/day for liver transplant patients (30 centers), and 7±3 mg/kg/day for heart transplant patients (24 centers). Total daily doses were divided into two equal daily doses. The Neoral® dose is subsequently adjusted to achieve a pre-defined cyclosporine blood concentration. *(See Blood Concentration Monitoring in Transplant Patients, below)* If cyclosporine trough blood concentrations are used, the target range is the same for Neoral® as for Sandimmune®. Using the same trough concentration target range for Neoral® as for Sandimmune® results in greater cyclosporine exposure when Neoral® is administered. *(See Pharmacokinetics, Absorption)* Dosing should be titrated based on clinical assessments of rejection and tolerability. Lower Neoral® doses may be sufficient as maintenance therapy.

Adjunct therapy with adrenal corticosteroids is recommended initially. Different tapering dosage schedules of prednisone appear to achieve similar results. A representative dosage schedule based on the patients weight started with 2.0 mg/kg/day for the first 4 days tapered to 1.0 mg/kg/day by 1 week, 0.6 mg/kg/day by 2 weeks, 0.3 mg/kg/day by 1 month, and 0.15 mg/kg/day by 2 months and thereafter as a maintenance dose. Steroid doses may be further tapered on an individualized basis depending on status of patient and function of graft. Adjustments in dosage of prednisone must be made according to the clinical situation.

Conversion from Sandimmune® to Neoral® in Transplant Patients: In transplanted patients who are considered for conversion to Neoral® from Sandimmune®, Neoral® should be started with the same daily dose as was previously used with Sandimmune® (1:1 dose conversion). The Neoral® dose should subsequently be adjusted to attain the pre-conversion cyclosporine blood trough concentration. Using the same trough concentration target range for Neoral® as for Sandimmune® results in greater cyclosporine exposure when Neoral® is administered. *(See Pharmacokinetics, Absorption)* Patients with suspected poor absorption of Sandimmune® require different dosing strategies. *(See Transplant Patients with Poor Absorption of Sandimmune®, below)* In some patients, the increase in blood trough concentration is more pronounced and may be of clinical significance.

Until the blood trough concentration attains the pre-conversion value, it is strongly recommended that the cyclosporine blood trough concentration be monitored every 4 to 7 days after conversion to Neoral®. In addition, clinical safety parameters such as serum creatinine and blood pressure should be monitored every two weeks during the first two months after conversion. If the blood trough concentrations are outside the desired range and/or if the clinical safety parameters worsen, the dosage of Neoral® must be adjusted accordingly.

Transplant Patients with Poor Absorption of Sandimmune®: Patients with lower than expected cyclosporine blood trough concentrations in relation to the oral dose of Sandimmune® may have poor or inconsistent absorption of cyclosporine from Sandimmune®. After conversion to Neoral®, patients tend to have higher cyclosporine concentrations. **Due to the increase in bioavailability of cyclosporine following conversion to Neoral®, the cyclosporine blood trough concentration may exceed the target range. Particular caution should be exercised when converting patients to Neoral® at doses greater than 10 mg/kg/day.** The dose of Neoral® should be titrated individually based on cyclosporine trough concentrations, tolerability, and clinical response. In this population the cyclosporine blood trough concentration should be measured more frequently, at least twice a week (daily, if initial dose exceeds 10 mg/kg/day) until the concentration stabilizes within the desired range.

Rheumatoid Arthritis: The initial dose of Neoral® is 2.5 mg/kg/day, taken twice daily as a divided (BID) oral dose. Salicylates, nonsteroidal anti-inflammatory agents, and oral corticosteroids may be continued. *(See WARNINGS and PRECAUTIONS: Drug Interactions)* Onset of action generally occurs between 4 and 8 weeks. If insufficient clinical benefit is seen and tolerability is good (including serum creatinine less than 30% above baseline), the dose may be increased by 0.5-0.75 mg/kg/day after 8 weeks and again after 12 weeks to a maximum of 4 mg/kg/day. If no benefit is seen by 16 weeks of therapy, Neoral® therapy should be discontinued.

Dose decreases by 25%-50% should be made at any time to control adverse events, e.g., hypertension elevations in serum creatinine (30% above patient's pretreatment level) or clinically significant laboratory abnormalities. *(See WARNINGS and PRECAUTIONS)*

If dose reduction is not effective in controlling abnormalities or if the adverse event or abnormality is severe, Neoral® should be discontinued. The same initial dose and dosage range should be used if Neoral® is combined with the recommended dose of methotrexate. Most patients can be treated with Neoral® doses of 3 mg/kg/day or below when combined with methotrexate doses of up to 15 mg/week. *(See CLINICAL PHARMACOLOGY, Clinical Trials)*

There is limited long-term treatment data. Recurrence of rheumatoid arthritis disease activity is generally apparent within 4 weeks after stopping cyclosporine.

Psoriasis: The initial dose of Neoral® should be 2.5 mg/kg/day. Neoral® should be taken twice daily, as a divided (1.25 mg/kg BID) oral dose. Patients should be kept at that dose for at least 4 weeks, barring adverse events. If significant clinical improvement has not occurred in patients by that time, the patient's dosage should be increased at 2 week intervals. Based on patient response, dose increases of approximately 0.5 mg/kg/day should be made to a maximum of 4.0 mg/kg/day.

Dose decreases by 25%-50% should be made at any time to control adverse events, e.g., hypertension, elevations in serum creatinine (≥25% above the patient's pretreatment level), or clinically significant laboratory abnormalities. If dose reduction is not effective in controlling abnormalities, or if the adverse event or abnormality is severe, Neoral® should be discontinued. *(See Special Monitoring of Psoriasis Patients)*

Patients generally show some improvement in the clinical manifestations of psoriasis in 2 weeks. Satisfactory control and stabilization of the disease may take 12-16 weeks to achieve. Results of a dose-titration clinical trial with Neoral® indicate that an improvement of psoriasis by 75% or more (based on PASI) was achieved in 51% of the patients after 8 weeks and in 79% of the patients after 12 weeks. Treatment should be discontinued if satisfactory response cannot be achieved after 6 weeks at 4 mg/kg/day or the patient's maximum tolerated dose. Once a patient is adequately controlled and appears stable the dose of Neoral® should be lowered, and the patient treated with the lowest dose that maintains an adequate response (this should not necessarily be total clearing of the patient). In clinical trials, cyclosporine doses at the lower end of the recommended dosage range were effective in maintaining a satisfactory response in 60% of the patients. Doses below 2.5 mg/kg/day may also be equally effective.

Upon stopping treatment with cyclosporine, relapse will occur in approximately 6 weeks (50% of the patients) to 16 weeks (75% of the patients). In the majority of patients rebound does not occur after cessation of treatment with cyclosporine. Thirteen cases of transformation of chronic plaque psoriasis to more severe forms of psoriasis have been reported. There were 9 cases of pustular and 4 cases of erythrodermic psoriasis. Long term experience with Neoral® in psoriasis patients is limited and continuous treatment for extended periods greater than one year is not recommended. Alternation with other forms of treatment should be considered in the long term management of patients with this life long disease.

Adverse Events Occurring in 3% or More of Psoriasis Patients in Controlled Clinical Trials

Body System*	Preferred Term	Neoral® (N=182)	Sandimmune® (N=185)
Infection or Potential Infection		24.7%	24.3%
	Influenza-like Symptoms	9.9%	8.1%
	Upper Respiratory Tract Infections	7.7%	11.3%
Cardiovascular System		28.0%	25.4%
	Hypertension**	27.5%	25.4%
Urinary System		24.2%	16.2%
	Increased Creatinine	19.8%	15.7%
Central and Peripheral Nervous System		26.4%	20.5%
	Headache	15.9%	14.0%
	Paresthesia	7.1%	4.8%
Musculoskeletal System		13.2%	8.7%
	Arthralgia	6.0%	1.1%
Body As A Whole–General		29.1%	22.2%
	Pain	4.4%	3.2%
Metabolic and Nutritional		9.3%	9.7%
Reproductive, female		8.5% (4 of 47 females)	11.5% (6 of 52 females)
Resistance Mechanism		18.7%	21.1%
Skin and Appendages		17.6%	15.1%
	Hypertrichosis	6.6%	5.4%
Respiratory System		5.0%	6.5%
	Bronchospasm, coughing, dyspnea, rhinitis	5.0%	4.9%
Psychiatric		5.0%	3.8%
Gastrointestinal System		19.8%	28.7%
	Abdominal pain	2.7%	6.0%
	Diarrhea	5.0%	5.9%
	Dyspepsia	2.2%	3.2%
	Gum hyperplasia	3.8%	6.0%
	Nausea	5.5%	5.9%
White cell and RES		4.4%	2.7%

*Total percentage of events within the system

**Newly occurring hypertension = SBP≥160 mm Hg and/or DBP≥90 mm Hg

Neoral® Oral Solution (cyclosporine oral solution, USP) MODIFIED—Recommendations for Administration: To make Neoral® Oral Solution (cyclosporine oral solution, USP) MODIFIED more palatable, it should be diluted preferably with orange or apple juice that is at room temperature. Grapefruit juice affects metabolism of cyclosporine and should be avoided. The combination of Neoral® solution with milk can be unpalatable.

Take the prescribed amount of Neoral® Oral Solution (cyclosporine oral solution, USP) MODIFIED from the container using the dosing syringe supplied, after removal of the protective cover, and transfer the solution to a glass of orange or apple juice. Stir well and drink at once. Do not allow diluted oral solution to stand before drinking. Use a glass container (not plastic). Rinse the glass with more diluent to ensure that the total dose is consumed. After use, dry the outside of the dosing syringe with a clean towel and replace the protective cover. Do not rinse the dosing syringe with water or other cleaning agents. If the syringe requires cleaning, it must be completely dry before resuming use.

Blood Concentration Monitoring in Transplant Patients: Transplant centers have found blood concentration monitoring of cyclosporine to be an essential component of patient management. Of importance to blood concentration analysis are the type of assay used, the transplanted organ, and other immunosuppressant agents being administered. While no fixed relationship has been established, blood concentration monitoring may assist in the clinical evaluation of rejection and toxicity, dose adjustments, and the assessment of compliance.

Various assays have been used to measure blood concentrations of cyclosporine. Older studies using a nonspecific assay often cited concentrations that were roughly twice those of the specific assays. Therefore, comparison between concentrations in the published literature and an individual patient concentration using current assays must be made with detailed knowledge of the assay methods employed. Current assay results are also not interchangeable and their use should be guided by their approved labeling. A discussion of the different assay methods is contained in *Annals of Clinical Biochemistry* 1994;31:420-446. While several assays and assay matrices are available, there is a consensus that parent-compound-specific assays correlate best with clinical events. Of these, HPLC is the standard reference, but the monoclonal antibody RIAs and the monoclonal antibody FPIA offer sensitivity, reproducibility, and convenience. Most clinicians base their monitoring on trough cyclosporine concentrations. *Applied Pharmacokinetics, Principles of Therapeutic Drug Monitoring* (1992) contains a broad discussion of cyclosporine pharmacokinetics and drug monitoring techniques. Blood concentration monitoring is not a replacement for renal function monitoring or tissue biopsies.

HOW SUPPLIED

Neoral® Soft Gelatin Capsules (cyclosporine capsules, USP) MODIFIED

25 mg

Oval, blue-gray imprinted in red, "Neoral" over "25 mg."
Packages of 30 unit-dose blisters (NDC 0078-0246-15).

100 mg

Oblong, blue-gray imprinted in red, "NEORAL" over "100 mg."
Packages of 30 unit-dose blisters (NDC 0078-0248-15).

Store and Dispense: In the original unit-dose container at controlled room temperature 68°-77°F (20°-25°C).

Neoral® Oral Solution (cyclosporine oral solution, USP) MODIFIED: A clear, yellow liquid supplied in 50 mL bottles containing 100 mg/mL (NDC 0078-0274-22).

Store and Dispense: In the original container at controlled room temperature 68°-77°F (20°-25°C). Do not store in the refrigerator. Once opened, the contents must be used within two months. At temperatures below 68°F (20°C) the solution may gel; light flocculation or the formation of a light sediment may also occur. There is no impact on product performance or dosing using the syringe provided. Allow to warm to room temperature 77°F (25°C) to reverse these changes.

Neoral® Soft Gelatin Capsules (cyclosporine capsules, USP) MODIFIED

Manufactured by R.P. Scherer GmbH, EBERBACH/BADEN, GERMANY

Manufactured for Novartis Pharmaceuticals Corporation, East Hanover, NJ 07936

Neoral® Oral Solution (cyclosporine oral solution, USP) MODIFIED

Continued on next page

Neoral—Cont.

Manufactured by NOVARTIS PHARMA AG, Basle, Switzerland
Manufactured for Novartis Pharmaceuticals Corporation, East Hanover, NJ 07936

T2001-18
REV: JANUARY 2001 PRINTED IN USA 89005005

RITALIN® hydrochloride Ⓒ℞
[*rit ' ah-lin*]
methylphenidate hydrochloride tablets USP

RITALIN-SR® Ⓒ℞
methylphenidate hydrochloride USP sustained-release tablets
Rx only

Prescribing information for this product, which appears on page(s) 2206–2207 of the 2001 PDR, has been completely revised as follows. Please write "See Supplement A" next to the product heading.

Prescribing Information

DESCRIPTION

Ritalin hydrochloride, methylphenidate hydrochloride USP, is a mild central nervous system (CNS) stimulant, available as tablets of 5, 10, and 20 mg for oral administration; Ritalin-SR is available as sustained-release tablets of 20 mg for oral administration. Methylphenidate hydrochloride is methyl α-phenyl-2-piperidineacetate hydrochloride, and its structural formula is

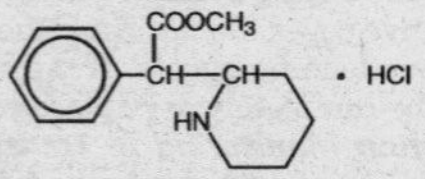

Methylphenidate hydrochloride USP is a white, odorless, fine crystalline powder. Its solutions are acid to litmus. It is freely soluble in water and in methanol, soluble in alcohol, and slightly soluble in chloroform and in acetone. Its molecular weight is 269.77.

Inactive Ingredients. Ritalin tablets: D&C Yellow No. 10 (5-mg and 20-mg tablets), FD&C Green No. 3 (10-mg tablets), lactose, magnesium stearate, polyethylene glycol, starch (5-mg and 10-mg tablets), sucrose, talc, and tragacanth (20-mg tablets).

Ritalin-SR tablets: Cellulose compounds, cetostearyl alcohol, lactose, magnesium stearate, mineral oil, povidone, titanium dioxide, and zein.

CLINICAL PHARMACOLOGY

Ritalin is a mild central nervous system stimulant.

The mode of action in man is not completely understood, but Ritalin presumably activates the brain stem arousal system and cortex to produce its stimulant effect.

There is neither specific evidence which clearly establishes the mechanism whereby Ritalin produces its mental and behavioral effects in children, nor conclusive evidence regarding how these effects relate to the condition of the central nervous system.

Ritalin in the SR tablets is more slowly but as extensively absorbed as in the regular tablets. Relative bioavailability of the SR tablet compared to the Ritalin tablet, measured by the urinary excretion of Ritalin major metabolite (α-phenyl-2-piperidine acetic acid) was 105% (49%-168%) in children and 101% (85%-152%) in adults. The time to peak rate in children was 4.7 hours (1.3-8.2 hours) for the SR tablets and 1.9 hours (0.3-4.4 hours) for the tablets. An average of 67% of SR tablet dose was excreted in children as compared to 86% in adults.

In a clinical study involving adult subjects who received SR tablets, plasma concentrations of Ritalin's major metabolite appeared to be greater in females than in males. No gender differences were observed for Ritalin plasma concentration in the same subjects.

INDICATIONS

Attention Deficit Disorders, Narcolepsy

Attention Deficit Disorders (previously known as Minimal Brain Dysfunction in Children). Other terms being used to describe the behavioral syndrome below include: Hyperkinetic Child Syndrome, Minimal Brain Damage, Minimal Cerebral Dysfunction, Minor Cerebral Dysfunction.

Ritalin is indicated as an integral part of a total treatment program which typically includes other remedial measures (psychological, educational, social) for a stabilizing effect in children with a behavioral syndrome characterized by the following group of developmentally inappropriate symptoms: moderate-to-severe distractibility, short attention span, hyperactivity, emotional lability, and impulsivity. The diagnosis of this syndrome should not be made with finality when these symptoms are only of comparatively recent origin. Nonlocalizing (soft) neurological signs, learning disability, and abnormal EEG may or may not be present, and a diagnosis of central nervous system dysfunction may or may not be warranted.

Special Diagnostic Considerations

Specific etiology of this syndrome is unknown, and there is no single diagnostic test. Adequate diagnosis requires the use not only of medical but of special psychological, educational, and social resources.

Characteristics commonly reported include: chronic history of short attention span, distractibility, emotional lability, impulsivity, and moderate-to-severe hyperactivity; minor neurological signs and abnormal EEG. Learning may or may not be impaired. The diagnosis must be based upon a complete history and evaluation of the child and not solely on the presence of one or more of these characteristics.

Drug treatment is not indicated for all children with this syndrome. Stimulants are not intended for use in the child who exhibits symptoms secondary to environmental factors and/or primary psychiatric disorders, including psychosis. Appropriate educational placement is essential and psychosocial intervention is generally necessary. When remedial measures alone are insufficient, the decision to prescribe stimulant medication will depend upon the physician's assessment of the chronicity and severity of the child's symptoms.

CONTRAINDICATIONS

Marked anxiety, tension, and agitation are contraindications to Ritalin, since the drug may aggravate these symptoms. Ritalin is contraindicated also in patients known to be hypersensitive to the drug, in patients with glaucoma, and in patients with motor tics or with a family history or diagnosis of Tourette's syndrome.

Ritalin is contraindicated during treatment with monoamine oxidase inhibitors, and also within a minimum of 14 days following discontinuation of a monoamine oxidase inhibitor (hypertensive crises may result).

WARNINGS

Ritalin should not be used in children under six years, since safety and efficacy in this age group have not been established.

Sufficient data on safety and efficacy of long-term use of Ritalin in children are not yet available. Although a causal relationship has not been established, suppression of growth (i.e., weight gain, and/or height) has been reported with the long-term use of stimulants in children. Therefore, patients requiring long-term therapy should be carefully monitored.

Ritalin should not be used for severe depression of either exogenous or endogenous origin. Clinical experience suggests that in psychotic children, administration of Ritalin may exacerbate symptoms of behavior disturbance and thought disorder.

Ritalin should not be used for the prevention or treatment of normal fatigue states.

There is some clinical evidence that Ritalin may lower the convulsive threshold in patients with prior history of seizures, with prior EEG abnormalities in absence of seizures, and, very rarely, in absence of history of seizures and no prior EEG evidence of seizures. Safe concomitant use of anticonvulsants and Ritalin has not been established. In the presence of seizures, the drug should be discontinued.

Use cautiously in patients with hypertension. Blood pressure should be monitored at appropriate intervals in all patients taking Ritalin, especially those with hypertension.

Symptoms of visual disturbances have been encountered in rare cases. Difficulties with accommodation and blurring of vision have been reported.

Drug Interactions

Ritalin may decrease the hypotensive effect of guanethidine. Use cautiously with pressor agents.

Human pharmacologic studies have shown that Ritalin may inhibit the metabolism of coumarin anticoagulants, anticonvulsants (phenobarbital, diphenylhydantoin, primidone), phenylbutazone, and tricyclic drugs (imipramine, clomipramine, desipramine). Downward dosage adjustments of these drugs may be required when given concomitantly with Ritalin.

Serious adverse events have been reported in concomitant use with clonidine, although no causality for the combination has been established. The safety of using methylphenidate in combination with clonidine or other centrally acting alpha-2 agonists has not been systematically evaluated.

Usage in Pregnancy

Adequate animal reproduction studies to establish safe use of Ritalin during pregnancy have not been conducted. However, in a recently conducted study, methylphenidate has been shown to have teratogenic effects in rabbits when given in doses of 200 mg/kg/day, which is approximately 167 times and 78 times the maximum recommended human dose on a mg/kg and a mg/m^2 basis, respectively. In rats, teratogenic effects were not seen when the drug was given in doses of 75 mg/kg/day, which is approximately 62.5 and 13.5 times the maximum recommended human dose on a mg/kg and a mg/m^2 basis, respectively. Therefore, until more information is available, Ritalin should not be prescribed for women of childbearing age unless, in the opinion of the physician, the potential benefits outweigh the possible risks.

Drug Dependence

Ritalin should be given cautiously to emotionally unstable patients, such as those with a history of drug dependence or alcoholism, because such patients may increase dosage on their own initiative.

Chronically abusive use can lead to marked tolerance and psychic dependence with varying degrees of abnormal behavior. Frank psychotic episodes can occur, especially with parenteral abuse. Careful supervision is required during drug withdrawal, since severe depression as well as the effects of chronic overactivity can be unmasked. Long-term follow-up may be required because of the patient's basic personality disturbances.

PRECAUTIONS

Patients with an element of agitation may react adversely; discontinue therapy if necessary.

Periodic CBC, differential, and platelet counts are advised during prolonged therapy.

Drug treatment is not indicated in all cases of this behavioral syndrome and should be considered only in light of the complete history and evaluation of the child. The decision to prescribe Ritalin should depend on the physician's assessment of the chronicity and severity of the child's symptoms and their appropriateness for his/her age. Prescription should not depend solely on the presence of one or more of the behavioral characteristics.

When these symptoms are associated with acute stress reactions, treatment with Ritalin is usually not indicated.

Long-term effects of Ritalin in children have not been well established.

Carcinogenesis/Mutagenesis

In a lifetime carcinogenicity study carried out in B6C3F1 mice, methylphenidate caused an increase in hepatocellular adenomas and, in males only, an increase in hepatoblastomas, at a daily dose of approximately 60 mg/kg/day. This dose is approximately 30 times and 2.5 times the maximum recommended human dose on a mg/kg and mg/m^2 basis, respectively. Hepatoblastoma is a relatively rare rodent malignant tumor type. There was no increase in total malignant hepatic tumors. The mouse strain used is sensitive to the development of hepatic tumors, and the significance of these results to humans is unknown.

Methylphenidate did not cause any increases in tumors in a lifetime carcinogenicity study carried out in F344 rats; the highest dose used was approximately 45 mg/kg/day, which is approximately 22 times and 4 times the maximum recommended human dose on a mg/kg and mg/m^2 basis, respectively.

Methylphenidate was not mutagenic in the in vitro Ames reverse mutation assay or in the in vitro mouse lymphoma cell forward mutation assay. Sister chromatid exchanges and chromosome aberrations were increased, indicative of a weak clastogenic response, in an in vitro assay in cultured Chinese Hamster Ovary (CHO) cells. The genotoxic potential of methylphenidate has not been evaluated in an in vivo assay.

ADVERSE REACTIONS

Nervousness and insomnia are the most common adverse reactions but are usually controlled by reducing dosage and omitting the drug in the afternoon or evening. Other reactions include hypersensitivity (including skin rash, urticaria, fever, arthralgia, exfoliative dermatitis, erythema multiforme with histopathological findings of necrotizing vasculitis, and thrombocytopenic purpura); anorexia; nausea; dizziness; palpitations; headache; dyskinesia; drowsiness; blood pressure and pulse changes, both up and down; tachycardia; angina; cardiac arrhythmia; abdominal pain; weight loss during prolonged therapy. There have been rare reports of Tourette's syndrome. Toxic psychosis has been reported. Although a definite causal relationship has not been established, the following have been reported in patients taking this drug: instances of abnormal liver function, ranging from transaminase elevation to hepatic coma; isolated cases of cerebral arteritis and/or occlusion; leukopenia and/or anemia; transient depressed mood; a few instances of scalp hair loss. Very rare reports of neuroleptic malignant syndrome (NMS) have been received, and, in most of these, patients were concurrently receiving therapies associated with NMS. In a single report, a ten year old boy who had been taking methylphenidate for approximately 18 months experienced an NMS-like event within 45 minutes of ingesting his first dose of venlafaxine. It is uncertain whether this case represented a drug-drug interaction, a response to either drug alone, or some other cause.

In children, loss of appetite, abdominal pain, weight loss during prolonged therapy, insomnia, and tachycardia may occur more frequently; however, any of the other adverse reactions listed above may also occur.

DOSAGE AND ADMINISTRATION

Dosage should be individualized according to the needs and responses of the patient.

Adults

Tablets: Administer in divided doses 2 or 3 times daily, preferably 30 to 45 minutes before meals. Average dosage is 20 to 30 mg daily. Some patients may require 40 to 60 mg daily. In others, 10 to 15 mg daily will be adequate. Patients who are unable to sleep if medication is taken late in the day should take the last dose before 6 p.m.

SR Tablets: Ritalin-SR tablets have a duration of action of approximately 8 hours. Therefore, Ritalin-SR tablets may be used in place of Ritalin tablets when the 8-hour dosage of Ritalin-SR corresponds to the titrated 8-hour dosage of Ritalin. Ritalin-SR tablets must be swallowed whole and never crushed or chewed.

Children (6 years and over)

Ritalin should be initiated in small doses, with gradual weekly increments. Daily dosage above 60 mg is not recommended.

If improvement is not observed after appropriate dosage adjustment over a one-month period, the drug should be discontinued.

Tablets: Start with 5 mg twice daily (before breakfast and lunch) with gradual increments of 5 to 10 mg weekly.
SR Tablets: Ritalin-SR tablets have a duration of action of approximately 8 hours. Therefore, Ritalin-SR tablets may be used in place of Ritalin tablets when the 8-hour dosage of Ritalin-SR corresponds to the titrated 8-hour dosage of Ritalin. Ritalin-SR tablets must be swallowed whole and never crushed or chewed.
If paradoxical aggravation of symptoms or other adverse effects occur, reduce dosage, or, if necessary, discontinue the drug.
Ritalin should be periodically discontinued to assess the child's condition. Improvement may be sustained when the drug is either temporarily or permanently discontinued.
Drug treatment should not and need not be indefinite and usually may be discontinued after puberty.

OVERDOSAGE

Signs and symptoms of acute overdosage, resulting principally from overstimulation of the central nervous system and from excessive sympathomimetic effects, may include the following: vomiting, agitation, tremors, hyperreflexia, muscle twitching, convulsions (may be followed by coma), euphoria, confusion, hallucinations, delirium, sweating, flushing, headache, hyperpyrexia, tachycardia, palpitations, cardiac arrhythmias, hypertension, mydriasis, and dryness of mucous membranes.
Consult with a Certified Poison Control Center regarding treatment for up-to-date guidance and advice.
Treatment consists of appropriate supportive measures. The patient must be protected against self-injury and against external stimuli that would aggravate overstimulation already present. Gastric contents may be evacuated by gastric lavage. In the presence of severe intoxication, use a carefully titrated dosage of a *short-acting* barbiturate before performing gastric lavage. Other measures to detoxify the gut include administration of activated charcoal and a cathartic. Intensive care must be provided to maintain adequate circulation and respiratory exchange; external cooling procedures may be required for hyperpyrexia.
Efficacy of peritoneal dialysis or extracorporeal hemodialysis for Ritalin overdosage has not been established.

HOW SUPPLIED

Tablets 5 mg — round, yellow (imprinted CIBA 7)
Bottles of 100 .... NDC 0083-0007-30
Tablets 10 mg — round, pale green, scored (imprinted CIBA 3)
Bottles of 100 .... NDC 0083-0003-30
Tablets 20 mg — round, pale yellow, scored (imprinted CIBA 34)
Bottles of 100 .... NDC 0083-0034-30
Do not store above 30°C (86°F). Protect from light.
Dispense in tight, light-resistant container (USP).
SR Tablets 20 mg — round, white, coated (imprinted CIBA 16)
Bottles of 100 .... NDC 0083-0016-30
Note: SR Tablets are color-additive free.
Do not store above 30°C (86°F). Protect from moisture.
Dispense in tight, light-resistant container (USP).

T2001-08
REV: JANUARY 2001 Printed in U.S.A. 89002403
NOVARTIS
Novartis Pharmaceuticals Corporation
East Hanover, New Jersey 07936

SANDIMMUNE® Soft Gelatin Capsules ℞
(cyclosporine capsules, USP)
SANDIMMUNE® Oral Solution ℞
(cyclosporine oral solution, USP)
SANDIMMUNE® Injection ℞
(cyclosporine injection, USP)
FOR INFUSION ONLY
Rx only

Prescribing information for this product, which appears on pages 2207–2210 of the 2001 PDR, has been completely revised as follows. Please write "See Supplement A" next to the product heading.

WARNING
Only physicians experienced in immunosuppressive therapy and management of organ transplant patients should prescribe Sandimmune® (cyclosporine). Patients receiving the drug should be managed in facilities equipped and staffed with adequate laboratory and supportive medical resources. The physician responsible for maintenance therapy should have complete information requisite for the follow-up of the patient.
Sandimmune® (cyclosporine) should be administered with adrenal corticosteroids but not with other immunosuppressive agents. Increased susceptibility to infection and the possible development of lymphoma may result from immunosuppression.

Sandimmune® soft gelatin capsules (cyclosporine capsules, USP) and Sandimmune® oral solution (cyclosporine oral solution, USP) have decreased bioavailability in comparison to Neoral® soft gelatin capsules (cyclosporine capsules, USP) MODIFIED and Neoral® oral solution (cyclosporine oral solution, USP) MODIFIED.
Sandimmune® and Neoral® are not bioequivalent and cannot be used interchangeably without physician supervision.
The absorption of cyclosporine during chronic administration of Sandimmune® soft gelatin capsules and oral solution was found to be erratic. It is recommended that patients taking the soft gelatin capsules or oral solution over a period of time be monitored at repeated intervals for cyclosporine blood levels and subsequent dose adjustments be made in order to avoid toxicity due to high levels and possible organ rejection due to low absorption of cyclosporine. This is of special importance in liver transplants. Numerous assays are being developed to measure blood levels of cyclosporine. Comparison of levels in published literature to patient levels using current assays must be done with detailed knowledge of the assay methods employed. *(See Blood Level Monitoring under DOSAGE AND ADMINISTRATION)*

DESCRIPTION

Cyclosporine, the active principle in Sandimmune® (cyclosporine) is a cyclic polypeptide immunosuppressant agent consisting of 11 amino acids. It is produced as a metabolite by the fungus species *Beauveria nivea*.
Chemically, cyclosporine is designated as [*R*-[*R**,*R**-(*E*)]]-cyclic (L-alanyl-D-alanyl-*N*-methyl-L-leucyl-*N*-methyl-L-leucyl-*N*-methyl-L-valyl-3-hydroxy-*N*,4-dimethyl-L-2-amino-6-octenoyl-L-α-amino-butyryl-*N*-methylglycyl-*N*-methyl-L-leucyl-L-valyl-*N*-methyl-L-leucyl).
Sandimmune® Soft Gelatin Capsules (cyclosporine capsules, USP) are available in 25 mg and 100 mg strengths.
Each 25 mg capsule contains:
cyclosporine, USP .... 25 mg
alcohol, USP dehydrated .... max 12.7% by volume
Each 100 mg capsule contains:
cyclosporine, USP .... 100 mg
alcohol, USP dehydrated .... max 12.7% by volume
Inactive Ingredients: corn oil, gelatin, glycerol, Labrafil M 2125 CS (polyoxyethylated glycolysed glycerides), red iron oxide (25 mg and 100 mg capsule only), sorbitol, titanium dioxide, and other ingredients.
Sandimmune® Oral Solution (cyclosporine oral solution, USP) is available in 50 mL bottles.
Each mL contains:
cyclosporine, USP .... 100 mg
alcohol, Ph. Helv. .... 12.5% by volume
dissolved in an olive oil, Ph. Helv./Labrafil M 1944 CS (polyoxyethylated oleic glycerides) vehicle which must be further diluted with milk, chocolate milk, or orange juice before oral administration.
Sandimmune® Injection (cyclosporine injection, USP) is available in a 5 mL sterile ampul for I.V. administration.
Each mL contains:
cyclosporine, USP .... 50 mg
Cremophor® EL (polyoxyethylated castor oil) ...... 650 mg
alcohol, Ph. Helv. .... 32.9% by volume
nitrogen .... qs
which must be diluted further with 0.9% Sodium Chloride Injection or 5% Dextrose Injection before use.
The chemical structure of cyclosporine (also known as cyclosporin A) is:

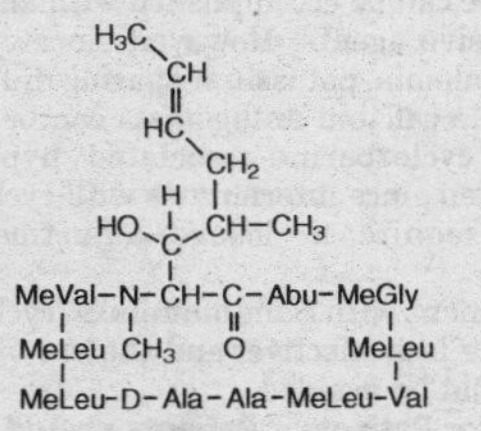

$C_{62}H_{111}N_{11}O_{12}$ Mol. Wt. 1202.63

CLINICAL PHARMACOLOGY

Sandimmune® (cyclosporine) is a potent immunosuppressive agent which in animals prolongs survival of allogeneic transplants involving skin, heart, kidney, pancreas, bone marrow, small intestine, and lung. Sandimmune® (cyclosporine) has been demonstrated to suppress some humoral immunity and to a greater extent, cell-mediated reactions such as allograft rejection, delayed hypersensitivity, experimental allergic encephalomyelitis, Freund's adjuvant arthritis, and graft vs. host disease in many animal species for a variety of organs.
Successful kidney, liver, and heart allogeneic transplants have been performed in man using Sandimmune® (cyclosporine).
The exact mechanism of action of Sandimmune® (cyclosporine) is not known. Experimental evidence suggests that the effectiveness of cyclosporine is due to specific and reversible inhibition of immunocompetent lymphocytes in the G_0- or G_1-phase of the cell cycle. T-lymphocytes are preferentially inhibited. The T-helper cell is the main target, although the T-suppressor cell may also be suppressed. Sandimmune® (cyclosporine) also inhibits lymphokine production and release including interleukin-2 or T-cell growth factor (TCGF).
No functional effects on phagocytic (changes in enzyme secretions not altered, chemotactic migration of granulocytes, macrophage migration, carbon clearance *in vivo*) or tumor cells (growth rate, metastasis) can be detected in animals. Sandimmune® (cyclosporine) does not cause bone marrow suppression in animal models or man.
The absorption of cyclosporine from the gastrointestinal tract is incomplete and variable. Peak concentrations (C_{max}) in blood and plasma are achieved at about 3.5 hours. C_{max} and area under the plasma or blood concentration/time curve (AUC) increase with the administered dose; for blood the relationship is curvilinear (parabolic) between 0 and 1400 mg. As determined by a specific assay, C_{max} is approximately 1.0 ng/mL/mg of dose for plasma and 2.7-1.4 ng/mL/mg of dose for blood (for low to high doses). Compared to an intravenous infusion, the absolute bioavailability of the oral solution is approximately 30% based upon the results in 2 patients. The bioavailability of Sandimmune® soft gelatin capsules (cyclosporine capsules, USP) is equivalent to Sandimmune® oral solution (cyclosporine oral solution, USP).
Cyclosporine is distributed largely outside the blood volume. In blood the distribution is concentration dependent. Approximately 33%-47% is in plasma, 4%-9% in lymphocytes, 5%-12% in granulocytes, and 41%-58% in erythrocytes. At high concentrations, the uptake by leukocytes and erythrocytes becomes saturated. In plasma, approximately 90% is bound to proteins, primarily lipoproteins.
The disposition of cyclosporine from blood is biphasic with a terminal half-life of approximately 19 hours (range: 10-27 hours). Elimination is primarily biliary with only 6% of the dose excreted in the urine.
Cyclosporine is extensively metabolized but there is no major metabolic pathway. Only 0.1% of the dose is excreted in the urine as unchanged drug. Of 15 metabolites characterized in human urine, 9 have been assigned structures. The major pathways consist of hydroxylation of the Cγ-carbon of 2 of the leucine residues, Cη-carbon hydroxylation, and cyclic ether formation (with oxidation of the double bond) in the side chain of the amino acid 3-hydroxyl-*N*,4-dimethyl-L-2-amino-6-octenoic acid and *N*-demethylation of *N*-methyl leucine residues. Hydrolysis of the cyclic peptide chain or conjugation of the aforementioned metabolites do not appear to be important biotransformation pathways.

INDICATIONS AND USAGE

Sandimmune® (cyclosporine) is indicated for the prophylaxis of organ rejection in kidney, liver, and heart allogeneic transplants. It is always to be used with adrenal corticosteroids. The drug may also be used in the treatment of chronic rejection in patients previously treated with other immunosuppressive agents.
Because of the risk of anaphylaxis, Sandimmune® injection (cyclosporine injection, USP) should be reserved for patients who are unable to take the soft gelatin capsules or oral solution.

CONTRAINDICATIONS

Sandimmune® injection (cyclosporine injection, USP) is contraindicated in patients with a hypersensitivity to Sandimmune® (cyclosporine) and/or Cremophor® EL (polyoxyethylated castor oil).

WARNINGS: *(See boxed WARNINGS)*

Sandimmune® (cyclosporine), when used in high doses, can cause hepatotoxicity and nephrotoxicity.
It is not unusual for serum creatinine and BUN levels to be elevated during Sandimmune® (cyclosporine) therapy. These elevations in renal transplant patients do not necessarily indicate rejection, and each patient must be fully evaluated before dosage adjustment is initiated.
Nephrotoxicity has been noted in 25% of cases of renal transplantation, 38% of cases of cardiac transplantation, and 37% of cases of liver transplantation. Mild nephrotoxicity was generally noted 2-3 months after transplant and consisted of an arrest in the fall of the preoperative elevations of BUN and creatinine at a range of 35-45 mg/dl and 2.0-2.5 mg/dl respectively. These elevations were often responsive to dosage reduction.
More overt nephrotoxicity was seen early after transplantation and was characterized by a rapidly rising BUN and creatinine. Since these events are similar to rejection episodes care must be taken to differentiate between them. This form of nephrotoxicity is usually responsive to Sandimmune® (cyclosporine) dosage reduction.
Although specific diagnostic criteria which reliably differentiate renal graft rejection from drug toxicity have not been found, a number of parameters have been significantly associated to one or the other. It should be noted however, that up to 20% of patients may have simultaneous nephrotoxicity and rejection.
[See table at top of next page]
A form of chronic progressive cyclosporine-associated nephrotoxicity is characterized by serial deterioration in renal function and morphologic changes in the kidneys. From 5%-15% of transplant recipients will fail to show a reduction in a rising serum creatinine despite a decrease or discontinuation of cyclosporine therapy. Renal biopsies from these patients will demonstrate an interstitial fibrosis with tubular atrophy. In addition, toxic tubulopathy, peritubular capillary congestion, arteriolopathy, and a striped form of interstitial fibrosis with tubular atrophy may be present. Though none of these morphologic changes is entirely specific, a histologic diagnosis of chronic progressive cyclosporine-associated nephrotoxicity requires evidence of these.

Continued on next page

Sandimmune—Cont.

When considering the development of chronic nephrotoxicity it is noteworthy that several authors have reported an association between the appearance of interstitial fibrosis and higher cumulative doses or persistently high circulating trough levels of cyclosporine. This is particularly true during the first 6 posttransplant months when the dosage tends to be highest and when, in kidney recipients, the organ appears to be most vulnerable to the toxic effects of cyclosporine. Among other contributing factors to the development of interstitial fibrosis in these patients must be included, prolonged perfusion time, warm ischemia time, as well as episodes of acute toxicity, and acute and chronic rejection. The reversibility of interstitial fibrosis and its correlation to renal function have not yet been determined.

Impaired renal function at any time requires close monitoring, and frequent dosage adjustment may be indicated. In patients with persistent high elevations of BUN and creatinine who are unresponsive to dosage adjustments, consideration should be given to switching to other immunosuppressive therapy. In the event of severe and unremitting rejection, it is preferable to allow the kidney transplant to be rejected and removed rather than increase the Sandimmune® (cyclosporine) dosage to a very high level in an attempt to reverse the rejection.

Occasionally patients have developed a syndrome of thrombocytopenia and microangiopathic hemolytic anemia which may result in graft failure. The vasculopathy can occur in the absence of rejection and is accompanied by avid platelet consumption within the graft as demonstrated by Indium 111 labeled platelet studies. Neither the pathogenesis nor the management of this syndrome is clear. Though resolution has occurred after reduction or discontinuation of Sandimmune® (cyclosporine) and 1) administration of streptokinase and heparin or 2) plasmapheresis, this appears to depend upon early detection with Indium 111 labeled platelet scans. *(See ADVERSE REACTIONS)*

Significant hyperkalemia (sometimes associated with hyperchloremic metabolic acidosis) and hyperuricemia have been seen occasionally in individual patients.

Hepatotoxicity has been noted in 4% of cases of renal transplantation, 7% of cases of cardiac transplantation, and 4% of cases of liver transplantation. This was usually noted during the first month of therapy when high doses of Sandimmune® (cyclosporine) were used and consisted of elevations of hepatic enzymes and bilirubin. The chemistry elevations usually decreased with a reduction in dosage.

As in patients receiving other immunosuppressants, those patients receiving Sandimmune® (cyclosporine) are at increased risk for development of lymphomas and other malignancies, particularly those of the skin. The increased risk appears related to the intensity and duration of immunosuppression rather than to the use of specific agents. Because of the danger of oversuppression of the immune system, which can also increase susceptibility to infection, Sandimmune® (cyclosporine) should not be administered with other immunosuppressive agents except adrenal corticosteroids. The efficacy and safety of cyclosporine in combination with other immunosuppressive agents have not been determined.

There have been reports of convulsions in adult and pediatric patients receiving cyclosporine, particularly in combination with high dose methylprednisolone.

Encephalopathy has been described both in post-marketing reports and in the literature. Manifestations include impaired consciousness, convulsions, visual disturbances (including blindness), loss of motor function, movement disorders and psychiatric disturbances. In many cases, changes in the white matter have been detected using imaging techniques and pathologic specimens. Predisposing factors such as hypertension, hypomagnesemia, hypocholesterolemia, high-dose corticosteroids, high cyclosporine blood concentrations, and graft-versus-host disease have been noted in many but not all of the reported cases. The changes in most cases have been reversible upon discontinuation of cyclosporine, and in some cases improvement was noted after reduction of dose. It appears that patients receiving liver transplant are more susceptible to encephalopathy than those receiving kidney transplant.

Rarely (approximately 1 in 1000), patients receiving Sandimmune® injection (cyclosporine injection, USP) have experienced anaphylactic reactions. Although the exact cause of these reactions is unknown, it is believed to be due to the Cremophor® EL (polyoxyethylated castor oil) used as the vehicle for the I.V. formulation. These reactions have consisted of flushing of the face and upper thorax, acute respiratory distress with dyspnea and wheezing, blood pressure changes, and tachycardia. One patient died after respiratory arrest and aspiration pneumonia. In some cases, the reaction subsided after the infusion was stopped.

Patients receiving Sandimmune® Injection (cyclosporine injection, USP) should be under continuous observation for at least the first 30 minutes following the start of the infusion and at frequent intervals thereafter. If anaphylaxis occurs, the infusion should be stopped. An aqueous solution of epinephrine 1:1000 should be available at the bedside as well as a source of oxygen.

Anaphylactic reactions have not been reported with the soft gelatin capsules or oral solution which lack Cremophor® EL (polyoxyethylated castor oil). In fact, patients experiencing anaphylactic reactions have been treated subsequently with the soft gelatin capsules or oral solution without incident.

Care should be taken in using Sandimmune® (cyclosporine) with nephrotoxic drugs. *(See PRECAUTIONS)*

Nephrotoxicity vs Rejection

Parameter	Nephrotoxicity	Rejection
History	Donor > 50 years old or hypotensive Prolonged kidney preservation Prolonged anastomosis time Concomitant nephrotoxic drugs	Antidonor immune response Retransplant patient
Clinical	Often > 6 weeks postop[b] Prolonged initial nonfunction (acute tubular necrosis)	Often < 4 weeks postop[b] Fever > 37.5°C Weight gain > 0.5 kg Graft swelling and tenderness Decrease in daily urine volume > 500 mL (or 50%)
Laboratory	CyA serum trough level > 200 ng/mL Gradual rise in Cr (< 0.15 mg/dl/day)[a] Cr plateau < 25% above baseline BUN/Cr ≥ 20	CyA serum trough level < 150 ng/mL Rapid rise in Cr (> 0.3 mg/dl/day)[a] Cr > 25% above baseline BUN/Cr < 20
Biopsy	Arteriolopathy (medial hypertrophy[a], hyalinosis, nodular deposits, intimal thickening, endothelial vacuolization, progressive scarring)	Endovasculitis[c] (proliferation[a], intimal arteritis[b], necrosis, sclerosis)
	Tubular atrophy, isometric vacuolization, isolated calcifications	Tubulitis with RBC[b] and WBC[b] casts, some irregular vacuolization
	Minimal edema	Interstitial edema[c] and hemorrhage[b]
	Mild focal infiltrates[c]	Diffuse moderate to severe mononuclear infiltrates[d]
	Diffuse interstitial fibrosis, often striped form	Glomerulitis (mononuclear cells)[c]
Aspiration Cytology	CyA deposits in tubular and endothelial cells Fine isometric vacuolization of tubular cells	Inflammatory infiltrate with mononuclear phagocytes, macrophages, lymphoblastoid cells, and activated T-cells These strongly express HLA-DR antigens
Urine Cytology	Tubular cells with vacuolization and granularization	Degenerative tubular cells, plasma cells, and lymphocyturia > 20% of sediment
Manometry	Intracapsular pressure < 40 mm Hg[b]	Intracapsular pressure > 40 mm Hg[b]
Ultrasonography	Unchanged graft cross sectional area	Increase in graft cross sectional area AP diameter ≥ Transverse diameter
Magnetic Resonance Imagery	Normal appearance	Loss of distinct corticomedullary junction, swelling, image intensity of parachyma approaching that of psoas, loss of hilar fat
Radionuclide Scan	Normal or generally decreased perfusion Decrease in tubular function (^{131} I-hippuran) > decrease in perfusion (^{99}m Tc DTPA)	Patchy arterial flow Decrease in perfusion > decrease in tubular function Increased uptake of Indium 111 labeled platelets or Tc-99m in colloid
Therapy	Responds to decreased Sandimmune® (cyclosporine)	Responds to increased steroids or antilymphocyte globulin

$^a p < 0.05$, $^b p < 0.01$, $^c p < 0.001$, $^d p < 0.0001$

Because Sandimmune® is not bioequivalent to Neoral®, conversion from Neoral® to Sandimmune® using a 1:1 ratio (mg/kg/day) may result in a lower cyclosporine blood concentration. Conversion from Neoral® to Sandimmune® should be made with increased blood concentration monitoring to avoid the potential of underdosing.

PRECAUTIONS

General: Patients with malabsorption may have difficulty in achieving therapeutic levels with Sandimmune® soft gelatin capsules or oral solution.

Hypertension is a common side effect of Sandimmune® (cyclosporine) therapy. *(See ADVERSE REACTIONS)* Mild or moderate hypertension is more frequently encountered than severe hypertension and the incidence decreases over time. Antihypertensive therapy may be required. Control of blood pressure can be accomplished with any of the common antihypertensive agents. However, since cyclosporine may cause hyperkalemia, potassium-sparing diuretics should not be used. While calcium antagonists can be effective agents in treating cyclosporine-associated hypertension, care should be taken since interference with cyclosporine metabolism may require a dosage adjustment. *(See Drug Interactions)*

During treatment with Sandimmune® (cyclosporine), vaccination may be less effective; and the use of live attenuated vaccines should be avoided.

Information for Patients: Patients should be advised that any change of cyclosporine formulation should be made cautiously and only under physician supervision because it may result in the need for a change in dosage.

Patients should be informed of the necessity of repeated laboratory tests while they are receiving the drug. They should be given careful dosage instructions, advised of the potential risks during pregnancy, and informed of the increased risk of neoplasia.

Patients using cyclosporine oral solution with its accompanying syringe for dosage measurement should be cautioned not to rinse the syringe either before or after use. Introduction of water into the product by any means will cause variation in dose.

Laboratory Tests: Renal and liver functions should be assessed repeatedly by measurement of BUN, serum creatinine, serum bilirubin, and liver enzymes.

Drug Interactions: All of the individual drugs cited below are well substantiated to interact with cyclosporine. In addition, concomitant non-steroidal anti-inflammatory drugs, particularly in the setting of dehydration, may potentiate renal dysfunction.

Drugs That May Potentiate Renal Dysfunction

Antibiotics	Antineoplastic
gentamicin	melphalan
tobramycin	*Antifungals*
vancomycin	amphotericin B
trimethoprim with sulfamethoxazole	ketoconazole

Anti-Inflammatory Drugs	Gastrointestinal Agents
azapropazon	cimetidine
diclofenac	ranitidine
naproxen	*Immunosuppressives*
sulindac	tacrolimus
colchicine	

Drugs That Alter Cyclosporine Concentrations:

Compounds that decrease cyclosporine absorption such as orlistat should be avoided. Cyclosporine is extensively metabolized by cytochrome P-450 3A. Substances that inhibit this enzyme could decrease metabolism and increase cyclosporine concentrations. Substances that are inducers of cytochrome P-450 activity could increase metabolism and decrease cyclosporine concentrations. Monitoring of circulating cyclosporine concentrations and appropriate Neoral® dosage adjustment are essential when these drugs are used concomitantly. *(See Blood Concentration Monitoring)*

Drugs That Increase Cyclosporine Concentrations

Calcium Channel Blockers	Antifungals
diltiazem	fluconazole
nicardipine	itraconazole
verapamil	ketoconazole
Antibiotics	*Other Drugs*
clarithromycin	allopurinol
erythromycin	bromocriptine
quinupristin/dalfopristin	danazol
	metoclopramide
Glucorticoids	colchicine
methylprednisolone	amiodarone

The HIV protease inhibitors (e.g., indinavir, nelfinavir, ritonavir, and saquinavir) are known to inhibit cytochrome P-450 3A and thus could potentially increase the concentrations of cyclosporine, however no formal studies of the interaction are available. Care should be exercised when these drugs are administered concomitantly.

Grapefruit and grapefruit juice affect metabolism, increasing blood concentrations of cyclosporine, thus should be avoided.

Drugs/Dietary Supplements That Decrease Cyclosporine Concentrations

Antibiotics	Other Drugs/Dietary Supplements
nafcillin	octreotide
rifampin	ticlopidine
Anticonvulsants	orlistat
carbamazepine	St. John's Wort
phenobarbital	
phenytoin	

There have been reports of a serious drug interaction between cyclosporine and the herbal dietary supplement, St. John's Wort. This interaction has been reported to produce a marked reduction in the blood concentrations of cyclosporine, resulting in subtherapeutic levels, rejection of transplanted organs, and graft loss.

Rifabutin is known to increase the metabolism of other drugs metabolized by the cytochrome P-450 system. The interaction between rifabutin and cyclosporine has not been studied. Care should be exercised when these two drugs are administered concomitantly.

Nonsteroidal Anti-inflammatory Drug (NSAID) Interactions: Clinical status and serum creatinine should be closely monitored when cyclosporine is used with nonsteroidal anti-inflammatory agents in rheumatoid arthritis patients. *(See WARNINGS)*

Pharmacodynamic interactions have been reported to occur between cyclosporine and both naproxen and sulindac, in that concomitant use is associated with additive decreases in renal function, as determined by ^{99m}Tc-diethylenetri-aminepentaacetic acid (DTPA) and (*p*-aminohippuric acid) PAH clearances. Although concomitant administration of diclofenac does not affect blood levels of cyclosporine, it has been associated with approximate doubling of diclofenac blood levels and occasional reports of reversible decreases in renal function. Consequently, the dose of diclofenac should be in the lower end of the therapeutic range.

Methotrexate Interaction: Preliminary data indicate that when methotrexate and cyclosporine were co-administered to rheumatoid arthritis patients (N=20), methotrexate concentrations (AUCs) were increased approximately 30% and the concentrations (AUCs) of its metabolite, 7-hydroxy methotrexate, were decreased by approximately 80%. The clinical significance of this interaction is not known. Cyclosporine concentrations do not appear to have been altered (N=6).

Other Drug Interactions: Reduced clearance of prednisolone, digoxin, and lovastatin has been observed when these drugs are administered with cyclosporine. In addition, a decrease in the apparent volume of distribution of digoxin has been reported after cyclosporine administration. Severe digitalis toxicity has been seen within days of starting cyclosporine in several patients taking digoxin. Cyclosporine should not be used with potassium-sparing diuretics because hyperkalemia can occur.

During treatment with cyclosporine, vaccination may be less effective. The use of live vaccines should be avoided.

Myositis has occurred with concomitant lovastatin, frequent gingival hyperplasia with nifedipine, and convulsions with high dose methylprednisolone.

Psoriasis patients receiving other immunosuppressive agents or radiation therapy (including PUVA and UVB) should not receive concurrent cyclosporine because of the possibility of excessive immunosuppression.

For additional information on Cyclosporine Drug Interactions please contact Novartis Medical Affairs Department at 888-NOW-NOVA (888-669-6682).

Carcinogenesis, Mutagenesis, and Impairment of Fertility: Cyclosporine gave no evidence of mutagenic or teratogenic effects in appropriate test systems. Only at dose levels toxic to dams, were adverse effects seen in reproduction studies in rats. *(See Pregnancy)*

Carcinogenicity studies were carried out in male and female rats and mice. In the 78-week mouse study, at doses of 1, 4, and 16 mg/kg/day, evidence of a statistically significant trend was found for lymphocytic lymphomas in females, and the incidence of hepatocellular carcinomas in mid-dose males significantly exceeded the control value. In the 24-month rat study, conducted at 0.5, 2, and 8 mg/kg/day, pancreatic islet cell adenomas significantly exceeded the control rate in the low dose level. The hepatocellular carcinomas and pancreatic islet cell adenomas were not dose related.

No impairment in fertility was demonstrated in studies in male and female rats.

Cyclosporine has not been found mutagenic/genotoxic in the Ames Test, the V79-HGPRT Test, the micronucleus test in mice and Chinese hamsters, the chromosome-aberration tests in Chinese hamster bone-marrow, the mouse dominant lethal assay, and the DNA-repair test in sperm from treated mice. A recent study analyzing sister chromatid exchange (SCE) induction by cyclosporine using human lymphocytes *in vitro* gave indication of a positive effect (i.e., induction of SCE), at high concentrations in this system.

An increased incidence of malignancy is a recognized complication of immunosuppression in recipients of organ transplants. The most common forms of neoplasms are non-Hodgkin's lymphoma and carcinomas of the skin. The risk of malignancies in cyclosporine recipients is higher than in the normal, healthy population but similar to that in patients receiving other immunosuppressive therapies. It has been reported that reduction or discontinuance of immunosuppression may cause the lesions to regress.

Pregnancy: *Pregnancy Category C.* Sandimmune® oral solution (cyclosporine oral solution, USP) has been shown to be embryo- and fetotoxic in rats and rabbits when given in doses 2-5 times the human dose. At toxic doses (rats at 30 mg/kg/day and rabbits at 100 mg/kg/day), Sandimmune® oral solution (cyclosporine oral solution, USP) was embryo- and fetotoxic as indicated by increased pre- and postnatal mortality and reduced fetal weight together with related skeletal retardations. In the well-tolerated dose range (rats at up to 17 mg/kg/day and rabbits at up to 30 mg/kg/day), Sandimmune® oral solution (cyclosporine oral solution, USP) proved to be without any embryolethal or teratogenic effects. There are no adequate and well-controlled studies in pregnant women. Sandimmune® (cyclosporine) should be used during pregnancy only if the potential benefit justifies the potential risk to the fetus.

The following data represent the reported outcomes of 116 pregnancies in women receiving Sandimmune® (cyclosporine) during pregnancy, 90% of whom were transplant patients, and most of whom received Sandimmune® (cyclosporine) throughout the entire gestational period. Since most of the patients were not prospectively identified, the results are likely to be biased toward negative outcomes.

Body System/ Adverse Reactions	Randomized Kidney Patients		All Sandimmune® (cyclosporine) Patients		
	Sandimmune® (N=227) %	Azathioprine (N=228) %	Kidney (N=705) %	Heart (N=112) %	Liver (N=75) %
Genitourinary					
Renal Dysfunction	32	6	25	38	37
Cardiovascular					
Hypertension	26	18	13	53	27
Cramps	4	<1	2	<1	0
Skin					
Hirsutism	21	<1	21	28	45
Acne	6	8	2	2	1
Central Nervous System					
Tremor	12	0	21	31	55
Convulsions	3	1	1	4	5
Headache	2	<1	2	15	4
Gastrointestinal					
Gum Hyperplasia	4	0	9	5	16
Diarrhea	3	<1	3	4	8
Nausea/Vomiting	2	<1	4	10	4
Hepatotoxicity	<1	<1	4	7	4
Abdominal Discomfort	<1	0	<1	7	0
Autonomic Nervous System					
Paresthesia	3	0	1	2	1
Flushing	<1	0	4	0	4
Hematopoietic					
Leukopenia	2	19	<1	6	0
Lymphoma	<1	0	1	6	1
Respiratory					
Sinusitis	<1	0	4	3	7
Miscellaneous					
Gynecomastia	<1	0	<1	4	3

Renal Transplant Patients In Whom Therapy Was Discontinued			
	Randomized Patients		All Sandimmune® Patients
Reason for Discontinuation	Sandimmune® (N=227) %	Azathioprine (N=228) %	(N=705) %
Renal Toxicity	5.7	0	5.4
Infection	0	0.4	0.9
Lack of Efficacy	2.6	0.9	1.4
Acute Tubular Necrosis	2.6	0	1.0
Lymphoma/Lymphoproliferative Disease	0.4	0	0.3
Hypertension	0	0	0.3
Hematological Abnormalities	0	0.4	0
Other	0	0	0.7

Infectious Complications in the Randomized Renal Transplant Patients		
Complication	Sandimmune® Treatment (N=227) % of Complications	Standard Treatment* (N=228) % of Complications
Septicemia	5.3	4.8
Abscesses	4.4	5.3
Systemic Fungal Infection	2.2	3.9
Local Fungal Infection	7.5	9.6
Cytomegalovirus	4.8	12.3
Other Viral Infections	15.9	18.4
Urinary Tract Infections	21.1	20.2
Wound and Skin Infections	7.0	10.1
Pneumonia	6.2	9.2

*Some patients also received ALG.

The only consistent patterns of abnormality were premature birth (gestational period of 28 to 36 weeks) and low birth weight for gestational age. It is not possible to separate the effects of Sandimmune® (cyclosporine) on these pregnancies from the effects of the other immunosuppressants, the underlying maternal disorders, or other aspects of the transplantation milieu. Sixteen fetal losses occurred. Most of the pregnancies (85 of 100) were complicated by disorders; including pre-eclampsia, eclampsia, premature labor, abruptio placentae, oligohydramnios, Rh incompatibility and fetoplacental dysfunction. Preterm delivery occurred in 47%. Seven malformations were reported in 5 viable infants and in 2 cases of fetal loss. Twenty-eight percent of the infants were small for gestational age. Neonatal complications occurred in 27%. In a report of 23 children followed up to 4 years, postnatal development was said to be normal. More information on cyclosporine use in pregnancy is available from Novartis Pharmaceuticals Corporation.

Nursing Mothers: Since Sandimmune® (cyclosporine) is excreted in human milk, nursing should be avoided.

Pediatric Use: Although no adequate and well controlled studies have been conducted in children, patients as young as 6 months of age have received the drug with no unusual adverse effects.

ADVERSE REACTIONS

The principal adverse reactions of Sandimmune® (cyclosporine) therapy are renal dysfunction, tremor, hirsutism, hypertension, and gum hyperplasia.

Hypertension, which is usually mild to moderate, may occur in approximately 50% of patients following renal transplantation and in most cardiac transplant patients.

Glomerular capillary thrombosis has been found in patients treated with cyclosporine and may progress to graft failure. The pathologic changes resemble those seen in the hemolytic-uremic syndrome and include thrombosis of the renal microvasculature, with platelet-fibrin thrombi occluding glomerular capillaries and afferent arterioles, microangiopathic hemolytic anemia, thrombocytopenia, and decreased renal function. Similar findings have been observed when other immunosuppressives have been employed posttransplantation.

Hypomagnesemia has been reported in some, but not all, patients exhibiting convulsions while on cyclosporine therapy. Although magnesium-depletion studies in normal subjects suggest that hypomagnesemia is associated with neurologic disorders, multiple factors, including hypertension, high dose methylprednisolone, hypocholesterolemia, and nephrotoxicity associated with high plasma concentrations of cyclosporine appear to be related to the neurological manifestations of cyclosporine toxicity.

The following reactions occurred in 3% or greater of 892 patients involved in clinical trials of kidney, heart, and liver transplants:

[See table above]

The following reactions occurred in 2% or less of patients: allergic reactions, anemia, anorexia, confusion, conjunctivitis, edema, fever, brittle fingernails, gastritis, hearing loss, hiccups, hyperglycemia, muscle pain, peptic ulcer, thrombocytopenia, tinnitus.

The following reactions occurred rarely: anxiety, chest pain, constipation, depression, hair breaking, hematuria, joint pain, lethargy, mouth sores, myocardial infarction, night sweats, pancreatitis, pruritus, swallowing difficulty, tingling, upper GI bleeding, visual disturbance, weakness, weight loss.

[See table above]

Sandimmune® (cyclosporine) was discontinued on a temporary basis and then restarted in 18 additional patients.

[See table above]

Continued on next page

Sandimmune—Cont.

Cremophor® EL (polyoxyethylated castor oil) is known to cause hyperlipemia and electrophoretic abnormalities of lipoproteins. These effects are reversible upon discontinuation of treatment but are usually not a reason to stop treatment.

OVERDOSAGE

There is a minimal experience with overdosage. Because of the slow absorption of Sandimmune® soft gelatin capsules or oral solution, forced emesis would be of value up to 2 hours after administration. Transient hepatotoxicity and nephrotoxicity may occur which should resolve following drug withdrawal. General supportive measures and symptomatic treatment should be followed in all cases of overdosage. Sandimmune® (cyclosporine) is not dialyzable to any great extent, nor is it cleared well by charcoal hemoperfusion. The oral LD_{50} is 2329 mg/kg in mice, 1480 mg/kg in rats, and > 1000 mg/kg in rabbits. The I.V. LD_{50} is 148 mg/kg in mice, 104 mg/kg in rats, and 46 mg/kg in rabbits.

DOSAGE AND ADMINISTRATION

Sandimmune® Soft Gelatin Capsules (cyclosporine capsules, USP) and Sandimmune® Oral Solution (cyclosporine oral solution, USP): Sandimmune® soft gelatin capsules (cyclosporine capsules, USP) and Sandimmune® oral solution (cyclosporine oral solution, USP) have decreased bioavailability in comparison to Neoral® soft gelatin capsules (cyclosporine capsules, USP) MODIFIED and Neoral® oral solution (cyclosporine oral solution, USP) MODIFIED. Sandimmune® and Neoral® are not bioequivalent and cannot be used interchangeably without physician supervision.

The initial oral dose of Sandimmune® (cyclosporine) should be given 4-12 hours prior to transplantation as a single dose of 15 mg/kg. Although a daily single dose of 14-18 mg/kg was used in most clinical trials, few centers continue to use the highest dose, most favoring the lower end of the scale. There is a trend towards use of even lower initial doses for renal transplantation in the ranges of 10-14 mg/kg/day. The initial single daily dose is continued postoperatively for 1-2 weeks and then tapered by 5% per week to a maintenance dose of 5-10 mg/kg/day. Some centers have successfully tapered the maintenance dose to as low as 3 mg/kg/day in selected *renal* transplant patients without an apparent rise in rejection rate.

(See Blood Level Monitoring below)

In pediatric usage, the same dose and dosing regimen may be used as in adults although in several studies children have required and tolerated higher doses than those used in adults.

Adjunct therapy with adrenal corticosteroids is recommended. Different tapering dosage schedules of prednisone appear to achieve similar results. A dosage schedule based on the patients weight started with 2.0 mg/kg/day for the first 4 days tapered to 1.0 mg/kg/day by 1 week, 0.6 mg/kg/day by 2 weeks, 0.3 mg/kg/day by 1 month, and 0.15 mg/kg/day by 2 months and thereafter as a maintenance dose. Another center started with an initial dose of 200 mg tapered by 40 mg/day until reaching 20 mg/day. After 2 months at this dose, a further reduction to 10 mg/day was made. Adjustments in dosage of prednisone must be made according to the clinical situation.

To make Sandimmune® oral solution (cyclosporine oral solution, USP) more palatable, the oral solution may be diluted with milk, chocolate milk, or orange juice preferably at room temperature. Patients should avoid switching diluents frequently. Sandimmune® soft gelatin capsules and oral solution should be administered on a consistent schedule with regard to time of day and relation to meals.

Take the prescribed amount of Sandimmune® (cyclosporine) from the container using the dosage syringe supplied after removal of the protective cover, and transfer the solution to a glass of milk, chocolate milk, or orange juice. Stir well and drink at once. Do not allow to stand before drinking. It is best to use a glass container and rinse it with more diluent to ensure that the total dose is taken. After use, replace the dosage syringe in the protective cover. Do not rinse the dosage syringe with water or other cleaning agents either before or after use. If the dosage syringe requires cleaning, it must be completely dry before resuming use. Introduction of water into the product by any means will cause variation in dose.

Sandimmune® Injection (cyclosporine injection, USP)
FOR INFUSION ONLY
Note: Anaphylactic reactions have occurred with Sandimmune® injection (cyclosporine injection, USP). *(See WARNINGS)*

Patients unable to take Sandimmune® soft gelatin capsules or oral solution pre- or postoperatively may be treated with the I.V. concentrate. **Sandimmune® Injection (cyclosporine injection, USP) is administered at 1/3 the oral dose.** The initial dose of Sandimmune® injection (cyclosporine injection, USP) should be given 4-12 hours prior to transplantation as a single I.V. dose of 5-6 mg/kg/day. This daily single dose is continued postoperatively until the patient can tolerate the soft gelatin capsules or oral solution. Patients should be switched to Sandimmune® soft gelatin capsules or oral solution as soon as possible after surgery. In pediatric usage, the same dose and dosing regimen may be used, although higher doses may be required.

Adjunct steroid therapy is to be used. *(See aforementioned)*

Immediately before use, the I.V. concentrate should be diluted 1 mL Sandimmune® injection (cyclosporine injection, USP) in 20 mL-100 mL 0.9% Sodium Chloride Injection or 5% Dextrose Injection and given in a slow intravenous infusion over approximately 2-6 hours.
Diluted infusion solutions should be discarded after 24 hours.
The Cremophor® EL (polyoxyethylated castor oil) contained in the concentrate for intravenous infusion can cause phthalate stripping from PVC.
Parenteral drug products should be inspected visually for particulate matter and discoloration prior to administration, whenever solution and container permit.
Blood Level Monitoring: Several study centers have found blood level monitoring of cyclosporine useful in patient management. While no fixed relationships have yet been established, in one series of 375 consecutive cadaveric renal transplant recipients, dosage was adjusted to achieve specific whole blood 24-hour trough levels of 100-200 ng/mL as determined by high-pressure liquid chromatography (HPLC). Of major importance to blood level analysis is the type of assay used. The above levels are specific to the parent cyclosporine molecule and correlate directly to the new monoclonal specific radioimmunoassays (mRIA-sp). Nonspecific assays are also available which detect the parent compound molecule and various of its metabolites. Older studies often cited levels using a nonspecific assay which were roughly twice those of specific assays. Assay results are not interchangeable and their use should be guided by their approved labeling. If plasma specimens are employed, levels will vary with the temperature at the time of separation from whole blood. Plasma levels may range from 1/2-1/5 of whole blood levels. Refer to individual assay labeling for complete instructions. In addition, *Transplantation Proceedings* (June 1990) contains position papers and a broad consensus generated at the Cyclosporine-Therapeutic Drug Monitoring conference that year. Blood level monitoring is not a replacement for renal function monitoring or tissue biopsies.

HOW SUPPLIED

Sandimmune® Soft Gelatin Capsules (cyclosporine capsules, USP)
25 mg: Oblong, pink, branded "⚕ 78/240". Unit dose packages of 30 capsules, 3 blister cards of 10 capsules (NDC 0078-0240-15).
100 mg: Oblong, dusty rose, branded "⚕ 78/241". Unit dose packages of 30 capsules, 3 blister cards of 10 capsules (NDC 0078-0241-15).
Store and Dispense: In the original unit dose container at temperatures below 86°F (30°C). An odor may be detected upon opening the unit dose container, which will dissipate shortly thereafter. This odor does not affect the quality of the product.
Sandimmune® Oral Solution (cyclosporine oral solution, USP): Supplied in 50 mL bottles containing 100 mg of cyclosporine per mL (NDC 0078-0110-22). A dosage syringe is provided for dispensing.
Store and Dispense: In the original container at temperatures below 86°F (30°C). Do not store in the refrigerator. Protect from freezing. Once opened, the contents must be used within 2 months.
Sandimmune® Injection (cyclosporine injection, USP)
FOR INTRAVENOUS INFUSION
Supplied as a 5 mL sterile ampul containing 50 mg of cyclosporine per mL, in boxes of 10 ampuls (NDC 0078-0109-01).
Store and Dispense: At temperatures below 86°F (30°C) and protected from light.
Sandimmune® Soft Gelatin Capsules (cyclosporine capsules, USP)
Manufactured by
R.P. Scherer GmbH, EBERBACH/BADEN, GERMANY
Manufactured for
Novartis Pharmaceuticals Corporation, East Hanover, NJ 07936
Sandimmune® Oral Solution (cyclosporine oral solution, USP) and
Sandimmune® Injection (cyclosporine injection, USP)
FOR INFUSION ONLY
Manufactured by
NOVARTIS PHARMA AG, Basle, Switzerland
Manufactured for
Novartis Pharmaceuticals Corporation, East Hanover, NJ 07936
Novartis Pharmaceuticals Corporation
East Hanover, New Jersey 07936

T2001-04
REV: JANUARY 2001 PRINTED IN U.S.A. 89005203
©2001 Novartis
*Cremophor is the registered trademark of BASF Aktiengesellschaft.

SIMULECT®
[sĭ mu lǝct]
(basiliximab)
For Injection
Rx only

Prescribing Information
Prescribing information for this product, which appears on pages 2218–2220 of the 2001 PDR, has been completely revised as follows. Please write "See Supplement A" next to the product heading.

WARNING
Only physicians experienced in immunosuppression therapy and management of organ transplantation patients should prescribe Simulect® (basiliximab). The physician responsible for Simulect® administration should have complete information requisite for the follow-up of the patient. Patients receiving the drug should be managed in facilities equipped and staffed with adequate laboratory and supportive medical resources.

DESCRIPTION

Simulect® (basiliximab) is a chimeric (murine/human) monoclonal antibody (IgG_{1k}), produced by recombinant DNA technology, that functions as an immunosuppressive agent, specifically binding to and blocking the interleukin-2 receptor α-chain (IL-2Rα, also known as CD25 antigen) on the surface of activated T-lymphocytes. Based on the amino acid sequence, the calculated molecular weight of the protein is 144 kilodaltons. It is a glycoprotein obtained from fermentation of an established mouse myeloma cell line genetically engineered to express plasmids containing the human heavy and light chain constant region genes and mouse heavy and light chain variable region genes encoding the RFT5 antibody that binds selectively to the IL-2Rα.
The active ingredient, basiliximab, is water soluble. The drug product, Simulect®, is a sterile lyophilisate which is available in 6 mL colorless glass vials. Each vial contains 20 mg basiliximab, 7.21 mg monobasic potassium phosphate, 0.99 mg disodium hydrogen phosphate (anhydrous), 1.61 mg sodium chloride, 20 mg sucrose, 80 mg mannitol and 40 mg glycine, to be reconstituted in 5 mL of Sterile Water for Injection, USP. No preservatives are added.

CLINICAL PHARMACOLOGY
General
Mechanism of action: Basiliximab functions as an IL-2 receptor antagonist by binding with high affinity ($K_a = 1 \times 10^{10}$ M^{-1}) to the alpha chain of the high affinity IL-2 receptor complex and inhibiting IL-2 binding. Basiliximab is specifically targeted against IL-2Rα, which is selectively expressed on the surface of activated T-lymphocytes. This specific high affinity binding of Simulect® (basiliximab) to IL-2Rα competitively inhibits IL-2-mediated activation of lymphocytes, a critical pathway in the cellular immune response involved in allograft rejection.
While in the circulation, Simulect® impairs the response of the immune system to antigenic challenges. Whether the ability to respond to repeated or ongoing challenges with those antigens returns to normal after Simulect® is cleared is unknown. *(See PRECAUTIONS)*
Pharmacokinetics
Adults: Single-dose and multiple-dose pharmacokinetic studies have been conducted in patients undergoing first kidney transplantation. Cumulative doses ranged from 15 mg up to 150 mg. Peak mean ± SD serum concentration following intravenous infusion of 20 mg over 30 minutes is 7.1 ± 5.1 mg/L. There is a dose-proportional increase in C_{max} and AUC up to the highest tested single dose of 60 mg. The volume of distribution at steady state is 8.6 ± 4.1 L. The extent and degree of distribution to various body compartments have not been fully studied. The terminal half-life is 7.2 ± 3.2 days. Total body clearance is 41 ± 19 mL/h. No clinically relevant influence of body weight or gender on distribution volume or clearance has been observed in adult patients. Elimination half-life was not influenced by age (20-69 years), gender or race. *(See DOSAGE AND ADMINISTRATION)*
Pediatric: The pharmacokinetics of Simulect® were assessed in 12 pediatric renal transplantation patients, children (2-11 years of age, n=8) and adolescents (12-15 years of age, n=4). These data indicate that in children, the volume of distribution at steady state was 5.2 ± 2.8 L, half-life was 11.5 ± 6.3 days and clearance was 17 ± 6 mL/h. Distribution volume and clearance are reduced by about 50% compared to adult renal transplantation patients. Disposition parameters were not influenced to a clinically relevant extent by age, body weight (9-37 kg) or body surface area (0.44-1.20 m²) in this age group. In adolescents, the volume of distribution at steady state was 10.1 ± 7.6 L, half-life was 7.2 ± 3.6 days and clearance was 45 ± 25 mL/h. Disposition in adolescents was similar to that in adult renal transplantation patients. *(See DOSAGE AND ADMINISTRATION)*
Pharmacodynamics
Complete and consistent binding to IL-2Rα in adults is maintained as long as serum Simulect® levels exceed 0.2 μg/mL. As concentrations fall below this threshold, the IL-2Rα sites are no longer fully bound and the number of T-cells expressing unbound IL-2Rα returns to pretherapy values within 1-2 weeks. The relationship between serum concentration and receptor saturation was assessed in two pediatric patients (2 and 12 years of age) and was similar to that characterized in adult renal transplantation patients. *In vitro* studies using human tissues indicate that Simulect® binds only to lymphocytes.
At the recommended dosing regimen, the mean ± SD duration of basiliximab saturation of IL-2Rα was 36 ± 14 days *(See DOSAGE AND ADMINISTRATION)*. The duration of clinically significant IL-2 receptor blockade after the recommended course of Simulect® is not known. No significant changes to circulating lymphocyte numbers or cell phenotypes were observed by flow cytometry.

Clinical Studies

The safety and efficacy of Simulect® for the prophylaxis of acute organ rejection in adults following first cadaveric- or living-donor renal transplantation were assessed in two randomized, double-blind, placebo-controlled, multicenter trials. These studies compared two 20-mg doses of Simulect® with placebo when each was administered intravenously as part of a standard immunosuppressive regimen comprised of cyclosporine oral solution USP (MODIFIED) and corticosteroids, administered starting on Day 0, to prevent acute renal allograft rejection. The first dose of Simulect® or placebo was administered within 2 hours prior to transplantation surgery (Day 0) and the second dose administered on Day 4 post-transplantation. The regimen of Simulect® was chosen to provide 30-45 days of IL-2Rα saturation. 729 patients were enrolled in the two studies, of which 363 Simulect®-treated patients and 358 placebo-treated patients underwent transplantation. One study was conducted at 21 sites in Europe and Canada (EU/CAN Study); the second was conducted at 21 sites in the USA (US Study). Patients 18-75 years of age undergoing first cadaveric (EU/CAN and US Studies) or living-donor (US only) renal transplantation, with ≥1 HLA mismatch, were enrolled. The primary efficacy endpoint in both studies was the incidence of death, graft loss or an episode of acute rejection during the first 6 months post-transplantation. Secondary efficacy endpoints included the primary efficacy variable measured during the first 12 months post-transplantation, the incidence of biopsy-confirmed acute rejection during the first 6 and 12 months post-transplantation, and patient survival and graft survival, each measured at 12 months post-transplantation. Table 1 summarizes the results of these studies. Figure 1 displays the Kaplan-Meier estimates of the percentage of patients by treatment group experiencing the primary efficacy endpoint during the first 12 months post-transplantation for the US study. Patients in both studies receiving Simulect® experienced a significantly lower incidence of biopsy-confirmed rejection episodes at both 6 and 12 months post-transplantation. There was no difference in the rate of delayed graft function, patient survival, or graft survival between Simulect®-treated patients and placebo-treated patients in either study.

There was no evidence that the clinical benefit of Simulect® was limited to specific subpopulations based on age, gender, race, donor type (cadaveric or living-donor allograft) or history of diabetes mellitus.
[See table above]

Table 1
Efficacy Parameters (Percentage of Patients)

	EU/CAN Study			US Study		
	Placebo (N=185)	Simulect® (N=190)	p-value	Placebo (N=173)	Simulect® (N=173)	p-value
Primary endpoint						
Death, graft loss or acute rejection episode (0-6 months)						
	57%	42%	0.003	55%	38%	0.002
Secondary endpoints						
Death, graft loss or acute rejection episode (0-12 months)						
	60%	46%	0.007	58%	41%	0.001
Biopsy-confirmed rejection episode (0-6 months)						
	44%	30%	0.007	46%	33%	0.015
Biopsy-confirmed rejection episode (0-12 months)						
	46%	32%	0.005	49%	35%	0.009
Patient survival (12 months)						
	97%	95%	0.29	96%	97%	0.56
Patients with functioning graft (12 months)						
	87%	88%	0.70	93%	95%	0.50

Figure 1
Kaplan-Meier Estimate of the Percentage of Subjects with Death, Graft Loss or First Rejection Episode
Month: 0 –12

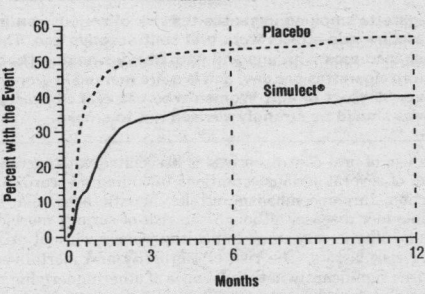

In a multicenter, randomized, double-blind, placebo-controlled trial of Simulect for the prevention of allograft rejection in liver transplant recipients (n=381) receiving concomitant cyclosporine, USP (MODIFIED) and steroids, the incidence of the combined endpoint of death, graft loss, or first biopsy-confirmed rejection episode at either 6 or 12 months was similar between patients randomized to receive Simulect and those randomized to receive placebo.

INDICATIONS AND USAGE

Simulect® (basiliximab) is indicated for the prophylaxis of acute organ rejection in patients receiving renal transplantation when used as part of an immunosuppressive regimen that includes cyclosporine and corticosteroids.

The efficacy of Simulect for the prophylaxis of acute rejection in recipients of other solid organ allografts has not been demonstrated.

CONTRAINDICATIONS

Simulect® (basiliximab) is contraindicated in patients with known hypersensitivity to basiliximab or any other component of the formulation. See composition of Simulect® under *DESCRIPTION*.

WARNINGS: See *Boxed WARNING*.

General

Simulect® (basiliximab) should be administered under qualified medical supervision. Patients should be informed of the potential benefits of therapy and the risks associated with administration of immunosuppressive therapy.

While neither the incidence of lymphoproliferative disorders nor opportunistic infections was higher in Simulect®-treated patients than in placebo-treated patients, patients on immunosuppressive therapy are at increased risk for developing these complications and should be monitored accordingly.

Hypersensitivity

Severe acute (onset within 24 hours) hypersensitivity reactions including anaphylaxis have been observed both on initial exposure to Simulect® and/or following re-exposure after several months. These reactions may include hypotension, tachycardia, cardiac failure, dyspnea, wheezing, bronchospasm, pulmonary edema, respiratory failure, urticaria, rash, pruritus, and/or sneezing. If a severe hypersensitivity reaction occurs, therapy with Simulect® should be permanently discontinued. Medications for the treatment of severe hypersensitivity reactions including anaphylaxis should be available for immediate use. Patients previously administered Simulect® should only be re-exposed to a subsequent course of therapy with extreme caution. The potential risks of such re-administration, specifically those associated with immunosuppression are not known.

PRECAUTIONS

General

It is not known whether Simulect® (basiliximab) use will have a long-term effect on the ability of the immune system to respond to antigens first encountered during Simulect®-induced immunosuppression.

Immunogenicity

Of renal transplantation patients treated with Simulect® (basiliximab) and tested for anti-idiotype antibodies, 1/246 developed an anti-idiotype antibody response, with no deleterious clinical effect upon the patient. In the US Study, the incidence of human anti-murine antibody (HAMA) in renal transplantation patients treated with Simulect® was 2/138 in patients not exposed to muromonab-CD3 and 4/34 in patients who subsequently received muromonab-CD3. The available clinical data on the use of muromonab-CD3 in patients previously treated with Simulect® suggest that subsequent use of muromonab-CD3 or other murine anti-lymphocytic antibody preparations is not precluded.

Drug Interactions

No formal drug-drug interaction studies have been conducted. The following medications have been administered in clinical trials with Simulect® (basiliximab) with no incremental increase in adverse reactions: ATG/ALG, azathioprine, corticosteroids, cyclosporine, mycophenolate mofetil, and muromonab-CD3.

Carcinogenesis, Mutagenesis and Impairment of Fertility

No mutagenic potential of Simulect® was observed in the *in vitro* assays with Salmonella (Ames) and V79 Chinese hamster cells. No long-term or fertility studies in laboratory animals have been performed to evaluate the potential of Simulect® to produce carcinogenicity or fertility impairment, respectively.

Pregnancy Category B

There are no adequate and well-controlled studies in pregnant women. No maternal toxicity, embryotoxicity, or teratogenicity was observed in cynomolgus monkeys 100 days post coitum following dosing with basiliximab during the organogenesis period; blood levels in pregnant monkeys were 13-fold higher than those seen in human patients. Immunotoxicology studies have not been performed in the offspring. Because IgG molecules are known to cross the placental barrier, because IL-2 receptor may play an important role in development of the immune system, and because animal reproduction studies are not always predictive of human response, Simulect® should only be used in pregnant women when the potential benefit justifies the potential risk to the fetus. Women of childbearing potential should use effective contraception before beginning Simulect® therapy, during therapy, and for 2 months after completion of Simulect® therapy.

Nursing Mothers

It is not known whether Simulect® is excreted in human milk. Because many drugs including human antibodies are excreted in human milk, and because of the potential for adverse reactions, a decision should be made to discontinue nursing or to discontinue the drug, taking into account the importance of the drug to the mother.

Pediatric Use

No adequate and well-controlled studies have been completed in pediatric patients. In an ongoing safety and pharmacokinetic study, pediatric patients [2-11 years of age (n=8), 12-15 years of age (n=4), median age 9.5 years] were treated with Simulect® via intravenous bolus injection in addition to standard immunosuppressive agents including cyclosporine, corticosteroids, azathioprine, and mycophenolate mofetil.

Preliminary results indicate that 16.7% (2/12) of patients had experienced an acute rejection episode by 3 months post-transplantation. The most frequently reported adverse events were fever and urinary tract infections (41.7% each). Overall, the adverse event profile was consistent with general clinical experience in the pediatric renal transplantation population and with the profile in the controlled adult renal transplantation studies. The available pharmacokinetic data in children and adolescents are described in *CLINICAL PHARMACOLOGY* and *DOSAGE AND ADMINISTRATION*.

It is not known whether the immune response to vaccines, infection, and other antigenic stimuli administered or encountered during Simulect® therapy is impaired or whether such response will remain impaired after Simulect® therapy.

Geriatric Use

Controlled clinical studies of Simulect® have included a small number of patients 65 years and older (Simulect® 15; placebo 19). From the available data comparing Simulect®- and placebo-treated patients, the adverse event profile in patients ≥65 years of age is not different from patients <65 years of age and no age-related dosing adjustment is required. Caution must be used in giving immunosuppressive drugs to elderly patients.

ADVERSE REACTIONS

The incidence of adverse events for Simulect® (basiliximab) was determined in two randomized comparative double-blind trials for the prevention of renal allograft rejection. A total of 721 patients received renal allografts, of which 363 received Simulect® and 358 received placebo. All patients received concomitant cyclosporine oral solution USP (MODIFIED) and corticosteroids.

Simulect® did not appear to add to the background of adverse events seen in organ transplantation patients as a consequence of their underlying disease and the concurrent administration of immunosuppressants and other medications. Adverse events were reported by 99% of the patients in the placebo-treated group and 99% of the patients in the Simulect®-treated group. Simulect® did not increase the incidence of serious adverse events observed compared with placebo. The most frequently reported adverse events were gastrointestinal disorders, reported in 75% of Simulect®-treated patients and 73% of placebo-treated patients.

The incidence and types of adverse events were similar in Simulect®-treated and placebo-treated patients. The following adverse events occurred in ≥10% of Simulect®-treated patients: *Gastrointestinal System:* constipation, nausea, diarrhea, abdominal pain, vomiting, dyspepsia, moniliasis; *Metabolic and Nutritional:* hyperkalemia, hypokalemia, hyperglycemia, hyperuricemia, hypophosphatemia, hypocalcemia, weight increase, hypercholesterolemia, acidosis; *Central and Peripheral Nervous System:* headache, tremor, dizziness; *Urinary System:* dysuria, increased non-protein nitrogen, urinary tract infection; *Body as a Whole–General:* pain, peripheral edema, edema, fever, viral infection, leg edema, asthenia; *Cardiovascular Disorders–General:* hypertension; *Respiratory System:* dyspnea, upper respiratory tract infection, coughing, rhinitis, pharyngitis; *Skin and Appendages:* surgical wound complications, acne; *Psychiatric:* insomnia; *Musculoskeletal System:* leg pain, back pain; *Red Blood Cell:* anemia.

The following adverse events, not mentioned above, were reported with an incidence of ≥3% and <10% in patients treated with Simulect® in the two controlled clinical trials: *Body as a Whole:* accidental trauma, chest pain, increased drug level, face edema, fatigue, infection, malaise, generalized edema, rigors, sepsis; *Cardiovascular:* angina pectoris, cardiac failure, chest pain, abnormal heart sounds, aggravated hypertension, hypotension; *Nervous System:* hypoesthesia, neuropathy, paraesthesia; *Endocrine:* increased glucocorticoids; *Gastrointestinal:* enlarged abdomen, flatulence, gastrointestinal disorder, gastroenteritis, GI hemorrhage, gum hyperplasia, melena, esophagitis, ulcerative stomatitis; *Heart Rate and Rhythm:* arrhythmia, atrial fibrillation, tachycardia; *Metabolic and Nutritional:* dehydration, diabetes mellitus, fluid overload, hypercalcemia, hyperlipemia, hypo-

Continued on next page

Simulect—Cont.

glycemia, hypoproteinemia, hypomagnesemia; ***Musculoskeletal:*** arthralgia, arthropathy, bone fracture, cramps, hernia, myalgia; ***Nervous System:*** paraesthesia, hypoesthesia; ***Platelet and Bleeding:*** hematoma, hemorrhage, purpura, thrombocytopenia, thrombosis; ***Psychiatric:*** agitation, anxiety, depression; ***Red Blood Cell:*** polycythemia; ***Reproductive Disorders, Male:*** impotence, genital edema; ***Respiratory:*** bronchitis, bronchospasm, abnormal chest sounds, pneumonia, pulmonary disorder, pulmonary edema, sinusitis; ***Skin and Appendages:*** cyst, herpes simplex, herpes zoster, hypertrichosis, pruritus, rash, skin disorder, skin ulceration; ***Urinary:*** albuminuria, bladder disorder, hematuria, frequent micturition, oliguria, abnormal renal function, renal tubular necrosis, surgery, ureteral disorder, urinary retention; ***Vascular Disorders:*** vascular disorder; ***Vision Disorders:*** cataract, conjunctivitis, abnormal vision.

Incidence of Malignancies: The overall incidence of malignancies among all patients in the two 12-month controlled trials was not significantly different between the Simulect® and placebo treatment groups. Overall, lymphoma/lymphoproliferative disease occurred in 1 patient (0.3%) in the Simulect® group compared with 2 patients (0.6%) in the placebo group. Other malignancies were reported among 5 patients (1.4%) in the Simulect® group compared with 7 patients (1.9%) in patients treated with placebo.

Incidence of Infectious Episodes: Cytomegalovirus infection was reported in 14% of Simulect®-treated patients and 18% of placebo-treated patients. The rates of infections, serious infections, and infectious organisms were similar in the Simulect® and placebo treatment groups.

Post-Marketing Experience

Severe acute hypersensitivity reactions including anaphylaxis characterized by hypotension, tachycardia, cardiac failure, dyspnea, wheezing, bronchospasm, pulmonary edema, respiratory failure, urticaria, rash, pruritus, and/or sneezing, as well as capillary leak syndrome and cytokine release syndrome, have been reported during post-marketing experience with Simulect®.

OVERDOSAGE

There have not been any reports of overdoses with Simulect® (basiliximab). A maximum tolerated dose has not been determined in patients. In clinical studies, Simulect® has been administered to renal transplantation patients in single doses of up to 60 mg without any associated serious adverse events.

DOSAGE AND ADMINISTRATION

Simulect® (basiliximab) is used as part of an immunosuppressive regimen that includes cyclosporine and corticosteroids. Simulect® is for central or peripheral intravenous administration only. Reconstituted Simulect® (20 mg in 5 mL) should be diluted to a volume of 50 mL with normal saline or dextrose 5% and administered as an intravenous infusion over 20 to 30 minutes.

Simulect® should only be administered once it has been determined that the patient will receive the graft and concomitant immunosuppression. Patients previously administered Simulect® should only be re-exposed to a subsequent course of therapy with extreme caution.

Adult: In adult patients, the recommended regimen is two doses of 20 mg each. The first 20 mg dose should be given within 2 hours prior to transplantation surgery. The recommended second 20 mg dose should be given 4 days after transplantation. The second dose should be withheld if complications such as severe hypersensitivity reactions to Simulect® or graft loss occur.

Pediatric: For children and adolescents from 2 up to 15 years of age, the recommended regimen is two doses of 12 mg/m^2 each, up to a maximum of 20 mg/dose. The first dose should be given within 2 hours prior to transplantation surgery. The recommended second dose should be given 4 days after transplantation. The second dose should be withheld if complications such as severe hypersensitivity reactions to Simulect® or graft loss occur.

RECONSTITUTION OF 20 mg Simulect® (basiliximab) VIAL

To prepare the infusion solution, add 5 mL of Sterile Water for Injection, USP, using aseptic technique, to the vial containing the Simulect® (basiliximab) powder. Shake the vial gently to dissolve the powder.

The reconstituted solution is isotonic and should be diluted to a volume of 50 mL with normal saline or dextrose 5% for infusion. When mixing the solution, gently invert the bag in order to avoid foaming; DO NOT SHAKE.

Parenteral drug products should be inspected visually for particulate matter and discoloration before administration. After reconstitution, Simulect® should be a clear to opalescent, colorless solution. If particulate matter is present or the solution is colored, do not use.

Care must be taken to assure sterility of the prepared solution because the drug product does not contain any antimicrobial preservatives or bacteriostatic agents.

It is recommended that after reconstitution the solution should be used immediately. If not used immediately, it can be stored at 2°C to 8°C for 24 hours or at room temperature for 4 hours. Discard the reconstituted solution if not used within 24 hours.

No incompatibility between Simulect® and polyvinyl chloride bags or infusion sets has been observed. No data are available on the compatibility of Simulect® with other intravenous substances. Other drug substances should not be added or infused simultaneously through the same intravenous line.

HOW SUPPLIED

Simulect® (basiliximab) is supplied in a single use glass vial containing 20 mg of basiliximab.

Each carton contains

1 Simulect® vial .... NDC 0078-0331-84

Store lyophilized Simulect® under refrigerated conditions (2°C to 8°C; 36°F to 46°F).

Do not use beyond the expiration date stamped on the vial.

REV: NOVEMBER 2000 PRINTED IN U.S.A. 89007802
US License No. 1244
Manufactured by
Novartis Pharma AG
Basel, Switzerland for
Novartis Pharmaceuticals Corporation
East Hanover, New Jersey 07936

Ortho-McNeil Pharmaceutical

RARITAN, NJ 08869-0602

www.ortho-mcneil.com
For Medical Information/Emergencies Contact:
Generally:
(800) 682-6532
In Emergencies:
(908) 218-7325

ORTHO-NOVUM® Tablets ℞
(norethindrone/ethinyl estradiol)
and MODICON® Tablets ℞
(norethindrone/ethinyl estradiol)

Prescribing information for this product, which appears on pages 2363–2370 of the 2001 PDR, has been completely revised as follows. Please write "See Supplement A" next to the product heading.

Prescribing Information

Patients should be counseled that this product does not protect against HIV infection (AIDS) and other sexually transmitted diseases.

COMBINATION ORAL CONTRACEPTIVES

Each of the following products is a combination oral contraceptive containing the progestational compound norethindrone and the estrogenic compound ethinyl estradiol.

ORTHO-NOVUM 7/7/7 □ 21 Tablets and ORTHO-NOVUM 7/7/7 □ 28 Tablets: Each white tablet contains 0.5 mg of norethindrone and 0.035 mg of ethinyl estradiol. Inactive ingredients include lactose, magnesium stearate and pregelatinized starch. Each light peach tablet contains 0.75 mg of norethindrone and 0.035 mg of ethinyl estradiol. Inactive ingredients include FD&C Yellow No. 6, lactose, magnesium stearate and pregelatinized starch. Each peach tablet contains 1 mg of norethindrone and 0.035 mg of ethinyl estradiol. Inactive ingredients include FD&C Yellow No. 6, lactose, magnesium stearate and pregelatinized starch. Each green tablet in the ORTHO-NOVUM 7/7/7 □ 28 package contains only inert ingredients, as follows: D&C Yellow No. 10 Aluminum Lake, FD&C Blue No. 2 Aluminum Lake, lactose, magnesium stearate, microcrystalline cellulose and pregelatinized starch.

ORTHO-NOVUM 10/11 □ 21 Tablets and ORTHO-NOVUM 10/11 □ 28 Tablets: Each white tablet contains 0.5 mg of norethindrone and 0.035 mg of ethinyl estradiol. Inactive ingredients include lactose, magnesium stearate and pregelatinized starch. Each peach tablet contains 1 mg norethindrone and 0.035 mg ethinyl estradiol. Inactive ingredients include FD&C Yellow No. 6, lactose, magnesium stearate and pregelatinized starch. Each green tablet in the ORTHO-NOVUM 10/11 □ 28 package contains only inert ingredients, as listed under green tablets in ORTHO-NOVUM 7/7/7 □ 28.

ORTHO-NOVUM 1/35 □ 21 Tablets and ORTHO-NOVUM 1/35 □ 28 Tablets: Each peach tablet contains 1 mg of norethindrone and 0.035 mg of ethinyl estradiol. Inactive ingredients include FD&C Yellow No. 6, lactose, magnesium stearate and pregelatinized starch. Each green tablet in the ORTHO-NOVUM 1/35 □ 28 package contains only inert ingredients, as listed under green tablets in ORTHO-NOVUM 7/7/7 □ 28.

MODICON 21 Tablets and MODICON 28 Tablets: Each white tablet contains 0.5 mg of norethindrone and 0.035 mg of ethinyl estradiol. Inactive ingredients include lactose, magnesium stearate and pregelatinized starch. Each green tablet in the MODICON 28 package contains only inert ingredients, as listed under green tablets in ORTHO-NOVUM 7/7/7 □ 28.

The chemical name for norethindrone is 17-hydroxy-19-nor-17α-pregn-4-en-20-yn-3-one, for ethinyl estradiol is 19-nor-17α-pregna-1,3,5(10)-trien-20-yne-3,17-diol. Their structural formulas are as follows:

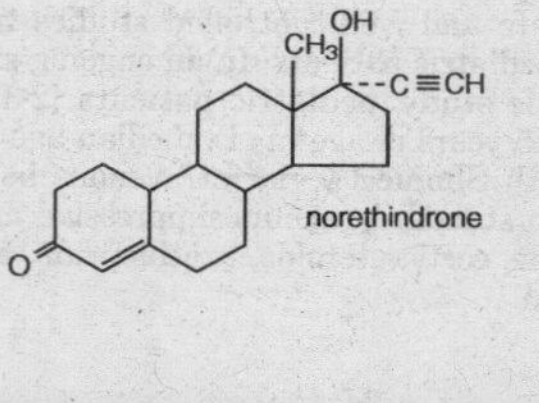

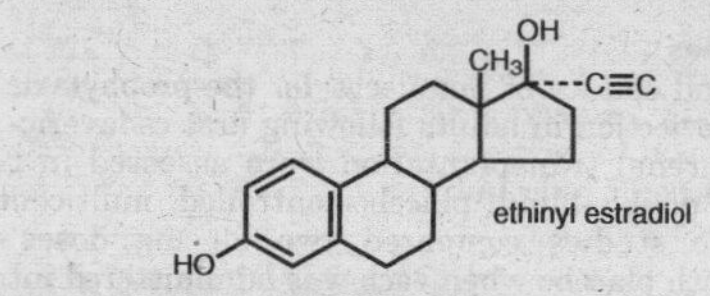

CLINICAL PHARMACOLOGY

COMBINATION ORAL CONTRACEPTIVES

Combination oral contraceptives act by suppression of gonadotropins. Although the primary mechanism of this action is inhibition of ovulation, other alterations include changes in the cervical mucus (which increase the difficulty of sperm entry into the uterus) and the endometrium (which reduce the likelihood of implantation).

INDICATIONS AND USAGE

ORTHO-NOVUM 7/7/7 □ 21, ORTHO-NOVUM 7/7/7 □ 28, ORTHO-NOVUM 10/11 □ 21, ORTHO-NOVUM 10/11 □ 28, ORTHO-NOVUM 1/35 □ 21, ORTHO-NOVUM 1/35 □ 28, MODICON 21, and **MODICON 28** are indicated for the prevention of pregnancy in women who elect to use this product as a method of contraception.

Oral contraceptives are highly effective. Table I lists the typical accidental pregnancy rates for users of combination oral contraceptives and other methods of contraception. The efficacy of these contraceptive methods, except sterilization, depends upon the reliability with which they are used. Correct and consistent use of methods can result in lower failure rates.

[See table at bottom of next page]

CONTRAINDICATIONS

Oral contraceptives should not be used in women who currently have the following conditions:

- Thrombophlebitis or thromboembolic disorders
- A past history of deep vein thrombophlebitis or thromboembolic disorders
- Cerebral vascular or coronary artery disease
- Migraine with focal aura
- Known or suspected carcinoma of the breast
- Carcinoma of the endometrium or other known or suspected estrogen-dependent neoplasia
- Undiagnosed abnormal genital bleeding
- Cholestatic jaundice of pregnancy or jaundice with prior pill use
- Acute or chronic hepatocellular disease with abnormal liver function
- Hepatic adenomas or carcinomas
- Known or suspected pregnancy
- Hypersensitivity to any component of this product

WARNINGS

Cigarette smoking increases the risk of serious cardiovascular side effects from oral contraceptive use. This risk increases with age and with heavy smoking (15 or more cigarettes per day) and is quite marked in women over 35 years of age. Women who use oral contraceptives should be strongly advised not to smoke.

The use of oral contraceptives is associated with increased risks of several serious conditions including myocardial infarction, thromboembolism, stroke, hepatic neoplasia, and gallbladder disease, although the risk of serious morbidity or mortality is very small in healthy women without underlying risk factors. The risk of morbidity and mortality increases significantly in the presence of other underlying risk factors such as hypertension, hyperlipidemias, obesity and diabetes.

Practitioners prescribing oral contraceptives should be familiar with the following information relating to these risks. The information contained in this package insert is principally based on studies carried out in patients who used oral contraceptives with higher formulations of estrogens and progestogens than those in common use today. The effect of long-term use of the oral contraceptives with lower formulations of both estrogens and progestogens remains to be determined.

Throughout this labeling, epidemiological studies reported are of two types: retrospective or case control studies and prospective or cohort studies. Case control studies provide a measure of the relative risk of a disease, namely, a *ratio* of the incidence of a disease among oral contraceptive users to that among nonusers. The relative risk does not provide information on the actual clinical occurrence of a disease. Cohort studies provide a measure of attributable risk, which is the *difference* in the incidence of disease between oral contraceptive users and nonusers. The attributable risk does provide information about the actual occurrence of a disease in the population (adapted from refs. 2 and 3 with the author's permission). For further information, the reader is referred to a text on epidemiological methods.

1. THROMBOEMBOLIC DISORDERS AND OTHER VASCULAR PROBLEMS

a. Myocardial Infarction

An increased risk of myocardial infarction has been attributed to oral contraceptive use. This risk is primarily in smokers or women with other underlying risk factors for coronary artery disease such as hypertension, hypercholesterolemia, morbid obesity, and diabetes. The relative risk of heart attack for current oral contraceptive users has been estimated to be two to six.[4–10] The risk is very low under the age of 30.

Smoking in combination with oral contraceptive use has been shown to contribute substantially to the incidence of myocardial infarctions in women in their mid-thirties or older with smoking accounting for the majority of excess cases.[11] Mortality rates associated with circulatory disease have been shown to increase substantially in smokers, especially in those 35 years of age and older among women who use oral contraceptives.

TABLE II: CIRCULATORY DISEASE MORTALITY RATES PER 100,000 WOMAN-YEARS BY AGE, SMOKING STATUS AND ORAL CONTRACEPTIVE USE

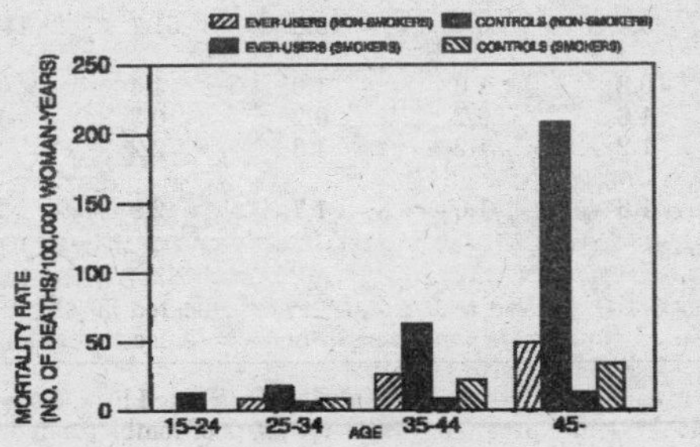

(Adapted from P.M. Layde and V. Beral, ref. #12.)

Oral contraceptives may compound the effects of well-known risk factors, such as hypertension, diabetes, hyperlipidemias, age and obesity.[13] In particular, some progestogens are known to decrease HDL cholesterol and cause glucose intolerance, while estrogens may create a state of hyperinsulinism.[14–18] Oral contraceptives have been shown to increase blood pressure among users (see Section 9 in WARNINGS). Similar effects on risk factors have been associated with an increased risk of heart disease. Oral contraceptives must be used with caution in women with cardiovascular disease risk factors.

b. Thromboembolism

An increased risk of thromboembolic and thrombotic disease associated with the use of oral contraceptives is well established. Case control studies have found the relative risk of users compared to nonusers to be 3 for the first episode of superficial venous thrombosis, 4 to 11 for deep vein thrombosis or pulmonary embolism, and 1.5 to 6 for women with predisposing conditions for venous thromboembolic disease.[2,3,19–24] Cohort studies have shown the relative risk to be somewhat lower, about 3 for new cases and about 4.5 for new cases requiring hospitalization.[25] The risk of thromboembolic disease associated with oral contraceptives is not related to length of use and disappears after pill use is stopped.[2]

A two- to four-fold increase in relative risk of post-operative thromboembolic complications has been reported with the use of oral contraceptives.[9] The relative risk of venous thrombosis in women who have predisposing conditions is twice that of women without such medical conditions.[26] If feasible, oral contraceptives should be discontinued at least four weeks prior to and for two weeks after elective surgery of a type associated with an increase in risk of thromboembolism and during and following prolonged immobilization. Since the immediate postpartum period is also associated with an increased risk of thromboembolism, oral contraceptives should be started no earlier than four weeks after delivery in women who elect not to breast feed. After an induced or spontaneous abortion that occurs at or after 20 weeks gestation, hormonal contraceptives may be started either on Day 21 post-abortion or on the first day of the first spontaneous menstruation, whichever comes first.[92]

c. Cerebrovascular diseases

Oral contraceptives have been shown to increase both the relative and attributable risks of cerebrovascular events (thrombotic and hemorrhagic strokes), although, in general, the risk is greatest among older (>35 years), hypertensive women who also smoke. Hypertension was found to be a risk factor for both users and nonusers, for both types of strokes, and smoking interacted to increase the risk of stroke.[27–29]

In a large study, the relative risk of thrombotic strokes has been shown to range from 3 for normotensive users to 14 for users with severe hypertension.[30] The relative risk of hemorrhagic stroke is reported to be 1.2 for non-smokers who used oral contraceptives, 2.6 for smokers who did not use oral contraceptives, 7.6 for smokers who used oral contraceptives, 1.8 for normotensive users and 25.7 for users with severe hypertension.[30] The attributable risk is also greater in older women.[3]

d. Dose-related risk of vascular disease from oral contraceptives

A positive association has been observed between the amount of estrogen and progestogen in oral contraceptives and the risk of vascular disease.[31–33] A decline in serum high density lipoproteins (HDL) has been reported with many progestational agents.[14–16] A decline in serum high density lipoproteins has been associated with an increased incidence of ischemic heart disease. Because estrogens increase HDL cholesterol, the net effect of an oral contraceptive depends on a balance achieved between doses of estrogen and progestogen and the activity of the progestogen used in the contraceptives. The activity and amount of both hormones should be considered in the choice of an oral contraceptive.

Minimizing exposure to estrogen and progestogen is in keeping with good principles of therapeutics. For any particular estrogen/progestogen combination, the dosage regimen prescribed should be one which contains the least amount of estrogen and progestogen that is compatible with a low failure rate and the needs of the individual patient. New acceptors of oral contraceptive agents should be started on preparations containing 0.035 mg or less of estrogen.

e. Persistence of risk of vascular disease

There are two studies which have shown persistence of risk of vascular disease for ever-users of oral contraceptives. In a study in the United States, the risk of developing myocardial infarction after discontinuing oral contraceptives persists for at least 9 years for women 40–49 years who had used oral contraceptives for five or more years, but this increased risk was not demonstrated in other age groups.[8] In another study in Great Britain, the risk of developing cerebrovascular disease persisted for at least 6 years after discontinuation of oral contraceptives, although excess risk was very small.[34] However, both studies were performed with oral contraceptive formulations containing 50 micrograms or higher of estrogens.

2. ESTIMATES OF MORTALITY FROM CONTRACEPTIVE USE

One study gathered data from a variety of sources which have estimated the mortality rate associated with different methods of contraception at different ages (Table III). These estimates include the combined risk of death associated with contraceptive methods plus the risk attributable to pregnancy in the event of method failure. Each method of contraception has its specific benefits and risks. The study concluded that with the exception of oral contraceptive users 35 and older who smoke, and 40 and older who do not smoke, mortality associated with all methods of birth control is low and below that associated with childbirth. The observation of an increase in risk of mortality with age for oral contraceptive users is based on data gathered in the 1970's.[35] Current clinical recommendation involves the use of lower estrogen dose formulations and a careful consideration of risk factors. In 1989, the Fertility and Maternal Health Drugs Advisory Committee was asked to review the use of oral contraceptives in women 40 years of age and over. The Committee concluded that although cardiovascular disease risks may be increased with oral contraceptive use after age 40 in healthy non-smoking women (even with the newer low-dose formulations), there are also greater potential health risks associated with pregnancy in older women and with the alternative surgical and medical procedures which may be necessary if such women do not have access to effective and acceptable means of contraception. The Committee recommended that the benefits of low-dose oral contraceptive use by healthy non-smoking women over 40 may outweigh the possible risks.

Of course, older women, as all women who take oral contraceptives, should take an oral contraceptive which contains the least amount of estrogen and progestogen that is compatible with a low failure rate and individual patient needs.

[See table at top of next page]

3. CARCINOMA OF THE REPRODUCTIVE ORGANS AND BREASTS

Numerous epidemiological studies have been performed on the incidence of breast, endometrial, ovarian and cervical cancer in women using oral contraceptives. While there are conflicting reports, most studies suggest that use of oral contraceptives is not associated with an overall increase in the risk of developing breast cancer. Some studies have reported an increased relative risk of developing breast cancer particularly at a younger age. This increased relative risk has been reported to be related to duration of use.[36–44,79–89]

A meta-analysis of 54 studies found a small increase in the frequency of having breast cancer diagnosed for women who were currently using combined oral contraceptives or had used them within the past ten years. This increase in the frequency of breast cancer diagnosis, within ten years of stopping use, was generally accounted for by cancers localized to the breast. There was no increase in the frequency of having breast cancer diagnosed ten or more years after cessation of use.[90]

Some studies suggest that oral contraceptive use has been associated with an increase in the risk of cervical intraepithelial neoplasia in some populations of women.[45–48] However, there continues to be controversy about the extent to which such findings may be due to differences in sexual behavior and other factors.

4. HEPATIC NEOPLASIA

Benign hepatic adenomas are associated with oral contraceptive use, although the incidence of benign tumors is rare in the United States. Indirect calculations have estimated the attributable risk to be in the range of 3.3 cases/100,000 for users, a risk that increases after four or more years of use especially with oral contraceptives of higher dose.[49] Rupture of benign, hepatic adenomas may cause death through intra-abdominal hemorrhage.[50,51]

TABLE I: PERCENTAGE OF WOMEN EXPERIENCING AN UNINTENDED PREGNANCY DURING THE FIRST YEAR OF TYPICAL USE AND THE FIRST YEAR OF PERFECT USE OF CONTRACEPTION AND THE PERCENTAGE CONTINUING USE AT THE END OF THE FIRST YEAR. UNITED STATES.

	% of Women Experiencing an Unintended Pregnancy within the First Year of Use		% of Women Continuing Use at One Year[3]
Method (1)	Typical Use[1] (2)	Perfect Use[2] (3)	(4)
Chance[4]	85	85	
Spermicides[5]	26	6	40
Periodic abstinence	25		63
Calender		9	
Ovulation Method		3	
Sympto-Thermal[6]		2	
Post-Ovulation		1	
Withdrawal	19	4	
Cap[7]			
Parous Women	40	26	42
Nulliparous Women	20	9	56
Sponge			
Parous Women	40	20	42
Nulliparous Women	20	9	56
Diaphragm[7]	20	6	56
Condom[8]			
Female (Reality)	21	5	56
Male	14	3	61
Pill	5		71
Progestin Only		0.5	
Combined		0.1	
IUD			
Progesterone T	2.0	1.5	81
Copper T380A	0.8	0.6	78
LNg 20	0.1	0.1	81
Depo-Provera	0.3	0.3	70
Norplant and Norplant-2	0.05	0.05	88
Female Sterilization	0.5	0.5	100
Male Sterilization	0.15	0.10	100

Adapted from Hatcher et al., 1998 Ref. #1.

[1]Among *typical* couples who initiate use of a method (not necessarily for the first time), the percentage who experience an accidental pregnancy during the first year if they do not stop use for any other reason.

[2]Among couples who initiate use of a method (not necessarily for the first time) and who use it *perfectly* (both consistently and correctly), the percentage who experience an accidental pregnancy during the first year if they do not stop use for any other reason.

[3]Among couples attempting to avoid pregnancy, the percentage who continue to use a method for one year.

[4]The percents becoming pregnant in columns (2) and (3) are based on data from populations where contraception is not used and from women who cease using contraception in order to become pregnant. Among such populations, about 89% become pregnant within one year. This estimate was lowered slightly (to 85%) to represent the percent who would become pregnant within one year among women now relying on reversible methods of contraception if they abandoned contraception altogether.

[5]Foams, creams, gels, vaginal suppositories, and vaginal film.

[6]Cervical mucus (ovulation) method supplemented by calendar in the pre-ovulatory and basal body temperature in the post-ovulatory phases.

[7]With spermicidal cream or jelly.

[8]Without spermicides.

Continued on next page

Ortho-Novum—Cont.

Studies have shown an increased risk of developing hepatocellular carcinoma[52–54, 91] in oral contraceptive users. However, these cancers are rare in the U.S.

5. OCULAR LESIONS
There have been clinical case reports of retinal thrombosis associated with the use of oral contraceptives. Oral contraceptives should be discontinued if there is unexplained partial or complete loss of vision; onset of proptosis or diplopia; papilledema; or retinal vascular lesions. Appropriate diagnostic and therapeutic measures should be undertaken immediately.

6. ORAL CONTRACEPTIVE USE BEFORE OR DURING EARLY PREGNANCY
Extensive epidemiological studies have revealed no increased risk of birth defects in women who have used oral contraceptives prior to pregnancy.[56,57] The majority of recent studies also do not indicate a teratogenic effect, particularly in so far as cardiac anomalies and limb reduction defects are concerned,[55,56,58,59] when taken inadvertently during early pregnancy.
The administration of oral contraceptives to induce withdrawal bleeding should not be used as a test for pregnancy. Oral contraceptives should not be used during pregnancy to treat threatened or habitual abortion.
It is recommended that for any patient who has missed two consecutive periods, pregnancy should be ruled out before continuing oral contraceptive use. If the patient has not adhered to the prescribed schedule, the possibility of pregnancy should be considered at the time of the first missed period. Oral contraceptive use should be discontinued until pregnancy is ruled out.

7. GALLBLADDER DISEASE
Earlier studies have reported an increased lifetime relative risk of gallbladder surgery in users of oral contraceptives and estrogens.[60,61] More recent studies, however, have shown that the relative risk of developing gallbladder disease among oral contraceptive users may be minimal.[62–64] The recent findings of minimal risk may be related to the use of oral contraceptive formulations containing lower hormonal doses of estrogens and progestogens.

8. CARBOHYDRATE AND LIPID METABOLIC EFFECTS
Oral contraceptives have been shown to cause a decrease in glucose tolerance in a significant percentage of users.[17] This effect has been shown to be directly related to estrogen dose.[65] Progestogens increase insulin secretion and create insulin resistance, this effect varying with different progestational agents.[17,66] However, in the non-diabetic woman, oral contraceptives appear to have no effect on fasting blood glucose.[67] Because of these demonstrated effects, prediabetic and diabetic women in particular should be carefully monitored while taking oral contraceptives.
A small proportion of women will have persistent hypertriglyceridemia while on the pill. As discussed earlier (see WARNINGS 1a and 1d), changes in serum triglycerides and lipoprotein levels have been reported in oral contraceptive users.

9. ELEVATED BLOOD PRESSURE
Women with significant hypertension should not be started on hormonal contraception.[92] An increase in blood pressure has been reported in women taking oral contraceptives[68] and this increase is more likely in older oral contraceptive users[69] and with extended duration of use.[61] Data from the Royal College of General Practitioners[12] and subsequent randomized trials have shown that the incidence of hypertension increases with increasing progestational activity.
Women with a history of hypertension or hypertension-related diseases, or renal disease[70] should be encouraged to use another method of contraception. If women elect to use oral contraceptives, they should be monitored closely and if significant elevation of blood pressure occurs, oral contraceptives should be discontinued. For most women, elevated blood pressure will return to normal after stopping oral contraceptives, and there is no difference in the occurrence of hypertension between former and never users.[68–71]

10. HEADACHE
The onset or exacerbation of migraine or development of headache with a new pattern which is recurrent, persistent or severe requires discontinuation of oral contraceptives and evaluation of the cause.

11. BLEEDING IRREGULARITIES
Breakthrough bleeding and spotting are sometimes encountered in patients on oral contraceptives, especially during the first three months of use. Nonhormonal causes should be considered and adequate diagnostic measures taken to rule out malignancy or pregnancy in the event of breakthrough bleeding, as in the case of any abnormal vaginal bleeding. If pathology has been excluded, time or a change to another formulation may solve the problem. In the event of amenorrhea, pregnancy should be ruled out.
Some women may encounter post-pill amenorrhea or oligomenorrhea, especially when such a condition was preexistent.

12. ECTOPIC PREGNANCY
Ectopic as well as intrauterine pregnancy may occur in contraceptive failures.

PRECAUTIONS

1. PHYSICAL EXAMINATION AND FOLLOW UP
It is good medical practice for all women to have annual history and physical examinations, including women using oral contraceptives. The physical examination, however, may be deferred until after initiation of oral contraceptives if requested by the woman and judged appropriate by the clinician. The physical examination should include special reference to blood pressure, breasts, abdomen and pelvic organs, including cervical cytology, and relevant laboratory tests. In case of undiagnosed, persistent or recurrent abnormal vaginal bleeding, appropriate measures should be conducted to rule out malignancy. Women with a strong family history of breast cancer or who have breast nodules should be monitored with particular care.

TABLE III: ANNUAL NUMBER OF BIRTH-RELATED OR METHOD-RELATED DEATHS ASSOCIATED WITH CONTROL OF FERTILITY PER 100,000 NONSTERILE WOMEN, BY FERTILITY CONTROL METHOD ACCORDING TO AGE

Method of control and outcome	15-19	20-24	25-29	30-34	35-39	40-44
No fertility control methods*	7.0	7.4	9.1	14.8	25.7	28.2
Oral contraceptives non-smoker**	0.3	0.5	0.9	1.9	13.8	31.6
Oral contraceptives smoker**	2.2	3.4	6.6	13.5	51.1	117.2
IUD**	0.8	0.8	1.0	1.0	1.4	1.4
Condom*	1.1	1.6	0.7	0.2	0.3	0.4
Diaphragm/ spermicide*	1.9	1.2	1.2	1.3	2.2	2.8
Periodic abstinence*	2.5	1.6	1.6	1.7	2.9	3.6

*Deaths are birth-related
**Deaths are method-related

Adapted from H.W. Ory, ref. #35.

2. LIPID DISORDERS
Women who are being treated for hyperlipidemias should be followed closely if they elect to use oral contraceptives. Some progestogens may elevate LDL levels and may render the control of hyperlipidemias more difficult.

3. LIVER FUNCTION
If jaundice develops in any woman receiving such drugs, the medication should be discontinued. Steroid hormones may be poorly metabolized in patients with impaired liver function.

4. FLUID RETENTION
Oral contraceptives may cause some degree of fluid retention. They should be prescribed with caution, and only with careful monitoring, in patients with conditions which might be aggravated by fluid retention.

5. EMOTIONAL DISORDERS
Women with a history of depression should be carefully observed and the drug discontinued if depression recurs to a serious degree.

6. CONTACT LENSES
Contact lens wearers who develop visual changes or changes in lens tolerance should be assessed by an ophthalmologist.

7. DRUG INTERACTIONS
Reduced efficacy and increased incidence of breakthrough bleeding and menstrual irregularities have been associated with concomitant use of rifampin. A similar association, though less marked, has been suggested with barbiturates, phenylbutazone, phenytoin sodium, carbamazepine, griseofulvin, topiramite, and possibly with ampicillin and tetracyclines.[72] A possible interaction has been suggested with hormonal contraceptives and the herbal supplement St. John's Wort based on some reports of oral contraceptive users experiencing breakthrough bleeding shortly after starting St. John's Wort. Pregnancies have been reported by users of combined hormonal contraceptives who also used some form of St. John's Wort. Healthcare prescribers are advised to consult the package inserts of medication administered concomitantly with oral contraceptives.

8. INTERACTIONS WITH LABORATORY TESTS
Certain endocrine and liver function tests and blood components may be affected by oral contraceptives:

a. Increased prothrombin and factors VII, VIII, IX, and X; decreased antithrombin 3; increased norepinephrine-induced platelet aggregability.
b. Increased thyroid binding globulin (TBG) leading to increased circulating total thyroid hormone, as measured by protein-bound iodine (PBI), T4 by column or by radioimmunoassay. Free T3 resin uptake is decreased, reflecting the elevated TBG, free T4 concentration is unaltered.
c. Other binding proteins may be elevated in serum.
d. Sex-binding globulins are increased and result in elevated levels of total circulating sex steroids and corticoids; however, free or biologically active levels remain unchanged.
e. Triglycerides may be increased.
f. Glucose tolerance may be decreased.
g. Serum folate levels may be depressed by oral contraceptive therapy. This may be of clinical significance if a woman becomes pregnant shortly after discontinuing oral contraceptives.

9. CARCINOGENESIS
See WARNINGS Section.

10. PREGNANCY
Pregnancy Category X. See CONTRAINDICATIONS and WARNINGS Sections.

11. NURSING MOTHERS
Small amounts of oral contraceptive steroids have been identified in the milk of nursing mothers and a few adverse effects on the child have been reported, including jaundice and breast enlargement. In addition, combination oral contraceptives given in the postpartum period may interfere with lactation by decreasing the quantity and quality of breast milk. If possible, the nursing mother should be advised not to use combination oral contraceptives but to use other forms of contraception until she has completely weaned her child.

12. PEDIATRIC USE
Safety and efficacy of ORTHO-NOVUM Tablets and MODICON Tablets has been established in women of reproductive age. Safety and efficacy are expected to be the same for postpubertal adolescents under the age of 16 and for users 16 years and older. Use of this product before menarche is not indicated.

13. SEXUALLY TRANSMITTED DISEASES
Patients should be counseled that this product does not protect against HIV infection (AIDS) and other sexually transmitted diseases.

INFORMATION FOR THE PATIENT
See Patient Labeling printed below.

ADVERSE REACTIONS

An increased risk of the following serious adverse reactions has been associated with the use of oral contraceptives (See WARNINGS Section).

- Thrombophlebitis and venous thrombosis with or without embolism
- Arterial thromboembolism
- Pulmonary embolism
- Myocardial infarction
- Cerebral hemorrhage
- Cerebral thrombosis
- Hypertension
- Gallbladder disease
- Hepatic adenomas or benign liver tumors

The following adverse reactions have been reported in patients receiving oral contraceptives and are believed to be drug-related:

- Nausea
- Vomiting
- Gastrointestinal symptoms (such as abdominal cramps and bloating)
- Breakthrough bleeding
- Spotting
- Change in menstrual flow
- Amenorrhea
- Temporary infertility after discontinuation of treatment
- Edema
- Melasma which may persist
- Breast changes: tenderness, enlargement, secretion
- Change in weight (increase or decrease)
- Change in cervical erosion and secretion
- Diminution in lactation when given immediately postpartum
- Cholestatic jaundice
- Migraine
- Rash (allergic)
- Mental depression
- Reduced tolerance to carbohydrates
- Vaginal candidiasis
- Change in corneal curvature (steepening)
- Intolerance to contact lenses

The following adverse reactions have been reported in users of oral contraceptives and the association has been neither confirmed nor refuted:

- Pre-menstrual syndrome
- Cataracts
- Changes in appetite
- Cystitis-like syndrome
- Headache
- Nervousness
- Dizziness
- Hirsutism
- Loss of scalp hair
- Erythema multiforme
- Erythema nodosum
- Hemorrhagic eruption
- Vaginitis
- Porphyria
- Impaired renal function
- Hemolytic uremic syndrome
- Acne

- Changes in libido
- Colitis
- Budd-Chiari Syndrome

OVERDOSAGE

Serious ill effects have not been reported following acute ingestion of large doses of oral contraceptives by young children. Overdosage may cause nausea, and withdrawal bleeding may occur in females.

NON-CONTRACEPTIVE HEALTH BENEFITS

The following non-contraceptive health benefits related to the use of combination oral contraceptives are supported by epidemiological studies which largely utilized oral contraceptive formulations containing estrogen doses exceeding 0.035 mg of ethinyl estradiol or 0.05 mg mestranol.[73–78]

Effects on menses:

- increased menstrual cycle regularity
- decreased blood loss and decreased incidence of iron deficiency anemia
- decreased incidence of dysmenorrhea

Effects related to inhibition of ovulation:

- decreased incidence of functional ovarian cysts
- decreased incidence of ectopic pregnancies

Other effects:

- decreased incidence of fibroadenomas and fibrocystic disease of the breast
- decreased incidence of acute pelvic inflammatory disease
- decreased incidence of endometrial cancer
- decreased incidence of ovarian cancer

DOSAGE AND ADMINISTRATION

To achieve maximum contraceptive effectiveness, ORTHO-NOVUM Tablets and MODICON Tablets must be taken exactly as directed and at intervals not exceeding 24 hours. ORTHO-NOVUM Tablets and MODICON Tablets are available in the DIALPAK® Tablet Dispenser which is preset for a Sunday Start. Day 1 Start is also available.

21-Day Regimen (Sunday Start)

When taking ORTHO-NOVUM 7/7/7 □ 21, ORTHO-NOVUM 10/11 □ 21, ORTHO-NOVUM 1/35 □ 21, and MODICON 21, the first tablet should be taken on the first Sunday after menstruation begins. If period begins on Sunday, the first tablet is taken on that day. One tablet is taken daily for 21 days. For subsequent cycles, no tablets are taken for 7 days, then a tablet is taken the next day (Sunday). For the first cycle of a Sunday Start regimen, another method of contraception should be used until after the first 7 consecutive days of administration.

If the patient misses one (1) active tablet in Weeks 1, 2, or 3, the tablet should be taken as soon as she remembers. If the patient misses two (2) active tablets in Week 1 or Week 2, the patient should take two (2) tablets the day she remembers and two (2) tablets the next day; and then continue taking one (1) tablet a day until she finishes the pack. The patient should be instructed to use a back-up method of birth control if she has sex in the seven (7) days after missing pills. If the patient misses two (2) active tablets in the third week or misses three (3) or more active tablets in a row, the patient should continue taking one tablet every day until Sunday. On Sunday the patient should throw out the rest of the pack and start a new pack that same day. The patient should be instructed to use a back-up method of birth control if she has sex in the seven (7) days after missing pills.

Complete instructions to facilitate patient counseling on proper pill usage may be found in the Detailed Patient Labeling ("How to Take the Pill" section).

21-Day Regimen (Day 1 Start)

The dosage of ORTHO-NOVUM 7/7/7 □ 21, ORTHO-NOVUM 10/11 □ 21, ORTHO-NOVUM 1/35 □ 21, and MODICON 21, for the initial cycle of therapy is one tablet administered daily from the 1st day through the 21st day of the menstrual cycle, counting the first day of menstrual flow as "Day 1." For subsequent cycles, no tablets are taken for 7 days, then a new course is started of one tablet a day for 21 days. The dosage regimen then continues with 7 days of no medication, followed by 21 days of medication, instituting a three-weeks-on, one-week-off dosage regimen.

If the patient misses one (1) active tablet in Weeks 1, 2, or 3, the tablet should be taken as soon as she remembers. If the patient misses two (2) active tablets in Week 1 or Week 2, the patient should take two (2) tablets the day she remembers and two (2) tablets the next day; and then continue taking one (1) tablet a day until she finishes the pack. The patient should be instructed to use a back-up method of birth control if she has sex in the seven (7) days after missing pills. If the patient misses two (2) active tablets in the third week or misses three (3) or more active tablets in a row, the patient should throw out the rest of the pack and start a new pack that same day. The patient should be instructed to use a back-up method of birth control if she has sex in the seven (7) days after missing pills.

Complete instructions to facilitate patient counseling on proper pill usage may be found in the Detailed Patient Labeling ("How to Take the Pill" section).

28-Day Regimen (Sunday Start)

When taking ORTHO-NOVUM 7/7/7 □ 28, ORTHO-NOVUM 10/11 □ 28, ORTHO-NOVUM 1/35 □ 28, and MODICON 28, the first tablet should be taken on the first Sunday after menstruation begins. If period begins on Sunday, the first tablet should be taken that day. Take one active tablet daily for 21 days followed by one green placebo tablet daily for 7 days. After 28 tablets have been taken, a new course is started the next day (Sunday). For the first cycle of a Sunday Start regimen, another method of contraception should be used until after the first 7 consecutive days of administration.

If the patient misses one (1) active tablet in Weeks 1, 2, or 3, the tablet should be taken as soon as she remembers. If the patient misses two (2) active tablets in Week 1 or Week 2, the patient should take two (2) tablets the day she remembers and two (2) tablets the next day; and then continue taking one (1) tablet a day until she finishes the pack. The patient should be instructed to use a back-up method of birth control if she has sex in the seven (7) days after missing pills. If the patient misses two (2) active tablets in the third week or misses three (3) or more active tablets in a row, the patient should continue taking one tablet every day until Sunday. On Sunday the patient should throw out the rest of the pack and start a new pack that same day. The patient should be instructed to use a back-up method of birth control if she has sex in the seven (7) days after missing pills.

Complete instructions to facilitate patient counseling on proper pill usage may be found in the Detailed Patient Labeling ("How to Take the Pill" section).

28-Day Regimen (Day 1 Start)

The dosage of ORTHO-NOVUM 7/7/7 □ 28, ORTHO-NOVUM 10/11 □ 28, ORTHO-NOVUM 1/35 □ 28, and MODICON 28, for the initial cycle of therapy is one active tablet administered daily from the 1st through the 21st day of the menstrual cycle, counting the first day of menstrual flow as "Day 1" followed by one green tablet daily for 7 days. Tablets are taken without interruption for 28 days. After 28 tablets have been taken, a new course is started the next day.

If the patient misses one (1) active tablet in Weeks 1, 2, or 3, the tablet should be taken as soon as she remembers. If the patient misses two (2) active tablets in Week 1 or Week 2, the patient should take two (2) tablets the day she remembers and two (2) tablets the next day; and then continue taking one (1) tablet a day until she finishes the pack. The patient should be instructed to use a back-up method of birth control if she has sex in the seven (7) days after missing pills. If the patient misses two (2) active tablets in the third week or misses three (3) or more active tablets in a row, the patient should throw out the rest of the pack and start a new pack that same day. The patient should be instructed to use a back-up method of birth control if she has sex in the seven (7) days after missing pills.

Complete instructions to facilitate patient counseling on proper pill usage may be found in the Detailed Patient Labeling ("How to Take the Pill" section).

The use of ORTHO-NOVUM 7/7/7, ORTHO-NOVUM 10/11, ORTHO-NOVUM 1/35, and MODICON for contraception may be initiated 4 weeks postpartum in women who elect not to breast feed. When the tablets are administered during the postpartum period, the increased risk of thromboembolic disease associated with the postpartum period must be considered. (See CONTRAINDICATIONS and WARNINGS concerning thromboembolic disease. See also PRECAUTIONS for "Nursing Mothers.") The possibility of ovulation and conception prior to initiation of medication should be considered.

(See Discussion of Dose-Related Risk of Vascular Disease from Oral Contraceptives.)

ADDITIONAL INSTRUCTIONS FOR ALL DOSING REGIMENS

Breakthrough bleeding, spotting, and amenorrhea are frequent reasons for patients discontinuing oral contraceptives. In breakthrough bleeding, as in all cases of irregular bleeding from the vagina, nonfunctional causes should be borne in mind. In undiagnosed persistent or recurrent abnormal bleeding from the vagina, adequate diagnostic measures are indicated to rule out pregnancy or malignancy. If pathology has been excluded, time or a change to another formulation may solve the problem. Changing to an oral contraceptive with a higher estrogen content, while potentially useful in minimizing menstrual irregularity, should be done only if necessary since this may increase the risk of thromboembolic disease.

Use of oral contraceptives in the event of a missed menstrual period:

1. If the patient has not adhered to the prescribed schedule, the possibility of pregnancy should be considered at the time of the first missed period and oral contraceptive use should be discontinued and a non-hormonal method should be used until pregnancy is ruled out.
2. If the patient has adhered to the prescribed regimen and misses two consecutive periods, pregnancy should be ruled out before continuing oral contraceptive use.

HOW SUPPLIED

ORTHO-NOVUM 7/7/7 □ 21 Tablets are available in a DIALPAK® Tablet Dispenser (NDC 0062-1780-15) containing 21 tablets, as follows: 7 white tablets (0.5 mg norethindrone and 0.035 mg ethinyl estradiol), 7 light peach tablets (0.75 mg norethindrone and 0.035 mg ethinyl estradiol) and 7 peach tablets (1 mg norethindrone and 0.035 mg ethinyl estradiol). The white tablets are unscored with "Ortho" and "535" debossed on each side; the light peach tablets are unscored with "Ortho" and "75" debossed on each side; the peach tablets are unscored with "Ortho" and "135" debossed on each side.

ORTHO-NOVUM 7/7/7 □ 21 is available for clinic usage in a VERIDATE® Tablet Dispenser (unfilled) and VERIDATE Refills (NDC 0062-1780-20).

ORTHO-NOVUM 7/7/7 □ 28 Tablets are available in a DIALPAK Tablet Dispenser (NDC 0062-1781-15) containing 28 tablets, as follows: 7 white, 7 light peach and 7 peach tablets as described under ORTHO-NOVUM 7/7/7 □ 21, and 7 green tablets containing inert ingredients.

ORTHO-NOVUM 7/7/7 □ 28 is available for clinic usage in a VERIDATE Tablet Dispenser (unfilled) and VERIDATE Refills (NDC 0062-1781-20).

ORTHO-NOVUM 10/11 □ 21 Tablets are available in a DIALPAK Tablet Dispenser (NDC 0062-1770-15) containing 21 tablets, as follows: 10 white tablets (0.5 mg norethindrone and 0.035 mg ethinyl estradiol) and 11 peach tablets (1 mg norethindrone and 0.035 mg ethinyl estradiol). The white tablets are unscored with "Ortho" and "535" debossed on each side; the peach tablets are unscored with "Ortho" and "135" debossed on each side.

ORTHO-NOVUM 10/11 □ 28 Tablets are available in a DIALPAK Tablet Dispenser (NDC 0062-1771-15) containing 28 tablets, as follows: 10 white and 11 peach tablets as described under ORTHO-NOVUM 10/11 □ 21, and 7 green tablets containing inert ingredients.

ORTHO-NOVUM 10/11 □ 28 is available for clinic usage in a VERIDATE Tablet Dispenser (unfilled) and VERIDATE Refills (NDC 0062-1771-20).

ORTHO-NOVUM 1/35 □ 21 Tablets are available in a DIALPAK Tablet Dispenser (NDC 0062-1760-15) containing 21 peach tablets (1 mg norethindrone and 0.035 mg ethinyl estradiol) which are unscored with "Ortho" and "135" debossed on each side.

ORTHO-NOVUM 1/35 □ 21 is available for clinic usage in a VERIDATE Tablet Dispenser (unfilled) and VERIDATE Refills (NDC 0062-1760-20).

ORTHO-NOVUM 1/35 □ 28 Tablets are available in a DIALPAK Tablet Dispenser (NDC 0062-1761-15) containing 28 tablets, as follows: 21 peach tablets as described under ORTHO-NOVUM 1/35 □ 21, and 7 green tablets containing inert ingredients.

ORTHO-NOVUM 1/35 □ 28 is available for clinic usage in a VERIDATE Tablet Dispenser (unfilled) and VERIDATE Refills (NDC 0062-1761-20).

MODICON 21 Tablets are available in a DIALPAK Tablet Dispenser (NDC 0062-1712-15) containing 21 white tablets (0.5 mg norethindrone and 0.035 mg ethinyl estradiol) which are unscored with "Ortho" and "535" debossed on each side.

MODICON 28 Tablets are available in a DIALPAK Tablet Dispenser (NDC 0062-1714-15) containing 28 tablets, as follows: 21 white tablets as described under MODICON 21, and 7 green tablets containing inert ingredients.

MODICON 28 is available for clinic usage in a VERIDATE Tablet Dispenser (unfilled) and VERIDATE Refills (NDC 0062-1714-20).

℞ only

REFERENCES

1. Trussel J. Contraceptive efficacy. In Hatcher RA, Trussel J, Stewart F, Cates W, Stewart GK, Kowal D, Guest F, Contraceptive Technology: Seventeenth Revised Edition. New York NY: Irvington Publishers, 1998, in press. **2.** Stadel BV, Oral contraceptives and cardiovascular disease. (Pt. 1). N Engl J Med 1981; 305:612–618. **3.** Stadel BV, Oral contraceptives and cardiovascular disease. (Pt. 2). N Engl J Med 1981; 305:672–677. **4.** Adam SA, Thorogood M. Oral contraception and myocardial infarction revisited: the effects of new preparations and prescribing patterns. Br J Obstet Gynaecol 1981; 88:838–845. **5.** Mann JI, Inman WH. Oral contraceptives and death from myocardial infarction. Br Med J 1975; 2(5965):245–248. **6.** Mann JI, Vessey MP, Thorogood M, Doll R. Myocardial infarction in young women with special reference to oral contraceptive practice. Br Med J 1975; 2(5956):241–245. **7.** Royal College of General Practitioners' Oral Contraception Study: further analyses of mortality in oral contraceptive users. Lancet 1981; 1:541–546. **8.** Slone D, Shapiro S, Kaufman DW, Rosenberg L, Miettinen OS, Stolley PD. Risk of myocardial infarction in relation to current and discontinued use of oral contraceptives. N Engl J Med 1981; 305:420–424. **9.** Vessey MP. Female hormones and vascular disease—an epidemiological overview. Br J Fam Plann 1980; 6 (Supplement): 1–12. **10.** Russell-Briefel RG, Ezzati TM, Fulwood R, Perlman JA, Murphy RS. Cardiovascular risk status and oral contraceptive use, United States, 1976–80. Prevent Med 1986; 15:352–362. **11.** Goldbaum GM, Kendrick JS, Hogelin GC, Gentry EM. The relative impact of smoking and oral contraceptive use on women in the United States. JAMA 1987; 258:1339–1342. **12.** Layde PM, Beral V. Further analyses of mortality in oral contraceptive users; Royal College of General Practitioners' Oral Contraception Study. (Table 5) Lancet 1981; 1:541–546. **13.** Knopp RH. Arteriosclerosis risk: the roles of oral contraceptives and postmenopausal estrogens. J Reprod Med 1986; 31(9) (Supplement): 913–921. **14.** Krauss RM, Roy S, Mishell DR, Casagrande J, Pike MC. Effects of two low-dose oral contraceptives on serum lipids and lipoproteins: Differential changes in high-density lipoproteins subclasses. Am J Obstet 1983; 145:446–452. **15.** Wahl P, Walden C, Knopp R, Hoover J, Wallace R, Heiss G, Rifkind B. Effect of estrogen/progestin potency on lipid/lipoprotein cholesterol. N Engl J Med 1983; 308:862–867. **16.** Wynn V, Niththyananthan R. The effect of progestin in combined oral contraceptives on serum lipids with special reference to high density lipoproteins. Am J Obstet Gynecol 1982; 142:766–771. **17.** Wynn V, Godsland I. Effects of oral contraceptives on carbohydrate metabolism. J Reprod Med 1986; 31(9)(Supplement):892–897. **18.** LaRosa JC. Atherosclerotic risk factors in cardiovascular disease. J Reprod Med 1986; 31(9)(Supple-

Continued on next page

Ortho-Novum—Cont.

ment):906–912. 19. Inman WH, Vessey MP. Investigation of death from pulmonary, coronary, and cerebral thrombosis and embolism in women of child-bearing age. Br Med J 1968; 2(5599):193–199. 20. Maguire MG, Tonascia J, Sartwell PE, Stolley PD, Tockman MS. Increased risk of thrombosis due to oral contraceptives: a further report. Am J Epidemiol 1979; 110(2):188–195. 21. Petitti DB, Wingerd J, Pellegrin F, Ramacharan S. Risk of vascular disease in women: smoking, oral contraceptives, noncontraceptive estrogens, and other factors. JAMA 1979; 242:1150–1154. 22. Vessey MP, Doll R. Investigation of relation between use of oral contraceptives and thromboembolic disease. Br Med J 1968; 2(5599):199–205. 23. Vessey MP, Doll R. Investigation of relation between use of oral contraceptives and thromboembolic disease. A further report. Br Med J 1969; 2(5658):651–657. 24. Porter JB, Hunter JR, Danielson DA, Jick H, Stergachis A. Oral contraceptives and non-fatal vascular disease—recent experience. Obstet Gynecol 1982; 59(3):299–302. 25. Vessey M, Doll R, Peto R, Johnson B, Wiggins P. A long-term follow-up study of women using different methods of contraception: an interim report. J Biosocial Sci 1976; 8:375–427. 26. Royal College of General Practitioners: Oral Contraceptives, venous thrombosis, and varicose veins. J Royal Coll Gen Pract 1978; 28:393–399. 27. Collaborative Group for the Study of Stroke in Young Women: Oral contraception and increased risk of cerebral ischemia or thrombosis. N Engl J Med 1973; 288:871–878. 28. Petitti DB, Wingerd J. Use of oral contraceptives, cigarette smoking, and risk of subarachnoid hemorrhage. Lancet 1978; 2:234–236. 29. Inman WH. Oral contraceptives and fatal subarachnoid hemorrhage. Br Med J 1979; 2(6203):1468–1470. 30. Collaborative Group for the Study of Stroke in Young Women: Oral Contraceptives and stroke in young women: associated risk factors. JAMA 1975; 231:718–722. 31. Inman WH, Vessey MP, Westerholm B, Engelund A. Thromboembolic disease and the steroidal content of oral contraceptives. A report to the Committee on Safety of Drugs. Br Med J 1970; 2:203–209. 32. Meade TW, Greenberg G, Thompson SG. Progestogens and cardiovascular reactions associated with oral contraceptives and a comparison of the safety of 50- and 35-mcg oestrogen preparations. Br Med J 1980; 280(6224):1157–1161. 33. Kay CR. Progestogens and arterial disease—evidence from the Royal College of General Practitioners' Study. Am J Obstet Gynecol 1982; 142:762–765. 34. Royal College of General Practitioners: Incidence of arterial disease among oral contraceptive users. J Royal Coll Gen Pract 1983; 33:75–82. 35. Ory HW. Mortality associated with fertility and fertility control: 1983. Family Planning Perspectives 1983; 15:50–56. 36. The Cancer and Steroid Hormone Study of the Centers for Disease Control and the National Institute of Child Health and Human Development: Oral contraceptive use and the risk of breast cancer. N Engl J Med 1986; 315:405–411. 37. Pike MC, Henderson BE, Krailo MD, Duke A, Roy S. Breast cancer in young women and use of oral contraceptives: possible modifying effect of formulation and age at use. Lancet 1983; 2:926–929. 38. Paul C, Skegg DG, Spears GFS, Kaldor JM. Oral contraceptives and breast cancer: A national study. Br Med J 1986; 293:723–725. 39. Miller DR, Rosenberg L, Kaufman DW, Schottenfeld D, Stolley PD, Shapiro S. Breast cancer risk in relation to early oral contraceptive use. Obstet Gynecol 1986; 68:863–868. 40. Olsson H, Olsson ML, Moller TR, Ranstam J, Holm P. Oral contraceptive use and breast cancer in young women in Sweden (letter). Lancet 1985; 1(8431):748–749. 41. McPherson K, Vessey M, Neil A, Doll R, Jones L, Roberts M. Early contraceptive use and breast cancer: Results of another case-control study. Br J Cancer 1987; 56:653–660. 42. Huggins GR, Zucker PF. Oral contraceptives and neoplasia: 1987 update. Fertil Steril 1987; 47:733–761. 43. McPherson K, Drife JO. The pill and breast cancer: why the uncertainty? Br Med J 1986; 293:709–710. 44. Shapiro S. Oral contraceptives—time to take stock. N Engl J Med 1987; 315:450–451. 45. Ory H, Naib Z, Conger SB, Hatcher RA, Tyler CW. Contraceptive choice and prevalence of cervical dysplasia and carcinoma in situ. Am J Obstet Gynecol 1976; 124:573–577. 46. Vessey MP, Lawless M, McPherson K, Yeates D. Neoplasia of the cervix uteri and contraception: a possible adverse effect of the pill. Lancet 1983; 2:930. 47. Brinton LA, Huggins GR, Lehman HF, Malli K, Savitz DA, Trapido E, Rosenthal J, Hoover R. Long term use of oral contraceptives and risk of invasive cervical cancer. Int J Cancer 1986; 38:339–344. 48. WHO Collaborative Study of Neoplasia and Steroid Contraceptives: Invasive cervical cancer and combined oral contraceptives. Br Med J 1985; 290:961–965 49. Rooks JB, Ory HW, Ishak KG, Strauss LT, Greenspan JR, Hill AP, Tyler CW. Epidemiology of hepatocellular adenoma: the role of oral contraceptive use. JAMA 1979; 242:644–648. 50. Bein NN, Goldsmith HS. Recurrent massive hemorrhage from benign hepatic tumors secondary to oral contraceptives. Br J Surg 1977; 64:433–435. 51. Klatskin G. Hepatic tumors: possible relationship to use of oral contraceptives. Gastroenterology 1977; 73:386–394. 52. Henderson BE, Preston-Martin S, Edmondson HA, Peters RL, Pike MC. Hepatocellular carcinoma and oral contraceptives. Br J Cancer 1983; 48:437–440. 53. Neuberger J, Forman D, Doll R, Williams R. Oral contraceptives and hepatocellular carcinoma. Br Med J 1986; 292:1355–1357. 54. Forman D, Vincent TJ, Doll R. Cancer of the liver and oral contraceptives. Br Med J 1986; 292:1357–1361. 55. Harlap S, Eldor J. Births following oral contraceptive failures. Obstet Gynecol 1980; 55:447–452. 56. Savolainen E, Saksela E, Saxen L. Teratogenic hazards of oral contraceptives analyzed in a national malformation register. Am J Obstet Gynecol 1981; 140:521–524. 57. Janerich DT, Piper JM, Glebatis DM. Oral contraceptives and birth defects. Am J Epidemiol 1980; 112:73–79. 58. Ferencz C, Matanoski GM, Wilson PD, Rubin JD, Neill CA, Gutberlet R. Maternal hormone therapy and congenital heart disease. Teratology 1980; 21:225–239. 59. Rothman KJ, Fyler DC, Goldblatt A, Kreidberg MB. Exogenous hormones and other drug exposures of children with congenital heart disease. Am J Epidemiol 1979; 109:433–439. 60. Boston Collaborative Drug Surveillance Program: Oral contraceptives and venous thromboembolic disease, surgically confirmed gallbladder disease, and breast tumors. Lancet 1973; 1:1399–1404. 61. Royal College of General Practitioners: Oral contraceptives and health. New York, Pittman 1974. 62. Layde PM, Vessey MP, Yeates D. Risk of gallbladder disease: a cohort study of young women attending family planning clinics. J Epidemiol Community Health 1982; 36:274–278. 63. Rome Group for Epidemiology and Prevention of Cholelithiasis (GREPCO): Prevalence of gallstone disease in an Italian adult female population. Am J Epidemiol 1984; 119:796–805. 64. Storm BL, Tamragouri RT, Morse ML, Lazar EL, West SL, Stolley PD, Jones JK. Oral contraceptives and other risk factors for gallbladder disease. Clin Pharmacol Ther 1986; 39:335–341. 65. Wynn V, Adams PW, Godsland IF, Melrose J, Niththyananthan R, Oakley NW, Seedj A. Comparison of effects of different combined oral contraceptive formulations on carbohydrate and lipid metabolism. Lancet 1979; 1:1045–1049. 66. Wynn V. Effect of progesterone and progestins on carbohydrate metabolism. In: Progesterone and Progestin. Bardin CW, Milgrom E, Mauvis-Jarvis P. eds. New York, Raven Press, 1983; pp. 395–410. 67. Perlman JA, Roussell-Briefel RG, Ezzati TM, Lieberknecht G. Oral glucose tolerance and the potency of oral contraceptive progestogens. J Chronic Dis 1985; 38:857–864. 68. Royal College of General Practitioners' Oral Contraception Study: Effect on hypertension and benign breast disease of progestogen component in combined oral contraceptives. Lancet 1977; 1:624. 69. Fisch IR, Frank J. Oral contraceptives and blood pressure. JAMA 1977; 237:2499–2503. 70. Laragh AJ. Oral contraceptive induced hypertension—nine years later. Am J Obstet Gynecol 1976; 126:141–147. 71. Ramcharan S, Peritz E, Pellegrin FA, Williams WT. Incidence of hypertension in the Walnut Creek Contraceptive Drug Study cohort: In: Pharmacology of steroid contraceptive drugs. Garattini S, Berendes HW. Eds. New York, Raven Press, 1977; pp. 277–288, (Monographs of the Mario Negri Institute for Pharmacological Research Milan.) 72. Stockley I. Interactions with oral contraceptives. J Pharm 1976; 216:140–143. 73. The Cancer and Steroid Hormone Study of the Centers for Disease Control and the National Institute of Child Health and Human Development: Oral contraceptive use and the risk of ovarian cancer. JAMA 1983; 249:1596–1599. 74. The Cancer and Steroid Hormone Study of the Centers for Disease Control and the National Institute of Child Health and Human Development: Combination oral contraceptive use and the risk of endometrial cancer. JAMA 1987; 257:796–800. 75. Ory HW. Functional ovarian cysts and oral contraceptives: negative association confirmed surgically. JAMA 1974; 228:68–69. 76. Ory HW, Cole P, MacMahon B, Hoover R. Oral contraceptives and reduced risk of benign breast disease. N Engl J Med 1976; 294:419–422. 77. Ory HW. The noncontraceptive health benefits from oral contraceptive use. Fam Plann Perspect 1982; 14:182–184. 78. Ory HW, Forrest JD, Lincoln R. Making choices: Evaluating the health risks and benefits of birth control methods. New York, The Alan Guttmacher Institute, 1983; p. 1. 79. Schlesselman J, Stadel BV, Murray P, Lai S. Breast cancer in relation to early use of oral contraceptives. JAMA 1988; 259:1828–1833. 80. Hennekens CH, Speizer FE, Lipnick RJ, Rosner B, Bain C, Belanger C, Stampfer MJ, Willett W, Peto R. A case-control study of oral contraceptive use and breast cancer. JNCI 1984; 72:39–42. 81. LaVecchia C, Decarli A, Fasoli M, Franceschi S, Gentile A, Negri E, Parazzini F, Tognoni G. Oral contraceptives and cancers of the breast and of the female genital tract. Interim results from a case-control study. Br J Cancer 1986; 54:311–317. 82. Meirik O, Lund E, Adami H, Bergstrom R, Christoffersen T, Bergsjo P. Oral contraceptive use and breast cancer in young women. A Joint National Case-control study in Sweden and Norway. Lancet 1986; 11:650–654. 83. Kay CR, Hannaford PC. Breast cancer and the pill—A further report from the Royal College of General Practitioners' oral contraception study. Br J Cancer 1988; 58:675–680. 84. Stadel BV, Lai S, Schlesselman JJ, Murray P. Oral contraceptives and premenopausal breast cancer in nulliparous women. Contraception 1988; 38:287–299. 85. Miller DR, Rosenberg L, Kaufman DW, Stolley P, Warshauer ME, Shapiro S. Breast cancer before age 45 and oral contraceptive use: New Findings. Am J Epidemiol 1989; 129:269–280. 86. The UK National Case-Control Study Group, Oral contraceptive use and breast cancer risk in young women. Lancet 1989; 1:973–982. 87. Schlesselman JJ. Cancer of the breast and reproductive tract in relation to use of oral contraceptives. Contraception 1989; 40:1–38. 88. Vessey MP, McPherson K, Villard-Mackintosh L, Yeates D. Oral contraceptives and breast cancer: latest findings in a large cohort study. Br J Cancer 1989; 59:613–617. 89. Jick SS, Walker AM, Stergachis A, Jick H. Oral contraceptives and breast cancer. Br J Cancer 1989; 59:618–621. 90. Collaborative Group on Hormonal Factors in Breast Cancer. Breast cancer and hormonal contraceptives: collaborative reanalysis of individual data on 53 297 women with breast cancer and 100 239 women without breast cancer from 54 epidemiological studies. Lancet 1996; 347:1713–1727. 91. Palmer JR, Rosenberg L, Kaufman DW, Warshauer ME, Stolley P, Shapiro S. Oral Contraceptive Use and Liver Cancer. Am J Epidemiol 1989; 130:878–882. 92. Improving access to quality care in family planning: Medical eligibility criteria for contraceptive use. Geneva, WHO, Family and Reproductive Health, 1996.

BRIEF SUMMARY PATIENT PACKAGE INSERT

Oral contraceptives, also known as "birth control pills" or "the pill," are taken to prevent pregnancy and when taken correctly, have a failure rate of less than 1% per year when used without missing any pills. The typical failure rate of large numbers of pill users is 5% per year when women who miss pills are included. For most women oral contraceptives are also free of serious or unpleasant side effects. However, forgetting to take pills considerably increases the chances of pregnancy.

For the majority of women, oral contraceptives can be taken safely. But there are some women who are at high risk of developing certain serious diseases that can be fatal or may cause temporary or permanent disability. The risks associated with taking oral contraceptives increase significantly if you:

• smoke
• have high blood pressure, diabetes, high cholesterol
• have or have had clotting disorders, heart attack, stroke, angina pectoris, cancer of the breast or sex organs, jaundice or malignant or benign liver tumors.

Although cardiovascular disease risks may be increased with oral contraceptive use after age 40 in healthy, non-smoking women (even with the newer low-dose formulations), there are also greater potential health risks associated with pregnancy in older women.

You should not take the pill if you suspect you are pregnant or have unexplained vaginal bleeding.

> Cigarette smoking increases the risk of serious cardiovascular side effects from oral contraceptive use. This risk increases with age and with heavy smoking (15 or more cigarettes per day) and is quite marked in women over 35 years of age. Women who use oral contraceptives are strongly advised not to smoke.

Most side effects of the pill are not serious. The most common such effects are nausea, vomiting, bleeding between menstrual periods, weight gain, breast tenderness, and difficulty wearing contact lenses. These side effects, especially nausea and vomiting, may subside within the first three months of use.

The serious side effects of the pill occur very infrequently, especially if you are in good health and are young. However, you should know that the following medical conditions have been associated with or made worse by the pill:

1. Blood clots in the legs (thrombophlebitis), lungs (pulmonary embolism), stoppage or rupture of a blood vessel in the brain (stroke), blockage of blood vessels in the heart (heart attack or angina pectoris) or other organs of the body. As mentioned above, smoking increases the risk of heart attacks and strokes and subsequent serious medical consequences.

2. In rare cases, oral contraceptives can cause benign but dangerous liver tumors. These benign liver tumors can rupture and cause fatal internal bleeding. In addition, some studies report an increased risk of developing liver cancer. However, liver cancers are rare.

3. High blood pressure, although blood pressure usually returns to normal when the pill is stopped.

The symptoms associated with these serious side effects are discussed in the detailed leaflet given to you with your supply of pills. Notify your doctor or health care provider if you notice any unusual physical disturbances while taking the pill. In addition, drugs such as rifampin, as well as some anticonvulsants and some antibiotics may decrease oral contraceptive effectiveness.

There is conflict among studies regarding breast cancer and oral contraceptive use. Some studies have reported an increase in the risk of developing breast cancer, particularly at a younger age. This increased risk appears to be related to duration of use. The majority of studies have found no overall increase in the risk of developing breast cancer. Some studies have found an increase in the incidence of cancer of the cervix in women who use oral contraceptives. However, this finding may be related to factors other than the use of oral contraceptives. There is insufficient evidence to rule out the possibility that pills may cause such cancers.

Taking the combination pill provides some important non-contraceptive benefits. These include less painful menstruation, less menstrual blood loss and anemia, fewer pelvic infections, and fewer cancers of the ovary and the lining of the uterus.

Be sure to discuss any medical condition you may have with your health care provider. Your health care provider will take a medical and family history before prescribing oral contraceptives and will examine you. The physical examination may be delayed to another time if you request it and the health care provider believes that it is a good medical practice to postpone it. You should be reexamined at least once a year while taking oral contraceptives. Your pharmacist should have given you the detailed patient information labeling which gives you further information which you should read and discuss with your health care provider. This product (like all oral contraceptives) is intended to prevent pregnancy. It does not protect against transmission of

HIV (AIDS) and other sexually transmitted diseases such as chlamydia, genital herpes, genital warts, gonorrhea, hepatitis B, and syphilis.

DETAILED PATIENT LABELING

PLEASE NOTE: This labeling is revised from time to time as important new medical information becomes available. Therefore, please review this labeling carefully.

The following oral contraceptive products contain a combination of an estrogen and progestogen, the two kinds of female hormones:

ORTHO-NOVUM 7/7/7 □ 21 Day Regimen and ORTHO-NOVUM 7/7/7 □ 28 Day Regimen
Each white tablet contains 0.5 mg norethindrone and 0.035 mg ethinyl estradiol. Each light peach tablet contains 0.75 mg norethindrone and 0.035 mg ethinyl estradiol. Each peach tablet contains 1 mg norethindrone and 0.035 mg ethinyl estradiol. Each green tablet in ORTHO-NOVUM 7/7/7 □ 28 Day Regimen contains inert ingredients.

ORTHO-NOVUM 10/11 □ 21 Day Regimen and ORTHO-NOVUM 10/11 □ 28 Day Regimen
Each white tablet contains 0.5 mg norethindrone and 0.035 mg ethinyl estradiol. Each peach tablet contains 1 mg norethindrone and 0.035 mg ethinyl estradiol. Each green tablet in ORTHO-NOVUM 10/11 □ 28 Day Regimen contains inert ingredients.

ORTHO-NOVUM 1/35 □ 21 Day Regimen and ORTHO-NOVUM 1/35 □ 28 Day Regimen
Each peach tablet contains 1 mg norethindrone and 0.035 mg ethinyl estradiol. Each green tablet in ORTHO-NOVUM 1/35 □ 28 Day Regimen contains inert ingredients.

MODICON 21 Day Regimen and MODICON 28 Day Regimen
Each white tablet contains 0.5 mg norethindrone and 0.035 mg ethinyl estradiol. Each green tablet in MODICON 28 Day Regimen contains inert ingredients.

INTRODUCTION

Any woman who considers using oral contraceptives (the birth control pill or the pill) should understand the benefits and risks of using this form of birth control. This patient labeling will give you much of the information you will need to make this decision and will also help you determine if you are at risk of developing any of the serious side effects of the pill. It will tell you how to use the pill properly so that it will be as effective as possible. However, this labeling is not a replacement for a careful discussion between you and your health care provider. You should discuss the information provided in this labeling with him or her, both when you first start taking the pill and during your revisits. You should also follow your health care provider's advice with regard to regular check-ups while you are on the pill.

EFFECTIVENESS OF ORAL CONTRACEPTIVES

Oral contraceptives or "birth control pills" or "the pill" are used to prevent pregnancy and are more effective than other non-surgical methods of birth control. When they are taken correctly, the chance of becoming pregnant is less than 1% (1 pregnancy per 100 women per year of use) when used perfectly, without missing any pills. Typical failure rates are actually 5% per year. The chance of becoming pregnant increases with each missed pill during a menstrual cycle.

In comparison, typical failure rates for other non-surgical methods of birth control during the first year of use are as follows:

Implant: <1%
Injection: <1%
IUD: 1 to 2%
Diaphragm with spermicides: 20%
Spermicides alone: 26%
Vaginal sponge: 20 to 40%
Female sterilization: <1%
Male sterilization: <1%
Cervical Cap with spermicides: 20 to 40%
Condom alone (male): 14%
Condom alone (female): 21%
Periodic abstinence: 25%
Withdrawal: 19%
No methods: 85%

WHO SHOULD NOT TAKE ORAL CONTRACEPTIVES

> **Cigarette smoking increases the risk of serious cardiovascular side effects from oral contraceptive use. This risk increases with age and with heavy smoking (15 or more cigarettes per day) and is quite marked in women over 35 years of age. Women who use oral contraceptives are strongly advised not to smoke.**

Some women should not use the pill. For example, you should not take the pill if you are pregnant or think you may be pregnant. You should also not use the pill if you have any of the following conditions:
- A history of heart attack or stroke
- Blood clots in the legs (thrombophlebitis), lungs (pulmonary embolism), or eyes
- A history of blood clots in the deep veins of your legs
- Chest pain (angina pectoris)
- Known or suspected breast cancer or cancer of the lining of the uterus, cervix or vagina
- Unexplained vaginal bleeding (until a diagnosis is reached by your doctor)
- Yellowing of the whites of the eyes or of the skin (jaundice) during pregnancy or during previous use of the pill
- Liver tumor (benign or cancerous)
- Known or suspected pregnancy

ANNUAL NUMBER OF BIRTH-RELATED OR METHOD-RELATED DEATHS ASSOCIATED WITH CONTROL OF FERTILITY PER 100,000 NONSTERILE WOMEN, BY FERTILITY CONTROL METHOD ACCORDING TO AGE

Method of control and outcome	15-19	20-24	25-29	30-34	35-39	40-44
No fertility control methods*	7.0	7.4	9.1	14.8	25.7	28.2
Oral contraceptives non-smoker**	0.3	0.5	0.9	1.9	13.8	31.6
Oral contraceptives smoker**	2.2	3.4	6.6	13.5	51.1	117.2
IUD**	0.8	0.8	1.0	1.0	1.4	1.4
Condom*	1.1	1.6	0.7	0.2	0.3	0.4
Diaphragm/ spermicide*	1.9	1.2	1.2	1.3	2.2	2.8
Periodic abstinence*	2.5	1.6	1.6	1.7	2.9	3.6

*Deaths are birth-related
**Deaths are method-related

Tell your health care provider if you have ever had any of these conditions. Your health care provider can recommend a safer method of birth control.

OTHER CONSIDERATIONS BEFORE TAKING ORAL CONTRACEPTIVES

Tell your health care provider if you have or have had:
- Breast nodules, fibrocystic disease of the breast, an abnormal breast x-ray or mammogram
- Diabetes
- Elevated cholesterol or triglycerides
- High blood pressure
- Migraine or other headaches or epilepsy
- Mental depression
- Gallbladder, liver, heart or kidney disease
- History of scanty or irregular menstrual periods

Women with any of these conditions should be checked often by their health care provider if they choose to use oral contraceptives.

Also, be sure to inform your doctor or health care provider if you smoke or are on any medications.

RISKS OF TAKING ORAL CONTRACEPTIVES

1. Risk of developing blood clots
Blood clots and blockage of blood vessels are one of the most serious side effects of taking oral contraceptives and can cause death or serious disability. In particular, a clot in the legs can cause thrombophlebitis and a clot that travels to the lungs can cause a sudden blocking of the vessel carrying blood to the lungs. Rarely, clots occur in the blood vessels of the eye and may cause blindness, double vision, or impaired vision.

If you take oral contraceptives and need elective surgery, need to stay in bed for a prolonged illness or injury or have recently delivered a baby, you may be at risk of developing blood clots. You should consult your doctor about stopping oral contraceptives three to four weeks before surgery and not taking oral contraceptives for two weeks after surgery or during bed rest. You should also not take oral contraceptives soon after delivery of a baby. It is advisable to wait for at least four weeks after delivery if you are not breast feeding or four weeks after a second trimester abortion. If you are breast feeding, you should wait until you have weaned your child before using the pill. (See also the section on Breast Feeding in General Precautions.)

The risk of circulatory disease in oral contraceptive users may be higher in users of high dose pills and may be greater with longer duration of oral contraceptive use. In addition, some of these increased risks may continue for a number of years after stopping oral contraceptives. The risk of abnormal blood clotting increases with age in both users and non-users of oral contraceptives, but the increased risk from the oral contraceptive appears to be present at all ages. For women aged 20 to 44, it is estimated that about 1 in 2,000 using oral contraceptives will be hospitalized each year because of abnormal clotting. Among nonusers in the same age group, about 1 in 20,000 would be hospitalized each year. For oral contraceptive users in general, it has been estimated that in women between the ages of 15 and 34 the risk of death due to a circulatory disorder is about 1 in 12,000 per year, whereas for nonusers the rate is about 1 in 50,000 per year. In the age group 35 to 44, the risk is estimated to be about 1 in 2,500 per year for oral contraceptive users and about 1 in 10,000 per year for nonusers.

2. Heart attacks and strokes
Oral contraceptives may increase the tendency to develop strokes (stoppage or rupture of blood vessels in the brain) and angina pectoris and heart attacks (blockage of blood vessels in the heart). Any of these conditions can cause death or serious disability.

Smoking greatly increases the possibility of suffering heart attacks and strokes. Furthermore, smoking and the use of oral contraceptives greatly increase the chances of developing and dying of heart disease.

3. Gallbladder disease
Oral contraceptive users probably have a greater risk than nonusers of having gallbladder disease, although this risk may be related to pills containing high doses of estrogens.

4. Liver tumors
In rare cases, oral contraceptives can cause benign but dangerous liver tumors. These benign liver tumors can rupture and cause fatal internal bleeding. In addition, some studies report an increased risk of developing liver cancer. However, liver cancers are rare.

5. Cancer of the reproductive organs and breasts
There is conflict among studies regarding breast cancer and oral contraceptive use. Some studies have reported an increase in the risk of developing breast cancer, particularly at a younger age. This increased risk appears to be related to duration of use. The majority of studies have found no overall increase in the risk of developing breast cancer.

A meta-analysis of 54 studies found a small increase in the frequency of having breast cancer diagnosed for women who were currently using combined oral contraceptives or had used them within the past ten years. This increase in the frequency of breast cancer diagnosis, within ten years of stopping use, was generally accounted for by cancers localized to the breast. There was no increase in the frequency of having breast cancer diagnosed ten or more years after cessation of use.

Some studies have found an increase in the incidence of cancer of the cervix in women who use oral contraceptives. However, this finding may be related to factors other than the use of oral contraceptives. There is insufficient evidence to rule out the possibility that pills may cause such cancers.

ESTIMATED RISK OF DEATH FROM A BIRTH CONTROL METHOD OR PREGNANCY

All methods of birth control and pregnancy are associated with a risk of developing certain diseases which may lead to disability or death. An estimate of the number of deaths associated with different methods of birth control and pregnancy has been calculated and is shown in the following table.

[See table above]

In the above table, the risk of death from any birth control method is less than the risk of childbirth, except for oral contraceptive users over the age of 35 who smoke and pill users over the age of 40 even if they do not smoke. It can be seen in the table that for women aged 15 to 39, the risk of death was highest with pregnancy (7-26 deaths per 100,000 women, depending on age). Among pill users who do not smoke, the risk of death was always lower than that associated with pregnancy for any age group, although over the age of 40, the risk increases to 32 deaths per 100,000 women, compared to 28 associated with pregnancy at that age. However, for pill users who smoke and are over the age of 35, the estimated number of deaths exceeds those for other methods of birth control. If a woman is over the age of 40 and smokes, her estimated risk of death is four times higher (117/100,000 women) than the estimated risk associated with pregnancy (28/100,000 women) in that age group. The suggestion that women over 40 who do not smoke should not take oral contraceptives is based on information from older, higher-dose pills. An Advisory Committee of the FDA discussed this issue in 1989 and recommended that the benefits of low-dose oral contraceptive use by healthy, non-smoking women over 40 years of age may outweigh the possible risks.

WARNING SIGNALS

If any of these adverse effects occur while you are taking oral contraceptives, call your doctor immediately:
- Sharp chest pain, coughing of blood, or sudden shortness of breath (indicating a possible clot in the lung)
- Pain in the calf (indicating a possible clot in the leg)
- Crushing chest pain or heaviness in the chest (indicating a possible heart attack)
- Sudden severe headache or vomiting, dizziness or fainting, disturbances of vision or speech, weakness, or numbness in an arm or leg (indicating a possible stroke)
- Sudden partial or complete loss of vision (indicating a possible clot in the eye)
- Breast lumps (indicating possible breast cancer or fibrocystic disease of the breast; ask your doctor or health care provider to show you how to examine your breasts)
- Severe pain or tenderness in the stomach area (indicating a possibly ruptured liver tumor)
- Difficulty in sleeping, weakness, lack of energy, fatigue, or change in mood (possibly indicating severe depression)

Continued on next page

Ortho-Novum—Cont.

- Jaundice or a yellowing of the skin or eyeballs, accompanied frequently by fever, fatigue, loss of appetite, dark colored urine, or light colored bowel movements (indicating possible liver problems)

SIDE EFFECTS OF ORAL CONTRACEPTIVES

1. Vaginal bleeding
Irregular vaginal bleeding or spotting may occur while you are taking the pills. Irregular bleeding may vary from slight staining between menstrual periods to breakthrough bleeding which is a flow much like a regular period. Irregular bleeding occurs most often during the first few months of oral contraceptive use, but may also occur after you have been taking the pill for some time. Such bleeding may be temporary and usually does not indicate any serious problems. It is important to continue taking your pills on schedule. If the bleeding occurs in more than one cycle or lasts for more than a few days, talk to your doctor or health care provider.

2. Contact lenses
If you wear contact lenses and notice a change in vision or an inability to wear your lenses, contact your doctor or health care provider.

3. Fluid retention
Oral contraceptives may cause edema (fluid retention) with swelling of the fingers or ankles and may raise your blood pressure. If you experience fluid retention, contact your doctor or health care provider.

4. Melasma
A spotty darkening of the skin is possible, particularly of the face, which may persist.

5. Other side effects
Other side effects may include nausea and vomiting, change in appetite, headache, nervousness, depression, dizziness, loss of scalp hair, rash, and vaginal infections.
If any of these side effects bother you, call your doctor or health care provider.

GENERAL PRECAUTIONS

1. Missed periods and use of oral contraceptives before or during early pregnancy
There may be times when you may not menstruate regularly after you have completed taking a cycle of pills. If you have taken your pills regularly and miss one menstrual period, continue taking your pills for the next cycle but be sure to inform your health care provider before doing so. If you have not taken the pills daily as instructed and missed a menstrual period, you may be pregnant. If you missed two consecutive menstrual periods, you may be pregnant. Check with your health care provider immediately to determine whether you are pregnant. Do not continue to take oral contraceptives until you are sure you are not pregnant, but continue to use another method of contraception.
There is no conclusive evidence that oral contraceptive use is associated with an increase in birth defects, when taken inadvertently during early pregnancy. Previously, a few studies had reported that oral contraceptives might be associated with birth defects, but these findings have not been seen in more recent studies. Nevertheless, oral contraceptives or any other drugs should not be used during pregnancy unless clearly necessary and prescribed by your doctor. You should check with your doctor about risks to your unborn child of any medication taken during pregnancy.

2. While breast feeding
If you are breast feeding, consult your doctor before starting oral contraceptives. Some of the drug will be passed on to the child in the milk. A few adverse effects on the child have been reported, including yellowing of the skin (jaundice) and breast enlargement. In addition, combination oral contraceptives may decrease the amount and quality of your milk. If possible, do not use combination oral contraceptives while breast feeding. You should use another method of contraception since breast feeding provides only partial protection from becoming pregnant and this partial protection decreases significantly as you breast feed for longer periods of time. You should consider starting combination oral contraceptives only after you have weaned your child completely.

3. Laboratory tests
If you are scheduled for any laboratory tests, tell your doctor you are taking birth control pills. Certain blood tests may be affected by birth control pills.

4. Drug interactions
Certain drugs may interact with birth control pills to make them less effective in preventing pregnancy or cause an increase in breakthrough bleeding. Such drugs include rifampin, drugs used for epilepsy such as barbiturates (for example, phenobarbital), anticonvulsants such as topiramate (TOPAMAX), carbamazepine (Tegretol is one brand of this drug), phenytoin (Dilantin is one brand of this drug), phenylbutazone (Butazolidin is one brand), certain drugs used in the treatment of HIV or AIDS, and possibly certain antibiotics. You may need to use additional contraception when you take drugs which can make oral contraceptives less effective. A possible interaction has been suggested with hormonal contraceptives and the herbal supplement St. John's Wort based on some reports of oral contraceptive users experiencing breakthrough bleeding shortly after starting St. John's Wort. Pregnancies have been reported by users of combined hormonal contraceptives who also used some form of St. John's Wort.

5. Sexually transmitted diseases
This product (like all oral contraceptives) is intended to prevent pregnancy. It does not protect against transmission of HIV (AIDS) and other sexually transmitted diseases such as chlamydia, genital herpes, genital warts, gonorrhea, hepatitis B, and syphilis.

HOW TO TAKE THE PILL
IMPORTANT POINTS TO REMEMBER
BEFORE YOU START TAKING YOUR PILLS:
1. BE SURE TO READ THESE DIRECTIONS:
Before you start taking your pills.
Anytime you are not sure what to do.
2. THE RIGHT WAY TO TAKE THE PILL IS TO TAKE ONE PILL EVERY DAY AT THE SAME TIME.
If you miss pills you could get pregnant. This includes starting the pack late.
The more pills you miss, the more likely you are to get pregnant.
3. MANY WOMEN HAVE SPOTTING OR LIGHT BLEEDING, OR MAY FEEL SICK TO THEIR STOMACH DURING THE FIRST 1–3 PACKS OF PILLS. If you feel sick to your stomach, do not stop taking the pill. The problem will usually go away. If it doesnt go away, check with your doctor or clinic.
4. MISSING PILLS CAN ALSO CAUSE SPOTTING OR LIGHT BLEEDING, even when you make up these missed pills.
On the days you take 2 pills to make up for missed pills, you could also feel a little sick to your stomach.
5. IF YOU HAVE VOMITING OR DIARRHEA, for any reason, or IF YOU TAKE SOME MEDICINES, including some antibiotics, your pills may not work as well. Use a back-up method (such as condoms, foam, or sponge) until you check with your doctor or clinic.
6. IF YOU HAVE TROUBLE REMEMBERING TO TAKE THE PILL, talk to your doctor or clinic about how to make pill-taking easier or about using another method of birth control.
7. IF YOU HAVE ANY QUESTIONS OR ARE UNSURE ABOUT THE INFORMATION IN THIS LEAFLET, call your doctor or clinic.

BEFORE YOU START TAKING YOUR PILLS
1. DECIDE WHAT TIME OF DAY YOU WANT TO TAKE YOUR PILL.
It is important to take it at about the same time every day.
2. LOOK AT YOUR PILL PACK TO SEE IF IT HAS 21 OR 28 PILLS:
The 21-pill pack has 21 "active" pills (with hormones) to take for 3 weeks. This is followed by 1 week without pills.
The 28-pill pack has 21 "active" pills (with hormones) to take for 3 weeks. This is followed by 1 week of "reminder" green pills (without hormones).
ORTHO-NOVUM 7/7/7: There are 7 white "active" pills, 7 light peach "active" pills, and 7 peach "active" pills.
ORTHO-NOVUM 10/11: There are 10 white "active" pills and 11 peach "active" pills.
ORTHO-NOVUM 1/35: There are 21 peach "active" pills.
MODICON: There are 21 white "active" pills.
3. ALSO FIND:
   1) where on the pack to start taking pills,
   2) in what order to take the pills.
CHECK PICTURE OF PILL PACK AND ADDITIONAL INSTRUCTIONS FOR USING THIS PACKAGE IN THE BRIEF SUMMARY PATIENT PACKAGE INSERT.
4. BE SURE YOU HAVE READY AT ALL TIMES:
ANOTHER KIND OF BIRTH CONTROL (such as condoms, foam, or sponge) to use as a back-up method in case you miss pills.
AN EXTRA, FULL PILL PACK.

WHEN TO START THE FIRST PACK OF PILLS
You have a choice of which day to start taking your first pack of pills. ORTHO-NOVUM 7/7/7, ORTHO-NOVUM 10/11, ORTHO-NOVUM 1/35, and MODICON are available in the DIALPAK® Tablet Dispenser which is preset for a Sunday Start. Day 1 Start is also provided. Decide with your doctor or clinic which is the best day for you. Pick a time of day which will be easy to remember.

SUNDAY START:
ORTHO-NOVUM 7/7/7: Take the first "active" white pill of the first pack on the Sunday after your period starts, even if you are still bleeding. If your period begins on Sunday, start the pack the same day.
ORTHO-NOVUM 10/11: Take the first "active" white pill of the first pack on the Sunday after your period starts, even if you are still bleeding. If your period begins on Sunday, start the pack the same day.
ORTHO-NOVUM 1/35: Take the first "active" peach pill of the first pack on the Sunday after your period starts, even if you are still bleeding. If your period begins on Sunday, start the pack the same day.
MODICON: Take the first "active" white pill of the first pack on the Sunday after your period starts, even if you are still bleeding. If your period begins on Sunday, start the pack the same day.
Use another method of birth control as a back-up method if you have sex anytime from the Sunday you start your first pack until the next Sunday (7 days). Condoms, foam, or the sponge are good back-up methods of birth control.

DAY 1 START:
ORTHO-NOVUM 7/7/7: Take the first "active" white pill of the first pack during the first 24 hours of your period.
ORTHO-NOVUM 10/11: Take the first "active" white pill of the first pack during the first 24 hours of your period.
ORTHO-NOVUM 1/35: Take the first "active" peach pill of the first pack during the first 24 hours of your period.
MODICON: Take the first active white pill of the first pack during the first 24 hours of your period.

You will not need to use a back-up method of birth control, since you are starting the pill at the beginning of your period.

WHAT TO DO DURING THE MONTH
1. TAKE ONE PILL AT THE SAME TIME EVERY DAY UNTIL THE PACK IS EMPTY.
Do not skip pills even if you are spotting or bleeding between monthly periods or feel sick to your stomach (nausea). Do not skip pills even if you do not have sex very often.
2. WHEN YOU FINISH A PACK OR SWITCH YOUR BRAND OF PILLS:
21 pills: Wait 7 days to start the next pack. You will probably have your period during that week. Be sure that no more than 7 days pass between 21-day packs.
28 pills: Start the next pack on the day after your last "reminder" pill. Do not wait any days between packs.

WHAT TO DO IF YOU MISS PILLS
ORTHO-NOVUM 7/7/7:
If you **MISS 1** white, light peach, or peach "active" pill:
1. Take it as soon as you remember. Take the next pill at your regular time. This means you may take 2 pills in 1 day.
2. You do not need to use a back-up birth control method if you have sex.
If you **MISS 2** white or light peach "active" pills in a row in **WEEK 1 OR WEEK** 2 of your pack:
1. Take 2 pills on the day you remember and 2 pills the next day.
2. Then take 1 pill a day until you finish the pack.
3. You MAY BECOME PREGNANT if you have sex in the 7 days after you miss pills. You MUST use another birth control method (such as condoms, foam, or sponge) as a back-up method for those 7 days.
If you **MISS 2** peach "active" pills in a row in **THE 3RD WEEK**:
1. **If you are a Sunday Starter:**
Keep taking 1 pill every day until Sunday. On Sunday, THROW OUT the rest of the pack and start a new pack of pills that same day.
If you are a Day 1 Starter:
THROW OUT the rest of the pill pack and start a new pack that same day.
2. You may not have your period this month but this is expected. However, if you miss your period 2 months in a row, call your doctor or clinic because you might be pregnant.
3. You MAY BECOME PREGNANT if you have sex in the 7 days after you miss pills. You MUST use another birth control method (such as condoms, foam, or sponge) as a back-up method for those 7 days.
If you **MISS 3 OR MORE** white, light peach, or peach "active" pills in a row (during the first 3 weeks):
1. **If you are a Sunday Starter:**
Keep taking 1 pill every day until Sunday. On Sunday, THROW OUT the rest of the pack and start a new pack of pills that same day.
If you are a Day 1 Starter:
THROW OUT the rest of the pill pack and start a new pack that same day.
2. You may not have your period this month but this is expected. However, if you miss your period 2 months in a row, call your doctor or clinic because you might be pregnant.
3. You MAY BECOME PREGNANT if you have sex in the 7 days after you miss pills. You MUST use another birth control method (such as condoms, foam, or sponge) as a back-up method for those 7 days.

ORTHO-NOVUM 10/11:
If you **MISS 1** white or peach "active" pill:
1. Take it as soon as you remember. Take the next pill at your regular time. This means you may take 2 pills in 1 day.
2. You do not need to use a back-up birth control method if you have sex.
If you **MISS 2** white or peach "active" pills in a row in **WEEK 1 OR WEEK 2** of your pack:
1. Take 2 pills on the day you remember and 2 pills the next day.
Then take 1 pill a day until you finish the pack.
You MAY BECOME PREGNANT if you have sex in the 7 days after you miss pills. You MUST use another birth control method (such as condoms, foam, or sponge) as a back-up method for those 7 days.
If you **MISS 2** peach "active" pills in a row in **THE 3RD WEEK**:
1. **If you are a Sunday Starter:**
Keep taking 1 pill every day until Sunday. On Sunday, THROW OUT the rest of the pack and start a new pack of pills that same day.
If you are a Day 1 Starter:
THROW OUT the rest of the pill pack and start a new pack that same day.
2. You may not have your period this month but this is expected. However, if you miss your period 2 months in a row, call your doctor or clinic because you might be pregnant.
3. You MAY BECOME PREGNANT if you have sex in the 7 days after you miss pills. You MUST use another birth control method (such as condoms, foam, or sponge) as a back-up method for those 7 days.
If you **MISS 3 OR MORE** white or peach "active" pills in a row (during the first 3 weeks):
1. **If you are a Sunday Starter:**
Keep taking 1 pill every day until Sunday. On Sunday, THROW OUT the rest of the pack and start a new pack of pills that same day.
If you are a Day 1 Starter:
THROW OUT the rest of the pill pack and start a new pack that same day.
2. You may not have your period this month but this is expected. However, if you miss your period 2 months in a row, call your doctor or clinic because you might be pregnant.

3. You MAY BECOME PREGNANT if you have sex in the 7 days after you miss pills. You MUST use another birth control method (such as condoms, foam, or sponge) as a back-up method for those 7 days.

ORTHO-NOVUM 1/35:

If you **MISS 1** peach "active" pill:

1. Take it as soon as you remember. Take the next pill at your regular time. This means you may take 2 pills in 1 day.
2. You do not need to use a back-up birth control method if you have sex.

If you **MISS 2** peach "active" pills in a row in **WEEK 1 OR WEEK 2** of your pack:

1. Take 2 pills on the day you remember and 2 pills the next day.
2. Then take 1 pill a day until you finish the pack.
3. You MAY BECOME PREGNANT if you have sex in the 7 days after you miss pills. You MUST use another birth control method (such as condoms, foam, or sponge) as a back-up method for those 7 days.

If you **MISS 2** peach "active" pills in a row in **THE 3RD WEEK:**

1. **If you are a Sunday Starter:**
Keep taking 1 pill every day until Sunday. On Sunday, THROW OUT the rest of the pack and start a new pack of pills that same day.
If you are a Day 1 Starter:
THROW OUT the rest of the pill pack and start a new pack that same day.
2. You may not have your period this month but this is expected. However, if you miss your period 2 months in a row, call your doctor or clinic because you might be pregnant.
3. You MAY BECOME PREGNANT if you have sex in the 7 days after you miss pills. You MUST use another birth control method (such as condoms, foam, or sponge) as a back-up method for those 7 days.

If you **MISS 3 OR MORE** peach "active" pills in a row (during the first 3 weeks):

1. **If you are a Sunday Starter:**
Keep taking 1 pill every day until Sunday. On Sunday, THROW OUT the rest of the pack and start a new pack of pills that same day.
If you are a Day 1 Starter:
THROW OUT the rest of the pill pack and start a new pack that same day.
2. You may not have your period this month but this is expected. However, if you miss your period 2 months in a row, call your doctor or clinic because you might be pregnant.
3. You MAY BECOME PREGNANT if you have sex in the 7 days after you miss pills. You MUST use another birth control method (such as condoms, foam, or sponge) as a back-up method for those 7 days.

MODICON:

If you **MISS 1** white "active" pill:

1. Take it as soon as you remember. Take the next pill at your regular time. This means you may take 2 pills in 1 day.
2. You do not need to use a back-up birth control method if you have sex.

If you **MISS 2** white "active" pills in a row in **WEEK 1 OR WEEK 2** of your pack:

1. Take 2 pills on the day you remember and 2 pills the next day.
2. Then take 1 pill a day until you finish the pack.
3. You MAY BECOME PREGNANT if you have sex in the 7 days after you miss pills. You MUST use another birth control method (such as condoms, foam, or sponge) as a back-up method for those 7 days.

If you **MISS 2** white "active" pills in a row in **THE 3RD WEEK:**

1. **If you are a Sunday Starter:**
Keep taking 1 pill every day until Sunday. On Sunday, THROW OUT the rest of the pack and start a new pack of pills that same day.
If you are a Day 1 Starter:
THROW OUT the rest of the pill pack and start a new pack that same day.
2. You may not have your period this month but this is expected. However, if you miss your period 2 months in a row, call your doctor or clinic because you might be pregnant.
3. You MAY BECOME PREGNANT if you have sex in the 7 days after you miss pills. You MUST use another birth control method (such as condoms, foam, or sponge) as a back-up method for those 7 days.

If you **MISS 3 OR MORE** white "active" pills in a row (during the first 3 weeks):

1. **If you are a Sunday Starter:**
Keep taking 1 pill every day until Sunday. On Sunday, THROW OUT the rest of the pack and start a new pack of pills that same day.
If you are a Day 1 Starter:
THROW OUT the rest of the pill pack and start a new pack that same day.
2. You may not have your period this month but this is expected. However, if you miss your period 2 months in a row, call your doctor or clinic because you might be pregnant.
3. You MAY BECOME PREGNANT if you have sex in the 7 days after you miss pills. You MUST use another birth control method (such as condoms, foam, or sponge) as a back-up method for those 7 days.

A REMINDER FOR THOSE ON 28-DAY PACKS:

If you forget any of the 7 green "reminder" pills in Week 4: THROW AWAY the pills you missed.

Keep taking 1 pill each day until the pack is empty.

You do not need a back-up method.

FINALLY, IF YOU ARE STILL NOT SURE WHAT TO DO ABOUT THE PILLS YOU HAVE MISSED:

Use a BACK-UP METHOD anytime you have sex.

KEEP TAKING ONE "ACTIVE" PILL EACH DAY until you can reach your doctor or clinic.

PREGNANCY DUE TO PILL FAILURE

Combination Oral Contraceptives

The incidence of pill failure resulting in pregnancy is approximately one percent (i.e., one pregnancy per 100 women per year) if taken every day as directed, but more typical failure rates are 5%. If failure does occur, the risk to the fetus is minimal.

PREGNANCY AFTER STOPPING THE PILL

There may be some delay in becoming pregnant after you stop using oral contraceptives, especially if you had irregular menstrual cycles before you used oral contraceptives. It may be advisable to postpone conception until you begin menstruating regularly once you have stopped taking the pill and desire pregnancy.

There does not appear to be any increase in birth defects in newborn babies when pregnancy occurs soon after stopping the pill.

OVERDOSAGE

Serious ill effects have not been reported following ingestion of large doses of oral contraceptives by young children. Overdosage may cause nausea and withdrawal bleeding in females. In case of overdosage, contact your health care provider or pharmacist.

OTHER INFORMATION

Your health care provider will take a medical and family history before prescribing oral contraceptives and will examine you. The physical examination may be delayed to another time if you request it and the health care provider believes that it is a good medical practice to postpone it. You should be reexamined at least once a year. Be sure to inform your health care provider if there is a family history of any of the conditions listed previously in this leaflet. Be sure to keep all appointments with your health care provider, because this is a time to determine if there are early signs of side effects of oral contraceptive use.

Do not use the drug for any condition other than the one for which it was prescribed. This drug has been prescribed specifically for you; do not give it to others who may want birth control pills.

HEALTH BENEFITS FROM ORAL CONTRACEPTIVES

In addition to preventing pregnancy, use of combination oral contraceptives may provide certain benefits. They are:

- menstrual cycles may become more regular
- blood flow during menstruation may be lighter and less iron may be lost. Therefore, anemia due to iron deficiency is less likely to occur.
- pain or other symptoms during menstruation may be encountered less frequently
- ectopic (tubal) pregnancy may occur less frequently
- noncancerous cysts or lumps in the breast may occur less frequently
- acute pelvic inflammatory disease may occur less frequently
- oral contraceptive use may provide some protection against developing two forms of cancer: cancer of the ovaries and cancer of the lining of the uterus.

If you want more information about birth control pills, ask your doctor or pharmacist. They have a more technical leaflet called the Professional Labeling, which you may wish to read. The professional labeling is also published in a book entitled *Physicians' Desk Reference*, available in many book stores and public libraries.

ORTHO-McNEIL PHARMACEUTICAL, INC.
Raritan, New Jersey 08869

© OMP 1998 REVISED DECEMBER 2000 635-50-700-4

ORTHO-PREFEST® ℞

[*orthō-prē-fēst*]
(estradiol/norgestimate)
tablets

Prescribing information for this product, which appears on pages 2370–2374 of the 2001 PDR, has been completely revised as follows. Please write "See Supplement A" next to the product heading.

Prescribing Information

DESCRIPTION

The ORTHO-PREFEST® regimen provides for a single oral tablet to be taken once daily. The pink tablet containing 1.0 mg estradiol is taken on days one through three of therapy; the white tablet containing 1.0 mg estradiol and 0.09 mg norgestimate is taken on days four through six of therapy. This pattern is then repeated continuously to produce the constant estrogen/intermittent progestogen regimen of ORTHO-PREFEST®.

The estrogenic component of ORTHO-PREFEST® is 17β-estradiol. It is a white, crystalline solid, chemically described as estra-1,3,5(10)-triene-3,17β-diol. It has an empirical formula of $C_{18}H_{24}O_2$ and molecular weight of 272.39. The structural formula is:

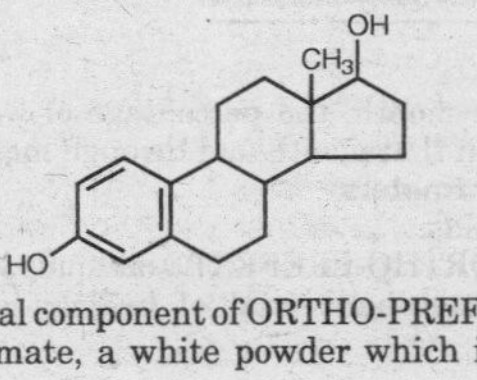

The progestational component of ORTHO-PREFEST® is micronized norgestimate, a white powder which is chemically described as (17α)-17-(Acetyloxyl)-13-ethyl-18, 19-dinorpregn-4-en-20-yn-3-one3-oxime. It has an empirical formula of $C_{23}H_{31}NO_3$ and a molecular weight of 369.50. The structural formula is:

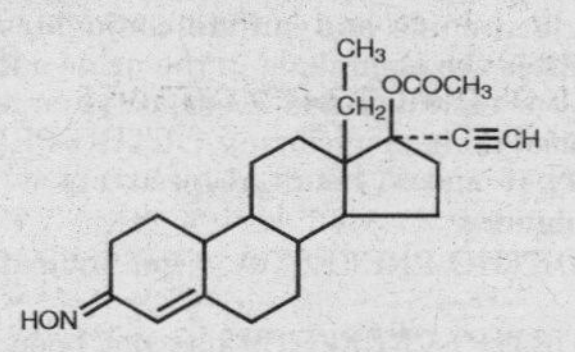

Each tablet for oral administration contains 1.0 mg estradiol alone or 1.0 mg estradiol and 0.09 mg of norgestimate, and the following inactive ingredients: croscarmellose sodium, microcrystalline cellulose, magnesium stearate, ferric oxide red, and lactose monohydrate.

CLINICAL PHARMACOLOGY

Estrogens are important in the development and maintenance of the female reproductive system and secondary sex characteristics. By a direct action, they cause growth and development of the uterus, fallopian tubes, and vagina. With other hormones, such as pituitary hormones and progesterone, they cause enlargement of the breasts through promotion of ductal growth, stromal development, and the accretion of fat. Estrogens are intricately involved with other hormones, especially progesterone, in the processes of the ovulatory menstrual cycle and pregnancy and affect the release of pituitary gonadotropins. They also contribute to the shaping of the skeleton, maintenance of tone and elasticity of urogenital structures, changes in the epiphyses of the long bones that allow for the pubertal growth spurt and its termination, and pigmentation of the nipples and genitals.

Although circulating estrogens exist in a dynamic equilibrium of metabolic interconversions, estradiol is the principal intracellular human estrogen and is substantially more potent than its metabolites, estrone and estriol at the receptor level. The primary source of estrogen in adult women with normal menstrual cycles is the ovarian follicle, which secretes 70 to 500 micrograms of estradiol daily, depending on the phase of the menstrual cycle. After menopause, most endogenous estrogens are produced by conversion of androstenedione, secreted by the adrenal cortex, to estrone by the peripheral tissues. Thus, estrone and the sulfate conjugated form, estrone sulfate, are the most abundant circulating estrogens in postmenopausal women.

Circulating estrogens modulate the pituitary secretion of the gonadotropins, luteinizing hormone (LH) and follicle stimulating hormone (FSH) through a negative feedback mechanism and estrogen replacement therapy acts to reduce the elevated levels of these hormones seen in postmenopausal women.

Norgestimate is a derivative of 19-nortestosterone and binds to androgen and progestogen receptors, similar to that of the natural hormone progesterone; it does not bind to estrogen receptors. Progestins counter the estrogenic effects by decreasing the number of nuclear estradiol receptors and suppressing epithelial DNA synthesis in endometrial tissue.

Pharmacokinetics

Absorption:

Estradiol reaches its peak serum concentration (C_{max}) at approximately 7 hours in postmenopausal women receiving ORTHO-PREFEST® (Table 1). Norgestimate is completely metabolized; its primary active metabolite, 17-deacetylnorgestimate, reaches C_{max} at approximately 2 hours after dose (Table 1). Upon co-administration of ORTHO-PREFEST® with a high fat meal, the C_{max} values for estrone and estrone sulfate were increased by 14% and 24% respectively, and the C_{max} for 17-deacetylnorgestimate was decreased by 16%. The AUC values for these analytes were not significantly affected by food.

Distribution:

The distribution of exogenous estrogens is similar to that of endogenous estrogens. Estrogens are widely distributed in the body and are generally found in higher concentrations in the sex hormone target organs. Estradiol is bound mainly to sex hormone binding globulin (SHBG), and to albumin. 17-deacetylnorgestimate, the primary active metabolite of norgestimate, does not bind to SHBG but to other serum proteins. The percent protein binding of 17-deacetylnorgestimate is approximately 99%.

Metabolism:

Exogenous estrogens are metabolized in the same manner as endogenous estrogens. Circulating estrogens exist in a dynamic equilibrium of metabolic interconversions. These transformations take place mainly in the liver. Estradiol is converted reversibly to estrone, and both can be converted to estriol, which is the major urinary metabolite. Estrogens also undergo enterohepatic recirculation via sulfate and glucuronide conjugation in the liver, biliary secretion of conjugates into the intestine, and hydrolysis in the gut followed by reabsorption. In postmenopausal women a significant portion of the circulating estrogens exist as sulfate conjugates, especially estrone sulfate, which serves as a circulating reservoir for the formation of more active estrogens. Norgestimate is extensively metabolized by first-pass mechanisms in gastrointestinal tract and/or liver. Norgestimate's primary active metabolite is 17-deacetylnorgestimate.

Continued on next page

Ortho-Prefest—Cont.

Excretion:
Estradiol, estrone, and estriol are excreted in the urine along with glucuronide and sulfate conjugates. Nonestimate metabolites are eliminated in the urine and feces. The half-life ($t_{1/2}$) of estradiol and 17-deacetylnorgestimate in postmenopausal women receiving ORTHO-PREFEST® is approximately 16 and 37 hours, respectively.

Special Populations
Pediatric: ORTHO-PREFEST® is not indicated in children.
Geriatric: ORTHO-PREFEST® has not been studied in geriatric patients.
Gender: ORTHO-PREFEST® is indicated in women only.
Effects of Race, Age, and Body Weight: The effects of race, age, and body weight on the pharmacokinetics of estradiol, norgestimate, and their metabolites were evaluated in 164 healthy postmenopausal women (100 Caucasians, 61 Hispanics, 2 Blacks, and 1 Asian). No significant pharmacokinetic difference was observed between the Caucasian and the Hispanic postmenopausal women. No significant difference due to age (40–66 years) was observed. No significant difference due to body weight was observed in women in the 60 to 80 kg weight range. Women with body weight higher than 80 kg, however, had approximately 40% lower peak serum levels of 17-deacetylnorgestimate, 30% lower AUC values for 17-deacetylnorgestimate and 30% lower C_{max} values for norgestrel. The clinical relevance of these observations is unknown.
Renal Insufficiency: It has been reported in the literature that at both baseline and after estradiol ingestion, postmenopausal women with end stage renal disease (ESRD) had higher free serum estradiol levels than the control subjects. No pharmacokinetic study with norgestimate or a hormone combination with norgestimate has been conducted in postmenopausal women with ESRD.
Hepatic Insufficiency: No pharmacokinetic study for ORTHO-PREFEST® has been conducted in postmenopausal women with hepatic impairment.
[See table 1 above]

Drug-Drug Interactions
Estradiol, norgestimate, and their metabolites inhibit a variety of P450 enzymes in human liver microsomes. However, the clinical and toxicological consequences of such interaction are likely to be insignificant because, under the recommended dosing regimen, the in vivo concentrations of these steroids, even at the peak serum levels, are relatively low compared to the inhibitory constant (Ki). Results of a subset population (n=24) from a clinical study conducted in 36 healthy postmenopausal women indicated that the steady state serum estradiol levels during the estradiol plus norgestimate phase of the regimen may be lower by 12–18% as compared with estradiol administered alone. The serum estrone levels may decrease by 4% and the serum estrone sulfate levels may increase by 17% during the estradiol plus norgestimate phase as compared with estradiol administered alone. The clinical relevance of these observations is unknown.

CLINICAL STUDIES

Efficacy on Postmenopausal Symptoms
The effect of the estrogen component of ORTHO-PREFEST® on vasomotor symptoms was confirmed in a 12-week placebo-controlled trial of healthy postmenopausal women with moderate-to-severe vasomotor symptoms (MSVS). The addition of norgestimate to estrogen (i.e., the ORTHO-PREFEST® regimen) was studied in two 12-month trials in healthy postmenopausal women (n=1212) for endometrial protection. Results from a subset population (n=119) of these 12-month trials (women with MSVS) are shown in Table 2.

Table 2: Change in the Mean Number of Moderate-to-Severe Vasomotor Symptoms (Subset of Subjects with ≥7 Moderate-to-Severe Hot Flushes per Day)

	1 mg E_2		ORTHO-PREFEST®	
	N	Mean	N	Mean
Baseline	29	11.0	26	10.9
Week 4	29	3.3	26	2.6
Week 8	29	1.1	23	0.9
Week 12	29	1.1	23	0.7

The effects of the addition of norgestimate on steady state estrogen levels and the clinical relevance thereof have been discussed in **CLINICAL PHARMACOLOGY** (see **Drug-Drug Interactions**).

Efficacy on Vulvar and Vaginal Atrophy
The effect of the estrogen component of ORTHO-PREFEST® on vulvovaginal atrophy was confirmed in a 12-week placebo-controlled trial of healthy postmenopausal women with moderate-to-severe vasomotor symptoms (MSVS). The addition of norgestimate to estrogen (i.e., the ORTHO-PREFEST® regimen) was studied in a 12-month trial in healthy postmenopausal women for endometrial protection. Results from a subset population (n=69) with paired tests for maturation index of the vaginal mucosa are shown in Table 3.
[See table 3 above]

Table 1: Mean Pharmacokinetic Parameters of E_2, E_1, E_1S, and 17d-NGM[1] Following Single and Multiple Dosing of ORTHO-PREFEST®

Analyte	Parameter[2]	Units	First Dose E_2	First Dose E_2/NGM	Multiple Dose E_2	Multiple Dose E_2/NGM
E_2	C_{max}	pg/mL	27.4	39.3	49.7	46.2
	t_{max}	h	7	7	7	7
	AUC(0–24 h)	pg. h/mL	424	681	864	779
E_1	C_{max}	pg/mL	210	285	341	325
	t_{max}	h	6	6	7	6
	AUC(0–24 h)	pg. h/mL	2774	4153	5429	4957
E_1S	C_{max}	ng/mL	11.1	13.9	14.9	14.5
	t_{max}	h	5	4	6	5
	AUC(0–24 h)	ng.h/mL	135	180	198	198
17d-NGM	C_{max}	pg/mL	NA[3]	515	NA	643
	t_{max}	h	NA	2	NA	2
	AUC(0–24 h)	pg. h/mL	NA	2146	NA	5322
	$t_{1/2}$	h	NA	37	NA	NA

[1] E_2 = Estradiol, E_1 = Estrone, E_1S = Estrone Sulfate, 17d-NGM = 17-deacetylnorgestimate. Baseline uncorrected data are reported for E_2, E_1 and E_1S.
[2] C_{max} = peak serum concentration, t_{max} = time to reach peak serum concentration, AUC(0–24 h) = area under serum concentration vs. time curve from 0 to 24 hours after dose, $t_{1/2}$ = half-life.
[3] NA= Not available or not applicable.

Table 3: Summary of Maturation Index Results in Subjects with Paired Tests Following 7 Months Treatment with ORTHO-PREFEST® or Estradiol

	Pretreatment Mean	Month 7 Mean	Mean Change
1 mg Estradiol (N=37)			
Parabasal Cells (%)	25.1	2.7	−22.4
Intermediate Cells (%)	69.2	76.4	7.2
Superficial Cells (%)	5.7	20.9	15.3
ORTHO-PREFEST® (N=32)			
Parabasal Cells (%)	31.9	0.0	−31.9
Intermediate Cells (%)	64.2	80.9	16.7
Superficial Cells (%)	3.9	19.1	15.2

Table 4: Incidence of Endometrial Hyperplasia After 12 Months of Treatment (Intent To Treat Population)

	Continuous 1 mg estradiol	ORTHO-PREFEST®
Total No. Subjects	265	242
Total No. Evaluable Biopsies	256 (97%)	227 (94%)
Normal endometrium	182 (71%)	227 (100%)
Simple hyperplasia	64 (25%)	0 (0%)
Complex hyperplasia	2 (0.8%)	0 (0%)
Hyperplasia with cytological atypia	8 (3%)	0 (0%)

Table 5: Effects on Blood Lipoproteins at Month 12

	1 mg E_2		ORTHO-PREFEST®	
		Mean %		Mean %
	N	Change	N	Change
Total Cholesterol	36	1.2	31	−1.9
HDL	36	12.0	31	9.7
LDL	31	1.7	30	1.2
Triglycerides	36	29.0	31	9.4

Effects on the Endometrium
The effect of ORTHO-PREFEST® on the endometrium was evaluated in two 12-month trials. The combined results are shown in Table 4.
[See table 4 above]
In another 12-month controlled clinical trial for endometrial protection an additional 190 postmenopausal women were treated with ORTHO-PREFEST®. No subject had a diagnosis of endometrial hyperplasia after treatment.

Control of Uterine Bleeding
The effect of ORTHO-PREFEST® on uterine bleeding was evaluated in two 12-month trials.
Combined results are shown in Figure 1.

Figure 1: Subjects with Cumulative Amenorrhea Over Time (Intent To Treat Population)

Legend:
— 1 mg E_2 (N=304)
—O— ORTHO-PREFEST (N=307)

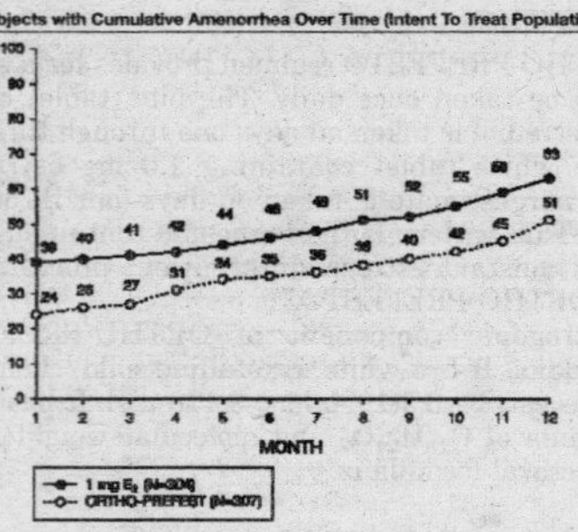

Note: At each month, the percentage of women who were amenorrheic in that month and through month 12 is shown.

Metabolic Parameters
Effects on Lipids:
The effect of ORTHO-PREFEST® on lipids was evaluated in a 12-month metabolic trial of healthy postmenopausal women.

Results are shown in Table 5.
[See table 5 above]

INDICATIONS AND USAGE
ORTHO-PREFEST® therapy is indicated in women with an intact uterus for the:
1. Treatment of moderate to severe vasomotor symptoms associated with the menopause.
2. Treatment of vulvar and vaginal atrophy.
3. Prevention of osteoporosis.
Most prospective studies of efficacy for this indication have been carried out in white postmenopausal women, without stratification by other risk factors, and tend to show a universally beneficial effect on bone. Since estrogen administration is associated with risk, patient selection must be individualized based on the balance of risks and benefits.
Case-control studies have shown an approximately 60-percent reduction in hip and wrist fractures in women whose estrogen replacement was begun within a few years after menopause. Studies also suggest that estrogen reduces the rate of vertebral fractures. When estrogen therapy is discontinued, bone mass declines at a rate comparable to the immediate postmenopausal period.
White and Asian women are at higher risk for osteoporosis than Black women, and thin women are at higher risk than heavier women, who generally have higher endogenous estrogen levels. Early menopause is one of the strongest predictors for the development of osteoporosis. Other factors associated with osteoporosis include genetic factors (small build, family history), lifestyle (cigarette smoking, alcohol abuse, sedentary exercise habits) and nutrition (below average body weight and dietary calcium intake).
The mainstays of prevention and management of osteoporosis are weight-bearing exercise, adequate lifetime calcium intake, and, when indicated, estrogen. Postmenopausal women absorb dietary calcium less efficiently than premenopausal women and require an average of 1500 mg/day of elemental calcium to remain in neutral calcium balance. The average calcium intake in the USA is 400–600 mg/day.

Therefore, when not contraindicated, calcium supplementation may be helpful for women with suboptimal dietary intake.

CONTRAINDICATIONS

Estrogens/progestins should not be used in individuals with any of the following conditions:
1. Known or suspected pregnancy.
2. Undiagnosed abnormal genital bleeding.
3. Known or suspected cancer of the breast.
4. Known or suspected estrogen-dependent neoplasia.
5. Active or past history of thrombophlebitis or thromboembolic disorders.
6. Hypersensitivity to any components of this product.

WARNINGS
Based on experience with estrogens and/or progestins:
1. Induction of Malignant Neoplasms
Endometrial Cancer:
The reported endometrial cancer risk among unopposed estrogen users is about 2 to 12-fold greater than in non-users, and appears dependent on duration of treatment and on estrogen dose. Most studies show no significant increased risk associated with the use of estrogens for less than one year. The greatest risk appears associated with prolonged use, with increased risks of 15 to 24-fold for five years to ten years or more, and this risk has been shown to persist for at least 8–15 years after estrogen therapy is discontinued. Using progestin therapy together with estrogen therapy significantly reduces but does not eliminate this risk.

Results from two 12-month clinical trials of the effects of ORTHO-PREFEST® on endometrial hyperplasia are shown in the Clinical Studies section of this label.

Appropriate diagnostic measures should be undertaken to rule out malignancy in all cases of undiagnosed, persistent, or recurring abnormal vaginal bleeding.

Breast Cancer:
While some epidemiologic studies suggest an increase in breast cancer for estrogen alone users versus non-users, other studies have not shown any increased risk. The addition of progestin to estrogen may further increase the risk of breast cancer. In the Nurse's Health Study of 121,700 women that examined the relationship between postmenopausal use of hormones and the risk of breast cancer, the risk of breast cancer was shown to be related to both dose and duration of use. In this study and others, the risk is not statistically significant until 5 years of use. In women without a uterus who are candidates for hormone replacement therapy, there is no demonstrated benefit from the addition of progestin to estrogen replacement therapy compared to estrogen alone therapy.

Women who are candidates for long-term use of hormone replacement therapy (either estrogen alone or estrogen/progestin) should be advised of potential benefits and risks (including the potential for an increased risk of breast cancer).

All women should receive yearly breast exams by a health-care provider and perform monthly breast-self examinations. In addition, mammography examinations should be scheduled as suggested by providers based on patient age and risk factors. Breast cancers found in current or recent users of hormone replacement therapy may be more likely to be localized to the breast than those in non-users.

2. Venous Thromboembolism
Epidemiologic studies have reported an increased risk of venous thromboembolism (VTE) in users of estrogen replacement therapy (ERT) who did not have predisposing conditions for VTE, such as past history of cardiovascular disease or a recent history of pregnancy, surgery, trauma, or serious illness. The increased risk was found only in current ERT users; it did not persist in former users. The findings were similar for ERT alone or with added progestin and pertain to commonly used ERT types and doses, including 0.625 mg or more per day orally of conjugated estrogens, 1 mg or more per day orally of estradiol, and 50 micrograms or more per day of transdermal estradiol. The studies found the VTE risk to be about one case per 10,000 women per year among women not using ERT and without predisposing conditions. The risk in current ERT users was increased to 2–3 cases per 10,000 women per year.

3. Cardiovascular Disease
Large doses of estrogens (5 mg conjugated estrogens per day), comparable to those used to treat cancer of the prostate and breast, have been shown to increase the risks of nonfatal myocardial infarction, pulmonary embolism, and thrombophlebitis in a large prospective clinical trial in men.

4. Hypercalcemia
Administration of estrogens may lead to severe hypercalcemia in patients with breast cancer and bone metastases. If this occurs, the drugs should be stopped and appropriate measures taken to reduce the serum calcium level.

5. Gallbladder Disease
A 2 to 4-fold increase in the risk of gallbladder disease requiring surgery in women receiving postmenopausal estrogens has been reported.

PRECAUTIONS
General
Data from the Heart and Estrogen/Progestin Replacement Study (HERS), a controlled clinical trial of secondary prevention of 2,763 post-menopausal women with documented heart disease, showed more coronary heart disease (CHD) events in the hormone treated group than in the placebo group in year 1. There were fewer events in years 4 and 5. During an average follow-up of 4.1 years, treatment with oral conjugated estrogen plus medroxyprogesterone acetate did not reduce the overall rate of CHD events in postmenopausal women with established coronary disease. The effects of estrogen replacement on the primary prevention of cardiovascular disease have not been adequately studied. Some studies have reported reduction in the risk of cardiovascular disease in women receiving estrogen alone therapy or combination estrogen/progestin therapy.

Based on experience with estrogens and/or progestins:
1. Addition of a progestin when a woman has not had a hysterectomy
Studies of the addition of a progestin for 10 or more days of a cycle of estrogen administration, or daily with estrogen in a continuous regimen, have reported a lowered incidence of endometrial hyperplasia than would be induced by estrogen treatment alone.

There are, however, possible risks that may be associated with the use of progestins in estrogen replacement regimens. These include:
a. adverse effects on lipoprotein metabolism (lowering HDL and raising LDL).
b. impairment of glucose tolerance;
and;
c. possible enhancement of mitotic activity in breast epithelial tissue. There is minimal epidemiological data available to address this point.
The choice of progestin, its dose, and its regimen may be important in minimizing these adverse effects.

2. Endometrial hyperplasia
In pharmacokinetic studies with ORTHO-PREFEST®, women with body weight greater than 80 kg, had approximately 40% lower peak serum levels of 17-deacetylnorgestimate, 30% lower AUC values for 17-deacetylnorgestimate and 30% lower C_{max} values for norgestrel. 17-deacetylnorgestimate and norgestrel are metabolites of the progestin norgestimate.

Although the clinical relevance of these observations is unknown, the underlying risk of endometrial hyperplasia is known to be higher in overweight women. Therefore, clinical surveillance is important. Appropriate diagnostic measures, including endometrial sampling when indicated, should be undertaken to rule out malignancy in all cases of undiagnosed persistent or recurring abnormal vaginal bleeding or in women with other risk factors for endometrial hyperplasia.

3. Elevated blood pressure
Occasional increases in blood pressure during estrogen replacement therapy have been attributed to idiosyncratic reactions to estrogens in a small number of case reports. A generalized effect of estrogen therapy on blood pressure was not found in the one randomized, placebo-controlled study that has been reported. This effect was also not observed in clinical studies with ORTHO-PREFEST®.

4. Familial hyperlipoproteinemia
Estrogen therapy may be associated with elevations of plasma triglycerides leading to pancreatitis and other complications in patients with familial defects of lipoprotein metabolism.

5. Impaired liver function
Estrogens may be poorly metabolized in patients with impaired liver function.

Information For The Patient
See text of PATIENT LABELING, below.
Drug/Laboratory Test Interactions
1. Accelerated prothrombin time, partial thromboplastin time, and platelet aggregation time; increased platelet count; increased factors II, VII antigen, VIII antigen, VIII coagulant activity, IX, X, XII, VII-X complex, II-VII-X complex, and beta-thromboglobulin; decreased levels of anti-factor Xa and antithrombin III, decreased antithrombin III activity; increased levels of fibrinogen and fibrinogen activity; increased plasminogen antigen and activity.
2. Increased thyroid-binding globulin (TBG) leading to increased circulating total thyroid hormone, as measured by protein-bound iodine (PBI), T4 levels (by column or by radioimmunoassay) or T3 levels by radioimmunoassay. T3 resin uptake is decreased, reflecting the elevated TBG. Free T4 and free T3 concentrations are unaltered.
3. Other binding proteins may be elevated in serum, i.e., corticosteroid binding globulin (CBG), sex hormone-binding globulin (SHBG), leading to increased circulating corticosteroids and sex steroids respectively. Free or biologically active hormone concentrations are unchanged. Other plasma proteins may be increased (angiotensinogen/renin substrate, alpha-1-antitrypsin, ceruloplasmin).
4. Increased plasma HDL and HDL-2 subfraction concentrations, reduced LDL cholesterol concentration, increased triglycerides levels.
5. Impaired glucose tolerance. For this reason, diabetic patients should be carefully observed while receiving estrogen/progestin therapy.
6. Reduced response to metyrapone test.
7. Reduced serum folate concentration.
Carcinogenesis, Mutagenesis, and Impairment of Fertility
Long-term continuous administration of natural and synthetic estrogens in certain animal species increases the frequency of carcinomas of the breasts, uterus, cervix, vagina, testis, and liver. (See CONTRAINDICATIONS and WARNINGS.)
Pregnancy Category X
ORTHO-PREFEST® should not be used during pregnancy. (See CONTRAINDICATIONS.)
Nursing Mothers
As a general principle, the administration of any drug to nursing mothers should be done only when clearly necessary since many drugs are excreted in human milk. Estrogen administration to nursing mothers has been shown to decrease the quantity and quality of the milk. Estrogens are not indicated for the prevention of postpartum breast engorgement.

ADVERSE REACTIONS
In four 12-month trials that included 579 healthy postmenopausal women treated with ORTHO-PREFEST® the following treatment-emergent adverse events occurred at a rate ≥ 5% (Table 6):

Table 6: All Treatment-Emergent Adverse Events Regardless of Drug Relationship Reported at a Frequency of ≥ 5% with ORTHO-PREFEST®

Four 12-Month Clinical Trials

	ORTHO-PREFEST® (estradiol and NGM) (N = 579) n (%)
Body as a Whole	
Back pain	69 (12%)
Fatigue	32 (6%)
Influenza-like symptoms	64 (11%)
Pain	37 (6%)
Digestive System	
Abdominal pain	70 (12%)
Flatulence	29 (5%)
Nausea	34 (6%)
Tooth disorder	27 (5%)
Musculoskeletal System	
Arthralgia	51 (9%)
Myalgia	30 (5%)
Nervous System	
Dizziness	27 (5%)
Headache	132 (23%)
Psychiatric Disorders	
Depression	27 (5%)
Reproductive System	
Breast pain	92 (16%)
Dysmenorrhea	48 (8%)
Vaginal bleeding (all)	52 (9%)
Vaginitis	42 (7%)
Resistance Mechanism Disorders	
Viral infection	35 (6%)
Respiratory System	
Coughing	28 (5%)
Pharyngitis	38 (7%)
Sinusitis	44 (8%)
Upper respiratory-tract infection	121 (21%)

Endometrial Hyperplasia
See Table 4 for incidence of endometrial hyperplasia in clinical trials for efficacy.

In all clinical studies, endometrial biopsy specimens initially were read for safety by a single pathologist. All biopsies were subsequently evaluated by at least 2 blinded expert pathologists as per study protocol. Those biopsy specimens initially read as hyperplasia were reported in the safety database, were evaluated by the expert pathologist panel, and were determined not to be cases of hyperplasia. The following additional adverse reactions have been reported with estrogen therapy (see WARNINGS and PRECAUTIONS regarding induction of neoplasia, increased incidence of gallbladder disease, cardiovascular disease, elevated blood pressure, and hypercalcemia).

1. Genitourinary System. Changes in vaginal bleeding pattern and abnormal withdrawal bleeding or flow; breakthrough bleeding, spotting; increase in size of uterine leiomyomata; vaginal candidiasis; change in amount of cervical secretion.
2. Breasts. Tenderness, enlargement, galactorrhea.
3. Gastrointestinal. Cholestatic jaundice, nausea, vomiting, abdominal cramps, bloating, increased incidence of gallbladder disease.
4. Skin. Chloasma or melasma; which may persist when drug is discontinued; erythema multiforme; erythema nodosum; hemorrhagic eruption; loss of scalp hair; hirsutism.
5. Central Nervous System. Headache, migraine, dizziness; mental depression; chorea.
6. Eyes. Steepening of corneal curvature; intolerance to contact lenses.
7. Miscellaneous. Increase or decrease in weight; reduced carbohydrate tolerance; aggravation of porphyria; edema; changes in libido.

Continued on next page

Ortho-Prefest—Cont.

OVERDOSAGE

No serious ill effects have been reported following acute ingestion of large doses of estrogen/progestin-containing oral contraceptives by young children. Overdosage may cause nausea and vomiting, and withdrawal bleeding may occur in females.

DOSAGE AND ADMINISTRATION

ORTHO-PREFEST® regimen consists of the daily administration of a single tablet containing 1 mg estradiol (pink color) for three days followed by a single tablet of 1 mg estradiol combined with 0.09 mg norgestimate (white color) for three days. This regimen is repeated continuously without interruption.

1. For treatment of moderate to severe vasomotor symptoms and vulvar and vaginal atrophy associated with menopause, the patient should start with the first tablet in the first row, and place the weekday schedule sticker which starts with the weekday of first tablet intake in the appropriate space. After all tablets from the blister card have been used, the first tablet from a new blister card should be taken on the following day.
   This dose may not be the lowest effective dose for treatment of vulvar and vaginal atrophy.
   Patients should be re-evaluated at three-month to six-month intervals to determine if treatment for symptoms is still necessary.
2. For prevention of osteoporosis, the patient should start with the first tablet in the first row, and place the weekday schedule sticker which starts with the weekday of first tablet intake in the appropriate space. After all tablets from the blister card have been used, the first tablet from a new blister card should be taken on the following day.
   This dose may not be the lowest effective dose for the prevention of osteoporosis.

Missed Tablets

If a tablet is missed for one or more days, therapy should be resumed with the next available tablet. The patient should continue to take only one tablet each day in sequence.

HOW SUPPLIED

ORTHO-PREFEST® is available as two separate, round-shaped tablets for oral administration supplied in a blister card with the following configuration: 3 pink tablets, followed by 3 white tablets for a total of 30 tablets per blister card.

Each blister card contains 15 tablets of each of the following components:

1 mg estradiol: pink tablets embossed with "1" and "J-C" on one side and "E2" and "O-M" on the other side.

1 mg estradiol/0.09 mg norgestimate: white tablets embossed with "1/90" and "J-C" on one side and "E2/N" and "O-M" on the other side.

NDC: 0062-1840-01 ORTHO-PREFEST®, 30 Tablets/Blister

This product is stable for 24 months. Store at 25°C (77°F); excursions permitted to 15°–30°C (59°–86°F).

PATIENT INSTRUCTIONS

INFORMATION FOR THE PATIENT

INTRODUCTION

This leaflet describes when and how to use estrogens/progestins, and the risks and benefits of estrogen/progestin treatment.

Estrogens/progestins have important benefits but also some risks. You must decide, with your doctor, whether the risks are acceptable in comparison to the benefits. If you use estrogens, make sure you are using the lowest possible dose that works, and that you don't use them longer than necessary. How long you need to use estrogens will depend on the reason for use.

ESTROGENS INCREASE THE RISK OF CANCER OF THE UTERUS

THIS FINDING REFERS TO ESTROGENS GIVEN WITHOUT PROGESTIN

Progestin drugs taken with estrogen-containing drugs significantly reduce, but do not eliminate, this risk.

If you use any drug containing estrogen, it is important to visit your doctor regularly and report any unusual vaginal bleeding right away. Vaginal bleeding after menopause may be a warning sign of uterine cancer. Your doctor should evaluate any unusual vaginal bleeding to find out the cause.

If you take ORTHO-PREFEST® and later find you were pregnant when you took it, be sure to discuss this with your doctor as soon as possible.

USES OF ESTROGEN

Not every estrogen drug is approved for every use listed in this section. If you want to know which of these uses are approved for the medicine prescribed for you, ask your doctor or pharmacist to show you the professional labeling.

To reduce moderate or severe menopausal symptoms. Estrogens are hormones made by the ovaries of normal women. Between ages 45 and 55, the ovaries normally stop making estrogens. This leads to a drop in body estrogen levels, which causes the "change of life" or menopause (the end of monthly menstrual periods). If both ovaries are removed during an operation before natural menopause takes place, the sudden drop in estrogen levels causes "surgical menopause."

When the estrogen levels begin dropping some women develop very uncomfortable symptoms such as feelings of warmth in the face, neck, and chest, or sudden intense episodes of heat and sweating ("hot flashes" or "hot flushes"). Using estrogen drugs can help the body adjust to lower estrogen levels and reduce these symptoms. Most women have only mild menopausal symptoms or none at all and do not need to use estrogen drugs for these symptoms. Others may need to take estrogens for a few months while their bodies adjust to lower estrogen levels. The majority of women do not need estrogen replacement for longer than six months for these symptoms.

To treat vulvar and vaginal atrophy (itching, burning, dryness in or around the vagina, difficulty or burning on urination) associated with menopause.

To prevent thinning of bones (osteoporosis). Osteoporosis is a thinning of the bones that makes them weaker and allows them to break more easily. The bones of the spine, wrists and hips break most often in osteoporosis. Both men and women start to lose bone mass after about age 40, but women lose bone mass faster after the menopause. Using estrogens after the menopause slows down bone thinning and may prevent bones from breaking. Lifelong adequate calcium intake, either in the diet (such as dairy products) or by calcium supplements (to reach a total daily intake of 1000 milligrams per day before menopause or 1500 milligrams per day after menopause), may help to prevent osteoporosis. Regular weight-bearing exercise may also help to prevent osteoporosis. Before you change your calcium intake or exercise habits, it is important to discuss these lifestyle changes with your doctor to find out if they are safe for you.

The decision to treat a woman with estrogens for the prevention of osteoporosis depends on the woman's risk of developing osteoporosis without treatment and the risks of estrogen use. Women who are likely to develop osteoporosis often have one or more of the following characteristics: White or Asian race, slim, cigarette smokers, and a family history of osteoporosis in a mother, sister, or aunt. Women who have relatively early menopause, often because their ovaries were removed during an operation (surgical menopause), are also more likely to develop osteoporosis than women whose menopause happens at the average age.

WHO SHOULD NOT USE ESTROGENS

Estrogens should not be used:

During pregnancy

If you think you may be pregnant, do not use any form of estrogen-containing drug. Using some types of estrogens while you are pregnant may cause your unborn child to have birth defects. Estrogens do not prevent miscarriage.

If you have unusual vaginal bleeding which has not been evaluated by your doctor

Unusual vaginal bleeding can be a warning sign of cancer of the uterus, especially if it happens after menopause. Your doctor must find out the cause of the bleeding so that he or she can recommend the proper treatment.

If you have had cancer

Since estrogens may increase the risk of certain types of breast and uterine cancer, you should not use estrogens unless your doctor recommends that you take it. (For certain patients with breast or prostate cancer, estrogens may help.)

If you have any circulation problems

Women with abnormal blood clotting conditions should avoid estrogen use (see **RISKS OF ESTROGENS AND/OR PROGESTINS,** below).

After childbirth or when breast-feeding a baby

Estrogens should not be used to try to stop the breasts from filling with milk after a baby is born. Such treatment may increase the risk of developing blood clots (see **RISKS OF ESTROGENS AND/OR PROGESTINS,** below).

RISKS OF ESTROGENS AND/OR PROGESTINS

Cancer of the uterus

Your risk of developing cancer of the uterus gets higher the longer you use estrogens and the larger the dose you use. Because of this risk, it is important to take the lowest dose that works and to take it only as long as you need it.

Using progestin therapy together with estrogen therapy reduces, but does not eliminate, the higher risk of uterine cancer related to estrogen use (see also **OTHER INFORMATION,** below).

If you have had your uterus removed (total hysterectomy), there is no danger of developing cancer of the uterus.

Cancer of the breast

Studies examining the risk of breast cancer among women using estrogen alone and combined estrogen/progestin therapy report an increased risk of breast cancer over the estrogen alone therapy.

If you do not have your uterus, there is no need for combined estrogen/progestin therapy since estrogen alone therapy is sufficient and may pose less risk for breast cancer.

If you do have your uterus, you should discuss the benefits and risks of combined estrogen/progestin therapy with your health care provider. Regular breast exams by a health professional and monthly self-exams are recommended for all women. Mammography may also be recommended depending on your age and risk factors.

Abnormal blood clotting

Taking estrogens may cause changes in your blood clotting system. These changes allow the blood to clot more easily, possibly allowing clots to form in your bloodstream. If blood clots do form in your bloodstream, they can cut off the blood supply to vital organs, causing serious problems. These problems may include a stroke (by cutting off blood to the brain), heart attack (by cutting off blood to the heart), a pulmonary clot (by cutting off blood to the lungs), or other problems. Any of these conditions may cause death or serious long-term disability.

Gallbladder disease

Women who use estrogens after menopause are more likely to develop gallbladder disease needing surgery than women who do not use estrogens.

SIDE EFFECTS

In addition to the risks listed above, the following side effects have been reported with estrogen and/or progestin use:

- Nausea and vomiting
- Breast tenderness or enlargement
- Enlargement of benign tumors of the uterus ("fibroids")
- Retention of excess fluid
- A spotty darkening of the skin, particularly on the face
- Irregular vaginal bleeding or spotting
- Headache, migraine, dizziness, faintness or change in vision including intolerance to contact lenses
- Mental depression
- Vaginal yeast infections

USE IN CHILDREN

Estrogen treatment has not been shown either effective or safe for use by infants, children or adolescent boys or girls.

REDUCING THE RISKS OF ESTROGEN USE

While you are using ORTHO-PREFEST®:

See your doctor regularly

Visit your doctor regularly for a check-up. If you develop vaginal bleeding, you may need further evaluation.

Reassess your need for treatment

You and your doctor should reevaluate whether or not you still need ORTHO-PREFEST® every six months.

Be alert for signs of trouble

If any of these warning signals (or any other unusual symptoms) happen while you are using ORTHO-PREFEST®, call your doctor immediately:

- Abnormal bleeding from the vagina (possible uterine cancer).
- Pains in the calves or chest, a sudden shortness of breath or coughing blood (indicating possible clots in the legs, heart, or lungs).
- Severe headache or vomiting, dizziness, faintness, or changes in vision or speech, weakness or numbness of an arm or leg (indicating possible clots in the brain or eye).
- Breast lumps (possible breast cancer; ask your doctor or health professional to show you how to examine your breasts monthly).
- Yellowing of the skin and/or whites of the eyes (possible liver problems).
- Pain, swelling, or tenderness in the abdomen (possible gallbladder problem).

OTHER INFORMATION

Estrogens increase the risk of developing a condition (endometrial hyperplasia) that may lead to cancer of the lining of the uterus. Taking progestins, another hormonal drug, with estrogens lowers the risk of developing this condition. Since you still have your uterus, your doctor has prescribed ORTHO-PREFEST® which has both an estrogen and progestin.

In studies of ORTHO-PREFEST® users, women weighing more than 176 pounds (80 kg) had lower blood levels of progestin than women weighing less than 176 pounds. The clinical relevance of this finding is unknown.

Your doctor has prescribed this drug for you and you alone. Do not give the drug to anyone else.

Keep this and all drugs out of the reach of children. In case of overdose, call your doctor, hospital, or poison control center immediately.

HOW SUPPLIED

ORTHO-PREFEST® therapy consists of the daily administration of a single tablet containing 1 mg estradiol (pink color) for three days followed by a single tablet of 1 mg estradiol combined with 0.09 mg norgestimate (white color) for three days. The three days of pink tablets followed by 3-days of white tablets are repeated continuously during treatment.

ORTHO-PREFEST® is available as two separate, round-shaped tablets for oral administration and is supplied in a blister card with the following configuration: 4 rows of 7 tablets each and one row with 2 tablets, with space on the blister to place one of 7 weekday schedules.

ORTHO-McNEIL PHARMACEUTICAL, INC.
Raritan, NJ 08869

 Revised November 2000 638-10-785-3

ORTHO TRI-CYCLEN® Tablets ℞
ORTHO-CYCLEN® Tablets
(norgestimate/ethinyl estradiol)

Prescribing information for this product, which appears on pages 2374–2381 of the 2001 PDR, has been completely revised as follows. Please write "See Supplement A" next to the product heading.

Prescribing Information

Patients should be counseled that this product does not protect against HIV infection (AIDS) and other sexually transmitted diseases.

DESCRIPTION

Each of the following products is a combination oral contraceptive containing the progestational compound norgestimate and the estrogenic compound ethinyl estradiol.

ORTHO TRI-CYCLEN ☐ 21 Tablets and ORTHO TRI-CYCLEN ☐ 28 Tablets.

Each white tablet contains 0.180 mg of the progestational compound, norgestimate (18,19-Dinor-17-pregn-4-en-20-

yn-3-one,17-(acetyloxy)-13-ethyl-,oxime,(17α)-(+)-) and 0.035 mg of the estrogenic compound, ethinyl estradiol (19-nor-17α-pregna,1,3,5(10)-trien-20-yne-3,17-diol). Inactive ingredients include lactose, magnesium stearate, and pregelatinized starch.

Each light blue tablet contains 0.215 mg of the progestational compound norgestimate (18,19-Dinor-17-pregn-4-en-20-yn-3-one,17-(acetyloxy)-13-ethyl-,oxime,(17α)-(+)-) and 0.035 mg of the estrogenic compound, ethinyl estradiol (19-nor-17α-pregna,1,3,5(10)-trien-20-yne-3,17-diol). Inactive ingredients include FD&C Blue No. 2 Aluminum Lake, lactose, magnesium stearate, and pregelatinized starch.

Each blue tablet contains 0.250 mg of the progestational compound norgestimate (18,19-Dinor-17-pregn-4-en-20-yn-3-one,17-(acetyloxy)-13-ethyl-,oxime,(17α)-(+)-) and 0.035 mg of the estrogenic compound, ethinyl estradiol (19-nor-17α-pregna,1,3,5(10)-trien-20-yne-3,17-diol). Inactive ingredients include FD&C Blue No. 2 Aluminum Lake, lactose, magnesium stearate, and pregelatinized starch.

Each green tablet in the ORTHO TRI-CYCLEN □ 28 package contains only inert ingredients, as follows: D&C Yellow No. 10 Aluminum Lake, FD&C Blue No. 2 Aluminum Lake, lactose, magnesium stearate, microcrystalline cellulose and pregelatinized starch.

ORTHO-CYCLEN □ 21 Tablets and ORTHO-CYCLEN □ 28 Tablets.

Each blue tablet contains 0.250 mg of the progestational compound norgestimate (18,19-Dinor-17-pregn-4-en-20-yn-3-one,17-(acetyloxy)-13-ethyl-,oxime,(17α)-(+)-) and 0.035 mg of the estrogenic compound, ethinyl estradiol (19-nor-17α-pregna,1,3,5(10)-trien-20-yne-3,17-diol). Inactive ingredients include FD&C Blue No. 2 Aluminum Lake, lactose, magnesium stearate, and pregelatinized starch.

Each green tablet in the ORTHO-CYCLEN □ 28 package contains only inert ingredients, as follows: D&C Yellow No. 10 Aluminum Lake, FD&C Blue No. 2 Aluminum Lake, lactose, magnesium stearate, microcrystalline cellulose and pregelatinized starch.

Norgestimate

Ethinyl Estradiol

CLINICAL PHARMACOLOGY
ORAL CONTRACEPTION
Combination oral contraceptives act by suppression of gonadotropins. Although the primary mechanism of this action is inhibition of ovulation, other alterations include changes in the cervical mucus (which increase the difficulty of sperm entry into the uterus) and the endometrium (which reduce the likelihood of implantation).

Receptor binding studies, as well as studies in animals and humans, have shown that norgestimate and 17-deacetyl norgestimate, the major serum metabolite, combine high progestational activity with minimal intrinsic androgenicity.[90-93] Norgestimate, in combination with ethinyl estradiol, does not counteract the estrogen-induced increases in sex hormone binding globulin (SHBG), resulting in lower serum testosterone.[90,91,94]

ACNE
Acne is a skin condition with a multifactorial etiology. The combination of ethinyl estradiol and norgestimate may increase sex hormone binding globulin (SHBG) and decrease free testosterone resulting in a decrease in the severity of facial acne in otherwise healthy women with this skin condition.

Norgestimate and ethinyl estradiol are well absorbed following oral administration of ORTHO-CYCLEN and ORTHO TRI-CYCLEN. On the average, peak serum concentrations of norgestimate and ethinyl estradiol are observed within two hours (0.5–2.0 hr for norgestimate and 0.75–3.0 hr for ethinyl estradiol) after administration followed by a rapid decline due to distribution and elimination. Although norgestimate serum concentrations following single or multiple dosing were generally below assay detection within 5 hours, a major norgestimate serum metabolite, 17-deacetyl norgestimate, (which exhibits a serum half-life ranging from 12 to 30 hours) appears rapidly in serum with concentrations greatly exceeding that of norgestimate. The 17-deacetylated metabolite is pharmacologically active and the pharmacologic profile is similar to that of norgestimate. The elimination half-life of ethinyl estradiol ranged from approximately 6 to 14 hours.

Both norgestimate and ethinyl estradiol are extensively metabolized and eliminated by renal and fecal pathways. Following administration of ^{14}C-norgestimate, 47% (45–49%) and 37% (16–49%) of the administered radioactivity was eliminated in the urine and feces, respectively. Unchanged

norgestimate was not detected in the urine. In addition to 17-deacetyl norgestimate, a number of metabolites of norgestimate have been identified in human urine following administration of radiolabeled norgestimate. These include 18,19-Dinor-17-pregn-4-en-20-yn-3-one,17-hydroxy-13-ethyl,(17α)-(-);18,19-Dinor-5β-17-pregnan-20-yn,3α,17β-dihydroxy-13-ethyl,(17α), various hydroxylated metabolites and conjugates of these metabolites. Ethinyl estradiol is metabolized to various hydroxylated products and their glucuronide and sulfate conjugates.

INDICATIONS AND USAGE
ORTHO-CYCLEN and ORTHO TRI-CYCLEN Tablets are indicated for the prevention of pregnancy in women who elect to use oral contraceptives as a method of contraception.

ORTHO TRI-CYCLEN is indicated for the treatment of moderate acne vulgaris in females, ≥ 15 years of age, who have no known contraindications to oral contraceptive therapy, desire contraception, have achieved menarche and are unresponsive to topical anti-acne medications.

Oral contraceptives are highly effective. Table I lists the typical accidental pregnancy rates for users of combination oral contraceptives and other methods of contraception. The efficacy of these contraceptive methods, except sterilization, depends upon the reliability with which they are used. Correct and consistent use of methods can result in lower failure rates.

[See table above]

In clinical trials with ORTHO-CYCLEN, 1,651 subjects completed 24,272 cycles and a total of 18 pregnancies were reported. This represents an overall use-efficacy (typical user efficacy) pregnancy rate of 0.96 per 100 women-years. This rate includes patients who did not take the drug correctly.

In four clinical trials with ORTHO TRI-CYCLEN, the use-efficacy pregnancy rate ranged from 0.68 to 1.47 per 100 women-years. In total, 4,756 subjects completed 45,244 cycles and a total of 42 pregnancies were reported. This represents an overall use-efficacy rate of 1.21 per 100 women-years. One of these 4 studies was a randomized comparative clinical trial in which 4,633 subjects completed 22,312 cycles. Of the 2,312 patients on ORTHO TRI-CYCLEN, 8 pregnancies were reported. This represents an overall use-efficacy pregnancy rate of 0.94 per 100 women-years.

In two double-blind, placebo-controlled, six month, multicenter clinical trials, ORTHO TRI-CYCLEN showed a statistically significant decrease in inflammatory lesion count and total lesion count (Table II). The adverse reaction profile of ORTHO TRI-CYCLEN from these two controlled clinical trials is consistent with what has been noted from previous studies involving ORTHO TRI-CYCLEN and are the known risks associated with oral contraceptives.

TABLE II: Acne Vulgaris Indication
Combined Results: Two Multicenter, Placebo-Controlled Trials
Primary Efficacy Variables: Evaluable-for-Efficacy Population

	ORTHO TRI-CYCLEN®	Placebo
	N = 163	N = 161
Mean Age at Enrollment	27.3 years	28.0
Inflammatory Lesions – Mean Percent Reduction	56.6	36.6
Total Lesions – Mean Percent Reduction	49.6	30.3

CONTRAINDICATIONS
Oral contraceptives should not be used in women who currently have the following conditions:
- Thrombophlebitis or thromboembolic disorders
- A past history of deep vein thrombophlebitis or thromboembolic disorders
- Cerebral vascular or coronary artery disease
- Migraine with focal aura
- Known or suspected carcinoma of the breast
- Carcinoma of the endometrium or other known or suspected estrogen dependent neoplasia
- Undiagnosed abnormal genital bleeding
- Cholestatic jaundice of pregnancy or jaundice with prior pill use
- Acute or chronic hepatocellular disease with abnormal liver function

TABLE I: PERCENTAGE OF WOMEN EXPERIENCING AN UNINTENDED PREGNANCY DURING THE FIRST YEAR OF TYPICAL USE AND THE FIRST YEAR OF PERFECT USE OF CONTRACEPTION AND THE PERCENTAGE CONTINUING USE AT THE END OF THE FIRST YEAR, UNITED STATES.

Method (1)	% of Women Experiencing an Unintended Pregnancy within the First Year of Use		% of Women Continuing Use at One Year[3]
	Typical Use[1] (2)	Perfect Use[2] (3)	(4)
Chance[4]	85	85	
Spermicides[5]	26	6	40
Periodic abstinence	25		63
Calendar		9	
Ovulation Method		3	
Sympto-Thermal[6]		2	
Post-Ovulation		1	
Withdrawal	19	4	
Cap[7]			
Parous Women	40	26	42
Nulliparous Women	20	9	56
Sponge			
Parous Women	40	20	42
Nulliparous Women	20	9	56
Diaphragm[7]	20	6	56
Condom[8]			
Female (Reality)	21	5	56
Male	14	3	61
Pill	5		71
Progestin Only		0.5	
Combined		0.1	
IUD			
Progesterone T	2.0	1.5	81
Copper T380A	0.8	0.6	78
LNg 20	0.1	0.1	81
Depo-Provera	0.3	0.3	70
Norplant and Norplant-2	0.05	0.05	88
Female Sterilization	0.5	0.5	100
Male Sterilization	0.15	0.10	100

Adapted from Hatcher et al., 1998 Ref. #1.

[1]Among *typical* couples who initiate use of a method (not necessarily for the first time), the percentage who experience an accidental pregnancy during the first year if they do not stop use for any other reason.

[2]Among couples who initiate use of a method (not necessarily for the first time) and who use it *perfectly* (both consistently and correctly), the percentage who experience an accidental pregnancy during the first year if they do not stop use for any other reason.

[3]Among couples attempting to avoid pregnancy, the percentage who continue to use a method for one year.

[4]The percents becoming pregnant in columns (2) and (3) are based on data from populations where contraception is not used and from women who cease using contraception in order to become pregnant. Among such populations, about 89% become pregnant within one year. This estimate was lowered slightly (to 85%) to represent the percent who would become pregnant within one year among women now relying on reversible methods of contraception if they abandoned contraception altogether.

[5]Foams, creams, gels, vaginal suppositories, and vaginal film.

[6]Cervical mucus (ovulation) method supplemented by calendar in the pre-ovulatory and basal body temperature in the post-ovulatory phases.

[7]With spermicidal cream or jelly.

[8]Without spermicides.

Continued on next page

Ortho Tri-Cyclen—Cont.

- Hepatic adenomas or carcinomas
- Known or suspected pregnancy
- Hypersensitivity to any component of this product

WARNINGS

Cigarette smoking increases the risk of serious cardiovascular side effects from oral contraceptive use. This risk increases with age and with heavy smoking (15 or more cigarettes per day) and is quite marked in women over 35 years of age. Women who use oral contraceptives should be strongly advised not to smoke.

The use of oral contraceptives is associated with increased risks of several serious conditions including myocardial infarction, thromboembolism, stroke, hepatic neoplasia, and gallbladder disease, although the risk of serious morbidity or mortality is very small in healthy women without underlying risk factors. The risk of morbidity and mortality increases significantly in the presence of other underlying risk factors such as hypertension, hyperlipidemias, obesity and diabetes.

Practitioners prescribing oral contraceptives should be familiar with the following information relating to these risks.

The information contained in this package insert is principally based on studies carried out in patients who used oral contraceptives with higher formulations of estrogens and progestogens than those in common use today. The effect of long-term use of the oral contraceptives with lower formulations of both estrogens and progestogens remains to be determined.

Throughout this labeling, epidemiological studies reported are of two types: retrospective or case control studies and prospective or cohort studies. Case control studies provide a measure of the relative risk of a disease, namely, a *ratio* of the incidence of a disease among oral contraceptive users to that among nonusers. The relative risk does not provide information on the actual clinical occurrence of a disease. Cohort studies provide a measure of attributable risk, which is the *difference* in the incidence of disease between oral contraceptive users and nonusers. The attributable risk does provide information about the actual occurrence of a disease in the population (adapted from refs. 2 and 3 with the author's permission). For further information, the reader is referred to a text on epidemiological methods.

1. THROMBOEMBOLIC DISORDERS AND OTHER VASCULAR PROBLEMS

a. Myocardial Infarction

An increased risk of myocardial infarction has been attributed to oral contraceptive use. This risk is primarily in smokers or women with other underlying risk factors for coronary artery disease such as hypertension, hypercholesterolemia, morbid obesity, and diabetes. The relative risk of heart attack for current oral contraceptive users has been estimated to be two to six.[4–10] The risk is very low under the age of 30.

Smoking in combination with oral contraceptive use has been shown to contribute substantially to the incidence of myocardial infarctions in women in their mid-thirties or older with smoking accounting for the majority of excess cases.[11] Mortality rates associated with circulatory disease have been shown to increase substantially in smokers, especially in those 35 years of age and older among women who use oral contraceptives.

CIRCULATORY DISEASE MORTALITY RATES PER 100,000 WOMAN-YEARS BY AGE, SMOKING STATUS AND ORAL CONTRACEPTIVE USE

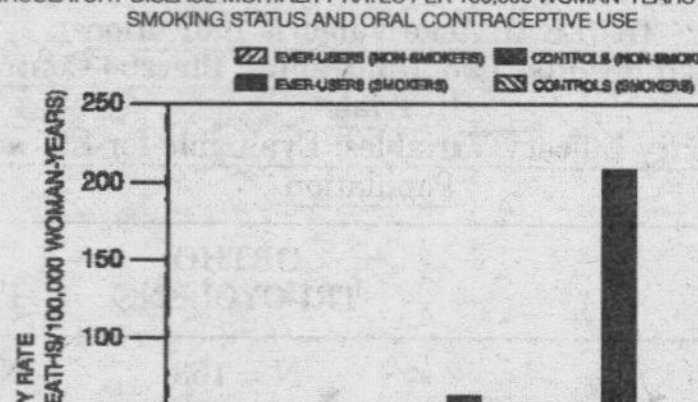

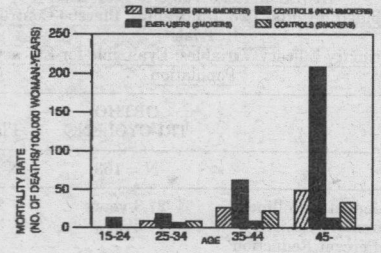

TABLE III. (Adapted from P.M. Layde and V. Beral, ref. #12.)

Oral contraceptives may compound the effects of well-known risk factors, such as hypertension, diabetes, hyperlipidemias, age and obesity.[13] In particular, some progestogens are known to decrease HDL cholesterol and cause glucose intolerance, while estrogens may create a state of hyperinsulinism.[14–18] Oral contraceptives have been shown to increase blood pressure among users (see Section 9 in WARNINGS). Similar effects on risk factors have been associated with an increased risk of heart disease. Oral contraceptives must be used with caution in women with cardiovascular disease risk factors.

Norgestimate has minimal androgenic activity (see CLINICAL PHARMACOLOGY), and there is some evidence that the risk of myocardial infarction associated with oral contraceptives is lower when the progestogen has minimal androgenic activity than when the activity is greater [97].

b. Thromboembolism

An increased risk of thromboembolic and thrombotic disease associated with the use of oral contraceptives is well established. Case control studies have found the relative risk of users compared to nonusers to be 3 for the first episode of superficial venous thrombosis, 4 to 11 for deep vein thrombosis or pulmonary embolism, and 1.5 to 6 for women with predisposing conditions for venous thromboembolic disease.[2,3,19–24] Cohort studies have shown the relative risk to be somewhat lower, about 3 for new cases and about 4.5 for new cases requiring hospitalization.[25] The risk of thromboembolic disease associated with oral contraceptives is not related to length of use and disappears after pill use is stopped.[2]

A two- to four-fold increase in relative risk of post-operative thromboembolic complications has been reported with the use of oral contraceptives.[9] The relative risk of venous thrombosis in women who have predisposing conditions is twice that of women without such medical conditions.[26] If feasible, oral contraceptives should be discontinued at least four weeks prior to and for two weeks after elective surgery of a type associated with an increase in risk of thromboembolism and during and following prolonged immobilization. Since the immediate postpartum period is also associated with an increased risk of thromboembolism, oral contraceptives should be started no earlier than four weeks after delivery in women who elect not to breast feed. After an induced or spontaneous abortion that occurs at or after 20 weeks gestation, hormonal contraceptives may be started either on Day 21 post-abortion or on the first day of the first spontaneous menstruation, whichever comes first [98].

c. Cerebrovascular diseases

Oral contraceptives have been shown to increase both the relative and attributable risks of cerebrovascular events (thrombotic and hemorrhagic strokes), although, in general, the risk is greatest among older (>35 years), hypertensive women who also smoke. Hypertension was found to be a risk factor for both users and nonusers, for both types of strokes, and smoking interacted to increase the risk of stroke.[27–29]

In a large study, the relative risk of thrombotic strokes has been shown to range from 3 for normotensive users to 14 for users with severe hypertension.[30] The relative risk of hemorrhagic stroke is reported to be 1.2 for non-smokers who used oral contraceptives, 2.6 for smokers who did not use oral contraceptives, 7.6 for smokers who used oral contraceptives, 1.8 for normotensive users and 25.7 for users with severe hypertension.[30] The attributable risk is also greater in older women.[3]

d. Dose-related risk of vascular disease from oral contraceptives

A positive association has been observed between the amount of estrogen and progestogen in oral contraceptives and the risk of vascular disease.[31–33] A decline in serum high density lipoproteins (HDL) has been reported with many progestational agents.[14–16] A decline in serum high density lipoproteins has been associated with an increased incidence of ischemic heart disease. Because estrogens increase HDL cholesterol, the net effect of an oral contraceptive depends on a balance achieved between doses of estrogen and progestogen and the activity of the progestogen used in the contraceptives. The activity and amount of both hormones should be considered in the choice of an oral contraceptive.

Minimizing exposure to estrogen and progestogen is in keeping with good principles of therapeutics. For any particular estrogen/progestogen combination, the dosage regimen prescribed should be one which contains the least amount of estrogen and progestogen that is compatible with a low failure rate and the needs of the individual patient. New acceptors of oral contraceptive agents should be started on preparations containing 0.035 mg or less of estrogen.

e. Persistence of risk of vascular disease

There are two studies which have shown persistence of risk of vascular disease for ever-users of oral contraceptives. In a study in the United States, the risk of developing myocardial infarction after discontinuing oral contraceptives persists for at least 9 years for women 40–49 years who had used oral contraceptives for five or more years, but this increased risk was not demonstrated in other age groups.[8] In another study in Great Britain, the risk of developing cerebrovascular disease persisted for at least 6 years after discontinuation of oral contraceptives, although excess risk was very small.[34] However, both studies were performed with oral contraceptive formulations containing 50 micrograms or higher of estrogens.

2. ESTIMATES OF MORTALITY FROM CONTRACEPTIVE USE

One study gathered data from a variety of sources which have estimated the mortality rate associated with different methods of contraception at different ages (Table IV). These estimates include the combined risk of death associated with contraceptive methods plus the risk attributable to pregnancy in the event of method failure. Each method of contraception has its specific benefits and risks. The study concluded that with the exception of oral contraceptive users 35 and older who smoke, and 40 and older who do not smoke, mortality associated with all methods of birth control is low and below that associated with childbirth. The observation of an increase in risk of mortality with age for oral contraceptive users is based on data gathered in the 1970's.[35] Current clinical recommendation involves the use of lower estrogen dose formulations and a careful consideration of risk factors. In 1989, the Fertility and Maternal Health Drugs Advisory Committee was asked to review the use of oral contraceptives in women 40 years of age and over. The Committee concluded that although cardiovascular disease risks may be increased with oral contraceptive use after age 40 in healthy non-smoking women (even with the newer low-dose formulations), there are also greater potential health risks associated with pregnancy in older women and with the alternative surgical and medical procedures which may be necessary if such women do not have access to effective and acceptable means of contraception. The Committee recommended that the benefits of low-dose oral contraceptive use by healthy non-smoking women over 40 may outweigh the possible risks.

Of course, older women, as all women, who take oral contraceptives, should take an oral contraceptive which contains the least amount of estrogen and progestogen that is compatible with a low failure rate and individual patient needs. [See table below]

TABLE IV: ANNUAL NUMBER OF BIRTH-RELATED OR METHOD-RELATED DEATHS ASSOCIATED WITH CONTROL OF FERTILITY PER 100,000 NON-STERILE WOMEN, BY FERTILITY CONTROL METHOD ACCORDING TO AGE

Method of control and outcome	15-19	20-24	25-29	30-34	35-39	40-44
No fertility control methods*	7.0	7.4	9.1	14.8	25.7	28.2
Oral contraceptives non-smoker**	0.3	0.5	0.9	1.9	13.8	31.6
Oral contraceptives smoker**	2.2	3.4	6.6	13.5	51.1	117.2
IUD**	0.8	0.8	1.0	1.0	1.4	1.4
Condom*	1.1	1.6	0.7	0.2	0.3	0.4
Diaphragm/spermicide*	1.9	1.2	1.2	1.3	2.2	2.8
Periodic abstinence*	2.5	1.6	1.6	1.7	2.9	3.6

*Deaths are birth-related
**Deaths are method-related

Adapted from H.W. Ory, ref. #35.

3. CARCINOMA OF THE REPRODUCTIVE ORGANS AND BREASTS

Numerous epidemiological studies have been performed on the incidence of breast, endometrial, ovarian, and cervical cancer in women using oral contraceptives. While there are conflicting reports, most studies suggest that use of oral contraceptives is not associated with an overall increase in the risk of developing breast cancer. Some studies have reported an increased relative risk of developing breast cancer, particularly at a younger age. This increased relative risk has been reported to be related to duration of use.[36–44,79–89]

A meta-analysis of 54 studies found a small increase in the frequency of having breast cancer diagnosed for women who were currently using combined oral contraceptives or had used them within the past ten years. This increase in the frequency of breast cancer diagnosis, within ten years of stopping use, was generally accounted for by cancers localized to the breast. There was no increase in the frequency of having breast cancer diagnosed ten or more years after cessation of use.[95]

Some studies suggest that oral contraceptive use has been associated with an increase in the risk of cervical intraepithelial neoplasia in some populations of women.[45–48] However, there continues to be controversy about the extent to which such findings may be due to differences in sexual behavior and other factors.

4. HEPATIC NEOPLASIA

Benign hepatic adenomas are associated with oral contraceptive use, although the incidence of benign tumors is rare in the United States. Indirect calculations have estimated the attributable risk to be in the range of 3.3 cases/100,000 for users, a risk that increases after four or more years of use especially with oral contraceptives of higher dose.[49] Rupture of benign, hepatic adenomas may cause death through intra-abdominal hemorrhage.[50,51]

Studies have shown an increased risk of developing hepatocellular carcinoma[52–54,96] in oral contraceptive users. However, these cancers are rare in the U.S.

5. OCULAR LESIONS

There have been clinical case reports of retinal thrombosis associated with the use of oral contraceptives. Oral contraceptives should be discontinued if there is unexplained partial or complete loss of vision; onset of proptosis or diplopia; papilledema; or retinal vascular lesions. Appropriate diagnostic and therapeutic measures should be undertaken immediately.

6. ORAL CONTRACEPTIVE USE BEFORE OR DURING EARLY PREGNANCY

Extensive epidemiological studies have revealed no increased risk of birth defects in women who have used oral

contraceptives prior to pregnancy.[56,57] The majority of recent studies also do not indicate a teratogenic effect, particularly in so far as cardiac anomalies and limb reduction defects are concerned,[55,56,58,59] when taken inadvertently during early pregnancy.

The administration of oral contraceptives to induce withdrawal bleeding should not be used as a test for pregnancy. Oral contraceptives should not be used during pregnancy to treat threatened or habitual abortion.

It is recommended that for any patient who has missed two consecutive periods, pregnancy should be ruled out before continuing oral contraceptive use. If the patient has not adhered to the prescribed schedule, the possibility of pregnancy should be considered at the time of the first missed period. Oral contraceptive use should be discontinued until pregnancy is ruled out.

7. GALLBLADDER DISEASE

Earlier studies have reported an increased lifetime relative risk of gallbladder surgery in users of oral contraceptives and estrogens.[60,61] More recent studies, however, have shown that the relative risk of developing gallbladder disease among oral contraceptive users may be minimal.[62-64] The recent findings of minimal risk may be related to the use of oral contraceptive formulations containing lower hormonal doses of estrogens and progestogens.

8. CARBOHYDRATE AND LIPID METABOLIC EFFECTS

Oral contraceptives have been shown to cause a decrease in glucose tolerance in a significant percentage of users.[17] This effect has been shown to be directly related to estrogen dose.[65] Progestogens increase insulin secretion and create insulin resistance, this effect varying with different progestational agents.[17,66] However, in the non-diabetic woman, oral contraceptives appear to have no effect on fasting blood glucose.[67] Because of these demonstrated effects, prediabetic and diabetic women in particular should be carefully monitored while taking oral contraceptives.

A small proportion of women will have persistent hypertriglyceridemia while on the pill. As discussed earlier (see WARNINGS 1a and 1d), changes in serum triglycerides and lipoprotein levels have been reported in oral contraceptive users.

In clinical studies with ORTHO-CYCLEN there were no clinically significant changes in fasting blood glucose levels. No statistically significant changes in mean fasting blood glucose levels were observed over 24 cycles of use. Glucose tolerance tests showed minimal, clinically insignificant changes from baseline to cycles 3, 12, and 24.

In clinical studies with ORTHO TRI-CYCLEN there were no clinically significant changes in fasting blood glucose levels. Minimal statistically significant changes were noted in glucose levels over 24 cycles of use. Glucose tolerance tests showed no clinically significant changes from baseline to cycles 3, 12, and 24.

9. ELEVATED BLOOD PRESSURE

Women with significant hypertension should not be started on hormonal contraception.[98] An increase in blood pressure has been reported in women taking oral contraceptives[68] and this increase is more likely in older oral contraceptive users[69] and with extended duration of use.[61] Data from the Royal College of General Practitioners[12] and subsequent randomized trials have shown that the incidence of hypertension increases with increasing progestational activity. Women with a history of hypertension or hypertension-related diseases, or renal disease[70] should be encouraged to use another method of contraception. If women elect to use oral contraceptives, they should be monitored closely and if significant elevation of blood pressure occurs, oral contraceptives should be discontinued. For most women, elevated blood pressure will return to normal after stopping oral contraceptives, and there is no difference in the occurrence of hypertension between former and never users.[68-71] It should be noted that in two separate large clinical trials (N = 633 and N = 911), no statistically significant changes in mean blood pressure were observed with ORTHO-CYCLEN.

10. HEADACHE

The onset or exacerbation of migraine or development of headache with a new pattern which is recurrent, persistent or severe requires discontinuation of oral contraceptives and evaluation of the cause.

11. BLEEDING IRREGULARITIES

Breakthrough bleeding and spotting are sometimes encountered in patients on oral contraceptives, especially during the first three months of use. Non-hormonal causes should be considered and adequate diagnostic measures taken to rule out malignancy or pregnancy in the event of breakthrough bleeding, as in the case of any abnormal vaginal bleeding. If pathology has been excluded, time or a change to another formulation may solve the problem. In the event of amenorrhea, pregnancy should be ruled out.

Some women may encounter post-pill amenorrhea or oligomenorrhea, especially when such a condition was preexistent.

12. ECTOPIC PREGNANCY

Ectopic as well as intrauterine pregnancy may occur in contraceptive failures.

PRECAUTIONS

1. PHYSICAL EXAMINATION AND FOLLOW UP

It is good medical practice for all women to have annual history and physical examinations, including women using oral contraceptives. The physical examination, however, may be deferred until after initiation of oral contraceptives if requested by the woman and judged appropriate by the clinician. The physical examination should include special reference to blood pressure, breasts, abdomen and pelvic organs, including cervical cytology, and relevant laboratory tests. In case of undiagnosed, persistent or recurrent abnormal vaginal bleeding, appropriate measures should be conducted to rule out malignancy. Women with a strong family history of breast cancer or who have breast nodules should be monitored with particular care.

2. LIPID DISORDERS

Women who are being treated for hyperlipidemias should be followed closely if they elect to use oral contraceptives. Some progestogens may elevate LDL levels and may render the control of hyperlipidemias more difficult.

3. LIVER FUNCTION

If jaundice develops in any woman receiving such drugs, the medication should be discontinued. Steroid hormones may be poorly metabolized in patients with impaired liver function.

4. FLUID RETENTION

Oral contraceptives may cause some degree of fluid retention. They should be prescribed with caution, and only with careful monitoring, in patients with conditions which might be aggravated by fluid retention.

5. EMOTIONAL DISORDERS

Women with a history of depression should be carefully observed and the drug discontinued if depression recurs to a serious degree.

6. CONTACT LENSES

Contact lens wearers who develop visual changes or changes in lens tolerance should be assessed by an ophthalmologist.

7. DRUG INTERACTIONS

Reduced efficacy and increased incidence of breakthrough bleeding and menstrual irregularities have been associated with concomitant use of rifampin. A similar association, though less marked, has been suggested with barbiturates, phenylbutazone, phenytoin sodium, carbamazepine, griseofulvin, topiramate, and possibly with ampicillin and tetracyclines.[72] A possible interaction has been suggested with hormonal contraceptives and the herbal supplement St. Johns Wort based on some reports of oral contraceptive users experiencing breakthrough bleeding shortly after starting St. Johns Wort. Pregnancies have been reported by users of combined hormonal contraceptives who also used some form of St. Johns Wort. Healthcare prescribers are advised to consult the package inserts of medication administered concomitantly with oral contraceptives.

8. INTERACTIONS WITH LABORATORY TESTS

Certain endocrine and liver function tests and blood components may be affected by oral contraceptives:

a. Increased prothrombin and factors VII, VIII, IX, and X; decreased antithrombin 3; increased norepinephrine-induced platelet aggregability.

b. Increased thyroid binding globulin (TBG) leading to increased circulating total thyroid hormone, as measured by protein-bound iodine (PBI), T4 by column or by radioimmunoassay. Free T3 resin uptake is decreased, reflecting the elevated TBG, free T4 concentration is unaltered.

c. Other binding proteins may be elevated in serum.

d. Sex hormone binding globulins are increased and result in elevated levels of total circulating sex steroids; however, free or biologically active levels either decrease or remain unchanged.

e. High-density lipoprotein (HDL-C) and total cholesterol (Total-C) may be increased, low-density lipoprotein (LDL-C) may be increased or decreased, while LDL-C/HDL-C ratio may be decreased and triglycerides may be unchanged.

f. Glucose tolerance may be decreased.

g. Serum folate levels may be depressed by oral contraceptive therapy. This may be of clinical significance if a woman becomes pregnant shortly after discontinuing oral contraceptives.

9. CARCINOGENESIS

See WARNINGS Section.

10. PREGNANCY

Pregnancy Category X. See CONTRAINDICATIONS and WARNINGS Sections.

11. NURSING MOTHERS

Small amounts of oral contraceptive steroids have been identified in the milk of nursing mothers and a few adverse effects on the child have been reported, including jaundice and breast enlargement. In addition, combination oral contraceptives given in the postpartum period may interfere with lactation by decreasing the quantity and quality of breast milk. If possible, the nursing mother should be advised not to use combination oral contraceptives but to use other forms of contraception until she has completely weaned her child.

12. PEDIATRIC USE

Safety and efficacy of ORTHO-CYCLEN Tablets and ORTHO TRI-CYCLEN Tablets have been established in women of reproductive age. Safety and efficacy are expected to be the same for postpubertal adolescents under the age of 16 and for users 16 years and older. Use of this product before menarche is not indicated.

13. SEXUALLY TRANSMITTED DISEASES

Patients should be counseled that this product does not protect against HIV infection (AIDS) and other sexually transmitted diseases.

INFORMATION FOR THE PATIENT

See Patient Labeling printed below.

ADVERSE REACTIONS

An increased risk of the following serious adverse reactions has been associated with the use of oral contraceptives (See WARNINGS Section).

- Thrombophlebitis and venous thrombosis with or without embolism
- Arterial thromboembolism
- Pulmonary embolism
- Myocardial infarction
- Cerebral hemorrhage
- Cerebral thrombosis
- Hypertension
- Gallbladder disease
- Hepatic adenomas or benign liver tumors

The following adverse reactions have been reported in patients receiving oral contraceptives and are believed to be drug-related:

- Nausea
- Vomiting
- Gastrointestinal symptoms (such as abdominal cramps and bloating)
- Breakthrough bleeding
- Spotting
- Change in menstrual flow
- Amenorrhea
- Temporary infertility after discontinuation of treatment
- Edema
- Melasma which may persist
- Breast changes: tenderness, enlargement, secretion
- Change in weight (increase or decrease)
- Change in cervical erosion and secretion
- Diminution in lactation when given immediately postpartum
- Cholestatic jaundice
- Migraine
- Rash (allergic)
- Mental depression
- Reduced tolerance to carbohydrates
- Vaginal candidiasis
- Change in corneal curvature (steepening)
- Intolerance to contact lenses

The following adverse reactions have been reported in users of oral contraceptives and the association has been neither confirmed nor refuted:

- Pre-menstrual syndrome
- Cataracts
- Changes in appetite
- Cystitis-like syndrome
- Headache
- Nervousness
- Dizziness
- Hirsutism
- Loss of scalp hair
- Erythema multiforme
- Erythema nodosum
- Hemorrhagic eruption
- Vaginitis
- Porphyria
- Impaired renal function
- Hemolytic uremic syndrome
- Acne
- Changes in libido
- Colitis
- Budd-Chiari Syndrome

OVERDOSAGE

Serious ill effects have not been reported following acute ingestion of large doses of oral contraceptives by young children. Overdosage may cause nausea and withdrawal bleeding may occur in females.

NON-CONTRACEPTIVE HEALTH BENEFITS

The following non-contraceptive health benefits related to the use of combination oral contraceptives are supported by epidemiological studies which largely utilized oral contraceptive formulations containing estrogen doses exceeding 0.035 mg of ethinyl estradiol or 0.05 mg mestranol.[73-78]

Effects on menses:

- increased menstrual cycle regularity
- decreased blood loss and decreased incidence of iron deficiency anemia
- decreased incidence of dysmenorrhea

Effects related to inhibition of ovulation:

- decreased incidence of functional ovarian cysts
- decreased incidence of ectopic pregnancies

Other effects:

- decreased incidence of fibroadenomas and fibrocystic disease of the breast
- decreased incidence of acute pelvic inflammatory disease
- decreased incidence of endometrial cancer
- decreased incidence of ovarian cancer

DOSAGE AND ADMINISTRATION

ORAL CONTRACEPTION

To achieve maximum contraceptive effectiveness, ORTHO TRI-CYCLEN Tablets and ORTHO-CYCLEN Tablets must be taken exactly as directed and at intervals not exceeding 24 hours. ORTHO TRI-CYCLEN and ORTHO-CYCLEN are available in the DIALPAK® Tablet Dispenser which is preset for a Sunday Start. Day 1 Start is also provided.

21-Day Regimen (Sunday Start)

When taking ORTHO TRI-CYCLEN □ 21 and ORTHO-CYCLEN □ 21, the first tablet should be taken on the first Sunday after menstruation begins. If period begins

Continued on next page

Ortho Tri-Cyclen—Cont.

on Sunday, the first tablet is taken on that day. One tablet is taken daily for 21 days. For subsequent cycles, no tablets are taken for 7 days, then a tablet is taken the next day (Sunday). For the first cycle of a Sunday Start regimen, another method of contraception should be used until after the first 7 consecutive days of administration.

If the patient misses one (1) active tablet in Weeks 1, 2, or 3, the tablet should be taken as soon as she remembers. If the patient misses two (2) active tablets in Week 1 or Week 2, the patient should take two (2) tablets the day she remembers and two (2) tablets the next day; and then continue taking one (1) tablet a day until she finishes the pack. The patient should be instructed to use a back-up method of birth control if she has sex in the seven (7) days after missing pills. If the patient misses two (2) active tablets in the third week or misses three (3) or more active tablets in a row, the patient should continue taking one tablet every day until Sunday. On Sunday the patient should throw out the rest of the pack and start a new pack that same day. The patient should be instructed to use a back-up method of birth control if she has sex in the seven (7) days after missing pills.

Complete instructions to facilitate patient counseling on proper pill usage may be found in the Detailed Patient Labeling ("How to Take the Pill" section).

21-Day Regimen (Day 1 Start)

The dosage of ORTHO TRI-CYCLEN □ 21 and ORTHO-CYCLEN □ 21, for the initial cycle of therapy is one tablet administered daily from the 1st day through the 21st day of the menstrual cycle, counting the first day of menstrual flow as "Day 1." For subsequent cycles, no tablets are taken for 7 days, then a new course is started of one tablet a day for 21 days. The dosage regimen then continues with 7 days of no medication, followed by 21 days of medication, instituting a three-weeks-on, one-week-off dosage regimen.

If the patient misses one (1) active tablet in Weeks 1, 2, or 3, the tablet should be taken as soon as she remembers. If the patient misses two (2) active tablets in Week 1 or Week 2, the patient should take two (2) tablets the day she remembers and two (2) tablets the next day; and then continue taking one (1) tablet a day until she finishes the pack. The patient should be instructed to use a back-up method of birth control if she has sex in the seven (7) days after missing pills. If the patient misses two (2) active tablets in the third week or misses three (3) or more active tablets in a row, the patient should throw out the rest of the pack and start a new pack that same day. The patient should be instructed to use a back-up method of birth control if she has sex in the seven (7) days after missing pills.

Complete instructions to facilitate patient counseling on proper pill usage may be found in the Detailed Patient Labeling ("How to Take the Pill" section).

28-Day Regimen (Sunday Start)

When taking ORTHO TRI-CYCLEN □ 28 and ORTHO-CYCLEN □ 28 the first tablet should be taken on the first Sunday after menstruation begins. If period begins on Sunday, the first tablet should be taken that day. Take one active tablet daily for 21 days followed by one green tablet daily for 7 days. After 28 tablets have been taken, a new course is started the next day (Sunday). For the first cycle of a Sunday Start regimen, another method of contraception should be used until after the first 7 consecutive days of administration.

If the patient misses one (1) active tablet in Weeks 1, 2, or 3, the tablet should be taken as soon as she remembers. If the patient misses two (2) active tablets in Week 1 or Week 2, the patient should take two (2) tablets the day she remembers and two (2) tablets the next day; and then continue taking one (1) tablet a day until she finishes the pack. The patient should be instructed to use a back-up method of birth control if she has sex in the seven (7) days after missing pills. If the patient misses two (2) active tablets in the third week or misses three (3) or more active tablets in a row, the patient should continue taking one tablet every day until Sunday. On Sunday the patient should throw out the rest of the pack and start a new pack that same day. The patient should be instructed to use a back-up method of birth control if she has sex in the seven (7) days after missing pills.

Complete instructions to facilitate patient counseling on proper pill usage may be found in the Detailed Patient Labeling ("How to Take the Pill" section).

28-Day Regimen (Day 1 Start)

The dosage of ORTHO TRI-CYCLEN □ 28 and ORTHO-CYCLEN □ 28, for the initial cycle of therapy is one active tablet administered daily from the 1st day through the 21st day of the menstrual cycle, counting the first day of menstrual flow as "Day 1" followed by one green tablet daily for 7 days. Tablets are taken without interruption for 28 days. After 28 tablets have been taken, a new course is started the next day.

If the patient misses one (1) active tablet in Weeks 1, 2, or 3, the tablet should be taken as soon as she remembers. If the patient misses two (2) active tablets in Week 1 or Week 2, the patient should take two (2) tablets the day she remembers and two (2) tablets the next day; and then continue taking one (1) tablet a day until she finishes the pack. The patient should be instructed to use a back-up method of birth control if she has sex in the seven (7) days after missing pills. If the patient misses two (2) active tablets in the third week or misses three (3) or more active tablets in a row, the patient should throw out the rest of the pack and start a new pack that same day. The patient should be instructed to use a back-up method of birth control if she has sex in the seven (7) days after missing pills.

Complete instructions to facilitate patient counseling on proper pill usage may be found in the Detailed Patient Labeling ("How to Take the Pill" section).

The use of ORTHO TRI-CYCLEN and ORTHO-CYCLEN for contraception may be initiated 4 weeks postpartum in women who elect not to breast feed. When the tablets are administered during the postpartum period, the increased risk of thromboembolic disease associated with the postpartum period must be considered. (See CONTRAINDICATIONS and WARNINGS concerning thromboembolic disease. See also PRECAUTIONS for "Nursing Mothers.") The possibility of ovulation and conception prior to initiation of medication should be considered.

(See Discussion of Dose-Related Risk of Vascular Disease from Oral Contraceptives.)

ADDITIONAL INSTRUCTIONS FOR ALL DOSING REGIMENS

Breakthrough bleeding, spotting, and amenorrhea are frequent reasons for patients discontinuing oral contraceptives. In breakthrough bleeding, as in all cases of irregular bleeding from the vagina, nonfunctional causes should be borne in mind. In undiagnosed persistent or recurrent abnormal bleeding from the vagina, adequate diagnostic measures are indicated to rule out pregnancy or malignancy. If pathology has been excluded, time or a change to another formulation may solve the problem. Changing to an oral contraceptive with a higher estrogen content, while potentially useful in minimizing menstrual irregularity, should be done only if necessary since this may increase the risk of thromboembolic disease.

Use of oral contraceptives in the event of a missed menstrual period:

1. If the patient has not adhered to the prescribed schedule, the possibility of pregnancy should be considered at the time of the first missed period and oral contraceptive use should be discontinued and a non-hormonal method should be used until pregnancy is ruled out.
2. If the patient has adhered to the prescribed regimen and misses two consecutive periods, pregnancy should be ruled out before continuing oral contraceptive use.

ACNE

The timing of initiation of dosing with ORTHO TRI-CYCLEN for acne should follow the guidelines for use of ORTHO TRI-CYCLEN as an oral contraceptive. **Consult the DOSAGE AND ADMINISTRATION section for oral contraceptives.** The dosage regimen for ORTHO TRI-CYCLEN for treatment of facial acne, as available in a DIALPAK® Tablet Dispenser, utilizes a 21-day active and a 7-day placebo schedule. Take one active tablet daily for 21 days followed by one green tablet for 7 days. After 28 tablets have been taken, a new course is started the next day.

HOW SUPPLIED

ORTHO TRI-CYCLEN □ 21 Tablets are available in a DIALPAK® Tablet Dispenser (NDC 0062-1902-15) containing 21 tablets. Each white tablet contains 0.180 mg of the progestational compound, norgestimate, together with 0.035 mg of the estrogenic compound, ethinyl estradiol. Each light blue tablet contains 0.215 mg of the progestational compound, norgestimate, together with 0.035 mg of the estrogenic compound, ethinyl estradiol. Each blue tablet contains 0.250 mg of the progestational compound, norgestimate, together with 0.035 mg of the estrogenic compound, ethinyl estradiol.

The white tablets are unscored, with "Ortho" and "180" debossed on each side; the light blue tablets are unscored with "Ortho" and "215" debossed on each side; the blue tablets are unscored with "Ortho" and "250" debossed on each side.

ORTHO TRI-CYCLEN □ 28 Tablets are available in a DIALPAK® Tablet Dispenser (NDC 0062-1903-15) containing 28 tablets. Each white tablet contains 0.180 mg of the progestational compound, norgestimate, together with 0.035 mg of the estrogenic compound, ethinyl estradiol. Each light blue tablet contains 0.215 mg of the progestational compound, norgestimate, together with 0.035 mg of the estrogenic compound, ethinyl estradiol. Each blue tablet contains 0.250 mg of the progestational compound, norgestimate, together with 0.035 mg of the estrogenic compound, ethinyl estradiol. Each green tablet contains inert ingredients.

The white tablets are unscored, with "Ortho" and "180" debossed on each side; the light blue tablets are unscored with "Ortho" and "215" debossed on each side; the blue tablets are unscored with "Ortho" and "250" debossed on each side.

ORTHO TRI-CYCLEN □ 28 Tablets are available for clinic usage in a VERIDATE® Tablet Dispenser (unfilled) and VERIDATE Refills (NDC 0062-1903-20).

ORTHO-CYCLEN □ 21 Tablets are available in a DIALPAK® Tablet Dispenser (NDC 0062-1900-15) containing 21 tablets. Each blue tablet contains 0.250 mg of the progestational compound, norgestimate, together with 0.035 mg of the estrogenic compound, ethinyl estradiol which are unscored with "Ortho" and "250" debossed on each side.

ORTHO-CYCLEN □ 28 Tablets are available in a DIALPAK® Tablet Dispenser (NDC 0062-1901-15) containing 28 tablets as follows: 21 blue tablets as described under ORTHO-CYCLEN □ 21 Tablets, and 7 green tablets containing inert ingredients.

ORTHO-CYCLEN □ 28 Tablets are available for clinic usage in a VERIDATE® Tablet Dispenser (unfilled) and VERIDATE Refills (NDC 0062-1901-20).

℞ only

REFERENCES

1. Trussel J. Contraceptive efficacy. In Hatcher RA, Trussel J, Stewart F, Cates W, Stewart GK, Kowal D, Guest F, Contraceptive Technology: Seventeenth Revised Edition. New York NY: Irvington Publishers, 1998, in press. **2.** Stadel BV, Oral contraceptives and cardiovascular disease. (Pt. 1). N Engl J Med 1981; 305:612–618. **3.** Stadel BV, Oral contraceptives and cardiovascular disease. (Pt. 2). N Engl J Med 1981; 305:672–677. **4.** Adam SA, Thorogood M. Oral contraception and myocardial infarction revisited: the effects of new preparations and prescribing patterns. Br J Obstet Gynaecol 1981; 88:838–845. **5.** Mann JI, Inman WH. Oral contraceptives and death from myocardial infarction. Br Med J 1975; 2(5965):245–248. **6.** Mann JI, Vessey MP, Thorogood M, Doll R. Myocardial infarction in young women with special reference to oral contraceptive practice. Br Med J 1975; 2(5956):241–245. **7.** Royal College of General Practitioners' Oral Contraception Study: further analyses of mortality in oral contraceptive users. Lancet 1981; 1:541–546. **8.** Slone D, Shapiro S, Kaufman DW, Rosenberg L, Miettinen OS, Stolley PD. Risk of myocardial infarction in relation to current and discontinued use of oral contraceptives. N Engl J Med 1981; 305:420–424. **9.** Vessey MP. Female hormones and vascular disease—an epidemiological overview. Br J Fam Plann 1980; 6 (Supplement): 1–12. **10.** Russell-Briefel RG, Ezzati TM, Fulwood R, Perlman JA, Murphy RS. Cardiovascular risk status and oral contraceptive use, United States, 1976-80. Prevent Med 1986; 15:352–362. **11.** Goldbaum GM, Kendrick JS, Hogelin GC, Gentry EM. The relative impact of smoking and oral contraceptive use on women in the United States. JAMA 1987; 258:1339–1342. **12.** Layde PM, Beral V. Further analyses of mortality in oral contraceptive users: Royal College of General Practitioners' Oral Contraception Study. (Table 5) Lancet 1981; 1:541–546. **13.** Knopp RH. Arteriosclerosis risk: the roles of oral contraceptives and postmenopausal estrogens. J Reprod Med 1986; 31(9)(Supplement): 913–921. **14.** Krauss RM, Roy S, Mishell DR, Casagrande J, Pike MC. Effects of two low-dose oral contraceptives on serum lipids and lipoproteins: Differential changes in high-density lipoprotein subclasses. Am J Obstet 1983; 145:446–452. **15.** Wahl P, Walden C, Knopp R, Hoover J, Wallace R, Heiss G, Rifkind B. Effect of estrogen/progestin potency on lipid/lipoprotein cholesterol. N Engl J Med 1983; 308:862–867. **16.** Wynn V, Niththyananthan R. The effect of progestin in combined oral contraceptives on serum lipids with special reference to high density lipoproteins. Am J Obstet Gynecol 1982; 142:766–771. **17.** Wynn V, Godsland I. Effects of oral contraceptives on carbohydrate metabolism. J Reprod Med 1986; 31(9)(Supplement):892–897. **18.** LaRosa JC. Atherosclerotic risk factors in cardiovascular disease. J Reprod Med 1986; 31(9)(Supplement): 906–912. **19.** Inman WH, Vessey MP. Investigation of death from pulmonary, coronary, and cerebral thrombosis and embolism in women of child-bearing age. Br Med J 1968; 2(5599):193–199. **20.** Maguire MG, Tonascia J, Sartwell PE, Stolley PD, Tockman MS. Increased risk of thrombosis due to oral contraceptives: a further report. Am J Epidemiol 1979; 110(2):188–195. **21.** Petitti DB, Wingerd J, Pellegrin F, Ramacharan S. Risk of vascular disease in women: smoking, oral contraceptives, noncontraceptive estrogens, and other factors. JAMA 1979; 242:1150–1154. **22.** Vessey MP, Doll R. Investigation of relation between use of oral contraceptives and thromboembolic disease. Br Med J 1968; 2(5599):199–205. **23.** Vessey MP, Doll R. Investigation of relation between use of oral contraceptives and thromboembolic disease. A further report. Br Med J 1969; 2(5658):651–657. **24.** Porter JB, Hunter JR, Danielson DA, Jick H, Stergachis A. Oral contraceptives and non-fatal vascular disease—recent experience. Obstet Gynecol 1982; 59(3):299–302. **25.** Vessey M, Doll R, Peto R, Johnson B, Wiggins P. A long-term follow-up study of women using different methods of contraception: an interim report. J Biosocial Sci 1976; 8:375–427. **26.** Royal College of General Practitioners: Oral Contraceptives, venous thrombosis, and varicose veins. J Royal Coll Gen Pract 1978; 28:393–399. **27.** Collaborative Group for the Study of Stroke in Young Women: Oral contraception and increased risk of cerebral ischemia or thrombosis. N Engl J Med 1973; 288:871–878. **28.** Petitti DB, Wingerd J. Use of oral contraceptives, cigarette smoking, and risk of subarachnoid hemorrhage. Lancet 1978; 2:234–236. **29.** Inman WH. Oral contraceptives and fatal subarachnoid hemorrhage. Br Med J 1979; 2(6203):1468–1470. **30.** Collaborative Group for the Study of Stroke in Young Women: Oral Contraceptives and stroke in young women: associated risk factors. JAMA 1975; 231:718–722. **31.** Inman WH, Vessey MP, Westerholm B, Engelund A. Thromboembolic disease and the steroidal content of oral contraceptives. A report to the Committee on Safety of Drugs. Br Med J 1970; 2:203–209. **32.** Meade TW, Greenberg G, Thompson SG. Progestogens and cardiovascular reactions associated with oral contraceptives and a comparison of the safety of 50- and 35-mcg oestrogen preparations. Br Med J 1980; 280(6224):1157–1161. **33.** Kay CR. Progestogens and arterial disease—evidence from the Royal College of General Practitioners' Study. Am J Obstet Gynecol 1982; 142:762–765. **34.** Royal College of General Practitioners: Incidence of arterial disease among oral contraceptive users. J Royal Coll Gen Pract 1983; 33:75–82. **35.** Ory HW. Mortality associated with fertility and fertility control: 1983. Family Planning Perspectives 1983; 15:50–56. **36.** The Cancer and Steroid Hormone Study of the Centers for Disease Control and the National Institute of Child Health and Human Development: Oral contraceptive use and the risk of breast cancer. N Engl J Med 1986; 315:405–411. **37.** Pike MC, Henderson BE, Krailo MD, Duke A, Roy S. Breast cancer in young women and use of oral contraceptives: possible modifying effect of formulation and age at use. Lancet 1983; 2:926–929. **38.** Paul C, Skegg DG, Spears GFS, Kaldor JM. Oral contraceptives and breast cancer: A national study. Br Med J 1986; 293:723–725. **39.** Miller DR, Rosenberg L, Kaufman DW, Schottenfeld D, Stolley PD, Shapiro S. Breast cancer risk in relation to early oral contraceptive use. Obstet Gynecol 1986; 68:863–868. **40.** Olsson H, Olsson ML, Moller TR, Ranstam J, Holm P. Oral contraceptive use and breast cancer in young women in Sweden (letter). Lancet 1985; 1(8431):748–749. **41.** McPherson K, Vessey M, Neil A, Doll R, Jones L, Roberts M. Early contraceptive use and breast cancer: Results of another case-control study. Br J Cancer 1987; 56:653–660. **42.** Huggins GR, Zucker PF. Oral contraceptives and neoplasia: 1987 update. Fertil Steril 1987; 47:733–761. **43.** McPherson K, Drife JO. The pill and breast cancer: why the uncertainty? Br Med J 1986; 293:709–710. **44.** Shapiro S. Oral contraceptives—time to take stock. N Engl J Med 1987; 315:450–451. **45.** Ory H, Naib Z, Conger SB, Hatcher RA, Tyler CW. Contraceptive choice and prevalence of cervical dysplasia and carcinoma in situ. Am J Obstet Gynecol 1976; 124:573–577. **46.** Vessey MP, Lawless M, McPherson K, Yeates D. Neoplasia of the cervix uteri and contraception: a possible adverse effect of the pill. Lancet 1983; 2:930. **47.** Brinton LA, Huggins GR, Lehman HF, Malli K, Savitz DA, Trapido E, Rosenthal J, Hoover R. Long term use of oral contraceptives and risk of invasive cervical cancer. Int J Cancer 1986; 38:339–344. **48.** WHO Collaborative Study of Neoplasia and Steroid Contraceptives: Invasive cervical cancer and combined oral contraceptives. Br Med J 1985; 290:961–965. **49.** Rooks JB, Ory HW, Ishak KG, Strauss LT, Greenspan JR, Hill AP, Tyler CW. Epidemiology of hepatocellular adenoma: the role of oral contraceptive use. JAMA 1979; 242:644–648. **50.** Bein NN, Goldsmith HS. Recurrent massive hemorrhage from benign hepatic tumors secondary to oral contraceptives. Br J Surg 1977; 64:433–435. **51.** Klatskin G. Hepatic tumors: possible relationship to use of oral contraceptives. Gastroenterology 1977; 73:386–394. **52.** Henderson BE, Preston-Martin S, Edmondson HA, Peters RL, Pike MC. Hepatocellular carcinoma and oral contraceptives. Br J Cancer 1983; 48:437–440. **53.** Neuberger J, Forman D, Doll R, Williams R. Oral contraceptives and hepatocellular carcinoma. Br Med J 1986; 292:1355–1357. **54.** Forman D, Vincent TJ, Doll R. Cancer of the liver and oral contraceptives. Br Med J 1986; 292:1357–1361. **55.** Harlap S, Eldor J. Births following oral contraceptive failures. Obstet Gynecol 1980; 55:447–452. **56.** Savolainen E, Saksela E, Saxen L. Teratogenic hazards of oral contraceptives analyzed in a national malformation register. Am J Obstet Gynecol 1981; 140:521–524. **57.** Janerich DT, Piper JM, Glebatis DM. Oral contraceptives and birth defects. Am J Epidemiol 1980; 112:73–79. **58.** Ferencz C, Matanoski GM, Wilson PD, Rubin JD, Neill CA, Gutberlet R. Maternal hormone therapy and congenital heart disease. Teratology 1980; 21:225–239. **59.** Rothman KJ, Fyler DC, Goldblatt A, Kreidberg MB. Exogenous hormones and other drug exposures of children with congenital heart disease. Am J Epidemiol 1979; 109:433–439. **60.** Boston Collaborative Drug Surveillance Program: Oral contraceptives and venous thromboembolic disease, surgically confirmed gallbladder disease, and breast tumors. Lancet 1973; 1:1399–1404. **61.** Royal College of General Practitioners: Oral contraceptives and health. New York, Pittman 1974. **62.** Layde PM, Vessey MP, Yeates D. Risk of gallbladder disease: a cohort study of young women attending family planning clinics. J Epidemiol Community Health 1982; 36:274–278. **63.** Rome Group for Epidemiology and Prevention of Cholelithiasis (GREPCO): Prevalence of gallstone disease in an Italian adult female population. Am J Epidemiol 1984; 119:796–805. **64.** Storm BL, Tamragouri RT, Morse ML, Lazar EL, West SL, Stolley PD, Jones JK. Oral contraceptives and other risk factors for gallbladder disease. Clin Pharmacol Ther 1986; 39:335–341. **65.** Wynn V, Adams PW, Godsland IF, Melrose J, Niththyananthan R, Oakley NW, Seedj A. Comparison of effects of different combined oral contraceptive formulations on carbohydrate and lipid metabolism. Lancet 1979; 1:1045–1049. **66.** Wynn V. Effect of progesterone and progestins on carbohydrate metabolism. In: Progesterone and Progestin. Bardin CW, Milgrom E, Mauvis-Jarvis P. eds. New York, Raven Press 1983; pp. 395–410. **67.** Perlman JA, Roussell-Briefel RG, Ezzati TM, Lieberknecht G. Oral glucose tolerance and the potency of oral contraceptive progestogens. J Chronic Dis 1985; 38:857–864. **68.** Royal College of General Practitioners' Oral Contraception Study: Effect on hypertension and benign breast disease of progestogen component in combined oral contraceptives. Lancet 1977; 1:624. **69.** Fisch IR, Frank J. Oral contraceptives and blood pressure. JAMA 1977; 237:2499–2503. **70.** Laragh AJ. Oral contraceptive induced hypertension—nine years later. Am J Obstet Gynecol 1976; 126:141–147. **71.** Ramcharan S, Peritz E, Pellegrin FA, Williams WT. Incidence of hypertension in the Walnut Creek Contraceptive Drug Study cohort: In: Pharmacology of steroid contraceptive drugs. Garattini S, Berendes HW. eds. New York, Raven Press, 1977; pp. 277–288, (Monographs of the Mario Negri Institute for Pharmacological Research Milan.) **72.** Stockley I. Interactions with oral contraceptives. J Pharm 1976; 216:140–143. **73.** The Cancer and Steroid Hormone Study of the Centers for Disease Control and the National Institute of Child Health and Human Development: Oral contraceptive use and the risk of ovarian cancer. JAMA 1983; 249:1596–1599. **74.** The Cancer and Steroid Hormone Study of the Centers for Disease Control and the National Institute of Child Health and Human Development: Combination oral contraceptive use and the risk of endometrial cancer. JAMA 1987; 257:796–800. **75.** Ory HW. Functional ovarian cysts and oral contraceptives: negative association confirmed surgically. JAMA 1974; 228:68–69. **76.** Ory HW, Cole P, MacMahon B, Hoover R. Oral contraceptives and reduced risk of benign breast disease. N Engl J Med 1976; 294:419–422. **77.** Ory HW. The noncontraceptive health benefits from oral contraceptive use. Fam Plann Perspect 1982; 14:182–184. **78.** Ory HW, Forrest JD, Lincoln R. Making choices: evaluating the health risks and benefits of birth control methods. New York, The Alan Guttmacher Institute, 1983; p. 1. **79.** Schlesselman J, Stadel BV, Murray P, Lai S. Breast cancer in relation to early use of oral contraceptives. JAMA 1988; 259:1828–1833. **80.** Hennekens CH, Speizer FE, Lipnick RJ, Rosner B, Bain C, Belanger C, Stampfer MJ, Willett W, Peto R. A case-control study of oral contraceptive use and breast cancer. JNCI 1984; 72:39–42. **81.** LaVecchia C, Decarli A, Fasoli M, Franceschi S, Gentile A, Negri E, Parazzini F, Tognoni G. Oral contraceptives and cancers of the breast and of the female genital tract. Interim results from a case-control study. Br J Cancer 1986; 54:311–317. **82.** Meirik O, Lund E, Adami H, Bergstrom R, Christoffersen T, Bergsjo P. Oral contraceptive use and breast cancer in young women. A Joint National Case-control study in Sweden and Norway. Lancet 1986; 11:650–654. **83.** Kay CR, Hannaford PC. Breast cancer and the pill—A further report from the Royal College of General Practitioners' oral contraception study. Br J Cancer 1988; 58:675–680. **84.** Stadel BV, Lai S, Schlesselman JJ, Murray P. Oral contraceptives and premenopausal breast cancer in nulliparous women. Contraception 1988; 38:287–299. **85.** Miller DR, Rosenberg , Kaufman DW, Stolley P, Warshauer ME, Shapiro S. Breast cancer before age 45 and oral contraceptive use: New findings. Am J Epidemiol 1989; 129:269–280. **86.** The UK National Case-Control Study Group, Oral contraceptive use and breast cancer risk in young women. Lancet 1989; 1:973–982. **87.** Schlesselman JJ. Cancer of the breast and reproductive tract in relation to use of oral contraceptives. Contraception 1989; 40:1–38. **88.** Vessey MP, McPherson K, Villard-Mackintosh L, Yeates D. Oral contraceptives and breast cancer: latest findings in a large cohort study. Br J Cancer 1989; 59:613–617. **89.** Jick SS, Walker AM, Stergachis A, Jick H. Oral contraceptives and breast cancer. Br J Cancer 1989; 59:618–621. **90.** Anderson FD. Selectivity and minimal androgenicity of norgestimate in monophasic and triphasic oral contraceptives. Acta Obstet Gynecol Scand 1992; 156 (Supplement):15–21. **91.** Chapdelaine A, Desmaris J-L, Derman RJ. Clinical evidence of minimal androgenic activity of norgestimate. Int J Fertil 1989; 34(51):347–352. **92.** Phillips A, Demarest K, Hahn DW, Wong F, McGuire JL. Progestational and androgenic receptor binding affinities and in vivo activities of norgestimate and other progestins. Contraception 1989; 41(4):399–409. **93.** Phillips A, Hahn DW, Klimek S, McGuire JL. A comparison of the potencies and activities of progestogens used in contraceptives. Contraception 1987; 36(2):181–192. **94.** Janaud A, Rouffy J, Upmalis D, Dain M-P. A comparison study of lipid and androgen metabolism with triphasic oral contraceptive formulations containing norgestimate or levonorgestrel. Acta Obstet Gynecol Scand 1992; 156 (Supplement):34–38. **95.** Collaborative Group on Hormonal Factors in Breast Cancer. Breast cancer and hormonal contraceptives: collaborative reanalysis of individual data on 53 297 women with breast cancer and 100 239 women without breast cancer from 54 epidemiological studies. Lancet 1996; 347:1713–1727. **96.** Palmer JR, Rosenberg L, Kaufman DW, Warshauer ME, Stolley P, Shapiro S. Oral Contraceptive Use and Liver Cancer. Am J Epidemiol 1989; 130:878–882. **97.** Lewis M, Spitzer WO, Heinemann LAJ, MacRae KD, Bruppacher R, Thorogood M, on behalf of Transnational Research Group on Oral Contraceptives and Health of Young Women. Third generation oral contraceptives and risk of myocardial infarction: an international case-control study. Br Med J 1996;312:88–90. **98.** Improving access to quality care in family planning: Medical eligibility criteria for contraceptive use. Geneva, WHO, Family and Reproductive Health, 1996.

BRIEF SUMMARY PATIENT PACKAGE INSERT

Oral contraceptives, also known as "birth control pills" or "the pill," are taken to prevent pregnancy. ORTHO TRI-CYCLEN may also be taken to treat moderate acne in females who are able to use the pill. When taken correctly to prevent pregnancy, oral contraceptives have a failure rate of less than 1% per year when used without missing any pills. The typical failure rate of large numbers of pill users is 5% per year when women who miss pills are included. For most women oral contraceptives are also free of serious or unpleasant side effects. However, forgetting to take pills considerably increases the chances of pregnancy. For the majority of women, oral contraceptives can be taken safely. But there are some women who are at high risk of developing certain serious diseases that can be fatal or may cause temporary or permanent disability. The risks associated with taking oral contraceptives increase significantly if you:

- smoke
- have high blood pressure, diabetes, high cholesterol
- have or have had clotting disorders, heart attack, stroke, angina pectoris, cancer of the breast or sex organs, jaundice or malignant or benign liver tumors.

Although cardiovascular disease risks may be increased with oral contraceptive use after age 40 in healthy, non-smoking women (even with the newer low-dose formulations), there are also greater potential health risks associated with pregnancy in older women.

You should not take the pill if you suspect you are pregnant or have unexplained vaginal bleeding.

Cigarette smoking increases the risk of serious cardiovascular side effects from oral contraceptive use. This risk increases with age and with heavy smoking (15 or more cigarettes per day) and is quite marked in women over 35 years of age. Women who use oral contraceptives are strongly advised not to smoke.

Most side effects of the pill are not serious. The most common such effects are nausea, vomiting, bleeding between menstrual periods, weight gain, breast tenderness, and difficulty wearing contact lenses. These side effects, especially nausea and vomiting, may subside within the first three months of use.

The serious side effects of the pill occur very infrequently, especially if you are in good health and are young. However, you should know that the following medical conditions have been associated with or made worse by the pill:

1. Blood clots in the legs (thrombophlebitis), lungs (pulmonary embolism), stoppage or rupture of a blood vessel in the brain (stroke), blockage of blood vessels in the heart (heart attack or angina pectoris) or other organs of the body. As mentioned above, smoking increases the risk of heart attacks and strokes and subsequent serious medical consequences.
2. In rare cases, oral contraceptives can cause benign but dangerous liver tumors. These benign liver tumors can rupture and cause fatal internal bleeding. In addition, some studies report an increased risk of developing liver cancer. However, liver cancers are rare.
3. High blood pressure, although blood pressure usually returns to normal when the pill is stopped.

The symptoms associated with these serious side effects are discussed in the detailed leaflet given to you with your supply of pills. Notify your doctor or health care provider if you notice any unusual physical disturbances while taking the pill. In addition, drugs such as rifampin, as well as some anticonvulsants and some antibiotics may decrease oral contraceptive effectiveness.

There is conflict among studies regarding breast cancer and oral contraceptive use. Some studies have reported an increase in the risk of developing breast cancer, particularly at a younger age. This increased risk appears to be related to duration of use. The majority of studies have found no overall increase in the risk of developing breast cancer. Some studies have found an increase in the incidence of cancer of the cervix in women who use oral contraceptives. However, this finding may be related to factors other than the use of oral contraceptives. There is insufficient evidence to rule out the possibility pills may cause such cancers.

Taking the combination pill provides some important non-contraceptive benefits. These include less painful menstruation, less menstrual blood loss and anemia, fewer pelvic infections, and fewer cancers of the ovary and the lining of the uterus.

Be sure to discuss any medical condition you may have with your health care provider. Your health care provider will take a medical and family history before prescribing oral contraceptives and will examine you. The physical examination may be delayed to another time if you request it and the health care provider believes that it is a good medical practice to postpone it. You should be reexamined at least once a year while taking oral contraceptives. Your pharmacist should have given you the detailed patient information labeling which gives you further information which you should read and discuss with your health care provider.

ORTHO-CYCLEN and ORTHO TRI-CYCLEN (like all oral contraceptives) are intended to prevent pregnancy. ORTHO TRI-CYCLEN is also used to treat moderate acne in females who are able to take oral contraceptives. Oral contraceptives do not protect against transmission of HIV (AIDS) and other sexually transmitted diseases such as chlamydia, genital herpes, genital warts, gonorrhea, hepatitis B, and syphilis.

DETAILED PATIENT LABELING

PLEASE NOTE: This labeling is revised from time to time as important new medical information becomes available. Therefore, please review this labeling carefully.

ORTHO TRI-CYCLEN ☐ 21 Day Regimen and
ORTHO TRI-CYCLEN ☐ 28 Day Regimen

Each white tablet contains 0.180 mg norgestimate and 0.035 mg ethinyl estradiol. Each light blue tablet contains 0.215 mg norgestimate and 0.035 mg ethinyl estradiol. Each blue tablet contains 0.250 mg norgestimate and 0.035 mg ethinyl estradiol. Each green tablet in ORTHO TRI-CYCLEN ☐ 28 Day Regimen contains inert ingredients.

ORTHO-CYCLEN ☐ 21 Day Regimen and
ORTHO-CYCLEN ☐ 28 Day Regimen

Each blue tablet contains 0.250 mg norgestimate and 0.035 mg ethinyl estradiol. Each green tablet in ORTHO-CYCLEN ☐ 28 Day Regimen contains inert ingredients.

INTRODUCTION

Any woman who considers using oral contraceptives (the birth control pill or the pill) should understand the benefits

Continued on next page

Ortho Tri-Cyclen—Cont.

and risks of using this form of birth control. This patient labeling will give you much of the information you will need to make this decision and will also help you determine if you are at risk of developing any of the serious side effects of the pill. It will tell you how to use the pill properly so that it will be as effective as possible. However, this labeling is not a replacement for a careful discussion between you and your health care provider. You should discuss the information provided in this labeling with him or her, both when you first start taking the pill and during your revisits. You should also follow your health care providers advice with regard to regular check-ups while you are on the pill.

EFFECTIVENESS OF ORAL CONTRACEPTIVES FOR CONTRACEPTION

Oral contraceptives or "birth control pills" or "the pill" are used to prevent pregnancy and are more effective than other non-surgical methods of birth control. When they are taken correctly, the chance of becoming pregnant is less than 1% (1 pregnancy per 100 women per year of use) when used perfectly, without missing any pills. Typical failure rates are actually 5% per year. The chance of becoming pregnant increases with each missed pill during a menstrual cycle.

In comparison, typical failure rates for other non-surgical methods of birth control during the first year of use are as follows:

Implant: <1%
Injection: <1%
IUD: 1 to 2%
Diaphragm with spermicides: 20%
Spermicides alone: 26%
Vaginal sponge: 20 to 40%
Female sterilization: <1%
Male sterilization: <1%
Cervical Cap with spermicides: 20 to 40%
Condom alone (male): 14%
Condom alone (female): 21%
Periodic abstinence: 25%
Withdrawal: 19%
No methods: 85%

WHO SHOULD NOT TAKE ORAL CONTRACEPTIVES

> Cigarette smoking increases the risk of serious cardiovascular side effects from oral contraceptive use. This risk increases with age and with heavy smoking (15 or more cigarettes per day) and is quite marked in women over 35 years of age. Women who use oral contraceptives are strongly advised not to smoke.

Some women should not use the pill. For example, you should not take the pill if you are pregnant or think you may be pregnant. You should also not use the pill if you have any of the following conditions:

• A history of heart attack or stroke
• Blood clots in the legs (thrombophlebitis), lungs (pulmonary embolism), or eyes
• A history of blood clots in the deep veins of your legs
• Chest pain (angina pectoris)
• Known or suspected breast cancer or cancer of the lining of the uterus, cervix or vagina
• Unexplained vaginal bleeding (until a diagnosis is reached by your doctor)
• Yellowing of the whites of the eyes or of the skin (jaundice) during pregnancy or during previous use of the pill
• Liver tumor (benign or cancerous)
• Known or suspected pregnancy

Tell your health care provider if you have ever had any of these conditions. Your health care provider can recommend a safer method of birth control.

OTHER CONSIDERATIONS BEFORE TAKING ORAL CONTRACEPTIVES

Tell your health care provider if you have or have had:
• Breast nodules, fibrocystic disease of the breast, an abnormal breast x-ray or mammogram
• Diabetes
• Elevated cholesterol or triglycerides
• High blood pressure
• Migraine or other headaches or epilepsy
• Mental depression
• Gallbladder, liver, heart or kidney disease

• History of scanty or irregular menstrual periods
Women with any of these conditions should be checked often by their health care provider if they choose to use oral contraceptives.
Also, be sure to inform your doctor or health care provider if you smoke or are on any medications.

RISKS OF TAKING ORAL CONTRACEPTIVES
1. Risk of developing blood clots

Blood clots and blockage of blood vessels are one of the most serious side effects of taking oral contraceptives and can cause death or serious disability. In particular, a clot in the legs can cause thrombophlebitis and a clot that travels to the lungs can cause a sudden blocking of the vessel carrying blood to the lungs. Rarely, clots occur in the blood vessels of the eye and may cause blindness, double vision, or impaired vision.

If you take oral contraceptives and need elective surgery, need to stay in bed for a prolonged illness or injury or have recently delivered a baby, you may be at risk of developing blood clots. You should consult your doctor about stopping oral contraceptives four weeks before surgery and not taking oral contraceptives for two weeks after surgery or during bed rest. You should also not take oral contraceptives soon after delivery of a baby. It is advisable to wait for at least four weeks after delivery if you are not breast feeding or four weeks after a second trimester abortion. If you are breast feeding, you should wait until you have weaned your child before using the pill. (See also the section on Breast Feeding in General Precautions.)

The risk of circulatory disease in oral contraceptive users may be higher in users of high-dose pills and may be greater with longer duration of oral contraceptive use. In addition, some of these increased risks may continue for a number of years after stopping oral contraceptives. The risk of abnormal blood clotting increases with age in both users and nonusers of oral contraceptives, but the increased risk from the oral contraceptive appears to be present at all ages. For women aged 20 to 44 it is estimated that about 1 in 2,000 using oral contraceptives will be hospitalized each year because of abnormal clotting. Among nonusers in the same age group, about 1 in 20,000 would be hospitalized each year. For oral contraceptive users in general, it has been estimated that in women between the ages of 15 and 34 the risk of death due to a circulatory disorder is about 1 in 12,000 per year, whereas for nonusers the rate is about 1 in 50,000 per year. In the age group 35 to 44, the risk is estimated to be about 1 in 2,500 per year for oral contraceptive users and about 1 in 10,000 per year for nonusers.

2. Heart attacks and strokes

Oral contraceptives may increase the tendency to develop strokes (stoppage or rupture of blood vessels in the brain) and angina pectoris and heart attacks (blockage of blood vessels in the heart). Any of these conditions can cause death or serious disability.

Smoking greatly increases the possibility of suffering heart attacks and strokes. Furthermore, smoking and the use of oral contraceptives greatly increase the chances of developing and dying of heart disease.

3. Gallbladder disease

Oral contraceptive users probably have a greater risk than nonusers of having gallbladder disease, although this risk may be related to pills containing high doses of estrogens.

4. Liver tumors

In rare cases, oral contraceptives can cause benign but dangerous liver tumors. These benign liver tumors can rupture and cause fatal internal bleeding. In addition, some studies report an increased risk of developing liver cancer. However, liver cancers are rare.

5. Cancer of the reproductive organs and breasts

There is conflict among studies regarding breast cancer and oral contraceptive use. Some studies have reported an increase in the risk of developing breast cancer, particularly at a younger age. This increased risk appears to be related to duration of use. The majority of studies have found no overall increase in the risk of developing breast cancer.

A meta-analysis of 54 studies found a small increase in the frequency of having breast cancer diagnosed for women who were currently using combined oral contraceptives or had used them within the past ten years. This increase in the frequency of breast cancer diagnosis, within ten years of stopping use, was generally accounted for by cancers localized to the breast. There was no increase in the frequency of having breast cancer diagnosed ten or more years after cessation of use.

Some studies have found an increase in the incidence of cancer of the cervix in women who use oral contraceptives. However, this finding may be related to factors other than the use of oral contraceptives. There is insufficient evidence to rule out the possibility that pills may cause such cancers.

ESTIMATED RISK OF DEATH FROM A BIRTH CONTROL METHOD OR PREGNANCY

All methods of birth control and pregnancy are associated with a risk of developing certain diseases which may lead to disability or death. An estimate of the number of deaths associated with different methods of birth control and pregnancy has been calculated and is shown in the following table.

[See table below]

In the above table, the risk of death from any birth control method is less than the risk of childbirth, except for oral contraceptive users over the age of 35 who smoke and pill users over the age of 40 even if they do not smoke. It can be seen in the table that for women aged 15 to 39, the risk of death was highest with pregnancy (7–26 deaths per 100,000 women, depending on age). Among pill users who do not smoke, the risk of death was always lower than that associated with pregnancy for any age group, although over the age of 40, the risk increases to 32 deaths per 100,000 women, compared to 28 associated with pregnancy at that age. However, for pill users who smoke and are over the age of 35, the estimated number of deaths exceeds those for other methods of birth control. If a woman is over the age of 40 and smokes, her estimated risk of death is four times higher (117/100,000 women) than the estimated risk associated with pregnancy (28/100,000 women) in that age group. The suggestion that women over 40 who do not smoke should not take oral contraceptives is based on information from older, higher-dose pills. An Advisory Committee of the FDA discussed this issue in 1989 and recommended that the benefits of low-dose oral contraceptive use by healthy, non-smoking women over 40 years of age may outweigh the possible risks.

WARNING SIGNALS

If any of these adverse effects occur while you are taking oral contraceptives, call your doctor immediately:
• Sharp chest pain, coughing of blood, or sudden shortness of breath (indicating a possible clot in the lung)
• Pain in the calf (indicating a possible clot in the leg)
• Crushing chest pain or heaviness in the chest (indicating a possible heart attack)
• Sudden severe headache or vomiting, dizziness or fainting, disturbances of vision or speech, weakness, or numbness in an arm or leg (indicating a possible stroke)
• Sudden partial or complete loss of vision (indicating a possible clot in the eye)
• Breast lumps (indicating possible breast cancer or fibrocystic disease of the breast; ask your doctor or health care provider to show you how to examine your breasts)
• Severe pain or tenderness in the stomach area (indicating a possibly ruptured liver tumor)
• Difficulty in sleeping, weakness, lack of energy, fatigue, or change in mood (possibly indicating severe depression)
• Jaundice or a yellowing of the skin or eyeballs, accompanied frequently by fever, fatigue, loss of appetite, dark colored urine, or light colored bowel movements (indicating possible liver problems)

SIDE EFFECTS OF ORAL CONTRACEPTIVES
1. Vaginal bleeding

Irregular vaginal bleeding or spotting may occur while you are taking the pills. Irregular bleeding may vary from slight staining between menstrual periods to breakthrough bleeding which is a flow much like a regular period. Irregular bleeding occurs most often during the first few months of oral contraceptive use, but may also occur after you have been taking the pill for some time. Such bleeding may be temporary and usually does not indicate any serious problems. It is important to continue taking your pills on schedule. If the bleeding occurs in more than one cycle or lasts for more than a few days, talk to your doctor or health care provider.

2. Contact lenses

If you wear contact lenses and notice a change in vision or an inability to wear your lenses, contact your doctor or health care provider.

3. Fluid retention

Oral contraceptives may cause edema (fluid retention) with swelling of the fingers or ankles and may raise your blood pressure. If you experience fluid retention, contact your doctor or health care provider.

4. Melasma

A spotty darkening of the skin is possible, particularly of the face, which may persist.

5. Other side effects

Other side effects may include nausea and vomiting, change in appetite, headache, nervousness, depression, dizziness, loss of scalp hair, rash, and vaginal infections.

If any of these side effects bother you, call your doctor or health care provider.

GENERAL PRECAUTIONS
1. Missed periods and use of oral contraceptives before or during early pregnancy

There may be times when you may not menstruate regularly after you have completed taking a cycle of pills. If you have taken your pills regularly and miss one menstrual period, continue taking your pills for the next cycle but be sure to inform your health care provider before doing so. If you

ANNUAL NUMBER OF BIRTH-RELATED OR METHOD-RELATED DEATHS ASSOCIATED WITH CONTROL OF FERTILITY PER 100,000 NON-STERILE WOMEN, BY FERTILITY CONTROL METHOD ACCORDING TO AGE

Method of control and outcome	15-19	20-24	25-29	30-34	35-39	40-44
No fertility control methods*	7.0	7.4	9.1	14.8	25.7	28.2
Oral contraceptives non-smoker**	0.3	0.5	0.9	1.9	13.8	31.6
Oral contraceptives smoker**	2.2	3.4	6.6	13.5	51.1	117.2
IUD**	0.8	0.8	1.0	1.0	1.4	1.4
Condom*	1.1	1.6	0.7	0.2	0.3	0.4
Diaphragm/spermicide*	1.9	1.2	1.2	1.3	2.2	2.8
Periodic abstinence*	2.5	1.6	1.6	1.7	2.9	3.6

*Deaths are birth-related
**Deaths are method-related

Adapted from H.W. Ory, ref. #35.

have not taken the pills daily as instructed and missed a menstrual period, you may be pregnant. If you missed two consecutive menstrual periods, you may be pregnant. Check with your health care provider immediately to determine whether you are pregnant. Do not continue to take oral contraceptives until you are sure you are not pregnant, but continue to use another method of contraception.

There is no conclusive evidence that oral contraceptive use is associated with an increase in birth defects, when taken inadvertently during early pregnancy. Previously, a few studies had reported that oral contraceptives might be associated with birth defects, but these findings have not been seen in more recent studies. Nevertheless, oral contraceptives or any other drugs should not be used during pregnancy unless clearly necessary and prescribed by your doctor. You should check with your doctor about risks to your unborn child of any medication taken during pregnancy.

2. While breast feeding
If you are breast feeding, consult your doctor before starting oral contraceptives. Some of the drug will be passed on to the child in the milk. A few adverse effects on the child have been reported, including yellowing of the skin (jaundice) and breast enlargement. In addition, combination oral contraceptives may decrease the amount and quality of your milk. If possible, do not use combination oral contraceptives while breast feeding. You should use another method of contraception since breast feeding provides only partial protection from becoming pregnant and this partial protection decreases significantly as you breast feed for longer periods of time. You should consider starting combination oral contraceptives only after you have weaned your child completely.

3. Laboratory tests
If you are scheduled for any laboratory tests, tell your doctor you are taking birth control pills. Certain blood tests may be affected by birth control pills.

4. Drug interactions
Certain drugs may interact with birth control pills to make them less effective in preventing pregnancy or cause an increase in breakthrough bleeding. Such drugs include rifampin, drugs used for epilepsy such as barbiturates (for example, phenobarbital), anticonvulsants such as topiramate (TOPAMAX), carbamazepine (Tegretol is one brand of this drug), phenytoin (Dilantin is one brand of this drug), phenylbutazone (Butazolidin is one brand), certain drugs used in the treatment of HIV or AIDS, and possibly certain antibiotics. You may need to use additional contraception when you take drugs which can make oral contraceptives less effective. A possible interaction has been suggested with hormonal contraceptives and the herbal supplement St. Johns Wort based on some reports of oral contraceptive users experiencing breakthrough bleeding shortly after starting St. Johns Wort. Pregnancies have been reported by users of combined hormonal contraceptives who also used some form of St. Johns Wort.

5. Sexually transmitted diseases
ORTHO-CYCLEN and ORTHO TRI-CYCLEN (like all oral contraceptives) are intended to prevent pregnancy. ORTHO TRI-CYCLEN is also used to treat moderate acne in females who are able to take oral contraceptives. Oral contraceptives do not protect against transmission of HIV (AIDS) and other sexually transmitted diseases such as chlamydia, genital herpes, genital warts, gonorrhea, hepatitis B, and syphilis.

HOW TO TAKE THE PILL
IMPORTANT POINTS TO REMEMBER
BEFORE YOU START TAKING YOUR PILLS:
1. BE SURE TO READ THESE DIRECTIONS:
Before you start taking your pills.
Anytime you are not sure what to do.
2. THE RIGHT WAY TO TAKE THE PILL IS TO TAKE ONE PILL EVERY DAY AT THE SAME TIME.
If you miss pills you could get pregnant. This includes starting the pack late. The more pills you miss, the more likely you are to get pregnant.
3. MANY WOMEN HAVE SPOTTING OR LIGHT BLEEDING, OR MAY FEEL SICK TO THEIR STOMACH DURING THE FIRST 1-3 PACKS OF PILLS. If you feel sick to your stomach, do not stop taking the pill. The problem will usually go away. If it doesnt go away, check with your doctor or clinic.
4. MISSING PILLS CAN ALSO CAUSE SPOTTING OR LIGHT BLEEDING, even when you make up these missed pills.
On the days you take 2 pills to make up for missed pills, you could also feel a little sick to your stomach.
5. IF YOU HAVE VOMITING OR DIARRHEA, for any reason, or IF YOU TAKE SOME MEDICINES, including some antibiotics, your pills may not work as well. Use a back-up method (such as condoms, foam, or sponge) until you check with your doctor or clinic.
6. IF YOU HAVE TROUBLE REMEMBERING TO TAKE THE PILL, talk to your doctor or clinic about how to make pill-taking easier or about using another method of birth control.
7. IF YOU HAVE ANY QUESTIONS OR ARE UNSURE ABOUT THE INFORMATION IN THIS LEAFLET, call your doctor or clinic.
BEFORE YOU START TAKING YOUR PILLS
1. DECIDE WHAT TIME OF DAY YOU WANT TO TAKE YOUR PILL.
It is important to take it at about the same time every day.
2. LOOK AT YOUR PILL PACK TO SEE IF IT HAS 21 OR 28 PILLS:
The 21-pill pack has 21 "active" pills (with hormones) to take for 3 weeks. This is followed by 1 week without pills.

The 28-pill pack has 21 "active" pills (with hormones) to take for 3 weeks. This is followed by 1 week of reminder green pills (without hormones).
ORTHO TRI-CYCLEN: There are 7 white "active" pills, 7 light blue "active" pills, and 7 blue "active" pills.
ORTHO-CYCLEN: There are 21 blue "active" pills.
3. ALSO FIND:
1) where on the pack to start taking pills,
2) in what order to take the pills.
CHECK PICTURE OF PILL PACK AND ADDITIONAL INSTRUCTIONS FOR USING THIS PACKAGE IN THE BRIEF SUMMARY PATIENT PACKAGE INSERT.
4. BE SURE YOU HAVE READY AT ALL TIMES:
ANOTHER KIND OF BIRTH CONTROL (such as condoms, foam, or sponge) to use as a back-up method in case you miss pills.
AN EXTRA, FULL PILL PACK.
WHEN TO START THE FIRST PACK OF PILLS
You have a choice of which day to start taking your first pack of pills. ORTHO TRI-CYCLEN and ORTHO- CYCLEN are available in the DIALPAK® Tablet Dispenser which is preset for a Sunday Start. Day 1 Start is also provided. Decide with your doctor or clinic which is the best day for you. Pick a time of day which will be easy to remember.
SUNDAY START:
ORTHO TRI-CYCLEN: Take the first "active" white pill of the first pack on the Sunday after your period starts, even if you are still bleeding. If your period begins on Sunday, start the pack that same day.
ORTHO-CYCLEN: Take the first "active" blue pill of the first pack on the Sunday after your period starts, even if you are still bleeding. If your period begins on Sunday, start the pack that same day.
Use another method of birth control as a back-up method if you have sex anytime from the Sunday you start your first pack until the next Sunday (7 days). Condoms, foam, or the sponge are good back-up methods of birth control.
DAY 1 START:
ORTHO TRI-CYCLEN: Take the first "active" white pill of the first pack during the first 24 hours of your period.
ORTHO-CYCLEN: Take the first "active" blue pill of the first pack during the first 24 hours of your period.
You will not need to use a back-up method of birth control, since you are starting the pill at the beginning of your period.
WHAT TO DO DURING THE MONTH
1. TAKE ONE PILL AT THE SAME TIME EVERY DAY UNTIL THE PACK IS EMPTY.
Do not skip pills even if you are spotting or bleeding between monthly periods or feel sick to your stomach (nausea). Do not skip pills even if you do not have sex very often.
2. WHEN YOU FINISH A PACK OR SWITCH YOUR BRAND OF PILLS:
21 pills: Wait 7 days to start the next pack. You will probably have your period during that week. Be sure that no more than 7 days pass between 21-day packs.
28 pills: Start the next pack on the day after your last "reminder" pill. Do not wait any days between packs.
WHAT TO DO IF YOU MISS PILLS
ORTHO TRI-CYCLEN:
If you **MISS 1** white, light blue, or blue "active" pill:
1. Take it as soon as you remember. Take the next pill at your regular time. This means you may take 2 pills in 1 day.
2. You do not need to use a back-up birth control method if you have sex.
If you **MISS 2** white or light blue "active" pills in a row in WEEK 1 OR WEEK 2 of your pack:
1. Take 2 pills on the day you remember and 2 pills the next day.
2. Then take 1 pill a day until you finish the pack.
3. You MAY BECOME PREGNANT if you have sex in the 7 days after you miss pills. You MUST use another birth control method (such as condoms, foam, or sponge) as a back-up method for those 7 days.
If you **MISS 2** blue "active" pills in a row in THE 3RD WEEK:
1. **If you are a Sunday Starter:**
Keep taking 1 pill every day until Sunday. On Sunday, THROW OUT the rest of the pack and start a new pack of pills that same day.
If you are a Day 1 Starter:
THROW OUT the rest of the pill pack and start a new pack that same day.
2. You may not have your period this month but this is expected. However, if you miss your period 2 months in a row, call your doctor or clinic because you might be pregnant.
3. You MAY BECOME PREGNANT if you have sex in the 7 days after you miss pills. You MUST use another birth control method (such as condoms, foam, or sponge) as a back-up method for those 7 days.
If you **MISS 3 OR MORE** white, light blue, or blue "active" pills in a row (during the first 3 weeks):
1. **If you are a Sunday Starter:**
Keep taking 1 pill every day until Sunday. On Sunday, THROW OUT the rest of the pack and start a new pack of pills that same day.
If you are a Day 1 Starter:
THROW OUT the rest of the pill pack and start a new pack that same day.
2. You may not have your period this month but this is expected. However, if you miss your period 2 months in a row, call your doctor or clinic because you might be pregnant.
3. You MAY BECOME PREGNANT if you have sex in the 7 days after you miss pills. You MUST use another birth control method (such as condoms, foam, or sponge) as a back-up method for those 7 days.

ORTHO-CYCLEN:
If you **MISS 1** blue "active" pill:
1. Take it as soon as you remember. Take the next pill at your regular time. This means you may take 2 pills in 1 day.
2. You do not need to use a back-up birth control method if you have sex.
If you **MISS 2** blue "active" pills in a row in WEEK 1 OR WEEK 2 of your pack:
1. Take 2 pills on the day you remember and 2 pills the next day.
2. Then take 1 pill a day until you finish the pack.
3. You MAY BECOME PREGNANT if you have sex in the 7 days after you miss pills. You MUST use another birth control method (such as condoms, foam, or sponge) as a back-up method for those 7 days.
If you **MISS 2** blue "active" pills in a row in THE 3RD WEEK:
1. **If you are a Sunday Starter:**
Keep taking 1 pill every day until Sunday. On Sunday, THROW OUT the rest of the pack and start a new pack of pills that same day.
If you are a Day 1 Starter:
THROW OUT the rest of the pill pack and start a new pack that same day.
2. You may not have your period this month but this is expected. However, if you miss your period 2 months in a row, call your doctor or clinic because you might be pregnant.
3. You MAY BECOME PREGNANT if you have sex in the 7 days after you miss pills. You MUST use another birth control method (such as condoms, foam, or sponge) as a back-up method for those 7 days.
If you **MISS 3 OR MORE** blue "active" pills in a row (during the first 3 weeks):
1. **If you are a Sunday Starter:**
Keep taking 1 pill every day until Sunday. On Sunday, THROW OUT the rest of the pack and start a new pack of pills that same day.
If you are a Day 1 Starter:
THROW OUT the rest of the pill pack and start a new pack that same day.
2. You may not have your period this month but this is expected. However, if you miss your period 2 months in a row, call your doctor or clinic because you might be pregnant.
3. You MAY BECOME PREGNANT if you have sex in the 7 days after you miss pills. You MUST use another birth control method (such as condoms, foam, or sponge) as a back-up method for those 7 days.
A REMINDER FOR THOSE ON 28-DAY PACKS:
If you forget any of the 7 green "reminder" pills in Week 4: THROW AWAY the pills you missed.
Keep taking 1 pill each day until the pack is empty.
You do not need a back-up method.

FINALLY, IF YOU ARE STILL NOT SURE WHAT TO DO ABOUT THE PILLS YOU HAVE MISSED:
Use a BACK-UP METHOD anytime you have sex.
KEEP TAKING ONE "ACTIVE" PILL EACH DAY until you can reach your doctor or clinic.

PREGNANCY DUE TO PILL FAILURE
The incidence of pill failure resulting in pregnancy is approximately one percent (i.e., one pregnancy per 100 women per year) if taken every day as directed, but more typical failure rates are 5%. If failure does occur, the risk to the fetus is minimal.

PREGNANCY AFTER STOPPING THE PILL
There may be some delay in becoming pregnant after you stop using oral contraceptives, especially if you had irregular menstrual cycles before you used oral contraceptives. It may be advisable to postpone conception until you begin menstruating regularly once you have stopped taking the pill and desire pregnancy.
There does not appear to be any increase in birth defects in newborn babies when pregnancy occurs soon after stopping the pill.

OVERDOSAGE
Serious ill effects have not been reported following ingestion of large doses of oral contraceptives by young children. Overdosage may cause nausea and withdrawal bleeding in females. In case of overdosage, contact your health care provider or pharmacist.

OTHER INFORMATION
Your health care provider will take a medical and family history before prescribing oral contraceptives and will examine you. The physical examination may be delayed to another time if you request it and the health care provider believes that it is a good medical practice to postpone it. You should be reexamined at least once a year. Be sure to inform your health care provider if there is a family history of any of the conditions listed previously in this leaflet. Be sure to keep all appointments with your health care provider, because this is a time to determine if there are early signs of side effects of oral contraceptive use.
Do not use the drug for any condition other than the one for which it was prescribed. This drug has been prescribed specifically for you; do not give it to others who may want birth control pills.

HEALTH BENEFITS FROM ORAL CONTRACEPTIVES
In addition to preventing pregnancy, use of combination oral contraceptives may provide certain benefits. They are:
• menstrual cycles may become more regular

Continued on next page

Ortho Tri-Cyclen—Cont.

- blood flow during menstruation may be lighter and less iron may be lost. Therefore, anemia due to iron deficiency is less likely to occur.
- pain or other symptoms during menstruation may be encountered less frequently
- ectopic (tubal) pregnancy may occur less frequently
- noncancerous cysts or lumps in the breast may occur less frequently
- acute pelvic inflammatory disease may occur less frequently
- oral contraceptive use may provide some protection against developing two forms of cancer: cancer of the ovaries and cancer of the lining of the uterus.

If you want more information about birth control pills, ask your doctor/health care provider or pharmacist. They have a more technical leaflet called the Professional Labeling, which you may wish to read. The professional labeling is also published in a book entitled *Physicians Desk Reference*, available in many book stores and public libraries.

ORTHO-McNEIL PHARMACEUTICAL, INC.
Raritan, New Jersey 08869
© OMP 1998 REVISED JUNE 2000 635-50-900-6

PARAGARD® T 380A ℞

Intrauterine Copper Contraceptive

Prescribing information for this product, which appears on pages 2383–2387 of the 2001 PDR, has been completely revised as follows. Please write "See Supplement A" next to the product heading.

Prescribing Information

Patients should be counseled that this product does not protect against HIV infection (AIDS) and other sexually transmitted diseases.

The ParaGard® T380A should only be inserted, managed, and removed by clinicians that have demonstrated clinical competence for these procedures received under supervision.

NOTICE

You have received a Patient Package Insert that Federal Regulations (21 CFR 310.502) require you to furnish to each patient who is considering the use of the ParaGard® T 380A.

The Patient Package Insert contains information on the safety and efficacy of the ParaGard® T 380A. Before inserting the ParaGard® T 380A:

- You should read the physician prescription labeling and be familiar with all the information it contains.
- You should counsel the patient and answer her questions about contraception, the ParaGard® T 380A, and the information in the Patient Package Insert.
- You and the patient should read each section of the Patient Package Insert, and if the patient agrees, she may sign a consent form provided for your convenience.

The Patient Package Insert is also available in Spanish and other foreign languages. Address requests to Ortho-McNeil Pharmaceutical, Inc. or telephone 1-800-322-4966.

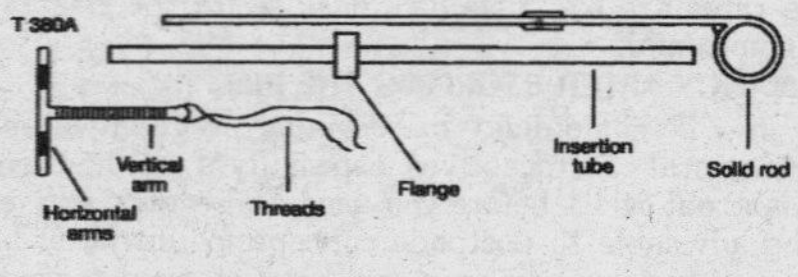

DESCRIPTION

The polyethylene body of the ParaGard® T 380A is wound with approximately 176 mg of copper wire and carries a copper collar of approximately 68.7 mg of copper on each of its transverse arms. The exposed surface areas of copper are 380 ± 23 mm.[2] The dimensions of the ParaGard® T 380A are 36 mm in the vertical direction and 32 mm in the horizontal direction. The tip of the vertical arm of the ParaGard® T 380A is enlarged to form a bulb having a diameter of 3 mm. The ParaGard® T 380A is equipped with a monofilament polyethylene thread which is tied through the bulb, resulting in two threads at the tip to aid in removal of the IUD. The ParaGard® T 380A contains barium sulfate to render it radiopaque.

The ParaGard® T 380A is packaged together with an insertion tube and solid rod in a Tyvek®- polyethylene pouch and then sterilized. The insertion tube is equipped with a movable flange to aid in gauging the depth to which the insertion tube is inserted through the cervical canal and into the uterine cavity.

CLINICAL PHARMACOLOGY

Available data indicate that the contraceptive effectiveness of the ParaGard® T 380A is enhanced by copper being released continuously from the copper coil and sleeves into the uterine cavity. The exact mechanism by which metallic copper enhances the contraceptive effect of an IUD has not been conclusively demonstrated. Various hypotheses have been advanced, including interference with sperm transport, fertilization, and implantation. Clinical studies with copper-bearing IUDs also suggest that fertilization is prevented either due to an altered number or lack of viability of spermatozoa.[1]

INDICATIONS AND USAGE

The ParaGard® T 380A is indicated for intrauterine contraception. ParaGard® T 380A is highly effective. Table II and Table III list an expected pregnancy rate for one year between 0.7 and 0.5, respectively. ParaGard® T 380A should not be kept in place longer than 10 years.

RECOMMENDED PATIENT PROFILE

The ParaGard® T 380A is recommended for women who have had at least one child, are in a stable, mutually monogamous relationship, and have no history of pelvic inflammatory disease.

CONTRAINDICATIONS

The ParaGard® T 380A should not be inserted when one or more of the following conditions exist:

1. Pregnancy or suspicion of pregnancy.
2. Abnormalities of the uterus resulting in distortion of the uterine cavity.
3. Acute pelvic inflammatory disease or a history of pelvic inflammatory disease.
4. Postpartum endometritis or infected abortion in the past 3 months.
5. Known or suspected uterine or cervical malignancy, including unresolved, abnormal "Pap" smear.
6. Genital bleeding of unknown etiology.
7. Untreated acute cervicitis or vaginitis, including bacterial vaginosis, until infection is controlled.
8. Copper-containing IUDs should not be inserted in the presence of diagnosed Wilson's disease.
9. Known allergy to copper.
10. Patient or her partner has multiple sexual partners.
11. Conditions associated with increased susceptibility to infections with microorganisms. Such conditions include, but are not limited to, leukemia, acquired immune deficiency syndrome (AIDS), and I.V. drug abuse.
12. Genital actinomycosis.
13. A previously inserted IUD that has not been removed.

WARNINGS

1. PREGNANCY

Effects on the offspring when pregnancy occurs with the ParaGard® T 380A in place are unknown.

a. **Septic Abortion**
Reports indicate an increased incidence of septic abortion with septicemia, septic shock, and death in patients becoming pregnant with an IUD in place. Most of these reports have been associated with, but are not limited to, the mid-trimester of pregnancy. In some cases, the initial symptoms have been insidious and not easily recognized. If pregnancy should occur with an IUD *in situ*, the IUD should be removed if the string is visible and removal is easily accomplished. Of course, manipulation may result in spontaneous abortion. If removal proves to be difficult, or if threads are not visible, interruption of the pregnancy should be considered and offered as an option. Rates of mortality with and without contraception are shown in Table I.

b. **Continuation of Pregnancy**
If the patient elects to maintain the pregnancy and the IUD remains *in situ*, she should be warned that there is an increased risk of spontaneous abortion and sepsis. In addition, she is at increased risk of premature labor and delivery. As a consequence of premature birth, the fetus is at increased risk of damage. She should be followed more closely than the usual obstetrical patient. The patient must be advised to report immediately all abnormal symptoms, such as flu-like syndrome, fever, abdominal cramping or pain, bleeding or vaginal discharge, because generalized symptoms of septicemia may be insidious.

2. ECTOPIC PREGNANCY

a. Patients with a history of ectopic pregnancy are at an increased risk of subsequent pregnancies being ectopic. Although current data indicate that there is no increased risk of ectopic pregnancy in patients using the ParaGard® T 380A and some data suggest there may be a lower risk than the general population using no method of contraception, a pregnancy which occurs with the ParaGard® T 380A in place is more likely to be ectopic than a pregnancy occurring without ParaGard® T 380A.[2–4] Therefore, patients who become pregnant while using the ParaGard® T 380A should be carefully evaluated for the possibility of an ectopic pregnancy.

b. Special attention should be directed to patients with delayed menses, slight metrorrhagia and/or unilateral pelvic pain, and to those patients who wish to terminate a pregnancy because of IUD failure, to determine whether ectopic pregnancy has occurred.

3. PELVIC INFECTION (PELVIC INFLAMMATORY DISEASE, PID)

The ParaGard® T 380A is contraindicated in the presence of PID or in women with a history of PID. Use of all IUDs, including the ParaGard® T 380A, has been associated with an increased incidence of PID. Therefore, a decision to use the ParaGard® T 380A must include consideration of the risks of PID. The highest rate of PID has been reported to occur after insertion and up to four months thereafter. A study suggests that the highest incidence occurs within 20 days postinsertion, then falls, remaining constant thereafter.[5] Administration of prophylactic antibiotics has been reported, although studies do not confirm the utility of this prophylactic measure in reducing PID. PID can necessitate hysterectomy and can also lead to tubo-ovarian abscesses, tubal occlusion and infertility, and tubal damage that can predispose to ectopic pregnancy. PID can result in peritonitis and, infrequently, in death. The effect of PID on fertility is especially important for women who may wish to have children at a later date.

a. **Women at special risk of PID**
The risk of PID appears to be greater for women who have multiple sexual partners and also for those women whose sexual partners have multiple sexual partners, as PID is most frequently caused by sexually transmitted diseases.

b. **PID warning to ParaGard® T 380A users**
All women who choose the ParaGard® T 380A must be informed prior to insertion that IUD use has been associated with an increased incidence of PID and that PID can necessitate hysterectomy, can cause tubal damage leading to ectopic pregnancy or infertility or, in infrequent cases, can cause death. Patients must be taught to recognize and report to their physician promptly any symptoms of pelvic inflammatory disease. These symptoms include development of menstrual disorders (prolonged or heavy bleeding), unusual vaginal discharge, abdominal or pelvic pain or tenderness, dyspareunia, chills, and fever.

c. **Asymptomatic PID**
PID may be asymptomatic but still result in tubal damage and its sequelae.[6,7]

d. **Treatment of PID**
Following diagnosis of PID, or suspected PID, bacteriologic specimens should be obtained and antibiotic therapy should be initiated promptly. Removal of the ParaGard® T 380A after initiation of antibiotic therapy is usually appropriate. Time should be allowed for therapeutic blood levels to be reached prior to removal. Guidelines for PID treatment are available from the Center for Disease Control (CDC), Atlanta, Georgia. A copy of the printed guidelines has been provided to you by Ortho-McNeil Pharmaceutical, Inc. The guidelines were established after deliberation by a group of experts and staff of the CDC, but they should not be construed as rules suitable for use in all patients. Adequate PID treatment requires the application of current standards of therapy prevailing at the time of occurrence of the infection with reference to the prescription labeling of the antibiotic selected.

Genital actinomycosis has been associated primarily with long-term IUD use. If actinomycosis occurs, promptly institute appropriate antibiotic therapy and remove the ParaGard® T 380A.

4. EMBEDMENT

Partial penetration or embedment of the ParaGard® T 380A in the endometrium or myometrium can result in difficult removal. In some cases this can result in breakage of the IUD, necessitating surgical removal.

5. PERFORATION

Partial or total perforation of the uterine wall or cervix may occur with use of the ParaGard® T 380A. The rate of perforation in randomized trials of the ParaGard® T 380A has been 1 in 1,360. Insertions immediately after the expulsion of the placenta are not known to be associated with increased risks of perforation, but insertion later in the first postpartum month, particularly during lactation, has been associated with an increased risk of perforation.[8,9] Thus, unless performed immediately postpartum, insertion should be delayed to the second postpartum month. IUD insertion immediately postabortion in the first trimester is not known to be associated with increased risks of perforation, but insertion after second trimester abortion should be delayed until the second postabortion month.

The possibility of perforation must be kept in mind during insertion and at the time of any subsequent examination. If perforation occurs, the ParaGard® T 380A should be removed as soon as possible. A surgical procedure may be required. Abdominal adhesions, intestinal penetration, intestinal obstruction, and local inflammatory reaction with abscess formation and erosion of adjacent viscera may result if the ParaGard® T 380A is left in the peritoneal cavity. There are reports of migration after insertion.

6. MEDICAL DIATHERMY

The use of medical diathermy (short-wave and microwave) in a patient with a metal-containing IUD may cause heat injury to the surrounding tissue. Therefore, medical diathermy to the abdominal and sacral areas should not be used on patients with a ParaGard® T 380A in place.

7. EFFECTS OF COPPER

Additional amounts of copper available to the body from the ParaGard® T 380A may precipitate symptoms in women with Wilson's disease. The incidence of Wilson's disease is approximately 1 in 200,000. The long term effects of intrauterine copper to a child conceived in the presence of an IUD are unknown.

8. RISKS OF MORTALITY

The available data from a variety of sources have been analyzed to estimate the risk of death associated with various methods of contraception. The estimates of risk of death include the combined risk of the contraceptive method plus the risk of pregnancy or abortion in the event of method failure. The findings of the analysis are shown in Table I.[10]

[See table I at top of next page]

PRECAUTIONS

Patients should be counseled that this product does not protect against HIV infection (AIDS) and other sexually transmitted diseases.

1. Patient Counseling

Prior to the insertion, the physician, nurse, or other trained health professional must provide the patient with the Patient Package Insert. The patient should be given the opportunity to read the information and discuss fully any questions she may have concerning the ParaGard® T 380A as well as other methods of contraception.

2. Patient Evaluation and Clinical Considerations

a. A complete medical and social history, including that of the partner, should be obtained to determine conditions that might influence the selection of an IUD. A physical examination should include a pelvic examination, a "Pap" smear, and appropriate tests for any other forms of genital disease, such as gonorrhea and chlamydia laboratory evaluations, if indicated. If actinomyces-like organisms are detected on the Pap smear, they should be cultured to determine whether genital actinomyces is present. The physician should determine that the patient is not pregnant.

b. The uterus should be carefully sounded prior to the insertion to determine the degree of patency of the endocervical canal and the internal os, and the direction and depth of the uterine cavity. In occasional cases, severe cervical stenosis may be encountered. Do not use excessive force to overcome this resistance.

c. The uterus should sound to a depth of 6 to 9 centimeters (cm). Insertion of an IUD into a uterine cavity measuring less than 6.0 cm by sounding may increase the incidence of expulsion, bleeding, pain, perforation, and possibly, pregnancy.

d. Clinicians are cautioned that it is imperative for them to become thoroughly familiar with the instructions for use before attempting placement of the ParaGard® T 380A. To reduce the possibility of insertion in the presence of an existing undetermined pregnancy, the optimal time for insertion is the latter part of the menstrual period, or one or two days thereafter. The ParaGard® T 380A should not be inserted postpartum or postabortion until involution of the uterus is complete. The incidence of perforation and expulsion is greater if involution is not complete. Data also suggest that there may be an increased risk of perforation and expulsion if the woman is lactating.[8,9] Other recent studies report no increased incidence of perforation or expulsion in lactating women.[11,12]
The ParaGard® T 380A should be placed at the fundus of the uterine cavity. Proper placement enhances contraceptive effectiveness and helps avoid perforation and partial or complete expulsion that could result in pregnancy.

e. Patients experiencing menorrhagia and/or metrorrhagia following IUD insertion may be at risk for the development of hypochromic microcytic anemia. Careful consideration of this risk must be given before insertion in patients with anemia or a history of menorrhagia or hypermenorrhea. Patients receiving anticoagulants or having a coagulopathy may have a greater risk of menorrhagia or hypermenorrhea.

f. Syncope, bradycardia, or other neurovascular episodes may occur during insertion or removal of IUDs, especially in patients with a previous disposition to these conditions or cervical stenosis.

g. Use of an IUD in patients with cervicitis should be postponed until treatment has eradicated the infection.

h. Patients with valvular or congenital heart disease are more prone to develop subacute bacterial endocarditis than patients who do not have valvular or congenital heart disease. Use of an IUD in these patients may represent a potential source of septic emboli. Patients with known congenital heart disease who may be at increased risk should be treated with appropriate antibiotics at the time of insertion.

i. Patients requiring chronic corticosteroid therapy or insulin for diabetes should be monitored with special care for infection.

j. Since the ParaGard® T 380A may be partially or completely expelled, patients should be reexamined and evaluated shortly after the first postinsertion menses, but no later than 3 months afterwards. Thereafter, annual examination with appropriate evaluation, including a "Pap" smear, should be carried out. The ParaGard® T 380A should be kept in place no longer than 10 years.

k. The patient should be told that some bleeding or cramps may occur during the first few weeks after insertion. If these symptoms continue or are severe she should report them to her physician. She should be instructed on how to check to make certain that the threads still protrude from the cervix and cautioned that there is no contraceptive protection if the ParaGard® T 380A has been expelled. She should check frequently, at least after each menstrual period. She should be cautioned not to dislodge the ParaGard® T 380A by pulling on the thread. If a partial expulsion occurs, removal is indicated.

l. Rarely, a copper-induced urticarial allergic skin reaction may develop in women using a copper-containing IUD. If the symptoms of such an allergic response occur, the patient should be instructed to tell the consulting physician that a copper-containing device is being used.

m. The effect of magnetic resonance imaging of the pelvis was investigated in one study[13] in women with the CU-7® (Intrauterine Copper Contraceptive) and the LIPPES LOOP™ IUD. The CU-7® has a different configuration and contains less copper than the ParaGard® T 380A. The results of the study indicate that neither the CU-7® nor the LIPPES LOOP™ were moved under the influence of the magnetic field nor did they heat during the spin-echo sequences usually employed for pelvic imaging.

TABLE I—Annual Number of Birth-Related or Method-Related Deaths Associated with Control of Fertility per 100,000 Non-sterile Women, by Fertility Control Method According to Age.

	Age Group					
Methods	**15–19**	**20–24**	**25–29**	**30–34**	**35–39**	**40–44**
No Birth Control Method/Term	4.7	5.4	4.8	6.3	11.7	20.6
No Birth Control Method/AB	2.1	2.0	1.6	1.9	2.8	5.3
IUD	0.2	0.3	0.2	0.1	0.3	0.6
Periodic Abstinence	1.4	1.3	0.7	1.0	1.0	1.9
Withdrawal	0.9	1.7	0.9	1.3	0.8	1.5
Condom	0.6	1.2	0.6	0.9	0.5	1.0
Diaphragm/Cap	0.6	1.1	0.6	0.9	1.6	3.1
Sponge	0.8	1.5	0.8	1.1	2.2	4.1
Spermicides	1.6	1.9	1.4	1.9	1.5	2.7
Oral Contraceptives	0.8	1.3	1.1	1.8	1.0	1.9
Implants/Injectables	0.2	0.6	0.5	0.8	0.5	0.6
Tubal Sterilization	1.3	1.2	1.1	1.1	1.2	1.3
Vasectomy	0.1	0.1	0.1	0.1	0.1	0.2

TABLE II GROSS ANNUAL TERMINATION AND CONTINUATION RATES PER 100* USERS
All Copper T 380A IUD Acceptors
Combined Population Council and WHO Studies

	YEAR									
Rate of Item	1	2	3	4	5	6	7	8	9	10
Pregnancy	0.7	0.3	0.6	0.2	0.3	0.2	0.0	0.4	0.0	0.0
Expulsion	5.7	2.5	1.6	1.2	0.3	0.0	0.6	1.7	0.2	0.4
Bleeding/Pain	11.9	9.8	7.0	3.5	3.7	2.7	3.0	2.5	2.2	3.7
Other Medical	2.5	2.1	1.6	1.7	0.1	0.3	1.0	0.4	0.7	0.3
Continuation	76.8	78.3	81.2	86.2	89.0	91.9	87.9	88.1	92.0	91.8
No. of Women:										
At Start of Year	4932	3149	2018	1121	872	621	563	483	423	325
At End of Year	3149	2018	1121	872	621	563	483	423	325	230

* Rates were calculated by weighing the annual rates by the number of subjects starting each year for each of the Population Council (3536 acceptors) and the World Health Organization (1396 acceptors) trials.

3. Insertion Prophylaxis

Observe strict asepsis at insertion; clean the endocervix with an antiseptic solution, because the presence of organisms capable of establishing PID cannot be determined by appearance, and because IUD insertion may be associated with introduction of vaginal bacteria into the uterus. Data do not confirm the utility of prophylactic administration of antibiotics in reducing the incidence of PID, and their use in nursing women is not recommended.

4. Requirements for Continuation and Removal

a. The ParaGard® T 380A must be replaced before the end of the tenth year of use. There is no evidence of decreasing contraceptive efficacy with time before ten years, but the contraceptive effectiveness at longer times has not been established; therefore, the patient should be informed of the known duration of contraceptive efficacy and be advised to return in 10 years for removal and possible insertion of a new ParaGard® T 380A.

b. The ParaGard® T 380A should be removed for the following medical reasons: menorrhagia- and/or metrorrhagia-producing anemia; pelvic infection; genital actinomycosis; intractable pelvic pain; dyspareunia; pregnancy, endometrial or cervical malignancy; uterine or cervical perforation; increase in length of the threads extending from the cervix, or any other indication of partial expulsion. Insertions immediately following placental delivery or first trimester abortion may result in threads becoming slightly longer as the uterus involutes and may not represent expulsion or partial expulsion.

c. If the retrieval threads cannot be visualized, they may have retracted into the uterus or have been broken, or the ParaGard® T 380A may have been broken, or the ParaGard® T 380A may have been expelled. Localization may be made by feeling with a probe, X-ray, or sonography. When the physician elects to recover a ParaGard® T 380A with the threads not visible, the removal instructions should be reviewed.

d. Should the patient's relationship cease to be mutually monogamous, or should her partner become HIV positive, or acquire a sexually transmitted disease, she should be instructed to report this change to her clinician immediately. It may be advisable to recommend the use of a barrier method as a partial protection against acquiring sexually transmitted diseases until the ParaGard® T 380A can be removed.

5. Continuing Care of Patients Using ParaGard® T 380A

a. Any inquiries regarding pain, odorous discharge, bleeding, fever, genital lesions or sores, or a missed period should be promptly responded to and prompt examination is recommended.

b. If examination during visits subsequent to insertion reveals that the length of the threads has visibly or palpably changed from the length at time of insertion, the ParaGard® T 380A should be considered displaced and should be removed. A new ParaGard® T 380A may be inserted at that time or during the next menses if it is certain that conception has not occurred. Under no circumstances should reinsertion with an expelled ParaGard® T 380A be attempted. A new ParaGard® T 380A should be inserted.

c. Since the ParaGard® T 380A may be partially or completely expelled, patients should be reexamined and evaluated shortly after the first postinsertion menses, but no later than 3 months afterwards. Thereafter, at least annual examination with appropriate evaluation, including a "Pap" smear, and if indicated, gonococcal and chlamydial laboratory evaluations, should be carried out. The ParaGard® T 380A should be kept in place no longer than 10 years.

d. In the event a pregnancy is confirmed during ParaGard T 380A use, the following steps should be taken:

- Determine whether the pregnancy is ectopic and take appropriate measures if it is.
- Inform patient of the risks of leaving an IUD *in situ* or removing it during pregnancy, and of the lack of data on the long term effects of the ParaGard® T 380A on the offspring of women who have had it *in utero* during conception or gestation (see WARNINGS). This information should include the risk of septic spontaneous abortion with the IUD *in situ*.
- If possible, the ParaGard® T 380A should be removed after the patient has been warned of the risks of removal. If removal is difficult, the patient should be counseled about and offered pregnancy termination.
- If the ParaGard® T 380A is left in place, the patient's course should be followed closely.

ADVERSE REACTIONS

These adverse reactions are not listed in any order of frequency or severity.

Reported adverse reactions with intrauterine contraceptives include: endometritis; spontaneous abortion; septic abortion; septicemia; perforation of the uterus and cervix; embedment; fragmentation of the IUD; pelvic infection; tubo-ovarian abscess; tubal damage; vaginitis; leukorrhea; cervical erosion; pregnancy; ectopic pregnancy; fetal damage; difficult removal; complete or partial expulsion of the IUD, particularly in those patients with uteri measuring less than 6.0 cm by sounding; menstrual spotting; prolongation of menstrual flow; anemia; amenorrhea or delayed menses; pain and cramping; dysmenorrhea; backaches; dyspareunia; neurovascular episodes, including bradycardia and syncope secondary to insertion. Uterine perforation and IUD displacement into the abdomen have been followed by peritonitis, abdominal adhesions, intestinal penetration, intestinal obstruction, and cystic masses in the pelvis. (Certain of these adverse reactions can lead to loss of fertility, partial or total removal of reproductive organs, hormonal imbalance, or death.) Urticarial allergic skin reaction may occur.

CLINICAL STUDIES

Different event rates have been reported with the use of different intrauterine contraceptives. Inasmuch as these rates are usually derived from separate studies conducted by different investigators in several populations, they cannot be compared with precision. Considerably different rates are likely to be obtained because event rates per unit of time tend to decrease as studies are extended, since more suscep-

Continued on next page

Paragard T 380A—Cont.

tible subjects discontinue due to expulsions, adverse reactions, or pregnancy, leaving the study population richer in less susceptible subjects. In clinical trials conducted by The Population Council[14,15] and WHO, use-effectiveness of the ParaGard® T 380A as calculated by the life table method was determined through ten (10) years of use.

Data suggest a higher pregnancy rate in women under 20.[14,15,17]

[See table II at top of previous page]

TABLE III GROSS ANNUAL EVENT RATES PER 100 CONTINUING USERS BY YEAR AND PARITY

	1 Year Parous
Pregnancy	0.5
Expulsion	2.3
Bleeding/Pain	3.4
Infection	0.3
Other Medical	0.5
Planning Pregnancy	0.6
Other Personal	0.7
Continuation	92.1
No. Completed	1842.0

Rates were calculated by combining the experience on a weighted basis from both an international study by the World Health Organization (2110 women) and a U.S. study by GynoPharma Inc. (230 women).

The lowest expected and typical failure rates during the first year of continuous use of all contraceptive methods are listed in Table IV (Adapted from Reference 16).

[See table IV above]

HOW SUPPLIED

Available in cartons of one (NDC 54765-380-01) or five (NDC 54765-380-05) sterile units. Each ParaGard® T 380A is packaged in a Tyvek®-polyethylene pouch, together with an insertion tube and solid rod.

CLINICIANS SHOULD HAVE DEMONSTRATED CLINICAL COMPETENCE IN PARAGARD® T 380A INSERTIONS, MANAGEMENT, AND REMOVAL RECEIVED UNDER SUPERVISION. PREVIOUS EDUCATION RE: SURGICAL PROCEDURES WILL REQUIRE VARYING LEVELS OF EXPERIENCE.

The ParaGard® T 380A (Intrauterine Copper Contraceptive) represents a different design in intrauterine contraceptives. Physicians are, therefore, cautioned that they should become thoroughly familiar with instructions for insertion before attempting placement of the ParaGard® T 380A. The insertion technique is different in several respects from that employed with other intrauterine contraceptives and the physician should pay particular attention to the drawings and commentary accompanying these instructions.

A single ParaGard® T 380A is placed at the fundus of the uterine cavity.

The ParaGard® T 380A may be inserted at any time during the cycle. However, it is essential that pregnancy be ruled out before insertion.

The ParaGard® T 380A is indicated for use up to 10 years. Therefore, the ParaGard® T 380A must be removed and a new one inserted on or before 10 years from the date of insertion.

PRELIMINARY PREPARATION AND INSERTION

1. Before insertion, you and the patient will want to review the Patient Package Insert. If the patient agrees, she may sign the Consent Form provided for your records.
2. Take a medical and social history.
3. Refer to CONTRAINDICATIONS, WARNINGS, and PRECAUTIONS.
4. Pelvic examination is to be performed prior to insertion of the ParaGard® T 380A, including a cervical "Pap" smear, and gonococcal and chlamydial evaluations, if indicated, and any other necessary specific tests.
5. If appropriate, commence antibiotic prophylaxis one hour before insertion.
6. Use of aseptic technique during insertion is essential.
7. The endocervix should be cleansed with an antiseptic solution and a tenaculum applied to the cervix with downward traction for correction of the angulation as well as stabilization of the cervix.
8. With a speculum in place, gently insert a sterile sound to determine the depth and direction of the uterine canal. Be sure to determine the position of the uterus before insertion.

CAUTION

Any intrauterine procedure can result in severe pain, bradycardia, and syncope.

It is generally believed that perforations, if they occur, are encountered at the time of insertion, although the perforation may not be detected until some time later. The position of the uterus should be determined during the preinsertion examination. Great care must be exercised during the preinsertion sounding and subsequent insertion. No attempt should be made to force the insertion.

TABLE IV—Percentage of women experiencing a contraceptive failure during the first year of typical use and the first year of perfect use and the percentage continuing use at the end of the first year, United States.[16]

Method	% of Women Experiencing an Accidental Pregnancy Within the First Year of Use		% of Women Continuing Use at One Year[3]
	Typical Use[1]	Perfect Use[2]	
Chance[4]	85	85	
Spermicides[5]	21	6	43
Periodic Abstinence	20		67
Calendar		9	
Ovulation Method		3	
Sympto-Thermal[6]		2	
Post-Ovulation		1	
Withdrawal	19	4	
Cap[7]			
Parous Women	36	26	45
Nulliparous Women	18	9	58
Sponge			
Parous Women	36	20	45
Nulliparous Women	18	9	58
Diaphragm[7]	18	6	58
Condom[8]			
Female (Reality)	21	5	56
Male	12	3	63
Pill	3		72
Progestin Only		0.5	
Combined		0.1	
IUD			
Progesterone T	2.0	1.5	81
Copper T 380A (ParaGard® T 380A)	0.8	0.6	78
Depo-Provera®	0.3	0.3	70
Norplant® (6 Capsules)	0.09	0.09	85
Female Sterilization	0.4	0.4	100
Male Sterilization	0.15	0.10	100

Emergency Contraceptive Pills: Treatment initiated within 72 hours after unprotected intercourse reduces the risk of pregnancy by at least 75%.[9]

Lactational Amenorrhea Method: LAM is a highly effective temporary method of contraception.[10]

Footnotes to Table IV

1. Among *typical* couples who initiate use of a method (not necessarily for the first time), the percentage who experience an accidental pregnancy during the first year if they do not stop use for any other reason.
2. Among couples who initiate use of a method (not necessarily for the first time) and who use it *perfectly* (both consistently and correctly), the percentage who experience an accidental pregnancy during the first year if they do not stop use for any other reason.
3. Among couples attempting to avoid pregnancy, the percentage who continue to use a method for one year.
4. The percentages failing in columns (2) and (3) are based on data from populations where contraception is not used and from women who cease using contraception in order to become pregnant. Among such populations, about 89% become pregnant within one year. This estimate was lowered slightly (to 85%) to represent the percentage who would become pregnant within 1 year among women now relying on reversible methods of contraception if they abandoned contraception altogether.
5. Foams, creams, gels, vaginal suppositories, and vaginal film.
6. Cervical mucus (ovulation) method supplemented by calendar in the pre-ovulatory and basal body temperature in the post-ovulatory phases.
7. With spermicidal cream or jelly.
8. Without spermicides.
9. The treatment schedule is one dose as soon as possible (but no more than 72 hours) after unprotected intercourse, and a second dose 12 hours after the first dose. The hormones that have been studied in the clinical trials of postcoital hormonal contraception are found in Nordette, Levlen, Lo/Orval (1 dose is 4 pills), Triphasil, Tri-Levlin (1 dose is 4 yellow pills), and Ovral (1 dose is 2 pills).
10. However, to maintain effective protection against pregnancy, another method of contraception must be used as soon as menstruation resumes, the frequency or duration of breastfeeds is reduced, bottle feeds are introduced, or the baby reaches 6 months of age.

HOW TO LOAD AND INSERT ParaGard® T 380A

STEP 1

To minimize the chance of introducing contamination, do not remove the ParaGard® T 380A from the insertion tube prior to placement in the uterus. Do not bend the arms of the ParaGard® T 380A earlier than 5 minutes before it is to be introduced into the uterus.

In the absence of sterile gloves, this can be accomplished without destroying sterility by folding the arms in the partially opened package. Place the partially opened package on a flat surface and pull the solid rod partially from the package so it will not interfere with assembly. Place thumb and index finger on top of package on ends of the horizontal arms. Push insertion tube against arms of ParaGard® T 380A as indicated by arrow in Fig. 1A to start arms folding.

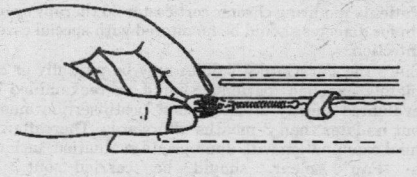

Fig. 1B

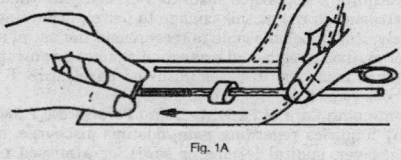

Fig. 1A

Complete the bending by bringing the thumb and index finger together using the other hand to maneuver the insertion tube to pick up the arms of the ParaGard® T 380A (Fig. 1B). Insert no further than necessary to insure retention of the arms. Introduce the solid rod into the insertion tube from the bottom alongside the threads until it touches the bottom of the ParaGard® T 380A.

[See figure at top of next column]

STEP 2

Adjust the movable flange so that it indicates the depth to which the ParaGard® T 380A should be inserted and the direction in which the arms of the ParaGard® T 380A will

open. At this point, make certain that the horizontal arms of the ParaGard® T 380A and the long axis of the flange lie in the same horizontal plane. Introduce the loaded insertion tube through the cervical canal and upwards until the ParaGard® T 380A lies in contact with the fundus. The movable flange should be at the cervix (Fig. 2).

DO NOT FORCE THE INSERTION.

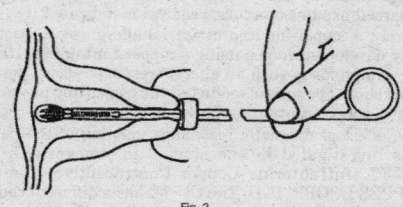

Fig. 2

STEP 3

To release the arms of the ParaGard® T 380A, withdraw the insertion tube not more than ½ inch while the solid rod is not permitted to move. This releases the arms of the ParaGard® T 380A (Fig. 3).

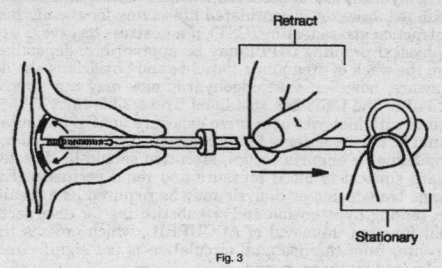

Fig. 3

STEP 4
After the arms are released, the insertion tube should be moved upward gently, until the resistance of the fundus is felt. This will assure placement of the T at the highest possible position within the endometrial cavity (Fig. 4).

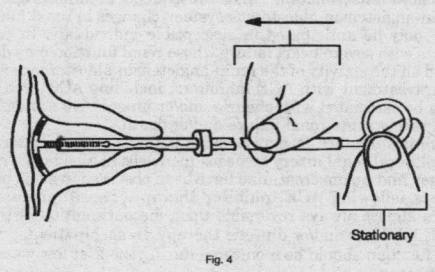

Fig. 4

STEP 5
Withdraw the solid rod while holding the insertion tube stationary (Fig. 5).

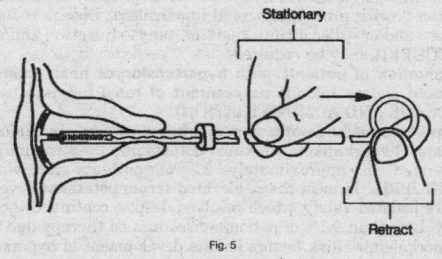

Fig. 5

STEP 6
Withdraw the insertion tube from the cervix. Be sure sufficient length of the threads are visible (approximately 1 in. or 2.5 cm.) to facilitate checking for the presence of the ParaGard® T 380A (Fig. 6). Notation of length of the threads should be made in patient record.

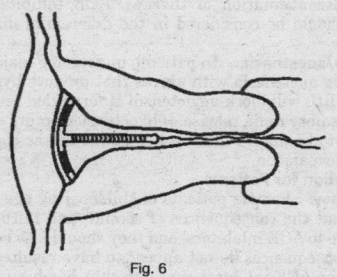

Fig. 6

HOW TO REMOVE ParaGard® T 380A
To remove the ParaGard® T 380A, pull gently on the exposed threads. The arms of the ParaGard® T 380A will fold upwards as it is withdrawn from the uterus. Even if removal proves difficult, the ParaGard® T 380A should not remain in the uterus after 10 years.

REFERENCES
1. Alvarez F et al: New insights on the mode of action on intrauterine contraceptives in women. *Fertil Steril* 1988; 49:768–773.
2. World Health Organization's Special Programme of Research, Development and Research Training in Human Reproduction: A multinational case-control study of ectopic pregnancy. *Clin Reprod Fertil* 1985; 3:131–143.
3. Ory HW, Women's Health Study: Ectopic pregnancy and intrauterine contraceptive devices: New perspectives. *Obstet Gynecol* 1981; 57:137–144.
4. Marchbanks PA et al: Risk factors for ectopic pregnancy: A population-based study. *JAMA* 1988; 259:1823–1827.
5. Farley TMM et al: Intrauterine devices and pelvic inflammatory disease: An international perspective. *Lancet* 1992; 339:785–788.
6. Cramer DW et al: Tubal infertility and the intrauterine device. *N Engl J Med* 1985; 312:941–947.
7. Daling JR et al: Primary tubal infertility in relation to the use of an intrauterine device. *N Engl J Med* 1985; 312:937–941.
8. Heartwell SF, Schlesselman S: Risk of uterine perforation among users of intrauterine devices. *Obstet Gynecol* 1983; 61:31–36.
9. Chi I-C, Kelly E: Is lactation a risk factor of IUD and sterilization-related uterine perforations? A hypothesis. *Int J Gynaecol Obstet* 1984; 22:315–317.
10. Harlap S, Kost K, Forrest JD: Preventing pregnancy, protecting health: a new look at birth control choices in the United States. The Alan Guttmacher Institute 1991; 1–129.
11. Chi I-C et al: Performance of the Copper T 380A Intrauterine device in breast feeding women. *Contraception* 1989; 39:603–618.
12. Farr G, Rivera R: Interactions between intrauterine contraceptive device use and breast-feeding status at time of intrauterine contraceptive device insertion. Analysis of TCu-380A acceptors in developing countries. *Am J Obstet Gynecol* 1992; 167:144–151.
13. Mark AS, Hricak H: Intrauterine contraceptive devices: MR imaging. *Radiology* 1987; 311–314.
14. Sivin I, Stern J: Long-acting, more effective Copper T IUDs: A summary of US experience, 1970–1975. *Stud Fam Plann* 1979; 10:263–281.
15. Sivin I, Schmidt F: Effectiveness of IUDs: A review. *Contraception* 1987; 36:55–84.
16. Trussell J: The Essentials of Contraception, in R.A. Hatcher, et al: *Contraceptive Technology*, 16th Revised Ed., New York, Irvington, 1994, p. 113–114.
17. World Health Organization (WHO): Mechanism of action, safety, and efficacy of intrauterine devices. Report of a WHO Scientific Group. Technical Report Series 753. Geneva; World Health Organization, 1987, p. 22.

Manufactured for
ORTHO-McNEIL PHARMACEUTICAL, INC.
Raritan, New Jersey 08869
by FEI Products, Inc.
N. Tonawanda, New York 14120

10U0732

©OMP 1998   Revised September 2000   631-40-410-5

Parke-Davis
**A Warner-Lambert Division
A Pfizer Company
201 TABOR ROAD
MORRIS PLAINS, NEW JERSEY 07950**

For Medical Information Contact:
During working hours:
Customer Service
Product/Medical Information
(800) 223-0432
FAX: (973) 385-2248
After Hours and Weekend Emergencies:
(973) 385-6089

Distribution:
1855 Shelby Oaks Drive North
Memphis, TN 38134
(901) 387-5200
Customer Service:
(800) 533-4535

EXPORT INQUIRIES:
Pfizer International Inc.
(212) 573-2323

ACCUPRIL®   ℞
(Quinapril Hydrochloride Tablets)

Prescribing information for this product, which appears on pages 2414–2417 of the 2001 PDR, has been completely revised as follows. Please write "See Supplement A" next to the product heading.

> **USE IN PREGNANCY**
> When used in pregnancy during the second and third trimesters, ACE inhibitors can cause injury and even death to the developing fetus. When pregnancy is detected, ACCUPRIL should be discontinued as soon as possible. See WARNINGS, Fetal/Neonatal Morbidity and Mortality.

DESCRIPTION
ACCUPRIL® (quinapril hydrochloride) is the hydrochloride salt of quinapril, the ethyl ester of a non-sulfhydryl, angiotensin-converting enzyme (ACE) inhibitor, quinaprilat. Quinapril hydrochloride is chemically described as [3S-[2[R*(R*)], 3R*]]-2-[2-[[1-(ethoxycarbonyl)-3-phenylpropyl]amino]-1-oxopropyl]-1,2,3,4-tetrahydro-3-isoquinolinecarboxylic acid, monohydrochloride. Its empirical formula is $C_{25}H_{30}N_2O_5 \cdot HCl$ and its structural formula is:
[See chemical structure at top of next column]
Quinapril hydrochloride is a white to off-white amorphous powder that is freely soluble in aqueous solvents.
ACCUPRIL tablets contain 5 mg, 10 mg, 20 mg, or 40 mg of quinapril for oral administration. Each tablet also contains

M.W.=474.98

candelilla wax, crospovidone, gelatin, lactose, magnesium carbonate, magnesium stearate, synthetic red iron oxide, and titanium dioxide.

CLINICAL PHARMACOLOGY
Mechanism of Action: Quinapril is deesterified to the principal metabolite, quinaprilat, which is an inhibitor of ACE activity in human subjects and animals. ACE is a peptidyl dipeptidase that catalyzes the conversion of angiotensin I to the vasoconstrictor, angiotensin II. The effect of quinapril in hypertension and in congestive heart failure (CHF) appears to result primarily from the inhibition of circulating and tissue ACE activity, thereby reducing angiotensin II formation. Quinapril inhibits the elevation in blood pressure caused by intravenously administered angiotensin I, but has no effect on the pressor response to angiotensin II, norepinephrine or epinephrine. Angiotensin II also stimulates the secretion of aldosterone from the adrenal cortex, thereby facilitating renal sodium and fluid reabsorption. Reduced aldosterone secretion by quinapril may result in a small increase in serum potassium. In controlled hypertension trials, treatment with ACCUPRIL alone resulted in mean increases in potassium of 0.07 mmol/L (see PRECAUTIONS). Removal of angiotensin II negative feedback on renin secretion leads to increased plasma renin activity (PRA).
While the principal mechanism of antihypertensive effect is thought to be through the renin-angiotensin-aldosterone system, quinapril exerts antihypertensive actions even in patients with low renin hypertension. ACCUPRIL was an effective antihypertensive in all races studied, although it was somewhat less effective in blacks (usually a predominantly low renin group) than in nonblacks. ACE is identical to kininase II, an enzyme that degrades bradykinin, a potent peptide vasodilator; whether increased levels of bradykinin play a role in the therapeutic effect of quinapril remains to be elucidated.
Pharmacokinetics and Metabolism: Following oral administration, peak plasma quinapril concentrations are observed within one hour. Based on recovery of quinapril and its metabolites in urine, the extent of absorption is at least 60%. The rate and extent of quinapril absorption are diminished moderately (approximately 25–30%) when ACCUPRIL tablets are administered during a high-fat meal. Following absorption, quinapril is deesterified to its major active metabolite, quinaprilat (about 38% of oral dose), and to other minor inactive metabolites. Following multiple oral dosing of ACCUPRIL, there is an effective accumulation half-life of quinaprilat of approximately 3 hours, and peak plasma quinaprilat concentrations are observed approximately 2 hours post-dose. Quinaprilat is eliminated primarily by renal excretion, up to 96% of an IV dose, and has an elimination half-life in plasma of approximately 2 hours and a prolonged terminal phase with a half-life of 25 hours. The pharmacokinetics of quinapril and quinaprilat are linear over a single-dose range of 5–80 mg doses and 40–160 mg in multiple daily doses. Approximately 97% of either quinapril or quinaprilat circulating in plasma is bound to proteins.
In patients with renal insufficiency, the elimination half-life of quinaprilat increases as creatinine clearance decreases. There is a linear correlation between plasma quinaprilat clearance and creatinine clearance. In patients with end-stage renal disease, chronic hemodialysis or continuous ambulatory peritoneal dialysis has little effect on the elimination of quinapril and quinaprilat. Elimination of quinaprilat may be reduced in elderly patients (≥65 years) and in those with heart failure; this reduction is attributable to decrease in renal function (see DOSAGE AND ADMINISTRATION). Quinaprilat concentrations are reduced in patients with alcoholic cirrhosis due to impaired deesterification of quinapril. Studies in rats indicate that quinapril and its metabolites do not cross the blood-brain barrier.
Pharmacodynamics and Clinical Effects
Hypertension: Single doses of 20 mg of ACCUPRIL provide over 80% inhibition of plasma ACE for 24 hours. Inhibition of the pressor response to angiotensin I is shorter-lived, with a 20 mg dose giving 75% inhibition for about 4 hours, 50% inhibition for about 8 hours, and 20% inhibition at 24 hours. With chronic dosing, however, there is substantial inhibition of angiotensin II levels at 24 hours by doses of 20–80 mg. Administration of 10 to 80 mg of ACCUPRIL to patients with mild to severe hypertension results in a reduction of sitting and standing blood pressure to about the same extent with minimal effect on heart rate. Symptomatic postural hypotension is infrequent although it can occur in patients who are salt-and/or volume-depleted (see WARNINGS). Antihypertensive activity commences within 1 hour with peak effects usually achieved by 2 to 4 hours after dosing. During chronic therapy, most of the blood pressure lowering effect of a given dose is obtained in 1–2 weeks. In multiple-dose studies, 10–80 mg per day in single or divided doses lowered systolic and diastolic blood pressure throughout the dosing interval, with a trough effect of about 5–11/3–7 mm Hg. The trough effect represents about 50% of the peak effect. While the dose-response relationship is relatively flat, doses of 40–80 mg were somewhat more effec-

Continued on next page

Accupril—Cont.

tive at trough than 10–20 mg, and twice daily dosing tended to give a somewhat lower trough blood pressure than once daily dosing with the same total dose. The antihypertensive effect of ACCUPRIL continues during long-term therapy, with no evidence of loss of effectiveness.

Hemodynamic assessments in patients with hypertension indicate that blood pressure reduction produced by quinapril is accompanied by a reduction in total peripheral resistance and renal vascular resistance with little or no change in heart rate, cardiac index, renal blood flow, glomerular filtration rate, or filtration fraction.

Use of ACCUPRIL with a thiazide diuretic gives a blood-pressure lowering effect greater than that seen with either agent alone.

In patients with hypertension, ACCUPRIL 10–40 mg was similar in effectiveness to captopril, enalapril, propranolol, and thiazide diuretics.

Therapeutic effects appear to be the same for elderly (≥65 years of age) and younger adult patients given the same daily dosages, with no increase in adverse events in elderly patients.

Heart Failure: In a placebo-controlled trial involving patients with congestive heart failure treated with digitalis and diuretics, parenteral quinaprilat, the active metabolite of quinapril, reduced pulmonary capillary wedge pressure and systemic vascular resistance and increased cardiac output/index. Similar favorable hemodynamic effects were seen with oral quinapril in baseline-controlled trials, and such effects appeared to be maintained during chronic oral quinapril therapy. Quinapril reduced renal hepatic vascular resistance and increased renal and hepatic blood flow with glomerular filtration rate remaining unchanged.

A significant dose response relationship for improvement in maximal exercise tolerance has been observed with ACCUPRIL therapy. Beneficial effects on the severity of heart failure as measured by New York Heart Association (NYHA) classification and Quality of Life and on symptoms of dyspnea, fatigue, and edema were evident after 6 months in a double blind, placebo controlled study. Favorable effects were maintained for up to two years of open label therapy. The effects of quinapril on long-term mortality in heart failure have not been evaluated.

INDICATIONS AND USAGE

Hypertension

ACCUPRIL is indicated for the treatment of hypertension. It may be used alone or in combination with thiazide diuretics.

Heart Failure

ACCUPRIL is indicated in the management of heart failure as adjunctive therapy when added to conventional therapy including diuretics and/or digitalis.

In using ACCUPRIL, consideration should be given to the fact that another angiotensin-converting enzyme inhibitor, captopril, has caused agranulocytosis, particularly in patients with renal impairment or collagen vascular disease. Available data are insufficient to show that ACCUPRIL does not have a similar risk (see WARNINGS).

Angioedema in black patients: Black patients receiving ACE inhibitor monotherapy have been reported to have a higher incidence of angioedema compared to non-blacks. It should also be noted that in controlled clinical trials ACE inhibitors have an effect on blood pressure that is less in black patients than in non-blacks.

CONTRAINDICATIONS

ACCUPRIL is contraindicated in patients who are hypersensitive to this product and in patients with a history of angioedema related to previous treatment with an ACE inhibitor.

WARNINGS

Anaphylactoid and Possibly Related Reactions

Presumably because angiotensin-converting inhibitors affect the metabolism of eicosanoids and polypeptides, including endogenous bradykinin, patients receiving ACE inhibitors (including Accupril) may be subject to a variety of adverse reactions, some of them serious.

Angioedema:

Angioedema of the face, extremities, lips, tongue, glottis, and larynx has been reported in patients treated with ACE inhibitors and has been seen in 0.1% of patients receiving ACCUPRIL.

In two similarly sized U.S. postmarketing trials that, combined, enrolled over 3,000 black patients and over 19,000 non-blacks, angioedema was reported in 0.30% and 0.55% of blacks (in study 1 and 2 respectively) and 0.39% and 0.17% of non-blacks.

Angioedema associated with laryngeal edema can be fatal. If laryngeal stridor or angioedema of the face, tongue, or glottis occurs, treatment with ACCUPRIL should be discontinued immediately, the patient treated in accordance with accepted medical care, and carefully observed until the swelling disappears. In instances where swelling is confined to the face and lips, the condition generally resolves without treatment; antihistamines may be useful in relieving symptoms. **Where there is involvement of the tongue, glottis, or larynx likely to cause airway obstruction, emergency therapy including, but not limited to, subcutaneous epinephrine solution 1:1000 (0.3 to 0.5 mL) should be promptly administered** (see ADVERSE REACTIONS).

Patients with a history of angioedema: Patients with a history of angioedema unrelated to ACE inhibitor therapy may be at increased risk of angioedema while receiving an ACE inhibitor (see also CONTRAINDICATIONS).

Anaphylactoid reactions during desensitization: Two patients undergoing desensitizing treatment with hymenoptera venom while receiving ACE inhibitors sustained life-threatening anaphylactoid reactions. In the same patients, these reactions were avoided when ACE inhibitors were temporarily withheld, but they reappeared upon inadvertent rechallenge.

Anaphylactoid reactions during membrane exposure: Anaphylactoid reactions have been reported in patients dialyzed with high-flux membranes and treated concomitantly with an ACE inhibitor. Anaphylactoid reactions have also been reported in patients undergoing low-density lipoprotein apheresis with dextran sulfate absorption.

Hepatic Failure: Rarely, ACE inhibitors have been associated with a syndrome that starts with cholestatic jaundice and progresses to fulminant hepatic necrosis and (sometimes) death. The mechanism of this syndrome is not understood. Patients receiving ACE inhibitors who develop jaundice or marked elevations of hepatic enzymes should discontinue the ACE inhibitor and receive appropriate medical follow-up.

Hypotension: Excessive hypotension is rare in patients with uncomplicated hypertension treated with ACCUPRIL alone. Patients with heart failure given ACCUPRIL commonly have some reduction in blood pressure, but discontinuation of therapy because of continuing symptomatic hypotension usually is not necessary when dosing instructions are followed. Caution should be observed when initiating therapy in patients with heart failure (see DOSAGE AND ADMINISTRATION). In controlled studies, syncope was observed in 0.4% of patients (N=3203); this incidence was similar to that observed for captopril (1%) and enalapril (0.8%). Patients at risk of excessive hypotension, sometimes associated with oliguria and/or progressive azotemia, and rarely with acute renal failure and/or death, include patients with the following conditions or characteristics: heart failure, hyponatremia, high dose diuretic therapy, recent intensive diuresis or increase in diuretic dose, renal dialysis, or severe volume and/or salt depletion of any etiology. It may be advisable to eliminate the diuretic (except in patients with heart failure), reduce the diuretic dose or cautiously increase salt intake (except in patients with heart failure) before initiating therapy with ACCUPRIL in patients at risk for excessive hypotension who are able to tolerate such adjustments.

In patients at risk of excessive hypotension, therapy with ACCUPRIL should be started under close medical supervision. Such patients should be followed closely for the first two weeks of treatment and whenever the dose of ACCUPRIL and/or diuretic is increased. Similar considerations may apply to patients with ischemic heart or cerebrovascular disease in whom an excessive fall in blood pressure could result in a myocardial infarction or a cerebrovascular accident.

If excessive hypotension occurs, the patient should be placed in the supine position and, if necessary, receive an intravenous infusion of normal saline. A transient hypotensive response is not a contraindication to further doses of ACCUPRIL, which usually can be given without difficulty once the blood pressure has stabilized. If symptomatic hypotension develops a dose reduction or discontinuation of ACCUPRIL or concomitant diuretic may be necessary.

Neutropenia/Agranulocytosis: Another ACE inhibitor, captopril, has been shown to cause agranulocytosis and bone marrow depression rarely in patients with uncomplicated hypertension, but more frequently in patients with renal impairment, especially if they also have a collagen vascular disease, such as systemic lupus erythematosus or scleroderma. Agranulocytosis did occur during ACCUPRIL treatment in one patient with a history of neutropenia during previous captopril therapy. Available data from clinical trials of ACCUPRIL are insufficient to show that, in patients without prior reactions to other ACE inhibitors, ACCUPRIL does not cause agranulocytosis at similar rates. As with other ACE inhibitors, periodic monitoring of white blood cell counts in patients with collagen vascular disease and/or renal disease should be considered.

Fetal/Neonatal Morbidity and Mortality: ACE inhibitors can cause fetal and neonatal morbidity and death when administered to pregnant women. Several dozen cases have been reported in the world literature. When pregnancy is detected, ACE inhibitors should be discontinued as soon as possible.

The use of ACE inhibitors during the second and third trimesters of pregnancy has been associated with fetal and neonatal injury, including hypotension, neonatal skull hypoplasia, anuria, reversible or irreversible renal failure, and death. Oligohydramnios has also been reported, presumably resulting from decreased fetal renal function; oligohydramnios in this setting has been associated with fetal limb contractures, craniofacial deformation, and hypoplastic lung development. Prematurity, intrauterine growth retardation, and patent ductus arteriosus have also been reported, although it is not clear whether these occurrences were due to the ACE inhibitor exposure.

These adverse effects do not appear to have resulted from intrauterine ACE inhibitor exposure that has been limited to the first trimester. Mothers whose embryos and fetuses are exposed to ACE inhibitors only during the first trimester should be so informed. Nonetheless, when patients become pregnant, physicians should make every effort to discontinue the use of ACCUPRIL as soon as possible.

Rarely (probably less often than once in every thousand pregnancies), no alternative to ACE inhibitors will be found. In these rare cases, the mothers should be apprised of the potential hazards to their fetuses, and serial ultrasound examinations should be performed to assess the intraamniotic environment.

If oligohydramnios is observed, ACCUPRIL should be discontinued unless it is considered life-saving for the mother. Contraction stress testing (CST), a non-stress test (NST), or biophysical profiling (BPP) may be appropriate, depending upon the week of pregnancy. Patients and physicians should be aware, however, that oligohydramnios may not appear until after the fetus has sustained irreversible injury.

Infants with histories of *in utero* exposure to ACE inhibitors should be closely observed for hypotension, oliguria, and hyperkalemia. If oliguria occurs, attention should be directed toward support of blood pressure and renal perfusion. Exchange transfusion or dialysis may be required as a means of reversing hypotension and/or substituting for disordered renal function. Removal of ACCUPRIL, which crosses the placenta, from the neonatal circulation is not significantly accelerated by these means.

No teratogenic effects of ACCUPRIL were seen in studies of pregnant rats and rabbits. On a mg/kg basis, the doses used were up to 180 times (in rats) and one time (in rabbits) the maximum recommended human dose.

PRECAUTIONS

General

Impaired renal function: As a consequence of inhibiting the renin-angiotensin-aldosterone system, changes in renal function may be anticipated in susceptible individuals. In patients with severe heart failure whose renal function may depend on the activity of the renin-angiotensin-aldosterone system, treatment with ACE inhibitors, including ACCUPRIL, may be associated with oliguria and/or progressive azotemia and rarely acute renal failure and/or death.

In clinical studies in hypertensive patients with unilateral or bilateral renal artery stenosis, increases in blood urea nitrogen and serum creatinine have been observed in some patients following ACE inhibitor therapy. These increases were almost always reversible upon discontinuation of the ACE inhibitor and/or diuretic therapy. In such patients, renal function should be monitored during the first few weeks of therapy.

Some patients with hypertension or heart failure with no apparent preexisting renal vascular disease have developed increases in blood urea and serum creatinine, usually minor and transient, especially when ACCUPRIL has been given concomitantly with a diuretic. This is more likely to occur in patients with preexisting renal impairment. Dosage reduction and/or discontinuation of any diuretic and/or ACCUPRIL may be required.

Evaluation of patients with hypertension or heart failure should always include assessment of renal function (see DOSAGE AND ADMINISTRATION).

Hyperkalemia and potassium-sparing diuretics: In clinical trials, hyperkalemia (serum potassium ≥5.8 mmol/L) occurred in approximately 2% of patients receiving ACCUPRIL. In most cases, elevated serum potassium levels were isolated values which resolved despite continued therapy. Less than 0.1% of patients discontinued therapy due to hyperkalemia. Risk factors for the development of hyperkalemia include renal insufficiency, diabetes mellitus, and the concomitant use of potassium-sparing diuretics, potassium supplements, and/or potassium-containing salt substitutes, which should be used cautiously, if at all, with ACCUPRIL (see PRECAUTIONS, Drug Interactions).

Cough: Presumably due to the inhibition of the degradation of endogenous bradykinin, persistent non-productive cough has been reported with all ACE inhibitors, always resolving after discontinuation of therapy. ACE inhibitor-induced cough should be considered in the differential diagnosis of cough.

Surgery/anesthesia: In patients undergoing major surgery or during anesthesia with agents that produce hypotension, ACCUPRIL will block angiotensin II formation secondary to compensatory renin release. If hypotension occurs and is considered to be due to this mechanism, it can be corrected by volume expansion.

Information for Patients

Pregnancy: Female patients of childbearing age should be told about the consequences of second- and third-trimester exposure to ACE inhibitors, and they should also be told that these consequences do not appear to have resulted from intrauterine ACE-inhibitor exposure that has been limited to the first trimester. These patients should be asked to report pregnancies to their physicians as soon as possible.

Angioedema: Angioedema, including laryngeal edema can occur with treatment with ACE inhibitors, especially following the first dose. Patients should be so advised and told to report immediately any signs or symptoms suggesting angioedema (swelling of face, extremities, eyes, lips, tongue, difficulty in swallowing or breathing) and to stop taking the drug until they have consulted with their physician (see WARNINGS).

Symptomatic hypotension: Patients should be cautioned that lightheadedness can occur, especially during the first few days of ACCUPRIL therapy, and that it should be reported to a physician. If actual syncope occurs, patients should be told to not take the drug until they have consulted with their physician (see WARNINGS).

All patients should be cautioned that inadequate fluid intake or excessive perspiration, diarrhea, or vomiting can lead to an excessive fall in blood pressure because of reduction in fluid volume, with the same consequences of lightheadedness and possible syncope.

Patients planning to undergo any surgery and/or anesthesia should be told to inform their physician that they are taking an ACE inhibitor.

Hyperkalemia: Patients should be told not to use potassium supplements or salt substitutes containing potassium without consulting their physician (see PRECAUTIONS).

Neutropenia: Patients should be told to report promptly any indication of infection (eg, sore throat, fever) which could be a sign of neutropenia.

NOTE: As with many other drugs, certain advice to patients being treated with ACCUPRIL is warranted. This information is intended to aid in the safe and effective use of this medication. It is not a disclosure of all possible adverse or intended effects.

Drug Interactions

Concomitant diuretic therapy: As with other ACE inhibitors, patients on diuretics, especially those on recently instituted diuretic therapy, may occasionally experience an excessive reduction of blood pressure after initiation of therapy with ACCUPRIL. The possibility of hypotensive effects with ACCUPRIL may be minimized by either discontinuing the diuretic or cautiously increasing salt intake prior to initiation of treatment with ACCUPRIL. If it is not possible to discontinue the diuretic, the starting dose of quinapril should be reduced (see DOSAGE AND ADMINISTRATION).

Agents increasing serum potassium: Quinapril can attenuate potassium loss caused by thiazide diuretics and increase serum potassium when used alone. If concomitant therapy of ACCUPRIL with potassium-sparing diuretics (eg, spironolactone, triamterene, or amiloride), potassium supplements, or potassium-containing salt substitutes is indicated, they should be used with caution along with appropriate monitoring of serum potassium (see PRECAUTIONS).

Tetracycline and other drugs that interact with magnesium: Simultaneous administration of tetracycline with ACCUPRIL reduced the absorption of tetracycline by approximately 28% to 37%, possibly due to the high magnesium content in ACCUPRIL tablets. This interaction should be considered if coprescribing ACCUPRIL and tetracycline or other drugs that interact with magnesium.

Lithium: Increased serum lithium levels and symptoms of lithium toxicity have been reported in patients receiving concomitant lithium and ACE inhibitor therapy. These drugs should be coadministered with caution and frequent monitoring of serum lithium levels is recommended. If a diuretic is also used, it may increase the risk of lithium toxicity.

Other agents: Drug interaction studies of ACCUPRIL with other agents showed:

- Multiple dose therapy with propranolol or cimetidine has no effect on the pharmacokinetics of single doses of ACCUPRIL.
- The anticoagulant effect of a single dose of warfarin (measured by prothrombin time) was not significantly changed by quinapril coadministration twice-daily.
- ACCUPRIL treatment did not affect the pharmacokinetics of digoxin.
- No pharmacokinetic interaction was observed when single doses of ACCUPRIL and hydrochlorothiazide were administered concomitantly.

Carcinogenesis, Mutagenesis, Impairment of Fertility

Quinapril hydrochloride was not carcinogenic in mice or rats when given in doses up to 75 or 100 mg/kg/day (50 to 60 times the maximum human daily dose, respectively, on an mg/kg basis and 3.8 to 10 times the maximum human daily dose when based on an mg/m² basis) for 104 weeks. Female rats given the highest dose level had an increased incidence of mesenteric lymph node hemangiomas and skin/subcutaneous lipomas. Neither quinapril nor quinaprilat were mutagenic in the Ames bacterial assay with or without metabolic activation. Quinapril was also negative in the following genetic toxicology studies: *in vitro* mammalian cell point mutation, sister chromatid exchange in cultured mammalian cells, micronucleus test with mice, *in vitro* chromosome aberration with V79 cultured lung cells, and in an *in vivo* cytogenetic study with rat bone marrow. There were no adverse effects on fertility or reproduction in rats at doses up to 100 mg/kg/day (60 and 10 times the maximum daily human dose when based on mg/kg and mg/m², respectively).

Pregnancy

Pregnancy Categories C (first trimester) and D (second and third trimesters): See WARNINGS, Fetal/Neonatal Morbidity and Mortality.

Nursing Mothers

Because ACCUPRIL is secreted in human milk, caution should be exercised when this drug is administered to a nursing woman.

Pediatric Use

The safety and effectiveness of ACCUPRIL in pediatric patients have not been established.

Geriatric Use

Of the total number of subjects in clinical studies of ACCUPRIL, 21% were 65 and over. (There was no distinction between patients over 65 or over 75 years.) No overall differences in safety or effectiveness were observed between these subjects and younger subjects, and other reported clinical experience has not identified differences in responses between the elderly and younger patients, but greater sensitivity of some older individuals cannot be ruled out.

This drug is known to be substantially excreted by the kidney, and the risk of toxic reactions to this drug may be greater in patients with impaired renal function. Because elderly patients are more likely to have decreased renal function, care should be taken in dose selection, and it may be useful to monitor renal function.

Elderly patients exhibited increased area under the plasma concentration time curve and peak levels for quinaprilat compared to values observed in younger patients; this appeared to relate to decreased renal function rather than to age itself.

ADVERSE REACTIONS

Hypertension

ACCUPRIL has been evaluated for safety in 4960 subjects and patients. Of these, 3203 patients, including 655 elderly patients, participated in controlled clinical trials. ACCUPRIL has been evaluated for long-term safety in over 1400 patients treated for 1 year or more.

Adverse experiences were usually mild and transient.

In placebo-controlled trials, discontinuation of therapy because of adverse events was required in 4.7% of patients with hypertension.

Adverse experiences probably or possibly related to therapy or of unknown relationship to therapy occurring in 1% or more of the 1563 patients in placebo-controlled hypertension trials who were treated with ACCUPRIL are shown below.

Adverse Events in Placebo-Controlled Trials

	Accupril (N=1563) Incidence (Discontinuance)	Placebo (N=579) Incidence (Discontinuance)
Headache	5.6 (0.7)	10.9 (0.7)
Dizziness	3.9 (0.8)	2.6 (0.2)
Fatigue	2.6 (0.3)	1.0
Coughing	2.0 (0.5)	0.0
Nausea and/or Vomiting	1.4 (0.3)	1.9 (0.2)
Abdominal Pain	1.0 (0.2)	0.7

Heart Failure

Accupril has been evaluated for safety in 1222 ACCUPRIL treated patients. Of these, 632 patients participated in controlled clinical trials. In placebo-controlled trials, discontinuation of therapy because of adverse events was required in 6.8% of patients with congestive heart failure.

Adverse experiences probably or possibly related or of unknown relationship to therapy occurring in 1% or more of the 585 patients in placebo-controlled congestive heart failure trials who were treated with ACCUPRIL are shown below.

	Accupril (N=585) Incidence (Discontinuance)	Placebo (N=295) Incidence (Discontinuance)
Dizziness	7.7 (0.7)	5.1 (1.0)
Coughing	4.3 (0.3)	1.4
Fatigue	2.6 (0.2)	1.4
Nausea and/or Vomiting	2.4 (0.2)	0.7
Chest Pain	2.4	1.0
Hypotension	2.9 (0.5)	1.0
Dyspnea	1.9 (0.2)	2.0
Diarrhea	1.7	1.0
Headache	1.7	1.0 (0.3)
Myalgia	1.5	2.0
Rash	1.4 (0.2)	1.0
Back Pain	1.2	0.3

See PRECAUTIONS, Cough.

Hypertension and/or Heart Failure

Clinical adverse experiences probably, possibly, or definitely related, or of uncertain relationship to therapy occurring in 0.5% to 1.0% (except as noted) of the patients with CHF or hypertension treated with ACCUPRIL (with or without concomitant diuretic) in controlled or uncontrolled trials (N=4847) and less frequent, clinically significant events seen in clinical trials or post-marketing experience (the rarer events are in italics) include (listed by body system):

General: back pain, malaise, viral infections

Cardiovascular: palpitation, vasodilation, tachycardia, *heart failure, hyperkalemia, myocardial infarction, cerebrovascular accident, hypertensive crisis, angina pectoris, orthostatic hypotension, cardiac rhythm disturbances, cardiogenic shock*

Hematology: *hemolytic anemia*

Gastrointestinal: flatulence, dry mouth or throat, constipation, *gastrointestinal hemorrhage, pancreatitis, abnormal liver function tests*

Nervous/Psychiatric: somnolence, vertigo, syncope, nervousness, depression, insomnia, paresthesia

Integumentary: alopecia, increased sweating, pemphigus, pruritus, *exfoliative dermatitis, photosensitivity reaction, dermatopolymyositis*

Urogenital: urinary tract infection, impotence, *acute renal failure, worsening renal failure*

Respiratory: *eosinophilic pneumonitis*

Other: amblyopia, edema, arthralgia, pharyngitis, *agranulocytosis, hepatitis, thrombocytopenia*

Fetal/Neonatal Morbidity and Mortality

See WARNINGS, Fetal/Neonatal Morbidity and Mortality.

Angioedema

Angioedema has been reported in patients receiving ACCUPRIL (0.1%). Angioedema associated with laryngeal edema may be fatal. If angioedema of the face, extremities, lips, tongue, glottis, and/or larynx occurs, treatment with ACCUPRIL should be discontinued and appropriate therapy instituted immediately. (See WARNINGS.)

Clinical Laboratory Test Findings

Hematology: (See WARNINGS)

Hyperkalemia: (See PRECAUTIONS)

Creatinine and Blood Urea Nitrogen: Increases (>1.25 times the upper limit of normal) in serum creatinine and blood urea nitrogen were observed in 2% and 2%, respectively, of all patients treated with ACCUPRIL alone. Increases are more likely to occur in patients receiving concomitant diuretic therapy than in those on ACCUPRIL alone. These increases often remit on continued therapy. In controlled studies of heart failure, increases in blood urea nitrogen and serum creatinine were observed in 11% and 8%, respectively, of patients treated with ACCUPRIL; most often these patients were receiving diuretics with or without digitalis.

OVERDOSAGE

No data are available with respect to overdosage in humans. Doses of 1440 to 4280 mg/kg of quinapril cause significant lethality in mice and rats.

The most likely clinical manifestation would be symptoms attributable to severe hypotension.

Laboratory determinations of serum levels of quinapril and its metabolites are not widely available, and such determinations have, in any event, no established role in the management of quinapril overdose.

No data are available to suggest physiological maneuvers (eg, maneuvers to change pH of the urine) that might accelerate elimination of quinapril and its metabolites. Hemodialysis and peritoneal dialysis have little effect on the elimination of quinapril and quinaprilat. Angiotensin II could presumably serve as a specific antagonist-antidote in the setting of quinapril overdose, but angiotensin II is essentially unavailable outside of scattered research facilities. Because the hypotensive effect of quinapril is achieved through vasodilation and effective hypovolemia, it is reasonable to treat quinapril overdose by infusion of normal saline solution.

DOSAGE AND ADMINISTRATION

Hypertension

Monotherapy: The recommended initial dosage of ACCUPRIL in patients not on diuretics is 10 or 20 mg once daily. Dosage should be adjusted according to blood pressure response measured at peak (2–6 hours after dosing) and trough (predosing). Generally, dosage adjustments should be made at intervals of at least 2 weeks. Most patients have required dosages of 20, 40, or 80 mg/day, given as a single dose or in two equally divided doses. In some patients treated once daily, the antihypertensive effect may diminish toward the end of the dosing interval. In such patients an increase in dosage or twice daily administration may be warranted. In general, doses of 40–80 mg and divided doses give a somewhat greater effect at the end of the dosing interval.

Concomitant Diuretics: If blood pressure is not adequately controlled with ACCUPRIL monotherapy, a diuretic may be added. In patients who are currently being treated with a diuretic, symptomatic hypotension occasionally can occur following the initial dose of ACCUPRIL. To reduce the likelihood of hypotension, the diuretic should, if possible, be discontinued 2 to 3 days prior to beginning therapy with ACCUPRIL (see WARNINGS). Then, if blood pressure is not controlled with ACCUPRIL alone, diuretic therapy should be resumed.

If the diuretic cannot be discontinued, an initial dose of 5 mg ACCUPRIL should be used with careful medical supervision for several hours and until blood pressure has stabilized. The dosage should subsequently be titrated (as described above) to the optimal response (see WARNINGS, PRECAUTIONS, and Drug Interactions.)

Renal Impairment: Kinetic data indicate that the apparent elimination half-life of quinaprilat increases as creatinine clearance decreases. Recommended starting doses, based on clinical and pharmacokinetic data from patients with renal impairment, are as follows:

Creatinine Clearance	Maximum Recommended Initial Dose
>60 mL/min	10 mg
30–60 mL/min	5 mg
10–30 mL/min	2.5 mg
<10 mL/min	Insufficient data for dosage recommendation

Patients should subsequently have their dosage titrated (as described above) to the optimal response.

Elderly (≥65 years): The recommended initial dosage of ACCUPRIL in elderly patients is 10 mg given once daily followed by titration (as described above) to the optimal response.

Heart Failure

ACCUPRIL is indicated as adjunctive therapy when added to conventional therapy including diuretics and/or digitalis. The recommended starting dose is 5 mg twice daily. This dose may improve symptoms of heart failure, but increases in exercise duration have generally required higher doses. Therefore, if the initial dosage of ACCUPRIL is well tolerated, patients should then be titrated at weekly intervals until an effective dose, usually 20 to 40 mg daily given in two equally divided doses, is reached or undesirable hypotension, orthostatis, or azotemia (see WARNINGS) prohibit reaching this dose.

Following the initial dose of ACCUPRIL, the patient should be observed under medical supervision for at least two

Continued on next page

Accupril—Cont.

hours for the presence of hypotension or orthostatis and, if present, until blood pressure stabilizes. The appearance of hypotension, orthostasis, or azotemia early in dose titration should not preclude further careful dose titration. Consideration should be given to reducing the dose of concomitant diuretics.

DOSE ADJUSTMENTS IN PATIENTS WITH HEART FAILURE AND RENAL IMPAIRMENT OR HYPONATREMIA

Pharmacokinetic data indicate that quinapril elimination is dependent on level of renal function. In patients with heart failure and renal impairment, the recommended initial dose of ACCUPRIL is 5 mg in patients with a creatinine clearance above 30 mL/min and 2.5 mg in patients with a creatinine clearance of 10 to 30 mL/min. There is insufficient data for dosage recommendation in patients with a creatinine clearance less than 10 mL/min. (See DOSAGE AND ADMINISTRATION, Heart Failure, WARNINGS, and PRECAUTIONS, Drug Interactions.)

If the initial dose is well tolerated, ACCUPRIL may be administered the following day as a twice daily regimen. In the absence of excessive hypotension or significant deterioration of renal function, the dose may be increased at weekly intervals based on clinical and hemodynamic response.

HOW SUPPLIED

ACCUPRIL tablets are supplied as follows:

5-mg tablets: brown, film-coated, elliptical scored tablets, coded "PD 527" on one side and "5" on the other.
N0071-0527-23 bottles of 90 tablets
N0071-0527-40 10 × 10 unit dose blisters

10-mg tablets: brown, film-coated, triangular tablets, coded "PD 530" on one side and "10" on the other.
N0071-0530-23 bottles of 90 tablets
N0071-0530-40 10 × 10 unit dose blisters

20-mg tablets: brown, film-coated, round tablets, coded "PD 532" on one side and "20" on the other.
N0071-0532-23 bottles of 90 tablets
N0071-0532-40 10 × 10 unit dose blisters

40-mg tablets: brown, film-coated, elliptical tablets, coded "PD 535" on one side and "40" on the other.
N0071-0535-23 bottles of 90 tablets

Dispense in well-closed containers as defined in the USP.

Storage: Store at controlled room temperature 15°–30°C (59°–86°F).

Protect from light.

Rx only

Revised July 2000

Manufactured by:
Parke Davis Pharmaceuticals, Ltd.
Vega Baja, PR 00694
Distributed by:
PARKE-DAVIS
Div of Warner-Lambert Co
Morris Plains, NJ 07950 USA
0527G078

CEREBYX® ℞

(Fosphenytoin Sodium Injection)

Prescribing information for this product, which appears on pages 2422–2425 of the 2001 PDR, has been completely revised as follows. Please write "See Supplement A" next to the product heading.

DESCRIPTION

Cerebyx® (fosphenytoin sodium injection) is a prodrug intended for parenteral administration; its active metabolite is phenytoin. Each Cerebyx vial contains 75 mg/mL fosphenytoin sodium (hereafter referred to as fosphenytoin) **equivalent to 50 mg/mL phenytoin sodium** after administration. Cerebyx is supplied in vials as a ready-mixed solution in Water for Injection, USP, and Tromethamine, USP (TRIS), buffer adjusted to pH 8.6 to 9.0 with either Hydrochloric Acid, NF, or Sodium Hydroxide, NF. Cerebyx is a clear, colorless to pale yellow, sterile solution.

The chemical name of fosphenytoin is 5,5-diphenyl-3-[(phosphonooxy)methyl]-2,4-imidazolidinedione disodium salt. The molecular structure of fosphenytoin is:

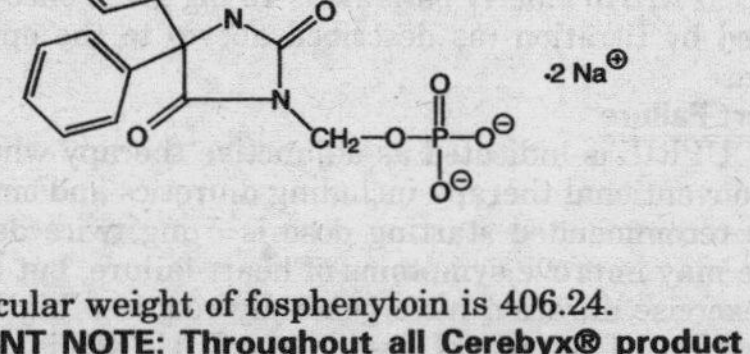

The molecular weight of fosphenytoin is 406.24.

IMPORTANT NOTE: Throughout all Cerebyx® product labeling, the amount and concentration of fosphenytoin is expressed in terms of phenytoin sodium equivalents (PE). Fosphenytoin's weight is expressed as phenytoin sodium equivalents to avoid the need to perform molecular weight-based adjustments when converting between fosphenytoin and phenytoin sodium doses. Cerebyx should always be prescribed and dispensed in phenytoin sodium equivalent units (PE) (see DOSAGE AND ADMINISTRATION).

CLINICAL PHARMACOLOGY

Introduction

Following parenteral administration of Cerebyx, fosphenytoin is converted to the anticonvulsant phenytoin. For every mmol of fosphenytoin administered, one mmol of phenytoin is produced. The pharmacological and toxicological effects of fosphenytoin include those of phenytoin. However, the hydrolysis of fosphenytoin to phenytoin yields two metabolites, phosphate and formaldehyde. Formaldehyde is subsequently converted to formate, which is in turn metabolized via a folate dependent mechanism. Although phosphate and formaldehyde (formate) have potentially important biological effects, these effects typically occur at concentrations considerably in excess of those obtained when Cerebyx is administered under conditions of use recommended in this labeling.

Mechanism of Action

Fosphenytoin is a prodrug of phenytoin and accordingly, its anticonvulsant effects are attributable to phenytoin.

After IV administration to mice, fosphenytoin blocked the tonic phase of maximal electroshock seizures at doses equivalent to those effective for phenytoin. In addition to its ability to suppress maximal electroshock seizures in mice and rats, phenytoin exhibits anticonvulsant activity against kindled seizures in rats, audiogenic seizures in mice, and seizures produced by electrical stimulation of the brainstem in rats. The cellular mechanisms of phenytoin thought to be responsible for its anticonvulsant actions include modulation of voltage-dependent sodium channels of neurons, inhibition of calcium flux across neuronal membranes, modulation of voltage-dependent calcium channels of neurons, and enhancement of the sodium-potassium ATPase activity of neurons and glial cells. The modulation of sodium channels may be a primary anticonvulsant mechanism because this property is shared with several other anticonvulsants in addition to phenytoin.

Pharmacokinetics and Drug Metabolism

Fosphenytoin

Absorption/Bioavailability: *Intravenous:* When Cerebyx is administered by IV infusion, maximum plasma fosphenytoin concentrations are achieved at the end of the infusion. Fosphenytoin has a half-life of approximately 15 minutes.

Intramuscular: Fosphenytoin is completely bioavailable following IM administration of Cerebyx. Peak concentrations occur at approximately 30 minutes postdose. Plasma fosphenytoin concentrations following IM administration are lower but more sustained than those following IV administration due to the time required for absorption of fosphenytoin from the injection site.

Distribution: Fosphenytoin is extensively bound (95% to 99%) to human plasma proteins, primarily albumin. Binding to plasma proteins is saturable with the result that the percent bound decreases as total fosphenytoin concentrations increase. Fosphenytoin displaces phenytoin from protein binding sites. The volume of distribution of fosphenytoin increases with Cerebyx dose and rate, and ranges from 4.3 to 10.8 liters.

Metabolism and Elimination: The conversion half-life of fosphenytoin to phenytoin is approximately 15 minutes. The mechanism of fosphenytoin conversion has not been determined, but phosphatases probably play a major role. Fosphenytoin is not excreted in urine. Each mmol of fosphenytoin is metabolized to 1 mmol of phenytoin, phosphate, and formate (see CLINICAL PHARMACOLOGY, Introduction and PRECAUTIONS, Phosphate Load for Renally Impaired Patients).

Phenytoin (after Cerebyx administration)

In general, IM administration of Cerebyx generates systemic phenytoin concentrations that are similar enough to oral phenytoin sodium to allow essentially interchangeable use.

The pharmacokinetics of fosphenytoin following IV administration of Cerebyx, however, are complex, and when used in an emergency setting (eg, status epilepticus), differences in rate of availability of phenytoin could be critical. Studies have therefore empirically determined an infusion rate for Cerebyx that gives a rate and extent of phenytoin systemic availability similar to that of a 50 mg/min phenytoin sodium infusion.

A dose of 15 to 20 mg PE/kg of Cerebyx infused at 100 to 150 mg PE/min yields plasma free phenytoin concentrations over time that approximate those achieved when an equivalent dose of phenytoin sodium (eg, parenteral Dilantin®) is administered at 50 mg/min (see DOSAGE AND ADMINISTRATION, WARNINGS).

[See figure at top of next column]

Following administration of single IV Cerebyx doses of 400 to 1200 mg PE, mean maximum total phenytoin concentrations increase in proportion to dose, but do not change appreciably with changes in infusion rate. In contrast, mean maximum unbound phenytoin concentrations increase with both dose and rate.

Absorption/Bioavailability: Fosphenytoin is completely converted to phenytoin following IV administration, with a half-life of approximately 15 minutes. Fosphenytoin is also completely converted to phenytoin following IM administration and plasma total phenytoin concentrations peak in approximately 3 hours.

Distribution: Phenytoin is highly bound to plasma proteins, primarily albumin, although to a lesser extent than fosphenytoin. In the absence of fosphenytoin, approximately 12% of total plasma phenytoin is unbound over the clinically relevant concentration range. However, fosphenytoin displaces phenytoin from plasma protein binding sites. This increases the fraction of phenytoin unbound (up to 30% unbound) during the period required for conversion of fosphenytoin to phenytoin (approximately 0.5 to 1 hour postinfusion).

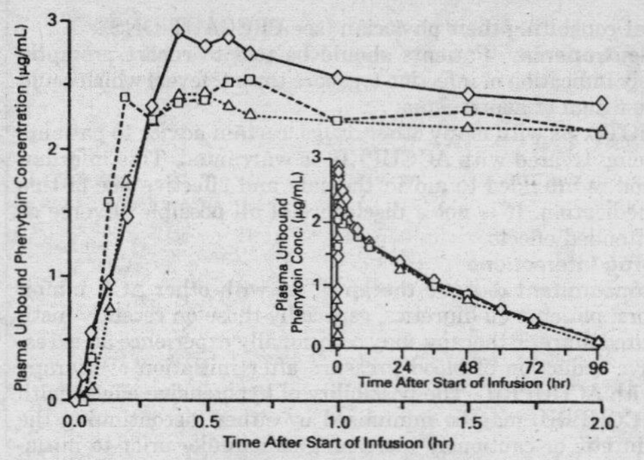

FIGURE 1. Mean plasma unbound phenytoin concentrations following IV administration of 1200 mg PE Cerebyx infused at 100 mg PE/min (triangles) or 150 mg PE/min (squares) and 1200 mg Dilantin infused at 50 mg/min (diamonds) to healthy subjects (N = 12). Inset shows time course for the entire 96-hour sampling period.

Metabolism and Elimination: Phenytoin derived from administration of Cerebyx is extensively metabolized in the liver and excreted in urine primarily as 5-(p-hydroxyphenyl)-5-phenylhydantoin and its glucuronide; little unchanged phenytoin (1%–5% of the Cerebyx dose) is recovered in urine. Phenytoin hepatic metabolism is saturable, and following administration of single IV Cerebyx doses of 400 to 1200 mg PE, total and unbound phenytoin AUC values increase disproportionately with dose. Mean total phenytoin half-life values (12.0 to 28.9 hr) following Cerebyx administration at these doses are similar to those after equal doses of parenteral Dilantin and tend to be greater at higher plasma phenytoin concentrations.

Special Populations

Patients with Renal or Hepatic Disease: Due to an increased fraction of unbound phenytoin in patients with renal or hepatic disease, or in those with hypoalbuminemia, the interpretation of total phenytoin plasma concentrations should be made with caution (see DOSAGE AND ADMINISTRATION). Unbound phenytoin concentrations may be more useful in these patient populations. After IV administration of Cerebyx to patients with renal and/or hepatic disease, or in those with hypoalbuminemia, fosphenytoin clearance to phenytoin may be increased without a similar increase in phenytoin clearance. This has the potential to increase the frequency and severity of adverse events (see PRECAUTIONS).

Age: The effect of age was evaluated in patients 5 to 98 years of age. Patient age had no significant impact on fosphenytoin pharmacokinetics. Phenytoin clearance tends to decrease with increasing age (20% less in patients over 70 years of age relative to that in patients 20–30 years of age). Phenytoin dosing requirements are highly variable and must be individualized (see DOSAGE AND ADMINISTRATION).

Gender and Race: Gender and race have no significant impact on fosphenytoin or phenytoin pharmacokinetics.

Pediatrics: Only limited pharmacokinetic data are available in children (N=8; age 5 to 10 years). In these patients with status epilepticus who received loading doses of Cerebyx, the plasma fosphenytoin, total phenytoin, and unbound phenytoin concentration-time profiles did not signal any major differences from those in adult patients with status epilepticus receiving comparable doses.

Clinical Studies

Infusion tolerance was evaluated in clinical studies. One double-blind study assessed infusion-site tolerance of equivalent loading doses (15–20 mg PE/kg) of Cerebyx infused at 150 mg PE/min or phenytoin infused at 50 mg/min. The study demonstrated better local tolerance (pain and burning at the infusion site), fewer disruptions of the infusion, and a shorter infusion period for Cerebyx-treated patients (Table 1).

TABLE 1. Infusion Tolerance of Equivalent Loading Doses of IV Cerebyx and IV Phenytoin

	IV Cerebyx N=90	IV Phenytoin N=22
Local Intolerance	9%[a]	90%
Infusion Disrupted	21%	67%
Average Infusion Time	13 min	44 min

[a]Percent of patients

Cerebyx-treated patients, however, experienced more systemic sensory disturbances (see PRECAUTIONS, Sensory Disturbances).

Infusion disruptions in Cerebyx-treated patients were primarily due to systemic burning, pruritus, and/or paresthesia while those in phenytoin-treated patients were primarily due to pain and burning at the infusion site (see Table 1).

In a double-blind study investigating temporary substitution of Cerebyx for oral phenytoin, IM Cerebyx was as well-tolerated as IM placebo. IM Cerebyx resulted in a slight increase in transient, mild to moderate local itching (23% of patients vs 11% of IM placebo-treated patients at any time during the study). This study also demonstrated that equimolar doses of IM Cerebyx may be substituted for oral phenytoin sodium with no dosage adjustments needed when initiating IM or returning to oral therapy. In contrast, switching between IM and oral phenytoin requires dosage adjustments because of slow and erratic phenytoin absorption from muscle.

INDICATIONS AND USAGE

Cerebyx is indicated for short-term parenteral administration when other means of phenytoin administration are unavailable, inappropriate or deemed less advantageous. The safety and effectiveness of Cerebyx in this use has not been systematically evaluated for more than 5 days.

Cerebyx can be used for the control of generalized convulsive status epilepticus and prevention and treatment of seizures occurring during neurosurgery. It can also be substituted, short-term, for oral phenytoin.

CONTRAINDICATIONS

Cerebyx is contraindicated in patients who have demonstrated hypersensitivity to Cerebyx or its ingredients, or to phenytoin or other hydantoins.

Because of the effect of parenteral phenytoin on ventricular automaticity, Cerebyx is contraindicated in patients with sinus bradycardia, sino-atrial block, second and third degree A-V block, and Adams-Stokes syndrome.

WARNINGS

DOSES OF CEREBYX ARE EXPRESSED AS THEIR PHENYTOIN SODIUM EQUIVALENTS IN THIS LABELING (PE=phenytoin sodium equivalent).

DO NOT, THEREFORE, MAKE ANY ADJUSTMENT IN THE RECOMMENDED DOSES WHEN SUBSTITUTING CEREBYX FOR PHENYTOIN SODIUM OR VICE VERSA.

The following warnings are based on experience with Cerebyx or phenytoin.

Status Epilepticus Dosing Regimen

- **Do not administer Cerebyx at a rate greater than 150 mg PE/min.**

The dose of IV Cerebyx (15 to 20 mg PE/kg) that is used to treat status epilepticus is administered at a maximum rate of 150 mg PE/min. The typical Cerebyx infusion administered to a 50 kg patient would take between 5 and 7 minutes. Note that the delivery of an identical molar dose of phenytoin using parenteral Dilantin or generic phenytoin sodium injection cannot be accomplished in less than 15 to 20 minutes because of the untoward cardiovascular effects that accompany the direct intravenous administration of phenytoin at rates greater than 50 mg/min.

If rapid phenytoin loading is a primary goal, IV administration of Cerebyx is preferred because the time to achieve therapeutic plasma phenytoin concentrations is greater following IM than that following IV administration (see DOSAGE AND ADMINISTRATION).

Withdrawal Precipitated Seizure, Status Epilepticus

Antiepileptic drugs should not be abruptly discontinued because of the possibility of increased seizure frequency, including status epilepticus. When, in the judgement of the clinician, the need for dosage reduction, discontinuation, or substitution of alternative antiepileptic medication arises, this should be done gradually. However, in the event of an allergic or hypersensitivity reaction, rapid substitution of alternative therapy may be necessary. In this case, alternative therapy should be an antiepileptic drug not belonging to the hydantoin chemical class.

Cardiovascular Depression

Hypotension may occur, especially after IV administration at high doses and high rates of administration. Following administration of phenytoin, severe cardiovascular reactions and fatalities have been reported with atrial and ventricular conduction depression and ventricular fibrillation. Severe complications are most commonly encountered in elderly or gravely ill patients. Therefore, careful cardiac monitoring is needed when administering IV loading doses of Cerebyx. Reduction in rate of administration or discontinuation of dosing may be needed.

Cerebyx should be used with caution in patients with hypotension and severe myocardial insufficiency.

Rash

Cerebyx should be discontinued if a skin rash appears. If the rash is exfoliative, purpuric, or bullous, or if lupus erythematosus, Stevens-Johnson syndrome, or toxic epidermal necrolysis is suspected, use of this drug should not be resumed and alternative therapy should be considered. If the rash is of a milder type (measles-like or scarlatiniform), therapy may be resumed after the rash has completely disappeared. If the rash recurs upon reinstitution of therapy, further Cerebyx or phenytoin administration is contraindicated.

Hepatic Injury

Cases of acute hepatotoxicity, including infrequent cases of acute hepatic failure, have been reported with phenytoin. These incidents have been associated with a hypersensitivity syndrome characterized by fever, skin eruptions, and lymphadenopathy, and usually occur within the first 2 months of treatment. Other common manifestations include jaundice, hepatomegaly, elevated serum transaminase levels, leukocytosis, and eosinophilia. The clinical course of acute phenytoin hepatotoxicity ranges from prompt recovery to fatal outcomes. In these patients with acute hepatotoxicity, Cerebyx should be immediately discontinued and not readministered.

Hemopoietic System

Hemopoietic complications, some fatal, have occasionally been reported in association with administration of phenytoin. These have included thrombocytopenia, leukopenia, granulocytopenia, agranulocytosis, and pancytopenia with or without bone marrow suppression.

There have been a number of reports that have suggested a relationship between phenytoin and the development of lymphadenopathy (local or generalized), including benign lymph node hyperplasia, pseudolymphoma, lymphoma, and Hodgkin's disease. Although a cause and effect relationship has not been established, the occurrence of lymphadenopathy indicates the need to differentiate such a condition from other types of lymph node pathology. Lymph node involvement may occur with or without symptoms and signs resembling serum sickness, eg, fever, rash, and liver involvement. In all cases of lymphadenopathy, follow-up observation for an extended period is indicated and every effort should be made to achieve seizure control using alternative antiepileptic drugs.

Alcohol Use

Acute alcohol intake may increase plasma phenytoin concentrations while chronic alcohol use may decrease plasma concentrations.

Usage in Pregnancy

Clinical:

A. *Risks to Mother.* An increase in seizure frequency may occur during pregnancy because of altered phenytoin pharmacokinetics. Periodic measurement of plasma phenytoin concentrations may be valuable in the management of pregnant women as a guide to appropriate adjustment of dosage (see PRECAUTIONS, Laboratory Tests). However, postpartum restoration of the original dosage will probably be indicated.

B. *Risks to the Fetus.* If this drug is used during pregnancy, or if the patient becomes pregnant while taking the drug, the patient should be apprised of the potential harm to the fetus.

Prenatal exposure to phenytoin may increase the risks for congenital malformations and other adverse developmental outcomes. Increased frequencies of major malformations (such as orofacial clefts and cardiac defects), minor anomalies (dysmorphic facial features, nail and digit hypoplasia), growth abnormalities (including microcephaly), and mental deficiency have been reported among children born to epileptic women who took phenytoin alone or in combination with other antiepileptic drugs during pregnancy. There have also been several reported cases of malignancies, including neuroblastoma, in children whose mothers received phenytoin during pregnancy. The overall incidence of malformations for children of epileptic women treated with antiepileptic drugs (phenytoin and/or others) during pregnancy is about 10%, or two-to three-fold that in the general population. However, the relative contributions of antiepileptic drugs and other factors associated with epilepsy to this increased risk are uncertain and in most cases it has not been possible to attribute specific developmental abnormalities to particular antiepileptic drugs.

Patients should consult with their physicians to weigh the risks and benefits of phenytoin during pregnancy.

C. *Postpartum Period.* A potentially life-threatening bleeding disorder related to decreased levels of vitamin K-dependent clotting factors may occur in newborns exposed to phenytoin *in utero*. This drug-induced condition can be prevented with vitamin K administration to the mother before delivery and to the neonate after birth.

Preclinical: Increased frequencies of malformations (brain, cardiovascular, digit, and skeletal anomalies), death, growth retardation, and functional impairment (chromodacryorrhea, hyperactivity, circling) were observed among the offspring of rats receiving fosphenytoin during pregnancy. Most of the adverse effects on embryo-fetal development occurred at doses of 33 mg PE/kg or higher (approximately 30% of the maximum human loading dose or higher on a mg/m^2 basis), which produced peak maternal plasma phenytoin concentrations of approximately 20 µg/mL or greater. Maternal toxicity was often associated with these doses and plasma concentrations, however, there is no evidence to suggest that the developmental effects were secondary to the maternal effects. The single occurrence of a rare brain malformation at a non-maternotoxic dose of 17 mg PE/kg (approximately 10% of the maximum human loading dose on a mg/m^2 basis) was also considered drug-induced. The developmental effects of fosphenytoin in rats were similar to those which have been reported following administration of phenytoin to pregnant rats.

No effects on embryo-fetal development were observed when rabbits were given up to 33 mg PE/kg of fosphenytoin (approximately 50% of the maximum human loading dose on a mg/m^2 basis) during pregnancy. Increased resorption and malformation rates have been reported following administration of phenytoin doses of 75 mg/kg or higher (approximately 120% of the maximum human loading dose or higher on a mg/m^2 basis) to pregnant rabbits.

PRECAUTIONS

General: (Cerebyx specific)

Sensory Disturbances

Severe burning, itching, and/or paresthesia were reported by 7 of 16 normal volunteers administered IV Cerebyx at a dose of 1200 mg PE at the maximum rate of administration (150 mg PE/min). The severe sensory disturbance lasted from 3 to 50 minutes in 6 of these subjects and for 14 hours in the seventh subject. In some cases, milder sensory disturbances persisted for as long as 24 hours. The location of the discomfort varied among subjects with the groin mentioned most frequently as an area of discomfort. In a separate cohort of 16 normal volunteers (taken from 2 other studies) who were administered IV Cerebyx at a dose of 1200 mg PE at the maximum rate of administration (150 mg PE/min), none experienced severe disturbances, but most experienced mild to moderate itching or tingling.

Patients administered Cerebyx at doses of 20 mg PE/kg at 150 mg PE/min are expected to experience discomfort of some degree. The occurrence and intensity of the discomfort can be lessened by slowing or temporarily stopping the infusion.

The effect of continuing infusion unaltered in the presence of these sensations is unknown. No permanent sequelae have been reported thus far. The pharmacologic basis for these positive sensory phenomena is unknown, but other phosphate ester drugs, which deliver smaller phosphate loads, have been associated with burning, itching, and/or tingling predominantly in the groin area.

Phosphate Load

The phosphate load provided by Cerebyx (0.0037 mmol phosphate/mg PE Cerebyx) should be considered when treating patients who require phosphate restriction, such as those with severe renal impairment.

IV Loading in Renal and/or Hepatic Disease or in Those With Hypoalbuminemia

After IV administration to patients with renal and/or hepatic disease, or in those with hypoalbuminemia, fosphenytoin clearance to phenytoin may be increased without a similar increase in phenytoin clearance. This has the potential to increase the frequency and severity of adverse events (see CLINICAL PHARMACOLOGY: Special Populations, and DOSAGE AND ADMINISTRATION: Dosing in Special Populations).

General: (phenytoin associated)

Cerebyx is *not* indicated for the treatment of *absence seizures*.

A small percentage of individuals who have been treated with phenytoin have been shown to metabolize the drug slowly. *Slow metabolism* may be due to limited enzyme availability and lack of induction; it appears to be genetically determined.

Phenytoin and other hydantoins are contraindicated in patients who have experienced phenytoin hypersensitivity. Additionally, caution should be exercised if using structurally similar (eg, barbiturates, succinimides, oxazolidinediones, and other related compounds) in these same patients.

Phenytoin has been infrequently associated with the exacerbation of *porphyria*. Caution should be exercised when Cerebyx is used in patients with this disease.

Hyperglycemia, resulting from phenytoin's inhibitory effect on insulin release, has been reported. Phenytoin may also raise the serum glucose concentrations in diabetic patients.

Plasma concentrations of phenytoin sustained above the optimal range may produce confusional states referred to as "delirium," "psychosis," or "encephalopathy," or rarely, irreversible cerebellar dysfunction. Accordingly, at the first sign of *acute toxicity*, determination of plasma phenytoin concentrations is recommended (see PRECAUTIONS: Laboratory Tests). Cerebyx dose reduction is indicated if phenytoin concentrations are excessive; if symptoms persist, administration of Cerebyx should be discontinued.

The liver is the primary site of biotransformation of phenytoin; patients with impaired liver function, elderly patients, or those who are gravely ill may show early signs of toxicity.

Phenytoin and other hydantoins are not indicated for seizures due to hypoglycemic or other metabolic causes. Appropriate diagnostic procedures should be performed as indicated.

Phenytoin has the potential to lower serum folate levels.

Laboratory Tests

Phenytoin doses are usually selected to attain therapeutic plasma total phenytoin concentrations of 10 to 20 µg/mL, (unbound phenytoin concentrations of 1 to 2 µg/mL). Following Cerebyx administration, it is recommended that phenytoin concentrations not be monitored until conversion to phenytoin is essentially complete. This occurs within approximately 2 hours after the end of IV infusion and 4 hours after IM injection.

Prior to complete conversion, commonly used immunoanalytical techniques, such as TDx®/TDxFLx™ (fluorescence polarization) and Emit® 2000 (enzyme multiplied), may significantly overestimate plasma phenytoin concentrations because of cross-reactivity with fosphenytoin. The error is dependent on plasma phenytoin and fosphenytoin concentration (influenced by Cerebyx dose, route and rate of administration, and time of sampling relative to dosing), and analytical method. Chromatographic assay methods accurately quantitate phenytoin concentrations in biological fluids in the presence of fosphenytoin. Prior to complete conversion, blood samples for phenytoin monitoring should be collected in tubes containing EDTA as an anticoagulant to minimize *ex vivo* conversion of fosphenytoin to phenytoin. However, even with specific assay methods, phenytoin concentrations measured before conversion of fosphenytoin is complete will not reflect phenytoin concentrations ultimately achieved.

Drug Interactions

No drugs are known to interfere with the conversion of fosphenytoin to phenytoin. Conversion could be affected by alterations in the level of phosphatase activity, but given the abundance and wide distribution of phosphatases in the body it is unlikely that drugs would affect this activity enough to affect conversion of fosphenytoin to phenytoin. Drugs highly bound to albumin could increase the unbound fraction of fosphenytoin. Although, it is unknown whether this could result in clinically significant effects, caution is advised when administering Cerebyx with other drugs that significantly bind to serum albumin.

Continued on next page

Cerebyx—Cont.

The pharmacokinetics and protein binding of fosphenytoin, phenytoin, and diazepam were not altered when diazepam and Cerebyx were concurrently administered in single submaximal doses.
The most significant drug interactions following administration of Cerebyx are expected to occur with drugs that interact with phenytoin. Phenytoin is extensively bound to serum plasma proteins and is prone to competitive displacement. Phenytoin is metabolized by hepatic cytochrome P450 enzymes and is particularly susceptible to inhibitory drug interactions because it is subject to saturable metabolism. Inhibition of metabolism may produce significant increases in circulating phenytoin concentrations and enhance the risk of drug toxicity. Phenytoin is a potent inducer of hepatic drug-metabolizing enzymes.
The most commonly occurring drug interactions are listed below:

- Drugs that may increase plasma phenytoin concentrations include: acute alcohol intake, amiodarone, chloramphenicol, chlordiazepoxide, cimetidine, diazepam, dicumarol, disulfiram, estrogens, ethosuximide, fluoxetine, H_2-antagonists, halothane, isoniazid, methylphenidate, phenothiazines, phenylbutazone, salicylates, succinimides, sulfonamides, tolbutamide, trazodone.
- Drugs that may decrease plasma phenytoin concentrations include: carbamazepine, chronic alcohol abuse, reserpine.
- Drugs that may either increase or decrease plasma phenytoin concentrations include: phenobarbital, valproic acid, and sodium valproate. Similarly, the effects of phenytoin on phenobarbital, valproic acid and sodium plasma valproate concentrations are unpredictable.
- Although not a true drug interaction, tricyclic antidepressants may precipitate seizures in susceptible patients and Cerebyx dosage may need to be adjusted.
- Drugs whose efficacy is impaired by phenytoin include: anticoagulants, corticosteroids, coumarin, digitoxin, doxycycline, estrogens, furosemide, oral contraceptives, rifampin, quinidine, theophylline, vitamin D.

Monitoring of plasma phenytoin concentrations may be helpful when possible drug interactions are suspected (see Laboratory Tests).

Drug/Laboratory Test Interactions
Phenytoin may decrease serum concentrations of T_4. It may also produce artifactually low results in dexamethasone or metyrapone tests. Phenytoin may also cause increased serum concentrations of glucose, alkaline phosphatase, and gamma glutamyl transpeptidase (GGT).
Care should be taken when using immunoanalytical methods to measure plasma phenytoin concentrations following Cerebyx administration (see Laboratory Tests).

Carcinogenesis, Mutagenesis, Impairment of Fertility
The carcinogenic potential of fosphenytoin has not been studied. Assessment of the carcinogenic potential of phenytoin in mice and rats is ongoing.
Structural chromosome aberration frequency in cultured V79 Chinese hamster lung cells was increased by exposure to fosphenytoin in the presence of metabolic activation. No evidence of mutagenicity was observed in bacteria (Ames test) or Chinese hamster lung cells *in vitro*, and no evidence for clastogenic activity was observed in an *in vivo* mouse bone marrow micronucleus test.
No effects on fertility were noted in rats of either sex given fosphenytoin. Maternal toxicity and altered estrous cycles, delayed mating, prolonged gestation length, and developmental toxicity were observed following administration of fosphenytoin during mating, gestation, and lactation at doses of 50 mg PE/kg or higher (approximately 40% of the maximum human loading dose or higher on a mg/m^2 basis).

Pregnancy—Category D: (see WARNINGS)

Use in Nursing Mothers
It is not known whether fosphenytoin is excreted in human milk.
Following administration of Dilantin, phenytoin appears to be excreted in low concentrations in human milk. Therefore, breast-feeding is not recommended for women receiving Cerebyx.

Pediatric Use
The safety of Cerebyx in pediatric patients has not been established.

Geriatric Use
No systematic studies in geriatric patients have been conducted. Phenytoin clearance tends to decrease with increasing age (see CLINICAL PHARMACOLOGY: Special Populations).

ADVERSE REACTIONS

The more important adverse clinical events caused by the IV use of Cerebyx or phenytoin are cardiovascular collapse and/or central nervous system depression. Hypotension can occur when either drug is administered rapidly by the IV route. The rate of administration is very important; for Cerebyx, it should not exceed 150 mg PE/min.
The adverse clinical events most commonly observed with the use of Cerebyx in clinical trials were nystagmus, dizziness, pruritus, paresthesia, headache, somnolence, and ataxia. With two exceptions, these events are commonly associated with the administration of IV phenytoin. Paresthesia and pruritus, however, were seen much more often following Cerebyx administration and occurred more often with IV Cerebyx administration than with IM Cerebyx administration. These events were dose and rate related; most alert patients (41 of 64; 64%) administered doses of ≥15 mg PE/kg at 150 mg PE/min experienced discomfort of some degree. These sensations, generally described as itching, burning, or tingling, were usually not at the infusion site. The location of the discomfort varied with the groin mentioned most frequently as a site of involvement. The paresthesia and pruritus were transient events that occurred within several minutes of the start of infusion and generally resolved within 10 minutes after completion of Cerebyx infusion. Some patients experienced symptoms for hours. These events did not increase in severity with repeated administration. Concurrent adverse events or clinical laboratory change suggesting an allergic process were not seen (see PRECAUTIONS, Sensory Disturbances).
Approximately 2% of the 859 individuals who received Cerebyx in premarketing clinical trials discontinued treatment because of an adverse event. The adverse events most commonly associated with withdrawal were pruritus (0.5%), hypotension (0.3%), and bradycardia (0.2%).
Dose and Rate Dependency of Adverse Events Following IV Cerebyx: The incidence of adverse events tended to increase as both dose and infusion rate increased. In particular, at doses of ≥15mg PE/kg and rates ≥150 mg PE/min, transient pruritus, tinnitus, nystagmus, somnolence, and ataxia occurred 2 to 3 times more often than at lower doses or rates.

Incidence in Controlled Clinical Trials
All adverse events were recorded during the trials by the clinical investigators using terminology of their own choosing. Similar types of events were grouped into standardized categories using modified COSTART dictionary terminology. These categories are used in the tables and listings below with the frequencies representing the proportion of individuals exposed to Cerebyx or comparative therapy.
The prescriber should be aware that these figures cannot be used to predict the frequency of adverse events in the course of usual medical practice where patient characteristics and other factors may differ from those prevailing during clinical studies. Similarly, the cited frequencies cannot be directly compared with figures obtained from other clinical investigations involving different treatments, uses or investigators. An inspection of these frequencies, however, does provide the prescribing physician with one basis to estimate the relative contribution of drug and nondrug factors to the adverse event incidences in the population studied.
Incidence in Controlled Clinical Trials—IV Administration To Patients With Epilepsy or Neurosurgical Patients: Table 2 lists treatment-emergent adverse events that occurred in at least 2% of patients treated with IV Cerebyx at the maximum dose and rate in a randomized, double-blind, controlled clinical trial where the rates for phenytoin and Cerebyx administration would have resulted in equivalent systemic exposure to phenytoin.

TABLE 2. Treatment-Emergent Adverse Event Incidence Following IV Administration at the Maximum Dose and Rate to Patients With Epilepsy or Neurosurgical Patients (Events in at Least 2% of Cerebyx-Treated Patients)

BODY SYSTEM Adverse Event	IV Cerebyx N=90	IV Phenytoin N=22
BODY AS A WHOLE		
Pelvic Pain	4.4	0.0
Asthenia	2.2	0.0
Back Pain	2.2	0.0
Headache	2.2	4.5
CARDIOVASCULAR		
Hypotension	7.7	9.1
Vasodilatation	5.6	4.5
Tachycardia	2.2	0.0
DIGESTIVE		
Nausea	8.9	13.6
Tongue Disorder	4.4	0.0
Dry Mouth	4.4	4.5
Vomiting	2.2	9.1
NERVOUS		
Nystagmus	44.4	59.1
Dizziness	31.1	27.3
Somnolence	20.0	27.3
Ataxia	11.1	18.2
Stupor	7.7	4.5
Incoordination	4.4	4.5
Paresthesia	4.4	0.0
Extrapyramidal Syndrome	4.4	0.0
Tremor	3.3	9.1
Agitation	3.3	0.0
Hypesthesia	2.2	9.1
Dysarthria	2.2	0.0
Vertigo	2.2	0.0
Brain Edema	2.2	4.5
SKIN AND APPENDAGES		
Pruritus	48.9	4.5
SPECIAL SENSES		
Tinnitus	8.9	9.1
Diplopia	3.3	0.0
Taste Perversion	3.3	0.0
Amblyopia	2.2	9.1
Deafness	2.2	0.0

Incidence in Controlled Trials—IM Administration to Patients With Epilepsy: Table 3 lists treatment-emergent adverse events that occurred in at least 2% of Cerebyx-treated patients in a double-blind, randomized, controlled clinical trial of adult epilepsy patients receiving either IM Cerebyx substituted for oral Dilantin or continuing oral Dilantin. Both treatments were administered for 5 days.

TABLE 3. Treatment-Emergent Adverse Event Incidence Following Substitution of IM Cerebyx for Oral Dilantin in Patients With Epilepsy (Events in at Least 2% of Cerebyx-Treated Patients)

BODY SYSTEM Adverse Event	IM Cerebyx N=179	Oral Dilantin N=61
BODY AS A WHOLE		
Headache	8.9	4.9
Asthenia	3.9	3.3
Accidental Injury	3.4	6.6
DIGESTIVE		
Nausea	4.5	0.0
Vomiting	2.8	0.0
HEMATOLOGIC AND LYMPHATIC		
Ecchymosis	7.3	4.9
NERVOUS		
Nystagmus	15.1	8.2
Tremor	9.5	13.1
Ataxia	8.4	8.2
Incoordination	7.8	4.9
Somnolence	6.7	9.8
Dizziness	5.0	3.3
Paresthesia	3.9	3.3
Reflexes Decreased	2.8	4.9
SKIN AND APPENDAGES		
Pruritus	2.8	0.0

Adverse Events During All Clinical Trials
Cerebyx has been administered to 859 individuals during all clinical trials. All adverse events seen at least twice are listed in the following, except those already included in previous tables and listings. Events are further classified within body system categories and enumerated in order of decreasing frequency using the following definitions: frequent adverse events are defined as those occurring in greater than 1/100 individuals; infrequent adverse events are those occurring in 1/100 to 1/1000 individuals.
Body As a Whole: *Frequent:* fever, injection-site reaction, infection, chills, face edema, injection-site pain; *Infrequent:* sepsis, injection-site inflammation, injection-site edema, injection-site hemorrhage, flu syndrome, malaise, generalized edema, shock, photosensitivity reaction, cachexia, cryptococcosis.
Cardiovascular: *Frequent:* hypertension; *Infrequent:* cardiac arrest, migraine, syncope, cerebral hemorrhage, palpitation, sinus bradycardia, atrial flutter, bundle branch block, cardiomegaly, cerebral infarct, postural hypotension, pulmonary embolus, QT interval prolongation, thrombophlebitis, ventricular extrasystoles, congestive heart failure.
Digestive: *Frequent:* constipation; *Infrequent:* dyspepsia, diarrhea, anorexia, gastrointestinal hemorrhage, increased salivation, liver function tests abnormal, tenesmus, tongue edema, dysphagia, flatulence, gastritis, ileus.
Endocrine: *Infrequent:* diabetes insipidus.
Hematologic and Lymphatic: *Infrequent:* thrombocytopenia, anemia, leukocytosis, cyanosis, hypochromic anemia, leukopenia, lymphadenopathy, petechia.
Metabolic and Nutritional: *Frequent:* hypokalemia; *Infrequent:* hyperglycemia, hypophosphatemia, alkalosis, acidosis, dehydration, hyperkalemia, ketosis.
Musculoskeletal: *Frequent:* myasthenia; *Infrequent:* myopathy, leg cramps, arthralgia, myalgia.
Nervous: *Frequent:* reflexes increased, speech disorder, dysarthria, intracranial hypertension, thinking abnormal, nervousness, hypesthesia; *Infrequent:* confusion, twitching, Babinski sign positive, circumoral paresthesia, hemiplegia, hypotonia, convulsion, extrapyramidal syndrome, insomnia, meningitis, depersonalization, CNS depression, depression, hypokinesia, hyperkinesia, brain edema, paralysis, psychosis, aphasia, emotional lability, coma, hyperesthesia, myoclonus, personality disorder, acute brain syndrome, encephalitis, subdural hematoma, encephalopathy, hostility, akathisia, amnesia, neurosis.
Respiratory: *Frequent:* pneumonia; *Infrequent:* pharyngitis, sinusitis, hyperventilation, rhinitis, apnea, aspiration pneumonia, asthma, dyspnea, atelectasis, cough increased, sputum increased, epistaxis, hypoxia, pneumothorax, hemoptysis, bronchitis.
Skin and Appendages: *Frequent:* rash; *Infrequent:* maculopapular rash, urticaria, sweating, skin discoloration, contact dermatitis, pustular rash, skin nodule.
Special Senses: *Frequent:* taste perversion; *Infrequent:* deafness, visual field defect, eye pain, conjunctivitis, photophobia, hyperacusis, mydriasis, parosmia, ear pain, taste loss.
Urogenital: *Infrequent:* urinary retention, oliguria, dysuria, vaginitis, albuminuria, genital edema, kidney failure, polyuria, urethral pain, urinary incontinence, vaginal moniliasis.

OVERDOSAGE

Nausea, vomiting, lethargy, tachycardia, bradycardia, asystole, cardiac arrest, hypotension, syncope, hypocalcemia, metabolic acidosis, and death have been reported in cases of overdosage with fosphenytoin.
The median lethal dose of fosphenytoin given intravenously in mice and rats was 156 mg PE/kg and approximately 250 mg PE/kg, or about 0.6 and 2 times, respectively, the maximum human loading dose on a mg/m^2 basis. Signs of acute toxicity in animals included ataxia, labored breathing, ptosis, and hypoactivity.

Because Cerebyx is a prodrug of phenytoin, the following information may be helpful. Initial symptoms of acute phenytoin toxicity are nystagmus, ataxia, and dysarthria. Other signs include tremor, hyperreflexia, lethargy, slurred speech, nausea, vomiting, coma, and hypotension. Depression of respiratory and circulatory systems leads to death. There are marked variations among individuals with respect to plasma phenytoin concentrations where toxicity occurs. Lateral gaze nystagmus usually appears at 20 µg/mL, ataxia at 30 µg/mL, and dysarthria and lethargy appear when the plasma concentration is over 40 µg/mL. However, phenytoin concentrations as high as 50 µg/mL have been reported without evidence of toxicity. As much as 25 times the therapeutic phenytoin dose has been taken, resulting in plasma phenytoin concentrations over 100 µg/mL, with complete recovery.

Treatment is nonspecific since there is no known antidote to Cerebyx or phenytoin overdosage. The adequacy of the respiratory and circulatory systems should be carefully observed, and appropriate supportive measures employed. Hemodialysis can be considered since phenytoin is not completely bound to plasma proteins. Total exchange transfusion has been used in the treatment of severe intoxication in children. In acute overdosage the possibility of other CNS depressants, including alcohol, should be borne in mind.

Formate and phosphate are metabolites of fosphenytoin and therefore may contribute to signs of toxicity following overdosage. Signs of formate toxicity are similar to those of methanol toxicity and are associated with severe anion-gap metabolic acidosis. Large amounts of phosphate, delivered rapidly, could potentially cause hypocalcemia with paresthesia, muscle spasms, and seizures. Ionized free calcium levels can be measured and, if low, used to guide treatment.

DOSAGE AND ADMINISTRATION

The dose, concentration in dosing solutions, and infusion rate of IV Cerebyx is expressed as phenytoin sodium equivalents (PE) to avoid the need to perform molecular weight-based adjustments when converting between fosphenytoin and phenytoin sodium doses. Cerebyx should always be prescribed and dispensed in phenytoin sodium equivalent units (PE). Cerebyx has important differences in administration from those for parenteral phenytoin sodium (see below).

Products with particulate matter or discoloration should not be used. Prior to IV infusion, dilute Cerebyx in 5% dextrose or 0.9% saline solution for injection to a concentration ranging from 1.5 to 25 mg PE/mL.

Status Epilepticus

- The loading dose of Cerebyx is 15 to 20 mg PE/kg administered at 100 to 150 mg PE/min.
- Because of the risk of hypotension, fosphenytoin should be administered no faster than 150 mg PE/min. Continuous monitoring of the electrocardiogram, blood pressure, and respiratory function is essential and the patient should be observed throughout the period where maximal serum phenytoin concentrations occur, approximately 10 to 20 minutes after the end of Cerebyx infusions.
- Because the full antiepileptic effect of phenytoin, whether given as Cerebyx or parenteral phenytoin, is not immediate, other measures, including concomitant administration of an IV benzodiazepine, will usually be necessary for the control of status epilepticus.
- The loading dose should be followed by maintenance doses of Cerebyx, or phenytoin either orally or parenterally.

If administration of Cerebyx does not terminate seizures, the use of other anticonvulsants and other appropriate measures should be considered.

IM Cerebyx should not be used in the treatment of status epilepticus because therapeutic phenytoin concentrations may not be reached as quickly as with IV administration. If IV access is impossible, loading doses of Cerebyx have been given by the IM route for other indications.

Nonemergent Loading and Maintenance Dosing

The loading dose of Cerebyx is 10–20 mg PE/kg given IV or IM. The rate of administration for IV Cerebyx should be no greater than 150 mg PE/min. Continuous monitoring of the electrocardiogram, blood pressure, and respiratory function is essential and the patient should be observed throughout the period where maximal serum phenytoin concentrations occur, approximately 10 to 20 minutes after the end of Cerebyx infusions.

The initial daily maintenance dose of Cerebyx is 4–6 mg PE/kg/day.

IM or IV Substitution For Oral Phenytoin Therapy

Cerebyx can be substituted for oral phenytoin sodium therapy at the same total daily dose.

Dilantin capsules are approximately 90% bioavailable by the oral route. Phenytoin, supplied as Cerebyx, is 100% bioavailable by both the IM and IV routes. For this reason, plasma phenytoin concentrations may increase modestly when IM or IV Cerebyx is substituted for oral phenytoin sodium therapy.

The rate of administration for IV Cerebyx should be no greater than 150 mg PE/min.

In controlled trials, IM Cerebyx was administered as a single daily dose utilizing either 1 or 2 injection sites. Some patients may require more frequent dosing.

Dosing in Special Populations

Patients with Renal or Hepatic Disease: Due to an increased fraction of unbound phenytoin in patients with renal or hepatic disease, or in those with hypoalbuminemia, the interpretation of total phenytoin plasma concentrations should be made with caution (see CLINICAL PHARMACOLOGY: Special Populations). Unbound phenytoin concentrations may be more useful in these patient populations. After IV Cerebyx administration to patients with renal and/or hepatic disease, or in those with hypoalbuminemia, fosphenytoin clearance to phenytoin may be increased without a similar increase in phenytoin clearance. This has the potential to increase the frequency and severity of adverse events (see PRECAUTIONS).

Elderly Patients: Age does not have a significant impact on the pharmacokinetics of fosphenytoin following Cerebyx administration. Phenytoin clearance is decreased slightly in elderly patients and lower or less frequent dosing may be required.

Pediatric: The safety of Cerebyx in pediatric patients has not been established.

HOW SUPPLIED

Cerebyx Injection is supplied as follows:

10 mL per vial—Each vial contains fosphenytoin sodium 750 mg equivalent to 500 mg of phenytoin sodium:
N 0071-4008-10. Packages of 10.

2 mL per vial—Each vial contains fosphenytoin sodium 150 mg equivalent to 100 mg of phenytoin sodium:
N 0071-4007-05. Packages of 25.

Both sizes of vials contain Tromethamine, USP (TRIS), Hydrochloric Acid, NF, or Sodium Hydroxide, NF, and Water for Injection, USP.

Cerebyx should always be prescribed in phenytoin sodium equivalent units (PE) (see DOSAGE AND ADMINISTRATION).

Storage

Store under refrigeration at 2°C to 8°C (36°F to 46°F). The product should not be stored at room temperature for more than 48 hours. Vials that develop particulate matter should not be used.

Rx only.

Revised May 1999

PARKE-DAVIS
Div of Warner-Lambert Co
Morris Plains, NJ 07950 USA
MADE IN IRELAND
4007G211

FEMHRT® ℞

[fĕm-härt]

(norethindrone acetate/ethinyl estradiol tablets)

Prescribing information for this product, which appears on pages 2438–2442 of the 2001 PDR, has been completely revised as follows. Please write "See Supplement A" next to the product heading.

DESCRIPTION

femhrt® 1/5 is a continuous dosage regimen of a progestin-estrogen combination for oral administration.

Each white D-shaped tablet contains 1 **mg** norethindrone acetate [19-Norpregn-4-en-20-yn-3-one, 17-(acetyloxy)-, (17α)-] and 5 **mcg** ethinyl estradiol [19-Norpregna-1,3,5(10)-trien-20-yne-3,17-diol, (17α)-]. Each tablet also contains calcium stearate, lactose monohydrate, microcrystalline cellulose, and cornstarch.

The structural formulas are as follows:

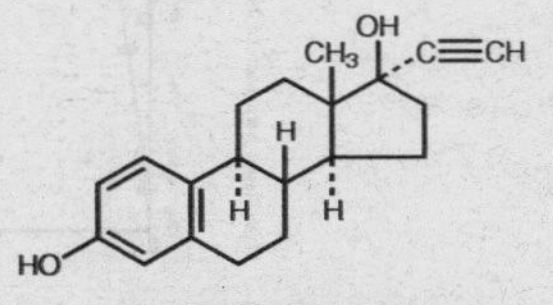

Ethinyl Estradiol
Molecular Weight: 296.41
Molecular Formula: $C_{20}H_{24}O_2$

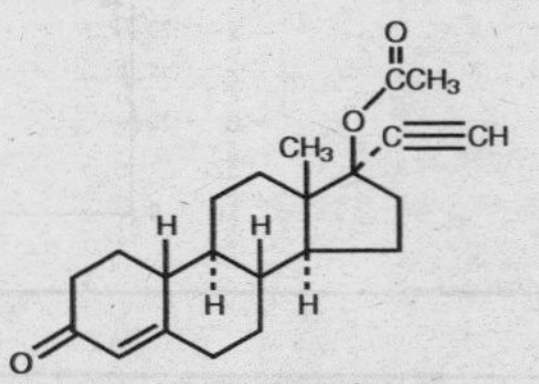

Norethindrone Acetate
Molecular Weight: 340.47
Molecular Formula: $C_{22}H_{28}O_3$

CLINICAL PHARMACOLOGY

Estrogens are largely responsible for the development and maintenance of the female reproductive system and secondary sex characteristics. Although circulating estrogens exist in a dynamic equilibrium of metabolic interconversions, estradiol is the principal intracellular human estrogen and is substantially more potent than estrone and estriol at the receptor level. The primary source of estrogen in normally cycling adult women is the ovarian follicle, which secretes 70 to 500 mcg of estradiol daily, depending on the phase of the menstrual cycle. After menopause, most endogenous estrogen is produced by conversion of androstenedione, secreted by the adrenal cortex, to estrone by peripheral tissues. Thus, estrone and the sulphate conjugated form, estrone sulphate, are the most abundant circulating estrogens in postmenopausal women. The pharmacologic effects of ethinyl estradiol are similar to those of endogenous estrogens.

Circulating estrogens modulate the pituitary secretion of the gonadotropins, luteinizing hormone (LH) and follicle stimulating hormone (FSH) through a negative feedback mechanism. Estrogen replacement therapy acts to reduce the elevated levels of these hormones seen in postmenopausal women.

Progestin compounds enhance cellular differentiation and generally oppose the actions of estrogens by decreasing estrogen receptor levels, increasing local metabolism of estrogens to less active metabolites, or inducing gene products that blunt cellular responses to estrogen. Progestins exert their effects in target cells by binding to specific progesterone receptors that interact with progesterone response elements in target genes. Progesterone receptors have been identified in the female reproductive tract, breast, pituitary, hypothalamus, bone, skeletal tissue and central nervous system. Progestins produce similar endometrial changes to those of the naturally occurring hormone progesterone.

The use of unopposed estrogen therapy has been associated with an increased risk of endometrial hyperplasia, a possible precursor of endometrial adenocarcinoma. The addition of continuous administration of progestin to an estrogen replacement regimen reduced the incidence of endometrial hyperplasia, and the attendant risk of carcinoma in women with intact uteri.

Pharmacokinetics

Absorption and Bioavailability

Norethindrone acetate (NA) is completely and rapidly deacetylated to norethindrone after oral administration, and the disposition of norethindrone acetate is indistinguishable from that of orally administered norethindrone. Norethindrone acetate and ethinyl estradiol (EE) are rapidly absorbed from *femhrt* 1/5 tablets, with maximum plasma concentrations of norethindrone and ethinyl estradiol generally occurring 1 to 2 hours postdose. Both are subject to first-pass metabolism after oral dosing, resulting in an absolute bioavailability of approximately 64% for norethindrone and 55% for ethinyl estradiol. Bioavailability of *femhrt* 1/5 tablets is similar to that from solution for norethindrone and slightly less for ethinyl estradiol. Administration of norethindrone acetate/ethinyl estradiol (NA/EE) tablets with a high fat meal decreases rate but not extent of ethinyl estradiol absorption. The extent of norethindrone absorption is increased by 27% following administration of NA/EE tablets with food.

The full pharmacokinetic profile of *femhrt* 1/5 (1 **mg** norethindrone acetate/5 **mcg** ethinyl estradiol) was not characterized due to assay sensitivity limitations. However, the multiple-dose pharmacokinetics were studied at a dose of 1 **mg** NA/10 **mcg** EE in 18 post-menopausal women. Mean plasma concentrations are shown below (Figure 1) and pharmacokinetic parameters are found in Table 1. Based on a population pharmacokinetic analysis, mean steady-state concentrations of norethindrone for 1 **mg** NA/5 **mcg** EE and 1/10 are slightly more than proportional to dose when compared to 0.5 **mg** NA/2.5 **mcg** EE tablets. It can be explained by higher sex hormone binding globulin (SHBG) concentrations. Mean steady-state plasma concentrations of ethinyl estradiol for the 0.5 **mg** NA/2.5 **mcg** EE tablets and *femhrt* 1/5 tablets are proportional to dose, but there is a less than proportional increase in steady-state concentrations for the NA/EE 1/10 tablet.

[See figure 1 at bottom of next page]

[See table 1 at bottom of next page]

Based on a population pharmacokinetic analysis, average steady-state concentrations (Css) of norethindrone and ethinyl estradiol for *femhrt* 1/5 (1 **mg** NA/5 **mcg** EE) tablets are estimated to be 2.6 ng/mL and 11.4 pg/mL, respectively. The pharmacokinetics of ethinyl estradiol and norethindrone acetate were not affected by age, (age range 40–62 years), in the postmenopausal population studied.

Distribution

Volume of distribution of norethindrone and ethinyl estradiol ranges from 2 to 4 L/kg. Plasma protein binding of both steroids is extensive (>95%); norethindrone binds to both albumin and sex hormone binding globulin (SHBG), whereas ethinyl estradiol binds only to albumin. Although ethinyl estradiol does not bind to SHBG, it induces SHBG synthesis.

Metabolism

Norethindrone undergoes extensive biotransformation, primarily via reduction, followed by sulfate and glucuronide conjugation. The majority of metabolites in the circulation are sulfates, with glucuronides accounting for most of the urinary metabolites. A small amount of norethindrone acetate is metabolically converted to ethinyl estradiol, such that exposure to ethinyl estradiol following administration of 1 **mg** of norethindrone acetate is equivalent to oral administration of 2.8 **mcg** ethinyl estradiol. Ethinyl estradiol is also extensively metabolized, both by oxidation and by conjugation with sulfate and glucuronide. Sulfates are the major circulating conjugates of ethinyl estradiol and glucuronides predominate in urine. The primary oxidative metabolite is 2-hydroxy ethinyl estradiol, formed by the CYP3A4 isoform of cytochrome P450. Part of the first-pass metabolism of ethinyl estradiol is believed to occur in gastrointestinal mucosa. Ethinyl estradiol may undergo enterohepatic circulation.

Continued on next page

femhrt—Cont.

Excretion

Norethindrone and ethinyl estradiol are excreted in both urine and feces, primarily as metabolites. Plasma clearance values for norethindrone and ethinyl estradiol are similar (approximately 0.4 L/hr/kg). Steady-state elimination half-lives of norethindrone and ethinyl estradiol following administration of 1 **mg** NA/10 **mcg** EE tablets are approximately 13 hours and 24 hours, respectively.

Special Populations

Pediatric

femhrt 1/5 is not indicated in children.

Geriatrics

The pharmacokinetics of *femhrt* 1/5 have not been studied in a geriatric population.

Race

The effect of race on the pharmacokinetics of *femhrt* 1/5 has not been studied.

Patients with Renal Insufficiency

The effect of renal disease on the disposition of *femhrt* 1/5 has not been evaluated. In premenopausal women with chronic renal failure undergoing peritoneal dialysis who received multiple doses of an oral contraceptive containing ethinyl estradiol and norethindrone, plasma ethinyl estradiol concentrations were higher and norethindrone concentrations were unchanged compared to concentrations in premenopausal women with normal renal function (see **PRECAUTIONS, Fluid Retention**).

Patients with Hepatic Impairment

The effect of hepatic disease on the disposition of *femhrt* 1/5 has not been evaluated. However, ethinyl estradiol and norethindrone may be poorly metabolized in patients with impaired liver function (see **PRECAUTIONS**).

Drug Interactions

See **PRECAUTIONS, Drug Interactions.**

Clinical Studies

Effects on Vasomotor Symptoms

A 12-week placebo-controlled, multicenter, randomized clinical trial was conducted in 266 symptomatic women who had at least 56 moderate to severe hot flashes during the week prior to randomization. On average, patients had 12 hot flashes per day upon study entry.

A total of 65 women were randomized to receive *femhrt* 1/5 and 66 women were randomized to the placebo group. The efficacy of *femhrt* 1/5 for the treatment of moderate to severe vasomotor symptoms (VMS) is demonstrated in Figure 2.

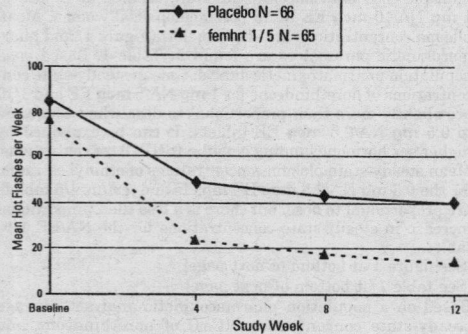

FIGURE 2.   Mean Hot Flash Frequencies by Treatment Group: Baseline Through Week 12 (Intent-to-Treat Population, Last Observation Carried Forward)

Endometrial Hyperplasia

A 2-year, placebo-controlled, multicenter, randomized clinical trial was conducted to determine the safety and efficacy of *femhrt* 1/5 on maintaining bone mineral density, protecting the endometrium, and to determine effects on lipids. A total of 1265 women were enrolled and randomized to either placebo, 0.2 **mg** NA/1 **mcg** EE, 0.5 **mg** NA/2.5 **mcg** EE, *femhrt* 1/5 and 1 **mg** NA/10 **mcg** EE or matching unopposed EE doses (1, 2.5, 5, or 10 **mcg**) for a total of 9 treatment groups. All participants received 1000 mg of calcium supplementation daily. Of the 1265 women randomized to the various treatment arms of this study, 137 were randomized to placebo, 146 to *femhrt* 1/5, and 141 to EE 5 **mcg**. Of these, 134 placebo, 143 *femhrt* 1/5, and 139 EE 5 **mcg** had a baseline endometrial result. Baseline biopsies were classified as normal (in approximately 95% of subjects), or insufficient tissue (in approximately 5% of subjects). Follow-up biopsies were obtained in approximately 70-80% of patients in each arm after 12 and 24 months of therapy. Results are shown in Table 2.

Table 2. Endometrial Biopsy Results After 12 and 24 Months of Treatment

	Placebo	*femhrt* 1/5	5 mcg ethinyl estradiol
Number of Patients Biopsied at Baseline	N=134	N=143	N=139
MONTH 12			
Patients Biopsied (%)	113 (84)	110 (77)	114 (82)
Insufficient Tissue	30	45	20
Atrophic Tissue	60	41	2
Proliferative Tissue	23	24	91
Endometrial Hyperplasia[a]	0	0	1
MONTH 24			
Patients Biopsied (%)	94 (70)	102 (71)	107 (77)
Insufficient Tissue	35	37	17
Atrophic Tissue	38	33	2
Proliferative Tissue	20	32	86
Endometrial Hyperplasia[a]	1	0	2

[a] All patients with endometrial hyperplasia were carried forward for all time points

Irregular Bleeding/Spotting

The cumulative incidence of amenorrhea, defined as no bleeding or spotting, was evaluated over 12 months for *femhrt* 1/5 and placebo arms. Results are shown in Figure 3.

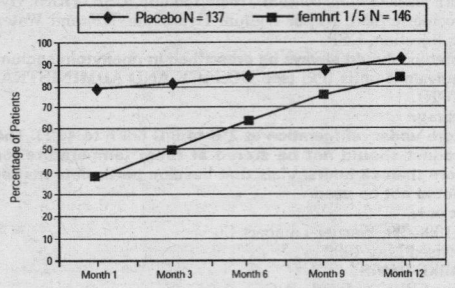

FIGURE 3.   Patients With Cumulative Amenorrhea Over Time: Intent-to-Treat Population, Last Observation Carried Forward

Effect on Bone Mineral Density

In the 2 year study, trabecular bone mineral density (BMD) was assessed at lumbar spine using quantitative computed tomography. A total of 283 postmenopausal women with intact uteri and normal baseline bone mineral density (124.14 mg/cc ± 9.60 mg/cc) were randomized to *femhrt* 1/5 (1 **mg** norethindrone acetate/5 **mcg** ethinyl estradiol) or placebo, and 87% contributed data to the Intent-To-Treat analysis. All patients received 1000 mg calcium in divided doses. Vitamin D was not supplemented. *femhrt* 1/5 resulted in significant increases in BMD at each assessment. There was a significant decrease in BMD in the placebo group (see Figure 4).

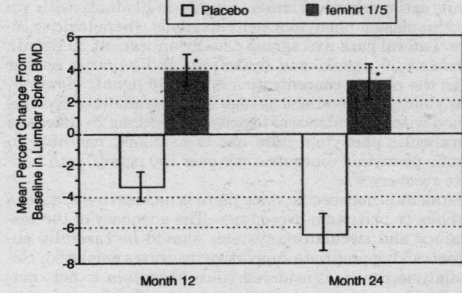

FIGURE.4   Mean Percent Change (±SE) From Baseline in Lumbar Spine BMD at Months 12 and 24 (Intent-to-Treat Population)

* Mean percent changes in BMD statistically significantly more positive than mean percent changes in placebo group at each time point.

Information Regarding Lipid Effects

Patients enrolled in the 2-year osteoporosis and endometrial protection trial were evaluated for changes in lipid parameters after 24 months of therapy. All subjects were postmenopausal women at low risk for cardiovascular disease. Results for *femhrt* 1/5 and placebo arms are shown in Table 3.

Table 3. Mean % Change From Baseline Lipid Profile. Values After 24 Months of Treatment

Lipid Parameter	Placebo N = 129	*femhrt* 1/5 (mg NA/mcg EE) N = 132
Total Cholesterol (mg/dL)	1.6	−7.0
HDL-C (mg/dL)	1.3	−6.7
LDL-C (mg/dL)	1.0	−7.5
Triglycerides (mg/dL)	19.1	12.1

NA = Norethindrone acetate. EE = Ethinyl estradiol.

INDICATIONS AND USAGE

femhrt 1/5 is indicated in women with an intact uterus for the:

1. Treatment of moderate to severe vasomotor symptoms associated with menopause.

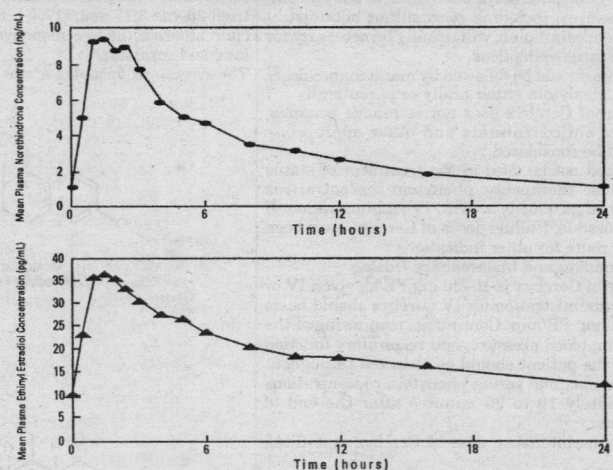

FIGURE 1.   Mean Steady-State (Day 87) Plasma Norethindrone and Ethinyl Estradiol Concentrations Following Continuous Oral Administration of 1 mg NA/10 mcg EE Tablets

Table 1. Mean (SD) Single-Dose (Day 1) and Steady-State (Day 87) Pharmacokinetic Parameters[a] Following Administration of 1 mg NA/10 mcg EE Tablets

	C_{max}	t_{max}	AUC(0–24)	CL/F	$t_{1/2}$
Norethindrone	ng/mL	hr	ng•hr/mL	mL/min	hr
Day 1	6.0 (3.3)	1.8 (0.8)	29.7 (16.5)	588 (416)	10.3 (3.7)
Day 87	10.7 (3.6)	1.8 (0.8)	81.8 (36.7)	226 (139)	13.3 (4.5)
Ethinyl Estradiol	pg/mL	hr	pg•hr/mL	mL/min	hr
Day 1	33.5 (13.7)	2.2 (1.0)	339 (113)	ND[b]	ND[b]
Day 87	38.3 (11.9)	1.8 (0.7)	471 (132)	383 (119)	23.9 (7.1)

[a] C_{max} = Maximum plasma concentration; t_{max} = time of C_{max}; AUC(0-24) = Area under the plasma concentration-time curve over the dosing interval; and CL/F = Apparent oral clearance; $t_{1/2}$ = Elimination half-life
[b] ND=Not determined

2. Prevention of osteoporosis.

Since estrogen administration is associated with risks as well as benefits, selection of patients ideally should be based on prospective identification of risk factors for developing osteoporosis. Unfortunately, there is no certain way to identify those women who will develop osteoporotic fractures. Thus, patient selection must be individualized based on the balance of risks and benefits.

Estrogen replacement therapy reduces bone resorption and retards or halts postmenopausal bone loss. Case-control studies have shown an approximately 60% reduction in hip and wrist fractures in women whose estrogen replacement was begun within a few years of menopause. Studies also suggest that estrogen reduces the rate of vertebral fractures. Even when started as late as 6 years after menopause, estrogen may prevent further loss of bone mass for as long as the treatment is continued. When estrogen therapy is discontinued, bone mass declines at a rate comparable to that in the immediate postmenopausal period. There is no evidence that estrogen replacement therapy restores bone mass to premenopausal levels.

Early menopause is one of the strongest predictors for the development of osteoporosis.

The mainstays of prevention and management of postmenopausal osteoporosis are estrogen, an adequate lifetime calcium intake, vitamin D and exercise. Postmenopausal women absorb dietary calcium less efficiently than premenopausal women and require an average of 1500 mg/day of elemental calcium to remain in neutral calcium balance. By comparison, premenopausal women require about 1000 mg/day and the average calcium intake in the USA is 400 to 600 mg/day. Therefore, when not contraindicated, calcium supplementation and adequate daily intake of vitamin D (400 IU) may be helpful.

CONTRAINDICATIONS

Progestogens/estrogens should not be used in individuals with any of the following conditions or circumstances:

1. Known or suspected pregnancy, including use for missed abortion or as a diagnostic test for pregnancy. Progestin or estrogen may cause fetal harm when administered to a pregnant woman.
2. Known or suspected cancer of the breast.
3. Known or suspected estrogen-dependent neoplasia.
4. Undiagnosed abnormal genital bleeding.
5. Active or past history of thrombophlebitis or thromboembolic disorders.
6. Known sensitivity to *femhrt* 1/5 or other estrogen and progestin containing products.

WARNINGS

1. Induction of Malignant Neoplasms
Endometrial Cancer
The reported endometrial cancer risk among users of unopposed estrogen is about 2- to 12-fold greater than in nonusers, and appears dependent on duration of treatment and on estrogen dose. Most studies show no significant increased risk associated with the use of estrogens for less than 1 year. The greatest risk appears associated with prolonged use, with increased risks of 15- to 24-fold for use of 5 to 10 years or more, and this risk has been shown to persist for at least 15 years after cessation of estrogen treatment. Results from a 2-year clinical study of the effects of *femhrt* 1/5 on endometrial hyperplasia are shown in the **Clinical Studies** section of this label.

Clinical surveillance of all women taking progestin/estrogen combinations is important. Adequate diagnostic measures, including endometrial sampling when indicated, should be undertaken to rule out malignancy in all cases of undiagnosed persistent or recurring abnormal vaginal bleeding. There is no evidence that "natural" estrogens are more or less hazardous than "synthetic" estrogens at equivalent doses.

Breast Cancer
While the majority of studies have not shown an increased risk of breast cancer in women who have ever used estrogen replacement therapy, some have reported a moderately increased risk (relative risks of 1.3–2.0) in those taking higher doses or those taking lower doses for prolonged periods of time, especially in excess of 10 years.

The effect of added progestins on the risk of breast cancer is unknown.

2. Gallbladder Disease
A 2- to 4-fold increase in the risk of gallbladder disease requiring surgery in women receiving postmenopausal estrogen has been reported.

3. Hypercalcemia
Administration of estrogens may lead to severe hypercalcemia in patients with breast cancer and bone metastases (see **CONTRAINDICATIONS**). If this occurs, the drugs should be stopped and appropriate measures taken to reduce the serum calcium level.

4. Pregnancy
Use in pregnancy is not recommended (see **CONTRAINDICATIONS**).

5. Venous Thromboembolism
Five epidemiologic studies have found an increased risk of venous thromboembolism (VTE) in users of estrogen replacement therapy (ERT) who did not have predisposing conditions for VTE, such as a past history of cardiovascular disease or a recent history of pregnancy, surgery, trauma, or serious illness. The increased risk was found only in current ERT users; it did not persist in former users. The risk appeared to be higher in the first year of use and decreased thereafter. The findings were similar for ERT alone or with added progestin and pertain to commonly used oral and transdermal doses, with a possible dose-dependent effect on risk. The studies found the VTE risk to be about one case per 10,000 women per year among women not using ERT and without predisposing conditions. The risk in current ERT users was increased to 2–3 cases per 10,000 women per year.

6. Visual Disturbances
Medication should be discontinued pending examination if there is a sudden partial or complete loss of vision, or if there is a sudden onset of proptosis, diplopia or migraine. If examination reveals papilledema or retinal vascular lesions, medication should be withdrawn.

PRECAUTIONS

A. General
Based on experience with estrogens and/or progestins:

1. Cardiovascular Risk
A causal relationship between estrogen replacement therapy and reduction of cardiovascular disease in postmenopausal women has not been proven. Furthermore, the effect of added progestins on this putative benefit is not yet known.

In recent years many published studies have suggested that there may be a cause-effect relationship between postmenopausal oral estrogen replacement therapy without cyclical progestins and a decrease in cardiovascular disease in women. Although most of the observational studies which assessed this statistical association have reported a 20% to 50% reduction in coronary heart disease risk and associated mortality in estrogen takers, the following should be considered when interpreting these reports:

(1) Because only one of these studies was randomized and it was too small to yield statistically significant results, all relevant studies were subject to selection bias. Thus, the apparently reduced risk of coronary artery disease cannot be attributed with certainty to estrogen replacement therapy. It may instead have been caused by life-style and medical characteristics of the women studied with the result that healthier women were selected for estrogen therapy. In general, treated women were of higher socioeconomic and educational status, more slender, more physically active, more likely to have undergone surgical menopause, and less likely to have diabetes than the untreated women. Although some studies attempted to control for these selection factors, it is common for properly designed randomized trials to fail to confirm benefits suggested by less rigorous study designs. Ongoing and future large-scale randomized trials may help to clarify the apparent benefit.

(2) Current medical practice often includes the use of concomitant progestin therapy in women with intact uteri (see **PRECAUTIONS** and **WARNINGS**). While the effects of added progestins on the risk of ischemic heart disease are not known, all available progestins reverse at least some of the favorable effects of estrogens on HDL and LDL levels (see **Clinical Studies**).

(3) While the effects of added progestins on the risk of breast cancer are also unknown, available epidemiological evidence suggests that progestins do not reduce, and may enhance the moderately increased breast cancer incidence that has been reported with prolonged estrogen replacement therapy (see **WARNINGS**).

2. Elevated Blood Pressure
Occasional blood pressure increases during estrogen replacement therapy have been attributed to idiosyncratic reactions to estrogens. More often, blood pressure has remained the same or has dropped. One study showed that postmenopausal estrogen users have higher blood pressure than nonusers.

Two other studies showed slightly lower blood pressure among estrogen users compared to nonusers. The data on the risk of estrogen use in postmenopausal women and the risk of stroke have not been considered conclusive. Nonetheless, blood pressure should be monitored at regular intervals with estrogen use.

3. Use in Hysterectomized Women
Existing data do not support the use of the combination of progestin and estrogen in postmenopausal women without a uterus.

4. Physical Examination
A complete medical and family history should be taken prior to the initiation of *femhrt* 1/5 and annually thereafter. These examinations should include special reference to blood pressure, breasts, abdomen, and pelvic organs, and should include a Papanicolaou smear.

5. Fluid Retention
Progestin/estrogen therapy may cause some degree of fluid retention. Conditions which might be exacerbated by this factor, such as asthma, epilepsy, migraine, and cardiac or renal dysfunction, require careful observation.

6. Uterine Bleeding and Mastodynia
Certain patients may develop undesirable manifestations of estrogenic stimulation, such as abnormal uterine bleeding and mastodynia. In cases of undiagnosed abnormal uterine bleeding, adequate diagnostic measures are indicated (see **WARNINGS**).

7. Impaired Liver Function
Estrogens and progestins may be poorly metabolized in patients with impaired liver function. If needed, therapy should be administered with caution.

8. Pathology Specimens
The pathologist should be advised of progestin/estrogen therapy when relevant specimens are submitted.

9. Hypercoagulability
Some studies have shown that women taking estrogen replacement therapy have hypercoagulability, primarily related to decreased antithrombin activity. This effect appears dose- and duration-dependent and is less pronounced than that associated with oral contraceptive use. Also, postmenopausal women tend to have changes in coagulation parameters at baseline compared to premenopausal women. There is some suggestion that low dose postmenopausal mestranol may increase the risk of thromboembolism, although the majority of studies (of primarily conjugated estrogen users) report no such increase. There is insufficient information on hypercoagulability in women who have had previous thromboembolic disease, therefore, *femhrt* 1/5 is contraindicated in such women.

10. Familial Hyperlipoproteinemia
Estrogen therapy may be associated with massive elevations of plasma triglycerides leading to pancreatitis and other complications in patients with familial defects of lipoprotein metabolism.

11. Depression
Patients who have a history of depression should be carefully observed and the drug discontinued if the depression recurs to a serious degree.

12. Impaired Glucose Tolerance
Diabetic patients should be carefully observed while receiving progestin/estrogen therapy. The effects of *femhrt* 1/5 on glucose tolerance have not been studied.

13. Lipoprotein Metabolism
(See **Clinical Studies**.)

B. Information for Patients
See text of Patient Package Insert which appears after the **HOW SUPPLIED** section.

C. Drug/Laboratory Test Interactions
The following drug/laboratory interactions have been observed with estrogen therapy, and/or *femhrt* 1/5:

1. In a 12-week study, *femhrt* 1/5 decreased Factor VII and plasminogen activator inhibitor-1 from baseline in a dose-related manner, but remained within the laboratory reference range for postmenopausal women. Mean levels of fibrinogen and partial thromboplastin time did not change from baseline for *femhrt* 1/5.
2. Estrogen therapy may increase thyroxine-binding globulin (TBG), leading to increased circulating total thyroid hormone (T4) as measured by protein-bound iodine (PBI), T4 levels (by column or radioimmunoassay), or T3 levels by radioimmunoassay. T3 resin uptake is decreased, reflecting the elevated TBG. Free T4 and free T3 concentrations are unaltered.
3. Estrogen therapy may elevate other binding proteins in serum, ie, corticosteroid binding globulin (CBG), sex hormone-binding globulin (SHBG), leading to increased circulating corticosteroids and sex steroids, respectively. Free or biologically active hormone concentrations are unchanged. Other plasma proteins may be increased (angiotensinogen/renin substrate, alpha-1-antitrypsin, ceruloplasmin).
   femhrt 1/5 was associated with a SHBG increase of 22%.
4. Estrogen therapy increases plasma HDL and HDL-2 subfraction concentrations, reduces LDL cholesterol concentration and increases triglyceride levels. (For effects during *femhrt* 1/5 treatment, see **Clinical Studies**.)
5. Estrogen therapy is associated with impaired glucose tolerance.
6. Estrogen therapy reduces response to metyrapone test.
7. Estrogen therapy reduces serum folate concentration.

D. Drug/Drug Interactions
No drug-drug interaction studies have been conducted with *femhrt* 1/5.

The following section contains information on drug interactions with ethinyl estradiol-containing products (specifically, oral contraceptives) that have been reported in the public literature. It is unknown whether such interactions occur with *femhrt* 1/5 or drug products containing other types of estrogens.

The Effects of Other Drugs on Ethinyl Estradiol
The metabolism of ethinyl estradiol is increased by rifampin and anticonvulsants such as phenobarbital, phenytoin, and carbamazepine. Coadministration of troglitazone and certain ethinyl-estradiol containing drug products (eg, oral contraceptives containing ethinyl estradiol) reduce the plasma concentrations of ethinyl estradiol by 30 percent.

Ascorbic acid and acetaminophen may increase AUC and/or plasma concentrations of ethinyl estradiol. Coadministration of atorvastatin and certain ethinyl-estradiol containing drug products (eg, oral contraceptives containing ethinyl estradiol) increase AUC values for ethinyl estradiol by 20 percent.

Clinical pharmacokinetic studies have not demonstrated any consistent effect of antibiotics (other than rifampin) on plasma concentrations of synthetic steroids.

The Effect of Ethinyl Estradiol on Other Drugs
Drug products containing ethinyl estradiol may inhibit the metabolism of other compounds. Increased plasma concentrations of cyclosporin, prednisolone, and theophylline have been reported with concomitant administration of certain drugs containing ethinyl estradiol (eg, oral contraceptives containing ethinyl estradiol). In addition, drugs containing ethinyl estradiol may induce the conjugation of other compounds.

Decreased plasma concentrations of acetaminophen and increased clearance of temazapam, salicylic acid, morphine, and clofibric acid have been noted when these drugs were

Continued on next page

femhrt—Cont.

administered with certain ethinyl-estradiol containing drug products (eg, oral contraceptives containing ethinyl estradiol).

E. Carcinogenesis, Mutagenesis, Impairment of Fertility
Long-term continuous administration of natural and synthetic estrogens in certain animal species increase the frequency of carcinomas of the breast, uterus, cervix, vagina, testis, and liver (see CONTRAINDICATIONS AND WARNINGS).

F. Pregnancy Category X
Estrogens/progestins should not be used during pregnancy (see CONTRAINDICATIONS AND WARNINGS).

G. Nursing Mothers
As a general principle, the administration of any drug to nursing mothers should be done only when clearly necessary since many drugs are excreted in human milk. Estrogen administration to nursing mothers has been shown to decrease the quantity and quality of the milk. Detectable amounts of drug have been identified in the milk of mothers receiving progestational drugs. The effect of this on the nursing infant has not been determined.

ADVERSE REACTIONS
Adverse events reported in controlled clinical studies of femhrt 1/5 are shown in Table 4 below.

Table 4. All Treatment-Emergent Adverse Events Reported at a Frequency of > 5% of Patients with femhrt 1/5
% of Patients

BODY SYSTEM/ Adverse Event	Placebo N = 247	femhrt 1/5 N = 258
BODY AS A WHOLE	40.1	39.5
Headache	14.6	18.2
Back Pain	5.3	4.7
Viral Infection	7.7	7.0
DIGESTIVE SYSTEM	24.4	33.0
Nausea and/or Vomiting	5.3	7.4
Abdominal Pain	4.5	8.1
MUSCULOSKELETAL SYSTEM	21.7	20.4
Arthralgia	6.9	5.8
Myalgia	8.5	7.8
PSYCHOBIOLOGIC FUNCTION	8.3	14.1
Nervousness	1.6	5.4
Depression	3.6	5.8
RESPIRATORY SYSTEM	37.2	35.6
Rhinitis	15.4	15.1
Sinusitis	9.7	8.1
UROGENITAL SYSTEM	25.0	40.8
Breast Pain	5.3	8.1
Urinary Tract Infection	3.2	6.2
Vaginitis	4.9	5.4

The following adverse events have been reported with estrogen and/or progestin therapy:

Genitourinary system: changes in vaginal bleeding pattern and abnormal withdrawal bleeding or flow, breakthrough bleeding, spotting, increase in size of uterine leiomyomata, vaginal candidiasis, changes in amount of cervical secretion, pre-menstrual-like syndrome, cystitis-like syndrome.
Breasts: tenderness, enlargement, fibrocystic disease of the breast.
Gastrointestinal: cholestatic jaundice, pancreatitis, flatulence, bloating, abdominal cramps.
Skin: chloasma or melasma that may persist when drug is discontinued, erythema multiforme, erythema nodosum, hemorrhagic eruption, loss of scalp hair, hirsutism, itching, skin rash and pruritus.
CNS: headache, migraine, dizziness, chorea, insomnia.
Cardiovascular: changes in blood pressure, cerebrovascular accidents, deep venous thrombosis, and pulmonary embolism.
Eyes: intolerance to contact lenses, sudden partial or complete loss of vision, proptosis, diplopia, otosclerosis.
Miscellaneous: increase or decrease in weight, reduced carbohydrate tolerance, aggravation of porphyria, changes in libido, fatigue, allergic or anaphylactoid reactions, leiomyoma, fibromyoma of the uterus, endometriosis.

OVERDOSAGE
ACUTE OVERDOSAGE
Serious ill effects have not been reported following acute ingestion of large doses of progestin/estrogen-containing oral contraceptives by young children. Overdosage of estrogen may cause nausea and vomiting, and withdrawal bleeding may occur.

DOSAGE AND ADMINISTRATION
femhrt 1/5 therapy consists of a single tablet taken once daily.
1. For the Treatment of Vasomotor Symptoms
femhrt 1/5 should be given once daily for the treatment of moderate to severe vasomotor symptoms associated with the menopause. Patients should be reevaluated at 3 to 6 month intervals to determine if treatment is still necessary.
2. Prevention of Osteoporosis
femhrt 1/5 should be given once daily to prevent postmenopausal osteoporosis (see Clinical Studies: Effect on Bone Mineral Density). Response to therapy can be assessed by measurement of bone mineral density.
Treated patients with an intact uterus should be monitored closely for signs of endometrial cancer, and appropriate di-

agnostic measures should be taken to rule out malignancy in the event of persistent or recurring vaginal bleeding. Patients should be evaluated at least annually for breast abnormalities and more often if there are any symptoms.

HOW SUPPLIED
femhrt 1/5 tablets are white and available in the following strength and package sizes:
N 0071-0144-23 Bottle of 90 D-shaped tablets with 1 mg norethindrone acetate and 5 mcg ethinyl estradiol
N 0071-0144-45 Blister card of 28 D-shaped tablets with 1 mg norethindrone acetate and 5 mcg ethinyl estradiol
Rx only
Keep this drug and all drugs out of the reach of children.
Store at 25°C (77°F); excursions permitted to 15-30°C (59-86°F)[see USP Controlled Room Temperature].

INFORMATION FOR THE PATIENT
What is femhrt® 1/5?
Your healthcare provider has prescribed femhrt 1/5, a combination of two hormones, a progestin (1 mg norethindrone acetate) and an estrogen (5 mcg ethinyl estradiol) intended for use once a day. This insert describes the major benefits and risks of your treatment, as well as how and when treatment may be taken. If you have any questions, please contact your physician, nurse or pharmacist.

femhrt 1/5 is approved for use in the following ways:
- **To reduce moderate to severe menopausal symptoms.** Estrogens are hormones produced by the ovaries of menstruating women. When a woman is between the ages of 45 and 55, the ovaries normally stop making estrogens. This drop in body estrogen levels causes the "change of life" or menopause, the end of monthly menstrual periods.
When estrogen levels begin dropping, some women develop very uncomfortable symptoms, such as feelings of warmth in the face, neck, and chest, or sudden intense episodes of heat and sweating ("hot flashes" or "hot flushes"). In some women the symptoms are mild; in others they can be severe. These symptoms may last only a few months or longer. Taking femhrt 1/5 can help reduce these symptoms. If you are not taking hormones for other reasons, such as the prevention of osteoporosis, you should take femhrt 1/5 only as long as you need it for relief from your menopausal symptoms.
- **To prevent thinning bones (osteoporosis).** Osteoporosis is a thinning of the bones that makes them weaker and allows them to break more easily. The bones of the spine, wrists, and hips may be affected by osteoporosis. femhrt 1/5 may be used as part of a program including weight-bearing exercise, such as walking or running, and calcium supplements.
Women likely to develop osteoporosis often have the following characteristics: white or Asian race, slim, cigarette smokers, and a family history of osteoporosis in a mother, sister or aunt. Women who have menopause at an earlier age, either naturally or because their ovaries were removed during an operation, are more likely to develop osteoporosis than women whose menopause happens later in life.

Who should not take femhrt 1/5?
femhrt 1/5 should not be taken in the following situations:
- **During pregnancy.** If you think you may be pregnant, do not take femhrt 1/5. Taking estrogens while you are pregnant may cause your unborn child to have birth defects. Do not take femhrt 1/5 to prevent miscarriage.
- **If you have unusual vaginal bleeding that has not been checked by your healthcare provider.** Unusual vaginal bleeding can be a warning sign of a serious condition, including cancer of the uterus, especially if bleeding happens after menopause. Your doctor must find out the cause of the bleeding to recommend the right treatment.
- **If you have had certain cancers.** Estrogens increase the risk of certain types of cancers, including cancer of the breast and uterus. If you have had cancer, talk with your doctor about whether you should take femhrt 1/5.
- **If you have any circulation problems.** Generally, estrogens should not be taken if you have ever had a blood-clotting condition or other circulatory problem. In special situations, some doctors may decide that estrogen therapy is so necessary that the risks of taking femhrt 1/5 are acceptable (see "What are the possible risks and side effects of femhrt 1/5?").
- **After childbirth or when breast-feeding a baby.** femhrt 1/5 should not be taken to try to stop the breasts from filling with milk after a baby is born. Taking femhrt 1/5 may increase your risk of developing blood clots (see "What are the possible risks and side effects of femhrt 1/5?").
- **If you have had a hysterectomy (uterus removed).** femhrt 1/5 contains a progestin to decrease the risk of developing endometrial hyperplasia (an overgrowth of the lining of the uterus that may lead to cancer). If you do not have a uterus, you do not need a progestin, and you should not take femhrt 1/5.

How should I take femhrt 1/5?
Take your femhrt 1/5 pill once a day at about the same time each day. If you miss a dose, take it as soon as you remember. If it is almost time for your next dose, skip the missed dose and take only your next regularly scheduled dose. Do not take two doses at the same time.
The length of treatment with estrogens varies from woman to woman. You and your healthcare provider should reevaluate every 3 to 6 months whether or not you still need femhrt 1/5 to control your hot flashes.

What are the possible risks and side effects of femhrt 1/5?
- **Cancer of the uterus.** femhrt 1/5 has estrogen and progestin in it. If you take any drug that contains estrogen, including femhrt, you should see your doctor for regular check-ups and report any unusual vaginal bleeding right away. Vaginal bleeding after menopause may be a warning sign of a serious condition, including cancer of the uterus. Your doctor should identify the cause of any unusual vaginal bleeding.
The risk of cancer of the uterus increases when estrogens are used without a progestin. The risk also increases the longer estrogens are taken and the larger the doses. You are more likely to get cancer of the uterus if you are overweight, diabetic, or have high blood pressure. femhrt 1/5, which contains a progestin, reduces the estrogen-related risk of getting a condition of the uterine lining called endometrial hyperplasia. This condition may lead to cancer of the uterus (see "Other Information").
- **Cancer of the breast.** Most studies have not shown a higher risk of breast cancer in women who have used estrogens. However, some studies report that breast cancer developed more often (up to twice the usual rate) in women who used estrogens for longer time periods, especially more than 10 years, or who used high doses for a shorter time period. The effects of added progestin on the risk of breast cancer are unknown. You should have regular breast examinations by a health professional and examine your own breasts monthly. Ask your health care provider to show you how to do a breast exam yourself. If you are over 50 years of age, you should have a mammogram every year.
- **Gallbladder disease.** Women who use estrogens after menopause are more likely to develop gallbladder disease that leads to surgery than women who do not use estrogens.
- **Abnormal blood clotting.** Taking estrogens may cause changes in your blood clotting system that allow the blood to clot more easily. If blood clots form in your bloodstream, they can cut off the blood supply to vital organs, causing serious problems. These problems may include a stroke (by cutting off blood to the brain), a heart attack (by cutting of blood to the heart), or a pulmonary embolus (by cutting off blood supply to the lungs). Any of these conditions may cause death or serious long-term disability.
- **Vaginal bleeding.** With femhrt 1/5, menstrual-like vaginal bleeding may occur. If bleeding occurs, it is frequently light spotting or bleeding, but it may be moderate or heavy. If you experience vaginal bleeding while taking femhrt 1/5, discuss your bleeding pattern with your healthcare provider.

In addition to the risks and side effects just listed, patients taking estrogen or progestin have reported the following side effects:
- nausea and vomiting
- breast tenderness or enlargement
- headache
- retention of extra fluid (edema), which may make some conditions worse, such as asthma, epilepsy, migraine, heart disease, or kidney disease
- runny nose
- abdominal pain
- enlargement of non-cancerous tumors (fibroids) of the uterus
- spotty darkening of the skin, particularly on the face; reddening of the skin; skin rashes

How can I reduce the risks associated with taking femhrt 1/5?
If you take femhrt 1/5, you can reduce your risks by carefully monitoring your treatment.
- **See your healthcare provider regularly.** While you take femhrt 1/5, see your doctor at least once a year for a checkup. If you develop vaginal bleeding while taking femhrt 1/5, you might need further evaluation. If members of your family have had breast cancer or if you have ever had breast lumps or an abnormal mammogram (breast x-ray), you may need more frequent breast examinations.
- **Reassess your need for treatment.** Every 3–6 months, you and your doctor should discuss whether or not you still need femhrt 1/5 for control of your hot flashes.
- **Be alert for signs of trouble.** If any of the following warning signs (or any other unusual symptoms) happen while you are taking femhrt 1/5, call your doctor right away:
  - pains in the calves or chest, sudden shortness of breath, or coughing blood (possible clots in the legs, heart, or lungs)
  - severe headache or vomiting, dizziness, faintness, or changes in vision or speech, weakness or numbness of an arm or leg (possible clots in the brain or eye)
  - breast lumps (possible breast cancer)
  - yellowing of the skin or whites of the eyes (possible liver problem)
  - pain, swelling, or tenderness in the abdomen (possible gallbladder problem)

Other Information
- Discuss carefully with your doctor or health care provider all the possible risks and benefits of long-term estrogen and progestin treatment as they affect you personally.
- If you take calcium supplements as part of your treatment to help prevent osteoporosis, ask your doctor about the amounts recommended. A daily intake of 1500 mg of calcium is often recommended for postmenopausal women. Vitamin D (400 IU daily) may help your body use more of the calcium.
- Taking estrogens with progestins may have unhealthy effects on blood sugar, which might make a diabetic condition worse.

- Your doctor has prescribed this drug for you and you alone. Do not give your *femhrt* 1/5 to anyone else. Do not take *femhrt* 1/5 for conditions for which it was not prescribed.
- Keep all drugs out of the reach of children. In case of overdose, call your doctor, hospital, or poison control center right away.

This leaflet provides the most important information about *femhrt* 1/5. If you want more information, ask your doctor or pharmacist for the professional labeling. The professional labeling is published in a book called "The Physicians' Desk Reference" or PDR, available in bookstores and public libraries.
Revised July 2000
Manufactured by:
DURAMED PHARMACEUTICALS, INC.
CINCINNATI, OH 45213 USA
Distributed by:
PARKE-DAVIS
Division of Warner-Lambert Co. ©1999–'00
Morris Plains, NJ 07950 USA
0132G032

LIPITOR® ℞
(Atorvastatin Calcium) Tablets

Prescribing information for this product, which appears on pages 2442–2445 of the 2001 PDR, has been completely revised as follows. Please write "See Supplement A" next to the product heading.

DESCRIPTION
Lipitor® (atorvastatin calcium) is a synthetic lipid-lowering agent. Atorvastatin is an inhibitor of 3-hydroxy-3-methylglutaryl-coenzyme A (HMG-CoA) reductase. This enzyme catalyzes the conversion of HMG-CoA to mevalonate, an early and rate-limiting step in cholesterol biosynthesis.
Atorvastatin calcium is [R-(R*, R*)]-2-(4-fluorophenyl)-β, δ-dihydroxy-5-(1-methylethyl)-3-phenyl-4-[(phenylamino) carbonyl]-1H-pyrrole-1-heptanoic acid, calcium salt (2:1) trihydrate. The empirical formula of atorvastatin calcium is $(C_{33}H_{34}FN_2O_5)_2Ca \bullet 3H_2O$ and its molecular weight is 1209.42. Its structural formula is:

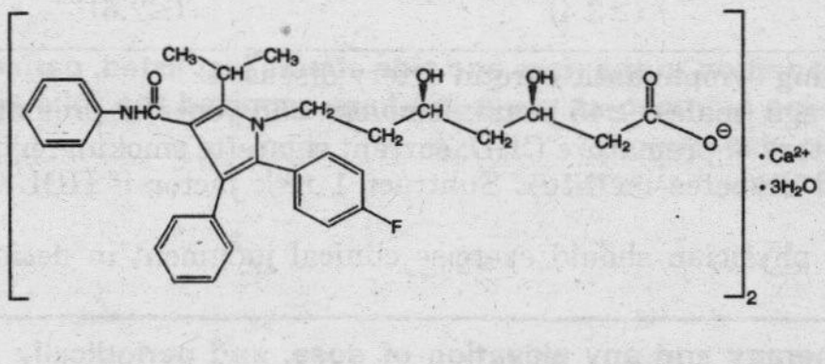

Atorvastatin calcium is a white to off-white crystalline powder that is insoluble in aqueous solutions of pH 4 and below. Atorvastatin calcium is very slightly soluble in distilled water, pH 7.4 phosphate buffer, and acetonitrile, slightly soluble in ethanol, and freely soluble in methanol.
Lipitor tablets for oral administration contain 10, 20, 40, or 80 mg atorvastatin and the following inactive ingredients: calcium carbonate, USP; candelilla wax, FCC; croscarmellose sodium, NF; hydroxypropyl cellulose, NF; lactose monohydrate, NF; magnesium stearate, NF; microcrystalline cellulose, NF; Opadry White YS-1-7040 (hydroxypropylmethylcellulose, polyethylene glycol, talc, titanium dioxide); polysorbate 80, NF; simethicone emulsion.

CLINICAL PHARMACOLOGY
Mechanism of Action
Atorvastatin is a selective, competitive inhibitor of HMG-CoA reductase, the rate-limiting enzyme that converts 3-hydroxy-3-methylglutaryl-coenzyme A to mevalonate, a precursor of sterols, including cholesterol. Cholesterol and triglycerides circulate in the bloodstream as part of lipoprotein complexes. With ultracentrifugation, these complexes separate into HDL (high-density lipoprotein), IDL (intermediate-density lipoprotein), LDL (low-density lipoprotein), and VLDL (very-low-density lipoprotein) fractions. Triglycerides (TG) and cholesterol in the liver are incorporated into VLDL and released into the plasma for delivery to peripheral tissues. LDL is formed from VLDL and is catabolized primarily through the high-affinity LDL receptor. Clinical and pathologic studies show that elevated plasma levels of total cholesterol (total-C), LDL-cholesterol (LDL-C), and apolipoprotein B (apo B) promote human atherosclerosis and are risk factors for developing cardiovascular disease, while increased levels of HDL-C are associated with a decreased cardiovascular risk.
In animal models, Lipitor lowers plasma cholesterol and lipoprotein levels by inhibiting HMG-CoA reductase and cholesterol synthesis in the liver and by increasing the number of hepatic LDL receptors on the cell-surface to enhance uptake and catabolism of LDL; Lipitor also reduces LDL production and the number of LDL particles. Lipitor reduces LDL-C in some patients with homozygous familial hypercholesterolemia (FH), a population that rarely responds to other lipid-lowering medication(s).
A variety of clinical studies have demonstrated that elevated levels of total-C, LDL-C, and apo B (a membrane complex for LDL-C) promote human atherosclerosis. Similarly, decreased levels of HDL-C (and its transport complex, apo

TABLE 1. Dose-Response in Patients With Primary Hypercholesterolemia (Adjusted Mean % Change from Baseline)[a]

Dose	N	TC	LDL-C	ApoB	TG	HDL-C	Non-HDL-C/ HDL-C
Placebo	21	4	4	3	10	-3	7
10	22	−29	−39	−32	−19	6	−34
20	20	−33	−43	−35	−26	9	−41
40	21	−37	−50	−42	−29	6	−45
80	23	−45	−60	−50	−37	5	−53

[a]Results are pooled from 2 dose-response studies

TABLE 2. Mean Percent Change From Baseline at End Point (Double-Blind, Randomized, Active-Controlled Trials)

Treatment (Daily Dose)	N	Total-C	LDL-C	ApoB	TG	HDL-C	Non-HDL-C/ HDL-C
Study 1							
Atorvastatin 10 mg	707	-27[a]	-36[a]	-28[a]	-17[a]	+7	-37[a]
Lovastatin 20 mg	191	−19	−27	−20	−6	+7	−28
95% CI for Diff[1]		−9.2,-6.5	−10.7,-7.1	−10.0,-6.5	−15.2,-7.1	−1.7,2.0	−11.1,-7.1
Study 2							
Atorvastatin 10 mg	222	-25[b]	-35[b]	-27[b]	-17[b]	+6	-36[b]
Pravastatin 20 mg	77	−17	−23	−17	−9	+8	−28
95% CI for Diff[1]		−10.8,-6.1	−14.5,-8.2	−13.4,-7.4	−14.1,-0.7	−4.9,1.6	−11.5,-4.1
Study 3							
Atorvastatin 10 mg	132	-29[c]	-37[c]	-34[c]	-23[c]	+7	-39[c]
Simvastatin 10 mg	45	−24	−30	−30	−15	+7	−33
95% CI for Diff[1]		−8.7,-2.7	−10.1,-2.6	−8.0,-1.1	−15.1,-0.7	−4.3,3.9	−9.6,-1.9

[1]A negative value for the 95% CI for the difference between treatments favors atorvastatin for all except HDL-C, for which a positive value favors atorvastatin. If the range does not include 0, this indicates a statistically significant difference.
[a]Significantly different from lovastatin, ANCOVA, $p \leq 0.05$
[b]Significantly different from pravastatin, ANCOVA, $p \leq 0.05$
[c]Significantly different from simvastatin, ANCOVA, $p \leq 0.05$

A) are associated with the development of atherosclerosis. Epidemiologic investigations have established that cardiovascular morbidity and mortality vary directly with the level of total-C and LDL-C, and inversely with the level of HDL-C.
Lipitor reduces total-C, LDL-C, and apo B in patients with homozygous and heterozygous FH, nonfamilial forms of hypercholesterolemia, and mixed dyslipidemia. Lipitor also reduces VLDL-C and TG and produces variable increases in HDL-C and apolipoprotein A-1. Lipitor reduces total-C, LDL-C, VLDL-C, apo B, TG, and non-HDL-C, and increases HDL-C in patients with isolated hypertriglyceridemia. Lipitor reduces intermediate density lipoprotein cholesterol (IDL-C) in patients with dysbetalipoproteinemia. The effect of Lipitor on cardiovascular morbidity and mortality has not been determined.
Like LDL, cholesterol-enriched triglyceride-rich lipoproteins, including VLDL, intermediate density lipoprotein (IDL), and remnants, can also promote atherosclerosis. Elevated plasma triglycerides are frequently found in a triad with low HDL-C levels and small LDL particles, as well as in association with non-lipid metabolic risk factors for coronary heart disease. As such, total plasma TG has not consistently been shown to be an independent risk factor for CHD. Furthermore, the independent effect of raising HDL or lowering TG on the risk of coronary and cardiovascular morbidity and mortality has not been determined.
Pharmacodynamics
Atorvastatin as well as some of its metabolites are pharmacologically active in humans. The liver is the primary site of action and the principal site of cholesterol synthesis and LDL clearance. Drug dosage rather than systemic drug concentration correlates better with LDL-C reduction. Individualization of drug dosage should be based on therapeutic response (see DOSAGE AND ADMINISTRATION).
Pharmacokinetics and Drug Metabolism
Absorption: Atorvastatin is rapidly absorbed after oral administration; maximum plasma concentrations occur within 1 to 2 hours. Extent of absorption increases in proportion to atorvastatin dose. The absolute bioavailability of atorvastatin (parent drug) is approximately 14% and the systemic availability of HMG-CoA reductase inhibitory activity is approximately 30%. The low systemic availability is attributed to presystemic clearance in gastrointestinal mucosa and/or hepatic first-pass metabolism. Although food decreases the rate and extent of drug absorption by approximately 25% and 9%, respectively, as assessed by C_{max} and AUC, LDL-C reduction is similar whether atorvastatin is given with or without food. Plasma atorvastatin concentrations are lower (approximately 30% for C_{max} and AUC) following evening drug administration compared with morning. However, LDL-C reduction is the same regardless of the time of day of drug administration (see DOSAGE AND ADMINISTRATION).
Distribution: Mean volume of distribution of atorvastatin is approximately 381 liters. Atorvastatin is ≥98% bound to plasma proteins. A blood/plasma ratio of approximately 0.25 indicates poor drug penetration into red blood cells. Based on observations in rats, atorvastatin is likely to be secreted in human milk (see CONTRAINDICATIONS, Pregnancy and Lactation, and PRECAUTIONS, Nursing Mothers).
Metabolism: Atorvastatin is extensively metabolized to ortho- and parahydroxylated derivatives and various beta-oxidation products. *In vitro* inhibition of HMG-CoA reductase by ortho- and parahydroxylated metabolites is equivalent to that of atorvastatin. Approximately 70% of circulating inhibitory activity for HMG-CoA reductase is attributed to active metabolites. *In vitro* studies suggest the importance of atorvastatin metabolism by cytochrome P450 3A4, consistent with increased plasma concentrations of atorvastatin in humans following coadministration with erythromycin, a known inhibitor of this isozyme (see PRECAUTIONS, Drug Interactions). In animals, the ortho-hydroxy metabolite undergoes further glucuronidation.
Excretion: Atorvastatin and its metabolites are eliminated primarily in bile following hepatic and/or extra-hepatic metabolism; however, the drug does not appear to undergo enterohepatic recirculation. Mean plasma elimination half-life of atorvastatin in humans is approximately 14 hours, but the half-life of inhibitory activity for HMG-CoA reductase is 20 to 30 hours due to the contribution of active metabolites. Less than 2% of a dose of atorvastatin is recovered in urine following oral administration.
Special Populations
Geriatric: Plasma concentrations of atorvastatin are higher (approximately 40% for C_{max} and 30% for AUC) in healthy elderly subjects (age ≥65 years) than in young adults. LDL-C reduction is comparable to that seen in younger patient populations given equal doses of Lipitor.
Pediatric: Pharmacokinetic data in the pediatric population are not available.
Gender: Plasma concentrations of atorvastatin in women differ from those in men (approximately 20% higher for C_{max} and 10% lower for AUC); however, there is no clinically significant difference in LDL-C reduction with Lipitor between men and women.
Renal Insufficiency: Renal disease has no influence on the plasma concentrations or LDL-C reduction of atorvastatin; thus, dose adjustment in patients with renal dysfunction is not necessary (see DOSAGE AND ADMINISTRATION).
Hemodialysis: While studies have not been conducted in patients with end-stage renal disease, hemodialysis is not expected to significantly enhance clearance of atorvastatin since the drug is extensively bound to plasma proteins.
Hepatic Insufficiency: In patients with chronic alcoholic liver disease, plasma concentrations of atorvastatin are markedly increased. C_{max} and AUC are each 4-fold greater in patients with Childs-Pugh A disease. C_{max} and AUC are approximately 16-fold and 11-fold increased, respectively, in patients with Childs-Pugh B disease (see CONTRAINDICATIONS).

Clinical Studies
Hypercholesterolemia (Heterozygous Familial and Nonfamilial) and Mixed Dyslipidemia (*Fredrickson* Types IIa and IIb)
Lipitor reduces total-C, LDL-C, VLDL-C, apo B, and TG, and increases HDL-C in patients with hypercholesterolemia and mixed dyslipidemia. Therapeutic response is seen within 2 weeks, and maximum response is usually achieved within 4 weeks and maintained during chronic therapy.
Lipitor is effective in a wide variety of patient populations with hypercholesterolemia, with and without hypertriglyceridemia, in men and women, and in the elderly. Experience in pediatric patients has been limited to patients with homozygous FH.
In two multicenter, placebo-controlled, dose-response studies in patients with hypercholesterolemia, Lipitor given as a

Continued on next page

Lipitor—Cont.

single dose over 6 weeks significantly reduced total-C, LDL-C, apo B, and TG (Pooled results are provided in Table 1).

[See table 1 at top of previous page]

In patients with *Fredrickson* Types IIa and IIb hyperlipoproteinemia pooled from 24 controlled trials, the median (25th and 75th percentile) percent changes from baseline in HDL-C for atorvastatin 10, 20, 40, and 80 mg were 6.4 (–1.4, 14), 8.7 (0, 17), 7.8 (0, 16), and 5.1 (–2.7, 15), respectively. Additionally, analysis of the pooled data demonstrated consistent and significant decreases in total-C , LDL-C, TG, total-C/HDL-C, and LDL-C/HDL-C.

In three multicenter, double-blind studies in patients with hypercholesterolemia, Lipitor was compared to other HMG-CoA reductase inhibitors. After randomization, patients were treated for 16 weeks with either Lipitor 10 mg per day or a fixed dose of the comparative agent (Table 2).

[See table 2 at top of previous page]

The impact on clinical outcomes of the differences in lipid-altering effects between treatments shown in Table 2 is not known. Table 2 does not contain data comparing the effects of atorvastatin 10 mg and higher doses of lovastatin, pravastatin, and simvastatin. The drugs compared in the studies summarized in the table are not necessarily interchangeable.

In a large clinical study, the number of patients meeting their National Cholesterol Education Program-Adult Treatment Panel (NCEP-ATP) II target LDL-C levels on 10 mg of Lipitor daily was assessed. After 16 weeks, 156/167 (93%) of patients with less than 2 risk factors for CHD and baseline LDL-C ≥190 mg/dL reached a target of ≤160 mg/dL; 141/218 (65%) of patients with 2 or more risk factors for CHD and LDL-C ≥160 mg/dL achieved a level of ≤130 mg/dL LDL-C; and 21/113 (19%) of patients with CHD and LDL-C ≥130 mg/dL reached a target level of ≤100 mg/dL LDL-C.

Hypertriglyceridemia (*Fredrickson* Type IV)

The response to Lipitor in 64 patients with isolated hypertriglyceridemia treated across several clinical trials is shown in the table below. For the atorvastatin-treated patients, median (min, max) baseline TG level was 565 (267–1502).

[See table 3 above]

Dysbetalipoproteinemia (*Fredrickson* Type III)

The results of an open-label crossover study of 16 patients (genotypes: 14 apo E2/E2 and 2 apo E3/E2) with dysbetalipoproteinemia (*Fredrickson* Type III) are shown in the table below.

[See table 4 above]

Homozygous Familial Hypercholesterolemia

In a study without a concurrent control group, 29 patients ages 6 to 37 years with homozygous FH received maximum daily doses of 20 to 80 mg of Lipitor. The mean LDL-C reduction in this study was 18%. Twenty-five patients with a reduction in LDL-C had a mean response of 20% (range of 7% to 53%, median of 24%); the remaining 4 patients had 7% to 24% increases in LDL-C. Five of the 29 patients had absent LDL-receptor function. Of these, 2 patients also had a portacaval shunt and had no significant reduction in LDL-C. The remaining 3 receptor-negative patients had a mean LDL-C reduction of 22%.

INDICATIONS AND USAGE

Lipitor is indicated:

1. as an adjunct to diet to reduce elevated total-C, LDL-C, apo B, and TG levels and to increase HDL-C in patients with primary hypercholesterolemia (heterozygous familial and nonfamilial) and mixed dyslipidemia (*Fredrickson* Types IIa and IIb);
2. as an adjunct to diet for the treatment of patients with elevated serum TG levels (*Fredrickson* Type IV);
3. for the treatment of patients with primary dysbetalipoproteinemia (*Fredrickson* Type III) who do not respond adequately to diet;
4. to reduce total-C and LDL-C in patients with homozygous familial hypercholesterolemia as an adjunct to other lipid-lowering treatments (eg, LDL apheresis) or if such treatments are unavailable.

Therapy with lipid-altering agents should be a component of multiple-risk-factor intervention in individuals at increased risk for atherosclerotic vascular disease due to hypercholesterolemia. Lipid-altering agents should be used in addition to a diet restricted in saturated fat and cholesterol only when the response to diet and other nonpharmacological measures has been inadequate (see *National Cholesterol Education Program (NCEP) Guidelines*, summarized in Table 5).

[See table 5 above]

At the time of hospitalization for an acute coronary event, consideration can be given to initiating drug therapy at discharge if the LDL-C level is ≥130 mg/dL (NCEP-ATP II).

Prior to initiating therapy with Lipitor, secondary causes for hypercholesterolemia (eg, poorly controlled diabetes mellitus, hypothyroidism, nephrotic syndrome, dysproteinemias, obstructive liver disease, other drug therapy, and alcoholism) should be excluded, and a lipid profile performed to measure total-C, LDL-C, HDL-C, and TG. For patients with TG <400 mg/dL (<4.5 mmol/L), LDL-C can be estimated using the following equation: LDL-C = total-C - (0.20 × [TG] + HDL-C). For TG levels >400 mg/dL (>4.5 mmol/L), this equation is less accurate and LDL-C concentrations should be determined by ultracentrifugation.

TABLE 3. Combined Patients With Isolated Elevated TG: Median (min, max) Percent Changes From Baseline

	Placebo (N=12)	Atorvastatin 10 mg (N=37)	Atorvastatin 20 mg (N=13)	Atorvastatin 80 mg (N=14)
Triglycerides	-12.4 (-36.6, 82.7)	-41.0 (-76.2, 49.4)	-38.7 (-62.7, 29.5)	-51.8 (-82.8, 41.3)
Total-C	-2.3 (-15.5, 24.4)	-28.2 (-44.9, -6.8)	-34.9 (-49.6, -15.2)	-44.4 (-63.5, -3.8)
LDL-C	3.6 (-31.3, 31.6)	-26.5 (-57.7, 9.8)	-30.4 (-53.9, 0.3)	-40.5 (-60.6, -13.8)
HDL-C	3.8 (-18.6, 13.4)	13.8 (-9.7, 61.5)	11.0 (-3.2, 25.2)	7.5 (-10.8, 37.2)
VLDL-C	-1.0 (-31.9, 53.2)	-48.8 (-85.8, 57.3)	-44.6 (-62.2, -10.8)	-62.0 (-88.2, 37.6)
non-HDL-C	-2.8 (-17.6, 30.0)	-33.0 (-52.1, -13.3)	-42.7 (-53.7, -17.4)	-51.5 (-72.9, -4.3)

TABLE 4. Open-Label Crossover Study of 16 Patients With Dysbetalipoproteinemia (*Fredrickson* Type III)

		Median % Change (min, max)	
	Median (min, max) at Baseline mg/dL)	Atorvastatin 10 mg	Atorvastatin 80 mg
Total-C	442 (225, 1320)	-37 (-85, 17)	-58 (-90, -31)
Triglycerides	678 (273, 5990)	-39 (-92, -8)	-53 (-95, -30)
IDL-C + VLDL-C	215 (111, 613)	-32 (-76, 9)	-63 (-90, -8)
non-HDL-C	411 (218, 1272)	-43 (-87, -19)	-64 (-92, -36)

TABLE 5. NCEP Guidelines for Lipid Management

Definite Atherosclerotic Disease[a]	Two or More Other Risk Factors[b]	LDL-Cholesterol mg/dL (mmol/L)	
		Initiation Level	Minimum Goal
No	No	≥190 (≥4.9)	<160 (<4.1)
No	Yes	≥160 (≥4.1)	<130 (<3.4)
Yes	Yes or No	≥130[c] (≥3.4)	≤100 (≤2.6)

[a] Coronary heart disease or peripheral vascular disease (including symptomatic carotid artery disease).

[b] Other risk factors for coronary heart disease (CHD) include: age (males: ≥45 years; females: ≥55 years or premature menopause without estrogen replacement therapy); family history of premature CHD; current cigarette smoking; hypertension; confirmed HDL-C<35 mg/dL (<0.91 mmol/L); and diabetes mellitus. Subtract 1 risk factor if HDL-C is ≥60 mg/dL (≥1.6 mmol/L).

[c] In CHD patients with LDL-C levels 100 to 129 mg/dL, the physician should exercise clinical judgment in deciding whether to initiate drug treatment.

Lipitor has not been studied in conditions where the major lipoprotein abnormality is elevation of chylomicrons (*Fredrickson* Types I and V).

CONTRAINDICATIONS

Active liver disease or unexplained persistent elevations of serum transaminases.

Hypersensitivity to any component of this medication.

Pregnancy and Lactation

Atherosclerosis is a chronic process and discontinuation of lipid-lowering drugs during pregnancy should have little impact on the outcome of long-term therapy of primary hypercholesterolemia. Cholesterol and other products of cholesterol biosynthesis are essential components for fetal development (including synthesis of steroids and cell membranes). Since HMG-CoA reductase inhibitors decrease cholesterol synthesis and possibly the synthesis of other biologically active substances derived from cholesterol, they may cause fetal harm when administered to pregnant women. Therefore, HMG-CoA reductase inhibitors are contraindicated during pregnancy and in nursing mothers. ATORVASTATIN SHOULD BE ADMINISTERED TO WOMEN OF CHILDBEARING AGE ONLY WHEN SUCH PATIENTS ARE HIGHLY UNLIKELY TO CONCEIVE AND HAVE BEEN INFORMED OF THE POTENTIAL HAZARDS. If the patient becomes pregnant while taking this drug, therapy should be discontinued and the patient apprised of the potential hazard to the fetus.

WARNINGS

Liver Dysfunction

HMG-CoA reductase inhibitors, like some other lipid-lowering therapies, have been associated with biochemical abnormalities of liver function. **Persistent elevations (>3 times the upper limit of normal [ULN] occurring on 2 or more occasions) in serum transaminases occurred in 0.7% of patients who received atorvastatin in clinical trials. The incidence of these abnormalities was 0.2%, 0.2%, 0.6%, and 2.3% for 10, 20, 40, and 80 mg, respectively.**

One patient in clinical trials developed jaundice. Increases in liver function tests (LFT) in other patients were not associated with jaundice or other clinical signs or symptoms. Upon dose reduction, drug interruption, or discontinuation, transaminase levels returned to or near pretreatment levels without sequelae. Eighteen of 30 patients with persistent LFT elevations continued treatment with a reduced dose of atorvastatin.

It is recommended that liver function tests be performed prior to and at 12 weeks following both the initiation of therapy and any elevation of dose, and periodically (eg, semiannually) thereafter. Liver enzyme changes generally occur in the first 3 months of treatment with atorvastatin. Patients who develop increased transaminase levels should be monitored until the abnormalities resolve. Should an increase in ALT or AST of >3 times ULN persist, reduction of dose or withdrawal of atorvastatin is recommended.

Atorvastatin should be used with caution in patients who consume substantial quantities of alcohol and/or have a history of liver disease. Active liver disease or unexplained persistent transaminase elevations are contraindications to the use of atorvastatin (see CONTRAINDICATIONS).

Skeletal Muscle

Rare cases of rhabdomyolysis with acute renal failure secondary to myoglobinuria have been reported with atorvastatin and with other drugs in this class.

Uncomplicated myalgia has been reported in atorvastatin-treated patients (see ADVERSE REACTIONS). Myopathy, defined as muscle aches or muscle weakness in conjunction with increases in creatine phosphokinase (CPK) values >10 times ULN, should be considered in any patient with diffuse myalgias, muscle tenderness or weakness, and/or marked elevation of CPK. Patients should be advised to report promptly unexplained muscle pain, tenderness or weakness, particularly if accompanied by malaise or fever. Atorvastatin therapy should be discontinued if markedly elevated CPK levels occur or myopathy is diagnosed or suspected.

The risk of myopathy during treatment with drugs in this class is increased with concurrent administration of cyclosporine, fibric acid derivatives, erythromycin, niacin, or azole antifungals. Physicians considering combined therapy with atorvastatin and fibric acid derivatives, erythromycin, immunosuppressive drugs, azole antifungals, or lipid-lowering doses of niacin should carefully weigh the potential benefits and risks and should carefully monitor patients for any signs or symptoms of muscle pain, tenderness, or weakness, particularly during the initial months of therapy and during any periods of upward dosage titration of either drug. Periodic creatine phosphokinase (CPK) determinations may be considered in such situations, but there is no assurance that such monitoring will prevent the occurrence of severe myopathy.

Atorvastatin therapy should be temporarily withheld or discontinued in any patient with an acute, serious condition suggestive of a myopathy or having a risk factor predisposing to the development of renal failure secondary to rhabdomyolysis (eg, severe acute infection, hypotension, major surgery, trauma, severe metabolic, endocrine and electrolyte disorders, and uncontrolled seizures).

PRECAUTIONS

General

Before instituting therapy with atorvastatin, an attempt should be made to control hypercholesterolemia with appropriate diet, exercise, and weight reduction in obese patients, and to treat other underlying medical problems (see INDICATIONS AND USAGE).

Information for Patients

Patients should be advised to report promptly unexplained muscle pain, tenderness, or weakness, particularly if accompanied by malaise or fever.

Drug Interactions

The risk of myopathy during treatment with drugs of this class is increased with concurrent administration of cyclosporine, fibric acid derivatives, niacin (nicotinic acid), erythromycin, azole antifungals (see WARNINGS, Skeletal Muscle).

Antacid: When atorvastatin and Maalox® TC suspension were coadministered, plasma concentrations of atorvastatin decreased approximately 35%. However, LDL-C reduction was not altered.

Antipyrine: Because atorvastatin does not affect the pharmacokinetics of antipyrine, interactions with other drugs metabolized via the same cytochrome isozymes are not expected.

Colestipol: Plasma concentrations of atorvastatin decreased approximately 25% when colestipol and atorvastatin were coadministered. However, LDL-C reduction was greater when atorvastatin and colestipol were coadministered than when either drug was given alone.

Cimetidine: Atorvastatin plasma concentrations and LDL-C reduction were not altered by coadministration of cimetidine.

Digoxin: When multiple doses of atorvastatin and digoxin were coadministered, steady-state plasma digoxin concentrations increased by approximately 20%. Patients taking digoxin should be monitored appropriately.

Erythromycin: In healthy individuals, plasma concentrations of atorvastatin increased approximately 40% with coadministration of atorvastatin and erythromycin, a known inhibitor of cytochrome P450 3A4 (see WARNINGS, Skeletal Muscle).

Oral Contraceptives: Coadministration of atorvastatin and an oral contraceptive increased AUC values for norethindrone and ethinyl estradiol by approximately 30% and 20%. These increases should be considered when selecting an oral contraceptive for a woman taking atorvastatin.

Warfarin: Atorvastatin had no clinically significant effect on prothrombin time when administered to patients receiving chronic warfarin treatment.

Endocrine Function

HMG-CoA reductase inhibitors interfere with cholesterol synthesis and theoretically might blunt adrenal and/or gonadal steroid production. Clinical studies have shown that atorvastatin does not reduce basal plasma cortisol concentration or impair adrenal reserve. The effects of HMG-CoA reductase inhibitors on male fertility have not been studied in adequate numbers of patients. The effects, if any, on the pituitary-gonadal axis in premenopausal women are unknown. Caution should be exercised if an HMG-CoA reductase inhibitor is administered concomitantly with drugs that may decrease the levels or activity of endogenous steroid hormones, such as ketoconazole, spironolactone, and cimetidine.

CNS Toxicity

Brain hemorrhage was seen in a female dog treated for 3 months at 120 mg/kg/day. Brain hemorrhage and optic nerve vacuolation were seen in another female dog that was sacrificed in moribund condition after 11 weeks of escalating doses up to 280 mg/kg/day. The 120 mg/kg dose resulted in a systemic exposure approximately 16 times the human plasma area-under-the-curve (AUC, 0–24 hours) based on the maximum human dose of 80 mg/day. A single tonic convulsion was seen in each of 2 male dogs (one treated at 10 mg/kg/day and one at 120 mg/kg/day) in a 2-year study. No CNS lesions have been observed in mice after chronic treatment for up to 2 years at doses up to 400 mg/kg/day or in rats at doses up to 100 mg/kg/day. These doses were 6 to 11 times (mouse) and 8 to 16 times (rat) the human AUC (0–24) based on the maximum recommended human dose of 80 mg/day.

CNS vascular lesions, characterized by perivascular hemorrhages, edema, and mononuclear cell infiltration of perivascular spaces, have been observed in dogs treated with other members of this class. A chemically similar drug in this class produced optic nerve degeneration (Wallerian degeneration of retinogeniculate fibers) in clinically normal dogs in a dose-dependent fashion at a dose that produced plasma drug levels about 30 times higher than the mean drug level in humans taking the highest recommended dose.

Carcinogenesis, Mutagenesis, Impairment of Fertility

In a 2-year carcinogenicity study in rats at dose levels of 10, 30, and 100 mg/kg/day, 2 rare tumors were found in muscle in high-dose females: in one, there was a rhabdomyosarcoma and, in another, there was a fibrosarcoma. This dose represents a plasma AUC (0–24) value of approximately 16 times the mean human plasma drug exposure after an 80 mg oral dose.

A 2-year carcinogenicity study in mice given 100, 200, or 400 mg/kg/day resulted in a significant increase in liver adenomas in high-dose males and liver carcinomas in high-dose females. These findings occurred at plasma AUC (0–24) values of approximately 6 times the mean human plasma drug exposure after an 80 mg oral dose.

In vitro, atorvastatin was not mutagenic or clastogenic in the following tests with and without metabolic activation: the Ames test with *Salmonella typhimurium* and *Escherichia coli*, the HGPRT forward mutation assay in Chinese hamster lung cells, and the chromosomal aberration assay in Chinese hamster lung cells. Atorvastatin was negative in the *in vivo* mouse micronucleus test.

Studies in rats performed at doses up to 175 mg/kg (15 times the human exposure) produced no changes in fertility. There was aplasia and aspermia in the epididymis of 2 of 10 rats treated with 100 mg/kg/day of atorvastatin for 3 months (16 times the human AUC at the 80 mg dose); testis weights were significantly lower at 30 and 100 mg/kg and epididymal weight was lower at 100 mg/kg. Male rats given 100 mg/kg/day for 11 weeks prior to mating had decreased sperm motility, spermatid head concentration, and increased abnormal sperm. Atorvastatin caused no adverse effects on semen parameters, or reproductive organ histopathology in dogs given doses of 10, 40, or 120 mg/kg for two years.

Pregnancy

Pregnancy Category X

See CONTRAINDICATIONS

Safety in pregnant women has not been established. Atorvastatin crosses the rat placenta and reaches a level in fetal liver equivalent to that of maternal plasma. Atorvastatin was not teratogenic in rats at doses up to 300 mg/kg/day or in rabbits at doses up to 100 mg/kg/day. These doses resulted in multiples of about 30 times (rat) or 20 times (rabbit) the human exposure based on surface area (mg/m²).

In a study in rats given 20, 100, or 225 mg/kg/day, from gestation day 7 through to lactation day 21 (weaning), there was decreased pup survival at birth, neonate, weaning, and maturity in pups of mothers dosed with 225 mg/kg/day. Body weight was decreased on days 4 and 21 in pups of mothers dosed at 100 mg/kg/day; pup body weight was decreased at birth and at days 4, 21, and 91 at 225 mg/kg/day. Pup development was delayed (rotorod performance at 100 mg/kg/day and acoustic startle at 225 mg/kg/day; pinnae detachment and eye opening at 225 mg/kg/day). These doses correspond to 6 times (100 mg/kg) and 22 times (225 mg/kg) the human AUC at 80 mg/day.

Rare reports of congenital anomalies have been received following intrauterine exposure to HMG-CoA reductase inhibitors. There has been one report of severe congenital bony deformity, tracheo-esophageal fistula, and anal atresia (VATER association) in a baby born to a woman who took lovastatin with dextroamphetamine sulfate during the first trimester of pregnancy. Lipitor should be administered to women of child-bearing potential only when such patients are highly unlikely to conceive and have been informed of the potential hazards. If the woman becomes pregnant while taking Lipitor, it should be discontinued and the patient advised again as to the potential hazards to the fetus.

Nursing Mothers

Nursing rat pups had plasma and liver drug levels of 50% and 40%, respectively, of that in their mother's milk. Because of the potential for adverse reactions in nursing infants, women taking Lipitor should not breast-feed (see CONTRAINDICATIONS).

Pediatric Use

Treatment experience in a pediatric population is limited to doses of Lipitor up to 80 mg/day for 1 year in 8 patients with homozygous FH. No clinical or biochemical abnormalities were reported in these patients. None of these patients was below 9 years of age.

Geriatric Use

Treatment experience in adults age ≥70 years with doses of Lipitor up to 80 mg/day has been evaluated in 221 patients. The safety and efficacy of Lipitor in this population were similar to those of patients <70 years of age.

ADVERSE REACTIONS

Lipitor is generally well-tolerated. Adverse reactions have usually been mild and transient. In controlled clinical studies of 2502 patients, <2% of patients were discontinued due to adverse experiences attributable to atorvastatin. The most frequent adverse events thought to be related to atorvastatin were constipation, flatulence, dyspepsia, and abdominal pain.

Clinical Adverse Experiences

Adverse experiences reported in ≥2% of patients in placebo-controlled clinical studies of atorvastatin, regardless of causality assessment, are shown in Table 6.

[See table above]

TABLE 6. Adverse Events in Placebo-Controlled Studies (% of Patients)

BODY SYSTEM/ Adverse Event	Placebo N=270	Atorvastatin 10 mg N=863	Atorvastatin 20 mg N=36	Atorvastatin 40 mg N=79	Atorvastatin 80 mg N=94
BODY AS A WHOLE					
Infection	10.0	10.3	2.8	10.1	7.4
Headache	7.0	5.4	16.7	2.5	6.4
Accidental Injury	3.7	4.2	0.0	1.3	3.2
Flu Syndrome	1.9	2.2	0.0	2.5	3.2
Abdominal Pain	0.7	2.8	0.0	3.8	2.1
Back Pain	3.0	2.8	0.0	3.8	1.1
Allergic Reaction	2.6	0.9	2.8	1.3	0.0
Asthenia	1.9	2.2	0.0	3.8	0.0
DIGESTIVE SYSTEM					
Constipation	1.8	2.1	0.0	2.5	1.1
Diarrhea	1.5	2.7	0.0	3.8	5.3
Dyspepsia	4.1	2.3	2.8	1.3	2.1
Flatulence	3.3	2.1	2.8	1.3	1.1
RESPIRATORY SYSTEM					
Sinusitis	2.6	2.8	0.0	2.5	6.4
Pharyngitis	1.5	2.5	0.0	1.3	2.1
SKIN AND APPENDAGES					
Rash	0.7	3.9	2.8	3.8	1.1
MUSCULOSKELETAL SYSTEM					
Arthralgia	1.5	2.0	0.0	5.1	0.0
Myalgia	1.1	3.2	5.6	1.3	0.0

The following adverse events were reported, regardless of causality assessment in patients treated with atorvastatin in clinical trials. The events in italics occurred in ≥2% of patients and the events in plain type occurred in <2% of patients.

Body as a Whole: *Chest pain*, face edema, fever, neck rigidity, malaise, photosensitivity reaction, generalized edema.

Digestive System: *Nausea*, gastroenteritis, liver function tests abnormal, colitis, vomiting, gastritis, dry mouth, rectal hemorrhage, esophagitis, eructation, glossitis, mouth ulceration, anorexia, increased appetite, stomatitis, biliary pain, cheilitis, duodenal ulcer, dysphagia, enteritis, melena, gum hemorrhage, stomach ulcer, tenesmus, ulcerative stomatitis, hepatitis, pancreatitis, cholestatic jaundice.

Respiratory System: *Bronchitis, rhinitis*, pneumonia, dyspnea, asthma, epistaxis.

Nervous System: *Insomnia, dizziness*, paresthesia, somnolence, amnesia, abnormal dreams, libido decreased, emotional lability, incoordination, peripheral neuropathy, torticollis, facial paralysis, hyperkinesia, depression, hypesthesia, hypertonia.

Musculoskeletal System: *Arthritis*, leg cramps, bursitis, tenosynovitis, myasthenia, tendinous contracture, myositis.

Skin and Appendages: Pruritus, contact dermatitis, alopecia, dry skin, sweating, acne, urticaria, eczema, seborrhea, skin ulcer.

Urogenital System: *Urinary tract infection*, urinary frequency, cystitis, hematuria, impotence, dysuria, kidney calculus, nocturia, epididymitis, fibrocystic breast, vaginal hemorrhage, albuminuria, breast enlargement, metrorrhagia, nephritis, urinary incontinence, urinary retention, urinary urgency, abnormal ejaculation, uterine hemorrhage.

Special Senses: Amblyopia, tinnitus, dry eyes, refraction disorder, eye hemorrhage, deafness, glaucoma, parosmia, taste loss, taste perversion.

Cardiovascular System: Palpitation, vasodilatation, syncope, migraine, postural hypotension, phlebitis, arrhythmia, angina pectoris, hypertension.

Metabolic and Nutritional Disorders: *Peripheral edema*, hyperglycemia, creatine phosphokinase increased, gout, weight gain, hypoglycemia.

Hemic and Lymphatic System: Ecchymosis, anemia, lymphadenopathy, thrombocytopenia, petechia.

Postintroduction Reports

Adverse events associated with Lipitor therapy reported since market introduction, that are not listed above, regardless of causality assessment, include the following: anaphylaxis, angioneurotic edema, bullous rashes (including erythema multiforme, Stevens-Johnson syndrome, and toxic epidermal necrolysis), and rhabdomyolysis.

OVERDOSAGE

There is no specific treatment for atorvastatin overdosage. In the event of an overdose, the patient should be treated symptomatically, and supportive measures instituted as required. Due to extensive drug binding to plasma proteins, hemodialysis is not expected to significantly enhance atorvastatin clearance.

DOSAGE AND ADMINISTRATION

The patient should be placed on a standard cholesterol-lowering diet before receiving Lipitor and should continue on this diet during treatment with Lipitor.

Continued on next page

Lipitor—Cont.

Hypercholesterolemia (Heterozygous Familial and Nonfamilial) and Mixed Dyslipidemia (*Fredrickson* Types IIa and IIb)

The recommended starting dose of Lipitor is 10 mg once daily. The dosage range is 10 to 80 mg once daily. Lipitor can be administered as a single dose at any time of the day, with or without food. Therapy should be individualized according to goal of therapy and response (see *NCEP Guidelines,* summarized in Table 5). After initiation and/or upon titration of Lipitor, lipid levels should be analyzed within 2 to 4 weeks and dosage adjusted accordingly.

Since the goal of treatment is to lower LDL-C, the NCEP recommends that LDL-C levels be used to initiate and assess treatment response. Only if LDL-C levels are not available, should total-C be used to monitor therapy.

Homozygous Familial Hypercholesterolemia

The dosage of Lipitor in patients with homozygous FH is 10 to 80 mg daily. Lipitor should be used as an adjunct to other lipid-lowering treatments (eg, LDL apheresis) in these patients or if such treatments are unavailable.

Concomitant Therapy

Atorvastatin may be used in combination with a bile acid binding resin for additive effect. The combination of HMG-CoA reductase inhibitors and fibrates should generally be avoided (see WARNINGS, Skeletal Muscle, and PRECAUTIONS, Drug Interactions for other drug-drug interactions).

Dosage in Patients With Renal Insufficiency

Renal disease does not affect the plasma concentrations nor LDL-C reduction of atorvastatin; thus, dosage adjustment in patients with renal dysfunction is not necessary (see CLINICAL PHARMACOLOGY, Pharmacokinetics).

HOW SUPPLIED

Lipitor is supplied as white, elliptical, film-coated tablets of atorvastatin calcium containing 10, 20, 40, and 80 mg atorvastatin.

10 mg tablets: coded "PD 155" on one side and "10" on the other.

N0071-0155-23 bottles of 90
N0071-0155-34 bottles of 5000
N0071-0155-40 10 × 10 unit dose blisters

20 mg tablets: coded "PD 156" on one side and "20" on the other.

N0071-0156-23 bottles of 90
N0071-0156-40 10 × 10 unit dose blisters

40 mg tablets: coded "PD 157" on one side and "40" on the other.

N0071-0157-23 bottles of 90

80 mg tablets: coded "PD 158" on one side and "80" on the other.

N0071-0158-23 bottles of 90

Storage

Store at controlled room temperature 20°–25°C (68°–77°F) [see USP].

Rx only

Revised March 2000

Manufactured by:
Warner-Lambert Export, Ltd. ©1998–'00
Dublin, Ireland
Distributed by:
PARKE-DAVIS
Div of Warner-Lambert Co
Morris Plains, NJ 07950 USA
MADE IN PUERTO RICO
Marketed by:
PARKE-DAVIS
Div of Warner-Lambert Co and
PFIZER Inc.
New York, NY 10017
0155G247

NEURONTIN® ℞
(Gabapentin) Capsules
NEURONTIN® ℞
(Gabapentin) Tablets
NEURONTIN® ℞
(Gabapentin) Oral Solution

Prescribing information for this product, which appears on pages 2458–2461 of the 2001 PDR, has been completely revised as follows. Please write "See Supplement A" next to the product heading.

DESCRIPTION

Neurontin® (gabapentin) capsules, Neurontin® (gabapentin) tablets, and Neurontin® (gabapentin) oral solution are supplied as imprinted hard shell capsules containing 100 mg, 300 mg, and 400 mg of gabapentin, elliptical film-coated tablets containing 600 mg and 800 mg of gabapentin or an oral solution containing 250 mg/5 mL of gabapentin.

The inactive ingredients for the capsules are lactose, cornstarch, and talc. The 100 mg capsule shell contains gelatin and titanium dioxide. The 300 mg capsule shell contains gelatin, titanium dioxide, and yellow iron oxide. The 400 mg capsule shell contains gelatin, red iron oxide, titanium dioxide, and yellow iron oxide. The imprinting ink contains FD&C Blue No. 2 and titanium dioxide.

The inactive ingredients for the tablets are poloxamer 407, copolyvidonum, cornstarch, magnesium stearate, hydroxypropyl cellulose, talc, candelilla wax and purified water. The imprinting ink for the 600 mg tablets contains synthetic black iron oxide, pharmaceutical shellac, pharmaceutical glaze, propylene glycol, ammonium hydroxide, isopropyl alcohol and n-butyl alcohol. The imprinting ink for the 800 mg tablets contains synthetic yellow iron oxide, synthetic red iron oxide, hydroxypropyl methylcellulose, propylene glycol, methanol, isopropyl alcohol and deionized water.

The inactive ingredients for the oral solution are glycerin, xylitol, purified water and artificial cool strawberry anise flavor.

Gabapentin is described as 1-(aminomethyl)cyclohexaneacetic acid with an empirical formula of $C_9H_{17}NO_2$ and a molecular weight of 171.24. The molecular structure of gabapentin is:

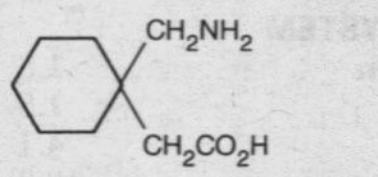

Gabapentin is a white to off-white crystalline solid. It is freely soluble in water and both basic and acidic aqueous solutions.

CLINICAL PHARMACOLOGY

Mechanism of Action

The mechanism by which gabapentin exerts its anticonvulsant action is unknown, but in animal test systems designed to detect anticonvulsant activity, gabapentin prevents seizures as do other marketed anticonvulsants. Gabapentin exhibits antiseizure activity in mice and rats in both the maximal electroshock and pentylenetetrazole seizure models and other preclinical models (e.g., strains with genetic epilepsy, etc.). The relevance of these models to human epilepsy is not known.

Gabapentin is structurally related to the neurotransmitter GABA (gamma-aminobutyric acid) but it does not interact with GABA receptors, it is not converted metabolically into GABA or a GABA agonist, and it is not an inhibitor of GABA uptake or degradation. Gabapentin was tested in radioligand binding assays at concentrations up to 100 µM and did not exhibit affinity for a number of other common receptor sites, including benzodiazepine, glutamate, N-methyl-D-aspartate (NMDA), quisqualate, kainate, strychnine-insensitive or strychnine-sensitive glycine, alpha 1, alpha 2, or beta adrenergic, adenosine A1 or A2, cholinergic muscarinic or nicotinic, dopamine D1 or D2, histamine H1, serotonin S1 or S2, opiate mu, delta or kappa, voltage-sensitive calcium channel sites labeled with nitrendipine or diltiazem, or at voltage-sensitive sodium channel sites with batrachotoxinin A 20-alpha-benzoate.

Several test systems ordinarily used to assess activity at the NMDA receptor have been examined. Results are contradictory. Accordingly, no general statement about the effects, if any, of gabapentin at the NMDA receptor can be made.

In vitro studies with radiolabeled gabapentin have revealed a gabapentin binding site in areas of rat brain including neocortex and hippocampus. A high-affinity binding protein in animal brain tissue has been identified as an auxiliary subunit of voltage-activated calcium channels. However, functional correlates of gabapentin binding, if any, remain to be elucidated.

Pharmacokinetics and Drug Metabolism

All pharmacological actions following gabapentin administration are due to the activity of the parent compound; gabapentin is not appreciably metabolized in humans.

Oral Bioavailability: Gabapentin bioavailability is not dose proportional; i.e., as dose is increased, bioavailability decreases. A 400 mg dose, for example, is about 25% less bioavailable than a 100 mg dose. Over the recommended dose range of 300 to 600 mg T.I.D., however, the differences in bioavailability are not large, and bioavailability is about 60 percent. Food has only a slight effect on the rate and extent of absorption of gabapentin (14% increase in AUC and C_{max}).

Distribution: Gabapentin circulates largely unbound (<3%) to plasma protein. The apparent volume of distribution of gabapentin after 150 mg intravenous administration is 58±6 L (Mean ±SD). In patients with epilepsy, steady-state predose (Cmin) concentrations of gabapentin in cerebrospinal fluid were approximately 20% of the corresponding plasma concentrations.

Elimination: Gabapentin is eliminated from the systemic circulation by renal excretion as unchanged drug. Gabapentin is not appreciably metabolized in humans.

Gabapentin elimination half-life is 5 to 7 hours and is unaltered by dose or following multiple dosing. Gabapentin elimination rate constant, plasma clearance, and renal clearance are directly proportional to creatinine clearance (see Special Populations: Patients With Renal Insufficiency, below). In elderly patients, and in patients with impaired renal function, gabapentin plasma clearance is reduced. Gabapentin can be removed from plasma by hemodialysis.

Dosage adjustment in patients with compromised renal function or undergoing hemodialysis is recommended (see DOSAGE AND ADMINISTRATION, Table 2).

Special Populations: *Adult Patients With Renal Insufficiency:* Subjects (N=60) with renal insufficiency (mean creatinine clearance ranging from 13–114 mL/min) were administered single 400 mg oral doses of gabapentin. The mean gabapentin half-life ranged from about 6.5 hours (patients with creatinine clearance >60 mL/min) to 52 hours (creatinine clearance <30 mL/min) and gabapentin renal clearance from about 90 mL/min (>60 mL/min group) to about 10 mL/min (<30 mL/min). Mean plasma clearance (CL/F) decreased from approximately 190 mL/min to 20 mL/min.

Dosage adjustment in adult patients with compromised renal function is necessary (see DOSAGE AND ADMINISTRATION). Pediatric patients with renal insufficiency have not been studied.

Hemodialysis: In a study in anuric subjects (N=11), the apparent elimination half-life of gabapentin on nondialysis days was about 132 hours; dialysis three times a week (4 hours duration) lowered the apparent half-life of gabapentin by about 60%, from 132 hours to 51 hours. Hemodialysis thus has a significant effect on gabapentin elimination in anuric subjects.

Dosage adjustment in patients undergoing hemodialysis is necessary (see DOSAGE AND ADMINISTRATION).

Hepatic Disease: Because gabapentin is not metabolized, no study was performed in patients with hepatic impairment.

Age: The effect of age was studied in subjects 20–80 years of age. Apparent oral clearance (CL/F) of gabapentin decreased as age increased, from about 225 mL/min in those under 30 years of age to about 125 mL/min in those over 70 years of age. Renal clearance (CLr) and CLr adjusted for body surface area also declined with age; however, the decline in the renal clearance of gabapentin with age can largely be explained by the decline in renal function. Reduction of gabapentin dose may be required in patients who have age related compromised renal function. (See PRECAUTIONS, Geriatric Use, and DOSAGE AND ADMINISTRATION.)

Pediatric: Gabapentin pharmacokinetics were determined in 48 pediatric subjects between the ages of 1 month and 12 years following a dose of approximately 10 mg/kg. Peak plasma concentrations were similar across the entire age group and occurred 2 to 3 hours postdose. In general, pediatric subjects between 1 month and <5 years of age achieved approximately 30% lower exposure (AUC) than that observed in those 5 years of age and older. Accordingly, oral clearance normalized per body weight was higher in the younger children. Apparent oral clearance of gabapentin was directly proportional to creatinine clearance. Gabapentin elimination half-life averaged 4.7 hours and was similar across the age groups studied.

A population pharmacokinetic analysis was performed in 253 pediatric subjects between 1 month and 13 years of age. Patients received 10 to 65 mg/kg/day given T.I.D. Apparent oral clearance (CL/F) was directly proportional to creatinine clearance and this relationship was similar following a single dose and at steady state. Higher oral clearance values were observed in children <5 years of age compared to those observed in children 5 years of age and older, when normalized per body weight. The clearance was highly variable in infants <1 year of age. The normalized CL/F values observed in pediatric patients 5 years of age and older were consistent with values observed in adults after a single dose. The oral volume of distribution normalized per body weight was constant across the age range.

These pharmacokinetic data indicate that the effective daily dose in pediatric patients ages 3 and 4 years should be 40 mg/kg/day to achieve average plasma concentrations similar to those achieved in patients 5 years of age and older receiving gabapentin at 30 mg/kg/day. (See DOSAGE AND ADMINISTRATION.)

Gender: Although no formal study has been conducted to compare the pharmacokinetics of gabapentin in men and women, it appears that the pharmacokinetic parameters for males and females are similar and there are no significant gender differences.

Race: Pharmacokinetic differences due to race have not been studied. Because gabapentin is primarily renally excreted and there are no important racial differences in creatinine clearance, pharmacokinetic differences due to race are not expected.

Clinical Studies

The effectiveness of Neurontin® as adjunctive therapy (added to other antiepileptic drugs) was established in multicenter placebo-controlled, double-blind, parallel-group clinical trials in adult and pediatric patients (3 years and older) with refractory partial seizures.

Evidence of effectiveness was obtained in three trials conducted in 705 patients (age 12 years and above) and one trial conducted in 247 pediatric patients (3 to 12 years of age). The patients enrolled had a history of at least 4 partial seizures per month in spite of receiving one or more antiepileptic drugs at therapeutic levels and were observed on their established antiepileptic drug regimen during a 12-week baseline period (6 weeks in the study of pediatric patients). In patients continuing to have at least 2 (or 4 in some studies) seizures per month, Neurontin® or placebo was then added on to the existing therapy during a 12-week treatment period. Effectiveness was assessed primarily on the basis of the percent of patients with a 50% or greater reduction in seizure frequency from baseline to treatment (the "responder rate") and a derived measure called response ratio, a measure of change defined as $(T - B)/(T + B)$, where B is the patient's baseline seizure frequency and T is the patient's seizure frequency during treatment. Response ratio is distributed within the range -1 to $+1$. A zero value indicates no change while complete elimination of seizures would give a value of -1; increased seizure rates would give positive values. A response ratio of -0.33 corresponds to a 50% reduction in seizure frequency. The results given below are for all partial seizures in the intent-to-treat (all patients who received any doses of treatment) population in each study, unless otherwise indicated.

One study compared Neurontin® 1200 mg/day T.I.D. with placebo. Responder rate was 23% (14/61) in the Neurontin® group and 9% (6/66) in the placebo group; the difference between groups was statistically significant. Response ratio was also better in the Neurontin® group (−0.199) than in the placebo group (−0.044), a difference that also achieved statistical significance.

A second study compared primarily 1200 mg/day T.I.D. Neurontin® (N=101) with placebo (N=98). Additional smaller Neurontin® dosage groups (600 mg/day, N=53; 1800 mg/day, N=54) were also studied for information regarding dose response. Responder rate was higher in the Neurontin® 1200 mg/day group (16%) than in the placebo group (8%), but the difference was not statistically significant. The responder rate at 600 mg (17%) was also not significantly higher than in the placebo, but the responder rate in the 1800 mg group (26%) was statistically significantly superior to the placebo rate. Response ratio was better in the Neurontin® 1200 mg/day group (−0.103) than in the placebo group (−0.022); but this difference was also not statistically significant (p = 0.224). A better response was seen in the Neurontin® 600 mg/day group (−0.105) and 1800 mg/day group (−0.222) than in the 1200 mg/day group, with the 1800 mg/day group achieving statistical significance compared to the placebo group.

A third study compared Neurontin® 900 mg/day T.I.D. (N=111) and placebo (N=109). An additional Neurontin® 1200 mg/day dosage group (N=52) provided dose-response data. A statistically significant difference in responder rate was seen in the Neurontin® 900 mg/day group (22%) compared to that in the placebo group (10%). Response ratio was also statistically significantly superior in the Neurontin® 900 mg/day group (−0.119) compared to that in the placebo group (−0.027), as was response ratio in 1200 mg/day Neurontin® (−0.184) compared to placebo.

Analyses were also performed in each study to examine the effect of Neurontin® on preventing secondarily generalized tonic-clonic seizures. Patients who experienced a secondarily generalized tonic-clonic seizure in either the baseline or in the treatment period in all three placebo-controlled studies were included in these analyses. There were several response ratio comparisons that showed a statistically significant advantage for Neurontin® compared to placebo and favorable trends for almost all comparisons.

Analysis of responder rate using combined data from all three studies and all doses (N=162, Neurontin®; N=89, placebo) also showed a significant advantage for Neurontin® over placebo in reducing the frequency of secondarily generalized tonic-clonic seizures.

In two of the three controlled studies, more than one dose of Neurontin® was used. Within each study the results did not show a consistently increased response to dose. However, looking across studies, a trend toward increasing efficacy with increasing dose is evident (see Figure 1).

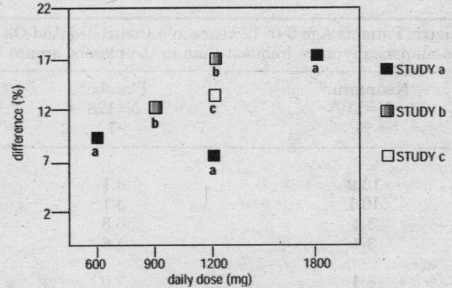

FIGURE 1. Responder Rate in Patients Receiving Neurontin® Expressed as a Difference from Placebo by Dose and Study

In the figure, treatment effect magnitude, measured on the Y axis in terms of the difference in the proportion of gabapentin and placebo assigned patients attaining a 50% or greater reduction in seizure frequency from baseline, is plotted against the daily dose of gabapentin administered (X axis).

Although no formal analysis by gender has been performed, estimates of response (Response Ratio) derived from clinical trials (398 men, 307 women) indicate no important gender differences exist. There was no consistent pattern indicating that age had any effect on the response to Neurontin®. There were insufficient numbers of patients of races other than Caucasian to permit a comparison of efficacy among racial groups.

A fourth study in pediatric patients age 3 to 12 years compared 25–35 mg/kg/day Neurontin (N=118) with placebo (N=127). For all partial seizures in the intent-to-treat population, the response ratio was statistically significantly better for the Neurontin group (−0.146) than for the placebo group (−0.079). For the same population, the responder rate for Neurontin (21%) was not significantly different from placebo (18%).

A study in pediatric patients age 1 month to 3 years compared 40 mg/kg/day Neurontin (N=38) with placebo (N=38) in patients who were receiving at least one marketed antiepileptic drug and had at least one partial seizure during the screening period (within 2 weeks prior to baseline). Patients had up to 48 hours of baseline and up to 72 hours of double-blind video EEG monitoring to record and count the occurrence of seizures. There were no statistically significant differences between treatments in either the response ratio or responder rate.

INDICATIONS AND USAGE

Neurontin® (gabapentin) is indicated as adjunctive therapy in the treatment of partial seizures with and without secondary generalization in patients over 12 years of age with epilepsy. Neurontin is also indicated as adjunctive therapy in the treatment of partial seizures in pediatric patients age 3–12 years.

CONTRAINDICATIONS

Neurontin® is contraindicated in patients who have demonstrated hypersensitivity to the drug or its ingredients.

WARNINGS

Neuropsychiatric Adverse Events—Pediatric Patients 3–12 years of age

Gabapentin use in pediatric patients with epilepsy 3–12 years of age is associated with the occurrence of central nervous system related adverse events. The most significant of these can be classified into the following categories: 1) emotional lability (primarily behavioral problems), 2) hostility, including aggressive behaviors, 3) thought disorder, including concentration problems and change in school performance, and 4) hyperkinesia (primarily restlessness and hyperactivity). Among the gabapentin-treated patients, most of the events were mild to moderate in intensity.

In controlled trials in pediatric patients 3–12 years of age the incidence of these adverse events was: emotional lability 6% (gabapentin-treated patients) vs 1.3% (placebo-treated patients); hostility 5.2% vs 1.3%; hyperkinesia 4.7% vs 2.9%; and thought disorder 1.7% vs 0%. One of these events, a report of hostility, was considered serious. Discontinuation of gabapentin treatment occurred in 1.3% of patients reporting emotional lability and hyperkinesia and 0.9% of gabapentin-treated patients reporting hostility and thought disorder. One placebo-treated patient (0.4%) withdrew due to emotional lability.

Withdrawal Precipitated Seizure, Status Epilepticus

Antiepileptic drugs should not be abruptly discontinued because of the possibility of increasing seizure frequency.

In the placebo-controlled studies in patients >12 years of age, the incidence of status epilepticus in patients receiving Neurontin® was 0.6% (3 of 543) versus 0.5% in patients receiving placebo (2 of 378). Among the 2074 patients >12 years of age treated with Neurontin® across all studies (controlled and uncontrolled) 31 (1.5%) had status epilepticus. Of these, 14 patients had no prior history of status epilepticus either before treatment or while on other medications. Because adequate historical data are not available, it is impossible to say whether or not treatment with Neurontin® is associated with a higher or lower rate of status epilepticus than would be expected to occur in a similar population not treated with Neurontin®.

Tumorigenic Potential

In standard preclinical in vivo lifetime carcinogenicity studies, an unexpectedly high incidence of pancreatic acinar adenocarcinomas was identified in male, but not female, rats. (See PRECAUTIONS: Carcinogenesis, Mutagenesis, Impairment of Fertility.) The clinical significance of this finding is unknown. Clinical experience during gabapentin's premarketing development provides no direct means to assess its potential for inducing tumors in humans.

In clinical studies comprising 2085 patient-years of exposure in patients >12 years of age, new tumors were reported in 10 patients (2 breast, 3 brain, 2 lung, 1 adrenal, 1 non-Hodgkin's lymphoma, 1 endometrial carcinoma in situ), and preexisting tumors worsened in 11 patients (9 brain, 1 breast, 1 prostate) during or up to 2 years following discontinuation of Neurontin®. Without knowledge of the background incidence and recurrence in a similar population not treated with Neurontin®, it is impossible to know whether the incidence seen in this cohort is or is not affected by treatment.

Sudden and Unexplained Deaths

During the course of premarketing development of Neurontin®, 8 sudden and unexplained deaths were recorded among a cohort of 2203 patients treated (2103 patient-years of exposure).

Some of these could represent seizure-related deaths in which the seizure was not observed, e.g., at night. This represents an incidence of 0.0038 deaths per patient-year. Although this rate exceeds that expected in a healthy population matched for age and sex, it is within the range of estimates for the incidence of sudden unexplained deaths in patients with epilepsy not receiving Neurontin® (ranging from 0.0005 for the general population of epileptics to 0.003 for a clinical trial population similar to that in the Neurontin® program, to 0.005 for patients with refractory epilepsy). Consequently, whether these figures are reassuring or raise further concern depends on comparability of the populations reported upon to the Neurontin® cohort and the accuracy of the estimates provided.

PRECAUTIONS

Information for Patients

Patients should be instructed to take Neurontin® only as prescribed.

Patients should be advised that Neurontin® may cause dizziness, somnolence and other symptoms and signs of CNS depression. Accordingly, they should be advised neither to drive a car nor to operate other complex machinery until they have gained sufficient experience on Neurontin® to gauge whether or not it affects their mental and/or motor performance adversely.

Laboratory Tests

Clinical trials data do not indicate that routine monitoring of clinical laboratory parameters is necessary for the safe use of Neurontin®. The value of monitoring Neurontin® blood concentrations has not been established. Neurontin® may be used in combination with other antiepileptic drugs without concern for alteration of the blood concentrations of gabapentin or of other antiepileptic drugs.

Drug Interactions

Gabapentin is not appreciably metabolized nor does it interfere with the metabolism of commonly coadministered antiepileptic drugs.

The drug interaction data described in this section were obtained from studies involving healthy adults and adult patients with epilepsy.

Phenytoin: In a single and multiple dose study of Neurontin® (400 mg T.I.D.) in epileptic patients (N=8) maintained on phenytoin monotherapy for at least 2 months, gabapentin had no effect on the steady-state trough plasma concentrations of phenytoin and phenytoin had no effect on gabapentin pharmacokinetics.

Carbamazepine: Steady-state trough plasma carbamazepine and carbamazepine 10, 11 epoxide concentrations were not affected by concomitant gabapentin (400 mg T.I.D.; N=12) administration. Likewise, gabapentin pharmacokinetics were unaltered by carbamazepine administration.

Valproic Acid: The mean steady-state trough serum valproic acid concentrations prior to and during concomitant gabapentin administration (400 mg T.I.D.; N=17) were not different and neither were gabapentin pharmacokinetic parameters affected by valproic acid.

Phenobarbital: Estimates of steady-state pharmacokinetic parameters for phenobarbital or gabapentin (300 mg T.I.D.; N=12) are identical whether the drugs are administered alone or together.

Cimetidine: In the presence of cimetidine at 300 mg Q.I.D. (N=12) the mean apparent oral clearance of gabapentin fell by 14% and creatinine clearance fell by 10%. Thus cimetidine appeared to alter the renal excretion of both gabapentin and creatinine, an endogenous marker of renal function. This small decrease in excretion of gabapentin by cimetidine is not expected to be of clinical importance. The effect of gabapentin on cimetidine was not evaluated.

Oral Contraceptive: Based on AUC and half-life, multiple-dose pharmacokinetic profiles of norethindrone and ethinyl estradiol following administration of tablets containing 2.5 mg of norethindrone acetate and 50 mcg of ethinyl estradiol were similar with and without coadministration of gabapentin (400 mg T.I.D.; N=13). The Cmax of norethindrone was 13% higher when it was coadministered with gabapentin; this interaction is not expected to be of clinical importance.

Antacid (Maalox®): Maalox reduced the bioavailability of gabapentin (N=16) by about 20%. This decrease in bioavailability was about 5% when gabapentin was administered 2 hours after Maalox. It is recommended that gabapentin be taken at least 2 hours following Maalox administration.

Effect of Probenecid: Probenecid is a blocker of renal tubular secretion. Gabapentin pharmacokinetic parameters without and with probenecid were comparable. This indicates that gabapentin does not undergo renal tubular secretion by the pathway that is blocked by probenecid.

Drug/Laboratory Tests Interactions

Because false positive readings were reported with the Ames N-Multistix SG® dipstick test for urinary protein when gabapentin was added to other antiepileptic drugs, the more specific sulfosalicylic acid precipitation procedure is recommended to determine the presence of urine protein.

Carcinogenesis, Mutagenesis, Impairment of Fertility

Gabapentin was given in the diet to mice at 200, 600, and 2000 mg/kg/day and to rats at 250, 1000, and 2000 mg/kg/day for 2 years. A statistically significant increase in the incidence of pancreatic acinar cell adenomas and carcinomas was found in male rats receiving the high dose; the no-effect dose for the occurrence of carcinomas was 1000 mg/kg/day. Peak plasma concentrations of gabapentin in rats receiving the high dose of 2000 mg/kg were 10 times higher than plasma concentrations in humans receiving 3600 mg per day, and in rats receiving 1000 mg/kg/day peak plasma concentrations were 6.5 times higher than in humans receiving 3600 mg/day. The pancreatic acinar cell carcinomas did not affect survival, did not metastasize and were not locally invasive. The relevance of this finding to carcinogenic risk in humans is unclear.

Studies designed to investigate the mechanism of gabapentin-induced pancreatic carcinogenesis in rats indicate that gabapentin stimulates DNA synthesis in rat pancreatic acinar cells in vitro and, thus, may be acting as a tumor promoter by enhancing mitogenic activity. It is not known whether gabapentin has the ability to increase cell proliferation in other cell types or in other species, including humans.

Gabapentin did not demonstrate mutagenic or genotoxic potential in three in vitro and four in vivo assays. It was negative in the Ames test and the in vitro HGPRT forward mutation assay in Chinese hamster lung cells; it did not produce significant increases in chromosomal aberrations in the in vitro Chinese hamster lung cell assay; it was negative in the in vivo chromosomal aberration assay and in the in vivo micronucleus test in Chinese hamster bone marrow; it was negative in the in vivo mouse micronucleus assay; and it did not induce unscheduled DNA synthesis in hepatocytes from rats given gabapentin.

No adverse effects on fertility or reproduction were observed in rats at doses up to 2000 mg/kg (approximately 5 times the maximum recommended human dose on an mg/m² basis).

Continued on next page

Neurontin—Cont.

Pregnancy

Pregnancy Category C: Gabapentin has been shown to be fetotoxic in rodents, causing delayed ossification of several bones in the skull, vertebrae, forelimbs, and hindlimbs. These effects occurred when pregnant mice received oral doses of 1000 or 3000 mg/kg/day during the period of organogenesis, or approximately 1 to 4 times the maximum dose of 3600 mg/day given to epileptic patients on a mg/m² basis. The no-effect level was 500 mg/kg/day or approximately _ of the human dose on a mg/m² basis.

When rats were dosed prior to and during mating, and throughout gestation, pups from all dose groups (500, 1000 and 2000 mg/kg/day) were affected. These doses are equivalent to less than approximately 1 to 5 times the maximum human dose on a mg/m² basis. There was an increased incidence of hydroureter and/or hydronephrosis in rats in a study of fertility and general reproductive performance at 2000 mg/kg/day with no effect at 1000 mg/kg/day, in a teratology study at 1500 mg/kg/day with no effect at 300 mg/kg/day, and in a perinatal and postnatal study at all doses studied (500, 1000 and 2000 mg/kg/day). The doses at which the effects occurred are approximately 1 to 5 times the maximum human dose of 3600 mg/day on a mg/m² basis; the no-effect doses were approximately 3 times (Fertility and General Reproductive Performance study) and approximately equal to (Teratogenicity study) the maximum human dose on a mg/m² basis. Other than hydroureter and hydronephrosis, the etiologies of which are unclear, the incidence of malformations was not increased compared to controls in offspring of mice, rats, or rabbits given doses up to 50 times (mice), 30 times (rats), and 25 times (rabbits) the human daily dose on a mg/kg basis, or 4 times (mice), 5 times (rats), or 8 times (rabbits) the human daily dose on a mg/m² basis. In a teratology study in rabbits, an increased incidence of postimplantation fetal loss occurred in dams exposed to 60, 300 and 1500 mg/kg/day, or less than approximately _ to 8 times the maximum human dose on a mg/m² basis. There are no adequate and well-controlled studies in pregnant women. Because animal reproduction studies are not always predictive of human response, this drug should be used during pregnancy only if the potential benefit justifies the potential risk to the fetus.

Use in Nursing Mothers

Gabapentin is secreted into human milk following oral administration. A nursed infant could be exposed to a maximum dose of approximately 1 mg/kg/day of gabapentin. Because the effect on the nursing infant is unknown, Neurontin® should be used in women who are nursing only if the benefits clearly outweigh the risks.

Pediatric Use

Effectiveness in pediatric patients below the age of 3 years has not been established (see CLINICAL PHARMACOLOGY, Clinical Studies).

Geriatric Use

Clinical studies of Neurontin did not include sufficient numbers of subjects aged 65 and over to determine whether they responded differently from younger subjects. Other reported clinical experience has not identified differences in responses between the elderly and younger patients. In general, dose selection for an elderly patient should be cautious, usually starting at the low end of the dosing range, reflecting the greater frequency of decreased hepatic, renal, or cardiac function, and of concomitant disease or other drug therapy.

This drug is known to be substantially excreted by the kidney, and the risk of toxic reactions to this drug may be greater in patients with impaired renal function. Because elderly patients are more likely to have decreased renal function, care should be taken in dose selection, and it may be useful to monitor renal function (see CLINICAL PHARMACOLOGY, ADVERSE REACTIONS, and DOSAGE AND ADMINISTRATION sections).

ADVERSE REACTIONS

The most commonly observed adverse events associated with the use of Neurontin® in combination with other antiepileptic drugs in patients >12 years of age, not seen at an equivalent frequency among placebo-treated patients, were somnolence, dizziness, ataxia, fatigue, and nystagmus. The most commonly observed adverse events reported with the use of Neurontin in combination with other antiepileptic drugs in pediatric patients 3 to 12 years of age, not seen at an equal frequency among placebo-treated patients, were viral infection, fever, nausea and/or vomiting, somnolence, and hostility (see WARNINGS, Neuropsychiatric Adverse Events).

Approximately 7% of the 2074 patients >12 years of age and approximately 7% of the 449 pediatric patients 3 to 12 years of age who received Neurontin® in premarketing clinical trials discontinued treatment because of an adverse event. The adverse events most commonly associated with withdrawal in patients >12 years of age were somnolence (1.2%), ataxia (0.8%), fatigue (0.6%), nausea and/or vomiting (0.6%), and dizziness (0.6%). The adverse events most commonly associated with withdrawal in pediatric patients were emotional lability (1.6%), hostility (1.3%), and hyperkinesia (1.1%).

Incidence in Controlled Clinical Trials

Table 1 lists treatment-emergent signs and symptoms that occurred in at least 1% of Neurontin®-treated patients >12 years of age with epilepsy participating in placebo-controlled trials and were numerically more common in the Neurontin® group. In these studies, either Neurontin® or placebo was added to the patient's current antiepileptic drug therapy. Adverse events were usually mild to moderate in intensity.

The prescriber should be aware that these figures, obtained when Neurontin® was added to concurrent antiepileptic drug therapy, cannot be used to predict the frequency of adverse events in the course of usual medical practice where patient characteristics and other factors may differ from those prevailing during clinical studies. Similarly, the cited frequencies cannot be directly compared with figures obtained from other clinical investigations involving different treatments, uses, or investigators. An inspection of these frequencies, however, does provide the prescribing physician with one basis to estimate the relative contribution of drug and nondrug factors to the adverse event incidences in the population studied.

[See table 1 above]

Other events in more than 1% of patients >12 years of age but equally or more frequent in the placebo group included: headache, viral infection, fever, nausea and/or vomiting, abdominal pain, diarrhea, convulsions, confusion, insomnia, emotional lability, rash, acne.

Among the treatment-emergent adverse events occurring at an incidence of at least 10% of Neurontin-treated patients, somnolence and ataxia appeared to exhibit a positive dose-response relationship.

The overall incidence of adverse events and the types of adverse events seen were similar among men and women treated with Neurontin®. The incidence of adverse events increased slightly with increasing age in patients treated with either Neurontin® or placebo. Because only 3% of patients (28/921) in placebo-controlled studies were identified as nonwhite (black or other), there are insufficient data to support a statement regarding the distribution of adverse events by race.

Table 2 lists treatment-emergent signs and symptoms that occurred in at least 2% of Neurontin-treated patients age 3 to 12 years of age with epilepsy participating in placebo-controlled trials and were numerically more common in the Neurontin group. Adverse events were usually mild to moderate in intensity.

[See table 2 above]

Other events in more than 2% of pediatric patients 3 to 12 years of age but equally or more frequent in the placebo

---

TABLE 1. Treatment-Emergent Adverse Event Incidence in Controlled Add-On Trials In Patients >12 years of age
(Events in at least 1% of Neurontin patients and numerically more frequent than in the placebo group)

Body System/ Adverse Event	Neurontin®[a] N=543 %	Placebo[a] N=378 %
Body As A Whole		
Fatigue	11.0	5.0
Weight Increase	2.9	1.6
Back Pain	1.8	0.5
Peripheral Edema	1.7	0.5
Cardiovascular		
Vasodilatation	1.1	0.3
Digestive System		
Dyspepsia	2.2	0.5
Mouth or Throat Dry	1.7	0.5
Constipation	1.5	0.8
Dental Abnormalities	1.5	0.3
Increased Appetite	1.1	0.8
Hematologic and Lymphatic Systems		
Leukopenia	1.1	0.5
Musculoskeletal System		
Myalgia	2.0	1.9
Fracture	1.1	0.8
Nervous System		
Somnolence	19.3	8.7
Dizziness	17.1	6.9
Ataxia	12.5	5.6
Nystagmus	8.3	4.0
Tremor	6.8	3.2
Nervousness	2.4	1.9
Dysarthria	2.4	0.5
Amnesia	2.2	0.0
Depression	1.8	1.1
Thinking Abnormal	1.7	1.3
Twitching	1.3	0.5
Coordination Abnormal	1.1	0.3
Respiratory System		
Rhinitis	4.1	3.7
Pharyngitis	2.8	1.6
Coughing	1.8	1.3
Skin and Appendages		
Abrasion	1.3	0.0
Pruritus	1.3	0.5
Urogenital System		
Impotence	1.5	1.1
Special Senses		
Diplopia	5.9	1.9
Amblyopia[b]	4.2	1.1
Laboratory Deviations		
WBC Decreased	1.1	0.5

[a] Plus background antiepileptic drug therapy
[b] Amblyopia was often described as blurred vision.

TABLE 2. Treatment-Emergent Adverse Event Incidence in Pediatric Patients Age 3 to 12 Years in a Controlled Add-On Trial (Events in at least 2% of Neurontin patients and numerically more frequent than in the placebo group)

Body System/ Adverse Event	Neurontin[a] N=119 %	Placebo[a] N=128 %
Body As A Whole		
Viral Infection	10.9	3.1
Fever	10.1	3.1
Weight Increase	3.4	0.8
Fatigue	3.4	1.6
Digestive System		
Nausea and/or Vomiting	8.4	7.0
Nervous System		
Somnolence	8.4	4.7
Hostility	7.6	2.3
Emotional Lability	4.2	1.6
Dizziness	2.5	1.6
Hyperkinesia	2.5	0.8
Respiratory System		
Bronchitis	3.4	0.8
Respiratory Infection	2.5	0.8

[a] Plus background antiepileptic drug therapy

group included: pharyngitis, upper respiratory infection, headache, rhinitis, convulsions, diarrhea, anorexia, coughing, and otitis media.

Other Adverse Events Observed During All Clinical Trials
Neurontin® has been administered to 2074 patients >12 years of age during all clinical trials, only some of which were placebo-controlled. During these trials, all adverse events were recorded by the clinical investigators using terminology of their own choosing. To provide a meaningful estimate of the proportion of individuals having adverse events, similar types of events were grouped into a smaller number of standardized categories using modified COSTART dictionary terminology. These categories are used in the listing below. The frequencies presented represent the proportion of the 2074 patients >12 years of age exposed to Neurontin® who experienced an event of the type cited on at least one occasion while receiving Neurontin®. All reported events are included except those already listed in the previous table, those too general to be informative, and those not reasonably associated with the use of the drug.

Events are further classified within body system categories and enumerated in order of decreasing frequency using the following definitions: frequent adverse events are defined as those occurring in at least 1/100 patients; infrequent adverse events are those occurring in 1/100 to 1/1000 patients; rare events are those occurring in fewer than 1/1000 patients.

Body As A Whole: *Frequent:* asthenia, malaise, face edema; *Infrequent:* allergy, generalized edema, weight decrease, chill; *Rare:* strange feelings, lassitude, alcohol intolerance, hangover effect.

Cardiovascular System: *Frequent:* hypertension; *Infrequent:* hypotension, angina pectoris, peripheral vascular disorder, palpitation, tachycardia, migraine, murmur; *Rare:* atrial fibrillation, heart failure, thrombophlebitis, deep thrombophlebitis, myocardial infarction, cerebrovascular accident, pulmonary thrombosis, ventricular extrasystoles, bradycardia, premature atrial contraction, pericardial rub, heart block, pulmonary embolus, hyperlipidemia, hypercholesterolemia, pericardial effusion, pericarditis.

Digestive System: *Frequent:* anorexia, flatulence, gingivitis; *Infrequent:* glossitis, gum hemorrhage, thirst, stomatitis, increased salivation, gastroenteritis, hemorrhoids, bloody stools, fecal incontinence, hepatomegaly; *Rare:* dysphagia, eructation, pancreatitis, peptic ulcer, colitis, blisters in mouth, tooth discolor, perlèche, salivary gland enlarged, lip hemorrhage, esophagitis, hiatal hernia, hematemesis, proctitis, irritable bowel syndrome, rectal hemorrhage, esophageal spasm.

Endocrine System: *Rare:* hyperthyroid, hypothyroid, goiter, hypoestrogen, ovarian failure, epididymitis, swollen testicle, cushingoid appearance.

Hematologic and Lymphatic System: *Frequent:* purpura most often described as bruises resulting from physical trauma; *Infrequent:* anemia, thrombocytopenia, lymphadenopathy; *Rare:* WBC count increased, lymphocytosis, non-Hodgkin's lymphoma, bleeding time increased.

Musculoskeletal System: *Frequent:* arthralgia; *Infrequent:* tendinitis, arthritis, joint stiffness, joint swelling, positive Romberg test; *Rare:* costochondritis, osteoporosis, bursitis, contracture.

Nervous System: *Frequent:* vertigo, hyperkinesia, paresthesia, decreased or absent reflexes, increased reflexes, anxiety, hostility; *Infrequent:* CNS tumors, syncope, dreaming abnormal, aphasia, hypesthesia, intracranial hemorrhage, hypotonia, dysesthesia, paresis, dystonia, hemiplegia, facial paralysis, stupor, cerebellar dysfunction, positive Babinski sign, decreased position sense, subdural hematoma, apathy, hallucination, decrease or loss of libido, agitation, paranoia, depersonalization, euphoria, feeling high, doped-up sensation, suicidal, psychosis; *Rare:* choreoathetosis, orofacial dyskinesia, encephalopathy, nerve palsy, personality disorder, increased libido, subdued temperament, apraxia, fine motor control disorder, meningismus, local myoclonus, hyperesthesia, hypokinesia, mania, neurosis, hysteria, antisocial reaction, suicide gesture.

Respiratory System: *Frequent:* pneumonia; *Infrequent:* epistaxis, dyspnea, apnea; *Rare:* mucositis, aspiration pneumonia, hyperventilation, hiccup, laryngitis, nasal obstruction, snoring, bronchospasm, hypoventilation, lung edema.

Dermatological: *Infrequent:* alopecia, eczema, dry skin, increased sweating, urticaria, hirsutism, seborrhea, cyst, herpes simplex; *Rare:* herpes zoster, skin discolor, skin papules, photosensitive reaction, leg ulcer, scalp seborrhea, psoriasis, desquamation, maceration, skin nodules, subcutaneous nodule, melanosis, skin necrosis, local swelling.

Urogenital System: *Infrequent:* hematuria, dysuria, urination frequency, cystitis, urinary retention, urinary incontinence, vaginal hemorrhage, amenorrhea, dysmenorrhea, menorrhagia, breast cancer, unable to climax, ejaculation abnormal; *Rare:* kidney pain, leukorrhea, pruritus genital, renal stone, acute renal failure, anuria, glycosuria, nephrosis, nocturia, pyuria, urination urgency, vaginal pain, breast pain, testicle pain.

Special Senses: *Frequent:* abnormal vision; *Infrequent:* cataract, conjunctivitis, eyes dry, eye pain, visual field defect, photophobia, bilateral or unilateral ptosis, eye hemorrhage, hordeolum, hearing loss, earache, tinnitus, inner ear infection, otitis, taste loss, unusual taste, eye twitching, ear fullness; *Rare:* eye itching, abnormal accommodation, perforated ear drum, sensitivity to noise, eye focusing problem, watery eyes, retinopathy, glaucoma, iritis, corneal disorders, lacrimal dysfunction, degenerative eye changes, blindness, retinal degeneration, miosis, chorioretinitis, strabismus, eustachian tube dysfunction, labyrinthitis, otitis externa, odd smell.

Adverse events occurring during clinical trials in 449 pediatric patients 3 to 12 years of age treated with gabapentin that were not reported in adjunctive trials in adults are:

Body as a Whole: dehydration, infectious mononucleosis
Digestive System: hepatitis
Hemic and Lymphatic System: coagulation defect
Nervous System: aura disappeared, occipital neuralgia
Psychobiologic Function: sleepwalking
Respiratory System: pseudocroup, hoarseness

Postmarketing and Other Experience
In addition to the adverse experiences reported during clinical testing of Neurontin®, the following adverse experiences have been reported in patients receiving marketed Neurontin®. These adverse experiences have not been listed above and data are insufficient to support an estimate of their incidence or to establish causation. The listing is alphabetized: angioedema, blood glucose fluctuation, erythema multiforme, elevated liver function tests, fever, hyponatremia, jaundice, Stevens-Johnson syndrome.

DRUG ABUSE AND DEPENDENCE

The abuse and dependence potential of Neurontin® has not been evaluated in human studies.

OVERDOSAGE

A lethal dose of gabapentin was not identified in mice and rats receiving single oral doses as high as 8000 mg/kg. Signs of acute toxicity in animals included ataxia, labored breathing, ptosis, sedation, hypoactivity, or excitation.

Acute oral overdoses of Neurontin® up to 49 grams have been reported. In these cases, double vision, slurred speech, drowsiness, lethargy and diarrhea were observed. All patients recovered with supportive care.

Gabapentin can be removed by hemodialysis. Although hemodialysis has not been performed in the few overdose cases reported, it may be indicated by the patient's clinical state or in patients with significant renal impairment.

DOSAGE AND ADMINISTRATION

Neurontin® is recommended for add-on therapy in patients 3 years of age and older. Effectiveness in pediatric patients below the age of 3 years has not been established.

Neurontin® is given orally with or without food.

Patients >12 years of age: The effective dose of Neurontin® is 900 to 1800 mg/day and given in divided doses (three times a day) using 300 or 400 mg capsules, or 600 or 800 mg tablets. The starting dose is 300 mg three times a day. If necessary, the dose may be increased using 300 or 400 mg capsules, or 600 or 800 mg tablets three times a day up to 1800 mg/day. Dosages up to 2400 mg/day have been well tolerated in long-term clinical studies. Doses of 3600 mg/day have also been administered to a small number of patients for a relatively short duration, and have been well tolerated. The maximum time between doses in the T.I.D. schedule should not exceed 12 hours.

Pediatric Patients Age 3–12 years: The starting dose should range from 10–15 mg/kg/day in 3 divided doses, and the effective dose reached by upward titration over a period of approximately 3 days. The effective dose of Neurontin in patients 5 years of age and older is 25–35 mg/kg/day and given in divided doses (three times a day). The effective dose in pediatric patients ages 3 and 4 years is 40 mg/kg/day and given in divided doses (three times a day). (See CLINICAL PHARMACOLOGY, Pediatrics.) Neurontin® may be administered as the oral solution, capsule, or tablet, or using combinations of these formulations. Dosages up to 50 mg/kg/day have been well-tolerated in a long-term clinical study. The maximum time interval between doses should not exceed 12 hours.

It is not necessary to monitor gabapentin plasma concentrations to optimize Neurontin® therapy. Further, because there are no significant pharmacokinetic interactions among Neurontin® and other commonly used antiepileptic drugs, the addition of Neurontin® does not alter the plasma levels of these drugs appreciably.

If Neurontin® is discontinued and/or an alternate anticonvulsant medication is added to the therapy, this should be done gradually over a minimum of 1 week.

Creatinine clearance is difficult to measure in outpatients. In patients with stable renal function, creatinine clearance (C_{Cr}) can be reasonably well estimated using the equation of Cockcroft and Gault:

for females C_{Cr}=(0.85)(140-age)(weight)/[(72)(S_{Cr})]
for males C_{Cr}=(140-age)(weight)/[(72)(S_{Cr})]

where age is in years, weight is in kilograms and S_{Cr} is serum creatinine in mg/dL.

Dosage adjustment in patients ≥12 years of age with compromised renal function or undergoing hemodialysis is recommended as follows:

TABLE 3. Neurontin® Dosage Based on Renal Function

Renal Function Creatinine Clearance (mL/min)	Total Daily Dose (mg/day)	Dose Regimen (mg)
>60	1200	400 T.I.D.
30–60	600	300 B.I.D.
15–30	300	300 Q.D.
<15	150	300 Q.O.D.[a]
Hemodialysis	—	200–300[b]

[a] Every other day
[b] Loading dose of 300 to 400 mg in patients who have never received Neurontin®, then 200 to 300 mg Neurontin® following each 4 hours of hemodialysis.

The use of Neurontin® in patients <12 years of age with compromised renal function has not been studied.

HOW SUPPLIED

Neurontin® (gabapentin) capsules, tablets and oral solution are supplied as follows:

100 mg capsules;
White hard gelatin capsules printed with "PD" on one side and "Neurontin®/100 mg" on the other; available in:
Bottles of 100: N 0071-0803-24
Unit dose 50's: N 0071-0803-40

300 mg capsules;
Yellow hard gelatin capsules printed with "PD" on one side and "Neurontin®/300 mg" on the other; available in:
Bottles of 100: N 0071-0805-24
Unit dose 50's: N 0071-0805-40

400 mg capsules;
Orange hard gelatin capsules printed with "PD" on one side and "Neurontin®/400 mg" on the other; available in:
Bottles of 100: N 0071-0806-24
Unit dose 50's: N 0071-0806-40

600 mg tablets;
White elliptical film-coated tablets printed in black ink with "Neurontin® 600" on one side; available in:
Bottles of 100: N 0071-0416-24
Bottles of 500: N 0071-0416-30
Unit dose 50's: N 0071-0416-40

800 mg tablets;
White elliptical film-coated tablets printed in orange with "Neurontin® 800" on one side; available in:
Bottles of 100: N 0071-0426-24
Bottles of 500: N 0071-0426-30
Unit dose 50's: N 0071-0426-40

250 mg/5 mL oral solution;
Clear colorless to slightly yellow solution; each 5 mL of oral solution contains 250 mg of gabapentin; available in:
Bottles containing 470 mL: N 0071-2012-23

Storage (Capsules)
Store at Controlled Room Temperature 15°–30°C (59°–86°F).
Storage (Tablets)
Store at 25°C (77°F); excursions permitted to 15°–30°C (59°–86°F) [see USP Controlled Room Temperature].
Storage (Oral Solution)
Store refrigerated, 2°–8°C (36°–46°F)
Rx only
Revised November 2000
Capsules and Tablets:
Manufactured by:
Parke Davis Pharmaceuticals, Ltd.
Vega Baja, PR 00694
Oral Solution:
Manufactured for:
Parke Davis Pharmaceuticals, Ltd.
Vega Baja, PR 00694
Distributed by:
PARKE-DAVIS
Div of Warner-Lambert Co
Morris Plains, NJ 07950 USA

0416G641

ZARONTIN® ℞

[ză "rŏn 'tĭn]
(ethosuximide, USP)
Capsules

Prescribing information for this product, which appears on pages 2462–2463 of the 2001 PDR, has been completely revised as follows. Please write "See Supplement A" next to the product heading.

DESCRIPTION

Zarontin (ethosuximide) is an anticonvulsant succinimide, chemically designated as alpha-ethyl-alpha-methyl-succinimide, with the following structural formula:

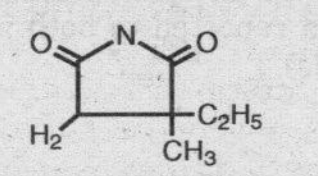

Each Zarontin capsule contains 250 mg ethosuximide, USP. Also contains: polyethylene glycol 400, NF. The capsule contains D&C yellow No. 10; FD&C red No. 3; gelatin, NF; glycerin, USP; and sorbitol.

CLINICAL PHARMACOLOGY

Ethosuximide suppresses the paroxysmal three cycle per second spike and wave activity associated with lapses of consciousness which is common in absence (petit mal) seizures. The frequency of epileptiform attacks is reduced, apparently by depression of the motor cortex and elevation of the threshold of the central nervous system to convulsive stimuli.

INDICATIONS AND USAGE

Zarontin is indicated for the control of absence (petit mal) epilepsy.

CONTRAINDICATION

Ethosuximide should not be used in patients with a history of hypersensitivity to succinimides.

Continued on next page

Zarontin Capsules—Cont.

WARNINGS

Blood dyscrasias, including some with fatal outcome, have been reported to be associated with the use of ethosuximide; therefore, periodic blood counts should be performed. Should signs and/or symptoms of infection (eg, sore throat, fever) develop, blood counts should be considered at that point.

Ethosuximide is capable of producing morphological and functional changes in the animal liver. In humans, abnormal liver and renal function studies have been reported.

Ethosuximide should be administered with extreme caution to patients with known liver or renal disease. Periodic urinalysis and liver function studies are advised for all patients receiving the drug.

Cases of systemic lupus erythematosus have been reported with the use of ethosuximide. The physician should be alert to this possibility.

Usage in Pregnancy: Reports suggest an association between the use of anticonvulsant drugs by women with epilepsy and an elevated incidence of birth defects in children born to these women. Data are more extensive with respect to phenytoin and phenobarbital, but these are also the most commonly prescribed anticonvulsants; less systematic or anecdotal reports suggest a possible similar association with the use of all known anticonvulsant drugs.

The reports suggesting an elevated incidence of birth defects in children of drug-treated epileptic women cannot be regarded as adequate to prove a definite cause and effect relationship. There are intrinsic methodological problems in obtaining adequate data on drug teratogenicity in humans; the possibility also exists that other factors, eg, genetic factors or the epileptic condition itself, may be more important than drug therapy in leading to birth defects. The great majority of mothers on anticonvulsant medication deliver normal infants. It is important to note that anticonvulsant drugs should not be discontinued in patients in whom the drug is administered to prevent major seizures because of the strong possibility of precipitating status epilepticus with attendant hypoxia and threat to life. In individual cases where the severity and frequency of the seizure disorder are such that the removal of medication does not pose a serious threat to the patient, discontinuation of the drug may be considered prior to and during pregnancy, although it cannot be said with any confidence that even minor seizures do not pose some hazard to the developing embryo or fetus.

The prescribing physician will wish to weigh these considerations in treating or counseling epileptic women of childbearing potential.

PRECAUTIONS

General:

Ethosuximide, when used alone in mixed types of epilepsy, may increase the frequency of grand mal seizures in some patients.

As with other anticonvulsants, it is important to proceed slowly when increasing or decreasing dosage, as well as when adding or eliminating other medication. Abrupt withdrawal of anticonvulsant medication may precipitate absence (petit mal) status.

Information for Patients:

Ethosuximide may impair the mental and/or physical abilities required for the performance of potentially hazardous tasks, such as driving a motor vehicle or other such activity requiring alertness; therefore, the patient should be cautioned accordingly.

Patients taking ethosuximide should be advised of the importance of adhering strictly to the prescribed dosage regimen.

Patients should be instructed to promptly contact their physician if they develop signs and/or symptoms (eg, sore throat, fever), suggesting an infection.

Drug Interactions:

Since Zarontin (ethosuximide) may interact with concurrently administered antiepileptic drugs, periodic serum level determinations of these drugs may be necessary (eg, ethosuximide may elevate phenytoin serum levels and valproic acid has been reported to both increase and decrease ethosuximide levels).

Pregnancy:

See WARNINGS.

Pediatric Use:

Safety and effectiveness in pediatric patients below the age of 3 years have not been established. (See DOSAGE AND ADMINISTRATION section.)

ADVERSE REACTIONS

Gastrointestinal System: Gastrointestinal symptoms occur frequently and include anorexia, vague gastric upset, nausea and vomiting, cramps, epigastric and abdominal pain, weight loss, and diarrhea. There have been reports of gum hypertrophy and swelling of the tongue.

Hemopoietic System: Hemopoietic complications associated with the administration of ethosuximide have included leukopenia, agranulocytosis, pancytopenia, with or without bone marrow suppression, and eosinophilia.

Nervous System: Neurologic and sensory reactions reported during therapy with ethosuximide have included drowsiness, headache, dizziness, euphoria, hiccups, irritability, hyperactivity, lethargy, fatigue, and ataxia. Psychiatric or psychological aberrations associated with ethosuximide administration have included disturbances of sleep, night terrors, inability to concentrate, and aggressiveness. These effects may be noted particularly in patients who have previously exhibited psychological abnormalities. There have been rare reports of paranoid psychosis, increased libido, and increased state of depression with overt suicidal intentions.

Integumentary System: Dermatologic manifestations which have occurred with the administration of ethosuximide have included urticaria, Stevens-Johnson syndrome, systemic lupus erythematosus, pruritic erythematous rashes, and hirsutism.

Special Senses: Myopia.

Genitourinary System: Vaginal bleeding, microscopic hematuria.

OVERDOSAGE

Acute overdoses may produce nausea, vomiting, and CNS depression including coma with respiratory depression. A relationship between ethosuximide toxicity and its plasma levels has not been established. The therapeutic range of serum levels is 40 mcg/mL to 100 mcg/mL, although levels as high as 150 mcg/mL have been reported without signs of toxicity.

Treatment:

Treatment should include emesis (unless the patient is or could rapidly become obtunded, comatose, or convulsing) or gastric lavage, activated charcoal, cathartics, and general supportive measures. Hemodialysis may be useful to treat ethosuximide overdose. Forced diuresis and exchange transfusions are ineffective.

DOSAGE AND ADMINISTRATION

Zarontin is administered by the oral route. The *initial* dose for patients 3 to 6 years of age is one capsule (250 mg) per day; for patients 6 years of age and older, 2 capsules (500 mg) per day. The dose thereafter must be individualized according to the patient's response. Dosage should be increased by small increments. One useful method is to increase the daily dose by 250 mg every four to seven days until control is achieved with minimal side effects. Dosages exceeding 1.5 g daily, in divided doses, should be administered only under the strictest supervision of the physician. The *optimal* dose for most pediatric patients is 20 mg/kg/day. This dose has given average plasma levels within the accepted therapeutic range of 40 to 100 mcg/mL. Subsequent dose schedules can be based on effectiveness and plasma level determinations.

Zarontin may be administered in combination with other anticonvulsants when other forms of epilepsy coexist with absence (petit mal). The *optimal* dose for most pediatric patients is 20 mg/kg/day.

HOW SUPPLIED

Zarontin is supplied as:

N 0071-0237-24—Bottles of 100. Each capsule contains 250 mg ethosuximide.

Store at 25°C (77°F); excursions permitted to 15–30°C (59–86°F) [see USP Controlled Room Temperature].

Zarontin is also supplied as:

N 0071-2418-23—1 pint bottles. Each 5 mL of syrup contains 250 mg ethosuximide in a raspberry flavored base.

Rx only

0237G210

Revised October 2000

Manufactured by:
R.P. Scherer North America
St. Petersburg, FL 33716 USA
Distributed by:
Parke-Davis
Div of Warner-Lambert Co
Morris Plains, NJ 07950 USA

Pfizer Inc.

235 EAST 42nd STREET
NEW YORK, NY 10017–5755

For Medical Information Contact:
(800) 438-1985
24 hours a day, seven days a week.

ARICEPT® ℞

(Donepezil Hydrochloride Tablets)

Prescribing information for this product, which appears on pages 2469–2472 of the 2001 PDR, has been completely revised as follows. Please write "See Supplement A" next to the product heading.

DESCRIPTION

ARICEPT® (donepezil hydrochloride) is a reversible inhibitor of the enzyme acetylcholinesterase, known chemically as (±)-2,3-dihydro-5,6-dimethoxy-2-[[1-(phenylmethyl)-4-piperidinyl]methyl]-1*H*-inden-1-one hydrochloride. Donepezil hydrochloride is commonly referred to in the pharmacological literature as E2020. It has an empirical formula of $C_{24}H_{29}NO_3HCl$ and a molecular weight of 415.96. Donepezil hydrochloride is a white crystalline powder and is freely soluble in chloroform, soluble in water and in glacial acetic acid, slightly soluble in ethanol and in acetonitrile and practically insoluble in ethyl acetate and in n-hexane.

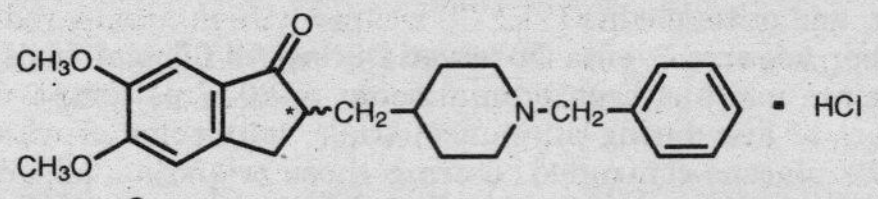

ARICEPT® is available for oral administration in film-coated tablets containing 5 or 10 mg of donepezil hydrochloride. Inactive ingredients are lactose monohydrate, corn starch, microcrystalline cellulose, hydroxypropyl cellulose, and magnesium stearate. The film coating contains talc, polyethylene glycol, hydroxypropyl methylcellulose and titanium dioxide. Additionally, the 10 mg tablet contains yellow iron oxide (synthetic) as a coloring agent.

CLINICAL PHARMACOLOGY

Current theories on the pathogenesis of the cognitive signs and symptoms of Alzheimer's Disease attribute some of them to a deficiency of cholinergic neurotransmission.

Donepezil hydrochloride is postulated to exert its therapeutic effect by enhancing cholinergic function. This is accomplished by increasing the concentration of acetylcholine through reversible inhibition of its hydrolysis by acetylcholinesterase. If this proposed mechanism of action is correct, donepezil's effect may lessen as the disease process advances and fewer cholinergic neurons remain functionally intact. There is no evidence that donepezil alters the course of the underlying dementing process.

Clinical Trial Data

The effectiveness of ARICEPT® as a treatment for Alzheimer's Disease is demonstrated by the results of two randomized, double-blind, placebo-controlled clinical investigations in patients with Alzheimer's Disease (diagnosed by NINCDS and DSM III-R criteria, Mini-Mental State Examination ≥ 10 and ≤ 26 and Clinical Dementia Rating of 1 or 2). The mean age of patients participating in ARICEPT® trials was 73 years with a range of 50 to 94. Approximately 62% of patients were women and 38% were men. The racial distribution was white 95%, black 3% and other races 2%.

Study Outcome Measures: In each study, the effectiveness of treatment with ARICEPT® was evaluated using a dual outcome assessment strategy.

The ability of ARICEPT® to improve cognitive performance was assessed with the cognitive subscale of the Alzheimer's Disease Assessment Scale (ADAS-cog), a multi-item instrument that has been extensively validated in longitudinal cohorts of Alzheimer's Disease patients. The ADAS-cog examines selected aspects of cognitive performance including elements of memory, orientation, attention, reasoning, language and praxis. The ADAS-cog scoring range is from 0 to 70, with higher scores indicating greater cognitive impairment. Elderly normal adults may score as low as 0 or 1, but it is not unusual for non-demented adults to score slightly higher.

The patients recruited as participants in each study had mean scores on the Alzheimer's Disease Assessment Scale (ADAS-cog) of approximately 26 units, with a range from 4 to 61. Experience gained in longitudinal studies of ambulatory patients with mild to moderate Alzheimer's Disease suggest that they gain 6 to 12 units a year on the ADAS-cog. However, lesser degrees of change are seen in patients with very mild or very advanced disease because the ADAS-cog is not uniformly sensitive to change over the course of the disease. The annualized rate of decline in the placebo patients participating in ARICEPT® trials was approximately 2 to 4 units per year.

The ability of ARICEPT® to produce an overall clinical effect was assessed using a Clinician's Interview Based Impression of Change that required the use of caregiver information, the CIBIC plus. The CIBIC plus is not a single instrument and is not a standardized instrument like the ADAS-cog. Clinical trials for investigational drugs have used a variety of CIBIC formats, each different in terms of depth and structure.

As such, results from a CIBIC plus reflect clinical experience from the trial or trials in which it was used and cannot be compared directly with the results of CIBIC plus evaluations from other clinical trials. The CIBIC plus used in ARICEPT® trials was a semi-structured instrument that was intended to examine four major areas of patient function: General, Cognitive, Behavioral and Activities of Daily Living. It represents the assessment of a skilled clinician based upon his/her observations at an interview with the patient, in combination with information supplied by a caregiver familiar with the behavior of the patient over the interval rated. The CIBIC plus is scored as a seven point categorical rating, ranging from a score of 1, indicating "markedly improved," to a score of 4, indicating "no change" to a score of 7, indicating "markedly worse." The CIBIC plus has not been systematically compared directly to assessments not using information from caregivers (CIBIC) or other global methods.

Thirty-Week Study

In a study of 30 weeks duration, 473 patients were randomized to receive single daily doses of placebo, 5 mg/day or 10 mg/day of ARICEPT®. The 30-week study was divided into a 24-week double-blind active treatment phase followed by a 6-week single-blind placebo washout period. The study was designed to compare 5 mg/day or 10 mg/day fixed doses of ARICEPT® to placebo. However, to reduce the likelihood of cholinergic effects, the 10 mg/day treatment was started following an initial 7-day treatment with 5 mg/day doses.

Effects on the ADAS-cog: Figure 1 illustrates the time course for the change from baseline in ADAS-cog scores for all three dose groups over the 30 weeks of the study. After 24 weeks of treatment, the mean differences in the ADAS-cog change scores for ARICEPT® treated patients compared to the patients on placebo were 2.8 and 3.1 units for the 5 mg/day and 10 mg/day treatments, respectively. These differences were statistically significant. While the treatment effect size may appear to be slightly greater for the 10 mg/day treatment, there was no statistically significant difference between the two active treatments.

Following 6 weeks of placebo washout, scores on the ADAS-cog for both the ARICEPT® treatment groups were indistinguishable from those patients who had received only placebo for 30 weeks. This suggests that the beneficial effects of ARICEPT® abate over 6 weeks following discontinuation of treatment and do not represent a change in the underlying disease. There was no evidence of a rebound effect 6 weeks after abrupt discontinuation of therapy.

Figure 1. Time-course of the Change from Baseline in ADAS-cog Score for Patients Completing 24 Weeks of Treatment.

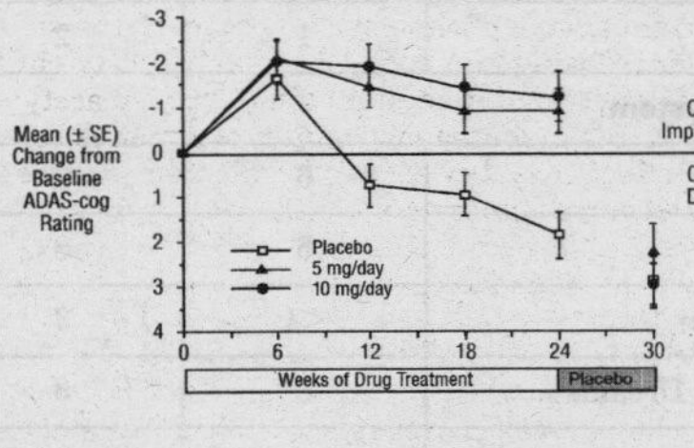

Figure 2 illustrates the cumulative percentages of patients from each of the three treatment groups who had attained the measure of improvement in ADAS-cog score shown on the X axis. Three change scores, (7-point and 4-point reductions from baseline or no change in score) have been identified for illustrative purposes and the percent of patients in each group achieving that result is shown in the inset table. The curves demonstrate that both patients assigned to placebo and ARICEPT® have a wide range of responses, but that the active treatment groups are more likely to show the greater improvements. A curve for an effective treatment would be shifted to the left of the curve for placebo, while an ineffective or deleterious treatment would be superimposed upon or shifted to the right of the curve for placebo, respectively.

Figure 2. Cumulative Percentage of Patients Completing 24 Weeks of Double-blind Treatment with Specified Changes from Baseline ADAS-cog Scores. The Percentages of Randomized Patients who Completed the Study were: Placebo 80%, 5 mg/day 85% and 10 mg/day 68%.

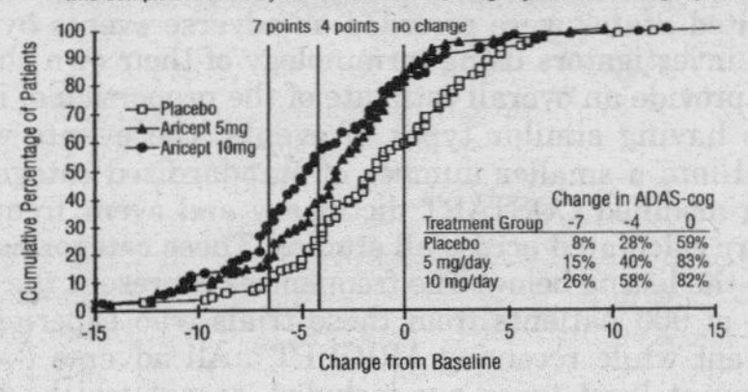

Effects on the CIBIC plus: Figure 3 is a histogram of the frequency distribution of CIBIC plus scores attained by patients assigned to each of the three treatment groups who completed 24 weeks of treatment. The mean drug-placebo differences for these groups of patients were 0.35 units and 0.39 units for 5 mg/day and 10 mg/day of ARICEPT®, respectively. These differences were statistically significant. There was no statistically significant difference between the two active treatments.

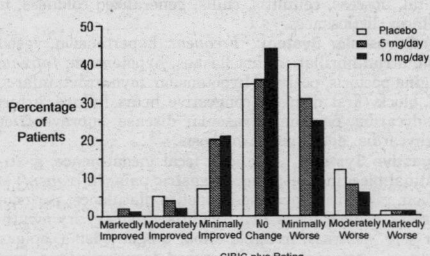

Figure 3. Frequency Distribution of CIBIC plus Scores at Week 24

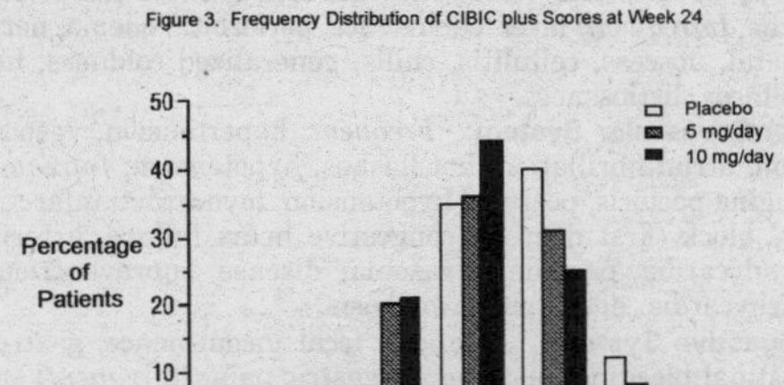

Fifteen-Week Study

In a study of 15 weeks duration, patients were randomized to receive single daily doses of placebo or either 5 mg/day or 10 mg/day of ARICEPT® for 12 weeks, followed by a 3-week placebo washout period. As in the 30-week study, to avoid acute cholinergic effects, the 10 mg/day treatment followed an initial 7-day treatment with 5 mg/day doses.

Effects on the ADAS-Cog: Figure 4 illustrates the time course of the change from baseline in ADAS-cog scores for all three dose groups over the 15 weeks of the study. After 12 weeks of treatment, the differences in mean ADAS-cog change scores for the ARICEPT® treated patients compared to the patients on placebo were 2.7 and 3.0 units each, for the 5 and 10 mg/day ARICEPT® treatment groups respectively. These differences were statistically significant. The effect size for the 10 mg/day group may appear to be slightly larger than that for 5 mg/day. However, the differences between active treatments were not statistically significant.

Figure 4. Time-course of the Change from Baseline in ADAS-cog Score for Patients Completing the 15-week Study.

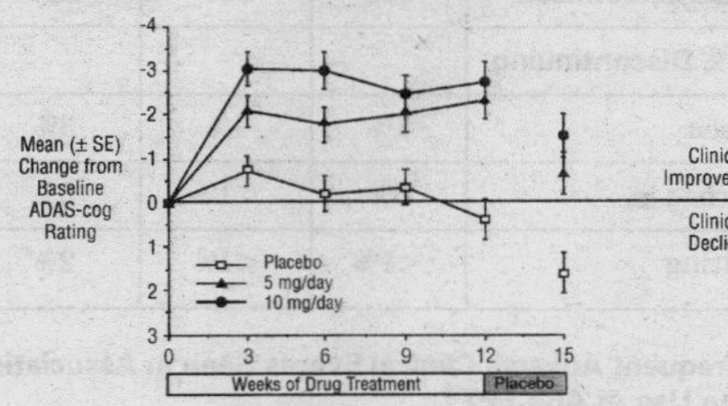

Following 3 weeks of placebo washout, scores on the ADAS-cog for both the ARICEPT® treatment groups increased, indicating that discontinuation of ARICEPT® resulted in a loss of its treatment effect. The duration of this placebo washout period was not sufficient to characterize the rate of loss of the treatment effect, but, the 30-week study (see above) demonstrated that treatment effects associated with the use of ARICEPT® abate within 6 weeks of treatment discontinuation.

Figure 5 illustrates the cumulative percentages of patients from each of the three treatment groups who attained the measure of improvement in ADAS-cog score shown on the X axis. The same three change scores, (7-point and 4-point reductions from baseline or no change in score) as selected for the 30-week study have been used for this illustration. The percentages of patients achieving those results are shown in the inset table.

As observed in the 30-week study, the curves demonstrate that patients assigned to either placebo or to ARICEPT® have a wide range of responses, but that the ARICEPT® treated patients are more likely to show the greater improvements in cognitive performance.

Figure 5. Cumulative Percentage of Patients with Specified Changes from Baseline ADAS-cog Scores. The Percentages of Randomized Patients Within Each Treatment Group Who Completed the Study Were: Placebo 93%, 5 mg/day 90% and 10 mg/day 82%.

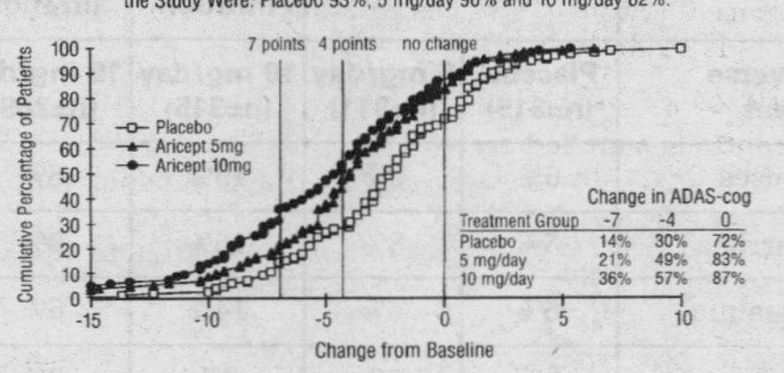

Effects on the CIBIC plus: Figure 6 is a histogram of the frequency distribution of CIBIC plus scores attained by patients assigned to each of the three treatment groups who completed 12 weeks of treatment. The differences in mean scores for ARICEPT® treated patients compared to the patients on placebo at Week 12 were 0.36 and 0.38 units for the 5 mg/day and 10 mg/day treatment groups, respectively. These differences were statistically significant.

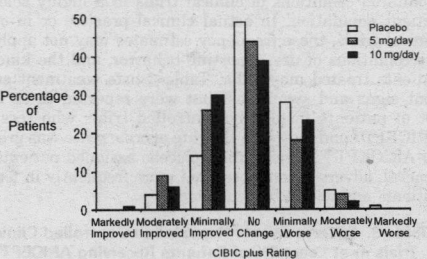

Figure 6 Frequency Distribution of CIBIC plus Scores at Week 12

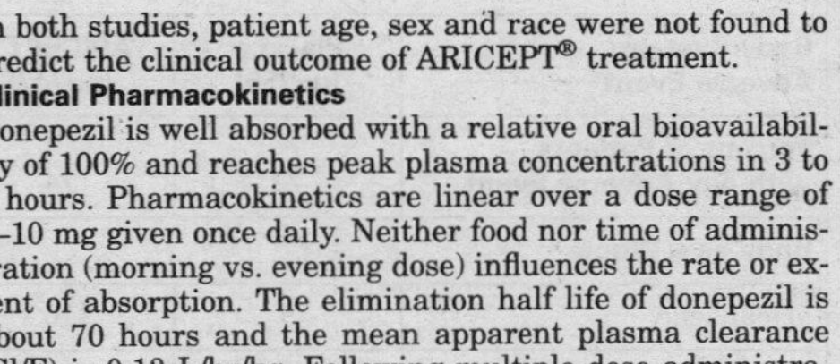

In both studies, patient age, sex and race were not found to predict the clinical outcome of ARICEPT® treatment.

Clinical Pharmacokinetics

Donepezil is well absorbed with a relative oral bioavailability of 100% and reaches peak plasma concentrations in 3 to 4 hours. Pharmacokinetics are linear over a dose range of 1–10 mg given once daily. Neither food nor time of administration (morning vs. evening dose) influences the rate or extent of absorption. The elimination half life of donepezil is about 70 hours and the mean apparent plasma clearance (Cl/F) is 0.13 L/hr/kg. Following multiple dose administration, donepezil accumulates in plasma by 4–7 fold and steady state is reached within 15 days. The steady state volume of distribution is 12 L/kg. Donepezil is approximately 96% bound to human plasma proteins, mainly to albumins (about 75%) and alpha$_1$-acid glycoprotein (about 21%) over the concentration range of 2–1000 ng/mL.

Donepezil is both excreted in the urine intact and extensively metabolized to four major metabolites, two of which are known to be active, and a number of minor metabolites, not all of which have been identified. Donepezil is metabolized by CYP 450 isoenzymes 2D6 and 3A4 and undergoes glucuronidation. Following administration of ^{14}C-labeled donepezil, plasma radioactivity, expressed as a percent of the administered dose, was present primarily as intact donepezil (53%) and as 6-O-desmethyl donepezil (11%), which has been reported to inhibit AChE to the same extent as donepezil *in vitro* and was found in plasma at concentrations equal to about 20% of donepezil. Approximately 57% and 15% of the total radioactivity was recovered in urine and feces, respectively, over a period of 10 days, while 28% remained unrecovered, with about 17% of the donepezil dose recovered in the urine as unchanged drug.

Special Populations:

Hepatic Disease: In a study of 10 patients with stable alcoholic cirrhosis, the clearance of ARICEPT® was decreased by 20% relative to 10 healthy age and sex matched subjects.

Renal Disease: In a study of 4 patients with moderate to severe renal impairment (Cl_{Cr} < 22 mL/min/1.73 m^2) the clearance of ARICEPT® did not differ from 4 age and sex matched healthy subjects.

Age: No formal pharmacokinetic study was conducted to examine age related differences in the pharmacokinetics of ARICEPT®. However, mean plasma ARICEPT® concentrations measured during therapeutic drug monitoring of elderly patients with Alzheimer's Disease are comparable to those observed in young healthy volunteers.

Gender and Race: No specific pharmacokinetic study was conducted to investigate the effects of gender and race on the disposition of ARICEPT®. However, retrospective pharmacokinetic analysis indicates that gender and race (Japanese and Caucasians) did not affect the clearance of ARICEPT®.

Drug-Drug Interactions

Drugs Highly Bound to Plasma Proteins: Drug displacement studies have been performed *in vitro* between this highly bound drug (96%) and other drugs such as furosemide, digoxin, and warfarin. ARICEPT® at concentrations of 0.3–10 µg/mL did not affect the binding of furosemide (5 µg/mL), digoxin (2 ng/mL), and warfarin (3 µg/mL) to human albumin. Similarly, the binding of ARICEPT® to human albumin was not affected by furosemide, digoxin and warfarin.

Effect of ARICEPT® on the Metabolism of Other Drugs: No *in vivo* clinical trials have investigated the effect of ARICEPT® on the clearance of drugs metabolized by CYP 3A4 (e.g. cisapride, terfenadine) or by CYP 2D6 (e.g. imipramine). However, *in vitro* studies show a low rate of binding to these enzymes (mean K_i about 50–130 µM), that, given the therapeutic plasma concentrations of donepezil (164 nM), indicates little likelihood of interference.

Whether ARICEPT® has any potential for enzyme induction is not known.

Formal pharmacokinetic studies evaluated the potential of ARICEPT® for interaction with theophylline, cimetidine, warfarin and digoxin. No significant effects on the pharmacokinetics of these drugs were observed.

Effect of Other Drugs on the Metabolism of ARICEPT®: Ketoconazole and quinidine, inhibitors of CYP450, 3A4 and 2D6, respectively, inhibit donepezil metabolism *in vitro*. Whether there is a clinical effect of these inhibitors is not known. Inducers of CYP 2D6 and CYP 3A4 (e.g., phenytoin, carbamazepine, dexamethasone, rifampin, and phenobarbital) could increase the rate of elimination of ARICEPT®.

Formal pharmacokinetic studies demonstrated that the metabolism of ARICEPT® is not significantly affected by concurrent administration of digoxin or cimetidine.

INDICATIONS AND USAGE

ARICEPT® is indicated for the treatment of mild to moderate dementia of the Alzheimer's type.

CONTRAINDICATIONS

ARICEPT® is contraindicated in patients with known hypersensitivity to donepezil hydrochloride or to piperidine derivatives.

WARNINGS

Anesthesia: ARICEPT®, as a cholinesterase inhibitor, is likely to exaggerate succinylcholine-type muscle relaxation during anesthesia.

Cardiovascular Conditions: Because of their pharmacological action, cholinesterase inhibitors may have vagotonic effects on the sinoatrial and atrioventricular nodes. This effect may manifest as bradycardia or heart block in patients both with and without known underlying cardiac conduction abnormalities. Syncopal episodes have been reported in association with the use of ARICEPT®.

Gastrointestinal Conditions: Through their primary action, cholinesterase inhibitors may be expected to increase gastric acid secretion due to increased cholinergic activity. Therefore, patients should be monitored closely for symptoms of active or occult gastrointestinal bleeding, especially those at increased risk for developing ulcers, e.g., those with a history of ulcer disease or those receiving concurrent nonsteroidal anti-inflammatory drugs (NSAIDS). Clinical studies of ARICEPT® have shown no increase, relative to placebo, in the incidence of either peptic ulcer disease or gastrointestinal bleeding.

Continued on next page

Aricept—Cont.

ARICEPT®, as a predictable consequence of its pharmacological properties, has been shown to produce diarrhea, nausea and vomiting. These effects, when they occur, appear more frequently with the 10 mg/day dose than with the 5 mg/day dose. In most cases, these effects have been mild and transient, sometimes lasting one to three weeks, and have resolved during continued use of ARICEPT®.

Genitourinary: Although not observed in clinical trials of ARICEPT®, cholinomimetics may cause bladder outflow obstruction.

Neurological Conditions: Seizures: Cholinomimetics are believed to have some potential to cause generalized convulsions. However, seizure activity also may be a manifestation of Alzheimer's Disease.

Pulmonary Conditions: Because of their cholinomimetic actions, cholinesterase inhibitors should be prescribed with care to patients with a history of asthma or obstructive pulmonary disease.

PRECAUTIONS

Drug-Drug Interactions (see Clinical Pharmacology: Clinical Pharmacokinetics: Drug-drug Interactions)

Effect of ARICEPT® on the Metabolism of Other Drugs: No *in vivo* clinical trials have investigated the effect of ARICEPT® on the clearance of drugs metabolized by CYP 3A4 (e.g. cisapride, terfenadine) or by CYP 2D6 (e.g. imipramine). However, *in vitro* studies show a low rate of binding to these enzymes (mean K_i about 50–130 µM), that, given the therapeutic plasma concentrations of donepezil (164 nM), indicates little likelihood of interference.

Whether ARICEPT® has any potential for enzyme induction is not known.

Effect of Other Drugs on the Metabolism of ARICEPT®: Ketoconazole and quinidine, inhibitors of CYP450, 3A4 and 2D6, respectively, inhibit donepezil metabolism *in vitro*. Whether there is a clinical effect of these inhibitors is not known. Inducers of CYP 2D6 and CYP 3A4 (e.g., phenytoin, carbamazepine, dexamethasone, rifampin, and phenobarbital) could increase the rate of elimination of ARICEPT®.

Use with Anticholinergics: Because of their mechanism of action, cholinesterase inhibitors have the potential to interfere with the activity of anticholinergic medications.

Use with Cholinomimetics and Other Cholinesterase Inhibitors: A synergistic effect may be expected when cholinesterase inhibitors are given concurrently with succinylcholine, similar neuromuscular blocking agents or cholinergic agonists such as bethanechol.

Carcinogenesis, Mutagenesis, Impairment of Fertility

Carcinogenicity studies of donepezil have not been completed.

Donepezil was not mutagenic in the Ames reverse mutation assay in bacteria. In the chromosome aberration test in cultures of Chinese hamster lung (CHL) cells, some clastogenic effects were observed. Donepezil was not clastogenic in the *in vivo* mouse micronucleus test.

Donepezil had no effect on fertility in rats at doses up to 10 mg/kg/day (approximately 8 times the maximum recommended human dose on a mg/m² basis).

Pregnancy

Pregnancy Category C: Teratology studies conducted in pregnant rats at doses up to 16 mg/kg/day (approximately 13 times the maximum recommended human dose on a mg/m² basis) and in pregnant rabbits at doses up to 10 mg/kg/day (approximately 16 times the maximum recommended human dose on a mg/m² basis) did not disclose any evidence for a teratogenic potential of donepezil. However, in a study in which pregnant rats were given up to 10 mg/kg/day (approximately 8 times the maximum recommended human dose on a mg/m² basis) from day 17 of gestation through day 20 postpartum, there was a slight increase in still births and a slight decrease in pup survival through day 4 postpartum at this dose; the next lower dose tested was 3 mg/kg/day. There are no adequate or well-controlled studies in pregnant women. ARICEPT® should be used during pregnancy only if the potential benefit justifies the potential risk to the fetus.

Nursing Mothers

It is not known whether donepezil is excreted in human breast milk. ARICEPT® has no indication for use in nursing mothers.

Pediatric Use

There are no adequate and well-controlled trials to document the safety and efficacy of ARICEPT® in any illness occurring in children.

ADVERSE REACTIONS

Adverse Events Leading to Discontinuation

The rates of discontinuation from controlled clinical trials of ARICEPT® due to adverse events for the ARICEPT® 5 mg/day treatment groups were comparable to those of placebo-treatment groups at approximately 5%. The rate of discontinuation of patients who received 7-day escalations from 5 mg/day to 10 mg/day, was higher at 13%.

The most common adverse events leading to discontinuation, defined as those occurring in at least 2% of patients and at twice the incidence seen in placebo patients, are shown in Table 1.

Table 1. Most Frequent Adverse Events Leading to Withdrawal from Controlled Clinical Trials by Dose Group

Dose Group	Placebo	5 mg/day ARICEPT®	10 mg/day ARICEPT®
Patients Randomized	355	350	315
Event/% Discontinuing			
Nausea	1%	1%	3%
Diarrhea	0%	<1%	3%
Vomiting	<1%	<1%	2%

Most Frequent Adverse Clinical Events Seen in Association with the Use of ARICEPT®

The most common adverse events, defined as those occurring at a frequency of at least 5% in patients receiving 10 mg/day and twice the placebo rate, are largely predicted by ARICEPT®'s cholinomimetic effects. These include nausea, diarrhea, insomnia, vomiting, muscle cramp, fatigue and anorexia. These adverse events were often of mild intensity and transient, resolving during continued ARICEPT® treatment without the need for dose modification.

There is evidence to suggest that the frequency of these common adverse events may be affected by the rate of titration. An open-label study was conducted with 269 patients who received placebo in the 15 and 30-week studies. These patients were titrated to a dose of 10 mg/day over a 6-week period. The rates of common adverse events were lower than those seen in patients titrated to 10 mg/day over one week in the controlled clinical trials and were comparable to those seen in patients on 5 mg/day.

See Table 2 for a comparison of the most common adverse events following one and six week titration regimens.

Table 2. Comparison of rates of adverse events in patients titrated to 10 mg/day over 1 and 6 weeks

	No titration		One week titration	Six week titration
Adverse Event	**Placebo (n=315)**	**5 mg/day (n=311)**	**10 mg/day (n=315)**	**10 mg/day (n=269)**
Nausea	6%	5%	19%	6%
Diarrhea	5%	8%	15%	9%
Insomnia	6%	6%	14%	6%
Fatigue	3%	4%	8%	3%
Vomiting	3%	3%	8%	5%
Muscle cramps	2%	6%	8%	3%
Anorexia	2%	3%	7%	3%

Adverse Events Reported in Controlled Trials

The events cited reflect experience gained under closely monitored conditions of clinical trials in a highly selected patient population. In actual clinical practice or in other clinical trials, these frequency estimates may not apply, as the conditions of use, reporting behavior, and the kinds of patients treated may differ. Table 3 lists treatment emergent signs and symptoms that were reported in at least 2% of patients in placebo-controlled trials who received ARICEPT® and for which the rate of occurrence was greater for ARICEPT® assigned than placebo assigned patients. In general, adverse events occurred more frequently in female patients and with advancing age.

Table 3. Adverse Events Reported in Controlled Clinical Trials in at Least 2% of Patients Receiving ARICEPT® and at a Higher Frequency than Placebo-treated Patients

Body System/ Adverse Event	Placebo (n=355)	ARICEPT® (n=747)
Percent of Patients with any Adverse Event	72	74
Body as a Whole		
Headache	9	10
Pain, various locations	8	9
Accident	6	7
Fatigue	3	5
Cardiovascular System		
Syncope	1	2
Digestive System		
Nausea	6	11
Diarrhea	5	10
Vomiting	3	5
Anorexia	2	4
Hemic and Lymphatic System		
Ecchymosis	3	4
Metabolic and Nutritional Systems		
Weight Decrease	1	3
Musculoskeletal System		
Muscle Cramps	2	6
Arthritis	1	2
Nervous System		
Insomnia	6	9
Dizziness	6	8
Depression	<1	3
Abnormal Dreams	0	3
Somnolence	<1	2
Urogenital System		
Frequent Urination	1	2

Other Adverse Events Observed During Clinical Trials

ARICEPT® has been administered to over 1700 individuals during clinical trials worldwide. Approximately 1200 of these patients have been treated for at least 3 months and more than 1000 patients have been treated for at least 6 months. Controlled and uncontrolled trials in the United States included approximately 900 patients. In regards to the highest dose of 10 mg/day, this population includes 650 patients treated for 3 months, 475 patients treated for 6 months and 116 patients treated for over 1 year. The range of patient exposure is from 1 to 1214 days.

Treatment emergent signs and symptoms that occurred during 3 controlled clinical trials and two open-label trials in the United States were recorded as adverse events by the clinical investigators using terminology of their own choosing. To provide an overall estimate of the proportion of individuals having similar types of events, the events were grouped into a smaller number of standardized categories using a modified COSTART dictionary and event frequencies were calculated across all studies. These categories are used in the listing below. The frequencies represent the proportion of 900 patients from these trials who experienced that event while receiving ARICEPT®. All adverse events occurring at least twice are included, except for those already listed in Tables 2 or 3, COSTART terms too general to be informative, or events less likely to be drug caused. Events are classified by body system and listed using the following definitions: *frequent adverse events*—those occurring in at least 1/100 patients; *infrequent adverse events*—those occurring in 1/100 to 1/1000 patients. These adverse events are not necessarily related to ARICEPT® treatment and in most cases were observed at a similar frequency in placebo-treated patients in the controlled studies. No important additional adverse events were seen in studies conducted outside the United States.

Body as a Whole: *Frequent:* influenza, chest pain, toothache; *Infrequent:* fever, edema face, periorbital edema, hernia hiatal, abscess, cellulitis, chills, generalized coldness, head fullness, listlessness.

Cardiovascular System: *Frequent:* hypertension, vasodilation, atrial fibrillation, hot flashes, hypotension; *Infrequent:* angina pectoris, postural hypotension, myocardial infarction, AV block (first degree), congestive heart failure, arteritis, bradycardia, peripheral vascular disease, supraventricular tachycardia, deep vein thrombosis.

Digestive System: *Frequent:* fecal incontinence, gastrointestinal bleeding, bloating, epigastric pain; *Infrequent:* eructation, gingivitis, increased appetite, flatulence, periodontal abscess, cholelithiasis, diverticulitis, drooling, dry mouth, fever sore, gastritis, irritable colon, tongue edema, epigastric distress, gastroenteritis, increased transaminases, hemorrhoids, ileus, increased thirst, jaundice, melena, polydipsia, duodenal ulcer, stomach ulcer.

Endocrine System: *Infrequent:* diabetes mellitus, goiter.

Hemic and Lymphatic System: *Infrequent:* anemia, thrombocythemia, thrombocytopenia, eosinophilia, erythrocytopenia.

Metabolic and Nutritional Disorders: *Frequent:* dehydration; *Infrequent:* gout, hypokalemia, increased creatine kinase, hyperglycemia, weight increase, increased lactate dehydrogenase.

Musculoskeletal System: *Frequent:* bone fracture; *Infrequent:* muscle weakness, muscle fasciculation.

Nervous System: *Frequent:* delusions, tremor, irritability, paresthesia, aggression, vertigo, ataxia, increased libido, restlessness, abnormal crying, nervousness, aphasia; *Infrequent:* cerebrovascular accident, intracranial hemorrhage, transient ischemic attack, emotional lability, neuralgia, coldness (localized), muscle spasm, dysphoria, gait abnormality, hypertonia, hypokinesia, neurodermatitis, numbness (localized), paranoia, dysarthria, dysphasia, hostility, decreased libido, melancholia, emotional withdrawal, nystagmus, pacing.

Respiratory System: *Frequent:* dyspnea, sore throat, bronchitis; *Infrequent:* epistaxis, post nasal drip, pneumonia, hyperventilation, pulmonary congestion, wheezing, hypoxia, pharyngitis, pleurisy, pulmonary collapse, sleep apnea, snoring.

Skin and Appendages: *Frequent:* pruritus, diaphoresis, urticaria; *Infrequent:* dermatitis, erythema, skin discoloration, hyperkeratosis, alopecia, fungal dermatitis, herpes zoster, hirsutism, skin striae, night sweats, skin ulcer.

Special Senses: *Frequent:* cataract, eye irritation, vision blurred; *Infrequent:* dry eyes, glaucoma, earache, tinnitus, blepharitis, decreased hearing, retinal hemorrhage, otitis externa, otitis media, bad taste, conjunctival hemorrhage, ear buzzing, motion sickness, spots before eyes.

Urogenital System: *Frequent:* urinary incontinence, nocturia; *Infrequent:* dysuria, hematuria, urinary urgency, metrorrhagia, cystitis, enuresis, prostate hypertrophy, pyelonephritis, inability to empty bladder, breast fibroadenosis, fibrocystic breast, mastitis, pyuria, renal failure, vaginitis.

Postintroduction Reports

Voluntary reports of adverse events temporally associated with ARICEPT® that have been received since market introduction that are not listed above, and that there is inadequate data to determine the causal relationship with the drug include the following: abdominal pain, agitation, cholecystitis, confusion, convulsions, hallucinations, heart block (all types), hemolytic anemia, hepatitis, hyponatremia, neuroleptic malignant syndrome, pancreatitis, and rash.

OVERDOSAGE

Because strategies for the management of overdose are continually evolving, it is advisable to contact a Poison Control Center to determine the latest recommendations for the management of an overdose of any drug.

As in any case of overdose, general supportive measures should be utilized. Overdosage with cholinesterase inhibitors can result in cholinergic crisis characterized by severe nausea, vomiting, salivation, sweating, bradycardia, hypotension, respiratory depression, collapse and convulsions. Increasing muscle weakness is a possibility and may result in death if respiratory muscles are involved. Tertiary anticholinergics such as atropine may be used as an antidote for ARICEPT® overdosage. Intravenous atropine sulfate titrated to effect is recommended: an initial dose of 1.0 to 2.0 mg IV with subsequent doses based upon clinical response. Atypical responses in blood pressure and heart rate have been reported with other cholinomimetics when co-administered with quaternary anticholinergics such as glycopyrrolate. It is not known whether ARICEPT® and/or its metabolites can be removed by dialysis (hemodialysis, peritoneal dialysis, or hemofiltration).

Dose-related signs of toxicity in animals included reduced spontaneous movement, prone position, staggering gait, lacrimation, clonic convulsions, depressed respiration, salivation, miosis, tremors, fasciculation and lower body surface temperature.

DOSAGE AND ADMINISTRATION

The dosages of ARICEPT® shown to be effective in controlled clinical trials are 5 mg and 10 mg administered once per day.

The higher dose of 10 mg did not provide a statistically significantly greater clinical benefit than 5 mg. There is a suggestion, however, based upon order of group mean scores and dose trend analyses of data from these clinical trials, that a daily dose of 10 mg of ARICEPT® might provide additional benefit for some patients. Accordingly, whether or not to employ a dose of 10 mg is a matter of prescriber and patient preference.

Evidence from the controlled trials indicates that the 10 mg dose, with a one week titration, is likely to be associated with a higher incidence of cholinergic adverse events than the 5 mg dose. In open label trials using a 6 week titration, the frequency of these same adverse events was similar between the 5 mg and 10 mg dose groups. Therefore, because steady state is not achieved for 15 days and because the incidence of untoward effects may be influenced by the rate of dose escalation, treatment with a dose of 10 mg should not be contemplated until patients have been on a daily dose of 5 mg for 4 to 6 weeks.

ARICEPT® should be taken in the evening, just prior to retiring. ARICEPT® can be taken with or without food.

HOW SUPPLIED

ARICEPT® is supplied as film-coated, round tablets containing either 5 mg or 10 mg of donepezil hydrochloride.

The 5 mg tablets are white. The strength, in mg (5), is debossed on one side and ARICEPT is debossed on the other side.

The 10 mg tablets are yellow. The strength, in mg (10), is debossed on one side and ARICEPT is debossed on the other side.

5 mg (White)   Bottles of 30 (NDC# 62856-245-30)
                 Bottles of 90 (NDC# 62856-245-90)
                 Unit Dose Blister Package 100 (10×10)
                 (NDC# 62856-245-41)

10 mg (Yellow)   Bottles of 30 (NDC# 62856-246-30)

Bottles of 90 (NDC# 62856-246-90)
Unit Dose Blister Package 100 (10×10)
(NDC# 62856-246-41)

Storage: Store at controlled room temperature, 15°C to 30°C (59°F to 86°F).

Rx only

ARICEPT® is a registered trademark of
Eisai Co., Ltd, Tokyo, Japan
Manufactured and Marketed by
Eisai Inc., Teaneck, NJ 07666
Distributed/Marketed by
Pfizer Inc, New York, NY 10017

©2000 Eisai Inc.
Printed in U.S.A.
200176   Revised December 2000

CARDURA®   ℞
(doxazosin mesylate)
Tablets

Prescribing information for this product, which appears on pages 2473–2477 of the 2001 PDR, has been completely revised as follows. Please write "See Supplement A" next to the product heading.

DESCRIPTION

CARDURA® (doxazosin mesylate) is a quinazoline compound that is a selective inhibitor of the alpha$_1$ subtype of alpha adrenergic receptors. The chemical name of doxazosin mesylate is 1-(4-amino-6,7-dimethoxy-2-quinazolinyl)-4-(1,4-benzodioxan-2-ylcarbonyl) piperazine methanesulfonate. The empirical formula for doxazosin mesylate is $C_{23}H_{25}N_5O_5 \cdot CH_4O_3S$ and the molecular weight is 547.6. It has the following structure:

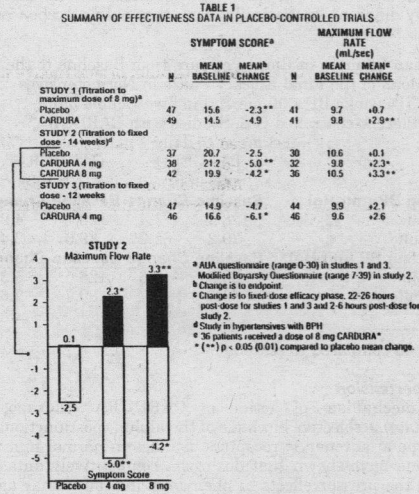

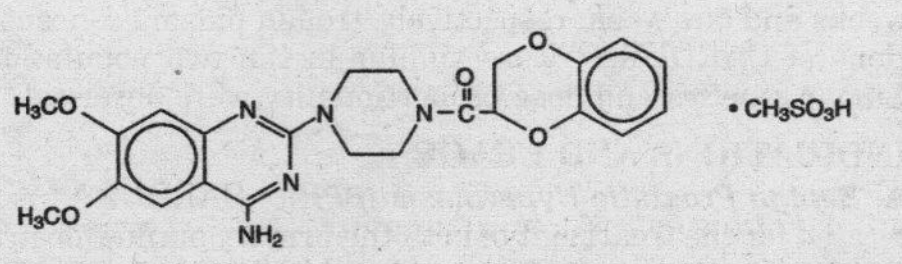

CARDURA® (doxazosin mesylate) is freely soluble in dimethylsulfoxide, soluble in dimethylformamide, slightly soluble in methanol, ethanol, and water (0.8% at 25°C), and very slightly soluble in acetone and methylene chloride. CARDURA® is available as colored tablets for oral use and contains 1 mg (white), 2 mg (yellow), 4 mg (orange) and 8 mg (green) of doxazosin as the free base.

The inactive ingredients for all tablets are: microcrystalline cellulose, lactose, sodium starch glycolate, magnesium stearate and sodium lauryl sulfate. The 2 mg tablet contains D & C yellow 10 and FD & C yellow 6; the 4 mg tablet contains FD & C yellow 6; the 8 mg tablet contains FD & C blue 10 and D & C yellow 10.

CLINICAL PHARMACOLOGY
Pharmacodynamics
A. Benign Prostatic Hyperplasia (BPH)

Benign prostatic hyperplasia (BPH) is a common cause of urinary outflow obstruction in aging males. Severe BPH may lead to urinary retention and renal damage. A static and a dynamic component contribute to the symptoms and reduced urinary flow rate associated with BPH. The static component is related to an increase in prostate size caused, in part, by a proliferation of smooth muscle cells in the prostatic stroma. However, the severity of BPH symptoms and the degree of urethral obstruction do not correlate well with the size of the prostate. The dynamic component of BPH is associated with an increase in smooth muscle tone in the prostate and bladder neck. The degree of tone in this area is mediated by the alpha$_1$ adrenoceptor, which is present in high density in the prostatic stroma, prostatic capsule and bladder neck. Blockade of the alpha$_1$ receptor decreases urethral resistance and may relieve the obstruction and BPH symptoms. In the human prostate, CARDURA® antagonizes phenylephrine (alpha$_1$ agonist)-induced contractions, *in vitro*, and binds with high affinity to the alpha$_{1c}$ adrenoceptor. The receptor subtype is thought to be the predominant functional type in the prostate. CARDURA® acts within 1–2 weeks to decrease the severity of BPH symptoms and improve urinary flow rate. Since alpha$_1$ adrenoceptors are of low density in the urinary bladder (apart from the bladder neck), CARDURA® should maintain bladder contractility.

The efficacy of CARDURA® was evaluated extensively in over 900 patients with BPH in double-blind, placebo-controlled trials. CARDURA® treatment was superior to placebo in improving patient symptoms and urinary flow rate. Significant relief with CARDURA® was seen as early as one week into the treatment regimen, with CARDURA® treated patients (N=173) showing a significant (p<0.01) increase in maximum flow rate of 0.8 mL/sec compared to a decrease of 0.5 mL/sec in the placebo group (N=41). In long-term studies improvement was maintained for up to 2 years of treatment. In 66–71% of patients, improvements above baseline were seen in both symptoms and maximum urinary flow rate.

In three placebo-controlled studies of 14–16 weeks duration obstructive symptoms (hesitation, intermittency, dribbling, weak urinary stream, incomplete emptying of the bladder) and irritative symptoms (nocturia, daytime frequency, urgency, burning) of BPH were evaluated at each visit by pa-

tient-assessed symptom questionnaires. The bothersomeness of symptoms was measured with a modified Boyarsky questionnaire. Symptom severity/frequency was assessed using a modified Boyarsky questionnaire or an AUA-based questionnaire. Uroflowmetric evaluations were performed at times of peak (2–6 hours post-dose) and/or trough (24 hours post-dose) plasma concentrations of CARDURA®. The results from the three placebo-controlled studies (N=609) showing significant efficacy with 4 mg and 8 mg doxazosin are summarized in Table 1. In all three studies, CARDURA® resulted in statistically significant relief of obstructive and irritative symptoms compared to placebo. Statistically significant improvements of 2.3–3.3 mL/sec in maximum flow rate were seen with CARDURA® in Studies 1 and 2, compared to 0.1–0.7 mL/sec with placebo.

TABLE 1
SUMMARY OF EFFECTIVENESS DATA IN PLACEBO-CONTROLLED TRIALS

	SYMPTOM SCORE[a]				MAXIMUM FLOW RATE (mL/sec)		
	N	MEAN BASELINE	MEAN[b] CHANGE	N	MEAN BASELINE	MEAN[c] CHANGE
STUDY 1 (Titration to maximum dose of 8 mg)[d]						
Placebo	47	15.6	-2.3**	41	9.7	+0.7
CARDURA	49	14.5	-4.9	41	9.8	+2.9**
STUDY 2 (Titration to fixed dose - 14 weeks)[e]						
Placebo	37	20.7	-2.5	30	10.6	+0.1
CARDURA 4 mg	38	21.2	-5.0**	32	9.8	+2.3*
CARDURA 8 mg	42	19.9	-4.2*	36	10.5	+3.3**
STUDY 3 (Titration to fixed dose - 12 weeks)						
Placebo	47	14.9	-4.7	44	9.9	+2.1
CARDURA 4 mg	46	16.6	-6.1*	46	9.6	+2.6

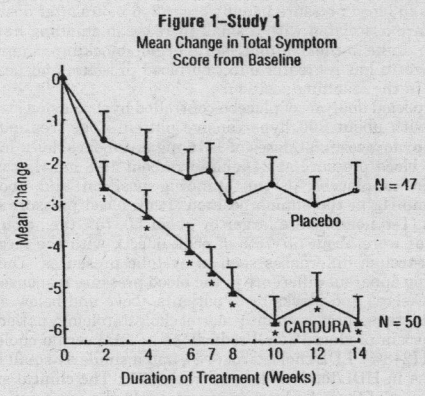

STUDY 2
Maximum Flow Rate

[a] AUA questionnaire (range 0-30) in studies 1 and 3. Modified Boyarsky Questionnaire (range 7-39) in study 2.
[b] Change is to endpoint.
[c] Change is to fixed-dose efficacy phase. 22-26 hours post-dose for studies 1 and 3 and 2-6 hours post-dose for study 2.
[d] Study in hypertensives with BPH
[e] 36 patients received a dose of 8 mg CARDURA®.
*(**) p < 0.05 (0.01) compared to placebo mean change.

In one fixed dose study (Study 2) CARDURA® (doxazosin mesylate) therapy (4–8 mg, once daily) resulted in a significant and sustained improvement in maximum urinary flow rate of 2.3–3.3 mL/sec (Table 1) compared to placebo (0.1 mL/sec). In this study, the only study in which weekly evaluations were made, significant improvement with CARDURA® vs. placebo was seen after one week. The proportion of patients who responded with a maximum flow rate improvement of ≥3 mL/sec was significantly larger with CARDURA® (34–42%) than placebo (13–17%). A significantly greater improvement was also seen in average flow rate with CARDURA® (1.6 mL/sec) than with placebo (0.2 mL/sec). The onset and time course of symptom relief and increased urinary flow from Study 1 are illustrated in Figure 1.

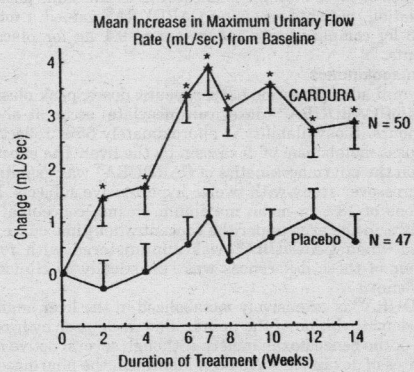

Figure 1–Study 1
Mean Change in Total Symptom Score from Baseline

Mean Increase in Maximum Urinary Flow Rate (mL/sec) from Baseline

---

* p < 0.05 Compared to Placebo; + p < 0.05 Compared to Baseline; Doxazosin Titration to Maximum of 8 mg.

Continued on next page

Cardura—Cont.

In BPH patients (N=450) treated for up to 2 years in open-label studies, CARDURA® therapy resulted in significant improvement above baseline in urinary flow rates and BPH symptoms. The significant effects of CARDURA® were maintained over the entire treatment period.

Although blockade of alpha₁ adrenoceptors also lowers blood pressure in hypertensive patients with increased peripheral vascular resistance, CARDURA® treatment of normotensive men with BPH did not result in a clinically significant blood pressure lowering effect (Table 2). The proportion of normotensive patients with a sitting systolic blood pressure less than 90 mmHg and/or diastolic blood pressure less than 60 mmHg at any time during treatment with CARDURA® 1–8 mg once daily was 6.7% with doxazosin and not significantly different (statistically) from that with placebo (5%).

TABLE 2
Mean Changes in Blood Pressure from Baseline to the Mean of the Final Efficacy Phase in Normotensives (Diastolic BP <90 mmHg) in Two Double-blind, Placebo-controlled U.S. Studies with CARDURA® 1-8 mg once daily.

	PLACEBO (N=85)		CARDURA® (N=183)	
Sitting BP (mmHg)	Baseline	Change	Baseline	Change
Systolic	128.4	−1.4	128.8	−4.9*
Diastolic	79.2	−1.2	79.6	−2.4*
Standing BP (mmHg)	Baseline	Change	Baseline	Change
Systolic	128.5	−0.6	128.5	−5.3*
Diastolic	80.5	−0.7	80.4	−2.6*

*p≤0.05 compared to placebo

B. Hypertension

The mechanism of action of CARDURA® (doxazosin mesylate) is selective blockade of the alpha₁ (postjunctional) subtype of adrenergic receptors. Studies in normal human subjects have shown that doxazosin competitively antagonized the pressor effects of phenylephrine (an alpha₁ agonist) and the systolic pressor effect of norepinephrine. Doxazosin and prazosin have similar abilities to antagonize phenylephrine. The antihypertensive effect of CARDURA® results from a decrease in systemic vascular resistance. The parent compound doxazosin is primarily responsible for the antihypertensive activity. The low plasma concentrations of known active and inactive metabolites of doxazosin (2-piperazinyl, 6′- and 7′-hydroxy and 6- and 7-O-desmethyl compounds) compared to parent drug indicate that the contribution of even the most potent compound (6′-hydroxy) to the antihypertensive effect of doxazosin in man is probably small. The 6′- and 7′-hydroxy metabolites have demonstrated antioxidant properties at concentrations of 5 μM, in vitro.

Administration of CARDURA® results in a reduction in systemic vascular resistance. In patients with hypertension there is little change in cardiac output. Maximum reductions in blood pressure usually occur 2–6 hours after dosing and are associated with a small increase in standing heart rate. Like other alpha₁-adrenergic blocking agents, doxazosin has a greater effect on blood pressure and heart rate in the standing position.

In a pooled analysis of placebo-controlled hypertension studies with about 300 hypertensive patients per treatment group, doxazosin, at doses of 1–16 mg given once daily, lowered blood pressure at 24 hours by about 10/8 mmHg compared to placebo in the standing position and about 9/5 mmHg in the supine position. Peak blood pressure effects (1–6 hours) were larger by about 50–75% (i.e., trough values were about 55–70% of peak effect), with the larger peak-trough differences seen in systolic pressures. There was no apparent difference in the blood pressure response of Caucasians and blacks or of patients above and below age 65. In these predominantly normocholesterolemic patients doxazosin produced small reductions in total serum cholesterol (2–3%), LDL cholesterol (4%), and a similarly small increase in HDL/total cholesterol ratio (4%). The clinical significance of these findings is uncertain. In the same patient population, patients receiving CARDURA® gained a mean of 0.6 kg compared to a mean loss of 0.1 kg for placebo patients.

Pharmacokinetics

After oral administration of therapeutic doses, peak plasma levels of CARDURA® (doxazosin mesylate) occur at about 2–3 hours. Bioavailability is approximately 65%, reflecting first pass metabolism of doxazosin by the liver. The effect of food on the pharmacokinetics of CARDURA® was examined in a crossover study with twelve hypertensive subjects. Reductions of 18% in mean maximum plasma concentration and 12% in the area under the concentration-time curve occurred when CARDURA® was administered with food. Neither of these differences was statistically or clinically significant.

CARDURA® is extensively metabolized in the liver, mainly by O-demethylation of the quinazoline nucleus or hydroxylation of the benzodioxan moiety. Although several active metabolites of doxazosin have been identified, the pharmacokinetics of these metabolites have not been characterized. In a study of two subjects administered radiolabelled doxazosin 2 mg orally and 1 mg intravenously on two separate occasions, approximately 63% of the dose was eliminated in the feces and 9% of the dose was found in the urine. On average only 4.8% of the dose was excreted as unchanged drug in the

feces and only a trace of the total radioactivity in the urine was attributed to unchanged drug. At the plasma concentrations achieved by therapeutic doses approximately 98% of the circulating drug is bound to plasma proteins.

Plasma elimination of doxazosin is biphasic, with a terminal elimination half-life of about 22 hours. Steady-state studies in hypertensive patients given doxazosin doses of 2–16 mg once daily showed linear kinetics and dose proportionality. In two studies, following the administration of 2 mg orally once daily, the mean accumulation ratios (steady-state AUC vs. first dose AUC) were 1.2 and 1.7. Enterohepatic recycling is suggested by secondary peaking of plasma doxazosin concentrations.

In a crossover study in 24 normotensive subjects, the pharmacokinetics and safety of doxazosin were shown to be similar with morning and evening dosing regimens. The area under the curve after morning dosing was, however, 11% less than that after evening dosing and the time to peak concentration after evening dosing occurred significantly later than that after morning dosing (5.6 hr vs. 3.5 hr).

The pharmacokinetics of CARDURA® (doxazosin mesylate) in young (<65 years) and elderly (≥65 years) subjects were similar for plasma half-life values and oral clearance. Pharmacokinetic studies in elderly patients and patients with renal impairment have shown no significant alterations compared to younger patients with normal renal function. Administration of a single 2 mg dose to patients with cirrhosis (Child-Pugh Class A) showed a 40% increase in exposure to doxazosin. There are only limited data on the effects of drugs known to influence the hepatic metabolism of doxazosin [e.g., cimetidine (see PRECAUTIONS)]. As with any drug wholly metabolized by the liver, use of CARDURA® in patients with altered liver function should be undertaken with caution.

In two placebo-controlled studies, of normotensive and hypertensive BPH patients, in which doxazosin was administered in the morning and the titration interval was two weeks and one week, respectively, trough plasma concentrations of CARDURA® were similar in the two populations. Linear kinetics and dose proportionality were observed.

INDICATIONS AND USAGE

A. Benign Prostatic Hyperplasia (BPH). CARDURA® is indicated for the treatment of both the urinary outflow obstruction and obstructive and irritative symptoms associated with BPH: obstructive symptoms (hesitation, intermittency, dribbling, weak urinary stream, incomplete emptying of the bladder) and irritative symptoms (nocturia, daytime frequency, urgency, burning). CARDURA® may be used in all BPH patients whether hypertensive or normotensive. In patients with hypertension and BPH, both conditions were effectively treated with CARDURA® monotherapy. CARDURA® provides rapid improvement in symptoms and urinary flow rate in 66–71% of patients. Sustained improvements with CARDURA® were seen in patients treated for up to 14 weeks in double-blind studies and up to 2 years in open-label studies.

B. Hypertension. CARDURA® (doxazosin mesylate) is also indicated for the treatment of hypertension. CARDURA® may be used alone or in combination with diuretics, beta-adrenergic blocking agents, calcium channel blockers or angiotensin-converting enzyme inhibitors.

CONTRAINDICATIONS

CARDURA® is contraindicated in patients with a known sensitivity to quinazolines (e.g., prazosin, terazosin), doxazosin, or any of the inert ingredients.

WARNINGS

Syncope and "First-dose" Effect: Doxazosin, like other alpha-adrenergic blocking agents, can cause marked hypotension, especially in the upright position, with syncope and other postural symptoms such as dizziness. Marked orthostatic effects are most common with the first dose but can also occur when there is a dosage increase, or if therapy is interrupted for more than a few days. To decrease the likelihood of excessive hypotension and syncope, it is essential that treatment be initiated with the 1 mg dose. The 2, 4, and 8 mg tablets are not for initial therapy. Dosage should then be adjusted slowly (see DOSAGE AND ADMINISTRATION section) with evaluations and increases in dose every two weeks to the recommended dose. Additional antihypertensive agents should be added with caution.

Patients being titrated with doxazosin should be cautioned to avoid situations where injury could result should syncope occur, during both the day and night.

In an early investigational study of the safety and tolerance of increasing daily doses of doxazosin in normotensives beginning at 1 mg/day, only 2 of 6 subjects could tolerate more than 2 mg/day without experiencing symptomatic postural hypotension. In another study of 24 healthy normotensive male subjects receiving initial doses of 2 mg/day of doxazosin, seven (29%) of the subjects experienced symptomatic postural hypotension between 0.5 and 6 hours after the first dose necessitating termination of the study. In this study, 2 of the normotensive subjects experienced syncope. Subsequent trials in hypertensive patients always began doxazosin dosing at 1 mg/day resulting in a 4% incidence of postural side effects at 1 mg/day with no cases of syncope.

In multiple dose clinical trials in hypertension involving over 1500 hypertensive patients with dose titration every one to two weeks, syncope was reported in 0.7% of patients. None of these events occurred at the starting dose of 1 mg and 1.2% (8/664) occurred at 16 mg/day.

In placebo-controlled, clinical trials in BPH, 3 out of 665 patients (0.5%) taking doxazosin reported syncope. Two of the patients were taking 1 mg doxazosin, while one patient was taking 2 mg doxazosin when syncope occurred. In the open-label, long-term extension follow-up of approximately 450 BPH patients, there were 3 reports of syncope (0.7%). One patient was taking 2 mg, one patient was taking 8 mg and one patient was taking 12 mg when syncope occurred. In a clinical pharmacology study, one subject receiving 2 mg experienced syncope.

If syncope occurs, the patient should be placed in a recumbent position and treated supportively as necessary.

Priapism: Rarely (probably less frequently than once in every several thousand patients), alpha₁ antagonists, including doxazosin, have been associated with priapism (painful penile erection, sustained for hours and unrelieved by sexual intercourse or masturbation). Because this condition can lead to permanent impotence if not promptly treated, patients must be advised about the seriousness of the condition (see PRECAUTIONS: Information for Patients).

PRECAUTIONS

General:

Prostate Cancer: Carcinoma of the prostate causes many of the symptoms associated with BPH and the two disorders frequently co-exist. Carcinoma of the prostate should therefore be ruled out prior to commencing therapy with CARDURA®.

Orthostatic Hypotension: While syncope is the most severe orthostatic effect of CARDURA®, other symptoms of lowered blood pressure, such as dizziness, lightheadedness, or vertigo can occur, especially at initiation of therapy or at the time of dose increases.

a) Hypertension

These symptoms were common in clinical trials in hypertension, occurring in up to 23% of all patients treated and causing discontinuation of therapy in about 2%.

In placebo-controlled titration trials in hypertension, orthostatic effects were minimized by beginning therapy at 1 mg per day and titrating every two weeks to 2, 4, or 8 mg per day. There was an increased frequency of orthostatic effects in patients given 8 mg or more, 10%, compared to 5% at 1–4 mg and 3% in the placebo group.

b) Benign Prostatic Hyperplasia

In placebo-controlled trials in BPH, the incidence of orthostatic hypotension with doxazosin was 0.3% and did not increase with increasing dosage (to 8 mg/day). The incidence of discontinuations due to hypotensive or orthostatic symptoms was 3.3% with doxazosin and 1% with placebo. The titration interval in these studies was one to two weeks.

Patients in occupations in which orthostatic hypotension could be dangerous should be treated with particular caution. As alpha₁ antagonists can cause orthostatic effects, it is important to evaluate standing blood pressure two minutes after standing and patients should be advised to exercise care when arising from a supine or sitting position.

If hypotension occurs, the patient should be placed in the supine position and, if this measure is inadequate, volume expansion with intravenous fluids or vasopressor therapy may be used. A transient hypotensive response is not a contraindication to further doses of CARDURA® (doxazosin mesylate).

Information for Patients (See patient package insert): Patients should be made aware of the possibility of syncopal and orthostatic symptoms, especially at the initiation of therapy, and urged to avoid driving or hazardous tasks for 24 hours after the first dose, after a dosage increase, and after interruption of therapy when treatment is resumed. They should be cautioned to avoid situations where injury could result should syncope occur during initiation of doxazosin therapy. They should also be advised of the need to sit or lie down when symptoms of lowered blood pressure occur, although these symptoms are not always orthostatic, and to be careful when rising from a sitting or lying position. If dizziness, lightheadedness, or palpitations are bothersome they should be reported to the physician, so that dose adjustment can be considered. Patients should also be told that drowsiness or somnolence can occur with CARDURA® (doxazosin mesylate) or any selective alpha₁ adrenoceptor antagonist, requiring caution in people who must drive or operate heavy machinery.

Patients should be advised about the possibility of priapism as a result of treatment with alpha₁ antagonists. Patients should know that this adverse event is very rare. If they experience priapism, it should be brought to immediate medical attention for if not treated promptly it can lead to permanent erectile dysfunction (impotence).

Drug/Laboratory Test Interactions: CARDURA® does not affect the plasma concentration of prostate specific antigen in patients treated for up to 3 years. Both doxazosin, an alpha₁ inhibitor, and finasteride, a 5-alpha reductase inhibitor, are highly protein bound and hepatically metabolized. There is no definitive controlled clinical experience on the concomitant use of alpha₁ inhibitors and 5-alpha reductase inhibitors at this time.

Impaired Liver Function: CARDURA® should be administered with caution to patients with evidence of impaired hepatic function or to patients receiving drugs known to influence hepatic metabolism (see CLINICAL PHARMACOLOGY).

Leukopenia/Neutropenia: Analysis of hematologic data from hypertensive patients receiving CARDURA® in controlled hypertension clinical trials showed that the mean WBC (N=474) and mean neutrophil counts (N= 419) were decreased by 2.4% and 1.0%, respectively, compared to placebo, a phenomenon seen with other alpha blocking drugs. In BPH patients the incidence of clinically significant WBC abnormalities was 0.4% (2/459) with CARDURA® and 0% (0/147) with placebo, with no statistically significant difference between the two treatment groups. A search through a data base of 2400 hypertensive patients and 665 BPH patients revealed 4 hypertensives in which drug-related neutropenia could not be ruled out and one BPH patient in which drug related leukopenia could not be ruled out. Two hypertensives had a single low value on the last day of treatment. Two hypertensives had stable, non-progressive neutrophil counts in the 1000/mm^3 range over periods of 20 and 40 weeks. One BPH patient had a decrease from a WBC count of 4800/mm^3 to 2700/mm^3 at the end of the study; there was no evidence of clinical impairment. In cases where follow-up was available the WBCs and neutrophil counts returned to normal after discontinuation of CARDURA®. No patients became symptomatic as a result of the low WBC or neutrophil counts.

Drug Interactions: Most (98%) of plasma doxazosin is protein bound. *In vitro* data in human plasma indicate that CARDURA® has no effect on protein binding of digoxin, warfarin, phenytoin or indomethacin. There is no information on the effect of other highly plasma protein bound drugs on doxazosin binding. CARDURA® has been administered without any evidence of an adverse drug interaction to patients receiving thiazide diuretics, beta-blocking agents, and nonsteroidal anti-inflammatory drugs. In a placebo-controlled trial in normal volunteers, the administration of a single 1 mg dose of doxazosin on day 1 of a four-day regimen of oral cimetidine (400 mg twice daily) resulted in a 10% increase in mean AUC of doxazosin (p=0.006), and a slight but not statistically significant increase in mean C_{max} and mean half-life of doxazosin. The clinical significance of this increase in doxazosin AUC is unknown.

In clinical trials, CARDURA® tablets have been administered to patients on a variety of concomitant medications; while no formal interaction studies have been conducted, no interactions were observed. CARDURA® tablets have been used with the following drugs or drug classes: 1) analgesic/anti-inflammatory (e.g., acetaminophen, aspirin, codeine and codeine combinations, ibuprofen, indomethacin); 2) antibiotics (e.g., erythromycin, trimethoprim and sulfamethoxazole, amoxicillin); 3) antihistamines (e.g., chlorpheniramine); 4) cardiovascular agents (e.g., atenolol, hydrochlorothiazide, propranolol); 5) corticosteroids; 6) gastrointestinal agents (e.g., antacids); 7) hypoglycemics and endocrine drugs; 8) sedatives and tranquilizers (e.g., diazepam); 9) cold and flu remedies.

Cardiac Toxicity in Animals: An increased incidence of myocardial necrosis or fibrosis was displayed by Sprague-Dawley rats after 6 months of dietary administration at concentrations calculated to provide 80 mg doxazosin/kg/day and after 12 months of dietary administration at concentrations calculated to provide 40 mg doxazosin/kg/day (AUC exposure in rats 8 times the human AUC exposure with a 12 mg/day therapeutic dose). Myocardial fibrosis was observed in both rats and mice treated in the same manner with 40 mg doxazosin/kg/day for 18 months (exposure 8 times human AUC exposure in rats and somewhat equivalent to human C_{max} exposure in mice). No cardiotoxicity was observed at lower doses (up to 10 or 20 mg/kg/day, depending on the study) in either species. These lesions were not observed after 12 months of oral dosing in dogs at maximum doses of 20 mg/kg/day [maximum plasma concentrations (C_{max}) in dogs 14 times the C_{max} exposure in humans receiving a 12 mg/day therapeutic dose] and in Wistar rats at doses of 100 mg/kg/day (C_{max} exposures 15 times human C_{max} exposure with a 12 mg/day therapeutic dose). There is no evidence that similar lesions occur in humans.

Carcinogenesis, Mutagenesis, Impairment of Fertility: Chronic dietary administration (up to 24 months) of doxazosin mesylate at maximally tolerated doses of 40 mg/kg/day in rats and 120 mg/kg/day in mice revealed no evidence of carcinogenic potential. The highest doses evaluated in the rat and mouse studies are associated with AUCs (a measure of systemic exposure) that are 8 times and 4 times, respectively, the human AUC at a dose of 16 mg/day. Mutagenicity studies revealed no drug- or metabolite-related effects at either chromosomal or subchromosomal levels.

Studies in rats showed reduced fertility in males treated with doxazosin at oral doses of 20 (but not 5 or 10) mg/kg/day, about 4 times the AUC exposures obtained with a 12 mg/day human dose. This effect was reversible within two weeks of drug withdrawal. There have been no reports of any effects of doxazosin on male fertility in humans.

Pregnancy: Teratogenic Effects, Pregnancy Category C. Studies in pregnant rabbits and rats at daily oral doses of up to 41 and 20 mg/kg, respectively (plasma drug concentrations 10 and 4 times human C_{max} and AUC exposures with a 12 mg/day therapeutic dose), have revealed no evidence of harm to the fetus. A dosage regimen of 82 mg/kg/day in the rabbit was associated with reduced fetal survival. There are no adequate and well-controlled studies in pregnant women. Because animal reproduction studies are not always predictive of human response, CARDURA® should be used during pregnancy only if clearly needed.

Radioactivity was found to cross the placenta following oral administration of labelled doxazosin to pregnant rats.

Nonteratogenic Effects: In peri-postnatal studies in rats, postnatal development at maternal doses of 40 or 50 mg/kg/day of doxazosin (8 times human AUC exposure with a 12 mg/day therapeutic dose) was delayed as evidenced by slower body weight gain and a slightly later appearance of anatomical features and reflexes.

Nursing Mothers: Studies in lactating rats given a single oral dose of 1 mg/kg of [2-^{14}C]-CARDURA® indicate that doxazosin accumulates in rat breast milk with a maximum concentration about 20 times greater than the maternal plasma concentration. It is not known whether this drug is excreted in human milk. Because many drugs are excreted in human milk, caution should be exercised when CARDURA® is administered to a nursing mother.

Pediatric Use: The safety and effectiveness of CARDURA® as an antihypertensive agent have not been established in children.

Use in Elderly: The safety and effectiveness profile of CARDURA® in BPH was similar in the elderly (age ≥65 years) and younger (age <65 years) patients.

ADVERSE REACTIONS

A. Benign Prostatic Hyperplasia

The incidence of adverse events has been ascertained from worldwide clinical trials in 965 BPH patients. The incidence rates presented below (Table 3) are based on combined data from seven placebo-controlled trials involving once daily administration of CARDURA® (doxazosin mesylate) in doses of 1–16 mg in hypertensives and 0.5–8 mg in normotensives. The adverse events when the incidence in the CARDURA® group was at least 1% are summarized in Table 3. No significant difference in the incidence of adverse events compared to placebo was seen except for dizziness, fatigue, hypotension, edema and dyspnea. Dizziness and dyspnea appeared to be dose-related.

TABLE 3
ADVERSE REACTIONS DURING
PLACEBO-CONTROLLED STUDIES
BENIGN PROSTATIC HYPERPLASIA

Body System	CARDURA® (N=665)	PLACEBO (N=300)
BODY AS A WHOLE		
Back pain	1.8%	2.0%
Chest pain	1.2%	0.7%
Fatigue	8.0%*	1.7%
Headache	9.9%	9.0%
Influenza-like symptoms	1.1%	1.0%
Pain	2.0%	1.0%
CARDIOVASCULAR SYSTEM		
Hypotension	1.7%*	0.0%
Palpitation	1.2%	0.3%
DIGESTIVE SYSTEM		
Abdominal Pain	2.4%	2.0%
Diarrhea	2.3%	2.0%
Dyspepsia	1.7%	1.7%
Nausea	1.5%	0.7%
METABOLIC AND NUTRITIONAL DISORDERS		
Edema	2.7%*	0.7%
NERVOUS SYSTEM		
Dizziness†	15.6%*	9.0%
Mouth Dry	1.4%	0.3%
Somnolence	3.0%	1.0%
RESPIRATORY SYSTEM		
Dyspnea	2.6%*	0.3%
Respiratory Disorder	1.1%	0.7%
SPECIAL SENSES		
Vision Abnormal	1.4%	0.7%
UROGENITAL SYSTEM		
Impotence	1.1%	1.0%
Urinary Tract Infection	1.4%	2.3%
SKIN & APPENDAGES		
Sweating Increased	1.1%	1.0%
PSYCHIATRIC DISORDERS		
Anxiety	1.1%	0.3%
Insomnia	1.2%	0.3%

*p≤0.05 for treatment differences
†Includes vertigo

In these placebo-controlled studies of 665 CARDURA® patients, treated for a mean of 85 days, additional adverse reactions have been reported. These are less than 1% and not distinguishable from those that occurred in the placebo group. Adverse reactions with an incidence of less than 1% but of clinical interest are (CARDURA® vs. placebo): *Cardiovascular System:* angina pectoris (0.6% vs. 0.7%), postural hypotension (0.3% vs. 0.3%), syncope (0.5% vs. 0.0%), tachycardia (0.9% vs. 0.0%); *Urogenital System:* dysuria (0.5% vs. 1.3%), and *Psychiatric Disorders:* libido decreased (0.8% vs. 0.3%). The safety profile in patients treated for up to three years was similar to that in the placebo-controlled studies. The majority of adverse experiences with CARDURA® were mild.

B. Hypertension

CARDURA® has been administered to approximately 4000 hypertensive patients, of whom 1679 were included in the hypertension clinical development program. In that program, minor adverse effects were frequent, but led to discontinuation of treatment in only 7% of patients. In placebo-controlled studies adverse effects occurred in 49% and 40% of patients in the doxazosin and placebo groups, respectively, and led to discontinuation in 2% of patients in each group. The major reasons for discontinuation were postural effects (2%), edema, malaise/fatigue, and some heart rate disturbance, each about 0.7%.

In controlled hypertension clinical trials directly comparing CARDURA® to placebo there was no significant difference in the incidence of side effects, except for dizziness (including postural), weight gain, somnolence and fatigue/malaise. Postural effects and edema appeared to be dose related. The prevalence rates presented below are based on combined data from placebo-controlled studies involving once daily administration of doxazosin at doses ranging from 1–16 mg. Table 4 summarizes those adverse experiences (possibly/probably related) reported for patients in these hypertension studies where the prevalence rate in the doxazosin group was at least 0.5% or where the reaction is of particular interest.

TABLE 4
ADVERSE REACTIONS DURING
PLACEBO-CONTROLLED STUDIES

	HYPERTENSION	
	DOXAZOSIN (N=339)	PLACEBO (N=336)
CARDIOVASCULAR SYSTEM		
Dizziness	19%	9%
Vertigo	2%	1%
Postural Hypotension	0.3%	0%
Edema	4%	3%
Palpitation	2%	3%
Arrhythmia	1%	0%
Hypotension	1%	0%
Tachycardia	0.3%	1%
Peripheral Ischemia	0.3%	0%
SKIN & APPENDAGES		
Rash	1%	1%
Pruritus	1%	1%
MUSCULOSKELETAL SYSTEM		
Arthralgia/Arthritis	1%	0%
Muscle Weakness	1%	0%
Myalgia	1%	0%
CENTRAL & PERIPHERAL N.S.		
Headache	14%	16%
Paresthesia	1%	1%
Kinetic Disorders	1%	0%
Ataxia	1%	0%
Hypertonia	1%	0%
Muscle Cramps	1%	0%
AUTONOMIC		
Mouth Dry	2%	2%
Flushing	1%	0%
SPECIAL SENSES		
Vision Abnormal	2%	1%
Conjunctivitis/Eye Pain	1%	1%
Tinnitus	1%	0.3%
PSYCHIATRIC		
Somnolence	5%	1%
Nervousness	2%	2%
Depression	1%	1%
Insomnia	1%	1%
Sexual Dysfunction	2%	1%
GASTROINTESTINAL		
Nausea	3%	4%
Diarrhea	2%	3%
Constipation	1%	1%
Dyspepsia	1%	1%
Flatulence	1%	1%
Abdominal Pain	0%	2%
Vomiting	0%	1%
RESPIRATORY		
Rhinitis	3%	1%
Dyspnea	1%	1%
Epistaxis	1%	0%
URINARY		
Polyuria	2%	0%
Urinary Incontinence	1%	0%
Micturition Frequency	0%	2%
GENERAL		
Fatigue/Malaise	12%	6%
Chest Pain	2%	2%
Asthenia	1%	1%
Face Edema	1%	0%
Pain	2%	2%

Additional adverse reactions have been reported, but these are, in general, not distinguishable from symptoms that might have occurred in the absence of exposure to doxazosin. The following adverse reactions occurred with a frequency of between 0.5% and 1%: syncope, hypoesthesia,

Continued on next page

Cardura—Cont.

increased sweating, agitation, increased weight. The following additional adverse reactions were reported by <0.5% of 3960 patients who received doxazosin in controlled or open, short- or long-term clinical studies, including international studies. *Cardiovascular System:* angina pectoris, myocardial infarction, cerebrovascular accident; *Autonomic Nervous System:* pallor; *Metabolic:* thirst, gout, hypokalemia; *Hematopoietic:* lymphadenopathy, purpura; *Reproductive System:* breast pain; *Skin Disorders:* alopecia, dry skin, eczema; *Central Nervous System:* paresis, tremor, twitching, confusion, migraine, impaired concentration; *Psychiatric:* paroniria, amnesia, emotional lability, abnormal thinking, depersonalization; *Special Senses:* parosmia, earache, taste perversion, photophobia, abnormal lacrimation; *Gastrointestinal System:* increased appetite, anorexia, fecal incontinence, gastroenteritis; *Respiratory System:* bronchospasm, sinusitis, coughing, pharyngitis; *Urinary System:* renal calculus; *General Body System:* hot flushes, back pain, infection, fever/rigors, decreased weight, influenza-like symptoms.

CARDURA® has not been associated with any clinically significant changes in routine biochemical tests. No clinically relevant adverse effects were noted on serum potassium, serum glucose, uric acid, blood urea nitrogen, creatinine or liver function tests. CARDURA® has been associated with decreases in white blood cell counts (see PRECAUTIONS).

In post-marketing experience the following additional adverse reactions have been reported: *Autonomic Nervous System:* priapism; *Central Nervous System:* hypoesthesia; *Endocrine System:* gynecomastia; *Gastrointestinal System:* vomiting; *General Body System:* allergic reaction; *Heart Rate/Rhythm:* bradycardia; *Hematopoietic:* leukopenia, thrombocytopenia; *Liver/Biliary System:* hepatitis, hepatitis cholestatic; *Respiratory System:* bronchospasm aggravated; *Urinary System:* hematuria, micturition disorder, micturition frequency, nocturia.

OVERDOSAGE

Experience with CARDURA® overdosage is limited. Two adolescents who each intentionally ingested 40 mg CARDURA® with diclofenac or paracetamol, were treated with gastric lavage with activated charcoal and made full recoveries. A two-year-old child who accidently ingested 4 mg CARDURA® was treated with gastric lavage and remained normotensive during the five-hour emergency room observation period. A six-month-old child accidentally received a crushed 1 mg tablet of CARDURA® and was reported to have been drowsy. A 32-year-old female with chronic renal failure, epilepsy and depression intentionally ingested 60 mg CARDURA® (blood level 0.9 µg/mL; normal values in hypertensives=0.02 µg/mL); death was attributed to a grand mal seizure resulting from hypotension. A 39-year-old female who ingested 70 mg CARDURA,® alcohol and Dalmane® (flurazepam) developed hypotension which responded to fluid therapy.

The oral LD_{50} of doxazosin is greater than 1000 mg/kg in mice and rats. The most likely manifestation of overdosage would be hypotension, for which the usual treatment would be intravenous infusion of fluid. As doxazosin is highly protein bound, dialysis would not be indicated.

DOSAGE AND ADMINISTRATION

DOSAGE MUST BE INDIVIDUALIZED. The initial dosage of CARDURA® in patients with hypertension and/or BPH is 1 mg given once daily in the a.m. or p.m. This starting dose is intended to minimize the frequency of postural hypotension and first dose syncope associated with CARDURA®. Postural effects are most likely to occur between 2 and 6 hours after a dose. Therefore blood pressure measurements should be taken during this time period after the first dose and with each increase in dose. If CARDURA® administration is discontinued for several days, therapy should be restarted using the initial dosing regimen.

A. *BENIGN PROSTATIC HYPERPLASIA 1–8 mg once daily.* The initial dosage of CARDURA® is 1 mg, given once daily in the a.m. or p.m. Depending on the individual patient's urodynamics and BPH symptomatology, dosage may then be increased to 2 mg and thereafter to 4 mg and 8 mg once daily, the maximum recommended dose for BPH. The recommended titration interval is 1–2 weeks. Blood pressure should be evaluated routinely in these patients.

B. *HYPERTENSION 1–16 mg once daily.* The initial dosage of CARDURA® is 1 mg given once daily. Depending on the individual patient's standing blood pressure response (based on measurements taken at 2–6 hours post-dose and 24 hours post-dose), dosage may then be increased to 2 mg and thereafter if necessary to 4 mg, 8 mg and 16 mg to achieve the desired reduction in blood pressure.

Increases in dose beyond 4 mg increase the likelihood of excessive postural effects including syncope, postural dizziness/vertigo and postural hypotension. At a titrated dose of 16 mg once daily the frequency of postural effects is about 12% compared to 3% for placebo.

HOW SUPPLIED

CARDURA® (doxazosin mesylate) is available as colored tablets for oral administration. Each tablet contains doxazosin mesylate equivalent to 1 mg (white), 2 mg (yellow), 4 mg (orange) or 8 mg (green) of the active constituent, doxazosin.

CARDURA® TABLETS (doxazosin mesylate) are available as 1 mg (white), 2 mg (yellow), 4 mg (orange) and 8 mg (green) scored tablets.

Bottles of 100:	1 mg (NDC 0049-2750-66)
	2 mg (NDC 0049-2760-66)
	4 mg (NDC 0049-2770-66)
	8 mg (NDC 0049-2780-66)
Unit Dose Packages of 100:	1 mg (NDC 0049-2750-41)
	2 mg (NDC 0049-2760-41)
	4 mg (NDC 0049-2770-41)
	8 mg (NDC 0049-2780-41)

Recommended Storage: Store below 86°F (30°C).

Rx only

Pfizer Roerig

Division of Pfizer Inc, NY, NY 10017

Printed in U.S.A.

69-4538-00-7 Revised June 2000

PROCARDIA® ℞

[*pro-car 'dē-ă*]

nifedipine

CAPSULES

For Oral Use

Prescribing information for this product, which appears on pages 2510–2512 of the 2001 PDR, has been completely revised as follows. Please write "See Supplement A" next to the product heading.

DESCRIPTION

PROCARDIA® (nifedipine) is an antianginal drug belonging to a class of pharmacological agents, the calcium channel blockers. Nifedipine is 3,5-pyridinedicarboxylic acid, 1,4-dihydro-2, 6-dimethyl-4-(2-nitrophenyl)-, dimethyl ester, $C_{17}H_{18}N_2O_6$, and has the structural formula:

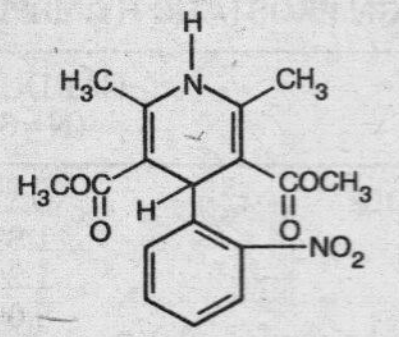

Nifedipine is a yellow crystalline substance, practically insoluble in water but soluble in ethanol. It has a molecular weight of 346.3. PROCARDIA capsules are formulated as soft gelatin capsules for oral administration each containing 10 mg or 20 mg nifedipine.

Inert ingredients in the formulations are: glycerin; peppermint oil; polyethylene glycol; soft gelatin capsules (which contain Yellow 6, and may contain Red Ferric Oxide and other inert ingredients), and water. The 10 mg capsules also contain saccharin sodium.

CLINICAL PHARMACOLOGY

PROCARDIA is a calcium ion influx inhibitor (slow-channel blocker or calcium ion antagonist) and inhibits the transmembrane influx of calcium ions into cardiac muscle and smooth muscle. The contractile processes of cardiac muscle and vascular smooth muscle are dependent upon the movement of extracellular calcium ions into these cells through specific ion channels. PROCARDIA selectively inhibits calcium ion influx across the cell membrane of cardiac muscle and vascular smooth muscle without changing serum calcium concentrations.

Mechanism of Action

The precise means by which this inhibition relieves angina has not been fully determined, but includes at least the following two mechanisms:

1) Relaxation and Prevention of Coronary Artery Spasm

PROCARDIA dilates the main coronary arteries and coronary arterioles, both in normal and ischemic regions, and is a potent inhibitor of coronary artery spasm, whether spontaneous or ergonovine-induced. This property increases myocardial oxygen delivery in patients with coronary artery spasm, and is responsible for the effectiveness of PROCARDIA in vasospastic (Prinzmetal's or variant) angina. Whether this effect plays any role in classical angina is not clear, but studies of exercise tolerance have not shown an increase in the maximum exercise rate-pressure product, a widely accepted measure of oxygen utilization. This suggests that, in general, relief of spasm or dilation of coronary arteries is not an important factor in classical angina.

2) Reduction of Oxygen Utilization

PROCARDIA regularly reduces arterial pressure at rest and at a given level of exercise by dilating peripheral arterioles and reducing the total peripheral resistance (afterload) against which the heart works. This unloading of the heart reduces myocardial energy consumption and oxygen requirements and probably accounts for the effectiveness of PROCARDIA in chronic stable angina.

Pharmacokinetics and Metabolism

PROCARDIA is rapidly and fully absorbed after oral administration. The drug is detectable in serum 10 minutes after oral administration, and peak blood levels occur in approximately 30 minutes. Bioavailability is proportional to dose from 10 to 30 mg; half-life does not change significantly with dose. There is little difference in relative bioavailability when PROCARDIA capsules are given orally and either swallowed whole, bitten and swallowed, or bitten and held sublingually. However, biting through the capsule prior to swallowing does result in slightly earlier plasma concentrations (27 ng/mL 10 minutes after 10 mg) than if capsules are swallowed intact. It is highly bound by serum proteins. PROCARDIA is extensively converted to inactive metabolites and approximately 80 percent of PROCARDIA and metabolites are eliminated via the kidneys. The half-life of nifedipine in plasma is approximately two hours. Since hepatic biotransformation is the predominant route for the disposition of nifedipine, the pharmacokinetics may be altered in patients with chronic liver disease. Patients with hepatic impairment (liver cirrhosis) have a longer disposition half-life and higher bioavailability of nifedipine than healthy volunteers. The degree of serum protein binding of nifedipine is high (92–98%). Protein binding may be greatly reduced in patients with renal or hepatic impairment.

In healthy subjects, the elimination half-life of a BID sustained release nifedipine formulation [that was neither Procardia Capsules nor Procardia XL (nifedipine) Extended Release Tablets] was longer in elderly subjects (6.7 h) compared to young subjects (3.8 h) following oral administration. A decreased clearance was also observed in the elderly (348 ml/min) following intravenous administration.

Co-administration of nifedipine with grapefruit juice resulted in approximately a 2-fold increase in nifedipine AUC and Cmax with no change in half-life. The increased plasma concentrations are most likely due to inhibition of CYP 3A4 related first-pass metabolism.

Hemodynamics

Like other slow-channel blockers, PROCARDIA exerts a negative inotropic effect on isolated myocardial tissue. This is rarely, if ever, seen in intact animals or man, probably because of reflex responses to its vasodilating effects. In man, PROCARDIA causes decreased peripheral vascular resistance and a fall in systolic and diastolic pressure, usually modest (5–10mm Hg systolic), but sometimes larger. There is usually a small increase in heart rate, a reflex response to vasodilation. Measurements of cardiac function in patients with normal ventricular function have generally found a small increase in cardiac index without major effects on ejection fraction, left ventricular end diastolic pressure (LVEDP) or volume (LVEDV). In patients with impaired ventricular function, most acute studies have shown some increase in ejection fraction and reduction in left ventricular filling pressure.

Electrophysiologic Effects

Although, like other members of its class, PROCARDIA decreases sinoatrial node function and atrioventricular conduction in isolated myocardial preparations, such effects have not been seen in studies in intact animals or in man. In formal electrophysiologic studies, predominantly in patients with normal conduction systems, PROCARDIA has had no tendency to prolong atrioventricular conduction, prolong sinus node recovery time, or slow sinus rate.

INDICATIONS AND USAGE

I. Vasospastic Angina

PROCARDIA (nifedipine) is indicated for the management of vasospastic angina confirmed by any of the following criteria: 1) classical pattern of angina at rest accompanied by ST segment elevation, 2) angina or coronary artery spasm provoked by ergonovine, or 3) angiographically demonstrated coronary artery spasm. In those patients who have had angiography, the presence of significant fixed obstructive disease is not incompatible with the diagnosis of vasospastic angina, provided that the above criteria are satisfied. PROCARDIA may also be used where the clinical presentation suggests a possible vasospastic component but where vasospasm has not been confirmed, e.g., where pain has a variable threshold on exertion or when angina is refractory to nitrates and/or adequate doses of beta blockers.

II. Chronic Stable Angina
(Classical Effort-Associated Angina)

PROCARDIA is indicated for the management of chronic stable angina (effort-associated angina) without evidence of vasospasm in patients who remain symptomatic despite adequate doses of beta blockers and /or organic nitrates or who cannot tolerate those agents.

In chronic stable angina (effort-associated angina) PROCARDIA has been effective in controlled trials of up to eight weeks duration in reducing angina frequency and increasing exercise tolerance, but confirmation of sustained effectiveness and evaluation of long-term safety in these patients are incomplete.

Controlled studies in small numbers of patients suggest concomitant use of PROCARDIA and beta-blocking agents may be beneficial in patients with chronic stable angina, but available information is not sufficient to predict with confidence the effects of concurrent treatment, especially in patients with compromised left ventricular function or cardiac conduction abnormalities. When introducing such concomitant therapy, care must be taken to monitor blood pressure closely since severe hypotension can occur from the combined effects of the drugs. (See WARNINGS.)

CONTRAINDICATIONS

Known hypersensitivity reaction to PROCARDIA.

WARNINGS

Excessive Hypotension

Although, in most patients, the hypotensive effect of PROCARDIA is modest and well tolerated, occasional patients have had excessive and poorly tolerated hypotension. These responses have usually occurred during initial titration or at the time of subsequent upward dosage adjustment. Although patients have rarely experienced excessive hypotension on PROCARDIA alone, this may be more common in patients on concomitant beta-blocker therapy. Although not approved for this purpose, PROCARDIA and other immediate-release nifedipine capsules have been used (orally and sublingually) for acute reduction of blood pres-

sure. Several well-documented reports describe cases of profound hypotension, myocardial infarction, and death when immediate-release nifedipine was used in this way. **PROCARDIA capsules should not be used for the acute reduction of blood pressure.**
PROCARDIA and other immediate-release nifedipine capsules have also been used for the long-term control of essential hypertension, although no properly-controlled studies have been conducted to define an appropriate dose or dose interval for such treatment. **PROCARDIA capsules should not be used for the control of essential hypertension.**
Several well-controlled, randomized trials studied the use of immediate-release nifedipine in patients who had just sustained myocardial infarctions. In none of these trials did immediate-release nifedipine appear to provide any benefit. In some of the trials, patients who received immediate-release nifedipine had significantly worse outcomes than patients who received placebo. **PROCARDIA capsules should not be administered within the first week or two after myocardial infarction, and they should also be avoided in the setting of acute coronary syndrome (when infarction may be imminent).**
Severe hypotension and/or increased fluid volume requirements have been reported in patients receiving PROCARDIA together with a beta-blocking agent who underwent coronary artery bypass surgery using high dose fentanyl anesthesia. The interaction with high dose fentanyl appears to be due to the combination of PROCARDIA and a beta blocker, but the possibility that it may occur with PROCARDIA alone, with low doses of fentanyl, in other surgical procedures, or with other narcotic analgesics cannot be ruled out. In PROCARDIA treated patients where surgery using high dose fentanyl anesthesia is contemplated, the physician should be aware of these potential problems and, if the patient's condition permits, sufficient time (at least 36 hours) should be allowed for PROCARDIA to be washed out of the body prior to surgery.
Increased Angina and/or Myocardial Infarction
Rarely, patients, particularly those who have severe obstructive coronary artery disease, have developed well documented increased frequency, duration and/or severity of angina or acute myocardial infarction on starting PROCARDIA or at the time of dosage increase. The mechanism of this effect is not established.
Beta Blocker Withdrawal
Patients recently withdrawn from beta blockers may develop a withdrawal syndrome with increased angina, probably related to increased sensitivity to catecholamines. Initiation of PROCARDIA treatment will not prevent this occurrence and might be expected to exacerbate it by provoking reflex catecholamine release. There have been occasional reports of increased angina in a setting of beta blocker withdrawal and PROCARDIA initiation. It is important to taper beta blockers if possible, rather than stopping them abruptly before beginning PROCARDIA.
Congestive Heart Failure
Rarely, patients, usually receiving a beta blocker, have developed heart failure after beginning PROCARDIA. Patients with tight aortic stenosis may be at greater risk for such an event, as the unloading effect of PROCARDIA would be expected to be of less benefit to these patients, owing to their fixed impedance to flow across the aortic valve.

PRECAUTIONS
General: Hypotension: Because PROCARDIA decreases peripheral vascular resistance, careful monitoring of blood pressure during the initial administration and titration of PROCARDIA is suggested. Close observation is especially recommended for patients already taking medications that are known to lower blood pressure. (See WARNINGS.)
Peripheral Edema: Mild to moderate peripheral edema, typically associated with arterial vasodilation and not due to left ventricular dysfunction, occurs in about one in ten patients treated with PROCARDIA (nifedipine). This edema occurs primarily in the lower extremities and usually responds to diuretic therapy. With patients whose angina is complicated by congestive heart failure, care should be taken to differentiate this peripheral edema from the effects of increasing left ventricular dysfunction.
Laboratory Tests: Rare, usually transient, but occasionally significant elevations of enzymes such as alkaline phosphatase, CPK, LDH, SGOT and SGPT have been noted. The relationship to PROCARDIA therapy is uncertain in most cases, but probable in some. These laboratory abnormalities have rarely been associated with clinical symptoms; however, cholestasis with or without jaundice has been reported. Rare instances of allergic hepatitis have been reported.
PROCARDIA, like other calcium channel blockers, decreases platelet aggregation in vitro. Limited clinical studies have demonstrated a moderate but statistically significant decrease in platelet aggregation and an increase in bleeding time in some PROCARDIA patients. This is thought to be a function of inhibition of calcium transport across the platelet membrane. No clinical significance for these findings has been demonstrated.
Positive direct Coombs Test with/without hemolytic anemia has been reported but a causal relationship between PROCARDIA administration and positivity of this laboratory test, including hemolysis, could not be determined.
Although PROCARDIA has been used safely in patients with renal dysfunction and has been reported to exert a beneficial effect, in certain cases, rare, reversible elevations in BUN and serum creatinine have been reported in patients with pre-existing chronic renal insufficiency. The relationship to PROCARDIA therapy is uncertain in most cases but probable in some.

Drug Interactions: Beta-adrenergic blocking agents: (See INDICATIONS AND USAGE and WARNINGS.) Experience in over 1400 patients in a non-comparative clinical trial has shown that concomitant administration of PROCARDIA and beta-blocking agents is usually well tolerated, but there have been occasional literature reports suggesting that the combination may increase the likelihood of congestive heart failure, severe hypotension or exacerbation of angina.
Long-acting nitrates: PROCARDIA may be safely co-administered with nitrates, but there have been no controlled studies to evaluate the antianginal effectiveness of this combination.
Digitalis: Since there have been isolated reports of patients with elevated digoxin levels, and there is a possible interaction between digoxin and nifedipine, it is recommended that digoxin levels be monitored when initiating, adjusting, and discontinuing nifedipine to avoid possible over- or underdigitalization.
Quinidine: There have been rare reports of an interaction between quinidine and nifedipine (with a decreased plasma level of quinidine).
Coumarin anticoagulants: There have been rare reports of increased prothrombin time in patients taking coumarin anticoagulants to whom PROCARDIA was administered. However, the relationship to PROCARDIA therapy is uncertain.
Cimetidine: A study in six healthy volunteers has shown a significant increase in peak nifedipine plasma levels (80%) and area-under-the-curve (74%) after a one week course of cimetidine at 1000 mg per day and nifedipine at 40 mg per day. Ranitidine produced smaller, non-significant increases. The effect may be mediated by the known inhibition of cimetidine on hepatic cytochrome P-450, the enzyme system probably responsible for the first-pass metabolism of nifedipine. If nifedipine therapy is initiated in a patient currently receiving cimetidine, cautious titration is advised.
Other Interactions
Grapefruit Juice: Co-administration of nifedipine with grapefruit juice resulted in approximately a 2-fold increase in nifedipine AUC and Cmax with no change in half-life. The increased plasma concentrations are most likely due to inhibition of CYP 3A4 related first-pass metabolism. Co-administration of nifedipine with grapefruit juice is to be avoided.
Carcinogenesis, Mutagenesis, Impairment of Fertility: Nifedipine was administered orally to rats for two years and was not shown to be carcinogenic. When given to rats prior to mating, nifedipine caused reduced fertility at a dose approximately 30 times the maximum recommended human dose. There is a literature report of reversible reduction in the ability of human sperm obtained from a limited number of infertile men taking recommended doses of nifedipine to bind to and fertilize an ovum in vitro. In vivo mutagenicity studies were negative.
Pregnancy: Pregnancy Category C: Nifedipine has been shown to produce teratogenic findings in rats and rabbits, including digital anomalies similar to those reported for phenytoin. Digital anomalies have been reported to occur with other members of the dihydropyridine class and are possibly a result of compromised uterine blood flow. Nifedipine administration was associated with a variety of embryotoxic, placentotoxic, and fetotoxic effects, including stunted fetuses (rats, mice, rabbits), rib deformities (mice), cleft palate (mice), small placentas and underdeveloped chorionic villi (monkeys), embryonic and fetal deaths (rats, mice, rabbits), and prolonged pregnancy/decreased neonatal survival (rats; not evaluated in other species). On a mg/kg basis, all of the doses associated with the teratogenic embryotoxic or fetotoxic effects in animals were higher (3.5 to 42 times) than the maximum recommended human dose of 120 mg/day. On a mg/m² basis, some doses were higher and some were lower than the maximum recommended human dose but all are within an order of magnitude of it. The doses associated with placentotoxic effects in monkeys were equivalent to or lower than the maximum recommended human dose on a mg/m² basis.
There are no adequate and well-controlled studies in pregnant women. PROCARDIA should be used during pregnancy only if the potential benefit justifies the potential risk to the fetus.
Pediatric Use: Safety and effectiveness in pediatric patients have not been established. Use in pediatric population is not recommended.
Geriatric Use: Although small pharmacokinetic studies have identified an increased half-life and increased Cmax and AUC (see CLINICAL PHARMACOLOGY: Pharmacokinetics and Metabolism), clinical studies of nifedipine did not include sufficient numbers of subjects aged 65 and over to determine whether they respond differently from younger subjects. Other reported clinical experience has not identified differences in response between the elderly and younger patients. In general, dose selection for an elderly patient should be cautious, usually starting at the low end of the dosing range, reflecting the greater frequency of decreased hepatic, renal or cardiac function, and of concomitant disease or other drug therapy.

ADVERSE REACTIONS
In multiple-dose U.S. and foreign controlled studies in which adverse reactions were reported spontaneously, adverse effects were frequent but generally not serious and rarely required discontinuation of therapy or dosage adjustment. Most were expected consequences of the vasodilator effects of PROCARDIA.

Adverse Effect	PROCARDIA (%) (N=226)	Placebo (%) (N=235)
Dizziness, lightheadedness, giddiness	27	15
Flushing, heat sensation	25	8
Headache	23	20
Weakness	12	10
Nausea, heartburn	11	8
Muscle cramps, tremor	8	3
Peripheral edema	7	1
Nervousness, mood changes	7	4
Palpitation	7	5
Dyspnea, cough, wheezing	6	3
Nasal congestion, sore throat	6	8

There is also a large uncontrolled experience in over 2100 patients in the United States. Most of the patients had vasospastic or resistant angina pectoris, and about half had concomitant treatment with beta-adrenergic blocking agents. The most common adverse events were:
Incidence Approximately 10%
Cardiovascular: peripheral edema
Central Nervous System: dizziness or lightheadedness
Gastrointestinal: nausea
Systemic: headache and flushing, weakness
Incidence Approximately 5%
Cardiovascular: transient hypotension
Incidence 2% or Less
Cardiovascular: palpitation
Respiratory: nasal and chest congestion, shortness of breath
Gastrointestinal: diarrhea, constipation, cramps, flatulence
Musculoskeletal: inflammation, joint stiffness, muscle cramps
Central Nervous System: shakiness, nervousness, jitteriness, sleep disturbances, blurred vision, difficulties in balance
Other: dermatitis, pruritus, urticaria, fever, sweating, chills, sexual difficulties
Incidence Approximately 0.5%
Cardiovascular: syncope (mostly with initial dosing and/or an increase in dose), erythromelalgia
Incidence Less Than 0.5%
Hematologic: thrombocytopenia, anemia, leukopenia, purpura
Gastrointestinal: allergic hepatitis
Face and Throat: angioedema (mostly oropharyngeal edema with breathing difficulty in a few patients), gingival hyperplasia
CNS: depression, paranoid syndrome
Special Senses: transient blindness at the peak of plasma level, tinnitus
Urogenital: nocturia, polyuria
Other: arthritis with ANA (+), exfoliative dermatitis, gynecomastia
Musculoskeletal: myalgia
Several of these side effects appear to be dose related. Peripheral edema occurred in about one in 25 patients at doses less than 60 mg per day and in about one patient in eight at 120 mg per day or more. Transient hypotension, generally of mild to moderate severity and seldom requiring discontinuation of therapy, occurred in one of 50 patients at less than 60 mg per day and in one of 20 patients at 120 mg per day or more.
Very rarely, introduction of PROCARDIA therapy was associated with an increase in anginal pain, possibly due to associated hypotension. Transient unilateral loss of vision has also occurred.
In addition, more serious adverse events were observed, not readily distinguishable from the natural history of the disease in these patients. It remains possible, however, that some or many of these events were drug related. Myocardial infarction occurred in about 4% of patients and congestive heart failure or pulmonary edema in about 2%. Ventricular arrhythmias or conduction disturbances each occurred in fewer than 0.5% of patients.
In a subgroup of over 1000 patients receiving PROCARDIA with concomitant beta blocker therapy, the pattern and incidence of adverse experiences was not different from that of the entire group of PROCARDIA (nifedipine) treated patients. (See PRECAUTIONS.)
In a subgroup of approximately 250 patients with a diagnosis of congestive heart failure as well as angina pectoris (about 10% of the total patient population), dizziness or lightheadedness, peripheral edema, headache or flushing each occurred in one in eight patients. Hypotension occurred in about one in 20 patients. Syncope occurred in approximately one patient in 250. Myocardial infarction or symptoms of congestive heart failure each occurred in about one patient in 15. Atrial or ventricular dysrhythmias each occurred in about one patient in 150.
In post-marketing experience, there have been rare reports of exfoliative dermatitis caused by nifedipine. There have been rare reports of exfoliative or bullous skin adverse events (such as erythema multiforme, Stevens-Johnson Syndrome, and toxic epidermal necrolysis) and photosensitivity reactions.

Continued on next page

Procardia—Cont.

OVERDOSAGE

Experience with nifedipine overdosage is limited. Generally, overdosage with nifedipine leading to pronounced hypotension calls for active cardiovascular support including monitoring of cardiovascular and respiratory function, elevation of extremities, and judicious use of calcium infusion, pressor agents and fluids. Clearance of nifedipine would be expected to be prolonged in patients with impaired liver function. Since nifedipine is highly protein bound, dialysis is not likely to be of any benefit; however, plasmapheresis may be beneficial.

DOSAGE AND ADMINISTRATION

The dosage of PROCARDIA needed to suppress angina and that can be tolerated by the patient must be established by titration. Excessive doses can result in hypotension.

Therapy should be initiated with the 10 mg capsule. The starting dose is one 10 mg capsule, swallowed whole, 3 times/day. The usual effective dose range is 10–20 mg three times daily. Some patients, especially those with evidence of coronary artery spasm, respond only to higher doses, more frequent administration, or both. In such patients, doses of 20–30 mg three or four times daily may be effective. Doses above 120 mg daily are rarely necessary. More than 180 mg per day is not recommended.

In most cases, PROCARDIA titration should proceed over a 7–14 day period so that the physician can assess the response to each dose level and monitor the blood pressure before proceeding to higher doses.

If symptoms so warrant, titration may proceed more rapidly provided that the patient is assessed frequently. Based on the patient's physical activity level, attack frequency, and sublingual nitroglycerin consumption, the dose of PROCARDIA may be increased from 10 mg t.i.d. to 20 mg t.i.d. and then to 30 mg t.i.d. over a three-day period.

In hospitalized patients under close observation, the dose may be increased in 10 mg increments over four- to six-hour periods as required to control pain and arrhythmias due to ischemia. A single dose should rarely exceed 30 mg.

Co-administration of nifedipine with grapefruit juice is to be avoided **(see CLINICAL PHARMACOLOGY and PRECAUTIONS: Other Interactions).**

No rebound effect has been observed upon discontinuation of PROCARDIA. However, if discontinuation of PROCARDIA is necessary, sound clinical practice suggests that the dosage should be decreased gradually with close physician supervision.

Co-Administration with Other Antianginal Drugs

Sublingual nitroglycerin may be taken as required for the control of acute manifestations of angina, particularly during PROCARDIA titration. See **PRECAUTIONS, Drug Interactions,** for information on co-administration of PROCARDIA with beta blockers or long-acting nitrates.

HOW SUPPLIED

PROCARDIA® soft gelatin capsules are supplied in:

Bottles of 100:	10 mg	(NDC 0069-2600-66)
	20 mg	(NDC 0069-2610-66)
Bottles of 300:	10 mg	(NDC 0069-2600-72)

The capsules should be protected from light and moisture and stored at controlled room temperature 59° to 77°F (15° to 25°C) in the manufacturer's original container.

Rx only

Manufactured by Pfizer Inc.
Encapsulated by
R. P. Scherer
Clearwater, FL 33518
Pfizer Labs
Division of Pfizer Inc, NY, NY 10017
Printed in U.S.A.
69-4990-00-1 Revised September 2000

SINEQUAN® ℞

[sin 'a-kwon]
(doxepin HCl)
Capsules
Oral Concentrate

Prescribing information for this product, which appears on pages 2515–2516 of the 2001 PDR, has been completely revised as follows. Please write "See Supplement A" next to the product heading.

DESCRIPTION

SINEQUAN® (doxepin hydrochloride) is one of a class of psychotherapeutic agents known as dibenzoxepin tricyclic compounds. The molecular formula of the compound is $C_{19}H_{21}NO \bullet HCl$ having a molecular weight of 316. It is a white crystalline solid readily soluble in water, lower alcohols and chloroform.

Inert ingredients for the capsule formulations are: hard gelatin capsules (which may contain Blue 1, Red 3, Red 40, Yellow 10, and other inert ingredients); magnesium stearate; sodium lauryl sulfate; starch.

Inert ingredients for the oral concentrate formulation are: glycerin; methylparaben; peppermint oil; propylparaben; water.

CHEMISTRY

SINEQUAN (doxepin HCl) is a dibenzoxepin derivative and is the first of a family of tricyclic psychotherapeutic agents. Specifically, it is an isomeric mixture of:

1-Propanamine, 3-dibenz[*b,e*]oxepin-11 (6*H*)ylidene-*N,N*-dimethyl-, hydrochloride.

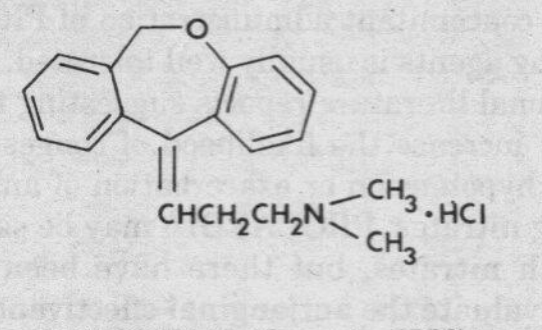

SINEQUAN (doxepin HCl)

ACTIONS

The mechanism of action of SINEQUAN (doxepin HCl) is not definitely known. It is not a central nervous system stimulant nor a monoamine oxidase inhibitor. The current hypothesis is that the clinical effects are due, at least in part, to influences on the adrenergic activity at the synapses so that deactivation of norepinephrine by reuptake into the nerve terminals is prevented. Animal studies suggest that doxepin HCl does not appreciably antagonize the antihypertensive action of guanethidine. In animal studies anticholinergic, antiserotonin and antihistamine effects on smooth muscle have been demonstrated. At higher than usual clinical doses, norepinephrine response was potentiated in animals. This effect was not demonstrated in humans.

At clinical dosages up to 150 mg per day, SINEQUAN can be given to man concomitantly with guanethidine and related compounds without blocking the antihypertensive effect. At dosages above 150 mg per day blocking of the antihypertensive effect of these compounds has been reported.

SINEQUAN is virtually devoid of euphoria as a side effect. Characteristic of this type of compound, SINEQUAN has not been demonstrated to produce the physical tolerance or psychological dependence associated with addictive compounds.

INDICATIONS

SINEQUAN is recommended for the treatment of:

1. Psychoneurotic patients with depression and/or anxiety.
2. Depression and/or anxiety associated with alcoholism (not to be taken concomitantly with alcohol).
3. Depression and/or anxiety associated with organic disease (the possibility of drug interaction should be considered if the patient is receiving other drugs concomitantly).
4. Psychotic depressive disorders with associated anxiety including involutional depression and manic-depressive disorders.

The target symptoms of psychoneurosis that respond particularly well to SINEQUAN include anxiety, tension, depression, somatic symptoms and concerns, sleep disturbances, guilt, lack of energy, fear, apprehension and worry.

Clinical experience has shown that SINEQUAN is safe and well tolerated even in the elderly patient. Owing to lack of clinical experience in the pediatric population, SINEQUAN is not recommended for use in children under 12 years of age.

CONTRAINDICATIONS

SINEQUAN is contraindicated in individuals who have shown hypersensitivity to the drug. Possibility of cross sensitivity with other dibenzoxepines should be kept in mind. SINEQUAN is contraindicated in patients with glaucoma or a tendency to urinary retention. These disorders should be ruled out, particularly in older patients.

WARNINGS

The once-a-day dosage regimen of SINEQUAN in patients with intercurrent illness or patients taking other medications should be carefully adjusted. This is especially important in patients receiving other medications with anticholinergic effects.

Usage in Geriatrics: The use of SINEQUAN on a once-a-day dosage regimen in geriatric patients should be adjusted carefully based on the patient's condition (see PRECAUTIONS—Geriatric Use).

Usage in Pregnancy: Reproduction studies have been performed in rats, rabbits, monkeys and dogs and there was no evidence of harm to the animal fetus. The relevance to humans is not known. Since there is no experience in pregnant women who have received this drug, safety in pregnancy has not been established. There has been a report of apnea and drowsiness occurring in a nursing infant whose mother was taking SINEQUAN.

Usage in Children: The use of SINEQUAN in children under 12 years of age is not recommended because safe conditions for its use have not been established.

PRECAUTIONS

Drug Interactions: *Drugs Metabolized by P450 2D6:* The biochemical activity of the drug metabolizing isozyme cytochrome P450 2D6 (debrisoquin hydroxylase) is reduced in a subset of the Caucasian population (about 7–10% of Caucasians are so-called "poor metabolizers"); reliable estimates of the prevalence of reduced P450 2D6 isozyme activity among Asian, African and other populations are not yet available. Poor metabolizers have higher than expected plasma concentrations of tricyclic antidepressants (TCAs) when given usual doses. Depending on the fraction of drug metabolized by P450 2D6, the increase in plasma concentration may be small, or quite large (8-fold increase in plasma AUC of the TCA).

In addition, certain drugs inhibit the activity of this isozyme and make normal metabolizers resemble poor metabolizers. An individual who is stable on a given dose of TCA may become abruptly toxic when given one of these inhibiting drugs as concomitant therapy. The drugs that inhibit cytochrome P450 2D6 include some that are not metabolized by the enzyme (quinidine; cimetidine) and many that are substrates for P450 2D6 (many other antidepressants, phenothiazines, and the Type 1C antiarrhythmics propafenone and flecainide). While all the selective serotonin reuptake inhibitors (SSRIs), e.g., fluoxetine, sertraline, and paroxetine, inhibit P450 2D6, they may vary in the extent of inhibition. The extent to which SSRI-TCA interactions may pose clinical problems will depend on the degree of inhibition and the pharmacokinetics of the SSRI involved. Nevertheless, caution is indicated in the co-administration of TCAs with any of the SSRIs and also in switching from one class to the other. Of particular importance, sufficient time must elapse before initiating TCA treatment in a patient being withdrawn from fluoxetine, given the long half-life of the parent and active metabolite (at least 5 weeks may be necessary).

Concomitant use of tricyclic antidepressants with drugs that can inhibit cytochrome P450 2D6 may require lower doses than usually prescribed for either the tricyclic antidepressant or the other drug. Furthermore, whenever one of these other drugs is withdrawn from co-therapy, an increased dose of tricyclic antidepressant may be required. It is desirable to monitor TCA plasma levels whenever a TCA is going to be co-administered with another drug known to be an inhibitor of P450 2D6.

MAO Inhibitors: Serious side effects and even death have been reported following the concomitant use of certain drugs with MAO inhibitors. Therefore, MAO inhibitors should be discontinued at least two weeks prior to the cautious initiation of therapy with SINEQUAN. The exact length of time may vary and is dependent upon the particular MAO inhibitor being used, the length of time it has been administered, and the dosage involved.

Cimetidine: Cimetidine has been reported to produce clinically significant fluctuations in steady-state serum concentrations of various tricyclic antidepressants. Serious anticholinergic symptoms (i.e., severe dry mouth, urinary retention and blurred vision) have been associated with elevations in the serum levels of tricyclic antidepressant when cimetidine therapy is initiated. Additionally, higher than expected tricyclic antidepressant levels have been observed when they are begun in patients already taking cimetidine. In patients who have been reported to be well controlled on tricyclic antidepressants receiving concurrent cimetidine therapy, discontinuation of cimetidine has been reported to decrease established steady-state serum tricyclic antidepressant levels and compromise their therapeutic effects.

Alcohol: It should be borne in mind that alcohol ingestion may increase the danger inherent in any intentional or unintentional SINEQUAN overdosage. This is especially important in patients who may use alcohol excessively.

Tolazamide: A case of severe hypoglycemia has been reported in a type II diabetic patient maintained on tolazamide (1 gm/day) 11 days after the addition of doxepin (75 mg/day).

Drowsiness: Since drowsiness may occur with the use of this drug, patients should be warned of the possibility and cautioned against driving a car or operating dangerous machinery while taking the drug. Patients should also be cautioned that their response to alcohol may be potentiated.

Sedating drugs may cause confusion and oversedation in the elderly; elderly patients generally should be started on low doses of SINEQUAN and observed closely. (See PRECAUTIONS—Geriatric Use.)

Suicide: Since suicide is an inherent risk in any depressed patient and may remain so until significant improvement has occurred, patients should be closely supervised during the early course of therapy. Prescriptions should be written for the smallest feasible amount.

Psychosis: Should increased symptoms of psychosis or shift to manic symptomatology occur, it may be necessary to reduce dosage or add a major tranquilizer to the dosage regimen.

Geriatric Use: A determination has not been made whether controlled clinical studies of SINEQUAN included sufficient numbers of subjects aged 65 and over to define a difference in response from younger subjects. Other reported clinical experience has not identified differences in responses between the elderly and younger patients. In general, dose selection for an elderly patient should be cautious, usually starting at the low end of the dosing range, reflecting the greater frequency of decreased hepatic, renal or cardiac function, and of concomitant disease or other drug therapy.

The extent of renal excretion of SINEQUAN has not been determined. Because elderly patients are more likely to have decreased renal function, care should be taken in dose selections.

Sedating drugs may cause confusion and oversedation in the elderly; elderly patients generally should be started on low doses of SINEQUAN and observed closely. (See WARNINGS.)

ADVERSE REACTIONS

NOTE: Some of the adverse reactions noted below have not been specifically reported with SINEQUAN use. However, due to the close pharmacological similarities among the tricyclics, the reactions should be considered when prescribing SINEQUAN (doxepin HCl).

Anticholinergic Effects: Dry mouth, blurred vision, constipation, and urinary retention have been reported. If they do not subside with continued therapy, or become severe, it may be necessary to reduce the dosage.

Central Nervous System Effects: Drowsiness is the most commonly noticed side effect. This tends to disappear as therapy is continued. Other infrequently reported CNS side effects are confusion, disorientation, hallucinations, numbness, paresthesias, ataxia, extrapyramidal symptoms, seizures, tardive dyskinesia, and tremor.

Cardiovascular: Cardiovascular effects including hypotension, hypertension, and tachycardia have been reported occasionally.

Allergic: Skin rash, edema, photosensitization, and pruritus have occasionally occurred.

Hematologic: Eosinophilia has been reported in a few patients. There have been occasional reports of bone marrow depression manifesting as agranulocytosis, leukopenia, thrombocytopenia, and purpura.

Gastrointestinal: Nausea, vomiting, indigestion, taste disturbances, diarrhea, anorexia, and aphthous stomatitis have been reported. (See Anticholinergic Effects.)

Endocrine: Raised or lowered libido, testicular swelling, gynecomastia in males, enlargement of breasts and galactorrhea in the female, raising or lowering of blood sugar levels, and syndrome of inappropriate antidiuretic hormone secretion have been reported with tricyclic administration.

Other: Dizziness, tinnitus, weight gain, sweating, chills, fatigue, weakness, flushing, jaundice, alopecia, headache, exacerbation of asthma, and hyperpyrexia (in association with chlorpromazine) have been occasionally observed as adverse effects.

Withdrawal Symptoms: The possibility of development of withdrawal symptoms upon abrupt cessation of treatment after prolonged SINEQUAN administration should be borne in mind. These are not indicative of addiction and gradual withdrawal of medication should not cause these symptoms.

DOSAGE AND ADMINISTRATION

For most patients with illness of mild to moderate severity, a starting daily dose of 75 mg is recommended. Dosage may subsequently be increased or decreased at appropriate intervals and according to individual response. The usual optimum dose range is 75 mg/day to 150 mg/day.

In more severely ill patients higher doses may be required with subsequent gradual increase to 300 mg/day if necessary. Additional therapeutic effect is rarely to be obtained by exceeding a dose of 300 mg/day.

In patients with very mild symptomatology or emotional symptoms accompanying organic disease, lower doses may suffice. Some of these patients have been controlled on doses as low as 25–50 mg/day.

The total daily dosage of SINEQUAN may be given on a divided or once-a-day dosage schedule. If the once-a-day schedule is employed, the maximum recommended dose is 150 mg/day. This dose may be given at bedtime. **The 150 mg capsule strength is intended for maintenance therapy only and is not recommended for initiation of treatment.**

Anti-anxiety effect is apparent before the antidepressant effect. Optimal antidepressant effect may not be evident for two to three weeks.

OVERDOSAGE

Deaths may occur from overdosage with this class of drugs. Multiple drug ingestion (including alcohol) is common in deliberate tricyclic antidepressant overdose. As the management is complex and changing, it is recommended that the physician contact a poison control center for current information on treatment. Signs and symptoms of toxicity develop rapidly after tricyclic antidepressant overdose; therefore, hospital monitoring is required as soon as possible.

Manifestations: Critical manifestations of overdose include: cardiac dysrhythmias, severe hypotension, convulsions, and CNS depression, including coma. Changes in the electrocardiogram, particularly in QRS axis or width, are clinically significant indicators of tricyclic antidepressant toxicity.

Other signs of overdose may include: confusion, disturbed concentration, transient visual hallucinations, dilated pupils, agitation, hyperactive reflexes, stupor, drowsiness, muscle rigidity, vomiting, hypothermia, hyperpyrexia, or any of the symptoms listed under ADVERSE REACTIONS.

General Recommendations:

General: Obtain an ECG and immediately initiate cardiac monitoring. Protect the patient's airway, establish an intravenous line and initiate gastric decontamination. A minimum of six hours of observation with cardiac monitoring and observation for signs of CNS or respiratory depression, hypotension, cardiac dysrhythmias and/or conduction blocks, and seizures is strongly advised. If signs of toxicity occur at any time during this period, extended monitoring is recommended. There are case reports of patients succumbing to fatal dysrhythmias late after overdose; these patients had clinical evidence of significant poisoning prior to death and most received inadequate gastrointestinal decontamination. Monitoring of plasma drug levels should not guide management of the patient.

Gastrointestinal Decontamination: All patients suspected of tricyclic antidepressant overdose should receive gastrointestinal decontamination. This should include large volume gastric lavage followed by activated charcoal. If consciousness is impaired, the airway should be secured prior to lavage. Emesis is contraindicated.

Cardiovascular: A maximal limb-lead QRS duration of ≥0.10 seconds may be the best indication of the severity of the overdose. Intravenous sodium bicarbonate should be used to maintain the serum pH in the range of 7.45 to 7.55. If the pH response is inadequate, hyperventilation may also be used. Concomitant use of hyperventilation and sodium bicarbonate should be done with extreme caution, with frequent pH monitoring. A pH>7.60 or a pCO_2 <20 mm Hg is undesirable. Dysrhythmias unresponsive to sodium bicarbonate therapy/hyperventilation may respond to lidocaine, bretylium or phenytoin. Type 1A and 1C antiarrhythmics are generally contraindicated (e.g., quinidine, disopyramide, and procainamide).

In rare instances, hemoperfusion may be beneficial in acute refractory cardiovascular instability in patients with acute toxicity. However, hemodialysis, peritoneal dialysis, exchange transfusions, and forced diuresis generally have been reported as ineffective in tricyclic antidepressant poisoning.

CNS: In patients with CNS depression, early intubation is advised because of the potential for abrupt deterioration. Seizures should be controlled with benzodiazepines, or if these are ineffective, other anticonvulsants (e.g., phenobarbital, phenytoin). Physostigmine is not recommended except to treat life-threatening symptoms that have been unresponsive to other therapies, and then only in consultation with a poison control center.

Psychiatric Follow-up: Since overdosage is often deliberate, patients may attempt suicide by other means during the recovery phase. Psychiatric referral may be appropriate.

Pediatric Management: The principles of management of child and adult overdosages are similar. It is strongly recommended that the physician contact the local poison control center for specific pediatric treatment.

HOW SUPPLIED

SINEQUAN® is available as capsules containing doxepin HCl equivalent to:

10 mg	—100's	(NDC 0049-5340-66)
25 mg	—100's	(NDC 0049-5350-66)
50 mg	—100's	(NDC 0049-5360-66)
	5000's	(NDC 0049-5360-94)
75 mg	—100's	(NDC 0049-5390-66)
100 mg	—100's	(NDC 0049-5380-66)
150 mg	—50's	(NDC 0049-5370-50)

SINEQUAN® Oral Concentrate is available in 120 mL bottles (NDC 0049-5100-47) with an accompanying dropper calibrated at 5 mg, 10 mg, 15 mg, 20 mg, and 25 mg. Each mL contains doxepin HCl equivalent to 10 mg doxepin. Just prior to administration, SINEQUAN® Oral Concentrate should be diluted with approximately 120 mL of water, whole or skimmed milk, or orange, grapefruit, tomato, prune or pineapple juice. SINEQUAN® Oral Concentrate is not physically compatible with a number of carbonated beverages. For those patients requiring antidepressant therapy who are on methadone maintenance, SINEQUAN® Oral Concentrate and methadone syrup can be mixed together with Gatorade®, lemonade, orange juice, sugar water, Tang®, or water; but not with grape juice. Preparation and storage of bulk dilutions is not recommended.

Rx only

Distributed by
Pfizer Roerig
Division of Pfizer Inc, NY, NY 10017

Printed in U.S.A.
69-2135-00-1 Revised April 2000

TROVAN® Tablets ℞
[*trō-văn*]
(trovafloxacin mesylate)
TROVAN® I.V. ℞
(alatrofloxacin mesylate injection)
For Intravenous Infusion

Prescribing information for this product, which appears on pages 2525–2531 of the 2001 PDR, has been completely revised as follows. Please write "See Supplement A" next to the product heading.

TROVAN® HAS BEEN ASSOCIATED WITH SERIOUS LIVER INJURY LEADING TO LIVER TRANSPLANTATION AND/OR DEATH. TROVAN-ASSOCIATED LIVER INJURY HAS BEEN REPORTED WITH BOTH SHORT-TERM AND LONG-TERM DRUG EXPOSURE. TROVAN USE EXCEEDING 2 WEEKS IN DURATION IS ASSOCIATED WITH A SIGNIFICANTLY INCREASED RISK OF SERIOUS LIVER INJURY. LIVER INJURY HAS ALSO BEEN REPORTED FOLLOWING TROVAN RE-EXPOSURE. TROVAN SHOULD BE RESERVED FOR USE IN PATIENTS WITH SERIOUS, LIFE- OR LIMB-THREATENING INFECTIONS WHO RECEIVE THEIR INITIAL THERAPY IN AN IN-PATIENT HEALTH CARE FACILITY (I.E., HOSPITAL OR LONG-TERM NURSING CARE FACILITY). TROVAN SHOULD NOT BE USED WHEN SAFER, ALTERNATIVE ANTIMICROBIAL THERAPY WILL BE EFFECTIVE. (SEE WARNINGS.)

TROVAN® is available as TROVAN Tablets (trovafloxacin mesylate) for oral administration and as TROVAN I.V. (alatrofloxacin mesylate injection), a prodrug of trovafloxacin, for intravenous administration.

DESCRIPTION

TROVAN Tablets

TROVAN Tablets contain trovafloxacin mesylate, a synthetic broad-spectrum antibacterial agent for oral administration. Chemically, trovafloxacin mesylate, a fluoronaphthyridone related to the fluoroquinolone antibacterials, is (1α, 5α, 6α)-7-(6-amino-3-azabicyclo[3.1.0]hex-3-yl)-1-(2,4-difluorophenyl)-6-fluoro-1,4-dihydro-4-oxo-1,8-naphthyridine-3-carboxylic acid, monomethanesulfonate. Trovafloxacin mesylate differs from other quinolone derivatives by having a 1,8-naphthyridine nucleus.

The chemical structure is:

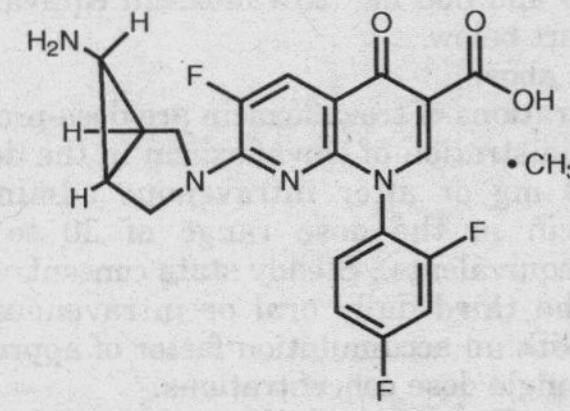

Its empirical formula is $C_{20}H_{15}F_3N_4O_3 \bullet CH_3SO_3H$ and its molecular weight is 512.46.

Trovafloxacin mesylate is a white to off-white powder.

Trovafloxacin mesylate is available in 100 mg and 200 mg (trovafloxacin equivalent) blue, film-coated tablets. TROVAN Tablets contain microcrystalline cellulose, cross-linked sodium carboxymethylcellulose and magnesium stearate. The tablet coating is a mixture of hydroxypropylcellulose, hydroxypropylmethylcellulose, titanium dioxide, polyethylene glycol and FD&C blue #2 aluminum lake.

TROVAN I.V.

TROVAN I.V. contains alatrofloxacin mesylate, the L-alanyl-L-alanyl prodrug of trovafloxacin mesylate. Chemically, alatrofloxacin mesylate is (1α, 5α, 6α)-L-alanyl-*N*-[3-[6-carboxy-8-(2,4-difluorophenyl)-3-fluoro-5,8-dihydro-5-oxo-1,8-naphthyridine-2-yl]-3-azabicyclo[3.1.0]hex-6-yl]-L-alaninamide, monomethanesulfonate. It is intended for administration by intravenous infusion.

Following intravenous administration, the alanine substituents in alatrofloxacin are rapidly hydrolyzed *in vivo* to yield trovafloxacin. (See CLINICAL PHARMACOLOGY.)

The chemical structure is:

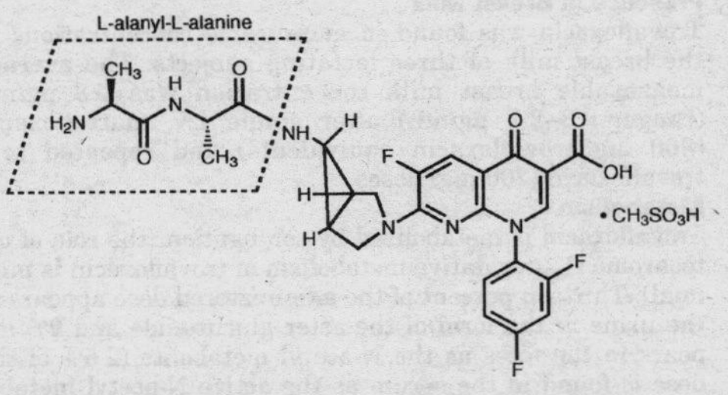

Its empirical formula is $C_{26}H_{25}F_3N_6O_5 \bullet CH_3SO_3H$ and its molecular weight is 654.62.

Alatrofloxacin mesylate is a white to light yellow powder.

TROVAN I.V. is available in 40 mL and 60 mL single use vials as a sterile, preservative-free aqueous concentrate of 5 mg trovafloxacin/mL as alatrofloxacin mesylate intended for dilution prior to intravenous administration of doses of 200 mg or 300 mg of trovafloxacin, respectively. (See **HOW SUPPLIED.**)

The formulation contains Water for Injection, and may contain sodium hydroxide or hydrochloric acid for pH adjustment. The pH range for the 5 mg/mL aqueous concentrate is 3.5 to 4.3.

CLINICAL PHARMACOLOGY

After intravenous administration, alatrofloxacin is rapidly converted to trovafloxacin. Plasma concentrations of alatrofloxacin are below quantifiable levels within 5 to 10 minutes of completion of a 1 hour infusion.

Absorption

Trovafloxacin is well-absorbed from the gastrointestinal tract after oral administration. The absolute bioavailability is approximately 88%. For comparable dosages, no dosage adjustment is necessary when switching from parenteral to oral administration (Figure 1). (See **DOSAGE AND ADMINISTRATION.**)

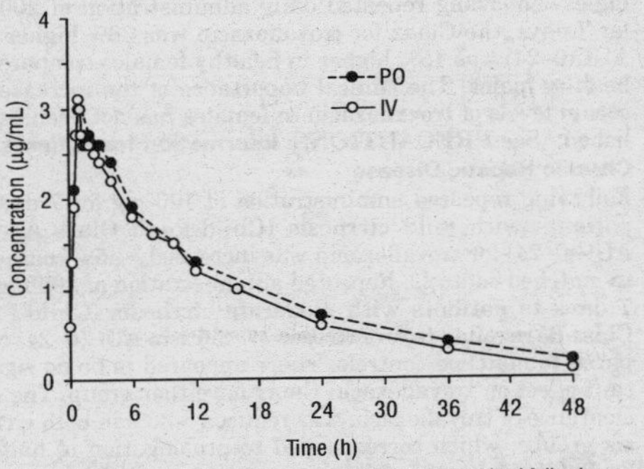

Figure 1. Mean trovafloxacin serum concentrations determined following 1 hour intravenous infusions of alatrofloxacin at daily doses of 200 mg (trovafloxacin equivalents) to healthy male volunteers and following daily oral administration of 200 mg trovafloxacin for 7 days to six male and six female healthy young volunteers.

Continued on next page

Trovan—Cont.

Pharmacokinetics
The mean pharmacokinetic parameters (±SD) of trovafloxacin after single and multiple 100 mg and 200 mg oral doses and 1 hour intravenous infusions of alatrofloxacin in doses of 200 and 300 mg (trovafloxacin equivalents) appear in the chart below.
[See first table above]

Serum concentrations of trovafloxacin are dose-proportional after oral administration of trovafloxacin in the dose range of 30 to 1000 mg or after intravenous administration of alatrofloxacin in the dose range of 30 to 400 mg (trovafloxacin equivalents). Steady state concentrations are achieved by the third daily oral or intravenous dose of trovafloxacin with an accumulation factor of approximately 1.3 times the single dose concentrations.

Oral absorption of trovafloxacin is not altered by concomitant food intake; therefore, it can be administered without regard to food.

The systemic exposure to trovafloxacin ($AUC_{0-\infty}$) administered as crushed tablets via nasogastric tube into the stomach was identical to that of orally administered intact tablets. Administration of concurrent enteral feeding solutions had no effect on the absorption of trovafloxacin given via nasogastric tube into the stomach. When trovafloxacin was administered as crushed tablets into the duodenum via nasogastric tube, the $AUC_{0-\infty}$ and peak serum concentration (C_{max}) were reduced by 30% relative to the orally administered intact tablets. Time to peak serum level (T_{max}) was also decreased from 1.7 hrs to 1.1 hrs.

Distribution
The mean plasma protein bound fraction is approximately 76%, and is concentration-independent. Trovafloxacin is widely distributed throughout the body. Rapid distribution of trovafloxacin into tissues results in significantly higher trovafloxacin concentrations in most target tissues than in plasma or serum.
[See second table above]

Presence in Breast Milk
Trovafloxacin was found in measurable concentrations in the breast milk of three lactating subjects. The average measurable breast milk concentration was 0.8 µg/mL (range: 0.3–2.1 µg/mL) after single I.V. alatrofloxacin (300 mg trovafloxacin equivalents) and repeated oral trovafloxacin (200 mg) doses.

Metabolism
Trovafloxacin is metabolized by conjugation (the role of cytochrome P_{450} oxidative metabolism of trovafloxacin is minimal). Thirteen percent of the administered dose appears in the urine in the form of the ester glucuronide and 9% appears in the feces as the N-acetyl metabolite (2.5% of the dose is found in the serum as the active N-acetyl metabolite). Other minor metabolites (diacid, sulfamate, hydroxycarboxylic acid) have been identified in both urine and feces in small amounts (<4% of the administered dose).

Excretion
Approximately 50% of an oral dose is excreted unchanged (43% in the feces and 6% in the urine).
After multiple 200 mg doses, to healthy subjects, mean (±SD) cumulative urinary trovafloxacin concentrations were 12.1±3.4 µg/mL. With these levels of trovafloxacin in urine, crystals of trovafloxacin have not been observed in the urine of human subjects.

Special Populations
Geriatric
In adult subjects, the pharmacokinetics of trovafloxacin are not affected by age (range 19–78 years).
Pediatric
Limited information is available in the pediatric population (see **Distribution**). The pharmacokinetics of trovafloxacin have not been fully characterized in pediatric populations less than 18 years of age.
Gender
There are no significant differences in trovafloxacin pharmacokinetics between males and females when differences in body weight are taken into account. After single 200 mg doses, trovafloxacin Cmax and AUC(0–∞) were 60% and 32% higher, respectively, in healthy females compared to healthy males. Following repeated daily administration of 200 mg for 7 days, the Cmax for trovafloxacin was 38% higher and AUC(0–24) was 16% higher in healthy females compared to healthy males. The clinical importance of the increases in serum levels of trovafloxacin in females has not been established. (See **PRECAUTIONS: Information for Patients.**)

Chronic Hepatic Disease
Following repeated administration of 100 mg for 7 days to patients with mild cirrhosis (Child-Pugh Class A), the AUC(0–24) for trovafloxacin was increased ~45% compared to matched controls. Repeated administration of 200 mg for 7 days to patients with moderate cirrhosis (Child-Pugh Class B) resulted in an increase of ~50% in AUC(0–24) compared to matched controls. There appeared to be no significant effect on trovafloxacin Cmax for either group. The oral clearance of trovafloxacin was reduced ~30% in both cirrhosis groups, which corresponded to prolongation of half-life by 2–2.5 hours (25–30% increase) compared to controls. There are no data in patients with severe cirrhosis (Child-Pugh Class C). Dosage adjustment is recommended in patients with mild to moderate cirrhosis. (See **DOSAGE AND ADMINISTRATION**.)

Renal Insufficiency
The pharmacokinetics of trovafloxacin are not affected by renal impairment. Trovafloxacin serum concentrations are not significantly altered in subjects with severe renal insufficiency (creatinine clearance <20 mL/min), including patients on hemodialysis.

Photosensitivity Potential
In a study of the skin response to ultraviolet and visible radiation conducted in 48 healthy volunteers (12 per group), the minimum erythematous dose (MED) was measured for ciprofloxacin, lomefloxacin, trovafloxacin and placebo before and after drug administration for 5 days. In this study, trovafloxacin (200 mg q.d.) was shown to have a lower potential for producing delayed photosensitivity skin reactions than ciprofloxacin (500 mg b.i.d.) or lomefloxacin (400 mg q.d.), although greater than placebo. (See **PRECAUTIONS: Information for Patients.**)

Drug-drug Interactions
The systemic availability of trovafloxacin following oral tablet administration is significantly reduced by the concomitant administration of antacids containing aluminum and magnesium salts, sucralfate, vitamins or minerals containing iron, and concomitant intravenous morphine administration.

Administration of trovafloxacin (300 mg p.o.) 30 minutes after administration of an antacid containing magnesium hydroxide and aluminum hydroxide resulted in reductions in systemic exposure to trovafloxacin (AUC) of 66% and peak serum concentration (Cmax) of 60%. (See **PRECAUTIONS: Drug Interactions, DOSAGE AND ADMINISTRATION.**)

Concomitant sucralfate administration (1g) with trovafloxacin 200 mg p.o. resulted in a 70% decrease in trovafloxacin systemic exposure (AUC) and a 77% reduction in peak serum concentration (Cmax). (See **PRECAUTIONS: Drug Interactions, DOSAGE AND ADMINISTRATION.**)

Concomitant administration of ferrous sulfate (120 mg elemental iron) with trovafloxacin 200 mg p.o. resulted in a 40% reduction in trovafloxacin systemic exposure (AUC) and a 48% decrease in trovafloxacin Cmax. (See **PRECAUTIONS: Drug Interactions, DOSAGE AND ADMINISTRATION.**)

Concomitant administration of intravenous morphine (0.15 mg/kg) with oral trovafloxacin (200 mg) resulted in a

TROVAFLOXACIN PHARMACOKINETIC PARAMETERS

	C_{max} (µg/mL)	T_{max} (hrs)	$AUC^{1,2}$ (µg•h/mL)	$T_{1/2}$ (hrs)	Vd_{ss} (L/Kg)	CL (mL/hr/Kg)	CL_r (mL/hr/Kg)
Trovafloxacin 100 mg							
Single dose	1.0±0.3	0.9±0.4	11.2±2.2	9.1	—	—	—
Multiple dose	1.1±0.2	1.0±0.5	11.8±1.8	10.5	—	—	—
Trovafloxacin 200 mg							
Single dose	2.1±0.5	1.8±0.9	26.7±7.5	9.6	—	—	—
Multiple dose	3.1±1.0	1.2±0.5	34.4±5.7	12.2	—	—	—
Alatrofloxacin 200 mg*							
Single dose	2.7±0.4	1.0±0.0	28.1±5.1	9.4	1.2±0.2	93.0±17.4	6.5±3.5
Multiple dose	3.1±0.6	1.0±0.0	32.2±7.3	11.7	1.3±0.1	81.7±17.8	8.6±2.4
Alatrofloxacin 300 mg*							
Single dose	3.6±0.6	1.3±0.4	46.1±5.2	11.2	1.2±0.1	84.6±6.0	6.9±0.5
Multiple dose	4.4±0.6	1.2±0.2	46.3±3.9	12.7	1.4±0.1	84.5±11.1	8.4±1.8

* trovafloxacin equivalents
[1,2] Single dose: AUC(0—∞), multiple dose: AUC(0—24)
C_{max}= Maximum serum concentration; T_{max}=Time to C_{max}; AUC=Area under concentration vs. time curve; $T_{1/2}$=serum half-life; Vd_{ss}=Volume of distribution; CL=Total clearance; CL_r=Renal clearance

Fluid or Tissue	Tissue-Fluid/Serum Ratio* (Range)
Respiratory	
bronchial macrophages	
(multiple dose)	24.1 (9.6–41.8)
lung mucosa	1.1 (0.7–1.5)
lung epithelial lining fluid	
(multiple dose)	5.8 (1.1–17.5)
whole lung	2.1 (0.42–5.03)
Skin, Musculoskeletal	
skin	1.0 (0.20–1.88)
subcutaneous tissue	0.4 (0.15–0.68)
skin blister fluid	0.7–0.9 (blister/plasma)
skeletal muscle	1.5 (0.50–2.90)
bone	1.0 (0.55–1.67)
Gastrointestinal	
colonic tissue	0.7 (0.0–1.47)
peritoneal fluid	0.4 (0.0–1.25)
bile	15.4 (11.9–21.0)
Central Nervous System	
cerebrospinal fluid (CSF), adults	0.25 (0.03–0.33)
cerebrospinal fluid (CSF), children	0.28**
Reproductive	
prostatic tissue	1.0 (0.5–1.6)
cervix (multiple dose)	0.6 (0.5–0.7)
ovary	1.6 (0.3–2.2)
fallopian tube	0.7 (0.2–1.1)
myometrium (multiple dose)	0.6 (0.4–0.8)
uterus	0.6 (0.3–0.8)
vaginal fluid (multiple dose)	4.7 (0.8–20.8)

*Mean values in adults over 2–29 hours following drug administration, except individual lung tissues, which were single time points of 6 hours following drug administration
**Ratio of composite AUC(0–24) in CSF/composite AUC (0–24) in serum in 22 pediatric patients aged 1 to 12 years after 1 hour I.V. infusion of single dose alatrofloxacin (equivalent trovafloxacin dose range: 4.5–9.9 mg/kg)

36% reduction in trovafloxacin AUC and a 46% decrease in trovafloxacin Cmax. Trovafloxacin administration had no effect on the pharmacokinetics of morphine or its pharmacologically active metabolite, morphine-6-β-glucuronide. (See **PRECAUTIONS: Drug Interactions, DOSAGE AND ADMINISTRATION.**)

Minor pharmacokinetic interactions that are most likely without clinical significance include calcium carbonate, omeprazole and caffeine.

Concomitant administration of calcium carbonate (1000 mg) with trovafloxacin 200 mg p.o. resulted in a 20% reduction in trovafloxacin AUC and a 17% reduction in peak serum trovafloxacin concentration (Cmax).

A 40 mg dose of omeprazole given 2 hours prior to trovafloxacin (300 mg p.o.) resulted in a 17% reduction in trovafloxacin AUC and a 17% reduction in trovafloxacin peak serum concentration (Cmax).

Administration of trovafloxacin (200 mg) concomitantly with caffeine (200 mg) resulted in a 17% increase in caffeine AUC and a 15% increase in caffeine Cmax. These changes in caffeine exposure are not considered clinically significant.

No significant pharmacokinetic interactions were seen when TROVAN was co-administered with cimetidine, theophylline, digoxin, warfarin and cyclosporine.

Cimetidine co-administration (400 mg twice daily for 5 days) with trovafloxacin (200 mg p.o. daily for 3 days) resulted in changes in trovafloxacin AUC and Cmax of less than 5%.

Trovafloxacin (200 mg p.o. daily for 7 days) co-administration with theophylline (300 mg twice daily for 14 days) resulted in no change in theophylline AUC and Cmax.

Trovafloxacin (200 mg p.o. daily for 10 days) co-administration with digoxin (0.25 mg daily for 20 days) did not significantly alter systemic exposure (AUC) to digoxin or the renal clearance of digoxin.

Trovafloxacin (200 mg p.o. daily for 7 days) did not interfere with either the pharmacokinetics or the pharmacodynamics of warfarin (daily for 21 days).

Concomitant oral administration of trovafloxacin did not affect the systemic exposure (AUC) or peak plasma concentrations (Cmax) of the S or R isomers of warfarin, nor did it influence prothrombin times. (See **PRECAUTIONS: Drug Interactions.**)

Trovafloxacin (200 mg p.o. daily for 7 days) co-administration with cyclosporine (daily doses from 150–450 mg for 7 days) resulted in decreases of 10% or less in systemic exposure to cyclosporine (AUC) and in the peak blood concentrations of cyclosporine.

Microbiology

Trovafloxacin is a fluoronaphthyridone related to the fluoroquinolones with *in vitro* activity against a wide range of gram-negative and gram-positive aerobic, and anaerobic microorganisms. The bactericidal action of trovafloxacin results from inhibition of DNA gyrase and topoisomerase IV. DNA gyrase is an essential enzyme that is involved in the replication, transcription and repair of bacterial DNA. Topoisomerase IV is an enzyme known to play a key role in the partitioning of the chromosomal DNA during bacterial cell division. Mechanism of action of fluoroquinolones including trovafloxacin is different from that of penicillins, cephalosporins, aminoglycosides, macrolides, and tetracyclines. Therefore, fluoroquinolones may be active against pathogens that are resistant to these antibiotics. There is no cross-resistance between trovafloxacin and the mentioned classes of antibiotics. The overall results obtained from *in vitro* synergy studies, testing combinations of trovafloxacin with beta-lactams and aminoglycosides, indicate that synergy is strain specific and not commonly encountered. This agrees with results obtained previously with other fluoroquinolones. Resistance to trovafloxacin *in vitro* develops slowly via multiple-step mutation in a manner similar to other fluoroquinolones. Resistance to trovafloxacin *in vitro* occurs at a general frequency of between 1×10^{-7} to 10^{-10}. Although cross-resistance has been observed between trovafloxacin and some other fluoroquinolones, some microorganisms resistant to other fluoroquinolones may be susceptible to trovafloxacin.

Trovafloxacin has been shown to be active against most strains of the following microorganisms, both *in vitro* and in clinical infections as described in the **INDICATIONS AND USAGE** section:

Aerobic gram-positive microorganisms
Enterococcus faecalis (many strains are only moderately susceptible)
Staphylococcus aureus (methicillin-susceptible strains)
Streptococcus agalactiae
Streptococcus pneumoniae (penicillin-susceptible strains)
Viridans group streptococci
Aerobic gram-negative microorganisms
Escherichia coli
Gardnerella vaginalis
Haemophilus influenzae
Klebsiella pneumoniae
Moraxella catarrhalis
Proteus mirabilis
Pseudomonas aeruginosa
Anaerobic microorganisms
Bacteroides fragilis
Peptostreptococcus species
Prevotella species
Other microorganisms
Chlamydia pneumoniae
Legionella pneumophila
Mycoplasma pneumoniae

Microorganism	MIC Range (μg/mL)
Escherichia coli ATCC 25922	0.004–0.016
Staphylococcus aureus ATCC 29213	0.008–0.03
Pseudomonas aeruginosa ATCC 27853	0.25–2.0
Enterococcus faecalis ATCC 29212	0.06–0.25
Haemophilus influenzae[d] ATCC 49247	0.004–0.016
Streptococcus pneumoniae[e] ATCC 49619	0.06–0.25

[d]This quality control range is applicable to only *H. influenzae* ATCC 49247 tested by a microdilution procedure using HTM[1].
[e]This quality control range is applicable to only *S. pneumoniae* ATCC 49619 tested by a microdilution procedure using cation-adjusted Mueller-Hinton broth with 2–5% lysed horse blood.

The following *in vitro* data are available, **but their clinical significance is unknown.**

Trovafloxacin exhibits *in vitro* minimum inhibitory concentrations (MICs) of ≤2 μg/mL against most (90%) strains of the following microorganisms; however, the safety and effectiveness of trovafloxacin in treating clinical infections due to these microorganisms have not been established in adequate and well-controlled clinical trials.

Aerobic gram-positive microorganisms
Streptococcus pneumoniae (penicillin-resistant strains)
Aerobic gram-negative microorganisms
Citrobacter freundii
Enterobacter aerogenes
Morganella morganii
Proteus vulgaris
Anaerobic microorganisms
Bacteroides distasonis
Bacteroides ovatus
Clostridium perfringens
Other microorganisms
Mycoplasma hominis
Ureaplasma urealyticum

NOTE: *Mycobacterium tuberculosis* and *Mycobacterium avium-intracellulare* complex organisms are commonly resistant to trovafloxacin.

NOTE: The activity of trovafloxacin against *Treponema pallidum* has not been evaluated; however, other quinolones are not active against *Treponema pallidum*. (See **WARNINGS**.)

Susceptibility Tests:
Dilution Techniques: Quantitative methods are used to determine antimicrobial minimum inhibitory concentrations (MICs). These MICs provide estimates of the susceptibility of bacteria to antimicrobial compounds. The MICs should be determined using a standardized procedure. Standardized procedures are based on dilution methods[1] (broth or agar) or equivalent with standardized inoculum concentrations and standardized concentrations of trovafloxacin mesylate powder. The MIC values should be interpreted according to the following criteria:

For testing non-fastidious aerobic organisms:

MIC (μg/mL)	Interpretation
≤2.0	Susceptible (S)
4.0	Intermediate (I)
≥8.0	Resistant (R)

For testing *Haemophilus* spp.[a]:

MIC (μg/mL)	Interpretation[b]
≤1.0	Susceptible (S)

[a]This interpretive standard is applicable only to broth microdilution susceptibility tests with *Haemophilus* spp. using Haemophilus Test Medium (HTM)[1].
[b]The current absence of data on resistant strains precludes defining any results other than "Susceptible". Strains yielding MIC results suggestive of a "nonsusceptible" category should be submitted to a reference laboratory for further testing.

For testing *Streptococcus* spp. including *Streptococcus pneumoniae*[c]:

MIC (μg/mL)	Interpretation
≤1.0	Susceptible (S)
2.0	Intermediate (I)
≥4.0	Resistant (R)

[c]These interpretive standards are applicable only to broth microdilution susceptibility tests using cation-adjusted Mueller-Hinton broth with 2–5% lysed horse blood.

A report of "Susceptible" indicates that the pathogen is likely to be inhibited if the antimicrobial compound in the blood reaches the concentration usually achievable. A report of "Intermediate" indicates that the result should be considered equivocal, and, if the microorganism is not fully susceptible to alternative, clinically feasible drugs, the test should be repeated. This category implies possible clinical applicability in body sites where the drug is physiologically concentrated or in situations where high dosage of drug can be used. This category also provides a buffer zone which prevents small uncontrolled technical factors from causing major discrepancies in interpretation. A report of "Resistant" indicates that the pathogen is not likely to be inhibited if the antimicrobial compound in the blood reaches the concentration usually achievable; other therapy should be selected.

Standardized susceptibility test procedures require the use of laboratory control microorganisms to control the technical aspects of the laboratory procedures. Standard trovafloxacin mesylate powder should provide the following MIC values:
[See table above]

Diffusion Techniques: Quantitative methods that require measurement of zone diameters also provide reproducible estimates of the susceptibility of bacteria to antimicrobial compounds. One such standardized procedure[2] requires the use of standardized inoculum concentrations. This procedure

---

uses paper disks impregnated with trovafloxacin mesylate equivalent to 10 μg trovafloxacin to test the susceptibility of microorganisms to trovafloxacin.

Reports from the laboratory providing results of the standard single-disk susceptibility test with a trovafloxacin mesylate disk (equivalent to 10 μg trovafloxacin) should be interpreted according to the following criteria:

The following zone diameter interpretive criteria should be used for testing non-fastidious aerobic organisms:

Zone Diameter (mm)	Interpretation
≥17	Susceptible (S)
14–16	Intermediate (I)
≤13	Resistant (R)

For testing *Haemophilus* spp.[f]:

Zone Diameter (mm)	Interpretation[g]
≥22	Susceptible (S)

[f]This zone diameter standard is applicable only to tests with *Haemophilus* spp. using HTM[2].
[g]The current absence of data on resistant strains precludes defining any results other than "Susceptible". Strains yielding MIC results suggestive of a "nonsusceptible" category should be submitted to a reference laboratory for further testing.

For testing *Streptococcus* spp. including *Streptococcus pneumoniae*[h]:

Zone Diameter (mm)	Interpretation
≥19	Susceptible (S)
18–16	Intermediate (I)
≤15	Resistant (R)

[h]These zone diameter standards only apply to tests performed using Mueller-Hinton agar supplemented with 5% sheep blood incubated in 5% CO_2.

Interpretation should be as stated above for results using dilution techniques. Interpretation involves correlation of the diameter obtained in the disk test with the MIC for trovafloxacin.

As with standardized dilution techniques, diffusion methods require the use of laboratory control microorganisms that are used to control the technical aspects of the laboratory procedures. For the diffusion technique, the trovafloxacin mesylate equivalent to 10-μg trovafloxacin disk should provide the following zone diameters in these laboratory quality control strains:
[See table at top of next page]

Anaerobic Techniques: For anaerobic bacteria, the susceptibility to trovafloxacin as MICs can be determined by standardized test methods[3]. The MIC values obtained should be interpreted according to the following criteria:

MIC (μg/mL)	Interpretation
≤2.0	Susceptible (S)
4.0	Intermediate (I)
≥8.0	Resistant (R)

Interpretation is identical to that stated above for results using dilution techniques.

As with other susceptibility techniques, the use of laboratory control microorganisms is required to control the technical aspects of the laboratory standardized procedures. Standardized trovafloxacin mesylate powder should provide the following MIC values:

Microorganism	MIC[k] (μg/mL)
Bacteroides fragilis ATCC 25285	0.125–0.5
Bacteroides thetaiotamicron ATCC 29741	0.25–1.0
Eubacterium lentum ATCC 43055	0.25–1.0

[k]These quality control ranges were derived from tests performed in the broth formulation of Wilkins-Chalgren agar.

INDICATIONS AND USAGE

TROVAN is indicated for the treatment of patients initiating therapy in in-patient health care facilities (i.e., hospitals and long term nursing care facilities) with serious, life- or limb-threatening infections caused by susceptible strains of the designated microorganisms in the conditions listed below. (See **DOSAGE AND ADMINISTRATION**.)

Nosocomial pneumonia caused by *Escherichia coli*, *Pseudomonas aeruginosa*, *Haemophilus influenzae*, or *Staphylococcus aureus*. As with other antimicrobials, where *Pseudomonas aeruginosa* is a documented or presumptive pathogen, combination therapy with either an aminoglycoside or aztreonam may be clinically indicated.

Community acquired pneumonia caused by *Streptococcus pneumoniae*, *Haemophilus influenzae*, *Klebsiella pneumoniae*, *Staphylococcus aureus*, *Mycoplasma pneumoniae*, *Moraxella catarrhalis*, *Legionella pneumophila*, or *Chlamydia pneumoniae*.

Continued on next page

Trovan—Cont.

Microorganism	Zone Diameter Range (mm)
Escherichia coli ATCC 25922	29–36
Staphylococcus aureus ATCC 25923	29–35
Pseudomonas aeruginosa ATCC 27853	21–27
Haemophilus influenzae[i] ATCC 49247	32–39
Streptococcus pneumoniae[j] ATCC 49619	25–32

[i] This quality control limit applies to tests conducted with *Haemophilus influenzae* ATCC 49247 using HTM[2].
[j] This quality control range is applicable only to tests performed by disk diffusion using Mueller-Hinton agar supplemented with 5% defibrinated sheep blood.

Complicated intra-abdominal infections, including post-surgical infections caused by *Escherichia coli, Bacteroides fragilis,* viridans group streptococci, *Pseudomonas aeruginosa, Klebsiella pneumoniae, Peptostreptococcus* species, or *Prevotella species.*
Gynecologic and pelvic infections including endomyometritis, parametritis, septic abortion and post-partum infections caused by *Escherichia coli, Bacteroides fragilis,* viridans group streptococci, *Enterococcus faecalis, Streptococcus agalactiae, Peptostreptococcus* species, *Prevotella* species, or *Gardnerella vaginalis.*
Complicated skin and skin structure infections, including diabetic foot infections, caused by *Staphylococcus aureus, Streptococcus agalactiae, Pseudomonas aeruginosa, Enterococcus faecalis, Escherichia coli,* or *Proteus mirabilis.* **NOTE:** TROVAN has not been studied in the treatment of osteomyelitis. (See **WARNINGS.**)

CONTRAINDICATIONS

TROVAN is contraindicated in persons with a history of hypersensitivity to trovafloxacin, alatrofloxacin, quinolone antimicrobial agents or any other components of these products.

WARNINGS

(See boxed **WARNING.**) **TROVAN-ASSOCIATED LIVER ENZYME ABNORMALITIES, SYMPTOMATIC HEPATITIS, JAUNDICE, AND LIVER FAILURE (INCLUDING RARE REPORTS OF ACUTE HEPATIC NECROSIS WITH EOSINOPHILIC INFILTRATION, LIVER TRANSPLANTATION AND/OR DEATH) HAVE BEEN REPORTED WITH BOTH SHORT-TERM AND LONG-TERM DRUG EXPOSURE IN MEN AND WOMEN. TROVAN USE EXCEEDING 2 WEEKS IN DURATION IS ASSOCIATED WITH A SIGNIFICANTLY INCREASED RISK OF SERIOUS LIVER INJURY. LIVER INJURY HAS ALSO BEEN REPORTED FOLLOWING TROVAN RE-EXPOSURE. CLINICIANS SHOULD MONITOR LIVER FUNCTION TESTS (e.g., AST, ALT, BILIRUBIN) IN TROVAN RECIPIENTS WHO DEVELOP SIGNS OR SYMPTOMS CONSISTENT WITH HEPATITIS. CLINICIANS SHOULD CONSIDER DISCONTINUING TROVAN IN THOSE PATIENTS WHO DEVELOP LIVER FUNCTION TEST ABNORMALITIES.**
THE SAFETY AND EFFECTIVENESS OF TROVAFLOXACIN IN PEDIATRIC PATIENTS AND ADOLESCENTS LESS THAN 18 YEARS OF AGE, PREGNANT WOMEN, AND NURSING WOMEN HAVE NOT BEEN ESTABLISHED. (See **PRECAUTIONS: Pediatric Use, Pregnancy,** and **Nursing Mothers** subsections.)
As with other members of the quinolone class, trovafloxacin has caused arthropathy and/or chondrodysplasia in immature rats and dogs. The significance of these findings to humans is unknown. (See **ANIMAL PHARMACOLOGY.**)
Convulsions, increased intracranial pressure and psychosis have been reported in patients receiving quinolones. Quinolones may also cause central nervous system stimulation which may lead to tremors, restlessness, lightheadedness, confusion, hallucinations, paranoia, depression, nightmares and insomnia. These reactions may occur following the first dose. If these reactions occur in patients receiving trovafloxacin or alatrofloxacin, the drug should be discontinued and appropriate measures instituted. (See **PRECAUTIONS: General, Information for Patients, Drug Interactions** and **ADVERSE REACTIONS.**)
As with other quinolones, TROVAN should be used with caution in patients with known or suspected CNS disorders, such as severe cerebral atherosclerosis, epilepsy, and other factors that predispose to seizures. (See **ADVERSE REACTIONS.**)
Serious and occasionally fatal hypersensitivity and/or anaphylactic reactions have been reported in patients receiving therapy with TROVAN. These reactions may occur following the first dose. Some reactions have been accompanied by cardiovascular collapse, hypotension/shock, seizure, loss of consciousness, tingling, angioedema (including tongue, laryngeal, throat or facial edema/swelling), airway obstruction (including bronchospasm, shortness of breath and acute respiratory distress), dyspnea, urticaria, itching and other serious skin reactions, including generalized erythema.
Life-threatening hypotension has been reported with alatrofloxacin administration. This has occurred in patients receiving alatrofloxacin at either the recommended rate of infusion or if given more rapidly. Hypotension may be potentiated with the concomitant administration of anesthetic agents. Alatrofloxacin should only be administered by slow intravenous infusion over a period of 60 minutes. Blood pressure should be monitored closely during infusion.
TROVAN should be discontinued at the first appearance of a skin rash or any other sign of hypersensitivity. Serious acute hypersensitivity reactions may require treatment with epinephrine and other resuscitative measures, including oxygen, intravenous fluids, antihistamines, corticosteroids, pressor amines and airway management, as clinically indicated. (See **PRECAUTIONS** and **ADVERSE REACTIONS.**)
Serious and sometimes fatal events, some due to hypersensitivity and some due to uncertain etiology, have been reported in patients receiving therapy with all antibiotics. These events may be severe and generally occur following the administration of multiple doses. Clinical manifestations may include one or more of the following: fever, rash or severe dermatologic reactions (e.g., toxic epidermal necrolysis, Stevens-Johnson Syndrome); vasculitis, arthralgia, myalgia, serum sickness; allergic pneumonitis, interstitial nephritis; acute renal insufficiency or failure; hepatitis, jaundice, acute hepatic necrosis or failure; anemia, including hemolytic and aplastic; thrombocytopenia, including thrombotic thrombocytopenic purpura; leukopenia; agranulocytosis; pancytopenia; and/or other hematologic abnormalities.
Pseudomembranous colitis has been reported with nearly all antibacterial agents, including TROVAN, and may range in severity from mild to life-threatening. Therefore, it is important to consider this diagnosis in patients who present with diarrhea subsequent to the administration of any antibacterial agent.
Treatment with antibacterial agents alters the flora of the colon and may permit overgrowth of clostridia. Studies indicate that a toxin produced by *Clostridium difficile* is the primary cause of "antibiotic-associated colitis."
After the diagnosis of pseudomembranous colitis has been established, therapeutic measures should be initiated. Mild cases of pseudomembranous colitis usually respond to drug discontinuation alone. In moderate to severe cases, consideration should be given to management with fluids and electrolytes, protein supplementation, and treatment with an antibacterial drug clinically effective against *C. difficile* colitis. (See **ADVERSE REACTIONS.**)
Although not seen in TROVAN clinical trials, ruptures of the shoulder, hand, and Achilles tendons that required surgical repair or resulted in prolonged disability have been reported in patients receiving quinolones. TROVAN should be discontinued if the patient experiences pain, inflammation or rupture of a tendon. Patients should rest and refrain from exercise until the diagnosis of tendinitis or tendon rupture has been confidently excluded. Tendon rupture can occur during or after therapy with quinolones.
Trovafloxacin has not been shown to be effective in the treatment of syphilis. Antimicrobial agents used in high doses for short periods of time to treat gonorrhea may mask or delay the symptoms of incubating syphilis. All patients with gonorrhea should have a serologic test for syphilis at the time of diagnosis.

PRECAUTIONS

General:
Moderate to severe phototoxicity reactions have been observed in patients who are exposed to direct sunlight while receiving some drugs in this class. Therapy should be discontinued if phototoxicity (e.g., a skin eruption, etc.) occurs.
The safety and efficacy of TROVAN in patients with severe cirrhosis (Child-Pugh Class C) have not been studied.
Symptomatic pancreatitis has been reported on therapy. Clinicians should monitor pancreatic tests in patients who develop symptoms consistent with pancreatitis as clinically indicated.
Because a rapid or bolus intravenous injection may result in life-threatening hypotension, alatrofloxacin should only be administered by slow intravenous infusion over a period of 60 minutes. Profound hypotension has also been reported in patients receiving alatrofloxacin at the recommended rate of infusion. (See **WARNINGS** and **DOSAGE AND ADMINISTRATION: Intravenous Administration.**)
Information for Patients:
Patients should be advised:
- to discontinue therapy and to inform their physician immediately if they develop symptoms suggestive of hepatic dysfunction including fatigue, anorexia, vomiting, abdominal pain, jaundice, dark urine or pale stool. (See **WARNINGS.**)
- to inform their physician if they develop symptoms suggestive of pancreatitis including abdominal pain and/or nausea and vomiting. (See **PRECAUTIONS: General.**)
- that TROVAN Tablets may be taken without regard to meals;
- that vitamins or minerals containing iron, aluminum- or magnesium-base antacids, antacids containing citric acid buffered with sodium citrate, or sucralfate or Videx®, (Didanosine), chewable/buffered tablets or the pediatric powder for oral solution, should be taken at least 2 hours before or 2 hours after taking TROVAN tablets. (See **PRECAUTIONS: Drug Interactions.**);
- that TROVAN may cause lightheadedness and/or dizziness. Dizziness and/or lightheadedness was the most common adverse reaction reported, and for females under 45 years, it was reported significantly more frequently than in other groups. The incidence of dizziness may be substantially reduced if TROVAN Tablets are taken at bedtime or with food. Patients should know how they react to trovafloxacin before they operate an automobile or machinery or engage in activities requiring mental alertness and coordination. (See **WARNINGS** and **ADVERSE REACTIONS.**);
- to discontinue treatment and inform their physician if they experience pain, inflammation or rupture of a tendon, and to rest and refrain from exercise until the diagnosis of tendinitis or tendon rupture has been confidently excluded;
- that TROVAN may be associated with hypersensitivity reactions, even following the first dose, and to discontinue the drug at the first sign of a skin rash, hives or other skin reactions, difficulty in swallowing or breathing, any swelling suggesting angioedema (e.g., swelling of the lips, tongue, face, tightness of the throat, hoarseness), or other symptoms of an allergic reaction. (See **WARNINGS** and **ADVERSE REACTIONS.**);
- to avoid excessive sunlight or artificial ultraviolet light (e.g., tanning beds) while taking TROVAN and to discontinue therapy if phototoxicity (e.g., sunburn-like reaction or skin eruption) occurs.
- that convulsions have been reported in patients taking quinolones, including trovafloxacin, and to notify their physician before taking this drug if there is a history of this condition.

Drug Interactions:
Antacids, Sucralfate, and Iron: The absorption of oral trovafloxacin is significantly reduced by the concomitant administration of some antacids containing magnesium or aluminum, citric acid/sodium citrate (Bicitra®), as well as sucralfate and iron (ferrous ions). These agents as well as formulations containing divalent and trivalent cations such as Videx®, (Didanosine), chewable/buffered tablets or the pediatric powder for oral solution, should be taken at least 2 hours before or 2 hours after oral trovafloxacin administration. (See **CLINICAL PHARMACOLOGY.**)
Morphine: Co-administration of intravenous morphine significantly reduces the absorption of oral trovafloxacin. Intravenous morphine should be administered at least 2 hours after oral TROVAN dosing in the fasted state and at least 4 hours after oral TROVAN is taken with food. Trovafloxacin administration had no effect on the pharmacokinetics of morphine or its metabolite, morphine-6-β-glucuronide. (See **CLINICAL PHARMACOLOGY.**)
Warfarin: There have been reports during the post-marketing experience that trovafloxacin/alatrofloxacin enhance the effects of warfarin, including cases of bleeding. The mechanism for this reaction is unknown. Prothrombin time, International Normalized Ratio (INR) or other suitable anticoagulation tests should be closely monitored if trovafloxacin/alatrofloxacin is administered concomitantly with warfarin. Patients should also be monitored for evidence of bleeding.
Minor pharmacokinetic interactions without clinical significance have been observed with co-administration of TROVAN Tablets with caffeine, omeprazole and calcium carbonate. (See **CLINICAL PHARMACOLOGY.**)
No significant pharmacokinetic interactions with theophylline, cimetidine, digoxin, warfarin, or cyclosporine have been observed with TROVAN Tablets. (See **CLINICAL PHARMACOLOGY.**)
Alatrofloxacin should not be co-administered with any solution containing multivalent cations, e.g., magnesium, through the same intravenous line. (See **DOSAGE AND ADMINISTRATION.**)
Laboratory Test Interactions:
There are no reported laboratory test interactions.
Carcinogenesis, Mutagenesis, Impairment of Fertility:
Long term studies in animals to determine the carcinogenic potential of trovafloxacin or alatrofloxacin have not been conducted.
TROVAN did not shorten the time to development of UV-induced skin tumors in hairless albino (Skh-1) mice; thus, it was not photo co-carcinogenic in this model. These mice received oral trovafloxacin and concurrent irradiation with simulated sunlight 5 days per week for 40 weeks followed by a 12-week treatment-free observation period. The daily dose of UV radiation used in this study was approximately 30% of the minimal dose of UV radiation that would induce erythema in Caucasian humans. The median time to the development of skin tumors in the hairless mice (42–43 weeks) was similar in the vehicle control group and those given 10 or 30 mg/kg of trovafloxacin daily. At a dose level of 30 mg/kg/day, the mice had skin trovafloxacin concentrations of approximately 7 μg/g. Following multiple 200 mg daily doses of trovafloxacin, the amount in human skin is estimated to be about 3 μg/g, based upon plasma concentrations measured at this dose level.
Trovafloxacin was not mutagenic in the Ames Salmonella reversion assay or CHO/HGPRT mammalian cell gene mutation assay and it was not clastogenic in mitogen-stimulated human lymphocytes or mouse bone marrow cells. A mouse micronucleus test conducted with alatrofloxacin was also negative. The positive response observed in the *E. coli* bacterial mutagenicity assay may be due to the inhibition of DNA gyrase by trovafloxacin.
Trovafloxacin and alatrofloxacin did not affect the fertility of male or female rats at oral and I.V. doses of 75 mg/kg/day and 50 mg/kg/day, respectively. These doses are 15 and 10 times the recommended maximum human dose based on mg/kg or approximately 2 times based on mg/m^2. However, oral doses of trovafloxacin at 200 mg/kg/day (40 times the recommended maximum human dose based on mg/kg or about 6 times based on mg/m^2) were associated with increased preimplantation loss in rats.

Pregnancy: Teratogenic Effects. Pregnancy Category C:
An increase in skeletal variations was observed in rat fetuses after daily oral 75 mg/kg maternal doses of trovafloxacin (approximately 15 times the highest recommended human dose based on mg/kg or 2 times based upon body surface area) were administered during organogenesis. However, fetal skeletal variations were not observed in rats dosed orally with 15 mg/kg trovafloxacin. Evidence of fetotoxicity (increased perinatal mortality and decreased body weights) was also observed in rats at 75 mg/kg. Daily oral doses of trovafloxacin at 45 mg/kg (approximately 9 times the highest recommended human dose based on mg/kg or 2.7 times based upon body surface area) in the rabbit were not associated with an increased incidence of fetal skeletal variations or malformations.
An increase in skeletal variations and malformations was observed in rat fetuses after daily intravenous doses of alatrofloxacin at ≥20 mg/kg/day (approximately 4 times the highest recommended human dose based on mg/kg or 0.6 times based upon body surface area) were administered to dams during organogenesis. In the rabbit, an increase in fetal skeletal malformations was also observed when 20 mg/kg/day (approximately equal to the highest recommended human dose based upon body surface area) of alatrofloxacin was given intravenously during the period of organogenesis. Intravenous dosing of alatrofloxacin at 6.5 mg/kg in the rat or rabbit was not associated with an increased incidence of skeletal variations or malformations. Fetotoxicity and fetal skeletal malformations have been associated with other quinolones.
Oral doses of trovafloxacin >5mg/kg were associated with an increased gestation time in rats, and several dams at 75 mg/kg experienced uterine dystocia.
There are no adequate and well-controlled studies in pregnant women. TROVAN should be used during pregnancy only if the potential benefit justifies the potential risk to the fetus. (See **WARNINGS.**)

Nursing Mothers:
Trovafloxacin is excreted in human milk and was found in measurable concentrations in the breast milk of lactating subjects. (See **CLINICAL PHARMACOLOGY, Distribution.**)
Because of the potential for unknown effects from trovafloxacin in nursing infants from mothers taking trovafloxacin, a decision should be made either to discontinue nursing or to discontinue the drug, taking into account the importance of the drug to the mother.

Pediatric Use:
The safety and effectiveness of trovafloxacin in pediatric patients and adolescents less than 18 years of age have not been established. Quinolones, including trovafloxacin, cause arthropathy and osteochondrosis in juvenile animals of several species. (See **WARNINGS.**)

Geriatric Use:
In multiple-dose clinical trials of trovafloxacin, 27% of patients were ≥65 years of age and 12% of patients were ≥75 years of age. The overall incidence of drug-related adverse reactions, including central nervous system and gastrointestinal side effects, was less in the ≥65 year group than the other age groups.

ADVERSE REACTIONS

Over 6000 patients have been treated with TROVAN in multidose clinical efficacy trials worldwide.
In TROVAN studies the majority of adverse reactions were described as mild in nature (over 90% were described as mild or moderate). TROVAN was discontinued for adverse events thought related to drug in 5% of patients (dizziness 2.4%, nausea 1.9%, headache 1.1%, and vomiting 1.0%).
[See table above]

TROVAN Drug-Related Adverse Reactions (frequency ≥1%) in Multiple-Dose Clinical Trials

	200 mg oral qd (N=3259)	200 mg I.V.→ 200 mg oral qd (N=634)	300 mg I.V.→ 200 mg oral qd (N=623)
Dizziness	11%	2%	2%
Lightheadedness	4%	2%	<1%
Nausea	8%	5%	4%
Headache	5%	5%	1%
Vomiting	3%	1%	3%
Diarrhea	2%	2%	2%
Abdominal pain	1%	1%	0%
Application/injection/ insertion site reaction	n/a	5%	2%
Vaginitis	2%	2%	<1%
Pruritus	<1%	2%	2%
Rash	<1%	2%	2%

Dizziness/lightheadedness on TROVAN is generally mild, lasts for a few hours following a dose, and in most cases, resolves with continued dosing. The incidence of dizziness and lightheadedness in TROVAN patients over 65 years is 3.1% and 0.6%, respectively. (See **PRECAUTIONS: Information for Patients.**)
TROVAN appears to have a low potential for phototoxicity. In clinical trials with TROVAN, only mild, treatment-related phototoxicity was observed in less than 0.03% (2/7096) of patients.
Additional reported drug-related events in clinical trials (remotely, possibly, probably or unknown) that occurred in <1% of TROVAN-treated patients are:
APPLICATION/INJECTION/INSERTION SITE: Application/injection/insertion site device complications, inflammation, pain, edema
AUTONOMIC NERVOUS: flushing, increased sweating, dry mouth, cold clammy skin, increased saliva
CARDIOVASCULAR: peripheral edema, chest pain, thrombophlebitis, hypotension, palpitation, periorbital edema, hypertension, syncope, tachycardia, angina pectoris, bradycardia, peripheral ischemia, edema, dizziness postural
CENTRAL & PERIPHERAL NERVOUS SYSTEM: confusion, paresthesia, vertigo, hypoesthesia, ataxia, convulsions, dysphonia, hypertonia, migraine, involuntary muscle contractions, speech disorder, encephalopathy, abnormal gait, hyperkinesia, hypokinesia, tongue paralysis, abnormal coordination, tremor, dyskinesia
GASTROINTESTINAL: altered bowel habit, constipation, diarrhea-*Clostridium difficile*, dyspepsia, flatulence, loose stools, gastritis, dysphagia, increased appetite, gastroenteritis, rectal disorder, colitis, pseudomembranous colitis, enteritis, eructation, gastrointestinal disorder, melena, hiccup
ORAL CAVITY: gingivitis, stomatitis, altered saliva, tongue disorder, tongue edema, tooth disorder, cheilitis, halitosis
GENERAL/OTHER: fever, fatigue, pain, asthenia, moniliasis, hot flushes, back pain, chills, infection (bacterial, fungal), malaise, sepsis, alcohol intolerance, allergic reaction, anaphylactoid reaction, drug (other) toxicity/reaction, weight increase, weight decrease
HEMATOPOIETIC: anemia, granulocytopenia, hemorrhage unspecified, leukopenia, prothrombin decreased, thrombocythemia, thrombocytopenia
LIVER/BILIARY: increased hepatic enzymes, hepatic function abnormal, bilirubinemia, discolored feces, jaundice
METABOLIC/NUTRITIONAL: hyperglycemia, thirst
MUSCULOSKELETAL: arthralgia, muscle cramps, myalgia, muscle weakness, skeletal pain, tendinitis, arthropathy
PSYCHIATRIC: anxiety, anorexia, agitation, nervousness, somnolence, insomnia, depression, amnesia, concentration impaired, depersonalization, dreaming abnormal, emotional lability, euphoria, hallucination, impotence, libido decreased-male, paroniria, thinking abnormal
REPRODUCTIVE: Female: leukorrhea, menstrual disorder; Male: balanoposthitis
RESPIRATORY: dyspnea, rhinitis, sinusitis, bronchospasm, coughing, epistaxis, respiratory insufficiency, upper respiratory tract infection, respiratory disorder, asthma, hemoptysis, hypoxia, stridor
SKIN/APPENDAGES: pruritus ani, skin disorder, skin ulceration, angioedema, dermatitis, dermatitis fungal, photosensitivity skin reaction, seborrhea, skin exfoliation, urticaria
SPECIAL SENSES: taste perversion, eye pain, abnormal vision, conjunctivitis, photophobia, conjunctival hemorrhage, hyperacusis, scotoma, tinnitus, visual field defect, diplopia, xerophthalmia
URINARY SYSTEM: dysuria, face edema, micturition frequency, interstitial nephritis, renal failure acute, renal function abnormal, urinary incontinence
LABORATORY CHANGES: Changes in laboratory parameters, without regard to drug relationship, occurring in ≥1% of TROVAN-treated patients were: decreased hemoglobin and hematocrit; increased platelets; decreased and increased WBC; eosinophilia; increased ALT (SGPT), AST (SGOT), and alkaline phosphatase; decreased protein and albumin; increased BUN and creatinine; decreased sodium; and bicarbonate. It is not known whether these abnormalities were caused by the drug or the underlying condition being treated. The incidence and magnitude of liver function abnormalities with TROVAN were the same as comparator agents except in the only study in which oral TROVAN was administered for 28 days. In this study (chronic bacterial prostatitis) nine percent (13/140) of TROVAN-treated patients experienced elevations of serum transaminases (AST and/or ALT) of ≥3 times the upper limit of normal. These liver function test abnormalities generally developed at the end of, or following completion of, the planned 28-day course of therapy, but were not associated with concurrent elevations of related laboratory measures of hepatic function (such as serum bilirubin, alkaline phosphatase, or lactate dehydrogenase). Patients were asymptomatic with these abnormalities, which generally returned to normal within 1–2 months after discontinuation of therapy. (See **ADVERSE REACTIONS: POST-MARKETING EXPERIENCE** subsection.)

POST-MARKETING EXPERIENCE:
Adverse reactions reported with TROVAN during the post-marketing period include:
GASTROINTESTINAL: symptomatic pancreatitis.
GENERAL/OTHER: anaphylaxis, Stevens-Johnson Syndrome.
HEMATOPOIETIC: agranulocytosis, aplastic anemia, pancytopenia.
LIVER/BILIARY: symptomatic hepatitis (some patients experienced an associated peripheral eosinophilia), liver failure (including acute hepatic necrosis with eosinophilic infiltration). TROVAN-associated liver enzyme abnormalities and/or symptomatic hepatitis have occurred during short-term or long-term therapy. (See **WARNINGS.**)

OVERDOSAGE

Trovafloxacin has a low order of acute toxicity. The minimum lethal oral dose in mice and rats was 2000 mg/kg or greater. The minimum lethal I.V. dose for the prodrug, alatrofloxacin, was 50–125 mg/kg for mice and greater than 75 mg/kg for rats. Clinical signs observed included decreased activity and respiration, ataxia, ptosis, tremors and convulsions.
In the event of acute oral overdosage, the stomach should be emptied by inducing vomiting or by gastric lavage. The patient should be carefully observed and given symptomatic and supportive treatment. Adequate hydration should be maintained. Trovafloxacin is not efficiently removed from the body by hemodialysis.

DOSAGE AND ADMINISTRATION

The recommended dosage for TROVAN for the treatment of serious, life- or limb-threatening infections is described in the table below. Doses of TROVAN are administered once every 24 hours. TROVAN should not usually be administered for more than 2 weeks. It should only be administered for longer than 2 weeks if the treating physician believes the benefits to the individual patients clearly outweigh the risks of such longer-term treatment. (See boxed **WARNING.**)
Oral doses should be administered at least 2 hours before or 2 hours after antacids containing magnesium or aluminum, as well as sucralfate, citric acid buffered with sodium citrate (e.g., Bicitra®), metal cations (e.g., ferrous sulfate) and Videx®, (Didanosine), chewable/buffered tablets or the pediatric powder for oral solution.
Intravenous morphine should be administered at least 2 hours after oral TROVAN dosing in the fasted state and at least 4 hours after oral TROVAN is taken with food.
Patients whose therapy is started with TROVAN I.V. may be switched to TROVAN Tablets to complete the course of therapy, if deemed appropriate by the treating physician. In certain patients with serious and life- or limb-threatening infections as described in the **INDICATIONS AND USAGE** Section, TROVAN Tablets may be considered appropriate initial therapy, when the treating physician believes that the benefit of the product for the patient outweighs the potential risk.
TROVAN I.V. (alatrofloxacin mesylate injection) should only be administered by INTRAVENOUS infusion. It is not for intramuscular, intrathecal, intraperitoneal, or subcutaneous administration.
Single-use vials require dilution prior to administration. (See **PREPARATION OF ALATROFLOXACIN MESYLATE INJECTION FOR ADMINISTRATION.**)
[See first table at top of next page]
NOTE: As with other antimicrobials, where *Pseudomonas aeruginosa* is a documented or presumptive pathogen, combination therapy with either an aminoglycoside or aztreonam may be clinically indicated.
IMPAIRED RENAL FUNCTION: No adjustment in the dosage of TROVAN is necessary in patients with impaired renal function. Trovafloxacin is eliminated primarily by biliary excretion. Trovafloxacin is not efficiently removed from the body by hemodialysis.
CHRONIC HEPATIC DISEASE (cirrhosis): The following table provides dosing guidelines for patients with mild or moderate cirrhosis (Child-Pugh Class A and B). There are no data in patients with severe cirrhosis (Child-Pugh Class C).

INDICATED DOSE (Normal hepatic function)	CHRONIC HEPATIC DISEASE DOSE
300 mg I.V.	200 mg I.V.
200 mg I.V. or oral	100 mg I.V. or oral

Continued on next page

Trovan—Cont.

INTRAVENOUS ADMINISTRATION

AFTER DILUTION WITH AN APPROPRIATE DILUENT, TROVAN I.V. SHOULD BE ADMINISTERED BY INTRAVENOUS INFUSION OVER A PERIOD OF 60 MINUTES. CAUTION: RAPID OR BOLUS INTRAVENOUS INFUSION SHOULD BE AVOIDED. (See **PRECAUTIONS**.)

TROVAN I.V. is supplied in single-use vials containing a concentrated solution of alatrofloxacin mesylate in Water for Injection (equivalent of 200 mg or 300 mg as trovafloxacin). Each mL contains alatrofloxacin mesylate equivalent to 5 mg trovafloxacin. (See **HOW SUPPLIED** for container sizes.) THESE TROVAN I.V. SINGLE-USE VIALS MUST BE FURTHER DILUTED WITH AN APPROPRIATE SOLUTION PRIOR TO INTRAVENOUS ADMINISTRATION. This parenteral drug product should be inspected visually for discoloration and particulate matter prior to dilution and administration. Since no preservative or bacteriostatic agent is present in this product, aseptic technique must be used in preparation of the final parenteral solution.

PREPARATION OF ALATROFLOXACIN MESYLATE INJECTION FOR ADMINISTRATION

The intravenous dose should be prepared by aseptically withdrawing the appropriate volume of concentrate from the vials of TROVAN I.V. This should be diluted with a suitable intravenous solution to a final concentration of 1–2 mg/mL. (See **Compatible Intravenous Solutions**.) The resulting solution should be infused over a period of 60 minutes by direct infusion or through a Y-type intravenous infusion set which may already be in place.

Since the vials are for single use only, any unused portion should be discarded.

Since only limited data are available on the compatibility of alatrofloxacin intravenous injection with other intravenous substances, additives or other medications should not be added to TROVAN I.V. in single-use vials or infused simultaneously through the same intravenous line.

If the same intravenous line is used for sequential infusion of several different drugs, the line should be flushed before and after infusion of TROVAN I.V. with an infusion solution compatible with TROVAN I.V. and with any other drug(s) administered via this common line.

If TROVAN I.V. is to be given concomitantly with another drug, each drug should be given separately in accordance with the recommended dosage and route of administration for each drug.

The desired dosage of TROVAN I.V. may be prepared according to the following chart:

[See second table above]

For example, to prepare a 200 mg dose at an infusion concentration of 2 mg/mL (as trovafloxacin), 40 mL of TROVAN I.V. is withdrawn from a vial and diluted with 60 mL of a compatible intravenous fluid to produce a total infusion solution volume of 100 mL.

Compatible Intravenous Solutions:
5% Dextrose Injection, USP
0.45% Sodium Chloride Injection, USP
5% Dextrose and 0.45% Sodium Chloride Injection, USP
5% Dextrose and 0.2% Sodium Chloride Injection, USP
Lactated Ringer's and 5% Dextrose Injection, USP

TROVAN I.V. should not be diluted with 0.9% Sodium Chloride Injection, USP (normal saline), alone or in combination with other diluents. A precipitate may form under these conditions. In addition, TROVAN I.V. should not be diluted with Lactated Ringer's, USP.

Normal saline, 0.9% Sodium Chloride Injection, USP can be used for flushing I.V. lines prior to or after administration of TROVAN I.V.

Stability of TROVAN I.V. as Supplied:
When stored under recommended conditions, TROVAN I.V., as supplied in 40 mL or 60 mL vials, is stable through the expiration date printed on the label.

Stability of TROVAN I.V. Following Dilution:
TROVAN I.V., when diluted with compatible intravenous solutions to concentrations of 0.5 to 2.0 mg/mL (as trovafloxacin), is physically and chemically stable for up to 7 days when refrigerated or up to 3 days at room temperature stored in glass bottles or plastic (PVC type) intravenous containers.

HOW SUPPLIED

Trovan Tablets and Injection are being distributed only to hospitals and long term nursing care facilities for patients initiating therapy in these facilities.

Tablets
TROVAN® (trovafloxacin mesylate) Tablets are available as blue, film-coated tablets. The 100 mg tablets are round and contain trovafloxacin mesylate equivalent to 100 mg trovafloxacin. The 200 mg tablets are modified oval-shaped and contain trovafloxacin mesylate equivalent to 200 mg trovafloxacin.

TROVAN Tablets are packaged and in unit dose blister strips in the following configurations:

100-mg tablets: color: blue; shape: round; debossing: "PFIZER" on one side and "378" on the other

  Bottles of 30 (NDC 0049-3780-30)

  Unit Dose/40 tablets (NDC 0049-3780-43)

200-mg tablets: color: blue; shape: modified oval; debossing: "PFIZER" on one side and "379" on the other

  Bottles of 30 (NDC 0049-3790-30)

  Unit Dose/40 tablets (NDC 0049-3790-43)

DOSAGE GUIDELINES

INFECTION*/LOCATION AND TYPE	DAILY UNIT DOSE AND ROUTE OF ADMINISTRATION	TOTAL DURATION (See **WARNINGS**.)
Nosocomial Pneumonia (See NOTE 1 below.)	300 mg I.V.† followed by 200 mg oral	10–14 days
Community Acquired Pneumonia	200 mg oral or 200 mg I.V. followed by 200 mg oral	7–14 days
Complicated Intra-Abdominal Infections, including post-surgical infections	300 mg I.V.† followed by 200 mg oral	7–14 days
Gynecologic and Pelvic Infections	300 mg I.V.† followed by 200 mg oral	7–14 days
Skin and Skin Structure Infections, Complicated, including diabetic foot infections	200 mg oral or 200 mg I.V. followed by 200 mg oral	10–14 days

*due to the designated pathogens (See **INDICATIONS AND USAGE**.)
† Where the 300 mg TROVAN I.V. dose is indicated, therapy should be decreased to the 200 mg dose as soon as clinically indicated.

DOSAGE STRENGTH (mg) (trovafloxacin equivalent)	VOLUME TO WITHDRAW (mL)	DILUENT VOLUME (mL)	TOTAL VOLUME (mL)	INFUSION CONC (mg/mL)
100 mg	20	30	50	2
100 mg	20	80	100	1
200 mg	40	60	100	2
200 mg	40	160	200	1
300 mg	60	90	150	2
300 mg	60	240	300	1

Pathogen	End of Treatment TROVAN	End of Treatment Comparators	End of Study TROVAN	End of Study Comparators
S. pneumoniae	89% (63/71)	95% (62/65)	87% (55/63)	91% (50/55)
H. influenzae	97% (35/36)	94% (46/49)	90% (28/31)	94% (44/47)
M. catarrhalis	100% (8/8)	100% (4/4)	100% (6/6)	100% (4/4)
S. aureus	100% (8/8)	93% (13/14)	100% (6/6)	91% (10/11)
K. pneumoniae	100% (3/3)	89% (8/9)	100% (3/3)	86% (6/7)
L. pneumophila	77% (10/13)	86% (12/14)	75% (9/12)	86% (12/14)
M. pneumoniae	100% (20/20)	87% (13/15)	94% (17/18)	79% (11/14)
C. pneumoniae	75% (6/8)	100% (18/18)	67% (4/6)	94% (16/17)

Pathogen	End of Treatment TROVAN	End of Treatment Ciprofloxacin	End of Study TROVAN	End of Study Ciprofloxacin
P. aeruginosa	67% (10/15)	55% (6/11)	62% (8/13)	25% (2/8)
H. influenzae	88% (7/8)	89% (8/9)	83% (5/6)	86% (6/7)
E. coli	71% (5/7)	80% (4/5)	50% (3/6)	80% (4/5)
S. aureus	64% (7/11)	80% (8/10)	50% (4/8)	67% (4/6)

Storage
TROVAN Tablets should be stored at 15°C to 30°C (59°F to 86°F) in airtight containers (USP).

Injection
TROVAN is also available for intravenous administration as the prodrug, TROVAN® I.V. (alatrofloxacin mesylate injection), in the following configurations:
Single-use vials containing a clear, colorless to pale-yellow concentrated solution of alatrofloxacin mesylate equivalent to 5 mg trovafloxacin/mL.
  5 mg/mL, 40 mL, 200 mg
  Unit dose package (NDC 0049-3890-28)
  5 mg/mL, 60 mL, 300 mg
  Unit dose package (NDC 0049-3900-28)

Storage
TROVAN I.V. should be stored at 15°C to 30°C (59°F to 86°F). Protect From Light. Do Not Freeze.

ANIMAL PHARMACOLOGY

Quinolones have been shown to cause arthropathy in immature animals.

Arthropathy and chondrodysplasia were observed in immature animals given trovafloxacin. (See **WARNINGS**.)

At doses from 10 to 15 times the human dose based on mg/kg or approximately 3 to 5 times based on mg/m², trovafloxacin has been shown to cause arthropathy in immature rats and dogs. In addition, these drugs are associated with an increased incidence of chondrodysplasia in rats compared to controls. There is no evidence of arthropathies in fully mature rats and dogs at doses from 40 or 10 times the human dose based on mg/kg or approximately 5 times based on mg/m² for a 6 month exposure period.

Unlike some other members of the quinolone class, crystalluria and ocular toxicity were not observed in chronic safety studies with rats or dogs with either trovafloxacin or its prodrug, alatrofloxacin.

Quinolones have been reported to have proconvulsant activity that is exacerbated with concomitant use of non-steroidal anti-inflammatory drugs (NSAIDS). Neither trovafloxacin administered orally at 500 mg/kg, nor alatrofloxacin administered intravenously at 75 mg/kg, showed an increase in measures of seizure activity in mice at doses when used in combination with the active metabolite of the NSAID, fenbufen.

As with other members of the quinolone class, trovafloxacin at doses 5 to 10 times the human dose based on mg/kg or 1 to 5 times the human dose based on mg/m² produces testicular degeneration in rats and dogs dosed for 6 months.

At a dose of trovafloxacin 10 times the highest human dose based on mg/kg or approximately 5 times based on mg/m², elevated liver enzyme levels which correlated with centrilobular hepatocellular vacuolar degeneration and necrosis were observed in dogs in a 6 month study. A subsequent study demonstrated reversibility of these effects when trovafloxacin was discontinued.

Pathogen	End of Treatment		End of Study	
	TROVAN	Imipenem/Cila Amox/Clav	TROVAN	Imipenem/Cila Amox/Clav
E. coli	94% (72/77)	90% (52/58)	86% (66/77)	86% (51/59)
Bacteroides fragilis	97% (30/31)	82% (28/34)	84% (26/31)	75% (27/36)
viridans group streptococci	90% (18/20)	83% (19/23)	90% (18/20)	78% (18/23)
Pseudomonas aeruginosa	94% (15/16)	82% (14/17)	88% (14/16)	83% (15/18)
Klebsiella pneumoniae	80% (12/15)	71% (10/14)	67% (10/15)	71% (10/14)
Peptostreptococcus spp.	86% (12/14)	88% (7/8)	79% (11/14)	75% (6/8)
Prevotella spp.	77% (10/13)	50% (2/4)	77% (10/13)	60% (3/5)

CLINICAL STUDIES

Hospitalized Community Acquired Pneumonia

Adult patients with clinically and radiologically documented community acquired pneumonia, requiring hospitalization and initial intravenous therapy, participated in two randomized, multicenter, double-blind, double-dummy trials. The first trial compared intravenous alatrofloxacin (200 mg once daily for 2 to 7 days) followed by oral trovafloxacin (200 mg once daily) for a total of 7 to 14 days of therapy to intravenous ciprofloxacin (400 mg BID) plus ampicillin (500 mg QID) for 2 to 7 days followed by oral ciprofloxacin (500 mg BID) plus amoxicillin (500 mg TID) for a total of 7 to 14 days of therapy. The second study compared intravenous alatrofloxacin (200 mg once daily for 2 to 7 days) followed by oral trovafloxacin (200 mg once daily) for a total of 7 to 14 days of therapy to intravenous ceftriaxone (1000 mg once daily for 2 to 7 days) followed by oral cefpodoxime (400 mg BID) for 7 to 14 days of total therapy with optional blinded erythromycin added to the ceftriaxone/cefpodoxime arm if an atypical pneumonia was suspected.

The clinical success rate (cure + improvement with no need for further antibiotic therapy) at the End of Treatment was 90% (311/346) and 90% (325/363) for TROVAN and the comparator agents, respectively. The clinical success rate at the End of Study (Day 30) was 86% (256/299) and 85% (283/334) for TROVAN and the comparator agents, respectively. All cause mortality (Day 1–35) was 2.45% (10/408) on TROVAN and 5.45% (23/422) on the comparator agents.

The following outcomes are the clinical success rates for the clinically evaluable patient groups by pathogen in these two studies:

[See third table at middle of previous page]

Of the above patients with clinical failure at end of treatment or study, only one alatrofloxacin patient (*H. influenzae* + *S. pneumoniae*) and one ceftriaxone + erythromycin patient (*Legionella*) had a microbiologically confirmed persistent pathogen at the time of failure with no emergence of resistance in either study.

Nosocomial Pneumonia

Adult patients with clinically and radiologically documented nosocomial pneumonia participated in a randomized, multicenter, double-blind, double-dummy trial comparing intravenous alatrofloxacin (300 mg once daily for 2 to 7 days) followed by oral trovafloxacin (200 mg once daily) for a total of 7 to 14 days of therapy to intravenous ciprofloxacin (400 mg BID) for 2 to 7 days followed by oral ciprofloxacin (750 mg BID) for a total of 7 to 14 days of therapy with optional blinded clindamycin or metronidazole added to the ciprofloxacin arm if an anaerobic pneumonia was suspected. In subjects with documented Pseudomonas infection or methicillin-resistant *S. aureus*, aztreonam or vancomycin, respectively, could have been added to either treatment regimen.

The clinical success rate (cure + improvement with no need for further antibiotic therapy) at the End of Treatment was 77% (68/88) and 78% (79/101) for TROVAN and ciprofloxacin, respectively. The clinical success rate at the End of Study (Day 30) was 69% (50/72) and 68% (54/79) for TROVAN and ciprofloxacin, respectively.

The following outcomes are the clinical success rates for the clinically evaluable patient groups by pathogen:

[See fourth table at middle of previous page]

Of the above patients with clinical failure at end of treatment or study, 2 alatrofloxacin patients (*S. aureus*, *P. aeruginosa*) and 4 ciprofloxacin patients (all *P. aeruginosa*) had a microbiologically confirmed persistent pathogen at the time of failure. Three of the 4 ciprofloxacin patients with clinical failure and persistence had emergence of resistance with none on alatrofloxacin.

Complicated Intra-Abdominal Infections

Patients hospitalized with clinically documented, complicated intra-abdominal infections, including post-surgical infections, participated in a randomized, double-blind, multicenter trial comparing intravenous alatrofloxacin (300 mg once daily) followed by oral trovafloxacin (200 mg once daily) to intravenous imipenem/cilastatin (1g q8h) followed by oral amoxicillin/clavulanic acid (500 mg TID) for a maximum of 14 days of therapy. The clinical success rate (cure + improvement) at the End of Treatment was 88% (136/155) and 86% (122/142) for alatrofloxacin→trovafloxacin and imipenem/cilastatin→amoxicillin/clavulanic acid, respectively. The clinical success rate at the End of Study (Day 30) was 83% (129/156) and 84% (127/152) for alatrofloxacin→trovafloxacin and imipenem/cilastatin→amoxicillin/clavulanic acid, respectively.

The following are the clinical success rates for the clinically evaluable patient groups by pathogen:

[See table above]

Of patients with a baseline pathogen and a clinical response of failure at the End of Study, 9 of 26 on TROVAN and 10 of 21 on imipenem/cilastatin had microbiologically-confirmed persistence of the baseline pathogen with no emergence of resistance in either group.

REFERENCES:

1. National Committee for Clinical Laboratory Standards, Methods for Dilution Antimicrobial Susceptibility Tests for Bacteria That Grow Aerobically—Fourth Edition; Approved Standard, NCCLS Document M7-A4, Vol. 17, No. 2, NCCLS, Wayne, PA, January, 1997.
2. National Committee for Clinical Laboratory Standards. Performance Standards for Antimicrobial Disk Susceptibility Tests—Sixth Edition; Approved Standard, NCCLS Document M2-A6, Vol. 17, No. 1, NCCLS, Wayne, PA, January, 1997.
3. National Committee for Clinical Laboratory Standards. Methods for Antimicrobial Susceptibility Testing of Anaerobic Bacteria—Fourth Edition; Approved Standard, NCCLS Document M11-A4, Vol. 17, No. 22, NCCLS, Wayne, PA, December, 1997.

U.S. Patent No. 5,164,402

Rx only

TROVAN is manufactured and distributed by
Pfizer Roerig
Division of Pfizer Inc, NY NY 10017

Printed in U.S.A.
69-5328-00-6 Revised April 2000

ZITHROMAX® ℞

(azithromycin tablets)
(azithromycin capsules)
and
(azithromycin for oral suspension)

Prescribing information for this product, which appears on pages 2542–2546 of the 2001 PDR, has been completely revised as follows. Please write "See Supplement A" next to the product heading.

DESCRIPTION

ZITHROMAX® (azithromycin tablets, azithromycin capsules and azithromycin for oral suspension) contains the active ingredient azithromycin, an azalide, a subclass of macrolide antibiotics, for oral administration. Azithromycin has the chemical name *(2R,3S,4R,5R,8R,10R,11R,12S,13S,14R)*-13-[(2,6-dideoxy-3-*C*-methyl-3-*O*-methyl-α-*L*-*ribo*-hexopyranosyl)oxy]-2-ethyl-3,4,10-trihydroxy-3,5,6,8,10,12,14-heptamethyl-11-[[3,4,6-trideoxy-3-(dimethylamino)-β-*D*-*xylo*-hexopyranosyl]oxy]-1-oxa-6-azacyclopentadecan-15-one. Azithromycin is derived from erythromycin; however, it differs chemically from erythromycin in that a methyl-substituted nitrogen atom is incorporated into the lactone ring. Its molecular formula is $C_{38}H_{72}N_2O_{12}$, and its molecular weight is 749.00. Azithromycin has the following structural formula:

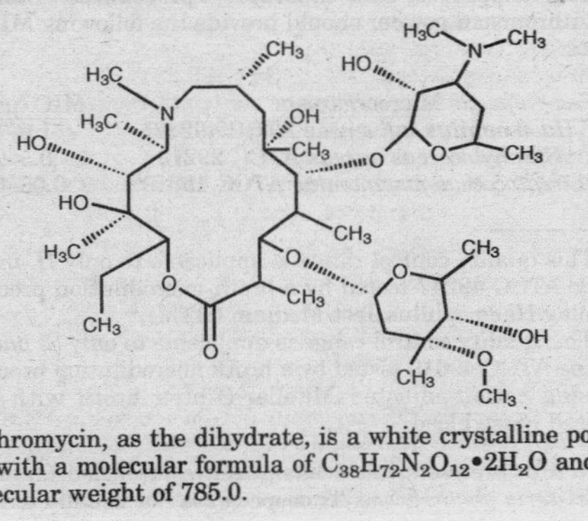

Azithromycin, as the dihydrate, is a white crystalline powder with a molecular formula of $C_{38}H_{72}N_2O_{12}•2H_2O$ and a molecular weight of 785.0.

ZITHROMAX® is supplied for oral administration as film-coated, modified capsular shaped tablets containing azithromycin dihydrate equivalent to 250 mg azithromycin and the following inactive ingredients: dibasic calcium phosphate anhydrous, pregelatinized starch, sodium croscarmellose, magnesium stearate, sodium lauryl sulfate, hydroxypropyl methylcellulose, lactose, titanium dioxide, triacetin and D&C Red #30 aluminum lake.

ZITHROMAX® capsules contain azithromycin dihydrate equivalent to 250 mg of azithromycin. The capsules are supplied in red opaque hard-gelatin capsules (containing FD&C Red #40). They also contain the following inactive ingredients: anhydrous lactose, corn starch, magnesium stearate, and sodium lauryl sulfate.

It is also supplied as a powder for oral suspension.

ZITHROMAX® for oral suspension is supplied in bottles containing azithromycin dihydrate powder equivalent to 300 mg, 600 mg, 900 mg, or 1200 mg azithromycin per bottle and the following inactive ingredients: sucrose; sodium phosphate, tribasic, anhydrous; hydroxypropyl cellulose; xanthan gum; FD&C Red #40; and spray dried artificial cherry, creme de vanilla and banana flavors. After constitution, each 5 mL of suspension contains 100 mg or 200 mg of azithromycin.

CLINICAL PHARMACOLOGY

Adult Pharmacokinetics: Following oral administration, azithromycin is rapidly absorbed and widely distributed throughout the body. Rapid distribution of azithromycin into tissues and high concentration within cells result in significantly higher azithromycin concentrations in tissues than in plasma or serum.

The pharmacokinetic parameters of azithromycin capsules in plasma after a loading dose of 500 mg (2–250 mg capsules) on day one followed by 250 mg (1–250 mg capsules) q.d. on days two through five in healthy young adults (age 18–40 years old) are portrayed in the following chart:

Pharmacokinetic Parameters (Mean)	Total n = 12	
	Day 1	Day 5
C_{max} (μg/mL)	0.41	0.24
T_{max} (h)	2.5	3.2
AUC_{0-24} (μg•h/mL)	2.6	2.1
C_{min} (μg/mL)	0.05	0.05
Urinary Excret. (% dose)	4.5	6.5

In this study, there was no significant difference in the disposition of azithromycin between male and female subjects. Plasma concentrations of azithromycin following single 500 mg oral and i.v. doses declined in a polyphasic pattern resulting in an average terminal half-life of 68 hours. With a regimen of 500 mg on Day 1 and 250 mg/day on Days 2–5, C_{min} and C_{max} remained essentially unchanged from Day 2 through Day 5 of therapy. However, without a loading dose, azithromycin C_{min} levels required 5 to 7 days to reach steady-state.

In an open, randomized, two-way crossover study, pharmacokinetic parameters (AUC_{0-72}, C_{max}, T_{max}) determined from 36 fasted healthy male volunteers who received two 250-mg commercial capsules and two 250-mg tablets were:

[See first table at top of next page]

When azithromycin capsules were administered with food to 11 adult healthy male subjects, the rate of absorption (C_{max}) of azithromycin from the capsule formulation was reduced by 52% and the extent of absorption (AUC) by 43%.

In an open label, randomized, two-way crossover study in 12 healthy subjects to assess the effect of a high fat standard meal on the serum concentrations of azithromycin resulting from the oral administration of two 250-mg film-coated tablets, it was shown that food increased C_{max} by 23% while there was no change in AUC.

When azithromycin suspension was administered with food to 28 adult healthy male subjects, the rate of absorption (C_{max}) was increased by 56% while the extent of absorption (AUC) was unchanged.

The AUC of azithromycin was unaffected by co-administration of an antacid containing aluminum and magnesium hydroxide with ZITHROMAX® capsules (azithromycin); however, the C_{max} was reduced by 24%. Administration of cimetidine (800 mg) two hours prior to azithromycin had no effect on azithromycin absorption.

When studied in healthy elderly subjects from age 65 to 85 years, the pharmacokinetic parameters of azithromycin in elderly men were similar to those in young adults; however, in elderly women, although higher peak concentrations (increased by 30 to 50%) were observed, no significant accumulation occurred.

The high values in adults for apparent steady-state volume of distribution (31.1 L/kg) and plasma clearance (630 mL/min) suggest that the prolonged half-life is due to extensive uptake and subsequent release of drug from tissues.

The serum protein binding of azithromycin is variable in the concentration range approximating human exposure, decreasing from 51% at 0.02 μg/mL to 7% at 2 μg/mL.

Biliary excretion of azithromycin, predominantly as unchanged drug, is a major route of elimination. Over the course of a week, approximately 6% of the administered dose appears as unchanged drug in urine.

There are no pharmacokinetic data available from studies in hepatically- or renally-impaired individuals.

Continued on next page

Zithromax—Cont.

The effect of azithromycin on the plasma levels or pharmacokinetics of theophylline administered in multiple doses adequate to reach therapeutic steady-state plasma levels is not known. (See **PRECAUTIONS**.)

Selected tissue (or fluid) concentration and tissue (or fluid) to plasma/serum concentration ratios are shown in the following table:

[See second table above]

The extensive tissue distribution was confirmed by examination of additional tissues and fluids (bone, ejaculum, prostate, ovary, uterus, salpinx, stomach, liver, and gallbladder). As there are no data from adequate and well-controlled studies of azithromycin treatment of infections in these additional body sites, the clinical significance of these tissue concentration data is unknown.

Following a regimen of 500 mg on the first day and 250 mg daily for 4 days, only very low concentrations were noted in cerebrospinal fluid (less than 0.01 μg/mL) in the presence of non-inflamed meninges.

Pediatric Pharmacokinetics:

In two clinical studies, azithromycin for oral suspension was dosed at 10 mg/kg on day 1, followed by 5 mg/kg on days 2 through 5 to two groups of children (aged 1–5 years and 5–15 years, respectively). The mean pharmacokinetic parameters at Day 5 were C_{max}=0.216 μg/mL, T_{max}=1.9 hours, and AUC_{0-24}=1.822 μg•hr/mL for the 1- to 5-year-old group and were C_{max}=0.383 μg/mL, T_{max}=2.4 hours, and AUC_{0-24}=3.109 μg•hr/mL for the 5- to 15-year-old group.

There are no pharmacokinetic data on azithromycin suspension when administered at a dose of 12 mg/kg/day in the presence or absence of food. (For the pediatric pharyngitis/tonsillitis dose, see **DOSAGE AND ADMINISTRATION**.)

Microbiology: Azithromycin acts by binding to the 50S ribosomal subunit of susceptible microorganisms and, thus, interfering with microbial protein synthesis. Nucleic acid synthesis is not affected.

Azithromycin concentrates in phagocytes and fibroblasts as demonstrated by *in vitro* incubation techniques. Using such methodology, the ratio of intracellular to extracellular concentration was >30 after one hour incubation. *In vivo* studies suggest that concentration in phagocytes may contribute to drug distribution to inflamed tissues.

Azithromycin has been shown to be active against most strains of the following microorganisms, both *in vitro* and in clinical infections as described in the **INDICATIONS AND USAGE** section.

Aerobic gram-positive microorganisms

Staphylococcus aureus
Streptococcus agalactiae
Streptococcus pneumoniae
Streptococcus pyogenes

NOTE: Azithromycin demonstrates cross-resistance with erythromycin-resistant gram-positive strains. Most strains of *Enterococcus faecalis* and methicillin-resistant staphylococci are resistant to azithromycin.

Aerobic gram-negative microorganisms

Haemophilus ducreyi
Haemophilus influenzae
Moraxella catarrhalis
Neisseria gonorrhoeae

"Other" microorganisms

Chlamydia pneumoniae
Chlamydia trachomatis
Mycoplasma pneumoniae

Beta-lactamase production should have no effect on azithromycin activity.

The following *in vitro* data are available, **but their clinical significance is unknown**.

Azithromycin exhibits *in vitro* minimum inhibitory concentrations (MIC's) of 0.5 μg/mL or less against most (≥90%) strains of streptococci and MIC's of 2.0 μg/mL or less against most (≥90%) strains of other listed microorganisms. However, the safety and effectiveness of azithromycin in treating clinical infections due to these microorganisms have not been established in adequate and well-controlled trials.

Aerobic gram-positive microorganisms

Streptococci (Groups C, F, G)
Viridans group streptococci

Aerobic gram-negative microorganisms

Bordetella pertussis
Legionella pneumophila

Anaerobic microorganisms

Peptostreptococcus species
Prevotella bivia

"Other" microorganisms

Ureaplasma urealyticum

Susceptibility Tests

Azithromycin can be solubilized for *in vitro* susceptibility testing using dilution techniques by dissolving in a minimum amount of 95% ethanol and diluting to the working stock concentration with broth. Further dilutions may be made in water.

Dilution Techniques:

Quantitative methods are used to determine antimicrobial minimum inhibitory concentrations (MIC's). These MIC's provide estimates of the susceptibility of bacteria to antimicrobial compounds. The MIC's should be determined using a standardized procedure. Standardized procedures are based on a dilution method[1] (broth or agar) or equivalent with standardized inoculum concentrations and standardized

	Capsule	Tablet	90% CI
AUC_{0-72} (μg•h/mL)	4.1 (1.2)	4.3 (1.2)	(99–113%)
C_{max} (μg/mL)	0.5 (0.2)	0.5 (0.2)	(96–121%)
T_{max} (hours)	2.1 (0.8)	2.2 (0.9)	

AZITHROMYCIN CONCENTRATIONS FOLLOWING TWO–250 mg (500 mg) CAPSULES IN ADULTS

TISSUE OR FLUID	TIME AFTER DOSE (h)	TISSUE OR FLUID CONCENTRATION (μg/g or μg/mL)[1]	CORRESPONDING PLASMA OR SERUM LEVEL (μg/mL)	TISSUE (FLUID) PLASMA (SERUM) RATIO[1]
SKIN	72–96	0.4	0.012	35
LUNG	72–96	4.0	0.012	>100
SPUTUM*	2–4	1.0	0.64	2
SPUTUM**	10–12	2.9	0.1	30
TONSIL***	9–18	4.5	0.03	>100
TONSIL***	180	0.9	0.006	>100
CERVIX****	19	2.8	0.04	70

[1] High tissue concentrations should not be interpreted to be quantitatively related to clinical efficacy. The antimicrobial activity of azithromycin is pH related. Azithromycin is concentrated in cell lysosomes which have a low intraorganelle pH, at which the drug's activity is reduced. However, the extensive distribution of drug to tissues may be relevant to clinical activity.
* Sample was obtained 2–4 hours after the first dose.
** Sample was obtained 10–12 hours after the first dose.
*** Dosing regimen of 2 doses of 250 mg each, separated by 12 hours.
**** Sample was obtained 19 hours after a single 500 mg dose.

concentrations of azithromycin powder. The MIC values should be interpreted according to the following criteria:

For testing aerobic microorganisms other than *Haemophilus* species, *Neisseria gonorrhoeae*, and streptococci:

MIC (μg/mL)	Interpretation
≤ 2	Susceptible (S)
4	Intermediate (I)
≥ 8	Resistant (R)

For testing *Haemophilus* species:[a]

MIC (μg/mL)	Interpretation
≤ 4	Susceptible (S)

[a]These interpretive standards are applicable only to broth microdilution susceptibility testing with *Haemophilus* species using Haemophilus Test Medium.[1]

The current absence of data on resistant strains precludes defining any categories other than "Susceptible." Strains yielding MIC results suggestive of a "nonsusceptible" category should be submitted to a reference laboratory for further testing.

For testing Streptococci including *S. pneumoniae*:[b]

MIC (μg/mL)	Interpretation
≤ 0.5	Susceptible (S)
1	Intermediate (I)
≥ 2	Resistant (R)

[b]These interpretive standards are applicable only to broth microdilution susceptibility tests using cation-adjusted Mueller-Hinton broth with 2–5% lysed horse blood.

No interpretive criteria have been established for testing *Neisseria gonorrhoeae*. This species is not usually tested.

A report of "Susceptible" indicates that the pathogen is likely to respond to monotherapy with azithromycin. A report of "Intermediate" indicates that the result should be considered equivocal, and, if the microorganism is not fully susceptible to alternative, clinically feasible drugs, the test should be repeated. This category implies possible clinical applicability in body sites where the drug is physiologically concentrated or in situations where high dosage of drug can be used. This category also provides a buffer zone which prevents small uncontrolled technical factors from causing major discrepancies in interpretation. A report of "Resistant" indicates that achievable drug concentrations are unlikely to be inhibitory; other therapy should be selected.

Standardized susceptibility test procedures require the use of laboratory control microorganisms to control the technical aspects of the laboratory procedures. Standard azithromycin powder should provide the following MIC values:

Microorganism	MIC (μg/mL)
Haemophilus influenzae ATCC 49247[a]	1.0–4.0
Staphylococcus aureus ATCC 29213	0.5–2.0
Streptococcus pneumoniae ATCC 49619[b]	0.06–0.25

[a]This quality control range is applicable to only *H. influenzae* ATCC 49247 tested by a broth microdilution procedure using Haemophilus Test Medium (HTM).[1]

[b]This quality control range is applicable to only *S. pneumoniae* ATCC 49619 tested by a broth microdilution procedure using cation-adjusted Mueller-Hinton broth with 2–5% lysed horse blood.

No interpretive criteria have been established for testing *Neisseria gonorrhoeae*. This species is not usually tested.

Diffusion Techniques:

Quantitative methods that require measurement of zone diameters also provide reproducible estimates of the susceptibility of bacteria to antimicrobial compounds. One such standardized procedure[2] requires the use of standardized inoculum concentrations. This procedure uses paper disks impregnated with 15-μg azithromycin to test the susceptibility of microorganisms to azithromycin.

Reports from the laboratory providing results of the standard single-disk susceptibility test with a 15-μg azithromycin disk should be interpreted according to the following criteria:

For testing aerobic microorganisms (including streptococci)[a] except *Haemophilus* species and *Neisseria gonorrhoeae*:

Zone Diameter (mm)	Interpretation
≥ 18	Susceptible (S)
14–17	Intermediate (I)
≤ 13	Resistant (R)

[a]These zone diameter standards for streptococci apply only to tests performed using Mueller-Hinton agar supplemented with 5% sheep blood and incubated in 5% CO_2.

For testing *Haemophilus* species:[b]

Zone Diameter (mm)	Interpretation
≥ 12	Susceptible (S)

[b]These zone diameter standards apply only to tests with *Haemophilus* species using Haemophilus Test Medium (HTM).[2]

The current absence of data on resistant strains precludes defining any categories other than "Susceptible." Strains yielding zone diameter results suggestive of a "nonsusceptible" category should be submitted to a reference laboratory for further testing.

No interpretive criteria have been established for testing *Neisseria gonorrhoeae*. This species is not usually tested.

Interpretation should be as stated above for results using dilution techniques. Interpretation involves correlation of the diameter obtained in the disk test with the MIC for azithromycin.

As with standardized dilution techniques, diffusion methods require the use of laboratory control microorganisms that are used to control the technical aspects of the laboratory procedures. For the diffusion technique, the 15-μg azithromycin disk should provide the following zone diameters in these laboratory test quality control strains:

Microorganism	Zone Diameter (mm)
Haemophilus influenzae ATCC 49247[a]	13–21
Staphylococcus aureus ATCC 25923	21–26
Streptococcus pneumoniae ATCC 49619[b]	19–25

[a]These quality control limits apply only to tests conducted with *H. influenzae* ATCC 49247 using Haemophilus Test Medium (HTM).[2]

[b]These quality control limits apply only to tests conducted with *S. pneumoniae* ATCC 49619 using Mueller-Hinton agar supplemented with 5% sheep blood incubated in 5% CO_2.

INDICATIONS AND USAGE

ZITHROMAX® (azithromycin) is indicated for the treatment of patients with mild to moderate infections (pneumonia: see **WARNINGS**) caused by susceptible strains of the designated microorganisms in the specific conditions listed below. As recommended dosages, durations of therapy, and applicable patient populations vary among these infections, please see **DOSAGE AND ADMINISTRATION** for specific dosing recommendations.

Adults:

Acute bacterial exacerbations of chronic obstructive pulmonary disease due to *Haemophilus influenzae, Moraxella catarrhalis,* or *Streptococcus pneumoniae.*

Community-acquired pneumonia due to *Chlamydia pneumoniae, Haemophilus influenzae, Mycoplasma pneumoniae,* or *Streptococcus pneumoniae* in patients appropriate for oral therapy.

NOTE: Azithromycin should not be used in patients with pneumonia who are judged to be inappropriate for oral therapy because of moderate to severe illness or risk factors such as any of the following:

patients with cystic fibrosis,

patients with nosocomially acquired infections,

patients with known or suspected bacteremia,

patients requiring hospitalization,

elderly or debilitated patients, or

patients with significant underlying health problems that may compromise their ability to respond to their illness (including immunodeficiency or functional asplenia).

Pharyngitis/tonsillitis caused by *Streptococcus pyogenes* as an alternative to first-line therapy in individuals who cannot use first-line therapy.

NOTE: Penicillin by the intramuscular route is the usual drug of choice in the treatment of *Streptococcus pyogenes* infection and the prophylaxis of rheumatic fever. ZITHROMAX® is often effective in the eradication of susceptible strains of *Streptococcus pyogenes* from the nasopharynx. Because some strains are resistant to ZITHROMAX®, susceptibility tests should be performed when patients are treated with ZITHROMAX®. Data establishing efficacy of azithromycin in subsequent prevention of rheumatic fever are not available.

Uncomplicated skin and skin structure infections due to *Staphylococcus aureus, Streptococcus pyogenes,* or *Streptococcus agalactiae.* Abscesses usually require surgical drainage.

Urethritis and cervicitis due to *Chlamydia trachomatis* or *Neisseria gonorrhoeae.*

Genital ulcer disease in men due to *Haemophilus ducreyi* (chancroid). Due to the small number of women included in clinical trials, the efficacy of azithromycin in the treatment of chancroid in women has not been established.

ZITHROMAX®, at the recommended dose, should not be relied upon to treat syphilis. Antimicrobial agents used in high doses for short periods of time to treat non-gonococcal urethritis may mask or delay the symptoms of incubating syphilis. All patients with sexually-transmitted urethritis or cervicitis should have a serologic test for syphilis and appropriate cultures for gonorrhea performed at the time of diagnosis. Appropriate antimicrobial therapy and follow-up tests for these diseases should be initiated if infection is confirmed.

Appropriate culture and susceptibility tests should be performed before treatment to determine the causative organism and its susceptibility to azithromycin. Therapy with ZITHROMAX® may be initiated before results of these tests are known; once the results become available, antimicrobial therapy should be adjusted accordingly.

Children: (See **Pediatric Use** and **CLINICAL STUDIES IN PEDIATRIC PATIENTS.**)

Acute otitis media caused by *Haemophilus influenzae, Moraxella catarrhalis,* or *Streptococcus pneumoniae.* (For specific dosage recommendation, see **DOSAGE AND ADMINISTRATION.**)

Community-acquired pneumonia due to *Chlamydia pneumoniae, Haemophilus influenzae, Mycoplasma pneumoniae,* or *Streptococcus pneumoniae* in patients appropriate for oral therapy. (For specific dosage recommendation, see **DOSAGE AND ADMINISTRATION.**)

NOTE: Azithromycin should not be used in pediatric patients with pneumonia who are judged to be inappropriate for oral therapy because of moderate to severe illness or risk factors such as any of the following:

patients with cystic fibrosis,

patients with nosocomially acquired infections,

patients with known or suspected bacteremia,

patients requiring hospitalization, or

patients with significant underlying health problems that may compromise their ability to respond to their illness (including immunodeficiency or functional asplenia).

Pharyngitis/tonsillitis caused by *Streptococcus pyogenes* as an alternative to first-line therapy in individuals who cannot use first-line therapy. (For specific dosage recommendation, see **DOSAGE AND ADMINISTRATION.**)

NOTE: Penicillin by the intramuscular route is the usual drug of choice in the treatment of *Streptococcus pyogenes* infection and the prophylaxis of rheumatic fever. ZITHROMAX® is often effective in the eradication of susceptible strains of *Streptococcus pyogenes* from the nasopharynx. Because some strains are resistant to ZITHROMAX®, susceptibility tests should be performed when patients are treated with ZITHROMAX®. Data establishing efficacy of azithromycin in subsequent prevention of rheumatic fever are not available.

Appropriate culture and susceptibility tests should be performed before treatment to determine the causative organism and its susceptibility to azithromycin. Therapy with ZITHROMAX® may be initiated before results of these tests are known; once the results become available, antimicrobial therapy should be adjusted accordingly.

CONTRAINDICATIONS

ZITHROMAX® is contraindicated in patients with known hypersensitivity to azithromycin, erythromycin, or any macrolide antibiotic.

WARNINGS

Serious allergic reactions, including angioedema, anaphylaxis, and dermatologic reactions including Stevens Johnson Syndrome and toxic epidermal necrolysis have been reported rarely in patients on azithromycin therapy. Although rare, fatalities have been reported. (See **CONTRAINDICATIONS.**) Despite initially successful symptomatic treatment of the allergic symptoms, when symptomatic therapy was discontinued, the allergic symptoms **recurred soon thereafter in some patients without further azithromycin exposure.** These patients required prolonged periods of observation and symptomatic treatment. The relationship of these episodes to the long tissue half-life of azithromycin and subsequent prolonged exposure to antigen is unknown at present.

If an allergic reaction occurs, the drug should be discontinued and appropriate therapy should be instituted. Physicians should be aware that reappearance of the allergic symptoms may occur when symptomatic therapy is discontinued.

In the treatment of pneumonia, azithromycin has only been shown to be safe and effective in the treatment of community-acquired pneumonia due to *Chlamydia pneumoniae, Haemophilus influenzae, Mycoplasma pneumoniae,* or *Streptococcus pneumoniae* in patients appropriate for oral therapy. Azithromycin should not be used in patients with pneumonia who are judged to be inappropriate for oral therapy because of moderate to severe illness or risk factors such as any of the following: patients with cystic fibrosis, patients with nosocomially acquired infections, patients with known or suspected bacteremia, patients requiring hospitalization, elderly or debilitated patients, or patients with significant underlying health problems that may compromise their ability to respond to their illness (including immunodeficiency or functional asplenia).

Pseudomembranous colitis has been reported with nearly all antibacterial agents and may range in severity from mild to life-threatening. Therefore, it is important to consider this diagnosis in patients who present with diarrhea subsequent to the administration of antibacterial agents.

Treatment with antibacterial agents alters the normal flora of the colon and may permit overgrowth of clostridia. Studies indicate that a toxin produced by *Clostridium difficile* is a primary cause of "antibiotic-associated colitis."

After the diagnosis of pseudomembranous colitis has been established, therapeutic measures should be initiated. Mild cases of pseudomembranous colitis usually respond to discontinuation of the drug alone. In moderate to severe cases, consideration should be given to management with fluids and electrolytes, protein supplementation, and treatment with an antibacterial drug clinically effective against *Clostridium difficile* colitis.

PRECAUTIONS

General: Because azithromycin is principally eliminated via the liver, caution should be exercised when azithromycin is administered to patients with impaired hepatic function. There are no data regarding azithromycin usage in patients with renal impairment; thus, caution should be exercised when prescribing azithromycin in these patients.

The following adverse events have not been reported in clinical trials with azithromycin, an azalide; however, they have been reported with macrolide products: ventricular arrhythmias, including ventricular tachycardia and *torsade de pointes,* in individuals with prolonged QT intervals.

There has been a spontaneous report from the post-marketing experience of a patient with previous history of arrhythmias who experienced *torsade de pointes* and subsequent myocardial infarction following a course of azithromycin therapy.

Information for Patients:

Patients should be cautioned to take ZITHROMAX® capsules and ZITHROMAX® suspension at least one hour prior to a meal or at least two hours after a meal. These medications should not be taken with food.

ZITHROMAX® tablets can be taken with or without food.

Patients should also be cautioned not to take aluminum- and magnesium-containing antacids and azithromycin simultaneously.

The patient should be directed to discontinue azithromycin immediately and contact a physician if any signs of an allergic reaction occur.

Drug Interactions: Aluminum- and magnesium-containing antacids reduce the peak serum levels (rate) but not the AUC (extent) of azithromycin absorption.

Administration of cimetidine (800 mg) two hours prior to azithromycin had no effect on azithromycin absorption.

Azithromycin did not affect the plasma levels or pharmacokinetics of theophylline administered as a single intravenous dose. The effect of azithromycin on the plasma levels or pharmacokinetics of theophylline administered in multiple doses resulting in therapeutic steady-state levels of theophylline is not known. However, concurrent use of macrolides and theophylline has been associated with increases in the serum concentrations of theophylline. Therefore, until further data are available, prudent medical practice dictates careful monitoring of plasma theophylline levels in patients receiving azithromycin and theophylline concomitantly.

Azithromycin did not affect the prothrombin time response to a single dose of warfarin. However, prudent medical practice dictates careful monitoring of prothrombin time in all patients treated with azithromycin and warfarin concomitantly. Concurrent use of macrolides and warfarin in clinical practice has been associated with increased anticoagulant effects.

The following drug interactions have not been reported in clinical trials with azithromycin; however, no specific drug interaction studies have been performed to evaluate potential drug-drug interaction. Nonetheless, they have been observed with macrolide products. Until further data are developed regarding drug interactions when azithromycin and these drugs are used concomitantly, careful monitoring of patients is advised:

Digoxin-elevated digoxin levels.

Ergotamine or dihydroergotamine-acute ergot toxicity characterized by severe peripheral vasospasm and dysesthesia.

Triazolam-decrease the clearance of triazolam and thus may increase the pharmacologic effect of triazolam.

Drugs metabolized by the cytochrome P^{450} system-elevations of serum carbamazepine, terfenadine, cyclosporine, hexobarbital, and phenytoin levels.

Laboratory Test Interactions: There are no reported laboratory test interactions.

Carcinogenesis, Mutagenesis, Impairment of Fertility: Long-term studies in animals have not been performed to evaluate carcinogenic potential. Azithromycin has shown no mutagenic potential in standard laboratory tests: mouse lymphoma assay, human lymphocyte clastogenic assay, and mouse bone marrow clastogenic assay. No evidence of impaired fertility due to azithromycin was found.

Pregnancy: Teratogenic Effects. Pregnancy Category B: Reproduction studies have been performed in rats and mice at doses up to moderately maternally toxic dose levels (i.e., 200 mg/kg/day). These doses, based on a mg/m^2 basis, are estimated to be 4 and 2 times, respectively, the human daily dose of 500 mg. In the animal studies, no evidence of harm to the fetus due to azithromycin was found. There are, however, no adequate and well-controlled studies in pregnant women. Because animal reproduction studies are not always predictive of human response, azithromycin should be used during pregnancy only if clearly needed.

Nursing Mothers: It is not known whether azithromycin is excreted in human milk. Because many drugs are excreted in human milk, caution should be exercised when azithromycin is administered to a nursing woman.

Pediatric Use: (See **CLINICAL PHARMACOLOGY, INDICATIONS AND USAGE,** and **DOSAGE AND ADMINISTRATION.**)

Acute Otitis Media (dosage regimen: 10 mg/kg on Day 1 followed by 5 mg/kg on Days 2–5): Safety and effectiveness in the treatment of children with otitis media under 6 months of age have not been established.

Community-Aquired Pneumonia (dosage regimen: 10 mg/kg on Day 1 followed by 5 mg/kg on Days 2–5): Safety and effectiveness in the treatment of children with community-acquired pneumonia under 6 months of age have not been established. Safety and effectiveness for pneumonia due to *Chlamydia pneumoniae* and *Mycoplasma pneumoniae* were documented in pediatric clinical trials. Safety and effectiveness for pneumonia due to *Haemophilus influenzae* and *Streptococcus pneumoniae* were not documented bacteriologically in the pediatric clinical trial due to difficulty in obtaining specimens. Use of azithromycin for these two microorganisms is supported, however, by evidence from adequate and well-controlled studies in adults.

Pharyngitis/Tonsillitis (dosage regimen: 12 mg/kg on Days 1–5): Safety and effectiveness in the treatment of children with pharyngitis/tonsillitis under 2 years of age have not been established.

Studies evaluating the use of repeated courses of therapy have not been conducted. (See CLINICAL PHARMACOLOGY and ANIMAL TOXICOLOGY.)

Geriatric Use: Pharmacokinetic parameters in older volunteers (65–85 years old) were similar to those in younger volunteers (18–40 years old) for the 5-day therapeutic regimen. Dosage adjustment does not appear to be necessary for older patients with normal renal and hepatic function receiving treatment with this dosage regimen. (See **CLINICAL PHARMACOLOGY.**)

ADVERSE REACTIONS

In clinical trials, most of the reported side effects were mild to moderate in severity and were reversible upon discontinuation of the drug. Approximately 0.7% of the patients (adults and children) from the multiple-dose clinical trials discontinued ZITHROMAX® (azithromycin) therapy because of treatment-related side effects. Most of the side effects leading to discontinuation were related to the gastrointestinal tract, e.g., nausea, vomiting, diarrhea, or abdominal pain. Potentially serious side effects of angioedema and cholestatic jaundice were reported rarely.

Clinical:

Adults:

Multiple-dose regimen: Overall, the most common side effects in adult patients receiving a multiple-dose regimen of ZITHROMAX® were related to the gastrointestinal system with diarrhea/loose stools (5%), nausea (3%), and abdominal pain (3%) being the most frequently reported.

No other side effects occurred in patients on the multiple-dose regimen of ZITHROMAX® with a frequency greater than 1%. Side effects that occurred with a frequency of 1% or less included the following:

Continued on next page

Zithromax—Cont.

Cardiovascular: Palpitations, chest pain.
Gastrointestinal: Dyspepsia, flatulence, vomiting, melena, and cholestatic jaundice.
Genitourinary: Monilia, vaginitis, and nephritis.
Nervous System: Dizziness, headache, vertigo, and somnolence.
General: Fatigue.
Allergic: Rash, photosensitivity, and angioedema.
Single 1-gram dose regimen: Overall, the most common side effects in patients receiving a single-dose regimen of 1 gram of ZITHROMAX® were related to the gastrointestinal system and were more frequently reported than in patients receiving the multiple-dose regimen.
Side effects that occurred in patients on the single one-gram dosing regimen of ZITHROMAX® with a frequency of 1% or greater included diarrhea/loose stools (7%), nausea (5%), abdominal pain (5%), vomiting (2%), dyspepsia (1%), and vaginitis (1%).
Single 2-gram dose regimen: Overall, the most common side effects in patients receiving a single 2-gram dose of ZITHROMAX® were related to the gastrointestinal system. Side effects that occurred in patients in this study with a frequency of 1% or greater included nausea (18%), diarrhea/loose stools (14%), vomiting (7%), abdominal pain (7%), vaginitis (2%), dyspepsia (1%), and dizziness (1%). The majority of these complaints were mild in nature.
Children:
Multiple-dose regimens: The types of side effects in children were comparable to those seen in adults, with different incidence rates for the two dosage regimens recommended in children.
Acute Otitis Media: For the recommended dosage regimen of 10 mg/kg on Day 1 followed by 5 mg/kg on Days 2–5, the most frequent side effects attributed to treatment were diarrhea/loose stools (2%), abdominal pain (2%), vomiting (1%), and nausea (1%).
Community-Acquired Pneumonia: For the recommended dosage regimen of 10 mg/kg on Day 1 followed by 5 mg/kg on Days 2–5, the most frequent side effects attributed to treatment were diarrhea/loose stools (5.8%), abdominal pain, vomiting, and nausea (1.9% each), and rash (1.6%).
Pharyngitis/tonsillitis: For the recommended dosage regimen of 12 mg/kg on Days 1–5, the most frequent side effects attributed to treatment were diarrhea/loose stools (6%), vomiting (5%), abdominal pain (3%), nausea (2%), and headache (1%).
With either treatment regimen, no other side effects occurred in children treated with ZITHROMAX® with a frequency greater than 1%. Side effects that occurred with a frequency of 1% or less included the following:
Cardiovascular: Chest pain.
Gastrointestinal: Dyspepsia, constipation, anorexia, flatulence, and gastritis.
Nervous System: Headache (otitis media dosage), hyperkinesia, dizziness, agitation, nervousness, insomnia.
General: Fever, fatigue, malaise.
Allergic: Rash.
Skin and Appendages: Pruritus, urticaria.
Special Senses: Conjunctivitis.
Post-Marketing Experience:
Adverse events reported with azithromycin during the post-marketing period in adult and/or pediatric patients for which a causal relationship may not be established include:
Allergic: Arthralgia, edema, urticaria, angioedema.
Cardiovascular: Arrhythmias including ventricular tachycardia.
Gastrointestinal: Anorexia, constipation, dyspepsia, flatulence, vomiting/diarrhea rarely resulting in dehydration, pseudomembranous colitis and rare reports of tongue discoloration.
General: Asthenia, paresthesia and anaphylaxis (rarely fatal).
Genitourinary: Interstitial nephritis and acute renal failure, oral candidiasis, vaginitis.
Hematopoietic: Thrombocytopenia.
Liver/Biliary: Abnormal liver function including hepatitis and cholestatic jaundice, as well as rare cases of hepatic necrosis and hepatic failure, some of which have resulted in death.
Nervous System: Convulsions, dizziness/vertigo, headache, somnolence, hyperactivity, nervousness, and agitation.
Psychiatric: Aggressive reaction and anxiety.
Skin/Appendages: Pruritus, rarely serious skin reactions including erythema multiforme, Stevens Johnson Syndrome, and toxic epidermal necrolysis.
Special Senses: Hearing disturbances including hearing loss, deafness, and/or tinnitus, rare reports of taste perversion.
Laboratory Abnormalities:
Adults:
Significant abnormalities (irrespective of drug relationship) occurring during the clinical trials were reported as follows: with an incidence of 1–2%, elevated serum creatine phosphokinase, potassium, ALT (SGPT), GGT, and AST (SGOT); with an incidence of less than 1%, leukopenia, neutropenia, decreased platelet count, elevated serum alkaline phosphatase, bilirubin, BUN, creatinine, blood glucose, LDH, and phosphate.
When follow-up was provided, changes in laboratory tests appeared to be reversible.

PEDIATRIC DOSAGE GUIDELINES FOR OTITIS MEDIA AND COMMUNITY-ACQUIRED PNEUMONIA
(Age 6 months and above, see Pediatric Use.)
Based on Body Weight

OTITIS MEDIA AND COMMUNITY-ACQUIRED PNEUMONIA

Dosing Calculated on 10 mg/kg on Day 1 dose, followed by 5 mg/kg on Days 2 to 5.

Weight		100 mg/5 mL Suspension		200 mg/5 mL Suspension		
Kg	lbs	Day 1	Days 2–5	Day 1	Days 2–5	Total mL per Treatment Course
10	22	5 mL (1 tsp)	2.5 mL (½ tsp)			15 mL
20	44			5 mL (1 tsp)	2.5 mL (½ tsp)	15 mL
30	66			7.5 mL (1½ tsp)	3.75 mL (¾ tsp)	22.5 mL
40	88			10 mL (2 tsp)	5 mL (1 tsp)	30 mL

PEDIATRIC DOSAGE GUIDELINES FOR PHARYNGITIS/TONSILLITIS
(Age 2 years and above, see Pediatric Use.)
Based on Body Weight

PHARYNGITIS/TONSILLITIS

Dosing Calculated on 12 mg/kg once daily Days 1 to 5.

Weight		200 mg/5 mL Suspension Day 1–5	Total mL per Treatment Course
Kg	lbs		
8	18	2.5 mL (½ tsp)	12.5 mL
17	37	5 mL (1 tsp)	25 mL
25	55	7.5 mL (1½ tsp)	37.5 mL
33	73	10 mL (2 tsp)	50 mL
40	88	12.5 mL (2½ tsp)	62.5 mL

Amount of water to be added	Total volume after constitution (azithromycin content)	Azithromycin concentration after constitution
9 mL (300 mg)	15 mL (300 mg)	100 mg/5 mL
9 mL (600 mg)	15 mL (600 mg)	200 mg/5 mL
12 mL (900 mg)	22.5 mL (900 mg)	200 mg/5 mL
5 mL (1200 mg)	30 mL (1200 mg)	200 mg/5 mL

In multiple-dose clinical trials involving more than 3000 patients, 3 patients discontinued therapy because of treatment-related liver enzyme abnormalities and 1 because of a renal function abnormality.
Children:
Significant abnormalities (irrespective of drug relationship) occurring during clinical trials were all reported at a frequency of less than 1%, but were similar in type to the adult pattern.
In multiple-dose clinical trials involving almost 3300 pediatric patients, no patients discontinued therapy because of treatment-related laboratory abnormalities.

DOSAGE AND ADMINISTRATION
(See INDICATIONS AND USAGE and CLINICAL PHARMACOLOGY.)
Adults:
The recommended dose of ZITHROMAX® for the treatment of mild to moderate acute bacterial exacerbations of chronic obstructive pulmonary disease, community-acquired pneumonia of mild severity, pharyngitis/tonsillitis (as second-line therapy), and uncomplicated skin and skin structure infections due to the indicated organisms is: 500 mg as a single dose on the first day followed by 250 mg once daily on days 2 through 5.
ZITHROMAX® capsules should be given at least 1 hour before or 2 hours after a meal. ZITHROMAX® capsules should not be taken with food.
ZITHROMAX® tablets can be taken with or without food.
The recommended dose of ZITHROMAX® for the treatment of genital ulcer disease due to *Haemophilus ducreyi* (chancroid), non-gonococcal urethritis and cervicitis due to *C. trachomatis* is: a single 1 gram (1000 mg) dose of ZITHROMAX®.
The recommended dose of ZITHROMAX® for the treatment of urethritis and cervicitis due to *Neisseria gonorrhoeae* is a single 2 gram (2000 mg) dose of ZITHROMAX®.
Children:
Acute Otitis Media and Community-Acquired Pneumonia:
The recommended dose of ZITHROMAX® for oral suspension for the treatment of children with acute otitis media and community-acquired pneumonia is 10 mg/kg as a single dose on the first day (not to exceed 500 mg/day) followed by 5 mg/kg on days 2 through 5 (not to exceed 250 mg/day). (See chart below.)
ZITHROMAX® for oral suspension should be given at least 1 hour before or 2 hours after a meal.
ZITHROMAX® for oral suspension should not be taken with food.
[See first table above]

Pharyngitis/Tonsillitis: The recommended dose for children with pharyngitis/tonsillitis is 12 mg/kg once a day for 5 days (not to exceed 500 mg/day). (See chart below.)
ZITHROMAX® for oral suspension should be given at least 1 hour before or 2 hours after a meal.
ZITHROMAX® for oral suspension should not be taken with food.
[See second table above]
Constituting instructions for ZITHROMAX® Oral Suspension, 300, 600, 900, 1200 mg bottles. The table below indicates the volume of water to be used for constitution:
[See third table above]
Shake well before each use. Oversized bottle provides shake space. Keep tightly closed.
After mixing, store at 5° to 30°C (41° to 86°F) and use within 10 days. Discard after full dosing is completed.

HOW SUPPLIED
ZITHROMAX® tablets are supplied as red modified capsular shaped, engraved, film-coated tablets containing azithromycin dihydrate equivalent to 250 mg of azithromycin.
ZITHROMAX® tablets are engraved with "PFIZER" on one side and "306" on the other. These are packaged in bottles and blister cards of 6 tablets (Z-PAKS®) as follows:

Bottles of 30	NDC 0069-3060-30
Boxes of 3 (Z-PAKS® of 6)	NDC 0069-3060-75
Unit Dose package of 50	NDC 0069-3060-86

ZITHROMAX® tablets should be stored between 15° to 30°C (59° to 86°F).
ZITHROMAX® for oral suspension after constitution contains a flavored suspension.
ZITHROMAX® for oral suspension is supplied in bottles with accompanying calibrated dropper as follows:

Azithromycin contents per bottle	NDC
300 mg	NDC 0069-3110-19
600 mg	NDC 0069-3120-19
900 mg	NDC 0069-3130-19
1200 mg	NDC 0069-3140-19

Storage: Store dry powder below 30°C (86°F). Store constituted suspension between 5° to 30°C (41° to 86°F) and discard when full dosing is completed.

CLINICAL STUDIES IN PEDIATRIC PATIENTS
(See INDICATIONS AND USAGE and Pediatric Use.)
From the perspective of evaluating pediatric clinical trials, Days 11–14 (6–9 days after completion of the five-day regi-

Bacteriologic Eradication:

	Day 11 Azithromycin	Day 30 Azithromycin
S. pneumoniae	61/74 (82%)	40/56 (71%)
H. influenzae	43/54 (80%)	30/47 (64%)
M. catarrhalis	28/35 (80%)	19/26 (73%)
S. pyogenes	11/11 (100%)	7/7
Overall	177/217 (82%)	97/137 (73%)

Bacteriologic Eradication:

	Day 11		Day 30	
	Azithromycin	Control	Azithromycin	Control
S. pneumoniae	25/29 (86%)	26/26 (100%)	22/28 (79%)	18/22 (82%)
H. influenzae	9/11 (82%)	9/9	8/10 (80%)	6/8
M. catarrhalis	7/7	5/5	5/5	2/3
S. pyogenes	2/2	5/5	2/2	4/4
Overall	43/49 (88%)	45/45 (100%)	37/45 (82%)	30/37 (81%)

Three U.S. Streptococcal Pharyngitis Studies
Azithromycin vs. Penicillin V
EFFICACY RESULTS

	Day 14	Day 30
Bacteriologic Eradication:		
Azithromycin	323/340 (95%)	255/330 (77%)
Penicillin V	242/332 (73%)	206/325 (63%)
Clinical Success (Cure plus improvement):		
Azithromycin	336/343 (98%)	310/330 (94%)
Penicillin V	284/338 (84%)	241/325 (74%)

men) were considered on-therapy evaluations because of the extended half-life of azithromycin. Day 11–14 data are provided for clinical guidance. Day 30 evaluations were considered the primary test of cure endpoint.

Acute Otitis Media

Efficacy Protocol 1

In a double-blind, controlled clinical study of acute otitis media performed in the United States, azithromycin (10 mg/kg on Day 1 followed by 5 mg/kg on Days 2–5) was compared to an antimicrobial/beta-lactamase inhibitor. In this study, very strict evaluability criteria were used to determine clinical response and safety results were obtained. For the 553 patients who were evaluated for clinical efficacy, the clinical success rate (i.e., cure plus improvement) at the Day 11 visit was 88% for azithromycin and 88% for the control agent. For the 521 patients who were evaluated at the Day 30 visit, the clinical success rate was 73% for azithromycin and 71% for the control agent.

In the safety analysis of the above study, the incidence of adverse events, primarily gastrointestinal, in all patients treated was 9% with azithromycin and 31% with the control agent. The most common side effects were diarrhea/loose stools (4% azithromycin vs. 20% control), vomiting (2% azithromycin vs. 7% control), and abdominal pain (2% azithromycin vs. 5% control).

Efficacy Protocol 2

In a noncomparative clinical and microbiologic trial performed in the United States, where significant rates of beta-lactamase producing organisms (35%) were found, 131 patients were evaluable for clinical efficacy. The combined clinical success rate (i.e., cure and improvement) at the Day 11 visit was 84% for azithromycin. For the 122 patients who were evaluated at the Day 30 visit, the clinical success rate was 70% for azithromycin.

Microbiologic determinations were made at the pre-treatment visit. Microbiology was not reassessed at later visits. The following presumptive bacterial/clinical cure outcomes (i.e., clinical success) were obtained from the evaluable group:

[See first table above]

In the safety analysis of this study, the incidence of adverse events, primarily gastrointestinal, in all patients treated was 9%. The most common side effect was diarrhea (4%).

Efficacy Protocol 3

In another controlled comparative clinical and microbiologic study of otitis media performed in the United States, azithromycin was compared to an antimicrobial/beta-lactamase inhibitor. This study utilized two of the same investigators as Efficacy Protocol 2 (above), and these two investigators enrolled 90% of the patients in Efficacy Protocol 3. For this reason, Efficacy Protocol 3 was not considered to be an independent study. Significant rates of beta-lactamase producing organisms (20%) were found. Ninety-two (92) patients were evaluable for clinical and microbiologic efficacy. The combined clinical success rate (i.e., cure and improvement) of those patients with a baseline pathogen at the Day 11 visit was 88% for azithromycin vs. 100% for control; at the Day 30 visit, the clinical success rate was 82% for azithromycin vs. 80% for control.

Microbiologic determinations were made at the pre-treatment visit. Microbiology was not reassessed at later visits. At the Day 11 and Day 30 visits, the following presumptive bacterial/clinical cure outcomes (i.e., clinical success) were obtained from the evaluable group:

[See second table above]

In the safety analysis of the above study, the incidence of adverse events, primarily gastrointestinal, in all patients treated was 4% with azithromycin and 31% with the control agent. The most common side effect was diarrhea/loose stools (2% azithromycin vs. 29% control).

Pharyngitis/Tonsillitis

In 3 double-blind controlled studies, conducted in the United States, azithromycin (12 mg/kg once a day for 5 days) was compared to penicillin V (250 mg three times a day for 10 days) in the treatment of pharyngitis due to documented Group A β-hemolytic streptococci (GABHS or *S. pyogenes*). Azithromycin was clinically and microbiologically statistically superior to penicillin at Day 14 and Day 30 with the following clinical success (i.e., cure and improvement) and bacteriologic efficacy rates (for the combined evaluable patient with documented GABHS):

[See third table above]

Approximately 1% of azithromycin-susceptible *S. pyogenes* isolates were resistant to azithromycin following therapy.

The incidence of adverse events, primarily gastrointestinal, in all patients treated was 18% on azithromycin and 13% on penicillin. The most common side effects were diarrhea/loose stools (6% azithromycin vs. 2% penicillin), vomiting (6% azithromycin vs. 4% penicillin), and abdominal pain (3% azithromycin vs. 1% penicillin).

ANIMAL TOXICOLOGY

Phospholipidosis (intracellular phospholipid accumulation) has been observed in some tissues of mice, rats, and dogs given multiple doses of azithromycin. It has been demonstrated in numerous organ systems (e.g., eye, dorsal root ganglia, liver, gallbladder, kidney, spleen, and pancreas) in dogs treated with azithromycin at doses which, expressed on a mg/kg basis, are only 2 times greater than the recommended adult human dose and in rats at doses comparable to the recommended adult human dose. This effect has been reversible after cessation of azithromycin treatment. Phospholipidosis has been observed to a similar extent in the tissues of neonatal rats and dogs given daily doses of azithromycin ranging from 10 days to 30 days. Based on the pharmacokinetic data, phospholipidosis has been seen in the rat (30 mg/kg dose) at observed C_{max} value of 1.3 μg/mL (6 times greater than the observed C_{max} of 0.216 μg/mL at the pediatric dose of 10 mg/kg). Similarly, it has been shown in the dog (10 mg/kg dose) at observed C_{max} value of 1.5 μg/mL (7 times greater than the observed same C_{max} and drug dose in the studied pediatric population). On mg/m^2 basis, 30 mg/kg dose in the rat (135 mg/m^2) and 10 mg/kg dose in the dog (79 mg/m^2) are approximately 0.4 and 0.6 times, respectively, the recommended dose in the pediatric patients with an average body weight of 25 kg. This effect, similar to that seen in the adult animals, is reversible after cessation of azithromycin treatment. The significance of these findings for animals and for humans is unknown.

REFERENCES:

1. National Committee for Clinical Laboratory Standards. Methods for Dilution Antimicrobial Susceptibility Tests for Bacteria that Grow Aerobically–Third Edition. Approved Standard NCCLS Document M7-A3, Vol. 13, No. 25, NCCLS, Villanova, PA, December 1993.
2. National Committee for Clinical Laboratory Standards. Performance Standards for Antimicrobial Disk Susceptibility Tests–Fifth Edition. Approved Standard NCCLS Document M2-A5, Vol. 13, No. 24, NCCLS, Villanova, PA, December 1993.

Rx only

Licensed from Pliva

Pfizer Labs
Division of Pfizer Inc, NY, NY 10017
Printed in U.S.A.
70-5179-00-8
Revised January 2001

ZITHROMAX® ℞

(azithromycin for injection)

For IV infusion only

Prescribing information for this product, which appears on pages 2550–2553 of the 2001 PDR, has been completely revised as follows. Please write "See Supplement A" next to the product heading.

DESCRIPTION

ZITHROMAX® (azithromycin for injection) contains the active ingredient azithromycin, an azalide, a subclass of macrolide antibiotics, for intravenous injection. Azithromycin has the chemical name (*2R,3S,4R,5R,8R,10R,11R,12S,13S,14R*)-13-[(2,6-dideoxy-3-*C*-methyl-3-*O*-methyl-α-*L*-*ribo*-hexopyranosyl)oxy]-2-ethyl-3,4,10-trihydroxy-3,5,6,8,10,12,14-heptamethyl-11-[[3,4,6-trideoxy-3-(dimethylamino)-β-*D*-*xylo*-hexopyranosyl]oxy]-1-oxa-6-azacyclopentadecan-15-one. Azithromycin is derived from erythromycin; however, it differs chemically from erythromycin in that a methyl-substituted nitrogen atom is incorporated into the lactone ring. Its molecular formula is $C_{38}H_{72}N_2O_{12}$, and its molecular weight is 749.00. Azithromycin has the following structural formula:

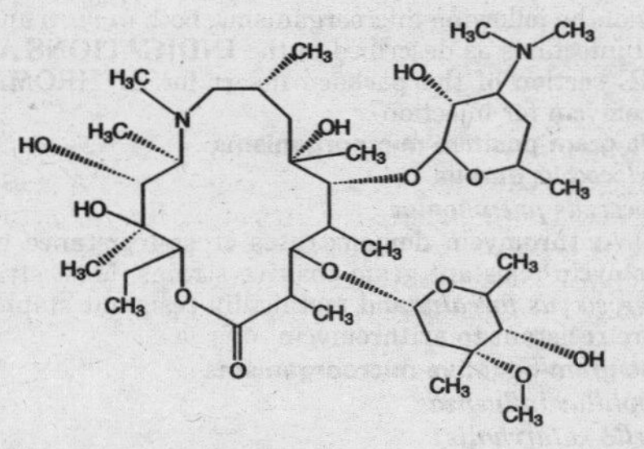

Azithromycin, as the dihydrate, is a white crystalline powder with a molecular formula of $C_{38}H_{72}N_2O_{12} \cdot 2H_2O$ and a molecular weight of 785.0.

ZITHROMAX® (azithromycin for injection) consists of azithromycin dihydrate and the following inactive ingredients: citric acid and sodium hydroxide. ZITHROMAX® (azithromycin for injection) is supplied in lyophilized form in a 10-mL vial equivalent to 500 mg of azithromycin for intravenous administration. Reconstitution, according to label directions, results in approximately 5 mL of ZITHROMAX® for intravenous injection with each mL containing azithromycin dihydrate equivalent to 100 mg of azithromycin.

CLINICAL PHARMACOLOGY

In patients hospitalized with community-acquired pneumonia receiving single daily one-hour intravenous infusions for 2 to 5 days of 500 mg azithromycin at a concentration of 2 mg/mL, the mean C_{max} ± S.D. achieved was 3.63 ± 1.60 μg/mL, while the 24-hour trough level was 0.20 ± 0.15 μg/mL, and the AUC_{24} was 9.60 ± 4.80 μg•h/mL.

The mean C_{max}, 24-hour trough and AUC_{24} values were 1.14 ± 0.14 μg/mL, 0.18 ± 0.02 μg/mL, and 8.03 ± 0.86 μg•h/mL, respectively, in normal volunteers receiving a 3-hour intravenous infusion of 500 mg azithromycin at a concentration of 1 mg/mL. Similar pharmacokinetic values were obtained in patients hospitalized with community-acquired pneumonia that received the same 3-hour dosage regimen for 2–5 days.

[See first table at top of next page]

The average CL_t and V_d values were 10.18 mL/min/kg and 33.3 L/kg, respectively, in 18 normal volunteers receiving 1000 to 4000-mg doses given as 1 mg/mL over 2 hours.

Comparison of the plasma pharmacokinetic parameters following the 1st and 5th daily doses of 500 mg intravenous azithromycin showed only an 8% increase in C_{max} but a 61% increase in AUC_{24} reflecting a threefold rise in C_{24} trough levels.

Following single oral doses of 500 mg azithromycin to 12 healthy volunteers, C_{max}, trough level, and AUC_{24} were reported to be 0.41 μg/mL, 0.05 μg/mL, and 2.6 μg•h/mL, respectively. These oral values are approximately 38%, 83%, and 52% of the values observed following a single 500-mg I.V. 3-hour infusion (C_{max}: 1.08 μg/mL, trough: 0.06 μg/mL, and AUC_{24}: 5.0 μg•h/mL). Thus, plasma concentrations are higher following the intravenous regimen throughout the 24-hour interval. The pharmacokinetic parameters on day 5 of azithromycin 250-mg capsules following a 500-mg oral loading dose to healthy young adults (age 18-40 years old) were as follows: C_{max}: 0.24 μg/mL, AUC_{24}: 2.1 μg•h/mL. Tissue levels have not been obtained following intravenous infusions of azithromycin. Selected tissue (or fluid) concentration and tissue (or fluid) to plasma/serum concentration ratios following oral administration of azithromycin are shown in the following table:

[See second table at top of next page]

Tissue levels were determined following a single oral dose of 500 mg azithromycin in 7 gynecological patients. Approximately 17 hours after dosing, azithromycin concentrations were 2.7 μg/g in ovarian tissue, 3.5 μg/g in uterine tissue, and 3.3 μg/g in salpinx. Tissue levels have not been obtained following intravenous infusion of azithromycin.

In a multiple-dose study in 12 normal volunteers utilizing a 500-mg (1 mg/mL) one-hour intravenous-dosage regimen for five days, the amount of administered azithromycin dose excreted in urine in 24 hours was about 11% after the 1st dose and 14% after the 5th dose. These values are greater than the reported 6% excreted unchanged in urine after oral administration of azithromycin. Biliary excretion is a major route of elimination for unchanged drug, following oral administration.

Continued on next page

Zithromax IV—Cont.

The serum protein binding of azithromycin is variable in the concentration range approximating human exposure decreasing from 51% at 0.02 µg/mL to 7% at 2 µg/mL.

Microbiology: Azithromycin acts by binding to the 50S ribosomal subunit of susceptible microorganisms and, thus, interfering with microbial protein synthesis. Nucleic acid synthesis is not affected.

Azithromycin concentrates in phagocytes and fibroblasts as demonstrated by *in vitro* incubation techniques. Using such methodology, the ratio of intracellular to extracellular concentration was >30 after one hour incubation. *In vivo* studies suggest that concentration in phagocytes may contribute to drug distribution to inflamed tissues.

Azithromycin has been shown to be active against most strains of the following microorganisms, both *in vitro* and in clinical infections as described in the **INDICATIONS AND USAGE** section of the package insert for ZITHROMAX® (azithromycin for injection).

Aerobic gram-positive microorganisms
Staphylococcus aureus
Streptococcus pneumoniae
NOTE: Azithromycin demonstrates cross-resistance with erythromycin-resistant gram-positive strains. Most strains of *Enterococcus faecalis* and methicillin-resistant staphylococci are resistant to azithromycin.

Aerobic gram-negative microorganisms
Haemophilus influenzae
Moraxella catarrhalis
Neisseria gonorrhoeae

"Other" microorganisms
Chlamydia pneumoniae
Chlamydia trachomatis
Legionella pneumophila
Mycoplasma hominis
Mycoplasma pneumoniae
Beta-lactamase production should have no effect on azithromycin activity.

Azithromycin has been shown to be active against most strains of the following microorganisms, both *in vitro* and in clinical infections as described in the **INDICATIONS AND USAGE** section of the package insert for ZITHROMAX® (azithromycin tablets) and ZITHROMAX® (azithromycin for oral suspension).

Aerobic gram-positive microorganisms
Staphylococcus aureus
Streptococcus agalactiae
Streptococcus pneumoniae
Streptococcus pyogenes

Aerobic gram-negative microorganisms
Haemophilus ducreyi
Haemophilus influenzae
Moraxella catarrhalis
Neisseria gonorrhoeae

"Other" microorganisms
Chlamydia pneumoniae
Chlamydia trachomatis
Mycoplasma pneumoniae
The following *in vitro* data are available, **but their clinical significance is unknown.**

Azithromycin exhibits *in vitro* minimum inhibitory concentrations (MIC's) of 0.5 µg/mL or less against most (≥90%) strains of streptococci listed below and MIC's of 2.0 µg/mL or less against most (≥90%) strains of other listed microorganisms. However, the safety and effectiveness of azithromycin in treating clinical infections due to these microorganisms have not been established in adequate and well-controlled clinical trials.

Aerobic gram-positive microorganisms
Streptococci (Groups C, F, G)
Viridans group streptococci

Anaerobic microorganisms
Peptostreptococcus species
Prevotella bivia

Aerobic gram-negative microorganisms
Bordetella pertussis

"Other" microorganisms
Ureaplasma urealyticum

Susceptibility Tests
Azithromycin can be solubilized for *in vitro* susceptibility testing using dilution techniques by dissolving in a minimum amount of 95% ethanol and diluting to the working stock concentration with broth.

Dilution Techniques:
Quantitative methods are used to determine antimicrobial minimum inhibitory concentrations (MIC's). These MIC's provide estimates of the susceptibility of bacteria to antimicrobial compounds. The MIC's should be determined using a standardized procedure. Standardized procedures are based on a dilution method[1] (broth or agar) or equivalent with standardized inoculum concentrations and standardized concentrations of azithromycin powder. The MIC values should be interpreted according to the following criteria:
For testing aerobic microorganisms other than *Haemophilus* species, *Neisseria gonorrhoeae*, and streptococci:

MIC (µg/mL)	Interpretation
≤ 2	Susceptible (S)
4	Intermediate (I)
≥ 8	Resistant (R)

Plasma concentrations (µg/mL ± S.D.) after the last daily intravenous infusion of 500 mg azithromycin

Infusion Concentration, Duration	Time after starting the infusion (hr)									
	0.5	1	2	3	4	6	8	12	24	
2 mg/mL, 1 hr[a]	2.98	3.63	0.60	0.40	0.33	0.26	0.27	0.20	0.20	
	±1.12	±1.73	±0.31	±0.23	±0.16	±0.14	±0.15	±0.12	±0.15	
1 mg/mL, 3 hr[b]	0.91	1.02	1.14	1.13	0.32	0.28	0.27	0.22	0.18	
	±0.13	±0.11	±0.13	±0.16	±0.05	±0.04	±0.03	±0.02	±0.02	

a=500 mg (2 mg/mL) for 2–5 days in Community-acquired pneumonia patients.
b=500 mg (1 mg/mL) for 5 days in healthy subjects.

AZITHROMYCIN CONCENTRATIONS FOLLOWING
TWO—250 mg (500 mg) CAPSULES IN ADULTS

TISSUE OR FLUID	TIME AFTER DOSE (h)	TISSUE OR FLUID CONCENTRATION (µg/g or µg/mL)[1]	CORRESPONDING PLASMA OR SERUM LEVEL (µg/mL)	TISSUE (FLUID) PLASMA (SERUM) RATIO[1]
SKIN	72–96	0.4	0.012	35
LUNG	72–96	4.0	0.012	>100
SPUTUM*	2–4	1.0	0.64	2
SPUTUM**	10–12	2.9	0.1	30
TONSIL***	9–18	4.5	0.03	>100
TONSIL***	180	0.9	0.006	>100
CERVIX****	19	2.8	0.04	70

[1] High tissue concentrations should not be interpreted to be quantitatively related to clinical efficacy. The antimicrobial activity of azithromycin is pH related. Azithromycin is concentrated in cell lysosomes which have a low intraorganelle pH, at which the drug's activity is reduced. However, the extensive distribution of drug to tissues may be relevant to clinical activity.
* Sample was obtained 2–4 hours after the first dose.
** Sample was obtained 10–12 hours after the first dose.
*** Dosing regimen of 2 doses of 250 mg each, separated by 12 hours.
**** Sample was obtained 19 hours after a single 500 mg dose.

For testing *Haemophilus* species[a]:

MIC (µg/mL)	Interpretation
≤ 4	Susceptible (S)

[a]This interpretive standard is applicable only to broth microdilution susceptibility testing with *Haemophilus* species using *Haemophilus* Test Medium (HTM)[1].

The current absence of data on resistant strains precludes defining any categories other than "Susceptible". Strains yielding MIC results suggestive of a "nonsusceptible" category should be submitted to a reference laboratory for further testing.
For testing streptococci including *S. pneumoniae*[b]:

MIC (µg/mL)	Interpretation
≤ 0.5	Susceptible (S)
1	Intermediate (I)
≥ 2	Resistant (R)

[b]These interpretive standards are applicable only to broth microdilution susceptibility tests using cation-adjusted Mueller-Hinton broth with 2–5% lysed horse blood[1].

No interpretive criteria have been established for testing *Neisseria gonorrhoeae*. This species is not usually tested.
A report of "Susceptible" indicates that the pathogen is likely to respond to monotherapy with azithromycin. A report of "Intermediate" indicates that the result should be considered equivocal, and, if the microorganism is not fully susceptible to alternative, clinically feasible drugs, the test should be repeated. This category implies possible clinical applicability in body sites where the drug is physiologically concentrated or in situations where high dosage of drug can be used. This category also provides a buffer zone which prevents small uncontrolled technical factors from causing major discrepancies in interpretation. A report of "Resistant" indicates that achievable drug concentrations are unlikely to be inhibitory; other therapy should be selected.
Standardized susceptibility test procedures require the use of laboratory control microorganisms to control the technical aspects of the laboratory procedures. Standard azithromycin powder should provide the following MIC values:

Microorganism	MIC (µg/mL)
Haemophilus influenzae ATCC 49247[a]	1.0–4.0
Staphylococcus aureus ATCC 29213	0.5–2.0
Streptococcus pneumoniae ATCC 49619[b]	0.06–0.25

[a]This quality control range is applicable to only *H. influenzae* ATCC 49247 tested by a broth microdilution procedure using *Haemophilus* Test Medium (HTM)[1].
[b]This quality control range is applicable to only *S. pneumoniae* ATCC 49619 tested by a broth microdilution procedure using cation-adjusted Mueller-Hinton broth with 2–5% lysed horse blood.[1]

Diffusion Techniques:
Quantitative methods that require measurement of zone diameters also provide reproducible estimates of the suscepti-

---

bility of bacteria to antimicrobial compounds. One such standardized procedure[2] requires the use of standardized inoculum concentrations. This procedure uses paper disks impregnated with 15-µg azithromycin to test the susceptibility of microorganisms to azithromycin.
Reports from the laboratory providing results of the standard single-disk susceptibility test with a 15-µg azithromycin disk should be interpreted according to the following criteria:
For testing aerobic microorganisms (including streptococci)[a] except *Haemophilus* species and *Neisseria gonorrhoeae*:

Zone Diameter (mm)	Interpretation
≥ 18	Susceptible (S)
14–17	Intermediate (I)
≤ 13	Resistant (R)

[a]These zone diameter standards for streptococci apply only to tests performed using Mueller-Hinton agar supplemented with 5% sheep blood and incubated in 5% CO_2[2].

For testing *Haemophilus* species[b]:

Zone Diameter (mm)	Interpretation
≥ 12	Susceptible (S)

[b]This zone diameter standard is applicable only to tests with *Haemophilus* species using *Haemophilus* Test Medium (HTM)[2].

The current absence of data on resistant strains precludes defining any categories other than "Susceptible". Strains yielding zone diameter results suggestive of a "nonsusceptible" category should be submitted to a reference laboratory for further testing.
No interpretive criteria have been established for testing *Neisseria gonorrhoeae*. This species is not usually tested.
Interpretation should be as stated above for results using dilution techniques. Interpretation involves correlation of the diameter obtained in the disk test with the MIC for azithromycin.
As with standardized dilution techniques, diffusion methods require the use of laboratory control microorganisms that are used to control the technical aspects of the laboratory procedures. For the diffusion technique, the 15-µg azithromycin disk should provide the following zone diameters in these laboratory test quality control strains:

Microorganism	Zone Diameter (mm)
Haemophilus influenzae ATCC 49247[a]	13–21
Staphylococcus aureus ATCC 25923	21–26
Streptococcus pneumoniae ATCC 49619[b]	19–25

[a]These quality control limits are applicable only to tests conducted with *H. influenzae* ATCC 49247 using *Haemophilus* Test Medium (HTM)[2].
[b]These quality control limits are applicable only to tests conducted with *S. pneumoniae* ATCC 49619 using Mueller-Hinton agar supplemented with 5% sheep blood incubated in 5% CO_2[2].

INDICATIONS AND USAGE

ZITHROMAX® (azithromycin for injection) is indicated for the treatment of patients with infections caused by susceptible strains of the designated microorganisms in the conditions listed below. As recommended dosages, durations of therapy, and applicable patient populations vary among these infections, please see **DOSAGE AND ADMINISTRATION** for dosing recommendations.

Community-acquired pneumonia due to *Chlamydia pneumoniae, Haemophilus influenzae, Legionella pneumophila, Moraxella catarrhalis, Mycoplasma pneumoniae, Staphylococcus aureus,* or *Streptococcus pneumoniae* in patients who require initial intravenous therapy.

Pelvic inflammatory disease due to *Chlamydia trachomatis, Neisseria gonorrhoeae,* or *Mycoplasma hominis* in patients who require initial intravenous therapy. If anaerobic microorganisms are suspected of contributing to the infection, an antimicrobial agent with anaerobic activity should be administered in combination with ZITHROMAX®.

ZITHROMAX® (azithromycin for injection) should be followed by ZITHROMAX® by the oral route as required. (See **DOSAGE AND ADMINISTRATION.**)

Appropriate culture and susceptibility tests should be performed before treatment to determine the causative microorganism and its susceptibility to azithromycin. Therapy with ZITHROMAX® may be initiated before results of these tests are known; once the results become available, antimicrobial therapy should be adjusted accordingly.

CONTRAINDICATIONS

ZITHROMAX® is contraindicated in patients with known hypersensitivity to azithromycin, erythromycin, or any macrolide antibiotic.

WARNINGS

Serious allergic reactions, including angioedema, anaphylaxis, and dermatologic reactions including Stevens Johnson Syndrome and toxic epidermal necrolysis have been reported rarely in patients on azithromycin therapy. Although rare, fatalities have been reported. (See **CONTRAINDICATIONS.**) Despite initially successful symptomatic treatment of the allergic symptoms, when symptomatic therapy was discontinued, the allergic symptoms **recurred soon thereafter in some patients without further azithromycin exposure.** These patients required prolonged periods of observation and symptomatic treatment. The relationship of these episodes to the long tissue half-life of azithromycin and subsequent prolonged exposure to antigen is unknown at present.

If an allergic reaction occurs, the drug should be discontinued and appropriate therapy should be instituted. Physicians should be aware that reappearance of the allergic symptoms may occur when symptomatic therapy is discontinued.

Pseudomembranous colitis has been reported with nearly all antibacterial agents and may range in severity from mild to life-threatening. Therefore, it is important to consider this diagnosis in patients who present with diarrhea subsequent to the administration of antibacterial agents.

Treatment with antibacterial agents alters the normal flora of the colon and may permit overgrowth of clostridia. Studies indicate that a toxin produced by *Clostridium difficile* is a primary cause of "antibiotic-associated colitis."

After the diagnosis of pseudomembranous colitis has been established, therapeutic measures should be initiated. Mild cases of pseudomembranous colitis usually respond to discontinuation of the drug alone. In moderate to severe cases, consideration should be given to management with fluids and electrolytes, protein supplementation, and treatment with an antibacterial drug clinically effective against *Clostridium difficile* colitis.

PRECAUTIONS

General: Because azithromycin is principally eliminated via the liver, caution should be exercised when azithromycin is administered to patients with impaired hepatic function. There are no data regarding azithromycin usage in patients with renal impairment; therefore, caution should be exercised when prescribing azithromycin in these patients.

ZITHROMAX® (azithromycin for injection) should be reconstituted and diluted as directed and administered as an intravenous infusion over not less than 60 minutes. (See **DOSAGE AND ADMINISTRATION.**)

Local I.V. site reactions have been reported with the intravenous administration of azithromycin. The incidence and severity of these reactions were the same when 500 mg azithromycin were given over 1 hour (2 mg/mL as 250 mL infusion) or over 3 hours (1 mg/mL as 500 mL infusion). (See **ADVERSE REACTIONS.**) All volunteers who received infusate concentrations above 2.0 mg/mL experienced local I.V. site reactions and, therefore, higher concentrations should be avoided.

The following adverse events have not been reported in clinical trials with azithromycin; however, they have been reported with macrolide products: ventricular arrhythmias, including ventricular tachycardia, and *torsades de pointes,* in individuals with prolonged QT intervals. There has been a spontaneous report from the post-marketing experience of a patient with previous history of arrhythmias who experienced *torsades de pointes* and subsequent myocardial infarction following a course of oral azithromycin therapy.

Information for Patients:

Patients should be cautioned not to take aluminum- and magnesium-containing antacids and azithromycin by the oral route simultaneously.

Patients should be directed to discontinue azithromycin and contact a physician if any signs of an allergic reaction occur.

Drug Interactions: Aluminum- and magnesium-containing antacids reduce the peak serum levels (rate) but not the AUC (extent) of orally administered azithromycin.

Administration of cimetidine (800 mg) two hours prior to orally administered azithromycin had no effect on azithromycin absorption.

Azithromycin given by the oral route did not affect the plasma levels or pharmacokinetics of theophylline administered as a single intravenous dose. The effect of azithromycin on the plasma levels or pharmacokinetics of theophylline administered in multiple doses resulting in therapeutic steady-state levels of theophylline is not known. However, concurrent use of macrolides and theophylline has been associated with increases in the serum concentrations of theophylline. Therefore, until further data are available, prudent medical practice dictates careful monitoring of plasma theophylline levels in patients receiving azithromycin and theophylline concomitantly.

Azithromycin given by the oral route did not affect the prothrombin time response to a single dose of warfarin. However, prudent medical practice dictates careful monitoring of prothrombin time in all patients treated with azithromycin and warfarin concomitantly. Concurrent use of macrolides and warfarin in clinical practice has been associated with increased anticoagulant effects.

The following drug interactions have not been reported in clinical trials with azithromycin; however, no specific drug interaction studies have been performed to evaluate potential drug-drug interaction. Nonetheless, they have been observed with macrolide products. Until further data are developed regarding drug interactions when azithromycin and these drugs are used concomitantly, careful monitoring of patients is advised:

Digoxin—elevated digoxin levels.

Ergotamine or dihydroergotamine—acute ergot toxicity characterized by severe peripheral vasospasm and dysesthesia.

Triazolam—Increased pharmacologic effect of triazolam by decreasing the clearance of triazolam.

Drugs metabolized by the cytochrome P^{450} system—elevations of serum carbamazepine, terfenadine, cyclosporine, hexobarbital, and phenytoin levels.

Laboratory Test Interactions: There are no reported laboratory test interactions.

Carcinogenesis, Mutagenesis, Impairment of Fertility: Long-term studies in animals have not been performed to evaluate carcinogenic potential. Azithromycin has shown no mutagenic potential in standard laboratory tests: mouse lymphoma assay, human lymphocyte clastogenic assay, and mouse bone marrow clastogenic assay. No evidence of impaired fertility due to azithromycin was found.

Pregnancy: Teratogenic Effects. Pregnancy Category B: Reproduction studies have been performed in rats and mice at doses up to moderately maternally toxic dose levels (i.e., 200 mg/kg/day by the oral route). These doses, based on a mg/m² basis, are estimated to be 4 and 2 times, respectively, the human daily dose of 500 mg by the oral route. In the animal studies, no evidence of harm to the fetus due to azithromycin was found. There are, however, no adequate and well-controlled studies in pregnant women. Because animal reproduction studies are not always predictive of human response, azithromycin should be used during pregnancy only if clearly needed.

Nursing Mothers: It is not known whether azithromycin is excreted in human milk. Because many drugs are excreted in human milk, caution should be exercised when azithromycin is administered to a nursing woman.

Pediatric Use: Safety and effectiveness of azithromycin for intravenous injection in children or adolescents under 16 years have not been established. In controlled clinical studies, azithromycin has been administered to pediatric patients (age 6 months to 16 years) by the oral route. For information regarding the use of ZITHROMAX® (azithromycin for oral suspension) in the treatment of pediatric patients, refer to the **INDICATIONS AND USAGE** and **DOSAGE AND ADMINISTRATION** sections of the prescribing information for ZITHROMAX® (azithromycin for oral suspension) 100 mg/5 mL and 200 mg/5 mL bottles.

Geriatric Use: Pharmacokinetic studies with intravenous azithromycin have not been performed in older volunteers. Pharmacokinetics of azithromycin following oral administration in older volunteers (65–85 years old) were similar to those in younger volunteers (18–40 years old) for the 5-day therapeutic regimen.

ADVERSE REACTIONS

In clinical trials of intravenous azithromycin for community-acquired pneumonia, in which 2–5 I.V. doses were given, most of the reported side effects were mild to moderate in severity and were reversible upon discontinuation of the drug. The majority of patients in these trials had one or more comorbid diseases and were receiving concomitant medications. Approximately 1.2% of the patients discontinued intravenous ZITHROMAX® therapy, and a total of 2.4% discontinued azithromycin therapy by either the intravenous or oral route because of clinical or laboratory side effects.

In clinical trials conducted in patients with pelvic inflammatory disease, in which 1–2 I.V. doses were given, 2% of women who received monotherapy with azithromycin and 4% who received azithromycin plus metronidazole discontinued therapy due to clinical side effects.

Clinical side effects leading to discontinuations from these studies were most commonly gastrointestinal (abdominal pain, nausea, vomiting, diarrhea), and rashes; laboratory side effects leading to discontinuation were increases in transaminase levels and/or alkaline phosphatase levels.

Clinical:

Overall, the most common side effects associated with treatment in adult patients who received I.V./P.O. ZITHROMAX® in studies of community-acquired pneumonia were related to the gastrointestinal system with diarrhea/loose stools (4.3%), nausea (3.9%), abdominal pain (2.7%), and vomiting (1.4%) being the most frequently reported. Approximately 12% of patients experienced a side effect related to the intravenous infusion; most common were pain at the injection site (6.5%) and local inflammation (3.1%).

The most common side effects associated with treatment in adult women who received I.V./P.O. ZITHROMAX® in studies of pelvic inflammatory disease were related to the gastrointestinal system. Diarrhea (8.5%) and nausea (6.6%) were most commonly reported, followed by vaginitis (2.8%), abdominal pain (1.9%), anorexia (1.9%), rash and pruritus (1.9%). When azithromycin was co-administered with metronidazole in these studies, a higher proportion of women experienced side effects of nausea (10.3%), abdominal pain (3.7%), vomiting (2.8%), application site reaction, stomatitis, dizziness, or dyspnea (all at 1.9%).

No other side effects occurred in patients on the multiple dose I.V./P.O. regimen of ZITHROMAX® in these studies with a frequency greater than 1%.

Side effects that occurred with a frequency of 1% or less included the following:

Gastrointestinal: dyspepsia, flatulence, mucositis, oral moniliasis, and gastritis

Nervous System: headache, somnolence

Allergic: bronchospasm

Special Senses: taste perversion

Post-Marketing Experience:

Adverse events reported with orally administered azithromycin during the post-marketing period in adult and/or pediatric patients for which a causal relationship could not be established include:

Allergic: arthralgia, edema, urticaria, angioedema

Cardiovascular: arrhythmias, including ventricular tachycardia

Gastrointestinal: anorexia, constipation, dyspepsia, flatulence, vomiting/diarrhea rarely resulting in dehydration, pseudomembranous colitis and rare reports of tongue discoloration

General: asthenia, paresthesia and anaphylaxis (rarely fatal)

Genitourinary: interstitial nephritis and acute renal failure, moniliasis, vaginitis

Hematopoietic: thrombocytopenia

Liver/Biliary: abnormal liver function including hepatitis and cholestatic jaundice, as well as rare cases of hepatic necrosis and hepatic failure, which have rarely resulted in death

Nervous System: convulsions, dizziness/vertigo, headache, somnolence, hyperactivity, nervousness, and agitation

Psychiatric: aggressive reaction and anxiety

Skin/Appendages: pruritus, rarely serious skin reactions including erythema multiforme, Stevens Johnson Syndrome, and toxic epidermal necrolysis

Special Senses: hearing disturbances including hearing loss, deafness, and/or tinnitus, rare reports of taste perversion

Laboratory Abnormalities:

Significant abnormalities (irrespective of drug relationship) occurring during the clinical trials were reported as follows: with an incidence of 4–6%, elevated ALT (SGPT), AST (SGOT), creatinine

with an incidence of 1–3%, elevated LDH, bilirubin

with an incidence of less than 1%, leukopenia, neutropenia, decreased platelet count, and elevated serum alkaline phosphatase

When follow-up was provided, changes in laboratory tests appeared to be reversible.

In multiple-dose clinical trials involving more than 750 patients treated with ZITHROMAX® (I.V./P.O.), less than 2% of patients discontinued azithromycin therapy because of treatment-related liver enzyme abnormalities.

DOSAGE AND ADMINISTRATION

(See **INDICATIONS AND USAGE and CLINICAL PHARMACOLOGY.**)

The recommended dose of ZITHROMAX® (azithromycin for injection) for the treatment of adult patients with community-acquired pneumonia due to the indicated organisms is: 500 mg as a single daily dose by the intravenous route for at least two days. Intravenous therapy should be followed by azithromycin by the oral route at a single, daily dose of 500 mg, administered as two 250-mg tablets to complete a 7- to 10-day course of therapy. The timing of the switch to oral therapy should be done at the discretion of the physician and in accordance with clinical response.

The recommended dose of ZITHROMAX® (azithromycin) for the treatment of adult patients with pelvic inflammatory disease due to the indicated organisms is: 500 mg as a single daily dose by the intravenous route for one or two days. Intravenous therapy should be followed by azithromycin by the oral route at a single, daily dose of 250 mg to complete a 7-day course of therapy. The timing of the switch to oral

Continued on next page

Zithromax IV—Cont.

therapy should be done at the discretion of the physician and in accordance with clinical response. If anaerobic microorganisms are suspected of contributing to the infection, an antimicrobial agent with anaerobic activity should be administered in combination with ZITHROMAX®.

The infusate concentration and rate of infusion for ZITHROMAX® (azithromycin for injection) should be either 1 mg/mL over 3 hours or 2 mg/mL over 1 hour.

Preparation of the solution for intravenous administration is as follows:

Reconstitution

Prepare the initial solution of ZITHROMAX® (azithromycin for injection) by adding 4.8 mL of Sterile Water For Injection to the 500 mg vial and shaking the vial until all of the drug is dissolved. Since ZITHROMAX® (azithromycin for injection) is supplied under vacuum, it is recommended that a standard 5 mL (non-automated) syringe be used to ensure that the exact amount of 4.8 mL of Sterile Water is dispensed. Each mL of reconstituted solution contains 100 mg azithromycin. Reconstituted solution is stable for 24 hours when stored below 30°C or 86°F.

Parenteral drug products should be inspected visually for particulate matter prior to administration. If particulate matter is evident in reconstituted fluids, the drug solution should be discarded.

Dilute this solution further prior to administration as instructed below.

Dilution

To provide azithromycin over a concentration range of 1.0–2.0 mg/mL, transfer 5 mL of the 100 mg/mL azithromycin solution into the appropriate amount of any of the diluents listed below:

Normal Saline (0.9% sodium chloride)
½ Normal Saline (0.45% sodium chloride)
5% Dextrose in Water
Lactated Ringer's Solution
5% Dextrose in ½ Normal Saline (0.45% sodium chloride) with 20 mEq KCl
5% Dextrose in Lactated Ringer's Solution
5% Dextrose in 1/3 Normal Saline (0.3% sodium chloride)
5% Dextrose in ½ Normal Saline (0.45% sodium chloride)
Normosol®-M in 5% Dextrose
Normosol®-R in 5% Dextrose

Final Infusion Solution Concentration (mg/mL)	Amount of Diluent (mL)
1.0 mg/mL	500 mL
2.0 mg/mL	250 mL

It is recommended that a 500-mg dose of ZITHROMAX® (azithromycin for injection), diluted as above, be infused over a period of not less than 60 minutes.

ZITHROMAX® (azithromycin for injection) should not be given as a bolus or as an intramuscular injection.

Other intravenous substances, additives, or medications should not be added to ZITHROMAX® (azithromycin for injection), or infused simultaneously through the same intravenous line.

Storage

When diluted according to the instructions (1.0 mg/mL to 2.0 mg/mL), ZITHROMAX® (azithromycin for injection) is stable for 24 hours at or below room temperature (30°C or 86°F), or for 7 days if stored under refrigeration (5°C or 41°F).

HOW SUPPLIED

ZITHROMAX® (azithromycin for injection) is supplied in lyophilized form under a vacuum in a 10-mL vial equivalent to 500 mg of azithromycin for intravenous administration. Each vial also contains sodium hydroxide and 413.6 mg citric acid.

These are packaged as follows:

10 vials of 500 mg NDC 0069-3150-83

CLINICAL STUDIES

Community-Acquired Pneumonia

In a controlled study of community-acquired pneumonia performed in the U.S., azithromycin (500 mg as a single daily dose by the intravenous route for 2–5 days, followed by 500 mg/day by the oral route to complete 7–10 days therapy) was compared to cefuroxime (2250 mg/day in three divided doses by the intravenous route for 2–5 days followed by 1000 mg/day in two divided doses by the oral route to complete 7–10 days therapy), with or without erythromycin. For the 291 patients who were evaluable for clinical efficacy, the clinical outcome rates, i.e., cure, improved, and success (cure + improved) among the 277 patients seen at 10–14 days post-therapy were as follows:

Clinical Outcome	Azithromycin	Comparator
Cure	46%	44%
Improved	32%	30%
Success (Cure + Improved)	78%	74%

In a separate, uncontrolled clinical and microbiological trial performed in the U.S., 94 patients with community-acquired pneumonia who received azithromycin in the same regimen were evaluable for clinical efficacy. The clinical outcome rates, i.e., cure, improved, and success (cure + improved) among the 84 patients seen at 10–14 days post-therapy were as follows:

Clinical Outcome	Azithromycin
Cure	60%
Improved	29%
Success (Cure + Improved)	89%

Microbiological determinations in both trials were made at the pre-treatment visit and, where applicable, were reassessed at later visits. Serological testing was done on baseline and final visit specimens. The following combined presumptive bacteriological eradication rates were obtained from the evaluable groups:

Combined Bacteriological Eradication Rates for Azithromycin:

(at last completed visit)	Azithromycin
S. pneumoniae	64/67 (96%)[a]
H. influenzae	41/43 (95%)
M. catarrhalis	9/10
S. aureus	9/10

[a]Nineteen of twenty-four patients (79%) with positive blood cultures for *S. pneumoniae* were cured (intent to treat analysis) with eradication of the pathogen.

The presumed bacteriological outcomes at 10–14 days post-therapy for patients treated with azithromycin with evidence (serology and/or culture) of atypical pathogens for both trials were as follows:

[See table below]

Evidence of Infection	Total	Cure	Improved	Cure + Improved
Mycoplasma pneumoniae	18	11 (61%)	5 (28%)	16 (89%)
Chlamydia pneumoniae	34	15 (44%)	13 (38%)	28 (82%)
Legionella pneumophila	16	5 (31%)	8 (50%)	13 (81%)

ANIMAL TOXICOLOGY

Phospholipidosis (intracellular phospholipid accumulation) has been observed in some tissues of mice, rats, and dogs given multiple doses of azithromycin. It has been demonstrated in numerous organ systems (e.g., eye, dorsal root ganglia, liver, gallbladder, kidney, spleen, and pancreas) in dogs treated with azithromycin at doses which, expressed on a mg/kg basis, are only 2 times greater than the recommended adult human dose and in rats at doses comparable to the recommended adult human dose. This effect has been reversible after cessation of azithromycin treatment. Phospholipidosis has been observed to a similar extent in the tissues of neonatal rats and dogs given daily doses of azithromycin ranging from 10 days to 30 days. Based on the pharmacokinetic data, phospholipidosis has been seen in the rat (30 mg/kg dose) at observed C_{max} value of 1.3 μg/mL (6 times greater than the observed C_{max} of 0.216 μg/mL at the pediatric dose of 10 mg/kg). Similarly, it has been shown in the dog (10 mg/kg dose) at observed C_{max} value of 1.5 μg/mL (7 times greater than the observed same C_{max} and drug dose in the studied pediatric population). On mg/m^2 basis, 30 mg/kg dose in the rat (135 mg/m^2) and 10 mg/kg dose in the dog (79 mg/m^2) are approximately 0.4 and 0.6 times, respectively, the recommended dose in the pediatric patients with an average body weight of 25 kg. This effect, similar to that seen in the adult animals, is reversible after cessation of azithromycin treatment. The significance of these findings for animals and for humans is unknown.

REFERENCES:

1. National Committee for Clinical Laboratory Standards. Methods for Dilution Antimicrobial Susceptibility Tests for Bacteria that Grow Aerobically—Third Edition. Approved Standard NCCLS Document M7-A3, Vol. 13, No. 25, NCCLS, Villanova, PA, December, 1993.
2. National Committee for Clinical Laboratory Standards. Performance Standards for Antimicrobial Disk Susceptibility Tests—Fifth Edition. Approved Standard NCCLS Document M2-A5, Vol. 13, No. 24, NCCLS, Villanova, PA, December, 1993.

Rx only

Licensed from Pliva

Pfizer Labs
Division of Pfizer Inc, NY, NY 10017

Printed in U.S.A.
70-5191-00-4 Revised July 2000

ZOLOFT® ℞

(sertraline hydrochloride)
Tablets and Oral Concentrate

Prescribing information for this product, which appears on pages 2553–2558 of the 2001 PDR, has been completely revised as follows. Please write "See Supplement A" next to the product heading.

DESCRIPTION

ZOLOFT® (sertraline hydrochloride) is a selective serotonin reuptake inhibitor (SSRI) for oral administration. It is chemically unrelated to other SSRIs, tricyclic, tetracyclic, or other available antidepressant agents. It has a molecular weight of 342.7. Sertraline hydrochloride has the following chemical name: (1S-cis)-4-(3,4-dichlorophenyl)-1,2,3,4-tetrahydro-N-methyl-1-naphthalenamine hydrochloride. The empirical formula $C_{17}H_{17}NCl_2 \cdot HCl$ is represented by the following structural formula:

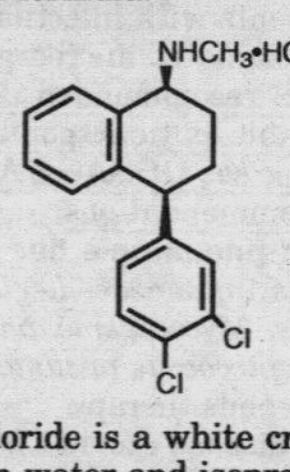

Sertraline hydrochloride is a white crystalline powder that is slightly soluble in water and isopropyl alcohol, and sparingly soluble in ethanol.

ZOLOFT is supplied for oral administration as scored tablets containing sertraline hydrochloride equivalent to 25, 50 and 100 mg of sertraline and the following inactive ingredients: dibasic calcium phosphate dihydrate, D & C Yellow #10 aluminum lake (in 25 mg tablet), FD & C Blue #1 aluminum lake (in 25 mg tablet), FD & C Red #40 aluminum lake (in 25 mg tablet), FD & C Blue #2 aluminum lake (in 50 mg tablet), hydroxypropyl cellulose, hydroxypropyl methylcellulose, magnesium stearate, microcrystalline cellulose, polyethylene glycol, polysorbate 80, sodium starch glycolate, synthetic yellow iron oxide (in 100 mg tablet), and titanium dioxide.

ZOLOFT oral concentrate is available in a multidose 60 mL bottle. Each mL of solution contains sertraline hydrochloride equivalent to 20 mg of sertraline. The solution contains the following inactive ingredients: glycerin, alcohol (12%), menthol, butylated hydroxytoluene (BHT). The oral concentrate must be diluted prior to administration (see PRECAUTIONS, Information for Patients and DOSAGE AND ADMINISTRATION).

CLINICAL PHARMACOLOGY

Pharmacodynamics

The mechanism of action of sertraline is presumed to be linked to its inhibition of CNS neuronal uptake of serotonin (5HT). Studies at clinically relevant doses in man have demonstrated that sertraline blocks the uptake of serotonin into human platelets. *In vitro* studies in animals also suggest that sertraline is a potent and selective inhibitor of neuronal serotonin reuptake and has only very weak effects on norepinephrine and dopamine neuronal reuptake. *In vitro* studies have shown that sertraline has no significant affinity for adrenergic ($alpha_1$, $alpha_2$, beta), cholinergic, GABA, dopaminergic, histaminergic, serotonergic ($5HT_{1A}$, $5HT_{1B}$, $5HT_2$), or benzodiazepine receptors; antagonism of such receptors has been hypothesized to be associated with various anticholinergic, sedative, and cardiovascular effects for other psychotropic drugs. The chronic administration of sertraline was found in animals to downregulate brain norepinephrine receptors, as has been observed with other clinically effective antidepressants. Sertraline does not inhibit monoamine oxidase.

Pharmacokinetics

Systemic Bioavailability—In man, following oral once-daily dosing over the range of 50 to 200 mg for 14 days, mean peak plasma concentrations (Cmax) of sertraline occurred between 4.5 to 8.4 hours post-dosing. The average terminal elimination half-life of plasma sertraline is about 26 hours. Based on this pharmacokinetic parameter, steady-state sertraline plasma levels should be achieved after approximately one week of once-daily dosing. Linear dose-proportional pharmacokinetics were demonstrated in a single dose study in which the Cmax and area under the plasma concentration time curve (AUC) of sertraline were proportional to dose over a range of 50 to 200 mg. Consistent with the terminal elimination half-life, there is an approximately two-fold accumulation, compared to a single dose, of sertraline with repeated dosing over a 50 to 200 mg dose range. The single dose bioavailability of sertraline tablets is approximately equal to an equivalent dose of solution.

In a relative bioavailability study comparing the pharmacokinetics of 100 mg sertraline as the oral solution to a 100 mg sertraline tablet in 16 healthy adults, the solution to tablet ratio of geometric mean AUC and Cmax values were 114.8% and 120.6%, respectively. 90% confidence intervals (CI) were within the range of 80–125% with the exception of the upper 90% CI limit for Cmax which was 126.5%.

The effects of food on the bioavailability of the sertraline tablet and oral concentrate were studied in subjects administered a single dose with and without food. For the tablet, AUC was slightly increased when drug was administered with food but the Cmax was 25% greater, while the time to reach peak plasma concentration (Tmax) decreased from 8 hours post-dosing to 5.5 hours. For the oral concentrate, Tmax was slightly prolonged from 5.9 hours to 7.0 hours with food.

Metabolism—Sertraline undergoes extensive first pass metabolism. The principal initial pathway of metabolism for sertraline is N-demethylation. N-desmethylsertraline has a plasma terminal elimination half-life of 62 to 104 hours. Both *in vitro* biochemical and *in vivo* pharmacological testing have shown N-desmethylsertraline to be substantially less active than sertraline. Both sertraline and N-desmethylsertraline undergo oxidative deamination and subsequent reduction, hydroxylation, and glucuronide conjugation. In a study of radiolabeled sertraline involving two healthy male subjects, sertraline accounted for less than 5% of the plasma radioactivity. About 40–45% of the administered radioactivity was recovered in urine in 9 days. Unchanged sertraline was not detectable in the urine. For the same period, about 40–45% of the administered radioactivity was accounted for in feces, including 12–14% unchanged sertraline.

Desmethylsertraline exhibits time-related, dose dependent increases in AUC (0–24 hour), Cmax and Cmin, with about a 5–9 fold increase in these pharmacokinetic parameters between day 1 and day 14.

Protein Binding—In vitro protein binding studies performed with radiolabeled ^{3}H-sertraline showed that sertraline is highly bound to serum proteins (98%) in the range of 20 to 500 ng/mL. However, at up to 300 and 200 ng/mL concentrations, respectively, sertraline and N-desmethylsertraline did not alter the plasma protein binding of two other highly protein bound drugs, viz., warfarin and propranolol (see PRECAUTIONS).

Pediatric Pharmacokinetics—Sertraline pharmacokinetics were evaluated in a group of 61 pediatric patients (29 aged 6–12 years, 32 aged 13–17 years) with a DSM-III-R diagnosis of depression or obsessive-compulsive disorder. Patients included both males (N=28) and females (N=33). During 42 days of chronic sertraline dosing, sertraline was titrated up to 200 mg/day and maintained at that dose for a minimum of 11 days. On the final day of sertraline 200 mg/day, the 6–12 year old group exhibited a mean sertraline AUC (0–24 hr) of 3107 ng-hr/mL, mean Cmax of 165 ng/mL, and mean half-life of 26.2 hr. The 13–17 year old group exhibited a mean sertraline AUC (0–24 hr) of 2296 ng-hr/mL, mean Cmax of 123 ng/mL, and mean half-life of 27.8 hr. Higher plasma levels in the 6–12 year old group were largely attributable to patients with lower body weights. No gender associated differences were observed. By comparison, a group of 22 separately studied adults between 18 and 45 years of age (11 male, 11 female) received 30 days of 200 mg/day sertraline and exhibited a mean sertraline AUC (0–24 hr) of 2570 ng-hr/mL, mean Cmax of 142 ng/mL, and mean half-life of 27.2 hr. Relative to the adults, both the 6–12 year olds and the 13–17 year olds showed about 22% lower AUC (0–24 hr) and Cmax values when plasma concentration was adjusted for weight. These data suggest that pediatric patients metabolize sertraline with slightly greater efficiency than adults. Nevertheless, lower doses may be advisable for pediatric patients given their lower body weights, especially in very young patients, in order to avoid excessive plasma levels (see DOSAGE AND ADMINISTRATION).

Age—Sertraline plasma clearance in a group of 16 (8 male, 8 female) elderly patients treated for 14 days at a dose of 100 mg/day was approximately 40% lower than in a similarly studied group of younger (25 to 32 y.o.) individuals. Steady-state, therefore, should be achieved after 2 to 3 weeks in older patients. The same study showed a decreased clearance of desmethylsertraline in older males, but not in older females.

Liver Disease—As might be predicted from its primary site of metabolism, liver impairment can affect the elimination of sertraline. In patients with chronic mild liver impairment (N=10, 8 patients with Child-Pugh scores of 5–6 and 2 patients with Child-Pugh scores of 7–8) who received 50 mg sertraline per day maintained for 21 days, sertraline clearance was reduced, resulting in approximately 3-fold greater exposure compared to age-matched volunteers with no hepatic impairment (N=10). The exposure to desmethylsertraline was approximately 2-fold greater compared to age-matched volunteers with no hepatic impairment. There were no significant differences in plasma protein binding observed between the two groups. The effects of sertraline in patients with moderate and severe hepatic impairment have not been studied. The results suggest that the use of sertraline in patients with liver disease must be approached with caution. If sertraline is administered to patients with liver impairment, a lower or less frequent dose should be used (see PRECAUTIONS and DOSAGE AND ADMINISTRATION).

Renal Disease—Sertraline is extensively metabolized and excretion of unchanged drug in urine is a minor route of elimination. In volunteers with mild to moderate (CLcr=30–60 mL/min), moderate to severe (CLcr=10–29 mL/min) or severe (receiving hemodialysis) renal impairment (N=10 each group), the pharmacokinetics and protein binding of 200 mg sertraline per day maintained for 21 days were not altered compared to age-matched volunteers (N=12) with no renal impairment. Thus sertraline multiple dose pharmacokinetics appear to be unaffected by renal impairment (see PRECAUTIONS).

Clinical Trials

Depression—The efficacy of ZOLOFT as a treatment for depression was established in two placebo-controlled studies in adult outpatients meeting DSM-III criteria for major depression. Study 1 was an 8-week study with flexible dosing of ZOLOFT in a range of 50 to 200 mg/day; the mean dose for completers was 145 mg/day. Study 2 was a 6-week fixed-dose study, including ZOLOFT doses of 50, 100, and 200 mg/day. Overall, these studies demonstrated ZOLOFT to be superior to placebo on the Hamilton Depression Rating Scale and the Clinical Global Impression Severity and Improvement scales. Study 2 was not readily interpretable regarding a dose response relationship for effectiveness.

Study 3 involved depressed outpatients who had responded by the end of an initial 8-week open treatment phase on ZOLOFT 50–200 mg/day. These patients (N=295) were randomized to continuation for 44 weeks on double-blind ZOLOFT 50–200 mg/day or placebo. A statistically significantly lower relapse rate was observed for patients taking ZOLOFT compared to those on placebo. The mean dose for completers was 70 mg/day.

Analyses for gender effects on outcome did not suggest any differential responsiveness on the basis of sex.

Obsessive-Compulsive Disorder (OCD)—The effectiveness of ZOLOFT in the treatment of OCD was demonstrated in three multicenter placebo-controlled studies of adult outpatients (Studies 1–3). Patients in all studies had moderate to severe OCD (DSM-III or DSM-III-R) with mean baseline ratings on the Yale Brown Obsessive-Compulsive Scale (YBOCS) total score ranging from 23 to 25.

Study 1 was an 8-week study with flexible dosing of ZOLOFT in a range of 50 to 200 mg/day; the mean dose for completers was 186 mg/day. Patients receiving ZOLOFT experienced a mean reduction of approximately 4 points on the YBOCS total score which was significantly greater than the mean reduction of 2 points in placebo-treated patients.

Study 2 was a 12-week fixed-dose study, including ZOLOFT doses of 50, 100, and 200 mg/day. Patients receiving ZOLOFT doses of 50 and 200 mg/day experienced mean reductions of approximately 6 points on the YBOCS total score which were significantly greater than the approximately 3 point reduction in placebo-treated patients.

Study 3 was a 12-week study with flexible dosing of ZOLOFT in a range of 50 to 200 mg/day; the mean dose for completers was 185 mg/day. Patients receiving ZOLOFT experienced a mean reduction of approximately 7 points on the YBOCS total score which was significantly greater than the mean reduction of approximately 4 points in placebo-treated patients.

Analyses for age and gender effects on outcome did not suggest any differential responsiveness on the basis of age or sex.

The effectiveness of ZOLOFT for the treatment of OCD was also demonstrated in a 12-week, multicenter, parallel group study in a pediatric outpatient population (children and adolescents, ages 6–17). Patients in this study were initiated at doses of either 25 mg/day (children, ages 6–12) or 50 mg/day (adolescents, ages 13–17), and then titrated over the next four weeks to a maximum dose of 200 mg/day, as tolerated. The mean dose for completers was 178 mg/day. Dosing was once a day in the morning or evening. Patients in this study had moderate to severe OCD (DSM-III-R) with mean baseline ratings on the Children's Yale-Brown Obsessive-Compulsive Scale (CYBOCS) total score of 22. Patients receiving sertraline experienced a mean reduction of approximately 7 units on the CYBOCS total score which was significantly greater than the 3 unit reduction for placebo patients. Analyses for age and gender effects on outcome did not suggest any differential responsiveness on the basis of age or sex.

Panic Disorder—The effectiveness of ZOLOFT in the treatment of panic disorder was demonstrated in three double-blind, placebo-controlled studies (Studies 1–3) of adult outpatients who had a primary diagnosis of panic disorder (DSM-III-R), with or without agoraphobia.

Studies 1 and 2 were 10-week flexible dose studies. ZOLOFT was initiated at 25 mg/day for the first week, and then patients were dosed in a range of 50–200 mg/day on the basis of clinical response and toleration. The mean ZOLOFT doses for completers to 10 weeks were 131 mg/day and 144 mg/day, respectively, for Studies 1 and 2. In these studies, ZOLOFT was shown to be significantly more effective than placebo on change from baseline in panic attack frequency and on the Clinical Global Impression Severity of Illness and Global Improvement scores. The difference between ZOLOFT and placebo in reduction from baseline in the number of full panic attacks was approximately 2 panic attacks per week in both studies.

Study 3 was a 12-week fixed-dose study, including ZOLOFT doses of 50, 100, and 200 mg/day. Patients receiving ZOLOFT experienced a significantly greater reduction in panic attack frequency than patients receiving placebo. Study 3 was not readily interpretable regarding a dose response relationship for effectiveness.

Subgroup analyses did not indicate that there were any differences in treatment outcomes as a function of age, race, or gender.

Posttraumatic Stress Disorder (PTSD)—The effectiveness of ZOLOFT in the treatment of PTSD was established in two multicenter placebo-controlled studies (Studies 1–2) of adult outpatients who met DSM-III-R criteria for PTSD. The mean duration of PTSD for these patients was 12 years (Studies 1 and 2 combined) and 44% of patients (169 of the 385 patients treated) had secondary depressive disorder.

Studies 1 and 2 were 12-week flexible dose studies. ZOLOFT was initiated at 25 mg/day for the first week, and patients were then dosed in the range of 50–200 mg/day on the basis of clinical response and toleration. The mean ZOLOFT dose for completers was 146 mg/day and 151 mg/day, respectively for Studies 1 and 2. Study outcome was assessed by the Clinician-Administered PTSD Scale Part 2 (CAPS) which is a multi-item instrument that measures the three PTSD diagnostic symptom clusters of reexperiencing/intrusion, avoidance/numbing, and hyperarousal as well as the patient-rated Impact of Event Scale (IES) which measures intrusion and avoidance symptoms. ZOLOFT was shown to be significantly more effective than placebo on change from baseline to endpoint on the CAPS, IES and on the Clinical Global Impressions (CGI) Severity of Illness and Global Improvement scores. In two additional placebo-controlled PTSD trials, the difference in response to treatment between patients receiving ZOLOFT and patients receiving placebo was not statistically significant. One of these additional studies was conducted in patients similar to those recruited for Studies 1 and 2, while the second additional study was conducted in predominantly male veterans.

As PTSD is a more common disorder in women than men, the majority (76%) of patients in these trials were women (152 and 139 women on sertraline and placebo versus 39 and 55 men on sertraline and placebo; Studies 1 and 2 com-

bined). Post hoc exploratory analyses revealed a significant difference between ZOLOFT and placebo on the CAPS, IES and CGI in women, regardless of baseline diagnosis of comorbid depression, but essentially no effect in the relatively smaller number of men in these studies. The clinical significance of this apparent gender interaction is unknown at this time. There was insufficient information to determine the effect of race or age on outcome.

INDICATIONS AND USAGE

Depression—ZOLOFT® (sertraline hydrochloride) is indicated for the treatment of depression.

The efficacy of ZOLOFT in the treatment of a major depressive episode was established in six to eight week controlled trials of outpatients whose diagnoses corresponded most closely to the DSM-III category of major depressive disorder (see Clinical Trials under CLINICAL PHARMACOLOGY). A major depressive episode implies a prominent and relatively persistent depressed or dysphoric mood that usually interferes with daily functioning (nearly every day for at least 2 weeks); it should include at least 4 of the following 8 symptoms: change in appetite, change in sleep, psychomotor agitation or retardation, loss of interest in usual activities or decrease in sexual drive, increased fatigue, feelings of guilt or worthlessness, slowed thinking or impaired concentration, and a suicide attempt or suicidal ideation.

The antidepressant action of ZOLOFT in hospitalized depressed patients has not been adequately studied.

The efficacy of ZOLOFT in maintaining an antidepressant response for up to 44 weeks following 8 weeks of open-label acute treatment (52 weeks total) was demonstrated in a placebo-controlled trial. The usefulness of the drug in patients receiving ZOLOFT for extended periods should be reevaluated periodically (see Clinical Trials under CLINICAL PHARMACOLOGY).

Obsessive-Compulsive Disorder—ZOLOFT is indicated for the treatment of obsessions and compulsions in patients with obsessive-compulsive disorder (OCD), as defined in the DSM-III-R; i.e., the obsessions or compulsions cause marked distress, are time-consuming, or significantly interfere with social or occupational functioning.

The efficacy of ZOLOFT was established in 12-week trials with obsessive-compulsive outpatients having diagnoses of obsessive-compulsive disorder as defined according to DSM-III or DSM-III-R criteria (see Clinical Trials under CLINICAL PHARMACOLOGY).

Obsessive-compulsive disorder is characterized by recurrent and persistent ideas, thoughts, impulses, or images (obsessions) that are ego-dystonic and/or repetitive, purposeful, and intentional behaviors (compulsions) that are recognized by the person as excessive or unreasonable.

The effectiveness of ZOLOFT in long-term use for OCD, i.e., for more than 12 weeks, has not been systematically evaluated in placebo-controlled trials. Therefore, the physician who elects to use ZOLOFT for extended periods should periodically reevaluate the long-term usefulness of the drug for the individual patient (see DOSAGE AND ADMINISTRATION).

Panic Disorder—ZOLOFT is indicated for the treatment of panic disorder, with or without agoraphobia, as defined in DSM-IV. Panic disorder is characterized by the occurrence of unexpected panic attacks and associated concern about having additional attacks, worry about the implications or consequences of the attacks, and/or a significant change in behavior related to the attacks.

The efficacy of ZOLOFT was established in three 10–12 week trials in panic disorder patients whose diagnoses corresponded to the DSM-III-R category of panic disorder (see Clinical Trials under CLINICAL PHARMACOLOGY).

Panic disorder (DSM-IV) is characterized by recurrent unexpected panic attacks, i.e., a discrete period of intense fear or discomfort in which four (or more) of the following symptoms develop abruptly and reach a peak within 10 minutes: (1) palpitations, pounding heart, or accelerated heart rate; (2) sweating; (3) trembling or shaking; (4) sensations of shortness of breath or smothering; (5) feeling of choking; (6) chest pain or discomfort; (7) nausea or abdominal distress; (8) feeling dizzy, unsteady, lightheaded, or faint; (9) derealization (feelings of unreality) or depersonalization (being detached from oneself); (10) fear of losing control; (11) fear of dying; (12) paresthesias (numbness or tingling sensations); (13) chills or hot flushes.

The effectiveness of ZOLOFT® (sertraline hydrochloride) in long-term use, that is, for more than 12 weeks, has not been systematically evaluated in controlled trials. Therefore, the physician who elects to use ZOLOFT for extended periods should periodically re-evaluate the long-term usefulness of the drug for the individual patient (see DOSAGE AND ADMINISTRATION).

Posttraumatic Stress Disorder (PTSD)—ZOLOFT® (sertraline hydrochloride) is indicated for the treatment of posttraumatic stress disorder.

The efficacy of ZOLOFT in the treatment of PTSD was established in two 12-week placebo-controlled trials of outpatients whose diagnosis met criteria for the DSM-III-R category of PTSD (see Clinical Trials under CLINICAL PHARMACOLOGY).

PTSD, as defined by DSM-III-R/IV, requires exposure to a traumatic event that involved actual or threatened death or serious injury, or threat to the physical integrity of self or others, and a response which involves intense fear, helplessness, or horror. Symptoms that occur as a result of exposure to the traumatic event include reexperiencing of the event in the form of intrusive thoughts, flashbacks or dreams, and intense psychological distress and physiological reactivity on exposure to cues to the event; avoidance of situations reminiscent of the traumatic event, inability to recall details of the event, and/or numbing of general responsiveness

Continued on next page

Zoloft—Cont.

TABLE 1
MOST COMMON TREATMENT-EMERGENT ADVERSE EVENTS: INCIDENCE IN PLACEBO-CONTROLLED CLINICAL TRIALS

	Percentage of Patients Reporting Event							
	Depression/Other*		OCD		Panic Disorder		PTSD	
Body System/ Adverse Event	**ZOLOFT (N=861)**	**Placebo (N=853)**	**ZOLOFT (N=533)**	**Placebo (N=373)**	**ZOLOFT (N=430)**	**Placebo (N=275)**	**ZOLOFT (N=374)**	**Placebo (N=376)**
Autonomic Nervous System Disorders								
Ejaculation Failure(1)	7	<1	17	2	19	1	11	1
Mouth Dry	16	9	14	9	15	10	11	6
Sweating Increased	8	3	6	1	5	1	4	2
Centr. & Periph. Nerv. System Disorders								
Somnolence	13	6	15	8	15	9	13	9
Tremor	11	3	8	1	5	1	5	1
General								
Fatigue	11	8	14	10	11	6	10	5
Gastrointestinal Disorders								
Anorexia	3	2	11	2	7	2	8	2
Constipation	8	6	6	4	7	3	3	3
Diarrhea/Loose Stools	18	9	24	10	20	9	24	15
Dyspepsia	6	3	10	4	10	8	6	6
Nausea	26	12	30	11	29	18	21	11
Psychiatric Disorders								
Agitation	6	4	6	3	6	2	5	5
Insomnia	16	9	28	12	25	18	20	11
Libido Decreased	1	<1	11	2	7	1	7	2

(1)Primarily ejaculatory delay. Denominator used was for male patients only (N=271 ZOLOFT depression/other*; N=271 placebo depression/other*; N=296 ZOLOFT OCD; N=219 placebo OCD; N=216 ZOLOFT panic disorder; N=134 placebo panic disorder; N=130 ZOLOFT PTSD; N=149 placebo PTSD).
*Depression and other premarketing controlled trials.

manifested as diminished interest in significant activities, estrangement from others, restricted range of affect, or sense of foreshortened future; and symptoms of autonomic arousal including hypervigilance, exaggerated startle response, sleep disturbance, impaired concentration, and irritability or outbursts of anger. A PTSD diagnosis requires that the symptoms are present for at least a month and that they cause clinically significant distress or impairment in social, occupational, or other important areas of functioning. The effectiveness of ZOLOFT in long-term use for PTSD, i.e., for more than 12 weeks, has not been systematically evaluated in placebo-controlled trials; therefore, the physician who elects to use ZOLOFT for extended periods should periodically reevaluate the long-term usefulness of the drug for the individual patient (see DOSAGE AND ADMINISTRATION).

CONTRAINDICATIONS

All Dosage Forms of ZOLOFT:
Concomitant use in patients taking monoamine oxidase inhibitors (MAOIs) is contraindicated (see WARNINGS).
Oral Concentrate:
ZOLOFT oral concentrate is contraindicated with ANTABUSE (disulfiram) due to the alcohol content of the concentrate.

WARNINGS

Cases of serious sometimes fatal reactions have been reported in patients receiving ZOLOFT® (sertraline hydrochloride), a selective serotonin reuptake inhibitor (SSRI), in combination with a monoamine oxidase inhibitor (MAOI). Symptoms of a drug interaction between an SSRI and an MAOI include: hyperthermia, rigidity, myoclonus, autonomic instability with possible rapid fluctuations of vital signs, mental status changes that include confusion, irritability, and extreme agitation progressing to delirium and coma. These reactions have also been reported in patients who have recently discontinued an SSRI and have been started on an MAOI. Some cases presented with features resembling neuroleptic malignant syndrome. Therefore, ZOLOFT should not be used in combination with an MAOI, or within 14 days of discontinuing treatment with an MAOI. Similarly, at least 14 days should be allowed after stopping ZOLOFT before starting an MAOI.

PRECAUTIONS

General

Activation of Mania/Hypomania—During premarketing testing, hypomania or mania occurred in approximately 0.4% of ZOLOFT® (sertraline hydrochloride) treated patients.

Weight Loss—Significant weight loss may be an undesirable result of treatment with sertraline for some patients, but on average, patients in controlled trials had minimal, 1 to 2 pound weight loss, versus smaller changes on placebo. Only rarely have sertraline patients been discontinued for weight loss.

Seizure—ZOLOFT has not been evaluated in patients with a seizure disorder. These patients were excluded from clinical studies during the product's premarket testing. No seizures were observed among approximately 3000 patients treated with ZOLOFT in the development program for depression. However, 4 patients out of approximately 1800 (220 <18 years of age) exposed during the development program for obsessive-compulsive disorder experienced seizures, representing a crude incidence of 0.2%. Three of these patients were adolescents, two with a seizure disorder and one with a family history of seizure disorder, none of whom were receiving anticonvulsant medication. Accordingly, ZOLOFT should be introduced with care in patients with a seizure disorder.

Suicide—The possibility of a suicide attempt is inherent in depression and may persist until significant remission occurs. Close supervision of high risk patients should accompany initial drug therapy. Prescriptions for ZOLOFT should be written for the smallest quantity of tablets consistent with good patient management, in order to reduce the risk of overdose.

Because of the well-established comorbidity between OCD and depression, panic disorder and depression, and PTSD and depression, the same precautions observed when treating patients with depression should be observed when treating patients with OCD, panic disorder or PTSD.

Weak Uricosuric Effect—ZOLOFT® (sertraline hydrochloride) is associated with a mean decrease in serum uric acid of approximately 7%. The clinical significance of this weak uricosuric effect is unknown.

Use in Patients with Concomitant Illness—Clinical experience with ZOLOFT in patients with certain concomitant systemic illness is limited. Caution is advisable in using ZOLOFT in patients with diseases or conditions that could affect metabolism or hemodynamic responses.

ZOLOFT has not been evaluated or used to any appreciable extent in patients with a recent history of myocardial infarction or unstable heart disease. Patients with these diagnoses were excluded from clinical studies during the product's premarket testing. However, the electrocardiograms of 774 patients who received ZOLOFT in double-blind trials were evaluated and the data indicate that ZOLOFT is not associated with the development of significant ECG abnormalities.

ZOLOFT is extensively metabolized by the liver. In patients with chronic mild liver impairment, sertraline clearance was reduced, resulting in increased AUC, Cmax and elimination half-life. The effects of sertraline in patients with moderate and severe hepatic impairment have not been studied. The use of sertraline in patients with liver disease must be approached with caution. If sertraline is administered to patients with liver impairment, a lower or less frequent dose should be used (see CLINICAL PHARMACOLOGY and DOSAGE AND ADMINISTRATION).

Since ZOLOFT is extensively metabolized, excretion of unchanged drug in urine is a minor route of elimination. A clinical study comparing sertraline pharmacokinetics in healthy volunteers to that in patients with renal impairment ranging from mild to severe (requiring dialysis) indicated that the pharmacokinetics and protein binding are unaffected by renal disease. Based on the pharmacokinetic results, there is no need for dosage adjustment in patients with renal impairment (see CLINICAL PHARMACOLOGY).

Interference with Cognitive and Motor Performance—In controlled studies, ZOLOFT did not cause sedation and did not interfere with psychomotor performance. (See **Information for Patients.**)

Hyponatremia—Several cases of hyponatremia have been reported and appeared to be reversible when ZOLOFT was discontinued. Some cases were possibly due to the syndrome of inappropriate antidiuretic hormone secretion. The majority of these occurrences have been in elderly individuals, some in patients taking diuretics or who were otherwise volume depleted.

Platelet Function—There have been rare reports of altered platelet function and/or abnormal results from laboratory studies in patients taking ZOLOFT. While there have been reports of abnormal bleeding or purpura in several patients taking ZOLOFT, it is unclear whether ZOLOFT had a causative role.

Information for Patients

Physicians are advised to discuss the following issues with patients for whom they prescribe ZOLOFT:

Patients should be told that although ZOLOFT has not been shown to impair the ability of normal subjects to perform tasks requiring complex motor and mental skills in laboratory experiments, drugs that act upon the central nervous system may affect some individuals adversely. Therefore, patients should be told that until they learn how they respond to ZOLOFT they should be careful doing activities when they need to be alert, such as driving a car or operating machinery.

Patients should be told that although ZOLOFT has not been shown in experiments with normal subjects to increase the mental and motor skill impairments caused by alcohol, the concomitant use of ZOLOFT and alcohol is not advised.

Patients should be told that while no adverse interaction of ZOLOFT with over-the-counter (OTC) drug products is known to occur, the potential for interaction exists. Thus, the use of any OTC product should be initiated cautiously according to the directions of use given for the OTC product.

Patients should be advised to notify their physician if they become pregnant or intend to become pregnant during therapy.

Patients should be advised to notify their physician if they are breast feeding an infant.

ZOLOFT oral concentrate is contraindicated with ANTABUSE (disulfiram) due to the alcohol content of the concentrate.

ZOLOFT Oral Concentrate contains 20 mg/mL of sertraline (as the hydrochloride) as the active ingredient and 12% alcohol. ZOLOFT Oral Concentrate must be diluted before use. Just before taking, use the dropper provided to remove the required amount of ZOLOFT Oral Concentrate and mix with 4 oz (1/2 cup) of water, ginger ale, lemon/lime soda, lemonade or orange juice ONLY. Do not mix ZOLOFT Oral Concentrate with anything other than the liquids listed. The dose should be taken immediately after mixing. Do not mix in advance. At times, a slight haze may appear after mixing; this is normal. Note that caution should be exercised for persons with latex sensitivity, as the dropper dispenser contains dry natural rubber.

Laboratory Tests

None.

Drug Interactions

Potential Effects of Coadministration of Drugs Highly Bound to Plasma Proteins—Because sertraline is tightly bound to plasma protein, the administration of ZOLOFT® (sertraline hydrochloride) to a patient taking another drug which is tightly bound to protein (e.g., warfarin, digitoxin) may cause a shift in plasma concentrations potentially resulting in an adverse effect. Conversely, adverse effects may result from displacement of protein bound ZOLOFT by other tightly bound drugs.

In a study comparing prothrombin time AUC (0–120 hr) following dosing with warfarin (0.75 mg/kg) before and after 21 days of dosing with either ZOLOFT (50–200 mg/day) or placebo, there was a mean increase in prothrombin time of 8% relative to baseline for ZOLOFT compared to a 1% decrease for placebo ($p<0.02$). The normalization of prothrombin time for the ZOLOFT group was delayed compared to the placebo group. The clinical significance of this change is unknown. Accordingly, prothrombin time should be carefully monitored when ZOLOFT therapy is initiated or stopped.

Cimetidine—In a study assessing disposition of ZOLOFT (100 mg) on the second of 8 days of cimetidine administration

(800 mg daily), there were significant increases in ZOLOFT mean AUC (50%), Cmax (24%) and half-life (26%) compared to the placebo group. The clinical significance of these changes is unknown.

CNS Active Drugs—In a study comparing the disposition of intravenously administered diazepam before and after 21 days of dosing with either ZOLOFT (50 to 200 mg/day escalating dose) or placebo, there was a 32% decrease relative to baseline in diazepam clearance for the ZOLOFT group compared to a 19% decrease relative to baseline for the placebo group (p<0.03). There was a 23% increase in Tmax for desmethyldiazepam in the ZOLOFT group compared to a 20% decrease in the placebo group (p<0.03). The clinical significance of these changes is unknown.

In a placebo-controlled trial in normal volunteers, the administration of two doses of ZOLOFT did not significantly alter steady-state lithium levels or the renal clearance of lithium.

Nonetheless, at this time, it is recommended that plasma lithium levels be monitored following initiation of ZOLOFT therapy with appropriate adjustments to the lithium dose. The risk of using ZOLOFT in combination with other CNS active drugs has not been systematically evaluated. Consequently, caution is advised if the concomitant administration of ZOLOFT and such drugs is required.

There is limited controlled experience regarding the optimal timing of switching from other antidepressants to ZOLOFT. Care and prudent medical judgment should be exercised when switching, particularly from long-acting agents. The duration of an appropriate washout period which should intervene before switching from one selective serotonin reuptake inhibitor (SSRI) to another has not been established.

Monoamine Oxidase Inhibitors—See CONTRAINDICATIONS and WARNINGS.

Drugs Metabolized by P450 3A4—In two separate *in vivo* interaction studies, sertraline was co-administered with cytochrome P450 3A4 substrates, terfenadine or carbamazepine, under steady-state conditions. The results of these studies demonstrated that sertraline co-administration did not increase plasma concentrations of terfenadine or carbamazepine. These data suggest that sertraline's extent of inhibition of P450 3A4 activity is not likely to be of clinical significance.

Drugs Metabolized by P450 2D6—Many antidepressants, e.g., the SSRIs, including sertraline, and most tricyclic antidepressants inhibit the biochemical activity of the drug metabolizing isozyme cytochrome P450 2D6 (debrisoquin hydroxylase), and, thus, may increase the plasma concentrations of co-administered drugs that are metabolized by P450 2D6. The drugs for which this potential interaction is of greatest concern are those metabolized primarily by 2D6 and which have a narrow therapeutic index, e.g., the tricyclic antidepressants and the Type 1C antiarrhythmics propafenone and flecainide. The extent to which this interaction is an important clinical problem depends on the extent of the inhibition of P450 2D6 by the antidepressant and the therapeutic index of the co-administered drug. There is variability among the antidepressants in the extent of clinically important 2D6 inhibition, and in fact sertraline at lower doses has a less prominent inhibitory effect on 2D6 than some others in the class. Nevertheless, even sertraline has the potential for clinically important 2D6 inhibition. Consequently, concomitant use of a drug metabolized by P450 2D6 with ZOLOFT may require lower doses than usually prescribed for the other drug. Furthermore, whenever ZOLOFT is withdrawn from co-therapy, an increased dose of the co-administered drug may be required (see Tricyclic Antidepressants under PRECAUTIONS).

Sumatriptan—There have been rare postmarketing reports describing patients with weakness, hyperreflexia, and incoordination following the use of a selective serotonin reuptake inhibitor (SSRI) and sumatriptan. If concomitant treatment with sumatriptan and an SSRI (e.g., citalopram, fluoxetine, fluvoxamine, paroxetine, sertraline) is clinically warranted, appropriate observation of the patient is advised.

Tricyclic Antidepressants (TCAs)—The extent to which SSRI–TCA interactions may pose clinical problems will depend on the degree of inhibition and the pharmacokinetics of the SSRI involved. Nevertheless, caution is indicated in the co-administration of TCAs with ZOLOFT, because sertraline may inhibit TCA metabolism. Plasma TCA concentrations may need to be monitored, and the dose of TCA may need to be reduced, if a TCA is co-administered with ZOLOFT (see Drugs Metabolized by P450 2D6 under PRECAUTIONS).

Hypoglycemic Drugs—In a placebo-controlled trial in normal volunteers, administration of ZOLOFT for 22 days (including 200 mg/day for the final 13 days) caused a statistically significant 16% decrease from baseline in the clearance of tolbutamide following an intravenous 1000 mg dose. ZOLOFT administration did not noticeably change either the plasma protein binding or the apparent volume of distribution of tolbutamide, suggesting that the decreased clearance was due to a change in the metabolism of the drug. The clinical significance of this decrease in tolbutamide clearance is unknown.

Atenolol—ZOLOFT (100 mg) when administered to 10 healthy male subjects had no effect on the beta-adrenergic blocking ability of atenolol.

Digoxin—In a placebo-controlled trial in normal volunteers, administration of ZOLOFT for 17 days (including 200 mg/day for the last 10 days) did not change serum digoxin levels or digoxin renal clearance.

Microsomal Enzyme Induction—Preclinical studies have shown ZOLOFT to induce hepatic microsomal enzymes. In clinical studies, ZOLOFT was shown to induce hepatic enzymes minimally as determined by a small (5%) but statistically significant decrease in antipyrine half-life following administration of 200 mg/day for 21 days. This small change in antipyrine half-life reflects a clinically insignificant change in hepatic metabolism.

Electroconvulsive Therapy—There are no clinical studies establishing the risks or benefits of the combined use of electroconvulsive therapy (ECT) and ZOLOFT.

Alcohol—Although ZOLOFT did not potentiate the cognitive and psychomotor effects of alcohol in experiments with normal subjects, the concomitant use of ZOLOFT and alcohol is not recommended.

Carcinogenesis—Lifetime carcinogenicity studies were carried out in CD-1 mice and Long-Evans rats at doses up to 40 mg/kg/day. These doses correspond to 1 times (mice) and 2 times (rats) the maximum recommended human dose (MRHD) on a mg/m² basis. There was a dose-related increase of liver adenomas in male mice receiving sertraline at 10–40 mg/kg (0.25–1.0 times the MRHD on a mg/m² basis). No increase was seen in female mice or in rats of either sex receiving the same treatments, nor was there an increase in hepatocellular carcinomas. Liver adenomas have a variable rate of spontaneous occurrence in the CD-1 mouse and are of unknown significance to humans. There was an increase in follicular adenomas of the thyroid in female rats receiving sertraline at 40 mg/kg (2 times the MRHD on a mg/m² basis); this was not accompanied by thyroid hyperplasia. While there was an increase in uterine adenocarcinomas in rats receiving sertraline at 10–40 mg/kg (0.5–2.0 times the MRHD on a mg/m² basis) compared to placebo controls, this effect was not clearly drug related.

Mutagenesis—Sertraline had no genotoxic effects, with or without metabolic activation, based on the following assays: bacterial mutation assay; mouse lymphoma mutation assay; and tests for cytogenetic aberrations *in vivo* in mouse bone marrow and *in vitro* in human lymphocytes.

Impairment of Fertility—A decrease in fertility was seen in one of two rat studies at a dose of 80 mg/kg (4 times the maximum recommended human dose on a mg/m² basis).

Pregnancy—Pregnancy Category C—Reproduction studies have been performed in rats and rabbits at doses up to 80 mg/kg/day and 40 mg/kg/day, respectively. These doses correspond to approximately 4 times the maximum recommended human dose (MRHD) on a mg/m² basis. There was no evidence of teratogenicity at any dose level. When pregnant rats and rabbits were given sertraline during the period of organogenesis, delayed ossification was observed in fetuses at doses of 10 mg/kg (0.5 times the MRHD on a mg/m² basis) in rats and 40 mg/kg (4 times the MRHD on a mg/m² basis) in rabbits. When female rats received sertraline during the last third of gestation and throughout lactation, there was an increase in the number of stillborn pups and in the number of pups dying during the first 4 days after birth. Pup body weights were also decreased during the first four days after birth. These effects occurred at a dose of 20 mg/kg (1 times the MRHD on a mg/m² basis). The no effect dose for rat pup mortality was 10 mg/kg (0.5 times the MRHD on a mg/m² basis). The decrease in pup survival was shown to be due to *in utero* exposure to sertraline. The clinical significance of these effects is unknown. There are no adequate and well-controlled studies in pregnant women. ZOLOFT® (sertraline hydrochloride) should be used during pregnancy only if the potential benefit justifies the potential risk to the fetus.

TABLE 2
TREATMENT-EMERGENT ADVERSE EVENTS: INCIDENCE IN PLACEBO-CONTROLLED CLINICAL TRIALS
Percentage of Patients Reporting Event
Depression/Other*, OCD, Panic Disorder and PTSD combined

Body System/Adverse Event**	ZOLOFT (N=2198)	Placebo (N=1877)
Autonomic Nervous System Disorders		
Ejaculation Failure[1]	14	1
Mouth Dry	15	9
Sweating Increased	6	2
Centr. & Periph. Nerv. System Disorders		
Somnolence	14	7
Dizziness	12	7
Headache	26	24
Paresthesia	3	2
Tremor	8	2
Disorders of Skin and Appendages		
Rash	3	2
Gastrointestinal Disorders		
Anorexia	6	2
Constipation	7	5
Diarrhea/Loose Stools	21	11
Dyspepsia	8	4
Flatulence	4	3
Nausea	27	13
Vomiting	4	2
General		
Fatigue	11	7
Hot Flushes	2	1
Psychiatric Disorders		
Agitation	6	4
Anxiety	4	3
Insomnia	22	11
Libido Decreased	6	1
Nervousness	6	4
Special Senses		
Vision Abnormal	4	2

[1]Primarily ejaculatory delay. Denominator used was for male patients only (N=913 ZOLOFT; N=773 placebo).
*Depression and other premarketing controlled trials.
**Included are events reported by at least 2% of patients taking ZOLOFT except the following events, which had an incidence on placebo greater than or equal to ZOLOFT: abdominal pain and pharyngitis.

Continued on next page

Zoloft—Cont.

Labor and Delivery—The effect of ZOLOFT on labor and delivery in humans is unknown.

Nursing Mothers—It is not known whether, and if so in what amount, sertraline or its metabolites are excreted in human milk. Because many drugs are excreted in human milk, caution should be exercised when ZOLOFT is administered to a nursing woman.

Pediatric Use—The efficacy of ZOLOFT for the treatment of obsessive-compulsive disorder was demonstrated in a 12-week, multicenter, placebo-controlled study with 187 outpatients ages 6–17 (see Clinical Trials under CLINICAL PHARMACOLOGY). The effectiveness of ZOLOFT in pediatric patients with depression or panic disorder has not been systematically evaluated.

Sertraline pharmacokinetics were evaluated in 61 pediatric patients between 6 and 17 years of age with depression or OCD and revealed similar drug exposures to those of adults when plasma concentration was adjusted for weight (see Pharmacokinetics under CLINICAL PHARMACOLOGY).

More than 250 patients with depression or OCD between 6 and 17 years of age have received ZOLOFT in clinical trials. The adverse event profile observed in these patients was generally similar to that observed in adult studies with ZOLOFT (see ADVERSE REACTIONS). As with other SSRIs, decreased appetite and weight loss have been observed in association with the use of ZOLOFT. Consequently, regular monitoring of weight and growth is recommended if treatment of a child with an SSRI is to be continued long term. Safety and effectiveness in pediatric patients below the age of 6 have not been established.

The risks, if any, that may be associated with sertraline's extended use in children and adolescents with OCD have not been systematically assessed. The prescriber should be mindful that the evidence relied upon to conclude that sertraline is safe for use in children and adolescents derives from relatively short-term clinical studies and from extrapolation of experience gained with adult patients. In particular, there are no studies that directly evaluate the effects of long-term sertraline use on the growth, development, and maturation of children and adolescents. Although there is no affirmative finding to suggest that sertraline possesses a capacity to adversely affect growth, development or maturation, the absence of such findings is not compelling evidence of the absence of the potential of sertraline to have adverse effects in chronic use.

Geriatric Use—U.S. geriatric clinical studies of ZOLOFT in depression included 663 ZOLOFT-treated subjects ≥65 years of age, of those, 180 were ≥75 years of age. No overall differences in the pattern of adverse reactions were observed in the geriatric clinical trial subjects relative to those reported in younger subjects (see ADVERSE REACTIONS), and other reported experience has not identified differences in safety patterns between the elderly and younger subjects. As with all medications, greater sensitivity of some older individuals cannot be ruled out. There were 947 subjects in placebo-controlled geriatric clinical studies of ZOLOFT in depression. No overall differences in the pattern of efficacy were observed in the geriatric clinical trial subjects relative to those reported in younger subjects.

Other Adverse Events in Geriatric Patients. In 354 geriatric subjects treated with ZOLOFT in placebo-controlled trials, the overall profile of adverse events was generally similar to that shown in Tables 1 and 2. Urinary tract infection was the only adverse event not appearing in Tables 1 and 2 and reported at an incidence of at least 2% and at a rate greater than placebo in placebo-controlled trials.

As with other SSRIs, ZOLOFT has been associated with cases of clinically significant hyponatremia in elderly patients (see Hyponatremia under PRECAUTIONS).

ADVERSE REACTIONS

During its premarketing assessment, multiple doses of ZOLOFT were administered to over 4000 adult subjects as of February 26, 1998. The conditions and duration of exposure to ZOLOFT varied greatly, and included (in overlapping categories) clinical pharmacology studies, open and double-blind studies, uncontrolled and controlled studies, inpatient and outpatient studies, fixed-dose and titration studies, and studies for multiple indications, including depression, OCD, panic disorder and PTSD.

Untoward events associated with this exposure were recorded by clinical investigators using terminology of their own choosing. Consequently, it is not possible to provide a meaningful estimate of the proportion of individuals experiencing adverse events without first grouping similar types of untoward events into a smaller number of standardized event categories.

In the tabulations that follow, a World Health Organization dictionary of terminology has been used to classify reported adverse events. The frequencies presented, therefore, represent the proportion of the over 4000 adult individuals exposed to multiple doses of ZOLOFT who experienced a treatment-emergent adverse event of the type cited on at least one occasion while receiving ZOLOFT. An event was considered treatment-emergent if it occurred for the first time or worsened while receiving therapy following baseline evaluation. It is important to emphasize that events reported during therapy were not necessarily caused by it.

The prescriber should be aware that the figures in the tables and tabulations cannot be used to predict the incidence of side effects in the course of usual medical practice where patient characteristics and other factors differ from those that prevailed in the clinical trials. Similarly, the cited frequencies cannot be compared with figures obtained from other clinical investigations involving different treatments, uses, and investigators. The cited figures, however, do provide the prescribing physician with some basis for estimating the relative contribution of drug and nondrug factors to the side effect incidence rate in the population studied.

Incidence in Placebo-Controlled Trials—Table 1 enumerates the most common treatment-emergent adverse events associated with the use of ZOLOFT (incidence of at least 5% for ZOLOFT and at least twice that for placebo within at least one of the indications) for the treatment of adult patients with depression/other*, OCD, panic disorder and PTSD in placebo-controlled clinical trials. Most patients received doses of 50 to 200 mg/day. Table 2 enumerates treatment-emergent adverse events that occurred in 2% or more of adult patients treated with ZOLOFT and with incidence greater than placebo who participated in controlled clinical trials comparing ZOLOFT with placebo in the treatment of depression/other*, OCD, panic disorder and PTSD. Table 2 provides combined data for the pool of studies that are provided separately by indication in Table 1.

[See table at top of page 316]
[See table at top of previous page]

Associated with Discontinuation in Placebo-Controlled Clinical Trials

Table 3 lists the adverse events associated with discontinuation of ZOLOFT® (sertraline hydrochloride) treatment (incidence at least twice that for placebo and at least 1% for ZOLOFT in clinical trials) in depression/other*, OCD, panic disorder and PTSD.

[See table 3 above]

TABLE 3
MOST COMMON ADVERSE EVENTS ASSOCIATED WITH DISCONTINUATION IN PLACEBO-CONTROLLED CLINICAL TRIALS

Adverse Event	Depression/Other*, OCD, Panic Disorder and PTSD combined (N=2198)	Depression/Other* (N=861)	OCD (N=533)	Panic Disorder (N=430)	PTSD (N=374)
Agitation	1%	1%	—	2%	—
Diarrhea	2%	2%	2%	1%	—
Dizziness	1%	—	1%	—	—
Dry Mouth	—	1%	—	—	—
Dyspepsia	—	—	—	1%	—
Ejaculation Failure(1)	1%	1%	1%	2%	—
Headache	1%	2%	—	—	1%
Insomnia	2%	1%	3%	2%	—
Nausea	3%	4%	3%	3%	2%
Nervousness	—	—	—	2%	—
Somnolence	2%	1%	2%	2%	—
Tremor	—	2%	—	—	—

(1)Primarily ejaculatory delay. Denominator used was for male patients only (N=271 depression/other*; N=296 OCD; N=216 panic disorder; N=130 PTSD).
*Depression and other premarketing controlled trials.

Male and Female Sexual Dysfunction with SSRIs

Although changes in sexual desire, sexual performance and sexual satisfaction often occur as manifestations of a psychiatric disorder, they may also be a consequence of pharmacologic treatment. In particular, some evidence suggests that selective serotonin reuptake inhibitors (SSRIs) can cause such untoward sexual experiences. Reliable estimates of the incidence and severity of untoward experiences involving sexual desire, performance and satisfaction are difficult to obtain, however, in part because patients and physicians may be reluctant to discuss them. Accordingly, estimates of the incidence of untoward sexual experience and performance cited in product labeling, are likely to underestimate their actual incidence.

Table 4 below displays the incidence of sexual side effects reported by at least 2% of patients taking ZOLOFT in placebo-controlled trials.

[See table 4 above]

TABLE 4

Treatment	Ejaculation failure (primarily delayed ejaculation)		Decreased libido	
	N (males only)	Incidence	N (males and females)	Incidence
ZOLOFT	913	14%	2198	6%
Placebo	773	1%	1877	1%

There are no adequate and well-controlled studies examining sexual dysfunction with sertraline treatment.

Priapism has been reported with all SSRIs.

While it is difficult to know the precise risk of sexual dysfunction associated with the use of SSRIs, physicians should routinely inquire about such possible side effects.

Other Adverse Events in Pediatric Patients—In approximately N=250 pediatric patients treated with ZOLOFT, the overall profile of adverse events was generally similar to that seen in adult studies, as shown in Tables 1 and 2. However, the following adverse events, not appearing in Tables 1 and 2, were reported at an incidence of at least 2% and occurred at a rate of at least twice the placebo rate in a controlled trial (N=187): hyperkinesia, twitching, fever, malaise, purpura, weight decrease, concentration impaired, manic reaction, emotional lability, thinking abnormal, and epistaxis.

Other Events Observed During the Premarketing Evaluation of ZOLOFT® (sertraline hydrochloride)—Following is a list of treatment-emergent adverse events reported during premarketing assessment of ZOLOFT in clinical trials (over 4000 adult subjects) except those already listed in the previous tables or elsewhere in labeling.

In the tabulations that follow, a World Health Organization dictionary of terminology has been used to classify reported adverse events. The frequencies presented, therefore, represent the proportion of the over 4000 adult individuals exposed to multiple doses of ZOLOFT who experienced an event of the type cited on at least one occasion while receiving ZOLOFT. All events are included except those already listed in the previous tables or elsewhere in labeling and those reported in terms so general as to be uninformative and those for which a causal relationship to ZOLOFT treatment seemed remote. It is important to emphasize that although the events reported occurred during treatment with ZOLOFT, they were not necessarily caused by it.

Events are further categorized by body system and listed in order of decreasing frequency according to the following definitions: frequent adverse events are those occurring on one or more occasions in at least 1/100 patients; infrequent adverse events are those occurring in 1/100 to 1/1000 patients; rare events are those occurring in fewer than 1/1000 patients. Events of major clinical importance are also described in the PRECAUTIONS section.

Autonomic Nervous System Disorders—*Frequent:* impotence; *Infrequent:* flushing, increased saliva, cold clammy skin, mydriasis; *Rare:* pallor, glaucoma, priapism, vasodilation.

Body as a Whole—General Disorders—*Rare:* allergic reaction, allergy.

Cardiovascular—*Frequent:* palpitations, chest pain; *Infrequent:* hypertension, tachycardia, postural dizziness, postural hypotension, periorbital edema, peripheral edema, hypotension, peripheral ischemia, syncope, edema, dependent edema; *Rare:* precordial chest pain, substernal chest pain, aggravated hypertension, myocardial infarction, cerebrovascular disorder.

Central and Peripheral Nervous System Disorders—*Frequent:* hypertonia, hypoesthesia; *Infrequent:* twitching, confusion, hyperkinesia, vertigo, ataxia, migraine, abnormal coordination, hyperesthesia, leg cramps, abnormal gait, nystagmus, hypokinesia; *Rare:* dysphonia, coma, dyskinesia, hypotonia, ptosis, choreoathetosis, hyporeflexia.
Disorders of Skin and Appendages—*Infrequent:* pruritus, acne, urticaria, alopecia, dry skin, erythematous rash, photosensitivity reaction, maculopapular rash; *Rare:* follicular rash, eczema, dermatitis, contact dermatitis, bullous eruption, hypertrichosis, skin discoloration, pustular rash.
Endocrine Disorders—*Rare:* exophthalmos, gynecomastia.
Gastrointestinal Disorders—*Frequent:* appetite increased; *Infrequent:* dysphagia, tooth caries aggravated, eructation, esophagitis, gastroenteritis; *Rare:* melena, glossitis, gum hyperplasia, hiccup, stomatitis, tenesmus, colitis, diverticulitis, fecal incontinence, gastritis, rectum hemorrhage, hemorrhagic peptic ulcer, proctitis, ulcerative stomatitis, tongue edema, tongue ulceration.
General—*Frequent:* back pain, asthenia, malaise, weight increase; *Infrequent:* fever, rigors, generalized edema; *Rare:* face edema, aphthous stomatitis.
Hearing and Vestibular Disorders—*Rare:* hyperacusis, labyrinthine disorder.
Hematopoietic and Lymphatic—*Rare:* anemia, anterior chamber eye hemorrhage.
Liver and Biliary System Disorders—*Rare:* abnormal hepatic function.
Metabolic and Nutritional Disorders—*Infrequent:* thirst; *Rare:* hypoglycemia, hypoglycemia reaction.
Musculoskeletal System Disorders—*Frequent:* myalgia; *Infrequent:* arthralgia, dystonia, arthrosis, muscle cramps, muscle weakness.
Psychiatric Disorders—*Frequent:* yawning, other male sexual dysfunction, other female sexual dysfunction; *Infrequent:* depression, amnesia, paroniria, teeth-grinding, emotional lability, apathy, abnormal dreams, euphoria, paranoid reaction, hallucination, aggressive reaction, aggravated depression, delusions; *Rare:* withdrawal syndrome, suicide ideation, libido increased, somnambulism, illusion.
Reproductive—*Infrequent:* menstrual disorder, dysmenorrhea, intermenstrual bleeding, vaginal hemorrhage, amenorrhea, leukorrhea; *Rare:* female breast pain, menorrhagia, balanoposthitis, breast enlargement, atrophic vaginitis, acute female mastitis.
Respiratory System Disorders—*Frequent:* rhinitis; *Infrequent:* coughing, dyspnea, upper respiratory tract infection, epistaxis, bronchospasm, sinusitis; *Rare:* hyperventilation, bradypnea, stridor, apnea, bronchitis, hemoptysis, hypoventilation, laryngismus, laryngitis.
Special Senses—*Frequent:* tinnitus; *Infrequent:* conjunctivitis, earache, eye pain, abnormal accommodation; *Rare:* xerophthalmia, photophobia, diplopia, abnormal lacrimation, scotoma, visual field defect.
Urinary System Disorders—*Infrequent:* micturition frequency, polyuria, urinary retention, dysuria, nocturia, urinary incontinence; *Rare:* cystitis, oliguria, pyelonephritis, hematuria, renal pain, strangury.
Laboratory Tests—In man, asymptomatic elevations in serum transaminases (SGOT [or AST] and SGPT [or ALT]) have been reported infrequently (approximately 0.8%) in association with ZOLOFT® (sertraline hydrochloride) administration. These hepatic enzyme elevations usually occurred within the first 1 to 9 weeks of drug treatment and promptly diminished upon drug discontinuation.
ZOLOFT therapy was associated with small mean increases in total cholesterol (approximately 3%) and triglycerides (approximately 5%), and a small mean decrease in serum uric acid (approximately 7%) of no apparent clinical importance.
The safety profile observed with ZOLOFT treatment in patients with depression, OCD, panic disorder and PTSD is similar.
Other Events Observed During the Postmarketing Evaluation of ZOLOFT—Reports of adverse events temporally associated with ZOLOFT that have been received since market introduction, that are not listed above and that may have no causal relationship with the drug, include the following: acute renal failure, anaphylactoid reaction, angioedema, blindness, optic neuritis, cataract, increased coagulation times, bradycardia, AV block, atrial arrhythmias, QT-interval prolongation, ventricular tachycardia (including torsade de pointes-type arrhythmias), hypothyroidism, agranulocytosis, aplastic anemia and pancytopenia, leukopenia, thrombocytopenia, lupus-like syndrome, serum sickness, hyperglycemia, galactorrhea, hyperprolactinemia, neuroleptic malignant syndrome-like events, extrapyramidal symptoms, oculogyric crisis, serotonin syndrome, psychosis, pulmonary hypertension, severe skin reactions, which potentially can be fatal, such as Stevens-Johnson syndrome, vasculitis, photosensitivity and other severe cutaneous disorders, rare reports of pancreatitis, and liver events—clinical features (which in the majority of cases appeared to be reversible with discontinuation of ZOLOFT) occurring in one or more patients include: elevated enzymes, increased bilirubin, hepatomegaly, hepatitis, jaundice, abdominal pain, vomiting, liver failure and death.

DRUG ABUSE AND DEPENDENCE

Controlled Substance Class—ZOLOFT® (sertraline hydrochloride) is not a controlled substance.
Physical and Psychological Dependence—In a placebo-controlled, double-blind, randomized study of the comparative abuse liability of ZOLOFT, alprazolam, and d-amphetamine in humans, ZOLOFT did not produce the positive subjective effects indicative of abuse potential, such as euphoria or drug liking, that were observed with the other two drugs. Premarketing clinical experience with ZOLOFT did not reveal any tendency for a withdrawal syndrome or any drug-seeking behavior. In animal studies ZOLOFT does not demonstrate stimulant or barbiturate-like (depressant) abuse potential. As with any CNS active drug, however, physicians should carefully evaluate patients for history of drug abuse and follow such patients closely, observing them for signs of ZOLOFT misuse or abuse (e.g., development of tolerance, incrementation of dose, drug-seeking behavior).

OVERDOSAGE

Human Experience—Of 1,027 cases of overdose involving sertraline hydrochloride worldwide, alone or with other drugs, there were 72 deaths (circa 1999).
Among 634 overdoses in which sertraline hydrochloride was the only drug ingested, 8 resulted in fatal outcome, 75 completely recovered, and 27 patients experienced sequelae after overdosage to include alopecia, decreased libido, diarrhea, ejaculation disorder, fatigue, insomnia, somnolence and serotonin syndrome. The remaining 524 cases had an unknown outcome. The most common signs and symptoms associated with non-fatal sertraline hydrochloride overdosage were somnolence, vomiting, tachycardia, nausea, dizziness, agitation and tremor.
The largest known ingestion was 13.5 grams in a patient who took sertraline hydrochloride alone and subsequently recovered. However, another patient who took 2.5 grams of sertraline hydrochloride alone experienced a fatal outcome.
Other important adverse events reported with sertraline hydrochloride overdose (single or multiple drugs) include bradycardia, bundle branch block, coma, convulsions, delirium, hallucinations, hypertension, hypotension, manic reaction, pancreatitis, QT-interval prolongation, serotonin syndrome, stupor and syncope.
Overdose Management—Treatment should consist of those general measures employed in the management of overdosage with any antidepressant.
Ensure an adequate airway, oxygenation and ventilation. Monitor cardiac rhythm and vital signs. General supportive and symptomatic measures are also recommended. Induction of emesis is not recommended. Gastric lavage with a large-bore orogastric tube with appropriate airway protection, if needed, may be indicated if performed soon after ingestion, or in symptomatic patients.
Activated charcoal should be administered. Due to large volume of distribution of this drug, forced diuresis, dialysis, hemoperfusion and exchange transfusion are unlikely to be of benefit. No specific antidotes for sertraline are known.
In managing overdosage, consider the possibility of multiple drug involvement. The physician should consider contacting a poison control center on the treatment of any overdose. Telephone numbers for certified poison control centers are listed in the *Physicians' Desk Reference* (PDR®).

DOSAGE AND ADMINISTRATION

Initial Treatment

Dosage for Adults

Depression and Obsessive-Compulsive Disorder—ZOLOFT treatment should be administered at a dose of 50 mg once daily.
Panic Disorder and Posttraumatic Stress Disorder—ZOLOFT treatment should be initiated with a dose of 25 mg once daily. After one week, the dose should be increased to 50 mg once daily.
While a relationship between dose and effect has not been established for depression, OCD, panic disorder or PTSD, patients were dosed in a range of 50–200 mg/day in the clinical trials demonstrating the effectiveness of ZOLOFT for the treatment of these indications. Consequently, a dose of 50 mg, administered once daily, is recommended as the initial dose. Patients not responding to a 50 mg dose may benefit from dose increases up to a maximum of 200 mg/day. Given the 24 hour elimination half-life of ZOLOFT, dose changes should not occur at intervals of less than 1 week.
ZOLOFT should be administered once daily, either in the morning or evening.

Dosage for Pediatric Population (Children and Adolescents)

Obsessive-Compulsive Disorder—ZOLOFT treatment should be initiated with a dose of 25 mg once daily in children (ages 6–12) and at a dose of 50 mg once daily in adolescents (ages 13–17).
While a relationship between dose and effect has not been established for OCD, patients were dosed in a range of 25–200 mg/day in the clinical trials demonstrating the effectiveness of ZOLOFT for pediatric patients (6–17 years) with OCD. Patients not responding to an initial dose of 25 or 50 mg/day may benefit from dose increases up to a maximum of 200 mg/day. For children with OCD, their generally lower body weights compared to adults should be taken into consideration in advancing the dose, in order to avoid excess dosing. Given the 24 hour elimination half-life of ZOLOFT, dose changes should not occur at intervals of less than 1 week.
ZOLOFT should be administered once daily, either in the morning or evening.

Dosage for Hepatically Impaired Patients

The use of sertraline in patients with liver disease should be approached with caution. The effects of sertraline in patients with moderate and severe hepatic impairment have not been studied. If sertraline is administered to patients with liver impairment, a lower or less frequent dose should be used (see CLINICAL PHARMACOLOGY and PRECAUTIONS).

Maintenance/Continuation/Extended Treatment

Depression—It is generally agreed that acute episodes of depression require several months or longer of sustained pharmacologic therapy. Whether the dose of antidepressant needed to induce remission is identical to the dose needed to maintain and/or sustain euthymia is unknown. Systematic evaluation of ZOLOFT has shown that its antidepressant efficacy is maintained for periods of up to 44 weeks following 8 weeks of open-label acute treatment (52 weeks total) at a dose of 50–200 mg/day (mean dose of 70 mg/day) (see Clinical Trials under CLINICAL PHARMACOLOGY).
Obsessive-Compulsive Disorder, Panic Disorder and Posttraumatic Stress Disorder—Although the efficacy of ZOLOFT beyond 10–12 weeks of dosing for OCD, panic disorder and PTSD has not been documented in controlled trials, all are chronic conditions, and it is reasonable to consider continuation of a responding patient. Dosage adjustments may be needed to maintain the patient on the lowest effective dosage, and patients should be periodically reassessed to determine the need for continued treatment.
Switching Patients to or from a Monoamine Oxidase Inhibitor—At least 14 days should elapse between discontinuation of an MAOI and initiation of therapy with ZOLOFT. In addition, at least 14 days should be allowed after stopping ZOLOFT before starting an MAOI (see CONTRAINDICATIONS and WARNINGS).

ZOLOFT Oral Concentrate

ZOLOFT Oral Concentrate contains 20 mg/mL of sertraline (as the hydrochloride) as the active ingredient and 12% alcohol. ZOLOFT Oral Concentrate must be diluted before use. Just before taking, use the dropper provided to remove the required amount of ZOLOFT Oral Concentrate and mix with 4 oz (1/2 cup) of water, ginger ale, lemon/lime soda, lemonade or orange juice ONLY. Do not mix ZOLOFT Oral Concentrate with anything other than the liquids listed. The dose should be taken immediately after mixing. Do not mix in advance. At times, a slight haze may appear after mixing; this is normal. Note that caution should be exercised for patients with latex sensitivity, as the dropper dispenser contains dry natural rubber.
ZOLOFT oral concentrate is contraindicated with ANTABUSE (disulfiram) due to the alcohol content of the concentrate.

HOW SUPPLIED

ZOLOFT® (sertraline hydrochloride) capsular-shaped scored tablets, containing sertraline hydrochloride equivalent to 25, 50 and 100 mg of sertraline, are packaged in bottles.
ZOLOFT® 25 mg Tablets: light green film coated tablets engraved on one side with ZOLOFT and on the other side scored and engraved with 25 mg.

NDC 0049-4960-50	Bottles of 50

ZOLOFT® 50 mg Tablets: light blue film coated tablets engraved on one side with ZOLOFT and on the other side scored and engraved with 50 mg.

NDC 0049-4900-66	Bottles of 100
NDC 0049-4900-73	Bottles of 500
NDC 0049-4900-94	Bottles of 5000
NDC 0049-4900-41	Unit Dose Packages of 100

ZOLOFT® 100 mg Tablets: light yellow film coated tablets engraved on one side with ZOLOFT and on the other side scored and engraved with 100 mg.

NDC 0049-4910-66	Bottles of 100
NDC 0049-4910-73	Bottles of 500
NDC 0049-4910-94	Bottles of 5000
NDC 0049-4910-41	Unit Dose Packages of 100

Store at controlled room temperature, 59° to 86°F (15° to 30°C).
ZOLOFT® Oral Concentrate: ZOLOFT Oral Concentrate is a clear, colorless solution with a menthol scent containing sertraline hydrochloride equivalent to 20 mg of sertraline per mL and 12% alcohol. It is supplied as a 60 mL bottle with an accompanying calibrated dropper.

NDC 0049-4940-23	Bottles of 60 mL

Store at controlled room temperature, 59° to 86°F (15° to 30°C).

Rx only

Distributed by
Roerig
Division of Pfizer Inc, NY, NY 10017

Printed in U.S.A.
69-4721-00-8 Revised September 2000

To keep your **PDR** up to date throughout the year, note these revisions on the corresponding pages of the annual volume. Simply write **"See Supplement A"** next to the product heading.

Purdue Pharma L.P.
ONE STAMFORD FORUM
STAMFORD, CT 06901-3431

For Medical Inquiries:
888-726-7535
Adverse Drug Experiences:
888-726-7535
Customer Service:
800-877-5666
FAX 800-877-3210

OXYCONTIN® ©℞
(OXYCODONE HCl CONTROLLED-RELEASE) TABLETS
10 mg 20 mg 40 mg 80 mg* 160 mg*

> *80 mg and 160 mg for use in opioid-tolerant patients only

Prescribing information for this product, which appears on pages 2697–2701 of the 2001 PDR, has been completely revised as follows. Please write "See Supplement A" next to the product heading.

DESCRIPTION
OxyContin® (oxycodone hydrochloride controlled-release) tablets are an opioid analgesic supplied in 10 mg, 20 mg, 40 mg, 80 mg, and 160 mg tablet strengths for oral administration. The tablet strengths describe the amount of oxycodone per tablet as the hydrochloride salt. The structural formula for oxycodone hydrochloride is as follows:

$C_{18}H_{21}NO_4 \cdot HCl$ MW 351.83

The chemical formula is 4, 5-epoxy-14-hydroxy-3-methoxy-17-methylmorphinan-6-one hydrochloride.
Oxycodone is a white, odorless crystalline powder derived from the opium alkaloid, thebaine. Oxycodone hydrochloride dissolves in water (1 g in 6 to 7 mL). It is slightly soluble in alcohol (octanol water partition coefficient 0.7). The tablets contain the following inactive ingredients: ammonio methacrylate copolymer, hydroxypropyl methylcellulose, lactose, magnesium stearate, povidone, red iron oxide (20 mg strength tablet only), stearyl alcohol, talc, titanium dioxide, triacetin, yellow iron oxide (40 mg strength tablet only), yellow iron oxide with FD&C blue No. 2 (80 mg strength tablet only), FD&C blue No. 2 (160 mg strength tablet only) and other ingredients.
OxyContin® 80 mg and 160 mg Tablets ARE FOR USE IN OPIOID-TOLERANT PATIENTS ONLY.

CLINICAL PHARMACOLOGY
Central Nervous System
Oxycodone is a pure agonist opioid whose principal therapeutic action is analgesia. Other therapeutic effects of oxycodone include anxiolysis, euphoria, and feelings of relaxation. Like all pure opioid agonists, there is no ceiling effect to analgesia, such as is seen with partial agonists or non-opioid analgesics.
The precise mechanism of the analgesic action is unknown. However, specific CNS opioid receptors for endogenous compounds with opioid-like activity have been identified throughout the brain and spinal cord and play a role in the analgesic effects of this drug.
Oxycodone produces respiratory depression by direct action on brain stem respiratory centers. The respiratory depression involves both a reduction in the responsiveness of the brain stem respiratory centers to increases in carbon dioxide tension and to electrical stimulation.
Oxycodone depresses the cough reflex by direct effect on the cough center in the medulla. Antitussive effects may occur with doses lower than those usually required for analgesia. Oxycodone causes miosis, even in total darkness. Pinpoint pupils are a sign of opioid overdose but are not pathognomonic. Marked mydriasis rather than miosis may be seen due to hypoxia in overdose situations.
Gastrointestinal Tract and Other Smooth Muscle
Oxycodone causes a reduction in motility associated with an increase in smooth muscle tone in the antrum of the stomach and duodenum. Digestion of food in the small intestine is delayed and propulsive contractions are decreased. Propulsive peristaltic waves in the colon are decreased, while tone may be increased to the point of spasm resulting in constipation. Other opioid-induced effects may include a reduction in gastric, biliary and pancreatic secretions, spasm of sphincter of Oddi, and transient elevations in serum amylase.
Cardiovascular System
Oxycodone may produce release of histamine with or without associated peripheral vasodilation. Manifestations of histamine release and/or peripheral vasodilation may include pruritus, flushing, red eyes, sweating, and/or orthostatic hypotension.
Concentration—Efficacy Relationships (Pharmacodynamics)
Studies in normal volunteers and patients reveal predictable relationships between oxycodone dosage and plasma oxycodone concentrations, as well as between concentration and certain expected opioid effects. In normal volunteers these include pupillary constriction, sedation and overall "drug effect" and in patients, analgesia and feelings of "relaxation." In non-tolerant patients, analgesia is not usually seen at a plasma oxycodone concentration of less than 5–10 ng/mL.
As with all opioids, the minimum effective plasma concentration for analgesia will vary widely among patients, especially among patients who have been previously treated with potent agonist opioids. As a result, patients need to be treated with individualized titration of dosage to the desired effect. The minimum effective analgesic concentration of oxycodone for any individual patient may increase with repeated dosing due to an increase in pain and/or the development of tolerance.
Concentration—Adverse Experience Relationships
OxyContin tablets are associated with typical opioid-related adverse experiences similar to those seen with immediate-release oxycodone and all opioids. There is a general relationship between increasing oxycodone plasma concentration and increasing frequency of dose-related opioid adverse experiences such as nausea, vomiting, CNS effects, and respiratory depression. In opioid-tolerant patients, the situation is altered by the development of tolerance to opioid-related side effects, and the relationship is poorly understood.
As with all opioids, the dose must be individualized (see **DOSAGE AND ADMINISTRATION**), because the effective analgesic dose for some patients will be too high to be tolerated by other patients.

PHARMACOKINETICS AND METABOLISM
The activity of OxyContin® (oxycodone hydrochloride controlled-release) tablets is primarily due to the parent drug oxycodone. OxyContin tablets are designed to provide controlled delivery of oxycodone over 12 hours. Oxycodone release from OxyContin tablets is pH independent. Oxycodone is well absorbed from OxyContin tablets with an oral bioavailability of from 60% to 87%. The relative oral bioavailability of OxyContin to immediate-release oral dosage forms is 100%. Upon repeated dosing in normal volunteers, steady-state levels were achieved within 24–36 hours. Dose proportionality and/or bioavailability has been established for the 10 mg, 20 mg, 40 mg, 80 mg, and 160 mg tablet strengths for both peak plasma levels (C_{max}) and extent of absorption (AUC). Oxycodone is extensively metabolized and eliminated primarily in the urine as both conjugated and unconjugated metabolites. The apparent elimination half-life of oxycodone following the administration of OxyContin was 4.5 hours compared to 3.2 hours for immediate-release oxycodone.
Absorption
About 60% to 87% of an oral dose of oxycodone reaches the central compartment in comparison to a parenteral dose. This high oral bioavailability is due to low pre-systemic and/or first-pass metabolism. In normal volunteers, the $t\frac{1}{2}$ of absorption is 0.4 hours for immediate-release oral oxycodone. In contrast, OxyContin tablets exhibit a biphasic absorption pattern with two apparent absorption half-times of 0.6 and 6.9 hours, which describes the initial release of oxycodone from the tablet followed by a prolonged release.
Plasma Oxycodone By Time
Dose proportionality has been established for the 10 mg, 20 mg, 40 mg, and 80 mg tablet strengths for both peak plasma concentrations (C_{max}) and extent of absorption (AUC) (see Table 1 below). Another study established that the 160 mg tablet is bioequivalent to 2 × 80 mg tablets as well as to 4 × 40 mg for both peak plasma concentrations (C_{max}) and extent of absorption (AUC) (see Table 2 below). Given the short half-life of elimination of oxycodone from OxyContin, steady-state plasma concentrations of oxycodone are achieved within 24–36 hours of initiation of

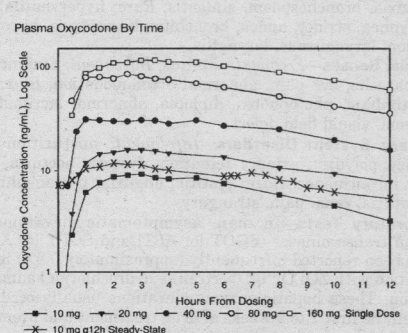

dosing with OxyContin tablets. In a study comparing 10 mg of OxyContin every 12 hours to 5 mg of immediate-release oxycodone every 6 hours, the two treatments were found to be equivalent for AUC and C_{max}, and similar for C_{min} (trough) concentrations. There was less fluctuation in plasma concentrations for the OxyContin tablets than for the immediate-release formulation.
[See table 1 above]
[See table 2 above]
Food Effects
Food has no significant effect on the extent of absorption of oxycodone from OxyContin. However, the peak plasma concentration of oxycodone increased by 25% when OxyContin 160 mg tablet was administered with a high fat meal.
Distribution
Following intravenous administration, the volume of distribution (Vss) for oxycodone was 2.6 L/kg. Oxycodone binding to plasma protein at 37°C and a pH of 7.4 was about 45%. Once absorbed, oxycodone is distributed to skeletal muscle, liver, intestinal tract, lungs, spleen, and brain. Oxycodone has been found in breast milk (see **PRECAUTIONS**).
Metabolism
Oxycodone hydrochloride is extensively metabolized to noroxycodone, oxymorphone, and their glucuronides. The major circulating metabolite is noroxycodone with an AUC ratio of 0.6 relative to that of oxycodone. Noroxycodone is reported to be a considerably weaker analgesic than oxycodone. Oxymorphone, although possessing analgesic activity, is present in the plasma only in low concentrations. The correlation between oxymorphone concentrations and opioid effects was much less than that seen with oxycodone plasma concentrations. The analgesic activity profile of other metabolites is not known at present.
The formation of oxymorphone, but not noroxycodone, is mediated by CYP2D6 and as such its formation can, in theory, be affected by other drugs (see **Drug-Drug Interactions**).
Excretion
Oxycodone and its metabolites are excreted primarily via the kidney. The amounts measured in the urine have been

Table 1
Mean [% coefficient variation]

Regimen/ Dosage Form	AUC (ng•hr/mL)†	C_{max} (ng/mL)	T_{max} (hrs)	Trough Conc. (ng/mL)
Single Dose				
10 mg OxyContin	100.7 [26.6]	10.6 [20.1]	2.7 [44.1]	n.a.
20 mg OxyContin	207.5 [35.9]	21.4 [36.6]	3.2 [57.9]	n.a.
40 mg OxyContin	423.1 [33.3]	39.3 [34.0]	3.1 [77.4]	n.a.
80 mg OxyContin*	1085.5 [32.3]	98.5 [32.1]	2.1 [52.3]	n.a.
Multiple Dose 10 mg OxyContin Tablets q12h	103.6 [38.6]	15.1 [31.0]	3.2 [69.5]	7.2 [48.1]
5 mg immediate-release q6h	99.0 [36.2]	15.5 [28.8]	1.6 [49.7]	7.4 [50.9]

Table 2
Mean [% coefficient variation]

Regimen/ Dosage Form	AUC_∞ (ng•hr/mL)†	C_{max} (ng/mL)	T_{max} (hrs)	Trough Conc. (ng/mL)
Single Dose				
4×40 mg OxyContin*	1935.3 [34.7]	152.0 [28.9]	2.56 [42.3]	n.a.
2×80 mg OxyContin*	1859.3 [30.1]	153.4 [25.1]	2.78 [69.3]	n.a.
1×160 mg OxyContin*	1856.4 [30.5]	156.4 [24.8]	2.54 [36.4]	n.a.

†for single-dose $AUC=AUC_{0-inf}$: for multiple-dose $AUC=AUC_{0-T}$
*data obtained while volunteers received naltrexone which can enhance absorption

reported as follows: free oxycodone up to 19%; conjugated oxycodone up to 50%; free oxymorphone 0%; conjugated oxymorphone ≤ 14%; both free and conjugated noroxycodone have been found in the urine but not quantified. The total plasma clearance was 0.8 L/min for adults.

Special Populations

Elderly

The plasma concentrations of oxycodone are only nominally affected by age, being 15% greater in elderly as compared to young subjects. There were no differences in adverse event reporting between young and elderly subjects.

Gender

Female subjects have, on average, plasma oxycodone concentrations up to 25% higher than males on a body weight adjusted basis. The reason for this difference is unknown.

Renal Impairment

Preliminary data from a study involving patients with mild to severe renal dysfunction (creatinine clearance <60 mL/min) show peak plasma oxycodone and noroxycodone concentrations 50% and 20% higher, respectively, and AUC values for oxycodone, noroxycodone, and oxymorphone 60%, 50%, and 40% higher than normal subjects, respectively. This is accompanied by an increase in sedation but not by differences in respiratory rate, pupillary constriction, or several other measures of drug effect. There was an increase in $t_{1/2}$ of elimination for oxycodone of only 1 hour (see **PRECAUTIONS**).

Hepatic Impairment

Preliminary data from a study involving patients with mild to moderate hepatic dysfunction show peak plasma oxycodone and noroxycodone concentrations 50% and 20% higher, respectively, than normal subjects. AUC values are 95% and 65% higher, respectively. Oxymorphone peak plasma concentrations and AUC values are lower by 30% and 40%. These differences are accompanied by increases in some, but not other, drug effects. The $t_{1/2}$ elimination for oxycodone increased by 2.3 hours (see **PRECAUTIONS**).

Rectal Administration

Rectal administration of OxyContin tablets is not recommended. Preliminary data from a study involving 21 normal volunteers show OxyContin tablets administered per rectum resulted in an AUC 39% greater and a C_{max} 9% higher than tablets administered by mouth (see **PRECAUTIONS**).

Drug-Drug Interactions (see PRECAUTIONS)

Oxycodone is metabolized in part via CYP2D6 to oxymorphone which represents less than 15% of the total administered dose. This route of elimination can be blocked by a variety of drugs (e.g., certain cardiovascular drugs and antidepressants). Patients receiving such drugs concomitantly with OxyContin do not appear to present different therapeutic profiles than other patients.

CLINICAL TRIALS

OxyContin® (oxycodone hydrochloride controlled-release) tablets were evaluated in studies involving 713 patients with either cancer or non-cancer pain. All patients receiving OxyContin were dosed q12h. Efficacy comparable to other forms of oral oxycodone was demonstrated in clinical studies using pharmacokinetic, pharmacodynamic, and efficacy outcomes. The outcome of these trials indicated: (1) a positive relationship between dose and plasma oxycodone concentration, (2) a positive relationship between plasma oxycodone concentration and analgesia, and (3) an observed peak to trough variation in plasma concentration with OxyContin lying within the observed range established with qid dosing of immediate-release oxycodone in clinical populations at the same total daily dose.

In clinical trials, OxyContin tablets were substituted for a wide variety of analgesics, including acetaminophen (APAP), aspirin (ASA), other non-steroidal anti-inflammatory drugs (NSAIDs), opioid combination products and single-entity opioids, primarily morphine. In cancer patients receiving adequate opioid therapy at baseline, pain intensity scores and acceptability of therapy remained unchanged by transfer to OxyContin. For non-cancer pain patients who had moderate to severe pain at baseline on prn opioid therapy, pain control and acceptability of therapy improved with the introduction of fixed-interval therapy with OxyContin.

Use in Cancer Pain

OxyContin was studied in three double-blind, controlled clinical trials involving 341 cancer patients and several open-label trials with therapy durations of over 10 months. Two, double-blind, controlled clinical studies indicated that OxyContin dosed q12h produced analgesic efficacy equivalent to immediate-release oxycodone dosed qid at the same total daily dose. Peak and trough plasma concentrations attained were similar to those attained with immediate-release oxycodone at equivalent total daily doses. With titration to analgesic effect and proper use of rescue medication, nearly every patient achieved adequate pain control with OxyContin.

In the third study, a double-blind, active-controlled, crossover trial, OxyContin dosed q12h was shown to be equivalent in efficacy and safety to immediate-release oxycodone dosed qid at the same total daily dose. Patients were able to be titrated to an acceptable analgesic effect with either OxyContin or immediate-release oxycodone with both treatments providing stable pain control within 2 days in most patients.

In patients with cancer pain, the total daily OxyContin doses tested ranged from 20 mg to 640 mg per day. The average total daily dose was approximately 105 mg per day.

Studies in Non-Cancer Pain

A double-blind, placebo-controlled, fixed-dose, parallel group study was conducted in 133 patients with moderate to severe osteoarthritis pain, who were judged as having inadequate pain control with prn opioids and maximal non-steroidal anti-inflammatory therapy. In this study, 20 mg OxyContin q12h significantly decreased pain and improved quality of life, mood, and sleep, relative to placebo. Both dose-concentration and concentration-effect relationships were noted with a minimum effective plasma oxycodone concentration of approximately 5–10 ng/mL.

In a double-blind, active-controlled, crossover study involving 57 patients with low-back pain inadequately controlled with prn opioids and non-opioid therapy, OxyContin administered q12h provided analgesia equivalent to immediate-release oxycodone administered qid. Patients could be titrated to an acceptable analgesic effect with either OxyContin or immediate-release forms of oxycodone.

Single-Dose Comparison with Standard Therapy

A single-dose, double-blind, placebo-controlled, post-operative study of 182 patients was conducted utilizing graded doses of OxyContin (10, 20, and 30 mg). Twenty and 30 mg of OxyContin gave equivalent peak analgesic effect compared to two oxycodone 5 mg/acetaminophen 325 mg tablets and to 15 mg immediate-release oxycodone, while the 10 mg dose of OxyContin was intermediate between both the immediate-release and combination products and placebo. The onset of analgesic action with OxyContin occurred within 1 hour in most patients following oral administration.

OxyContin is not recommended pre-operatively (pre-emptive analgesia) or for the management of pain in the immediate post-operative period (the first 12 to 24 hours following surgery) because the safety or appropriateness of fixed-dose, long-acting opioids in this setting has not been established.

Other Clinical Trials

In open-label trials involving approximately 200 patients with cancer-related and non-cancer pain, dosed according to the package insert recommendations, appropriate analgesic effectiveness was noted without regard to age, gender, race, or disease state. There were no unusual drug interactions observed in patients receiving a wide range of medications common in these populations.

For opioid-naive patients, the average total daily dose of OxyContin was approximately 40 mg per day. There was no evidence of oxycodone and metabolite accumulation during 8 months of therapy. For cancer pain patients the average total daily dose was 105 mg (range 20 to 720 mg) per day. There was a significant decrease in acute opioid-related side effects, except for constipation, during the first several weeks of therapy. Development of significant tolerance to analgesia was uncommon.

A cohort of patients have been treated with OxyContin 80 mg tablets. There were no differences in the efficacy or safety profiles than seen with the other tablet strengths.

INDICATIONS AND USAGE

OxyContin® tablets are a controlled-release oral formulation of oxycodone hydrochloride indicated for the management of moderate to severe pain where use of an opioid analgesic is appropriate for more than a few days (see **CLINICAL PHARMACOLOGY; CLINICAL TRIALS**).

CONTRAINDICATIONS

OxyContin® is contraindicated in patients with known hypersensitivity to oxycodone, or in any situation where opioids are contraindicated. This includes patients with significant respiratory depression (in unmonitored settings or the absence of resuscitative equipment), and patients with acute or severe bronchial asthma or hypercarbia. OxyContin is contraindicated in any patient who has or is suspected of having paralytic ileus.

WARNINGS

OxyContin® (oxycodone hydrochloride controlled-release) TABLETS ARE TO BE SWALLOWED WHOLE, AND ARE NOT TO BE BROKEN, CHEWED OR CRUSHED. TAKING BROKEN, CHEWED OR CRUSHED OxyContin TABLETS COULD LEAD TO THE RAPID RELEASE AND ABSORPTION OF A POTENTIALLY TOXIC DOSE OF OXYCODONE.

Respiratory Depression

Respiratory depression is the chief hazard from all opioid agonist preparations. Respiratory depression occurs most frequently in elderly or debilitated patients, usually following large initial doses in non-tolerant patients, or when opioids are given in conjunction with other agents that depress respiration.

Oxycodone should be used with extreme caution in patients with significant chronic obstructive pulmonary disease or cor pulmonale, and in patients having a substantially decreased respiratory reserve, hypoxia, hypercapnia, or preexisting respiratory depression. In such patients, even usual therapeutic doses of oxycodone may decrease respiratory drive to the point of apnea. In these patients alternative non-opioid analgesics should be considered, and opioids should be employed only under careful medical supervision at the lowest effective dose.

Head Injury

The respiratory depressant effects of opioids include carbon dioxide retention and secondary elevation of cerebrospinal fluid pressure, and may be markedly exaggerated in the presence of head injury, intracranial lesions, or other sources of pre-existing increased intracranial pressure. Oxycodone produces effects on pupillary response and consciousness which may obscure neurologic signs of further increases in intracranial pressure in patients with head injuries.

Hypotensive Effect

OxyContin®, like all opioid analgesics, may cause severe hypotension in an individual whose ability to maintain blood pressure has been compromised by a depleted blood volume, or after concurrent administration with drugs such as phenothiazines or other agents which compromise vasomotor tone. OxyContin may produce orthostatic hypotension in ambulatory patients. OxyContin, like all opioid analgesics, should be administered with caution to patients in circulatory shock, since vasodilation produced by the drug may further reduce cardiac output and blood pressure.

PRECAUTIONS

Special Precautions Regarding OxyContin® 80 mg and 160 mg Tablets

OxyContin® 80 mg and 160 mg Tablets are for use only in opioid-tolerant patients requiring daily oxycodone equivalent dosages of 160 mg or more for the 80 mg tablet and 320 mg or more for the 160 mg tablet. Care should be taken in the prescription of this tablet strength. Patients should be instructed against use by individuals other than the patient for whom it was prescribed, as such inappropriate use may have severe medical consequences.

One OxyContin® 160 mg tablet is comparable to two 80 mg tablets when taken on an empty stomach. With a high fat meal, however, there is a 25% greater peak plasma concentration following one 160 mg tablet. Dietary caution should be taken when patients are initially titrated to 160 mg tablets (see DOSAGE and ADMINISTRATION).

General

OxyContin® (oxycodone hydrochloride controlled-release) tablets are intended for use in patients who require oral pain therapy with an opioid agonist of more than a few days duration. As with any opioid analgesic, it is critical to adjust the dosing regimen individually for each patient (see **DOSAGE AND ADMINISTRATION**).

Selection of patients for treatment with OxyContin should be governed by the same principles that apply to the use of similar controlled-release opioid analgesics (see **INDICATIONS AND USAGE**). Opioid analgesics given on a fixed-dosage schedule have a narrow therapeutic index in certain patient populations, especially when combined with other drugs, and should be reserved for cases where the benefits of opioid analgesia outweigh the known risks of respiratory depression, altered mental state, and postural hypotension. Physicians should individualize treatment in every case, using non-opioid analgesics, prn opioids and/or combination products, and chronic opioid therapy with drugs such as OxyContin in a progressive plan of pain management such as outlined by the World Health Organization, the Agency for Health Care Policy and Research, and the American Pain Society.

Use of OxyContin is associated with increased potential risks and should be used only with caution in the following conditions: acute alcoholism; adrenocortical insufficiency (e.g., Addison's disease); CNS depression or coma; delirium tremens; debilitated patients; kyphoscoliosis associated with respiratory depression; myxedema or hypothyroidism; prostatic hypertrophy or urethral stricture; severe impairment of hepatic, pulmonary or renal function; and toxic psychosis.

The administration of oxycodone, like all opioid analgesics, may obscure the diagnosis or clinical course in patients with acute abdominal conditions. Oxycodone may aggravate convulsions in patients with convulsive disorders, and all opioids may induce or aggravate seizures in some clinical settings.

Interactions with other CNS Depressants

OxyContin, like all opioid analgesics, should be used with caution and started in a reduced dosage ($1/3$ to $1/2$ of the usual dosage) in patients who are concurrently receiving other central nervous system depressants including sedatives or hypnotics, general anesthetics, phenothiazines, other tranquilizers, and alcohol. Interactive effects resulting in respiratory depression, hypotension, profound sedation, or coma may result if these drugs are taken in combination with the usual doses of OxyContin.

Interactions with Mixed Agonist/Antagonist Opioid Analgesics

Agonist/antagonist analgesics (i.e., pentazocine, nalbuphine, butorphanol, and buprenorphine) should be administered with caution to a patient who has received or is receiving a course of therapy with a pure opioid agonist analgesic such as oxycodone. In this situation, mixed agonist/antagonist analgesics may reduce the analgesic effect of oxycodone and/or may precipitate withdrawal symptoms in these patients.

Ambulatory Surgery

OxyContin is not recommended pre-operatively (pre-emptive analgesia) or for the management of pain in the immediate post-operative period (the first 12 to 24 hours following surgery) for patients not previously taking the drug, because its safety in this setting has not been established. Patients who are already receiving OxyContin tablets as part of ongoing analgesic therapy may be safely continued on the drug if appropriate dosage adjustments are made considering the procedure, other drugs given, and the temporary changes in physiology caused by the surgical intervention (see **PRECAUTIONS; Drug-Drug Interactions**, and **DOSAGE AND ADMINISTRATION**).

Post-Operative Use

Morphine and other opioids have been shown to decrease bowel motility. Ileus is a common post-operative complica-

Continued on next page

OxyContin—Cont.

tion, especially after intra-abdominal surgery with opioid analgesia. Caution should be taken to monitor for decreased bowel motility in post-operative patients receiving opioids. Standard supportive therapy should be implemented.

Use in Pancreatic/Biliary Tract Disease

Oxycodone may cause spasm of the sphincter of Oddi and should be used with caution in patients with biliary tract disease, including acute pancreatitis. Opioids like oxycodone may cause increases in the serum amylase level.

Tolerance and Physical Dependence

Tolerance is the need for increasing doses of opioids to maintain a defined effect such as analgesia (in the absence of disease progression or other external factors). Physical dependence is the occurrence of withdrawal symptoms after abrupt discontinuation of a drug or upon administration of an antagonist. Physical dependence and tolerance are not unusual during chronic opioid therapy.

Significant tolerance should not occur in most of the patients treated with the lowest doses of oxycodone. It should be expected, however, that a fraction of cancer patients will develop some degree of tolerance and require progressively higher dosages of OxyContin to maintain pain control during chronic treatment. Regardless of whether this occurs as a result of increased pain secondary to disease progression or pharmacological tolerance, dosages can usually be increased safely by adjusting the patient's dose to maintain an acceptable balance between pain relief and side effects. The dosage should be selected according to the patient's individual analgesic response and ability to tolerate side effects. Tolerance to the analgesic effect of opioids is usually paralleled by tolerance to side effects, except for constipation.

Physical dependence results in withdrawal symptoms in patients who abruptly discontinue the drug or may be precipitated through the administration of drugs with opioid antagonist activity (see **OVERDOSAGE**). If OxyContin is abruptly discontinued in a physically dependent patient, an abstinence syndrome may occur. This is characterized by some or all of the following: restlessness, lacrimation, rhinorrhea, yawning, perspiration, chills, myalgia, and mydriasis. Other symptoms also may develop, including: irritability, anxiety, backache, joint pain, weakness, abdominal cramps, insomnia, nausea, anorexia, vomiting, diarrhea, or increased blood pressure, respiratory rate, or heart rate.

If signs and symptoms of withdrawal occur, patients should be treated by reinstitution of opioid therapy followed by a gradual, tapered dose reduction of OxyContin combined with symptomatic support (see **DOSAGE AND ADMINISTRATION: Cessation of Therapy**).

Information for Patients/Caregivers

If clinically advisable, patients receiving OxyContin (oxycodone hydrochloride controlled-release) tablets or their caregivers should be given the following information by the physician, nurse, pharmacist, or caregiver:

1. Patients should be advised that OxyContin tablets were designed to work properly only if swallowed whole. They may release all their contents at once if broken, chewed or crushed, resulting in a risk of overdose.

2. Patients should be advised to report episodes of breakthrough pain and adverse experiences occurring during therapy. Individualization of dosage is essential to make optimal use of this medication.

3. Patients should be advised not to adjust the dose of OxyContin without consulting the prescribing professional.

4. Patients should be advised that OxyContin may impair mental and/or physical ability required for the performance of potentially hazardous tasks (e.g., driving, operating heavy machinery).

5. Patients should not combine OxyContin with alcohol or other central nervous system depressants (sleep aids, tranquilizers) except by the orders of the prescribing physician, because additive effects may occur.

6. Women of childbearing potential who become, or are planning to become, pregnant should be advised to consult their physician regarding the effects of analgesics and other drug use during pregnancy on themselves and their unborn child.

7. Patients should be advised that OxyContin is a potential drug of abuse. They should protect it from theft, and it should never be given to anyone other than the individual for whom it was prescribed.

8. Patients should be advised that they may pass empty matrix "ghosts" (tablets) via colostomy or in the stool, and that this is of no concern since the active medication has already been absorbed.

9. Patients should be advised that if they have been receiving treatment with OxyContin for more than a few weeks and cessation of therapy is indicated, it may be appropriate to taper the OxyContin dose, rather than abruptly discontinue it, due to the risk of precipitating withdrawal symptoms. Their physician can provide a dose schedule to accomplish a gradual discontinuation of the medication.

Laboratory Monitoring

Due to the broad range of plasma concentrations seen in clinical populations, the varying degrees of pain, and the development of tolerance, plasma oxycodone measurements are usually not helpful in clinical management. Plasma concentrations of the active drug substance may be of value in selected, unusual or complex cases.

Interactions with Alcohol and Drugs of Abuse

Oxycodone may be expected to have additive effects when used in conjunction with alcohol, other opioids or illicit drugs which cause central nervous system depression.

Use in Drug and Alcohol Addiction

OxyContin is an opioid with no approved use in the management of addictive disorders. Its proper usage in individuals with drug or alcohol dependence, either active or in remission, is for the management of pain requiring opioid analgesia.

Drug-Drug Interactions

Opioid analgesics, including OxyContin, may enhance the neuromuscular blocking action of skeletal muscle relaxants and produce an increased degree of respiratory depression. Oxycodone is metabolized in part to oxymorphone via CYP2D6. While this pathway may be blocked by a variety of drugs (e.g., certain cardiovascular drugs and antidepressants), such blockade has not yet been shown to be of clinical significance with this agent. Clinicians should be aware of this possible interaction, however.

Use with CNS Depressants

OxyContin, like all opioid analgesics, should be started at $^1/_3$ to $^1/_2$ of the usual dosage in patients who are concurrently receiving other central nervous system depressants including sedatives or hypnotics, general anesthetics, phenothiazines, centrally acting anti-emetics, tranquilizers, and alcohol because respiratory depression, hypotension, and profound sedation or coma may result. No specific interaction between oxycodone and monoamine oxidase inhibitors has been observed, but caution in the use of any opioid in patients taking this class of drugs is appropriate.

Mutagenicity/Carcinogenicity

Oxycodone was not mutagenic in the following assays: Ames Salmonella and E. Coli test with and without metabolic activation at doses of up to 5000 µg, chromosomal aberration test in human lymphocytes in the absence of metabolic activation at doses of up to 1500 µg/mL and with activation 48 hours after exposure at doses of up to 5000 µg/mL, and in the in vivo bone marrow micronucleus test in mice (at plasma levels of up to 48 µg/mL). Mutagenic results occurred in the presence of metabolic activation in the human chromosomal aberration test (at greater than or equal to 1250 µg/mL) at 24 but not 48 hours of exposure and in the mouse lymphoma assay at doses of 50 µg/mL or greater with metabolic activation and at 400 µg/mL or greater without metabolic activation. The data from these tests indicate that the genotoxic risk to humans may be considered low.

Studies of oxycodone in animals to evaluate its carcinogenic potential have not been conducted owing to the length of clinical experience with the drug substance.

Pregnancy

Teratogenic Effects—Category B: Reproduction studies have been performed in rats and rabbits by oral administration at doses up to 8 mg/kg (48 mg/m^2) and 125 mg/kg (1375 mg/m^2), respectively. These doses are 3 and 47 times a human dose of 160 mg/day (90 mg/m^2), based on mg/kg of a 60 kg adult (0.5 and 15 times this human dose based upon mg/m^2). The results did not reveal evidence of harm to the fetus due to oxycodone. There are, however, no adequate and well-controlled studies in pregnant women. Because animal reproduction studies are not always predictive of human response, this drug should be used during pregnancy only if clearly needed.

Nonteratogenic Effects—Neonates whose mothers have been taking oxycodone chronically may exhibit respiratory depression and/or withdrawal symptoms, either at birth and/or in the nursery.

Labor and Delivery

OxyContin is not recommended for use in women during and immediately prior to labor and delivery because oral opioids may cause respiratory depression in the newborn.

Nursing Mothers

Low concentrations of oxycodone have been detected in breast milk. Withdrawal symptoms can occur in breast-feeding infants when maternal administration of an opioid analgesic is stopped. Ordinarily, nursing should not be undertaken while a patient is receiving OxyContin since oxycodone may be excreted in the milk.

Pediatric Use

Safety and effectiveness in pediatric patients below the age of 18 have not been established with this dosage form of oxycodone. However, oxycodone has been used extensively in the pediatric population in other dosage forms, as have the excipients used in this formulation. No specific increased risk is expected from the use of this form of oxycodone in pediatric patients old enough to safely take tablets if dosing is adjusted for the patient's weight (see **DOSAGE AND ADMINISTRATION**). **It must be remembered that OxyContin tablets cannot be crushed or divided for administration.**

Geriatric Use

In controlled pharmacokinetic studies in elderly subjects (greater than 65 years) the clearance of oxycodone appeared to be slightly reduced. Compared to young adults, the plasma concentrations of oxycodone were increased approximately 15% (see **PHARMACOKINETCS AND METABOLISM**). Of the total number of subjects (445) in clinical studies of OxyContin, 148 (33.3%) were age 65 and older (including those age 75 and older) while 40 (9.0%) were age 75 and older. In clinical trials with appropriate initiation of therapy and dose titration, no untoward or unexpected side effects were seen based on age, and the usual doses and dosing intervals are appropriate for the geriatric patient. As with all opioids, the starting dose should be reduced to $^1/_3$ to $^1/_2$ of the usual dosage in debilitated, non-tolerant patients.

Hepatic Impairment

A study of OxyContin in patients with hepatic impairment indicates greater plasma concentrations than those with normal function. The initiation of therapy at $^1/_3$ to $^1/_2$ the usual doses and careful dose titration is warranted.

Renal Impairment

In patients with renal impairment, as evidenced by decreased creatinine clearance (<60 mL/min), the concentrations of oxycodone in the plasma are approximately 50% higher than in subjects with normal renal function. Dose initiation should follow a conservative approach. Dosages should be adjusted according to the clinical situation.

Gender Differences

In pharmacokinetic studies, opioid-naive females demonstrate up to 25% higher average plasma concentrations and greater frequency of typical opioid adverse events than males, even after adjustment for body weight. The clinical relevance of a difference of this magnitude is low for a drug intended for chronic usage at individualized dosages, and there was no male/female difference detected for efficacy or adverse events in clinical trials.

Rectal Administration

OxyContin® Tablets are not recommended for administration per rectum. A study in normal volunteers showed a significantly greater AUC and higher C_{max} during this route of administration (see **PHARMACOKINETICS AND METABOLISM**).

ADVERSE REACTIONS

Serious adverse reactions which may be associated with OxyContin® (oxycodone hydrochloride controlled-release) tablet therapy in clinical use are those observed with other opioid analgesics, including: respiratory depression, apnea, respiratory arrest, and (to an even lesser degree) circulatory depression, hypotension, or shock (see **OVERDOSAGE**).

The non-serious adverse events seen on initiation of therapy with OxyContin are typical opioid side effects. These events are dose-dependent, and their frequency depends upon the dose, the clinical setting, the patient's level of opioid tolerance, and host factors specific to the individual. They should be expected and managed as a part of opioid analgesia. The most frequent (>5%) include: constipation, nausea, somnolence, dizziness, vomiting, pruritus, headache, dry mouth, sweating, and asthenia.

In many cases the frequency of these events during initiation of therapy may be minimized by careful individualization of starting dosage, slow titration, and the avoidance of large swings in the plasma concentrations of the opioid. Many of these adverse events will cease or decrease in intensity as OxyContin therapy is continued and some degree of tolerance is developed.

In clinical trials comparing OxyContin with immediate-release oxycodone and placebo, the most common adverse events (>5%) reported by patients (pts) at least once during therapy were:

Table 3

	OxyContin (n=227)		Immediate-Release (n=225)		Placebo (n=45)	
	# Pts	(%)	# Pts	(%)	# Pts	(%)
Constipation	52	(23)	58	(26)	3	(7)
Nausea	52	(23)	60	(27)	5	(11)
Somnolence	52	(23)	55	(24)	2	(4)
Dizziness	29	(13)	35	(16)	4	(9)
Pruritus	29	(13)	28	(12)	1	(2)
Vomiting	27	(12)	31	(14)	3	(7)
Headache	17	(7)	19	(8)	3	(7)
Dry Mouth	13	(6)	15	(7)	1	(2)
Asthenia	13	(6)	16	(7)	–	–
Sweating	12	(5)	13	(6)	1	(2)

The following adverse experiences were reported in OxyContin treated patients with an incidence between 1% and 5%. In descending order of frequency they were anorexia, nervousness, insomnia, fever, confusion, diarrhea, abdominal pain, dyspepsia, rash, anxiety, euphoria, dyspnea, postural hypotension, chills, twitching, gastritis, abnormal dreams, thought abnormalities, and hiccups.

The following adverse reactions occurred in less than 1% of patients involved in clinical trials or were reported in post marketing experience:

General: accidental injury, chest pain, facial edema, malaise, neck pain, pain

Cardiovascular: migraine, syncope, vasodilation, ST depression

Digestive: dysphagia, eructation, flatulence, gastrointestinal disorder, increased appetite, nausea and vomiting, stomatitis, ileus

Hemic and Lymphatic: lymphadenopathy

Metabolic and Nutritional: dehydration, edema, hyponatremia, peripheral edema, syndrome of inappropriate antidiuretic hormone secretion, thirst

Nervous: abnormal gait, agitation, amnesia, depersonalization, depression, emotional lability, hallucination, hyperkinesia, hypesthesia, hypotonia, malaise, paresthesia, seizures, speech disorder, stupor, tinnitus, tremor, vertigo, withdrawal syndrome with or without seizures

Respiratory: cough increased, pharyngitis, voice alteration

Skin: dry skin, exfoliative dermatitis, urticaria

Special Senses: abnormal vision, taste perversion

Urogenital: amenorrhea, decreased libido, dysuria, hematuria, impotence, polyuria, urinary retention, urination impaired

DRUG ABUSE AND DEPENDENCE (Addiction)

OxyContin® is a mu-agonist opioid with an abuse liability similar to morphine and is a Schedule II controlled substance. Oxycodone products are common targets for both drug abusers and drug addicts. Delayed absorption, as provided by OxyContin tablets when used properly for the management of pain, is believed to reduce the abuse liability of a drug.

Drug addiction (drug dependence, psychological dependence) is characterized by a preoccupation with the procurement, hoarding, and abuse of drugs for non-medicinal purposes. Drug dependence is treatable, utilizing a multi-disciplinary approach, but relapse is common. Iatrogenic "addiction" to opioids legitimately used in the management of pain is very rare. "Drug seeking" behavior is very common to addicts. Tolerance and physical dependence in pain patients are *not* signs of psychological dependence. Preoccupation with achieving adequate pain relief can be appropriate behavior in a patient with poor pain control. Most chronic pain patients limit their intake of opioids to achieve a balance between the benefits of the drug and dose-limiting side effects.

Physicians should be aware that psychological dependence may not be accompanied by concurrent tolerance and symptoms of physical dependence in all addicts. In addition, abuse of opioids can occur in the absence of true psychological dependence and is characterized by misuse for non-medical purposes, often in combination with other psychoactive substances.

OxyContin consists of a dual-polymer matrix, intended for oral use only. Parenteral venous injection of the tablet constituents, especially talc, can be expected to result in local tissue necrosis and pulmonary granulomas.

OVERDOSAGE

Acute overdosage with oxycodone can be manifested by respiratory depression, somnolence progressing to stupor or coma, skeletal muscle flaccidity, cold and clammy skin, constricted pupils, bradycardia, hypotension, and death.

In the treatment of oxycodone overdosage, primary attention should be given to the re-establishment of a patent airway and institution of assisted or controlled ventilation. Supportive measures (including oxygen and vasopressors) should be employed in the management of circulatory shock and pulmonary edema accompanying overdose as indicated. Cardiac arrest or arrhythmias may require cardiac massage or defibrillation.

The pure opioid antagonists such as naloxone or nalmefene are specific antidotes against respiratory depression from opioid overdose. Opioid antagonists should not be administered in the absence of clinically significant respiratory or circulatory depression secondary to oxycodone overdose. They should be administered cautiously to persons who are known, or suspected to be, physically dependent on any opioid agonist including OxyContin®. In such cases, an abrupt or complete reversal of opioid effects may precipitate an acute abstinence syndrome. The severity of the withdrawal syndrome produced will depend on the degree of physical dependence and the dose of the antagonist administered. Please see the prescribing information for the specific opioid antagonist for details of their proper use.

DOSAGE AND ADMINISTRATION
General Principles
OxyContin® (oxycodone hydrochloride controlled-release) TABLETS ARE TO BE SWALLOWED WHOLE, AND ARE NOT TO BE BROKEN, CHEWED OR CRUSHED. TAKING BROKEN, CHEWED OR CRUSHED OxyContin TABLETS COULD LEAD TO THE RAPID RELEASE AND ABSORPTION OF A POTENTIALLY TOXIC DOSE OF OXYCODONE.

ONE OxyContin® 160 MG TABLET IS COMPARABLE TO TWO 80 MG TABLETS WHEN TAKEN ON AN EMPTY STOMACH. WITH A HIGH FAT MEAL, HOWEVER, THERE IS A 25% GREATER PEAK PLASMA CONCENTRATION FOLLOWING ONE 160 MG TABLET. DIETARY CAUTION SHOULD BE TAKEN WHEN PATIENTS ARE INITIALLY TITRATED TO 160 MG TABLETS.

In treating pain it is vital to assess the patient regularly and systematically. Therapy should also be regularly reviewed and adjusted based upon the patient's own reports of pain and side effects and the health professional's clinical judgment.

OxyContin is intended for the management of moderate to severe pain in patients who require treatment with an oral opioid analgesic for more than a few days. The controlled-release nature of the formulation allows it to be effectively administered every 12 hours (see CLINICAL PHARMACOLOGY; PHARMACOKINETICS AND METABOLISM). While symmetric (same dose AM and PM), around-the-clock, q12h dosing is appropriate for the majority of patients, some patients may benefit from asymmetric (different dose given in AM than in PM) dosing, tailored to their pain pattern. It is usually appropriate to treat a patient with only one opioid for around-the-clock therapy.

Initiation of Therapy
It is critical to initiate the dosing regimen for each patient individually, taking into account the patient's prior opioid and non-opioid analgesic treatment. Attention should be given to:

(1) the general condition and medical status of the patient;
(2) the daily dose, potency, and kind of the analgesic(s) the patient has been taking;
(3) the reliability of the conversion estimate used to calculate the dose of oxycodone;
(4) the patient's opioid exposure and opioid tolerance (if any);
(5) special safety issues associated with conversion to OxyContin doses at or exceeding 160 mg q12h (see Special Instructions for OxyContin 80 mg and 160 mg Tablets); and

(6) the balance between pain control and adverse experiences.

Care should be taken to use low initial doses of OxyContin in patients who are not already opioid-tolerant, especially those who are receiving concurrent treatment with muscle relaxants, sedatives, or other CNS active medications (see PRECAUTIONS: Drug-Drug Interactions).

Patients Not Already Taking Opioids (opioid-naive)
Clinical trials have shown that patients may initiate analgesic therapy with OxyContin. A reasonable starting dose for most patients who are opioid-naive is 10 mg q12h. If a non-opioid analgesic [aspirin (ASA), acetaminophen (APAP) or a non-steroidal anti-inflammatory (NSAID)] is being provided, it may be continued. If the current non-opioid is discontinued, early upward dose titration may be necessary.

Conversion from Fixed-Ratio Opioid/APAP, ASA, or NSAID Combination Drugs
Patients who are taking 1 to 5 tablets/capsules/caplets per day of a regular strength fixed-combination opioid/non-opioid should be started on 10 to 20 mg OxyContin q12h. For patients taking 6 to 9 tablets/capsules/caplets, a starting dose of 20 to 30 mg q12h is suggested. For those taking 10 to 12 tablets/capsules/caplets a day, 30 to 40 mg q12h should be considered. The non-opioid may be continued as a separate drug. Alternatively, a different non-opioid analgesic may be selected. If the decision is made to discontinue the non-opioid analgesic, consideration should be given to early upward titration.

Patients Currently on Opioid Therapy
If a patient has been receiving opioid-containing medications prior to OxyContin therapy, the total daily (24-hour) dose of the other opioids should be determined.

1. Using standard conversion ratio estimates (see Table 4 below), multiply the mg/day of the previous opioids by the appropriate multiplication factors to obtain the equivalent total daily dose of oral oxycodone.
2. Divide this 24-hour oxycodone dose in half to obtain the twice a day (q12h) dose of OxyContin.
3. Round down to a dose which is appropriate for the tablet strengths available (10 mg, 20 mg, 40 mg, 80 mg, and 160 mg tablets).
4. Discontinue all other around-the-clock opioid drugs when OxyContin therapy is initiated.

No fixed conversion ratio is likely to be satisfactory in all patients, especially patients receiving large opioid doses. The recommended doses shown in Table 4 are only a starting point, and close observation and frequent titration are indicated until patients are stable on the new therapy.

Table 4
Multiplication Factors for Converting the Daily Dose of Prior Opioids to the Daily Dose of Oral Oxycodone*
(Mg/Day Prior Opioid × Factor = Mg/Day Oral Oxycodone)

	Oral Prior Opioid	Parenteral Prior Opioid
Oxycodone	1	—
Codeine	0.15	—
Fentanyl TTS	SEE BELOW	SEE BELOW
Hydrocodone	0.9	—
Hydromorphone	4	20
Levorphanol	7.5	15
Meperidine	0.1	0.4
Methadone	1.5	3
Morphine	0.5	3

*To be used only for conversion to oral oxycodone. For patients receiving high-dose parenteral opioids, a more conservative conversion is warranted. For example, for high-dose parenteral morphine, use 1.5 instead of 3 as a multiplication factor.

In all cases, supplemental analgesia (see below) should be made available in the form of immediate-release oral oxycodone or another suitable short-acting analgesic. OxyContin can be safely used concomitantly with usual doses of non-opioid analgesics and analgesic adjuvants, provided care is taken to select a proper initial dose (see PRECAUTIONS).

Conversion from Transdermal Fentanyl to OxyContin
Eighteen hours following the removal of the transdermal fentanyl patch, OxyContin treatment can be initiated. Although there has been no systematic assessment of such conversion, a conservative oxycodone dose, approximately 10 mg q12h of OxyContin, should be initially substituted for each 25 μg/hr fentanyl transdermal patch. The patient should be followed closely for early titration, as there is very limited clinical experience with this conversion.

Managing Expected Opioid Adverse Experiences
Most patients receiving opioids, especially those who are opioid-naive, will experience side effects. Frequently, the side effects from OxyContin are transient, but may require evaluation and management. Adverse events such as constipation should be anticipated and treated aggressively and prophylactically with a stimulant laxative and/or stool softener. Patients do not usually become tolerant to the constipating effects of opioids.

Other opioid-related side effects such as sedation and nausea are usually self-limited and often do not persist beyond the first few days. If nausea persists and is unacceptable to the patient, treatment with anti-emetics or other modalities may relieve these symptoms and should be considered.

Patients receiving OxyContin may pass an intact matrix "ghost" in the stool or via colostomy. These ghosts contain little or no residual oxycodone and are of no clinical consequence.

Individualization of Dosage
Once therapy is initiated, pain relief and other opioid effects should be frequently assessed. Patients should be titrated to adequate effect (generally mild or no pain with the regular use of no more than two doses of supplemental analgesia per 24 hours). Rescue medication should be available (see Supplemental Analgesia). Because steady-state plasma concentrations are approximated within 24 to 36 hours, dosage adjustment may be carried out every 1 to 2 days. It is most appropriate to increase the q12h dose, not the dosing frequency. There is no clinical information on dosing intervals shorter than q12h. As a guideline, except for the increase from 10 mg to 20 mg q12h, the total daily oxycodone dose usually can be increased by 25% to 50% of the current dose at each increase. If signs of excessive opioid-related adverse experiences are observed, the next dose may be reduced. If this adjustment leads to inadequate analgesia, a supplemental dose of immediate-release oxycodone may be given. Alternatively, non-opioid analgesic adjuvants may be employed. Dose adjustments should be made to obtain an appropriate balance between pain relief and opioid-related adverse experiences. If significant adverse events occur before the therapeutic goal of mild or no pain is achieved, the events should be treated aggressively. Once adverse events are under control, upward titration should continue to an acceptable level of pain control.

During periods of changing analgesic requirements, including initial titration, frequent contact is recommended between physician, other members of the health-care team, the patient, and the caregiver/family.

Special Instructions for OxyContin® 80 mg and 160 mg Tablets (For use in opioid-tolerant patients only)
OxyContin® 80 mg and 160 mg Tablets are for use only in opioid-tolerant patients requiring daily oxycodone equivalent dosages of 160 mg or more for the 80 mg tablet and 320 mg or more for the 160 mg tablet. Care should be taken in the prescription of this tablet strength. Patients should be instructed against use by individuals other than the patient for whom it was prescribed, as such inappropriate use may have severe medical consequences.

One OxyContin® 160 mg tablet is comparable to two 80 mg tablets when taken on an empty stomach. With a high fat meal, however, there is a 25% greater peak plasma concentration following one 160 mg tablet. Dietary caution should be taken when patients are initially titrated to 160 mg tablets.

Supplemental Analgesia
Most cancer patients given around-the-clock therapy with controlled-release opioids will need to have immediate-release medication available for "rescue" from breakthrough pain or to prevent pain that occurs predictably during certain patient activities (incident pain).

Rescue medication can be immediate-release oxycodone, either alone or in combination with acetaminophen, aspirin, or other NSAIDs as a supplemental analgesic. The supplemental analgesic should be prescribed at $\frac{1}{4}$ to $\frac{1}{3}$ of the 12-hour OxyContin dose as shown in Table 5. The rescue medication is dosed as needed for breakthrough pain and administered one hour before anticipated incident pain. If more than two doses of rescue medication are needed within 24 hours, the dose of OxyContin should be titrated upward. Caregivers and patients using prn rescue analgesia in combination with around-the-clock opioids should be advised to report incidents of breakthrough pain to the physician managing the patient's analgesia (see Information for Patients/Caregivers).

Table 5
Table of Appropriate Supplemental Analgesia

OxyContin q12h Dose (mg)	Rescue Dose (immediate-release oxycodone) (mg) dosed PRN
10 (1×10 mg)	5
20 (2×10 mg)	5
30 (3×10 mg)	10
40 (2×20 mg)	10
60 (3×20 mg)	15
80 (2×40 mg)	20
120 (3×40 mg)	30
160 (2×80 mg)	40
240 (3×80 mg)	60
320 (2×160 mg)	80
480 (3×160 mg)	120

Maintenance of Therapy
The intent of the titration period is to establish a patient-specific q12h dose that will maintain adequate analgesia with acceptable side effects for as long as pain relief is necessary. Should pain recur then the dose can be incrementally increased to re-establish pain control. The method of therapy adjustment outlined above should be employed to re-establish pain control.

During chronic therapy, especially for non-cancer pain syndromes, the continued need for around-the-clock opioid therapy should be reassessed periodically (e.g., every 6 to 12 months) as appropriate.

Cessation of Therapy
When the patient no longer requires therapy with OxyContin tablets, patients receiving doses of 20–60 mg/day can usually have the therapy stopped abruptly without incident. However, higher doses should be tapered over several days to prevent signs and symptoms of withdrawal in the physically dependent patient. The daily dose should be

Continued on next page

OxyContin—Cont.

reduced by approximately 50% for the first two days and then reduced by 25% every two days thereafter until the total dose reaches the dose recommended for opioid-naive patients (10 or 20 mg q12h). Therapy can then be discontinued.

If signs of withdrawal appear, tapering should be stopped. The dose should be slightly increased until the signs and symptoms of opioid withdrawal disappear. Tapering should then begin again but with longer periods of time between each dose reduction.

Conversion from OxyContin to Parenteral Opioids

To avoid overdose, conservative dose conversion ratios should be followed. Initiate treatment with about 50% of the estimated equianalgesic daily dose of parenteral opioid divided into suitable individual doses based on the appropriate dosing interval, and titrate based upon the patient's response.

SAFETY AND HANDLING

OxyContin® (oxycodone hydrochloride controlled-release) tablets are solid dosage forms that pose no known health risk to health-care providers beyond that of any controlled substance. As with all such drugs, care should be taken to prevent diversion or abuse by proper handling.

HOW SUPPLIED

OxyContin® (oxycodone hydrochloride controlled-release) 10 mg tablets are round, unscored, white-colored, convex tablets bearing the symbol OC on one side and 10 on the other. They are supplied as follows:

NDC 59011-100-10: child-resistant closure, opaque plastic bottles of 100

NDC 59011-100-25: unit dose packaging with 25 individually numbered tablets per card; one card per glue end carton

OxyContin® (oxycodone hydrochloride controlled-release) 20 mg tablets are round, unscored, pink-colored, convex tablets bearing the symbol OC on one side and 20 on the other. They are supplied as follows:

NDC 59011-103-10: child-resistant closure, opaque plastic bottles of 100

NDC 59011-103-25: unit dose packaging with 25 individually numbered tablets per card; one card per glue end carton

OxyContin® (oxycodone hydrochloride controlled-release) 40 mg tablets are round, unscored, yellow-colored, convex tablets bearing the symbol OC on one side and 40 on the other. They are supplied as follows:

NDC 59011-105-10: child-resistant closure, opaque plastic bottles of 100

NDC 59011-105-25: unit dose packaging with 25 individually numbered tablets per card; one card per glue end carton

OxyContin® (oxycodone hydrochloride controlled-release) 80 mg tablets are round, unscored, green-colored, convex tablets bearing the symbol OC on one side and 80 on the other. They are supplied as follows:

NDC 59011-107-10: child-resistant closure, opaque plastic bottles of 100

NDC 59011-107-25: unit dose packaging with 25 individually numbered tablets per card; one card per glue end carton

OxyContin® (oxycodone hydrochloride controlled-release) 160 mg tablets are caplet-shaped, unscored, blue-colored, convex tablets bearing the symbol OC on one side and 160 on the other. They are supplied as follows:

NDC 59011-109-10: child-resistant closure, opaque plastic bottles of 100

NDC 59011-109-25: unit dose packaging with 25 individually numbered tablets per card; one card per glue end carton

Store at 25°C (77°F); excursions permitted between 15°–30°C (59°–86°F).

Dispense in tight, light-resistant container.

CAUTION

DEA Order Form Required.

Purdue Pharma L.P.
Stamford, CT 06901-3431

Copyright© 1995, 2000 Purdue Pharma L.P.

U.S. Patent Numbers 4,861,598; 4,970,075; 5,266,331; 5,508,042; 5,549,912; and 5,656,295

November 27, 2000 N4909
065570-0E-001

In the PDR annual,
the **Brand and Generic Name Index**
(PINK section)
alphabetizes drugs under both
brand and generic names.

A. H. Robins Company

1407 CUMMINGS DRIVE
RICHMOND, VA 23220

Direct General Inquiries to:
(610) 688-4400

For Emergency Medical Information Contact:
Day: (800) 934-5556 8:30 AM to 4:30 PM (Eastern Standard Time), Weekdays only
Night: (610) 688-4400 (Emergencies only; non-emergencies should wait until the next day)

For Medical/Pharmacy Inquiries on Marketed Products Call:
Medical Affairs, (800) 934-5556 8:30 AM to 4:30 PM (Eastern Standard Time), Weekdays only

DOPRAM® INJECTABLE ℞

[do 'pram]
brand of Doxapram Hydrochloride Injection, USP

Prescribing information for this product, which appears on pages 2709–2710 of the 2001 PDR, has been revised. Please write "See Supplement A" next to the product heading.

In the **DESCRIPTION** section, the sentence "Due to its benzyl alcohol content, Dopram Injection should not be used in newborns.", which appears under the contents of each mL of Dopram Injection, should be deleted.

Under the subheading "***Postanesthesia***" in the **INDICATIONS** section, the second paragraph listed as item "b" should be deleted and replaced with the following:

b. To pharmacologically stimulate deep breathing in the postoperative patient. (A quantative method of assessing oxygenation, such as pulse oximetry, is recommended.)

In the second sentence of the paragraph under the subheading "***3. Chronic pulmonary disease associated with acute hypercapnea.***", the words "(approximately 2 hours)" should be deleted and replaced with "(see **DOSAGE AND ADMINISTRATION**)".

In the first sentence under the heading "**CONTRAINDICATIONS**", the word "newborns" should be deleted and replaced with the word "neonates," and the following should be added after the word "neonates":

(See **WARNINGS** and **PRECAUTIONS**, ***Pediatric use***)

The words "or any of the injection components" should be added to the end of the fourth paragraph after the word "drug" in the **CONTRAINDICATIONS** section.

The following paragraph should be added as the new first paragraph under the **WARNINGS** heading:

Doxapram should not be used in conjunction with mechanical ventilation. This product contains benzyl alcohol as a preservative. Benzyl alcohol has been associated with a fatal "gasping syndrome" in neonates (see **CONTRAINDICATIONS** and **PRECAUTIONS**, ***Pediatric use.***)

The second sentence of the first paragraph under the subheading "***1. In postanesthetic use***" in the **WARNINGS** section should be deleted and replaced with the following:

More specific tests (e.g., peripheral nerve stimulation, airway pressures, head lift, pulse oximetry, and end-tidal carbon dioxide) to assess adequacy of ventilation are recommended before administering doxapram.

The following paragraph should be added as the new fourth item under the subheading "***1. In postanesthetic use***" in the **WARNINGS** section:

d. In patients who have received general anesthesia utilizing a volatile agent known to sensitize the myocardium to catecholamines, administration of doxapram should be delayed until the volatile agent has been excreted in order to lessen the potential for arrhythmias, including ventricular tachycardia and ventricular fibrillation (see **PRECAUTIONS**, ***Drug interactions.***)

The second paragraph, which follows the letter "b", under the subheading "***3. In chronic obstructive pulmonary disease***" should be deleted.

The first sentence of the paragraph that follows the letter "g" under "***1. General***" in the **PRECAUTIONS** section should be deleted and replaced with the following sentence:

Anticonvulsants such as intravenous short-acting barbiturates, along with oxygen and resuscitative equipment should be readily available to manage overdosage manifested by excessive central nervous system stimulation.

In the last sentence of the paragraph described above, the word "or" should be inserted between the words "post-hyperventilation" and "hypoventilation."

In the sentence following the letter "b" under the subheading "***In postanesthetic use***" in the **PRECAUTIONS** section, the word "**PRECAUTIONS,**" should be inserted after the word "See."

In the second sentence of the paragraph following the letter "b" under the subheading "***In chronic obstructive pulmonary disease***" in the **PRECAUTIONS** section, the following should be added after "1/2 hour":

during the infusion period to prevent development of CO_2 retention and acidosis in patients with chronic obstructive pulmonary disease with acute hypercapnia

In the first sentence following the subheading "***Drug Interactions***" the word "***General***" should be added to the end after the word "Precautions."

The third paragraph under the subheading "***Drug Interactions***" should be deleted and replaced with the following paragraph:

In patients who have received general anesthesia utilizing a volatile agent known to sensitize the myocardium to catecholamines, administration of doxapram should be delayed until the volatile agent has been excreted in order to lessen the potential for arrhythmias, including ventricular tachycardia and ventricular fibrillation (see **WARNINGS**).

The paragraph following the subheading "***Pediatric use***" in the **PRECAUTIONS** section should be deleted and replaced with the following two paragraphs:

Pediatric use. Safety and effectiveness in pediatric patients below the age of 12 years have not been established. This product contains benzyl alcohol as a preservative. Benzyl alcohol has been associated with a fatal "gasping syndrome" in neonates (see **CONTRAINDICATIONS** and **WARNINGS**). The "gasping syndrome", characterized by central nervous system depression, metabolic acidosis, gasping respirations, and high levels of benzyl alcohol and its metabolites found in the blood and urine, has been associated with exposure to benzyl alcohol in neonates and low-birth-weight neonates. Additional symptoms may include gradual neurological deterioration, seizures, intracranial hemorrhage, hematologic abnormalities, skin breakdown, hepatic and renal failure, hypotension, bradycardia, and cardiovascular collapse.

Premature neonates given doxapram doses of 2 to 2.5 mg/kg/h have developed irritability, jitteriness, hyperglycemia, glucosuria, abdominal distension, increased gastric residuals, vomiting, erratic limb movements, excessive crying, disturbed sleep, and, in premature neonates with risk factors such as perinatal asphyxia and intracerebral hemorrhage, seizures, and second-degree heart block caused by QT prolongation. In all instances, doxapram was administered following administration of xanthine derivatives such as aminophylline or theophylline.

The first sentence under the **ADVERSE REACTIONS** heading should be deleted and replaced with the following sentence:

Adverse reactions reported coincident with the administration of Dopram include:

The words "(including ventricular tachycardia and ventricular fibrillation)" should be inserted after the word "arrhythmias" in the list of adverse reactions under the subheading "3. ***Cardiovascular***" in the **ADVERSE REACTIONS** section.

The following should be added after the word "retention" in the list of adverse reactions under the subheading "5. ***Genitourinary***" in the **ADVERSE REACTIONS** section:

Elevation of BUN and albuminuria

The subheading "6. ***Laboratory determinations***" in the **ADVERSE REACTIONS** section should be deleted and replaced with "6. ***Hemic and Lymphatic.***"

The last sentence, which begins with the words "Elevations of BUN...", of the paragraph under the old subheading "6. ***Laboratory determinations***" in the **ADVERSE REACTIONS** section should be deleted.

TENEX® ℞

[tĕn' ĕks]
(Guanfacine Hydrochloride)
Tablets

Prescribing information for this product, which appears on pages 2719–2720 of the 2001 PDR, has been revised. Please write "See Supplement A" next to the product heading.

The following sentence should be added to the end of the paragraph under the heading **Pediatric Use** in the **PRECAUTIONS** section:

There have been spontaneous postmarketing reports of mania and aggressive behavioral changes in pediatric patients with attention-deficit hyperactivity disorder (ADHD) receiving Tenex.

To keep your **PDR** up to date
throughout the year, note these revisions
on the corresponding pages of the annual
volume. Simply write **"See Supplement A"**
next to the product heading.

Roche Pharmaceuticals

Roche Laboratories Inc.
340 Kingsland Street
Nutley, NJ 07110-1199

Please note that there has been a change in the Medical Needs Program toll-free telephone number, which appears on page 2721 of the 2001 PDR.

For Medical Information
(Including routine inquiries, adverse drug events and product complaints)
Call: (800) 526-6367
In Emergencies: 24-hour service
For the Medical Needs Program:
Call: (800) 285-4484
Write: Professional Product Information

CYTOVENE®-IV ℞
(ganciclovir sodium for injection)
FOR INTRAVENOUS INFUSION ONLY

CYTOVENE®
(ganciclovir capsules)
FOR ORAL ADMINISTRATION

Prescribing information for this product, which appears on pages 2736–2742 of the 2001 PDR has been revised as follows. Please write "See Supplement A" next to the product heading.

In the PRECAUTIONS section, Geriatric Use subsection, the second paragraph has been revised and reads as follows:

Clinical studies of CYTOVENE-IV and CYTOVENE did not include sufficient numbers of subjects aged 65 and over to determine whether they respond differently from younger subjects. In general, dose selection for an elderly patient should be cautious, reflecting the greater frequency of decreased hepatic, renal, or cardiac function, and of concomitant disease or other drug therapy. CYTOVENE-IV and CYTOVENE are known to be substantially excreted by the kidney, and the risk of toxic reactions to this drug may be greater in patients with impaired renal function. Because elderly patients are more likely to have decreased renal function, care should be taken in dose selection. In addition, renal function should be monitored and dosage adjustments should be made accordingly (see *Use in Patients With Renal Impairment* and DOSAGE AND ADMINISTRATION).

*Revised: September 2000

FORTOVASE® ℞
(saquinavir)
SOFT GELATIN CAPSULES

Prescribing information for this product, which appears on pages 2747–2751 of the 2001 PDR, has been completely revised as follows. Please write "See Supplement A" next to the product heading.

DESCRIPTION

FORTOVASE brand of saquinavir is an inhibitor of the human immunodeficiency virus (HIV) protease. FORTOVASE is available as beige, opaque, soft gelatin capsules for oral administration in a 200-mg strength (as saquinavir free base). Each capsule also contains the inactive ingredients medium chain mono- and diglycerides, povidone and dl-alpha tocopherol. Each capsule shell contains gelatin and glycerol 85% with the following colorants: red iron oxide, yellow iron oxide and titanium dioxide. The chemical name for saquinavir is N-tert-butyl-decahydro-2-[2(R)-hydroxy-4-phenyl-3(S)-[[N-(2-quinolylcarbonyl)-L-asparaginyl]-amino]-butyl]-(4aS,8aS)-isoquinoline-3(S)-carboxamide which has a molecular formula $C_{38}H_{50}N_6O_5$ and a molecular weight of 670.86. Saquinavir has the following structural formula:

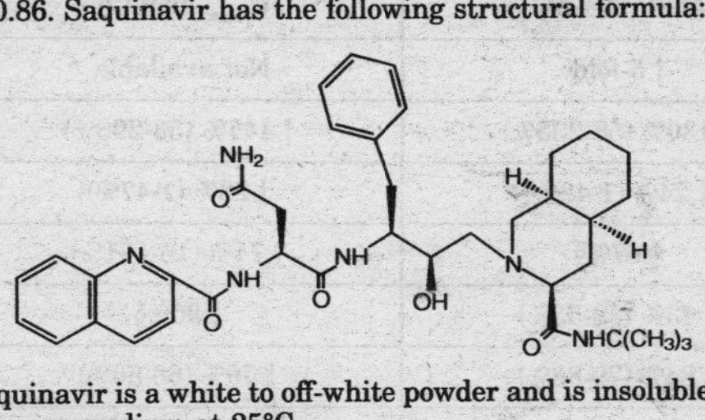

Saquinavir is a white to off-white powder and is insoluble in aqueous medium at 25°C.

MICROBIOLOGY

Mechanism of Action: Saquinavir is an inhibitor of HIV protease. HIV protease is an enzyme required for the proteolytic cleavage of viral polyprotein precursors into individual functional proteins found in infectious HIV. Saquinavir is a peptide-like substrate analogue that binds to the protease active site and inhibits the activity of the enzyme. Saquinavir inhibition prevents cleavage of the viral polyproteins resulting in the formation of immature noninfectious virus particles.

Antiviral Activity In Vitro: In vitro antiviral activity of saquinavir was assessed in lymphoblastoid and monocytic cell lines and in peripheral blood lymphocytes. Saquinavir inhibited HIV activity in both acutely and chronically infected cells. IC_{50} and IC_{90} values (50% and 90% inhibitory concentrations) were in the range of 1 to 30 nM and 5 to 80 nM, respectively; however, these concentrations may be altered in the presence of human plasma due to protein binding of saquinavir. In cell culture saquinavir demonstrated additive to synergistic effects against HIV in double- and triple-combination regimens with reverse transcriptase inhibitors zidovudine, zalcitabine, didanosine, lamivudine, stavudine and nevirapine, without enhanced cytotoxicity. The relationship between in vitro susceptibility of HIV to saquinavir and inhibition of HIV replication in humans has not been established.

Drug Resistance: HIV isolates with reduced susceptibility to saquinavir (4-fold or greater increase in IC_{50} from baseline; ie, phenotypic resistance) have been selected in vitro. Genotypic analyses of these HIV isolates showed several mutations in the HIV-protease gene but only those at codons 48 (Gly→Val) and/or 90 (Leu→Met) were consistently associated with saquinavir resistance.

Isolates from selected patients with loss of antiviral activity and prolonged (range: 24 to 147 weeks) therapy with INVIRASE® (saquinavir mesylate) (alone or in combination with nucleoside analogues) showed reduced susceptibility to saquinavir. Genotypic analysis of these isolates showed that mutations at amino acid positions 48 and/or 90 of the HIV-protease gene were most consistently associated with saquinavir resistance. Other mutations in the protease gene were also observed. Mutations at codons 48 and 90 have not been detected in isolates from protease inhibitor naive patients.

In a study (NV15107) of treatment-experienced patients receiving FORTOVASE monotherapy (1200 mg tid) for 8 weeks followed by antiretroviral combination therapy for a period of 4 to 48 weeks (median 32 weeks), 10 of 32 patients showed genotypic changes associated with reduced susceptibility to saquinavir. However, for resistance evaluation virus could not be recovered from 11 of 32 patients.

In a study (NV15355) of treatment-naive patients receiving FORTOVASE in combination with two nucleoside analogues for a period of 16 weeks, 1 of 28 patient isolates showed genotypic changes at codon 71 and 90 in the HIV-protease gene.

Cross-resistance: Among protease inhibitors variable cross-resistance has been recognized. Analysis of saquinavir-resistant isolates from patients following prolonged (24 to 147 weeks) therapy with INVIRASE showed that a majority of patients had resistance to at least one of four other protease inhibitors (indinavir, nelfinavir, ritonavir, 141W94).

CLINICAL PHARMACOLOGY

Pharmacokinetics: The pharmacokinetic properties of saquinavir when administered as FORTOVASE have been evaluated in healthy volunteers (n=207) and HIV-infected patients (n=91) after single-oral doses (range: 300 mg to 1200 mg) and multiple-oral doses (range: 400 mg to 1200 mg tid). The disposition properties of saquinavir have been studied in healthy volunteers after intravenous doses of 6, 12, 36 or 72 mg (n=21).

ABSORPTION AND BIOAVAILABILITY IN ADULTS: Following multiple dosing of FORTOVASE (1200 mg tid) in HIV-infected patients in study NV15107, the mean steady-state area under the plasma concentration versus time curve (AUC) at week 3 was 7249 ng·h/mL (n=31) compared to 866 ng·h/mL (n=10) following multiple dosing with 600 mg tid of INVIRASE (Table 1). Preliminary results from a pharmacokinetic substudy of NV15182 showed a mean saquinavir AUC of 3485 (CV 66%) ng·h/mL (n=11) in patients sampled between weeks 61 to 69 of therapy (see PRECAUTIONS: *General*). While this mean AUC value was lower than that of the week 3 steady-state value for FORTOVASE (1200 mg tid) from study NV15107, it remained higher than the mean AUC value for INVIRASE in study NV15107.

Table 1. Mean AUC_8 in Patients Treated With FORTOVASE and INVIRASE (Week 3)

Treatment	n	AUC_8 ng·h/mL	± SD
FORTOVASE			
1200 mg tid	31	7249	± 6174
INVIRASE			
600 mg tid	10	866	± 533

The absolute bioavailability of saquinavir administered as FORTOVASE has not been assessed. However, following single 600-mg doses, the relative bioavailability of saquinavir as FORTOVASE compared to saquinavir administered as INVIRASE was estimated as 331% (95% CI 207% to 530%). The absolute bioavailability of saquinavir administered as INVIRASE averaged 4% (CV 73%, range: 1% to 9%) in 8 healthy volunteers who received a single 600-mg dose of INVIRASE following a high-fat breakfast (48 g protein, 60 g carbohydrate, 57 g fat; 1006 kcal). In healthy volunteers receiving single doses of FORTOVASE (300 mg to 1200 mg) and in HIV-infected patients receiving multiple doses of FORTOVASE (400 mg to 1200 mg tid), a greater than dose-proportional increase in saquinavir plasma concentrations has been observed.

Comparison of pharmacokinetic parameters between single- and multiple-dose studies shows that following multiple dosing of FORTOVASE (1200 mg tid) in healthy male volunteers (n=18), the steady-state AUC was 80% (95% CI 22% to 176%) higher than that observed after a single 1200-mg dose (n=30).

HIV-infected patients administered FORTOVASE (1200 mg tid) had AUC and maximum plasma concentration (C_{max}) values approximately twice those observed in healthy volunteers receiving the same treatment regimen. The mean AUC values at week 1 were 4159 (CV 88%) and 8839 (CV 82%) ng·h/mL, and C_{max} values were 1420 (CV 81%) and 2477 (CV 76%) ng/mL for healthy volunteers and HIV-infected patients, respectively.

FOOD EFFECT: The mean 12-hour AUC after a single 800-mg oral dose of saquinavir in healthy volunteers (n=12) was increased from 167 ng·h/mL (CV 45%), under fasting conditions, to 1120 ng·h/mL (CV 54%) when FORTOVASE was given with breakfast (48 g protein, 60 g carbohydrate, 57 g fat; 1006 kcal).

DISTRIBUTION IN ADULTS: The mean steady-state volume of distribution following intravenous administration of a 12-mg dose of saquinavir (n=8) was 700 L (CV 39%), suggesting saquinavir partitions into tissues. It has been shown that saquinavir, up to 30 µg/mL is approximately 97% bound to plasma proteins.

METABOLISM AND ELIMINATION IN ADULTS: In vitro studies using human liver microsomes have shown that the metabolism of saquinavir is cytochrome P450 mediated with the specific isoenzyme, CYP3A4, responsible for more than 90% of the hepatic metabolism. Based on in vitro studies, saquinavir is rapidly metabolized to a range of mono- and di-hydroxylated inactive compounds. In a mass balance study using 600 mg ^{14}C-saquinavir mesylate (n=8), 88% and 1% of the orally administered radioactivity was recovered in feces and urine, respectively, within 5 days of dosing. In an additional 4 subjects administered 10.5 mg ^{14}C-saquinavir intravenously, 81% and 3% of the intravenously administered radioactivity was recovered in feces and urine, respectively, within 5 days of dosing. In mass balance studies, 13% of circulating radioactivity in plasma was attributed to unchanged drug after oral administration and the remainder attributed to saquinavir metabolites. Following intravenous administration, 66% of circulating radioactivity was attributed to unchanged drug and the remainder attributed to saquinavir metabolites, suggesting that saquinavir undergoes extensive first-pass metabolism.

Systemic clearance of saquinavir was rapid, 1.14 L/h/kg (CV 12%) after intravenous doses of 6, 36 and 72 mg. The mean residence time of saquinavir was 7 hours (n=8).

SPECIAL POPULATIONS: Hepatic or Renal Impairment: Saquinavir pharmacokinetics in patients with hepatic or renal insufficiency has not been investigated (see PRECAUTIONS). Only 1% of saquinavir is excreted in the urine, so the impact of renal impairment on saquinavir elimination should be minimal.

Gender, Race and Age: The effect of gender was investigated in healthy volunteers receiving single 1200-mg doses of FORTOVASE (n=12 females, 18 males). No effect of gender was apparent on the pharmacokinetics of saquinavir in this study.

The effect of race on the pharmacokinetics of saquinavir when administered as FORTOVASE is unknown.

The pharmacokinetics of saquinavir when administered as FORTOVASE has not been investigated in patients >65 years of age or in pediatric patients (<16 years of age).

DRUG INTERACTIONS (see PRECAUTIONS *Drug Interactions*): Several drug interaction studies have been completed with both INVIRASE and FORTOVASE. Results from studies conducted with INVIRASE may not be applicable to FORTOVASE. Table 2 summarizes the effect of FORTOVASE on the geometric mean AUC and C_{max} of coadministered drugs. Table 3 summarizes the effect of coadministered drugs on the geometric mean AUC and C_{max} of saquinavir.

[See table 2 at bottom of next page]
[See table 3 at bottom of next page]

For information regarding clinical recommendations, see PRECAUTIONS *Drug Interactions*.

INDICATIONS AND USAGE

FORTOVASE is indicated for use in combination with other antiretroviral agents for the treatment of HIV infection. This indication is based on a study that showed a reduction in both mortality and AIDS-defining clinical events for patients who received INVIRASE in combination with HIVID® (zalcitabine) compared to patients who received either HIVID or INVIRASE alone. This indication is also based on studies that showed increased saquinavir concentrations and improved antiviral activity for FORTOVASE 1200 mg tid compared to INVIRASE 600 mg tid.

Description of Clinical Studies: *STUDIES WITH FORTOVASE (saquinavir):*

Study NV15355: Efficacy Study

Study NV15355 is an ongoing, open-label, randomized, parallel study comparing FORTOVASE (n=90) and INVIRASE (n=81) in combination with two nucleoside reverse transcriptase inhibitors of choice in treatment-naive patients. The median age was 35 (range: 18 to 63), 92% of patients were male, and 68% were Caucasian. Mean baseline CD_4 cell count was 429 cells/mm^3, and mean baseline plasma HIV-RNA was 4.8 log_{10} copies/mL.

At week 16, 60 patients on the FORTOVASE arm compared to 30 patients on the INVIRASE arm had plasma HIV RNA levels below the limit of assay quantification (<400 copies/mL, Amplicor HIV-1 Monitor™ Test).

At week 16, mean changes from baseline in CD_4 cell counts and plasma HIV-RNA levels between the two treatment arms were statistically indistinguishable. The mean change in CD_4 cell count was 97 cells/mm^3 for the FORTOVASE arm and 115 cells/mm^3 for the INVIRASE arm. The mean

Continued on next page

Fortovase—Cont.

changes in plasma HIV-RNA levels are summarized in Figure 1.

Figure 1. Mean Change from Baseline in Plasma HIV-RNA Levels in Study NV15355*

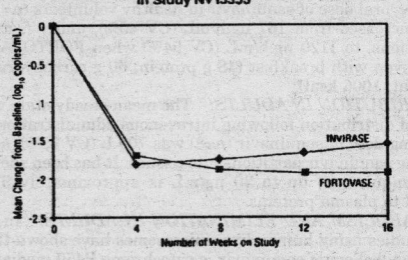

Number of Patients					
Week	0	4	8	12	16
INVIRASE	81	74	71	75	69†
FORTOVASE	90	83	79	78	75*

* Amplicor HIV-1 Monitor™ Test. Limit of quantification = 400 copies/mL.
† By 16 weeks of therapy, 15 patients receiving FORTOVASE and 7 receiving INVIRASE had discontinued study treatment: 5 patients on INVIRASE had missing data at week 16.

Study NV15182: Safety Study
Study NV15182 was an open-label safety study of FORTOVASE in combination with other antiretroviral agents in 442 patients (median age 39 [range: 15 to 71], 90% male and 73% Caucasian). The mean baseline CD_4 cell count was 227 cells/mm^3 and mean baseline HIV-RNA was 4.14 $\log_{10}$ copies/mL. The safety results from this study are displayed in the ADVERSE REACTIONS section.
STUDIES WITH INVIRASE (saquinavir mesylate):
Study NV14256: INVIRASE + HIVID Versus Either Monotherapy
Study NV14256 (North America) was a randomized, double-blind study comparing the combination of INVIRASE 600 mg tid + HIVID to HIVID monotherapy and INVIRASE monotherapy. The study accrued 970 patients, with median baseline CD_4 cell count at study entry of 170 cells/mm^3. Median duration of prior ZDV treatment was 17 months. Median duration of follow-up was 17 months. There were 88 first AIDS-defining events or deaths in the HIVID monotherapy group, 84 in the INVIRASE monotherapy group and 51 in the combination group. For survival there were 30 deaths in the HIVID group, 40 in the INVIRASE group and 11 deaths in the combination group.

The analysis of clinical endpoints from this study showed that the 18-month cumulative incidence of clinical disease progression to AIDS-defining event or death was 17.7% for patients randomized to INVIRASE + HIVID compared to 30.7% for patients randomized to HIVID monotherapy and 28.3% for patients randomized to INVIRASE monotherapy. The reduction in the number of clinical events for the combination regimen relative to both monotherapy regimens was statistically significant (see Figure 2 for Kaplan-Meier estimates of time to disease progression).

Figure 2. Time to First AIDS-Defining Event (or Death) (days) NV14256

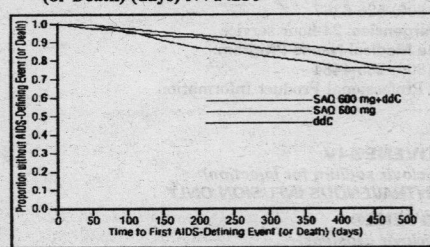

The 18-month cumulative mortality was 4% for patients randomized to INVIRASE + HIVID, 8.9% for patients ran-

---

Table 2. Effect of FORTOVASE on the Pharmacokinetics of Coadministered Drugs

Coadministered Drug	FORTOVASE Dose	N	% Change for Coadministered Drug	
			AUC (95%CI)	C_{max} (95%CI)
Clarithromycin 500 mg bid × 7 days Clarithromycin 14-OH clarithromycin metabolite	1200 mg tid × 7 days	12V	↑ 45% (17-81%) ↓ 24% (5-40%)	↑ 39% (10-76%) ↓ 34% (14-50%)
Nelfinavir 750-mg single dose	1200 mg tid × 4 days	14P	↑ 18% (5-33%)	↔
Ritonavir 400 mg bid × 14 days	400 mg bid × 14 days	8V	↔	↔
Sildenafil 100-mg single dose[1]	1200 mg tid × 8 days	27V	↑ 210% (150-300%)	↑ 140% (80-230%)
Terfenadine 60 mg bid × 11 days* Terfenadine Terfenadine acid metabolite	1200 mg tid × 4 days	12V	↑ 368% (257-514%) ↑ 120% (89-156%)	↑ 253% (164-373%) ↑ 93% (59-133%)

↑ Denotes an average increase in exposure by the percentage indicated.
↓ Denotes an average decrease in exposure by the percentage indicated.
↔ Denotes no statistically significant change in exposure was observed.
* FORTOVASE should not be coadministered with terfenadine (see PRECAUTIONS: *Drug Interactions*).
P Patient
V Healthy Volunteers.

Table 3. Effect of Coadministered Drugs on FORTOVASE and INVIRASE Pharmacokinetics

Coadministered Drug	FORTOVASE Dose	N	% Change for Saquinavir	
			AUC (95%CI)	C_{max} (95%CI)
Clarithromycin 500 mg bid × 7 days	1200 mg tid × 7 days	12V	↑ 177% (108-269%)	↑ 187% (105-300%)
Indinavir 800 mg q8h × 2 days	800-mg single dose 1200-mg single dose	6V 6V	↑ 620% (273-1288%) ↑ 364% (190-644%)	↑ 551% (320-908%) ↑ 299% (138-568%)
Nelfinavir 750 mg × 4 days	1200-mg single dose	14P	↑ 392% (271-553%)	↑ 179% (105-280%)
Ritonavir 400 mg bid × 14 days*	400 mg bid × 14 days†	8V	↑ 121% (7-359%)	↑ 64%§

Coadministered Drug	INVIRASE Dose	N	% Change for Saquinavir	
			AUC (95%CI)	C_{max} (95%CI)
Delavirdine 400 mg tid × 14 days	600 mg tid × 21 days	13V	↑ 5-fold	Not available
Ketoconazole 200 mg qd × 6 days	600 mg tid × 6 days	12V	↑ 130% (58-235%)	↑ 147% (53-298%)
Nevirapine 200 mg bid × 21 days	600 mg tid × 7 days	23P	↓ 24% (1-42%)	↓ 28% (1-47%)
Ranitidine 150 mg × 2 doses	600-mg single dose	12V	↑ 67%§	↑ 74% (16-161%)
Rifabutin 300 mg qd × 14 days	600 mg tid × 14 days	12P	↓ 43% (29-53%)	↓ 30%§
Rifampin 600 mg qd × 7 days	600 mg tid × 14 days	12V	↓ 84% (79-88%)	↓ 79% (68-86%)
Ritonavir 400 mg bid steady state*	400 mg bid steady state‡	7P	↑ 1587% (808-3034%)	↑ 1277% (577-2702%)
Zalcitabine (ddC) 0.75 mg tid × 7 days	600 mg tid × 7 days	27P	↔	↔
Zidovudine (ZDV) 200 mg tid × > 7 days	600 mg tid × > 7 days	20P	↔	↔

↑ Denotes an average increase in exposure by the percentage indicated.
↓ Denotes an average decrease in exposure by the percentage indicated.
↔ Denotes no statistically significant change in exposure was observed.
* When ritonavir was combined with the same dose of either INVIRASE or FORTOVASE, actual mean plasma exposures (AUC_{12}, 18.2 µg·h/mL, 20.0 µg·h/mL, respectively) were not significantly different.
† Compared to standard FORTOVASE 1200 mg tid regimen (n=33).
‡ Compared to standard INVIRASE 600 mg tid regimen (n=114).
§ Did not reach statistical significance.
P Patient
V Healthy Volunteers.

domized to HIVID monotherapy and 12.6% for patients randomized to INVIRASE monotherapy. The reduction in the number of deaths for the combination regimen relative to both monotherapy regimens was statistically significant (see Figure 3 for Kaplan-Meier estimates of time to death).

Figure 3. Time to Death (days) NV14256

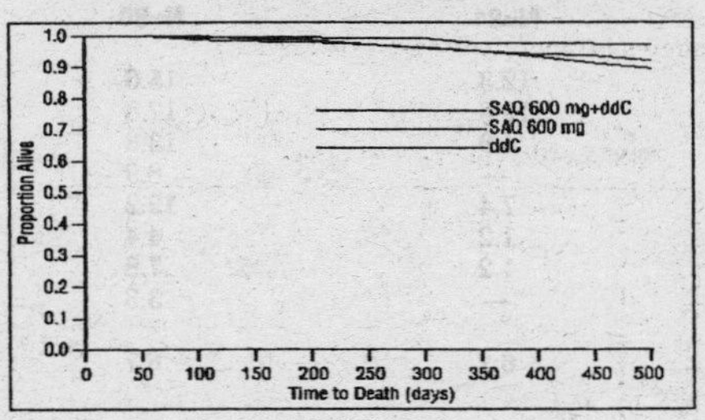

CONTRAINDICATIONS

FORTOVASE is contraindicated in patients with clinically significant hypersensitivity to saquinavir or to any of the components contained in the capsule. FORTOVASE should not be administered concurrently with terfenadine, cisapride, astemizole, triazolam, midazolam or ergot derivatives, because competition for CYP3A by saquinavir could result in inhibition of the metabolism of these drugs and create the potential for serious and/or life-threatening reactions such as cardiac arrhythmias or prolonged sedation (see PRECAUTIONS: *Drug Interactions*).

WARNINGS

New onset diabetes mellitus, exacerbation of pre-existing diabetes mellitus and hyperglycemia have been reported during postmarketing surveillance in HIV-infected patients receiving protease-inhibitor therapy. Some patients required either initiation or dose adjustments of insulin or oral hypoglycemic agents for the treatment of these events. In some cases diabetic ketoacidosis has occurred. In those patients who discontinued protease-inhibitor therapy, hyperglycemia persisted in some cases. Because these events have been reported voluntarily during clinical practice, estimates of frequency cannot be made and a causal relationship between protease-inhibitor therapy and these events has not been established.

Concomitant use of FORTOVASE with lovastatin or simvastatin is not recommended. Caution should be exercised if HIV protease inhibitors, including FORTOVASE, are used concurrently with other HMG-CoA reductase inhibitors that are also metabolized by the CYP3A4 pathway (eg, atorvastatin or cerivastatin). Since increased concentrations of statins can, in rare cases, cause severe adverse events such as myopathy including rhabdomyolysis, this risk may be increased when HIV protease inhibitors, including saquinavir, are used in combination with these drugs.[2, 3]

PRECAUTIONS

General: FORTOVASE (saquinavir) soft gelatin capsules and INVIRASE (saquinavir mesylate) capsules are not bioequivalent and cannot be used interchangeably. Only FORTOVASE should be used for the initiation of saquinavir therapy (see DOSAGE AND ADMINISTRATION) since FORTOVASE soft gelatin capsules provide greater bioavailability and efficacy than INVIRASE capsules. For patients taking INVIRASE capsules with a viral load below the limit of quantification, a switch to FORTOVASE is recommended to maintain a virologic response. For patients taking INVIRASE capsules who have not had an adequate response or are failing therapy, if saquinavir resistance is clinically suspected, then FORTOVASE should not be used.[4] If resistance to saquinavir is not clinically suspected, a switch to FORTOVASE may be considered.[5, 6]

If a serious or severe toxicity occurs during treatment with FORTOVASE, FORTOVASE should be interrupted until the etiology of the event is identified or the toxicity resolves. At that time, resumption of treatment with full-dose FORTOVASE may be considered.

Preliminary results from a pharmacokinetic substudy of NV15182 from patients sampled between weeks 61 to 69 of treatment showed that the mean saquinavir AUC was lower than the week 3 mean AUC from study NV15107. However, the mean AUC of saquinavir at week 61 to 69 remained higher than the mean AUC of INVIRASE in study NV15107 (see CLINICAL PHARMACOLOGY *Pharmacokinetics*). The clinical significance of this finding is unknown.

Hepatic Insufficiency: Saquinavir is principally metabolized by the liver. Therefore, caution should be exercised when administering FORTOVASE to patients with hepatic insufficiency since patients with baseline liver function tests >5 times the upper limit of normal were not included in clinical studies. Although a causal relationship has not been established, there have been reports of exacerbation of chronic liver dysfunction, including portal hypertension, in patients with underlying hepatitis B or C, cirrhosis or other underlying liver abnormalities.

Hemophilia: There have been reports of spontaneous bleeding in patients with hemophilia A and B treated with protease inhibitors. In some patients additional factor VIII was required. In the majority of reported cases treatment with protease inhibitors was continued or restarted. A causal relationship between protease-inhibitor therapy and these episodes has not been established.

Drugs That Should Not Be Coadministered With FORTOVASE

Antihistamines	Astemizole, Terfenadine
Antimigraine	Ergot Derivatives
GI Motility Agents	Cisapride
Sedatives/Hypnotics	Midazolam, Triazolam
Clinically Significant Drug Interactions Which Decrease Saquinavir Plasma Concentrations	
HIV Non-nucleoside Reverse Transcriptase Inhibitors	Nevirapine*
Antimycobacterial Agents	Rifabutin*, Rifampin*
Clinically Significant Drug Interactions Which Increase Saquinavir Plasma Concentrations	
Antibiotics	Clarithromycin†
HIV Protease Inhibitors	Indinavir†, Ritonavir*†, Nelfinavir†
HIV Non-nucleoside Reverse Transcriptase Inhibitors	Delavirdine*
Antifungal Agents	Ketoconazole*
Other Potential Drug Interactions‡	
Anticonvulsants: Carbamazepine, Phenobarbital, Phenytoin	May decrease saquinavir plasma concentrations
Corticosteroids: Dexamethasone	May decrease saquinavir plasma concentrations

*Studied with INVIRASE.
†Studied with FORTOVASE.
‡This table is not all inclusive.

Fat Redistribution: Redistribution/accumulation of body fat including central obesity, dorsocervical fat enlargement (buffalo hump), peripheral wasting, breast enlargement and "cushingoid appearance" have been observed in patients receiving protease inhibitors. A causal relationship between protease inhibitor therapy and these events has not been established and the long-term consequences are currently unknown.[7, 6, 8]

Resistance/Cross-resistance: Varying degrees of cross-resistance among protease inhibitors have been observed. Continued administration of saquinavir therapy following loss of viral suppression may increase the likelihood of cross-resistance to other protease inhibitors (see MICROBIOLOGY).

Information for Patients: Patients should be informed that any change from INVIRASE to FORTOVASE should be made only under the supervision of a physician.

Patients should be informed that FORTOVASE is not a cure for HIV infection and that they may continue to contract illnesses associated with advanced HIV infection, including opportunistic infections. They should be informed that FORTOVASE therapy has not been shown to reduce the risk of transmitting HIV to others through sexual contact or blood contamination.

FORTOVASE may interact with some drugs; therefore, patients should be advised to report to their physician the use of any other prescription or nonprescription medication.

Patients should be informed that redistribution or accumulation of body fat may occur in patients receiving protease inhibitors and that the cause and long-term health effects of these conditions are not known at this time.[7]

Patients should be advised that FORTOVASE should be taken within 2 hours after a full meal (see CLINICAL PHARMACOLOGY: *Pharmacokinetics*). Patients should be advised of the importance of taking their medication every day, as prescribed, to achieve maximum benefit. Patients should not alter the dose or discontinue therapy without consulting their physician. If a dose is missed, patients should take the next dose as soon as possible. However, the patient should not double the next dose.

Patients should be told that the long-term effects of FORTOVASE are unknown at this time.

Patients should be informed that refrigerated (36° to 46°F, 2° to 8°C) capsules of FORTOVASE remain stable until the expiration date printed on the label. Once brought to room temperature [at or below 77°F (25°C)], capsules should be used within 3 months.

Laboratory Tests: Clinical chemistry tests should be performed prior to initiating FORTOVASE therapy and at appropriate intervals thereafter. Elevated nonfasting triglyceride levels have been observed in patients in saquinavir trials. Triglyceride levels should be periodically monitored during therapy. For comprehensive information concerning laboratory test alterations associated with use of other antiretroviral therapies, physicians should refer to the complete product information for these drugs.

Drug Interactions: **Several drug interaction studies have been completed with both INVIRASE and FORTOVASE. Observations from drug interaction studies with INVIRASE may not be predictive for FORTOVASE.**
[See table above]

ANTIBIOTICS:

Clarithromycin: Coadministration of clarithromycin with FORTOVASE resulted in a 177% increase in saquinavir plasma AUC, a 45% increase in clarithromycin AUC and a 24% decrease in clarithromycin 14-OH metabolite AUC.

ANTIHISTAMINES:

Terfenadine: Coadministration of terfenadine with FORTOVASE resulted in increased terfenadine plasma levels; therefore, FORTOVASE should not be administered concurrently with terfenadine because of the potential for serious and/or life-threatening cardiac arrhythmias.

Astemizole: Because a similar interaction to that seen with terfenadine is likely from the coadministration of FORTOVASE and astemizole, FORTOVASE should not be administered concurrently with astemizole.

ERECTILE DYSFUNCTION AGENTS:[1]

Sildenafil: In a study performed in healthy male volunteers, coadministration of saquinavir, a CYP3A4 inhibitor, at steady state (1200 mg tid) with sildenafil (100 mg single dose) resulted in a 140% increase in sildenafil C_{max} and a 210% increase in sildenafil AUC. Sildenafil had no effect on saquinavir pharmacokinetics. When sildenafil is administered concomitantly with saquinavir a starting dose of 25 mg[1] of sildenafil should be considered.[9, 10]

HIV PROTEASE INHIBITORS:

Indinavir: Coadministration of indinavir with FORTOVASE (1200-mg single dose) resulted in a 364% increase in saquinavir plasma AUC. Currently, there are no safety and efficacy data available from the use of this combination.

Nelfinavir: Coadministration of nelfinavir with FORTOVASE resulted in an 18% increase in nelfinavir plasma AUC and a 392% increase in saquinavir plasma AUC. Currently, there are no safety and efficacy data available from the use of this combination.

Ritonavir: Following approximately 4 weeks of a combination regimen of saquinavir (400 mg or 600 mg bid) and ritonavir (400 mg or 600 mg bid) in HIV-infected patients, saquinavir AUC values were at least 17-fold greater than historical AUC values from patients who received saquinavir 600 mg tid without ritonavir. When used in combination therapy for up to 24 weeks, doses greater than 400 mg bid of either ritonavir or saquinavir were associated with an increase in adverse events. Plasma exposures achieved with INVIRASE (400 mg bid) and ritonavir (400 mg bid) are similar to those achieved with FORTOVASE (400 mg bid) and ritonavir (400 mg bid).

HIV REVERSE TRANSCRIPTASE INHIBITORS:

Based on known metabolic pathways and routes of elimination for nucleoside reverse transcriptase inhibitors, no interaction with saquinavir is expected.

HIV NON-NUCLEOSIDE REVERSE TRANSCRIPTASE INHIBITORS:

Delavirdine: Coadministration of delavirdine with INVIRASE resulted in a 5-fold increase in saquinavir plasma AUC. Currently there are limited safety and no efficacy data available from the use of this combination. In a small, preliminary study, hepatocellular enzyme elevations

Continued on next page

Fortovase—Cont.

occurred in 13% of subjects during the first several weeks of the delavirdine and saquinavir combination (6% Grade 3 or 4). Hepatocellular changes should be monitored frequently if this combination is prescribed.

Nevirapine: Coadministration of nevirapine with INVIRASE resulted in a 24% decrease in saquinavir plasma AUC. Currently, there are no safety and efficacy data available from the use of this combination.

ANTIFUNGAL AGENTS:

Ketoconazole: Coadministration of ketoconazole with INVIRASE resulted in a 130% increase in saquinavir plasma AUC.

ANTIMYCOBACTERIAL AGENTS:

Rifabutin: Coadministration of rifabutin with INVIRASE resulted in a 43% decrease in saquinavir plasma AUC. Physicians should consider using an alternative to rifabutin when a patient is taking FORTOVASE.

Rifampin: Coadministration of rifampin with INVIRASE resulted in an 84% decrease in saquinavir plasma AUC. Physicians should consider using an alternative to rifampin when a patient is taking FORTOVASE.

H₂ ANTAGONISTS:

Ranitidine: Little or no change in the pharmacokinetics of INVIRASE was observed when coadministered with ranitidine. No significant interaction would be expected between FORTOVASE and ranitidine.

GI MOTILITY AGENTS:

Cisapride: Although no interaction study has been conducted, cisapride should not be administered concurrently with FORTOVASE because of the potential for serious and/or life-threatening cardiac arrhythmias.

Carcinogenesis, Mutagenesis and Impairment of Fertility:
Carcinogenesis: Carcinogenicity studies in rats and mice have not yet been completed.

Mutagenesis: Mutagenicity and genotoxicity studies, with and without metabolic activation where appropriate, have shown that saquinavir has no mutagenic activity in vitro in either bacterial (Ames test) or mammalian cells (Chinese hamster lung V79/HPRT test). Saquinavir does not induce chromosomal damage in vivo in the mouse micronucleus assay or in vitro in human peripheral blood lymphocytes and does not induce primary DNA damage in vitro in the unscheduled DNA synthesis test.

Impairment of Fertility: Fertility and reproductive performance were not affected in rats at plasma exposures (AUC values) approximately 50% of those achieved in humans at the recommended dose.

Pregnancy: Teratogenic Effects: Category B. Reproduction studies conducted with saquinavir in rats have shown no embryotoxicity or teratogenicity at plasma exposures (AUC values) approximately 50% of those achieved in humans at the recommended dose or in rabbits at plasma exposures approximately 40% of those achieved at the recommended clinical dose of FORTOVASE. Distribution studies in these species showed that placental transfer of saquinavir is low (less than 5% of maternal plasma concentrations).

Studies in rats indicated that exposure to saquinavir from late pregnancy through lactation at plasma concentrations (AUC values) approximately 50% of those achieved in humans at the recommended dose of FORTOVASE had no effect on the survival, growth and development of offspring to weaning. Because animal reproduction studies are not always predictive of human response, FORTOVASE should only be used during pregnancy after taking into account the importance of the drug to the mother. Presently, there are no reports of women receiving FORTOVASE in clinical trials who became pregnant.

Antiretroviral Pregnancy Registry: To monitor maternal-fetal outcomes of pregnant women exposed to antiretroviral medications, including FORTOVASE, an Antiretroviral Pregnancy Registry has been established. Physicians are encouraged to register patients by calling 1-800-258-4263.[11]

Nursing Mothers: The Centers for Disease Control and Prevention recommend that HIV-infected mothers not breastfeed their infants to avoid risking postnatal transmission of HIV. It is not known whether saquinavir is excreted in human milk. Because of both the potential for HIV transmission and the potential for serious adverse reactions in nursing infants, **mothers should be instructed not to breastfeed if they are receiving antiretroviral medications, including FORTOVASE.**[11]

Pediatric Use: Safety and effectiveness of FORTOVASE in HIV-infected pediatric patients younger than 16 years of age have not been established.

Geriatric Use: Clinical studies of FORTOVASE did not include sufficient numbers of subjects aged 65 and over to determine whether they respond differently from younger subjects. In general, caution should be taken when dosing FORTOVASE in elderly patients due to the greater frequency of decreased hepatic, renal, or cardiac function, and of concomitant disease or other drug therapy.[12, 6]

ADVERSE REACTIONS (see PRECAUTIONS)

The safety of FORTOVASE was studied in more than 500 patients who received the drug either alone or in combination with other antiretroviral agents. The majority of treatment-related adverse events were of mild intensity. The most frequently reported treatment-emergent adverse events among patients receiving FORTOVASE in combination with other antiretroviral agents were diarrhea, nausea, abdominal discomfort and dyspepsia.

Table 4. Percentage of Patients WithTreatment-Emergent Adverse Events* of at Least Moderate Intensity, Occurring in ≥2% of Patients

ADVERSE EVENT	NV15182 (48 weeks) FORTOVASE + TOC† N=442	NV15355 (16 weeks) Naive Patients INVIRASE + 2 RTIs‡ N=81	NV15355 (16 weeks) Naive Patients FORTOVASE + 2 RTIs‡ N=90
GASTROINTESTINAL			
Diarrhea	19.9	12.3	15.6
Nausea	10.6	13.6	17.8
Abdominal Discomfort	8.6	4.9	13.3
Dyspepsia	8.4	—	8.9
Flatulence	5.7	7.4	12.2
Vomiting	2.9	1.2	4.4
Abdominal Pain	2.3	1.2	7.8
Constipation	—	—	3.3
BODY AS A WHOLE			
Fatigue	4.8	6.2	6.7
CENTRAL AND PERIPHERAL NERVOUS SYSTEM			
Headaches	5.0	4.9	8.9
PSYCHIATRIC DISORDERS			
Depression	2.7	—	—
Insomnia	—	1.2	5.6
Anxiety	—	2.5	2.2
Libido Disorder	—	—	2.2
SPECIAL SENSES DISORDERS			
Taste Alteration	—	1.2	4.4
MUSCULOSKELETAL DISORDERS			
Pain	—	3.7	3.3
DERMATOLOGICAL DISORDERS			
Eczema	—	2.5	—
Rash	—	2.5	—
Verruca	—	—	2.2

* Includes adverse events at least possibly related to study drug or of unknown intensity and/or relationship to treatment (corresponding to ACTG Grade 3 and 4).
† Antiretroviral Treatment of Choice.
‡ Reverse Transcriptase Inhibitor.

Table 5. Percentage of Patients With Marked Laboratory Abnormalities*

BIOCHEMISTRY	Limit	NV15182 (48 weeks) FORTOVASE + TOC† N=442	NV15355 (16 weeks) Naive Patients INVIRASE + 2 RTIs‡ N=81	NV15355 (16 weeks) Naive Patients FORTOVASE + 2 RTIs‡ N=90
Alkaline Phosphatase	>5 × ULN§	0.5	0.0	0.0
Calcium (high)	>12.5 mg/dL	0.2	0.0	0.0
Creatine Kinase	>4 × ULN§	7.8	0.0	4.8
Gamma GT	>5 × ULN§	5.7	2.6	7.1
Glucose (low)	<40 mg/dL	6.4	2.5	3.5
Glucose (high)	>250 mg/dL	1.4	1.3	1.2
Phosphate	<1.5 mg/dL	0.5	0.0	0.0
Potassium (high)	>6.5 mEq/L	2.7	0.0	1.2
Serum Amylase	>2 × ULN§	1.9	ND	ND
SGOT (AST)	>5 × ULN§	4.1	0.0	1.2
SGPT (ALT)	>5 × ULN§	5.7	1.3	2.3
Sodium (high)	>157 mEq/L	0.7	0.0	0.0
Total Bilirubin	>2.5 × ULN§	1.6	0.0	0.0
HEMATOLOGY				
Hemoglobin	<7.0 gm/dL	0.7	0.0	1.2
Absolute Neutrophil Count	<750 mm³	2.9	2.9	1.2
Platelets	<50,000 mm³	0.9	2.5	0.0

* ACTG Grade 3 or above.
† Antiretroviral Treatment of Choice.
‡ Reverse Transcriptase Inhibitor.
§ ULN = Upper limit of normal range.
ND Not done.

Clinical adverse events of at least moderate intensity which occurred in ≥2% of patients in studies NV15182 and NV15355 are summarized in Table 4. The median duration of treatment in studies NV15182 and NV15355 were 52 and 18 weeks, respectively. In NV15182, more than 300 patients were on treatment for approximately 1 year.

FORTOVASE did not appear to alter the pattern, frequency or severity of known major toxicities associated with the use of nucleoside analogues. Physicians should refer to the complete product information for other antiretroviral agents as appropriate for drug-associated adverse reactions to these other agents.

Rare occurrences of the following serious adverse experiences have been reported during clinical trials of FORTOVASE and/or INVIRASE and were considered at least possibly related to use of study drugs: confusion, ataxia and weakness; seizures; headache; acute myeloblastic leukemia; hemolytic anemia; thrombocytopenia; thrombocytopenia and intracranial hemorrhage leading to death; attempted suicide; Stevens-Johnson syndrome; bullous skin eruption and polyarthritis; severe cutaneous reaction associated with increased liver function tests; isolated elevation of transaminases; exacerbation of chronic liver disease with Grade 4 elevated liver function tests, jaundice, ascites, and right and left upper quadrant abdominal pain; pancreatitis

leading to death; intestinal obstruction; portal hypertension; thrombophlebitis; peripheral vasoconstriction; drug fever; nephrolithiasis; and acute renal insufficiency.

Table 5 summarizes the percentage of patients with marked laboratory abnormalities in study NV15182 and NV15355 (median duration of treatment was 52 and 18 weeks, respectively). In study NV15182, by 48 weeks <1% of patients discontinued treatment due to laboratory abnormalities.
[See table 4 above]
[See table 5 above]
Additional marked lab abnormalities have been observed with INVIRASE. These include: calcium (low), phosphate (low), potassium (low), sodium (low).

Monotherapy and Combination Studies: Other clinical adverse experiences of any intensity, at least remotely related to FORTOVASE and INVIRASE, including those in <2% of patients, are listed below by body system.

Autonomic Nervous System: Mouth dry, night sweats, sweating increased

Body as a Whole: Allergic reaction, anorexia, appetite decreased, appetite disturbances, asthenia, chest pain, edema, fever, intoxication, malaise, olfactory disorder, pain body, pain pelvic, retrosternal pain, shivering, trauma, wasting syndrome, weakness generalized, weight decrease, redistribution/accumulation of body fat (see PRECAUTIONS: *Fat Redistribution*)[7]

Cardiovascular/Cerebrovascular: Cyanosis, heart murmur, heart rate disorder, heart valve disorder, hypertension, hypotension, stroke, syncope, vein distended

Central and Peripheral Nervous System: Ataxia, cerebral hemorrhage, confusion, convulsions, dizziness, dysarthria, dysesthesia, hyperesthesia, hyperreflexia, hyporeflexia, light-headed feeling, myelopolyradiculoneuritis, neuropathy, numbness extremities, numbness face, paresis, paresthesia, peripheral neuropathy, poliomyelitis, prickly sensation, progressive multifocal leukoencephalopathy, spasms, tremor, unconsciousness

Dermatological: Acne, alopecia, chalazion, dermatitis, dermatitis seborrheic, erythema, folliculitis, furunculosis, hair changes, hot flushes, nail disorder, papillomatosis, papular rash, photosensitivity reaction, pigment changes skin, parasites external, pruritus, psoriasis, rash maculopapular, rash pruritic, red face, skin disorder, skin nodule, skin syndrome, skin ulceration, urticaria, verruca, xeroderma

Endocrine/Metabolic: Dehydration, diabetes mellitus, hyperglycemia, hypoglycemia, hypothyroidism, thirst, triglyceride increase, weight increase

Gastrointestinal: Abdominal distention, bowel movements frequent, buccal mucosa ulceration, canker sores oral, cheilitis, colic abdominal, dysphagia, esophageal ulceration, esophagitis, eructation, fecal incontinence, feces bloodstained, feces discolored, gastralgia, gastritis, gastroesophageal reflux, gastrointestinal inflammation, gingivitis, glossitis, hemorrhage rectum, hemorrhoids, infectious diarrhea, melena, painful defecation, parotid disorder, pruritus ani, pyrosis, salivary glands disorder, stomach upset, stomatitis, taste unpleasant, toothache, tooth disorder, ulcer gastrointestinal

Hematologic: Anemia, neutropenia, pancytopenia, splenomegaly

Liver and Biliary: Cholangitis sclerosing, cholelithiasis, hepatitis, hepatomegaly, hepatosplenomegaly, jaundice, liver enzyme disorder, pancreatitis

Musculoskeletal: Arthralgia, arthritis, back pain, cramps leg, cramps muscle, lumbago, musculoskeletal disorders, myalgia, myopathy, pain facial, pain jaw, pain leg, pain musculoskeletal, stiffness, tissue changes

Neoplasm: Kaposi's sarcoma, tumor

Platelet, Bleeding, Clotting: Bleeding dermal, hemorrhage, microhemorrhages, thrombocytopenia

Psychiatric: Agitation, amnesia, anxiety attack, behavior disturbances, dreaming excessive, euphoria, hallucination, intellectual ability reduced, irritability, lethargy, overdose effect, psychic disorder, psychosis, somnolence, speech disorder

Reproductive System: Epididymitis, erectile impotence, impotence, menstrual disorder, menstrual irregularity, penis disorder, prostate enlarged, vaginal discharge

Resistance Mechanism: Abscess, angina tonsillaris, candidiasis, cellulitis, herpes simplex, herpes zoster, infection bacterial, infection mycotic, infection staphylococcal, infestation parasitic, influenza, lymphadenopathy, molluscum contagiosum, moniliasis

Respiratory: Asthma bronchial, bronchitis, cough, dyspnea, epistaxis, hemoptysis, laryngitis, pharyngitis, pneumonia, pulmonary disease, respiratory disorder, rhinitis, rhinitis allergic atopic, sinusitis, upper respiratory tract infection

Special Senses: Blepharitis, conjunctivitis, cytomegalovirus retinitis, dry eye syndrome, earache, ear pressure, eye irritation, hearing decreased, otitis, taste unpleasant, tinnitus, visual disturbance, xerophthalmia

Urinary System: Micturition disorder, nocturia, renal calculus, renal colic, urinary tract bleeding, urinary tract infection

OVERDOSAGE

Overdosage with FORTOVASE has not been reported. There were 2 patients who had overdoses with INVIRASE. No sequelae were noted in the first patient after ingesting 8 grams of INVIRASE as a single dose. The patient was treated with induction of emesis within 2 to 4 hours after ingestion. The second patient ingested 2.4 grams of INVIRASE in combination with 600 mg of ritonavir and experienced pain in the throat that lasted for 6 hours and then resolved.

DOSAGE AND ADMINISTRATION

FORTOVASE (saquinavir) soft gelatin capsules and INVIRASE (saquinavir mesylate) capsules are not bioequivalent and cannot be used interchangeably. When using saquinavir as part of an antiviral regimen FORTOVASE is the recommended formulation. In rare circumstances, INVIRASE may be considered if it is to be combined with antiretrovirals that significantly inhibit saquinavir's metabolism (see CLINICAL PHARMACOLOGY: *DRUG INTERACTIONS*).[5, 6]

The recommended dose of FORTOVASE is six 200-mg capsules orally, three times a day (1200 mg tid). FORTOVASE should be taken with a meal or up to 2 hours after a meal. When used in combination with nucleoside analogues, the dosage of FORTOVASE should not be reduced as this will lead to greater than dose proportional decreases in saquinavir plasma levels.

Patients should be advised that FORTOVASE, like other protease inhibitors, is recommended for use in combination with active antiretroviral therapy. Greater activity has been observed when new antiretroviral therapies are begun at the same time as FORTOVASE. As with all protease inhibitors, adherence to the prescribed regimen is strongly recommended. Concomitant therapy should be based on a patient's prior drug exposure.

Monitoring of Patients: Clinical chemistry tests should be performed prior to initiating FORTOVASE therapy and at appropriate intervals thereafter. For comprehensive patient monitoring recommendations for other antiretroviral therapies, physicians should refer to the complete product information for these drugs.

Dose Adjustment for Combination Therapy With FORTOVASE: For toxicities that may be associated with FORTOVASE, the drug should be interrupted. For recipients of combination therapy with FORTOVASE and other antiretroviral agents, dose adjustment of the other antiretroviral agents should be based on the known toxicity profile of the individual drug. Physicians should refer to the complete product information for these drugs for comprehensive dose adjustment recommendations and drug-associated adverse reactions.

HOW SUPPLIED

FORTOVASE 200-mg capsules are beige, opaque, soft gelatin capsules with ROCHE and 0246 imprinted on the capsule shell—bottles of 180 (NDC 0004-0246-48).

The capsules should be refrigerated at 36° to 46°F (2° to 8°C) in tightly closed bottles until dispensed.

For patient use, refrigerated (36° to 46°F, 2° to 8°C) capsules of FORTOVASE remain stable until the expiration date printed on the label. Once brought to room temperature [at or below 77°F (25°C)], capsules should be used within 3 months.

Rx only

Manufactured by:
F. Hoffmann-La Roche Ltd., Basel, Switzerland
Distributed by:
Pharmaceuticals
Roche Laboratories Inc.
340 Kingsland Street
Nutley, New Jersey 07110-1199

Revised: October 2000

Copyright © 1997–2000 by Roche Laboratories Inc. All rights reserved.

Annotations

1. FDA fax dated September 18, 2000.
2. FDA letter dated October 6, 1999.
3. Weder S, Jorga K.
   Drug Safety issue work-up: Drug interaction between saquinavir and HMG-CoA reductase Inhibitors.
   Hoffmann-La Roche, Basel, September 14, 1999.
4. FDA fax dated June 14, 2000.
5. FDA letter dated June 25, 1998.
6. FDA fax dated January 28, 2000.
7. FDA letter dated August 31, 1998.
8. FDA fax dated April 14, 2000.
9. Hall MCS, Ahmad S.
   Interaction between sildenafil and HIV-1 combination therapy.
   Lancet 1999; 353: 2071–2072
10. Weder S, Jorga K.
    Drug Safety issue work-up: Drug interaction between saquinavir and sildenafil.
    Hoffmann-La Roche, Basel, August 30, 1999.
11. FDA fax dated May 26, 2000, transmitted June 1, 2000.
12. 21 CFR §201.57(f)(10)(ii)(A)

INVIRASE® ℞
(saquinavir mesylate)
CAPSULES

Prescribing information for this product, which appears on pages 2756–2759 of the 2001 PDR, has been completely revised as follows. Please write "See Supplement A" next to the product heading.

> **WARNING:**
> **INVIRASE® (saquinavir mesylate) capsules and FORTOVASE® (saquinavir) soft gelatin capsules are not bioequivalent and cannot be used interchangeably. When using saquinavir as part of an antiviral regimen FORTOVASE is the recommended formulation. In rare circumstances, INVIRASE may be considered if it is to be combined with antiretrovirals that significantly inhibit saquinavir's metabolism (see CLINICAL PHARMACOLOGY: *DRUG INTERACTIONS*).**[1, 2]

DESCRIPTION

INVIRASE brand of saquinavir mesylate is an inhibitor of the human immunodeficiency virus (HIV) protease. INVIRASE is available as light brown and green, opaque hard gelatin capsules for oral administration in a 200-mg strength (as saquinavir free base). Each capsule also contains the inactive ingredients lactose, microcrystalline cellulose, povidone K30, sodium starch glycolate, talc and magnesium stearate. Each capsule shell contains gelatin and water with the following dye systems: red iron oxide, yellow iron oxide, black iron oxide, FD&C Blue #2 and titanium dioxide. The chemical name for saquinavir mesylate is N-tert-butyl-decahydro-2-[2(R)-hydroxy-4-phenyl-3(S)-[[N-(2-quinolylcarbonyl)-L-asparaginyl]amino]butyl]-(4aS,8aS)-isoquinoline-3(S)-carboxamide methanesulfonate with a molecular formula $C_{38}H_{50}N_6O_5 \cdot CH_4O_3S$ and a molecular weight of 766.96. The molecular weight of the free base is 670.86. Saquinavir mesylate has the following structural formula:

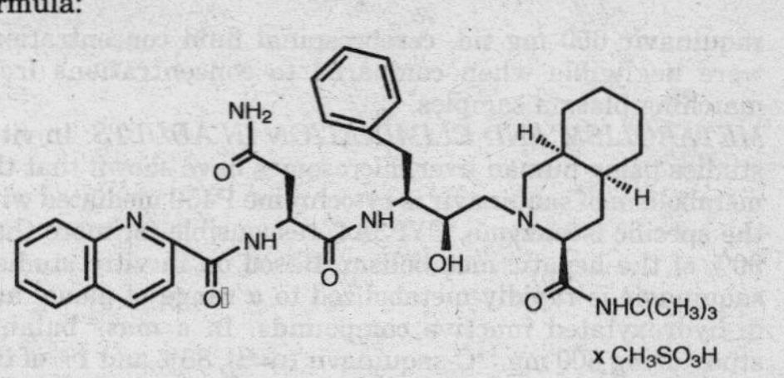

Saquinavir mesylate is a white to off-white, very fine powder with an aqueous solubility of 2.22 mg/mL at 25°C.

CLINICAL PHARMACOLOGY

Mechanism of Action: HIV protease cleaves viral polyprotein precursors to generate functional proteins in HIV-infected cells. The cleavage of viral polyprotein precursors is essential for maturation of infectious virus. Saquinavir mesylate, henceforth referred to as saquinavir, is a synthetic peptide-like substrate analogue that inhibits the activity of HIV protease and prevents the cleavage of viral polyproteins.

Microbiology: *Antiviral Activity In Vitro:* The in vitro antiviral activity of saquinavir was assessed in lymphoblastoid and monocytic cell lines and in peripheral blood lymphocytes. Saquinavir inhibited HIV activity in both acutely and chronically infected cells. IC50 values (50% inhibitory concentration) were in the range of 1 to 30 nM. In cell culture saquinavir demonstrated additive to synergistic effects against HIV in double- and triple-combination regimens with reverse transcriptase inhibitors zidovudine (ZDV), zalcitabine (ddC) and didanosine (ddI), without enhanced cytotoxicity.

Resistance: HIV isolates with reduced susceptibility to saquinavir have been selected in vitro. Genotypic analyses of these isolates showed substitution mutations in the HIV protease at amino acid positions 48 (Glycine to Valine) and 90 (Leucine to Methionine).

Phenotypic and genotypic changes in HIV isolates from patients treated with saquinavir were also monitored in Phase 1/2 clinical trials. Phenotypic changes were defined as a 10-fold decrease in sensitivity from baseline. Two viral protease mutations (L90M and/or G48V, the former predominating) were found in virus from treated, but not untreated, patients. The incidence across studies of phenotypic and genotypic changes in the subsets of patients studied for a period of 16 to 74 weeks (median observation time approximately 1 year) is shown in Table 1. However, the clinical relevance of phenotypic and genotypic changes associated with saquinavir therapy has not been established.

[See table 1 at top of next page]

Cross-resistance to Other Antiretrovirals: The potential for HIV cross-resistance between protease inhibitors has not been fully explored. Therefore, it is unknown what effect saquinavir therapy will have on the activity of subsequent protease inhibitors. Cross-resistance between saquinavir and reverse transcriptase inhibitors is unlikely because of the different enzyme targets involved. ZDV-resistant HIV isolates have been shown to be sensitive to saquinavir in vitro.

Pharmacokinetics: The pharmacokinetic properties of saquinavir have been evaluated in healthy volunteers (n=351) and HIV-infected patients (n=270) after single- and multiple-oral doses of 25, 75, 200 and 600 mg tid and in healthy volunteers after intravenous doses of 6, 12, 36 or 72 mg (n=21).

ABSORPTION AND BIOAVAILABILITY IN ADULTS: Following multiple dosing (600 mg tid) in HIV-infected patients (n=30), the steady-state area under the plasma concentration versus time curve (AUC) was 2.5 times (95% CI 1.6 to 3.8) higher than that observed after a single dose. HIV-infected patients administered saquinavir 600 mg tid, with the instructions to take saquinavir after a meal or substantial snack, had AUC and maximum plasma concentration (C_{max}) values which were about twice those observed in healthy volunteers receiving the same treatment regimen (Table 2).

[See table 2 at top of next page]

Absolute bioavailability averaged 4% (CV 73%, range: 1% to 9%) in 8 healthy volunteers who received a single 600-mg dose (3 × 200 mg) of saquinavir following a high fat breakfast (48 g protein, 60 g carbohydrate, 57 g fat; 1006 kcal). The low bioavailability is thought to be due to a combination of incomplete absorption and extensive first-pass metabolism.

FOOD EFFECT: The mean 24-hour AUC after a single 600-mg oral dose (6 × 100 mg) in healthy volunteers (n=6) was increased from 24 ng·h/mL (CV 33%), under fasting conditions, to 161 ng·h/mL (CV 35%) when saquinavir was given following a high fat breakfast (48 g protein, 60 g carbohydrate, 57 g fat; 1006 kcal). Saquinavir 24-hour AUC and C_{max} (n=6) following the administration of a higher calorie meal (943 kcal, 54 g fat) were on average two times higher than after a lower calorie, lower fat meal (355 kcal, 8 g fat). The effect of food has been shown to persist for up to 2 hours.

DISTRIBUTION IN ADULTS: The mean steady-state volume of distribution following intravenous administration of a 12-mg dose of saquinavir (n=8) was 700 L (CV 39%), suggesting saquinavir partitions into tissues. Saquinavir was approximately 98% bound to plasma proteins over a concentration range of 15 to 700 ng/mL. In 2 patients receiving

Continued on next page

Invirase—Cont.

saquinavir 600 mg tid, cerebrospinal fluid concentrations were negligible when compared to concentrations from matching plasma samples.

METABOLISM AND ELIMINATION IN ADULTS: In vitro studies using human liver microsomes have shown that the metabolism of saquinavir is cytochrome P450 mediated with the specific isoenzyme, CYP3A4, responsible for more than 90% of the hepatic metabolism. Based on in vitro studies, saquinavir is rapidly metabolized to a range of mono- and di-hydroxylated inactive compounds. In a mass balance study using 600 mg ^{14}C-saquinavir (n=8), 88% and 1% of the orally administered radioactivity was recovered in feces and urine, respectively, within 5 days of dosing. In an additional 4 subjects administered 10.5 mg ^{14}C-saquinavir intravenously, 81% and 3% of the intravenously administered radioactivity was recovered in feces and urine, respectively, within 5 days of dosing. In mass balance studies, 13% of circulating radioactivity in plasma was attributed to unchanged drug after oral administration and the remainder attributed to saquinavir metabolites. Following intravenous administration, 66% of circulating radioactivity was attributed to unchanged drug and the remainder attributed to saquinavir metabolites, suggesting that saquinavir undergoes extensive first-pass metabolism.
Systemic clearance of saquinavir was rapid, 1.14 L/h/kg (CV 12%) after intravenous doses of 6, 36 and 72 mg. The mean residence time of saquinavir was 7 hours (n=8).
SPECIAL POPULATIONS: Hepatic or Renal Impairment: Saquinavir pharmacokinetics in patients with hepatic or renal insufficiency has not been investigated (see PRECAUTIONS).
Gender, Race and Age: Pharmacokinetic data were available for 17 women in the Phase 1/2 studies. Pooled data did not reveal an apparent effect of gender on the pharmacokinetics of saquinavir.
The effect of race on the pharmacokinetics of saquinavir has not been evaluated, due to the small numbers of minorities for whom pharmacokinetic data were available.
Saquinavir pharmacokinetics has not been investigated in patients >65 years of age or in pediatric patients (<16 years).
DRUG INTERACTIONS: HIVID and ZDV: Concomitant use of INVIRASE with HIVID® (zalcitabine, ddC) and ZDV has been studied (as triple combination) in adults. Pharmacokinetic data suggest that the absorption, metabolism and elimination of each of these drugs are unchanged when they are used together.
Nelfinavir: In 14 HIV-positive patients, coadministration of nelfinavir (750 mg) with saquinavir [given as FORTOVASE™ (saquinavir), 1200 mg] resulted in an 18% (95% CI 5% to 33%) increase in nelfinavir plasma AUC and a 392% (95% CI 271% to 553%) increase in saquinavir plasma AUC (see PRECAUTIONS *Drug Interactions*).
Ritonavir: Following approximately 4 weeks of a combination regimen of saquinavir (400 or 600 mg bid) and ritonavir (400 or 600 mg bid) in HIV-positive patients, saquinavir AUC and C_{max} values increased at least 17-fold (95% CI 9- to 31-fold) and 14-fold, respectively (see PRECAUTIONS *Drug Interactions*).
Delavirdine: In 13 healthy volunteers, coadministration of saquinavir (600 mg tid) with delavirdine (400 mg tid) resulted in a 5-fold increase in saquinavir AUC. In 7 healthy volunteers, coadministration of saquinavir (600 mg tid) with delavirdine (400 mg tid) resulted in a 15% ± 16% decrease in delavirdine AUC (see PRECAUTIONS *Drug Interactions*).
Nevirapine: In 23 HIV-positive patients, coadministration of saquinavir (600 mg tid) with nevirapine (200 mg bid) resulted in a 24% (95% CI 1% to 42%) and 28% (95% CI 1% to 47%) decrease in saquinavir plasma AUC and C_{max}, respectively (see PRECAUTIONS *Drug Interactions*).
Ketoconazole: Concomitant administration of ketoconazole (200 mg qd) and saquinavir (600 mg tid) to 12 healthy volunteers resulted in steady-state saquinavir AUC and C_{max} values which were three times those seen with saquinavir alone. No dose adjustment is required when the two drugs are coadministered at the doses studied. Ketoconazole pharmacokinetics was unaffected by coadministration with saquinavir.
Rifampin: Coadministration of rifampin (600 mg qd) and saquinavir (600 mg tid) to 12 healthy volunteers decreased the steady-state AUC and C_{max} of saquinavir by approximately 80%.
Rifabutin: Preliminary data from 12 HIV-infected patients indicate that the steady-state AUC of saquinavir (600 mg tid) was decreased by 40% when saquinavir was coadministered with rifabutin (300 mg qd).

INDICATIONS AND USAGE

INVIRASE in combination with other antiretroviral agents is indicated for the treatment of HIV infection. This indication is based on results from studies of surrogate marker responses and from a clinical study that showed a reduction in both mortality and AIDS-defining clinical events for patients who received INVIRASE in combination with HIVID compared to patients who received either HIVID or INVIRASE alone.
Description of Clinical Studies: Patients With Advanced HIV Infection and Prior ZDV Therapy: Study NV14256 (North America) was a randomized, double-blind study comparing the combination of INVIRASE 600 mg tid + HIVID to HIVID monotherapy and INVIRASE monotherapy. The

study accrued 970 patients, with median baseline CD$_4$ cell count at study entry of 170 cells/mm^3. Median duration of prior ZDV treatment was 17 months. Median duration of follow-up was 17 months. There were 88 first AIDS-defining events or deaths in the HIVID monotherapy group, 84 in the INVIRASE monotherapy group and 51 in the combination group. For survival there were 30 deaths in the HIVID group, 40 in the INVIRASE group and 11 deaths in the combination group.
The analysis of clinical endpoints from this study showed that the 18-month cumulative incidence of clinical disease progression to AIDS-defining event or death was 17.7% for patients randomized to INVIRASE + HIVID compared to 30.7% for patients randomized to HIVID monotherapy and 28.3% for patients randomized to INVIRASE monotherapy. The reduction in the number of clinical events for the combination regimen relative to both monotherapy regimens was statistically significant (see Figure 1 for Kaplan-Meier estimates of time to disease progression).
The 18-month cumulative mortality was 4% for patients randomized to INVIRASE + HIVID, 8.9% for patients randomized to HIVID monotherapy and 12.6% for patients randomized to INVIRASE monotherapy. The reduction in the number of deaths for the combination regimen relative to both monotherapy regimens was statistically significant (see Figure 2 for Kaplan-Meier estimates of time to death).
Figure 5 shows mean CD$_4$ changes over 48 weeks for the three treatment arms in study NV14256. Table 3 displays log RNA reductions at 16, 24 and 48 weeks among INVIRASE combination treatment arms in three clinical trials, including NV14256. Monotherapy arms are included for reference.
In ACTG229/NV14255, 295 patients (mean baseline CD$_4$=165) with prolonged ZDV treatment (median 713 days) were randomized to receive either INVIRASE 600 mg tid + HIVID + ZDV (triple combination), INVIRASE 600 mg tid + ZDV or HIVID + ZDV. In analyses of average CD$_4$ changes over 24 weeks, the triple combination produced greater increases in CD$_4$ cell counts (see Figure 4) compared to that of HIVID + ZDV. There were no significant differences in CD$_4$ changes among patients receiving INVIRASE + ZDV and HIVID + ZDV.
Comparisons of data across studies (NV14256 compared to ACTG229/NV14255) suggest that when INVIRASE was added to a regimen of prolonged prior zidovudine, there was little activity contributed by continuing ZDV.
Advanced Patients Without Prior ZDV Therapy: A dose-ranging study (Italy, V13330) conducted in 92 ZDV-naive patients (mean baseline CD$_4$=179) studied INVIRASE at doses of 75 mg, 200 mg and 600 mg tid in combination with ZDV 200 mg tid compared to INVIRASE 600 mg tid alone and ZDV alone.
In analyses of average CD$_4$ changes over 16 weeks, treatment with the combination of INVIRASE 600 mg tid + ZDV produced greater CD$_4$ cell increases than ZDV monotherapy (see Figure 3). The CD$_4$ changes of ZDV in combination with doses of INVIRASE lower than 600 mg tid were no greater than that of ZDV alone.

Table 1. Frequency of Genotypic and Phenotypic Changes in Selected Patients Treated With Saquinavir

	Genotypic*		Phenotypic†	
	24 Week	1 Year	24 Week	1 Year
Monotherapy	3/8 (38%)	15/33 (45%)	2/22 (9%)	5/11 (45%)
Combination Therapy	5/30 (17%)	16/52 (31%)	0/23 (0%)	11/29 (38%)

*Double mutation (G48V and L90M) has occurred in 2 of 33 patients receiving monotherapy. The double mutation has not occurred with combination therapy.
†Phenotypic changes have been defined as at least a 10-fold change in sensitivity relative to baseline. In a few patients genotypic and phenotypic changes were unrelated.

Table 2. Mean (% CV) AUC and C_{max} in Patients and Healthy Volunteers

	AUC_8 (dose interval) (ng·h/mL)	C_{max} (ng/mL)
Healthy Volunteers (n=6)	359.0 (46)	90.39 (49)
Patients (n=113)	757.2 (84)	253.3 (99)

[See figure 4 at top of next column]
[See figure 5 at top of next column]
[See table 3 at top of next page]

Fig. 2. Time to Death (days) NV14256

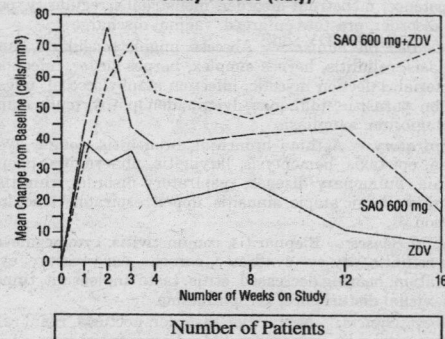

Fig. 3. Mean CD$_4$ Changes (cells/mm^3) from Baseline in Study V13330 (Italy)

Number of Patients		
Week	0	16
SAQ	15	14
ZDV	13	12
SAQ+ZDV	15	14

CONTRAINDICATIONS

INVIRASE is contraindicated in patients with clinically significant hypersensitivity to saquinavir or to any of the components contained in the capsule.
INVIRASE should not be administered concurrently with terfenadine, cisapride, astemizole, triazolam, midazolam or ergot derivatives. Inhibition of CYP3A4 by saquinavir could result in elevated plasma concentrations of these drugs, potentially causing serious or life-threatening reactions.

WARNINGS

New onset diabetes mellitus, exacerbation of preexisting diabetes mellitus and hyperglycemia have been reported during postmarketing surveillance in HIV-infected patients receiving protease inhibitor therapy. Some patients required either initiation or dose adjustments of insulin or oral hypoglycemic agents for treatment of these events. In some cases diabetic ketoacidosis has occurred. In those patients who discontinued protease inhibitor therapy, hyperglycemia persisted in some cases. Because these events have been reported voluntarily during clinical practice, estimates of frequency cannot be made and a causal relationship between protease inhibitor therapy and these events has not been established.

Fig. 1. Time to First AIDS-Defining Event (or Death) (days) NV14256

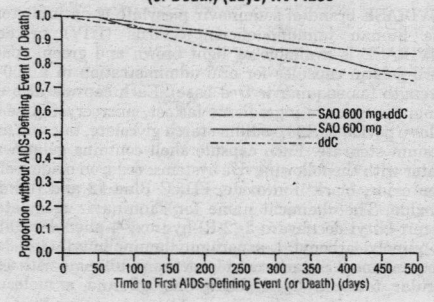

Table 3. Summary of Mean Log$_{10}$ Plasma RNA Results From Major INVIRASE Clinical Studies

	V13330 (Italy) Naive patients			NV14255/ACTG229 (USA) ZDV-experienced			NV14256 (North America) ZDV-experienced		
	ZDV	SAQ*	ZDV+SAQ	ZDV+ddC	ZDV+SAQ	ZDV+ddC+SAQ	ddC	SAQ	SAQ+ddC
n Enrolled	17	19	20	100	99	98	314	318	308
Prior ZDV									
n	—	—	—	99	98	97	305	315	304
Median Duration (days)	—	—	—	659	713	647	521	523	477
Log$_{10}$ Plasma RNA by PCR (copies/mL)									
n	17	19	20	100	97	96	300	307	294
Mean Baseline (n)	5.2 (17)	5.2 (19)	5.3 (20)	4.7 (100)	4.8 (97)	4.8 (96)	5.0 (300)	5.1 (307)	5.0 (294)
Mean Change from Baseline Week 16 (n)	−0.5 (15)	−0.2 (17)	−1.0 (17)	−0.3 (93)	0.0 (81)	−0.5 (86)	−0.4 (253)	−0.1 (262)	−0.6 (258)
Mean Change from Baseline Week 24 (n)	—	—	—	−0.2 (86)	0.0 (83)	−0.6 (84)	−0.3 (228)	−0.1 (244)	−0.6 (232)
Mean Change from Baseline Week 48 (n)	—	—	—	—	—	—	−0.3 (147)	−0.1 (167)	−0.6 (169)

* Saquinavir (SAQ) at 600 mg tid   — Indicates not applicable

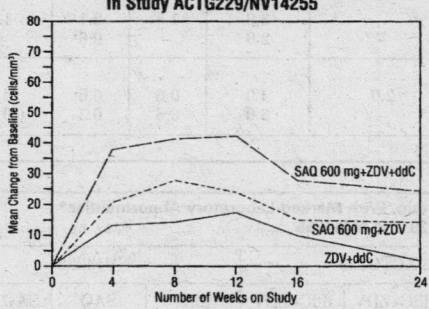

Fig. 4. Mean CD$_4$ Changes (cells/mm^3) from Baseline in Study ACTG229/NV14255

Number of Patients			
Week	0	12	24
ZDV+ddC	100	88	87
SAQ+ZDV	98	88	87
SAQ+ZDV+ddC	97	87	89

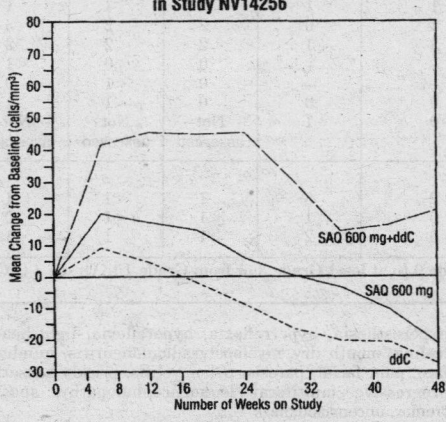

Fig. 5. Mean CD$_4$ Changes (cells/mm^3) from Baseline in Study NV14256

Number of Patients				
Week	0	12	24	48
ddC	313	258	235	154
SAQ+ddC	307	271	255	179
SAQ	317	263	242	175

Concomitant use of INVIRASE with lovastatin or simvastatin is not recommended. Caution should be exercised if HIV protease inhibitors, including INVIRASE, are used concurrently with other HMG-CoA reductase inhibitors that are also metabolized by the CYP3A4 pathway (eg, atorvastatin or cerivastatin). Since increased concentrations of statins can, in rare cases, cause severe adverse events such as myopathy including rhabdomyolysis, this risk may be increased when HIV protease inhibitors, including saquinavir, are used in combination with these drugs.[3, 4]

PRECAUTIONS
General: INVIRASE (saquinavir mesylate) capsules and FORTOVASE (saquinavir) soft gelatin capsules are not bioequivalent and cannot be used interchangeably. Only FORTOVASE should be used for the initiation of saquinavir therapy (see DOSAGE AND ADMINISTRATION) since

FORTOVASE soft gelatin capsules provide greater bioavailability and efficacy than INVIRASE capsules. For patients taking INVIRASE capsules with a viral load below the limit of quantification, a switch to FORTOVASE is recommended to maintain a virologic response. For patients taking INVIRASE capsules who have not had an adequate response or are failing therapy, if saquinavir resistance is clinically suspected, then FORTOVASE should not be used.[5] If resistance to saquinavir is not clinically suspected, a switch to FORTOVASE may be considered.[1, 2]
The safety profile of INVIRASE in pediatric patients younger than 16 years has not been established.
If a serious or severe toxicity occurs during treatment with INVIRASE, INVIRASE should be interrupted until the etiology of the event is identified or the toxicity resolves. At that time, resumption of treatment with full-dose INVIRASE may be considered. For nucleoside analogues used in combination with INVIRASE, physicians should refer to the complete product information for these drugs for dose adjustment recommendations and for information regarding drug-associated adverse reactions.
Caution should be exercised when administering INVIRASE to patients with hepatic insufficiency since patients with baseline liver function tests >5 times the upper limit of normal were not included in clinical studies. Although a causal relationship has not been established, exacerbation of chronic liver dysfunction, including portal hypertension, has been reported in patients with underlying hepatitis B or C, cirrhosis or other underlying liver abnormalities.
There have been reports of spontaneous bleeding in patients with hemophilia A and B treated with protease inhibitors. In some patients additional factor VIII was required. In the majority of reported cases treatment with protease inhibitors was continued or restarted. A causal relationship between protease inhibitor therapy and these episodes has not been established.
Fat Redistribution: Redistribution/accumulation of body fat including central obesity, dorsocervical fat enlargement (buffalo hump), peripheral wasting, breast enlargement, and "cushingoid appearance" have been observed in patients receiving protease inhibitors. A causal relationship between protease inhibitor therapy and these events has not been established and the long-term consequences are currently unknown.[6, 2, 7]
Resistance/Cross-resistance: The potential for HIV cross-resistance between protease inhibitors has not been fully explored. Therefore, it is unknown what effect saquinavir therapy will have on the activity of subsequent protease inhibitors (see *Microbiology*).
Information for Patients: Patients should be informed that INVIRASE is not a cure for HIV infection and that they may continue to acquire illnesses associated with advanced HIV infection, including opportunistic infections. Patients should be advised that INVIRASE should be used only in combination with an active nucleoside analogue regimen.
Patients should be informed that redistribution or accumulation of body fat may occur in patients receiving protease inhibitors and that the cause and long-term health effects of these conditions are not known at this time.[6]
Patients should be told that the long-term effects of INVIRASE are unknown at this time. They should be informed that INVIRASE therapy has not been shown to reduce the risk of transmitting HIV to others through sexual contact or blood contamination.
Patients should be advised that INVIRASE should be taken within 2 hours after a full meal (see *Pharmacokinetics*). When INVIRASE is taken without food, concentrations of saquinavir in the blood are substantially reduced and may result in no antiviral activity.
Laboratory Tests: Clinical chemistry tests should be performed prior to initiating INVIRASE therapy and at appropriate intervals thereafter. For comprehensive information concerning laboratory test alterations associated with use of individual nucleoside analogues, physicians should refer to the complete product information for these drugs.

Drug Interactions: METABOLIC ENZYME INDUCERS: INVIRASE should not be administered concomitantly with rifampin, since rifampin decreases saquinavir concentrations by 80% (see *Pharmacokinetics*). Rifabutin also substantially reduces saquinavir plasma concentrations by 40%. Other drugs that induce CYP3A4 (eg, phenobarbital, phenytoin, dexamethasone, carbamazepine) may also reduce saquinavir plasma concentrations. If therapy with such drugs is warranted, physicians should consider using alternatives when a patient is taking INVIRASE.
OTHER POTENTIAL INTERACTIONS: Coadministration of terfenadine, astemizole or cisapride with drugs that are known to be potent inhibitors of the cytochrome P4503A pathway (ie, ketoconazole, itraconazole, etc.) may lead to elevated plasma concentrations of terfenadine, astemizole or cisapride, which may in turn prolong QT intervals leading to rare cases of serious cardiovascular adverse events. Although INVIRASE is not a strong inhibitor of cytochrome P4503A, pharmacokinetic interaction studies with INVIRASE and terfenadine, astemizole or cisapride have not been conducted. Physicians should use alternatives to terfenadine, astemizole or cisapride when a patient is taking INVIRASE. Other compounds that are substrates of CYP3A4 (eg, calcium channel blockers, clindamycin, dapsone, quinidine, triazolam) may have elevated plasma concentrations when coadministered with INVIRASE; therefore, patients should be monitored for toxicities associated with such drugs.
ANTI-HIV COMPOUNDS: Nelfinavir: Coadministration of nelfinavir with saquinavir (given as FORTOVASE, 1200 mg) resulted in an 18% increase in nelfinavir plasma AUC and a 4-fold increase in saquinavir plasma AUC. If used in combination with saquinavir hard-gelatin capsules at the recommended dose of 600 mg tid, no dose adjustments are needed. Currently, there are no safety and efficacy data available from the use of this combination.
Ritonavir: Following approximately 4 weeks of a combination regimen of saquinavir (400 or 600 mg bid) and ritonavir (400 or 600 mg bid) in HIV-positive patients, saquinavir AUC values were at least 17-fold greater than historical AUC values from patients who received saquinavir 600 mg tid without ritonavir. When used in combination therapy for up to 24 weeks, doses greater than 400 mg bid of either ritonavir or saquinavir were associated with an increase in adverse events.
Delavirdine: Saquinavir AUC increased 5-fold when delavirdine (400 mg tid) and saquinavir (600 mg tid) were administered in combination. Currently, there are limited safety and no efficacy data available from the use of this combination. In a small, preliminary study, hepatocellular enzyme elevations occurred in 15% of subjects during the first several weeks of the delavirdine and saquinavir combination (6% Grade 3 or 4). Hepatocellular enzymes (ALT/AST) should be monitored frequently if this combination is prescribed.
Nevirapine: Coadministration of nevirapine with INVIRASE resulted in a 24% decrease in saquinavir plasma AUC. Currently, there are no safety and efficacy data available from the use of this combination.
ERECTILE DYSFUNCTION AGENTS:[8]
Sildenafil: In a study performed in healthy male volunteers, coadministration of saquinavir, a CYP3A4 inhibitor, at steady state (1200 mg tid) with sildenafil (100 mg single dose) resulted in a 140% increase in sildenafil C$_{max}$ and a 210% increase in sildenafil AUC. Sildenafil had no effect on saquinavir pharmacokinetics. When sildenafil is administered concomitantly with saquinavir a starting dose of 25 mg[8] of sildenafil should be considered.[9, 10]
Carcinogenesis, Mutagenesis and Impairment of Fertility:
Carcinogenesis: Carcinogenicity studies in rats and mice have not yet been completed.
Mutagenesis: Mutagenicity and genotoxicity studies, with and without metabolic activation where appropriate, have shown that saquinavir has no mutagenic activity in vitro in either bacterial (Ames test) or mammalian cells (Chinese hamster lung V79/HPRT test). Saquinavir does not induce chromosomal damage in vivo in the mouse micronucleus as-

Continued on next page

Invirase—Cont.

say or in vitro in human peripheral blood lymphocytes, and does not induce primary DNA damage in vitro in the unscheduled DNA synthesis test.

Impairment of Fertility: Fertility and reproductive performance were not affected in rats at plasma exposures (AUC values) up to five times those achieved in humans at the recommended dose.

Pregnancy: Teratogenic Effects: Category B. Reproduction studies conducted with saquinavir in rats have shown no embryotoxicity or teratogenicity at plasma exposures (AUC values) up to five times those achieved in humans at the recommended dose or in rabbits at plasma exposures four times those achieved at the recommended clinical dose. Studies in rats indicated that exposure to saquinavir from late pregnancy through lactation at plasma concentrations (AUC values) up to five times those achieved in humans at the recommended dose had no effect on the survival, growth and development of offspring to weaning. Because animal reproduction studies are not always predictive of human response, INVIRASE should be used during pregnancy after taking into account the importance of the drug to the mother. Presently, there are no reports of infants being born after women receiving INVIRASE in clinical trials became pregnant.

Antiretroviral Pregnancy Registry: To monitor maternal-fetal outcomes of pregnant women exposed to antiretroviral medications, including INVIRASE, an Antiretroviral Pregnancy Registry has been established. Physicians are encouraged to register patients by calling 1-800-258-4263.[11]

Nursing Mothers: **The Centers for Disease Control and Prevention recommend that HIV-infected mothers not breastfeed their infants to avoid risking postnatal transmission of HIV.** It is not known whether saquinavir is excreted in human milk. Because of both the potential for HIV transmission and the potential for serious adverse reactions in nursing infants, **mothers should be instructed not to breastfeed if they are receiving antiretroviral medications, including INVIRASE.[11]**

Pediatric Use: Safety and effectiveness of INVIRASE in HIV-infected pediatric patients younger than 16 years of age have not been established.

Geriatric Use: Clinical studies of INVIRASE did not include sufficient numbers of subjects aged 65 and over to determine whether they respond differently from younger subjects. In general, caution should be taken when dosing INVIRASE in elderly patients due to the greater frequency of decreased hepatic, renal, or cardiac function, and of concomitant disease or other drug therapy.[12, 2]

ADVERSE REACTIONS (see PRECAUTIONS)

The safety of INVIRASE was studied in patients who received the drug either alone or in combination with ZDV and/or HIVID (zalcitabine, ddC). The majority of adverse events were of mild intensity. The most frequently reported adverse events among patients receiving INVIRASE (excluding those toxicities known to be associated with ZDV and HIVID when used in combinations) were diarrhea, abdominal discomfort and nausea.

INVIRASE did not alter the pattern, frequency or severity of known major toxicities associated with the use of HIVID and/or ZDV. Physicians should refer to the complete product information for these drugs (or other antiretroviral agents as appropriate) for drug-associated adverse reactions to other nucleoside analogues.

In an open-label protocol, NV15114, in which 33 patients received treatment with INVIRASE, ZDV and lamivudine for 4 to 16 weeks, no unexpected toxicities were reported.

Table 4 lists clinical adverse events that occurred in ≥2% of patients receiving INVIRASE 600 mg tid alone or in combination with ZDV and/or HIVID in two trials. Median duration of treatment in NV14255/ACTG229 (triple-combination study) was 48 weeks; median duration of treatment in NV14256 (double-combination study) was approximately 1 year.

[See table 4 above]

Rare occurrences of the following serious adverse experiences have been reported during clinical trials of INVIRASE and were considered at least possibly related to use of study drugs: confusion, ataxia and weakness; acute myeloblastic leukemia; hemolytic anemia; attempted suicide; Stevens-Johnson syndrome; seizures; severe cutaneous reaction associated with increased liver function tests; isolated elevation of transaminases; thrombophlebitis; headache; thrombocytopenia; exacerbation of chronic liver disease with Grade 4 elevated liver function tests, jaundice, ascites, and right and left upper quadrant abdominal pain; drug fever; bullous skin eruption and polyarthritis; pancreatitis leading to death; nephrolithiasis; thrombocytopenia and intracranial hemorrhage leading to death; peripheral vasoconstriction; portal hypertension; intestinal obstruction. These events were reported from a database of >6000 patients. Over 100 patients on saquinavir therapy have been followed for >2 years.

Table 5 shows the percentage of patients with marked laboratory abnormalities in studies NV14255/ACTG229 and NV14256. Marked laboratory abnormalities are defined as a Grade 3 or 4 abnormality in a patient with a normal baseline value or a Grade 4 abnormality in a patient with a Grade 1 abnormality at baseline (ACTG Grading System). [See table 5 above]

Monotherapy and Combination Studies: Other clinical adverse experiences of any intensity, at least remotely related to INVIRASE, including those in <2% of patients on arms

Table 4. Percentage of Patients, by Study Arm, With Clinical Adverse Experiences Considered at Least Possibly Related to Study Drug or of Unknown Relationship and of Moderate, Severe or Life-threatening Intensity, Occurring in ≥2% of Patients in NV14255/ACTG229 and NV14256

ADVERSE EVENT	NV14255/ACTG229			NV14256		
	SAQ+ZDV n=99	SAQ+ddC+ZDV n=98	ddC+ZDV n=100	ddC n=325	SAQ n=327	SAQ+ddC n=318
GASTROINTESTINAL						
Diarrhea	3.0	1.0	–	0.9	4.9	4.4
Abdominal Discomfort	2.0	3.1	4.0	0.9	0.9	0.9
Nausea	–	3.1	3.0	1.5	2.4	0.9
Dyspepsia	1.0	1.0	2.0	0.6	0.9	0.9
Abdominal Pain	2.0	1.0	2.0	0.6	1.2	0.3
Mucosa Damage	–	–	4.0	–	–	0.3
Buccal Mucosa Ulceration	–	2.0	2.0	6.2	2.1	3.8
CENTRAL AND PERIPHERAL NERVOUS SYSTEM						
Headache	2.0	2.0	2.0	3.4	2.4	0.9
Paresthesia	2.0	3.1	4.0	1.2	0.3	0.3
Extremity Numbness	2.0	1.0	4.0	1.5	0.6	0.9
Dizziness	–	2.0	1.0	–	0.3	–
Peripheral Neuropathy	–	1.0	2.0	11.4	3.1	11.3
BODY AS A WHOLE						
Asthenia	6.1	9.2	10.0	–	0.3	–
Appetite Disturbances	–	1.0	2.0	–	–	–
SKIN AND APPENDAGES						
Rash	–	–	3.0	1.5	2.1	1.3
Pruritus	–	–	2.0	–	0.6	–
MUSCULOSKELETAL DISORDERS						
Musculoskeletal Pain	2.0	2.0	4.0	0.6	0.6	0.6
Myalgia	1.0	–	3.0	0.6	0.3	0.3

– Indicates no events reported

Table 5. Percentage of Patients, by Treatment Group, With Marked Laboratory Abnormalities* in NV14255/ACTG229 and NV14256

ADVERSE EVENT	NV14255/ACTG229			NV14256		
	SAQ+ZDV n=99	SAQ+ddC+ZDV n=98	ddC+ZDV n=100	ddC n=325	SAQ n=327	SAQ+ddC n=318
BIOCHEMISTRY						
Calcium (high)	1	0	0	<1	0	0
Calcium (low)	–	–	–	<1	<1	0
Creatinine Phosphokinase (high)	10	12	7	6	3	7
Glucose (high)	0	0	0	<1	1	1
Glucose (low)	0	0	0	5	5	5
Phosphate (low)	2	1	0	0	<1	<1
Potassium (high)	0	0	0	2	2	3
Potassium (low)	0	0	0	0	1	0
Serum Amylase (high)	2	1	1	2	1	1
SGOT (AST) (high)	2	2	0	2	2	3
SGPT (ALT) (high)	0	3	1	2	2	2
Sodium (high)	–	–	–	0	0	<1
Sodium (low)	–	–	–	0	<1	0
Total Bilirubin (high)	1	0	0	0	<1	1
Uric Acid	0	0	1	Not assessed	Not assessed	Not assessed
HEMATOLOGY						
Neutrophils (low)	2	2	8	1	1	1
Hemoglobin (low)	0	0	1	<1	<1	0
Platelets (low)	0	0	2	1	1	<1

*Marked Laboratory Abnormality defined as a shift from Grade 0 to at least Grade 3 or from Grade 1 to Grade 4 (ACTG Grading System)

containing INVIRASE in studies NV14255/ACTG229 and NV14256, and those in smaller clinical trials, are listed below by body system.

Body as a Whole: Allergic reaction, anorexia, chest pain, edema, fatigue, fever, intoxication, parasites external, retrosternal pain, shivering, wasting syndrome, weakness generalized, weight decrease, redistribution/accumulation of body fat (see PRECAUTIONS *Fat Redistribution*)[6]

Cardiovascular: Cyanosis, heart murmur, heart valve disorder, hypertension, hypotension, syncope, vein distended

Endocrine/Metabolic: Dehydration, diabetes mellitus, dry eye syndrome, hyperglycemia, weight increase, xerophthalmia

Gastrointestinal: Cheilitis, colic abdominal, constipation, dyspepsia, dysphagia, esophagitis, eructation, feces blood-stained, feces discolored, flatulence, gastralgia, gastritis, gastrointestinal inflammation, gingivitis, glossitis, hemorrhage rectum, hemorrhoids, hepatitis, hepatomegaly, hepatosplenomegaly, infectious diarrhea, jaundice, liver enzyme disorder, melena, pain pelvic, painful defecation, pancreatitis, parotid disorder, salivary glands disorder, stomach upset, stomatitis, toothache, tooth disorder, vomiting

Hematologic: Anemia, bleeding dermal, microhemorrhages, neutropenia, pancytopenia, splenomegaly, thrombocytopenia

Musculoskeletal: Arthralgia, arthritis, back pain, cramps leg, cramps muscle, creatine phosphokinase increased, musculoskeletal disorders, stiffness, tissue changes, trauma

Neurological: Ataxia, bowel movements frequent, confusion, convulsions, dysarthria, dysesthesia, heart rate disorder, hyperesthesia, hyperreflexia, hyporeflexia, light-headed feeling, mouth dry, myelopolyradiculoneuritis, numbness face, pain facial, paresis, poliomyelitis, prickly sensation, progressive multifocal leukoencephalopathy, spasms, tremor, unconsciousness

Psychological: Agitation, amnesia, anxiety, anxiety attack, depression, dreaming excessive, euphoria, hallucination, insomnia, intellectual ability reduced, irritability, lethargy, libido disorder, overdose effect, psychic disorder, psychosis, somnolence, speech disorder, suicide attempt

Reproductive System: Impotence, prostate enlarged, vaginal discharge

Resistance Mechanism: Abscess, angina tonsillaris, candidiasis, cellulitis, herpes simplex, herpes zoster, infection bacterial, infection mycotic, infection staphylococcal, influenza, lymphadenopathy, moniliasis, tumor

Respiratory: Bronchitis, cough, dyspnea, epistaxis, hemoptysis, laryngitis, pharyngitis, pneumonia, pulmonary disease, respiratory disorder, rhinitis, sinusitis, upper respiratory tract infection

Skin and Appendages: Acne, alopecia, chalazion, dermatitis, dermatitis seborrheic, eczema, erythema, folliculitis, furunculosis, hair changes, hot flushes, nail disorder, night sweats, papillomatosis, photosensitivity reaction, pigment changes skin, rash maculopapular, skin disorder, skin nodule, skin ulceration, sweating increased, urticaria, verruca, xeroderma

Special Senses: Blepharitis, earache, ear pressure, eye irritation, hearing decreased, otitis, taste alteration, tinnitus, visual disturbance

Urinary System: Micturition disorder, renal calculus, urinary tract bleeding, urinary tract infection

OVERDOSAGE

No acute toxicities or sequelae were noted in 1 patient who ingested 8 grams of INVIRASE as a single dose. The patient was treated with induction of emesis within 2 to 4 hours after ingestion. In an exploratory Phase 2 study of oral dosing with INVIRASE at 7200 mg/day (1200 mg q4h), there were no serious toxicities reported through the first 25 weeks of treatment.

DOSAGE AND ADMINISTRATION

INVIRASE (saquinavir mesylate) capsules and FORTOVASE (saquinavir) soft gelatin capsules are not bioequivalent and cannot be used interchangeably. When using saquinavir as part of an antiviral regimen FORTOVASE is the recommended formulation. In rare circumstances, INVIRASE may be considered if it is to be combined with antiretrovirals that significantly inhibit saquinavir's metabolism (see CLINICAL PHARMACOLOGY: *DRUG INTERACTIONS***).[1, 2]**
The recommended dose for INVIRASE in combination with a nucleoside analogue is three 200-mg capsules three times daily taken within 2 hours after a full meal. Please refer to the complete product information for each of the nucleoside analogues for the recommended doses of these agents.
INVIRASE should be used only in combination with an active antiretroviral nucleoside analogue regimen. Concomitant therapy should be based on a patient's prior drug exposure.
Monitoring of Patients: Clinical chemistry tests should be performed prior to initiating INVIRASE therapy and at appropriate intervals thereafter. For comprehensive patient monitoring recommendations for other nucleoside analogues, physicians should refer to the complete product information for these drugs.
Dose Adjustment for Combination Therapy With INVIRASE: For toxicities that may be associated with INVIRASE, the drug should be interrupted. INVIRASE at doses less than 600 mg tid are not recommended since lower doses have not shown antiviral activity. For recipients of combination therapy with INVIRASE and nucleoside analogues, dose adjustment of the nucleoside analogue should be based on the known toxicity profile of the individual drug. Physicians should refer to the complete product information for these drugs for comprehensive dose adjustment recommendations and drug-associated adverse reactions of nucleoside analogues.

HOW SUPPLIED

INVIRASE 200-mg capsules are light brown and green opaque capsules with ROCHE and 0245 imprinted on the capsule shell—bottles of 270 (NDC 0004-0245-15).
The capsules should be stored at 59° to 86°F (15° to 30°C) in tightly closed bottles.
Rx only
Manufactured by:
F. Hoffmann-La Roche Ltd., Basel, Switzerland or Hoffmann-La Roche Inc., Nutley, New Jersey
Distributed by:
Pharmaceuticals
Roche Laboratories Inc.
340 Kingsland Street
Nutley, New Jersey 07110-1199
Revised: October 2000
Printed in USA
Copyright © 1998-2000 by Roche Laboratories Inc. All rights reserved.

Annotations
1. FDA letter dated June 25, 1998.
2. FDA fax of January 28, 2000.
3. FDA letter dated October 6, 1999.
4. Weder S, Jorga K.
   Drug Safety issue work-up: Drug interaction between saquinavir and HMG-CoA reductase Inhibitors.
   Hoffmann-La Roche, Basel, September 14, 1999.
5. FDA fax dated June 14, 2000.
6. FDA letter dated August 31, 1998.
7. FDA fax dated April 14, 2000.
8. FDA fax dated September 18, 2000.
9. Hall MCS, Ahmad S.
   Interaction between sildenafil and HIV-1 combination therapy.
   Lancet 1999; 353: 2071-2072
10. Weder S, Jorga K.
    Drug Safety issue work-up: Drug interaction between saquinavir and sildenafil.
    Hoffmann-La Roche, Basel, August 30, 1999.
11. FDA fax dated May 26, 2000, transmitted June 1, 2000.
12. 21 CFR §201.57(f)(10)(ii)(A)

ROCEPHIN®   ℞
[ro-sef ' in]
(ceftriaxone sodium)
FOR INJECTION

Prescribing information for this product, which appears on pages 2765–2768 of the 2001 PDR, has been completely revised as follows. Please write "See Supplement A" next to the product heading.

TABLE 1. Ceftriaxone Plasma Concentrations After Single Dose Administration

Dose/Route	Average Plasma Concentrations (µg/mL)								
	0.5 hr	1 hr	2 hr	4 hr	6 hr	8 hr	12 hr	16 hr	24 hr
0.5 gm IV*	82	59	48	37	29	23	15	10	5
0.5 gm IM 250 mg/mL	22	33	38	35	30	26	16	ND	5
0.5 gm IM 350 mg/mL	20	32	38	34	31	24	16	ND	5
1 gm IV*	151	111	88	67	53	43	28	18	9
1 gm IM	40	68	76	68	56	44	29	ND	ND
2 gm IV*	257	192	154	117	89	74	46	31	15

*IV doses were infused at a constant rate over 30 minutes.
ND = Not determined.

TABLE 2. Urinary Concentrations of Ceftriaxone After Single Dose Administration

Dose/Route	Average Urinary Concentrations (µg/mL)					
	0–2 hr	2–4 hr	4–8 hr	8–12 hr	12–24 hr	24–48 hr
0.5 gm IV	526	366	142	87	70	15
0.5 gm IM	115	425	308	127	96	28
1 gm IV	995	855	293	147	132	32
1 gm IM	504	628	418	237	ND*	ND
2 gm IV	2692	1976	757	274	198	40

*ND = Not determined.

TABLE 3. Average Pharmacokinetic Parameters of Ceftriaxone in Pediatric Patients With Meningitis

	50 mg/kg IV	75 mg/kg IV
Maximum Plasma Concentrations (µg/mL)	216	275
Elimination Half-life (hr)	4.6	4.3
Plasma Clearance (mL/hr/kg)	49	60
Volume of Distribution (mL/kg)	338	373
CSF Concentration—inflamed meninges (µg/mL)	5.6	6.4
Range (µg/mL)	1.3–18.5	1.3–44
Time after dose (hr)	3.7 (± 1.6)	3.3 (± 1.4)

DESCRIPTION

Rocephin is a sterile, semisynthetic, broad-spectrum cephalosporin antibiotic for intravenous or intramuscular administration. Ceftriaxone sodium is (6*R*,7*R*)-7-[2-(2-Amino-4-thiazolyl)glyoxylamido]-8-oxo-3-[[(1,2,5,6-tetrahydro-2-methyl-5,6-dioxo-*as*-triazin-3-yl)thio]methyl]-5-thia-1-azabicyclo[4.2.0]oct-2-ene-2-carboxylic acid, 7^2-(*Z*)-(*O*-methyloxime), disodium salt, sesquaterhydrate.
The chemical formula of ceftriaxone sodium is $C_{18}H_{16}N_8Na_2O_7S_3$•3.5H$_2$O. It has a calculated molecular weight of 661.59 and the following structural formula:

Rocephin is a white to yellowish-orange crystalline powder which is readily soluble in water, sparingly soluble in methanol and very slightly soluble in ethanol. The pH of a 1% aqueous solution is approximately 6.7. The color of Rocephin solutions ranges from light yellow to amber, depending on the length of storage, concentration and diluent used.
Rocephin contains approximately 83 mg (3.6 mEq) of sodium per gram of ceftriaxone activity.

CLINICAL PHARMACOLOGY

Average plasma concentrations of ceftriaxone following a single 30-minute intravenous (IV) infusion of a 0.5, 1 or 2 gm dose and intramuscular (IM) administration of a single 0.5 (250 mg/mL or 350 mg/mL concentrations) or 1 gm dose in healthy subjects are presented in Table 1.
[See table 1 above]
Ceftriaxone was completely absorbed following IM administration with mean maximum plasma concentrations occurring between 2 and 3 hours postdosing. Multiple IV or IM doses ranging from 0.5 to 2 gm at 12- to 24-hour intervals resulted in 15% to 36% accumulation of ceftriaxone above single dose values.
Ceftriaxone concentrations in urine are high, as shown in Table 2.
[See table 2 above]
Thirty-three percent to 67% of a ceftriaxone dose was excreted in the urine as unchanged drug and the remainder was secreted in the bile and ultimately found in the feces as microbiologically inactive compounds. After a 1 gm IV dose, average concentrations of ceftriaxone, determined from 1 to 3 hours after dosing, were 581 µg/mL in the gallbladder bile, 788 µg/mL in the common duct bile, 898 µg/mL in the cystic duct bile, 78.2 µg/gm in the gallbladder wall and 62.1 µg/mL in the concurrent plasma.
Over a 0.15 to 3 gm dose range in healthy adult subjects, the values of elimination half-life ranged from 5.8 to 8.7 hours; apparent volume of distribution from 5.78 to 13.5 L; plasma clearance from 0.58 to 1.45 L/hour; and renal clearance from 0.32 to 0.73 L/hour. Ceftriaxone is reversibly bound to human plasma proteins, and the binding decreased from a value of 95% bound at plasma concentrations of <25 µg/mL to a value of 85% bound at 300 µg/mL. Ceftriaxone crosses the blood placenta barrier.
The average values of maximum plasma concentration, elimination half-life, plasma clearance and volume of distribution after a 50 mg/kg IV dose and after a 75 mg/kg IV dose in pediatric patients suffering from bacterial meningitis are shown in Table 3. Ceftriaxone penetrated the inflamed meninges of infants and pediatric patients; CSF concentrations after a 50 mg/kg IV dose and after a 75 mg/kg IV dose are also shown in Table 3.
[See table 3 above]
Compared to that in healthy adult subjects, the pharmacokinetics of ceftriaxone were only minimally altered in elderly subjects and in patients with renal impairment or hepatic dysfunction (Table 4); therefore, dosage adjustments are not necessary for these patients with ceftriaxone dosages up to 2 gm per day. Ceftriaxone was not removed to any significant extent from the plasma by hemodialysis. In 6 of 26 dialysis patients, the elimination rate of ceftriaxone was markedly reduced, suggesting that plasma concentrations of ceftriaxone should be monitored in these patients to determine if dosage adjustments are necessary.
[See table 4 at top of next page]
Pharmacokinetics in the Middle Ear Fluid: In one study, total ceftriaxone concentrations (bound and unbound) were measured in middle ear fluid obtained during the insertion of tympanostomy tubes in 42 pediatric patients with otitis media. Sampling times were from 1 to 50 hours after a single intramuscular injection of 50 mg/kg of ceftriaxone. Mean (± SD) ceftriaxone levels in the middle ear reached a peak of 35 (± 12) µg/mL at 24 hours, and remained at 19 (± 7) µg/mL at 48 hours. Based on middle ear fluid ceftriaxone concentrations in the 23 to 25 hour and the 46 to 50 hour sampling time intervals, a half-life of 25 hours was calculated. Ceftriaxone is highly bound to plasma proteins. The extent of binding to proteins in the middle ear fluid is unknown.
Microbiology: The bactericidal activity of ceftriaxone results from inhibition of cell wall synthesis. Ceftriaxone has a high degree of stability in the presence of beta-lactamases, both penicillinases and cephalosporinases, of gram-negative and gram-positive bacteria.
Ceftriaxone has been shown to be active against most strains of the following microorganisms, both in vitro and in clinical infections described in the INDICATIONS AND USAGE section.
Aerobic gram-negative microorganisms:
Acinetobacter calcoaceticus
Enterobacter aerogenes
Enterobacter cloacae
Escherichia coli
Haemophilus influenzae (including ampicillin-resistant and beta-lactamase producing strains)
Haemophilus parainfluenzae
Klebsiella oxytoca
Klebsiella pneumoniae
Moraxella catarrhalis (including beta-lactamase producing strains)

Continued on next page

Rocephin—Cont.

Morganella morganii
Neisseria gonorrhoeae (including penicillinase- and nonpenicillinase-producing strains)
Neisseria meningitidis
Proteus mirabilis
Proteus vulgaris
Serratia marcescens
Ceftriaxone is also active against many strains of *Pseudomonas aeruginosa*.
NOTE: Many strains of the above organisms that are multiply resistant to other antibiotics, eg, penicillins, cephalosporins, and aminoglycosides, are susceptible to ceftriaxone.
Aerobic gram-positive microorganisms:
Staphylococcus aureus (including penicillinase-producing strains)
Staphylococcus epidermidis
Streptococcus pneumoniae
Streptococcus pyogenes
Viridans group streptococci
NOTE: Methicillin-resistant staphylococci are resistant to cephalosporins, including ceftriaxone. Most strains of Group D streptococci and enterococci, eg, *Enterococcus (Streptococcus) faecalis*, are resistant.
Anaerobic microorganisms:
Bacteroides fragilis
Clostridium species
Peptostreptococcus species
NOTE: Most strains of *Clostridium difficile* are resistant.
The following in vitro data are available, **but their clinical significance is unknown**. Ceftriaxone exhibits in vitro minimal inhibitory concentrations (MICs) of • 8 µg/mL or less against most strains of the following microorganisms, however, the safety and effectiveness of ceftriaxone in treating clinical infections due to these microorganisms have not been established in adequate and well-controlled clinical trials.
Aerobic gram-negative microorganisms:
Citrobacter diversus
Citrobacter freundii
Providencia species (including *Providencia rettgeri*)
Salmonella species (including *Salmonella typhi*)
Shigella species
Aerobic gram-positive microorganisms:
Streptococcus agalactiae
Anaerobic microorganisms:
Prevotella (Bacteroides) bivius
Porphyromonas (Bacteroides) melaninogenicus

Susceptibility Tests:

Dilution Techniques: Quantitative methods are used to determine antimicrobial minimal inhibitory concentrations (MICs). These MICs provide estimates of the susceptibility of bacteria to antimicrobial compounds. The MICs should be determined using a standardized procedure.[1] Standardized procedures are based on a dilution method (broth or agar) or equivalent with standardized inoculum concentrations and standardized concentrations of ceftriaxone powder. The MIC values should be interpreted according to the following criteria[2] for aerobic organisms other than *Haemophilus* spp, *Neisseria gonorrhoeae*, and *Streptococcus* spp, including *Streptococcus pneumoniae:*

MIC (µg/mL)	Interpretation
• 8	(S) Susceptible
16–32	(I) Intermediate
• 64	(R) Resistant

The following interpretive criteria[2] should be used when testing *Haemophilus* species using Haemophilus Test Media (HTM).

MIC (µg/mL)	Interpretation
• 2	(S) Susceptible

The absence of resistant strains precludes defining any categories other than "Susceptible". Strains yielding results suggestive of a "Nonsusceptible" category should be submitted to a reference laboratory for further testing.
The following interpretive criteria[2] should be used when testing *Neisseria gonorrhoeae* when using GC agar base and 1% defined growth supplement.

MIC (µg/mL)	Interpretation
• 0.25	(S) Susceptible

The absence of resistant strains precludes defining any categories other than "Susceptible". Strains yielding results suggestive of a "Nonsusceptible" category should be submitted to a reference laboratory for further testing.
The following interpretive criteria[2] should be used when testing *Streptococcus* spp including *Streptococcus pneumoniae* using cation-adjusted Mueller-Hinton broth with 2 to 5% lysed horse blood.

MIC (µg/mL)	Interpretation
• 0.5	(S) Susceptible
1	(I) Intermediate
• 2	(R) Resistant

A report of "Susceptible" indicates that the pathogen is likely to be inhibited if the antimicrobial compound in the blood reaches the concentrations usually achievable. A report of "Intermediate" indicates that the results should be considered equivocal, and if the microorganism is not fully susceptible to alternative, clinically feasible drugs, the test should be repeated. This category implies possible clinical applicability in body sites where the drug is physiologically

TABLE 4. Average Pharmacokinetic Parameters of Ceftriaxone in Humans

Subject Group	Elimination Half-Life (hr)	Plasma Clearance (L/hr)	Volume of Distribution (L)
Healthy Subjects	5.8–8.7	0.58–1.45	5.8–13.5
Elderly Subjects (mean age, 70.5 yr)	8.9	0.83	10.7
Patients With Renal Impairment			
Hemodialysis Patients (0–5 mL/min)*	14.7	0.65	13.7
Severe (5–15 mL/min)	15.7	0.56	12.5
Moderate (16–30 mL/min)	11.4	0.72	11.8
Mild (31–60 mL/min)	12.4	0.70	13.3
Patients With Liver Disease	8.8	1.1	13.6

*Creatinine clearance.

Method	Microorganism	ATCC® #	MIC (µg/mL)
Agar	*Bacteroides fragilis*	25285	32–128
	Bacteroides thetaiotaomicron	29741	64–256
Broth	*Bacteroides thetaiotaomicron*	29741	32–128

concentrated or in situations where high dosage of the drug can be used. This category also provides a buffer zone which prevents small uncontrolled technical factors from causing major discrepancies in interpretation. A report of "Resistant" indicates that the pathogen is not likely to be inhibited if the antimicrobial compound in the blood reaches the concentrations usually achievable; other therapy should be selected.
Standardized susceptibility test procedures require the use of laboratory control microorganisms to control the technical aspects of the laboratory procedures. Standardized ceftriaxone powder should provide the following MIC values:[2]

Microorganism	ATCC® #	MIC (µg/mL)
Escherichia coli	25922	0.03–0.12
Staphylococcus aureus	29213	1–8*
Pseudomonas aeruginosa	27853	8–32
Haemophilus influenzae	49247	0.06–0.25
Neisseria gonorrhoeae	49226	0.004–0.015
Streptococcus pneumoniae	49619	0.03–0.12

*A bimodal distribution of MICs results at the extremes of the acceptable range should be suspect and control validity should be verified with data from other control strains.

Diffusion Techniques: Quantitative methods that require measurement of zone diameters also provide reproducible estimates of the susceptibility of bacteria to antimicrobial compounds. One such standardized procedure[3] requires the use of standardized inoculum concentrations. This procedure uses paper discs impregnated with 30 µg of ceftriaxone to test the susceptibility of microorganisms to ceftriaxone.
Reports from the laboratory providing results of the standard single-disc susceptibility test with a 30 µg ceftriaxone disc should be interpreted according to the following criteria for aerobic organisms other than *Haemophilus* spp, *Neisseria gonorrhoeae*, and *Streptococcus* spp:

Zone Diameter (mm)	Interpretation
• 21	(S) Susceptible
14–20	(I) Intermediate
• 13	(R) Resistant

The following interpretive criteria[3] should be used when testing *Haemophilus* species when using Haemophilus Test Media (HTM).

Zone Diameter (mm)	Interpretation
• 26	(S) Susceptible

The absence of resistant strains precludes defining any categories other than "Susceptible". Strains yielding results suggestive of a "Nonsusceptible" category should be submitted to a reference laboratory for further testing.
The following interpretive criteria[3] should be used when testing *Neisseria gonorrhoeae* when using GC agar base and 1% defined growth supplement.

Zone Diameter (mm)	Interpretation
• 35	(S) Susceptible

The absence of resistant strains precludes defining any categories other than "Susceptible". Strains yielding results suggestive of a "Nonsusceptible" category should be submitted to a reference laboratory for further testing.
The following interpretive criteria[3] should be used when testing *Streptococcus* spp other than *Streptococcus pneumoniae* when using Mueller-Hinton agar supplemented with 5% sheep blood incubated in 5% CO_2.

Zone Diameter (mm)	Interpretation
• 27	(S) Susceptible
25–26	(I) Intermediate
• 24	(R) Resistant

Interpretation should be as stated above for results using dilution techniques. Interpretation involves correlation of the diameter obtained in the disc test with the MIC for ceftriaxone.
Disc diffusion interpretive criteria for ceftriaxone discs against *Streptococcus pneumoniae* are not available, however, isolates of pneumococci with oxacillin zone diameters of >20 mm are susceptible (MIC • 0.06 µg/mL) to penicillin and can be considered susceptible to ceftriaxone. *Streptococcus pneumoniae* isolates should not be reported as penicillin (ceftriaxone) resistant or intermediate based solely on an oxacillin zone diameter of • 19 mm. The ceftriaxone MIC should be determined for those isolates with oxacillin zone diameters • 19 mm.
As with standardized dilution techniques, diffusion methods require the use of laboratory control microorganisms that are used to control the technical aspects of the laboratory procedures. For the diffusion technique, the 30 µg ceftriaxone disc should provide the following zone diameters in these laboratory test quality control strains:[3]

Microorganism	ATCC® #	Zone Diameter Ranges (mm)
Escherichia coli	25922	29–35
Staphylococcus aureus	25923	22–28
Pseudomonas aeruginosa	27853	17–23
Haemophilus influenzae	49247	31–39
Neisseria gonorrhoeae	49226	39–51
Streptococcus pneumoniae	49619	30–35

Anaerobic Techniques: For anaerobic bacteria, the susceptibility to ceftriaxone as MICs can be determined by standardized test methods.[4] The MIC values obtained should be interpreted according to the following criteria:

MIC (µg/mL)	Interpretation
• 16	(S) Susceptible
32	(I) Intermediate
• 64	(R) Resistant

As with other susceptibility techniques, the use of laboratory control microorganisms is required to control the technical aspects of the laboratory standardized procedures. Standardized ceftriaxone powder should provide the following MIC values for the indicated standardized anaerobic dilution[4] testing method:
[See second table above]
ATCC® is a registered trademark of the American Type Culture Collection.

INDICATIONS AND USAGE

Rocephin is indicated for the treatment of the following infections when caused by susceptible organisms:
LOWER RESPIRATORY TRACT INFECTIONS caused by *Streptococcus pneumoniae, Staphylococcus aureus, Haemophilus influenzae, Haemophilus parainfluenzae, Klebsiella pneumoniae, Escherichia coli, Enterobacter aerogenes, Proteus mirabilis* or *Serratia marcescens.*
ACUTE BACTERIAL OTITIS MEDIA caused by *Streptococcus pneumoniae, Haemophilus influenzae* (including beta-lactamase producing strains) or *Moraxella catarrhalis* (including beta-lactamase producing strains).
NOTE: In one study lower clinical cure rates were observed with a single dose of Rocephin compared to 10 days of oral therapy. In a second study comparable cure rates were observed between single dose Rocephin and the comparator. The potentially lower clinical cure rate of Rocephin should be balanced against the potential advantages of parenteral therapy (see CLINICAL STUDIES).
SKIN AND SKIN STRUCTURE INFECTIONS caused by *Staphylococcus aureus, Staphylococcus epidermidis, Streptococcus pyogenes,* Viridans group streptococci, *Escherichia coli, Enterobacter cloacae, Klebsiella oxytoea, Klebsiella pneumoniae, Proteus mirabilis, Morganella morganii,* *Pseudomonas aeruginosa, Serratia marcescens, Acinetobacter calcoaceticus, Bacteroides fragilis** or *Peptostreptococcus* species.
URINARY TRACT INFECTIONS (*complicated and uncomplicated*) caused by *Escherichia coli, Proteus mirabilis, Proteus vulgaris, Morganella morganii* or *Klebsiella pneumoniae.*
UNCOMPLICATED GONORRHEA (*cervical/urethral and rectal*) caused by *Neisseria gonorrhoeae*, including both penicillinase- and nonpenicillinase-producing strains, and pharyngeal gonorrhea caused by nonpenicillinase-producing strains of *Neisseria gonorrhoeae.*
PELVIC INFLAMMATORY DISEASE caused by *Neisseria gonorrhoeae*. Rocephin, like other cephalosporins, has no activity against *Chlamydia trachomatis*. Therefore, when cephalosporins are used in the treatment of patients with pelvic inflammatory disease and *Chlamydia trachomatis* is one of the suspected pathogens, appropriate antichlamydial coverage should be added.
BACTERIAL SEPTICEMIA caused by *Staphylococcus aureus, Streptococcus pneumoniae, Escherichia coli, Haemophilus influenzae* or *Klebsiella pneumoniae.*

BONE AND JOINT INFECTIONS caused by *Staphylococcus aureus, Streptococcus pneumoniae, Escherichia coli, Proteus mirabilis, Klebsiella pneumoniae* or *Enterobacter* species.

INTRA-ABDOMINAL INFECTIONS caused by *Escherichia coli, Klebsiella pneumoniae, Bacteroides fragilis, Clostridium* species (Note: most strains of *Clostridium difficile* are resistant) or *Peptostreptococcus* species.

MENINGITIS caused by *Haemophilus influenzae, Neisseria meningitidis* or *Streptococcus pneumoniae.* Rocephin has also been used successfully in a limited number of cases of meningitis and shunt infection caused by *Staphylococcus epidermidis** and *Escherichia coli.**

*Efficacy for this organism in this organ system was studied in fewer than ten infections.

SURGICAL PROPHYLAXIS: The preoperative administration of a single 1 gm dose of Rocephin may reduce the incidence of postoperative infections in patients undergoing surgical procedures classified as contaminated or potentially contaminated (eg, vaginal or abdominal hysterectomy or cholecystectomy for chronic calculous cholecystitis in high-risk patients, such as those over 70 years of age, with acute cholecystitis not requiring therapeutic antimicrobials, obstructive jaundice or common duct bile stones) and in surgical patients for whom infection at the operative site would present serious risk (eg, during coronary artery bypass surgery). Although Rocephin has been shown to have been as effective as cefazolin in the prevention of infection following coronary artery bypass surgery, no placebo-controlled trials have been conducted to evaluate any cephalosporin antibiotic in the prevention of infection following coronary artery bypass surgery.

When administered prior to surgical procedures for which it is indicated, a single 1 gm dose of Rocephin provides protection from most infections due to susceptible organisms throughout the course of the procedure.

Before instituting treatment with Rocephin, appropriate specimens should be obtained for isolation of the causative organism and for determination of its susceptibility to the drug. Therapy may be instituted prior to obtaining results of susceptibility testing.

CONTRAINDICATIONS

Rocephin is contraindicated in patients with known allergy to the cephalosporin class of antibiotics.

WARNINGS

BEFORE THERAPY WITH ROCEPHIN IS INSTITUTED, CAREFUL INQUIRY SHOULD BE MADE TO DETERMINE WHETHER THE PATIENT HAS HAD PREVIOUS HYPERSENSITIVITY REACTIONS TO CEPHALOSPORINS, PENICILLINS OR OTHER DRUGS. THIS PRODUCT SHOULD BE GIVEN CAUTIOUSLY TO PENICILLIN-SENSITIVE PATIENTS. ANTIBIOTICS SHOULD BE ADMINISTERED WITH CAUTION TO ANY PATIENT WHO HAS DEMONSTRATED SOME FORM OF ALLERGY, PARTICULARLY TO DRUGS. SERIOUS ACUTE HYPERSENSITIVITY REACTIONS MAY REQUIRE THE USE OF SUBCUTANEOUS EPINEPHRINE AND OTHER EMERGENCY MEASURES.

Pseudomembranous colitis has been reported with nearly all antibacterial agents, including ceftriaxone, and may range in severity from mild to life-threatening. Therefore, it is important to consider this diagnosis in patients who present with diarrhea subsequent to the administration of antibacterial agents.

Treatment with antibacterial agents alters the normal flora of the colon and may permit overgrowth of clostridia. Studies indicate that a toxin produced by *Clostridium difficile* is one primary cause of "antibiotic-associated colitis."

After the diagnosis of pseudomembranous colitis has been established, appropriate therapeutic measures should be initiated. Mild cases of pseudomembranous colitis usually respond to drug discontinuation alone. In moderate to severe cases, consideration should be given to management with fluids and electrolytes, protein supplementation and treatment with an antibacterial drug clinically effective against *Clostridium difficile* colitis.

PRECAUTIONS

General: Although transient elevations of BUN and serum creatinine have been observed, at the recommended dosages, the nephrotoxic potential of Rocephin is similar to that of other cephalosporins.

Ceftriaxone is excreted via both biliary and renal excretion (see CLINICAL PHARMACOLOGY). Therefore, patients with renal failure normally require no adjustment in dosage when usual doses of Rocephin are administered, but concentrations of drug in the serum should be monitored periodically. If evidence of accumulation exists, dosage should be decreased accordingly.

Dosage adjustments should not be necessary in patients with hepatic dysfunction; however, in patients with both hepatic dysfunction and significant renal disease, Rocephin dosage should not exceed 2 gm daily without close monitoring of serum concentrations.

Alterations in prothrombin times have occurred rarely in patients treated with Rocephin. Patients with impaired vitamin K synthesis or low vitamin K stores (eg, chronic hepatic disease and malnutrition) may require monitoring of prothrombin time during Rocephin treatment. Vitamin K administration (10 mg weekly) may be necessary if the prothrombin time is prolonged before or during therapy.

Prolonged use of Rocephin may result in overgrowth of nonsusceptible organisms. Careful observation of the patient is essential. If superinfection occurs during therapy, appropriate measures should be taken.

Rocephin should be prescribed with caution in individuals with a history of gastrointestinal disease, especially colitis. **There have been reports of sonographic abnormalities in the gallbladder of patients treated with Rocephin; some of these patients also had symptoms of gallbladder disease.** These abnormalities appear on sonography as an echo without acoustical shadowing suggesting sludge or as an echo with acoustical shadowing which may be misinterpreted as gallstones. The chemical nature of the sonographically detected material has been determined to be predominantly a ceftriaxone-calcium salt. **The condition appears to be transient and reversible upon discontinuation of Rocephin and institution of conservative management.** Therefore, Rocephin should be discontinued in patients who develop signs and symptoms suggestive of gallbladder disease and/or the sonographic findings described above.

Carcinogenesis, Mutagenesis, Impairment of Fertility: Carcinogenesis: Considering the maximum duration of treatment and the class of the compound, carcinogenicity studies with ceftriaxone in animals have not been performed. The maximum duration of animal toxicity studies was 6 months. *Mutagenesis:* Genetic toxicology tests included the Ames test, a micronucleus test and a test for chromosomal aberrations in human lymphocytes cultured in vitro with ceftriaxone. Ceftriaxone showed no potential for mutagenic activity in these studies.

Impairment of Fertility: Ceftriaxone produced no impairment of fertility when given intravenously to rats at daily doses up to 586 mg/kg/day, approximately 20 times the recommended clinical dose of 2 gm/day.

Pregnancy: Teratogenic Effects: Pregnancy Category B. Reproductive studies have been performed in mice and rats at doses up to 20 times the usual human dose and have no evidence of embryotoxicity, fetotoxicity or teratogenicity. In primates, no embryotoxicity or teratogenicity was demonstrated at a dose approximately 3 times the human dose.

There are, however, no adequate and well-controlled studies in pregnant women. Because animal reproductive studies are not always predictive of human response, this drug should be used during pregnancy only if clearly needed.

Nonteratogenic Effects: In rats, in the Segment I (fertility and general reproduction) and Segment III (perinatal and postnatal) studies with intravenously administered ceftriaxone, no adverse effects were noted on various reproductive parameters during gestation and lactation, including postnatal growth, functional behavior and reproductive ability of the offspring, at doses of 586 mg/kg/day or less.

Nursing Mothers: Low concentrations of ceftriaxone are excreted in human milk. Caution should be exercised when Rocephin is administered to a nursing woman.

Pediatric Use: Safety and effectiveness of Rocephin in neonates, infants and pediatric patients have been established for the dosages described in the DOSAGE and ADMINISTRATION section. In vitro studies have shown that ceftriaxone, like some other cephalosporins, can displace bilirubin from serum albumin. Rocephin should not be administered to hyperbilirubinemic neonates, especially prematures.

ADVERSE REACTIONS

Rocephin is generally well tolerated. In clinical trials, the following adverse reactions, which were considered to be related to Rocephin therapy or of uncertain etiology, were observed:

LOCAL REACTIONS—pain, induration and tenderness was 1% overall. Phlebitis was reported in <1% after IV administration. The incidence of warmth, tightness or induration was 17% (3/17) after IM administration of 350 mg/mL and 5% (1/20) after IM administration of 250 mg/mL.

HYPERSENSITIVITY—rash (1.7%). Less frequently reported (<1%) were pruritus, fever or chills.

HEMATOLOGIC—eosinophilia (6%), thrombocytosis (5.1%) and leukopenia (2.1%). Less frequently reported (<1%) were anemia, hemolytic anemia, neutropenia, lymphopenia, thrombocytopenia and prolongation of the prothrombin time.

GASTROINTESTINAL—diarrhea (2.7%). Less frequently reported (<1%) were nausea or vomiting, and dysgeusia. The onset of pseudomembranous colitis symptoms may occur during or after antibacterial treatment (see WARNINGS).

HEPATIC—elevations of SGOT (3.1%) or SGPT (3.3%). Less frequently reported (<1%) were elevations of alkaline phosphatase and bilirubin.

RENAL—elevations of the BUN (1.2%). Less frequently reported (<1%) were elevations of creatinine and the presence of casts in the urine.

CENTRAL NERVOUS SYSTEM—headache or dizziness were reported occasionally (<1%).

GENITOURINARY—moniliasis or vaginitis were reported occasionally (<1%).

MISCELLANEOUS—diaphoresis and flushing were reported occasionally (<1%).

Other rarely observed adverse reactions (<0.1%) include leukocytosis, lymphocytosis, monocytosis, basophilia, a decrease in the prothrombin time, jaundice, gallbladder sludge, glycosuria, hematuria, anaphylaxis, bronchospasm, serum sickness, abdominal pain, colitis, flatulence, dyspepsia, palpitations, epistaxis, biliary lithiasis, agranulocytosis, renal precipitations, and nephrolithiasis.

OVERDOSAGE

In the case of overdosage, drug concentration would not be reduced by hemodialysis or peritoneal dialysis. There is no specific antidote. Treatment of overdosage should be symptomatic.

DOSAGE AND ADMINISTRATION

Rocephin may be administered intravenously or intramuscularly.

ADULTS: The usual adult daily dose is 1 to 2 grams given once a day (or in equally divided doses twice a day) depending on the type and severity of infection. The total daily dose should not exceed 4 grams.

If *Chlamydia trachomatis* is a suspected pathogen, appropriate antichlamydial coverage should be added, because ceftriaxone sodium has no activity against this organism.

For the treatment of uncomplicated gonococcal infections, a single intramuscular dose of 250 mg is recommended.

For preoperative use (surgical prophylaxis), a single dose of 1 gram administered intravenously 1/2 to 2 hours before surgery is recommended.

PEDIATRIC PATIENTS: For the treatment of skin and skin structure infections, the recommended total daily dose is 50 to 75 mg/kg given once a day (or in equally divided doses twice a day). The total daily dose should not exceed 2 grams. For the treatment of acute bacterial otitis media, a single intramuscular dose of 50 mg/kg (not to exceed 1 gram) is recommended (see INDICATIONS AND USAGE).

For the treatment of serious miscellaneous infections other than meningitis, the recommended total daily dose is 50 to 75 mg/kg, given in divided doses every 12 hours. The total daily dose should not exceed 2 grams.

In the treatment of meningitis, it is recommended that the initial therapeutic dose be 100 mg/kg (not to exceed 4 grams). Thereafter, a total daily dose of 100 mg/kg/day (not to exceed 4 grams daily) is recommended. The daily dose may be administered once a day (or in equally divided doses every 12 hours). The usual duration of therapy is 7 to 14 days.

Generally, Rocephin therapy should be continued for at least 2 days after the signs and symptoms of infection have disappeared. The usual duration of therapy is 4 to 14 days; in complicated infections, longer therapy may be required.

When treating infections caused by *Streptococcus pyogenes*, therapy should be continued for at least 10 days.

No dosage adjustment is necessary for patients with impairment of renal or hepatic function; however, blood levels should be monitored in patients with severe renal impairment (eg, dialysis patients) and in patients with both renal and hepatic dysfunctions.

DIRECTIONS FOR USE

Intramuscular Administration: Reconstitute Rocephin powder with the appropriate diluent (see **COMPATIBILITY AND STABILITY**).

After reconstitution, each 1 mL of solution contains approximately 250 mg or 350 mg equivalent of ceftriaxone according to the amount of diluent indicated below. If required, more dilute solutions could be utilized. **A 350 mg/mL concentration is not recommended for the 250 mg vial since it may not be possible to withdraw the entire contents.** As with all intramuscular preparations, Rocephin should be injected well within the body of a relatively large muscle; aspiration helps to avoid unintentional injection into a blood vessel.

Vial Dosage Size	Amount of Diluent to be Added	
	250 mg/mL	350 mg/mL
250 mg	0.9 mL	—
500 mg	1.8 mL	1.0 mL
1 gm	3.6 mL	2.1 mL
2 gm	7.2 mL	4.2 mL

Intramuscular Convenience Kit: For the 500 mg vial, withdraw 1 mL of diluent, discard the remainder. Inject diluent into vial, shake vial thoroughly to form solution. Withdraw entire contents of vial into syringe to equal total labeled dose.

For 1 gm vial, withdraw entire contents of diluent (2.1 mL). Inject diluent into vial, shake vial thoroughly to form solution. Withdraw entire contents of vial into syringe to equal total labeled dose.

Intravenous Administration: Rocephin should be administered intravenously by infusion over a period of 30 minutes. Concentrations between 10 mg/mL and 40 mg/mL are recommended; however, lower concentrations may be used if desired. Reconstitute vials or "piggyback" bottles with an appropriate IV diluent (see **COMPATIBILITY AND STABILITY**).

Vial Dosage Size	Amount of Diluent to be Added
250 mg	2.4 mL
500 mg	4.8 mL
1 gm	9.6 mL
2 gm	19.2 mL

After reconstitution, each 1 mL of solution contains approximately 100 mg equivalent of ceftriaxone. Withdraw entire contents and dilute to the desired concentration with the appropriate IV diluent.

Piggyback Bottle Dosage Size	Amount of Diluent to be Added
1 gm	10 mL
2 gm	20 mL

After reconstitution, further dilute to 50 mL or 100 mL volumes with the appropriate IV diluent.

COMPATIBILITY AND STABILITY: Rocephin sterile powder should be stored at room temperature—77°F (25°C)—or below and protected from light. After reconstitution, protection from normal light is not necessary. The color

Continued on next page

Rocephin—Cont.

of solutions ranges from light yellow to amber, depending on the length of storage, concentration and diluent used.
Rocephin *intramuscular* solutions remain stable (loss of potency less than 10%) for the following time periods:
[See first table to the right]
Rocephin *intravenous* solutions, at concentrations of 10, 20 and 40 mg/mL, remain stable (loss of potency less than 10%) for the following time periods stored in glass or PVC containers:
[See second table to the right]
Similarly, Rocephin *intravenous* solutions, at concentrations of 100 mg/mL, remain stable in the IV piggyback glass containers for the above specified time periods.
The following *intravenous* Rocephin solutions are stable at room temperature (25°C) for 24 hours, at concentrations between 10 mg/mL and 40 mg/mL: Sodium Lactate (PVC container), 10% Invert Sugar (glass container), 5% Sodium Bicarbonate (glass container), Freamine III (glass container), Normosol-M in 5% Dextrose (glass and PVC containers), Ionosol-B in 5% Dextrose (glass container), 5% Mannitol (glass container), 10% Mannitol (glass container).
Ceftriaxone has been shown to be compatible with Flagyl® IV (metronidazole hydrochloride). The concentration should not exceed 5 to 7.5 mg/mL metronidazole hydrochloride with ceftriaxone 10 mg/mL as an admixture. The admixture is stable for 24 hours at room temperature only in 0.9% sodium chloride injection or 5% dextrose in water (D5W). No compatibility studies have been conducted with the Flagyl® IV RTU® (metronidazole) formulation or using other diluents. Metronidazole at concentrations greater than 8 mg/mL will precipitate. Do not refrigerate the admixture as precipitation will occur.
* Registered trademark of SCS Pharmaceuticals.
Vancomycin and fluconazole are physically incompatible with ceftriaxone in admixtures. When either of these drugs is to be administered concomitantly with ceftriaxone by intermittent intravenous infusion, it is recommended that they be given sequentially, with thorough flushing of the intravenous lines (with one of the compatible fluids) between the administrations.
After the indicated stability time periods, unused portions of solutions should be discarded.
NOTE: Parenteral drug products should be inspected visually for particulate matter before administration.
Rocephin reconstituted with 5% Dextrose or 0.9% Sodium Chloride solution at concentrations between 10 mg/mL and 40 mg/mL, and then stored in frozen state (–20°C) in PVC or polyolefin containers, remains stable for 26 weeks.
Frozen solutions should be thawed at room temperature before use. After thawing, unused portions should be discarded. **DO NOT REFREEZE.**
Rocephin solutions should *not* be physically mixed with or piggybacked into solutions containing other antimicrobial drugs or into diluent solutions other than those listed above, due to possible incompatibility.

ANIMAL PHARMACOLOGY
Concretions consisting of the precipitated calcium salt of ceftriaxone have been found in the gallbladder bile of dogs and baboons treated with ceftriaxone.
These appeared as a gritty sediment in dogs that received 100 mg/kg/day for 4 weeks. A similar phenomenon has been observed in baboons but only after a protracted dosing period (6 months) at higher dose levels (335 mg/kg/day or more). The likelihood of this occurrence in humans is considered to be low, since ceftriaxone has a greater plasma half-life in humans, the calcium salt of ceftriaxone is more soluble in human gallbladder bile and the calcium content of human gallbladder bile is relatively low.

HOW SUPPLIED
Rocephin is supplied as a sterile crystalline powder in glass vials and piggyback bottles. The following packages are available:
Vials containing 250 mg equivalent of ceftriaxone. Box of 1 (NDC 0004-1962-02) and box of 10 (NDC 0004-1962-01).
Vials containing 500 mg equivalent of ceftriaxone. Box of 1 (NDC 0004-1963-02) and box of 10 (NDC 0004-1963-01).
Vials containing 1 gm equivalent of ceftriaxone. Box of 1 (NDC 0004-1964-04) and box of 10 (NDC 0004-1964-01).
Piggyback bottles containing 1 gm equivalent of ceftriaxone. Box of 1 (NDC 0004-1964-02).
Vials containing 2 gm equivalent of ceftriaxone. Box of 10 (NDC 0004-1965-01).
Piggyback bottles containing 2 gm equivalent of ceftriaxone. Box of 1 (NDC 0004-1965-02).
Bulk pharmacy containers, containing 10 gm equivalent of ceftriaxone. Box of 1 (NDC 0004-1971-01). NOT FOR DIRECT ADMINISTRATION.
Rocephin is also supplied in an Intramuscular Convenience Kit, available in two strengths, consisting of a vial of ceftriaxone sodium as a sterile crystalline powder and a vial of Xylocaine®-MPF 1% (lidocaine HCl Injection, USP).
The following strengths are available:
Kit containing 1 vial of 500 mg equivalent of ceftriaxone, plus 1 vial of 2.1 mL Xylocaine (NDC 0004-2014-92).
Kit containing 1 vial of 1 gm equivalent of ceftriaxone, plus 1 vial of 2.1 mL Xylocaine (NDC 0004-2013-92).
Xylocaine®-MPF 1% (lidocaine HCl Injection, USP) is manufactured for Roche Laboratories Inc. by Astra USA, Inc., Westborough, MA 01581.
Rocephin is also supplied as a sterile crystalline powder in ADD-Vantage®* Vials as follows:

Diluent	Concentration mg/mL	Storage Room Temp. (25°C)	Refrigerated (4°C)
Sterile Water for	100	3 days	10 days
Injection	250, 350	24 hours	3 days
0.9% Sodium	100	3 days	10 days
Chloride Solution	250, 350	24 hours	3 days
5% Dextrose	100	3 days	10 days
Solution	250, 350	24 hours	3 days
Bacteriostatic Water + 0.9%	100	24 hours	10 days
Benzyl Alcohol	250, 350	24 hours	3 days
1% Lidocaine Solution	100	24 hours	10 days
(without epinephrine)	250, 350	24 hours	3 days

Diluent	Storage Room Temp. (25°C)	Refrigerated (4°C)
Sterile Water	3 days	10 days
0.9% Sodium Chloride Solution	3 days	10 days
5% Dextrose Solution	3 days	10 days
10% Dextrose Solution	3 days	10 days
5% Dextrose + 0.9% Sodium Chloride Solution*	3 days	Incompatible
5% Dextrose + 0.45% Sodium Chloride Solution	3 days	Incompatible

*Data available for 10 to 40 mg/mL concentrations in this diluent in PVC containers only.

Clinical Efficacy in Evaluable Population

Study Day	Ceftriaxone Single Dose	Comparator - 10 Days of Oral Therapy	95% Confidence Interval	Statistical Outcome
Study 1 - US		amoxicillin/clavulanate		
14	74% (220/296)	82% (247/302)	(–14.4%, –0.5%)	Ceftriaxone is lower than control at study day 14 and 28.
28	58% (167/288)	67% (200/297)	(–17.5%, –1.2%)	
Study 2 - US[5]		TMP-SMZ		
14	54% (113/210)	60% (124/206)	(–16.4%, 3.6%)	Ceftriaxone is equivalent to control at study day 14 and 28.
28	35% (73/206)	45% (93/205)	(–19.9%, 0.0%)	

	Study Day 13–15		Study Day 30+2	
Organism	No. Analyzed	No. Erad. (%)	No. Analyzed	No. Erad. (%)
Streptococcus pneumoniae	38	32 (84)	35	25 (71)
Haemophilus influenzae	33	28 (85)	31	22 (71)
Moraxella catarrhalis	15	12 (80)	15	9 (60)

ADD-Vantage Vials containing 1 gm equivalent of ceftriaxone. Box of 10 (NDC 0004-1964-05).
ADD-Vantage Vials containing 2 gm equivalent of ceftriaxone. Box of 10 (NDC 0004-1965-05).
Rocephin is also supplied premixed as a frozen, iso-osmotic, sterile, nonpyrogenic solution of ceftriaxone sodium in 50 mL single dose Galaxy®† containers (PL 2040 plastic), is manufactured for Roche Laboratories Inc. by Baxter Healthcare Corporation, Deerfield, Illinois 60015. The following strengths are available:
1 gm equivalent of ceftriaxone, iso-osmotic with approximately 1.9 gm Dextrose Hydrous, USP, added (NDC 0004-2002-78).
2 gm equivalent of ceftriaxone, iso-osmotic with approximately 1.2 gm Dextrose Hydrous, USP, added (NDC 0004-2003-78).
NOTE: Store Rocephin in the frozen state at or below –20°C/–4°F.
* Registered trademark of Abbott Laboratories, Inc.
† Registered trademark of Baxter International Inc.

CLINICAL STUDIES
Clinical Trials in Pediatric Patients With Acute Bacterial Otitis Media: In two adequate and well-controlled US clinical trials a single IM dose of ceftriaxone was compared with a 10 day course of oral antibiotic in pediatric patients between the ages of 3 months and 6 years. The clinical cure rates and statistical outcome appear in the table below:
[See third table above]
An open-label bacteriologic study of ceftriaxone without a comparator enrolled 108 pediatric patients, 79 of whom had positive baseline cultures for one or more of the common pathogens. The results of this study are tabulated as follows:
Week 2 and 4 Bacteriologic Eradication Rates in the Per Protocol Analysis in the Roche Bacteriologic Study by pathogen:
[See fourth table above]

REFERENCES
1. National Committee for Clinical Laboratory Standards, *Methods for Dilution Antimicrobial Susceptibility Tests for Bacteria that Grow Aerobically;* Approved Standard-Fifth Edition. NCCLS document M7-A5 (ISBN 1-56238-309-9). NCCLS, Wayne, PA 19087-1898, 2000.
2. National Committee for Clinical Laboratory Standards, Supplemental Tables. NCCLS document M100-S10(M7) (ISBN 1-56238-309-9). NCCLS, Wayne, PA 19087-1898, 2000.
3. National Committee for Clinical Laboratory Standards, *Performance Standards for Antimicrobial Disk Susceptibility Tests;* Approved Standard-Seventh Edition. NCCLS document M2-A7 (ISBN 1-56238-393-0). NCCLS, Wayne, PA 19087-1898, 2000.
4. National Committee for Clinical Laboratory Standards, *Methods for Antimicrobial Susceptibility Testing of Anaerobic Bacteria;* Approved Standard-Fourth Edition. NCCLS document M11-A4 (ISBN 1-56238-210-1). NCCLS, Wayne, PA 19087-1898, 1997.
5. Barnett ED, Teele DW, Klein JO, et al. *Comparison of Ceftriaxone and Trimethoprim-Sulfamethoxazole for Acute Otitis Media.* Pediatrics. Vol. 99, No. 1, January 1997.

Rx only
Pharmaceuticals
Roche Laboratories Inc.
340 Kingsland Street
Nutley, New Jersey 07110-1199
Revised: September 2000
Printed in USA

TAMIFLU®
(oseltamivir phosphate)
CAPSULES
AND FOR ORAL SUSPENSION

Prescribing information for this product, which appears on pages 2780–2782 of the 2001 PDR, has been completely revised as follows. Please write "See Supplement A" next to the product heading.

DESCRIPTION
TAMIFLU (oseltamivir phosphate) is available as a capsule containing 75 mg oseltamivir for oral use, in the form of oseltamivir phosphate, and as a powder for oral suspension, which when constituted with water as directed contains 12 mg/mL oseltamivir. In addition to the active ingredient, each capsule contains pregelatinized starch, talc, povidone K 30, croscarmellose sodium, and sodium stearyl fumarate. The capsule shell contains gelatin, titanium dioxide, yellow iron oxide, black iron oxide, and red iron oxide. Each capsule is printed with blue ink, which includes FD&C Blue No. 2 as the colorant. In addition to the active ingredient, the powder for oral suspension contains xanthan gum, monosodium citrate, sodium benzoate, sorbitol, saccharin sodium, titanium dioxide, and tutti-frutti flavoring.
Oseltamivir phosphate is a white crystalline solid with the chemical name (3R,4R,5S)-4-acetylamino-5-amino-3(1-ethylpropoxy)-1-cyclohexene-1-carboxylic acid, ethyl ester, phosphate (1:1). The chemical formula is $C_{16}H_{28}N_2O_4$ (free base). The molecular weight is 312.4 for oseltamivir free

base and 410.4 for oseltamivir phosphate salt. The structural formula is as follows:

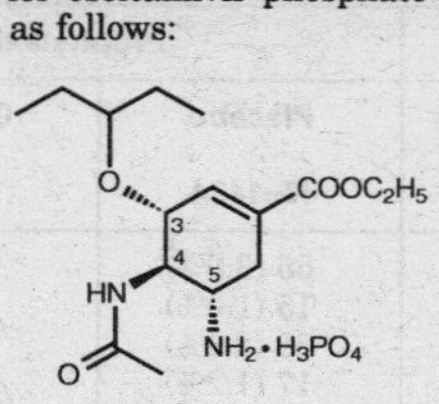

MICROBIOLOGY

Mechanism of Action: Oseltamivir is an ethyl ester prodrug requiring ester hydrolysis for conversion to the active form, oseltamivir carboxylate. The proposed mechanism of action of oseltamivir is via inhibition of influenza virus neuraminidase with the possibility of alteration of virus particle aggregation and release.

Antiviral Activity In Vitro: The antiviral activity of oseltamivir carboxylate against laboratory strains and clinical isolates of influenza virus was determined in cell culture assays. The concentrations of oseltamivir carboxylate required for inhibition of influenza virus were highly variable depending on the assay method used and the virus tested. The 50% and 90% inhibitory concentrations (IC50 and IC90) were in the range of 0.0008 µM to >35 µM and 0.004 µM to >100 µM, respectively (1 µM=0.284 µg/mL). The relationship between the in vitro antiviral activity in cell culture and the inhibition of influenza virus replication in humans has not been established.

Drug Resistance: Influenza A virus isolates with reduced susceptibility to oseltamivir carboxylate have been recovered in vitro by passage of virus in the presence of increasing concentrations of oseltamivir carboxylate. Genetic analysis of these isolates showed that reduced susceptibility to oseltamivir carboxylate is associated with mutations that result in amino acid changes in the viral neuraminidase or viral hemagglutinin or both.

In clinical studies of postexposure and seasonal prophylaxis, determination of resistance was limited by the low overall incidence rate of influenza infection and prophylactic effect of TAMIFLU.

In clinical studies in the treatment of naturally acquired infection with influenza virus, 1.3% (4/301) of posttreatment isolates in adult patients and adolescents, and 8.6% (9/105) in pediatric patients aged 1 to 12 years showed emergence of influenza variants with decreased neuraminidase susceptibility to oseltamivir carboxylate.

Genotypic analysis of these variants showed a specific mutation in the active site of neuraminidase compared to pretreatment isolates. The contribution of resistance due to alterations in the viral hemagglutinin has not been fully evaluated.

Cross-resistance: Cross-resistance between zanamivir-resistant influenza mutants and oseltamivir-resistant influenza mutants has been observed in vitro.

Due to limitations in the assays available to detect drug-induced shifts in virus susceptibility, an estimate of the incidence of oseltamivir resistance and possible cross-resistance to zanamivir in clinical isolates cannot be made. However, one of the three oseltamivir-induced mutations in the viral neuraminidase from clinical isolates is the same as one of the three mutations observed in zanamivir-resistant virus.

Insufficient information is available to fully characterize the risk of emergence of TAMIFLU resistance in clinical use.

Immune Response: No influenza vaccine interaction study has been conducted. In studies of naturally acquired and experimental influenza, treatment with TAMIFLU did not impair normal humoral antibody response to infection.

CLINICAL PHARMACOLOGY

PHARMACOKINETICS:

Absorption and Bioavailability: Oseltamivir is readily absorbed from the gastrointestinal tract after oral administration of oseltamivir phosphate and is extensively converted predominantly by hepatic esterases to oseltamivir carboxylate. At least 75% of an oral dose reaches the systemic circulation as oseltamivir carboxylate. Exposure to oseltamivir is less than 5% of the total exposure after oral dosing (Table 1).

[See table 1 above]

Table 1. Mean (% CV) Pharmacokinetic Parameters of Oseltamivir and Oseltamivir Carboxylate After a Multiple 75 mg Twice Daily Oral Dose (n=20)

Parameter	Oseltamivir	Oseltamivir Carboxylate
C_{max} (ng/mL)	65.2 (26)	348 (18)
AUC_{0-12h} (ng·h/mL)	112 (25)	2719 (20)

Plasma concentrations of oseltamivir carboxylate are proportional to doses up to 500 mg given twice daily (see DOSAGE AND ADMINISTRATION).

Coadministration with food has no significant effect on the peak plasma concentration (551 ng/mL under fasted conditions and 441 ng/mL under fed conditions) and the area under the plasma concentration time curve (6218 ng·h/mL under fasted conditions and 6069 ng·h/mL under fed conditions) of oseltamivir carboxylate.

Distribution: The volume of distribution (V_{ss}) of oseltamivir carboxylate, following intravenous administration in 24 subjects, ranged between 23 and 26 liters.

The binding of oseltamivir carboxylate to human plasma protein is low (3%). The binding of oseltamivir to human plasma protein is 42%, which is insufficient to cause significant displacement-based drug interactions.

Metabolism: Oseltamivir is extensively converted to oseltamivir carboxylate by esterases located predominantly in the liver. Neither oseltamivir nor oseltamivir carboxylate is a substrate for, or inhibitor of, cytochrome P450 isoforms.

Elimination: Absorbed oseltamivir is primarily (>90%) eliminated by conversion to oseltamivir carboxylate. Plasma concentrations of oseltamivir declined with a half-life of 1 to 3 hours in most subjects after oral administration. Oseltamivir carboxylate is not further metabolized and is eliminated in the urine. Plasma concentrations of oseltamivir carboxylate declined with a half-life of 6 to 10 hours in most subjects after oral administration. Oseltamivir carboxylate is eliminated entirely (>99%) by renal excretion. Renal clearance (18.8 L/h) exceeds glomerular filtration rate (7.5 L/h) indicating that tubular secretion occurs, in addition to glomerular filtration. Less than 20% of an oral radiolabeled dose is eliminated in feces.

Special Populations: *Renal Impairment:* Administration of 100 mg of oseltamivir phosphate twice daily for 5 days to patients with various degrees of renal impairment showed that exposure to oseltamivir carboxylate is inversely proportional to declining renal function. Oseltamivir carboxylate exposures in patients with normal and abnormal renal function administered various dose regimens of oseltamivir are described in Table 2.

[See table 2 above]

Table 2. Oseltamivir Carboxylate Exposures in Patients With Normal and Reduced Serum Creatinine Clearance

Parameter	Normal Renal Function			Impaired Renal Function				
	75 mg qd	75 mg bid	150 mg bid	Creatinine Clearance <10 mL/min		Creatinine Clearance >10 and <30 mL/min		
				CAPD	Hemodialysis			
				30 mg weekly	30 mg alternate HD cycle	75 mg daily	75 mg alternate days	30 mg daily
C_{max}	259*	348*	705*	766	850	1638	1175	655
C_{min}	39*	138*	288*	62	48	864	209	346
AUC_{0-48}	7476*	10876*	21864*	17381	12429	62636	21999	25054

*Observed values. All other values are predicted.

Pediatric Patients: The pharmacokinetics of oseltamivir and oseltamivir carboxylate have been evaluated in a single dose pharmacokinetic study in pediatric patients aged 5 to 16 years (n=18) and in a small number of pediatric patients aged 3 to 12 years (n=5) enrolled in a clinical trial. Younger pediatric patients cleared both the prodrug and the active metabolite faster than adult patients resulting in a lower exposure for a given mg/kg dose. For oseltamivir carboxylate, apparent total clearance decreases linearly with increasing age (up to 12 years). The pharmacokinetics of oseltamivir in pediatric patients over 12 years of age are similar to those in adult patients.

Geriatric Patients: Exposure to oseltamivir carboxylate at steady-state was 25% to 35% higher in geriatric patients (age range 65 to 78 years) compared to young adults given comparable doses of oseltamivir. Half-lives observed in the geriatric patients were similar to those seen in young adults. Based on drug exposure and tolerability, dose adjustments are not required for geriatric patients for either treatment or prophylaxis (see DOSAGE AND ADMINISTRATION: *Special Dosage Instructions*).

INDICATIONS AND USAGE

Treatment of Influenza: TAMIFLU is indicated for the treatment of uncomplicated acute illness due to influenza infection in patients older than 1 year of age who have been symptomatic for no more than 2 days.

Prophylaxis of Influenza: TAMIFLU is indicated for the prophylaxis of influenza in adult patients and adolescents 13 years and older.

TAMIFLU is not a substitute for early vaccination on an annual basis as recommended by the Centers for Disease Control's Immunization Practices Advisory Committee.

Description of Clinical Studies: Studies in Naturally Occurring Influenza:

Treatment of Influenza: Adult Patients: Two phase III placebo-controlled and double-blind clinical trials were conducted: one in the USA and one outside the USA. Patients were eligible for these trials if they had fever >100°F, accompanied by at least one respiratory symptom (cough, nasal symptoms or sore throat) and at least one systemic symptom (myalgia, chills/sweats, malaise, fatigue or headache) and influenza virus was known to be circulating in the community. In addition, all patients enrolled in the trials were allowed to take fever-reducing medications.

Of 1355 patients enrolled in these two trials, 849 (63%) patients were influenza-infected (age range 18 to 65 years; median age 34 years; 52% male; 90% Caucasian; 31% smokers). Of these 849 influenza-infected patients, 95% were infected with influenza A, 3% with influenza B, and 2% with influenza of unknown type.

TAMIFLU was started within 40 hours of onset of symptoms. Subjects participating in the trials were required to self-assess the influenza-associated symptoms as "none", "mild", "moderate" or "severe". Time to improvement was calculated from the time of treatment initiation to the time when all symptoms (nasal congestion, sore throat, cough, aches, fatigue, headaches, and chills/sweats) were assessed as "none" or "mild." In both studies, at the recommended dose of TAMIFLU 75 mg twice daily for 5 days, there was a 1.3 day reduction in the median time to improvement in influenza-infected subjects receiving TAMIFLU compared to subjects receiving placebo. Subgroup analyses of these studies by gender showed no differences in the treatment effect of TAMIFLU in men and women.

In the treatment of influenza, no increased efficacy was demonstrated in subjects receiving treatment of 150 mg TAMIFLU twice daily for 5 days.

Pediatric Patients: One double-blind placebo controlled treatment trial was conducted in pediatric patients aged 1 to 12 years (median age 5 years), who had fever (>100°F) plus one respiratory symptom (cough or coryza) when influenza virus was known to be circulating in the community. Of 698 patients enrolled in this trial, 452 (65%) were influenza-infected (50% male; 68% Caucasian). Of the 452 influenza-infected patients, 67% were infected with influenza A and 33% with influenza B.

The primary endpoint in this study was the time to freedom from illness, a composite endpoint which required 4 individual conditions to be met. These were: alleviation of cough, alleviation of coryza, resolution of fever, and parental opinion of a return to normal health and activity. TAMIFLU treatment of 2 mg/kg twice daily, started within 48 hours of onset of symptoms, significantly reduced the total composite time to freedom from illness by 1.5 days compared to placebo. Subgroup analyses of this study by gender showed no differences in the treatment effect of TAMIFLU in males and females.

Prophylaxis of Influenza: The efficacy of TAMIFLU in preventing naturally occurring influenza illness has been demonstrated in three seasonal prophylaxis studies and a postexposure prophylaxis study in households. The primary efficacy parameter for all these studies was the incidence of laboratory confirmed clinical influenza. Laboratory confirmed clinical influenza was defined as oral temperature ≥99.0°F/37.2°C plus at least one respiratory symptom (cough, sore throat, nasal congestion) and at least one constitutional symptom (aches and pain, fatigue, headache, chills/sweats), all recorded within 24 hours, plus either a positive virus isolation or a fourfold increase in virus antibody titers from baseline.

In a pooled analysis of two seasonal prophylaxis studies in healthy unvaccinated adults (aged 13 to 65 years), TAMIFLU 75 mg once daily taken for 42 days during a community outbreak reduced the incidence of laboratory confirmed clinical influenza from 4.8% (25/519) for the placebo group to 1.2% (6/520) for the TAMIFLU group.

In a seasonal prophylaxis study in elderly residents of skilled nursing homes, TAMIFLU 75 mg once daily taken for 42 days reduced the incidence of laboratory confirmed clinical influenza from 4.4% (12/272) for the placebo group to 0.4% (1/276) for the TAMIFLU group. About 80% of this elderly population were vaccinated, 14% of subjects had chronic airway obstructive disorders, and 43% had cardiac disorders.

In a study of postexposure prophylaxis in household contacts (aged ≥13 years) of an index case, TAMIFLU 75 mg once daily administered within 2 days of onset of symptoms in the index case and continued for 7 days reduced the incidence of laboratory confirmed clinical influenza from 12% (24/200) in the placebo group to 1% (2/205) for the TAMIFLU group. Index cases did not receive TAMIFLU in the study.

CONTRAINDICATIONS

TAMIFLU is contraindicated in patients with known hypersensitivity to any of the components of the product.

PRECAUTIONS

General: There is no evidence for efficacy of TAMIFLU in any illness caused by agents other than influenza viruses Types A and B.

Use of TAMIFLU should not affect the evaluation of individuals for annual influenza vaccination in accordance with guidelines of the Center for Disease Controls and Prevention Advisory Committee on Immunization Practices.

Continued on next page

Tamiflu—Cont.

Efficacy of TAMIFLU in patients who begin treatment after 40 hours of symptoms has not been established.

Efficacy of TAMIFLU in the treatment of subjects with chronic cardiac disease and/or respiratory disease has not been established. No difference in the incidence of complications was observed between the treatment and placebo groups in this population. No information is available regarding treatment of influenza in patients with any medical condition sufficiently severe or unstable to be considered at imminent risk of requiring hospitalization.

Safety and efficacy of repeated treatment or prophylaxis courses have not been studied.

Efficacy of TAMIFLU for treatment or prophylaxis has not been established in immunocompromised patients.

Serious bacterial infections may begin with influenza-like symptoms or may coexist with or occur as complications during the course of influenza. TAMIFLU has not been shown to prevent such complications.

Hepatic Impairment: The safety and pharmacokinetics in patients with hepatic impairment have not been evaluated.

Renal Impairment: Dose adjustment is recommended for patients with a serum creatinine clearance <30 mL/min (see DOSAGE AND ADMINISTRATION).

Information for Patients: Patients should be instructed to begin treatment with TAMIFLU as soon as possible from the first appearance of flu symptoms. Similarly, prevention should begin as soon as possible after exposure, at the recommendation of a physician.

Patients should be instructed to take any missed doses as soon as they remember, except if it is near the next scheduled dose (within 2 hours), and then continue to take TAMIFLU at the usual times.

TAMIFLU is not a substitute for a flu vaccination. Patients should continue receiving an annual flu vaccination according to guidelines on immunization practices.

Drug Interactions: Information derived from pharmacology and pharmacokinetic studies of oseltamivir suggests that clinically significant drug interactions are unlikely.

Oseltamivir is extensively converted to oseltamivir carboxylate by esterases, located predominantly in the liver. Drug interactions involving competition for esterases have not been extensively reported in literature. Low protein binding of oseltamivir and oseltamivir carboxylate suggests that the probability of drug displacement interactions is low.

In vitro studies demonstrate that neither oseltamivir nor oseltamivir carboxylate is a good substrate for P450 mixed-function oxidases or for glucuronyl transferases.

Cimetidine, a non-specific inhibitor of cytochrome P450 isoforms and competitor for renal tubular secretion of basic or cationic drugs, has no effect on plasma levels of oseltamivir or oseltamivir carboxylate.

Clinically important drug interactions involving competition for renal tubular secretion are unlikely due to the known safety margin for most of these drugs, the elimination characteristics of oseltamivir carboxylate (glomerular filtration and anionic tubular secretion) and the excretion capacity of these pathways. Coadministration of probenecid results in an approximate twofold increase in exposure to oseltamivir carboxylate due to a decrease in active anionic tubular secretion in the kidney. However, due to the safety margin of oseltamivir carboxylate, no dose adjustments are required when coadministering with probenecid.

Coadministration with amoxicillin does not alter plasma levels of either compound, indicating that competition for the anionic secretion pathway is weak.

In six subjects, multiple doses of oseltamivir did not affect the single-dose pharmacokinetics of acetaminophen.

Carcinogenesis, Mutagenesis, and Impairment of Fertility: Long-term carcinogenicity tests with oseltamivir are underway but have not been completed. However, a 26-week dermal carcinogenicity study of oseltamivir carboxylate in FVB/Tg.AC transgenic mice was negative. The animals were dosed at 40, 140, 400 or 780 mg/kg/day in two divided doses. The highest dose represents the maximum feasible dose based on the solubility of the compound in the control vehicle. A positive control, tetradecanoyl phorbol-13-acetate administered at 2.5 μg per dose three times per week gave a positive response.

Oseltamivir was found to be non-mutagenic in the Ames test and the human lymphocyte chromosome assay with and without enzymatic activation and negative in the mouse micronuleus test. It was found to be positive in a Syrian Hamster Embryo (SHE) cell transformation test. Oseltamivir carboxylate was non-mutagenic in the Ames test and the L5178Y mouse lymphoma assay with and without enzymatic activation and negative in the SHE cell transformation test.

In a fertility and early embryonic development study in rats, doses of oseltamivir at 50, 250, and 1500 mg/kg/day were administered to females for 2 weeks before mating, during mating and until day 6 of pregnancy. Males were dosed for 4 weeks before mating, during and for 2 weeks after mating. There were no effects on fertility, mating performance or early embryonic development at any dose level. The highest dose was approximately 100 times the human systemic exposure (AUC$_{0-24h}$) of oseltamivir carboxylate.

Pregnancy: Pregnancy Category C: There are insufficient human data upon which to base an evaluation of risk of TAMIFLU to the pregnant woman or developing fetus. Studies for effects on embryo-fetal development were conducted in rats (50, 250, and 1500 mg/kg/day) and rabbits (50, 150, and 500 mg/kg/day) by the oral route. Relative exposures at these

doses were, respectively, 2, 13, and 100 times human exposure in the rat and 4, 8, and 50 times human exposure in the rabbit. Pharmacokinetic studies indicated that fetal exposure was seen in both species. In the rat study, minimal maternal toxicity was reported in the 1500 mg/kg/day group. In the rabbit study, slight and marked maternal toxicities were observed, respectively, in the 150 and 500 mg/kg/day groups. There was a dose-dependent increase in the incidence rates of a variety of minor skeletal abnormalities and variants in the exposed offspring in these studies. However, the individual incidence rate of each skeletal abnormality or variant remained within the background rates of occurrence in the species studied.

Because animal reproductive studies may not be predictive of human response and there are no adequate and well-controlled studies in pregnant women, TAMIFLU should be used during pregnancy only if the potential benefit justifies the potential risk to the fetus.

Nursing Mothers: In lactating rats, oseltamivir and oseltamivir carboxylate are excreted in the milk. It is not known whether oseltamivir or oseltamivir carboxylate is excreted in human milk. TAMIFLU should, therefore, be used only if the potential benefit for the lactating mother justifies the potential risk to the breast-fed infant.

Pediatric Use: The safety and efficacy of TAMIFLU in pediatric patients younger than 1 year of age have not been established.

Geriatric Use: In an ongoing treatment study in otherwise healthy elderly patients, >65 years (n=168), given the recommended dosing regimen of TAMIFLU, there was a reduction in the median time to improvement in the subjects receiving TAMIFLU similar to that seen in younger adults. No overall difference in safety was observed between these subjects and younger adults. Safety and efficacy have been demonstrated in elderly residents of nursing homes who took TAMIFLU for up to 42 days for the prevention of influenza. Many of these individuals had cardiac and/or respiratory disease, and most had received vaccine that season (see INDICATIONS AND USAGE: *Description of Clinical Studies*).

ADVERSE REACTIONS

Treatment Studies in Adult Patients: A total of 1171 patients who participated in adult phase III controlled clinical trials for the treatment of influenza were treated with TAMIFLU. The most frequently reported adverse events in these studies were nausea and vomiting. These events were generally of mild to moderate degree and usually occurred on the first 2 days of administration. Less than 1% of subjects discontinued prematurely from clinical trials due to nausea and vomiting.

Adverse events that occurred with an incidence of ≥1% in 1440 patients taking placebo or TAMIFLU 75 mg twice daily in adult phase III treatment studies are shown in Table 3. This summary includes 945 healthy young adults and 495 "at risk" patients (elderly patients and patients with chronic cardiac or respiratory disease). Those events reported numerically more frequently in patients taking TAMIFLU compared with placebo were nausea, vomiting, bronchitis, insomnia, and vertigo.

[See table 3 above]

Adverse events included are: all events reported in the treatment studies with frequency ≥1% in the oseltamivir 75 mg bid group.

Additional adverse events occurring in <1% of patients receiving TAMIFLU for treatment included unstable angina, anemia, pseudomembranous colitis, humerus fracture, pneumonia, pyrexia, and peritonsillar abscess.

Prophylaxis Studies: A total of 3434 subjects (adolescents, healthy adults and elderly) participated in phase III prophylaxis studies, of whom 1480 received the recommended dose of 75 mg once daily for up to 6 weeks. Adverse events were qualitatively very similar to those seen in the treatment studies, despite a longer duration of dosing (Table 3). Events reported more frequently in subjects receiving TAMIFLU compared to subjects receiving placebo in prophylaxis studies, and more commonly than in treatment studies, were aches and pains, rhinorrhea, dyspepsia and upper respiratory tract infections. However, the difference in incidence between TAMIFLU and placebo for these events was less than 1%. There were no clinically relevant differences in the safety profile of the 942 elderly subjects who received TAMIFLU or placebo, compared with the younger population.

Treatment Studies in Pediatric Patients: A total of 1032 pediatric patients aged 1 to 12 years (including 698 otherwise healthy pediatric patients aged 1 to 12 years and 334 asthmatic pediatric patients aged 6 to 12 years) participated in phase III studies of TAMIFLU given for the treatment of influenza. A total of 515 pediatric patients received treatment with TAMIFLU oral suspension.

Adverse events occurring in >1% of pediatric patients receiving TAMIFLU treatment are listed in Table 4. The most frequently reported adverse event was vomiting. Other events reported more frequently by pediatric patients treated with TAMIFLU included abdominal pain, epistaxis, ear disorder, and conjunctivitis. These events generally occurred once and resolved despite continued dosing. They did not cause discontinuation of drug in the vast majority of cases.

The adverse event profile in adolescents is similar to that described for adult patients and pediatric patients aged 1 to 12 years.

[See table 4 above]

Observed During Clinical Practice for Treatment: The following adverse reactions have been identified during post-marketing use of TAMIFLU. Because these reactions are reported voluntarily from a population of uncertain size, it is not possible to reliably estimate their frequency or establish a causal relationship to TAMIFLU exposure.

General: Rash, swelling of the face or tongue
Cardiac: Arrhythmia
Neurologic: Seizure, confusion
Metabolic: Aggravation of diabetes

OVERDOSAGE

At present, there has been no experience with overdose. Single doses of up to 1000 mg of TAMIFLU have been associated with nausea and/or vomiting.

DOSAGE AND ADMINISTRATION

TAMIFLU may be taken with or without food (see *PHARMACOKINETICS*). However, when taken with food, tolerability may be enhanced in some patients.

Table 3. Most Frequent Adverse Events in Studies in Naturally Acquired Influenza

Adverse Event	Treatment		Prophylaxis	
	Placebo N=716	Oseltamivir 75 mg bid N=724	Placebo N=1434	Oseltamivir 75 mg bid N=1480
Nausea (without vomiting)	40 (5.6%)	72 (9.9%)	56 (3.9%)	104 (7.0%)
Vomiting	21 (2.9%)	68 (9.4%)	15 (1.0%)	31 (2.1%)
Diarrhea	70 (9.8%)	48 (6.6%)	38 (2.6%)	48 (3.2%)
Bronchitis	15 (2.1%)	17 (2.3%)	17 (1.2%)	11 (0.7%)
Abdominal pain	16 (2.2%)	16 (2.2%)	23 (1.6%)	30 (2.0%)
Dizziness	25 (3.5%)	15 (2.1%)	21 (1.5%)	24 (1.6%)
Headache	14 (2.0%)	13 (1.8%)	251 (17.5%)	298 (20.1%)
Cough	12 (1.7%)	9 (1.2%)	86 (6.0%)	83 (5.6%)
Insomnia	6 (0.8%)	8 (1.1%)	14 (1.0%)	18 (1.2%)
Vertigo	4 (0.6%)	7 (1.0%)	3 (0.2%)	4 (0.3%)
Fatigue	7 (1.0%)	7 (1.0%)	107 (7.5%)	117 (7.9%)

Table 4. Adverse Events Occurring On Treatment in >1% of Pediatric Patients Enrolled in Phase III Trials of TAMIFLU Treatment of Naturally Acquired Influenza

Adverse Event	Placebo N=517	TAMIFLU 2 mg/kg twice daily N=515
Vomiting	48 (9.3%)	77 (15.0%)
Diarrhea	55 (10.6%)	49 (9.5%)
Otitis media	58 (11.2%)	45 (8.7%)
Abdominal pain	20 (3.9%)	24 (4.7%)
Asthma (including aggravated)	19 (3.7%)	18 (3.5%)
Nausea	22 (4.3%)	17 (3.3%)
Epistaxis	13 (2.5%)	16 (3.1%)
Pneumonia	17 (3.3%)	10 (1.9%)
Ear disorder	6 (1.2%)	9 (1.7%)
Sinusitis	13 (2.5%)	9 (1.7%)
Bronchitis	11 (2.1%)	8 (1.6%)
Conjunctivitis	2 (0.4%)	5 (1.0%)
Dermatitis	10 (1.9%)	5 (1.0%)
Lymphadenopathy	8 (1.5%)	5 (1.0%)
Tympanic membrane disorder	6 (1.2%)	5 (1.0%)

Body Weight in kg	Body Weight in lbs	Recommended Dose for 5 days
≤15 kg	≤33 lbs	30 mg twice daily
>15 kg to 23 kg	>33 lbs to 51 lbs	45 mg twice daily
>23 kg to 40 kg	>51 lbs to 88 lbs	60 mg twice daily
>40 kg	>88 lbs	75 mg twice daily

Standard Dosage—Treatment of Influenza:

Adults and Adolescents: The recommended oral dose of TAMIFLU for treatment of influenza in adults and adolescents 13 years and older is 75 mg twice daily for 5 days. Treatment should begin within 2 days of onset of symptoms of influenza.

Pediatric Patients: The recommended oral dose of TAMIFLU oral suspension for pediatric patients 1 year and older or adult patients who cannot swallow a capsule is: [See table above]

An oral dosing dispenser with 30 mg, 45 mg, and 60 mg graduations is provided with the oral suspension; the 75 mg dose can be measured using a combination of 30 mg and 45 mg. It is recommended that patients use this dispenser. In the event that the dispenser provided is lost or damaged, another dosing syringe or other device may be used to deliver the following volumes: 2.5 mL (1/2 tsp) for children ≤15 kg, 3.8 mL (3/4 tsp) for >15 to 23 kg, 5.0 mL (1 tsp) for >23 to 40 kg, and 6.2 mL (1 1/4 tsp) for >40 kg.

Standard Dosage—Prophylaxis of Influenza: The recommended oral dose of TAMIFLU for prophylaxis of influenza in adults and adolescents 13 years and older following close contact with an infected individual is 75 mg once daily for at least 7 days. Therapy should begin within 2 days of exposure. The recommended dose for prophylaxis during a community outbreak of influenza is 75 mg once daily. Safety and efficacy have been demonstrated for up to 6 weeks. The duration of protection lasts for as long as dosing is continued.

Special Dosage Instructions: **Hepatic Impairment:** The safety and pharmacokinetics in patients with hepatic impairment have not been evaluated.

Renal Impairment: For plasma concentrations of oseltamivir carboxylate predicted to occur following various dosing schedules in patients with renal impairment, see CLINICAL PHARMACOLOGY: *PHARMACOKINETICS: Special Populations*.

Treatment of Influenza: Dose adjustment is recommended for patients with creatinine clearance between 10 and 30 mL/min receiving TAMIFLU for the treatment of influenza. In these patients it is recommended that the dose be reduced to 75 mg of TAMIFLU once daily for 5 days. No recommended dosing regimens are available for patients undergoing routine hemodialysis and continuous peritoneal dialysis treatment with end-stage renal disease.

Prophylaxis of Influenza: For the prophylaxis of influenza, dose adjustment is recommended for patients with creatinine clearance between 10 and 30 mL/min receiving TAMIFLU. In these patients it is recommended that the dose be reduced to 75 mg of TAMIFLU every other day. No recommended dosing regimens are available for patients undergoing routine hemodialysis and continuous peritoneal dialysis treatment with end-stage renal disease.

Pediatric Patients: The safety and efficacy of TAMIFLU for prophylaxis in pediatric patients younger than 13 years of age have not been established. The safety and efficacy of TAMIFLU for treatment in pediatric patients younger than 1 year of age have not been established.

Geriatric Patients: No dose adjustment is required for geriatric patients (see *PHARMACOKINETICS: Special Populations* and PRECAUTIONS).

Preparation of Oral Suspension:

It is recommended that TAMIFLU oral suspension be constituted by the pharmacist prior to dispensing to the patient:

1. Tap the closed bottle several times to loosen the powder.
2. Measure 52 mL of water in a graduated cylinder.
3. Add the total amount of water for constitution to the bottle and shake the closed bottle well for 15 seconds.
4. Remove the child-resistant cap and push bottle adapter into the neck of the bottle.
5. Close bottle with child-resistant cap tightly. This will assure the proper seating of the bottle adapter in the bottle and child-resistant status of the cap.

NOTE: SHAKE THE TAMIFLU ORAL SUSPENSION WELL BEFORE EACH USE.

The constituted oral suspension should be used within 10 days of preparation; the pharmacist should write the date of expiration of the constituted suspension on a pharmacy label. The patient package insert and oral dispenser should be dispensed to the patient.

HOW SUPPLIED

TAMIFLU Capsules: Supplied as 75-mg (75 mg free base equivalent of the phosphate salt) grey/light yellow hard gelatin capsules. "ROCHE" is printed in blue ink on the grey body and "75 mg" is printed in blue ink on the light yellow cap. Available in blister packages of 10 (NDC 0004-0800-85).

Storage: Store the capsules at 25°C (77°F); excursions permitted to 15° to 30°C (59° to 86°F). [See USP Controlled Room Temperature]

TAMIFLU Oral Suspension: Supplied as a white powder blend for constitution to a white tutti-frutti-flavored suspension. Available in 100 mL glass bottles with a bottle adapter and 1 oral dispenser (NDC 0004-0810-09).

Storage: Store dry powder at 25°C (77°F); excursions permitted to 15° to 30°C (59° to 86°F). [See USP Controlled Room Temperature]

Store constituted suspension at 25°C (77°F); excursions permitted to 15° to 30°C (59° to 86°F); or under refrigeration at 2° to 8°C (36° to 46°F). Do not freeze.

Rx only

Manufactured by:
F. Hoffmann-La Roche Ltd.
Basel, Switzerland

Distributed by:
Roche Pharmaceuticals
Roche Laboratories Inc.
340 Kingsland Street
Nutley, New Jersey 07110-1199

Licensor:
Gilead Sciences, Inc.
Foster City, California 94404

Revised: December 2000

Copyright © 1999–2000 by Roche Laboratories Inc. All rights reserved.

TICLID® ℞

[tye' klid]

(ticlopidine hydrochloride)

Tablets

Prescribing information for this product, which appears on pages 2786–2789 of the 2001 PDR, has been completely revised as follows. Please write "See Supplement A" next to the product heading.

WARNING: TICLID can cause life-threatening hematological adverse reactions, including neutropenia/agranulocytosis, thrombotic thrombocytopenic purpura (TTP) and aplastic anemia.

Neutropenia/Agranulocytosis: **Among 2048 patients in clinical trials in stroke patients, there were 50 cases (2.4%) of neutropenia (less than 1200 neutrophils/mm^3), and the neutrophil count was below 450/mm^3 in 17 of these patients (0.8% of the total population).**

TTP: **One case of thrombotic thrombocytopenic purpura was reported during clinical trials in stroke patients. Based on postmarketing data, US physicians reported about 100 cases between 1992 and 1997. Based on an estimated patient exposure of 2 million to 4 million, and assuming an event reporting rate of 10% (the true rate is not known), the incidence of ticlopidine-associated TTP may be as high as one case in every 2000 to 4000 patients exposed.**

Aplastic Anemia: **Aplastic anemia was not seen during clinical trials in stroke patients, but US physicians reported about 50 cases between 1992 and 1998. Based on an estimated patient exposure of 2 million to 4 million, and assuming an event reporting rate of 10% (the true rate is not known), the incidence of ticlopidine-associated aplastic anemia may be as high as one case in every 4000 to 8000 patients exposed.**

Monitoring of Clinical and Hematologic Status: **Severe hematological adverse reactions may occur within a few days of the start of therapy. The incidence of TTP peaks after about 3 to 4 weeks of therapy and neutropenia peaks at approximately 4 to 6 weeks. The incidence of aplastic anemia peaks after about 4 to 8 weeks of therapy. The incidence of the hematologic adverse reactions declines thereafter. Only a few cases of neutropenia, TTP, or aplastic anemia have arisen after more than 3 months of therapy.**

Hematological adverse reactions cannot be reliably predicted by any identified demographic or clinical characteristics. During the first 3 months of treatment, patients receiving TICLID must, therefore, be hematologically and clinically monitored for evidence of neutropenia or TTP. If any such evidence is seen, TICLID should be immediately discontinued.

The detection and treatment of ticlopidine-associated hematological adverse reactions are further described under WARNINGS.

DESCRIPTION

TICLID (ticlopidine hydrochloride) is a platelet aggregation inhibitor. Chemically it is 5-[(2-chlorophenyl)methyl]-4,5,6,7-tetrahydrothieno [3,2-c] pyridine hydrochloride. The structural formula is:

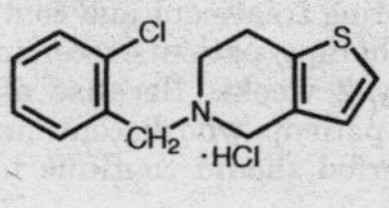

Ticlopidine hydrochloride is a white crystalline solid. It is freely soluble in water and self-buffers to a pH of 3.6. It also dissolves freely in methanol, is sparingly soluble in methylene chloride and ethanol, slightly soluble in acetone and insoluble in a buffer solution of pH 6.3. It has a molecular weight of 300.25.

TICLID tablets for oral administration are provided as white, oval, film-coated, blue-imprinted tablets containing 250 mg of ticlopidine hydrochloride. Each tablet also contains citric acid, magnesium stearate, microcrystalline cellulose, povidone, starch and stearic acid as inactive ingredients. The white film-coating contains hydroxypropylmethyl cellulose, polyethylene glycol and titanium dioxide. Each tablet is printed with blue ink, which includes FD&C Blue #1 aluminum lake as the colorant. The tablets are identified with Ticlid on one side and 250 on the reverse side.

CLINICAL PHARMACOLOGY

Mechanism of Action: When taken orally, ticlopidine hydrochloride causes a time- and dose-dependent inhibition of both platelet aggregation and release of platelet granule constituents, as well as a prolongation of bleeding time. The intact drug has no significant in vitro activity at the concentrations attained in vivo; and, although analysis of urine and plasma indicates at least 20 metabolites, no metabolite which accounts for the activity of ticlopidine has been isolated.

Ticlopidine hydrochloride, after oral ingestion, interferes with platelet membrane function by inhibiting ADP-induced platelet-fibrinogen binding and subsequent platelet-platelet interactions. The effect on platelet function is irreversible for the life of the platelet, as shown both by persistent inhibition of fibrinogen binding after washing platelets ex vivo and by inhibition of platelet aggregation after resuspension of platelets in buffered medium.

Pharmacokinetics and Metabolism: After oral administration of a single 250-mg dose, ticlopidine hydrochloride is rapidly absorbed with peak plasma levels occurring at approximately 2 hours after dosing and is extensively metabolized. Absorption is greater than 80%. Administration after meals results in a 20% increase in the AUC of ticlopidine.

Ticlopidine hydrochloride displays nonlinear pharmacokinetics and clearance decreases markedly on repeated dosing. In older volunteers the apparent half-life of ticlopidine after a single 250-mg dose is about 12.6 hours; with repeat dosing at 250 mg bid, the terminal elimination half-life rises to 4 to 5 days and steady-state levels of ticlopidine hydrochloride in plasma are obtained after approximately 14 to 21 days.

Ticlopidine hydrochloride binds reversibly (98%) to plasma proteins, mainly to serum albumin and lipoproteins. The binding to albumin and lipoproteins is nonsaturable over a wide concentration range. Ticlopidine also binds to alpha-1 acid glycoprotein. At concentrations attained with the recommended dose, only 15% or less ticlopidine in plasma is bound to this protein.

Ticlopidine hydrochloride is metabolized extensively by the liver; only trace amounts of intact drug are detected in the urine. Following an oral dose of radioactive ticlopidine hydrochloride administered in solution, 60% of the radioactivity is recovered in the urine and 23% in the feces. Approximately $^1/_3$ of the dose excreted in the feces is intact ticlopidine hydrochloride, possibly excreted in the bile. Ticlopidine hydrochloride is a minor component in plasma (5%) after a single dose, but at steady-state is the major component (15%). Approximately 40% to 50% of the radioactive metabolites circulating in plasma are covalently bound to plasma proteins, probably by acylation.

Clearance of ticlopidine decreases with age. Steady-state trough values in elderly patients (mean age 70 years) are about twice those in younger volunteer populations.

Hepatically Impaired Patients: The effect of decreased hepatic function on the pharmacokinetics of TICLID was studied in 17 patients with advanced cirrhosis. The average plasma concentration of ticlopidine in these subjects was slightly higher than that seen in older subjects in a separate trial (see CONTRAINDICATIONS).

Renally Impaired Patients: Patients with mildly (Ccr 50 to 80 mL/min) or moderately (Ccr 20 to 50 mL/min) impaired renal function were compared to normal subjects (Ccr 80 to 150 mL/min) in a study of the pharmacokinetic and platelet pharmacodynamic effects of TICLID (250 mg bid) for 11 days. Concentrations of unchanged TICLID were measured after a single 250-mg dose and after the final 250-mg dose on Day 11.

AUC values of ticlopidine increased by 28% and 60% in mild and moderately impaired patients, respectively, and plasma clearance decreased by 37% and 52%, respectively, but there were no statistically significant differences in ADP-induced platelet aggregation. In this small study (26 patients), bleeding times showed significant prolongation only in the moderately impaired patients.

Pharmacodynamics: In healthy volunteers over the age of 50, substantial inhibition (over 50%) of ADP-induced platelet aggregation is detected within 4 days after administration of ticlopidine hydrochloride 250 mg bid, and maximum platelet aggregation inhibition (60% to 70%) is achieved after 8 to 11 days. Lower doses cause less, and more delayed, platelet aggregation inhibition, while doses above 250 mg bid give little additional effect on platelet aggregation but an increased rate of adverse effects. The dose of 250 mg bid is the only dose that has been evaluated in controlled clinical trials.

Continued on next page

Ticlid—Cont.

After discontinuation of ticlopidine hydrochloride, bleeding time and other platelet function tests return to normal within 2 weeks, in the majority of patients.

At the recommended therapeutic dose (250 mg bid), ticlopidine hydrochloride has no known significant pharmacological actions in man other than inhibition of platelet function and prolongation of the bleeding time.

CLINICAL TRIALS: *Stroke Patients*

The effect of ticlopidine on the risk of stroke and cardiovascular events was studied in two multicenter, randomized, double-blind trials.

1. Study in Patients Experiencing Stroke Precursors: In a trial comparing ticlopidine and aspirin (The Ticlopidine Aspirin Stroke Study or TASS), 3069 patients (1987 men, 1082 women) who had experienced such stroke precursors as transient ischemic attack (TIA), transient monocular blindness (amaurosis fugax), reversible ischemic neurological deficit or minor stroke, were randomized to ticlopidine 250 mg bid or aspirin 650 mg bid. The study was designed to follow patients for at least 2 years and up to 5 years.

Over the duration of the study, TICLID significantly reduced the risk of fatal and nonfatal stroke by 24% (p = .011) from 18.1 to 13.8 per 100 patients followed for 5 years, compared to aspirin. During the first year, when the risk of stroke is greatest, the reduction in risk of stroke (fatal and nonfatal) compared to aspirin was 48%; the reduction was similar in men and women.

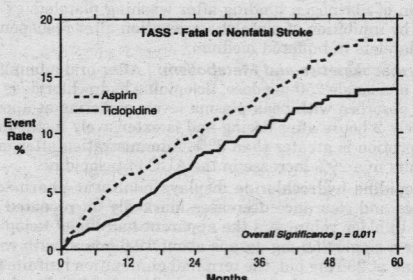

2. Study in Patients Who Had a Completed Atherothrombotic Stroke: In a trial comparing ticlopidine with placebo (The Canadian American Ticlopidine Study or CATS) 1073 patients who had experienced a previous atherothrombotic stroke were treated with TICLID 250 mg bid or placebo for up to 3 years.

TICLID significantly reduced the overall risk of stroke by 24% (p = .017) from 24.6 to 18.6 per 100 patients followed for 3 years, compared to placebo. During the first year the reduction in risk of fatal and nonfatal stroke over placebo was 33%.

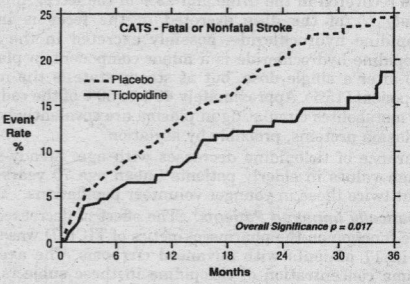

Stent Patients: The ability of TICLID to reduce the rate of thrombotic events after the placement of coronary artery stents has been studied in five randomized trials, one of substantial size (Stent Anticoagulation Restenosis Study or STARS) described below, and four smaller studies. In these trials, ticlopidine 250 mg bid with ASA (dose range from 100 mg bid to 325 mg qd) was compared to aspirin alone or to anticoagulant therapy plus aspirin. The trials enrolled patients undergoing both planned (elective) and unplanned coronary stent placement. The types of stents used, the use of intravascular ultrasound, and the use of high-pressure stent deployment varied among the trials, although all patients in STARS received a Palmaz-Schatz stent. The primary efficacy endpoints of the trials were similar, and included death, myocardial infarction and the need for repeat coronary angioplasty or CABG. All trials followed patients for at least 30 days.

In STARS, patients were randomized to receive one of three regimens for 4 weeks: aspirin alone, aspirin plus coumadin, or aspirin plus ticlopidine. Therapy was initiated following successful coronary stent placement. The primary endpoint was the incidence of stent thrombosis, defined as death, Q-Wave MI, or angiographic thrombus within the stented vessel demonstrated at the time of documented ischemia requiring emergent revascularization. The incidence rates for the primary endpoint and its components at 30 days are shown in the table below.

[See first table above]

TICLID® (ticlopidine hydrochloride)

STARS	TICLID + Aspirin N=546	Aspirin N=557	Coumadin + Aspirin N=550	Odds Ratio (95% C.I.)*	p-Value*
Primary Endpoint	3 (0.5%)	20 (3.6%)	15 (2.7%)	0.15 (0.03, 0.51)	<0.001
Deaths	0 (0%)	1 (0.2%)	0 (0%)	=	=
Q-Wave MI (Recurrent and Procedure Related)	1 (0.2%)	12 (2.2%)	8 (1.5%)	0.08 (0.002, 0.57)	0.004
Angiographically Evident Thrombosis	3 (0.5%)	16 (2.9%)	15 (2.7%)	0.19 (0.03, 0.66)	0.005

* Comparison of TICLID plus aspirin to aspirin alone.

STARS	TICLID + Aspirin N=546	Aspirin N=557	Coumadin + Aspirin N=550
Hemorrhagic Complications	30 (5.5%)	10 (1.8%)	34 (6.2%)
Cerebrovascular Accident	0 (0%)	2 (0.4%)	1 (0.2%)
Neutropenia (≤1200/mm^3)	3 (0.5%)	0 (0%)	1 (0.2%)

The use of ticlopidine plus aspirin did not affect the rate of non-Q-wave MIs when compared with aspirin alone or aspirin plus anticoagulants in STARS.

The use of ticlopidine plus aspirin was associated with a lower rate of recurrent cardiovascular events when compared with aspirin alone or aspirin plus anticoagulants in the other four randomized trials.

The rate of serious bleeding complications and neutropenia in STARS are shown in the table below. There were no cases of thrombotic thrombocytopenic purpura (TTP) or aplastic anemia reported in 1346 patients who received ticlopidine plus aspirin in the five randomized trials.

[See second table above]

INDICATIONS AND USAGE: TICLID is indicated:

- to reduce the risk of thrombotic stroke (fatal or nonfatal) in patients who have experienced stroke precursors, and in patients who have had a completed thrombotic stroke. Because TICLID is associated with a risk of life-threatening blood dyscrasias including thrombotic thrombocytopenic purpura (TTP), neutropenia/agranulocytosis and aplastic anemia (see BOXED WARNING and WARNINGS), TICLID should be reserved for patients who are intolerant or allergic to aspirin therapy or who have failed aspirin therapy.
- as adjunctive therapy with aspirin to reduce the incidence of subacute stent thrombosis in patients undergoing successful coronary stent implantation (see CLINICAL TRIALS).

CONTRAINDICATIONS

The use of TICLID is contraindicated in the following conditions:

- Hypersensitivity to the drug
- Presence of hematopoietic disorders such as neutropenia and thrombocytopenia or a past history of either TTP or aplastic anemia
- Presence of a hemostatic disorder or active pathological bleeding (such as bleeding peptic ulcer or intracranial bleeding)
- Patients with severe liver impairment

WARNINGS

Hematological Adverse Reactions: Neutropenia: Neutropenia may occur suddenly. Bone-marrow examination typically shows a reduction in white blood cell precursors. After withdrawal of ticlopidine, the neutrophil count usually rises to >1200/mm^3 within 1 to 3 weeks.

Thrombocytopenia: Rarely, thrombocytopenia may occur in isolation or together with neutropenia.

Thrombotic Thrombocytopenic Purpura (TTP): TTP is characterized by thrombocytopenia, microangiopathic hemolytic anemia (schistocytes [fragmented RBCs] seen on peripheral smear), neurological findings, renal dysfunction, and fever. The signs and symptoms can occur in any order, in particular, clinical symptoms may precede laboratory findings by hours or days. With prompt treatment (often including plasmapheresis), 70% to 80% of patients will survive with minimal or no sequelae. Because platelet transfusions may accelerate thrombosis in patients with TTP on ticlopidine, they should, if possible, be avoided.

Aplastic Anemia: Aplastic anemia is characterized by anemia, thrombocytopenia and neutropenia together with a bone marrow examination that shows decreases in the precursor cells for red blood cells, white blood cells, and platelets. Patients may present with signs or symptoms suggestive of infection, in association with low white blood cell and platelet counts. Prompt treatment, which may include the use of drugs to stimulate the bone marrow, can minimize the mortality associated with aplastic anemia.

Monitoring for Hematologic Adverse Reactions: Starting just before initiating treatment and continuing through the third month of therapy, patients receiving TICLID must be monitored every 2 weeks. Because of ticlopidine's long plasma half-life, patients who discontinue ticlopidine during this 3-month period should continue to be monitored for

2 weeks after discontinuation. More frequent monitoring, and monitoring after the first 3 months of therapy, is necessary only in patients with clinical signs (eg, signs or symptoms suggestive of infection) or laboratory signs (eg, neutrophil count less than 70% of the baseline count, decrease in hematocrit or platelet count) that suggest incipient hematological adverse reactions.

Clinically, fever might suggest neutropenia, TTP, or aplastic anemia; TTP might also be suggested by weakness, pallor, petechiae or purpura, dark urine (due to blood, bile pigments, or hemoglobin) or jaundice, or neurological changes. Patients should be told to discontinue TICLID and to contact the physician immediately upon the occurrence of any of these findings.

Laboratory monitoring should include a complete blood count, with special attention to the absolute neutrophil count (WBC × % neutrophils), platelet count, and the appearance of the peripheral smear. Ticlopidine is occasionally associated with thrombocytopenia unrelated to TTP or aplastic anemia. Any acute, unexplained reduction in hemoglobin or platelet count should prompt further investigation for a diagnosis of TTP, and the appearance of schistocytes (fragmented RBCs) on the smear should be treated as presumptive evidence of TTP. A simultaneous decrease in platelet count and WBC count should prompt further investigation for a diagnosis of aplastic anemia. If there are laboratory signs of TTP or aplastic anemia, or if the neutrophil count is confirmed to be <1200/mm^3, then TICLID should be discontinued immediately.

Other Hematological Effects: Rare cases of agranulocytosis, pancytopenia, or leukemia have been reported in postmarketing experience, some of which have been fatal. All forms of hematological adverse reactions are potentially fatal.

Cholesterol Elevation: TICLID therapy causes increased serum cholesterol and triglycerides. Serum total cholesterol levels are increased 8% to 10% within 1 month of therapy and persist at that level. The ratios of the lipoprotein subfractions are unchanged.

Anticoagulant Drugs: The tolerance and long-term safety of coadministration of TICLID with heparin, oral anticoagulants or fibrinolytic agents have not been established. In trials for cardiac stenting, patients received heparin and TICLID concomitantly for approximately 12 hours. If a patient is switched from an anticoagulant or fibrinolytic drug to TICLID, the former drug should be discontinued prior to TICLID administration.

PRECAUTIONS

General: TICLID should be used with caution in patients who may be at risk of increased bleeding from trauma, surgery or pathological conditions. If it is desired to eliminate the antiplatelet effects of TICLID prior to elective surgery, the drug should be discontinued 10 to 14 days prior to surgery. Several controlled clinical studies have found increased surgical blood loss in patients undergoing surgery during treatment with ticlopidine. In TASS and CATS it was recommended that patients have ticlopidine discontinued prior to elective surgery. Several hundred patients underwent surgery during the trials, and no excessive surgical bleeding was reported.

Prolonged bleeding time is normalized within 2 hours after administration of 20 mg methylprednisolone IV. Platelet transfusions may also be used to reverse the effect of TICLID on bleeding. Because platelet transfusions may accelerate thrombosis in patients with TTP on ticlopidine, they should, if possible, be avoided.

GI Bleeding: TICLID prolongs template bleeding time. The drug should be used with caution in patients who have lesions with a propensity to bleed (such as ulcers). Drugs that might induce such lesions should be used with caution in patients on TICLID (see CONTRAINDICATIONS).

Use in Hepatically Impaired Patients: Since ticlopidine is metabolized by the liver, dosing of TICLID or other drugs metabolized in the liver may require adjustment upon starting or stopping concomitant therapy. Because of limited experience in patients with severe hepatic disease, who may have bleeding diatheses, the use of TICLID is not recommended in this population (see CLINICAL PHARMACOLOGY and CONTRAINDICATIONS).

Use in Renally Impaired Patients: There is limited experience in patients with renal impairment. Decreased plasma clearance, increased AUC values and prolonged bleeding times can occur in renally impaired patients. In controlled clinical trials no unexpected problems have been encountered in patients having mild renal impairment, and there is no experience with dosage adjustment in patients with greater degrees of renal impairment. Nevertheless, for renally impaired patients, it may be necessary to reduce the dosage of ticlopidine or discontinue it altogether if hemorrhagic or hematopoietic problems are encountered (see CLINICAL PHARMACOLOGY).

***Information for the Patient* (see Patient Leaflet):** Patients should be told that a decrease in the number of white blood cells (neutropenia) or platelets (thrombocytopenia) can occur with TICLID, especially during the first 3 months of treatment and that neutropenia, if it is severe, can result in an increased risk of infection. They should be told it is critically important to obtain the scheduled blood tests to detect neutropenia or thrombocytopenia. Patients should also be reminded to contact their physicians if they experience any indication of infection such as fever, chills, or sore throat, any of which might be a consequence of neutropenia. Thrombocytopenia may be part of a syndrome called TTP. Symptoms and signs of TTP, such as fever, weakness, difficulty speaking, seizures, yellowing of skin or eyes, dark or bloody urine, pallor or petechiae (pinpoint hemorrhagic spots on the skin), should be reported immediately.

All patients should be told that it may take them longer than usual to stop bleeding when they take TICLID and that they should report any unusual bleeding to their physician. Patients should tell physicians and dentists that they are taking TICLID before any surgery is scheduled and before any new drug is prescribed.

Patients should be told to promptly report side effects of TICLID such as severe or persistent diarrhea, skin rashes or subcutaneous bleeding or any signs of cholestasis, such as yellow skin or sclera, dark urine, or light-colored stools.

Patients should be told to take TICLID with food or just after eating in order to minimize gastrointestinal discomfort.

Laboratory Tests: *Liver Function:* TICLID therapy has been associated with elevations of alkaline phosphatase, bilirubin, and transaminases, which generally occurred within 1 to 4 months of therapy initiation. In controlled clinical trials in stroke patients the incidence of elevated alkaline phosphatase (greater than two times upper limit of normal) was 7.6% in ticlopidine patients, 6% in placebo patients and 2.5% in aspirin patients. The incidence of elevated AST (SGOT) (greater than two times upper limit of normal) was 3.1% in ticlopidine patients, 4% in placebo patients and 2.1% in aspirin patients. No progressive increases were observed in closely monitored clinical trials (eg, no transaminase greater than 10 times the upper limit of normal was seen), but most patients with these abnormalities had therapy discontinued. Occasionally patients had developed minor elevations in bilirubin.

Postmarketing experience includes rare individuals with elevations in their transaminases and bilirubin to >10× above the upper limits of normal. Based on postmarketing and clinical trial experience, liver function testing, including ALT, AST, and GGT, should be considered whenever liver dysfunction is suspected, particularly during the first 4 months of treatment.

Drug Interactions: Therapeutic doses of TICLID caused a 30% increase in the plasma half-life of antipyrine and may cause analogous effects on similarly metabolized drugs. Therefore, the dose of drugs metabolized by hepatic microsomal enzymes with low therapeutic ratios or being given to patients with hepatic impairment may require adjustment to maintain optimal therapeutic blood levels when starting or stopping concomitant therapy with ticlopidine. Studies of specific drug interactions yielded the following results:

Aspirin and Other NSAIDs: Ticlopidine potentiates the effect of aspirin or other NSAIDs on platelet aggregation. The safety of concomitant use of ticlopidine and NSAIDs has not been established. The safety of concomitant use of ticlopidine and aspirin beyond 30 days has not been established (see CLINICAL TRIALS: *Stent Patients*). Aspirin did not modify the ticlopidine-mediated inhibition of ADP-induced platelet aggregation, but ticlopidine potentiated the effect of aspirin on collagen-induced platelet aggregation. Caution should be exercised in patients who have lesions with a propensity to bleed, such as ulcers. Long-term concomitant use of aspirin and ticlopidine is not recommended (see PRECAUTIONS: *GI Bleeding*).

Antacids: Administration of TICLID after antacids resulted in an 18% decrease in plasma levels of ticlopidine.

Cimetidine: Chronic administration of cimetidine reduced the clearance of a single dose of TICLID by 50%.

Digoxin: Coadministration of TICLID with digoxin resulted in a slight decrease (approximately 15%) in digoxin plasma levels. Little or no change in therapeutic efficacy of digoxin would be expected.

Theophylline: In normal volunteers, concomitant administration of TICLID resulted in a significant increase in the theophylline elimination half-life from 8.6 to 12.2 hours and a comparable reduction in total plasma clearance of theophylline.

Phenobarbital: In 6 normal volunteers, the inhibitory effects of TICLID on platelet aggregation were not altered by chronic administration of phenobarbital.

Phenytoin: In vitro studies demonstrated that ticlopidine does not alter the plasma protein binding of phenytoin. However, the protein binding interactions of ticlopidine and its metabolites have not been studied in vivo. Several cases of elevated phenytoin plasma levels with associated somnolence and lethargy have been reported following coadministration with TICLID. Caution should be exercised in coadministering this drug with TICLID, and it may be useful to remeasure phenytoin blood concentrations.

Propranolol: In vitro studies demonstrated that ticlopidine does not alter the plasma protein binding of propranolol. However, the protein binding interactions of ticlopidine and its metabolites have not been studied in vivo. Caution should be exercised in coadministering this drug with TICLID.

Other Concomitant Therapy: Although specific interaction studies were not performed, in clinical studies TICLID was used concomitantly with beta blockers, calcium channel blockers and diuretics without evidence of clinically significant adverse interactions (see PRECAUTIONS).

Food Interaction: The oral bioavailability of ticlopidine is increased by 20% when taken after a meal. Administration of TICLID with food is recommended to maximize gastrointestinal tolerance. In controlled trials in stroke patients TICLID was taken with meals.

Carcinogenesis, Mutagenesis, Impairment of Fertility: In a 2-year oral carcinogenicity study in rats, ticlopidine at daily doses of up to 100 mg/kg (610 mg/m^2) was not tumorigenic. For a 70-kg person (1.73 m^2 body surface area) the dose represents 14 times the recommended clinical dose on a mg/kg basis and two times the clinical dose on body surface area basis. In a 78-week oral carcinogenicity study in mice, ticlopidine at daily doses up to 275 mg/kg (1180 mg/m^2) was not tumorigenic. The dose represents 40 times the recommended clinical dose on a mg/kg basis and four times the clinical dose on body surface area basis.

Ticlopidine was not mutagenic in vitro in the Ames test, the rat hepatocyte DNA-repair assay, or the Chinese-hamster fibroblast chromosomal aberration test; or in vivo in the mouse spermatozoid morphology test, the Chinese-hamster micronucleus test, or the Chinese-hamster bone-marrow-cell sister-chromatid exchange test. Ticlopidine was found to have no effect on fertility of male and female rats at oral doses up to 400 mg/kg/day.

Pregnancy: *Teratogenic Effects:* Pregnancy: Category B. Teratology studies have been conducted in mice (doses up to 200 mg/kg/day), rats (doses up to 400 mg/kg/day) and rabbits (doses up to 200 mg/kg/day). Doses of 400 mg/kg in rats, 200 mg/kg/day in mice and 100 mg/kg in rabbits produced maternal toxicity, as well as fetal toxicity, but there was no evidence of a teratogenic potential of ticlopidine. There are, however, no adequate and well-controlled studies in pregnant women. Because animal reproduction studies are not always predictive of a human response, this drug should be used during pregnancy only if clearly needed.

Nursing Mothers: Studies in rats have shown ticlopidine is excreted in the milk. It is not known whether this drug is excreted in human milk. Because many drugs are excreted in human milk and because of the potential for serious adverse reactions in nursing infants from ticlopidine, a decision should be made whether to discontinue nursing or to discontinue the drug, taking into account the importance of the drug to the mother.

Pediatric Use: Safety and effectiveness in pediatric patients have not been established.

Geriatric Use: Clearance of ticlopidine is somewhat lower in elderly patients and trough levels are increased. The major clinical trials with TICLID in stroke patients were conducted in an elderly population with an average age of 64 years. Of the total number of patients in the therapeutic trials, 45% of patients were over 65 years old and 12% were over 75 years old. No overall differences in effectiveness or safety were observed between these patients and younger patients, and other reported clinical experience has not identified differences in responses between the elderly and younger patients, but greater sensitivity of some older individuals cannot be ruled out.

ADVERSE REACTIONS

Adverse reactions in stroke patients were relatively frequent with over 50% of patients reporting at least one. Most (30% to 40%) involved the gastrointestinal tract. Most adverse effects are mild, but 21% of patients discontinued therapy because of an adverse event, principally diarrhea, rash, nausea, vomiting, GI pain and neutropenia. Most adverse effects occur early in the course of treatment, but a new onset of adverse effects can occur after several months.

The incidence rates of adverse events listed in the following table were derived from multicenter, controlled clinical trials in stroke patients described above comparing TICLID, placebo and aspirin over study periods of up to 5.8 years. Adverse events considered by the investigator to be probably drug-related that occurred in at least 1% of patients treated with TICLID are shown in the following table:

[See table above]

Percent of Patients With Adverse Events in Controlled Studies
(TASS and CATS)

Event	TICLID (n= 2048) Incidence	Aspirin (n = 1527) Incidence	Placebo (n = 536) Incidence
Any Events	*60.0 (20.9)*	*53.2 (14.5)*	*34.3 (6.1)*
Diarrhea	12.5 (6.3)	5.2 (1.8)	4.5 (1.7)
Nausea	7.0 (2.6)	6.2 (1.9)	1.7 (0.9)
Dyspepsia	7.0 (1.1)	9.0 (2.0)	0.9 (0.2)
Rash	5.1 (3.4)	1.5 (0.8)	0.6 (0.9)
GI Pain	3.7 (1.9)	5.6 (2.7)	1.3 (0.4)
Neutropenia	2.4 (1.3)	0.8 (0.1)	1.1 (0.4)
Purpura	2.2 (0.2)	1.6 (0.1)	0.0 (0.0)
Vomiting	1.9 (1.4)	1.4 (0.9)	0.9 (0.4)
Flatulence	1.5 (0.1)	1.4 (0.3)	0.0 (0.0)
Pruritus	1.3 (0.8)	0.3 (0.1)	0.0 (0.0)
Dizziness	1.1 (0.4)	0.5 (0.4)	0.0 (0.0)
Anorexia	1.0 (0.4)	0.5 (0.3)	0.0 (0.0)
Abnormal Liver Function Test	1.0 (0.7)	0.3 (0.3)	0.0 (0.0)

Incidence of discontinuation, regardless of relationship to therapy, is shown in parentheses.

Hematological: Neutropenia/thrombocytopenia, TTP, aplastic anemia (see BOXED WARNING and WARNINGS), leukemia, agranulocytosis, eosinophilia, pancytopenia, thrombocytosis and bone-marrow depression have been reported.

Gastrointestinal: TICLID therapy has been associated with a variety of gastrointestinal complaints including diarrhea and nausea. The majority of cases are mild, but about 13% of patients discontinued therapy because of these. They usually occur within 3 months of initiation of therapy and typically are resolved within 1 to 2 weeks without discontinuation of therapy. If the effect is severe or persistent, therapy should be discontinued. In some cases of severe or bloody diarrhea, colitis was later diagnosed.

Hemorrhagic: TICLID has been associated with increased bleeding, spontaneous posttraumatic bleeding and perioperative bleeding including, but not limited to, gastrointestinal bleeding. It has also been associated with a number of bleeding complications such as ecchymosis, epistaxis, hematuria and conjunctival hemorrhage.

Intracerebral bleeding was rare in clinical trials in stroke patients with TICLID, with an incidence no greater than that seen with comparator agents (ticlopidine 0.5%, aspirin 0.6%, placebo 0.75%). It has also been reported postmarketing.

Rash: Ticlopidine has been associated with a maculopapular or urticarial rash (often with pruritus). Rash usually occurs within 3 months of initiation of therapy with a mean onset time of 11 days. If drug is discontinued, recovery occurs within several days. Many rashes do not recur on drug rechallenge. There have been rare reports of severe rashes, including Stevens-Johnson syndrome, erythema multiforme and exfoliative dermatitis.

Less Frequent Adverse Reactions (Probably Related): Clinical adverse experiences occurring in 0.5% to 1.0% of stroke patients in controlled trials include:

Digestive System: GI fullness
Skin and Appendages: urticaria
Nervous System: headache
Body as a Whole: asthenia, pain
Hemostatic System: epistaxis
Special Senses: tinnitus

In addition, rarer, relatively serious and potentially fatal events associated with the use of TICLID have also been reported from postmarketing experience: Hemolytic anemia with reticulocytosis, immune thrombocytopenia, hepatitis, hepatocellular jaundice, cholestatic jaundice, hepatic necrosis, hepatic failure, peptic ulcer, renal failure, nephrotic syndrome, hyponatremia, vasculitis, sepsis, allergic reactions (including angioedema, allergic pneumonitis, and anaphylaxis), systemic lupus (positive ANA), peripheral neuropathy, serum sickness, arthropathy and myositis.

OVERDOSAGE

One case of deliberate overdosage with TICLID has been reported by a foreign postmarketing surveillance program. A 38-year-old male took a single 6000-mg dose of TICLID (equivalent to 24 standard 250-mg tablets). The only abnormalities reported were increased bleeding time and increased SGPT. No special therapy was instituted and the patient recovered without sequelae.

Single oral doses of ticlopidine at 1600 mg/kg and 500 mg/kg were lethal to rats and mice, respectively. Symptoms of acute toxicity were GI hemorrhage, convulsions, hypothermia, dyspnea, loss of equilibrium and abnormal gait.

DOSAGE AND ADMINISTRATION

Stroke:

The recommended dose of TICLID is 250 mg bid taken with food. Other doses have not been studied in controlled trials for these indications.

Continued on next page

Ticlid—Cont.

Coronary Artery Stenting: The recommended dose of TICLID is 250 mg bid taken with food together with antiplatelet doses of aspirin for up to 30 days of therapy following successful stent implantation.

HOW SUPPLIED

TICLID is available in white, oval, film-coated 250-mg tablets, printed in blue with Ticlid on one side and 250 on the other. They are provided in unit of use bottles of 30 tablets (NDC 0004-0018-23) and 60 tablets (NDC 0004-0018-22) and 500 tablets (NDC 0004-0018-14).
Store at 15° to 30°C (59° to 86°F).

IMPORTANT INFORMATION ABOUT TICLID (ticlopidine HCl) TABLETS

The information in this leaflet is intended to help you use TICLID safely. Please read the leaflet carefully. Although it does not contain all the detailed medical information that is provided to your doctor, it provides facts about TICLID that are important for you to know. If you still have questions after reading this leaflet or if you have questions at any time during your treatment with TICLID, check with your doctor.

Why TICLID was Prescribed by Your Doctor:
Stroke Patients: TICLID is recommended to help reduce your risk of having a stroke, but only for patients who have had a stroke or early stroke warning symptoms while on aspirin, or for those who have these symptoms but are intolerant or allergic to aspirin.
Stent Patients: TICLID is recommended with aspirin for up to 30 days in patients who have had a stent implanted in their coronary arteries to reduce the risk of blood clots forming inside the stent.
Special Warning for Users of TICLID/Necessary Blood Tests:
TICLID is not prescribed for those who can take aspirin to reduce the risk of stroke because TICLID can cause life-threatening blood problems. **Getting your blood tests done and reporting symptoms to your doctor as soon as possible can avoid serious complications.**
The white cells of the blood that fight infection may drop to dangerous levels (a condition called neutropenia). This occurs in about 2.4% (1 in 40) of people on ticlopidine. You should be on the lookout for signs of infection such as fever, chills or sore throat. If this problem is caught early, it can almost always be reversed, but if undetected it can be fatal.
Another problem that has occurred in some patients taking ticlopidine is a decrease in cells called platelets (a condition called thrombocytopenia). This may occur as part of a syndrome that includes injury to red blood cells, causing anemia, kidney abnormalities, neurologic changes and fever. This condition is called TTP and can be fatal.
Things you should watch for as possible early signs of TTP are yellow skin or eye color, pinpoint dots (rash) on the skin, pale color, fever, weakness on a side of the body, or dark urine. **If any of these occur, contact your doctor immediately.**
Both complications occur most frequently in the first 90 days after TICLID is started. To make sure you don't develop either of these problems, your doctor will arrange for you to have your blood tested before you start taking TICLID and then every 2 weeks for the first 3 months you are on TICLID. If detected, neutropenia and thrombocytopenia can almost always be reversed. It is essential that you keep your appointments for the blood tests and that you call your doctor immediately if you have any indication that you may have TTP or neutropenia. If you stop taking TICLID for any reason within the first 3 months, you will still need to have your blood tested for an additional 2 weeks after you have stopped taking TICLID.
Rarely, decreases in the white blood cells, red blood cells and platelets can occur together. This condition is called aplastic anemia and can be fatal.
Things you should watch for as possible early signs of aplastic anemia are feeling of excessive weakness and tiredness, paleness, bruising, and bleeding from areas such as your nose or gums. You may also develop signs of infection such as fever. **If any of these occur, contact your doctor immediately.**
Other Warnings and Precautions: A few people may develop jaundice while being treated with TICLID. The signs of jaundice are yellowing of the skin or the whites of the eyes or consistent darkening of the urine or lightening in the color of the stools. These symptoms should be reported to your physician promptly.
If any of the symptoms described above for neutropenia, TTP, aplastic anemia or jaundice occur, contact your doctor immediately.
TICLID should be used only as directed by your doctor. Do not give TICLID to anyone else. **Keep TICLID out of reach of children!**
Some people may have such side effects as diarrhea, skin rash, stomach or intestinal discomfort. If any of these problems are persistent, or if you are concerned about them, bring them to your doctor's attention.
It may take longer than usual to stop bleeding when taking TICLID. Tell your doctor if you have any more bleeding or bruising than usual, and, if you have emergency surgery, be sure to let your doctor or dentist know that you are taking TICLID. Also, tell your doctor well in advance of any planned surgery (including tooth extraction), because he or she may recommend that you stop taking TICLID temporarily.
How TICLID Works: Stroke Patients: A stroke occurs when a clot (or thrombus) forms in a blood vessel in the brain or forms in another part of the body and breaks off, then travels to the brain (an embolus). In both cases the blood supply to part of the brain is blocked and that part of the brain is damaged. TICLID works by making the blood less likely to clot, although not so much less that it causes you to become likely to bleed, unless you have a bleeding disorder or some injury (such as a bleeding ulcer of the stomach or intestine) that is especially likely to bleed.
Stent Patients: A heart attack or angina (chest pain) can occur when fatty deposits block the arteries that carry oxygen and nutrient-rich blood to your heart. To decrease the chance of fatty deposits building up over time, your doctor may recommend the placement of a coronary stent. TICLID may be given to you with aspirin to make blood clots less likely to form inside the stent so that the artery remains open.
Who Should Not Take TICLID? Contact your doctor immediately and do not take TICLID if:

- you have an allergic reaction to TICLID
- you have a blood disorder or a serious bleeding problem, such as a bleeding stomach ulcer
- you have previously been told you had TTP or aplastic anemia
- you have severe liver disease or other liver problems
- you are pregnant or you are planning to become pregnant
- you are breastfeeding

Rx only

Distributed by:
Pharmaceuticals
Roche Laboratories Inc.
340 Kingsland Street
Nutley, New Jersey 07110-1199

Revised: March 2001

XELODA® ℞

[*xĕl-ōda*]
(capecitabine)
TABLETS

Prescribing information for this product, which appears on pages 2806–2809 of the 2001 PDR, has been completely revised as follows. Please write "See Supplement A" next to the product heading.

DESCRIPTION

XELODA (capecitabine) is a fluoropyrimidine carbamate with antineoplastic activity. It is an orally administered systemic prodrug of 5′-deoxy-5-fluorouridine (5′-DFUR) which is converted to 5-fluorouracil.
The chemical name for capecitabine is 5′-deoxy-5-fluoro-N-[(pentyloxy)carbonyl]-cytidine and has a molecular weight of 359.35. Capecitabine has the following structural formula:

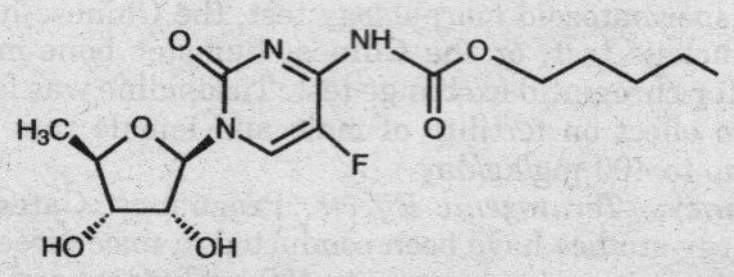

Capecitabine is a white to off-white crystalline powder with an aqueous solubility of 26 mg/mL at 20°C.
XELODA is supplied as biconvex, oblong film-coated tablets for oral administration. Each light peach-colored tablet contains 150 mg capecitabine and each peach-colored tablet contains 500 mg capecitabine. The inactive ingredients in XELODA include: anhydrous lactose, croscarmellose sodium, hydroxypropyl methylcellulose, microcrystalline cellulose, magnesium stearate and purified water. The peach or light peach film coating contains hydroxypropyl methylcellulose, talc, titanium dioxide, and synthetic yellow and red iron oxides.

CLINICAL PHARMACOLOGY

Capecitabine is relatively non-cytotoxic in vitro. This drug is enzymatically converted to 5-fluorouracil (5-FU) in vivo.
Bioactivation: Capecitabine is readily absorbed from the gastrointestinal tract. In the liver, a 60 kDa carboxyesterase hydrolyzes much of the compound to 5′-deoxy-5-fluorocytidine (5′-DFCR). Cytidine deaminase, an enzyme found in most tissues, including tumors, subsequently converts 5′-DFCR to 5′-deoxy-5-fluorouridine (5′-DFUR). The enzyme, thymidine phosphorylase (dThdPase), then hydrolyzes 5′-DFUR to the active drug 5-FU. Many tissues throughout the body express thymidine phosphorylase. Some human carcinomas express this enzyme in higher concentrations than surrounding normal tissues.
Metabolic Pathway of capecitabine to 5-FU
[See chemical structure at top of next column]

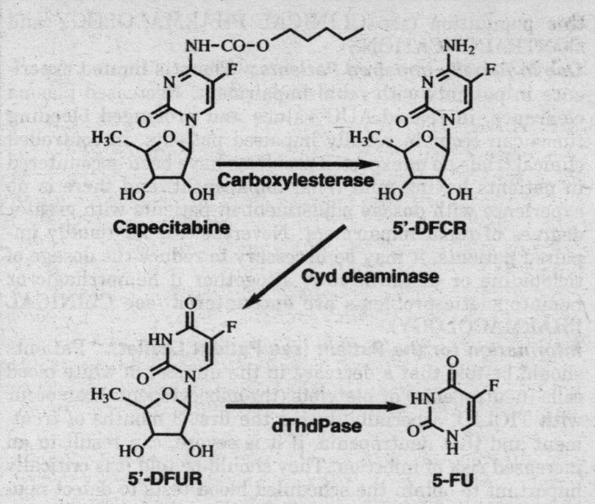

Mechanism of Action: Both normal and tumor cells metabolize 5-FU to 5-fluoro-2-deoxyuridine monophosphate (FdUMP) and 5-fluorouridine triphosphate (FUTP). These metabolites cause cell injury by two different mechanisms. First, FdUMP and the folate cofactor, N^{5-10}-methylenetetrahydrofolate, bind to thymidylate synthase (TS) to form a covalently bound ternary complex. This binding inhibits the formation of thymidylate from uracil. Thymidylate is the necessary precursor of thymidine triphosphate, which is essential for the synthesis of DNA, so that a deficiency of this compound can inhibit cell division. Second, nuclear transcriptional enzymes can mistakenly incorporate FUTP in place of uridine triphosphate (UTP) during the synthesis of RNA. This metabolic error can interfere with RNA processing and protein synthesis.
Pharmacokinetics in Colorectal Tumors and Adjacent Healthy Tissue: Following oral administration of capecitabine 7 days before surgery in patients with colorectal cancer, the median ratio of 5-FU concentration in colorectal tumors to adjacent tissues was 2.9 (range from 0.9 to 8.0). These ratios have not been evaluated in breast cancer patients or compared to 5-FU infusion.
Human Pharmacokinetics: The pharmacokinetics of XELODA and its metabolites have been evaluated in about 200 cancer patients over a dosage range of 500 to 3500 mg/m^2/day. Over this range, the pharmacokinetics of capecitabine and its metabolite, 5′-DFCR were dose proportional and did not change over time. The increases in the AUCs of 5′-DFUR and 5-FU, however, were greater than proportional to the increase in dose and the AUC of 5-FU was 34% higher on day 14 than on day 1. The elimination half-life of both parent capecitabine and 5-FU was about ¾ of an hour. The inter-patient variability in the C_{max} and AUC of 5-FU was greater than 85%.
Absorption, Distribution, Metabolism and Excretion: Capecitabine reached peak blood levels in about 1.5 hours (T_{max}) with peak 5-FU levels occurring slightly later, at 2 hours. Food reduced both the rate and extent of absorption of capecitabine with mean C_{max} and $AUC_{0-\infty}$ decreased by 60% and 35%, respectively. The C_{max} and $AUC_{0-\infty}$ of 5-FU were also reduced by food by 43% and 21%, respectively. Food delayed T_{max} of both parent and 5-FU by 1.5 hours (see PRECAUTIONS and DOSAGE AND ADMINISTRATION).
Plasma protein binding of capecitabine and its metabolites is less than 60% and is not concentration-dependent. Capecitabine was primarily bound to human albumin (approximately 35%).
Capecitabine is extensively metabolized enzymatically to 5-FU. The enzyme dihydropyrimidine dehydrogenase hydrogenates 5-FU, the product of capecitabine metabolism, to the much less toxic 5-fluoro-5,6-dihydro-fluorouracil (FUH_2). Dihydropyrimidinase cleaves the pyrimidine ring to yield 5-fluoro-ureido-propionic acid (FUPA). Finally, β-ureido-propionase cleaves FUPA to α-fluoro-β-alanine (FBAL) which is cleared in the urine.
Capecitabine and its metabolites are predominantly excreted in urine; 95.5% of administered capecitabine dose is recovered in urine. Fecal excretion is minimal (2.6%). The major metabolite excreted in urine is FBAL which represents 57% of the administered dose. About 3% of the administered dose is excreted in urine as unchanged drug.
Special Populations:
Age, Gender and Ethnicity: No formal studies were conducted to examine the effect of age or gender or ethnicity on the pharmacokinetics of capecitabine and its metabolites.
Hepatic Insufficiency: XELODA has been evaluated in 13 patients with mild to moderate hepatic dysfunction due to liver metastases defined by a composite score including bilirubin, AST/ALT and alkaline phosphatase following a single 1255 mg/m^2 dose of capecitabine. Both $AUC_{0-\infty}$ and C_{max} of capecitabine increased by 60% in patients with hepatic dysfunction compared to patients with normal hepatic function (n=14). The $AUC_{0-\infty}$ and C_{max} of 5-FU was not affected. In patients with mild to moderate hepatic dysfunction due to liver metastases, caution should be exercised when XELODA is administered. The effect of severe hepatic dysfunction on XELODA is not known (see PRECAUTIONS and DOSAGE AND ADMINISTRATION).
Drug-Drug Interactions:
Drugs Metabolized by Cytochrome P450 Enzymes: In vitro enzymatic studies with human liver microsomes indicated that capecitabine and 5′-DFUR had no inhibitory effects on substrates of cytochrome P450 for the major isoenzymes such as 1A2, 2A6, 3A4, 2C9, 2C19, 2D6, and 2E1, suggesting a low likelihood of interactions with drugs metabolized by cytochrome P450 enzymes.
Antacid: When Maalox®* (20 mL), an aluminum hydroxide- and magnesium hydroxide-containing antacid, was administered immediately after capecitabine (1250 mg/m^2, n=12 cancer patients), AUC and C_{max} increased by 16% and 35%, respectively, for capecitabine and by 18% and 22%, respectively, for 5′-DFCR. No effect was observed on the other

three major metabolites (5'-DFUR, 5-FU, FBAL) of capecitabine.

XELODA has a low potential for pharmacokinetic interactions related to plasma protein binding.

CLINICAL STUDIES

In a phase 1 study with XELODA in patients with solid tumors, the maximum tolerated dose as a single agent was 3000 mg/m^2 when administered daily for 2 weeks, followed by a 1-week rest period. The dose-limiting toxicities were diarrhea and leukopenia.

Breast Carcinoma: The antitumor activity of XELODA was evaluated in an open-label single-arm trial conducted in 24 centers in the US and Canada. A total of 162 patients with stage IV breast cancer were enrolled. The primary endpoint was tumor response rate in patients with measurable disease, with response defined as a ≥50% decrease in sum of the products of the perpendicular diameters of bidimensionally measurable disease for at least 1 month. XELODA was administered at a daily dose of 2510 mg/m^2 for 2 weeks followed by a 1-week rest period and given as 3-week cycles. The baseline demographics and clinical characteristics for all patients (n=162) and those with measurable disease (n=135) are shown in the table below. Resistance was defined as progressive disease while on treatment, with or without an initial response, or relapse within 6 months of completing treatment with an anthracycline-containing adjuvant chemotherapy regimen.

[See table 1 to the right]

Table 1. Baseline Demographics and Clinical Characteristics

	Patients with Measurable Disease (n=135)	All Patients (n=162)
Age (median, years)	55	56
Karnofsky PS	90	90
No. Disease Sites		
1–2	43 (32%)	60 (37%)
3–4	63 (46%)	69 (43%)
>5	29 (22%)	34 (21%)
Dominant Site of Disease		
Visceral[1]	101 (75%)	110 (68%)
Soft Tissue	30 (22%)	35 (22%)
Bone	4 (3%)	17 (10%)
Prior Chemotherapy		
Paclitaxel	135 (100%)	162 (100%)
Anthracycline[2]	122 (90%)	147 (91%)
5-FU	110 (81%)	133 (82%)
Resistance to Paclitaxel	103 (76%)	124 (77%)
Resistance to an Anthracycline[2]	55 (41%)	67 (41%)
Resistance to both Paclitaxel and an Anthracycline	43 (32%)	51 (31%)

[1]Lung, pleura, liver, peritoneum
[2]Includes 2 patients treated with an anthracenedione

Antitumor responses for patients with disease resistant to both paclitaxel and an anthracycline are shown in the table below.

Table 2. Response Rates in Doubly-Resistant Patients

	Resistance to Both Paclitaxel and an Anthracycline (n=43)
CR	0
PR[1]	11
CR + PR[1]	11
Response Rate[1] (95% C.I.)	25.6% (13.5, 41.2)
Duration of Response[1] Median in days[2] (Range)	154 (63 to 233)

[1]Includes 2 patients treated with an anthracenedione
[2]From date of first response

For the subgroup of 43 patients who were doubly resistant, the median time to progression was 102 days and the median survival was 255 days. The objective response rate in this population was supported by a response rate of 18.5% (1 CR, 24 PRs) in the overall population of 135 patients with measurable disease, who were less resistant to chemotherapy (see Table 1). The median time to progression was 90 days and the median survival was 306 days.

INDICATIONS AND USAGE

XELODA is indicated for the treatment of patients with metastatic breast cancer resistant to both paclitaxel and an anthracycline-containing chemotherapy regimen or resistant to paclitaxel and for whom further anthracycline therapy is not indicated, eg, patients who have received cumulative doses of 400 mg/m^2 of doxorubicin or doxorubicin equivalents. Resistance is defined as progressive disease while on treatment, with or without an initial response, or relapse within 6 months of completing treatment with an anthracycline-containing adjuvant regimen.

This indication is based on demonstration of a response rate. No results are available from controlled trials that demonstrate a clinical benefit resulting from treatment, such as improvement in disease-related symptoms, disease progression, or survival.

CONTRAINDICATIONS

XELODA is contraindicated in patients who have a known hypersensitivity to 5-fluorouracil.

XELODA is also contraindicated in patients with severe renal impairment (creatinine clearance below 30 mL/min [Cockroft and Gault]).

WARNINGS

Renal Insufficiency: In patients with moderate renal impairment (creatinine clearance 30–50 mL/min [Cockroft and Gault]) at baseline, a dose reduction to 75% of the XELODA starting dose is recommended. In patients with mild renal impairment (creatinine clearance 51–80 mL/min) no adjustment in starting dose is recommended (see DOSAGE AND ADMINISTRATION). Careful monitoring and prompt treatment interruption is recommended if the patient develops a grade 2, 3, or 4 adverse event with subsequent dose adjustments as outlined in the table in DOSAGE AND ADMINISTRATION.

Coagulopathy: Altered coagulation parameters and/or bleeding have been reported in patients taking XELODA concomitantly with coumarin-derivative anticoagulants such as warfarin and phenprocoumon. These events occurred within several days and up to several months after initiating XELODA therapy and, in a few cases, within one month after stopping XELODA. These events occurred in patients with and without liver metastases. Patients taking coumarin-derivative anticoagulants concomitantly with XELODA should be monitored regularly for alterations in their coagulation parameters (PT or INR) (see PRECAUTIONS: *Drug-Drug Interactions*).

Diarrhea: XELODA can induce diarrhea, sometimes severe. Patients with severe diarrhea should be carefully monitored and given fluid and electrolyte replacement if they become dehydrated. The median time to first occurrence of grade 2–4 diarrhea was 31 days (range from 1 to 322 days). National Cancer Institute of Canada (NCIC) grade 2 diarrhea is defined as an increase of 4 to 6 stools/day or nocturnal stools, grade 3 diarrhea as an increase of 7 to 9 stools/day or incontinence and malabsorption, and grade 4 diarrhea as an increase of ≥10 stools/day or grossly bloody diarrhea or the need for parenteral support. If grade 2, 3 or 4 diarrhea occurs, administration of XELODA should be immediately interrupted until the diarrhea resolves or decreases in intensity to grade 1. Following grade 3 or 4 diarrhea, subsequent doses of XELODA should be decreased (see DOSAGE AND ADMINISTRATION). Standard antidiarrheal treatments (eg, loperamide) are recommended.

Necrotizing enterocolitis (typhlitis) has been reported.

Geriatric Patients (gastrointestinal toxicity): Patients ≥80 years old may experience a greater incidence of gastrointestinal grade 3 or 4 adverse events (see PRECAUTIONS: *Geriatric Use*). Among the 14 patients 80 years of age and greater treated with capecitabine, three (21.4%), three (21.4%) and one (7.1%) patients experienced reversible grade 3 or 4 diarrhea, nausea and vomiting, respectively. Among the 313 patients age 60 to 79 years old, the incidence of gastrointestinal toxicity was similar to that in the overall population.

Pregnancy: XELODA may cause fetal harm when given to a pregnant woman. Capecitabine at doses of 198 mg/kg/day during organogenesis caused teratogenic malformations and embryo death in mice. In separate pharmacokinetic studies, this dose in mice produced 5'-DFUR AUC values about 0.2 times the corresponding values in patients administered the recommended daily dose. Teratogenic malformations in mice included cleft palate, anophthalmia, microphthalmia, oligodactyly, polydactyly, syndactyly, kinky tail and dilation of cerebral ventricles. At doses of 90 mg/kg/day, capecitabine given to pregnant monkeys during organogenesis caused fetal death. This dose produced 5'-DFUR AUC values about 0.6 times the corresponding values in patients administered the recommended daily dose. There are no adequate and well-controlled studies in pregnant women using XELODA. If the drug is used during pregnancy, or if the patient becomes pregnant while receiving this drug, the patient should be apprised of the potential hazard to the fetus. Women of childbearing potential should be advised to avoid becoming pregnant while receiving treatment with XELODA.

PRECAUTIONS

General: Patients receiving therapy with XELODA should be monitored by a physician experienced in the use of cancer chemotherapeutic agents. Most adverse events are reversible and do not need to result in discontinuation, although doses may need to be withheld or reduced (see DOSAGE AND ADMINISTRATION).

Hand-and-Foot Syndrome: Hand-and-foot syndrome (palmar-plantar erythrodysesthesia or chemotherapy induced acral erythema) is characterized by the following: numbness, dysesthesia/paresthesia, tingling, painless or painful swelling, erythema, desquamation, blistering and severe pain. Grade 2 hand-and-foot syndrome is defined as painful erythema and swelling of the hands and/or feet and/or discomfort affecting the patient's activities of daily living. Grade 3 hand-and-foot syndrome is defined as moist desquamation, ulceration, blistering and severe pain of the hands and/or feet and/or severe discomfort that causes the patient to be unable to work or perform activities of daily living. If grade 2 or 3 hand-and-foot syndrome occurs, administration of XELODA should be interrupted until the event resolves or decreases in intensity to grade 1. Following grade 3 hand-and-foot syndrome, subsequent doses of XELODA should be decreased (see DOSAGE AND ADMINISTRATION).

Cardiac: There has been cardiotoxicity associated with fluorinated pyrimidine therapy, including myocardial infarction, angina, dysrhythmias, cardiogenic shock, sudden death and electrocardiograph changes. These adverse events may be more common in patients with a prior history of coronary artery disease.

Hepatic Insufficiency: Patients with mild to moderate hepatic dysfunction due to liver metastases should be carefully monitored when XELODA is administered. The effect of severe hepatic dysfunction on the disposition of XELODA is not known (see CLINICAL PHARMACOLOGY and DOSAGE AND ADMINISTRATION).

Hyperbilirubinemia: Grade 3 or 4 hyperbilirubinemia occurred in 17% (n=97) of 570 patients with either metastatic breast or colorectal cancer who received a dose of 2510 mg/m^2 daily for 2 weeks followed by a 1-week rest period. Of 339 patients who had hepatic metastases at baseline and 231 patients without hepatic metastases at baseline, grade 3 or 4 hyperbilirubinemia occurred in 21.2% and 10.4%, respectively. Seventy-four (76%) of the 97 patients with grade 3 or 4 hyperbilirubinemia also had concurrent elevations in alkaline phosphatase and/or hepatic transaminases; 6% of these were grade 3 or 4. Only 4 patients (4%) had elevated hepatic transaminases without a concurrent elevation in alkaline phosphatase. If drug related grade 2–4 elevations in bilirubin occur, administration of XELODA should be immediately interrupted until the hyperbilirubinemia resolves or decreases in intensity to grade 1. NCIC grade 2 hyperbilirubinemia is defined as 1.5 × normal, grade 3 hyperbilirubinemia as 1.5-3 × normal and grade 4 hyperbilirubinemia as >3 × normal. (See recommended dose modifications under DOSAGE AND ADMINISTRATION.)

Hematologic: In 570 patients with either metastatic breast or colorectal cancer who received a dose of 2510 mg/m^2 administered daily for 2 weeks followed by a 1-week rest period, 4%, 2%, and 3% of patients had grade 3 or 4 neutropenia, thrombocytopenia and decreases in hemoglobin, respectively.

Carcinogenesis, Mutagenesis and Impairment of Fertility: Long-term studies in animals to evaluate the carcinogenic potential of capecitabine have not been conducted. Capecitabine was not mutagenic in vitro to bacteria (Ames test) or mammalian cells (Chinese hamster V79/HPRT gene mutation assay). Capecitabine was clastogenic in vitro to human peripheral blood lymphocytes but not clastogenic in vivo to mouse bone marrow (micronucleus test). Fluorouracil causes mutations in bacteria and yeast. Fluorouracil also causes chromosomal abnormalities in the mouse micronucleus test in vivo.

Impairment of Fertility: In studies of fertility and general reproductive performance in mice, oral capecitabine doses of 760 mg/kg/day disturbed estrus and consequently caused a decrease in fertility. In mice that became pregnant, no fetuses survived this dose. The disturbance in estrus was reversible. In males, this dose caused degenerative changes in the testes, including decreases in the number of spermatocytes and spermatids. In separate pharmacokinetic studies, this dose in mice produced 5'-DFUR AUC values about 0.7 times the corresponding values in patients administered the recommended daily dose.

Information for Patients (see Patient Package Insert): Patients and patients' caregivers should be informed of the expected adverse effects of XELODA, particularly nausea, vomiting, diarrhea, and hand-and-foot syndrome, and should be made aware that patient-specific dose adaptations during therapy are expected and necessary (see DOSAGE AND ADMINISTRATION). Patients should be encouraged to recog-

Continued on next page

Xeloda—Cont.

nize the common grade 2 toxicities associated with XELODA treatment.

Diarrhea: Patients experiencing grade 2 diarrhea (an increase of 4 to 6 stools/day or nocturnal stools) or greater should be instructed to stop taking XELODA immediately. Standard antidiarrheal treatments (eg, loperamide) are recommended.

Nausea: Patients experiencing grade 2 nausea (food intake significantly decreased but able to eat intermittently) or greater should be instructed to stop taking XELODA immediately. Initiation of symptomatic treatment is recommended.

Vomiting: Patients experiencing grade 2 vomiting (2 to 5 episodes in a 24-hour period) or greater should be instructed to stop taking XELODA immediately. Initiation of symptomatic treatment is recommended.

Hand-and-Foot Syndrome: Patients experiencing grade 2 hand-and-foot syndrome (painful erythema and swelling of the hands and/or feet and/or discomfort affecting the patients' activities of daily living) or greater should be instructed to stop taking XELODA immediately.

Stomatitis: Patients experiencing grade 2 stomatitis (painful erythema, edema or ulcers of the mouth or tongue, but able to eat) or greater should be instructed to stop taking XELODA immediately. Initiation of symptomatic treatment is recommended (see DOSAGE AND ADMINISTRATION).

Fever and Neutropenia: Patients who develop a fever of 100.5°F or greater or other evidence of potential infection should be instructed to call their physician.

Drug-Food Interaction: In all clinical trials, patients were instructed to administer XELODA within 30 minutes after a meal. Since current safety and efficacy data are based upon administration with food, it is recommended that XELODA be administered with food (see DOSAGE AND ADMINISTRATION).

Drug-Drug Interactions:

Antacid: The effect of an aluminum hydroxide- and magnesium hydroxide-containing antacid (Maalox)* on the pharmacokinetics of capecitabine was investigated in 12 cancer patients. There was a small increase in plasma concentrations of capecitabine and one metabolite (5'-DFCR); there was no effect on the 3 major metabolites (5'-DFUR, 5-FU and FBAL).

Coumarin Anticoagulants: Altered coagulation parameters and/or bleeding have been reported in patients taking capecitabine concomitantly with coumarin-derivative anticoagulants such as warfarin and phenprocoumon. Patients taking coumarin-derivative anticoagulants concomitantly with capecitabine should be monitored regularly for alterations in their coagulation parameters (PT or INR) (see WARNINGS: *Coagulopathy*).

Phenytoin: Postmarketing reports indicate that some patients receiving capecitabine and phenytoin had toxicity associated with elevated phenytoin levels. The level of phenytoin should be carefully monitored in patients taking XELODA and phenytoin dose may need to be reduced (see DOSAGE AND ADMINISTRATION: *Dose Modification Guidelines*).

Leucovorin: The concentration of 5-fluorouracil is increased and its toxicity may be enhanced by leucovorin. Deaths from severe enterocolitis, diarrhea, and dehydration have been reported in elderly patients receiving weekly leucovorin and fluorouracil.

Pregnancy: *Teratogenic Effects:* Category D (see WARNINGS). Women of childbearing potential should be advised to avoid becoming pregnant while receiving treatment with XELODA.

Nursing Women: It is not known whether the drug is excreted in human milk. Because many drugs are excreted in human milk and because of the potential for serious adverse reactions in nursing infants, it is recommended that nursing be discontinued when receiving XELODA therapy.

Pediatric Use: The safety and effectiveness of XELODA in persons <18 years of age have not been established.

Geriatric Use: No separate studies have been conducted to examine the effect of age on the pharmacokinetics of capecitabine and its metabolites. Patients ≥80 years old may experience a greater incidence of gastrointestinal grade 3 or 4 adverse events (see WARNINGS). Among the 14 patients 80 years of age and greater treated with capecitabine, 21.4%, 21.4% and 7.1% experienced grade 3 or 4 diarrhea, nausea and vomiting, respectively. Among the 313 patients 60 to 79 years old, the incidence was similar to the overall population. The elderly may be pharmacodynamically more sensitive to the toxic effects of 5-FU. Physicians should pay particular attention to monitoring the adverse effects of XELODA in the elderly.

ADVERSE REACTIONS

The following table shows the adverse events occurring in ≥5% of patients reported as at least remotely related to the administration of XELODA. Rates are rounded to the nearest whole number. The data are shown both for the study in stage IV breast cancer and for a group of 570 patients with breast and colorectal cancer who received a dose of 2510 mg/m² administered daily for 2 weeks followed by a 1-week rest period. The 570 patients were enrolled in 6 clinical trials (162 from the breast cancer trial described under CLINICAL STUDIES, 83 other patients with breast cancer and 325 patients with colorectal cancer). The mean duration of treatment was 121 days. A total of 71 patients (13%) discontinued treatment because of adverse events/intercurrent illness.

[See table below]

Shown below by body system are the adverse events in <5% of patients reported as related to the administration of XELODA and that were clinically at least remotely relevant. In parentheses is the incidence of grade 3 or 4 occurrences of each adverse event.

Gastrointestinal: intestinal obstruction (1.1), rectal bleeding (0.4), GI hemorrhage (0.2), esophagitis (0.4), gastritis, colitis, duodenitis, haematemesis, necrotizing enterocolitis
Skin: increased sweating (0.2), photosensitivity (0.2), radiation recall syndrome (0.2)
General: chest pain (0.2)
Neurological: ataxia (0.4), encephalopathy (0.2), depressed level of consciousness (0.2), loss of consciousness (0.2)
Metabolism: cachexia (0.4), hypertriglyceridemia (0.2)
Respiratory: dyspnea (0.5), epistaxis (0.2), bronchospasm (0.2), respiratory distress (0.2)
Infections: oral candidiasis (0.2), upper respiratory tract infection (0.2), urinary tract infection (0.2), bronchitis (0.2), pneumonia (0.2), sepsis (0.4), bronchopneumonia (0.2), gastroenteritis (0.2), gastrointestinal candidiasis (0.2), laryngitis (0.2), esophageal candidiasis (0.2)
Musculoskeletal: bone pain (0.2), joint stiffness (0.2)
Cardiac: angina pectoris (0.2), cardiomyopathy
Vascular: hypotension (0.2), hypertension (0.2), venous phlebitis and thrombophlebitis (0.2), deep venous thrombosis (0.7), lymphoedema (0.2), pulmonary embolism (0.4), cerebrovascular accident (0.2)
Blood: coagulation disorder (0.2), idiopathic thrombocytopenic purpura (0.2), pancytopenia (0.2)
Psychiatric: confusion (0.2)
Renal and Urinary: nocturia (0.2)
Hepatobiliary: hepatic fibrosis (0.2), cholestatic hepatitis (0.2), hepatitis (0.2)
Immune System: drug hypersensitivity (0.2)

OVERDOSAGE

Acute: Based on experience in animals and in humans treated up to doses of 3514 mg/m²/day, the anticipated manifestations of acute overdose would be nausea, vomiting, diarrhea, gastrointestinal irritation and bleeding, and bone marrow depression. Medical management of overdose should include customary supportive medical interventions aimed at correcting the presenting clinical manifestations. Although no clinical experience has been reported, dialysis may be of benefit in reducing circulating concentrations of 5'-DFUR, a low-molecular weight metabolite of the parent compound.

Single doses of XELODA were not lethal to mice, rats, and monkeys at doses up to 2000 mg/kg (2.4, 4.8, and 9.6 times the recommended human daily dose on a mg/m² basis).

DOSAGE AND ADMINISTRATION

The recommended dose of XELODA is 2500 mg/m² administered orally daily with food for 2 weeks followed by a 1-week rest period given as 3 week cycles. The XELODA daily dose is given orally in two divided doses (approximately 12 hours apart) at the end of a meal. XELODA tablets should be swallowed with water. The following table displays the total daily dose by body surface area and the number of tablets to be taken at each dose.

Table 4. XELODA Dose Calculation According to Body Surface Area

Dose level 2500 mg/m²/day		Number of tablets to be taken at each dose (morning and evening)	
Surface Area (m²)	Total Daily* Dose (mg)	150 mg	500 mg
• 1.24	3000	0	3
1.25–1.36	3300	1	3
1.37–1.51	3600	2	3
1.52–1.64	4000	0	4
1.65–1.76	4300	1	4
1.77–1.91	4600	2	4
1.92–2.04	5000	0	5
2.05–2.17	5300	1	5
• 2.18	5600	2	5

*Total Daily Dose divided by 2 to allow equal morning and evening doses.

Dose Modification Guidelines: Patients should be carefully monitored for toxicity. Toxicity due to XELODA administration may be managed by symptomatic treatment, dose interruptions and adjustment of XELODA dose. Once the dose has been reduced it should not be increased at a later time.
The phenytoin dose may need to be reduced when phenytoin is concomitantly administered with XELODA (see PRECAUTIONS: *Drug-Drug Interactions*).
[See table at top of next page]
Dosage modifications are not recommended for grade 1 events. Therapy with XELODA should be interrupted upon the occurrence of a grade 2 or 3 adverse experience. Once the adverse event has resolved or decreased in intensity to grade 1, then XELODA therapy may be restarted at full dose or as adjusted according to the above table. If a grade 4 experience occurs, therapy should be discontinued or interrupted until resolved or decreased to grade 1, and therapy should be restarted at 50% of the original dose. Doses of

Table 3. Percent Incidence of Adverse Events Considered Remotely, Possibly or Probably Related to Treatment in ≥5% of Patients

Adverse Event	Phase 2 Trial in Stage IV Breast Cancer (n=162)			Overall Savety Database (n=570)		
Body System/Adverse Event	Total	Grade 3	Grade 4	Total	Grade 3	Grade 4
GI						
Diarrhea	57	12	3	50	11	2
Nausea	53	4	–	44	4	–
Vomiting	37	4	–	26	3	–
Stomatitis	24	7	–	23	4	–
Abdominal pain	20	4	–	17	4	–
Constipation	15	1	–	9	1	–
Dyspepsia	8	–	–	6	–	–
Skin and Subcutaneous						
Hand-and-Foot Syndrome	57	11	–	45	13	–
Dermatitis	37	1	–	31	1	–
Nail disorder	7	–	–	4	–	–
General						
Fatigue	41	8	–	34	5	–
Pyrexia	12	1	–	10	–	–
Pain in limb	6	1	–	4	–	–
Neurological						
Paraesthesia	21	1	–	12	–	–
Headache	9	1	–	7	1	–
Dizziness	8	–	–	5	–	–
Insomnia	8	–	–	3	–	–
Metabolism						
Anorexia	23	3	–	20	2	–
Dehydration	7	4	1	5	2	1
Eye						
Eye Irritation	15	–	–	10	–	–
Musculoskeletal						
Myalgia	9	–	–	4	–	–
Cardiac						
Edema	9	1	–	6	–	–
Blood						
Neutropenia	26	2	2	22	3	2
Thrombocytopenia	24	3	1	21	1	1
Anemia	72	3	1	74	2	1
Lymphopenia	94	44	15	94	36	10
Hepatobiliary						
Hyperbilirubinemia	22	9	2	34	14	3

–Not observed or applicable

capecitabine omitted for toxicity are not replaced or restored; instead the patient should resume the planned treatment cycles.

Adjustment of Starting Dose in Special Populations:

Hepatic Impairment: In patients with mild to moderate hepatic dysfunction due to liver metastases, no starting dose adjustment is necessary; however, patients should be carefully monitored. Patients with severe hepatic dysfunction have not been studied.

Renal Impairment: In patients with moderate renal impairment (creatinine clearance 30-50 mL/min [Cockroft and Gault, as shown below]) at baseline, a dose reduction to 75% of the XELODA starting dose (from 2500 mg/m²/day to 1900 mg/m²/day) is recommended. In patients with mild renal impairment (creatinine clearance 51–80 mL/min) no adjustment in starting dose is recommended. Careful monitoring and prompt treatment interruption is recommended if the patient develops a grade 2, 3, or 4 adverse event with subsequent dose adjustments as outlined in the table above. XELODA is contraindicated in patients with severe renal impairment (creatinine clearance below 30 mL/min [Cockroft and Gault]).

[See table above]

Geriatrics: The elderly may be pharmacodynamically more sensitive to the toxic effects of 5-FU and therefore, physicians should exercise caution in monitoring the effects of XELODA in the elderly. Insufficient data are available to provide a dosage recommendation.

HOW SUPPLIED

XELODA is supplied as biconvex, oblong film-coated tablets, available in bottles as follows:

150 mg
color: light peach
engraving: XELODA on one side, 150 on the other
150 mg tablets packaged in bottles of 120 (NDC 0004-1100-51)

500 mg
color: peach
engraving: XELODA on one side, 500 on the other
500 mg tablets packaged in bottles of 240 (NDC 0004-1101-16)

Storage Conditions: Store at 25°C (77°F); excursions permitted to 15° to 30°C (59° to 86°F), keep tightly closed. [See USP Controlled Room Temperature]

*Maalox is a registered trademark of Novartis.
Rx only

Pharmaceuticals
Roche Laboratories Inc.
340 Kingsland Street
Nutley, New Jersey 07110-1199
Revised: November 2000
Printed in USA
Copyright © 1999-2000 by Roche Laboratories Inc. All rights reserved.

PATIENT PACKAGE INSERT (text only):

Patient Information About XELODA® (capecitabine) Tablets
This information will help you learn more about XELODA® (capecitabine) Tablets. It cannot, however, cover all possible precautions or side effects associated with XELODA nor does it list all the benefits and risks of XELODA. Your doctor should always be your first choice for detailed information about your medical condition and your treatment. Be sure to ask your doctor about any questions you may have.

What is XELODA?
• XELODA [zeh-LOE-duh] is an oral medication for the treatment of advanced breast cancer resistant to treatment with paclitaxel [pak-lih-TAK-sil] and an anthracycline [ann-thruh-SYE-kleen]-containing chemotherapy regimen. Paclitaxel is also known as Taxol®*. Anthracyclines include Adriamycin®† or doxorubicin.
• XELODA tablets come in two strengths: 150 mg (light peach) and 500 mg (peach).

How does XELODA work?
XELODA is converted in the body to the substance 5-fluorouracil. In some patients, this substance kills cancer cells and decreases the size of the tumor.

Who should not take XELODA?
• Patients allergic to 5-fluorouracil.
• Studies in animals suggest that XELODA may cause serious harm to an unborn child. No studies have been done with pregnant women. If you are pregnant, be sure to discuss with your doctor whether XELODA is right for you. Also, tell your doctor if you are nursing.
• Patients with severe renal impairment. Please inform your doctor if you know of any renal impairment that you may have. Your doctor may either prescribe a different drug or reduce the XELODA dose.

How should I take XELODA?
Your doctor will prescribe a dose and treatment regimen that is right for *you.* Your doctor may want you to take a combination of *150 mg* and *500 mg* tablets for each dose. If a combination of tablets is prescribed, it is very important that you correctly identify the tablets. Taking the wrong tablets could result in an overdose (too much medication) or underdose (too little medication). The 150 mg tablets are light peach in color and have 150 engraved on one side. The 500 mg tablets are peach in color and have 500 engraved on one side.
• Take the tablets in the combination prescribed by your doctor for your **morning and evening** doses.
• Take the tablets within **30 minutes after the end of a meal** (breakfast and dinner).
• XELODA tablets should be **swallowed with water.**

Table 5. Recommended Dose Modifications

Toxicity NCIC Grades*	During a Course of Therapy	Dose Adjustment for Next Cycle (% of starting dose)
• *Grade 1*	Maintain dose level	Maintain dose level
• *Grade 2*		
-1st appearance	Interrupt until resolved to grade 0–1	100%
-2nd appearance	Interrupt until resolved to grade 0–1	75%
-3rd appearance	Interrupt until resolved to grade 0–1	50%
-4th appearance	Discontinue treatment permanently	
• *Grade 3*		
-1st appearance	Interrupt until resolved to grade 0–1	75%
-2nd appearance	Interrupt until resolved to grade 0–1	50%
-3rd appearance	Discontinue treatment permanently	
• *Grade 4*		
-1st appearance	Discontinue permanently *or* If physician deems it to be in the patient's best interest to continue, interrupt until resolved to grade 0–1	50%

*National Cancer Institute of Canada Common Toxicity Criteria were used except for the Hand-and-Foot Syndrome (see PRECAUTIONS).

Cockroft and Gault Equation:

Creatinine clearance for males = $\dfrac{(140 - age) \,[yrs]) \,(body\ wt\ [kg])}{(72) \,(serum\ creatinine\ [mg/dL])}$

Creatinine clearance for females = $0.85 \times$ male value.

• It is important that you take all your medication as prescribed by your doctor.
• If you are taking the vitamin folic acid, please inform your doctor.
• If you are taking phenytoin (also known as Dilantin®‡), please inform your doctor. Your doctor may need to more frequently test the levels of phenytoin in your blood and/or change the dose of phenytoin that you are taking.
• If you are taking warfarin (also known as Coumadin®§), please inform your doctor. Your doctor may need to more frequently check how quickly your blood is clotting.

How long will I have to take XELODA?
It is recommended that XELODA be taken for 14 days followed by a 7-day rest period (no drug) given as a 21-day cycle. Your doctor will determine how many cycles of treatment you will need.

What if I miss a dose?
If you miss a dose of XELODA, do not take the missed dose at all and do not double the next one. Instead, continue your regular dosing schedule and check with your doctor.

What are the most common side effects of XELODA?
The most common side effects of XELODA are:
• diarrhea, nausea, vomiting, stomatitis (sores in mouth and throat), abdominal pain, constipation, loss of appetite or decreased appetite, and dehydration (excessive water loss from the body).
• hand-and-foot syndrome (palms of the hands or soles of the feet tingle, become numb, painful, swollen or red), rash, dry or itchy skin.
• tiredness, weakness, dizziness, headache, and fever.

When should I call my doctor?
It is important that you **CONTACT YOUR DOCTOR IMMEDIATELY** if you experience the following side effects. This will help reduce the likelihood that the side effect will continue or become serious. Your doctor may instruct you to decrease the dose and/or temporarily discontinue treatment with XELODA.
STOP taking XELODA immediately and contact your doctor if any of these symptoms occur:
• *Diarrhea:* if you have more than 4 bowel movements each day or any diarrhea at night.
• *Vomiting:* if you vomit more than once in a 24-hour time period.
• *Nausea:* if you lose your appetite, and the amount of food you eat each day is much less than usual.
• *Stomatitis:* if you have pain, redness, swelling, or sores in your mouth.
• *Hand-and-foot syndrome:* if you have pain, swelling or redness of hands and/or feet.
• *Fever or Infection:* if you have a temperature of 100.5°F or greater, or other evidence of infection.
If caught early, most of these side effects usually improve within 2 to 3 days after you stop taking XELODA. If they dont improve within 2 to 3 days, call your doctor again. After side effects have improved, your doctor will tell you whether to start taking XELODA again or what dose to use.

How should I store and use XELODA?
• Never share XELODA with anyone.
• XELODA should be stored at normal room temperature (about 65° to 85°F).
• Keep this and all other medications out of the reach of children.

• In case of accidental ingestion or if you suspect that more than the prescribed dose of this medication has been taken, contact your doctor or local poison control center or emergency room IMMEDIATELY.
• Medicines are sometimes prescribed for uses other than those listed in this leaflet. If you have any questions or concerns, or want more information about XELODA, contact your doctor or pharmacist.

*Taxol is a registered trademark of Bristol-Myers Squibb Company.
† Adriamycin is a registered trademark of Pharmacia & Upjohn Company.
‡ Dilantin is a registered trademark of Parke-Davis.
§ Coumadin is a registered trademark of DuPont Pharma.

DUE TO THE MERGER OF SCHEIN PHARMACEUTICAL, INC. AND WATSON, PLEASE REFER TO WATSON LABORATORIES, INC. FOR PRODUCT INFORMATION

Schering Corporation
a wholly-owned subsidiary of Schering-Plough Corporation
GALLOPING HILL ROAD
KENILWORTH, NJ 07033

Direct Inquiries to:
(908) 298-4000
CUSTOMER SERVICE:
(800) 222-7579
FAX: (908) 820-6400

For Medical Information Contact:
Schering Laboratories
Drug Information Services
2000 Galloping Hill Road
Kenilworth, NJ 07033
(800) 526-4099
FAX: (908) 298-2188

CLARITIN®
brand of loratadine
TABLETS, SYRUP, and
RAPIDLY-DISINTEGRATING TABLETS

Prescribing information for this product, which appears on pages 2884–2885 of the 2001 PDR, has been completely revised as follows. Please write "See Supplement A" next to the product heading.

Continued on next page

Claritin—Cont.

DESCRIPTION

Loratadine is a white to off-white powder not soluble in water, but very soluble in acetone, alcohol, and chloroform. It has a molecular weight of 382.89, and empirical formula of $C_{22}H_{23}ClN_2O_2$; its chemical name is ethyl 4-(8-chloro-5,6-dihydro-11*H*-benzo[5,6]cyclohepta [1,2-*b*]pyridin-11-ylidene)-1-piperidinecarboxylate and has the following structural formula:

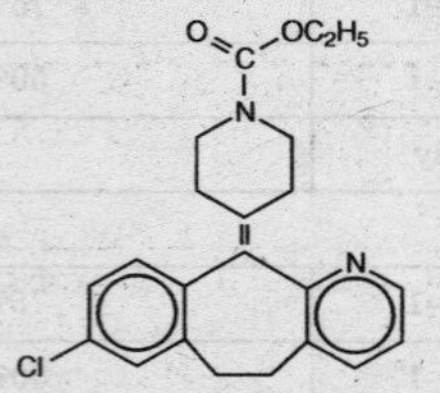

CLARITIN Tablets contain 10 mg micronized loratadine, an antihistamine, to be administered orally. It also contains the following inactive ingredients: corn starch, lactose, and magnesium stearate.

CLARITIN Syrup contains 1 mg/mL micronized loratadine, an antihistamine, to be administered orally. It also contains the following inactive ingredients: citric acid, edetate disodium, artificial flavor, glycerin, propylene glycol, sodium benzoate, sugar, and water. The pH is between 2.5 and 3.1.

CLARITIN REDITABS (loratadine rapidly-disintegrating tablets) contain 10 mg micronized loratadine, an antihistamine, to be administered orally. It disintegrates in the mouth within seconds after placement on the tongue, allowing its contents to be subsequently swallowed with or without water. CLARITIN REDITABS (loratadine rapidly-disintegrating tablets) also contain the following inactive ingredients: citric acid, gelatin, mannitol, and mint flavor.

CLINICAL PHARMACOLOGY

Loratadine is a long-acting tricyclic antihistamine with selective peripheral histamine H_1-receptor antagonistic activity.

Human histamine skin wheal studies following single and repeated 10 mg oral doses of CLARITIN have shown that the drug exhibits an antihistaminic effect beginning within 1 to 3 hours, reaching a maximum at 8 to 12 hours, and lasting in excess of 24 hours. There was no evidence of tolerance to this effect after 28 days of dosing with CLARITIN.

Whole body autoradiographic studies in rats and monkeys, radiolabeled tissue distribution studies in mice and rats, and *in vivo* radioligand studies in mice have shown that neither loratadine nor its metabolites readily cross the blood-brain barrier. Radioligand binding studies with guinea pig pulmonary and brain H_1-receptors indicate that there was preferential binding to peripheral versus central nervous system H_1-receptors.

Repeated application of CLARITIN REDITABS (loratadine rapidly-disintegrating tablets) to the hamster cheek pouch did not cause local irritation.

Pharmacokinetics: ***Absorption:*** Loratadine was rapidly absorbed following oral administration of 10 mg tablets, once daily for 10 days to healthy adult volunteers with times to maximum concentration (T_{max}) of 1.3 hours for loratadine and 2.5 hours for its major active metabolite, descarboethoxyloratadine. Based on a cross-study comparison of single doses of loratadine syrup and tablets given to healthy adult volunteers, the plasma concentration profile of descarboethoxyloratadine for the two formulations is comparable. The pharmacokinetics of loratadine and descarboethoxyloratadine are independent of dose over the dose range of 10 mg to 40 mg and are not altered by the duration of treatment. In a single-dose study, food increased the systemic bioavailability (AUC) of loratadine and descarboethoxyloratadine by approximately 40% and 15%, respectively. The time to peak plasma concentration (T_{max}) of loratadine and descarboethoxyloratadine was delayed by 1 hour. Peak plasma concentrations (C_{max}) were not affected by food.

Pharmacokinetic studies showed that CLARITIN REDITABS (loratadine rapidly-disintegrating tablets) provide plasma concentrations of loratadine and descarboethoxyloratadine similar to those achieved with CLARITIN Tablets. Following administration of 10 mg loratadine once daily for 10 days with each dosage form in a randomized crossover comparison in 24 normal adult subjects, similar mean exposures (AUC) and peak plasma concentrations (C_{max}) of loratadine were observed. CLARITIN REDITABS (loratadine rapidly-disintegrating tablets) mean AUC and C_{max} were 11% and 6% greater than that of the CLARITIN Tablet values, respectively. Descarboethoxyloratadine bioequivalence was demonstrated between the two formulations. After 10 days of dosing, mean peak plasma concentrations were attained at 1.3 hours and 2.3 hours (T_{max}) for parent and metabolite, respectively.

In a single-dose study with CLARITIN REDITABS (loratadine rapidly-disintegrating tablets), food increased the AUC of loratadine by approximately 48% and did not appreciably affect the AUC of descarboethoxyloratadine. The times to peak plasma concentration (T_{max}) of loratadine and descarboethoxyloratadine were delayed by approximately 2.4 and 3.7 hours, respectively, when food was consumed prior to CLARITIN REDITABS (loratadine rapidly-disintegrating tablets) administration. Parent and metabolite peak concentrations (C_{max}) were not affected by food.

In a single-dose study with CLARITIN REDITABS (loratadine rapidly-disintegrating tablets) in 24 subjects, the AUC of loratadine was increased by 26% when administered without water compared to administration with water, while C_{max} was not substantially affected. The bioavailability of descarboethoxyloratadine was not different when administered without water.

Metabolism: *In vitro* studies with human liver microsomes indicate that loratadine is metabolized to descarboethoxyloratadine predominantly by cytochrome P450 3A4 (CYP3A4) and, to a lesser extent, by cytochrome P450 2D6 (CYP2D6). In the presence of a CYP3A4 inhibitor ketoconazole, loratadine is metabolized to descarboethoxyloratadine predominantly by CYP2D6. Concurrent administration of loratadine with either ketoconazole, erythromycin (both CYP3A4 inhibitors), or cimetidine (CYP2D6 and CYP3A4 inhibitor) to healthy volunteers was associated with substantially increased plasma concentrations of loratadine (see **Drug Interactions** section).

Elimination: Approximately 80% of the total loratadine dose administered can be found equally distributed between urine and feces in the form of metabolic products within 10 days. In nearly all patients, exposure (AUC) to the metabolite is greater than to the parent loratadine. The mean elimination half-lives in normal adult subjects (n = 54) were 8.4 hours (range = 3 to 20 hours) for loratadine and 28 hours (range = 8.8 to 92 hours) for descarboethoxyloratadine. Loratadine and descarboethoxyloratadine reached steady-state in most patients by approximately the fifth dosing day. There was considerable variability in the pharmacokinetic data in all studies of CLARITIN Tablets and Syrup, probably due to the extensive first-pass metabolism.

Special Populations: ***Pediatric:*** The pharmacokinetic profile of loratadine in children in the 6- to 12-year age group is similar to that of adults. In a single-dose pharmacokinetic study of 13 pediatric volunteers (aged 8 to 12 years) given 10 mL of CLARITIN Syrup containing 10 mg loratadine, the ranges of individual subject values of pharmacokinetic parameters (AUC and C_{max}) were comparable to those following administration of a 10 mg tablet or syrup to adult volunteers.

The pharmacokinetic profile of loratadine in children in the 2 to 5-year age group (n = 18) is similar to that of adults. In a single-dose pharmacokinetic study of pediatric subjects (age 2 to 5 years) given 5 mL of CLARITIN Syrup containing 5 mg loratadine, the range of individual subject values of pharmacokinetic parameters (AUC and C_{max}) were comparable to those following administration of a 10 mg tablet or syrup to adult volunteers or children eight years of age and older.

Geriatric: In a study involving 12 healthy geriatric subjects (66 to 78 years old), the AUC and peak plasma levels (C_{max}) of both loratadine and descarboethoxyloratadine were approximately 50% greater than those observed in studies of younger subjects. The mean elimination half-lives for the geriatric subjects were 18.2 hours (range = 6.7 to 37 hours) for loratadine and 17.5 hours (range = 11 to 38 hours) for descarboethoxyloratadine.

Renal Impairment: In a study involving 12 subjects with chronic renal impairment (creatinine clearance ≤ 30 mL/min) both AUC and C_{max} increased by approximately 73% for loratadine and by 120% for descarboethoxyloratadine, as compared to six subjects with normal renal function (creatinine clearance ≥ 80 mL/min). The mean elimination half-lives of loratadine (7.6 hours) and descarboethoxyloratadine (23.9 hours) were not substantially different from that observed in normal subjects. Hemodialysis does not have an effect on the pharmacokinetics of loratadine or descarboethoxyloratadine in subjects with chronic renal impairment.

Hepatic Impairment: In seven patients with chronic alcoholic liver disease, the AUC and C_{max} of loratadine were double while the pharmacokinetic profile of descarboethoxyloratadine was not substantially different from that observed in other trials enrolling normal subjects. The elimination half-lives for loratadine and descarboethoxyloratadine were 24 hours and 37 hours, respectively, and increased with increasing severity of liver disease.

Clinical Trials: Clinical trials of CLARITIN Tablets involved over 10,700 patients, 12 years of age and older, who received either CLARITIN Tablets or another antihistamine and/or placebo in double-blind randomized controlled studies. In placebo-controlled trials, 10 mg once daily of CLARITIN Tablets was superior to placebo and similar to clemastine (1 mg BID) or terfenadine (60 mg BID) in effects on nasal and non-nasal symptoms of allergic rhinitis. In these studies, somnolence occurred less frequently with CLARITIN Tablets than with clemastine and at about the same frequency as terfenadine or placebo. In studies with CLARITIN Tablets at doses two to four times higher than the recommended dose of 10 mg, a dose-related increase in the incidence of somnolence was observed. Therefore, some patients, particularly those with hepatic or renal impairment and the elderly, or those on medications that impair clearance of loratadine and its metabolites, may experience somnolence. In addition, three placebo-controlled, double-blind, 2-week trials in 188 pediatric patients with seasonal allergic rhinitis aged 6 to 12 years, were conducted at doses of CLARITIN Syrup up to 10 mg once daily. In a double-blind, placebo-controlled study, the safety of 5 mg loratadine, administered in 5 mL of CLARITIN Syrup, was evaluated in 60 pediatric patients between 2 and 5 years of age. No unexpected adverse events were observed.

Clinical trials of CLARITIN REDITABS (loratadine rapidly-disintegrating tablets) involved over 1300 patients who received either CLARITIN REDITABS (loratadine rapidly-disintegrating tablets), CLARITIN Tablets, or placebo. In placebo-controlled trials, one CLARITIN REDITABS (loratadine rapidly-disintegrating tablets) once daily was superior to placebo and similar to CLARITIN Tablets in effects on nasal and non-nasal symptoms of seasonal allergic rhinitis.

Among those patients involved in double-blind, randomized, controlled studies of CLARITIN Tablets, approximately 1000 patients (age 12 and older), were enrolled in studies of chronic idiopathic urticaria. In placebo-controlled clinical trials, CLARITIN Tablets 10 mg once daily were superior to placebo in the management of chronic idiopathic urticaria, as demonstrated by reduction of associated itching, erythema, and hives. In these studies, the incidence of somnolence seen with CLARITIN Tablets was similar to that seen with placebo.

In a study in which CLARITIN Tablets were administered to adults at four times the clinical dose for 90 days, no clinically significant increase in the QT_c was seen on ECGs.

In a single-rising dose study in which doses up to 160 mg (16 times the clinical dose) were studied, loratadine did not cause any clinically significant changes on the QT_c interval in the ECGs.

INDICATIONS AND USAGE

CLARITIN is indicated for the relief of nasal and non-nasal symptoms of seasonal allergic rhinitis and for the treatment of chronic idiopathic urticaria in patients 2 years of age or older.

CONTRAINDICATIONS

CLARITIN is contraindicated in patients who are hypersensitive to this medication or to any of its ingredients.

PRECAUTIONS

General: Patients with liver impairment or renal insufficiency (GFR < 30 mL/min) should be given a lower initial dose (10 mg every other day). (See **CLINICAL PHARMACOLOGY: Special Populations.**)

Drug Interactions: Loratadine (10 mg once daily) has been coadministered with therapeutic doses of erythromycin, cimetidine, and ketoconazole in controlled clinical pharmacology studies in adult volunteers. Although increased plasma concentrations (AUC 0–24 hrs) of loratadine and/or descarboethoxyloratadine were observed following coadministration of loratadine with each of these drugs in normal volunteers (n = 24 in each study), there were no clinically relevant changes in the safety profile of loratadine, as assessed by electrocardiographic parameters, clinical laboratory tests, vital signs, and adverse events. There were no significant effects on QT_c intervals, and no reports of sedation or syncope. No effects on plasma concentrations of cimetidine or ketoconazole were observed. Plasma concentrations (AUC 0–24 hrs) of erythromycin decreased 15% with coadministration of loratadine relative to that observed with erythromycin alone. The clinical relevance of this difference is unknown. These above findings are summarized in the following table:

[See table below]

There does not appear to be an increase in adverse events in subjects who received oral contraceptives and loratadine.

Carcinogenesis, Mutagenesis, and Impairment of Fertility: In an 18-month carcinogenicity study in mice and a 2-year study in rats, loratadine was administered in the diet at doses up to 40 mg/kg (mice) and 25 mg/kg (rats). In the carcinogenicity studies, pharmacokinetic assessments were carried out to determine animal exposure to the drug. AUC data demonstrated that the exposure of mice given 40 mg/kg of loratadine was 3.6 (loratadine) and 18 (descarboethoxyloratadine) times the exposure in adults and 5 (loratadine) and 20 (descarboethoxyloratadine) times the exposure in children given the maximum recommended daily oral dose. Exposure of rats given 25 mg/kg of loratadine was 28 (loratadine) and 67 (descarboethoxyloratadine) times the exposure in adults and 40 (loratadine) and 80 (descarboethoxyloratadine) times the exposure in children given the maximum recommended daily oral dose. Male mice given 40 mg/kg had a significantly higher incidence of hepatocellular tumors (combined adenomas and carcinomas) than concurrent controls. In rats, a significantly higher incidence of hepatocellular tumors (combined adenomas and carcinomas) was observed in males given 10 mg/kg, and males and females given 25 mg/kg. Exposure of rats given 10 mg/kg of loratadine was 10 (loratadine) and 15 (descarboethoxyloratadine) times the exposure in adults and 15 (loratadine) and 20 (descarboethoxyloratadine) times the exposure in children given the maximum recommended daily oral dose. The clinical significance of these findings during long-term use of CLARITIN is not known.

In mutagenicity studies, there was no evidence of mutagenic potential in reverse (Ames) or forward point mutation

Effects on Plasma Concentrations (AUC 0-24 hrs) of Loratadine and Descarboethoxyloratadine After 10 Days of Coadministration (Loratadine 10 mg) in Normal Volunteers

	Loratadine	Descarboethoxyloratadine
Erythromycin (500 mg Q8h)	+ 40%	+46%
Cimetidine (300 mg QID)	+103%	+ 6%
Ketoconazole (200 mg Q12h)	+307%	+73%

(CHO-HGPRT) assays, or in the assay for DNA damage (rat primary hepatocyte unscheduled DNA assay) or in two assays for chromosomal aberrations (human peripheral blood lymphocyte clastogenesis assay and the mouse bone marrow erythrocyte micronucleus assay). In the mouse lymphoma assay, a positive finding occurred in the nonactivated but not the activated phase of the study.

Decreased fertility in male rats, shown by lower female conception rates, occurred at an oral dose of 64 mg/kg (approximately 50 times the maximum recommended human daily oral dose on a mg/m^2 basis) and was reversible with cessation of dosing. Loratadine had no effect on male or female fertility or reproduction in the rat at an oral dose of approximately 24 mg/kg (approximately 20 times the maximum recommended human daily oral dose on a mg/m^2 basis).

Pregnancy Category B: There was no evidence of animal teratogenicity in studies performed in rats and rabbits at oral doses up to 96 mg/kg (approximately 75 times and 150 times, respectively, the maximum recommended human daily oral dose on a mg/m^2 basis). There are, however, no adequate and well-controlled studies in pregnant women. Because animal reproduction studies are not always predictive of human response, CLARITIN should be used during pregnancy only if clearly needed.

Nursing Mothers: Loratadine and its metabolite, descarboethoxyloratadine, pass easily into breast milk and achieve concentrations that are equivalent to plasma levels with an AUC_{milk}/AUC_{plasma} ratio of 1.17 and 0.85 for loratadine and descarboethoxyloratadine, respectively. Following a single oral dose of 40 mg, a small amount of loratadine and descarboethoxyloratadine was excreted into the breast milk (approximately 0.03% of 40 mg over 48 hours). A decision should be made whether to discontinue nursing or to discontinue the drug, taking into account the importance of the drug to the mother. Caution should be exercised when CLARITIN is administered to a nursing woman.

Pediatric Use: The safety of CLARITIN Syrup at a daily dose of 10 mg has been demonstrated in 188 pediatric patients 6 to 12 years of age in placebo-controlled 2-week trials. The safety and tolerability of CLARITIN Syrup at a daily dose of 5 mg has been demonstrated in 60 pediatric patients 2 to 5 years of age in a double-blind, placebo-controlled, 2-week study. The effectiveness of CLARITIN for the treatment of seasonal allergic rhinitis and chronic idiopathic urticaria in children aged 2 to 12 years is based on an extrapolation of the demonstrated efficacy of CLARITIN in adults in these conditions and the likelihood that the disease course, pathophysiology, and the drug's effect are substantially similar to that of the adults. The recommended dose for the pediatric population is based on cross-study comparison of the pharmacokinetics of CLARITIN in adults and pediatric subjects and on the safety profile of loratadine in both adults and pediatric patients at doses equal to or higher than the recommended doses. The safety and effectiveness of CLARITIN in children under 2 years of age have not been established.

ADVERSE REACTIONS

CLARITIN Tablets: Approximately 90,000 patients, aged 12 and older, received CLARITIN Tablets 10 mg once daily in controlled and uncontrolled studies. Placebo-controlled clinical trials at the recommended dose of 10 mg once a day varied from 2 weeks' to 6 months' duration. The rate of premature withdrawal from these trials was approximately 2% in both the treated and placebo groups.

[See first table above]

Adverse events reported in placebo-controlled chronic idiopathic urticaria trials were similar to those reported in allergic rhinitis studies.

Adverse event rates did not appear to differ significantly based on age, sex, or race, although the number of nonwhite subjects was relatively small.

CLARITIN REDITABS (loratadine rapidly-disintegrating tablets): Approximately 500 patients received CLARITIN REDITABS (loratadine rapidly-disintegrating tablets) in controlled clinical trials of 2 weeks' duration. In these studies, adverse events were similar in type and frequency to those seen with CLARITIN Tablets and placebo.

Administration of CLARITIN REDITABS (loratadine rapidly-disintegrating tablets) did not result in an increased reporting frequency of mouth or tongue irritation.

CLARITIN Syrup: Approximately 300 pediatric patients 6 to 12 years of age received 10 mg loratadine once daily in controlled clinical trials for a period of 8 to 15 days. Among these, 188 children were treated with 10 mg loratadine syrup once daily in placebo-controlled trials. Adverse events in these pediatric patients were observed to occur with type and frequency similar to those seen in the adult population. The rate of premature discontinuance due to adverse events among pediatric patients receiving loratadine 10 mg daily was less than 1%.

[See second table above]

Sixty pediatric patients 2 to 5 years of age received 5 mg loratadine once daily in a double-blind, placebo-controlled clinical trial for a period of 14 days. No unexpected adverse events were seen given the known safety profile of loratadine and likely adverse reactions for this patient population. The following adverse events occurred with a frequency of 2 to 3 percent in the loratadine syrup-treated patients (2 to 5 years old) during the placebo-controlled trial, and more frequently than in the placebo group: diarrhea, epistaxis, pharyngitis, influenza-like symptoms, fatigue, stomatitis, tooth disorder, earache, viral infection, and rash.

In addition to those adverse events reported above (≥ 2%), the following adverse events have been reported in at least one patient in CLARITIN clinical trials in adult and pediatric patients:

Autonomic Nervous System: altered lacrimation, altered salivation, flushing, hypoesthesia, impotence, increased sweating, thirst.

REPORTED ADVERSE EVENTS WITH AN INCIDENCE OF MORE THAN 2% IN PLACEBO-CONTROLLED ALLERGIC RHINITIS CLINICAL TRIALS IN PATIENTS 12 YEARS OF AGE AND OLDER
PERCENT OF PATIENTS REPORTING

	LORATADINE 10 mg QD n = 1926	**PLACEBO** n = 2545	**CLEMASTINE** 1 mg BID n = 536	**TERFENADINE** 60 mg BID n = 684
Headache	12	11	8	8
Somnolence	8	6	22	9
Fatigue	4	3	10	2
Dry Mouth	3	2	4	3

ADVERSE EVENTS OCCURRING WITH A FREQUENCY OF ≥ 2% IN LORATADINE SYRUP-TREATED PATIENTS (6 TO 12 YEARS OLD) IN PLACEBO-CONTROLLED TRIALS, AND MORE FREQUENTLY THAN IN THE PLACEBO GROUP
PERCENT OF PATIENTS REPORTING

	LORATADINE 10 mg QD n = 188	**PLACEBO** n = 262	**CHLORPHENIRAMINE** 2-4 mg BID/TID n = 170
Nervousness	4	2	2
Wheezing	4	2	5
Fatigue	3	2	5
Hyperkinesia	3	1	1
Abdominal Pain	2	0	0
Conjunctivitis	2	<1	1
Dysphonia	2	<1	0
Malaise	2	0	1
Upper Respiratory Tract Infection	2	<1	0

Body as a Whole: angioneurotic edema, asthenia, back pain, blurred vision, chest pain, earache, eye pain, fever, leg cramps, malaise, rigors, tinnitus, weight gain.

Cardiovascular System: hypertension, hypotension, palpitations, supraventricular tachyarrhythmias, syncope, tachycardia.

Central and Peripheral Nervous System: blepharospasm, dizziness, dysphonia, hypertonia, migraine, paresthesia, tremor, vertigo.

Gastrointestinal System: altered taste, anorexia, constipation, diarrhea, dyspepsia, flatulence, gastritis, hiccup, increased appetite, loose stools, nausea, vomiting.

Musculoskeletal System: arthralgia, myalgia.

Psychiatric: agitation, amnesia, anxiety, confusion, decreased libido, depression, impaired concentration, insomnia, irritability, paroniria.

Reproductive System: breast pain, dysmenorrhea, menorrhagia, vaginitis.

Respiratory System: bronchitis, bronchospasm, coughing, dyspnea, hemoptysis, laryngitis, nasal dryness, sinusitis, sneezing.

Skin and Appendages: dermatitis, dry hair, dry skin, photosensitivity reaction, pruritus, purpura, urticaria.

Urinary System: altered micturition, urinary discoloration, urinary incontinence, urinary retention.

In addition, the following spontaneous adverse events have been reported rarely during the marketing of loratadine: abnormal hepatic function, including jaundice, hepatitis, and hepatic necrosis; alopecia; anaphylaxis; breast enlargement; erythema multiforme; peripheral edema; thrombocytopenia; and seizures.

DRUG ABUSE AND DEPENDENCE

There is no information to indicate that abuse or dependency occurs with CLARITIN.

OVERDOSAGE

In adults, somnolence, tachycardia, and headache have been reported with overdoses greater than 10 mg with the Tablet formulation (40 mg-180 mg). Extrapyramidal signs and palpitations have been reported in children with overdoses of greater than 10 mg of CLARITIN Syrup. In the event of overdosage, general symptomatic and supportive measures should be instituted promptly and maintained for as long as necessary.

Treatment of overdosage would reasonably consist of emesis (ipecac syrup), except in patients with impaired consciousness, followed by the administration of activated charcoal to absorb any remaining drug. If vomiting is unsuccessful, or contraindicated, gastric lavage should be performed with normal saline. Saline cathartics may also be of value for rapid dilution of bowel contents. Loratadine is not eliminated by hemodialysis. It is not known if loratadine is eliminated by peritoneal dialysis.

No deaths occurred at oral doses up to 5000 mg/kg in mice (approximately 1200 and 1400 times, respectively, the maximum recommended daily oral dose in adults and children on a mg/m^2 basis). No deaths occurred at oral doses up to 5000 mg/kg in matured rats (approximately 2400 and 2900 times, respectively, the maximum recommended daily oral dose in adults and children on a mg/m^2 basis). However, lethality occurred in juvenile rats at an oral dose of 125 mg/kg (approximately 100 and 70 times, respectively, the maximum recommended daily oral dose in adults and children on a mg/m^2 basis). No deaths occurred at oral doses up to 1280 mg/kg in monkeys (approximately 2100 and 1500 times, respectively, the maximum recommended daily oral dose in adults and children on a mg/m^2 basis).

DOSAGE AND ADMINISTRATION

Adults and children 6 years of age and over: The recommended dose of CLARITIN is one 10 mg tablet or reditab, or 2 teaspoonfuls (10 mg) of syrup once daily.

Children 2 to 5 years of age: The recommended dose of CLARITIN Syrup is 5 mg (1 teaspoonful) once daily.

In adults and children 6 years of age and over with liver failure or renal insufficiency (GFR < 30 mL/min), the starting dose should be 10 mg (one tablet or two teaspoonfuls) every other day. In children 2 to 5 years of age with liver failure or renal insufficiency, the starting dose should be 5 mg (one teaspoonful) every other day.

Administration of CLARITIN REDITABS (loratadine rapidly-disintegrating tablets): Place CLARITIN REDITABS (loratadine rapidly-disintegrating tablets) on the tongue. Tablet disintegration occurs rapidly. Administer with or without water.

HOW SUPPLIED

CLARITIN TABLETS: 10 mg, white to off-white compressed tablets; impressed with the product identification number "458" on one side and "CLARITIN 10" on the other; high-density polyethylene plastic bottles of 100 (NDC 0085-0458-03) and 500 (NDC 0085-0458-06). Also available, CLARITIN Unit-of-Use packages of 30 tablets (10 tablets per blister card) (NDC 0085-0458-05); and 10 × 10 tablet Unit Dose-Hospital Pack (NDC 0085-0458-04).

Protect Unit-of-Use packaging and Unit Dose-Hospital Pack from excessive moisture.

Store between 2° and 30°C (36° and 86°F).

CLARITIN Syrup: Clear, colorless to light-yellow liquid, containing 1 mg loratadine per mL; amber glass bottles of 16 fluid ounces (NDC 0085-1223-01).

Store between 2° and 25°C (36° and 77°F).

CLARITIN REDITABS (loratadine rapidly-disintegrating tablets): CLARITIN REDITABS (loratadine rapidly-disintegrating tablets), 10 mg, white to off-white blister-formed tablet; impressed with the letter "C" on one side; Unit-of-Use polyvinyl chloride blister packages of 30 tablets (three laminated foil pouches, each containing one blister card of 10 tablets) supplied with Patient's Instructions for Use (NDC 0085-1128-02).

Keep CLARITIN REDITABS (loratadine rapidly-disintegrating tablets) in a dry place.

Store between 2° and 25°C (36° and 77°F). Use within 6 months of opening laminated foil pouch, and immediately upon opening individual tablet blister.

Schering Corporation
Kenilworth, NJ 07033 USA
Rev. 9/00 19628477T

CLARITIN REDITABS (loratadine rapidly-disintegrating tablets) are manufactured for Schering Corporation by Scherer DDS, England.

U.S. Patent Nos. 4,282,233 and 4,371,516.

LOTRISONE® CREAM
LOTRISONE® LOTION

(clotrimazole and betamethasone dipropionate)

Prescribing information for this product, which appears on pages 2912–2914 of the 2001 PDR, has been completely revised as follows. Please write "See Supplement A" next to the product heading.

FOR TOPICAL USE ONLY, NOT FOR OPHTHALMIC, ORAL, OR INTRAVAGINAL USE, NOT RECOMMENDED FOR PATIENTS UNDER THE AGE OF 12 YEARS AND NOT RECOMMENDED FOR DIAPER DERMATITIS

Continued on next page

Lotrisone—Cont.

DESCRIPTION

LOTRISONE Cream and Lotion contain combinations of clotrimazole, a synthetic antifungal agent, and betamethasone dipropionate, a synthetic corticosteroid, for dermatologic use.

Chemically, clotrimazole is 1-(o-chloro-α,α-diphenylbenzyl) imidazole, with the empirical formula $C_{22}H_{17}ClN_2$, a molecular weight of 344.84, and the following structural formula:

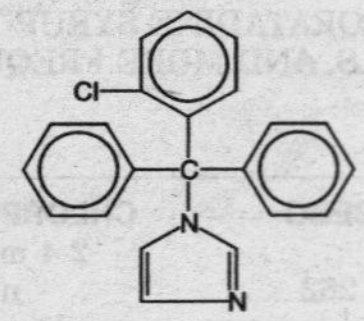

Clotrimazole is an odorless, white crystalline powder, insoluble in water and soluble in ethanol.

Betamethasone dipropionate has the chemical name 9-fluoro-11β,17,21-trihydroxy-16β-methylpregna-1,4-diene-3,20-dione 17,21-dipropionate, with the empirical formula $C_{28}H_{37}FO_7$, a molecular weight of 504.59, and the following structural formula:

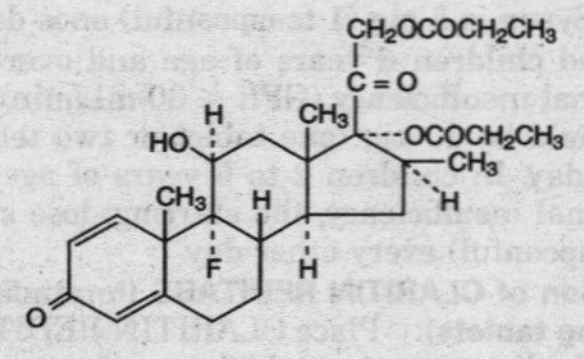

Betamethasone dipropionate is a white to creamy white, odorless crystalline powder, insoluble in water.

Each gram of LOTRISONE Cream contains 10 mg clotrimazole and 0.643 mg betamethasone dipropionate (equivalent to 0.5 mg betamethasone), in a hydrophilic cream consisting of purified water, mineral oil, white petrolatum, cetearyl alcohol 70/30, ceteareth-30, propylene glycol, sodium phosphate monobasic monohydrate, and phosphoric acid; benzyl alcohol as preservative.

LOTRISONE Cream is smooth, uniform, and white to off-white in color.

Each gram of LOTRISONE Lotion contains 10 mg clotrimazole and 0.643 mg betamethasone dipropionate (equivalent to 0.5 mg betamethasone), in a hydrophilic base of purified water, mineral oil, white petrolatum, cetearyl alcohol 70/30, ceteareth-30, propylene glycol, sodium phosphate monobasic monohydrate, and phosphoric acid; benzyl alcohol as a preservative.

LOTRISONE Lotion may contain sodium hydroxide. LOTRISONE Lotion is opaque and white in color.

CLINICAL PHARMACOLOGY

Clotrimazole and Betamethasone Dipropionate

LOTRISONE Cream has been shown to be least as effective as clotrimazole alone in a different cream vehicle. No comparative studies have been conducted with LOTRISONE Lotion and clotrimazole alone. Use of corticosteroids in the treatment of a fungal infection may lead to suppression of host inflammation leading to worsening or decreased cure rate.

Clotrimazole

Skin penetration and systemic absorption of clotrimazole following topical application of LOTRISONE Cream or Lotion have not been studied. The following information was obtained using 1% clotrimazole cream and solution formulations. Six hours after the application of radioactive clotrimazole 1% cream and 1% solution onto intact and acutely inflamed skin, the concentration of clotrimazole varied from 100 mcg/cm^3 in the stratum corneum, to 0.5 to 1 mcg/cm^3 in the reticular dermis, and 0.1 mcg/cm^3 in the subcutis. No measurable amount of radioactivity (<0.001 mcg/mL) was found in the serum within 48 hours after application under occlusive dressing of 0.5 mL of the solution or 0.8 g of the cream. Only 0.5% or less of the applied radioactivity was excreted in the urine.

Microbiology Mechanism of Action: Clotrimazole is an imidazole antifungal agent. Imidazoles inhibit 14-α-demethylation of lanosterol in fungi by binding to one of the cytochrome P-450 enzymes. This leads to the accumulation of 14-α-methylsterols and reduced concentrations of ergosterol, a sterol essential for a normal fungal cytoplasmic membrane. The methylsterols may affect the electron transport system, thereby inhibiting growth of fungi.

Activity *In Vivo*: Clotrimazole has been shown to be active against most strains of the following dermatophytes, both *in vitro* and in clinical infections as described in the **INDICATIONS AND USAGE** section: *Epidermophyton floccosum, Trichophyton mentagrophytes,* and *Trichophyton rubrum.*

Activity *In Vitro*: *In vitro,* clotrimazole has been shown to have activity against many dermatophytes, **but the clinical significance of this information is unknown.**

Drug Resistance: Strains of dermatophytes having a natural resistance to azoles including clotrimazole have not been reported. Resistance to azoles including clotrimazole has been reported in some *Candida* species.

No single-step or multiple-step resistance to clotrimazole has developed during successive passages of *Trichophyton mentagrophytes.*

Betamethasone Dipropionate

Betamethasone dipropionate, a corticosteroid, has been shown to have topical (dermatologic) and systemic pharmacologic and metabolic effects characteristic of this class of drugs.

Pharmacokinetics: The extent of percutaneous absorption of topical corticosteroids is determined by many factors, including the vehicle, the integrity of the epidermal barrier and the use of occlusive dressings. (See **DOSAGE AND ADMINISTRATION** section.) Topical corticosteroids can be absorbed from normal intact skin. Inflammation and/or other disease processes in the skin may increase percutaneous absorption of topical corticosteroids. Occlusive dressings substantially increase the percutaneous absorption of topical corticosteroids. (See **DOSAGE AND ADMINISTRATION** section.)

Once absorbed through the skin, the pharmacokinetics of topical corticosteroids are similar to systemically administered corticosteroids. Corticosteroids are bound to plasma proteins in varying degrees. Corticosteroids are metabolized primarily in the liver and are then excreted by the kidneys. Some of the topical corticosteroids and their metabolites are also excreted into the bile.

Studies performed with LOTRISONE Cream and Lotion indicate that these topical combination antifungal/corticosteroids may have vasoconstrictor potencies in a range that is comparable to high potency topical corticosteroids. Therefore, use is not recommended in patients less than 12 years of age, in diaper dermatitis, and under occlusion.

CLINICAL STUDIES (LOTRISONE Cream)

In clinical studies of tinea corporis, tinea cruris, and tinea pedis, patients treated with LOTRISONE Cream showed a better clinical response at the first return visit than patients treated with clotrimazole cream. In tinea corporis and tinea cruris, the patient returned 3 to 5 days after starting treatment, and in tinea pedis, after 1 week. Mycological cure rates observed in patients treated with LOTRISONE Cream were as good as or better than in those patients treated with clotrimazole cream. In these same clinical studies, patients treated with LOTRISONE Cream showed better clinical responses and mycological cure rates when compared with patients treated with betamethasone dipropionate cream.

CLINICAL STUDIES (LOTRISONE Lotion)

In the treatment of tinea pedis twice daily for 4 weeks, LOTRISONE Lotion was shown to be superior to vehicle in relieving symptoms of erythema, scaling, pruritus, and maceration at week 2. LOTRISONE Lotion was also shown to have a superior mycological cure rate compared to vehicle 2 weeks after discontinuation of treatment. It is unclear if the relief of symptoms at 2 weeks in this clinical study with LOTRISONE Lotion was due to the contribution of betamethasone dipropionate, clotrimazole, or both.

In the treatment of tinea cruris twice daily for 2 weeks, LOTRISONE Lotion was shown to be superior to vehicle in the relief of symptoms of erythema, scaling, and pruritus after 3 days. It is unclear if the relief of symptoms after 3 days in this clinical study with LOTRISONE Lotion was due to the contribution of betamethasone dipropionate, clotrimazole, or both.

The comparative efficacy and safety of LOTRISONE Lotion versus clotrimazole alone in a lotion vehicle have not been studied in the treatment of tinea pedis or tinea cruris or tinea corporis. The comparative efficacy and safety of LOTRISONE Lotion and LOTRISONE Cream have also not been studied.

INDICATIONS AND USAGE

LOTRISONE Cream and Lotion are indicated for the topical treatment of symptomatic inflammatory tinea pedis, tinea cruris, and tinea corporis due to *Epidermophyton floccosum, Trichophyton mentagrophytes,* and *Trichophyton rubrum.* Effective treatment without the risks associated with topical corticosteroid use may be obtained using a topical antifungal agent that does not contain a corticosteroid, especially for non-inflammatory tinea infections. The efficacy of LOTRISONE Cream or Lotion for the treatment of infections caused by zoophilic dermatophytes (eg, *Microsporum canis*) has not been established. Several cases of treatment failure of LOTRISONE Cream in the treatment of infections caused by *Microsporum canis* have been reported.

CONTRAINDICATIONS

LOTRISONE Cream or Lotion is contraindicated in patients who are sensitive to clotrimazole, betamethasone dipropionate, other corticosteroids or imidazoles, or to any ingredient in these preparations.

PRECAUTIONS

General Systemic absorption of topical corticosteroids can produce reversible hypothalamic-pituitary-adrenal (HPA) axis suppression with the potential for glucocorticosteroid insufficiency after withdrawal of treatment. Manifestations of Cushing's syndrome, hyperglycemia, and glucosuria can also be produced in some patients by systemic absorption of topical corticosteroids while on treatment.

Conditions which augment systemic absorption include use over large surface areas, prolonged use, and use under occlusive dressings. Patients applying LOTRISONE Cream or Lotion to a large surface area or to areas under occlusion should be evaluated periodically for evidence of HPA axis suppression. This may be done by using the ACTH stimulation, morning plasma cortisol, and urinary free cortisol tests.

LOTRISONE Cream was applied using large dosages, 7 g daily for 14 days (BID) to the crural area of normal subjects. Three of the eight normal subjects on whom LOTRISONE Cream was applied exhibited low morning plasma cortisol levels during treatment. One of these subjects has an abnormal Cortrosyn test. The effect on morning plasma cortisol was transient and subjects recovered one week after discontinuing dosing.

If HPA axis suppression is noted, an attempt should be made to withdraw the drug, to reduce the frequency of application, or to substitute a less potent corticosteroid. Recovery of HPA axis function is generally prompt upon discontinuation of topical corticosteroids. Infrequently, signs and symptoms of glucocorticosteroid insufficiency may occur, requiring supplemental systemic corticosteroids.

Pediatric patients may be more susceptible to systemic toxicity from equivalent doses due to their larger skin surface to body mass ratios. (See **PRECAUTIONS - Pediatric Use.**)

If irritation develops, LOTRISONE Cream or Lotion should be discontinued and appropriate therapy instituted.

THE SAFETY OF LOTRISONE CREAM OR LOTION HAS NOT BEEN DEMONSTRATED IN THE TREATMENT OF DIAPER DERMATITIS. ADVERSE EVENTS CONSISTENT WITH CORTICOSTEROID USE HAVE BEEN OBSERVED IN PATIENTS TREATED WITH LOTRISONE CREAM FOR DIAPER DERMATITIS. THE USE OF LOTRISONE CREAM OR LOTION IN THE TREATMENT OF DIAPER DERMATITIS IS NOT RECOMMENDED.

Information for Patients Patients using LOTRISONE Cream or Lotion should receive the following information and instructions:

1. The medication is to be used as directed by the physician and is not recommended for use longer than the prescribed time period. It is for external use only. Avoid contact with the eyes, mouth, or intravaginally.
2. This medication is to be used for the full prescribed treatment time, even though the symptoms may have improved. Notify the physician if there is no improvement after 1 week of treatment for tinea cruris or tinea corporis, or after 2 weeks for tinea pedis.
3. This medication should only be used for the disorder for which it was prescribed.
4. The treated skin area should not be bandaged, covered, or wrapped so as to be occluded. (See **DOSAGE AND ADMINISTRATION** section.)
5. Any signs of local adverse reactions should be reported to your physician.
6. Patients should avoid sources of infection or reinfection.
7. When using LOTRISONE Cream or Lotion in the groin area, patients should use the medication for 2 weeks only, and apply the cream or lotion sparingly. Patients should wear loose-fitting clothing. Notify the physician if the condition persists after 2 weeks.
8. The safety of LOTRISONE Cream or Lotion has not been demonstrated in the treatment of diaper dermatitis. Adverse events consistent with corticosteroid use have been observed in patients treated with LOTRISONE Cream for diaper dermatitis. The use of LOTRISONE Cream or Lotion in the treatment of diaper dermatitis is not recommended.

Laboratory Tests If there is a lack of response to LOTRISONE Cream or Lotion, appropriate confirmation of the diagnosis, including possible mycological studies, is indicated before instituting another course of therapy.

The following tests may be helpful in evaluating HPA-axis suppression due to the corticosteroid components:

Urinary free cortisol test

Morning plasma cortisol test

ACTH stimulation test

Carcinogenesis, Mutagenesis, Impairment of Fertility There are no laboratory animal studies with either the combination of clotrimazole and betamethasone dipropionate or with either component individually to evaluate carcinogenesis.

Betamethasone was negative in the bacterial mutagenicity assay (*Salmonella typhimurium* and *Escherichia coli*), and in the mammalian cell mutagenicity assay (CHO/HGPRT). It was positive in the *in vitro* human lymphocyte chromosome aberration assay, and equivocal in the *in vivo* mouse bone marrow micronucleus assay. This pattern of response is similar to that of dexamethasone and hydrocortisone.

In genotoxicity testing of clotrimazole, chromosomes of the spermatophores of Chinese hamsters, which had been exposed to five daily oral clotrimazole doses of 100 mg/kg body weight, were examined for structural changes during the metaphase. The results of this study showed that clotrimazole had no mutagenic effect.

Reproductive studies with betamethasone dipropionate carried out in rabbits at doses of 1.0 mg/kg by the intramuscular route and in mice up to 33 mg/kg by the intramuscular route indicated no impairment of fertility except for dose-related increases in fetal resorption rates in both species. These doses are approximately 5- and 38-fold the human dose based on a mg/m^2 comparison, respectively.

Oral doses of clotrimazole in mice resulted in decreased litter size at doses of 120 mg/kg and higher. This dose is approximately 10-fold the human dose based on a mg/m^2 comparison.

A Segment I (fertility and general reproduction) study of clotrimazole was conducted in rats. Males and females were dosed orally (diet admixture) at doses of 5, 10, 25, or 50 mg/kg/day for 10 weeks prior to mating. At 50 mg/kg (approximately 8 times the human dose based on a mg/m^2 comparison), there was an adverse effect on maternal body weight gain and rearing of the offspring. Doses of 25 mg/kg (approximately 4 times the human dose based on a mg/m² comparison) and lower were well tolerated and produced no adverse effects on fertility or reproduction.

Pregnancy Category C There have been no teratogenic studies performed in animals or humans with the combination of clotrimazole and betamethasone dipropionate.

A Segment II (teratology) study in pregnant rats with intravaginal doses up to 100 mg/kg clotrimazole have revealed no evidence of harm to the fetus. This dose is approximately 17-fold the human dose based on a mg/m² comparison.

Segment II (teratology) studies of clotrimazole were conducted by the oral (gavage) route in rats, mice, and rabbits. In rats administered 25, 50, 100, or 200 mg/kg/day, no increase in malformations was seen at doses up to 200 mg/kg. Doses of 100 and 200 mg/kg were embryotoxic (increased resorptions) as well as maternally toxic, while doses of 25 and 50 mg/kg were well tolerated by both the dams and the fetuses. These doses were approximately 4-, 8-, 17-, and 34-fold the human as well as maternally toxic, while doses of 25 and 50 mg/kg were well tolerated by both the dams and the fetuses. These doses were approximately 4-, 8-, 17-, and 34-fold the human dose based on a mg/m² comparison, respectively.

In pregnant mice, clotrimazole at oral doses of 25, 50, 100, or 200 mg/kg/day was not teratogenic and was well tolerated by both the dams and the fetuses. These doses were approximately 2-, 4-, 8-, and 17-fold the human dose based on a mg/m² comparison, respectively. No evidence of maternal toxicity or embryotoxicity was seen in pregnant rabbits dosed orally with 60, 120, or 180 mg/kg/day. These doses were approximately 20-, 40-, and 61-fold the human dose based on a mg/m² comparison, respectively.

Betamethasone dipropionate has been shown to be teratogenic in rabbits when given by the intramuscular route at doses of 0.05 mg/kg. This dose is approximately one-fifth the human dose based on a mg/m² comparison. The abnormalities observed included umbilical hernias, cephalocele and cleft palates.

Betamethasone dipropionate has not been tested for teratogenic potential by the dermal route of administration. Other corticosteroids have been shown to be teratogenic in laboratory animals when administered systemically at relatively low dosage levels. Some corticosteroids have been shown to be teratogenic after dermal application to laboratory animals.

Nursing Mothers Systemically administered corticosteroids appear in human milk and could suppress growth, interfere with endogenous corticosteroids production, or cause other untoward effects. It is not known whether topical administration of corticosteroids could result in sufficient systemic absorption to produce detectable quantities in human milk. Because many drugs are excreted in human milk, caution should be exercised when LOTRISONE Cream or Lotion is administered to a nursing woman.

Pediatric Use The safety of LOTRISONE Cream or Lotion has not been demonstrated in pediatric patients under 12 years of age. Adverse events consistent with corticosteroid use have been observed in patients under 12 years of age treated with LOTRISONE Cream. **THE USE OF LOTRISONE CREAM OR LOTION IN THE TREATMENT OF PATIENTS UNDER 12 YEARS OF AGE OR PATIENTS WITH DIAPER DERMATITIS IS NOT RECOMMENDED.**

Because of higher ratio of skin surface area to body mass, pediatric patients under the age of 12 years are at a higher risk with LOTRISONE Cream or Lotion. They are at increased risk of developing Cushing's syndrome while on treatment and adrenal insufficiency after withdrawal of treatment. Adverse effects, including striae and growth retardation, have been reported with inappropriate use of LOTRISONE Cream in infants and children. (See **PRECAUTIONS** and **ADVERSE REACTIONS** sections.)

Hypothalamic-pituitary-adrenal (HPA) axis suppression, Cushing's syndrome, linear growth retardation, delayed weight gain and intracranial hypertension have been reported in children receiving topical corticosteroids. Manifestations of adrenal suppression in children include low plasma cortisol levels and absence of response to ACTH stimulation. Manifestations of intracranial hypertension include bulging fontanelles, headaches, and bilateral papilledema.

Geriatric Use Clinical studies of LOTRISONE Cream and Lotion did not include sufficient numbers of subjects aged 65 and over to determine whether they respond differently from younger subjects. Postmarket adverse event reporting for LOTRISONE Cream in patients aged 65 and above includes reports of skin atrophy and extremely rare reports of skin ulceration. Caution should be exercised with the use of these corticosteroid-containing topical products on thinning skin. **THE USE OF LOTRISONE CREAM OR LOTION UNDER OCCLUSION, SUCH AS IN DIAPER DERMATITIS, IS NOT RECOMMENDED.**

ADVERSE REACTIONS

Adverse reactions reported for LOTRISONE Cream in clinical trials were paresthesia in 1.9% of patients, and rash, edema, and secondary infection, each in less than 1% of patients.

Adverse reactions reported for LOTRISONE Lotion in clinical trials were burning and dry skin in 1.6% of patients and stinging in less than 1% of patients.

The following local adverse reactions have been reported with topical corticosteroids and may occur more frequently with the use of occlusive dressings. These reactions are listed in an approximate decreasing order of occurrence:

itching, irritation, dryness, folliculitis, hypertrichosis, acneiform eruptions, hypopigmentation, perioral dermatitis, allergic contact dermatitis, maceration of the skin, secondary infection, skin atrophy, striae, and miliaria. In the pediatric population, reported adverse events for LOTRISONE Cream include growth retardation, benign intracranial hypertension, Cushing's syndrome (HPA axis suppression), and local cutaneous reactions, including skin atrophy.

Adverse reactions reported with the use of clotrimazole are as follows: erythema, stinging, blistering, peeling, edema, pruritus, urticaria and general irritation of the skin.

OVERDOSAGE

Amounts greater than 45 g/week of LOTRISONE Cream or 45 mL/week of LOTRISONE Lotion should not be used. Acute overdosage with topical solution of LOTRISONE Cream or Lotion is unlikely and would not be expected to lead to a life-threatening situation. LOTRISONE Cream or Lotion should not be used for longer than the prescribed time period.

Topically applied corticosteroids, such as the one contained in LOTRISONE Cream or Lotion can be absorbed in sufficient amounts to produce systemic effects. (See **PRECAUTIONS.**)

DOSAGE AND ADMINISTRATION

Gently massage sufficient LOTRISONE Cream or Lotion into the affected skin areas twice a day, in the morning and evening.

LOTRISONE Cream or Lotion should not be used longer than 2 weeks in the treatment of tinea corporis or tinea cruris, and amounts greater than 45 g per week of LOTRISONE Cream or amounts greater than 45 mL per week of LOTRISONE Lotion should not be used. If a patient with tinea corporis or tinea cruris shows no clinical improvement after 1 week of treatment with LOTRISONE Cream or Lotion, the diagnosis should be reviewed.

LOTRISONE Cream or Lotion should not be used longer than 4 weeks in the treatment of tinea pedis and amounts greater than 45 g per week of LOTRISONE Cream or amounts greater than 45 mL per week of LOTRISONE Lotion should not be used. If a patient with tinea pedis shows no clinical improvement after 2 weeks of treatment with LOTRISONE Cream or Lotion, the diagnosis should be reviewed.

LOTRISONE Cream or Lotion should not be used with occlusive dressings.

HOW SUPPLIED

LOTRISONE Cream is supplied in 15-g (NDC 0085-0924-01) and 45-g tubes (NDC 0085-0924-02); boxes of one. **Store between 2°C and 30°C (36°F and 86°F).**

LOTRISONE Lotion is supplied in 30-mL bottles (NDC 0085-0809-01), box of one. **Store at 25°C (77°F) in the upright position only; excursions permitted between 15°C and 30°C (59°F and 86°F).**

SHAKE WELL BEFORE EACH USE.

Rx only

Patient Information Leaflet
What is LOTRISONE Cream or Lotion?

LOTRISONE Cream and Lotion are medications used on the skin to treat fungal infections of the feet, groin and body, as diagnosed by your doctor. LOTRISONE Cream or Lotion should be used for fungal infections that are inflamed and have symptoms of redness and/or itching. Talk to your doctor if your fungal infection does not have these symptoms. LOTRISONE Cream and Lotion contain a corticosteroid. Notify your doctor if you notice side effects with the use of LOTRISONE Cream or Lotion (see **"What are the possible side effects of LOTRISONE Cream and Lotion?"** below). LOTRISONE Cream or Lotion is not to be used in the eyes, in the mouth, or in the vagina.

How do LOTRISONE Cream and Lotion work?

LOTRISONE Cream and Lotion are combinations or an antifungal agent (clotrimazole) and a corticosteroid (betamethasone dipropionate). Clotrimazole works against fungus. Betamethasone dipropionate, a corticosteroid, is used to help relieve redness, swelling, itching, and other discomforts of fungal infections.

LOTRISONE Cream and Lotion are not recommended for use in patients under the age of 12 years. LOTRISONE Cream or Lotion is not recommended for use in diaper rash. Patients who are sensitive to clotrimazole and betamethasone dipropionate, other corticosteroids or imidazoles, or any ingredients in the preparation should not use LOTRISONE Cream and Lotion.

How should I use LOTRISONE Cream or Lotion?

Gently massage sufficient LOTRISONE Cream or Lotion into the affected and surrounding skin areas twice a day, in the morning and evening. Treatment for 2 weeks on the groin or on the body, and for 4 weeks on the feet is recommended. The use of LOTRISONE Cream or Lotion for longer than 4 weeks is not recommended for any condition. Prolonged use of LOTRISONE Cream or Lotion may lead to unwanted side effects.

What other important information should I know about LOTRISONE Cream and Lotion?

1. This medication is to be used for the full prescribed treatment time, even though the symptoms may have improved. Notify your doctor if there is no improvement after 1 week of treatment on the groin or body or after 2 weeks on the feet.
2. This medication should only be used for the disorder for which it was prescribed.
3. The treated skin area should not be bandaged or otherwise covered or wrapped.

4. Any signs of side effects where LOTRISONE Cream or Lotion is applied should be reported to your doctor.
5. When using LOTRISONE Cream or Lotion in the groin area, it is especially important to use the medication for 2 weeks only, and to apply the cream or lotion sparingly. You should tell your doctor if your problem persists after 2 weeks. You should also wear loose-fitting clothing so as to avoid tightly covering the area where LOTRISONE Cream or Lotion is applied.
6. This medication is not recommended for use in diaper rash.

What are the possible side effects of LOTRISONE Cream and Lotion?

The following side effects have been reported with topical corticosteroid medications: itching, irritation, dryness, infection of the hair follicles, increased hair, acne, change in skin color, allergic skin reaction, skin thinning, and stretch marks. In children, reported adverse events for LOTRISONE Cream include slower growth, Cushing's syndrome (a type of hormone imbalance that can be very serious), and local skin reactions, including thinning skin and stretch marks.

Can LOTRISONE Cream or Lotion be used if I am pregnant or plan to become pregnant or if I am nursing?

Before using LOTRISONE Cream or Lotion, tell your doctor if you are pregnant or plan to become pregnant. Also, tell your doctor if you are nursing.

How should LOTRISONE Cream or Lotion be stored?

LOTRISONE Cream should be stored between 2°C and 30°C (36°F and 86°F). LOTRISONE Lotion should only be stored in an upright position between 15°C and 30°C (59°F and 86°F). Shake well before using LOTRISONE Lotion.

General advice about prescription medicines

This medicine was prescribed for your particular condition. Only use LOTRISONE Cream or Lotion to treat the condition for which your doctor has prescribed. Do not give LOTRISONE Cream or Lotion to other people. It may harm them.

This leaflet summarizes the most important information about LOTRISONE Cream and Lotion. If you would like more information, talk with your doctor. You can ask your pharmacist or doctor for information about LOTRISONE Cream and Lotion that is written for health professionals.

Rx only
Schering Corporation/
Key Pharmaceuticals, Inc.
Kenilworth, NJ 07033 USA
Copyright © 2000, Schering
Corporation. All rights reserved.
12/00
23623706
24441903T

NASONEX®   ℞
(mometasone furoate monohydrate)
Nasal Spray, 50 mcg*
FOR INTRANASAL USE ONLY
*calculated on the anhydrous basis

Prescribing information for this product, which appears on pages 2914–2917 of the 2001 PDR, has been completely revised as follows. Please write "See Supplement A" next to the product heading.

DESCRIPTION

Mometasone furoate monohydrate, the active component of NASONEX Nasal Spray, 50 mcg, is an anti-inflammatory corticosteroid having the chemical name, 9,21-Dichloro-11β,17-dihydroxy-16α-methylpregna-1,4-diene-3,20-dione 17-(2 furoate) monohydrate, and the following chemical structure:

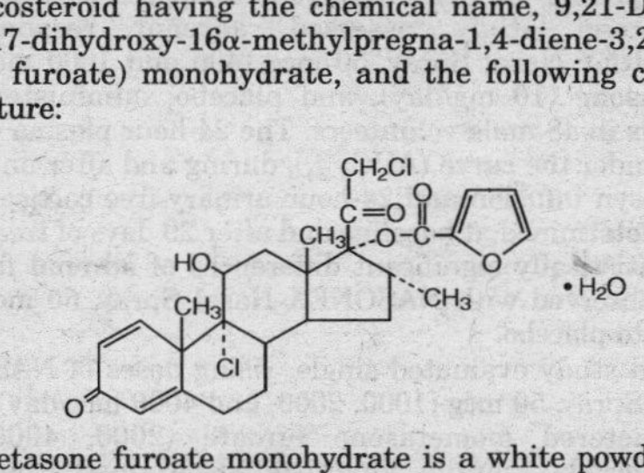

Mometasone furoate monohydrate is a white powder, with an empirical formula of $C_{27}H_{30}Cl_2O_6 \bullet H_2O$, and a molecular weight of 539.45. It is practically insoluble in water; slightly soluble in methanol, ethanol, and isopropanol; soluble in acetone and chloroform; and freely soluble in tetrahydrofuran. Its partition coefficient between octanol and water is greater than 5000.

NASONEX Nasal Spray, 50 mcg is a metered-dose, manual pump spray unit containing an aqueous suspension of mometasone furoate monohydrate equivalent to 0.05% w/w mometasone furoate calculated on the anhydrous basis; in an aqueous medium containing glycerin, microcrystalline cellulose and carboxymethylcellulose sodium, sodium citrate, 0.25% w/w phenylethyl alcohol, citric acid, benzalkonium chloride, and polysorbate 80. The pH is between 4.3 and 4.9.

After initial priming (10 actuations), each actuation of the pump delivers a metered spray containing 100 mg of suspension containing mometasone furoate monohydrate equivalent to 50 mcg of mometasone furoate calculated on the anhydrous basis. Each bottle of NASONEX Nasal Spray, 50 mcg provides 120 sprays.

Continued on next page

Nasonex—Cont.

CLINICAL PHARMACOLOGY

NASONEX Nasal Spray, 50 mcg is a corticosteroid demonstrating anti-inflammatory properties. The precise mechanism of corticosteroid action on allergic rhinitis is not known. Corticosteroids have been shown to have a wide range of effects on multiple cell types (eg, mast cells, eosinophils, neutrophils, macrophages, and lymphocytes) and mediators (eg, histamine, eicosanoids, leukotrienes, and cytokines) involved in inflammation.

In two clinical studies utilizing nasal antigen challenge, NASONEX Nasal Spray, 50 mcg decreased some markers of the early- and late-phase allergic response. These observations included decreases (vs placebo) in histamine and eosinophil cationic protein levels, and reductions (vs baseline) in eosinophils, neutrophils, and epithelial cell adhesion proteins. The clinical significance of these findings is not known.

The effect of NASONEX Nasal Spray, 50 mcg on nasal mucosa following 12 months of treatment was examined in 46 patients with allergic rhinitis. There was no evidence of atrophy and there was a marked reduction in intraepithelial eosinophilia and inflammatory cell infiltration (eg, eosinophils, lymphocytes, monocytes, neutrophils, and plasma cells).

Pharmacokinetics: ***Absorption:*** Mometasone furoate monohydrate administered as a nasal spray is virtually undetectable in plasma from adult and pediatric subjects despite the use of a sensitive assay with a lower quantitation limit (LOQ) of 50 pcg/mL.

Distribution: The *in vitro* protein binding for mometasone furoate was reported to be 98% to 99% in concentration range of 5 to 500 ng/mL.

Metabolism: Studies have shown that any portion of a mometasone furoate dose which is swallowed and absorbed undergoes extensive metabolism to multiple metabolites. There are no major metabolites detectable in plasma. Upon *in vitro* incubation, one of the minor metabolites formed is 6β-hydroxy-mometasone furoate. In human liver microsomes, the formation of the metabolite is regulated by cytochrome P-450 3A4 (CYP3A4).

Elimination: Following intravenous administration, the effective plasma elimination half-life of mometasone furoate is 5.8 hours. Any absorbed drug is excreted as metabolites mostly via the bile, and to a limited extent, into the urine.

Special Populations: The effects of renal impairment, hepatic impairment, age, or gender on mometasone furoate pharmacokinetics have not been adequately investigated.

Pharmacodynamics: Three clinical pharmacology studies have been conducted in humans to assess the effect of NASONEX Nasal Spray, 50 mcg at various doses on adrenal function. In one study, daily doses of 200 and 400 mcg of NASONEX Nasal Spray, 50 mcg and 10 mg of prednisone were compared to placebo in 64 patients with allergic rhinitis. Adrenal function before and after 36 consecutive days of treatment was assessed by measuring plasma cortisol levels following a 6-hour Cortrosyn (ACTH) infusion and by measuring 24-hour urinary-free cortisol levels. NASONEX Nasal Spray, 50 mcg, at both the 200- and 400-mcg dose, was not associated with a statistically significant decrease in mean plasma cortisol levels post-Cortrosyn infusion or a statistically significant decrease in the 24-hour urinary-free cortisol levels compared to placebo. A statistically significant decrease in the mean plasma cortisol levels post-Cortrosyn infusion and 24-hour urinary-free cortisol levels was detected in the prednisone treatment group compared to placebo.

A second study assessed adrenal response to NASONEX Nasal Spray, 50 mcg (400 and 1600 mcg/day), prednisone (10 mg/day), and placebo, administered for 29 days in 48 male volunteers. The 24-hour plasma cortisol area under the curve (AUC_{0-24}), during and after an 8-hour Cortrosyn infusion and 24-hour urinary-free cortisol levels were determined at baseline and after 29 days of treatment. No statistically significant differences of adrenal function were observed with NASONEX Nasal Spray, 50 mcg compared to placebo.

A third study evaluated single, rising doses of NASONEX Nasal Spray, 50 mcg (1000, 2000, and 4000 mcg/day), orally administered mometasone furoate (2000, 4000, and 8000 mcg/day), orally administered dexamethasone (200, 400, and 800 mcg/day), and placebo (administered at the end of each series of doses) in 24 male volunteers. Dose administrations were separated by at least 72 hours. Determination of serial plasma cortisol levels at 8 AM and for the 24-hour period following each treatment were used to calculate the plasma cortisol area under the curve (AUC_{0-24}). In addition, 24-hour urinary-free cortisol levels were collected prior to initial treatment administration and during the period immediately following each dose. No statistically significant decreases in the plasma cortisol AUC, 8 AM cortisol levels, or 24-hour urinary-free cortisol levels were observed in volunteers treated with either NASONEX Nasal Spray, 50 mcg or oral mometasone, as compared with placebo treatment. Conversely, nearly all volunteers treated with the three doses of dexamethasone demonstrated abnormal 8 AM cortisol levels (defined as a cortisol level <10 mcg/dL), reduced 24-hour plasma AUC values, and decreased 24-hour urinary-free cortisol levels, as compared to placebo treatment.

Two clinical pharmacology studies have been conducted in pediatric patients to assess the effect of mometasone furoate nasal spray, on the adrenal function at daily doses of 50, 100, and 200 mcg vs placebo. In one study, adrenal function before and after 7 consecutive days of treatment was assessed in 48 pediatric patients with allergic rhinitis (ages 6 to 11 years) by measuring morning plasma cortisol and 24-hour urinary-free cortisol levels. Mometasone furoate nasal spray, at all three doses, was not associated with a statistically significant decrease in mean plasma cortisol levels or a statistically significant decrease in the 24-hour urinary-free cortisol levels compared to placebo. In the second study, adrenal function before and after 14 consecutive days of treatment was assessed in 48 pediatric patients (ages 3 to 5 years) with allergic rhinitis by measuring plasma cortisol levels following a 30-minute Cortrosyn infusion. Mometasone furoate nasal spray, 50 mcg, at all three doses (50, 100, and 200 mcg/day), was not associated with a statistically significant decrease in mean plasma cortisol levels post-Cortrosyn infusion compared to placebo. All patients had a normal response to Cortrosyn.

Clinical Studies: The efficacy and safety of NASONEX Nasal Spray, 50 mcg in the prophylaxis and treatment of seasonal allergic rhinitis and the treatment of perennial allergic rhinitis have been evaluated in 18 controlled trials, and one uncontrolled clinical trial, in approximately 3000 adults (ages 17 to 85 years) and adolescents (ages 12 to 16 years). This included 1757 males and 1453 females, including a total of 283 adolescents (182 boys and 101 girls) with seasonal allergic or perennial allergic rhinitis, treated with NASONEX Nasal Spray, 50 mcg at doses ranging from 50 to 800 mcg/day. The majority of patients were treated with 200 mcg/day. These trials evaluated the total nasal symptom scores that included stuffiness, rhinorrhea, itching, and sneezing. Patients treated with NASONEX Nasal Spray, 50 mcg, 200 mcg/day had a significant decrease in total nasal symptom scores compared to placebo-treated patients. No additional benefit was observed for mometasone furoate doses greater than 200 mcg/day. A total of 350 patients have been treated with NASONEX Nasal Spray, 50 mcg for 1 year or longer.

The efficacy and safety of NASONEX Nasal Spray, 50 mcg in the treatment of seasonal allergic and perennial allergic rhinitis in pediatric patients (ages 3 to 11 years) have been evaluated in four controlled trials. This included approximately 990 pediatric patients ages 3 to 11 years (606 males and 384 females) with seasonal allergic or perennial allergic rhinitis treated with mometasone furoate nasal spray at doses ranging from 25 to 200 mcg/day. Pediatric patients treated with NASONEX Nasal Spray, 50 mcg (100 mcg total daily dose, 374 patients) had a significant decrease in total nasal symptom (congestion, rhinorrhea, itching, and sneezing) scores, compared to placebo-treated patients. No additional benefit was observed for the 200-mcg mometasone furoate total daily dose in pediatric patients (ages 3 to 11 years). A total of 163 pediatric patients have been treated for 1 year.

In patients with seasonal allergic rhinitis, NASONEX Nasal Spray, 50 mcg, demonstrated improvement in nasal symptoms (vs placebo) within 11 hours after the first dose based on one single-dose, parallel-group study of patients in an outdoor "park" setting (park study) and one environmental exposure unit (EEU) study, and within 2 days in two randomized, double-blind, placebo-controlled, parallel-group seasonal allergic rhinitis studies. Maximum benefit is usually achieved within 1 to 2 weeks after initiation of dosing.

Prophylaxis of seasonal allergic rhinitis for patients 12 years of age and older with NASONEX Nasal Spray, 50 mcg, given at a dose of 200 mcg/day, was evaluated in two clinical studies in 284 patients. These studies were designed such that patients received 4 weeks of prophylaxis with NASONEX Nasal Spray, 50 mcg prior to the anticipated onset of the pollen season; however, some patients received only 2 to 3 weeks of prophylaxis. Patients receiving 2 to 4 weeks of prophylaxis with NASONEX Nasal Spray, 50 mcg demonstrated a statistically significantly smaller mean increase in total nasal symptom scores with onset of the pollen season as compared to placebo patients.

INDICATIONS AND USAGE

NASONEX Nasal Spray, 50 mcg is indicated for the treatment of the nasal symptoms of seasonal allergic and perennial allergic rhinitis, in adults and pediatric patients 3 years of age and older. NASONEX Nasal Spray, 50 mcg is indicated for the prophylaxis of the nasal symptoms of seasonal allergic rhinitis in adult and adolescent patients 12 years and older. In patients with a known seasonal allergen that precipitates nasal symptoms of seasonal allergic rhinitis, initiation of prophylaxis with NASONEX Nasal Spray, 50 mcg is recommended 2 to 4 weeks prior to the anticipated start of the pollen season. Safety and effectiveness of NASONEX Nasal Spray, 50 mcg in pediatric patients less than 3 years of age have not been established.

CONTRAINDICATIONS

Hypersensitivity to any of the ingredients of this preparation contraindicates its use.

WARNINGS

The replacement of a systemic corticosteroid with a topical corticosteroid can be accompanied by signs of adrenal insufficiency and, in addition, some patients may experience symptoms of withdrawal; ie, joint and/or muscular pain, lassitude, and depression. Careful attention must be given when patients previously treated for prolonged periods with systemic corticosteroids are transferred to topical corticosteroids, with careful monitoring for acute adrenal insufficiency in response to stress. This is particularly important in those patients who have associated asthma or other clinical conditions where too rapid a decrease in systemic corticosteroid dosing may cause a severe exacerbation of their symptoms.

If recommended doses of intranasal corticosteroids are exceeded or if individuals are particularly sensitive or predisposed by virtue of recent systemic steroid therapy, symptoms of hypercorticism may occur, including very rare cases of menstrual irregularities, acneiform lesions, and cushingoid features. If such changes occur, topical corticosteroids should be discontinued slowly, consistent with accepted procedures for discontinuing oral steroid therapy.

Persons who are on drugs which suppress the immune system are more susceptible to infections than healthy individuals. Chickenpox and measles, for example, can have a more serious or even fatal course in nonimmune children or adults on corticosteroids. In such children or adults who have not had these diseases, particular care should be taken to avoid exposure. How the dose, route, and duration of corticosteroid administration affects the risk of developing a disseminated infection is not known. The contribution of the underlying disease and/or prior corticosteroid treatment to the risk is also not known. If exposed to chickenpox, prophylaxis with varicella zoster immune globin (VZIG) may be indicated. If exposed to measles, prophylaxis with pooled intramuscular immunoglobulin (IG) may be indicated. (See the respective package inserts for complete VZIG and IG prescribing information.) If chickenpox develops, treatment with antiviral agents may be considered.

PRECAUTIONS

General: Intranasal corticosteroids may cause a reduction in growth velocity when administered to pediatric patients (see **PRECAUTIONS, Pediatric Use** section). In clinical studies with NASONEX Nasal Spray, 50 mcg, the development of localized infections of the nose and pharynx with *Candida albicans* has occurred only rarely. When such an infection develops, use of NASONEX Nasal Spray, 50 mcg should be discontinued and appropriate local or systemic therapy instituted, if needed.

Nasal corticosteroids should be used with caution, if at all, in patients with active or quiescent tuberculous infection of the respiratory tract, or in untreated fungal, bacterial, systemic viral infections, or ocular herpes simplex.

Rarely, immediate hypersensitivity reactions may occur after the intranasal administration of mometasone furoate monohydrate. Extreme rare instances of wheezing have been reported.

Rare instances of nasal septum perforation and increased intraocular pressure have also been reported following the intranasal application of aerosolized corticosteroids. As with any long-term topical treatment of the nasal cavity, patients using NASONEX Nasal Spray, 50 mcg over several months or longer should be examined periodically for possible changes in the nasal mucosa.

Because of the inhibitory effect of corticosteroids on wound healing, patients who have experienced recent nasal septum ulcers, nasal surgery, or nasal trauma should not use a nasal corticosteroid until healing has occurred.

Glaucoma and cataract formation was evaluated in one controlled study of 12 weeks' duration and one uncontrolled study of 12 months' duration in patients treated with NASONEX Nasal Spray, 50 mcg at 200 mcg/day, using intraocular pressure measurements and slit lamp examination. No significant change from baseline was noted in the mean intraocular pressure measurements for the 141 NASONEX-treated patients in the 12-week study, as compared with 141 placebo-treated patients. No individual NASONEX-treated patient was noted to have developed a significant elevation in intraocular pressure or cataracts in this 12-week study. Likewise, no significant change from baseline was noted in the mean intraocular pressure measurements for the 139 NASONEX-treated patients in the 12-month study and again, no cataracts were detected in these patients. Nonetheless, nasal and inhaled corticosteroids have been associated with the development of glaucoma and/or cataracts. Therefore, close follow-up is warranted in patients with a change in vision and with a history of glaucoma and/or cataracts.

When nasal corticosteroids are used at excessive doses, systemic corticosteroid effects such as hypercorticism and adrenal suppression may appear. If such changes occur, NASONEX Nasal Spray, 50 mcg should be discontinued slowly, consistent with accepted procedures for discontinuing oral steroid therapy.

Information for Patients: Patients being treated with NASONEX Nasal Spray, 50 mcg should be given the following information and instructions. This information is intended to aid in the safe and effective use of this medication. It is not a disclosure of all intended or possible adverse effects. Patients should use NASONEX Nasal Spray, 50 mcg at regular intervals (once daily) since its effectiveness depends on regular use. Improvement in nasal symptoms of allergic rhinitis has been shown to occur within 11 hours after the first dose based on one single-dose, parallel-group study of patients in an outdoor "park" setting (park study) and one environmental exposure unit (EEU) study and within 2 days after the first dose in two randomized, double-blind, placebo-controlled, parallel-group seasonal allergic rhinitis studies. Maximum benefit is usually achieved within 1 to 2 weeks after initiation of dosing. Patients should take the medication as directed and should not increase the prescribed dosage by using it more than once a day in an attempt to increase its effectiveness. Patients should contact their physician if symptoms do not improve, or if the condition worsens. To assure proper use of this nasal spray, and to attain maximum benefit, patients should read and follow the accompanying Patient's Instructions for Use carefully.

Patients should be cautioned not to spray NASONEX Nasal Spray, 50 mcg into the eyes or directly onto the nasal septum.

Persons who are on immunosuppressant doses of corticosteroids should be warned to avoid exposure to chickenpox or measles, and patients should also be advised that if they are exposed, medical advice should be sought without delay.

Carcinogenesis, Mutagenesis, Impairment of Fertility: In a 2-year carcinogenicity study of Sprague Dawley rats, mometasone furoate demonstrated no statistically significant increase of tumors at inhalation doses up to 67 mcg/kg (approximately 3 and 2 times the maximum recommended daily intranasal dose in adults and children, respectively, on a mcg/m^2 basis). In a 19-month carcinogenicity study of Swiss CD-1 mice, mometasone furoate demonstrated no statistically significant increase in the incidence of tumors at inhalation doses up to 160 mcg/kg (approximately 4 and 3 times the maximum recommended daily intranasal dose in adults and children, respectively, on a mcg/m^2 basis).

At cytotoxic doses, mometasone furoate produced an increase in chromosome aberrations *in vitro* in Chinese hamster ovary-cell cultures in the nonactivation phase, but not in the presence of rat liver S9 fraction. Mometasone furoate was not mutagenic in the mouse-lymphoma assay and the *Salmonella/E. coli*/mammalian microsome mutation assay, a Chinese hamster lung cell (CHL) chromosomal-aberrations assay, an *in vivo* mouse bone-marrow erythrocyte-micronucleus assay, a rat bone-marrow clastogenicity assay, and the mouse male germ-cell clastogenicity assay. Mometasone furoate also did not induce unscheduled DNA synthesis *in vivo* in rat hepatocytes.

In reproductive studies in rats, impairment of fertility was not produced by subcutaneous doses up to 15 mcg/kg (less than the maximum recommended daily intranasal dose in adults on a mcg/m^2 basis). However, mometasone furoate caused prolonged gestation, prolonged and difficult labor, reduced offspring survival, and reduced maternal body weight gain at a dose of 15 mcg/kg.

Pregnancy: ***Teratogenic Effects: Pregnancy Category C:*** Mometasone furoate caused cleft palate in mice at subcutaneous doses of 60 mcg/kg and above (approximately 2 times the maximum recommended daily intranasal dose in adults on a mcg/m^2 basis). Offspring survival was reduced in the 180-mcg/kg group (approximately 4 times the maximum recommended daily intranasal dose in adults on a mcg/m^2 basis). No such effects were observed at 20 mcg/kg (less than the maximum recommended daily intranasal dose in adults on a mcg/m^2 basis).

In rabbits, mometasone furoate caused flexed front paws at a topical dermal dose of 150 mcg/kg (approximately 14 times the maximum recommended daily intranasal dose in adults on a mcg/m^2 basis).

In rats, mometasone furoate produced umbilical hernia, cleft palate, and delayed ossification at a topical dermal dose of 600 mcg/kg (approximately 30 times the maximum recommended daily intranasal dose in adults on a mcg/m^2 basis). At 1200 mcg/kg (approximately 60 times the maximum recommended daily intranasal dose in adults on a mcg/m^2 basis), microphthalmia, umbilical hernias, and delayed ossification were observed in rat pups.

In these developmental studies, there were also reductions in maternal body weight gain and effects on fetal growth (lower fetal body weights and/or delayed ossification) in mice (60 and 180 mcg/kg), rabbits (150 mcg/kg), and rats (600 mcg/kg).

In an oral developmental study in rabbits, at 700 mcg/kg, (approximately 70 times the maximum recommended daily intranasal dose in adults on a mcg/m^2 basis), increased incidences of resorptions and malformations, including cleft palate and/or head malformations (hydrocephaly or domed head) were observed. Pregnancy failure was observed in most rabbits at 2800 mcg/kg (approximately 270 times the maximum recommended daily intranasal dose in adults on a mcg/m^2 basis).

There are no adequate and well-controlled studies in pregnant women. NASONEX Nasal Spray, 50 mcg, like other corticosteroids, should be used during pregnancy only if the potential benefits justify the potential risk to the fetus. Experience with oral corticosteroids since their introduction in pharmacologic, as opposed to physiologic, doses suggests that rodents are more prone to teratogenic effects from corticosteroids than humans. In addition, because there is a natural increase in corticosteroid production during pregnancy, most women will require a lower exogenous corticosteroid dose and many will not need corticosteroid treatment during pregnancy.

Nonteratogenic Effects: Hypoadrenalism may occur in infants born to women receiving corticosteroids during pregnancy. Such infants should be carefully monitored.

Nursing Mothers: It is not known if mometasone furoate is excreted in human milk. Because other corticosteroids are excreted in human milk, caution should be used when NASONEX Nasal Spray, 50 mcg is administered to nursing women.

Pediatric Use: Controlled clinical studies have shown intranasal corticosteroids may cause a reduction in growth velocity in pediatric patients. This effect has been observed in the absence of laboratory evidence of hypothalamic-pituitary-adrenal (HPA) axis suppression, suggesting that growth velocity is a more sensitive indicator of systemic corticosteroid exposure in pediatric patients than some commonly used tests of HPA axis function. The long-term effects of this reduction in growth velocity associated with intranasal corticosteroids, including the impact on final adult height, are unknown. The potential for "catch up" growth following discontinuation of treatment with intranasal corticosteroids has not been adequately studied. The growth of pediatric patients receiving intranasal corticosteroids, including NASONEX Nasal Spray, 50 mcg should be monitored routinely (eg, via stadiometry). The potential growth effects of prolonged treatment should be weighed against clinical benefits obtained and the availability of safe and effective noncorticosteroid treatment alternatives. To minimize the systemic effects of intranasal corticosteroids, including NASONEX Nasal Spray, 50 mcg, each patient should be titrated to his/her lowest effective dose.

Seven hundred and twenty (720) patients 3 to 11 years of age were treated with mometasone furoate nasal spray, 50 mcg (100 mcg total daily dose) in controlled clinical trials. Safety and effectiveness in children less than 3 years of age have not been established.

A clinical study has been conducted for one year in pediatric patients (ages 3 to 9 years) to assess the effect of NASONEX Nasal Spray, 50 mcg (100 mcg total daily dose) on growth velocity. No statistically significant effect on growth velocity was observed for NASONEX Nasal Spray, 50 mcg compared to placebo. No evidence of clinically relevant HPA axis suppression was observed following a 30-minute Cosyntropin infusion.

The potential of NASONEX Nasal Spray to cause growth suppression in susceptible patients or when given at higher doses cannot be ruled out.

Geriatric Use: A total of 203 patients above 64 years of age (age range 64 to 85 years) have been treated with NASONEX Nasal Spray, 50 mcg for up to 3 months. The adverse reactions reported in this population were similar in type and incidence to those reported by younger patients.

ADVERSE REACTIONS

In controlled US and International clinical studies, a total of 3210 adult and adolescent patients aged 12 years and older received treatment with NASONEX Nasal Spray, 50 mcg at doses of 50 to 800 mcg/day. The majority of patients (n = 2103) were treated with 200 mcg/day. In controlled US and International studies, a total of 990 pediatric patients (ages 3 to 11 years) received treatment with NASONEX, 50 mcg, at doses of 25 to 200 mcg/day. The majority of pediatric patients (720) were treated with 100 mcg/day. A total of 513 adult, adolescent, and pediatric patients have been treated for 1 year or longer. The overall incidence of adverse events for patients treated with NASONEX Nasal Spray, 50 mcg was comparable to patients treated with the vehicle placebo. Also, adverse events did not differ significantly based on age, sex, or race. Three percent or less of patients in clinical trials discontinued treatment because of adverse events; this rate was similar for the vehicle and active comparators.

All adverse events (regardless of relationship to treatment) reported by 5% or more of adult and adolescent patients aged 12 years and older who received NASONEX Nasal Spray, 50 mcg, 200 mcg/day and by pediatric patients ages 3 to 11 years who received NASONEX Nasal Spray, 50 mcg, 100 mcg/day in clinical trials vs placebo and that were more common with NASONEX Nasal Spray, 50 mcg than placebo, are displayed in the table below.

[See table above]

ADVERSE EVENTS FROM CONTROLLED CLINICAL TRIALS IN SEASONAL ALLERGIC AND PERENNIAL ALLERGIC RHINITIS (PERCENT OF PATIENTS REPORTING)

	Adult and Adolescent Patients 12 years and older		Pediatric Patients Ages 3 to 11 years	
	NASONEX 200 mcg (N = 2103)	VEHICLE PLACEBO (N = 1671)	NASONEX 100 mcg (N = 374)	VEHICLE PLACEBO (N = 376)
Headache	26	22	17	18
Viral Infection	14	11	8	9
Pharyngitis	12	10	10	10
Epistaxis/Blood-Tinged Mucus	11	6	8	9
Coughing	7	6	13	15
Upper Respiratory Tract Infection	6	2	5	4
Dysmenorrhea	5	3	1	0
Musculoskeletal Pain	5	3	1	1
Sinusitis	5	3	4	4
Vomiting	1	1	5	4

Other adverse events which occurred in less than 5% but greater than or equal to 2% of mometasone furoate adult and adolescent patients (aged 12 years and older) treated with 200-mcg doses (regardless of relationship to treatment), and more frequently than in the placebo group included: arthralgia, asthma, bronchitis, chest pain, conjunctivitis, diarrhea, dyspepsia, earache, flu-like symptoms, myalgia, nausea, and rhinitis.

Other adverse events which occurred in less than 5% but greater or equal to 2% of mometasone furoate pediatric patients aged 3 to 11 years treated with 100-mcg doses vs placebo (regardless of relationship to treatment) and more frequently than in the placebo group included: diarrhea, nasal irritation, otitis media, and wheezing.

Rare cases of nasal ulcers and nasal and oral candidiasis were also reported in patients treated with NASONEX Nasal Spray, 50 mcg, primarily in patients treated for longer than 4 weeks.

In postmarketing surveillance of this product, cases of nasal burning and irritation, anaphylaxis and angioedema, and rare cases of nasal septal perforation have been reported.

OVERDOSAGE

There are no data available on the effects of acute or chronic overdosage with NASONEX Nasal Spray, 50 mcg. Because of low systemic bioavailability, and an absence of acute drug-related systemic findings in clinical studies, overdose is unlikely to require any therapy other than observation. Intranasal administration of 1600 mcg (8 times the recommended dose of NASONEX Nasal Spray, 50 mcg) daily for 29 days, to healthy human volunteers, was well tolerated with no increased incidence of adverse events. Single intranasal doses up to 4000 mcg have been studied in human volunteers with no adverse effects reported. Single oral doses up to 8000 mcg have been studied in human volunteers with no adverse effects reported. Chronic overdosage with any corticosteroid may result in signs or symptoms of hypercorticism (see **PRECAUTIONS**). Acute overdosage with this dosage form is unlikely since one bottle of NASONEX Nasal Spray, 50 mcg contains approximately 8500 mcg of mometasone furoate.

DOSAGE AND ADMINISTRATION

Adults and Children 12 Years of Age and Older: The usual recommended dose for prophylaxis and treatment of the nasal symptoms of seasonal allergic rhinitis and treatment of the nasal symptoms of perennial allergic rhinitis is two sprays (50 mcg of mometasone furoate in each spray) in each nostril once daily (total daily dose of 200 mcg).

In patients with a known seasonal allergen that precipitates nasal symptoms of seasonal allergic rhinitis, prophylaxis with NASONEX Nasal Spray, 50 mcg (200 mcg/day) is recommended 2 to 4 weeks prior to the anticipated start of the pollen season.

Children 3 to 11 Years of Age: The usual recommended dose for treatment of the nasal symptoms of seasonal allergic and perennial allergic rhinitis is one spray (50 mcg of mometasone furoate in each spray) in each nostril once daily (total daily dose of 100 mcg).

Improvement in nasal symptoms of allergic rhinitis has been shown to occur within 11 hours after the first dose based on one single-dose, parallel-group study of patients in an outdoor "park" setting (park study) and one environmental exposure unit (EEU) study and within 2 days after the first dose in two randomized, double-blind, placebo-controlled, parallel-group seasonal allergic rhinitis studies. Maximum benefit is usually achieved within 1 to 2 weeks. Patients should use NASONEX Nasal Spray, 50 mcg only once daily at a regular interval.

Prior to initial use of NASONEX Nasal Spray, 50 mcg, the pump must be primed by actuating ten times or until a fine spray appears. The pump may be stored unused for up to 1 week without repriming. If unused for more than 1 week, reprime by actuating two times, or until a fine spray appears.

Directions for Use: Illustrated Patient's Instructions for Use accompany each package of NASONEX Nasal Spray, 50 mcg.

Shake the bottle well before each use. Read complete instructions carefully and use only as directed.

1. Remove the teal-green plastic cap (Figure 1).
   [See figure at top of next column]
2. The very first time the spray is used, prime the pump by pressing downward on the shoulders of the white applicator using your forefinger and middle finger while supporting the base of the bottle with your thumb (Figure 2). Press down and release the pump ten times or until a fine spray appears. DO NOT spray into eyes. The pump is now

Continued on next page

Nasonex—Cont.

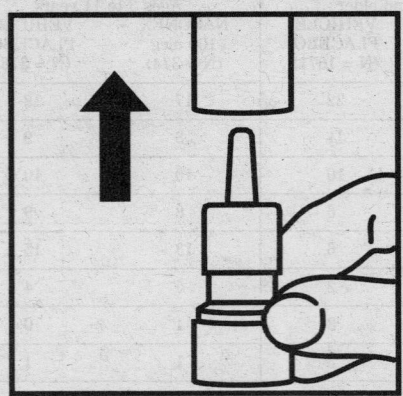

Figure 1

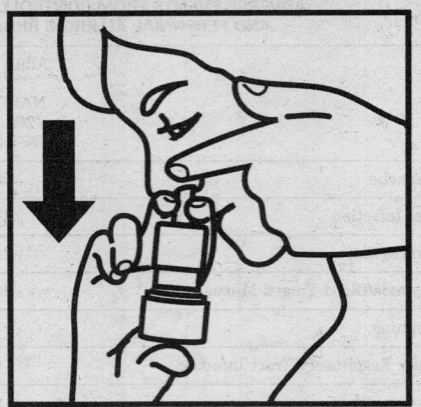

Figure 4

ready to use. The pump may be stored unused for up to 1 week without repriming. If unused for more than 1 week, reprime by spraying two times, or until a fine spray appears.

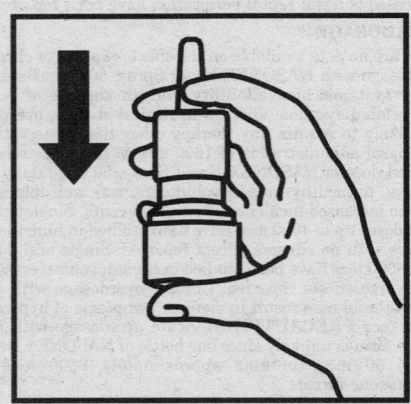

Figure 2

3. Gently blow your nose to clear the nostrils. Close one nostril. Tilt your head forward slightly and, keeping the bottle upright, carefully insert the nasal applicator into the other nostril (Figure 3). DO NOT spray directly onto nasal septum.

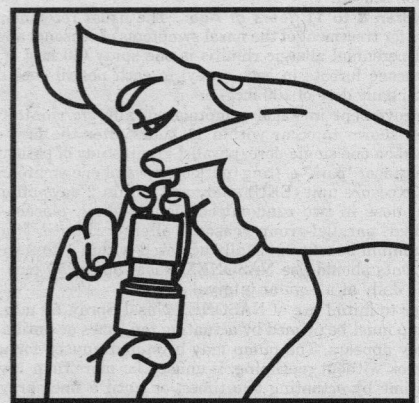

Figure 3

4. For each spray, press firmly downward once on the shoulders of the white applicator using your forefinger and middle finger while supporting the base of the bottle with your thumb. Breathe gently inward through the nostril (Figure 4).
   [See figure at top of next column]
5. Then breathe out through the mouth.
6. Repeat in the other nostril.
7. Replace the plastic cap.
The correct amount of medication in each spray can only be assured up to 120 sprays from the bottle even though the

bottle is not completely empty. You should keep track of the number of sprays used from each bottle of NASONEX Nasal Spray, 50 mcg and discard the bottle after using 120 sprays.

Cleaning: To clean the nasal applicator, remove the plastic cap and pull gently upward on the white nasal applicator so that it comes free. Wash the applicator and cap under a cold water tap. Dry and replace the nasal applicator followed by the plastic cap.

Caution: NASONEX Nasal Spray, 50 mcg is formulated for once-daily dosing. You should use NASONEX Nasal Spray, 50 mcg only once daily at a regular interval. Since NASONEX Nasal Spray, 50 mcg is not intended to give rapid relief of your nasal symptoms, the prescribed dosage should not be increased by using more often than once daily in an attempt to increase its effectiveness. NASONEX Nasal Spray, 50 mcg controls the underlying disorders responsible for your attacks, so it is important that you use it regularly at the time recommended by your physician. Based on single-day studies done in a park during pollen season or in a controlled pollen exposure room, improvement in nasal symptoms of allergic rhinitis has been shown to occur within 11 hours after the first dose. In other studies that lasted up to 2 weeks, improvement in nasal symptoms of seasonal allergic rhinitis was shown to occur within 2 days after the first dose. The full benefit of NASONEX Nasal Spray, 50 mcg is usually achieved within 1 to 2 weeks.

NASONEX Nasal Spray, 50 mcg should not be sprayed into the eyes.

Spraying NASONEX Nasal Spray, 50 mcg directly onto the nasal septum should be avoided.

Store between 2° and 25°C (36° and 77°F). Protect from light.

When NASONEX Nasal Spray, 50 mcg is removed from its cardboard container, prolonged exposure of the product to direct light should be avoided. Brief exposure to light, as with normal use, is acceptable.

SHAKE WELL BEFORE EACH USE.

HOW SUPPLIED

NASONEX (mometasone furoate monohydrate) Nasal Spray, 50 mcg is supplied in a white, high-density, polyethylene bottle fitted with a white metered-dose, manual spray pump, and teal-green cap. It contains 17 g of product formulation, 120 sprays, each delivering 50 mcg of mometasone furoate per actuation. Supplied with Patient's Instructions for Use (NDC 0085-1197-01).

Schering Corporation
Kenilworth, NJ 07033 USA
Rev. 7/00
20397942
20109866T

In the PDR annual,
the **Brand and Generic Name Index**
(PINK section)
alphabetizes drugs under both
brand and generic names.

SmithKline Beecham Pharmaceuticals
ONE FRANKLIN PLAZA
P.O. BOX 7929
PHILADELPHIA, PA 19101

For Medical Information Contact:
Medical Department
800-366-8900, ext. 5231

AVANDIA®   ℞
[ă-van-dee-ă]
brand of rosiglitazone maleate tablets

Prescribing information for this product, which appears on pages 3071–3075 of the 2001 PDR, has been completely revised as follows. Please write "See Supplement A" next to the product heading.

DESCRIPTION

Avandia (rosiglitazone maleate) is an oral antidiabetic agent which acts primarily by increasing insulin sensitivity. *Avandia* is used in the management of type 2 diabetes mellitus (also known as non-insulin-dependent diabetes mellitus [NIDDM] or adult-onset diabetes). *Avandia* improves glycemic control while reducing circulating insulin levels.

Pharmacological studies in animal models indicate that rosiglitazone improves sensitivity to insulin in muscle and adipose tissue and inhibits hepatic gluconeogenesis. Rosiglitazone maleate is not chemically or functionally related to the sulfonylureas, the biguanides, or the alpha-glucosidase inhibitors.

Chemically, rosiglitazone maleate is (±)-5-[[4-[2-(methyl-2-pyridinylamino)ethoxy]phenyl]methyl]-2,4-thiazolidinedione, (Z)-2-butenedioate (1:1) with a molecular weight of 473.52 (357.44 free base). The molecule has a single chiral center and is present as a racemate. Due to rapid interconversion, the enantiomers are functionally indistinguishable. The structural formula is:

rosiglitazone maleate

The molecular formula is $C_{18}H_{19}N_3O_3S \cdot C_4H_4O_4$. Rosiglitazone maleate is a white to off-white solid with a melting point range of 122° to 123°C. The pKa values of rosiglitazone maleate are 6.8 and 6.1. It is readily soluble in ethanol and a buffered aqueous solution with pH of 2.3; solubility decreases with increasing pH in the physiological range.

Each pentagonal film-coated Tiltab® tablet contains rosiglitazone maleate equivalent to rosiglitazone, 2 mg, 4 mg, or 8 mg, for oral administration. Inactive ingredients are: hydroxypropyl methylcellulose, lactose monohydrate, magnesium stearate, microcrystalline cellulose, polyethylene glycol 3000, sodium starch glycolate, titanium dioxide, triacetin, and one or more of the following: synthetic red and yellow iron oxides and talc.

CLINICAL PHARMACOLOGY

Mechanism of Action

Rosiglitazone, a member of the thiazolidinedione class of antidiabetic agents, improves glycemic control by improving insulin sensitivity. Rosiglitazone is a highly selective and potent agonist for the peroxisome proliferator-activated receptor-gamma (PPARγ). In humans, PPAR receptors are found in key target tissues for insulin action such as adipose tissue, skeletal muscle, and liver. Activation of PPARγ nuclear receptors regulates the transcription of insulin-responsive genes involved in the control of glucose production, transport, and utilization. In addition, PPARγ-responsive genes also participate in the regulation of fatty acid metabolism.

Insulin resistance is a common feature characterizing the pathogenesis of type 2 diabetes. The antidiabetic activity of rosiglitazone has been demonstrated in animal models of type 2 diabetes in which hyperglycemia and/or impaired glucose tolerance is a consequence of insulin resistance in target tissues. Rosiglitazone reduces blood glucose concentrations and reduces hyperinsulinemia in the ob/ob obese mouse, db/db diabetic mouse, and fa/fa fatty Zucker rat.

In animal models, rosiglitazone's antidiabetic activity was shown to be mediated by increased sensitivity to insulin's action in the liver, muscle, and adipose tissues. The expression of the insulin-regulated glucose transporter GLUT-4 was increased in adipose tissue. Rosiglitazone did not induce hypoglycemia in animal models of type 2 diabetes and/or impaired glucose tolerance.

Pharmacokinetics and Drug Metabolism

Maximum plasma concentration (C_{max}) and the area under the curve (AUC) of rosiglitazone increase in a dose-proportional manner over the therapeutic dose range (Table 1). The elimination half-life is 3 to 4 hours and is independent of dose.

Table 1. Mean (SD) Pharmacokinetic Parameters for Rosiglitazone Following Single Oral Doses (N=32)

Parameter	1 mg Fasting	2 mg Fasting	8 mg Fasting	8 mg Fed
AUC_{0-inf} [ng.hr./mL]	358 (112)	733 (184)	2971 (730)	2890 (795)
C_{max} [ng/mL]	76 (13)	156 (42)	598 (117)	432 (92)
Half-life [hr.]	3.16 (0.72)	3.15 (0.39)	3.37 (0.63)	3.59 (0.70)
CL/F* [L/hr.]	3.03 (0.87)	2.89 (0.71)	2.85 (0.69)	2.97 (0.81)

* CL/F = Oral Clearance.

Absorption
The absolute bioavailability of rosiglitazone is 99%. Peak plasma concentrations are observed about 1 hour after dosing. Administration of rosiglitazone with food resulted in no change in overall exposure (AUC), but there was an approximately 28% decrease in C_{max} and a delay in T_{max} (1.75 hours). These changes are not likely to be clinically significant; therefore, Avandia (rosiglitazone maleate) may be administered with or without food.

Distribution
The mean (CV%) oral volume of distribution (Vss/F) of rosiglitazone is approximately 17.6 (30%) liters, based on a population pharmacokinetic analysis. Rosiglitazone is approximately 99.8% bound to plasma proteins, primarily albumin.

Metabolism
Rosiglitazone is extensively metabolized with no unchanged drug excreted in the urine. The major routes of metabolism were N-demethylation and hydroxylation, followed by conjugation with sulfate and glucuronic acid. All the circulating metabolites are considerably less potent than parent and, therefore, are not expected to contribute to the insulin-sensitizing activity of rosiglitazone.
In vitro data demonstrate that rosiglitazone is predominantly metabolized by Cytochrome P_{450} (CYP) isoenzyme 2C8, with CYP2C9 contributing as a minor pathway.

Excretion
Following oral or intravenous administration of [14C]rosiglitazone maleate, approximately 64% and 23% of the dose was eliminated in the urine and in the feces, respectively. The plasma half-life of [14C]related material ranged from 103 to 158 hours.

Population Pharmacokinetics in Patients with Type 2 Diabetes
Population pharmacokinetic analyses from three large clinical trials including 642 men and 405 women with type 2 diabetes (aged 35 to 80 years) showed that the pharmacokinetics of rosiglitazone are not influenced by age, race, smoking, or alcohol consumption. Both oral clearance (CL/F) and oral steady-state volume of distribution (Vss/F) were shown to increase with increases in body weight. Over the weight range observed in these analyses (50 to 150 kg), the range of predicted CL/F and Vss/F values varied by <1.7-fold and <2.3-fold, respectively. Additionally, rosiglitazone CL/F was shown to be influenced by both weight and gender, being lower (about 15%) in female patients.

Special Populations
Age: Results of the population pharmacokinetic analysis (n=716 <65 years; n=331 ≥65 years) showed that age does not significantly affect the pharmacokinetics of rosiglitazone.
Gender: Results of the population pharmacokinetics analysis showed that the mean oral clearance of rosiglitazone in female patients (n=405) was approximately 6% lower compared to male patients of the same body weight (n=642).
As monotherapy and in combination with metformin, Avandia improved glycemic control in both males and females. In metformin combination studies, efficacy was demonstrated with no gender differences in glycemic response. In monotherapy studies, a greater therapeutic response was observed in females; however, in more obese patients, gender differences were less evident. For a given body mass index (BMI), females tend to have a greater fat mass than males. Since the molecular target PPARγ is expressed in adipose tissues, this differentiating characteristic may account, at least in part, for the greater response to Avandia in females. Since therapy should be individualized, no dose adjustments are necessary based on gender alone.
Hepatic Impairment: Unbound oral clearance of rosiglitazone was significantly lower in patients with moderate to severe liver disease (Child-Pugh Class B/C) compared to healthy subjects. As a result, unbound C_{max} and AUC_{0-inf} were increased 2- and 3-fold, respectively. Elimination half-life for rosiglitazone was about 2 hours longer in patients with liver disease, compared to healthy subjects.
Therapy with Avandia (rosiglitazone maleate) should not be initiated if the patient exhibits clinical evidence of active liver disease or increased serum transaminase levels (ALT >2.5X upper limit of normal) at baseline (see PRECAUTIONS, Hepatic Effects).
Renal Impairment: There are no clinically relevant differences in the pharmacokinetics of rosiglitazone in patients with mild to severe renal impairment or in hemodialysis-dependent patients compared to subjects with normal renal function. No dosage adjustment is therefore required in such patients receiving Avandia. Since metformin is contraindicated in patients with renal impairment, co-administration of metformin with Avandia is contraindicated in these patients.

Race: Results of a population pharmacokinetic analysis including subjects of Caucasian, black, and other ethnic origins indicate that race has no influence on the pharmacokinetics of rosiglitazone.
Pediatric Use: The safety and effectiveness of Avandia in pediatric patients have not been established.

CLINICAL STUDIES
In clinical studies, treatment with Avandia resulted in an improvement in glycemic control, as measured by fasting plasma glucose (FPG) and hemoglobin A1c (HbA1c), with a concurrent reduction in insulin and C-peptide. Postprandial glucose and insulin were also reduced. This is consistent with the mechanism of action of Avandia as an insulin sensitizer. The improvement in glycemic control was durable, with maintenance of effect for 52 weeks. The maximum recommended daily dose is 8 mg. Dose-ranging studies suggested that no additional benefit was obtained with a total daily dose of 12 mg.
The addition of Avandia to either metformin or a sulfonylurea resulted in significant reductions in hyperglycemia compared to any of these agents alone. These results are consistent with an additive effect on glycemic control when Avandia is used as combination therapy.

Patients with lipid abnormalities were not excluded from clinical trials of Avandia. In all 26-week controlled trials, across the recommended dose range, Avandia as monotherapy was associated with increases in total cholesterol, LDL, and HDL and decreases in free fatty acids. These changes were statistically significantly different from placebo or glyburide controls (Table 2).
Increases in LDL occurred primarily during the first 1 to 2 months of therapy with Avandia and LDL levels remained elevated above baseline throughout the trials. In contrast, HDL continued to rise over time. As a result, the LDL/HDL ratio peaked after 2 months of therapy and then appeared to decrease over time. Because of the temporal nature of lipid changes, the 52-week glyburide-controlled study is most

Continued on next page

Information on the SmithKline Beecham Pharmaceuticals products appearing here is based on the labeling in effect on May 15, 2001. Further information on these and other products may be obtained from the Medical Department, SmithKline Beecham Pharmaceuticals, One Franklin Plaza, Philadelphia, PA 19101.

Table 2. Summary of Mean Lipid Changes in 26-Week Placebo-Controlled and 52-Week Glyburide-Controlled Monotherapy Studies

| | Placebo-controlled Studies Week 26 | | | Glyburide-controlled Study Week 26 and Week 52 | | | |
| | | Avandia | | Glyburide titration | | Avandia 8 mg | |
	Placebo	4 mg daily*	8 mg daily*	Wk 26	Wk 52	Wk 26	Wk 52
Free Fatty Acids							
N	207	428	436	181	168	166	145
Baseline (mean)	18.1	17.5	17.9	26.4	26.4	26.9	26.6
% Change from baseline (mean)	+0.2%	−7.8%	−14.7%	−2.4%	−4.7%	−20.8%	−21.5%
LDL							
N	190	400	374	175	160	161	133
Baseline (mean)	123.7	126.8	125.3	142.7	141.9	142.1	142.1
% Change from baseline (mean)	+4.8%	+14.1%	+18.6%	−0.9%	−0.5%	+11.9%	+12.1%
HDL							
N	208	429	436	184	170	170	145
Baseline (mean)	44.1	44.4	43.0	47.2	47.7	48.4	48.3
% Change from baseline (mean)	+8.0%	+11.4%	+14.2%	+4.3%	+8.7%	+14.0%	+18.5%

*Once daily and twice daily dosing groups were combined.

Table 3. Glycemic Parameters in Two 26-Week Placebo-Controlled Trials

	Placebo	Avandia 2 mg twice daily	Avandia 4 mg twice daily
STUDY A			
N	158	166	169
FPG (mg/dL)			
Baseline (mean)	229	227	220
Change from baseline (mean)	19	−33	−54
Difference from placebo (adjusted mean)		−58*	−76*
Responders (≥30 mg/dL decrease from baseline)	16%	54%	64%
HbA1c (%)			
Baseline (mean)	9.0	9.0	8.8
Change from baseline (mean)	0.9	−0.3	−0.6
Difference from placebo (adjusted mean)		−1.2*	−1.5*
Responders (≥0.7% decrease from baseline)	6%	40%	42%

	Placebo	Avandia 4 mg once daily	Avandia 2 mg twice daily	Avandia 8 mg once daily	Avandia 4 mg twice daily
STUDY B					
N	173	180	186	181	187
FPG (mg/dL)					
Baseline (mean)	225	229	225	228	228
Change from baseline (mean)	8	−25	−35	−42	−55
Difference from placebo (adjusted mean)	−	−31*	−43*	−49*	−62*
Responders (≥30 mg/dL decrease from baseline)	19%	45%	54%	58%	70%
HbA1c (%)					
Baseline (mean)	8.9	8.9	8.9	8.9	9.0
Change from baseline (mean)	0.8	0.0	−0.1	−0.3	−0.7
Difference from placebo (adjusted mean)	−	−0.8*	−0.9*	−1.1*	−1.5*
Responders (≥0.7% decrease from baseline)	9%	28%	29%	39%	54%

*<0.0001 compared to placebo.

Avandia—Cont.

pertinent to assess long-term effects on lipids. At baseline, week 26, and week 52, mean LDL/HDL ratios were 3.1, 3.2, and 3.0, respectively, for *Avandia* 4 mg twice daily. The corresponding values for glyburide were 3.2, 3.1, and 2.9. The differences in change from baseline between *Avandia* and glyburide at week 52 were statistically significant.

The pattern of LDL and HDL changes following therapy with *Avandia* in combination with other hypoglycemic agents were generally similar to those seen with *Avandia* in monotherapy.

The changes in triglycerides during therapy with Avandia (rosiglitazone maleate) were variable and were generally not statistically different from placebo or glyburide controls.
[See table 2 at top of previous page]

Monotherapy
A total of 2315 patients with type 2 diabetes, previously treated with diet alone or antidiabetic medication(s), were treated with *Avandia* as monotherapy in six double-blind studies, which included two 26-week placebo-controlled studies, one 52-week glyburide-controlled study, and three placebo-controlled dose-ranging studies of 8 to 12 weeks duration. Previous antidiabetic medication(s) were withdrawn and patients entered a 2 to 4 week placebo run-in period prior to randomization.

Two 26-week, double-blind, placebo-controlled trials, in patients with type 2 diabetes with inadequate glycemic control (mean baseline FPG approximately 228 mg/dL and mean baseline HbA1c 8.9%), were conducted. Treatment with *Avandia* produced statistically significant improvements in FPG and HbA1c compared to baseline and relative to placebo (Table 3).
[See table 3 at top of previous page]

When administered at the same total daily dose, *Avandia* was generally more effective in reducing FPG and HbA1c when administered in divided doses twice daily compared to once daily doses. However, for HbA1c, the difference between the 4 mg once daily and 2 mg twice daily doses was not statistically significant.

Long-term maintenance of effect was evaluated in a 52-week, double-blind, glyburide-controlled trial in patients with type 2 diabetes. Patients were randomized to treatment with Avandia (rosiglitazone maleate) 2 mg twice daily (N=195) or *Avandia* 4 mg twice daily (N=189) or glyburide (N=202) for 52 weeks. Patients receiving glyburide were given an initial dosage of either 2.5 mg/day or 5.0 mg/day. The dosage was then titrated in 2.5 mg/day increments over the next 12 weeks, to a maximum dosage of 15.0 mg/day in order to optimize glycemic control. Thereafter the glyburide dose was kept constant.

The median titrated dose of glyburide was 7.5 mg. All treatments resulted in a statistically significant improvement in glycemic control from baseline (Figures 1 and 2). At the end of week 52, the reduction from baseline in FPG and HbA1c was −40.8 mg/dL and −0.53% with *Avandia* 4 mg twice daily; −25.4 mg/dL and −0.27% with *Avandia* 2 mg twice daily; and −30.0 mg/dL and −0.72% with glyburide. For HbA1c, the difference between *Avandia* 4 mg twice daily and glyburide was not statistically significant at week 52. The initial fall in FPG with glyburide was greater than with *Avandia*; however, this effect was less durable over time. The improvement in glycemic control seen with *Avandia* 4 mg twice daily at week 26 was maintained through week 52 of the study.

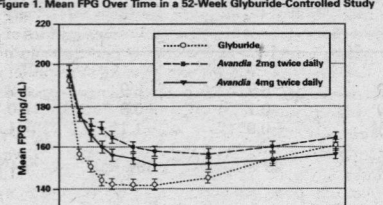

Figure 1. Mean FPG Over Time in a 52-Week Glyburide-Controlled Study

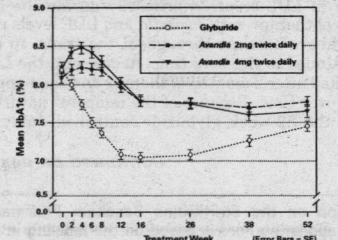

Figure 2. Mean HbA1c Over Time in a 52-Week Glyburide-Controlled Study

Hypoglycemia was reported in 12.1% of glyburide-treated patients versus 0.5% (2 mg twice daily) and 1.6% (4 mg

twice daily) of patients treated with *Avandia*. The improvements in glycemic control were associated with a mean weight gain of 1.75 kg and 2.95 kg for patients treated with 2 mg and 4 mg twice daily of *Avandia*, respectively, versus 1.9 kg in glyburide-treated patients. In patients treated with *Avandia*, C-peptide, insulin, pro-insulin, and pro-insulin split products were significantly reduced in a dose-ordered fashion, compared to an increase in the glyburide-treated patients.

Combination with Metformin
A total of 670 patients with type 2 diabetes participated in two 26-week, randomized, double-blind, placebo/active-controlled studies designed to assess the efficacy of Avandia (rosiglitazone maleate) in combination with metformin. *Avandia*, administered in either once daily or twice daily dosing regimens, was added to the therapy of patients who were inadequately controlled on a maximum dose (2.5 grams/day) of metformin.

In one study, patients inadequately controlled on 2.5 grams/day of metformin (mean baseline FPG 216 mg/dL and mean baseline HbA1c 8.8%) were randomized to receive *Avandia* 4 mg once daily, *Avandia* 8 mg once daily, or placebo in addition to metformin. A statistically significant improvement in FPG and HbA1c was observed in patients treated with the combinations of metformin and *Avandia* 4 mg once daily and *Avandia* 8 mg once daily, versus patients continued on metformin alone (Table 4).

Table 4. Glycemic Parameters in a 26-Week Combination Study

	Metformin	Avandia 4 mg once daily + metformin	Avandia 8 mg once daily + metformin
N	113	116	110
FPG (mg/dL)			
Baseline (mean)	214	215	220
Change from baseline (mean)	6	−33	−48
Difference from metformin alone (adjusted mean)		−40*	−53*
Responders (≥30 mg/dL decrease from baseline)	20%	45%	61%
HbA1c (%)			
Baseline (mean)	8.6	8.9	8.9
Change from baseline (mean)	0.5	−0.6	−0.8
Difference from metformin alone (adjusted mean)		−1.0*	−1.2*
Responders (≥0.7% decrease from baseline)	11%	45%	52%

*<0.0001 compared to metformin.

In a second 26-week study, patients with type 2 diabetes inadequately controlled on 2.5 grams/day of metformin who were randomized to receive the combination of *Avandia* 4 mg twice daily and metformin (N=105) showed a statistically significant improvement in glycemic control with a mean treatment effect for FPG of −56 mg/dL and a mean treatment effect for HbA1c of −0.8% over metformin alone. The combination of metformin and *Avandia* resulted in lower levels of FPG and HbA1c than either agent alone.

Patients who were inadequately controlled on a maximum dose (2.5 grams/day) of metformin and who were switched to monotherapy with Avandia (rosiglitazone maleate) demonstrated loss of glycemic control, as evidenced by increases in FPG and HbA1c. In this group, increases in LDL and VLDL were also seen.

Combination with a Sulfonylurea
A total of 1216 patients with type 2 diabetes participated in three 26-week randomized, double-blind, placebo/active-controlled studies designed to assess the efficacy and safety of *Avandia* in combination with a sulfonylurea. *Avandia* 2 mg or 4 mg daily, was administered either once daily or in divided doses twice daily, to patients inadequately controlled on a sulfonylurea.

In the two placebo-controlled studies, patients inadequately controlled on sulfonylureas that were randomized to single dose or divided doses of *Avandia* 4 mg daily plus a sulfonylurea showed significantly reduced FPG and HbA1c compared to sulfonylurea plus placebo (Table 5).

Table 5. Glycemic Parameters in Two 26-Week Combination Studies

Study C (patients on prior sulfonylurea monotherapy)	Sulfonylurea	Avandia 2 mg twice daily + sulfonylurea
N	192	183
FPG (mg/dL)		
Baseline (mean)	207	205
Change from baseline (mean)	+6	−38
Difference from sulfonylurea alone (adjusted mean)	–	−44*
Responders (≥30 mg/dL) decrease from baseline)	21%	56%
HbA1c (%)		
Baseline (mean)	9.2	9.2
Change from baseline (mean)	+0.2	−0.9
Difference from sulfonylurea alone (adjusted mean)	–	−1.0*

Study D (patients on prior single or multiple therapies)	Sulfonylurea	Avandia 4 mg once daily + sulfonylurea
N	115	116
FPG (mg/dL)		
Baseline (mean)	209	214
Change from baseline (mean)	+23	−25
Difference from sulfonylurea alone (adjusted mean)	–	−47*
Responders (≥30 mg/dL) decrease from baseline)	13%	46%
HbA1c (%)		
Baseline (mean)	8.9	9.1
Change from baseline (mean)	+0.6	−0.3
Difference from sulfonylurea alone (adjusted mean)	–	−0.9*

*≤0.0001 compared to sulfonylurea plus placebo.

In the third study, including patients on prior single or multiple therapies, in patients inadequately controlled on the maximal dose of glyburide (20 mg daily), *Avandia* 2 mg twice daily plus sulfonylurea significantly reduced FPG (n=98, mean change from baseline of −31 mg/dL) and HbA1c (mean change from baseline of −0.5%) compared to sulfonylurea plus placebo (n=99, mean change from baseline of FPG of +24 mg/dL and of HbA1c of +0.9%). The combination of sulfonylurea and *Avandia* resulted in lower levels of FPG and HbA1c than either agent alone. Patients who were switched from maximal dose of glyburide to 2 mg twice daily *Avandia* monotherapy demonstrated loss of glycemic control, as evidenced by increases in FPG and HbA1c.

INDICATIONS AND USAGE
Avandia is indicated as an adjunct to diet and exercise to improve glycemic control in patients with type 2 diabetes mellitus. *Avandia* is indicated as monotherapy. *Avandia* is also indicated for use in combination with a sulfonylurea or metformin when diet, exercise and a single agent do not result in adequate glycemic control. For patients inadequately controlled with a maximum dose of a sulfonylurea or metformin, *Avandia* should be added to, rather than substituted for, a sulfonylurea or metformin.

Management of type 2 diabetes should include diet control. Caloric restriction, weight loss, and exercise are essential for the proper treatment of the diabetic patient because they help improve insulin sensitivity. This is important not only in the primary treatment of type 2 diabetes, but also in maintaining the efficacy of drug therapy. Prior to initiation of therapy with Avandia (rosiglitazone maleate), secondary causes of poor glycemic control, e.g., infection, should be investigated and treated.

CONTRAINDICATIONS
Avandia is contraindicated in patients with known hypersensitivity to this product or any of its components.

WARNINGS
Cardiac Failure and Other Cardiac Effects: *Avandia*, like other thiazolidinediones, alone or in combination with other antidiabetic agents, can cause fluid retention, which may ex-

acerbate or lead to heart failure. Patients should be observed for signs and symptoms of heart failure. *Avandia* should be discontinued if any deterioration in cardiac status occurs.
Patients with New York Heart Association (NYHA) Class 3 and 4 cardiac status were not studied during the clinical trials. *Avandia* is not recommended in patients with NYHA Class 3 and 4 cardiac status.
In two 26-week U.S. trials involving 611 patients with type 2 diabetes, *Avandia* plus insulin therapy was compared with insulin therapy alone. These trials included patients with long-standing diabetes and a high prevalence of pre-existing medical conditions, including peripheral neuropathy (34%), retinopathy (19%), ischemic heart disease (14%), vascular disease (9%), and congestive heart failure (2.5%). In these clinical studies an increased incidence of cardiac failure and other cardiovascular adverse events were seen in patients on *Avandia* and insulin combination therapy compared to insulin and placebo. Patients who experienced heart failure were on average older, had a longer duration of diabetes, and were mostly on the higher 8 mg daily dose of *Avandia*. In this population, however, it was not possible to determine specific risk factors that could be used to identify all patients at risk of heart failure on combination therapy. Three of 10 patients who developed cardiac failure on combination therapy during the double blind part of the studies had no known prior evidence of congestive heart failure, or pre-existing cardiac condition. **The use of Avandia (rosiglitazone maleate) in combination therapy with insulin is not indicated (see ADVERSE REACTIONS).**

PRECAUTIONS

General

Due to its mechanism of action, *Avandia* is active only in the presence of endogenous insulin. Therefore, *Avandia* should not be used in patients with type 1 diabetes or for the treatment of diabetic ketoacidosis.

Hypoglycemia: Patients receiving *Avandia* in combination with other hypoglycemic agents may be at risk for hypoglycemia, and a reduction in the dose of the concomitant agent may be necessary.

Edema: *Avandia* should be used with caution in patients with edema. In a clinical study in healthy volunteers who received *Avandia* 8 mg once daily for 8 weeks, there was a statistically significant increase in median plasma volume compared to placebo.
Since thiazolidinediones, including rosiglitazone, can cause fluid retention, which can exacerbate or lead to congestive heart failure, *Avandia* should be used with caution in patients at risk for heart failure. Patients should be monitored for signs and symptoms of heart failure (see WARNINGS, Cardiac Failure and Other Cardiac Effects and PRECAUTIONS, Information for Patients).
In controlled clinical trials of patients with type 2 diabetes, mild to moderate edema was reported in patients treated with *Avandia*, and may be dose related. Patients with ongoing edema are more likely to have adverse events associated with edema if started on combination therapy with insulin and *Avandia* (see ADVERSE REACTIONS).

Weight Gain: Dose-related weight gain was seen with *Avandia* alone and in combination with other hypoglycemic agents (Table 6). The mechanism of weight gain is unclear but probably involves a combination of fluid retention and fat accumulation.
[See table above]

Table 6. Weight Changes (kg) from Baseline During Clinical Trials with *Avandia*

Monotherapy	Duration	Control Group		*Avandia* 4 mg	*Avandia* 8 mg
			Median (25th, 75th percentile)	Median (25th, 75th percentile)	Median (25th, 75th percentile)
	26 weeks	placebo	–0.9 (–2.8, 0.9)	1.0 (–0.9, 3.6)	3.1 (1.1, 5.8)
	52 weeks	sulfonylurea	2.0 (0, 4.0)	2.0 (–0.6, 4.0)	2.6 (0, 5.3)
Combination therapy					
sulfonylurea	26 weeks	sulfonylurea	0 (–1.3, 1.2)	1.8 (0, 3.1)	—
metformin	26 weeks	metformin	–1.4 (–3.2, 0.2)	0.8 (–1.0, 2.6)	2.1 (0, 4.3)
insulin	26 weeks	insulin	0.9 (–0.5, 2.7)	4.1 (1.4, 6.3)	5.4 (3.4, 7.3)

Hematologic: Across all controlled clinical studies, decreases in hemoglobin and hematocrit (mean decreases in individual studies ≤1.0 gram/dL and ≤3.3%, respectively) were observed for *Avandia* alone and in combination with other hypoglycemic agents. The changes occurred primarily during the first 3 months following initiation of *Avandia* therapy or following an increase in *Avandia* dose. White blood cell counts also decreased slightly in patients treated with *Avandia*. The observed changes may be related to the increased plasma volume observed with treatment with *Avandia* and may be dose related (see ADVERSE REACTIONS, Laboratory Abnormalities).

Ovulation: Therapy with *Avandia*, like other thiazolidinediones, may result in ovulation in some premenopausal anovulatory women. As a result, these patients may be at an increased risk for pregnancy while taking *Avandia* (see PRECAUTIONS, Pregnancy, Pregnancy Category C). Thus, adequate contraception in premenopausal women should be recommended. This possible effect has not been specifically investigated in clinical studies so the frequency of this occurrence is not known.
Although hormonal imbalance has been seen in preclinical studies (see PRECAUTIONS, Carcinogenesis, Mutagenesis, Impairment of Fertility), the clinical significance of this finding is not known. If unexpected menstrual dysfunction occurs, the benefits of continued therapy with *Avandia* should be reviewed.

Hepatic Effects: Another drug of the thiazolidinedione class, troglitazone, was associated with idiosyncratic hepatotoxicity, and very rare cases of liver failure, liver transplants, and death were reported during clinical use. In pre-approval controlled clinical trials in patients with type 2 diabetes, troglitazone was more frequently associated with clinically significant elevations in liver enzymes (ALT>3X upper limit of normal) compared to placebo. Very rare cases of reversible jaundice were also reported.
In pre-approval clinical studies in 4598 patients treated with *Avandia*, encompassing approximately 3600 patient years of exposure, there was no signal of drug-induced hepatotoxicity or elevation of ALT levels. In the pre-approval controlled trials, 0.2% of patients treated with *Avandia* had elevations in ALT >3X the upper limit of normal compared to 0.2% on placebo and 0.5% on active comparators. The ALT elevations in patients treated with *Avandia* were reversible and were not clearly causally related to therapy with Avandia (rosiglitazone maleate).
In postmarketing experience with *Avandia*, reports of hepatitis and of hepatic enzyme elevations to three or more times the upper limit of normal have been received. Very rarely, these reports have involved hepatic failure with and without fatal outcome, although causality has not been established. Rosiglitazone is structurally related to troglitazone, a thiazolidinedione no longer marketed in the United States, which was associated with idiosyncratic hepatotoxicity and rare cases of liver failure, liver transplants, and death during clinical use. Pending the availability of the results of additional large, long-term controlled clinical trials and additional postmarketing safety data, it is recommended that patients treated with *Avandia* undergo periodic monitoring of liver enzymes.
Liver enzymes should be checked prior to the initiation of therapy with *Avandia* in all patients. Therapy with *Avandia* should not be initiated in patients with increased baseline liver enzyme levels (ALT>2.5X upper limit of normal). In patients with normal baseline liver enzymes, following initiation of therapy with *Avandia*, it is recommended that liver enzymes be monitored every 2 months for the first 12 months, and periodically thereafter. Patients with mildly elevated liver enzymes (ALT levels ≤2.5X upper limit of normal) at baseline or during therapy with *Avandia* should be evaluated to determine the cause of the liver enzyme elevation. Initiation of, or continuation of, therapy with *Avandia* in patients with mild liver enzyme elevations should proceed with caution and include close clinical follow-up, including more frequent liver enzyme monitoring, to determine if the liver enzyme elevations resolve or worsen. If at any time ALT levels increase to >3X the upper limit of normal in patients on therapy with *Avandia*, liver enzyme levels should be rechecked as soon as possible. If ALT levels remain >3X the upper limit of normal, therapy with *Avandia* should be discontinued.
There are no data available from clinical trials to evaluate the safety of *Avandia* in patients who experienced liver abnormalities, hepatic dysfunction, or jaundice while on troglitazone. Avandia (rosiglitazone maleate) should not be used in patients who experienced jaundice while taking troglitazone.
If any patient develops symptoms suggesting hepatic dysfunction, which may include unexplained nausea, vomiting, abdominal pain, fatigue, anorexia and/or dark urine, liver enzymes should be checked. The decision whether to continue the patient on therapy with *Avandia* should be guided by clinical judgment pending laboratory evaluations. If jaundice is observed, drug therapy should be discontinued.

Laboratory Tests

Periodic fasting blood glucose and HbA1c measurements should be performed to monitor therapeutic response.
Liver enzyme monitoring is recommended prior to initiation of therapy with *Avandia* in all patients and periodically thereafter (see PRECAUTIONS, *Hepatic Effects* and ADVERSE REACTIONS, Serum Transaminase Levels).

Information for Patients

Patients should be informed of the following:
Management of type 2 diabetes should include diet control. Caloric restriction, weight loss, and exercise are essential for the proper treatment of the diabetic patient because they help improve insulin sensitivity. This is important not only in the primary treatment of type 2 diabetes, but in maintaining the efficacy of drug therapy.
It is important to adhere to dietary instructions and to regularly have blood glucose and glycosylated hemoglobin tested. Patients should be advised that it can take 2 weeks to see a reduction in blood glucose and 2 to 3 months to see full effect. Patients should be informed that blood will be drawn to check their liver function prior to the start of therapy and every 2 months for the first 12 months, and periodically thereafter. Patients with unexplained symptoms of nausea, vomiting, abdominal pain, fatigue, anorexia, or dark urine should immediately report these symptoms to their physician. Patients who experience an unusually rapid increase in weight or edema or who develop shortness of breath or other symptoms of heart failure while on *Avandia* should immediately report these symptoms to their physician.
Avandia can be taken with or without meals.
When using *Avandia* in combination with other hypoglycemic agents, the risk of hypoglycemia, its symptoms and treatment, and conditions that predispose to its development should be explained to patients and their family members.
Therapy with *Avandia*, like other thiazolidinediones, may result in ovulation in some premenopausal anovulatory women. As a result, these patients may be at an increased risk for pregnancy while taking *Avandia* (see PRECAUTIONS, Pregnancy, Pregnancy Category C). Thus, adequate contraception in premenopausal women should be recommended. This possible effect has not been specifically investigated in clinical studies so the frequency of this occurrence is not known.

Drug Interactions

Drugs Metabolized by Cytochrome P_{450}

In vitro drug metabolism studies suggest that rosiglitazone does not inhibit any of the major P_{450} enzymes at clinically relevant concentrations. *In vitro* data demonstrate that rosiglitazone is predominantly metabolized by CYP2C8, and to a lesser extent, 2C9.
Avandia (4 mg twice daily) was shown to have no clinically relevant effect on the pharmacokinetics of nifedipine and oral contraceptives (ethinylestradiol and norethindrone), which are predominantly metabolized by CYP3A4.
Glyburide: Avandia (2 mg twice daily) taken concomitantly with glyburide (3.75 to 10 mg/day) for 7 days did not alter the mean steady-state 24-hour plasma glucose concentrations in diabetic patients stabilized on glyburide therapy.
Metformin: Concurrent administration of *Avandia* (2 mg twice daily) and metformin (500 mg twice daily) in healthy volunteers for 4 days had no effect on the steady-state pharmacokinetics of either metformin or rosiglitazone.
Acarbose: Coadministration of acarbose (100 mg three times daily) for 7 days in healthy volunteers had no clinically relevant effect on the pharmacokinetics of a single oral dose of *Avandia*.
Digoxin: Repeat oral dosing of *Avandia* (8 mg once daily) for 14 days did not alter the steady-state pharmacokinetics of digoxin (0.375 mg once daily) in healthy volunteers.
Warfarin: Repeat dosing with *Avandia* had no clinically relevant effect on the steady-state pharmacokinetics of warfarin enantiomers.
Ethanol: A single administration of a moderate amount of alcohol did not increase the risk of acute hypoglycemia in type 2 diabetes mellitus patients treated with Avandia (rosiglitazone maleate).
Ranitidine: Pretreatment with ranitidine (150 mg twice daily for 4 days) did not alter the pharmacokinetics of either single oral or intravenous doses of rosiglitazone in healthy volunteers. These results suggest that the absorption of oral rosiglitazone is not altered in conditions accompanied by increases in gastrointestinal pH.

Carcinogenesis, Mutagenesis, Impairment of Fertility

Carcinogenesis: A 2-year carcinogenicity study was conducted in Charles River CD-1 mice at doses of 0.4, 1.5, and 6 mg/kg/day in the diet (highest dose equivalent to approximately 12 times human AUC at the maximum recommended human daily dose). Sprague-Dawley rats were dosed for 2 years by oral gavage at doses of 0.05, 0.3, and 2 mg/kg/day (highest dose equivalent to approximately 10 and 20 times human AUC at the maximum recommended human daily dose for male and female rats, respectively).
Rosiglitazone was not carcinogenic in the mouse. There was an increase in incidence of adipose hyperplasia in the mouse at doses ≥1.5 mg/kg/day (approximately 2 times human AUC at the maximum recommended human daily dose). In rats, there was a significant increase in the incidence of benign adipose tissue tumors (lipomas) at doses ≥0.3 mg/kg/day (approximately 2 times human AUC at the maximum recommended human daily dose). These proliferative changes in both species are considered due to the persistent pharmacological overstimulation of adipose tissue.

Continued on next page

Information on the SmithKline Beecham Pharmaceuticals products appearing here is based on the labeling in effect on May 15, 2001. Further information on these and other products may be obtained from the Medical Department, SmithKline Beecham Pharmaceuticals, One Franklin Plaza, Philadelphia, PA 19101.

Avandia—Cont.

Mutagenesis: Rosiglitazone was not mutagenic or clastogenic in the *in vitro* bacterial assays for gene mutation, the *in vitro* chromosome aberration test in human lymphocytes, the *in vivo* mouse micronucleus test, and the *iv vivo/in vitro* rat UDS assay. There was a small (about 2-fold) increase in mutation in the *in vitro* mouse lymphoma assay in the presence of metabolic activation.

Impairment of Fertility: Rosiglitazone had no effects on mating or fertility of male rats given up to 40 mg/kg/day (approximately 116 times human AUC at the maximum recommended human daily dose). Rosiglitazone altered estrous cyclicity (2 mg/kg/day) and reduced fertility (40 mg/kg/day) of female rats in association with lower plasma levels of progesterone and estradiol (approximately 20 and 200 times human AUC at the maximum recommended human daily dose, respectively). No such effects were noted at 0.2 mg/kg/day (approximately 3 times human AUC at the maximum recommended human daily dose). In monkeys, rosiglitazone (0.6 and 4.6 mg/kg/day; approximately 3 and 15 times human AUC at the maximum recommended human daily dose, respectively) diminished the follicular phase rise in serum estradiol with consequential reduction in the luteinizing hormone surge, lower luteal phase progesterone levels, and amenorrhea. The mechanism for these effects appears to be direct inhibition of ovarian steroidogenesis.

Animal Toxicology

Heart weights were increased in mice (3 mg/kg/day), rats (5 mg/kg/day), and dogs (2 mg/kg/day) with rosiglitazone treatments (approximately 5, 22, and 2 times human AUC at the maximum recommended human daily dose, respectively). Morphometric measurement indicated that there was hypertrophy in cardiac ventricular tissues, which may be due to increased heart work as a result of plasma volume expansion.

Pregnancy

Pregnancy Category C

There was no effect on implantation or the embryo with rosiglitazone treatment during early pregnancy in rats, but treatment during mid-late gestation was associated with fetal death and growth retardation in both rats and rabbits. Teratogenicity was not observed at doses up to 3 mg/kg in rats and 100 mg/kg in rabbits (approximately 20 and 75 times human AUC at the maximum recommended human daily dose, respectively). Rosiglitazone caused placental pathology in rats (3 mg/kg/day). Treatment of rats during gestation through lactation reduced litter size, neonatal viability, and postnatal growth, with growth retardation reversible after puberty. For effects on the placenta, embryo/fetus, and offspring, the no-effect dose was 0.2 mg/kg/day in rats and 15 mg/kg/day in rabbits. These no-effect levels are approximately 4 times human AUC at the maximum recommended human daily dose.

There are no adequate and well-controlled studies in pregnant women. Avandia (rosiglitazone maleate) should not be used during pregnancy unless the potential benefit justifies the potential risk to the fetus.

Because current information strongly suggests that abnormal blood glucose levels during pregnancy are associated with a higher incidence of congenital anomalies as well as increased neonatal morbidity and mortality, most experts recommend that insulin monotherapy be used during pregnancy to maintain blood glucose levels as close to normal as possible.

Labor and Delivery

The effect of rosiglitazone on labor and delivery in humans is not known.

Nursing Mothers

Drug-related material was detected in milk from lactating rats. It is not known whether *Avandia* is excreted in human milk. Because many drugs are excreted in human milk, *Avandia* should not be administered to a nursing woman.

ADVERSE REACTIONS

In clinical trials, approximately 4600 patients with type 2 diabetes have been treated with *Avandia*; 3300 patients were treated for 6 months or longer and 2000 patients were treated for 12 months or longer.

Trials of *Avandia* as Monotherapy and in Combination with Other Hypoglycemic Agents

The incidence and types of adverse events reported in clinical trials of *Avandia* as monotherapy are shown in Table 7. [See table below]

There were a small number of patients treated with *Avandia* who had adverse events of anemia and edema. Overall, these events were generally mild to moderate in severity and usually did not require discontinuation of treatment with Avandia (rosiglitazone maleate).

In double-blind studies, anemia was reported in 1.9% of patients receiving *Avandia* compared to 0.7% on placebo, 0.6% on sulfonylureas and 2.2% on metformin. Edema was reported in 4.8% of patients receiving *Avandia* compared to 1.3% on placebo, 1.0% on sulfonylureas, and 2.2% on metformin. Overall, the types of adverse experiences reported when *Avandia* was used in combination with a sulfonylurea or metformin were similar to those during monotherapy with *Avandia*. Reports of anemia (7.1%) were greater in patients treated with a combination of *Avandia* and metformin compared to monotherapy with *Avandia* or in combination with a sulfonylurea.

Lower pre-treatment hemoglobin/hematocrit levels in patients enrolled in the metformin combination clinical trials may have contributed to the higher reporting rate of anemia in these studies (see ADVERSE REACTIONS, Laboratory Abnormalities, Hematologic).

In 26-week double-blind studies, edema was reported with higher frequency in the *Avandia* plus insulin combination trials (insulin, 5.4%; and *Avandia* in combination with insulin, 14.7%). Reports of new onset or exacerbation of congestive heart failure occurred at rates of 1% for insulin alone, and 2% (4 mg) and 3% (8 mg) for insulin in combination with *Avandia* (see WARNINGS, Cardiac Failure and Other Cardiac Effects).

In postmarketing experience with *Avandia*, adverse events potentially related to volume expansion (e.g., congestive heart failure, pulmonary edema, and pleural effusions) have been reported.

Laboratory Abnormalities

Hematologic: Decreases in mean hemoglobin and hematocrit occurred in a dose-related fashion in patients treated with *Avandia* (mean decreases in individual studies up to 1.0 gram/dL hemoglobin and up to 3.3% hematocrit). The time course and magnitude of decreases were similar in patients treated with a combination of *Avandia* and other hypoglycemic agents or *Avandia* monotherapy. Pre-treatment levels of hemoglobin and hematocrit were lower in patients in metformin combination studies and may have contributed to the higher reporting rate of anemia. White blood cell counts also decreased slightly in patients treated with *Avandia*. Decreases in hematologic parameters may be related to increased plasma volume observed with treatment with *Avandia*.

Lipids: Changes in serum lipids have been observed following treatment with *Avandia* (see CLINICAL STUDIES).

Serum Transaminase Levels: In clinical studies in 4598 patients treated with Avandia (rosiglitazone maleate) encompassing approximately 3600 patient years of exposure, there was no evidence of drug-induced hepatotoxicity or elevated ALT levels.

In controlled trials, 0.2% of patients treated with *Avandia* had reversible elevations in ALT >3X the upper limit of normal compared to 0.2% on placebo and 0.5% on active comparators. Hyperbilirubinemia was found in 0.3% of patients treated with *Avandia* compared with 0.9% treated with placebo and 1% in patients treated with active comparators.

In the clinical program including long-term, open-label experience, the rate per 100 patient years exposure of ALT increase to >3X the upper limit of normal was 0.35 for patients treated with *Avandia*, 0.59 for placebo-treated patients, and 0.78 for patients treated with active comparator agents.

In pre-approval clinical trials, there were no cases of idiosyncratic drug reactions leading to hepatic failure. In postmarketing experience with Avandia (rosiglitazone maleate), reports of hepatic enzyme elevations three or more times the upper limit of normal and hepatitis have been received (see PRECAUTIONS, *Hepatic Effects*).

DOSAGE AND ADMINISTRATION

The management of antidiabetic therapy should be individualized. *Avandia* may be administered either at a starting dose of 4 mg as a single daily dose or divided and administered in the morning and evening. For patients who respond inadequately following 8 to 12 weeks of treatment, as determined by reduction in FPG, the dose may be increased to 8 mg daily as indicated below. Reductions in glycemic parameters by dose and regimen are described under CLINICAL STUDIES. *Avandia* may be taken with or without food.

Monotherapy

The usual starting dose of *Avandia* is 4 mg administered either as a single dose once daily or in divided doses twice daily. In clinical trials, the 4 mg twice daily regimen resulted in the greatest reduction in FPG and HbA1c.

Combination Therapy with a Sulfonylurea or Metformin

When *Avandia* is added to existing therapy, the current dose of sulfonylurea or metformin can be continued upon initiation of *Avandia* therapy.

Sulfonylurea:

When used in combination with sulfonylurea, the recommended dose of *Avandia* is 4 mg administered as either a single dose once daily or in divided doses twice daily. If patients report hypoglycemia, the dose of the sulfonylurea should be decreased.

Metformin:

The usual starting dose of *Avandia* in combination with metformin is 4 mg administered as either a single dose once daily or in divided doses twice daily. It is unlikely that the dose of metformin will require adjustment due to hypoglycemia during combination therapy with *Avandia*.

Maximum Recommended Dose:

The dose of *Avandia* should not exceed 8 mg daily, as a single dose or divided twice daily. The 8 mg daily dose has been shown to be safe and effective in clinical studies as monotherapy and in combination with metformin. Doses of *Avandia* greater than 4 mg daily in combination with a sulfonylurea have not been studied in adequate and well-controlled clinical trials.

Avandia may be taken with or without food.

No dosage adjustments are required for the elderly.

No dosage adjustment is necessary when *Avandia* is used as monotherapy in patients with renal impairment. Since metformin is contraindicated in such patients, concomitant administration of metformin and *Avandia* is also contraindicated in patients with renal impairment.

Therapy with *Avandia* should not be initiated if the patient exhibits clinical evidence of active liver disease or increased serum transaminase levels (ALT >2.5X upper limit of normal at start of therapy) (see PRECAUTIONS, *Hepatic Effects* and CLINICAL PHARMACOLOGY, Hepatic Impairment). Liver enzyme monitoring is recommended in all patients prior to initiation of therapy with *Avandia* and periodically thereafter (see PRECAUTIONS, *Hepatic Effects*).

There are no data on the use of *Avandia* in patients under 18 years of age; therefore, use of *Avandia* in pediatric patients is not recommended.

OVERDOSAGE

Limited data are available with regard to overdosage in humans. In clinical studies in volunteers, Avandia (rosiglitazone maleate) has been administered at single oral doses of up to 20 mg and was well-tolerated. In the event of an overdose, appropriate supportive treatment should be initiated as dictated by the patient's clinical status.

HOW SUPPLIED

Tablets: Each pentagonal film-coated Tiltab® tablet contains rosiglitazone as the maleate as follows: 2 mg-pink, debossed with SB on one side and 2 on the other; 4 mg-orange, debossed with SB on one side and 4 on the other; 8 mg-red-brown, debossed with SB on one side and 8 on the other.

2 mg bottles of 30: NDC 0029-3158-13
2 mg bottles of 60: NDC 0029-3158-18
2 mg bottles of 100: NDC 0029-3158-20
2 mg bottles of 500: NDC 0029-3158-25
2 mg SUP 100s: NDC 0029-3158-21
4 mg bottles of 30: NDC 0029-3159-13
4 mg bottles of 60: NDC 0029-3159-18
4 mg bottles of 100: NDC 0029-3159-20
4 mg bottles of 500: NDC 0029-3159-25
4 mg SUP 100s: NDC 0029-3159-21
8 mg bottles of 30: NDC 0029-3160-13
8 mg bottles of 100: NDC 0029-3160-20
8 mg bottles of 500: NDC 0029-3160-25
8 mg SUP 100s: NDC 0029-3160-21

STORAGE

Store at 25°C (77°F); excursions 15°–30°C (59°–86°F). Dispense in a tight, light-resistant container.

DATE OF ISSUANCE FEB. 2001

 ℞ only

SmithKline Beecham Pharmaceuticals
Philadelphia, PA 19101
AV:L6

Table 7. Adverse Events (≥5% in Any Treatment Group) Reported by Patients in Double-blind Clinical Trials with *Avandia* as Monotherapy

	Avandia Monotherapy N = 2526	Placebo N = 601	Metformin N = 225	Sulfonylureas* N = 626
Preferred Term	%	%	%	%
Upper respiratory tract infection	9.9	8.7	8.9	7.3
Injury	7.6	4.3	7.6	6.1
Headache	5.9	5.0	8.9	5.4
Back pain	4.0	3.8	4.0	5.0
Hyperglycemia	3.9	5.7	4.4	8.1
Fatigue	3.6	5.0	4.0	1.9
Sinusitis	3.2	4.5	5.3	3.0
Diarrhea	2.3	3.3	15.6	3.0
Hypoglycemia	0.6	0.2	1.3	5.9

*Includes patients receiving glyburide (N=514), gliclazide (N=91) or glipizide (N=21).

ENGERIX-B® ℞

[en 'jur-ix bee]

Hepatitis B Vaccine (Recombinant)

Prescribing information for this product, which appears on pages 3087–3090 of the 2001 PDR, has been completely revised as follows. Please write "See Supplement A" next to the product heading.

DESCRIPTION

Engerix-B [Hepatitis B Vaccine (Recombinant)] is a noninfectious recombinant DNA hepatitis B vaccine developed and manufactured by SmithKline Beecham Biologicals. It contains purified surface antigen of the virus obtained by culturing genetically engineered *Saccharomyces cerevisiae* cells, which carry the surface antigen gene of the hepatitis B virus. The surface antigen expressed in *Saccharomyces cerevisiae* cells is purified by several physicochemical steps and formulated as a suspension of the antigen adsorbed on aluminum hydroxide. The procedures used to manufacture *Engerix-B* result in a product that contains no more than 5% yeast protein. No substances of human origin are used in its manufacture.

Engerix-B is supplied as a sterile suspension for intramuscular administration. The vaccine is ready for use without reconstitution; it must be shaken before administration since a fine white deposit with a clear colorless supernatant may form on storage.

Pediatric/Adolescent

Each 0.5 mL of vaccine consists of 10 mcg of hepatitis B surface antigen adsorbed on 0.25 mg aluminum as aluminum hydroxide. The pediatric/adolescent vaccine is formulated without preservatives. The pediatric formulation contains a trace amount of thimerosal (<0.5 mcg mercury) from the manufacturing process, sodium chloride (9 mg/mL) and phosphate buffers (disodium phosphate dihydrate, 0.98 mg/mL; sodium dihydrogen phosphate dihydrate, 0.71 mg/mL).

Adult

Each 1 mL adult dose consists of 20 mcg of hepatitis B surface antigen adsorbed on 0.5 mg aluminum as aluminum hydroxide. The adult vaccine is formulated without preservatives. The adult formulation contains a trace amount of thimerosal (<1.0 mcg mercury) from the manufacturing process, sodium chloride (9 mg/mL) and phosphate buffers (disodium phosphate dihydrate, 0.98 mg/mL; sodium dihydrogen phosphate dihydrate, 0.71 mg/mL).

CLINICAL PHARMACOLOGY

Several hepatitis viruses are known to cause a systemic infection resulting in major pathologic changes in the liver (e.g., A,B,C,D,E,G). The estimated lifetime risk of HBV infection in the United States varies from almost 100% for the highest-risk groups to less than 20% for the population as a whole.[1] Hepatitis B infection can have serious consequences including acute massive hepatic necrosis, chronic active hepatitis and cirrhosis of the liver. Up to 90% of neonates and 6 to 10% of adults who are infected in the United States will become hepatitis B virus carriers.[1] It has been estimated that 200 to 300 million people in the world today are persistently infected with hepatitis B virus.[1] The Centers for Disease Control (CDC) estimates that there are approximately 1 to 1.25 million chronic carriers of hepatitis B virus in the United States.[1] Those patients who become chronic carriers can infect others and are at increased risk of developing primary hepatocellular carcinoma. Among other factors, infection with hepatitis B may be the single most important factor for development of this carcinoma.[1,2]

Reduced Risk of Hepatocellular Carcinoma: According to the CDC, the hepatitis B vaccine is recognized as the first anti-cancer vaccine because it can prevent primary liver cancer.[3]

A clear link has been demonstrated between chronic hepatitis B infection and the occurrence of hepatocellular carcinoma. In a Taiwanese study, the institution of universal childhood immunization against hepatitis B virus has been shown to decrease the incidence of hepatocellular carcinoma among children.[4] In a Korean study in adult males, vaccination against hepatitis B virus has been shown to decrease the incidence of, and risk of, developing hepatocellular carcinoma in adults.[5]

Considering the serious consequences of infection, immunization should be considered for all persons at potential risk of exposure to the hepatitis B virus. Mothers infected with hepatitis B virus can infect their infants at, or shortly after, birth if they are carriers of the HBsAg antigen or develop an active infection during the third trimester of pregnancy. Infected infants usually become chronic carriers. Therefore, screening of pregnant women for hepatitis B is recommended.[1] Because a vaccination strategy limited to high-risk individuals has failed to substantially lower the overall incidence of hepatitis B infection, the Advisory Committee on Immunization Practices (ACIP) recommends vaccination of all persons from birth to age 18.[6] The Committee on Infectious Diseases of the American Academy of Pediatrics (AAP) has also endorsed universal infant immunization as part of a comprehensive strategy for the control of hepatitis B infection.[7] The AAP, American Academy of Family Physicians (AAFP) and American Medical Association (AMA) also recommend routine vaccination of adolescents 11 to 12 years of age who have not been vaccinated previously.[8] The AAP further recommends that providers administer hepatitis B vaccine to all previously unvaccinated adolescents.[9] (See INDICATIONS AND USAGE.) There is no specific treatment for acute hepatitis B infection. However, those who develop anti-HBs antibodies after active infection are usually protected against subsequent infection. Antibody titers ≥10 mIU/mL against HBsAg are recognized as conferring protection against hepatitis B.[1] Seroconversion is defined as antibody titers ≥1 mIU/mL.

Protective Efficacy: Protective efficacy with Engerix-B [Hepatitis B Vaccine (Recombinant)] has been demonstrated in a clinical trial in neonates at high risk of hepatitis B infection.[10,11] Fifty-eight neonates born of mothers who were both HBsAg and HBeAg positive were given *Engerix-B* (10 mcg at 0, 1 and 2 months) without concomitant hepatitis B immune globulin. Two infants became chronic carriers in the 12-month follow-up period after initial inoculation. Assuming an expected carrier rate of 70%, the protective efficacy rate against the chronic carrier state during the first 12 months of life was 95%.

Immunogenicity in Neonates: Immunization with 10 mcg at 0, 1 and 6 months of age produced seroconversion in 100% of infants by month 7 with a GMT of 713 mIU/mL (N=52), and the seroprotection rate was 97%.

Clinical trials indicate that administration of hepatitis B immune globulin at birth does not alter the response to Engerix-B [Hepatitis B Vaccine (Recombinant)].

Immunization with 10 mcg at 0, 1 and 2 months of age produced a seroprotection rate of 96% in infants by month 4, with a GMT among seroconverters of 210 mIU/mL (N=311); an additional dose at month 12 produced a GMT among seroconverters of 2,941 mIU/mL at month 13 (N=126).

Immunogenicity in Pediatric Patients: In clinical trials with 242 children ages 6 months to, and including, 10 years given 10 mcg at months 0, 1 and 6, the seroprotection rate was 98% 1 to 2 months after the third dose; the GMT of seroconverters was 4,023 mIU/mL.

In a separate clinical trial including both children and adolescents aged 5 to 16 years, 10 mcg of *Engerix-B* was administered at 0, 1, and 6 months (N=181) or 0, 12, and 24 months (N=161). Immediately before the third dose of vaccine, seroprotection was achieved in 92.3% of subjects vaccinated on the 0, 1, 6-month schedule and 88.8% of subjects on the 0, 12, 24-month schedule (117.9 mIU/mL vs. 162.1 mIU/mL, respectively, p=0.18). One month following the third dose, seroprotection was achieved in 99.5% of children vaccinated on the 0, 1, 6-month schedule compared to 98.1% of those on the 0, 12, 24-month schedule. GMTs were higher (p=0.02) for children receiving vaccine on the 0, 1, 6-month schedule compared to those on the 0, 12, 24-month schedule (5,687.4 mIU/mL vs. 3,158.7 mIU/mL, respectively). The clinical relevance of this finding is unknown.

Immunogenicity in Adolescents: In clinical trials with healthy adolescent subjects 11 through 19 years of age, immunization with 10 mcg using a 0, 1, 6-month schedule produced a seroprotection rate of 97% at month 8 (N=119) with a GMT of 1,989 mIU/mL (N=118, 95% confidence intervals=1,318–3,020). Immunization with 20 mcg using a 0, 1, 6-month schedule produced a seroprotection rate of 99% at month 8 (N=122) with a GMT of 7,672 mIU/mL (N=122, 95% confidence intervals=5,248–10,965).

Immunogenicity in Healthy Adults and Adolescents: Clinical trials in healthy adult and adolescent subjects have shown that following a course of three doses of 20 mcg Engerix-B [Hepatitis B Vaccine (Recombinant)] given according to the ACIP recommended schedule of injections at months 0, 1 and 6, the seroprotection (antibody titers ≥10 mIU/mL) rate for all individuals was 79% at month 6 and 96% at month 7; the geometric mean antibody titer (GMT) for seroconverters at month 7 was 2,204 mIU/mL. On an alternate schedule (injections at months 0, 1 and 2) designed for certain populations (e.g., neonates born of hepatitis B infected mothers, individuals who have or might have been recently exposed to the virus, and certain travelers to high-risk areas. See INDICATIONS AND USAGE.), 99% of all individuals were seroprotected at month 3 and remained protected through month 12. On the alternate schedule, an additional dose at 12 months produced a GMT for seroconverters at month 13 of 9,163 mIU/mL.

Immunogenicity in Older Subjects: Among older subjects given 20 mcg at months 0, 1 and 6, the seroprotection rate 1 month after the third dose was 88%. However, as with other hepatitis B vaccines, in adults over 40 years of age, *Engerix-B* vaccine produced anti-HBs titers that were lower than those in younger adults (GMT among seroconverters 1 month after the third 20 mcg dose with a 0, 1, 6-month schedule: 610 mIU/mL for individuals over 40 years of age, N=50).

Immunogenicity in Subjects with Chronic Hepatitis C: In a clinical trial of subjects with chronic hepatitis C, 31 subjects received *Engerix-B* on the usual 0, 1, 6-month schedule. All subjects responded with seroprotective titers. The GMT of anti-HBs was 1,260 mIU/mL (95% CI:709–2237).

Hemodialysis Patients: Hemodialysis patients given hepatitis B vaccines respond with lower titers,[12] which remain at protective levels for shorter durations than in normal subjects. In a study in which patients on chronic hemodialysis (mean time on dialysis was 24 months; N=562) received 40 mcg of the plasma-derived vaccine at months 0, 1 and 6, approximately 50% of patients achieved antibody titers ≥10 mIU/mL.[12] Since a fourth dose of Engerix-B [Hepatitis B Vaccine (Recombinant)] given to healthy adults at month 12 following the 0, 1, 2-month schedule resulted in a substantial increase in the GMT (see above), a four-dose regimen was studied in hemodialysis patients. In a clinical trial of adults who had been on hemodialysis for a mean of 56 months (N=43), 67% of patients were seroprotected 2 months after the last dose of 40 mcg of *Engerix-B* (two × 20 mcg) given on a 0, 1, 2, 6-month schedule; the GMT among seroconverters was 93 mIU/mL.

Interchangeability with Other Hepatitis B Vaccines: Recombinant DNA vaccines are produced in yeast by expression of a hepatitis B virus gene sequence that codes for the hepatitis B surface antigen. Like plasma-derived vaccine, the yeast-derived vaccines are protein particles visible by electron microscopy and have hepatitis B surface antigen epitopes as determined by monoclonal antibody analyses. Yeast-derived vaccines have been shown by *in vitro* analyses to induce antibodies (anti-HBs) which are immunologically comparable by epitope specificity and binding affinity to antibodies induced by plasma-derived vaccine.[13] In cross absorption studies, no differences were detected in the spectra of antibodies induced in man to plasma-derived or to yeast-derived hepatitis B vaccines.[13]

Additionally, patients immunized approximately 3 years previously with plasma-derived vaccine and whose antibody titers were <100 mIU/mL (GMT: 35 mIU/mL; range: 9–94) were given a 20 mcg dose of Engerix-B [Hepatitis B Vaccine (Recombinant)]. All patients, including two who had not responded to the plasma-derived vaccine, showed a response to *Engerix-B* (GMT: 5,069 mIU/mL; range: 624–15,019). There have been no clinical studies in which a three-dose vaccine series was initiated with a plasma-derived hepatitis B vaccine and completed with *Engerix-B*, or vice versa. However, because the *in vitro* and *in vivo* studies described above indicate the comparability of the antibody produced in response to plasma-derived vaccine and *Engerix-B*, it should be possible to interchange the use of *Engerix-B* and plasma-derived vaccines (but see CONTRAINDICATIONS).

A controlled study (N=48) demonstrated that completion of a course of immunization with one dose of *Engerix-B* (20 mcg, month 6) following two doses of Recombivax HB®* (10 mcg, months 0 and 1) produced a similar GMT (4,077 mIU/mL) to immunization with three doses of *Recombivax HB* (10 mcg, months 0, 1 and 6; 2,654 mIU/mL). Thus, *Engerix-B* can be used to complete a vaccination course initiated with *Recombivax HB*.[14]

Other Clinical Studies: In one study,[15] four of 244 (1.6%) adults (homosexual men) at high risk of contracting hepatitis B virus became infected during the period prior to completion of three doses of *Engerix-B* (20 mcg at 0, 1, 6 months). No additional patients became infected during the 18-month follow-up period after completion of the immunization course.

INDICATIONS AND USAGE

Engerix-B is indicated for immunization against infection caused by all known subtypes of hepatitis B virus. As hepatitis D (caused by the delta virus) does not occur in the absence of hepatitis B infection, it can be expected that hepatitis D will also be prevented by *Engerix-B* vaccination.

Engerix-B will not prevent hepatitis caused by other agents, such as hepatitis A, C and E viruses, or other pathogens known to infect the liver.

Immunization is recommended in persons of all ages, especially those who are, or will be, at increased risk of exposure to hepatitis B virus,[1] for example:

Infants, Including Those Born of HBsAg-Positive Mothers (See DOSAGE AND ADMINISTRATION.)

Adolescents (See CLINICAL PHARMACOLOGY.)

Health Care Personnel: Dentists and oral surgeons. Dental, medical and nursing students. Physicians, surgeons and podiatrists. Nurses. Paramedical and ambulance personnel and custodial staff who may be exposed to the virus via blood or other patient specimens. Dental hygienists and dental nurses. Laboratory and blood-bank personnel handling blood, blood products, and other patient specimens. Hospital cleaning staff who handle waste.

Selected Patients and Patient Contacts: Patients and staff in hemodialysis units and hematology/oncology units. Patients requiring frequent and/or large volume blood transfusions or clotting factor concentrates (e.g., persons with hemophilia, thalassemia, sickle-cell anemia, cirrhosis). Clients (residents) and staff of institutions for the mentally handicapped. Classroom contacts of deinstitutionalized mentally handicapped persons who have persistent hepatitis B surface antigenemia and who show aggressive behavior. Household and other intimate contacts of persons with persistent hepatitis B surface antigenemia.

Subpopulations with a Known High Incidence of the Disease, such as: Alaskan Eskimos. Pacific Islanders. Indochinese immigrants. Haitian immigrants. Refugees from other HBV endemic areas. All infants of women born in areas where the infection is highly endemic.

Individuals with Chronic Hepatitis C: Risk factors for hepatitis C are similar to those for hepatitis B. Consequently, immunization with hepatitis B vaccine is recommended for individuals with chronic hepatitis C.

Persons Who May Be Exposed to the Hepatitis B Virus by Travel to High-Risk Areas (See ACIP Guidelines, 1990.)

Military Personnel Identified as Being at Increased Risk

Morticians and Embalmers

Persons at Increased Risk of the Disease Due to Their Sexual Practices,[1,16] such as: Persons with more than one sexual partner in a 6-month period. Persons who have contracted a sexually transmitted disease. Homosexually active males. Female prostitutes.

Prisoners

Users of Illicit Injectable Drugs

Others: Police and fire department personnel who render first aid or medical assistance, and any others who, through

Continued on next page

Information on the SmithKline Beecham Pharmaceuticals products appearing here is based on the labeling in effect on May 15, 2001. Further information on these and other products may be obtained from the Medical Department, SmithKline Beecham Pharmaceuticals, One Franklin Plaza, Philadelphia, PA 19101.

Engerix-B—Cont.

their work or personal life-style, may be exposed to the hepatitis B virus. Adoptees from countries of high HBV endemicity.
Use with Other Vaccines: The Immunization Practices Advisory Committee states that, in general, simultaneous administration of certain live and inactivated pediatric vaccines has not resulted in impaired antibody responses or increased rates of adverse reactions.[17] Separate sites and syringes should be used for simultaneous administration of injectable vaccines.

CONTRAINDICATIONS

Hypersensitivity to yeast or any other component of the vaccine is a contraindication for use of the vaccine. Patients experiencing hypersensitivity after an Engerix-B [Hepatitis B Vaccine (Recombinant)] injection should not receive further injections of *Engerix-B.*

WARNINGS

Hepatitis B has a long incubation period. Hepatitis B vaccination may not prevent hepatitis B infection in individuals who had an unrecognized hepatitis B infection at the time of vaccine administration. Additionally, it may not prevent infection in individuals who do not achieve protective antibody titers.

PRECAUTIONS

General As with other vaccines, although a moderate or severe febrile illness is sufficient reason to postpone vaccination, minor illnesses such as mild upper respiratory infections with or without low-grade fever are not contraindications.[17]

Prior to immunization, the patient's medical history should be reviewed. The physician should review the patient's immunization history for possible vaccine sensitivity, previous vaccination-related adverse reactions and occurrence of any adverse-event-related symptoms and/or signs, in order to determine the existence of any contraindication to immunization with *Engerix-B* and to allow an assessment of benefits and risks. Epinephrine injection (1:1000) and other appropriate agents used for the control of immediate allergic reactions must be immediately available should an acute anaphylactic reaction occur.

A separate sterile syringe and needle or a sterile disposable unit should be used for each individual patient to prevent transmission of hepatitis or other infectious agents from one person to another. Needles should be disposed of properly and should not be recapped.

Special care should be taken to prevent injection into a blood vessel.

As with any vaccine administered to immunosuppressed persons or persons receiving immunosuppressive therapy, the expected immune response may not be obtained. For individuals receiving immunosuppressive therapy, deferral of vaccination for at least 3 months after therapy may be considered.[17]

Multiple Sclerosis: Although no causal relationship has been established, rare instances of exacerbation of multiple sclerosis have been reported following administration of hepatitis B vaccines and other vaccines. In persons with multiple sclerosis, the benefit of immunization for prevention of hepatitis B infection and sequelae must be weighed against the risk of exacerbation of the disease.

Information for the Patient

Patients, parents or guardians should be informed of the potential benefits and risks of the vaccine, and of the importance of completing the immunization series. As with any vaccine, it is important when a subject returns for the next dose in a series that he/she be questioned concerning occurrence of any symptoms and/or signs of an adverse reaction after a previous dose of the same vaccine. Patients, parents or guardians should be told to report severe or unusual adverse reactions to their healthcare provider.

The parent or guardian should be given the Vaccine Information Materials, which are required by the National Childhood Vaccine Injury Act of 1986 to be given prior to immunization.

Drug Interactions

For information regarding simultaneous administration with other vaccines, refer to INDICATIONS AND USAGE.

Carcinogenesis, Mutagenesis, Impairment of Fertility

Engerix-B [Hepatitis B Vaccine (Recombinant)] has not been evaluated for carcinogenic or mutagenic potential, or for impairment of fertility.

Pregnancy Pregnancy Category C: Animal reproduction studies have not been conducted with *Engerix-B.* It is also not known whether *Engerix-B* can cause fetal harm when administered to a pregnant woman or can affect reproduction capacity. *Engerix-B* should be given to a pregnant woman only if clearly needed.

Nursing Mothers It is not known whether *Engerix-B* is excreted in human milk. Because many drugs are excreted in human milk, caution should be exercised when *Engerix-B* is administered to a nursing woman.

Pediatric Use *Engerix-B* has been shown to be well tolerated and highly immunogenic in infants and children of all ages. Newborns also respond well; maternally transferred antibodies do not interfere with the active immune response to the vaccine. (See CLINICAL PHARMACOLOGY for seroconversion rates and titers in neonates and children. See DOSAGE AND ADMINISTRATION for recommended pediatric dosage and for recommended dosage for infants born of HBsAg-positive mothers.)

Table 1. Recommended dosage and administration schedule

Group	Dose	Schedule
Infants born of:		
HBsAg-negative mothers	10 mcg/0.5mL	0, 1, 6 months
HBsAg-positive mothers	10 mcg/0.5 mL	0, 1, 6 months
Children:		
Birth through 10 years of age	10 mcg/0.5 mL	0, 1, 6 months
Adolescents:		
11 through 19 years of age	10 mcg/0.5 mL	0, 1, 6 months
Adults (>19 years)	20 mcg/1.0 mL	0, 1, 6 months
Adult hemodialysis	40 mcg/2.0 mL[a]	0, 1, 2, 6 months

[a]Two × 20 mcg in one or two injections.

Table 2. Alternate dosage and administration schedules

Group	Dose	Schedules
Infants born of:		
HBsAg-positive mothers	10 mcg/0.5 mL	0, 1, 2, 12 months[b]
Children:		
Birth through 10 years of age	10 mcg/0.5 mL	0, 1, 2, 12 months[b]
5 through 10 years of age	10 mcg/0.5 mL	0, 12, 24 months[c]
Adolescents:		
11 through 16 years of age	10 mcg/0.5 mL	0, 12, 24 months[c]
11 through 19 years of age	20 mcg/1.0 mL	0, 1, 6 months
11 through 19 years of age	20 mcg/1.0 mL	0, 1, 2, 12 months[b]
Adults (>19 years)	20 mcg/1.0 mL	0, 1, 2, 12 months[b]

[b] This schedule is designed for certain populations (e.g., neonates born of hepatitis B infected mothers, others who have or might have been recently exposed to the virus, certain travelers to high-risk areas. See INDICATIONS AND USAGE.). On this alternate schedule, an additional dose at 12 months is recommended for prolonged maintenance of protective titers.
[c] For children and adolescents for whom an extended administration schedule is acceptable based on risk of exposure.

ADVERSE REACTIONS

Engerix-B [Hepatitis B Vaccine (Recombinant)] is generally well tolerated. As with any vaccine, however, it is possible that expanded commercial use of the vaccine could reveal rare adverse reactions.

Ten double-blind studies involving 2,252 subjects showed no significant difference in the frequency or severity of adverse experiences between *Engerix-B* and plasma-derived vaccines. In 36 clinical studies a total of 13,495 doses of *Engerix-B* were administered to 5,071 healthy adults and children who were initially seronegative for hepatitis B markers, and healthy neonates. All subjects were monitored for 4 days post-administration. Frequency of adverse experiences tended to decrease with successive doses of *Engerix-B.* Using a symptom checklist,[†] the most frequently reported adverse reactions were injection site soreness (22%) and fatigue[†] (14%). Other reactions are listed below.

Incidence 1% to 10% of Injections

Local reactions at injection site: Induration; erythema; swelling.
Body as a whole: Fever (>37.5°C).
Nervous system: Headache;[†] dizziness.[†]

[†]Parent or guardian completed forms for children and neonates. Neonatal checklist did not include headache, fatigue or dizziness.

Incidence <1% of Injections

Local reactions at injection site: Pain; pruritus; ecchymosis.
Body as a whole: Sweating; malaise; chills; weakness; flushing; tingling.
Cardiovascular system: Hypotension.
Respiratory system: Influenza-like symptoms; upper respiratory tract illnesses.
Gastrointestinal system: Nausea; anorexia; abdominal pain/cramps; vomiting; constipation; diarrhea.
Lymphatic system: Lymphadenopathy.
Musculoskeletal system: Pain/stiffness in arm, shoulder or neck; arthralgia; myalgia; back pain.
Skin and appendages: Rash; urticaria; petechiae; pruritus; erythema.
Nervous system: Somnolence; insomnia; irritability; agitation.

Additional adverse experiences have been reported with the commercial use of *Energix-B.* Those listed below are to serve as alerting information to physicians.

Hypersensitivity: Anaphylaxis; erythema multiforme including Stevens-Johnson syndrome; angioedema; arthritis. An apparent hypersensitivity syndrome (serum-sickness-like) of delayed onset has been reported days to weeks after vaccination, including: arthralgia/arthritis (usually transient), fever and dermatologic reactions such as urticaria, erythema multiforme, ecchymoses and erythema nodosum (see CONTRAINDICATIONS).
Cardiovascular system: Tachycardia/palpitations.
Respiratory system: Bronchospasm including asthma-like symptoms.
Gastrointestinal system: Abnormal liver function tests; dyspepsia.

Nervous system: Migraine; syncope; paresis; neuropathy including hypoesthesia, paresthesia, Guillain-Barré syndrome and Bell's palsy, transverse myelitis; optic neuritis; multiple sclerosis; seizures.
Hematologic: Thrombocytopenia.
Skin and appendages: Eczema; purpura; herpes zoster; erythema nodosum; alopecia.
Special senses: Conjunctivitis; keratitis; visual disturbances; vertigo; tinnitus; earache.
Reporting Adverse Events
The National Childhood Vaccine Injury Act requires that the manufacturer and lot number of the vaccine administered be recorded by the healthcare provider in the vaccine recipient's permanent medical record, along with the date of administration of the vaccine and the name, address and title of the person administering the vaccine.[18] The Act further requires the healthcare provider to report to the U.S. Department of Health and Human Services via VAERS the occurrence following immunization of any event set forth in the Vaccine Injury Table including: anaphylaxis or anaphylactic shock within 4 hours, encephalopathy or encephalitis within 72 hours, or any sequelae thereof (including death).[18,19] In addition, any event considered a contraindication to further doses should be reported. The VAERS toll-free number is 1-800-822-7967.

DOSAGE AND ADMINISTRATION

Injection: Engerix-B [Hepatitis B Vaccine (Recombinant)] should be administered by intramuscular injection. *Do not inject intravenously or intradermally.* In adults, the injection should be given in the deltoid region but it may be preferable to inject in the anterolateral thigh in neonates and infants, who have smaller deltoid muscles. *Engerix-B* should not be administered in the gluteal region; such injections may result in suboptimal response. The attending physician should determine final selection of the injection site and needle size, depending upon the patient's age and the size of the target muscle. A 1-inch 23-gauge needle is sufficient to penetrate the anterolateral thigh in infants younger than 12 months of age. A 5/8-inch 25-gauge needle may be used to administer the vaccine in the deltoid region of toddlers and children up to, and including, 10 years of age. The 1-inch 23-gauge needle is appropriate for use in older children and adults.[17]

Engerix-B may be administered subcutaneously to persons at risk of hemorrhage (e.g., hemophiliacs). However, hepatitis B vaccines administered subcutaneously are known to result in lower GMTs. Additionally, when other aluminum-adsorbed vaccines have been administered subcutaneously, an increased incidence of local reactions including subcutaneous nodules has been observed. Therefore, subcutaneous administration should be used only in persons who are at risk of hemorrhage with intramuscular injections.

Preparation for Administration: Shake well before withdrawal and use. Parenteral drug products should be inspected visually for particulate matter or discoloration prior to administration. With thorough agitation, Engerix-B [Hepatitis B Vaccine (Recombinant)] is a slightly turbid white suspension. Discard if it appears otherwise. The vaccine should be used as supplied; no dilution is necessary.

The full recommended dose of the vaccine should be used. Any vaccine remaining in a single-dose vial should be discarded.

Dosing Schedules: The usual immunization regimen (see Table 1) consists of three doses of vaccine given according to the following schedule: 1st dose: at elected date; 2nd dose: 1 month later; 3rd dose: 6 months after first dose.

[See table 1 at top of previous page]

For hemodialysis patients, in whom vaccine-induced protection is less complete and may persist only as long as antibody levels remain above 10 mIU/mL, the need for booster doses should be assessed by annual antibody testing. 40 mcg (two × 20 mcg) booster doses with *Engerix-B* should be given when antibody levels decline below 10 mIU/mL.[1] Data show individuals given a booster with *Engerix-B* achieve high antibody titers. (See CLINICAL PHARMACOLOGY.) There are alternate dosing and administration schedules which may be used for specific populations (see Table 2 and accompanying explanations).

[See table 2 at top of previous page]

booster vaccinations: Whenever administration of a booster dose is appropriate, the dose of *Engerix-B* is 10 mcg for children 10 years of age and under; 20 mcg for adolescents 11 through 19 years of age and 20 mcg for adults. Studies have demonstrated a substantial increase in antibody titers after Engerix-B [Hepatitis B Vaccine (Recombinant)] booster vaccination following an initial course with both plasma- and yeast-derived vaccines. (See CLINICAL PHARMACOLOGY.)

See previous section for discussion on booster vaccination for adult hemodialysis patients.

Known or presumed exposure to hepatitis B virus: Unprotected individuals with known or presumed exposure to the hepatitis B virus (e.g., neonates born of infected mothers, others experiencing percutaneous or permucosal exposure) should be given hepatitis B immune globulin (HBIG) in addition to Engerix-B [Hepatitis B Vaccine (Recombinant)] in accordance with ACIP recommendations[1] and with the package insert for HBIG. Engerix-B [Hepatitis B Vaccine (Recombinant)] can be given on either dosing schedule (see above).

STORAGE
Store between 2° and 8°C (36° and 46°F). *Do not freeze*; discard if product has been frozen. Do not dilute to administer.

HOW SUPPLIED
Adult Dose
20 mcg/mL in Single-Dose Vials in packages of 1 and 25 vials.
   NDC 58160-857-01 (package of 1)
   NDC 58160-857-16 (package of 25)
20 mcg/mL in Single-Dose Prefilled Disposable Tip-Lok® Syringes with 1-inch 23-gauge needles.
   NDC 58160-857-35 (package of 5)
   NDC 58160-857-26 (package of 25)
Pediatric/Adolescent Doses
10 mcg/0.5 mL in Single-Dose Vials in packages of 1 and 10 vials.
   NDC 58160-856-01 (package of 1)
   NDC 58160-856-11 (package of 10)
10 mcg/0.5 mL in Single-Dose Prefilled Disposable Tip-Lok® Syringes with 1-inch 23-gauge needles.
   NDC 58160-856-35 (package of 5)
   NDC 58160-856-26 (package of 25)
10 mcg/0.5 mL in Single-Dose Prefilled Disposable Tip-Lok® Syringes with 5/8-inch 25-gauge needles.
   NDC 58160-856-36 (package of 5)
   NDC 58160-856-27 (package of 25)

REFERENCES
1. Centers for Disease Control and Prevention: Epidemiology and prevention of vaccine-preventable diseases. Atkinson, W., et al. (eds). 6th ed. 2000:207–229. 2. Beasley R.P., et al.: Efficacy of hepatitis B immune globulin for prevention of perinatal transmission of hepatitis B virus carrier state: final report of a randomized double-blind, placebo-controlled trial. *Hepatology* 3:135–141, 1983. 3. Centers for Disease Control and Prevention. *Federal Register*, Feb. 23, 1999, 64(35):9044–9045. 4. Chang M.H., Chen C.J., Lai M.S. Universal hepatitis B vaccination in Taiwan and the incidence of hepatocellular carcinoma in children. *N.Engl.J.Med.* 1997;336(26):1855–1859. 5. Lee M.S., Kim D.H., et al. Hepatitis B vaccination and reduced risk of primary liver cancer among male adults: A cohort study in Korea. *Int. J. Epidemiol.* 1998;27:316–319. 6. Centers for Disease Control and Prevention: Effectiveness of a Seventh Grade School Entry Vaccination Requirement—Statewide and Orange County, Florida, 1997–1998. *MMWR.* 1998;47(34):714. 7. Committee on Infectious Diseases: Universal hepatitis B immunization. *Pediatrics.* 89(4):795–800, 1992. 8. Centers for Control: Immunization of adolescents: recommendations of the Advisory Committee on Immunization Practices, the American Academy of Pediatrics, the American Academy of Family Physicians, and the American Medical Association. *MMWR.* 45(No. RR-13), 1996. 9. American Academy of Pediatrics: Immunization of adolescents: recommendations of the Advisory Committee on Immunization Practices, the American Academy of Pediatrics, the American Academy of Family Physicians, and the American Medical Association. *Pediatrics.* 1997;99(No.3):479–488. 10. Andre F.E., and Safary A.: Clinical experience with a yeast-derived hepatitis B vaccine. In Zuckerman A.J. (ed): *Viral hepatitis and liver disease*, Alan R. Liss, Inc., 1988, pp. 1025–1030. 11. Poovorawan Y., et al.: Protective efficacy of a recombinant DNA hepatitis B vaccine in neonates of HBe antigen-positive mothers. *JAMA.* 261(22):3278–3281, June 9, 1989.
12. Stevens C.E., et al.: Hepatitis B vaccine in patients receiving hemodialysis. *N. Engl. J. Med.* 311:496–501, 1984. 13. Hauser P., et al.: Immunological properties of recombinant HBsAg produced in yeast. *Postgrad. Med. J.* 63 (Suppl. 2):83–91, 1987. 14. Bush L.M., Moonsammy G.I., Boscia J.A. Evaluation of initiating a hepatitis B vaccination schedule with one vaccine and completing it with another. *Vaccine.* 1991:9(11):807–809. 15. Goilav C., et al.: Immunization of homosexual men with a recombinant DNA vaccine against hepatitis B: immunogenicity and protection. In Zuckerman, A.J. (ed): *Viral hepatitis and liver disease*, Alan R. Liss, Inc., 1988, pp. 1057–1058. 16. Centers for Disease Control and Prevention. 1998 Guidelines for treatment of sexually transmitted diseases. *MMWR.* 1998;47(RR-1):102. 17. Centers for Disease Control and Prevention: General Recommendations on Immunization: Recommendations of the Advisory Committee on Immunization Practices (ACIP). *MMWR.* 1994;43(RR-1):1–38. 18. Centers for Disease Control. National Childhood Vaccine Injury Act: Requirements for permanent vaccination records and for reporting of selected events after vaccination. *MMWR.* 1988;Vol. 37 (No. 13):197–200. 19. National Vaccine Injury Compensation Program: Revision of the vaccine injury table. *Federal Register.* Wednesday, February 8, 1995;Vol. 60 (No. 26):7694.

*yeast-derived, Hepatitis B Vaccine, MSD.
U.S. License No. 1090
Manufactured by
SmithKline Beecham Biologicals
Rixensart, Belgium
Distributed by
SmithKline Beecham Pharmaceuticals
Philadelphia, PA 19101
DATE OF ISSUANCE DEC. 2000
© SmithKline Beecham, 2000   ℞ only
Engerix-B and *Tip-Lok* are registered trademarks of SmithKline Beecham.
EB:L31A

INFANRIX®   ℞
**Diphtheria and
Tetanus Toxoids
and Acellular Pertussis
Vaccine Adsorbed**

Prescribing information for this product, which appears on pages 3100–3104 of the 2001 PDR, has been revised. Please write "See Supplement A" next to the product heading.
Under DESCRIPTION, replace the fifth paragraph with the following:
Each 0.5 mL dose also contains 2.5 mg 2-phenoxyethanol as a preservative, 4.5 mg sodium chloride, water for injection and not more than 0.02% (w/v) residual formaldehyde. Thimerosal is used in the early stages of manufacturing and is removed by subsequent purification steps to below the analytical detection limit, which upon calculation is <1 ng mercury/dose. Does not contain thimerosal as a preservative.
The vaccine contains polysorbate 80 (Tween 80) which is used in the production of the pertussis concentrate. The inactivated acellular pertussis components contribute less than 5 endotoxin units (EU) per 0.5 mL dose.
IN:L4

PAXIL®   ℞
[packs 'ill]
**brand of
paroxetine
hydrochloride
tablets and oral suspension**

Prescribing information for this product, which appears on pages 3114–3120 of the 2001 PDR, has been revised. Please write "See Supplement A" next to the product heading.
Replace CONTRAINDICATIONS and WARNINGS with the following:

CONTRAINDICATIONS
Concomitant use in patients taking either monoamine oxidase inhibitors (MAOIs) or thioridazine is contraindicated (see WARNINGS and PRECAUTIONS).
Paxil is contraindicated in patients with a hypersensitivity to paroxetine or any of the inactive ingredients in *Paxil*.

WARNINGS
Potential for Interaction with Monoamine Oxidase Inhibitors
In patients receiving another serotonin reuptake inhibitor drug in combination with a monoamine oxidase inhibitor (MAOI), there have been reports of serious, sometimes fatal, reactions including hyperthermia, rigidity, myoclonus, autonomic instability with possible rapid fluctuations of vital signs, and mental status changes that include extreme agitation progressing to delirium and coma. These reactions have also been reported in patients who have recently discontinued that drug and have been started on a MAOI. Some cases presented with features resembling neuroleptic malignant syndrome. While there are no human data showing such an interaction with *Paxil*, limited animal data on the effects of combined use of paroxetine and MAOIs suggest that these drugs may act synergistically to elevate blood pressure and evoke behavioral excitation. Therefore, it is recommended that Paxil (paroxetine hydrochloride) not be used in combination with a MAOI, or

within 14 days of discontinuing treatment with a MAOI. At least 2 weeks should be allowed after stopping *Paxil* before starting a MAOI.
Potential Interaction with Thioridazine
Thioridazine administration alone produces prolongation of the QTc interval, which is associated with serious ventricular arrhythmias, such as torsade de pointes-type arrhythmias, and sudden death. This effect appears to be dose-related.
An *in vivo* study suggests that drugs which inhibit P450IID6, such as paroxetine, will elevate plasma levels of thioridazine. Therefore, it is recommended that paroxetine not be used in combination with thioridazine (see CONTRAINDICATIONS and PRECAUTIONS).
Under PRECAUTIONS, insert the following after subsection Monoamine Oxidase Inhibitors:
Thioridazine: See CONTRAINDICATIONS and WARNINGS.
Also under PRECAUTIONS, replace subsection Drugs Metabolized by Cytochrome $P_{450}IID_6$ with the following:
Drugs Metabolized by Cytochrome $P_{450}IID_6$: Many drugs, including most antidepressants (paroxetine, other SSRIs and many tricyclics), are metabolized by the cytochrome P_{450} isozyme $P_{450}IID_6$. Like other agents that are metabolized by $P_{450}IID_6$, paroxetine may significantly inhibit the activity of this isozyme. In most patients (>90%), this $P_{450}IID_6$ isozyme is saturated early during *Paxil* dosing. In one study, daily dosing of *Paxil* (20 mg q.d.) under steady-state conditions increased single dose desipramine (100 mg) C_{max}, AUC and $T_{1/2}$ by an average of approximately two-, five- and three-fold, respectively. Concomitant use of *Paxil* with other drugs metabolized by cytochrome $P_{450}IID_6$ has not been formally studied but may require lower doses than usually prescribed for either *Paxil* or the other drug.
Therefore, co-administration of *Paxil* with other drugs that are metabolized by this isozyme, including certain antidepressants (e.g., nortriptyline, amitriptyline, imipramine, desipramine and fluoxetine), phenothiazines and Type 1C antiarrhythmics (e.g., propafenone, flecainide and encainide), or that inhibit this enzyme (e.g., quinidine), should be approached with caution.
However, due to the risk of serious ventricular arrhythmias and sudden death potentially associated with elevated plasma levels of thioridazine, paroxetine and thioridazine should not be co-administered (see CONTRAINDICATIONS and WARNINGS).
At steady state, when the $P_{450}IID_6$ pathway is essentially saturated, paroxetine clearance is governed by alternative P_{450} isozymes which, unlike $P_{450}IID_6$, show no evidence of saturation (see PRECAUTIONS—Tricyclic Antidepressants).
Under ADVERSE REACTIONS, replace subsection Postmarketing Reports with the following:
Postmarketing Reports
Voluntary reports of adverse events in patients taking Paxil (paroxetine hydrochloride) that have been received since market introduction and not listed above that may have no causal relationship with the drug include acute pancreatitis, elevated liver function tests (the most severe cases were deaths due to liver necrosis, and grossly elevated transaminases associated with severe liver dysfunction), Guillain-Barré syndrome, toxic epidermal necrolysis, priapism, syndrome of inappropriate ADH secretion, symptoms suggestive of prolactinemia and galactorrhea, neuroleptic malignant syndrome-like events; extrapyramidal symptoms which have included akathisia, bradykinesia, cogwheel rigidity, dystonia, hypertonia, oculogyric crisis which has been associated with concomitant use of pimozide, tremor and trismus, serotonin syndrome, associated in some cases with concomitant use of serotonergic drugs and with drugs which may have impaired *Paxil* metabolism (symptoms have included agitation, confusion, diaphoresis, hallucinations, hyperreflexia, myoclonus, shivering, tachycardia and tremor), status epilepticus, acute renal failure, pulmonary hypertension, allergic alveolitis, anaphylaxis, eclampsia, laryngismus, optic neuritis, porphyria, ventricular fibrillation, ventricular tachycardia (including torsade de pointes), thrombocytopenia, hemolytic anemia, and events related to impaired hematopoiesis (including aplastic anemia, pancytopenia, bone marrow aplasia, and agranulocytosis). There have been spontaneous reports that discontinuation (particularly when abrupt) may lead to symptoms such as dizziness, sensory disturbances, agitation or anxiety, nausea and sweating; these events are generally self-limiting. There has been a case report of an elevated phenytoin level after 4 weeks of *Paxil* and phenytoin co-administration. There has been a case report of severe hypotension when *Paxil* was added to chronic metoprolol treatment.
Under OVERDOSAGE, replace subsection Human Experience with the following:
Human Experience: Since the introduction of *Paxil* in the U.S., 342 spontaneous cases of deliberate or accidental overdosage during paroxetine treatment have been reported worldwide (circa 1999). These include overdoses with paroxetine alone and in combination with other substances. Of these, 48 cases were fatal and, of the fatalities, 17 appeared to involve paroxetine alone. Eight fatal cases which

Continued on next page

Information on the SmithKline Beecham Pharmaceuticals products appearing here is based on the labeling in effect on May 15, 2001. Further information on these and other products may be obtained from the Medical Department, SmithKline Beecham Pharmaceuticals, One Franklin Plaza, Philadelphia, PA 19101.

Paxil—Cont.

documented the amount of paroxetine ingested were generally confounded by the ingestion of other drugs or alcohol or the presence of significant comorbid conditions. Of 145 non-fatal cases with known outcome, most recovered without sequelae. The largest known ingestion involved 2000 mg of paroxetine (33 times the maximum recommended daily dose) in a patient who recovered.
Commonly reported adverse events associated with paroxetine overdosage include somnolence, coma, nausea, tremor, tachycardia, confusion, vomiting, and dizziness. Other notable signs and symptoms observed with overdoses involving paroxetine (alone or with other substances) include mydriasis, convulsions (including status epilepticus), ventricular dysrhythmias (including torsade de pointes), hypertension, aggressive reactions, syncope, hypotension, stupor, bradycardia, dystonia, rhabdomyolysis, symptoms of hepatic dysfunction (including hepatic failure, hepatic necrosis, jaundice, hepatitis, and hepatic steatosis), serotonin syndrome, manic reactions, myoclonus, acute renal failure, and urinary retention.
PX:L18

RELAFEN® ℞

[rel' ah-fen]
brand of nabumetone tablets

Prescribing information for this product, which appears on pages 3120–3122 of the 2001 PDR, has been revised as follows. Please write "See Supplement A" next to the product heading.

Under PRECAUTIONS, subsection Renal Effects, replace the third paragraph with the following:
Because nabumetone undergoes extensive hepatic metabolism, no adjustment of *Relafen* dosage is generally necessary in patients with renal insufficiency. However, as with all NSAIDs, patients with impaired renal function should be monitored more closely than patients with normal renal function (see CLINICAL PHARMACOLOGY, Renal Insufficiency). In patients with severe renal impairment (creatinine clearance ≤30 mL/min.), laboratory tests should be performed at baseline and within weeks of starting therapy. Further tests should be carried out as necessary; if the impairment worsens, discontinuation of therapy may be warranted. The oxidized and conjugated metabolites of 6MNA are eliminated primarily by the kidneys. The extent to which these largely inactive metabolites may accumulate in patients with renal failure has not been studied. As with other drugs whose metabolites are excreted by the kidneys, the possibility that adverse reactions (not listed in ADVERSE REACTIONS) may be attributable to these metabolites should be considered.
Under PRECAUTIONS, replace subsection Hepatic Function with the following:
Hepatic Function: As with other NSAIDs, borderline elevations of one or more liver function tests may occur in up to 15% of patients. These abnormalities may progress, may remain essentially unchanged, or may return to normal with continued therapy. The ALT (SGPT) test is probably the most sensitive indicator of liver dysfunction. Meaningful (3 times the upper limit of normal) elevations of ALT (SGPT) or AST (SGOT) have occurred in controlled clinical trials of Relafen (nabumetone) in less than 1% of patients. A patient with symptoms and/or signs suggesting liver dysfunction, or in whom an abnormal liver test has occurred, should be evaluated for evidence of the development of a more severe hepatic reaction while on *Relafen* therapy. Severe hepatic reactions, including jaundice and fatal hepatitis, have been reported with *Relafen* and other NSAIDs. Although such reactions are rare, if abnormal liver tests persist or worsen, if clinical signs and symptoms consistent with liver disease develop, or if systemic manifestations occur (e.g., eosinophilia, rash, etc.), *Relafen* should be discontinued. Because nabumetone's biotransformation to 6MNA is dependent upon hepatic function, the biotransformation could be decreased in patients with severe hepatic dysfunction. Therefore, *Relafen* should be used with caution in patients with severe hepatic impairment (see Pharmacokinetics, *Hepatic Impairment*).
Under ADVERSE REACTIONS, replace subsections Incidence <1%—Probably Causally Related and Incidence <1%—Causal Relationship Unknown with the following:

Incidence <1%—Probably Causally Related†

Gastrointestinal: Anorexia, jaundice, duodenal ulcer, dysphagia, gastric ulcer, gastroenteritis, gastrointestinal bleeding, increased appetite, liver function abnormalities, melena, *hepatic failure*.
Central Nervous System: Asthenia, agitation, anxiety, confusion, depression, malaise, paresthesia, tremor, vertigo.
Dermatologic: Bullous eruptions, photosensitivity, urticaria, pseudoporphyria cutanea tarda, *toxic epidermal necrolysis, erythema multiforme, Stevens-Johnson Syndrome.*
Cardiovascular: Vasculitis.
Metabolic: Weight gain.
Respiratory: Dyspnea, *eosinophilic pneumonia, hypersensitivity pneumonitis, idiopathic interstitial pneumonitis.*
Genitourinary: Albuminuria, azotemia, *hyperuricemia, interstitial nephritis, nephrotic syndrome, vaginal bleeding, renal failure.*
Special Senses: Abnormal vision.
Hematologic/Lymphatic: *Thrombocytopenia.*
Hypersensitivity: *Anaphylactoid reaction, anaphylaxis,* angioneurotic edema.

†Adverse reactions reported only in worldwide postmarketing experience or in the literature, not seen in clinical trials, are considered rarer and are italicized.

Incidence <1%—Causal Relationship Unknown‡

Gastrointestinal: Bilirubinuria, duodenitis, eructation, gallstones, gingivitis, glossitis, pancreatitis, rectal bleeding.
Central Nervous System: Nightmares.
Dermatologic: Acne, alopecia.
Cardiovascular: Angina, arrhythmia, hypertension, myocardial infarction, palpitations, syncope, thrombophlebitis.
Respiratory: Asthma, cough.
Genitourinary: Dysuria, hematuria, impotence, renal stones.
Special Senses: Taste disorder.
Body as a Whole: Fever, chills.
Hematologic/Lymphatic: Anemia, leukopenia, granulocytopenia.
Metabolic/Nutritional: Hyperglycemia, hypokalemia, weight loss.

‡Adverse reactions reported only in worldwide postmarketing experience or in the literature, not seen in clinical trials, are considered rarer and are italicized.

Replace OVERDOSAGE with the following:

OVERDOSAGE

Symptoms following acute NSAIDs overdoses are usually limited to lethargy, drowsiness, nausea, vomiting, and epigastric pain, which are generally reversible with supportive care. Gastrointestinal bleeding can occur. Hypertension, acute renal failure, respiratory depression and coma may occur, but are rare. Anaphylactoid reactions have been reported with therapeutic ingestion of NSAIDs, and may occur following an overdose.
Patients should be managed by symptomatic and supportive care following a NSAIDs overdose. There are no specific antidotes. Emesis and/or activated charcoal (60 to 100 grams in adults, 1 to 2 grams/kg in children) and/or osmotic cathartic may be indicated in patients seen within 4 hours of ingestion with symptoms or following a large overdose (5 to 10 times the usual dose). Forced diuresis, alkalinization of urine, hemodialysis, or hemoperfusion may not be useful due to high protein binding.
There have been overdoses of up to 25 grams of *Relafen* reported with no long-term sequelae following standard emergency treatment (i.e., activated charcoal, gastric lavage, IV H_2-blockers, etc.).
RL:L11

TIMENTIN® ℞

[tī 'mĕn-tĭn]
brand of sterile ticarcillin disodium and clavulanate potassium for Intravenous Administration

Prescribing information for this product, which appears on pages 3138–3140 of the 2001 PDR, has been revised. Please write "See Supplement A" next to the product heading.
Under ADVERSE REACTIONS, replace subsection Hypersensitivity reactions with the following:
Hypersensitivity reactions: skin rash, pruritus, urticaria, arthralgia, myalgia, drug fever, chills, chest discomfort, erythema multiforme, toxic epidermal necrolysis, Stevens-Johnson Syndrome and anaphylactic reactions
TI:L9IV

To keep your **PDR** up to date throughout the year, note these revisions on the corresponding pages of the annual volume. Simply write **"See Supplement A"** next to the product heading.

TAP Pharmaceuticals Inc.

LAKE FOREST, IL 60045

For Medical Information Contact:
Medical Department
(800) 622-2011 (LUPRON)
(800) 478-9526 (PREVACID)
In Emergencies:
(800) 622-2011 (LUPRON)
(800) 478-9526 (PREVACID)

PREVACID® ℞

[prĕ'-va-sĭd]
(lansoprazole)
Delayed-Release Capsules

Prescribing information for this product, which appears on pages 3189–3194 of the 2001 PDR, has been completely revised as follows. Please write "See Supplement A" next to the product heading.

DESCRIPTION

The active ingredient in PREVACID (lansoprazole) Delayed-Release Capsules is a substituted benzimidazole, 2-[[[3-methyl-4-(2,2,2-trifluoroethoxy)-2-pyridyl] methyl] sulfinyl] benzimidazole, a compound that inhibits gastric acid secretion. Its empirical formula is $C_{16}H_{14}F_3N_3O_2S$ with a molecular weight of 369.37. The structural formula is:

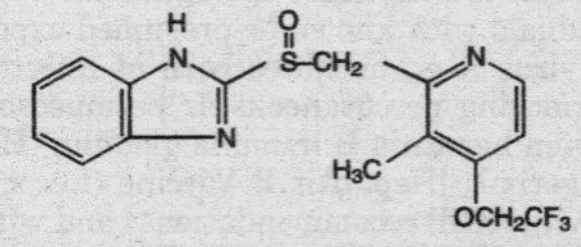

Lansoprazole is a white to brownish-white odorless crystalline powder which melts with decomposition at approximately 166°C. Lansoprazole is freely soluble in dimethylformamide; soluble in methanol; sparingly soluble in ethanol; slightly soluble in ethyl acetate, dichloromethane and acetonitrile; very slightly soluble in ether; and practically insoluble in hexane and water.

Lansoprazole is stable when exposed to light for up to two months. The compound degrades in aqueous solution, the rate of degradation increasing with decreasing pH. At 25°C the $t_{½}$ is approximately 0.5 hour at pH 5.0 and approximately 18 hours at pH 7.0.
PREVACID is supplied in delayed-release capsules for oral administration. The delayed-release capsules contain the active ingredient, lansoprazole, in the form of enteric-coated granules and are available in two dosage strengths: 15 mg and 30 mg of lansoprazole per capsule. Each delayed-release capsule contains enteric-coated granules consisting of lansoprazole, hydroxypropyl cellulose, low substituted hydroxypropyl cellulose, colloidal silicon dioxide, magnesium carbonate, methacrylic acid copolymer, starch, talc, sugar sphere, sucrose, polyethylene glycol, polysorbate 80, and titanium dioxide. Components of the gelatin capsule include gelatin, titanium dioxide, D&C Red No. 28, FD&C Blue No. 1, FD&C Green No. 3*, and FD&C Red No. 40.
* PREVACID 15-mg capsules only.

CLINICAL PHARMACOLOGY

Pharmacokinetics and Metabolism
PREVACID Delayed-Release Capsules contain an enteric-coated granule formulation of lansoprazole. Absorption of lansoprazole begins only after the granules leave the stomach. Absorption is rapid, with mean peak plasma levels of lansoprazole occurring after approximately 1.7 hours. Peak plasma concentrations of lansoprazole (C_{max}) and the area under the plasma concentration curve (AUC) of lansoprazole are approximately proportional in doses from 15 mg to 60 mg after single-oral administration. Lansoprazole does not accumulate and its pharmacokinetics are unaltered by multiple dosing.
Absorption
The absorption of lansoprazole is rapid, with mean C_{max} occurring approximately 1.7 hours after oral dosing, and relatively complete with absolute bioavailability over 80%. In healthy subjects, the mean (± SD) plasma half-life was 1.5 (± 1.0) hours. Both C_{max} and AUC are diminished by about 50% if the drug is given 30 minutes after food as opposed to the fasting condition. There is no significant food effect if the drug is given before meals.
Distribution
Lansoprazole is 97% bound to plasma proteins. Plasma protein binding is constant over the concentration range of 0.05 to 5.0 µg/mL.
Metabolism
Lansoprazole is extensively metabolized in the liver. Two metabolites have been identified in measurable quantities in plasma (the hydroxylated sulfinyl and sulfone derivatives of lansoprazole). These metabolites have very little or no antisecretory activity. Lansoprazole is thought to be transformed into two active species which inhibit acid secretion by (H^+,K^+)-ATPase within the parietal cell canaliculus, but are not present in the systemic circulation. The plasma elimination half-life of lansoprazole does not reflect its duration of suppression of gastric acid secretion. Thus, the plasma elimination half-life is less than two hours, while the acid inhibitory effect lasts more than 24 hours.

Elimination

Following single-dose oral administration of lansoprazole, virtually no unchanged lansoprazole was excreted in the urine. In one study, after a single oral dose of ^{14}C-lansoprazole, approximately one-third of the administered radiation was excreted in the urine and two-thirds was recovered in the feces. This implies a significant biliary excretion of the metabolites of lansoprazole.

Special Populations

Geriatric
The clearance of lansoprazole is decreased in the elderly, with elimination half-life increased approximately 50% to 100%. Because the mean half-life in the elderly remains between 1.9 to 2.9 hours, repeated once daily dosing does not result in accumulation of lansoprazole. Peak plasma levels were not increased in the elderly.

Pediatric
The pharmacokinetics of lansoprazole has not been investigated in patients <18 years of age.

Gender
In a study comparing 12 male and 6 female human subjects, no gender differences were found in pharmacokinetics and intragastric pH results. (Also see **Use in Women.**)

Renal Insufficiency
In patients with severe renal insufficiency, plasma protein binding decreased by 1.0%–1.5% after administration of 60 mg of lansoprazole. Patients with renal insufficiency had a shortened elimination half-life and decreased total AUC (free and bound). AUC for free lansoprazole in plasma, however, was not related to the degree of renal impairment, and C_{max} and T_{max} were not different from subjects with healthy kidneys.

Hepatic Insufficiency
In patients with various degrees of chronic hepatic disease, the mean plasma half-life of the drug was prolonged from 1.5 hours to 3.2–7.2 hours. An increase in mean AUC of up to 500% was observed at steady state in hepatically-impaired patients compared to healthy subjects. Dose reduction in patients with severe hepatic disease should be considered.

Race
The pooled mean pharmacokinetic parameters of lansoprazole from twelve U.S. Phase 1 studies (N=513) were compared to the mean pharmacokinetic parameters from two Asian studies (N=20). The mean AUCs of lansoprazole in Asian subjects were approximately twice those seen in pooled U.S. data; however, the inter-individual variability was high. The C_{max} values were comparable.

Pharmacodynamics

Mechanism of action
Lansoprazole belongs to a class of antisecretory compounds, the substituted benzimidazoles, that do not exhibit anticholinergic or histamine H_2-receptor antagonist properties, but that suppress gastric acid secretion by specific inhibition of the (H^+,K^+)-ATPase enzyme system at the secretory surface of the gastric parietal cell. Because this enzyme system is regarded as the acid (proton) pump within the parietal cell, lansoprazole has been characterized as a gastric acid-pump inhibitor, in that it blocks the final step of acid production. This effect is dose-related and leads to inhibition of both basal and stimulated gastric acid secretion irrespective of the stimulus.

Antisecretory activity
After oral administration, lansoprazole was shown to significantly decrease the basal acid output and significantly increase the mean gastric pH and percent of time the gastric pH was >3 and >4. Lansoprazole also significantly reduced meal-stimulated gastric acid output and secretion volume, as well as pentagastrin-stimulated acid output. In patients with hypersecretion of acid, lansoprazole significantly reduced basal and pentagastrin-stimulated gastric acid secretion. Lansoprazole inhibited the normal increases in secretion volume, acidity and acid output induced by insulin.

In a crossover study comparing lansoprazole 15 and 30 mg with omeprazole 20 mg for five days, the following effects on intragastric pH were noted. See Table 1.

[See table 1 above]

After the initial dose in this study, increased gastric pH was seen within 1–2 hours with lansoprazole 30 mg, 2–3 hours with lansoprazole 15 mg, and 3–4 hours with omeprazole 20 mg. After multiple daily dosing, increased gastric pH was seen within the first hour postdosing with lansoprazole 30 mg and within 1–2 hours postdosing with lansoprazole 15 mg and omeprazole 20 mg.

Acid suppression may enhance the effect of antimicrobials in eradicating Helicobacter pylori (H. pylori). The percentage of time gastric pH was elevated above 5 and 6 was evaluated in a crossover study of PREVACID given q.d., b.i.d. and t.i.d. See Table 2.

Table 2
Mean Antisecretory Effects After 5 Days of b.i.d. and t.i.d. Dosing

	PREVACID			
Parameter	30 mg q.d.	15 mg b.i.d.	30 mg b.i.d.	30 mg t.i.d.
% Time Gastric pH>5	43	47	59[+]	77*

Table 1
Mean Antisecretory Effects after Single and Multiple Daily Dosing

		PREVACID				Omeprazole	
		15 mg		30 mg		20 mg	
Parameter	Baseline Value	Day 1	Day 5	Day 1	Day 5	Day 1	Day 5
Mean 24-Hour pH	2.1	2.7[+]	4.0[+]	3.6*	4.9*	2.5	4.2[+]
Mean Nighttime pH	1.9	2.4	3.0[+]	2.6	3.8*	2.2	3.0[+]
% Time Gastric pH>3	18	33[+]	59[+]	51*	72*	30[+]	61[+]
% Time Gastric pH>4	12	22[+]	49[+]	41*	66*	19	51[+]

NOTE: An intragastric pH of >4 reflects a reduction in gastric acid by 99%.
*(p<0.05) versus baseline, lansoprazole 15 mg and omeprazole 20 mg.
[+](p<0.05) versus baseline only.

Table 3
Clarithromycin Susceptibility Test Results and Clinical/Bacteriological Outcomes[a]

Clarithromycin Pretreatment Results		Clarithromycin Post-treatment Results				
		H. pylori negative-eradicated	H. pylori positive-not eradicated			
			Post-treatment susceptibility results			
			S[b]	I[b]	R[b]	No MIC
Triple Therapy 14-Day (lansoprazole 30 mg b.i.d./amoxicillin 1 gm b.i.d./clarithromycin 500 mg b.i.d.) (M95-399, M93-131, M95-392)						
Susceptible[b]	112	105				7
Intermediate[b]	3	3				
Resistant[b]	17	6			7	4
Triple Therapy 10-Day (lansoprazole 30 mg b.i.d./amoxicillin 1 gm b.i.d./clarithromycin 500 mg b.i.d.) (M95-399)						
Susceptible[b]	42	40	1		1	
Intermediate[b]						
Resistant[b]	4	1			3	

[a] Includes only patients with pretreatment clarithromycin susceptibility test results
[b] Susceptibility (S) MIC ≤ 0.25 µg/mL, Intermediate (I) MIC 0.5–1.0 µg/mL, Resistant (R) MIC ≥ 2 µg/mL

% Time Gastric pH>6	20	23	28	45*

[+] (p<0.05) versus PREVACID 30 mg q.d.
*(p<0.05) versus PREVACID 30 mg q.d., 15 mg b.i.d. and 30 mg b.i.d.

The inhibition of gastric acid secretion as measured by intragastric pH returns gradually to normal over two to four days after multiple doses. There is no indication of rebound gastric acidity.

Enterochromaffin-like (ECL) cell effects
During lifetime exposure of rats with up to 150 mg/kg/day of lansoprazole dosed seven days per week, marked hypergastrinemia was observed followed by ECL cell proliferation and formation of carcinoid tumors, especially in female rats. (See **PRECAUTIONS, Carcinogenesis, Mutagenesis, Impairment of Fertility.**)

Gastric biopsy specimens from the body of the stomach from approximately 150 patients treated continuously with lansoprazole for at least one year did not show evidence of ECL cell effects similar to those seen in rat studies. Longer term data are needed to rule out the possibility of an increased risk of the development of gastric tumors in patients receiving long-term therapy with lansoprazole.

Other gastric effects in humans
Lansoprazole did not significantly affect mucosal blood flow in the fundus of the stomach. Due to the normal physiologic effect caused by the inhibition of gastric acid secretion, a decrease of about 17% in blood flow in the antrum, pylorus, and duodenal bulb was seen. Lansoprazole significantly slowed the gastric emptying of digestible solids. Lansoprazole increased serum pepsinogen levels and decreased pepsin activity under basal conditions and in response to meal stimulation or insulin injection. As with other agents that elevate intragastric pH, increases in gastric pH were associated with increases in nitrate-reducing bacteria and elevation of nitrite concentration in gastric juice in patients with gastric ulcer. No significant increase in nitrosamine concentrations was observed.

Serum gastrin effects
In over 2100 patients, median fasting serum gastrin levels increased 50% to 100% from baseline but remained within normal range after treatment with lansoprazole given orally in doses of 15 mg to 60 mg. These elevations reached a plateau within two months of therapy and returned to pretreatment levels within four weeks after discontinuation of therapy.

Endocrine effects
Human studies for up to one year have not detected any clinically significant effects on the endocrine system. Hormones studied include testosterone, luteinizing hormone (LH), follicle stimulating hormone (FSH), sex hormone binding globulin (SHBG), dehydroepiandrosterone sulfate (DHEA-S), prolactin, cortisol, estradiol, insulin, aldosterone, parathormone, glucagon, thyroid stimulating hormone (TSH), triiodothyronine (T_3), thyroxine (T_4), and somatotropic hormone (STH). Lansoprazole in oral doses of 15 to 60 mg for up to one year had no clinically significant effect on sexual function. In addition, lansoprazole in oral doses of 15 to 60 mg for two to eight weeks had no clinically significant effect on thyroid function.

In 24-month carcinogenicity studies in Sprague-Dawley rats with daily dosages up to 150 mg/kg, proliferative changes in the Leydig cells of the testes, including benign neoplasm, were increased compared to control rates.

Other effects
No systemic effects of lansoprazole on the central nervous system, lymphoid, hematopoietic, renal, hepatic, cardiovascular or respiratory systems have been found in humans. No visual toxicity was observed among 56 patients who had extensive baseline eye evaluations, were treated with up to 180 mg/day of lansoprazole and were observed for up to 58 months. Other rat-specific findings after lifetime exposure included focal pancreatic atrophy, diffuse lymphoid hyperplasia in the thymus, and spontaneous retinal atrophy.

CLINICAL PHARMACOLOGY

Microbiology
Lansoprazole, clarithromycin and/or amoxicillin have been shown to be active against most strains of Helicobacter pylori in vitro and in clinical infections as described in the **INDICATIONS AND USAGE** section.

Helicobacter
Helicobacter pylori

Pretreatment Resistance
Clarithromycin pretreatment resistance (≥ 2.0 µg/mL) was 9.5% (91/960) by E-test and 11.3% (12/106) by agar dilution in the dual and triple therapy clinical trials (M93-125, M93-130, M93-131, M95-392, and M95-399).

Amoxicillin pretreatment susceptible isolates (≤ 0.25 µg/mL) occurred in 97.8% (936/957) and 98.0% (98/100) of the patients in the dual and triple therapy clinical trials by E-test and agar dilution, respectively. Twenty-one of 957 patients (2.2%) by E-test and 2 of 100 patients (2.0%) by agar dilution had amoxicillin pretreatment MICs of > 0.25 µg/mL. One patient on the 14-day triple therapy regimen had an unconfirmed pretreatment amoxicillin minimum inhibitory concentration (MIC) of > 256 µg/mL by E-test and the patient was eradicated of H. pylori. See Table 3.

[See table 3 above]

Patients not eradicated of H. pylori following lansoprazole/amoxicillin/clarithromycin triple therapy will likely have clarithromycin resistant H. pylori. Therefore, for those patients who fail therapy, clarithromycin susceptibility testing should be done when possible. Patients with

Continued on next page

Prevacid—Cont.

clarithromycin resistant *H. pylori* should not be treated with lansoprazole/amoxicillin/clarithromycin triple therapy or with regimens which include clarithromycin as the sole antimicrobial agent.

Amoxicillin Susceptibility Test Results and Clinical/Bacteriological Outcomes

In the dual and triple therapy clinical trials, 82.6% (195/236) of the patients that had pretreatment amoxicillin susceptible MICs (≤ 0.25 µg/mL) were eradicated of *H. pylori*. Of those with pretreatment amoxicillin MICs of > 0.25 µg/mL, three of six had the *H. pylori* eradicated. A total of 30% (21/70) of the patients failed lansoprazole 30 mg t.i.d./amoxicillin 1 gm t.i.d. dual therapy and a total of 12.8% (22/172) of the patients failed the 10- and 14-day triple therapy regimens. Post-treatment susceptibility results were not obtained on 11 of the patients who failed therapy. Nine of the 11 patients with amoxicillin post-treatment MICs that failed the triple therapy regimen also had clarithromycin resistant *H. pylori* isolates.

Susceptibility Test for *Helicobacter pylori*

The reference methodology for susceptibility testing of *H. pylori* is agar dilution MICs.[1] One to three microliters of an inoculum equivalent to a No. 2 McFarland standard (1×10^7 - 1×10^8 CFU/mL for *H. pylori*) are inoculated directly onto freshly prepared antimicrobial containing Mueller-Hinton agar plates with 5% aged defibrinated sheep blood (≥ 2 weeks old). The agar dilution plates are incubated at 35°C in a microaerobic environment produced by a gas generating system suitable for campylobacters. After 3 days of incubation, the MICs are recorded as the lowest concentration of antimicrobial agent required to inhibit growth of the organism. The clarithromycin and amoxicillin MIC values should be interpreted according to the following criteria:

Clarithromycin MIC (µg/mL)[a]	Interpretation
≤ 0.25	Susceptible (S)
0.5–1.0	Intermediate (I)
≥ 2.0	Resistant (R)

Amoxicillin MIC (µg/mL)[b]	Interpretation
≤ 0.25	Susceptible (S)

[a] These are tentative breakpoints for the agar dilution methodology and they should not be used to interpret results obtained using alternative methods.

[b] There were not enough organisms with MICs > 0.25 µg/mL to determine a resistance breakpoint.

Standardized susceptibility test procedures require the use of laboratory control microorganisms to control the technical aspects of the laboratory procedures. Standard clarithromycin and amoxicillin powders should provide the following MIC values:

Microorganism	Antimicrobial Agent	MIC (µg/mL)[a]
H. pylori ATCC 43504	Clarithromycin	0.015–0.12 mcg/mL
H. pylori ATCC 43504	Amoxicillin	0.015–0.12 mcg/mL

[a] These are quality control ranges for the agar dilution methodology and they should not be used to control test results obtained using alternative methods.

Reference

1. National Committee for Clinical Laboratory Standards. Summary Minutes, Subcommittee on Antimicrobial Susceptibility Testing, Tampa, FL, January 11–13, 1998.

CLINICAL STUDIES

Duodenal Ulcer

In a U.S. multicenter, double-blind, placebo-controlled, dose-response (15, 30, and 60 mg of PREVACID once daily) study of 284 patients with endoscopically documented duodenal ulcer, the percentage of patients healed after two and four weeks was significantly higher with all doses of PREVACID than with placebo. There was no evidence of a greater or earlier response with the two higher doses compared with PREVACID 15 mg. Based on this study and the second study described below, the recommended dose of PREVACID in duodenal ulcer is 15 mg per day. See Table 4.
[See table 4 above]

PREVACID 15 mg was significantly more effective than placebo in relieving day and nighttime abdominal pain and in decreasing the amount of antacid taken per day.

In a second U.S. multicenter study, also double-blind, placebo-controlled, dose-comparison (15 and 30 mg of PREVACID once daily), and including a comparison with ranitidine, in 280 patients with endoscopically documented duodenal ulcer, the percentage of patients healed after four weeks was significantly higher with both doses of PREVACID than with placebo. There was no evidence of a greater or earlier response with the higher dose of PREVACID. Although the 15 mg dose of PREVACID was superior to ranitidine at 4 weeks, the lack of significant difference at 2 weeks and the absence of a difference between 30 mg of PREVACID and ranitidine leaves the comparative effectiveness of the two agents undetermined. See Table 5.
[See table 5 above]

H. pylori Eradication to Reduce the Risk of Duodenal Ulcer Recurrence

Randomized, double-blind clinical studies performed in the U.S. in patients with *H. pylori* and duodenal ulcer disease

Table 4
Duodenal Ulcer Healing Rates

	PREVACID			Placebo
Week	15 mg q.d. (N=68)	30 mg q.d. (N=74)	60 mg q.d. (N=70)	(N=72)
2	42.4%*	35.6%*	39.1%*	11.3%
4	89.4%*	91.7%*	89.9%*	46.1%

*(p≤0.001) versus placebo.

Table 5
Duodenal Ulcer Healing Rates

	PREVACID		Ranitidine	Placebo
Week	15 mg q.d. (N=80)	30 mg q.d. (N=77)	300 mg h.s. (N=82)	(N=41)
2	35.0%	44.2%	30.5%	34.2%
4	92.3%**	80.3%*	70.5%*	47.5%

*(p≤0.05) versus placebo.
**(p≤0.05) versus placebo and ranitidine.

Table 6
H. pylori Eradication Rates—Triple Therapy
(PREVACID/amoxicillin/clarithromycin)
Percent of Patients Cured
[95% Confidence Interval]
(Number of Patients)

Study	Duration	Triple Therapy Evaluable Analysis*	Triple Therapy Intent-to-Treat Analysis#
M93-131	14 days	92[†] [80.0–97.7] (N=48)	86[†] [73.3–93.5] (N=55)
M95-392	14 days	86[‡] [75.7–93.6] (N=66)	83[‡] [72.0–90.8] (N=70)
M95-399[+]	14 days	85 [77.0–91.0] (N=113)	82 [73.9–88.1] (N=126)
	10 days	84 [76.0–89.8] (N=123)	81 [73.9–87.6] (N=135)

* Based on evaluable patients with confirmed duodenal ulcer (active or within one year) and *H. pylori* infection at baseline defined as at least two of three positive endoscopic tests from CLOtest® (Delta West Ltd., Bentley, Australia), histology and/or culture. Patients were included in the analysis if they completed the study. Additionally, if patients dropped out of the study due to an adverse event related to the study drug, they were included in the evaluable analysis as failures of therapy.

Patients were included in the analysis if they had documented *H. pylori* infection at baseline as defined above and had a confirmed duodenal ulcer (active or within one year). All dropouts were included as failures of therapy.

† (p<0.05) versus PREVACID/amoxicillin and PREVACID/clarithromycin dual therapy

‡ (p<0.05) versus clarithromcyin/amoxicillin dual therapy

+ The 95% confidence interval for the difference in eradication rates, 10-day minus 14-day is (-10.5, 8.1) in the evaluable analysis and (-9.7, 9.1) in the intent-to-treat analysis.

Table 7
H. pylori Eradication Rates—14-Day Dual Therapy
(PREVACID/amoxicillin)
Percent of Patients Cured
[95% Confidence Interval]
(Number of Patients)

Study	Dual Therapy Evaluable Analysis*	Dual Therapy Intent-to-Treat Analysis#
M93-131	77[†] [62.5–87.2] (N=51)	70[†] [56.8–81.2] (N=60)
M93-125	66[‡] [51.9–77.5] (N=58)	61[‡] [48.5–72.9] (N=67)

* Based on evaluable patients with confirmed duodenal ulcer (active or within one year) and *H. pylori* infection at baseline defined as at least two of three positive endoscopic tests from CLOtest®, histology and/or culture. Patients were included in the analysis if they completed the study. Additionally, if patients dropped out of the study due to an adverse event related to the study drug, they were included in the analysis as failures of therapy.

Patients were included in the analysis if they had documented *H. pylori* infection at baseline as defined above and had a confirmed duodenal ulcer (active or within one year). All dropouts were included as failures of therapy.

† (p<0.05) versus PREVACID alone.

‡ (p<0.05) versus PREVACID alone or amoxicillin alone.

(defined as an active ulcer or history of an ulcer within one year) evaluated the efficacy of PREVACID in combination with amoxicillin capsules and clarithromycin tablets as triple 14-day therapy or in combination with amoxicillin capsules as dual 14-day therapy for the eradication of *H. pylori*. Based on the results of these studies, the safety and efficacy of two different eradication regimens were established:

Triple therapy: PREVACID 30 mg b.i.d./amoxicillin 1 gm b.i.d./clarithromycin 500 mg b.i.d.

Dual therapy: PREVACID 30 mg t.i.d./amoxicillin 1 gm t.i.d.

All treatments were for 14 days. *H. pylori* eradication was defined as two negative tests (culture and histology) at 4–6 weeks following the end of treatment.

Triple therapy was shown to be more effective than all possible dual therapy combinations. Dual therapy was shown to be more effective than both monotherapies. Eradication of *H. pylori* has been shown to reduce the risk of duodenal ulcer recurrence.

A randomized, double-blind clinical study performed in the U.S. in patients with *H. pylori* and duodenal ulcer disease (defined as an active ulcer or history of an ulcer within one year) compared the efficacy of PREVACID triple therapy for 10 and 14 days. This study established that the 10-day triple therapy was equivalent to the 14-day triple therapy in eradicating *H. pylori*. See Tables 6 and 7.
[See table 6 at middle of previous page]
[See table 7 at middle of previous page]

Long-Term Maintenance Treatment of Duodenal Ulcers
PREVACID has been shown to prevent the recurrence of duodenal ulcers. Two independent, double-blind, multicenter, controlled trials were conducted in patients with endoscopically confirmed healed duodenal ulcers. Patients remained healed significantly longer and the number of recurrences of duodenal ulcers was significantly less in patients treated with PREVACID than in patients treated with placebo over a 12-month period.
In trial #2, no significant difference was noted between PREVACID 15 mg and 30 mg in maintaining remission. See Table 8.
[See table 8 above]

Gastric Ulcer
In a U.S. multicenter, double-blind, placebo-controlled study of 253 patients with endoscopically documented gastric ulcer, the percentage of patients healed at four and eight weeks was significantly higher with PREVACID 15 mg and 30 mg once a day than with placebo.
Patients treated with any PREVACID dose reported significantly less day and night abdominal pain along with fewer days of antacid use and fewer antacid tablets used per day than the placebo group.
Independent substantiation of the effectiveness of PREVACID 30 mg was provided by a meta-analysis of published and unpublished data. See Table 9.
[See table 9 above]

Healing of NSAID-Associated Gastric Ulcer
In two U.S. and Canadian multicenter, double-blind, active-controlled studies in patients with endoscopically confirmed NSAID-associated gastric ulcer who continued their NSAID use, the percentage of patients healed after 8 weeks was statistically significantly higher with 30 mg of PREVACID than with the active control. A total of 711 patients were enrolled in the study, and 701 patients were treated. Patients ranged in age from 18 to 88 years (median age 59 years), with 67% female patients and 33% male patients. Race was distributed as follows: 87% Caucasian, 8% Black, 5% other. There was no statistically significant difference between PREVACID 30 mg q.d. and the active control on symptom relief (i.e., abdominal pain).
[See third table above]

Risk Reduction of NSAID-Associated Gastric Ulcer
In one large U.S., multicenter, double-blind, placebo- and misoprostol-controlled (misoprostol blinded only to the endoscopist) study in patients who required chronic use of an NSAID and who had a history of an endoscopically documented gastric ulcer, the proportion of patients remaining free from gastric ulcer at 4, 8, and 12 weeks was significantly higher with 15 or 30 mg of PREVACID than placebo. A total of 537 patients were enrolled in the study, and 535 patients were treated. Patients ranged in age from 23 to 89 years (median age 60 years), with 65% female patients and 35% male patients. Race was distributed as follows: 90% Caucasian, 6% Black, 4% other. The 30 mg dose of PREVACID demonstrated no additional benefit in risk reduction of the NSAID-associated gastric ulcer than the 15 mg dose.
[See fourth table above]

Gastroesophageal Reflux Disease (GERD)
Symptomatic GERD
In a U.S. multicenter, double-blind, placebo-controlled study of 214 patients with frequent GERD symptoms, but no esophageal erosions by endoscopy, significantly greater relief of heartburn associated with GERD was observed with the administration of lansoprazole 15 mg once daily up to 8 weeks than with placebo. No significant additional benefit from lansoprazole 30 mg once daily was observed.
The intent-to-treat analyses demonstrated significant reduction in frequency and severity of day and night heartburn. Data for frequency and severity for the 8-week treatment period are shown in Table 10 and Figures 1 and 2.
[See table 10 at top of next page]

Figure 1
Mean Severity of Day Heartburn By Study Day For Evaluable Patients
(3=Severe, 2=Moderate, 1=Mild, 0=None)

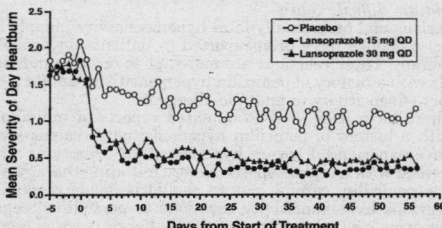

[See figure at top of next column]
In two U.S., multi-center double-blind, ranitidine-controlled studies of 925 total patients with frequent GERD symptoms, but no esophageal erosions by endoscopy, lansoprazole 15 mg was superior to ranitidine 150 mg (b.i.d.) in decreas-

Table 8
Endoscopic Remission Rates

Trial	Drug	No. of Pts.	Percent in Endoscopic Remission 0–3 mo.	0–6 mo.	0–12 mo.
#1	PREVACID 15 mg q.d.	86	90%*	87%*	84%*
	Placebo	83	49%	41%	39%
#2	PREVACID 30 mg q.d.	18	94%*	94%*	85%*
	PREVACID 15 mg q.d.	15	87%*	79%*	70%*
	Placebo	15	33%	0%	0%

%=Life Table Estimate
*(p≤0.001) versus placebo.

Table 9
Gastric Ulcer Healing Rates

Week	PREVACID 15 mg q.d. (N=65)	30 mg q.d. (N=63)	60 mg q.d. (N=61)	Placebo (N=64)
4	64.6%*	58.1%*	53.3%*	37.5%
8	92.2%*	96.8%*	93.2%*	76.7%

*(p≤0.05) versus placebo.

NSAID-Associated Gastric Ulcer Healing Rates[1]

	Study #1	
	PREVACID 30 mg q.d.	Active Control[2]
Week 4	60% (53/88)[3]	28% (23/83)
Week 8	79% (62/79)[3]	55% (41/74)
	Study #2	
	PREVACID 30 mg q.d.	Active Control[2]
Week 4	53% (40/75)	38% (31/82)
Week 8	77% (47/61)[3]	50% (33/66)

[1] Actual observed ulcer(s) healed at time points ±2 days
[2] Dose for healing of gastric ulcer
[3] (p≤0.05) versus the active control

NSAID-Associated Gastric Ulcer Risk Reduction Rates

	% of Patients Remaining Gastric Ulcer-Free[1]			
Week	PREVACID 15 mg q.d. (N=121)	PREVACID 30 mg q.d. (N=116)	Misoprostol 200 mcg q.i.d. (N=106)	Placebo (N=112)
4	90%	92%	96%	66%
8	86%	88%	95%	60%
12	80%	82%	93%	51%

[1] %=Life Table Estimate
(p<0.001) PREVACID 15 mg q.d. versus placebo; PREVACID 30 mg q.d. versus placebo; and misoprostol 200 mcg q.i.d. versus placebo.
(p<0.05) Misoprostol 200 mcg q.i.d. versus PREVACID 15 mg q.d.; and misoprostol 200 mcg q.i.d. versus PREVACID 30 mg q.d.

Figure 2
Mean Severity of Night Heartburn By Study Day For Evaluable Patients
(3=Severe, 2=Moderate, 1=Mild, 0=None)

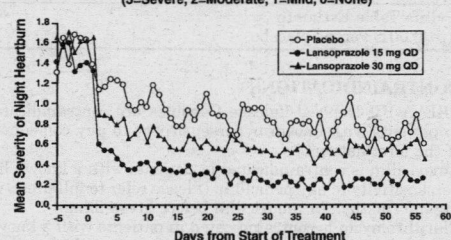

ing the frequency and severity of day and night heartburn associated with GERD for the 8 week treatment period. No significant additional benefit from lansoprazole 30 mg once daily was observed.

Erosive Esophagitis
In a U.S. multicenter, double-blind, placebo-controlled study of 269 patients entering with an endoscopic diagnosis of esophagitis with mucosal grading of 2 or more and grades 3 and 4 signifying erosive disease, the percentages of patients with healing were as shown in Table 11.
[See table 11 at top of next page]
In this study, all PREVACID groups reported significantly greater relief of heartburn and less day and night abdominal pain along with fewer days of antacid use and fewer antacid tablets taken per day than the placebo group.
Although all doses were effective, the earlier healing in the higher two doses suggests 30 mg q.d. as the recommended dose.
PREVACID was also compared in a U.S. multicenter, double-blind study to a low dose of ranitidine in 242 patients

with erosive reflux esophagitis. PREVACID at a dose of 30 mg was significantly more effective than ranitidine 150 mg b.i.d. as shown in Table 12.
[See table 12 at top of next page]
In addition, patients treated with PREVACID reported less day and nighttime heartburn and took less antacid tablets for fewer days than patients taking ranitidine 150 mg b.i.d. Although this study demonstrates effectiveness of PREVACID in healing erosive esophagitis, it does not represent an adequate comparison with ranitidine because the recommended ranitidine dose for esophagitis is 150 mg q.i.d., twice the dose used in this study.
In the two trials described and in several smaller studies involving patients with moderate to severe erosive esophagitis, PREVACID produced healing rates similar to those shown above.
In a U.S. multicenter, double-blind, active-controlled study, 30 mg of PREVACID was compared with ranitidine 150 mg b.i.d. in 151 patients with erosive reflux esophagitis that was poorly responsive to a minimum of 12 weeks of treatment with at least one H_2-receptor antagonist given at the dose indicated for symptom relief or greater, namely, cimetidine 800 mg/day, ranitidine 300 mg/day, famotidine 40 mg/day or nizatidine 300 mg/day. PREVACID 30 mg was more effective than ranitidine 150 mg b.i.d. in healing reflux esophagitis, and the percentage of patients with healing were as shown in Table 13. This study does not constitute a comparison of the effectiveness of histamine H_2-receptor antagonists with PREVACID, as all patients had demonstrated unresponsiveness to the histamine H_2-receptor antagonist mode of treatment. It does indicate, however, that PREVACID may be useful in patients failing on a histamine H_2-receptor antagonist.
[See table 13 at middle of next page]

Continued on next page

Prevacid—Cont.

Long-Term Maintenance Treatment of Erosive Esophagitis
Two independent, double-blind, multicenter, controlled trials were conducted in patients with endoscopically confirmed healed esophagitis. Patients remained in remission significantly longer and the number of recurrences of erosive esophagitis was significantly less in patients treated with PREVACID than in patients treated with placebo over a 12-month period. See Table 14.
[See table 14 to the right]
Regardless of initial grade of erosive esophagitis, PREVACID 15 mg and 30 mg were similar in maintaining remission.

Pathological Hypersecretory Conditions Including Zollinger-Ellison Syndrome
In open studies of 57 patients with pathological hypersecretory conditions, such as Zollinger-Ellison (ZE) syndrome with or without multiple endocrine adenomas, PREVACID significantly inhibited gastric acid secretion and controlled associated symptoms of diarrhea, anorexia and pain. Doses ranging from 15 mg every other day to 180 mg per day maintained basal acid secretion below 10 mEq/hr in patients without prior gastric surgery and below 5 mEq/hr in patients with prior gastric surgery.
Initial doses were titrated to the individual patient need, and adjustments were necessary with time in some patients. (See **DOSAGE AND ADMINISTRATION**.) PREVACID was well tolerated at these high dose levels for prolonged periods (greater than four years in some patients). In most ZE patients, serum gastrin levels were not modified by PREVACID. However, in some patients, serum gastrin increased to levels greater than those present prior to initiation of lansoprazole therapy.

INDICATIONS AND USAGE

Short-Term Treatment of Active Duodenal Ulcer
PREVACID Delayed-Release Capsules are indicated for short-term treatment (up to 4 weeks) for healing and symptom relief of active duodenal ulcer.

H. pylori Eradication to Reduce the Risk of Duodenal Ulcer Recurrence

Triple Therapy: PREVACID/amoxicillin/clarithromycin
PREVACID Delayed-Release Capsules, in combination with amoxicillin plus clarithromycin as triple therapy, are indicated for the treatment of patients with *H. pylori* infection and duodenal ulcer disease (active or one-year history of a duodenal ulcer) to eradicate *H. pylori*. Eradication of *H. pylori* has been shown to reduce the risk of duodenal ulcer recurrence. (See **CLINICAL STUDIES** and **DOSAGE AND ADMINISTRATION**.)

Dual Therapy: PREVACID/amoxicillin
PREVACID Delayed-Release Capsules, in combination with amoxicillin as dual therapy, are indicated for the treatment of patients with *H. pylori* infection and duodenal ulcer disease (active or one-year history of a duodenal ulcer) **who are either allergic or intolerant to clarithromycin or in whom resistance to clarithromycin is known or suspected.** (See the clarithromycin package insert, **MICROBIOLOGY** section.) Eradication of *H. pylori* has been shown to reduce the risk of duodenal ulcer recurrence. (See **CLINICAL STUDIES** and **DOSAGE AND ADMINISTRATION**.)

Maintenance of Healed Duodenal Ulcers
PREVACID Delayed-Release Capsules are indicated to maintain healing of duodenal ulcers. Controlled studies do not extend beyond 12 months.

Short-Term Treatment of Active Benign Gastric Ulcer
PREVACID Delayed-Release Capsules are indicated for short-term treatment (up to 8 weeks) for healing and symptom relief of active benign gastric ulcer.

Healing of NSAID-Associated Gastric Ulcer
PREVACID Delayed-Release Capsules are indicated for the treatment of NSAID-associated gastric ulcer in patients who continue NSAID use. Controlled studies did not extend beyond 8 weeks.

Risk Reduction of NSAID-Associated Gastric Ulcer
PREVACID Delayed-Release Capsules are indicated for reducing the risk of NSAID-associated gastric ulcers in patients with a history of a documented gastric ulcer who require the use of an NSAID. Controlled studies did not extend beyond 12 weeks.

Gastroesophageal Reflux Disease (GERD)

Short-Term Treatment of Symptomatic GERD
PREVACID Delayed-Release Capsules are indicated for the treatment of heartburn and other symptoms associated with GERD.

Short-Term Treatment of Erosive Esophagitis
PREVACID Delayed-Release Capsules are indicated for short-term treatment (up to 8 weeks) for healing and symptom relief of all grades of erosive esophagitis.
For patients who do not heal with PREVACID for 8 weeks (5-10%), it may be helpful to give an additional 8 weeks of treatment.
If there is a recurrence of erosive esophagitis an additional 8-week course of PREVACID may be considered.

Maintenance of Healing of Erosive Esophagitis
PREVACID Delayed-Release Capsules are indicated to maintain healing of erosive esophagitis. Controlled studies did not extend beyond 12 months.

Pathological Hypersecretory Conditions Including Zollinger-Ellison Syndrome
PREVACID Delayed-Release Capsules are indicated for the long-term treatment of pathological hypersecretory conditions, including Zollinger-Ellison syndrome.

Table 10
Frequency of Heartburn

Variable	Placebo (n=43)	PREVACID 15 mg (n=80)	PREVACID 30 mg (n=86)
		Median	
% of Days without Heartburn			
Week 1	0%	71%*	46%*
Week 4	11%	81%*	76%*
Week 8	13%	84%*	82%*
% of Nights without Heartburn			
Week 1	17%	86%*	57%*
Week 4	25%	89%*	73%*
Week 8	36%	92%*	80%*

*($p<0.01$) versus placebo.

Table 11
Erosive Esophagitis Healing Rates

Week	PREVACID 15 mg q.d. (N=69)	PREVACID 30 mg q.d. (N=65)	PREVACID 60 mg q.d. (N=72)	Placebo (N=63)
4	67.6%*	81.3%**	80.6%**	32.8%
6	87.7%*	95.4%*	94.3%*	52.5%
8	90.9%*	95.4%*	94.4%*	52.5%

*($p \leq 0.001$) versus placebo.
**($p \leq 0.05$) versus PREVACID 15 mg and placebo.

Table 12
Erosive Esophagitis Healing Rates

Week	PREVACID 30 mg q.d. (N=115)	Ranitidine 150 mg b.i.d. (N=127)
2	66.7%*	38.7%
4	82.5%*	52.0%
6	93.0%*	67.8%
8	92.1%*	69.9%

*($p \leq 0.001$) versus ranitidine.

Table 13
Reflux Esophagitis Healing Rates in Patients Poorly Responsive to Histamine H_2-Receptor Antagonist Therapy

Week	PREVACID 30 mg q.d. (N=100)	Ranitidine 150 mg b.i.d. (N=51)
4	74.7%*	42.6%
8	83.7%*	32.0%

*($p \leq 0.001$) versus ranitidine.

Table 14
Endoscopic Remission Rates

Trial	Drug	No. of Pts.	Percent in Endoscopic Remission 0–3 mo.	0–6 mo.	0–12 mo.
#1	PREVACID 15 mg q.d.	59	83%*	81%*	79%*
	PREVACID 30 mg q.d.	56	93%*	93%*	90%*
	Placebo	55	31%	27%	24%
#2	PREVACID 15 mg q.d.	50	74%*	72%*	67%*
	PREVACID 30 mg q.d.	49	75%*	72%*	55%*
	Placebo	47	16%	13%	13%

%=Life Table Estimate
*($p \leq 0.001$) versus placebo.

CONTRAINDICATIONS
PREVACID Delayed-Release Capsules are contraindicated in patients with known hypersensitivity to any component of the formulation.
Amoxicillin is contraindicated in patients with a known hypersensitivity to any penicillin. (Please refer to full prescribing information for amoxicillin before prescribing.)
Clarithromycin is contraindicated in patients with a known hypersensitivity to any macrolide antibiotic, and in patients receiving terfenadine therapy who have preexisting cardiac abnormalities or electrolyte disturbances. (Please refer to full prescribing information for clarithromycin before prescribing.)

WARNINGS
CLARITHROMYCIN SHOULD NOT BE USED IN PREGNANT WOMEN EXCEPT IN CLINICAL CIRCUMSTANCES WHERE NO ALTERNATIVE THERAPY IS APPROPRIATE. IF PREGNANCY OCCURS WHILE TAKING CLARITHROMYCIN, THE PATIENT SHOULD BE APPRISED OF THE POTENTIAL HAZARD TO THE FETUS. (SEE **WARNINGS** IN PRESCRIBING INFORMATION FOR CLARITHROMYCIN.)
Pseudomembranous colitis has been reported with nearly all antibacterial agents, including clarithromycin and amoxicillin, and may range in severity from mild to life threatening. Therefore, it is important to consider this diagnosis in patients who present with diarrhea subsequent to the administration of antibacterial agents.
Treatment with antibacterial agents alters the normal flora of the colon and may permit overgrowth of clostridia. Studies indicate that a toxin produced by *Clostridium difficile* is a primary cause of "antibiotic-associated colitis."
After the diagnosis of pseudomembranous colitis has been established, therapeutic measures should be initiated. Mild cases of pseudomembranous colitis usually respond to discontinuation of the drug alone. In moderate to severe cases, consideration should be given to management with fluids and electrolytes, protein supplementation, and treatment with an antibacterial drug clinically effective against *Clostridium difficile* colitis.
Serious and occasionally fatal hypersensitivity (anaphylactic) reactions have been reported in patients on penicillin therapy. These reactions are more apt to occur in individuals with a history of penicillin hypersensitivity and/or a history of sensitivity to multiple allergens.
There have been well-documented reports of individuals with a history of penicillin hypersensitivity reactions who have experienced severe hypersensitivity reactions when treated with a cephalosporin. Before initiating therapy with any penicillin, careful inquiry should be made concerning previous hypersensitivity reactions to penicillins, cephalosporins, and other allergens. If an allergic reaction occurs, amoxicillin should be discontinued and the appropriate therapy instituted.
SERIOUS ANAPHYLACTIC REACTIONS REQUIRE IMMEDIATE EMERGENCY TREATMENT WITH EPINEPHRINE. OXYGEN, INTRAVENOUS STEROIDS, AND AIRWAY MANAGEMENT, INCLUDING INTUBATION, SHOULD ALSO BE ADMINISTERED AS INDICATED.

PRECAUTIONS

General

Symptomatic response to therapy with lansoprazole does not preclude the presence of gastric malignancy.

Information for Patients

PREVACID Delayed-Release Capsules should be taken before eating.

Alternative Administration Options

For patients who have difficulty swallowing capsules, PREVACID Delayed-Release Capsules can be opened, and the intact granules contained within can be sprinkled on one tablespoon of either applesauce, ENSURE® pudding, cottage cheese, yogurt, or strained pears and swallowed immediately. The granules should not be chewed or crushed. Alternatively, PREVACID Delayed-Release Capsules may be emptied into a small volume of either orange juice or tomato juice (60 mL – approximately 2 ounces), mixed briefly and swallowed immediately. To insure complete delivery of the dose, the glass should be rinsed with two or more volumes of juice and the contents swallowed immediately. The granules have also been shown *in vitro* to remain intact when exposed to apple, cranberry, grape, orange, pineapple, prune, tomato, and V-8® vegetable juice and stored for up to 30 minutes.

For patients who have a nasogastric tube in place, PREVACID Delayed-Release Capsules can be opened and the intact granules mixed in 40 mL of apple juice and injected through the nasogastric tube into the stomach. After administering the granules, the nasogastric tube should be flushed with additional apple juice to clear the tube.

Drug Interactions

Lansoprazole is metabolized through the cytochrome P_{450} system, specifically through the CYP3A and CYP2C19 isozymes. Studies have shown that lansoprazole does not have clinically significant interactions with other drugs metabolized by the cytochrome P_{450} system, such as warfarin, antipyrine, indomethacin, ibuprofen, phenytoin, propranolol, prednisone, diazepam, clarithromycin, or terfenadine in healthy subjects. These compounds are metabolized through various cytochrome P_{450} isozymes including CYP1A2, CYP2C9, CYP2C19, CYP2D6, and CYP3A. When lansoprazole was administered concomitantly with theophylline (CYP1A2, CYP3A), a minor increase (10%) in the clearance of theophylline was seen. Because of the small magnitude and the direction of the effect on theophylline clearance, this interaction is unlikely to be of clinical concern. Nonetheless, individual patients may require additional titration of their theophylline dosage when lansoprazole is started or stopped to ensure clinically effective blood levels.

Lansoprazole has also been shown to have no clinically significant interaction with amoxicillin.

In a single-dose crossover study examining lansoprazole 30 mg and omeprazole 20 mg each administered alone and concomitantly with sucralfate 1 gram, absorption of the proton pump inhibitors was delayed and their bioavailability was reduced by 17% and 16%, respectively, when administered concomitantly with sucralfate. Therefore, proton pump inhibitors should be taken at least 30 minutes prior to sucralfate. In clinical trials, antacids were administered concomitantly with PREVACID Delayed-Release Capsules; this did not interfere with its effect.

Lansoprazole causes a profound and long-lasting inhibition of gastric acid secretion; therefore, it is theoretically possible that lansoprazole may interfere with the absorption of drugs where gastric pH is an important determinant of bioavailability (eg, ketoconazole, ampicillin esters, iron salts, digoxin).

Carcinogenesis, Mutagenesis, Impairment of Fertility

In two 24-month carcinogenicity studies, Sprague-Dawley rats were treated orally with doses of 5 to 150 mg/kg/day, about 1 to 40 times the exposure on a body surface (mg/m^2) basis, of a 50-kg person of average height (1.46 m^2 body surface area) given the recommended human dose of 30 mg/day (22.2 mg/m^2). Lansoprazole produced dose-related gastric enterochromaffin-like (ECL) cell hyperplasia and ECL cell carcinoids in both male and female rats. It also increased the incidence of intestinal metaplasia of the gastric epithelium in both sexes. In male rats, lansoprazole produced a dose-related increase of testicular interstitial cell adenomas. The incidence of these adenomas in rats receiving doses of 15 to 150 mg/kg/day (4 to 40 times the recommended human dose based on body surface area) exceeded the low background incidence (range = 1.4 to 10%) for this strain of rat. Testicular interstitial cell adenoma also occurred in 1 of 30 rats treated with 50 mg/kg/day (13 times the recommended human dose based on body surface area) in a 1-year toxicity study.

In a 24-month carcinogenicity study, CD-1 mice were treated orally with doses of 15 to 600 mg/kg/day, 2 to 80 times the recommended human dose based on body surface area. Lansoprazole produced a dose-related increased incidence of gastric ECL cell hyperplasia. It also produced an increased incidence of liver tumors (hepatocellular adenoma plus carcinoma). The tumor incidences in male mice treated with 300 and 600 mg/kg/day (40 to 80 times the recommended human dose based on body surface area) and female mice treated with 150 to 600 mg/kg/day (20 to 80 times the recommended human dose based on body surface area) exceeded the ranges of background incidences in historical controls for this strain of mice. Lansoprazole treatment produced adenoma of rete testis in male mice receiving 75 to 600 mg/kg/day (10 to 80 times the recommended human dose based on body surface area).

Table 15
Incidence of Possibly or Probably
Treatment-Related Adverse Events in Short-Term, Placebo-Controlled Studies

Body System/Adverse Event	PREVACID (N=1457) %	Placebo (N=467) %
Body as a Whole		
Abdominal Pain	1.8	1.3
Digestive System		
Diarrhea	3.6	2.6
Nausea	1.4	1.3

Lansoprazole was not genotoxic in the Ames test, the *ex vivo* rat hepatocyte unscheduled DNA synthesis (UDS) test, the *in vivo* mouse micronucleus test or the rat bone marrow cell chromosomal aberration test. It was positive in *in vitro* human lymphocyte chromosomal aberration assays.

Lansoprazole at oral doses up to 150 mg/kg/day (40 times the recommended human dose based on body surface area) was found to have no effect on fertility and reproductive performance of male and female rats.

Pregnancy: Teratogenic Effects.

Pregnancy Category B

Lansoprazole

Teratology studies have been performed in pregnant rats at oral doses up to 150 mg/kg/day (40 times the recommended human dose based on body surface area) and pregnant rabbits at oral doses up to 30 mg/kg/day (16 times the recommended human dose based on body surface area) and have revealed no evidence of impaired fertility or harm to the fetus due to lansoprazole.

There are, however, no adequate or well-controlled studies in pregnant women. Because animal reproduction studies are not always predictive of human response, this drug should be used during pregnancy only if clearly needed.

Pregnancy Category C

Clarithromycin

See **WARNINGS** (above) and full prescribing information for clarithromycin before using in pregnant women.

Nursing Mothers

Lansoprazole or its metabolites are excreted in the milk of rats. It is not known whether lansoprazole is excreted in human milk. Because many drugs are excreted in human milk, because of the potential for serious adverse reactions in nursing infants from lansoprazole, and because of the potential for tumorigenicity shown for lansoprazole in rat carcinogenicity studies, a decision should be made whether to discontinue nursing or to discontinue the drug, taking into account the importance of the drug to the mother.

Pediatric Use

Safety and effectiveness in pediatric patients have not been established.

Use in Women

Over 800 women were treated with lansoprazole. Ulcer healing rates in females were similar to those in males. The incidence rates of adverse events were also similar to those seen in males.

Use in Geriatric Patients

Ulcer healing rates in elderly patients are similar to those in a younger age group. The incidence rates of adverse events and laboratory test abnormalities are also similar to those seen in younger patients. For elderly patients, dosage and administration of lansoprazole need not be altered for a particular indication.

ADVERSE REACTIONS

Clinical

Worldwide, over 6100 patients have been treated with lansoprazole in Phase 2–3 clinical trials involving various dosages and durations of treatment. In general, lansoprazole treatment has been well-tolerated in both short-term and long-term trials.

The following adverse events shown in Table 15, were reported by the treating physician to have a possible or probable relationship to drug in 1% or more of PREVACID-treated patients and occurred at a greater rate in PREVACID-treated patients than placebo-treated patients:

[See table above]

Headache was also seen at greater than 1% incidence but was more common on placebo. The incidence of diarrhea was similar between patients who received placebo and patients who received lansoprazole 15 mg and 30 mg, but higher in the patients who received lansoprazole 60 mg (2.9%, 1.4%, 4.2%, and 7.4%, respectively).

The most commonly reported possibly or probably treatment-related adverse event during maintenance therapy was diarrhea.

In the risk reduction study of PREVACID for NSAID-associated gastric ulcers, the incidence of diarrhea for patients treated with PREVACID was 5%, misoprostol 22%, and placebo 3%.

Additional adverse experiences occurring in <1% of patients or subjects in domestic trials are shown below. Refer to **Postmarketing** for adverse reactions occurring since the drug was marketed.

Body as a Whole—asthenia, candidiasis, chest pain (not otherwise specified), edema, fever, flu syndrome, halitosis, infection (not otherwise specified), malaise; *Cardiovascular System*—angina, cerebrovascular accident, hypertension/hypotension, myocardial infarction, palpitations, shock (circulatory failure), vasodilation; *Digestive System*—anorexia, bezoar, cardiospasm, cholelithiasis, constipation, dry mouth/thirst, dyspepsia, dysphagia, eructation, esophageal stenosis, esophageal ulcer, esophagitis, fecal discoloration, flatulence, gastric nodules/fundic gland polyps, gastroenteritis, gastrointestinal hemorrhage, hematemesis, increased appetite, increased salivation, melena, rectal hemorrhage, stomatitis, tenesmus, ulcerative colitis; *Endocrine System*—diabetes mellitus, goiter, hyperglycemia/hypoglycemia; *Hemic and Lymphatic System*—anemia, hemolysis; *Metabolic and Nutritional Disorders*—gout, weight gain/loss; *Musculoskeletal System*—arthritis/arthralgia, musculoskeletal pain, myalgia; *Nervous System*—agitation, amnesia, anxiety, apathy, confusion, depression, dizziness/syncope, hallucinations, hemiplegia, hostility aggravated, libido decreased, nervousness, paresthesia, thinking abnormality; *Respiratory System*—asthma, bronchitis, cough increased, dyspnea, epistaxis, hemoptysis, hiccup, pneumonia, upper respiratory inflammation/infection; *Skin and Appendages*—acne, alopecia, pruritus, rash, urticaria; *Special Senses*—blurred vision, deafness, eye pain, otitis media, taste perversion, tinnitus, visual field defect; *Urogenital System*—abnormal menses, albuminuria, breast enlargement/gynecomastia, breast tenderness, glycosuria, hematuria, impotence, kidney calculus.

Postmarketing

On-going Safety Surveillance: Additional adverse experiences have been reported since lansoprazole has been marketed. The majority of these cases are foreign-sourced and a relationship to lansoprazole has not been established. Because these events were reported voluntarily from a population of unknown size, estimates of frequency cannot be made. These events are listed below by COSTART body system.

Body as a Whole—anaphylactoid-like reaction; *Digestive System*—hepatotoxicity, vomiting; *Hemic and Lymphatic System*—agranulocytosis, aplastic anemia, hemolytic anemia, leukopenia, neutropenia, pancytopenia, thrombocytopenia, and thrombotic thrombocytopenic purpura; *Special Senses*—speech disorder; *Urogenital System*—urinary retention.

Combination Therapy with Amoxicillin and Clarithromycin

In clinical trials using combination therapy with PREVACID plus amoxicillin and clarithromycin, and PREVACID plus amoxicillin, no adverse reactions peculiar to these drug combinations were observed. Adverse reactions that have occurred have been limited to those that had been previously reported with PREVACID, amoxicillin, or clarithromycin.

Triple Therapy: PREVACID/amoxicillin/clarithromycin

The most frequently reported adverse events for patients who received triple therapy for 14 days were diarrhea (7%), headache (6%), and taste perversion (5%). There were no statistically significant differences in the frequency of reported adverse events between the 10- and 14-day triple therapy regimens. No treatment-emergent adverse events were observed at significantly higher rates with triple therapy than with any dual therapy regimen.

Dual Therapy: PREVACID/amoxicillin

The most frequently reported adverse events for patients who received PREVACID t.i.d. plus amoxicillin t.i.d. dual therapy were diarrhea (8%) and headache (7%). No treatment-emergent adverse events were observed at significantly higher rates with PREVACID t.i.d. plus amoxicillin t.i.d. dual therapy than with PREVACID alone.

For more information on adverse reactions with amoxicillin or clarithromycin, refer to their package inserts, **ADVERSE REACTIONS** sections.

Laboratory Values

The following changes in laboratory parameters for lansoprazole were reported as adverse events:

Abnormal liver function tests, increased SGOT (AST), increased SGPT (ALT), increased creatinine, increased alkaline phosphatase, increased globulins, increased GGTP, increased/decreased/abnormal WBC, abnormal AG ratio, abnormal RBC, bilirubinemia, eosinophilia, hyperlipemia, increased/decreased electrolytes, increased/decreased cholesterol, increased glucocorticoids, increased LDH, increased/decreased/abnormal platelets, and increased gastrin levels. Additional isolated laboratory abnormalities were reported.

In the placebo controlled studies, when SGOT (AST) and SGPT (ALT) were evaluated, 0.4% (1/250) placebo patients and 0.3% (2/795) lansoprazole patients had enzyme elevations greater than three times the upper limit of normal range at the final treatment visit. None of these patients reported jaundice at any time during the study.

In clinical trials using combination therapy with PREVACID plus amoxicillin and clarithromycin, and

Continued on next page

Prevacid—Cont.

PREVACID plus amoxicillin, no increased laboratory abnormalities particular to these drug combinations were observed.

For more information on laboratory value changes with amoxicillin or clarithromycin, refer to their package inserts, **ADVERSE REACTIONS** section.

OVERDOSAGE

Oral doses up to 5000 mg/kg in rats (approximately 1300 times the recommended human dose based on body surface area) and mice (about 675.7 times the recommended human dose based on body surface area) did not produce deaths or any clinical signs.

Lansoprazole is not removed from the circulation by hemodialysis. In one reported case of overdose, the patient consumed 600 mg of lansoprazole' with no adverse reaction.

DOSAGE AND ADMINISTRATION
Short-Term Treatment of Duodenal Ulcer
The recommended adult oral dose is 15 mg once daily for 4 weeks. (See **INDICATIONS AND USAGE.**)
H. pylori Eradication to Reduce the Risk of Duodenal Ulcer Recurrence
Triple Therapy: PREVACID/amoxicillin/clarithromycin
The recommended adult oral dose is 30 mg PREVACID, 1 gram amoxicillin, and 500 mg clarithromycin, all given twice daily (q 12h) for 10 or 14 days. (See **INDICATIONS AND USAGE.**)
Dual Therapy: PREVACID/amoxicillin
The recommended adult oral dose is 30 mg PREVACID and 1 gram amoxicillin, each given three times daily (q 8h) for 14 days. (See **INDICATIONS AND USAGE.**)
Please refer to amoxicillin and clarithromycin full prescribing information for **CONTRAINDICATIONS** and **WARNINGS**, and for information regarding dosing in elderly and renally-impaired patients.
Maintenance of Healed Duodenal Ulcers
The recommended adult oral dose is 15 mg once daily. (See **CLINICAL STUDIES.**)
Short-Term Treatment of Gastric Ulcer
The recommended adult oral dose is 30 mg once daily for up to eight weeks. (See **CLINICAL STUDIES.**)
Healing of NSAID-Associated Gastric Ulcer
The recommended adult oral dose is 30 mg once daily for 8 weeks. Controlled studies did not extend beyond 8 weeks. (See **CLINICAL STUDIES.**)
Risk Reduction of NSAID-Associated Gastric Ulcer
The recommended adult oral dose is 15 mg once daily for up to 12 weeks. Controlled studies did not extend beyond 12 weeks. (See **CLINICAL STUDIES.**)
Gastroesophageal Reflux Disease (GERD)
Short-Term Treatment of Symptomatic GERD
The recommended adult oral dose is 15 mg once daily for up to 8 weeks.
Short-Term Treatment of Erosive Esophagitis
The recommended adult oral dose is 30 mg once daily for up to 8 weeks. For patients who do not heal with PREVACID for 8 weeks (5-10%), it may be helpful to give an additional 8 weeks of treatment. (See **INDICATIONS AND USAGE.**) If there is a recurrence of erosive esophagitis, an additional 8-week course of PREVACID may be considered.
Maintenance of Healing of Erosive Esophagitis
The recommended adult oral dose is 15 mg once daily. (See **CLINICAL STUDIES.**)
Pathological Hypersecretory Conditions Including Zollinger-Ellison Syndrome
The dosage of PREVACID in patients with pathologic hypersecretory conditions varies with the individual patient. The recommended adult oral starting dose is 60 mg once a day. Doses should be adjusted to individual patient needs and should continue for as long as clinically indicated. Dosages up to 90 mg twice daily have been administered. Daily dosages of greater than 120 mg should be administered in divided doses. Some patients with Zollinger-Ellison syndrome have been treated continuously with PREVACID for more than four years.
No dosage adjustment is necessary in patients with renal insufficiency or the elderly. For patients with severe liver disease, dosage adjustment should be considered.
PREVACID Delayed-Release Capsules should be taken before eating. In the clinical trials, antacids were used concomitantly with PREVACID.
Alternative Administration Options
For patients who have difficulty swallowing capsules, PREVACID Delayed-Release Capsules can be opened, and the intact granules contained within can be sprinkled on one tablespoon of either applesauce, ENSURE® pudding, cottage cheese, yogurt, or strained pears and swallowed immediately. The granules should not be chewed or crushed. Alternatively, PREVACID Delayed-Release Capsules may be emptied into a small volume of either orange juice or tomato juice (60 mL – approximately 2 ounces), mixed briefly and swallowed immediately. To insure complete delivery of the dose, the glass should be rinsed with two or more volumes of juice and the contents swallowed immediately. The granules have also been shown *in vitro* to remain intact when exposed to apple, cranberry, grape, orange, pineapple, prune, tomato, and V-8® vegetable juice and stored for up to 30 minutes.
For patients who have a nasogastric tube in place, PREVACID Delayed-Release Capsules can be opened and the intact granules mixed in 40 mL of apple juice and injected through the nasogastric tube into the stomach. After administering the granules, the nasogastric tube should be flushed with additional apple juice to clear the tube.

HOW SUPPLIED
PREVACID Delayed-Release Capsules, 15 mg, are opaque, hard gelatin, colored pink and green with the TAP logo and "PREVACID 15" imprinted on the capsules. The 30 mg are opaque, hard gelatin, colored pink and black with the TAP logo and "PREVACID 30" imprinted on the capsules. They are available as follows:
NDC 0300-1541-30
Unit of use bottles of 30: 15-mg capsules
NDC 0300-1541-13
Bottles of 100: 15-mg capsules
NDC 0300-1541-19
Bottles of 1000: 15-mg capsules
NDC 0300-1541-11
Unit dose package of 100: 15-mg capsules
NDC 0300-3046-13
Bottles of 100: 30-mg capsules
NDC 0300-3046-19
Bottles of 1000: 30-mg capsules
NDC 0300-3046-11
Unit dose package of 100: 30-mg capsules
Storage: PREVACID capsules should be stored in a tight container protected from moisture.
Store between 15°C and 30°C (59°F and 86°F).
Rx only
U.S. Patent Nos. 4,628,098; 4,689,333; 5,013,743; 5,026,560 and 5,045,321.
Manufactured for TAP Pharmaceuticals Inc. Lake Forest, Illinois 60045
ENSURE®is a registered trademark of Abbott Laboratories.
V-8® is a registered trademark of the Campbell Soup Company.
03-5073-R15, Rev. November, 2000
© 1995–2000 TAP Pharmaceutical Products Inc.
Shown in Product Identification Guide, page 338

PREVPAC®   Rx
(lansoprazole 30-mg capsules, amoxicillin 500-mg capsules, USP, and clarithromycin 500-mg tablets, USP)

Prescribing information for this product, which appears on pages 3194–3198 of the 2001 PDR, has been completely revised as follows. Please write "See Supplement A" next to the product heading.
THESE PRODUCTS ARE INTENDED ONLY FOR USE AS DESCRIBED. The individual products contained in this package should not be used alone or in combination for other purposes. The information described in this labeling concerns only the use of these products as indicated in this daily administration pack. For information on use of the individual components when dispensed as individual medications outside this combined use for treating *Helicobacter pylori* (*H. pylori*), please see the package inserts for each individual product.

DESCRIPTION
PREVPAC consists of a daily administration pack containing two PREVACID 30-mg capsules, four amoxicillin 500-mg capsules, USP, and two clarithromycin 500-mg tablets, USP, for oral administration.
PREVACID® (lansoprazole) Delayed-Release Capsules
The active ingredient in PREVACID capsules is a substituted benzimidazole, 2-[[[3-methyl-4-(2,2,2-trifluoroethoxy)-2-pyridyl] methyl]sulfinyl] benzimidazole, a compound that inhibits gastric acid secretion. Its empirical formula is $C_{16}H_{14}F_3N_3O_2S$ with a molecular weight of 369.37. The structural formula is:

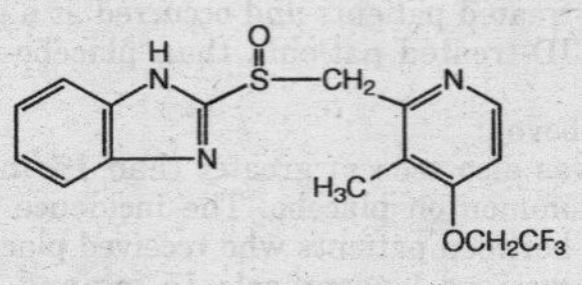

Lansoprazole is a white to brownish-white odorless crystalline powder which melts with decomposition at approximately 166°C. Lansoprazole is freely soluble in dimethylformamide; soluble in methanol; sparingly soluble in ethanol; slightly soluble in ethyl acetate, dichloromethane and acetonitrile; very slightly soluble in ether; and practically insoluble in hexane and water.
Each delayed-release capsule contains enteric-coated granules consisting of lansoprazole (30 mg), hydroxypropyl cellulose, low substituted hydroxypropyl cellulose, colloidal silicon dioxide, magnesium carbonate, methacrylic acid copolymer, starch, talc, sugar sphere, sucrose, polyethylene glycol, polysorbate 80, and titanium dioxide. Components of the gelatin capsule include gelatin, titanium dioxide, D&C Red No. 28, FD&C Blue No. 1, and FD&C Red No. 40.
TRIMOX® (amoxicillin, USP)
Amoxicillin, USP, (2S,5R,6R)-6-[(R)-(–)-2-Amino-2-(p-hydroxyphenyl) acetamido]-3,3-dimethyl-7-oxo-4-thia-1-azabicyclo[3.2.0]heptane-2-carboxylic acid trihydrate, is a semisynthetic penicillin, an analogue of ampicillin. It has the following chemical structure:

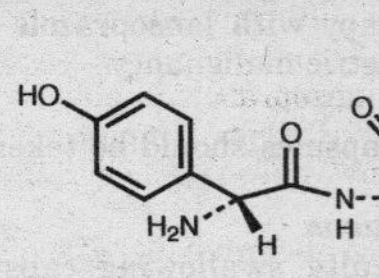

The empirical formula is $C_{16}H_{18}N_3O_5S \cdot 3H_2O$, and the molecular weight is 419.45.
The maroon and light-pink capsules contain amoxicillin trihydrate equivalent to 500 mg of amoxicillin. The inactive ingredient in the capsules is magnesium stearate.
BIAXIN® Filmtab® (clarithromycin tablets, USP)
Clarithromycin is a semi-synthetic macrolide antibiotic. Chemically, it is 6-0-methylerythromycin. The molecular formula is $C_{38}H_{69}NO_{13}$, and the molecular weight is 747.96. The structural formula is:

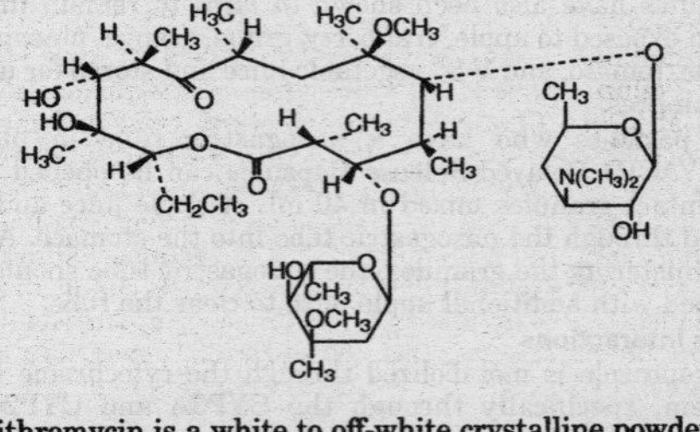

Clarithromycin is a white to off-white crystalline powder. It is soluble in acetone, slightly soluble in methanol, ethanol, and acetonitrile, and practically insoluble in water.
Each yellow oval film-coated immediate-release tablet contains 500 mg of clarithromycin and the following inactive ingredients: hydroxypropyl methylcellulose, hydroxypropyl cellulose, colloidal silicon dioxide, croscarmellose sodium, D&C Yellow No. 10, magnesium stearate, microcrystalline cellulose, povidone, propylene glycol, sorbic acid, sorbitan monooleate, titanium dioxide, and vanillin.

CLINICAL PHARMACOLOGY
Pharmacokinetics
Pharmacokinetics when all three of the PREVPAC components (PREVACID capsules, amoxicillin capsules, clarithromycin tablets) were coadministered has not been studied. Studies have shown no clinically significant interactions of PREVACID and amoxicillin or PREVACID and clarithromycin when administered together. There is no information about the gastric mucosal concentrations of PREVACID, amoxicillin and clarithromycin after administration of these agents concomitantly. The systemic pharmacokinetic information presented below is based on studies in which each product was administered alone.
PREVACID:
PREVACID capsules contain an enteric-coated granule formulation of lansoprazole. Absorption of lansoprazole begins only after the granules leave the stomach. Absorption is rapid, with mean peak plasma levels of lansoprazole occurring after approximately 1.7 hours. Peak plasma concentrations of lansoprazole (C_{max}) and the area under the plasma concentration curve (AUC) of lansoprazole are approximately proportional in doses from 15 mg to 60 mg after single-dose oral administration. Lansoprazole does not accumulate and its pharmacokinetics are unaltered by multiple dosing.
The absorption of lansoprazole is rapid, with mean C_{max} occurring approximately 1.7 hours after oral dosing, and relatively complete with absolute bioavailability over 80%. In healthy subjects, the mean (±SD) plasma half-life was 1.5 (±1.0) hours. Both C_{max} and AUC are diminished by about 50% if the drug is given 30 minutes after food as opposed to the fasting condition. There is no significant food effect if the drug is given before meals.
Lansoprazole is 97% bound to plasma proteins. Plasma protein binding is consistent over the concentration range of 0.05 to 5.0 mcg/mL.
Lansoprazole is extensively metabolized in the liver. Two metabolites have been identified in measurable quantities in plasma (the hydroxylated sulfinyl and sulfone derivatives of lansoprazole). These metabolites have very little or no antisecretory activity. Lansoprazole is thought to be transformed into two active species which inhibit acid secretion by (H^+,K^+)-ATPase within the parietal cell canaliculus, but are not present in the systemic circulation. The plasma elimination half-life of lansoprazole does not reflect its duration of suppression of gastric acid secretion. Thus, the plasma elimination half-life is less than two hours while the acid inhibitory effect lasts more than 24 hours.
Following single-dose oral administration of PREVACID, virtually no unchanged lansoprazole was excreted in the urine. In one study, after a single oral dose of ^{14}C-lansoprazole, approximately one-third of the administered radiation was excreted in the urine and two-thirds was recovered in the feces. This implies a significant biliary excretion of the metabolites of lansoprazole.
The clearance of lansoprazole is decreased in the elderly, with elimination half-life increased approximately 50% to 100%. Because the mean half-life in the elderly remains between 1.9 to 2.9 hours, repeated once daily dosing does not result in accumulation of lansoprazole. Peak plasma levels were not increased in the elderly.

In patients with severe renal insufficiency, plasma protein binding decreased by 1.0%–1.5% after administration of 60 mg of lansoprazole. Patients with renal insufficiency had a shortened elimination half-life and decreased total AUC (free and bound). AUC for free lansoprazole in plasma, however, was not related to the degree of renal impairment, and C_{max} and T_{max} were not different from subjects with healthy kidneys.

In patients with various degrees of chronic hepatic disease, the mean plasma half-life of the drug was prolonged from 1.5 hours to 3.2–7.2 hours. An increase in mean AUC of up to 500% was observed at steady state in hepatically-impaired patients compared to healthy subjects. Dose reduction in patients with severe hepatic disease should be considered.

The pooled pharmacokinetic parameters of PREVACID from twelve U.S. Phase I studies (N=513) were compared to the mean pharmacokinetic parameters from two Asian studies (N=20). The mean AUCs of PREVACID in Asian subjects are approximately twice that seen in pooled U.S. data; however, the inter-individual variability is high. The C_{max} values are comparable.

Amoxicillin:

Amoxicillin is stable in the presence of gastric acid and is well absorbed from the gastrointestinal tract and may be given with no regard to food. It diffuses readily into most body tissues and fluids, with the exception of brain and spinal fluid, except when meninges are inflamed. The half-life of amoxicillin is 61.3 minutes. Most of the amoxicillin is excreted unchanged in the urine; its excretion can be delayed by concurrent administration of probenecid. Amoxicillin is not highly protein-bound. In blood serum, amoxicillin is approximately 20% protein-bound as compared to 60% for penicillin G.

Orally administered doses of 500-mg amoxicillin capsules result in average peak blood levels 1 to 2 hours after administration in the range of 5.5 to 7.5 µg/mL.

Detectable serum levels are observed up to eight hours after an orally administered dose of amoxicillin. Approximately 60% of an orally administered dose of amoxicillin is excreted in the urine within 6 to 8 hours.

Clarithromycin:

Clarithromycin is rapidly absorbed from the gastrointestinal tract after oral administration. The absolute bioavailability of 250 mg clarithromycin tablets was approximately 50%. Food slightly delays both the onset of clarithromycin absorption and the formation of the antimicrobially active metabolite, 14-OH clarithromycin, but does not affect the extent of bioavailability. Therefore, clarithromycin tablets may be given without regard to food.

In fasting healthy human subjects, peak serum concentrations were attained within two hours after oral dosing. Steady-state peak serum clarithromycin concentrations were attained in two to three days and were approximately 2 to 3 µg/mL with a 500-mg dose administered every 12 hours. The elimination half-life of clarithromycin was 5 to 7 hours with 500 mg administered every 8 to 12 hours. The nonlinearity of clarithromycin pharmacokinetics is slight at the recommended dose of 500 mg administered every 12 hours. With a 500-mg dose every 8 to 12 hours, the peak steady-state concentration of 14-OH clarithromycin, the principal metabolite, is up to 1 µg/mL and its elimination half-life is about 7 to 9 hours. The steady-state concentration of this metabolite is generally attained within 2 to 3 days.

After a 500-mg tablet every 12 hours, the urinary excretion of clarithromycin is approximately 30%. The renal clearance of clarithromycin approximates the normal glomerular filtration rate. The major metabolite found in urine is 14-OH clarithromycin, which accounts for an additional 10% to 15% of the dose with a 500-mg tablet administered every 12 hours.

The steady-state concentrations of clarithromycin in subjects with impaired hepatic function did not differ from those in normal subjects; however, the 14-OH clarithromycin concentrations were lower in the hepatically impaired subjects. The decreased formation of 14-OH clarithromycin was at least partially offset by an increase in renal clearance of clarithromycin in the subjects with impaired hepatic function when compared to healthy subjects. The pharmacokinetics of clarithromycin was also altered in subjects with impaired renal function. (See **PRECAUTIONS** and **DOSAGE AND ADMINISTRATION.**)

Pharmacodynamics

MICROBIOLOGY

Lansoprazole, clarithromycin and/or amoxicillin have been shown to be active against most strains of *Helicobacter pylori in vitro* and in clinical infections as described in the **INDICATIONS AND USAGE** section.

Helicobacter

Helicobacter pylori

Pretreatment Resistance

Clarithromycin pretreatment resistance (≥2.0 µg/mL) was 9.5% (91/960) by E-test and 11.3% (12/106) by agar dilution in the dual and triple therapy clinical trials (M93-125, M93-130, M93-131, M95-392, and M95-399).

Amoxicillin pretreatment susceptible isolates (≤0.25 µg/mL) occurred in 97.8% (936/957) and 98.0% (98/100) of the patients in the dual and triple therapy clinical trials by E-test and agar dilution, respectively. Twenty-one of 957 patients (2.2%) by E-test and 2 of 100 patients (2.0%) by agar dilution had amoxicillin pretreatment MICs of >0.25 µg/mL. One patient on the 14-day triple therapy regimen had an unconfirmed pretreatment amoxicillin minimum inhibitory concentration (MIC) of >256 µg/mL by E-test and the patient was eradicated of *H. pylori*.

[See first table above]

Clarithromycin Susceptibility Test Results and Clinical/Bacteriological Outcomes[a]

Clarithromycin Pretreatment Results		Clarithromycin Post-treatment Results				
		H. pylori negative-eradicated	*H. pylori* positive- not eradicated Post-treatment susceptibility results S[b]	I[b]	R[b]	No MIC
Triple Therapy 14-Day (lansoprazole 30 mg b.i.d./amoxicillin 1 gm b.i.d./clarithromycin 500 mg b.i.d.) (M95-399, M93-131, M95-392)						
Susceptible[b]	112	105				7
Intermediate[b]	3	3				
Resistant[b]	17	6			7	4
Triple Therapy 10-Day (lansoprazole 30 mg b.i.d./amoxicillin 1 gm b.i.d./clarithromycin 500 mg b.i.d.) (M95-399)						
Susceptible[b]	42	40	1		1	
Intermediate[b]						
Resistant[b]	4	1			3	

[a] Includes only patients with pretreatment clarithromycin susceptibility test results

[b] Susceptible (S) MIC ≤0.25 µg/mL, Intermediate (I) MIC 0.5–1.0 µg/mL, Resistant (R) MIC ≥2 µg/mL

Patients not eradicated of *H. pylori* following lansoprazole/amoxicillin/clarithromycin triple therapy will likely have clarithromycin resistant *H. pylori*. Therefore, for those patients who fail therapy, clarithromycin susceptibility testing should be done when possible. Patients with clarithromycin resistant *H. pylori* should not be treated with lansoprazole/amoxicillin/clarithromycin triple therapy or with regimens which include clarithromycin as the sole antimicrobial agent.

Amoxicillin Susceptibility Test Results and Clinical/Bacteriological Outcomes

In the dual and triple therapy clinical trials, 82.6% (195/236) of the patients that had pretreatment amoxicillin susceptible MICs (≤0.25 µg/mL) were eradicated of *H. pylori*. Of those with pretreatment amoxicillin MICs of >0.25 µg/mL, three of six had the *H. pylori* eradicated. A total of 30% (21/70) of the patients failed lansoprazole 30 mg t.i.d./amoxicillin 1 gm t.i.d. dual therapy and a total of 12.8% (22/172) of the patients failed the 10- and 14-day triple therapy regimens. Post-treatment susceptibility results were not obtained on 11 of the patients who failed therapy. Nine of the 11 patients with amoxicillin post-treatment MICs that failed the triple therapy regimen also had clarithromycin resistant *H. pylori* isolates.

Susceptibility Test for *Helicobacter pylori*

The reference methodology for susceptibility testing of *H. pylori* is agar dilution MICs.[1] One to three microliters of an inoculum equivalent to a No. 2 McFarland standard ($1 \times 10^7 - 1 \times 10^8$ CFU/mL for *H. pylori*) are inoculated directly onto freshly prepared antimicrobial containing Mueller-Hinton agar plates with 5% aged defibrinated sheep blood (≥2 weeks old). The agar dilution plates are incubated at 35°C in a microaerobic environment produced by a gas generating system suitable for campylobacters. After 3 days of incubation, the MICs are recorded as the lowest concentration of antimicrobial agent required to inhibit growth of the organism. The clarithromycin and amoxicillin MIC values should be interpreted according to the following criteria:

Clarithromycin MIC (µg/mL)[a]	Interpretation
≤0.25	Susceptible (S)
0.5–1.0	Intermediate (I)
≥2.0	Resistant (R)

Amoxicillin MIC (µg/mL)[b]	Interpretation
≤0.25	Susceptible (S)

[a] These are tentative breakpoints for the agar dilution methodology and they should not be used to interpret results obtained using alternative methods.

[b] There were not enough organisms with MICs >0.25 µg/mL to determine a resistance breakpoint.

Standardized susceptibility test procedures require the use of laboratory control microorganisms to control the technical aspects of the laboratory procedures. Standard clarithromycin and amoxicillin powders should provide the following MIC values:

Microorganisms	Antimicrobial Agent	MIC (µg/mL)[a]
H. pylori ATCC 43504	Clarithromycin	0.015–0.12 mcg/mL
H. pylori ATCC 43504	Amoxicillin	0.015–0.12 mcg/mL

[a] These are quality control ranges for the agar dilution methodology and they should not be used to control test results obtained using alternative methods.

Reference

1. National Committee for Clinical Laboratory Standards. Summary Minutes, Subcommittee on Antimicrobial Susceptibility Testing, Tampa, FL, January 11–13, 1998.

Antisecretory activity

After oral administration, lansoprazole was shown to significantly decrease the basal acid output and significantly increase the mean gastric pH and percent of time the gastric pH was >3 and >4. Lansoprazole also significantly reduced meal-stimulated gastric acid output and secretion volume, as well as pentagastrin-stimulated acid output. In patients with hypersecretion of acid, lansoprazole significantly reduced basal and pentagastrin-stimulated gastric acid secretion. Lansoprazole inhibited the normal increases in secretion volume, acidity and acid output induced by insulin.

In a crossover study comparing lansoprazole 15 and 30 mg with omeprazole 20 mg for five days, the following effects on intragastric pH were noted:

[See second table above]

Mean Antisecretory Effects after Single and Multiple Daily Dosing

		PREVACID				Omeprazole	
	Baseline	15 mg		30 mg		20 mg	
Parameter	Value	Day 1	Day 5	Day 1	Day 5	Day 1	Day 5
Mean 24-Hour pH	2.1	2.7^{+}	4.0^{+}	3.6^{*}	4.9^{*}	2.5	4.2^{+}
Mean Nighttime pH	1.9	2.4	3.0^{+}	2.6	3.8^{*}	2.2	3.0^{+}
% Time Gastric pH>3	18	33^{+}	59^{+}	51^{*}	72^{*}	30^{+}	61^{+}
% Time Gastric pH>4	12	22^{+}	49^{+}	41^{*}	66^{*}	19	51^{+}

NOTE: An intragastric pH of >4 reflects a reduction in gastric acid by 99%.

*(p<0.05) versus baseline, lansoprazole 15 mg and omeprazole 20 mg.

+(p<0.05) versus baseline only.

After the initial dose in this study, increased gastric pH was seen within 1–2 hours with lansoprazole 30 mg, 2–3 hours with lansoprazole 15 mg, and 3–4 hours with omeprazole 20 mg. After multiple daily dosing, increased gastric pH was seen within the first hour postdosing with lansoprazole 30 mg and within 1–2 hours postdosing with lansoprazole 15 mg and omeprazole 20 mg.

The percentage of time gastric pH was elevated above 5 and 6 was evaluated in a crossover study of PREVACID given q.d., b.i.d. and t.i.d.

[See first table at top of next page]

The inhibition of gastric acid secretion as measured by intragastric pH returns gradually to normal over two to four days after multiple doses. There is no indication of rebound gastric acidity.

CLINICAL STUDIES

***H. pylori* Eradication to Reduce the Risk of Duodenal Ulcer Recurrence**

Randomized, double-blind clinical studies performed in the U.S. in patients with *H. pylori* and duodenal ulcer disease (defined as an active ulcer or history of an ulcer within one year) evaluated the efficacy of PREVPAC as triple 14-day therapy for the eradication of *H. pylori*. The triple therapy regimen (PREVACID 30 mg BID plus amoxicillin 1 gm BID plus clarithromycin 500 mg BID) produced statistically significantly higher eradication rates than PREVACID plus amoxicillin, PREVACID plus clarithromycin, and amoxicillin plus clarithromycin dual therapies.

Continued on next page

PREVPAC—Cont.

H. pylori eradication was defined as two negative tests (culture and histology) at 4 to 6 weeks following the end of treatment.
Triple therapy was shown to be more effective than all possible dual therapy combinations. The combination of PREVACID plus amoxicillin and clarithromycin as triple therapy was effective in eradicating *H. pylori*. Eradication of *H. pylori* has been shown to reduce the risk of duodenal ulcer recurrence.
A randomized, double-blind clinical study performed in the U.S. in patients with *H. pylori* and duodenal ulcer disease (defined as an active ulcer or history of an ulcer within one year) compared the efficacy of PREVACID triple therapy for 10 and 14 days. This study established that the 10-day triple therapy was equivalent to the 14-day triple therapy in eradicating *H. pylori*.
[See second table to the right]

Mean Antisecretory Effects After 5 Days of b.i.d. and t.i.d. Dosing

Parameter	PREVACID 30 mg q.d.	15 mg b.i.d.	30 mg b.i.d.	30 mg t.i.d.
% Time Gastric pH>5	43	47	59+	77*
% Time Gastric pH>6	20	23	28	45*

+(p<0.05) versus PREVACID 30 mg q.d.
*(p<0.05) versus PREVACID 30 mg q.d., 15 mg b.i.d. and 30 mg b.i.d.

***H. pylori* Eradication Rates—Triple Therapy**
(PREVACID/amoxicillin/clarithromycin)
Percent of Patients Cured
[95% Confidence Interval]
(Number of patients)

Study	Duration	Triple Therapy Evaluable Analysis*	Triple Therapy Intent-to-Treat Analysis#
M93-131	14 days	92† [80.0–97.7] (N=48)	86† [73.3–93.5] (N=55)
M95-392	14 days	86‡ [75.7–93.6] (N=66)	83‡ [72.0–90.8] (N=70)
M95-399+	14 days	85 [77.0–91.0] (N=113)	82 [73.9–88.1] (N=126)
	10 days	84 [76.0–89.8] (N=123)	81 [73.9–87.6] (N=135)

* Based on evaluable patients with confirmed duodenal ulcer (active or within one year) and *H. pylori* infection at baseline defined as at least two of three positive endoscopic tests from CLOtest® (Delta West Ltd., Bentley, Australia), histology and/or culture. Patients were included in the analysis if they completed the study. Additionally, if patients dropped out of the study due to an adverse event related to the study drug, they were included in the evaluable analysis as failures of therapy.
# Patients were included in the analysis if they had documented *H. pylori* infection at baseline as defined above and had a confirmed duodenal ulcer (active or within one year). All dropouts were included as failures of therapy.
† (p<0.05) versus PREVACID/amoxicillin and PREVACID/clarithromycin dual therapy
‡ (p<0.05) versus clarithromycin/amoxicillin dual therapy
+ The 95% confidence interval for the difference in eradication rates, 10-day minus 14-day is (-10.5, 8.1) in the evaluable analysis and (-9.7, 9.1) in the intent-to-treat analysis.

INDICATIONS AND USAGE

***H. pylori* Eradication to Reduce the Risk of Duodenal Ulcer Recurrence**
The components in PREVPAC (PREVACID, amoxicillin, and clarithromycin) are indicated for the treatment of patients with *H. pylori* infection and duodenal ulcer disease (active or one-year history of a duodenal ulcer) to eradicate *H. pylori*. Eradication of *H. pylori* has been shown to reduce the risk of duodenal ulcer recurrence (See **CLINICAL STUDIES** and **DOSAGE AND ADMINISTRATION**).

CONTRAINDICATIONS

PREVPAC is contraindicated in patients with known hypersensitivity to any component of the formulation of PREVACID, any macrolide antibiotic, or any penicillin.
Concomitant administration of PREVPAC with cisapride, pimozide, or terfenadine is contraindicated. There have been postmarketing reports of drug interactions when clarithromycin and/or erythromycin are co-administered with cisapride, pimozide, or terfenadine resulting in cardiac arrhythmias (QT prolongation, ventricular tachycardia, ventricular fibrillation, and torsades de pointes) most likely due to inhibition of hepatic metabolism of these drugs by erythromycin and clarithromycin. Fatalities have been reported.

WARNINGS

Amoxicillin:
Serious and occasionally fatal hypersensitivity (anaphylactoid) reactions have been reported in patients on penicillin therapy. Although anaphylaxis is more frequent following parenteral therapy, it has occurred in patients on oral penicillins. These reactions are more apt to occur in individuals with a history of penicillin hypersensitivity and/or a history of sensitivity to multiple allergens.
There have been well documented reports of individuals with a history of penicillin hypersensitivity reactions who have experienced severe hypersensitivity reactions when treated with a cephalosporin. Before initiating therapy with any penicillin, careful inquiry should be made concerning previous hypersensitivity reactions to penicillins, cephalosporins, and other allergens. If an allergic reaction occurs, amoxicillin should be discontinued and the appropriate therapy instituted.
SERIOUS ANAPHYLACTOID REACTIONS REQUIRE IMMEDIATE EMERGENCY TREATMENT WITH EPINEPHRINE. OXYGEN, INTRAVENOUS STEROIDS, AND AIRWAY MANAGEMENT, INCLUDING INTUBATION, SHOULD ALSO BE ADMINISTERED AS INDICATED.
Clarithromycin:
CLARITHROMYCIN SHOULD NOT BE USED IN PREGNANT WOMEN EXCEPT IN CLINICAL CIRCUMSTANCES WHERE NO ALTERNATIVE THERAPY IS APPROPRIATE. IF PREGNANCY OCCURS WHILE TAKING CLARITHROMYCIN, THE PATIENT SHOULD BE APPRISED OF THE POTENTIAL HAZARD TO THE FETUS. CLARITHROMYCIN HAS DEMONSTRATED ADVERSE EFFECTS OF PREGNANCY OUTCOME AND/OR EMBRYO-FETAL DEVELOPMENT IN MONKEYS, RATS, MICE, AND RABBITS AT DOSES THAT PRODUCED PLASMA LEVELS 2 TO 17 TIMES THE SERUM LEVELS ACHIEVED IN HUMANS TREATED AT THE MAXIMUM RECOMMENDED HUMAN DOSES. (See PRECAUTIONS - Pregnancy.)
Pseudomembranous colitis has been reported with nearly all antibacterial agents, including clarithromycin, and may range in severity from mild to life threatening. Therefore, it is important to consider this diagnosis in patients who present with diarrhea subsequent to the administration of antibacterial agents.
Treatment with antibacterial agents alters the normal flora of the colon and may permit overgrowth of clostridia. Studies indicate that a toxin produced by *Clostridium difficile* is a primary cause of "antibiotic-associated colitis."
After the diagnosis of pseudomembranous colitis has been established, therapeutic measures should be initiated. Mild cases of pseudomembranous colitis usually respond to discontinuation of the drug alone. In moderate to severe cases, consideration should be given to management with fluids and electrolytes, protein supplementation, and treatment with an antibacterial drug clinically effective against *Clostridium difficile* colitis.

PRECAUTIONS

Clarithromycin is principally excreted via the liver and kidney. Clarithromycin may be administered without dosage adjustment to patients with hepatic impairment and normal renal function. However, in the presence of severe renal impairment with or without coexisting hepatic impairment, decreased dosage or prolonged dosing intervals may be appropriate.
The possibility of superinfections with mycotic organisms or bacterial pathogens should be kept in mind during therapy. In such cases, discontinue PREVPAC and substitute appropriate treatment.
Symptomatic response to therapy with PREVACID does not preclude the presence of gastric malignancy.
Information for Patients: Each dose of PREVPAC contains four pills: one pink and black capsule (PREVACID), two maroon and light-pink capsules (amoxicillin) and one yellow tablet (clarithromycin). Each dose should be taken twice per day before eating. Patients should be instructed to swallow each pill whole.

Drug Interactions
PREVACID:
PREVACID is metabolized through the cytochrome P_{450} system, specifically through the CYP3A and CYP2C19 isozymes. Studies have shown that PREVACID does not have clinically significant interactions with other drugs metabolized by the cytochrome P_{450} system, such as warfarin, antipyrine, indomethacin, ibuprofen, phenytoin, propranolol, prednisone, diazepam, clarithromycin, or terfenadine in healthy subjects. These compounds are metabolized through various cytochrome P_{450} isozymes including CYP1A2, CYP2C9, CYP2C19, CYP2D6, and CYP3A. When PREVACID was administered concomitantly with theophylline (CYP1A2, CYP3A), a minor increase (10%) in the clearance of theophylline was seen. Because of the small magnitude and the direction of the effect on theophylline clearance, this interaction is unlikely to be of clinical concern. Nonetheless, individual patients may require additional titration of their theophylline dosage when PREVACID is started or stopped to ensure clinically effective blood levels.
PREVACID has also been shown to have no clinically significant interaction with amoxicillin.
In a single-dose crossover study examining PREVACID 30 mg and omeprazole 20 mg each administered alone and concomitantly with sucralfate 1 gram, absorption of the proton pump inhibitors was delayed and their bioavailability was reduced by 17% and 16%, respectively, when administered concomitantly with sucralfate. Therefore, proton pump inhibitors should be taken at least 30 minutes prior to sucralfate. In clinical trials, antacids were administered concomitantly with PREVACID Delayed-Release Capsules; this did not interfere with its effect.
PREVACID causes a profound and long-lasting inhibition of gastric acid secretion; therefore, it is theoretically possible that PREVACID may interfere with the absorption of drugs where gastric pH is an important determinant of bioavailability (eg, ketoconazole, ampicillin esters, iron salts, digoxin).

Clarithromycin:
Clarithromycin use in patients who are receiving theophylline may be associated with an increase of serum theophylline concentrations. Monitoring of serum theophylline concentrations should be considered for patients receiving high doses of theophylline or with baseline concentrations in the upper therapeutic range. In two studies in which theophylline was administered with clarithromycin (a theophylline sustained-release formulation was dosed at either 6.5 mg/kg or 12 mg/kg together with 250 or 500 mg q12h clarithromycin), the steady-state levels of C_{max}, C_{min}, and the area under the serum concentration time curve (AUC) of theophylline increased about 20%.
Concomitant administration of single doses of clarithromycin and carbamazepine has been shown to result in increased plasma concentrations of carbamazepine. Blood level monitoring of carbamazepine may be considered.
When clarithromycin and terfenadine were coadministered, plasma concentrations of the active acid metabolite of terfenadine were threefold higher, on average, than the values observed when terfenadine was administered alone. The pharmacokinetics of clarithromycin and the 14-hydroxy-clarithromycin were not significantly affected by coadministration of terfenadine once clarithromycin reached steady-state conditions. Concomitant administration of clarithromycin with terfenadine is contraindicated. (See **CONTRAINDICATIONS**.)
Spontaneous reports in the postmarketing period suggest that concomitant administration of clarithromycin and oral anticoagulants may potentiate the effects of the oral anticoagulants. Prothrombin times should be carefully monitored while patients are receiving clarithromycin and oral anticoagulants simultaneously.
Elevated digoxin serum concentrations in patients receiving clarithromycin and digoxin concomitantly have also been reported in postmarketing surveillance. Some patients have shown clinical signs consistent with digoxin toxicity, including potentially fatal arrhythmias. Serum digoxin levels should be carefully monitored while patients are receiving digoxin and clarithromycin simultaneously.
For information on interactions between clarithromycin in combination with other drugs which may be administered to HIV-infected patients, see the BIAXIN package insert, Drug Interactions, under the **PRECAUTIONS** section.
The following drug interactions, other than increased serum concentrations of carbamazepine and active acid metabolite of terfenadine, have not been reported in clinical trials with clarithromycin; however, they have been observed with erythromycin products and/or with clarithromycin in postmarketing experience.
Concurrent use of erythromycin or clarithromycin and ergotamine or dihydroergotamine has been associated in some patients with acute ergot toxicity characterized by severe peripheral vasospasm and dysesthesia.
Erythromycin has been reported to decrease the clearance of triazolam and, thus, may increase the pharmacologic effect of triazolam. There have been postmarketing reports

of drug interactions and CNS effects (e.g., somnolence and confusion) with the concomitant use of clarithromycin and triazolam.

There have been reports of an interaction between erythromycin and astemizole resulting in QT prolongation and torsades de pointes. Concomitant administration of erythromycin and astemizole is contraindicated. Because clarithromycin is also metabolized by cytochrome P_{450}, concomitant administration of clarithromycin with astemizole is not recommended.

As with other macrolides, clarithromycin has been reported to increase concentrations of HMG-CoA reductase inhibitors (e.g., lovastatin and simvastatin), through inhibition of cytochrome P_{450} metabolism of these drugs. Rare reports of rhabdomyolysis have been reported in patients taking these drugs concomitantly.

The use of erythromycin and clarithromycin in patients concurrently taking drugs metabolized by the cytochrome P_{450} system may be associated with elevations in serum levels of these other drugs. There have been reports of interactions of erythromycin and/or clarithromycin with carbamazepine, cyclosporine, tacrolimus, hexobarbital, phenytoin, alfentanil, disopyramide, lovastatin, bromocriptine, valproate, terfenadine, cisapride, pimozide, rifabutin, and astemizole. Serum concentrations of drugs metabolized by the cytochrome P_{450} system should be monitored closely in patients concurrently receiving these drugs.

Carcinogenesis, Mutagenesis, Impairment of Fertility

PREVACID:

In two 24-month carcinogenicity studies, Sprague-Dawley rats were treated orally with doses of 5 to 150 mg/kg/day, about 1 to 40 times the exposure on a body surface (mg/m^2) basis, of a 50-kg person of average height (1.46 m^2 body surface area) given the recommended human dose of 30 mg/day (22.2 mg/m^2). Lansoprazole produced dose-related gastric enterochromaffin-like (ECL) cell hyperplasia and ECL cell carcinoids in both male and female rats. It also increased the incidence of intestinal metaplasia of the gastric epithelium in both sexes. In male rats, lansoprazole produced a dose-related increase of testicular interstitial cell adenomas. The incidence of these adenomas in rats receiving doses of 15 to 150 mg/kg/day (4 to 40 times the recommended human dose based on body surface area) exceeded the low background incidence (range = 1.4 to 10%) for this strain of rat. Testicular interstitial cell adenoma also occurred in 1 of 30 rats treated with 50 mg/kg/day (13 times the recommended human dose based on body surface area) in a 1-year toxicity study.

In a 24-month carcinogenicity study, CD-1 mice were treated orally with doses of 15 to 600 mg/kg/day, 2 to 80 times the recommended human dose based on body surface area. Lansoprazole produced a dose-related increased incidence of gastric ECL cell hyperplasia. It also produced an increased incidence of liver tumors (hepatocellular adenoma plus carcinoma). The tumor incidences in male mice treated with 300 and 600 mg/kg/day (40 to 80 times the recommended human dose based on body surface area) and female mice treated with 150 to 600 mg/kg/day (20 to 80 times the recommended human dose based on body surface area) exceeded the ranges of background incidences in historical controls for this strain of mice. Lansoprazole treatment produced adenoma of rete testis in male mice receiving 75 to 600 mg/kg/day (10 to 80 times the recommended human dose based on body surface area).

Lansoprazole was not genotoxic in the Ames test, the *ex vivo* rat hepatocyte unscheduled DNA synthesis (UDS) test, the *in vivo* mouse micronucleus test or the rat bone marrow cell chromosomal aberration test. It was positive in *in vitro* human lymphocyte chromosomal aberration assays.

Lansoprazole at oral doses up to 150 mg/kg/day (40 times the recommended human dose based on body surface area) was found to have no effect on fertility and reproductive performance of male and female rats.

Amoxicillin:

Long-term studies in animals have not been performed with amoxicillin.

Clarithromycin:

The following *in vitro* mutagenicity tests have been conducted with clarithromycin:

- *Salmonella*/Mammalian Microsomes Test
- Bacterial Induced Mutation Frequency Test
- *In vitro* Chromosome Aberration Test
- Rat Hepatocyte DNA Synthesis Assay
- Mouse Lymphoma Assay
- Mouse Dominant Lethal Study
- Mouse Micronucleus Test

All tests had negative results except the *in vitro* Chromosome Aberration Test which was weakly positive in one test and negative in another.

In addition, a Bacterial Reverse-Mutation Test (Ames Test) has been performed on clarithromycin metabolites with negative results.

Fertility and reproduction studies have shown that daily doses of up to 160 mg/kg/day (1.3 times the recommended maximum human dose based on mg/m^2) to male and female rats caused no adverse effects on the estrous cycle, fertility, parturition, or number and viability of offspring. Plasma levels in rats after 150 mg/kg/day were 2 times the human serum levels.

In the 150 mg/kg/day monkey studies, plasma levels were 3 times the human serum levels. When given orally at 150 mg/kg/day (2.4 times the recommended maximum human dose based on mg/m^2), clarithromycin was shown to produce embryonic loss in monkeys. This effect has been attributed to marked maternal toxicity of the drug at this high dose.

In rabbits, *in utero* fetal loss occurred at an intravenous dose of 33 mg/m^2, which is 17 times less than the maximum proposed human oral daily dose of 618 mg/m^2.

Long-term studies in animals have not been performed to evaluate the carcinogenic potential of clarithromycin.

Pregnancy

Teratogenic Effects. Pregnancy Category C

Category C is based on the pregnancy category for clarithromycin.

Four teratogenicity studies in rats (three with oral doses and one with intravenous doses up to 160 mg/kg/day administered during the period of major organogenesis) and two in rabbits at oral doses up to 125 mg/kg/day (approximately 2 times the recommended maximum human dose based on mg/m^2) or intravenous doses of 30 mg/kg/day administered during gestation days 6 to 18 failed to demonstrate any teratogenicity from clarithromycin. Two additional oral studies in a different rat strain at similar doses and similar conditions demonstrated a low incidence of cardiovascular anomalies at doses of 150 mg/kg/day administered during gestation days 6 to 15. Plasma levels after 150 mg/kg/day were 2 times the human serum levels. Four studies in mice revealed a variable incidence of cleft palate following oral doses of 1000 mg/kg/day (2 and 4 times the recommended maximum human dose based on mg/m^2, respectively) during gestation days 6 to 15. Cleft palate was also seen at 500 mg/kg/day. The 1000 mg/kg/day exposure resulted in plasma levels 17 times the human serum levels. In monkeys, an oral dose of 70 mg/kg/day (an approximate equidose of the recommended maximum human dose based on mg/m^2) produced fetal growth retardation at plasma levels that were 2 times the human serum levels.

There were no adequate and well-controlled studies of PREVPAC in pregnant women. PREVPAC should be used during pregnancy only if the potential benefit justifies the potential risk to the fetus. (See **WARNINGS**.)

Labor and Delivery

Oral ampicillin-class antibiotics are poorly absorbed during labor. Studies in guinea pigs showed that intravenous administration of ampicillin slightly decreased the uterine tone and frequency of contractions, but moderately increased the height and duration of contractions. However, it is not known whether use of these drugs in humans during labor or delivery has immediate or delayed adverse effects on the fetus, prolongs the duration of labor, or increases the likelihood that forceps delivery or other obstetrical intervention or resuscitation of the newborn will be necessary.

Nursing Mothers

Amoxicillin is excreted in human milk in very small amounts. Because of the potential for serious adverse reactions in nursing infants from PREVPAC, a decision should be made whether to discontinue nursing or to discontinue the drug therapy, taking into account the importance of the therapy to the mother.

Pediatric Use

Safety and effectiveness of PREVPAC in pediatric patients infected with *H. pylori* have not been established. (See **CONTRAINDICATIONS** and **WARNINGS**.)

Geriatric Use

Elderly patients may suffer from asymptomatic renal and hepatic dysfunction. Care should be taken when administering PREVPAC to this patient population.

ADVERSE REACTIONS

The most common adverse reactions (≥3%) reported in clinical trials when all three components of this therapy were given concomitantly for 14 days are listed in the table below.

Adverse Reactions Most Frequently Reported in Clinical Trials (≥3%)

Adverse Reaction	Triple Therapy n=138 (%)
Diarrhea	7.0
Headache	6.0
Taste Perversion	5.0

The additional adverse reactions which were reported as possibly or probably related to treatment (<3%) in clinical trials when all three components of this therapy were given concomitantly are listed below and divided by body system: *Body as a Whole*—abdominal pain; *Digestive System*—dark stools, dry mouth/thirst, glossitis, rectal itching, nausea, oral moniliasis, stomatitis, tongue discoloration, tongue disorder, vomiting; *Musculoskeletal System*—myalgia; *Nervous System*—confusion, dizziness; *Respiratory System*—respiratory disorders; *Skin and Appendages*—skin reactions; *Urogenital System*—vaginitis, vaginal moniliasis. There were no statistically significant differences in the frequency of reported adverse events between the 10- and 14-day triple therapy regimens.

PREVACID:

The following adverse reactions from the labeling for lansoprazole are provided for information.

Worldwide, over 6100 patients have been treated with lansoprazole in Phase 2–3 clinical trials involving various dosages and durations of treatment. In general, lansoprazole treatment has been well tolerated in both short-term and long-term trials.

Incidence in Clinical Trials

The following adverse events were reported by the treating physician to have a possible or probable relationship to drug in 1% or more of patients treated with PREVACID capsules and occurred at a greater rate in patients treated with PREVACID capsules than placebo-treated patients:

Incidence of Possibly or Probably Treatment-Related Adverse Events in Short-term, Placebo-Controlled Studies

Body System/Adverse Event	PREVACID (N=1457) %	Placebo (N=467) %
Body as a Whole		
Abdominal Pain	1.8	1.3
Digestive System		
Diarrhea	3.6	2.6
Nausea	1.4	1.3

Headache was also seen at greater than 1% incidence but was more common on placebo. The incidence of diarrhea is similar between placebo and lansoprazole 15 mg and 30 mg patients, but higher in the lansoprazole 60 mg patients (2.9%, 1.4%, 4.2%, and 7.4%, respectively).

The most commonly reported possibly or probably treatment-related adverse event during maintenance therapy was diarrhea.

Additional adverse experiences occurring in <1% of patients or subjects in domestic trials are shown below.

Refer to ***Postmarketing*** for adverse reactions occuring since the drug was marketed.

Body as a Whole—asthenia, candidiasis, chest pain (not otherwise specified), edema, fever, flu syndrome, halitosis, infection (not otherwise specified), malaise; *Cardiovascular System*—angina, cerebrovascular accident, hypertension/hypotension, myocardial infarction, palpitations, shock (circulatory failure), vasodilation; *Digestive System*—anorexia, bezoar, cardiospasm, cholelithiasis, constipation, dry mouth/thirst, dyspepsia, dysphagia, eructation, esophageal stenosis, esophageal ulcer, esophagitis, fecal discoloration, flatulence, gastric nodules/fundic gland polyps, gastroenteritis, gastrointestinal hemorrhage, hematemesis, increased appetite, increased salivation, melena, rectal hemorrhage, stomatitis, tenesmus, ulcerative colitis, *Endocrine System*—diabetes mellitus, goiter, hyperglycemia/hypoglycemia; *Hemic and Lymphatic System*—anemia, hemolysis; *Metabolic and Nutritional Disorders*—gout, weight gain/loss; *Musculoskeletal System*—arthritis/arthralgia, musculoskeletal pain, myalgia; *Nervous System*—agitation, amnesia, anxiety, apathy, confusion, depression, dizziness/syncope, hallucinations, hemiplegia, hostility aggravated, libido decreased, nervousness, paresthesia, thinking abnormality; *Respiratory System*—asthma, bronchitis, cough increased, dyspnea, epistaxis, hemoptysis, hiccup, pneumonia, upper respiratory inflammation/infection; *Skin and Appendages*—acne, alopecia, pruritus, rash, urticaria; *Special Senses*—blurred vision, deafness, eye pain, otitis media, taste perversion, tinnitus, visual field defect; *Urogenital System*—abnormal menses, albuminuria, breast enlargement/gynecomastia, breast tenderness, glycosuria, hematuria, impotence, kidney calculus.

Postmarketing

Ongoing Safety Surveillance: Additional adverse experiences have been reported since lansoprazole has been marketed. The majority of these cases are foreign-sourced and a relationship of lansoprazole has not been established. Because these events were reported voluntarily form a population of unknown size, estimates of frequency cannot be made. These events are listed below by COSTART body system.

Body as a Whole—anaphylactoid-like reaction; *Digestive System*—hepatotoxicity, vomiting; *Hemic and Lymphatic System*—agranulocytosis, aplastic anemia, hemolytic anemia, leukopenia, neutropenia, pancytopenia, thrombocytopenia, and thrombotic thrombocytopenic purpura; *Special Senses*—speech disorder; *Urogenital System*—urinary retention.

Laboratory Values

The following changes in laboratory parameters were reported as adverse events.

Abnormal liver function tests, increased SGOT (AST), increased SGPT (ALT), increased creatinine, increased alkaline phosphatase, increased globulins, increased GGTP, increased/decreased/abnormal WBC, abnormal AG ratio, abnormal RBC, bilirubinemia, eosinophilia, hyperlipemia, increased/decreased electrolytes, increased/decreased cholesterol, increased glucocorticoids, increased LDH, increased/decreased/abnormal platelets, and increased gastrin levels. Additional isolated laboratory abnormalities were reported.

In the placebo-controlled studies, when SGOT (AST) and SGPT (ALT) were evaluated, 0.4% (1/250) placebo patients and 0.3% (2/795) lansoprazole patients had enzyme elevations greater than three times the upper limit of normal range at the final treatment visit. None of these patients reported jaundice at any time during the study.

Amoxicillin:

The following adverse reactions from the labeling for amoxicillin are provided for information.

As with other penicillins, it may be expected that untoward reactions will be essentially limited to sensitivity phenomena. They are more likely to occur in individuals who have

Continued on next page

PREVPAC—Cont.

previously demonstrated hypersensitivity to penicillins and in those with a history of allergy, asthma, hay fever, or urticaria.

The following adverse reactions have been reported as associated with the use of penicillin:

Gastrointestinal—Glossitis, stomatitis, black "hairy" tongue, nausea, vomiting, and diarrhea. (These reactions are usually associated with oral dosage forms.)

Hypersensitivity Reactions—Skin rashes and urticaria have been reported frequently. A few cases of exfoliative dermatitis and erythema multiforme have been reported. Anaphylaxis is the most serious reaction experienced and has usually been associated with the parenteral dosage form. **Note:** Urticaria, other skin rashes, and serum sickness-like reactions may be controlled with antihistamines and, if necessary, systemic corticosteroids. Whenever such reactions occur, penicillin should be discontinued unless, in the opinion of the physician, the condition being treated is life threatening and amenable only to penicillin therapy. Serious anaphylactic reactions require the immediate use of epinephrine, oxygen, and intravenous steroids.

Liver—A moderate rise in serum glutamic oxaloacetic transaminase (SGOT) has been noted, particularly in infants, but the significance of this finding is unknown.

Hemic and Lymphatic Systems—Anemia, thrombocytopenia, thrombocytopenic purpura, eosinophilia, leukopenia, and agranulocytosis have been reported during therapy with the penicillins. These reactions are usually reversible on discontinuation of therapy and are believed to be hypersensitivity phenomena.

Clarithromycin:

The following adverse reactions from the labeling for clarithromycin are provided for information.

The majority of side effects observed in clinical trials were of a mild and transient nature. Fewer than 3% of adult patients without mycobacterial infections discontinued therapy because of drug-related side effects.

The most frequently reported events in adults were diarrhea (3%), nausea (3%), abnormal taste (3%), dyspepsia (2%), abdominal pain/discomfort (2%), and headache (2%). Most of these events were described as mild or moderate in severity. Of the reported adverse events, only 1% was described as severe.

Postmarketing Experience:

Allergic reactions ranging from urticaria and mild skin eruptions to rare cases of anaphylaxis, Stevens-Johnson syndrome, and toxic epidermal necrolysis have occurred. Other spontaneously reported adverse events include glossitis, stomatitis, oral moniliasis, anorexia, vomiting, tongue discoloration, thrombocytopenia, leukopenia, neutropenia, and dizziness. There have been reports of tooth discoloration in patients treated with clarithromycin. Tooth discoloration is usually reversible with professional dental cleaning. There have been isolated reports of hearing loss, which is usually reversible, occurring chiefly in elderly women. Reports of alterations of the sense of smell, usually in conjunction with taste perversion or taste loss have also been reported.

Transient CNS events including anxiety, behavioral changes, confusional states, depersonalization, disorientation, hallucinations, insomnia, manic behavior, nightmares, psychosis, tinnitus, tremor, and vertigo have been reported during postmarketing surveillance. Events usually resolve with discontinuation of the drug.

Hepatic dysfunction, including increased liver enzymes and hepatocellular and/or cholestatic hepatitis, with or without jaundice, has been infrequently reported with clarithromycin. This hepatic dysfunction may be severe and is usually reversible. In very rare instances, hepatic failure with fatal outcome has been reported and generally has been associated with serious underlying diseases and/or concomitant medications.

There have been rare reports of hypoglycemia, some of which have occurred in patients taking oral hypoglycemic agents or insulin.

As with other macrolides, clarithromycin has been associated with QT prolongation and ventricular arrhythmias, including ventricular tachycardia and torsades de pointes.

Changes in Laboratory Values: Changes in laboratory values with possible clinical significance were as follows: *Hepatic*—elevated SGPT (ALT) <1%, SGOT (AST) <1%, GGT <1%, alkaline phosphatase <1%, LDH <1%, total bilirubin <1%; *Hematologic*—decreased WBC <1%, elevated prothrombin time 1%; *Renal*—elevated BUN 4%, elevated serum creatinine <1%. GGT, alkaline phosphatase, and prothrombin time are from adult studies only.

OVERDOSAGE

In case of an overdose, patients should contact a physician, poison control center, or emergency room. There is neither a pharmacologic basis nor data suggesting an increased toxicity of the combination compared to individual components.

Lansoprazole:

Oral doses up to 5000 mg/kg in rats (approximately 1300 times the 30 mg human dose based on body surface area) and mice (about 675.7 times the 30 mg human dose based on body surface area) did not produce deaths or any clinical signs.

Lansoprazole is not removed from the circulation by hemodialysis. In one reported case of overdose, the patient consumed 600 mg of lansoprazole with no adverse reaction.

Amoxicillin:

In case of overdosage, discontinue medication, treat symptomatically and institute supportive measures as required.

Amoxicillin can be removed from circulation by hemodialysis.

DOSAGE AND ADMINISTRATION

H. pylori Eradication to Reduce the Risk of Duodenal Ulcer Recurrence

The recommended adult oral dose is 30 mg PREVACID, 1 g amoxicillin, and 500 mg clarithromycin administered together twice daily (morning and evening) for 10 or 14 days. (See INDICATIONS AND USAGE.)

PREVPAC is not recommended in patients with creatinine clearance less than 30 mL/min.

HOW SUPPLIED

PREVPAC is supplied as an individual daily administration pack, each containing:

PREVACID:

– two opaque, hard gelatin, black and pink PREVACID 30-mg capsules, with the TAP logo and "PREVACID 30" imprinted on the capsules.

TRIMOX:

– four maroon and light pink amoxicillin 500-mg capsules, USP, with "BRISTOL 7279" imprinted on the capsules.

BIAXIN Filmtab:

– two yellow oval film-coated clarithromycin 500-mg tablets, USP, debossed with the Abbott logo on one side and "KL" on the other side of the tablets.

NDC 0300-3702-01   Daily administration pack
NDC 0300-3702-11   Daily administration card

Storage: Protect from light and moisture.

Store at a controlled room temperature between 20°C and 25°C (68°F and 77°F).

Rx only

U.S. Patent No. 5,013,743

PREVPAC is distributed by TAP Pharmaceuticals Inc.

PREVACID® (lansoprazole) Delayed-Release Capsules
Manufactured for TAP Pharmaceuticals Inc.
Lake Forest, Illinois 60045, U.S.A.
by Takeda Chemical Industries Limited
Osaka, Japan 541

TRIMOX® (amoxicillin, USP)
Manufactured by APOTHECON® A Bristol-Myers Squibb Company Princeton, NJ 08540, U.S.A.

BIAXIN® Filmtab® (clarithromycin tablets, USP)
Manufactured by Abbott Laboratories North Chicago, IL 60064, U.S.A.

Ref. 03-5062-R3; Revised: July, 2000
© 1997–2000 TAP Pharmaceutical Products Inc.

Shown in Product Identification Guide, page 338

Wallace Laboratories
P.O. BOX 1001
CRANBURY, NJ 08512

For Medical Information, Contact:
Generally:
Professional Services
800-526-3840
After Hours and Weekend Emergencies:
(609) 655-6474

Wallace Laboratories
Sales and Ordering:
Div. of Carter-Wallace, Inc
P.O. Box 1001
Cranbury, NJ 08512

ASTELIN®
(azelastine hydrochloride)
Nasal Spray, 137 mcg
For Intranasal Use Only

Prescribing information for this product, which appears on pages 3238–3239 of the 2001 PDR, has been completely revised as follows. Please write "See Supplement A" next to the product heading.

DESCRIPTION

Astelin® (azelastine hydrochloride) Nasal Spray, 137 micrograms (mcg), is an antihistamine formulated as a metered-spray solution for intranasal administration. Azelastine hydrochloride occurs as a white, almost odorless, crystalline powder with a bitter taste. It has a molecular weight of 418.37. It is sparingly soluble in water, methanol, and propylene glycol and slightly soluble in ethanol, octanol, and glycerine. It has a melting point of about 225°C and the pH of a saturated solution is between 5.0 and 5.4. Its chemical name is (±)-1-(2H)-phthalazinone,4-[(4-chlorophenyl) methyl]-2-(hexahydro-1-methyl-1H-azepin-4-yl)-, monohydrochloride. Its molecular formula is $C_{22}H_{24}CIN_3O \cdot HCl$ with the following chemical structure:

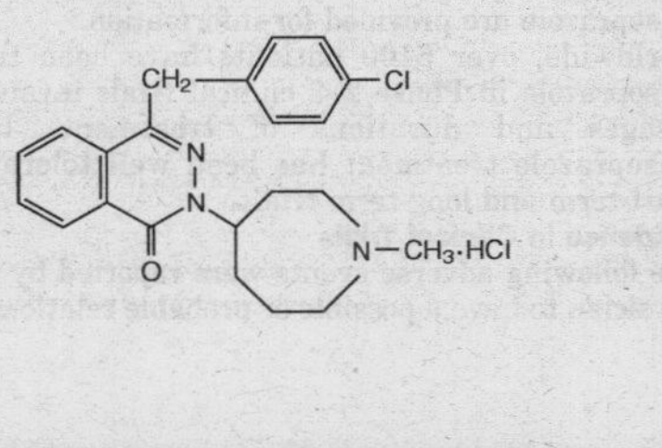

Astelin® Nasal Spray contains 0.1% azelastine hydrochloride in an aqueous solution at pH 6.8 ± 0.3. It also contains benzalkonium chloride (125 mcg/mL), edetate disodium, hydroxypropyl methyl cellulose, citric acid, dibasic sodium phosphate, sodium chloride, and purified water.

After priming, each metered spray delivers a 0.137 mL mean volume containing 137 mcg of azelastine hydrochloride (equivalent to 125 mcg of azelastine base). Each bottle can deliver 100 metered sprays.

CLINICAL PHARMACOLOGY

Azelastine hydrochloride, a phthalazinone derivative, exhibits histamine H_1-receptor antagonist activity in isolated tissues, animal models, and humans. Astelin® Nasal Spray is administered as a racemic mixture with no difference in pharmacologic activity noted between the enantiomers in *in vitro* studies. The major metabolite, desmethylazelastine, also possesses H_1-receptor antagonist activity.

Pharmacokinetics and Metabolism

After intranasal administration, the systemic bioavailability of azelastine hydrochloride is approximately 40%. Maximum plasma concentrations (Cmax) are achieved in 2–3 hours. Based on intravenous and oral administration, the elimination half-life, steady-state volume of distribution, and plasma clearance are 22 hours, 14.5 L/kg, and 0.5 L/h/kg, respectively. Approximately 75% of an oral dose of radiolabeled azelastine hydrochloride was excreted in the feces with less than 10% as unchanged azelastine. Azelastine is oxidatively metabolized to the principal active metabolite, desmethylazelastine, by the cytochrome P450 enzyme system. The specific P450 isoforms responsible for the biotransformation of azelastine have not been identified; however, clinical interaction studies with the known CYP3A4 inhibitor erythromycin failed to demonstrate a pharmacokinetic interaction. In a multiple-dose, steady-state drug interaction study in normal volunteers, cimetidine (400 mg twice daily), a nonspecific P450 inhibitor, raised orally administered mean azelastine (4 mg twice daily) concentrations by approximately 65%.

The major active metabolite, desmethylazelastine, was not measurable (below assay limits) after single-dose intranasal administration of azelastine hydrochloride. After intranasal dosing of azelastine hydrochloride to steady-state, plasma concentrations of desmethylazelastine range from 20–50% of azelastine concentrations. When azelastine hydrochloride is administered orally, desmethylazelastine has an elimination half-life of 54 hours. Limited data indicate that the metabolite profile is similar when azelastine hydrochloride is administered via the intranasal or oral route.

In vitro studies with human plasma indicate that the plasma protein building of azelastine and desmethylazelastine are approximately 88% and 97%, respectively.

Azelastine hydrochloride administered intranasally at doses above two sprays per nostril twice daily for 29 days resulted in greater than proportional increases in Cmax and area under the curve (AUC) for azelastine.

Studies in healthy subjects administered oral doses of azelastine hydrochloride demonstrated linear responses in Cmax and AUC.

Special Populations

Following oral administration, pharmacokinetic parameters were not influenced by age, gender, or hepatic impairment. Based on oral, single-dose studies, renal insufficiency (creatinine clearance <50 mL/min) resulted in a 70–75% higher Cmax and AUC compared to normal subjects. Time to maximum concentration was unchanged.

Oral azelastine has been safely administered to over 1400 asthmatic subjects, supporting the safety of administering Astelin® Nasal Spray to allergic rhinitis patients with asthma.

Pharmacodynamics

In a placebo-controlled study (95 subjects with allergic rhinitis), there was no evidence of an effect of Astelin® Nasal Spray (2 sprays per nostril twice daily for 56 days) on cardiac repolarization as represented by the corrected QT Interval (QTc) of the electrocardiogram. At higher oral exposures (≥4 mg twice daily), a nonclinically significant mean change on the QTc (3–7 millisecond increase) was observed. Interaction studies investigating the cardiac repolarization effects of concomitantly administered oral azelastine hydrochloride and erythromycin or ketoconazole were conducted. Oral erythromycin had no effect on azelastine pharmacokinetics or QTc based on analysis of serial electrocardiograms. Ketoconazole interfered with the measurement of azelastine plasma levels; however, no effects on QTc were observed (see PRECAUTIONS, Drug Interactions).

Clinical Trials

U.S. placebo-controlled clinical trials of Astelin® Nasal Spray included 322 patients with seasonal allergic rhinitis who received two sprays per nostril twice a day for up to 4 weeks. These trials included 55 pediatric patients ages 12 to 16 years. Astelin® Nasal Spray significantly improved a complex of symptoms, which included rhinorrhea, sneezing, and nasal pruritus.

In dose-ranging trials, Astelin® Nasal Spray administration resulted in a decrease in symptoms, which reached statistical significance from saline placebo within 3 hours after initial dosing and persisted over the 12-hour dosing interval. There were no findings on nasal examination in an 8-week study that suggested any adverse effect of azelastine on the nasal mucosa.

Two hundred sixteen patients with vasomotor rhinitis received Astelin® Nasal Spray two sprays per nostril twice a day in two U.S. placebo controlled trials. These patients had vasomotor rhinitis for at least one year, negative skin tests to indoor and outdoor aeroallergens, negative nasal smears for eosinophils, and negative sinus X-rays, Astelin® Nasal Spray significantly improved a symptom complex comprised of rhinorrhea, post nasal drip, nasal congestion, and sneezing.

INDICATIONS AND USAGE

Astelin® Nasal Spray is indicated for the treatment of the symptoms of seasonal allergic rhinitis such as rhinorrhea, sneezing, and nasal pruritus in adults and children 5 years and older, and for the treatment of the symptoms of vasomotor rhinitis, such as rhinorrhea, nasal congestion and post nasal drip in adults and children 12 years and older.

CONTRAINDICATIONS

Astelin® Nasal Spray is contraindicated in patients with a known hypersensitivity to azelastine hydrochloride or any of its components.

PRECAUTIONS

Activities Requiring Mental Alertness: In clinical trials, the occurrence of somnolence has been reported in some patients taking Astelin® Nasal Spray; due caution should therefore be exercised when driving a car or operating potentially dangerous machinery. Concurrent use of Astelin® Nasal Spray with alcohol or other CNS depressants should be avoided because additional reductions in alertness and additional impairment of CNS performance may occur.

Information for Patients: Patients should be instructed to use Astelin® Nasal Spray only as prescribed. For the proper use of the nasal spray and to attain maximum improvement, the patient should read and follow carefully the accompanying patient instructions. Patients should be instructed to prime the delivery system before initial use and after storage for 3 or more days (see PATIENT INSTRUCTIONS FOR USE). Patients should also be instructed to store the bottle upright at room temperature with the pump tightly closed and out of the reach of children. In case of accidental ingestion by a young child, seek professional assistance or contact a poison control center immediately.

Patients should be advised against the concurrent use of Astelin® Nasal Spray with other antihistamines without consulting a physician. Patients who are, or may become, pregnant should be told that this product should be used in pregnancy or during lactation only if the potential benefit justifies the potential risks to the fetus or nursing infant. Patients should be advised to assess their individual responses to Astelin® Nasal Spray before engaging in any activity requiring mental alertness, such as driving a car or operating machinery. Patients should be advised that the concurrent use of Astelin® Nasal Spray with alcohol or other CNS depressants may lead to additional reductions in alertness and impairment of CNS performance and should be avoided (see Drug Interactions).

Drug Interactions: Concurrent use of Astelin® Nasal Spray with alcohol or other CNS depressants should be avoided because additional reductions in alertness and additional impairment of CNS performance may occur.

Cimetidine (400 mg twice daily) increased the mean Cmax and AUC of orally administered azelastine hydrochloride (4 mg twice daily) by approximately 65%. Ranitidine hydrochloride (150 mg twice daily) had no effect on azelastine pharmacokinetics.

Interaction studies investigating the cardiac effects, as measured by the corrected QT interval (QTc), of concomitantly administered oral azelastine hydrochloride and erythromycin or ketoconazole were conducted. Oral erythromycin (500 mg three times daily for seven days) had no effect on azelastine pharmacokinetics or QTc based on analyses of serial electrocardiograms. Ketoconazole (200 mg twice daily for seven days) interfered with the measurement of azelastine plasma concentrations; however, no effects on QTc were observed.

No significant pharmacokinetic interaction was observed with the coadministration of an oral 4 mg dose of azelastine hydrochloride twice daily and theophylline 300 mg or 400 mg twice daily.

Carcinogenesis, Mutagenesis, Impairment of Fertility: In 2 year carcinogenicity studies in rats and mice azelastine hydrochloride did not show evidence of carcinogenicity at oral doses up to 30 mg/kg and 25 mg/kg, respectively (approximately 240 and 100 times the maximum recommended daily intranasal dose in adults and children on a mg/m² basis).

Azelastine hydrochloride showed no genotoxic effects in the Ames test, DNA repair test, mouse lymphoma forward mutation assay, mouse micronucleus test, or chromosomal aberration test in rat bone marrow.

Reproduction and fertility studies in rats showed no effects on male or female fertility at oral doses up to 30 mg/kg (approximately 240 times the maximum recommended daily intranasal dose in adults on a mg/m² basis). At 68.6 mg/kg (approximately 560 times the maximum recommended daily intranasal dose in adults on a mg/m² basis), the duration of estrous cycles was prolonged and copulatory activity and the number of pregnancies were decreased. The numbers of corpora lutea and implantations were decreased; however, preimplantation loss was not increased.

Pregnancy Category C: Azelastine hydrochloride has been shown to cause developmental toxicity. Treatment of mice with an oral dose of 68.6 mg/kg (approximately 280 times the maximum recommended daily intranasal dose in adults on a mg/m² basis) caused embryo-fetal death, malformations (cleft palate; short or absent tail; fused, absent or branched ribs), delayed ossification and decreased fetal weight. This dose also caused maternal toxicity as evidenced by decreased

body weight. Neither fetal nor maternal effects occurred at a dose of 3 mg/kg (approximately 10 times the maximum recommended daily intranasal dose in adults on a mg/m² basis). In rats, an oral dose of 30 mg/kg (approximately 240 times the maximum recommended daily intranasal dose in adults on a mg/m² basis) caused malformations (oligo-and brachydactylia), delayed ossification and skeletal variations, in the absence of maternal toxicity. At 68.6 mg/kg (approximately 560 times the maximum recommended daily intranasal dose in adults on a mg/m² basis) azelastine hydrochloride also caused embryo-fetal death and decreased fetal weight; however, the 68.6 mg/kg dose caused severe maternal toxicity. Neither fetal nor maternal effects occurred at a dose of 3 mg/kg (approximately 25 times the maximum recommended daily intranasal dose in adults on a mg/m² basis). In rabbits, oral doses of 30 mg/kg and greater (approximately 500 times the maximum recommended daily intranasal dose in adults on a mg/m² basis) caused abortion, delayed ossification and decreased fetal weight; however, these doses also resulted in severe maternal toxicity. Neither fetal nor maternal effects occurred at a dose of 0.3 mg/kg (approximately 5 times the maximum recommended daily intranasal dose in adults on a mg/m² basis).

There are no adequate and well-controlled clinical studies in pregnant women. Astelin® Nasal Spray should be used during pregnancy only if the potential benefit justifies the potential risk to the fetus.

Nursing Mothers: It is not known whether azelastine hydrochloride is excreted in human milk. Because many drugs are excreted in human milk, caution should be exercised when Astelin® Nasal Spray is administered to a nursing woman.

Pediatric Use: The safety and effectiveness of Astelin® Nasal Spray at a dose of 1 spray per nostril twice daily has been established for patients 5 through 11 years of age for the treatment of symptoms of seasonal allergic rhinitis. The safety of this dosage of Astelin® Nasal Spray was established in well-controlled studies of this dose in 176 patients 5 to 12 years of age treated for up to 6 weeks. The efficacy of Astelin® Nasal Spray at this dose is based on an extrapolation of the finding of efficacy in adults, on the likelihood that the disease course, pathophysiology and response to treatment are substantially similar in children compared to adults, and on supportive data from controlled clinical trials in patients 5 to 12 years of age at the dose of 1 spray per nostril twice daily. The safety and effectiveness of Astelin® Nasal Spray in patients below the age of 5 years have not been established.

Geriatric Use: Clinical studies of Astelin® Nasal Spray did not include sufficient numbers of subjects aged 65 and over to determine whether they respond differently from younger subjects. Other reported clinical experience has not identified differences in responses between the elderly and younger patients. In general, dose selection for an elderly patient should be cautious, usually starting at the low end of the dosing range, reflecting the greater frequency of decreased hepatic, renal, or cardiac function, and of concomitant disease or other drug therapy.

ADVERSE REACTIONS
Seasonal Allergic Rhinitis
Adverse experience information for Astelin® Nasal Spray is derived from six well-controlled, 2-day to 8-week clinical studies which included 391 patients who received Astelin® Nasal Spray at a dose of 2 sprays per nostril twice daily. In placebo-controlled efficacy trials, the incidence of discontinuation due to adverse reactions in patients receiving Astelin® Nasal Spray was not significantly different from vehicle placebo (2.2% vs 2.8%, respectively).

In these clinical studies, adverse events that occurred statistically significantly more often in patients treated with Astelin® Nasal Spray versus vehicle placebo included bitter taste (19.7% vs 0.6%), somnolence (11.5% vs 5.4%), weight increase (2.0% vs 0%), and myalgia (1.5% vs 0%).

The following adverse events were reported with frequencies ≥2% in the Astelin® Nasal Spray treatment group and more frequently than placebo in short-term (≤2 days) and long-term (2–8 weeks) clinical trials.

ADVERSE EVENT	Astelin® Nasal Spray n = 391	Vehicle Placebo n = 353
Bitter Taste	19.7	0.6
Headache	14.8	12.7
Somnolence	11.5	5.4
Nasal Burning	4.1	1.7
Pharyngitis	3.8	2.8
Dry Mouth	2.8	1.7
Paroxysmal Sneezing	3.1	1.1
Nausea	2.8	1.1
Rhinitis	2.3	1.4
Fatigue	2.3	1.4
Dizziness	2.0	1.4
Epistaxis	2.0	1.4
Weight Increase	2.0	0.0

A total of 176 patients 5 to 12 years of age were exposed to Astelin® Nasal Spray at a dose of 1 spray each nostril twice daily in 3 placebo-controlled studies. In these studies, adverse events that occurred more frequently in patients treated with Astelin® Nasal Spray than with placebo, and that were not represented in the adult adverse event table above include rhinitis/cold symptoms (17.0% vs 9.5%), cough (11.4% vs 8.3%), conjunctivitis (5.1% vs 1.8%), and asthma (4.5% vs 4.1%).

The following events were observed infrequently (<2% and exceeding placebo incidence) in patients who received Astelin® Nasal Spray (2 sprays/nostril twice daily) in U.S. clinical trials.
Cardiovascular: flushing, hypertension, tachycardia.
Dermatological: contact dermatitis, eczema, hair and follicle infection, furunculosis.
Digestive: constipation, gastroenteritis, glossitis, ulcerative stomatitis, vomiting, increased SGPT, aphthous stomatitis.
Metabolic and Nutritional: increased appetite.
Musculoskeletal: myalgia, temporomandibular dislocation.
Neurological: hyperkinesia, hypoesthesia, vertigo.
Psychological: anxiety, depersonalization, depression, nervousness, sleep disorder, thinking abnormal.
Respiratory: bronchospasm, coughing, throat burning, laryngitis.
Special Senses: conjunctivitis, eye abnormality, eye pain, watery eyes, taste loss.
Urogenital: albuminuria, amenorrhea, breast pain, hematuria, increased urinary frequency.
Whole Body: allergic reaction, back pain, herpes simplex, viral infection, malaise, pain in extremities, abdominal pain.

ADVERSE REACTIONS
Vasomotor Rhinitis
Adverse experience information for Astelin® Nasal Spray is derived from two placebo-controlled clinical studies which included 216 patients who received Astelin® Nasal Spray at a dose of 2 sprays per nostril twice daily for up to 28 days. The incidence of discontinuation due to adverse reactions in patients receiving Astelin® Nasal Spray was not different from vehicle placebo (2.8% vs 2.9%, respectively).

The following adverse events were reported with frequencies ≥2% in the Astelin® Nasal Spray treatment group and more frequently than placebo.

ADVERSE EVENT	Astelin® Nasal Spray n = 216	Vehicle Placebo n = 210
Bitter Taste	19.4	2.4
Headache	7.9	7.6
Dysesthesia	7.9	3.3
Rhinitis	5.6	2.4
Epistaxis	3.2	2.4
Sinusitis	3.2	1.9
Somnolence	3.2	1.0

Events observed infrequently (<2% and exceeding placebo incidence) in patients who received Astelin® Nasal Spray (2 sprays/nostril twice daily) in U.S. clinical trials in vasomotor rhinitis were similar to those observed in U.S. clinical trials in seasonal allergic rhinitis.

In controlled trials involving nasal and oral azelastine hydrochloride formulations, there were infrequent occurrences of hepatic transaminase elevations. The clinical relevance of these reports has not been established.

In addition, the following spontaneous adverse events have been reported during the marketing of Astelin® Nasal Spray and causal relationship with the drug is unknown: anaphylactoid reaction, application site irritation, chest pain, nasal congestion, confusion, diarrhea, dyspnea, facial edema, involuntary muscle contractions, paresthesia, parosmia, pruritus, rash, tolerance, urinary retention, vision abnormal and xerophthalmia.

OVERDOSAGE

There have been no reported overdosages with Astelin® Nasal Spray. Acute overdosage by adults with this dosage form is unlikely to result in clinically significant adverse events, other than increased somnolence, since one bottle of Astelin® Nasal Spray contains 17 mg of azelastine hydrochloride. Clinical studies in adults with single doses of the oral formulation of azelastine hydrochloride (up to 16 mg) have not resulted in increased incidence of serious adverse events. General supportive measures should be employed if overdosage occurs. There is no known antidote to Astelin® Nasal Spray. Oral ingestion of antihistamines has the potential to cause serious adverse effects in young children. Accordingly, Astelin® Nasal Spray should be kept out of the reach of children. Oral doses of 120 mg/kg and greater (approximately 460 times the maximum recommended daily intranasal dose in adults and children on a mg/m² basis) were lethal in mice. Responses seen prior to death were tremor, convulsions, decreased muscle tone, and salivation. In dogs,

Continued on next page

Astelin—Cont.

single oral doses as high as 10 mg/kg (approximately 260 times the maximum recommended daily intranasal dose in adults and children on a mg/m² basis) were well tolerated, but single oral doses of 20 mg/kg were lethal.

DOSAGE AND ADMINISTRATION

Seasonal Allergic Rhinitis
The recommended dose of Astelin® Nasal Spray in adults and children 12 years and older with seasonal allergic rhinitis is two sprays per nostril twice daily. The recommended dose of Astelin® Nasal Spray in children 5 years to 11 years of age is one spray per nostril twice daily.

Vasomotor Rhinitis
The recommended dose of Astelin® Nasal Spray in adults and children 12 years and older with vasomotor rhinitis is two sprays per nostril twice daily.
Before initial use, the screw cap on the bottle should be replaced with the pump unit and the delivery system should be primed with 4 sprays or until a fine mist appears. When 3 or more days have elapsed since the last use, the pump should be reprimed with 2 sprays or until a fine mist appears. **CAUTION: Avoid spraying in the eyes.**
Directions for Use: Illustrated patient instructions for proper use accompany each package of Astelin® Nasal Spray.

HOW SUPPLIED

Astelin® (azelastine hydrochloride) Nasal Spray, 137 mcg, (NDC 0037-0241-10) is supplied as a package containing a total of 200 metered sprays in two high-density polyethylene (HDPE) bottles fitted with screw caps. A separate metered-dose spray pump unit and a leaflet of patient instructions are also provided. The spray pump unit is packaged in a polyethylene wrapper and consists of a nasal spray pump fitted with a blue safety clip and a blue plastic dust cover.
Each Astelin® (azelastine hydrochloride) Nasal Spray, 137 mcg, bottle contains 17 mg (1mg/mL) of azelastine hydrochloride to be used with the supplied metered-dose spray pump unit. Each bottle can deliver 100 metered sprays. Each spray delivers a mean of 0.137 mL solution containing 137 mcg of azelastine hydrochloride.
ATTENTION: The imprinted expiration date applies to the product in the bottles with screw caps. After the spray pump is inserted into the first bottle of the dispensing package, both bottles of product should be discarded after 3 months, not to exceed the expiration date imprinted on the label.
Storage: Store at controlled room temperature 20°–25°C (68°–77°F). Protect from freezing.
Manufactured by
Wallace Laboratories
Division of Carter-Wallace, Inc.
Cranbury, NJ 08512-0181 for
Wallace Laboratories/ASTA Medica LLC
© 2000 Wallace Laboratories/ASTA Medica LLC
IN-023S3-11   Rev. 8/00

Watson Laboratories, Inc.
311 BONNIE CIRCLE
CORONA, CA 92880

Direct Inquiries to:
Customer Service Department
Telephone: 800/272-5525
FAX: 909/735-2871
For Medical Information Contact:
Telephone: 800/272-5525

FERRLECIT®   ℞
[fĕr "le'sit]
sodium ferric gluconate
complex in sucrose injection
62.5 mg/5 mL

Prescribing information for this product, which appears on pages 2878–2879 of the 2001 PDR, has been completely revised as follows. Please write "See Supplement A" next to the product heading.

DESCRIPTION

Ferrlecit® (sodium ferric gluconate complex in sucrose injection) is a stable macromolecular complex with an apparent molecular weight on gel chromatography of 289,000–440,000 daltons. The macromolecular complex is negatively charged at alkaline pH and is present in solution with sodium cations. The product has a deep red color indicative of ferric oxide linkages.
The structural formula is considered to be $[NaFe_2O_3(C_6H_{11}O_7)(C_{12}H_{22}O_{11})_5]_{n\sim200}$.
Each ampule of 5 mL of Ferrlecit® for intravenous injection contains 62.5 mg (12.5 mg/mL) of elemental iron as the sodium salt of a ferric ion carbohydrate complex in an alkaline aqueous solution with approximately 20% sucrose w/v (195 mg/mL) in water for injection, pH 7.7–9.7.
Each mL contains 9 mg of benzyl alcohol as an inactive ingredient.
Therapeutic Class: Hematinic

CLINICAL PHARMACOLOGY

Ferrlecit® is used to replete the total body content of iron. Iron is critical for normal hemoglobin synthesis to maintain

---

oxygen transport. Additionally, iron is necessary for metabolism and various enzymatic processes.
The total body iron content of an adult ranges from 2 to 4 grams. Approximately 2/3 is in hemoglobin and 1/3 is in reticuloendothelial (RE) storage (bone marrow, spleen, liver) bound to intracellular ferritin. The body highly conserves iron (daily loss of 0.03%) requiring supplementation of about 1 mg/day to replenish losses in healthy, non-menstruating adults. The etiology of iron deficiency in hemodialysis patients is varied and can include blood loss and/or increased iron utilization (e.g., from epoetin therapy). The administration of exogenous epoetin increases red blood cell production and iron utilization. The increased iron utilization and blood losses in the hemodialysis patient may lead to absolute or functional iron deficiency. Iron deficiency is absolute when hematological indicators of iron stores are low. Patients with functional iron deficiency do not meet laboratory criteria for absolute iron deficiency but demonstrate an increase in hemoglobin/hematocrit or a decrease in epoetin dosage with stable hemoglobin/hematocrit when parenteral iron is administered.

Pharmacokinetics
Multiple sequential single dose intravenous pharmacokinetic studies were performed on 14 healthy iron-deficient volunteers. Entry criteria included hemoglobin $\geq$10.5 gm/dL and transferrin saturation $\leq$15% (TSAT) or serum ferritin value $\leq$20 ng/mL. In the 1st stage, each subject was randomized 1:1 to undiluted Ferrlecit® injection of either 125 mg/hr or 62.5 mg/.5 hr (2.1 mg/min). Five days after the 1st stage, each subject was re-randomized 1:1 to undiluted Ferrlecit® injection of either 125 mg/7 min or 62.5 mg/4 min (>15.5 mg/min).
Peak drug levels (C_{max}) varied significantly by dosage and by rate of administration with the highest C_{max} observed in the regimen in which 125 mg was administered in 7 minutes (19 mg/L). The initial volume of distribution (V_{Ferr}) of 6 L corresponds well to calculated blood volume. V_{Ferr} did not vary by dosage or rate of administration. The terminal elimination half-life (λ_z-HL) for drug bound iron was approximately 1 hour. λ_z-HL varied by dose but not by rate of administration. The shortest value (0.85 h) occurred in the 62.5 mg/4 min regimen; the longest value (1.45 h) occurred in the 125 mg/7 min regimen. Total clearance of Ferrlecit® was 3.02 to 5.35 L/h. There was no significant variation by rate of administration. The AUC for Ferrlecit® bound iron varied by dose from 17.5 mg-h/L (62.5 mg) to 35.6 mg-h/L (125 mg). There was no significant variation by rate of administration. Approximately 80% of drug bound iron was delivered to transferrin as a mononuclear ionic iron species within 24 hours of administration in each dosage regimen. Direct movement of iron from Ferrlecit® to transferrin was not observed. Mean peak transferrin saturation did not exceed 100% and returned to near baseline by 40 hours.
In vitro experiments have shown that less than 1% of the iron species within Ferrlecit® can be dialyzed through membranes with pore sizes corresponding to 12,000 to 14,000 daltons over a period of up to 270 minutes. Human studies in renally competent subjects suggest the clinical insignificance of urinary excretion.
Drug-drug Interactions: Drug-drug interactions involving Ferrlecit® have not been studied. However, like other parenteral iron preparations, Ferrlecit® may be expected to reduce the absorption of concomitantly administered oral iron preparations.

CLINICAL STUDIES

Two clinical studies (Studies A and B) were conducted to assess the efficacy and safety of Ferrlecit®.

Study A
Study A was a three-center, randomized, open-label study of the safety and efficacy of two doses of Ferrlecit® administered intravenously to iron-deficient hemodialysis patients. The study included both a dose-response concurrent control and an historical control. Enrolled patients received a test dose of Ferrlecit® (25 mg of elemental iron) and were then randomly assigned to receive Ferrlecit® at cumulative doses of either 500 mg (low dose) or 1000 mg (high dose) of elemental iron. Ferrlecit® was given to both dose groups in eight divided doses during sequential dialysis sessions (a period of 16 to 17 days). At each dialysis session, patients in the low-dose group received Ferrlecit® 62.5 mg of elemental iron over 30 minutes, and those in the high-dose group received Ferrlecit® 125 mg of elemental iron over 60 minutes.

TABLE 1
Hemoglobin, Hematocrit, and Iron Studies

Study A	Mean Change from Baseline to Two Weeks After Cessation of Therapy		
	Ferrlecit® 1000 mg IV (N=44)	Ferrlecit® 500 mg IV (N=39)	Historical Control-Oral Iron (N=25)
Hemoglobin	1.1 g/dL*	0.3 g/dL	0.4 g/dL
Hematocrit	3.6%*	1.4%	0.8%
Transferrin Saturation	8.5%	2.8%	6.1%
Serum Ferritin	199 ng/mL	132 ng/mL	NA

*$p<0.01$ versus both the 500 mg group and the historical control group.

Cumulative Ferrlecit® Dose (mg of elemental iron)	62.5	250	375	562.5	625	750	1000	1125	1187.5
Patients (#)	1	1	2	1	10	4	12	6	1

The primary endpoint was the change in hemoglobin from baseline to the last available observation through Day 40. Eligibility for this study included chronic hemodialysis patients with a hemoglobin below 10 g/dL (or hematocrit at or below 32%) and either serum ferritin below 100 ng/mL or transferrin saturation below 18%. Exclusion criteria included significant underlying disease or inflammatory conditions or an epoetin requirement of greater than 10,000 unitsl three times per week. Parenteral iron and red cell transfusion were not allowed for two months before the study. Oral iron and red cell transfusion were not allowed during the study for Ferrlecit® treated patients.
The historical control population consisted of 25 chronic hemodialysis patients who received only oral iron supplementation for 14 months and did not receive red cell transfusion. All patients had stable epoetin doses and hematocrit values for at least two months before initiation of oral iron therapy. The evaluated population consisted of 39 patients in the low-dose Ferrlecit® group, 44 patients in the high-dose Ferrlecit® group, and 25 historical control patients.
The mean baseline hemoglobin and hematocrit were similar between treatment and historical control patients: 9.8 g/dL and 29% and 9.6 g/dL and 29% in low- and high-dose Ferrlecit® treated patients, respectively, and 9.4 g/dL and 29% in historical control patients. Baseline serum transferrin saturation was 20% in the low-dose group, 16% in the high-dose group, and 14% in the historical control. Baseline serum ferritin was 106 ng/mL in the low-dose group, 88 ng/mL in the high-dose group, and 606 ng/mL in the historical control.
Patients in the high-dose Ferrlecit® group achieved significantly higher increases in hemoglobin and hematocrit than either patients in the low-dose Ferrlecit® group or patients in the historical control group (oral iron). Patients in the low-dose Ferrlecit® group did not achieve significantly higher increases in hemoglobin and hematocrit than patients receiving oral iron. See Table 1.
[See table 1 above]

Study B
Study B was a single-center, non-randomized, open-label, historically-controlled, study of the safety and efficacy of variable, cumulative doses of intravenous Ferrlecit® in iron-deficient hemodialysis patients. Ferrlecit® administration was identical to Study A. The primary efficacy variable was the change in hemoglobin from baseline to the last available observation through Day 50.
Inclusion and exclusion criteria were identical to those of Study A as was the historical control population. Sixty-three patients were evaluated in this study: 38 in the Ferrlecit® treated group and 25 in the historical control group.
Ferrlecit® treated patients were considered to have completed the study per protocol if they received at least eight Ferrlecit® doses of either 62.5 mg or 125 mg of elemental iron. A total of 14 patients (37%) completed the study per protocol. Twelve (32%) Ferrlecit® treated patients received less than eight doses, and 12 (32%) patients had incomplete information on the sequence of dosing. Not all patients received Ferrlecit® at consecutive dialysis sessions and many received oral iron during the study.
[See second table above]
Baseline hemoglobin and hematocrit values were similar between the treatment and control groups, and were 9.1 g/dL and 27.3%, respectively, for Ferrlecit® treated patients. Serum iron studies were also similar between treatment and control groups, with the exception of serum ferritin, which was 606 ng/mL for historical control patients, compared to 77 ng/mL for Ferrlecit® treated patients.
In this patient population, only the Ferrlecit® treated group achieved significant increase in hemoglobin and hematocrit from baseline. This increase was significantly greater than that seen in the historical oral iron treatment group. See Table 2.
[See table 2 at bottom of next page]

INDICATIONS AND USAGE

Ferrlecit® is indicated for treatment of iron deficiency anemia in patients undergoing chronic hemodialysis who are receiving supplemental epoetin therapy.

CONTRAINDICATIONS

- All anemias not associated with iron deficiency.
- Hypersensitivity to Ferrlecit® or any of its inactive components.
- Evidence of iron overload.

WARNINGS

Hypersensitivity reactions have been reported with injectable iron products. See PRECAUTIONS.

PRECAUTIONS

General: Iron is not easily eliminated from the body and accumulation can be toxic. Unnecessary therapy with parenteral iron will cause excess storage of iron with consequent possibility of iatrogenic hemosiderosis. Iron overload is particularly apt to occur in patients with hemoglobinopathies and other refractory anemias. Ferrlecit® should not be administered to patients with iron overload. See OVERDOSAGE.

Hypersensitivity Reactions: Serious hypersensitivity reactions have been reported rarely in patients receiving Ferrlecit®. One case of a life-threatening hypersensitivity reaction has been observed in 1,097 patients who received a single dose of Ferrlecit® in a post-marketing safety study. Three serious hypersensitivity reactions have been reported from the spontaneous reporting system in the United States. See ADVERSE REACTIONS.

Hypotension: Hypotension associated with light-headedness, malaise, fatigue, weakness or severe pain in the chest, back, flanks, or groin has been associated with administration of intravenous iron. These hypotensive reactions are not associated with signs of hypersensitivity and have usually resolved within one or two hours. Successful treatment may consist of observation or, if the hypotension causes symptoms, volume expansion. See ADVERSE REACTIONS.

Carcinogenesis, mutagenesis, impairment of fertility: Long term carcinogenicity studies in animals were not performed. Studies to assess the effects of Ferrlecit® on fertility were not conducted. Ferrlecit® was not mutagenic in the Ames test and the rat micronucleus test. It produced a clastogenic effect in an *in vitro* chromosomal aberration assay in Chinese hamster ovary cells.

Pregnancy Category B: Ferrlecit® was not teratogenic at doses of elemental iron up to 100 mg/kg/day (300 mg/m²/day) in mice and 20 mg/kg/day (120 mg/m²/day) in rats. On a body surface area basis, these doses were 1.3 and 3.24 times the recommended human dose (125 mg/day or 92.5 mg/m²/day) for a person of 50 kg body weight, average height and body surface area of 1.46 m². There were no adequate and well-controlled studies in pregnant women. Ferrlecit® should be used during pregnancy only if the potential benefit justifies the potential risk to the fetus.

Nursing Mothers: It is not known whether this drug is excreted in human milk. Because many drugs are excreted in human milk, caution should be exercised when Ferrlecit® is administered to a nursing woman.

Pediatric Use: Safety and effectiveness of Ferrlecit® in pediatric patients have not been established. Ferrlecit® contains benzyl alcohol and therefore should not be used in neonates.

Geriatric Use: Clinical studies of Ferrlecit® did not include sufficient numbers of subjects aged 65 and over to determine whether they respond differently from younger subjects. Other reported clinical experience has not identified differences in responses between the elderly and younger patients. In particular, 51/159 hemodialysis patients in North American clinical studies were aged 65 years or older. Among these patients, no differences in safety or efficacy as a result of age were identified. In general, dose selection for an elderly patient should be cautious, usually starting at the low end of the dosing range, reflecting the greater frequency of decreased hepatic, renal, or cardiac function, and of concomitant disease or other drug therapy.

ADVERSE REACTIONS

Exposure to Ferrlecit® has been documented in over 1,400 patients on hemodialysis. This population included 1,097 Ferrlecit®-naïve patients who received a single-dose of Ferrlecit® in a placebo-controlled, cross-over, post-marketing safety study. Undiluted Ferrlecit was administered over ten minutes (125 mg of Ferrlecit® at 12.5 mg/min). No test dose was used. From a total of 1498 Ferrlecit®-treated patients in medical reports, North American trials, and post-marketing studies, twelve patients (0.8%) experienced serious reactions which precluded further therapy with Ferrlecit®.

Hypersensitivity Reactions: See PRECAUTIONS. In the single-dose, post-marketing, safety study, one patient experienced a life-threatening hypersensitivity reaction (diaphoresis, nausea, vomiting, severe lower back pain, dyspnea, and wheezing, for 20 minutes) following Ferrlecit® administration. Among 1097 patients who received Ferrlecit® in this study, there were 9 patients (0.82%) who had an adverse reaction that, in the view of the investigator, precluded further Ferrlecit® administration (drug intolerance). These included one life-threatening reaction, 6 allergic reactions (pruritus × 2, facial flushing, chills, dyspnea/chest pain, and rash), and 2 other reactions (hypotension and nausea). Another 2 patients (0.18%) experienced allergic reactions not deemed to represent drug intolerance (nausea/malaise and nausea/dizziness) following Ferrlecit® administration.

Seventy-two (7.0%) of the 1034 patients who had prior iron dextran exposure had a sensitivity to at least one form of iron dextran (INFeD® or Dexferrum®). The patient who experienced a life-threatening adverse event during the study had a previous severe anaphylactic reaction to dextran in both forms—INFeD® and Dexferrum®. The incidence of both drug intolerance and suspected allergic events following first dose Ferrlecit administration were 2.8% in patients with prior iron dextran sensitivity compared to 0.8% in patients without prior iron dextran sensitivity.

In this study, 28% of the patients received concomitant angiotensin converting enzyme inhibitor (ACEi) therapy. The incidences of both drug intolerance or suspected allergic events following first dose Ferrlecit® administration were 1.6% in patients with concomitant ACEi use compared to 0.7% in patients without concomitant ACEi use. The patient with a life-threatening event was not on ACEi therapy. One patient had facial flushing immediately on Ferrlecit® exposure. No hypotension occurred and the event resolved rapidly and spontaneously without intervention other than drug withdrawal.

In multiple dose Studies A and B, no fatal hypersensitivity reactions occurred among the 126 patients who received Ferrlecit®. Ferrlecit®-associated hypersensitivity events in Study A resulting in premature study discontinuation occurred in three out of a total 88 (3.4%) Ferrlecit®-treated patients. The first patient withdrew after the development of pruritus and chest pain following the test dose of Ferrlecit®. The second patient, in the high-dose group, experienced nausea, abdominal and flank pain, fatigue and rash following the first dose of Ferrlecit®. The third patient, in the low-dose group, experienced a "red blotchy rash" following the first dose of Ferrlecit®. Of the 38 patients exposed to Ferrlecit® in Study B, none reported hypersensitivity reactions.

Many chronic renal failure patients experience cramps, pain, nausea, rash, flushing, and pruritus.

Three cases of serious hypersensitivity reactions have been reported from the spontaneous reporting system in the United States.

Hypotension: See PRECAUTIONS. In the single dose safety study post-administration hypotensive events were observed in 22/1097 patients (2%) following Ferrlecit® administration. Hypotension has also been reported following administration of Ferrlecit® in European case reports. Of the 226 renal dialysis patients exposed to Ferrlecit® and reported in the literature, 3 (1.3%) patients experienced hypotensive events which were accompanied by flushing in two. All completely reversed after one hour without sequelae. Transient hypotension may occur during dialysis. Administration of Ferrlecit® may augment hypotension caused by dialysis.

Among the 126 patients who received Ferrlecit® in Studies A and B, one patient experienced a transient decreased level of consciousness without hypotension. Another patient discontinued treatment prematurely because of dizziness, lightheadedness, diplopia, malaise, and weakness without hypotension that resulted in a 3–4 hour hospitalization for observation following drug administration. The syndrome resolved spontaneously.

Adverse Laboratory Changes: No differences in laboratory findings associated with Ferrlecit® were reported in North American clinical trials when normalized against a National Institute of Health database on laboratory findings in 1,100 hemodialysis patients.

Most Frequent Adverse Reactions: In the single-dose, post-marketing safety study, 11% of patients who received Ferrlecit® and 9.4% of patients who received placebo reported adverse reactions. The most frequent adverse reactions following Ferrlecit® were: hypotension (2%), nausea, vomiting and/or diarrhea (2%), pain (0.7%), hypertension (0.6%), allergic reaction (0.5%), chest pain (0.5%), pruritus (0.5%), and back pain (0.4%). Similar adverse reactions were seen following placebo administration. However, because of the high baseline incidence of adverse events in the hemodialysis patient population, insufficient number of exposed patients, and limitations inherent to the cross-over, single dose study design, no comparison of event rates between Ferrlecit® and placebo treatments can be made.

In multiple-dose Studies A and B, the most frequent adverse reactions following Ferrlecit® were:

Body as a Whole: injection site reaction (33%), chest pain (10%), pain (10%), asthenia (7%), headache (7%), abdominal pain (6%), fatigue (6%), fever (5%), malaise, infection, abscess, back pain, chills, rigors, arm pain, carcinoma, flu-like syndrome, sepsis.

Nervous System: cramps (25%), dizziness (13%), paresthesias (6%), agitation, somnolence.

Respiratory System: dyspnea (11%), coughing (6%), upper respiratory infections (6%), rhinitis, pneumonia.

Cardiovascular System: hypotension (29%), hypertension (13%), syncope (6%), tachycardia (5%), bradycardia, vasodilatation, angina pectoris, myocardial infarction, pulmonary edema.

Gastrointestinal System: nausea, vomiting and/or diarrhea (35%), anorexia, rectal disorder, dyspepsia, eructation, flatulence, gastrointestinal disorder, melena.

Musculoskeletal System: leg cramps (10%), myalgia, arthralgia.

Skin and Appendages: pruritus (6%), rash, increased sweating.

Genitourinary System: urinary tract infection.

Special Senses: conjunctivitis, abnormal vision, ear disorder.

Metabolic and Nutritional Disorders: hyperkalemia (6%), generalized edema (5%), leg edema, peripheral edema, hypoglycemia, edema, hypervolemia, hypokalemia.

Hematologic System: abnormal erythrocytes (11%), anemia, leukocytosis, lymphadenopathy.

Other Adverse Reactions Observed During Clinical Trials: In the single-dose post-marketing safety study in 1,097 patients receiving Ferrlecit®, the following additional events were reported in two or more patients: hypertonia, nervousness, dry mouth, and hemorrhage.

OVERDOSAGE

Dosages in excess of iron needs may lead to accumulation of iron in iron storage sites and hemosiderosis. Periodic monitoring of laboratory parameters of iron storage may assist in recognition of iron accumulation. Ferrlecit® should not be administered in patients with iron overload.

Serum iron levels greater than 300 µg/dL may indicate iron poisoning which is characterized by abdominal pain, diarrhea, or vomiting which progresses to pallor or cyanosis, lassitude, drowsiness, hyperventilation due to acidosis, and cardiovascular collapse. Caution should be exercised in interpreting serum iron levels in the 24 hours following the administration of Ferrlecit® since many laboratory assays will falsely overestimate serum or transferrin bound iron by measuring iron still bound to the Ferrlecit® complex. Additionally, in the assessment of iron overload, caution should be exercised in interpreting serum ferritin levels in the week following Ferrlecit® administration since, in clinical studies, serum ferritin exhibited a non-specific rise which persisted for five days.

The Ferrlecit® iron complex is not dialyzable.

Ferrlecit® at elemental iron doses of 125 mg/kg, 78.8 mg/kg, 62.5 mg/kg and 250 mg/kg caused deaths to mice, rats, rabbits, and dogs respectively. The major symptoms of acute toxicity were decreased activity, staggering, ataxia, increases in the respiratory rate, tremor, and convulsions.

DOSAGE AND ADMINISTRATION

The dosage of Ferrlecit® is expressed in terms of mg of elemental iron. Each 5 mL ampule contains 62.5 mg of elemental iron (12.5 mg/mL).

The recommended dosage of Ferrlecit® for the repletion treatment of iron deficiency in hemodialysis patients is 10 mL of Ferrlecit® (125 mg of elemental iron). Ferrlecit® may be diluted in 100 mL of 0.9% sodium chloride administered by intravenous infusion over 1 hour. Ferrlecit® may also be administered undiluted as a slow IV injection (at a rate of up to 12.5 mg/min). Most patients will require a minimum cumulative dose of 1.0 gram of elemental iron, administered over eight sessions at sequential dialysis treatments, to achieve a favorable hemoglobin or hematocrit response. Patients may continue to require therapy with intravenous iron at the lowest dose necessary to maintain target levels of hemoglobin, hematocrit, and laboratory parameters of iron storage within acceptable limits. Ferrlecit® has been administered at sequential dialysis sessions by infusion or by slow IV injection during the dialysis session itself.

Note: Do not mix Ferrlecit® with other medications, or add to parenteral nutrition solutions for intravenous infusion. The compatibility of Ferrlecit® with intravenous infusion vehicles other than 0.9% sodium chloride has not been evaluated. Parenteral drug products should be inspected visually for particulate matter and discoloration before administration, whenever the solution and container permit.

If diluted in saline, use immediately after dilution.

HOW SUPPLIED

NDC# 0364-2791-23

Ferrlecit® is supplied in colorless glass ampules. Each ampule contains 62.5 mg of elemental iron in 5 mL for intravenous use, packaged in cartons of 10 ampules.

Store at 20°C–25°C (68°F–77°F); excursions permitted to 15°C–30°C (59°F–86°F). Do not freeze. See USP Controlled Room Temperature.

TABLE 2
Hemoglobin, Hematocrit, and Iron Studies

Mean Change from Baseline to One Month After Treatment

Study B	Ferrlecit® (N=38)	Oral Iron (N=25)
	change	change
Hemoglobin (g/dL)	1.3a,b	0.4
Hematocrit (%)	3.8a,b	0.2
Transferrin Saturation (%)	6.7b	1.7
Serum Ferritin (ng/mL)	73b	−145

a - p<0.05 on group comparison by the ANCOVA method.
b - p<0.001 from baseline by the paired t-test method.

Continued on next page

Ferrlecit—Cont.

Caution: Rx Only
© Watson Pharmaceuticals, Inc., and R&D Laboratories, Inc. 2001.

NORCO®   Ⓒ ℞
(Hydrocodone Bitartrate and Acetaminophen Tablets, USP)
Rx only

Prescribing information for this product, which appears on pages 3303–3304 of the 2001 PDR, has been completely revised as follows. Please write "See Supplement A" next to the product heading.

DESCRIPTION
NORCO® (Hydrocodone bitartrate and acetaminophen) is supplied in tablet form for oral administration.
Hydrocodone bitartrate is an opioid analgesic and antitussive and occurs as fine, white crystals or as a crystalline powder. It is affected by light. The chemical name is 4,5 α-epoxy-3-methoxy-17-methylmorphinan-6-one tartrate (1:1) hydrate (2:5). It has the following structural formula:

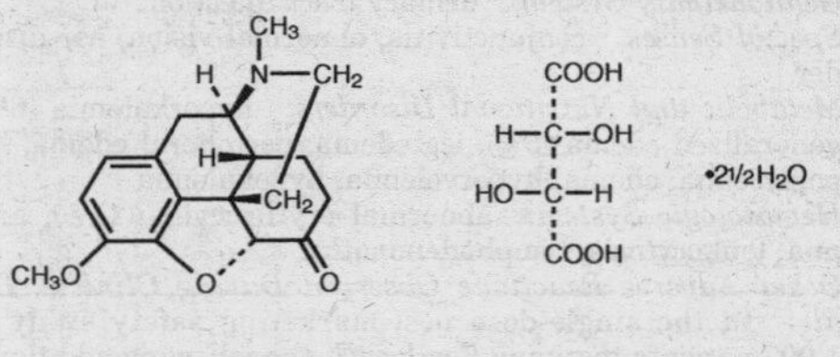

$C_{18}H_{21}NO_3 \cdot C_4H_6O_6 \cdot 2\frac{1}{2} H_2O$ M.W. = 494.50

Acetaminophen, 4-hydroxyacetanilide, a slightly bitter, white, odorless, crystalline powder, is a non-opiate, non-salicylate analgesic and antipyretic. It has the following structural formula:

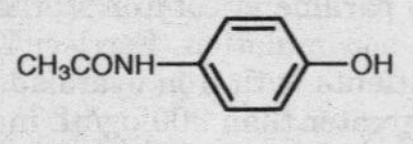

$C_8H_9NO_2$ M.W. = 151.17

NORCO®, for oral administration is available in the following strengths:

	Hydrocodone Bitartrate	Acetaminophen
NORCO® 7.5/325	7.5 mg	325 mg
NORCO® 10/325	10 mg	325 mg

In addition, each tablet contains the following inactive ingredients: croscarmellose sodium, crospovidone, magnesium stearate, microcrystalline cellulose, pregelatinized starch, povidone, and stearic acid; the 7.5 mg/325 mg tablets include FD&C Yellow #6 Aluminum Lake, the 10 mg/325 mg tablets include D&C Yellow #10 Aluminum Lake.

CLINICAL PHARMACOLOGY
Hydrocodone is a semisynthetic narcotic analgesic and antitussive with multiple actions qualitatively similar to those of codeine. Most of these involve the central nervous system and smooth muscle. The precise mechanism of action of hydrocodone and other opiates is not known, although it is believed to relate to the existence of opiate receptors in the central nervous system. In addition to analgesia, narcotics may produce drowsiness, changes in mood and mental clouding.
The analgesic action of acetaminophen involves peripheral influences, but the specific mechanism is as yet undetermined. Antipyretic activity is mediated through hypothalamic heat regulating centers. Acetaminophen inhibits prostaglandin synthetase. Therapeutic doses of acetaminophen have negligible effects on the cardiovascular or respiratory systems; however, toxic doses may cause circulatory failure and rapid, shallow breathing.
Pharmacokinetics: The behavior of the individual components is described below.
Hydrocodone: Following a 10 mg oral dose of hydrocodone administered to five adult male subjects, the mean peak concentration was 23.6 ± 5.2 ng/mL. Maximum serum levels were achieved at 1.3 ± 0.3 hours and the half-life was determined to be 3.8 ± 0.3 hours. Hydrocodone exhibits a complex pattern of metabolism including O-demethylation, N-demethylation and 6-ketoreduction to the corresponding 6-α- and 6-β-hydroxymetabolites. See **OVERDOSAGE** for toxicity information.
Acetaminophen: Acetaminophen is rapidly absorbed from the gastrointestinal tract and is distributed throughout most body tissues. The plasma half-life is 1.25 to 3 hours, but may be increased by liver damage and following overdosage. Elimination of acetaminophen is principally by liver metabolism (conjugation) and subsequent renal excretion of metabolites. Approximately 85% of an oral dose appears in the urine within 24 hours of administration, most as the glucuronide conjugate, with small amounts of other conjugates and unchanged drug. See **OVERDOSAGE** for toxicity information.

INDICATIONS AND USAGE
NORCO® is indicated for the relief of moderate to moderately severe pain.

CONTRAINDICATIONS
NORCO® should not be administered to patients who have previously exhibited hypersensitivity to hydrocodone or acetaminophen.

WARNINGS
Respiratory Depression: At high doses or in sensitive patients, hydrocodone may produce dose-related respiratory depression by acting directly on the brain stem respiratory center. Hydrocodone also affects the center that controls respiratory rhythm, and may produce irregular and periodic breathing.
Head Injury and Increased Intracranial Pressure: The respiratory depressant effects of narcotics and their capacity to elevate cerebrospinal fluid pressure may be markedly exaggerated in the presence of head injury, other intracranial lesions or a pre-existing increase in intracranial pressure. Furthermore, narcotics produce adverse reactions which may obscure the clinical course of patients with head injuries.
Acute Abdominal Conditions: The administration of narcotics may obscure the diagnosis or clinical course of patients with acute abdominal conditions.

PRECAUTIONS
General: Special Risk Patients: As with any narcotic analgesic agent, NORCO® should be used with caution in elderly or debilitated patients and those with severe impairment of hepatic or renal function, hypothyroidism, Addison's disease, prostatic hypertrophy or urethral stricture. The usual precautions should be observed and the possibility of respiratory depression should be kept in mind.
Cough Reflex: Hydrocodone suppresses the cough reflex; as with all narcotics, caution should be exercised when NORCO® is used postoperatively and in patients with pulmonary disease.
Information for Patients: Hydrocodone, like all narcotics, may impair the mental and/or physical abilities required for the performance of potentially hazardous tasks such as driving a car or operating machinery; patients should be cautioned accordingly.
Alcohol and other CNS depressants may produce an additive CNS depression, when taken with this combination product, and should be avoided.
Hydrocodone may be habit-forming. Patients should take the drug only for as long as it is prescribed, in the amounts prescribed, and no more frequently than prescribed.
Laboratory Tests: In patients with severe hepatic or renal disease, effects of therapy should be monitored with serial liver and/or renal function tests.
Drug Interactions: Patients receiving other narcotics, antihistamines, antipsychotics, antianxiety agents, or other CNS depressants (including alcohol) concomitantly with NORCO® may exhibit an additive CNS depression. When combined therapy is contemplated, the dose of one or both agents should be reduced.
The use of MAO inhibitors or tricyclic antidepressants with hydrocodone preparations may increase the effect of either the antidepressant or hydrocodone.
Drug/Laboratory Test Interactions: Acetaminophen may produce false-positive test results for urinary 5-hydroxyindoleacetic acid.
Carcinogenesis, Mutagenesis, Impairment of Fertility: No adequate studies have been conducted in animals to determine whether hydrocodone or acetaminophen have a potential for carcinogenesis, mutagenesis, or impairment of fertility.
Pregnancy: Teratogenic Effects: *Pregnancy Category C:* There are no adequate and well-controlled studies in pregnant women. NORCO® should be used during pregnancy only if the potential benefit justifies the potential risk to the fetus.
Nonteratogenic Effects: Babies born to mothers who have been taking opioids regularly prior to delivery will be physically dependent. The withdrawal signs include irritability and excessive crying, tremors, hyperactive reflexes, increased respiratory rate, increased stools, sneezing, yawning, vomiting, and fever. The intensity of the syndrome does not always correlate with the duration of maternal opioid use or dose. There is no consensus on the best method of managing withdrawal.
Labor and Delivery: As with all narcotics, administration of this product to the mother shortly before delivery may result in some degree of respiratory depression in the newborn, especially if higher doses are used.
Nursing Mothers: Acetaminophen is excreted in breast milk in small amounts, but the significance of its effects on nursing infants is not known. It is not known whether hydrocodone is excreted in human milk. Because many drugs are excreted in human milk and because of the potential for serious adverse reactions in nursing infants from hydrocodone and acetaminophen, a decision should be made whether to discontinue nursing or to discontinue the drug, taking into account the importance of the drug to the mother.
Pediatric Use: Safety and effectiveness in pediatric patients have not been established.

ADVERSE REACTIONS
The most frequently reported adverse reactions are lightheadedness, dizziness, sedation, nausea and vomiting. These effects seem to be more prominent in ambulatory than in nonambulatory patients, and some of these adverse reactions may be alleviated if the patient lies down.
Other adverse reactions include:
Central Nervous System: Drowsiness, mental clouding, lethargy, impairment of mental and physical performance, anxiety, fear, dysphoria, psychic dependence, mood changes.

Gastrointestinal System: Prolonged administration of NORCO® may produce constipation.
Genitourinary System: Ureteral spasm, spasm of vesical sphincters and urinary retention have been reported with opiates.
Respiratory Depression: Hydrocodone bitartrate may produce dose-related respiratory depression by acting directly on the brain stem respiratory centers (see **OVERDOSAGE**).
Dermatological: Skin rash, pruritus.
The following adverse drug events may be borne in mind as potential effects of acetaminophen: allergic reactions, rash, thrombocytopenia, agranulocytosis. Potential effects of high dosage are listed in the **OVERDOSAGE** section.

DRUG ABUSE AND DEPENDENCE
Controlled Substance: NORCO® is classified as a Schedule III controlled substance.
Abuse and Dependence: Psychic dependence, physical dependence, and tolerance may develop upon repeated administration of narcotics; therefore, this product should be prescribed and administered with caution. However, psychic dependence is unlikely to develop when NORCO® is used for a short time for the treatment of pain.
Physical dependence, the condition in which continued administration of the drug is required to prevent the appearance of a withdrawal syndrome, assumes clinically significant proportions only after several weeks of continued narcotic use, although some mild degree of physical dependence may develop after a few days of narcotic therapy. Tolerance, in which increasingly large doses are required in order to produce the same degree of analgesia, is manifested initially by a shortened duration of analgesic effect, and subsequently by decreases in the intensity of analgesia. The rate of development of tolerance varies among patients.

OVERDOSAGE
Following an acute overdosage, toxicity may result from hydrocodone or acetaminophen.
Signs and Symptoms: Hydrocodone: Serious overdose with hydrocodone is characterized by respiratory depression (a decrease in respiratory rate and/or tidal volume, Cheyne-Stokes respiration, cyanosis), extreme somnolence progressing to stupor or coma, skeletal muscle flaccidity, cold and clammy skin, and sometimes bradycardia and hypotension. In severe overdosage, apnea, circulatory collapse, cardiac arrest and death may occur.
Acetaminophen: In acetaminophen overdosage: dose-dependent, potentially fatal hepatic necrosis is the most serious adverse effect. Renal tubular necrosis, hypoglycemic coma, and thrombocytopenia may also occur.
Early symptoms following a potentially hepatotoxic overdose may include: nausea, vomiting, diaphoresis and general malaise. Clinical and laboratory evidence of hepatic toxicity may not be apparent until 48 to 72 hours postingestion.
In adults, hepatic toxicity has rarely been reported with acute overdoses of less than 10 grams, or fatalities with less than 15 grams.
Treatment: A single or multiple overdose with hydrocodone and acetaminophen is a potentially lethal polydrug overdose, and consultation with a regional poison control center is recommended.
Immediate treatment includes support of cardiorespiratory function and measures to reduce drug absorption. Vomiting should be induced mechanically, or with syrup of ipecac, if the patient is alert (adequate pharyngeal and laryngeal reflexes). Oral activated charcoal (1 g/kg) should follow gastric emptying. The first dose should be accompanied by an appropriate cathartic. If repeated doses are used, the cathartic might be included with alternate doses as required. Hypotension is usually hypovolemic and should respond to fluids. Vasopressors and other supportive measures should be employed as indicated. A cuffed endotracheal tube should be inserted before gastric lavage of the unconscious patient and, when necessary, to provide assisted respiration.
Meticulous attention should be given to maintaining adequate pulmonary ventilation. In severe cases of intoxication, peritoneal dialysis, or preferably hemodialysis may be considered. If hypoprothrombinemia occurs due to acetaminophen overdose, vitamin K should be administered intravenously.
Naloxone, a narcotic antagonist, can reverse respiratory depression and coma associated with opioid overdose. Naloxone hydrochloride 0.4 mg to 2 mg is given parenterally. Since the duration of action of hydrocodone may exceed that of the naloxone, the patient should be kept under continuous surveillance and repeated doses of the antagonist should be administered as needed to maintain adequate respiration. A narcotic antagonist should not be administered in the absence of clinically significant respiratory or cardiovascular depression.
If the dose of acetaminophen may have exceeded 140 mg/kg, acetylcysteine should be administered as early as possible. Serum acetaminophen levels should be obtained, since levels four or more hours following ingestion help predict acetaminophen toxicity. Do not await acetaminophen assay results before initiating treatment. Hepatic enzymes should be obtained initially, and repeated at 24-hour intervals.
Methemoglobinemia over 30% should be treated with methylene blue by slow intravenous administration.
The toxic dose for adults for acetaminophen is 10 g.

DOSAGE AND ADMINISTRATION
Dosage should be adjusted according to the severity of the pain and the response of the patient. However, it should be

kept in mind that tolerance to hydrocodone can develop with continued use and that the incidence of untoward effects is dose related.

The usual adult dosage is one tablet every four to six hours as needed for pain. The total daily dose should not exceed 6 tablets.

HOW SUPPLIED

NORCO® 7.5/325 is available as capsule-shaped, light orange tablets bisected on one side and debossed with "NORCO 729" on the other side. Each tablet contains 7.5 mg hydrocodone bitartrate and 325 mg acetaminophen. They are supplied as follows:

Bottles of 30   NDC 52544-729-30
Bottles of 100   NDC 52544-729-01
Bottles of 500   NDC 52544-729-05

NORCO® 10/325 is available as capsule-shaped, yellow tablets bisected on one side and debossed with "NORCO 539" on the other side. Each tablet contains 10 mg hydrocodone bitartrate and 325 mg acetaminophen. They are supplied as follows:

Bottles of 100   NDC 52544-539-01
Bottles of 500   NDC 52544-539-05

Store at controlled room temperature 15°C to 30°C (59°F to 86°F).

Dispense in a tight, light-resistant container with a child-resistant closure.

WATSON PHARMA

Watson Pharma, Inc.
a subsidiary of
Watson Laboratories, Inc., Corona CA 92880

13897
Revised: May 2000

Wyeth-Ayerst Pharmaceuticals

Division of American Home Products Corporation
P.O. BOX 8299
PHILADELPHIA, PA 19101

Direct General Inquiries to:
(610) 688-4400

For Medical Information Contact:
Medical Affairs
Day: (800) 934-5556
8:30 AM to 4:30 PM (Eastern Standard Time),
Weekdays only
In Emergencies:
Day: (800) 934-5556
Night: (610) 688-4400
(Emergencies only;
non-emergencies should wait until the next day)

ALESSE™-21 Tablets   ℞
[ă 'lĕs]
levonorgestrel and ethinyl estradiol tablets

Prescribing information for this product, which appears on pages 3337–3342 of the 2001 PDR, has been revised as follows. Please write "See Supplement A" next to the product heading.

Table II, which appears after the second paragraph of the **INDICATIONS AND USAGE** section should be deleted and replaced with the following:

TABLE II: PERCENTAGE OF WOMEN EXPERIENCING AN UNINTENDED PREGNANCY DURING THE FIRST YEAR OF USE OF A CONTRACEPTIVE METHOD

Method	Perfect Use	Typical Use
Levonorgestrel implants	0.05	0.05
Male sterilization	0.1	0.15
Female sterilization	0.5	0.5
Depo-Provera® (injectable progestogen)	0.3	0.3
Oral contraceptives		5
Combined	0.1	NA
Progestin only	0.5	NA
IUD		
Progesterone	1.5	2.0
Copper T 380A	0.6	0.8
Condom (male) without spermicide	3	14
(female) without spermicide	5	21
Cervical cap		
Nulliparous women	9	20
Parous women	26	40
Vaginal sponge		
Nulliparous women	9	20
Parous women	20	40
Diaphragm with spermicidal cream or jelly	6	20
Spermicides alone (foam, creams, jellies, and vaginal suppositories)	6	26
Periodic abstinence (all methods)	1–9*	25
Withdrawal	4	19
No contraception (planned pregnancy)	85	85

NA—not available
*Depending on method (calendar, ovulation, symptothermal, post-ovulation)
Adapted from Hatcher RA et al., *Contraceptive Technology, 17th Revised Edition.* New York, NY: Ardent Media, Inc., 1998.

The following should be added to the end of the **CONTRAINDICATIONS** section:

Hypersensitivity to any of the components of Alesse.

The words "certain inherited thrombophilias," should be inserted after the words "such as" just before the word "hypertension" in the last sentence of the first paragraph under the boxed warning at the beginning of the **WARNINGS** section.

The following sentence should be added as a new paragraph to the end of the subsection under the subheading "c. *Cerebrovascular diseases*" under the heading "1. THROMBOEMBOLIC DISORDERS AND OTHER VASCULAR PROBLEMS" in the **WARNINGS** section:

Women with migraine (particularly migraine with aura) who take combination oral contraceptives may be at an increased risk of stroke.

The first paragraph under the heading "3. CARCINOMA OF THE REPRODUCTIVE ORGANS" in the **WARNINGS** section should be deleted and replaced with the following:

A meta-analysis from 54 epidemiological studies reported that there is a slightly increased relative risk (RR=1.24) of having breast cancer diagnosed in women who are currently using combination oral contraceptives compared to never-users. The increased risk gradually disappears during the course of the 10 years after cessation of combination oral contraceptive use. These studies do not provide evidence for causation. The observed pattern of increased risk of breast cancer diagnosis may be due to earlier detection of breast cancer in combination oral contraceptive users, the biological effects of combination oral contraceptives, or a combination of both. Because breast cancer is rare in women under 40 years of age, the excess number of breast cancer diagnoses in current and recent combination oral contraceptive users is small in relation to the lifetime risk of breast cancer. Breast cancers diagnosed in ever-users tend to be less advanced clinically than the cancers diagnosed in never-users.

The following sentence should be added to the end of the paragraph under the subheading "10. HEADACHE" in the **WARNINGS** section:

(See "**WARNINGS**," 1c.)

The following sentence should be added as a new paragraph to the end of the subsection "2. LIPID DISORDERS" in the **PRECAUTIONS** section:

In patients with familial defects of lipoprotein metabolism receiving estrogen-containing preparations, there have been case reports of significant elevations of plasma triglycerides leading to pancreatitis.

The following sentence should be added as a new paragraph to the end of the subsection "7. DRUG INTERACTIONS" in the **PRECAUTIONS** section:

Troleandomycin may increase the risk of intrahepatic cholestasis during coadministration with combination oral contraceptives.

The following subheading and paragraph should be added after the paragraph under the subheading "11. NURSING MOTHERS" in the **PRECAUTIONS** section:

12. PEDIATRIC USE

Safety and efficacy of Alesse have been established in women of reproductive age. Safety and efficacy are expected to be the same for postpubertal adolescents under the age of 16 and users 16 and older. Use of this product before menarche is not indicated.

The adverse reaction "Pancreatitis" should be added to the end of the **ADVERSE REACTIONS** section.

The words ", or an inherited tendency to form blood clots" should be added after the word "cholesterol" to the end of the second bulleted point under the third paragraph of the **Brief Summary Patient Package Insert.**

The following sentence should be added to the end of the third paragraph, which starts "1. Blood clots in the legs...," under the boxed warning in the **Brief Summary Patient Package Insert.**

Women with migraine also may be at increased risk of stroke.

The seventh paragraph, which begins with the words "Studies to date...", under "3. High blood pressure," under the boxed warning in the **Brief Summary Patient Package Insert** should be deleted and replaced with the following two paragraphs:

Breast cancer has been diagnosed slightly more often in women who use the pill than in women of the same age who do not use the pill. This very small increase in the number of breast cancer diagnoses gradually disappears during the 10 years after stopping use of the pill. It is not known whether the difference is caused by the pill. It may be that women taking the pill were examined more often, so that breast cancer was more likely to be detected.

Some studies have found an increase in the incidence of cancer or precancerous lesions of the cervix in women who use the pill. However, this finding may be related to factors other than the use of the pill.

The list of typical failure rates under the third paragraph under the heading "EFFECTIVENESS OF ORAL CONTRACEPTIVES" in the **DETAILED PATIENT LABELING** section should be deleted and replaced with the following table:

TABLE: PERCENTAGE OF WOMEN EXPERIENCING AN UNINTENDED PREGNANCY DURING THE FIRST YEAR OF USE OF A CONTRACEPTIVE METHOD

Method	Perfect Use	Average Use
Levonorgestrel implants	0.05	0.05
Male sterilization	0.1	0.15
Female sterilization	0.5	0.5
Depo-Provera® (injectable progestogen)	0.3	0.3
Oral contraceptives		5
Combined	0.1	NA
Progestin only	0.5	NA
IUD		
Progesterone	1.5	2.0
Copper T 380A	0.6	0.8
Condom (male) without spermicide	3	14
(female) without spermicide	5	21
Cervical cap		
Never given birth	9	20
Given birth	26	40
Vaginal sponge		
Never given birth	9	20
Given birth	20	40
Diaphragm with spermicidal cream or jelly	6	20
Spermicides alone (foam, creams, jellies, and vaginal suppositories)	6	26
Periodic abstinence (all methods)	1–9*	25
Withdrawal	4	19
No contraception (planned pregnancy)	85	85

NA—not available
*Depending on method (calendar, ovulation, symptothermal, post-ovulation)
Adapted from Hatcher RA et al., *Contraceptive Technology, 17th Revised Edition.* New York, NY: Ardent Media, Inc., 1998.

The following bulleted item should be added to the end of the bulleted items under the boxed warning that appears under the heading "WHO SHOULD NOT TAKE ORAL CONTRACEPTIVES" in the **DETAILED PATIENT LABELING** section:

• Allergy or hypersensitivity to any of the components of Alesse.

The following should be added as the fifth bulleted point under the heading "OTHER CONSIDERATIONS BEFORE TAKING ORAL CONTRACEPTIVES" in the **DETAILED PATIENT LABELING** section:

• Inherited tendency to form blood clots

The following sentence should be added as a new paragraph under the heading "2. *Heart attacks and strokes*" under "RISKS OF TAKING ORAL CONTRACEPTIVES" in the **DETAILED PATIENT LABELING** section:

Women with migraine (particularly migraine with aura) who take oral contraceptives may be at higher risk of stroke.

Continued on next page

Alesse—Cont.

The two paragraphs under the heading "5. *Cancer of the reproductive organs*," under "RISKS OF TAKING ORAL CONTRACEPTIVES" in the **DETAILED PATIENT LABELING** section should be deleted and replaced with the following two paragraphs:

Breast cancer has been diagnosed slightly more often in women who use the pill than in women who do not use the pill. This very small increase in the number of breast cancer diagnoses gradually disappears after stopping the use of the pill. It is not known whether the difference is caused by the pill. It may be that women taking the pill were examined more often, so that breast cancer was more likely to be detected.

Some studies have found an increase in the incidence of cancer or precancerous lesions of the cervix in women who use oral contraceptives. However, this finding may be related to factors other than the use of oral contraceptives.

The following new section should be added to the end of the section "RISKS OF TAKING ORAL CONTRACEPTIVES" in the **DETAILED PATIENT LABELING** section:

6. *Lipid metabolism and inflammation of the pancreas*
In patients with inherited defects of lipid metabolism, there have been reports of significant elevations of plasma triglycerides during estrogen therapy. This has lead to pancreatitis in some cases.

The following should be added after the first paragraph under the subheading "4. *Drug interactions*" under GENERAL PRECAUTIONS in the **DETAILED PATIENT LABELING** section:

You may be at higher risk of a specific type of liver dysfunction if you take troleandomycin and oral contraceptives at the same time.

The paragraph, which starts "This product...", directly under the first paragraph under the subheading "4. *Drug interactions*" under GENERAL PRECAUTIONS in the **DETAILED PATIENT LABELING** section should be deleted.

CORDARONE® INTRAVENOUS
[kŏr′dă-rōn]
amiodarone hydrochloride

Prescribing information for this product, which appears on pages 3357–3360 of the 2001 PDR, has been revised as follows. Please write "See Supplement A" next to the product heading.

The paragraph under the heading **"Neonatal Hypo- or Hyperthyroidism"** in the WARNINGS section should be deleted and replaced with the following paragraph:

Although Cordarone use during pregnancy is uncommon, there have been a small number of published reports of congenital goiter/hypothyroidism and hyperthyroidism associated with its oral administration. If Cordarone I.V. is administered during pregnancy, the patient should be apprised of the potential hazard to the fetus.

The second sentence of the third paragraph under the heading **"Carcinogenesis, Mutagenesis, Impairment of Fertility"** in the PRECAUTIONS section should be deleted and replaced with the following:

However, in a study in which amiodarone HCl was orally administered to male and female rats, beginning 9 weeks prior to mating, reduced fertility was observed at a dose level of 90 mg/kg/day (approximately 1.4 times the maximum recommended human maintenance dose*).

The following paragraph should be added to the end of the section under the heading **Pediatric Use** in the PRECAUTIONS section:

Pediatric Use
The safety and efficacy of Cordarone in the pediatric population have not been established; therefore, its use in pediatric patients is not recommended.

Cordarone I.V. contains the preservative benzyl alcohol (see **DESCRIPTION**). There have been reports of fatal "gasping syndrome" in neonates (children less than one month of age) following the administration of intravenous solutions containing the preservative benzyl alcohol. Symptoms include a striking onset of gasping respiration, hypotension, bradycardia, and cardiovascular collapse.

The following paragraph and heading should be added to the end of the **PRECAUTIONS** section after the new paragraphs described above:

Geriatric Use
Clinical studies of Cordarone I.V. did not include sufficient numbers of subjects aged 65 and over to determine whether they respond differently from younger subjects. Other reported clinical experience has not identified differences in responses between the elderly and younger patients. In general, dose selection for an elderly patient should be cautious, usually starting at the low end of the dosing range, reflecting the greater frequency of decreased hepatic, renal, or cardiac function, and of concomitant disease or other drug therapy.

The last sentence, which begins with the words "The acute *oral* LD$_{50}$...", of the paragraph under the heading **OVERDOSAGE** should be deleted.

The following paragraph should be added after the eighth paragraph, which starts "It is well known that amiodarone...," of the **DOSAGE AND ADMINISTRATION** section:

Cordarone I.V. has been found to leach out plasticizers, including DEHP [di-(2-ethylhexyl) phthalate] from intra-venous tubing (including PVC tubing). The degree of leaching increases when infusing Cordarone I.V. at higher concentrations and lower flow rates than provided in **DOSAGE AND ADMINISTRATION**.

EFFEXOR® XR   ℞
[ĕf-fĕks′ŏr XR]
(venlafaxine hydrochloride)
Extended-Release Capsules

Prescribing information for this product, which appears on pages 3365–3370 of the 2001 PDR, has been revised. Please write "See Supplement A" next to the product heading.

The following paragraph should be added after the first paragraph under the heading *Vital Sign Changes* in the section **Adverse Findings Observed in Short-Term, Placebo-Controlled Studies with Effexor XR** in the ADVERSE REACTIONS section:

In a flexible-dose study, with Effexor doses in the range of 200–375 mg/day and mean dose greater than 300 mg/day, the mean pulse was increased by about 2 beats per minute compared with a decrease of about 1 beat per minute for placebo.

The following sentence should be inserted as the first paragraph under the heading *ECG Changes* in the section **Adverse Findings Observed in Short-Term, Placebo-Controlled Studies with Effexor XR** in the ADVERSE REACTIONS section:

In a flexible-dose study, with Effexor doses in the range of 200–375 mg/day and mean dose greater than 300 mg/day, the mean change in heart rate was 8.5 beats per minute compared with 1.7 beats per minute for placebo.

In the list of adverse reactions in the paragraph under the heading **Postmarketing Reports** in the **ADVERSE REACTIONS** section, the word "fatigue" should be added after the words "(including tardive dyskinesia)" and before the word "hemorrhage."

ENBREL®   ℞
[ĕn′ brĕl]
etanercept

Prescribing information for this product, which appears on pages 3370–3373 of the 2001 PDR, has been revised. Please write "See Supplement A" next to the product heading.

The first paragraph under the heading **WARNINGS** should be deleted and replaced with the following:

INFECTIONS
IN POST-MARKETING REPORTS, SERIOUS INFECTIONS AND SEPSIS, INCLUDING FATALITIES, HAVE BEEN REPORTED WITH THE USE OF ENBREL. MANY OF THE SERIOUS INFECTIONS HAVE OCCURRED IN PATIENTS ON CONCOMITANT IMMUNOSUPPRESSIVE THERAPY THAT, IN ADDITION TO THEIR UNDERLYING DISEASE, COULD PREDISPOSE THEM TO INFECTIONS. RARE CASES OF TUBERCULOSIS (TB) HAVE BEEN OBSERVED IN PATIENTS TREATED WITH TNF ANTAGONISTS, INCLUDING ENBREL. PATIENTS WHO DEVELOP A NEW INFECTION WHILE UNDERGOING TREATMENT WITH ENBREL SHOULD BE MONITORED CLOSELY. ADMINISTRATION OF ENBREL SHOULD BE DISCONTINUED IF A PATIENT DEVELOPS A SERIOUS INFECTION OR SEPSIS. TREATMENT WITH ENBREL SHOULD NOT BE INITIATED IN PATIENTS WITH ACTIVE INFECTIONS INCLUDING CHRONIC OR LOCALIZED INFECTIONS. PHYSICIANS SHOULD EXERCISE CAUTION WHEN CONSIDERING THE USE OF ENBREL IN PATIENTS WITH A HISTORY OF RECURRING INFECTIONS OR WITH UNDERLYING CONDITIONS WHICH MAY PREDISPOSE PATIENTS TO INFECTIONS, SUCH AS ADVANCED OR POORLY CONTROLLED DIABETES (see PRECAUTIONS and ADVERSE REACTIONS, Infections).

The following two subsections should be added after the new paragraph described above in the WARNINGS section:

Neurologic Events
Treatment with ENBREL and other agents that inhibit TNF have been associated with rare cases of new onset or exacerbation of central nervous system demyelinating disorders, some presenting with mental status changes and some associated with permanent disability. Rare cases of transverse myelitis, optic neuritis, and new onset or exacerbation of seizure disorders have been observed in association with ENBREL therapy. The causal relationship to ENBREL therapy remains unclear. While no clinical trials have been performed evaluating ENBREL therapy in patients with multiple sclerosis, other TNF antagonists administered to patients with multiple sclerosis have been associated with increases in disease activity.[12,13] Prescribers should exercise caution in considering the use of ENBREL in patients with preexisting or recent-onset central nervous system demyelinating disorders.

Hematologic Events
Rare reports of pancytopenia including aplastic anemia, some with a fatal outcome, have been reported in patients treated with ENBREL. The causal relationship to ENBREL therapy remains unclear. Although no high risk group has been identified, caution should be exercised in patients being treated with ENBREL who have a previous history of significant hematologic abnormalities. All patients should be advised to seek immediate medical attention if they develop signs and symptoms suggestive of blood dyscrasias or infection (e.g., persistent fever, bruising, bleeding, pallor) while on ENBREL. Discontinuation of ENBREL therapy should be considered in patients with confirmed significant hematologic abnormalities.

The following sentence should be added to the end of the paragraph under the heading **Injection Site Reactions** in the **ADVERSE REACTIONS** section:

In post-marketing experience, injection site bleeding and bruising have also been observed in conjunction with ENBREL therapy.

The following paragraph should be added to the end of the section under the heading **Infections** in the **ADVERSE REACTIONS** section:

In post-marketing experience, infections have been observed with various pathogens including viral, bacterial, fungal, and protozoal organisms. Infections have been noted in all organ systems and have been reported in patients receiving ENBREL alone or in combination with immunosuppressive agents.

The following sentence should be added to the end of the paragraph under the heading **Autoantibodies** in the **ADVERSE REACTIONS** section:

In post-marketing experience, very rare spontaneous adverse event reports have described patients with rheumatoid factor positive and/or erosive RA who have developed additional autoantibodies in conjunction with rash after ENBEL therapy.

The following section should be added after the section under the heading **Other Adverse Reactions** in the **ADVERSE REACTIONS** section:

Adverse Reaction Information from Spontaneous Reports
Adverse events have been reported during post-approval use of ENBREL. Because these events are reported voluntarily from a population of uncertain size, it is not always possible to reliably estimate their frequency or establish a causal relationship to ENBREL exposure.

Additional adverse events are listed by body system below:

Body as a whole:	angioedema, fatigue, fever, flu syndrome, generalized pain, weight gain
Cardiovascular:	chest pain, vasodilation (flushing)
Digestive:	altered sense of taste, anorexia, diarrhea, dry mouth, intestinal perforation
Hematologic/Lymphatic:	adenopathy, anemia, aplastic anemia, leukopenia, pancytopenia, thrombocytopenia, (see **WARNINGS**)
Musculoskeletal:	joint pain
Nervous:	paresthesias, stroke, seizures and central nervous system events suggestive of multiple sclerosis or isolated demyelinating conditions such as transverse myelitis or optic neuritis (see **WARNINGS**)
Ocular:	dry eyes, ocular inflammation
Respiratory:	dyspnea, interstitial lung disease, pulmonary disease, worsening of prior lung disorder
Skin:	cutaneous vasculitis, pruritis, subcutaneous nodules, urticaria

The words "(see **WARNINGS** and other sections under **ADVERSE REACTIONS**)" should be added after to the end of the first sentence after the word "patients" under the heading **Adverse Reactions in Pediatric Patients** in the **ADVERSE REACTIONS** section.

The following paragraph should be added to the end of the section under the heading **Adverse Reactions in Pediatric Patients** in the **ADVERSE REACTIONS** section:

In post-marketing experience, the following additional serious adverse events have been reported in pediatric patients: abscess with bacteremia, optic neuritis, pancytopenia, seizures, tuberculous arthritis, urinary tract infection (see **WARNINGS**), coagulopathy, cutaneous vasculitis, and transaminase elevations. The frequency of these events and their causal relationship to ENBREL therapy is unknown.

INDERIDE®   ℞
[ĭn ′dĕ-rīd]
(propranolol hydrochloride
[INDERAL®] and hydrochlorothiazide)

Prescribing information for this product, which appears on pages 3381–3383 of the 2001 PDR, has been revised. Please write "See Supplement A" next to the product heading.

The words "in patients on propranolol" should be added to end of the first paragraph following the subheading "Diabetes and Hypoglycemia" under **Propranolol hydrochloride (Inderal®)** in the WARNINGS section.

In the second sentence of the second paragraph following the subheading "Diabetes and Hypoglycemia" under **Propranolol hydrochloride (Inderal®)** in the WARNINGS section, the word "subjects" should be deleted and replaced with the word "patients."

The following should be added as the third paragraph paragraph following the subheading "Diabetes and Hypoglycemia" under **Propranolol hydrochloride (Inderal®)** in the WARNINGS section:

Acute increases in blood pressure have occurred after insulin-induced hypoglycemia in patients on propranolol.

INDERIDE® LA ℞

[ĭn 'de-rīde]

(propranolol hydrochloride and hydrochlorothiazide)
Long-Acting Capsules

Prescribing information for this product, which appears on pages 3383–3385 of the 2001 PDR, has been revised. Please write "See Supplement A" next to the product heading.

The words "in patients on propranolol" should be added to the end of the first paragraph after the subheading *"Diabetes and Hypoglycemia"* under **Propranolol Hydrochloride (Inderal®)** in the **WARNINGS** section.

The following paragraph should be added to the end of the section after the subheading *"Diabetes and Hypoglycemia"* under **Propranolol Hydrochloride (Inderal®)** in the **WARNINGS** section.

Acute increases in blood pressure have occurred after insulin-induced hypoglycemia in patients on propranolol.

The following paragraph should be added to the end of the subsection under the subheading **"Nursing Mothers"** in the **PRECAUTIONS** section:

Hydrochlorothiazide

Thiazides appear in breast milk. If the use of drug is deemed essential, the patient should stop nursing.

MYLOTARG™ ℞

[mī 'lō-tărg]

(gemtuzumab ozogamicin for injection)
FOR INTRAVENOUS USE ONLY

Prescribing information for this product, which appears on pages 3404–3407 of the 2001 PDR, has been revised. Please write "See Supplement A" next to the product heading.

The two paragraphs under the **WARNINGS** heading in the boxed warning should be deleted and replaced with the following five paragraphs:

Mylotarg should be administered under the supervision of physicians experienced in the treatment of acute leukemia and in facilities equipped to monitor and treat leukemia patients.

There are no controlled trials demonstrating efficacy and safety using Mylotarg in combination with other chemotherapeutic agents.

Severe myelosuppression occurs when Mylotarg is used at recommended doses.

HYPERSENSITIVITY REACTIONS INCLUDING ANAPHYLAXIS, INFUSION REACTIONS, PULMONARY EVENTS

Mylotarg administration can result in severe hypersensitivity reactions (including anaphylaxis), and other infusion-related reactions which may include severe pulmonary events. Infrequently, hypersensitivity reactions and pulmonary events have been fatal. In most cases, infusion-related symptoms occurred during the infusion or within 24 hours of administration of Mylotarg and resolved. Mylotarg infusion should be interrupted for patients experiencing dyspnea or clinically significant hypotension. Patients should be monitored until signs and symptoms completely resolve. Discontinuation of Mylotarg treatment should be strongly considered for patients who develop anaphylaxis, pulmonary edema, or acute respiratory distress syndrome. Since patients with high peripheral blast counts may be at greater risk for pulmonary events and tumor lysis syndrome, physicians should consider leukoreduction with hydroxyurea or leukapheresis to reduce the peripheral white count to below 30,000/μL prior to administration of Mylotarg. (See **WARNINGS**.)

HEPATOTOXICITY:

Hepatotoxicity, including severe hepatic veno-occlusive disease (VOD), has been reported in association with the use of Mylotarg. (See **WARNINGS** and **ADVERSE REACTIONS** sections.) Patients who receive Mylotarg either before or after hematopoietic stem-cell transplant (HSCT), and patients with underlying hepatic disease or abnormal liver function may be at increased risk for developing severe VOD. Death from liver failure and from VOD has been reported in patients who receive Mylotarg.

The first paragraph and sections under the headings **"Myelosuppression"**, **"Use in Patients with Hepatic Impairment,"** and **"Allergic Reactions"** in the **WARNINGS** section should be deleted and replaced with the following:

Mylotarg should be administered under the supervision of physicians experienced in the treatment of acute leukemia and in facilities equipped to monitor and treat leukemia patients.

There are no controlled trials demonstrating efficacy and safety using Mylotarg in combination with other chemotherapeutic agents.

Myelosuppression: Severe myelosuppression will occur in all patients given the recommended dose of this agent. Careful hematologic monitoring is required. Systemic infections should be treated.

Hypersensitivity Reactions Including Anaphylaxis, Infusion Reactions, Pulmonary Events: Mylotarg administration can result in severe hypersensitivity reactions (including anaphylaxis), and other infusion-related reactions which may include severe pulmonary events. Infrequently, hypersensitivity reactions and pulmonary events have been fatal. In most cases, infusion-related symptoms occurred during the infusion or within 24 hours of administration of Mylotarg and resolved.

Mylotarg (gemtuzumab ozogamicin for injection) infusion should be interrupted for patients experiencing dyspnea or clinically significant hypotension. Patients should be monitored until signs and symptoms completely resolve. Discontinuation of further Mylotarg treatment should be strongly considered for patients who develop anaphylaxis, pulmonary edema, or acute respiratory distress syndrome. Since patients with high peripheral blast counts may be at greater risk for such reactions, physicians should consider leukoreduction with hydroxyurea or leukapheresis to reduce the peripheral white count to below 30,000/μL prior to administration of Mylotarg.

Infusion Reactions: Mylotarg can produce a post-infusion symptom complex of fever and chills, and less commonly hypotension and dyspnea that may occur during the first 24 hours after administration. Grade 3 or 4 non-hematologic infusion-related adverse events included chills, fever, hypotension, hypertension, hyperglycemia, hypoxia, and dyspnea. Most patients received the following prophylactic medications before administration; diphenhydramine 50 mg po and acetaminophen 650–1000 mg po; thereafter, two additional doses of acetaminophen 650–1000 mg po, one every 4 hours as needed. Vital signs should be monitored during infusion and for the four hours following infusion.

In clinical studies, these symptoms generally occurred after the end of the 2-hour intravenous infusion and resolved after 2 to 4 hours with a supportive therapy of acetaminophen, diphenhydramine, and IV fluids. Fewer infusion-related events were observed after the second dose.

Pulmonary Events: Severe pulmonary events leading to death have been reported infrequently with the use of Mylotarg in the postmarketing setting. Signs, symptoms and clinical findings include dyspnea, pulmonary infiltrates, pleural effusions, non-cardiogenic pulmonary edema, pulmonary insufficiency and hypoxia, and acute respiratory distress syndrome. These events occur as sequelae of infusion reactions: patients with WBC counts > 30,000/μL may be at increased risk. (See Infusion Reactions section of **WARNINGS**.) Physicians should consider leukoreduction with hydroxyurea or leukapheresis to reduce the peripheral white count to below 30,000 μL prior to administration of Mylotarg. Patients with symptomatic intrinsic lung disease may also be at greater risk of severe pulmonary reactions.

Hepatotoxicity: Hepatotoxicity, including severe VOD, has been reported in association with the use of Mylotarg. Patients who receive Mylotarg either before or after HSCT, and patients with underlying hepatic disease or abnormal liver function may be at increased risk for developing severe VOD. Death from liver failure and from VOD has been reported in patients who received Mylotarg.

Use in Patients with Hepatic Impairment: Mylotarg has not been studied in patients with bilirubin > 2 mg/dL. Extra caution should be exercised when administering Mylotarg in patients with hepatic impairment (see **ADVERSE REACTIONS** section).

Tumor Lysis Syndrome (TLS): TLS may be a consequence of leukemia treatment with any chemotherapeutic agent including Mylotarg. Renal failure secondary to TLS has been reported in association with the use of Mylotarg. Appropriate measures, (e.g. hydration and allopurinol), must be taken to prevent hyperuricemia. Physicians should consider leukoreduction with hydroxyurea or leukapheresis to reduce the peripheral white blood count to < 30,000/μL prior to administration of Mylotarg (see **CLINICAL STUDIES** section).

The paragraph under the heading **"Treatment by Experienced Physicians"** in the **PRECAUTIONS** section should be deleted and replaced with the following:

Mylotarg should be administered under the supervision of physicians experienced in the treatment of acute leukemia and in facilities equipped to monitor and treat leukemia patients.

The subheading **"Tumor Lysis Syndrome"** and the paragraph following the subheading in the **WARNINGS** section should be deleted.

The paragraph following the heading **"Carcinogenesis, Mutagenesis, Impairment of Fertility"** in the **WARNINGS** section should be deleted and replaced with the following:

Carcinogenesis, Mutagenesis, Impairment of Fertility: No long-term studies in animals have been performed to evaluate the carcinogenic potential of Mylotarg. Gemtuzumab ozogamicin was clastogenic in the mouse *in vivo* micronucleus test. This positive result is consistent with the known ability of calicheamicin to cause double-stranded breaks in DNA. Gemtuzumab ozogamicin adversely affected male, but not female, fertility in rats. Following daily administration of gemtuzumab ozogamicin to male rats for 28 days at doses of 0.02 to 0.16 mg/kg/day (approximately 0.01 to 0.11 times the human dose on a mg/m^2 basis) gemtuzumab ozogamicin caused: decreased fertility rates, epididymal sperm counts, and sperm motility; increased incidence of sperm abnormalities; and microscopic evidence of decreased spermatogonia and spermatocyte count. These findings did not resolve following a 9-week recovery period.

The last sentence of the paragraph following the subheading **"Hepatotoxicity"** in the **ADVERSE REACTIONS** section should be deleted and replaced with the following sentence:

Among 27 patients who received hematopoietic stem cell transplantation following Mylotarg (gemtuzumab ozogamicin for injection), three (2 NRs and 1 CR) died of hepatic veno-occlusive disease (VOD) 22 to 35 days following transplantation.

The following section should be added to the end of the **ADVERSE REACTIONS** section:

Other Clinical Experience:

In postmarketing experience and other clinical trials, additional cases of VOD have been reported, some in association with the use of other chemotherapeutic agents, underlying hepatic disease/abnormal liver function, or a history of prior or subsequent HSCl. Renal failure secondary to TLS, hypersensitivity reactions, anaphylaxis, and pulmonary events, have also been reported in association with the use of Mylotarg (gemtuzumab ozogamicin for injection) (See **WARNINGS** section).

OVRAL®

[ŏh'vrăl]

norgestrel and ethinyl estradiol tablets

Prescribing information for this product, which appears on pages 3414–3415 of the 2001 PDR, has been revised as follows. Please write "See Supplement A" next to the product heading.

Table I and its footnotes should be deleted and replaced with the following:

TABLE I: PERCENTAGE OF WOMEN EXPERIENCING AN UNINTENDED PREGNANCY DURING THE FIRST YEAR OF USE OF A CONTRACEPTIVE METHOD

Method	Perfect Use	Typical Use
Levonorgestrel implants	0.05	0.05
Male sterilization	0.1	0.15
Female sterilization	0.5	0.5
Depo-Provera® (injectable progestogen)	0.3	0.3
Oral contraceptives		5
Combined	0.1	NA
Progestin only	0.5	NA
IUD		
Progesterone	1.5	2.0
Copper T 380A	0.6	0.8
Condom (male) without spermicide	3	14
(Female) without spermicide	5	21
Cervical cap		
Nulliparous women	9	20
Parous women	26	40
Vaginal sponge		
Nulliparous women	9	20
Parous women	20	40
Diaphragm with spermicidal cream or jelly	6	20
Spermicides alone (foam, creams, jellies, and vaginal suppositories)	6	26
Periodic abstinence (all methods)	1–9*	25
Withdrawal	4	19
No contraception (planned pregnancy)	85	85

NA—not available

*Depending on method (calendar, ovulation, symptothermal, post-ovulation)

Adapted from Hatcher RA et al, *Contraceptive Technology: 17th Revised Edition*, NY, NY: Ardent Media, Inc., 1998.

PHENERGAN® ℞

[fĕn 'ĕr-găn]

(promethazine HCl)
TABLETS •
SUPPOSITORIES

Prescribing information for this product, which appears on pages 3419–3420 of the 2001 PDR, has been revised as follows. Please write "See Supplement A" next to the product heading.

Continued on next page

Phenergan—Cont.

The following sentence should be added to the end of second paragraph of the **DESCRIPTION** section, which describes the rectal suppositories:

Phenergan Suppositories are for rectal administration only.

The first sentence of the **CONTRAINDICATIONS** section should be deleted and replaced with the following sentence:

Promethazine is contraindicated in comatose states, and in individuals known to be hypersensitive or to have had an idiosyncratic reaction to promethazine or to other phenothiazines.

The **WARNINGS** section should be deleted and replaced with the following:

WARNINGS

CNS Depression

Promethazine may impair the mental and/or physical abilities required for the performance of potentially hazardous tasks, such as driving a vehicle or operating machinery. The impairment may be amplified by concomitant use of other central-nervous-system depressants such as alcohol, sedatives/hypnotics (including barbiturates), narcotics, narcotic analgesics, general anesthetics, tricyclic antidepressants, and tranquilizers; therefore such agents should either be eliminated or given in reduced dosage in the presence of promethazine hydrochloride (see **PRECAUTIONS—Information for Patients** and **Drug Interactions**).

Respiratory Depression

Phenergan Tablets and Suppositories may lead to potentially fatal respiratory depression.

Use of Phenergan Tablets and Suppositories in patients with compromised respiratory function (e.g. COPD, sleep apnea) should be avoided.

Lower Seizure Threshold

Promethazine may lower seizure threshold. It should be used with caution in persons with seizure disorders or in persons who are using concomitant medications, such as narcotics or local anesthetics, which may also affect seizure threshold.

Bone-Marrow Depression

Phenergan Tablets and Suppositories should be used with caution in patients with bone-marrow depression. Leukopenia and agranulocytosis have been reported, usually when Phenergan has been used in association with other known marrow-toxic agents.

Use in Pediatric Patients

PHENERGAN TABLETS AND SUPPOSITORIES ARE NOT RECOMMENDED FOR USE IN PEDIATRIC PATIENTS LESS THAN TWO YEARS OF AGE.

CAUTION SHOULD BE EXERCISED WHEN ADMINISTERING PHENERGAN TABLETS AND SUPPOSITORIES TO PEDIATRIC PATIENTS 2 YEARS OF AGE AND OLDER BECAUSE OF THE POTENTIAL FOR FATAL RESPIRATORY DEPRESSION. ANTIEMETICS ARE NOT RECOMMENDED FOR TREATMENT OF UNCOMPLICATED VOMITING IN PEDIATRIC PATIENTS, AND THEIR USE SHOULD BE LIMITED TO PROLONGED VOMITING OF KNOWN ETIOLOGY. THE EXTRAPYRAMIDAL SYMPTOMS WHICH CAN OCCUR SECONDARY TO PHENERGAN TABLETS AND SUPPOSITORIES ADMINISTRATION MAY BE CONFUSED WITH THE CNS SIGNS OF UNDIAGNOSED PRIMARY DISEASE, e.g., ENCEPHALOPATHY OR REYE'S SYNDROME. THE USE OF PHENERGAN TABLETS AND SUPPOSITORIES SHOULD BE AVOIDED IN PEDIATRIC PATIENTS WHOSE SIGNS AND SYMPTOMS MAY SUGGEST REYE'S SYNDROME OR OTHER HEPATIC DISEASES.

Excessively large dosages of antihistamines, including promethazine in pediatric patients may cause hallucinations, convulsions, and sudden death. In pediatric patients who are actually ill associated with dehydration, there is an increased susceptibility to dystonias with the use of promethazine HCl.

Other Considerations

Administration of promethazine HCl has been associated with reported cholestatic jaundice.

The following paragraph should be inserted as the first paragraph under the heading **General** in the **PRECAUTIONS** section:

Drugs having anticholinergic properties should be used with caution in patients with narrow-angle glaucoma, prostatic hypertrophy, stenosing peptic ulcer, pyloroduodenal obstruction, and bladder-neck obstruction.

The three paragraphs under the heading **DRUG INTERACTIONS** should be deleted and replaced with the following:

CNS Depressants—Phenergan Tablets and Suppositories may increase, prolong, or intensify the sedative action of other central-nervous-system depressants, such as alcohol, sedatives/hypnotics (including barbiturates), narcotic analgesics, general anesthetics, tricyclic antidepressants, and tranquilizers; therefore, such agents should be avoided or administered in reduced dosage to patients receiving promethazine. When given concomitantly with Phenergan Tablets and Suppositories, the dose of barbiturates should be reduced by at least one-half, and the dose of narcotics should be reduced by at least one-half, and the dose of narcotics should be reduced by one-quarter to one-half. Dosage must be individualized. Excessive amounts of promethazine relative to a narcotic may lead to restlessness and motor hyperactivity in the patient with pain; these symptoms usually disappear with adequate control of the pain.

Epinephrine—Because of the potential for Phenergan to reverse epinephrine's vasopressor effect, epinephrine should NOT be used to treat hypotension associated with Phenergan overdose.

Anticholinergics—Concomitant use of other agents with anticholinergic properties should be undertaken with caution.

Monoamine Oxidase Inhibitors (MAOI)—Drug interactions, including an increased incidence of extrapyramidal effects, have been reported when some MAOI and phenothiazines are used concomitantly. This possibility should be considered with Phenergan Tablets and Suppositories.

The paragraph under the heading **Labor and Delivery** in the **PRECAUTIONS** section should be deleted and replaced with the following:

Promethazine HCl may be used alone or as an adjunct to narcotic analgesics during labor (see **DOSAGE AND ADMINISTRATION**).

Limited data suggest that use of Phenergan Tablets during labor and delivery does not have an appreciable effect on the duration of labor or delivery and does not increase the risk of need for intervention in the newborn. The effect on later growth and development of the newborn is unknown. (See also *Nonteratogenic Effects*.)

The second sentence of the paragraph under the heading **Nursing Mothers** in the **PRECAUTIONS** section should be deleted and replaced with the following:

Because many drugs are excreted in human milk and because of the potential for serious adverse reactions in nursing infants from Phenergan Tablets and Suppositories, a decision should be made whether to discontinue the drug, taking into account the importance of the drug to the mother.

The paragraph under the heading **Pediatric Use** should be deleted and replaced with the following two paragraphs:

Safety and effectiveness in children under 2 years of age have not been established.

Phenergan Tablets and Suppositories should be used with caution in pediatric patients 2 years of age and older (see **WARNINGS—Use in Pediatric Patients**).

The first paragraph following the heading *Nervous System* in the **ADVERSE REACTIONS** section should be deleted and replaced with the following:

Nervous System—Sedation, somnolence, blurred vision, dizziness; confusion, disorientation, and extrapyramidal symptoms such as oculogyric crisis, torticollis, and tongue protrusion; lassitude, tinnitus, incoordination, fatigue, euphoria, nervousness, diplopia, insomnia, tremors, convulsive seizures, excitation, catatonic-like states, hysteria. Hallucinations have also been reported.

The words "tachycardia, bradycardia, faintness" should be added to the end of the list of adverse reactions following the heading *"Cardiovascular"* in the **ADVERSE REACTIONS** section.

The list of adverse reactions following the heading *"Dermatologic"* in the **ADVERSE REACTIONS** section should be deleted and replaced with the following:

Dermatologic—Dermatitis, photosensitivity, urticaria.

The list of adverse reactions following the heading *"Gastrointestinal"* in the **ADVERSE REACTIONS** section should be deleted and replaced with the following:

Gastrointestinal—Dry mouth, nausea, vomiting, jaundice.

The following paragraphs should be added to the end of the **ADVERSE REACTIONS** section under the adverse reactions following the heading *"Gastrointestinal"*:

Respiratory—Asthma, nasal stuffiness, respiratory depression (potentially fatal) and apnea (potentially fatal). (See **WARNINGS—Respiratory Depression**).

Other—Angioneurotic edema.

Paradoxical Reactions (Overdosage)

Hyperexcitability and abnormal movements, which have been reported in pediatric patients following a single administration of promethazine, may be manifestations of relative overdosage, in which case, consideration should be given to the discontinuation of the promethazine and to the use of other drugs. Respiratory depression, nightmares, delirium, and agitated behavior have also been reported in some of these patients.

The second paragraph under the heading "TREATMENT" in the **OVERDOSAGE** section should be deleted and replaced with the following:

The treatment of choice for resulting hypotension is administration of intravenous fluids, accompanied by repositioning if indicated. In the event that vasopressors are considered for the management of severe hypotension which does not respond to intravenous fluids and repositioning, the administration of norepinephrine or phenylephrine should be considered. EPINEPHRINE SHOULD NOT BE USED, since its use in patients with partial adrenergic blockade may further lower the blood pressure. Extrapyramidal reactions may be treated with anticholinergic anti-parkinson agents, diphenhydramine, or barbiturates. Oxygen may also be administered.

The following paragraph should be added immediately after the **DOSAGE AND ADMINISTRATION** heading:

Phenergan Tablets and Phenergan Rectal Suppositories are not recommended for children under 2 years of age (see WARNINGS—Use in Pediatric Patients).

Phenergan Suppositories are for rectal administration only.

The first paragraph under the heading **Nausea and Vomiting** in the **DOSAGE AND ADMINISTRATION** section should be deleted and replaced with the following:

Antiemetics should not be used in vomiting of unknown etiology in children and adolescents (see **WARNINGS—Use in Pediatric Patients**).

The average effective dose of Phenergan for the active therapy of nausea and vomiting in children or adults is 25 mg. When oral medication cannot be tolerated, the dose should be given parenterally (cf. Phenergan Injection) or by rectal suppository. 12.5- to 25-mg doses may be repeated, as necessary, at 4- to 6-hour intervals.

The second and third paragraphs under the heading **Pre- and Postoperative Use** in the **DOSAGE AND ADMINISTRATION** section should be deleted and replaced with the following:

For preoperative medication children require doses of 0.5 mg per pound of body weight in combination with an appropriately reduced dose of narcotic or barbiturate and the appropriate dose of an atropine-like drug.

Usual adult dosage is 50 mg Phenergan with an appropriately reduced dose of narcotic or barbiturate and the required amount of a belladonna alkaloid.

PREMARIN® INTRAVENOUS   ℞
[*prĕm 'ă-rĭn*]
(conjugated estrogens, USP)
for Injection
Specially prepared for Intravenous & Intramuscular use

Prescribing information for this product, which appears on pages 3426–3429 of the 2001 PDR, has been revised. Please write "See Supplement A" next to the product heading.

The following paragraph should be added as the new item 1 under the heading **"A. General Precautions"** in the **PRECAUTIONS** section and the numbers 1 through 12 should be changed to 2–13, respectively:

1. The effects of estrogen replacement on the risk of cardiovascular disease have not been adequately studied. However, data from the Heart and Estrogen/Progestin Replacement Study (HERS), a controlled clinical trial of secondary prevention of 2,763 postmenopausal women with documented heart disease, demonstrated no benefit. During an average follow-up of 4.1 years, treatment with oral conjugated estrogens plus medroxyprogesterone acetate did not reduce the overall rate of coronary heart disease (CHD) events in postmenopausal women with established coronary disease. There were more CHD events in the hormone treated group than in the placebo group in year 1, but fewer events in years 3 through 5.

The following paragraph should be added as item 6 under the heading **The Dangers of Estrogen** in the **INFORMATION FOR THE PATIENT** section:

6. *Cardiovascular disease.* A recent 4-year study suggests that women with a history of coronary heart disease may have an increased risk of serious cardiac events during the first year of treatment with estrogen/progestin therapy. Therefore, if you have had a heart attack, or you have been told you have blocked coronary arteries (arteries to your heart) or have any heart problem, you should consult your physician regarding the potential benefits and risks of estrogen/progestin therapy.

PREMARIN®   ℞
[*prĕm 'ă-rĭn*]
(conjugated estrogens tablets, USP)

Rx only

Prescribing information for this product, which appears on pages 3429–3432 of the 2001 PDR, has been revised. Please write "See Supplement A" next to the product heading.

The second sentence, which begins with the words "There is insufficient…", of item 5 under **CONTRAINDICATIONS** should be deleted.

The subheading "3. *Thromboembolic disorders and other vascular problems*" in the **WARNINGS** section should be changed to just "3. *Thromboembolic disorders.*"

The paragraph under the old subheading "3. *Thromboembolic disorders and other vascular problems*" in the **WARNINGS** section should be deleted and replaced with the following paragraphs:

3. *Thromboembolic disorders*

Venous thromboembolism. Several epidemiologic studies have found an increased risk of venous thromboembolism (VTE) in users of estrogen replacement therapy (ERT) who did not have predisposing conditions for VTE, such as past history of cardiovascular disease or a recent history of pregnancy, surgery, trauma, or serious illness. The increased risk was found only in current ERT users; it did not persist in former users. The risk appeared to be higher in the first year of use and decreased thereafter. The findings were similar for ERT alone or with added progestins and pertain to commonly used oral and transdermal doses, with a possible dose-dependent effect on risk. The studies found the VTE risk to be about one case per 10,000 women per year among women not using ERT and without predisposing conditions. The risk in current ERT users was increased to 2–3 cases per 10,000 women per year.

Cardiovascular disease. Embolic cerebrovascular events have been reported in women receiving postmenopausal estrogens.

Large doses of estrogen (5 mg conjugated estrogens per day), comparable to those used to treat cancer of the proste and breast, have been shown in a large prospective inical trial in men to increase the risk of nonfatal myoardial infarction, pulmonary embolism, and thrombophlebitis.

The physician should be aware of the possibility of thrombotic disorders (thrombophlebitis, retinal thrombosis, cerebral embolism, and pulmonary embolism) during estrogen replacement therapy and be alert to their earliest manifestations. Should any of these occur or be suspected, estrogen replacement therapy should be discontinued immediately. Patients who have risk factors for thrombotic disorders should be kept under careful observation.

The following paragraph should be inserted as the first paragraph immediately following the subheading "2. *Cardiovascular risk*" under "**A. General**" in the **PRECAUTIONS** section:

2. *Cardiovascular risk.* The effects of estrogen replacement on the risk of cardiovascular disease have not been adequately studied. However, data from the Heart and Estrogen/Progestin Replacement Study (HERS), a controlled clinical trial of secondary prevention of 2,763 postmenopausal women with documented heart disease, demonstrated no benefit. During an average follow-up of 4.1 years, treatment with oral conjugated estrogens plus medroxyprogesterone acetate did not reduce the overall rate of coronary heart disease (CHD) events in postmenopausal women with established coronary disease. There were more CHD events in the hormone treated group than in the placebo group in year 1, but fewer events in years 3 through 5.

The paragraph that followed the subheading "2. *Cardiovascular risk*" under "**A. General**" in the **PRECAUTIONS** section and that begins with the words "A causal relationship..." should be underlined.

The following paragraph should be inserted as the new item 5 under "**A. General**" in the **PRECAUTIONS** section, and the numbers 5–11 should be changed to the numbers 6–12, respectively:

5. *Thromboembolism.* Based on data obtained with oral contraceptives, estrogens should be discontinued at least four weeks before surgery of the type associated with an increased risk of thromboembolism if feasible, or during periods of prolonged immobilization (see **WARNINGS**).

In the first paragraph under the **ADVERSE REACTIONS** heading, the words "and other vascular problems" should be deleted and the words "**WARNINGS** and" should be inserted just before the word "**PRECAUTIONS**."

The words ", retinal thrombosis (cutting off blood vessels in the eye)," should be inserted after the words "(cutting off blood to the lungs)" under the subheading "*Abnormal blood clotting*" under **RISKS OF ESTROGENS** in the **INFORMATION FOR THE PATIENT** section.

The following new subheading and subsection should be added to the end of the **RISKS OF ESTROGENS** in the **INFORMATION FOR THE PATIENT** section:

Cardiovascular disease

A recent 4 year study suggests that women with a history of coronary heart disease may have an increased risk of serious cardiac events during the first year of treatment with estrogen/progestin therapy. Therefore, if you have had a heart attack, or you have been told you have blocked coronary arteries (arteries to your heart) or have any heart problem, you should consult your physician regarding the potential benefits and risks of estrogen/progestin therapy.

PREMARIN® VAGINAL CREAM
[*prem'a-rin*]
conjugated estrogens
in a nonliquefying base

Prescribing information for this product, which appears on pages 3432–3434 of the 2001 PDR, has been revised as follows. Please write "See Supplement A" next to the product heading.

The boxed warning at the beginning of the prescribing information should be deleted and replaced with the following:

1. ESTROGENS HAVE BEEN REPORTED TO INCREASE THE RISK OF ENDOMETRIAL CARCINOMA IN POSTMENOPAUSAL WOMEN.

Close clinical surveillance of all women taking estrogens is important. Adequate diagnostic measures, including endometrial sampling when indicated, should be undertaken to rule out malignancy in all cases of undiagnosed persistent or recurring abnormal vaginal bleeding. There is no evidence that "natural" estrogens are more or less hazardous than "synthetic" estrogens at equiestrogenic doses.

2. ESTROGENS SHOULD NOT BE USED DURING PREGNANCY.

There is no indication for estrogen therapy during pregnancy or during the immediate postpartum period. Estrogens are ineffective for the prevention or treatment of threatened or habitual abortion. Estrogens are not indicated for the prevention of postpartum breast engorgement.

Estrogen therapy during pregnancy is associated with an increased risk of congenital defects in the reproductive organs of the fetus, and possibly other birth defects. Studies of women who received diethylstilbestrol (DES) during pregnancy have shown that female offspring have an increased risk of vaginal adenosis, squamous cell dysplasia of the uterine cervix, and clear cell vaginal cancer later in life; male offspring have an increased risk of urogenital abnormalities and possibly testicular cancer later in life. The 1985 DES Task Force concluded that use of DES during pregnancy is associated with a subsequent increased risk of breast cancer in the mothers, although a causal relationship remains unproven and the observed level of excess risk is similar to that for a number of other breast cancer risk factors.

Items 5 and 6 in the **CONTRAINDICATIONS** section should be deleted and replaced with the following:

5. Active or past history of thrombophlebitis or thromboembolic disorders.
6. Premarin Vaginal Cream should not be used in patients hypersensitive to its ingredients

The entire **WARNINGS** section should be deleted and replaced with the following:

WARNINGS

1. *Induction of malignant neoplasms.*

Breast cancer. While the majority of studies have not shown an increased risk of breast cancer in women who have ever used estrogen replacement therapy, some studies have reported a moderately increased risk (relative risks of 1.3 to 2.0) in those women taking higher doses or those taking lower doses for prolonged periods of time, especially in excess of 10 years. Other studies have not shown this relationship.

Women on this therapy should have regular breast examinations and should be instructed in breast self-examination, and women over the age of 40 should have regular mammograms.

Endometrial cancer. The reported endometrial cancer risk among unopposed estrogen users is about 2- to 12-fold greater than in non-users, and appears dependent on duration of treatment and on estrogen dose. Most studies show no significant increased risk associated with use of estrogens for less than one year. The greatest risk appears associated with prolonged use, with increased risks of 15- to 24-fold for five to ten years or more. In three studies, persistence of risk was demonstrated for 8 to over 15 years after cessation of estrogen treatment. In one study a significant decrease in the incidence of endometrial cancer occurred six months after estrogen withdrawal. Concurrent progestin therapy may offset this risk but the overall health impact in postmenopausal women is not known (see "**Precautions**").

Congenital lesions with malignant potential. Estrogen therapy during pregnancy is associated with an increased risk of fetal congenital reproductive tract disorders, and possibly other birth defects. Studies of women who received DES during pregnancy have shown that female offspring have an increased risk of vaginal adenosis, squamous cell dysplasia of the uterine cervix, and clear cell vaginal cancer later in life; male offspring have an increased risk of urogenital abnormalities and possibly testicular cancer later in life. Although some of these changes are benign, others are precursors of malignancy.

2. *Gallbladder disease.* A study has reported a 2- to 3-fold increase in the risk of surgically confirmed gallbladder disease in women receiving post-menopausal estrogens, similar to the 2-fold increase previously noted in users of oral contraceptives.

3. *Thromboembolic disorders*

Venous thromboembolism. Several epidemiologic studies have found an increased risk of venous thromboembolism (VTE) in users of estrogen replacement therapy (ERT) who did not have predisposing conditions for VTE, such as past history of cardiovascular disease or a recent history of pregnancy, surgery, trauma, or serious illness. The increased risk was found only in current ERT users; it did not persist in former users. The risk appeared to be higher in the first year of use and decreased thereafter. The findings were similar for ERT alone or with added progestins and pertain to commonly used oral and transdermal doses, with a possible dose-dependent effect on risk. The studies found the VTE risk to be about one case per 10,000 women per year among women not using ERT and without predisposing conditions. The risk in current ERT users was increased to 2–3 cases per 10,000 women per year.

If feasible, estrogen should be discontinued at least 4 weeks before surgery of the type associated with an increased risk of thromboembolism, or during periods of prolonged immobilization.

Cardiovascular disease. Embolic cerebrovascular events have been reported in women receiving postmenopausal estrogens.

Large doses of estrogen (5 mg conjugated estrogens per day), comparable to those used to treat cancer of the prostate and breast, have been shown in a large prospective clinical trial in men to increase the risk of nonfatal myocardial infarction, pulmonary embolism, and thrombophlebitis.

The physician should be aware of the possibility of thrombotic disorders (thrombophlebitis, retinal thrombosis, cerebral embolism, and pulmonary embolism) during estrogen replacement therapy and be alert to their earliest manifestations. Should any of these occur or be suspected, estrogen replacement therapy should be discontinued immediately. Patients who have risk factors for thrombotic disorders should be kept under careful observation.

4. *Elevated blood pressure.* Occasional blood pressure increases during estrogen replacement therapy have been attributed to idiosyncratic reactions to estrogens. More often, blood pressure has remained the same or has dropped. One study showed that postmenopausal estrogen users have higher blood pressure than nonusers. Two other studies showed slightly lower blood pressure among estrogen users compared to nonusers. Blood pressure should be monitored at regular intervals with estrogen use.

5. *Hypercalcemia.* Administration of estrogens may lead to severe hypercalcemia in patients with breast cancer and bone metastases. If this occurs, the drug should be stopped and appropriate measures taken to reduce the serum calcium level.

6. *Effects similar to those caused by estrogen-progestogen oral contraceptives*

a. *Hepatic adenoma.* Benign hepatic adenomas appear to be associated with the use of oral contraceptives. Although benign, and rare, these may rupture and may cause death through intra-abdominal hemorrhage. Such lesions have not yet been reported in association with other estrogen or progestogen preparations but should be considered in estrogen users having abdominal pain and tenderness, abdominal mass, or hypovolemic shock. Hepatocellular carcinoma has also been reported in women taking estrogen-containing oral contraceptives. The relationship of this malignancy to these drugs is not known at this time.

b. *Glucose tolerance.* A worsening of glucose tolerance has been observed in a significant percentage of patients on estrogen-containing oral contraceptives. For this reason, diabetic patients should be carefully observed while receiving estrogen.

The 13 items under the subheading **General Precautions** in the **PRECAUTIONS** section should be deleted and replaced with the following 15 items:

1. The effects of estrogen replacement on the risk of cardiovascular disease have not been adequately studied. However, data from the Heart and Estrogen/Progestin Replacement Study (HERS), a controlled clinical trial of secondary prevention of 2,763 postmenopausal women with documented heart disease, demonstrated no benefit. During an average follow-up of 4.1 years, treatment with oral conjugated estrogens plus medroxyprogesterone acetate did not reduce the overall rate of coronary heart disease (CHD) events in postmenopausal women with established coronary disease. There were more CHD events in the hormone treated group than in the placebo group in year 1, but fewer events in years 3 through 5.
2. A complete medical and family history should be taken prior to the initiation of any estrogen therapy. The pretreatment and periodic physical examinations should include special reference to blood pressure, breasts, abdomen, and pelvic organs, and should include a Papanicolaou smear. As a general rule, estrogens should not be prescribed for longer than one year without another physical examination being performed.
3. Fluid retention—Because estrogens may cause some degree of fluid retention, conditions which might be influenced by this factor, such as asthma, epilepsy, migraine, and cardiac or renal dysfunction, require careful observation.
4. Familial hyperlipoproteinemia—Estrogen therapy may be associated with massive elevations of plasma triglycerides leading to pancreatitis and other complications in patients with familial defects of lipoprotein metabolism.
5. Certain patients may develop undesirable manifestations of excessive estrogenic stimulation, such as abnormal or excessive uterine bleeding, mastodynia, etc.
6. Endometriosis may be exacerbated with administration of estrogen therapy.
7. Prolonged administration of unopposed estrogen therapy has been reported to increase the risk of endometrial hyperplasia in some patients.
8. Oral contraceptives appear to be associated with an increased incidence of mental depression. Although it is not clear whether this is due to the estrogenic or progestogenic component of the contraceptive, patients with a history of depression should be carefully observed.
9. Preexisting uterine leiomyomata may increase in size during estrogen use.
10. The pathologist should be advised of estrogen therapy when relevant specimens are submitted.
11. Patients with a past history of jaundice during pregnancy have an increased risk of recurrence of jaundice while receiving estrogen-containing oral-contraceptive therapy. If jaundice develops in any patient receiving estrogen, the medication should be discontinued while the cause is investigated.
12. Estrogens may be poorly metabolized in patients with impaired liver function and should be administered with caution in such patients.
13. Because estrogens influence the metabolism of calcium and phosphorus, they should be used with caution in patients with metabolic bone diseases that are associated with hypercalcemia or in patients with renal insufficiency.
14. Because of the effects of estrogens on epiphyseal closure, they should be used judiciously in young patients in whom bone growth is not yet complete.
15. Barrier contraceptives—Premarin Vaginal Cream exposure has been reported to weaken latex condoms. The potential for Premarin Vaginal Cream to weaken and contribute to the failure of condoms, diaphragms, or cervical caps made of latex or rubber should be considered.

The sentence under the subheading "**B. Information for Patients**" in the **PRECAUTIONS** section should be deleted and replaced with the following:

(See text which appears after the "**HOW SUPPLIED**" section.)

Continued on next page

Premarin Cream—Cont.

The first paragraph under the heading **ADVERSE REACTIONS** should be deleted and replaced with the following paragraph:
The following additional adverse reactions have been reported with estrogen therapy (See **"Warnings"** regarding induction of malignant neoplasms, gallbladder disease, thromboembolic disorders, elevated blood pressure, hypercalcemia, and effects similar to those caused by estrogen-progestogen oral contraceptives; see **"Warnings"** and **"Precautions"** regarding cardiovascular risk).
The words "; increased incidence of gallbladder disease" should be added to the end of the list of adverse reactions after the subheading "3. *Gastrointestinal:*" in the **ADVERSE REACTIONS** section.
The words "; anaphylactoid/anaphylactic reactions" should be added to the end of the list of adverse reactions after the subheading "8. *Miscellaneous:*" in the **ADVERSE REACTIONS** section.
The following boxed warning should be added after the second paragraph under the subheading **WHAT YOU SHOULD KNOW ABOUT ESTROGENS** in the **INFORMATION FOR THE PATIENT** section:

1. ESTROGENS INCREASE THE RISK OF CANCER OF THE UTERUS IN WOMEN WHO HAVE HAD THEIR MENOPAUSE ("CHANGE OF LIFE").
If you use any estrogen-containing drug, it is important to visit your doctor regularly and report any unusual vaginal bleeding right away. Vaginal bleeding after menopause may be a warning sign of uterine cancer. Your doctor should evaluate any unusual vaginal bleeding to find out the cause.
2. ESTROGNES SHOULD NOT BE USED DURING PREGNANCY.
Estrogens do not prevent miscarriage (spontaneous abortion) and are not needed in the days following childbirth. If you take estrogens during pregnancy, your unborn child has a greater than usual chance of having birth defects. The risk of developing these defects is small, but clearly larger than the risk in children whose mothers did not take estrogens during pregnancy. These birth defects may affect the baby's urinary system and sex organs. Daughters born to mothers who took DES (an estrogen drug) have a higher than usual chance of developing cancer of the vagina or cervix when they become teenagers or young adults. Sons may have a higher than usual chance of developing cancer of the testicles when they become teenagers or young adults.

The sentence "Estrogens are prescribed by doctors for a number of purposes, including:", which appears after the first sentence under the subheading **USES OF ESTROGEN** in the **INFORMATION FOR THE PATIENT** section should be deleted and replaced with the following paragraph:
If you want to know which of these possible uses are approved for the medicine prescribed for you, ask your doctor or pharmacist to show you the professional labeling. You can also look up the specific estrogen product in a book called *The Physicians' Desk Reference*, which is available in many book stores and public libraries. Generic drugs carry virtually the same labeling information as their brand name versions.
The fourth sentence, which begins with the words "In an attempt to avoid...", of the third paragraph under the subheading **ESTROGENS IN THE MENOPAUSE** in the **INFORMATION FOR THE PATIENT** should be deleted.
In the **INFORMATION FOR THE PATIENT** section, the subsections **THE DANGERS OF ESTROGENS, SPECIAL WARNING ABOUT PREGNANCY, OTHER EFFECTS OF ESTROGEN,** and **SUMMARY** should be deleted and replaced with the following new sections:
WHO SHOULD NOT USE ESTROGENS
Estrogens should not be used:
During pregnancy (see Boxed Warning).
If you think you may be pregnant, do not use any form of estrogen-containing drug. Using estrogens while you are pregnant may cause your unborn child to have birth defects. Estrogens do not prevent miscarriage.
If you have unusual vaginal bleeding which has not been evaluated by your doctor (see Boxed Warning).
Unusual vaginal bleeding can be a warning sign of cancer of the uterus, especially if it happens after menopause. Your doctor must find out the cause of the bleeding so that he or she can recommend the proper treatment. Taking estrogens without visiting your doctor can cause you serious harm if your vaginal bleeding is caused by cancer of the uterus.
If you have had cancer.
Since estrogens increase the risk of certain types of cancer, you should not use estrogens if you have had cancer of the breast or uterus, unless your doctor recommends that the drug may help in the cancer treatment. (For certain patients with breast or prostate cancer, estrogens may help.)
If you have any circulation problems.
Estrogen drugs should not be used except in unusually special situations in which your doctor judges that you need estrogen therapy so much that the risks are acceptable. Men and women with abnormal blood clotting conditions should avoid estrogen use (see **RISKS OF ESTROGENS**, below).
When they do not work.
During menopause, some women develop nervous symptoms or depression. Estrogens do not relieve these symptoms. You may have heard that taking estrogens for years after menopause will keep your skin soft and supple and keep you feeling young. There is no evidence for these claims and such long-term estrogen use may have serious risks.
After childbirth or when breastfeeding a baby.
Estrogens should not be used to try to stop the breasts from filling with milk after a baby is born. Such treatment may increase the risk of developing blood clots (see **RISKS OF ESTROGENS**, below).
If you are breastfeeding, you should avoid using any drugs because many drugs pass through to the baby in the milk. While nursing a baby, you should take drugs only on the advice of your health-care provider.
RISKS OF ESTROGENS
1. *Cancer of the uterus.* Your risk of developing cancer of the uterus gets higher the longer you use estrogens and the larger doses you use. One study showed that after women stop taking estrogens, this higher cancer risk quickly returns to the usual level of risk (as if you had never used estrogen therapy). Three other studies showed that the cancer risk stayed high for 8 to more than 15 years after stopping estrogen treatment. Because of this risk, **IT IS IMPORTANT TO TAKE THE LOWEST DOSE THAT WORKS AND TO TAKE IT ONLY AS LONG AS YOU NEED IT.**
Using progestin therapy together with estrogen therapy may reduce the higher risk of uterine cancer related to estrogen use (but see **OTHER INFORMATION**, below).
If you have had your uterus removed (total hysterectomy), there is no risk of developing cancer of the uterus.
2. *Cancer of the breast.* Most studies have not shown a higher risk of breast cancer in women who have ever used estrogens. However, some studies have reported that breast cancer developed more often (up to twice the usual rate) in women who used estrogens for long periods of time (especially more than 10 years), or who used higher doses for shorter time periods.
Regular breast examinations by a health professional and monthly self-examination are recommended for women receiving estrogen therapy, as they are for all women. Regular mammograms are recommended for all women over 40 years of age.
3. *Gallbladder disease.* Women who use estrogens after menopause are more likely to develop gallbladder disease needing surgery than women who do not use estrogens. Birth-control pills have a similar effect.
4. *Abnormal blood clotting.* Taking estrogens may increase the risk of blood clotting in various parts of the body. This can result in a stroke (if the clot is in the brain), a heart attack (a clot in a blood vessel of the heart), a pulmonary embolus (a clot which forms in the legs or pelvis, then breaks off and travels to the lungs), retinal thrombosis (a clot in the blood vessels in the eye), or other problems. Any of these conditions may cause death or serious long term disability.
5. *Inflammation of the pancreas (Pancreatitis).* Women with high triglyceride levels may have increased risk of developing inflammation of the pancreas.
6. *Endometriosis.* Administration of estrogens may worsen endometriosis. If you have had endometriosis, speak with your health professional.
7. *Cardiovascular disease.* A recent 4-year study suggests that women with a history of coronary heart disease may have an increased risk of serious cardiac events during the first year of treatment with estrogen/progestin therapy. Therefore, if you have had a heart attack, or you have been told you have blocked coronary arteries (arteries to your heart) or have any heart problem, you should consult your physician regarding the potential benefits and risks of estrogen/progestin therapy.
OTHER EFFECTS OF ESTROGENS
In addition to the serious known risks of estrogen described above, estrogens have the following side effects and potential risks:
1. *Nausea and vomiting.* The most common side effect of estrogen therapy is nausea. Vomiting is less common.
2. *Effects on breasts.* Estrogens may cause breast tenderness or enlargement and may cause the breast to secrete a liquid.
3. *Effects on the uterus.* Estrogens may cause benign fibroid tumors of the uterus to get larger.
4. *Effects on liver.* Women taking oral contraceptives develop, on rare occasions, a tumor of the liver which can rupture and bleed into the abdomen and may cause death. So far, these tumors have not been reported in women using estrogens in the menopause, but you should report any swelling or unusual pain or tenderness in the abdomen to your doctor immediately.
Women with a past history of jaundice (yellowing of the skin and white parts of the eye) may get jaundice again during estrogen use. If this occurs, stop taking estrogens and see your doctor.
5. *Other effects.* Estrogens may cause excessive fluid to be retained in the body. This may make some conditions worse, such as asthma, epilepsy, migraine, heart disease, or kidney disease.
REDUCING RISK OF ESTROGEN USE
If you use estrogens, you can reduce your risks by doing these things:
See your doctor regularly.
While you are using estrogens, it is important to visit your doctor at least once a year for a check-up. If you develop vaginal bleeding while taking estrogens, you may need further evaluation. If members of your family have had breast cancer or if you have ever had breast lumps or an abnor mammogram (breast X-ray), you may need to have more f quent breast examinations.
Reassess your need for estrogens.
You and your doctor should reevaluate whether or not you still need estrogens at least every six months.
Be alert for signs of trouble.
If any of these warning signals (or any other unusual symptoms) happen while you are using estrogens, call your doctor immediately:
- Abnormal bleeding from the vagina (possible uterine cancer)
- Pains in the calves or chest, sudden shortness of breath, or coughing blood (possible clot in the legs, heart, or lungs)
- Severe headache or vomiting, dizziness, faintness, changes in vision or speech, weakness or numbness of an arm or leg (possible clot in the brain or eye)
- Breast lumps (possible breast cancer; ask your doctor or health professional to show you how to examine your breasts monthly)
- Yellowing of the skin or eyes (possible liver problem)
- Pain, swelling, or tenderness in the abdomen (possible gallbladder problem)

OTHER INFORMATION
1. Estrogens increase the risk of developing a condition (endometrial hyperplasia) that may lead to cancer of the lining of the uterus. Taking progestins, another hormonal drug, with estrogens lowers the risk of developing this condition. Therefore, if your uterus has not been removed, your doctor may prescribe a progestin for you to take together with the estrogen.
You should know, however, that taking estrogens *with* progestins may have additional risks. These may include unhealthy effects on blood fats (especially the lowering of HDL blood cholesterol, the "good" blood fat which protects against heart disease). However, while it has been reported that some estrogen and progestin combinations have an unfavorable effect on blood fats, studies of Premarin given with medroxyprogesterone acetate (MPA) (0.625 mg Premarin with either 2.5 mg MPA continuously or 5 mg of MPA cyclically) have shown decreases in LDL ("bad" cholesterol) and increases in HDL ("good" cholesterol). Other risks include unhealthy effects on blood sugars, which might make a diabetic condition worse, and a possible further increase in breast cancer risk which may be associated with long-term estrogen use.
Some research has shown that estrogens taken *without* progestins may protect women against developing heart disease. However, this is not certain. The protection shown may have been caused by the characteristics of the estrogen-treated women, and not by the estrogen treatment itself. In general, treated women were slimmer, more physically active, and were less likely to have diabetes than the untreated women. These characteristics are known to protect against heart disease.
You are cautioned to discuss very carefully with your doctor or health-care provider all the possible risks and benefits of long-term estrogen and progestin treatment as they affect you personally.
2. Your doctor has prescribed this drug for you and you alone. Do not give the drug to anyone else.
3. If you will be taking calcium supplements as part of the treatment to help prevent osteoporosis, check with your doctor about the amount recommended.
4. Keep this and all drugs out of the reach of children. In case of overdose, call your doctor, hospital or poison control center immediately.
5. Premarin Vaginal Cream exposure has been reported to weaken latex condoms. The potential for Premarin Vaginal Cream to weaken and contribute to the failure of condoms, diaphragms, or cervical caps made of latex or rubber should be considered.
6. This leaflet provides a summary of the most important information about estrogens. If you want more information, ask your doctor or pharmacist to show you the professional labeling. The professional labeling is also published in a book called *The Physicians' Desk Reference*, which is available in bookstores and public libraries. Generic drugs carry virtually the same labeling information as their brand name versions.

PREMPRO™ ℞
[prĕm′ prō]
(conjugated estrogens/medroxyprogesterone acetate tablets)

PREMPHASE®
[prĕm′ fāz]
(conjugated estrogens/medroxyprogesterone acetate tablets)

Caution: Federal law prohibits dispensing without prescription.

Prescribing information for this product, which appears on pages 3434–3439 of the 2001 PDR, has been revised. Please write "See Supplement A" next to the product heading.
In Table 1 on page 3435, in the column under C_{max} under the 2 × 0.625 mg CE/5 mg MPA Combination Tablets column, the bottom entry across from MPA should be changed from "48" to "4.8".
The following should be added to the end of the contraindications section:

SIROLIMUS PHARMACOKINETIC PARAMETERS (MEAN ± SD) IN RENAL TRANSPLANT PATIENTS (MULTIPLE DOSE ORAL SOLUTION)[a,b]

n	Dose	$C_{max,ss}$[c] (ng/mL)	$t_{max,ss}$ (h)	$AUC_{\tau,ss}$[c] (ng•h/mL)	CL/F/WT[d] (mL/h/kg)
19	2 mg	12.2 ± 6.2	3.01 ± 2.40	158 ± 70	182 ± 72
23	5 mg	37.4 ± 21	1.84 ± 1.30	396 ± 193	221 ± 143

a: Sirolimus administered four hours after cyclosporine oral solution (MODIFIED) (e.g., Neoral® Oral Solution) and/or cyclosporine capsules (MODIFIED) (e.g., Neoral® Soft Gelatin Capsules).
b: As measured by the Liquid Chromatographic/Tandem Mass Spectrometric Method (LC/MS/MS).
c: These parameters were dose normalized prior to the statistical comparison.
d: CL/F/WT = oral dose clearance.

7. PREMPRO or PREMPHASE therapy should not be used in patients hypersensitive to the ingredients contained in the tablets.

The subheading *"Thromboembolic Disorders and Other Vascular Problems"* in the **WARNINGS** section should be changed to just *"Thromboembolic Disorders."*

The paragraph following the old subheading *"Thromboembolic Disorders and Other Vascular Problems"* in the **WARNINGS** section should be deleted and replaced with the following paragraphs:

Venous thromboembolism. Several epidemiological studies have found an increased risk of venous thromboembolism (VTE) in users of estrogen replacement therapy (ERT) who did not have predisposing conditions for VTE, such as past history of cardiovascular disease or a recent history of pregnancy, surgery, trauma, or serious illness. The increased risk was found only in current ERT users; it did not persist in former users. The risk appeared to be higher in the first year of use and decreased therafter. The findings were similar for ERT alone or with added progestin and pertain to commonly used oral and transdermal doses, with a possible dose-dependent effect on risk. The studies found the VTE risk to be about one case per 10,000 women per year among women not using ERT and without predisposing conditions. The risk in current ERT users was increased to 2–3 cases per 10,000 women per year.

Cardiovascular disease. Embolic cerebrovascular events have been reported in women receiving postmenopausal estrogens.

Large doses of estrogen (5 mg conjugated estrogens per day), comparable to those used to treat cancer of the prostate and breast, have been shown in a large prospective clinical trial in men to increase the risk of nonfatal myocardial infarction, pulmonary embolism, and thrombophlebitis.

The physician should be aware of the possibility of thrombotic disorders (thrombophlebitis, retinal thrombosis, cerebral embolism, and pulmonary embolism) during estrogen replacement therapy and be alert to their earliest manifestations. Should any of these occur or be suspected, estrogen replacement therapy should be discontinued immediately. Patients who have risk factors for thrombotic disorders should be kept under careful observation.

The sixth sentence, which starts with the words "Postmenopausal estrogen use...," of the paragraph following the subheading *"Elevated blood pressure"* in the **WARNINGS** section should be deleted, the word "Nonetheless," in the next sentence of the paragraph should also be deleted, and the "b" in the word "blood" should become a capital "B."

The first paragraph following the subheading *"Cardiovascular Risk"* under **"General"** in the **PRECAUTIONS** section should be underlined.

The words "(see **PRECAUTIONS** and **WARNINGS**)" should be added to the end of the first sentence, after the word "uteri", of the second paragraph following the subheading *"Cardiovascular Risk"* under **"General"** in the **PRECAUTIONS** section.

The following paragraph should be added as item 3 under "Based on experience with estrogens:" in the **PRECAUTIONS** section, and the number 3, which precedes the subheading *"Mastodynia,"* should be changed to the number 4:

3. *Thromboembolism.* Based on data obtained with oral contraceptives, estrogens should be discontinued at least four weeks before surgery of the type associated with an increased risk of thromboembolism if feasible, or during periods of prolonged immobilization (see **WARNINGS**).

The first paragraph under the heading **ADVERSE REACTIONS** should be deleted and replaced with the following paragraph:

(See **WARNINGS** regarding induction of malignant neoplasia, effects during pregnancy, increased incidence of gallbladder disease, elevated blood pressure, thromboembolic disorders, visual abnormalities, and hypercalcemia; see **WARNINGS** and **PRECAUTIONS** regarding cardiovascular disease.)

In the last line of the paragraph following the subheading *"Cancer of the breast"* under **RISKS OF ESTROGENS AND/OR PROGESTINS** in the **INFORMATION FOR THE PATIENT** section, the number "50" should be deleted and replaced with "40."

The words ", retinal thrombosis (cutting off blood vessels in the eye)," should be added after the phrase "(cutting off blood to the lungs)" in the paragraph following the subheading *"Abnormal blood clotting"* under **RISKS OF ESTROGENS AND/OR PROGESTINS** in the **INFORMATION FOR THE PATIENT** section.

RAPAMUNE® ORAL SOLUTION ℞

[*răp 'ă-mūn*]
sirolimus
Oral Solution
Tablets

Prescribing information for this product, which appears on pages 3443–3448 of the 2001 PDR, has been completely revised as follows. Please write "See Supplement A" next to the product heading.

WARNING:
Increased susceptibility to infection and the possible development of lymphoma may result from immunosuppression. Only physicians experienced in immunosuppressive therapy and management of renal transplant patients should use Rapamune®. Patients receiving the drug should be managed in facilities equipped and staffed with adequate laboratory and supportive medical resources. The physician responsible for maintenance therapy should have complete information requisite for the follow-up of the patient.

DESCRIPTION

Rapamune® (sirolimus) is an immunosuppressive agent. Sirolimus is a macrocyclic lactone produced by *Streptomyces hygroscopicus*. The chemical name of sirolimus (also known as rapamycin) is (3*S*,6*R*,7*E*,9*R*,10*R*,12*R*,14*S*,15*E*,17*E*,19*E*,21*S*,23*S*,26*R*,27*R*,34a*S*)-9,10,12,13,14,21,22,23,24,25,26,27,32,33,34,34a-hexadecahydro-9,27-dihydroxy-3-[(1*R*)-2-[(1*S*,3*R*,4*R*)-4-hydroxy-3-methoxycyclohexyl]-1-methylethyl]-10,21-dimethoxy-6,8,12,14,20,26-hexamethyl-23,27-epoxy-3*H*-pyrido[2,1-*c*][1,4] oxaazacyclohentri-acontine-1,5,11,28,29 (4*H*,6*H*,31*H*)-pentone. Its molecular formula is $C_{51}H_{79}NO_{13}$ and its molecular weight is 914.2. The structural formula of sirolimus is shown below.

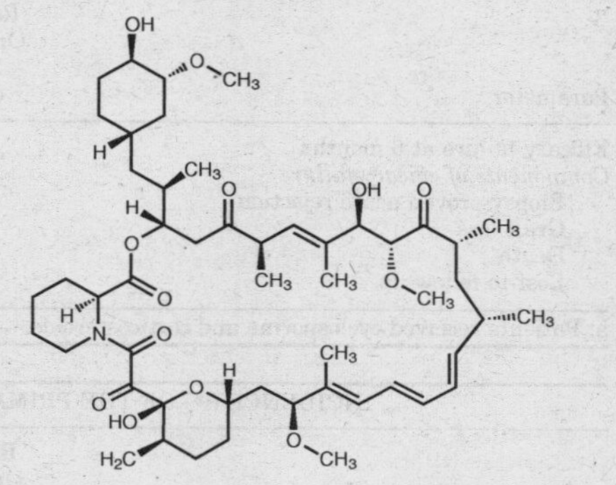

Sirolimus is a white to off-white powder and is insoluble in water, but freely soluble in benzyl alcohol, chloroform, acetone, and acetonitrile.

Rapamune® is available for administration as an oral solution containing 1 mg/mL sirolimus and as a white, triangular-shaped tablet containing 1 mg sirolimus.

The inactive ingredients in Rapamune® Oral Solution are Phosal 50 PG® (phosphatidylcholine, propylene glycol, mono- and di-glycerides, ethanol, soy fatty acids, and ascorbyl palmitate) and polysorbate 80. Rapamune Oral Solution contains 1.5%–2.5% ethanol.

The inactive ingredients in Rapamune® Tablets include sucrose, lactose, polyethylene glycol 8000, calcium sulfate, microcrystalline cellulose, pharmaceutical glaze, talc, titanium dioxide, magnesium stearate, povidone, poloxamer 188, polyethylene glycol 20,000, glyceryl monooleate, carnauba wax, and other ingredients.

CLINICAL PHARMACOLOGY

Mechanism of Action

Sirolimus inhibits T lymphocyte activation and proliferation that occurs in response to antigenic and cytokine (Interleukin [IL]-2, IL-4, and IL-15) stimulation by a mechanism that is distinct from that of other immunosuppressants. Sirolimus also inhibits antibody production. In cells, sirolimus binds to the immunophilin, FK Binding Protein-12 (FKBP-12), to generate an immunosuppressive complex. The sirolimus:FKBP-12 complex has no effect on calcineurin activity. This complex binds to and inhibits the activation of the mammalian Target Of Rapamycin (mTOR), a key regulatory kinase. This inhibition suppresses cytokine-driven T-cell proliferation, inhibiting the progression from the G_1 to the S phase of the cell cycle.

Studies in experimental models show that sirolimus prolongs allograft (kidney, heart, skin, islet, small bowel, pancreatico-duodenal, and bone marrow) surivival in mice, rats, pigs, and/or primates. Sirolimus reverses acute rejection of heart and kidney allografts in rats and prolonged the graft survival in presensitized rats. In some studies, the immunosuppressive effect of sirolimus lasted up to 6 months after discontinuation of therapy. This tolerization effect is alloantigen specific.

In rodent models of autoimmune disease, sirolimus suppresses immune-mediated events associated with systemic lupus erythematosus, collagen-induced arthritis, autoimmune type I diabetes, autoimmune myocarditis, experimental allergic encephalomyelitis, graft-versus-host disease, and autoimmune uveoretinitis.

Pharmacokinetics

Sirolimus pharmacokinetic activity has been determined following oral administration in healthy subjects, pediatric dialysis patients, hepatically-impaired patients, and renal transplant patients.

Absorption

Following administration of Rapamune® Oral Solution, sirolimus is rapidly absorbed, with a mean time-to-peak concentration (t_{max}) of approximately 1 hour after a single dose in healthy subjects and approximately 2 hours after multiple oral doses in renal transplant recipients. The systemic availability of sirolimus was estimated to be approximately 14% after the administration of Rapamune Oral Solution. The mean bioavailability of sirolimus after administration of the tablet is about 27% higher relative to the oral solution. Sirolimus oral tablets are not bioequivalent to the oral solution; however, clinical equivalence has been demonstrated at the 2-mg dose level. (See **CLINICAL STUDIES** and **DOSAGE AND ADMINISTRATION**). Sirolimus concentrations, following the administration of Rapamune Oral Solution to stable renal transplant patients, are dose proportional between 3 and 12 mg/m^2.

Food effects: In 22 healthy volunteers receiving Rapamune Oral Solution, a high-fat meal (1.88 kcal, 54.7% fat) altered the bioavailability characteristics of sirolimus. Compared to fasting, a 34% decrease in the peak blood sirolimus concentration (C_{max}), a 3.5-fold increase in the time-to-peak concentration (t_{max}), and a 35% increase in total exposure (AUC) was observed. After administration of Rapamune Tablets and a high-fat meal in 24 healthy volunteers, C_{max}, t_{max}, and AUC showed increases of 65%, 32%, and 23%, respectively. To minimize variability, both Rapamune Oral Solution and Tablets should be taken consistently with or without food (See **DOSAGE AND ADMINISTRATION**).

Distribution

The mean (±SD) blood-to-plasma ratio of sirolimus was 36 (± 17.9) in stable renal allograft recipients, indicating that sirolimus is extensively partitioned into formed blood elements. The mean volume of distribution (V_{ss}/F) of sirolimus is 12 ± 7.52 L/kg. Sirolimus is extensively bound (approximately 92%) to human plasma proteins. In man, the binding of sirolimus was shown mainly to be associated with serum albumin (97%), α_1-acid glycoprotein, and lipoproteins.

Metabolism

Sirolimus is a substrate for both cytochrome P450 IIIA4 (CYP3A4) and P-glycoprotein. Sirolimus is extensively metabolized by O-demethylation and/or hydroxylation. Seven (7) major metabolites, including hydroxy, demethyl, and hydroxydemethyl, are identifiable in whole blood. Some of these metabolites are also detectable in plasma, fecal, and urine samples. Glucuronide and sulfate conjugates are not present in any of the biologic matrices. Sirolimus is the major component in human whole blood and contributes to more than 90% of the immunosuppressive activity.

Excretion

After a single dose of [^{14}C]sirolimus in healthy volunteers, the majority (91%) of radioactivity was recovered from the feces, and only a minor amount (2.2%) was excreted in urine.

Pharmacokinetics in renal transplant patients

Rapamune Oral Solution: Pharmacokinetic parameters for sirolimus oral solution given daily in combination with cyclosporine and corticosteroids in renal transplant patients are summarized below based on data collected at months 1, 3, and 6 after transplantation. There were no significant differences in any of these parameters with respect to treatment group or month.

[See table above]

Whole blood sirolimus trough concentrations, as measured by immunoassay, (mean ± SD) for the 2 mg/day and 5 mg/day dose groups were 8.59 ± 4.01 ng/mL (n = 226) and 17.3 ± 7.4 ng/mL (n = 219), respectively. Whole blood trough sirolimus concentrations, as measured by LC/MS/MS, were significantly correlated (r^2 = 0.96) with $AUC_{\tau,ss}$. Upon repeated twice daily administration without an initial loading dose in a multiple-dose study, the average trough concentration of sirolimus increases approximately 2 to 3-fold over the initial 6 days of therapy at which time steady state is reached. A loading dose of 3 times the maintenance dose will provide near steady-state concentrations within 1 day in most patients. The mean ± SD terminal elimination half life ($t_{1/2}$) of sirolimus after multiple dosing in stable renal transplant patients was estimated to be about 62 ± 16 hours.

Rapamune Tablets: Pharmacokinetic parameters for sirolimus tablets administered daily in combination with cyclosporine and corticosteroids in renal transplant patients

Continued on next page

Rapamune—Cont.

are summarized below based on data collected at months 1 and 3 after transplantation.

[See first table above]

Whole blood sirolimus trough concentrations (mean ± SD), as measured by immunoassay, for the 2 mg oral solution and 2 mg tablets over 6 months, were 8.94 ± 4.36 ng/mL (n = 172) and 9.48 ± 3.85 ng/mL (n = 179), respectively. Whole blood trough sirolimus concentrations, as measured by LC/MS/MS, were significantly correlated (r^2 = 0.85) with $AUC_{\tau,ss}$. Mean whole blood sirolimus trough concentrations in patients receiving either Rapamune Oral Solution or Rapamune Tablets with a loading dose of three times the maintenance dose achieved steady-state concentrations within 24 hours after the start of dose administration.

Special Populations

Hepatic impairment: Sirolimus (15 mg) was administered as a single oral dose to 18 subjects with normal hepatic function and to 18 patients with Child-Pugh classification A or B hepatic impairment, in which hepatic impairment was primary and not related to an underlying systemic disease. Shown below are the mean ± SD pharmacokinetic parameters following the administration of sirolimus oral solution.

[See second table above]

Compared with the values in the normal hepatic group, the hepatic impairment group had higher mean values for sirolimus AUC (61%) and $t_{1/2}$ (43%) and had lower mean values for sirolimus CL/F/WT (33%). The mean $t_{1/2}$ increased from 79 ± 12 hours in subjects with normal hepatic function to 113 ± 41 hours in patients with impaired hepatic function. The rate of absorption of sirolimus was not altered by hepatic disease, as evidenced by C_{max} and t_{max} values. However, hepatic diseases with varying etiologies may show different effects and the pharmacokinetics of sirolimus in patients with severe hepatic dysfunction is unknown. Dosage adjustment is recommended for patients with mild to moderate hepatic impairment (see **DOSAGE AND ADMINISTRATION**).

Renal impairment: The effect of renal impairment on the pharmacokinetics of sirolimus is not known. However, there is minimal (2.2%) renal excretion of the drug or its metabolites.

Pediatric Limited pharmacokinetic data are available in pediatric patients. The table below summarizes pharmacokinetic data obtained in pediatric dialysis patients with chronically impaired renal function.

[See third table above]

Geriatric: Clinical studies of Rapamune did not include a sufficient number of patients > 65 years of age to determine whether they will respond differently than younger patients. After the administration of Rapamune Oral Solution, sirolimus trough concentration data in 35 renal transplant patients > 65 years of age were similar to those in the adult population (n = 822) 18 to 65 years of age. Similar results were obtained after the administration of Rapamune Tablets to 12 renal transplant patients > 65 years of age compared with adults (n = 167) 18 to 65 years of age.

Gender: After the administration of Rapamune Oral Solution, sirolimus oral dose clearance in males was 12% lower than that in females; male subjects had a significantly longer $t_{1/2}$ than did female subjects (72.3 hours versus 61.3 hours). A similar trend in the effect of gender on sirolimus oral dose clearance and $t_{1/2}$ was observed after the administration of Rapamune Tablets. Dose adjustments based on gender are not recommended.

Race: In large phase III trials using Rapamune Oral Solution and cyclosporine oral solution (MODIFIED) (e.g., Neoral® Oral Solution) and/or cyclosporine capsules (MODIFIED) (e.g., Neoral® Soft Gelatin Capsules), there were no significant differences in mean trough sirolimus concentrations over time between black (n = 139) and non-black (n = 724) patients during the first 6 months after transplantation at sirolimus doses of 2 mg/day and 5 mg/day. Similarly, after administration of Rapamune Tablets (2 mg/day) in a phase III trial, mean sirolimus trough concentrations over 6 months were not significantly different among black (n = 51) and non-black (n = 128) patients.

CLINICAL STUDIES

Rapamune® Oral Solution: The safety and efficacy of Rapamune® Oral Solution for the prevention of organ rejection following renal transplantation were assessed in two randomized, double-blind, multicenter, controlled trials. These studies compared two dose levels of Rapamune Oral Solution (2 mg and 5 mg, once daily) with azathioprine (Study 1) or placebo (Study 2) when administered in combination with cyclosporine and corticosteroids. Study 1 was conducted in the United States at 38 sites. Seven hundred nineteen (719) patients were enrolled in this trial and randomized following transplantation; 284 were randomized to receive Rapamune Oral Solution 2 mg/day, 274 were randomized to receive Rapamune Oral Solution 5 mg/day, and 161 to receive azathioprine 2–3 mg/kg/day. Study 2 was conducted in Australia, Canada, Europe, and the United States, at a total of 34 sites. Five hundred seventy-six (576) patients were enrolled in this trial and randomized before transplantation; 227 were randomized to receive Rapamune Oral Solution 2 mg/day, 219 were randomized to receive Rapamune Oral Solution 5 mg/day, and 130 to receive placebo. In both studies, the use of antilymphocyte antibody induction therapy was prohibited. In both studies, the primary efficacy endpoint was the rate of efficacy failure in the first 6 months after transplantation. Efficacy failure was de-

fined as the first occurrence of an acute rejection episode (confirmed by biopsy), graft loss, or death.

The tables below summarize the results of the primary efficacy analyses from these trials. Rapamune Oral Solution, at doses of 2 mg/day and 5 mg/day, significantly reduced the incidence of efficacy failure (statistically significant at the <0.025 level; nominal significance level adjusted for multiple [2] dose comparisons) at 6 months following transplantation compared to both azathioprine and placebo.

[See fourth table above]

[See fifth table above]

Patient and graft survival at 1 year were co-primary endpoints. The table below shows graft and patient survival at 1 year in Study 1 and Study 2. The graft and patient survival rates at 1 year were similar in the Rapamune- and comparator-treated patients.

[See sixth table above]

The reduction in the incidence of first biopsy-confirmed acute rejection episodes in Rapamune-treated patients compared to the control groups included a reduction in all grades of rejection.

[See first table at top of next page]

In Study 1, which was prospectively stratified by race within center, efficacy failure was similar for Rapamune Oral Solution 2 mg/day and lower for Rapamune Oral Solution 5 mg/day compared to azathioprine in black patients. In Study 2, which was not prospectively stratified by race, efficacy failure was similar for both Rapamune Oral Solution doses compared to placebo in black patients. The decision to use the higher dose of Rapamune Oral Solution in black patients must be weighed against the increased risk of dose-dependent adverse events that were observed with the Rapamune Oral Solution 5 mg dose (see **ADVERSE REACTIONS**).

[See second table at top of next page]

Mean glomerular filtration rates (GFR) at one year post transplant were calculated by using the Nankivell equation for all subjects in Studies 1 and 2 who had serum creatinine measured at 12 months. In Studies 1 and 2 mean GFR, at 12 months, were lower in patients treated with cyclosporine and Rapamune Oral Solution compared to those treated with cyclosporine and the respective azathioprine or placebo control.

SIROLIMUS PHARMACOKINETIC PARAMETERS (MEAN ± SD) IN RENAL TRANSPLANT PATIENTS (MULTIPLE DOSE TABLETS)[a,b]

n	Dose (2 mg/day)	$C_{max,ss}$[c] (ng/mL)	$t_{max,ss}$ (h)	$AUC_{\tau,ss}$[c] (ng•h/mL)	CL/F/WT[d] (mL/h/kg)
17	Oral solution	14.4 ± 5.3	2.12 ± 0.84	194 ± 78	173 ± 50
13	Tablets	15.0 ± 4.9	3.46 ± 2.40	230 ± 67	139 ± 63

a: Sirolimus administered four hours after cyclosporine oral solution (MODIFIED) (e.g., Neoral® Oral Solution) and/or cyclosporine capsules (MODIFIED) (e.g., Neoral® Soft Gelatin Capsules).
b: As measured by the Liquid Chromatographic/Tandem Mass Spectrometric Method (LC/MS/MS).
c: These parameters were dose normalized prior to the statistical comparison.
d: CL/F/WT = oral dose clearance.

SIROLIMUS PHARMACOKINETIC PARAMETERS (MEAN ± SD) IN 18 HEALTHY SUBJECTS AND 18 PATIENTS WITH HEPATIC IMPAIRMENT (15 MG SINGLE DOSE – ORAL SOLUTION)

Population	$C_{max,ss}$[a] (ng/mL)	t_{max} (h)	$AUC_{0-\infty}$ (ng•h/mL)	CL/F/WT (mL/h/kg)
Healthy subjects	78.2 ± 18.3	0.82 ± 0.17	970 ± 272	215 ± 76
Hepatic impairment	77.9 ± 23.1	0.84 ± 0.17	1567 ± 616	144 ± 62

a: As measured by (LC/MS/MS)

SIROLIMUS PHARMACOKINETIC PARAMETERS (MEAN ± SD) IN PEDIATRIC PATIENTS WITH STABLE CHRONIC RENAL FAILURE MAINTAINED ON HEMODIALYSIS OR PERITONEAL DIALYSIS (1, 3, 9, 15 MG/M² SINGLE DOSE)

Age Group (y)	n	t_{max} (h)	$t_{1/2}$ (h)	CL/F/WT (mL/h/kg)
5–11	9	1.1 ± 0.5	71 ± 40	580 ± 450
12–18	11	0.79 ± 0.17	55 ± 18	450 ± 232

INCIDENCE (%) OF THE PRIMARY ENDPOINT AT 6 MONTHS: STUDY 1[a]

Parameter	Rapamune® Oral Solution 2 mg/day (n = 284)	Rapamune® Oral Solution 5 mg/day (n = 274)	Azathioprine 2–3 mg/kg/day (n = 161)
Efficacy failure at 6 months	18.7	16.8	32.3
Components of efficacy failure			
Biopsy-proven acute rejection	16.5	11.3	29.2
Graft loss	1.1	2.9	2.5
Death	0.7	1.8	0
Lost to follow-up	0.4	0.7	0.6

a: Patients received cyclosporine and corticosteroids.

INCIDENCE (%) OF THE PRIMARY ENDPOINT AT 6 MONTHS: STUDY 2[a]

Parameter	Rapamune® Oral Solution 2 mg/day (n = 227)	Rapamune® Oral Solution 5 mg/day (n = 219)	Placebo (n = 130)
Efficacy failure at 6 months	30.0	25.6	47.7
Components of efficacy failure			
Biopsy-proven acute rejection	24.7	19.2	41.5
Graft loss	3.1	3.7	3.9
Death	2.2	2.7	2.3
Lost to follow-up	0	0	0

a: Patients received cyclosporine and corticosteroids.

---

1 YEAR GRAFT AND PATIENT SURVIVAL (%)[a]

Parameter	Rapamune® Oral Solution 2 mg/day	Rapamune® Oral Solution 5 mg/day	Azathioprine 2–3 mg/kg/day	Placebo
Study 1	(n = 284)	(n = 274)	(n = 161)	
Graft survival	94.7	92.7	93.8	
Patient survival	97.2	96.0	98.1	
Study 2	(n = 227)	(n = 219)		(n = 130)
Graft survival	89.9	90.9		87.7
Patient survival	96.5	95.0		94.6

a: Patients received cyclosporine and corticosteroids.

Within each treatment group in Studies 1 and 2, mean GFR at one year post transplant was lower in patients who experienced at least 1 episode of biopsy-proven acute rejection, compared to those who did not.

Renal function should be monitored and appropriate adjustment of the immunosuppression regimen should be considered in patients with elevated serum creatinine levels (see **PRECAUTIONS**).

Rapamune® Tablets: The safety and efficacy of Rapamune Oral Solution and Rapamune Tablets for the prevention of organ rejection following renal transplantation were compared in a randomized multicenter controlled trial (Study 3). This study compared a single dose level (2 mg, once daily) of Rapamune Oral Solution and Rapamune Tablets when administered in combination with cyclosporine and corticosteroids. The study was conducted at 30 centers in Australia, Canada, and the United States. Four hundred seventy-seven (477) patients were enrolled in this study and randomized before transplantation; 238 patients were randomized to receive Rapamune Oral Solution 2 mg/day and 239 patients were randomized to receive Rapamune Tablets 2 mg/day. In this study, the use of antilymphocyte antibody induction therapy was prohibited. The primary efficacy endpoint was the rate of efficacy failure in the first 3 months after transplantation. Efficacy failure was defined as the first occurrence of an acute rejection episode (confirmed by biopsy), graft loss, or death.

The table below summarizes the result of the primary efficacy analysis at 3 months from this trial. The overall rate of efficacy failure in the tablet treatment group was equivalent to the rate in the oral solution treatment group.
[See third table to the right]

The table below summarizes the results of the primary efficacy analysis at 6 months after transplantation.
[See fourth table to the right]

Graft and patient survival at 12 months were co-primary efficacy endpoints. There was no significant difference between the oral solution and tablet formulations for both graft and patient survival. Graft survival was 92.0% and 88.7% for the oral solution and tablet treatment groups, respectively. The patient survival rates in the oral solution and tablet treatment groups were 95.8% and 96.2%, respectively.

The mean GFR at 12 months, calculated by the Nankivell equation, were not significantly different for the oral solution group and for the tablet group.

The table below summarizes the mean GFR at one-year post-transplantation for all subjects in Study 3 who had serum creatinine measured at 12 months.

OVERALL CALCULATED GLOMERULAR FILTRATION RATES (CC/MIN) BY NANKIVELL EQUATION AT 12 MONTHS POST TRANSPLANT: STUDY 3

	Rapamune® Oral Solution	Rapamune® Tablets
Mean (SE)	58.3 (1.64)	58.5 (1.44)
	n = 166	n = 162

INDICATIONS AND USAGE

Rapamune is indicated for the prophylaxis of organ rejection in patients receiving renal transplants. It is recommended that Rapamune be used in a regimen with cyclosporine and corticosteroids.

CONTRAINDICATIONS

Rapamune is contraindicated in patients with a hypersensitivity to sirolimus or its derivatives or any component of the drug product.

WARNINGS

Increased susceptibility to infection and the possible development of lymphoma and other malignancies, particularly of the skin, may result from immunosuppression (see **ADVERSE REACTIONS**). Oversuppression of the immune system can also increase susceptibility to infection including opportunistic infections, fatal infections, and sepsis. Only physicians experienced in immunosuppressive therapy and management of organ transplant patients should use Rapamune. Patients receiving the drug should be managed in facilities equipped and staffed with adequate laboratory and supportive medical resources. The physician responsible for maintenance therapy should have complete information requisite for the follow-up of the patient. As usual for patients with increased risk for skin cancer, exposure to sunlight and UV light should be limited by wearing protective clothing and using a sunscreen with a high protection factor.

Increased serum cholesterol and triglycerides, that may require treatment, occurred more frequently in patients treated with Rapamune compared to azathioprine or placebo controls (see **PRECAUTIONS**).

In phase III studies, mean serum creatinine was increased and mean glomerular filtration rate was decreased in patients treated with Rapamune and cyclosporine compared to those treated with cyclosporine and placebo or azathioprine controls (see **CLINICAL STUDIES**). Renal function should be monitored during the administration of maintenance immunosuppression regimens including Rapamune in combination with cyclosporine, and appropriate adjustment of the

PERCENTAGE OF EFFICACY FAILURE BY RACE AT 6 MONTHS

Parameter	Rapamune® Oral Solution 2 mg/day	Rapamune® Oral Solution 5 mg/day	Azathioprine 2–3 mg/kg/day	Placebo
Study 1				
Black (n=166)	34.9 (n=63)	18.0 (n=61)	33.3 (n=42)	
Non-black (n=553)	14.0 (n=221)	16.4 (n=213)	31.9 (n=119)	
Study 2				
Black (n=66)	30.8 (n=26)	33.7 (n=27)		38.5 (n=13)
Non-black (n=510)	29.9 (n=201)	24.5 (n=192)		48.7 (n=117)

OVERALL CALCULATED GLOMERULAR FILTRATION RATES (CC/MIN) BY NANKIVELL EQUATION AT 12 MONTHS POST TRANSPLANT

Parameter	Rapamune® Oral Solution 2 mg/day	Rapamune® Oral Solution 5 mg/day	Azathioprine 2–3 mg/kg/day	Placebo
Study 1	(n=233)	(n=226)	(n=127)	
Mean (SE)	57.4 (1.28)	55.1 (1.28)	65.9 (1.69)	
Study 2	(n=190)	(n=175)		(n=101)
Mean (SE)	54.9 (1.26)	52.9 (1.46)		61.7 (1.81)

INCIDENCE (%) OF THE PRIMARY ENDPOINT AT 3 MONTHS: STUDY 3[a]

	Rapamune® Oral Solution (n = 238)	Rapamune® Tablets (n = 239)
Efficacy Failure at 3 months	23.5	24.7
Components of efficacy failure		
Biopsy-proven acute rejection	18.9	17.6
Graft loss	3.4	6.3
Death	1.3	0.8

a: Patients received cyclosporine and corticosteroids.

INCIDENCE (%) OF THE PRIMARY ENDPOINT AT 6 MONTHS: STUDY 3[a]

	Rapamune® Oral Solution (n = 238)	Rapamune® Tablets (n = 239)
Efficacy Failure at 6 months	26.1	27.2
Components of efficacy failure		
Biopsy-proven acute rejection	21.0	19.2
Graft loss	3.4	6.3
Death	1.7	1.7

a: Patients received cyclosporine and corticosteroids.

immunosuppression regimen should be considered in patients with elevated serum creatinine levels. Caution should be exercised when using agents which are known to impair renal function (see **PRECAUTIONS**).

In clinical trials, Rapamune has been administered concurrently with corticosteroids and with the following formulations of cyclosporine:

Sandimmune® Injection (cyclosporine injection)
Sandimmune® Oral Solution (cyclosporine oral solution)
Sandimmune® Soft Gelatin Capsules (cyclosporine capsules)
Neoral® Soft Gelatin Capsules (cyclosporine capsules [MODIFIED])
Neoral® Oral Solution (cyclosporine oral solution [MODIFIED])

The efficacy and safety of the use of Rapamune in combination with other immunosuppressive agents has not been determined.

PRECAUTIONS

General

Rapamune is intended for oral administration only.

Lymphocele, a known surgical complication of renal transplantation, occurred significantly more often in dose-related fashion in Rapamune-treated patients. Appropriate postoperative measures should be considered to minimize this complication.

Lipids

The use of Rapamune® in renal transplant patients was associated with increased serum cholesterol and triglycerides that may require treatment.

In phase III clinical trials, in *de novo* renal transplant recipients who began the study with normal, fasting, total serum cholesterol (fasting serum cholesterol < 200 mg/dL), there was an increased incidence of hypercholesterolemia (fasting serum cholesterol > 240 mg/dL) in patients receiving both Rapamune® 2 mg and Rapamune® 5 mg compared to azathioprine and placebo controls.

In phase III clinical trials, in *de novo* renal transplant recipients who began the study with normal, fasting, total serum triglycerides (fasting serum triglycerides < 200 mg/dL), there was an increased incidence of hypertriglyceridemia (fasting serum triglycerides > 500 mg/dL) in patients receiving Rapamune® 2 mg and Rapamune® 5 mg compared to azathioprine and placebo controls.

Treatment of new-onset hypercholesterolemia with lipid-lowering agents was required in 42–52% of patients enrolled in the Rapamune arms of the study compared to 16% of patients in the placebo arm and 22% of patients in the azathioprine arm.

Renal transplant patients have a higher prevalence of clinically significant hyperlipidemia. Accordingly, the risk/benefit should be carefully considered in patients with established hyperlipidemia before initiating an immunosuppressive regimen including Rapamune.

Any patient who is administered Rapamune should be monitored for hyperlipidemia using laboratory tests and if hyperlipidemia is detected, subsequent interventions such as diet, exercise, and lipid-lowering agents, as outlined by the National Cholesterol Education Program guidelines, should be initiated.

In the limited number of patients studied, the concomitant administration of Rapamune and HMG-CoA reductase inhibitors and/or fibrates appeared to be well tolerated. Nevertheless, all patients administered Rapamune with cyclosporine, in conjunction with an HMG-CoA reductase inhibitor, should be monitored for the development of rhabdomyolysis.

Renal Function

Patients treated with cyclosporine and Rapamune were noted to have higher serum creatinine levels and lower glomerular filtration rates compared with patients treated with cyclosporine and placebo or azathioprine controls. Renal function should be monitored during the administration of maintenance immunosuppression regimens including Rapamune in combination with cyclosporine, and appropriate adjustment of the immunosuppression regimen should be considered in patients with elevated serum creatinine levels. Caution should be exercised when using agents (e.g., aminoglycosides, and amphotericin B) that are known to have a deleterious effect on renal function.

Antimicrobial Prophylaxis

Cases of *Pneumocystis carinii* pneumonia have been reported in patients not receiving antimicrobial prophylaxis. Therefore, antimicrobial prophylaxis for *Pneumocystis carinii* pneumonia should be administered for 1 year following transplantation. Cytomegalovirus (CMV) prophylaxis is recommended for 3 months after transplantation, particularly for patients at increased risk for CMV disease.

Information for Patients

Patients should be given complete dosage instructions (see **Patient Instructions**). Women of childbearing potential should be informed of the potential risks during pregnancy and that they should use effective contraception prior to initiation of Rapamune therapy, during Rapamune therapy and for 12 weeks after Rapamune therapy has been stopped (see **PRECAUTIONS: Pregnancy**).

Continued on next page

Rapamune—Cont.

Patients should be told that exposure to sunlight and UV light should be limited by wearing protective clothing and using a sunscreen with a high protection factor because of the increased risk for skin cancer (see **WARNINGS**).

Laboratory Tests

It is prudent to monitor blood sirolimus levels in patients likely to have altered drug metabolism, in patients ≥13 years who weigh less than 40 kg, in patients with hepatic impairment, and during concurrent administration of potent CYP3A4 inducers and inhibitors (see **PRECAUTIONS: Drug Interactions**).

Drug Interactions

Sirolimus is known to be a substrate for both cytochrome CYP3A4 and P-glycoprotein. The pharmacokinetic interaction between sirolimus and concomitantly administered drugs is discussed below. Drug interaction studies have not been conducted with drugs other than those described below.

Cyclosporine capsules MODIFIED:

Rapamune Oral Solution: In a single dose drug-drug interaction study, 24 healthy volunteers were administered 10 mg sirolimus either simultaneously or 4 hours after a 300 mg dose of Neoral® Soft Gelatin Capsules (cyclosporine capsules [MODIFIED]). For simultaneous administration, the mean C_{max} and AUC of sirolimus were increased by 116% and 230%, respectively, relative to administration of sirolimus alone. However, when given 4 hours after Neoral® Soft Gelatin Capsules (cyclosporine capsules [MODIFIED]) administration, sirolimus C_{max} and AUC were increased by 37% and 80%, respectively, compared to administration of sirolimus alone.

Mean cyclosporine C_{max} and AUC were not significantly affected when sirolimus was given simultaneously or when administered 4 hours after Neoral® Soft Gelatin Capsules (cyclosporine capsules [MODIFIED]). However, after multiple-dose administration of sirolimus given 4 hours after Neoral® in renal post-transplant patients over 6 months, cyclosporine oral-dose clearance was reduced, and lower doses of Neoral® Soft Gelatin Capsules (cyclosporine capsules [MODIFIED]) were needed to maintain target cyclosporine concentration.

Rapamune Tablets: In a single-dose drug-drug interaction study, 24 healthy volunteers were administered 10 mg sirolimus (Rapamune Tablets) either simultaneously or 4 hours after a 300 mg dose of Neoral® Soft Gelatin Capsules (cyclosporine capsules [MODIFIED]). For simultaneous administration, mean C_{max} and AUC were increased by 512% and 148%, respectively, relative to administration of sirolimus alone. However, when given 4 hours after cyclosporine administration, sirolimus C_{max} and AUC were both increased by only 33% compared with administration of sirolimus alone.

Because of the effect of cyclosporine capsules (MODIFIED), it is recommended that sirolimus should be taken 4 hours after administration of cyclosporine oral solution (MODIFIED) and/or cyclosporine capsules (MODIFIED), (see DOSAGE AND ADMINISTRATION).

Cyclosporine oral solution: In a multiple-dose study in 150 psoriasis patients, sirolimus 0.5, 1.5, and 3 mg/m²/day was administered simultaneously with Sandimmune® Oral Solution (cyclosporine Oral Solution) 1.25 mg/kg/day. The increase in average sirolimus trough concentrations ranged between 67% to 86% relative to when sirolimus was administered without cyclosporine. The intersubject variability (%CV) for sirolimus trough concentrations ranged from 39.7% to 68.7%. There was no significant effect of multiple-dose sirolimus on cyclosporine trough concentrations following Sandimmune® Oral Solution (cyclosporine oral solution) administration. However, the %CV was higher (range 85.9%–165%) than those from previous studies.

Sandimmune® Oral Solution (cyclosporine oral solution) is not bioequivalent to Neoral® Oral Solution (cyclosporine oral solution MODIFIED), and should not be used interchangeably. Although there is no published data comparing Sandimmune® Oral Solution (cyclosporine oral solution) to SangCya® Oral Solution (cyclosporine oral solution [MODIFIED]), they should not be used interchangeably. Likewise, Sandimmune® Soft Gelatin Capsules (cyclosporine capsules) are not bioequivalent to Neoral® Soft Gelatin Capsules (cyclosporine capsules [MODIFIED]) and should not be used interchangeably.

Diltiazem: The simultaneous oral administration of 10 mg of sirolimus oral solution and 120 mg of diltiazem to 18 healthy volunteers significantly affected the bioavailability of sirolimus. Sirolimus C_{max}, t_{max}, and AUC were increased 1.4-, 1.3-, and 1.6-fold, respectively. Sirolimus did not affect the pharmacokinetics of either diltiazem or its metabolites desacetyldiltiazem and desmethyldiltiazem. If diltiazem is administered, sirolimus should be monitored and a dose adjustment may be necessary.

Ketoconazole: Multiple-dose ketoconazole administration significantly affected the rate and extent of absorption and sirolimus exposure after administration of Rapamune Oral Solution, as reflected by increases in sirolimus C_{max}, t_{max}, and AUC of 4.3-fold, 38%, and 10.9-fold, respectively. However, the terminal $t_{1/2}$ of sirolimus was not changed. Single-dose sirolimus did not affect steady-state 12-hour plasma ketoconazole concentrations. It is recommended that sirolimus oral solution and oral tablets should not be administered with ketoconazole.

Rifampin: Pretreatment of 14 healthy volunteers with multiple doses of rifampin, 600 mg daily for 14 days, followed by a single 20 mg-dose of sirolimus, greatly increased sirolimus oral-dose clearance by 5.5-fold (range = 2.8 to 10), which represents mean decreases in AUC and C_{max} of about 82% and 71%, respectively. In patients where rifampin is indicated, alternative therapeutic agents with less enzyme induction potential should be considered.

Drugs which may be coadministered without dose adjustment

Clinically significant pharmacokinetic drug-drug interactions were not observed in studies of drugs listed below. A synopsis of the type of study performed for each drug is provided. Sirolimus and these drugs may be coadministered without dose adjustments.

Acyclovir: Acyclovir, 200 mg, was administered once daily for 3 days followed by a single 10-mg dose of sirolimus oral solution on day 3 in 20 adult healthy volunteers.

Digoxin: Digoxin, 0.25 mg, was administered daily for 8 days and a single 10-mg dose of sirolimus oral solution was given on day 8 to 24 healthy volunteers.

Glyburide: A single 5-mg dose of glyburide and a single 10-mg dose of sirolimus oral solution were administered to 24 healthy volunteers. Sirolimus did not affect the hypoglycemic action of glyburide.

Nifedipine: A single 60-mg dose of nifedipine and a single 10-mg dose of sirolimus oral solution were administered to 24 healthy volunteers.

Norgestrel/ethinyl estradiol (Lo/Ovral®): Sirolimus oral solution, 2 mg, was given daily for 7 days to 21 healthy female volunteers on norgestrel/ethinyl estradiol.

Prednisolone: Pharmacokinetic information was obtained from 42 stable renal transplant patients receiving daily doses of prednisone (5–20 mg/day) and either single or multiple doses of sirolimus oral solution (0.5–5 mg/m² q 12h).

Sulfamethoxazole/trimethoprim (Bactrim®): A single oral dose of sulfamethoxazole (40 mg)/trimethoprim, (80 mg) was given to 15 renal transplant patients receiving daily oral doses of sirolimus (8 to 25 mg/m²).

Other drug interactions

Sirolimus is extensively metabolized by the CYP3A4 isoenzyme in the gut wall and liver. Therefore, absorption and the subsequent elimination of systemically absorbed sirolimus may be influenced by drugs that affect this isoenzyme. Inhibitors of CYP3A4 may decrease the metabolism of sirolimus and increase sirolimus levels, while inducers of CYP3A4 may increase the metabolism of sirolimus and decrease sirolimus levels.

Drugs that may increase sirolimus blood concentrations include:

- Calcium channel blockers: nicardipine, verapamil.
- Antifungal agents: clotrimazole, fluconazole, itraconazole.
- Macrolide antibiotics: clarithromycin, erythromycin, troleandomycin.
- Gastrointestinal prokinetic agents: cisapride, metoclopramide.
- Other drugs: bromocriptine, cimetidine, danazol, HIV-protease inhibitors (e.g., ritonavir, indinavir).

Drugs that may decrease sirolimus levels include:

- Anticonvulsants: carbamazepine, phenobarbital, phenytoin.
- Antibiotics: rifabutin, rifapentine.

This list is not all inclusive.

Care should be exercised when drugs or other substances that are metabolized by CYP3A4 are administered concomitantly with Rapamune. Grapefruit juice reduces CYP3A4-mediated metabolism of Rapamune and must not be used for dilution (see **DOSAGE AND ADMINISTRATION**).

Herbal Preparations

St. John's Wort (*hypericum perforatum*) induces CYP3A4 and P-glycoprotein. Since sirolimus is a substrate for both cytochrome CYP3A4 and P-glycoprotein, there is the potential that the use of St. John's Wort in patients receiving Rapamune could result in reduced sirolimus levels.

Vaccination

Immunosuppressants may affect response to vaccination. Therefore, during treatment with Rapamune, vaccination may be less effective. The use of live vaccines should be avoided; live vaccines may include, but are not limited to measles, mumps, rubella, oral polio, BCG, yellow fever, varicella, and TY21a typhoid.

Drug-Laboratory Test Interactions

There are no studies on the interactions of sirolimus in commonly employed clinical laboratory tests.

Carcinogenesis, Mutagenesis, and Impairment of Fertility

Sirolimus was not genotoxic in the *in vitro* bacterial reverse mutation assay, the Chinese hamster ovary cell chromosomal aberration assay, the mouse lymphoma cell forward mutation assay, or the *in vivo* mouse micronucleus assay.

Carcinogenicity studies were conducted in mice and rats. In an 86-week female mouse study at dosages of 0, 12.5, 25 and 50/6 (dosage lowered from 50 to 6 mg/kg/day at week 31 due to infection secondary to immunosuppression) there was a statistically significant increase in malignant lymphoma at all dose levels (approximately 16 to 135 times the clinical doses adjusted for body surface area) compared to controls. In a second mouse study at dosages of 0, 1, 3 and 6 mg/kg (approximately 3 to 16 times the clinical dose adjusted for body surface area), hepatocellular adenoma and carcinoma (males), were considered Rapamune related. In the 104-week rat study at dosages of 0, 0.05, 0.1, and 0.2 mg/kg/day (approximately 0.4 to 1 times the clinical dose adjusted for body surface area), there was a statistically significant increased incidence of testicular adenoma in the 0.2 mg/kg/day group.

There was no effect on fertility in female rats following the administration of sirolimus at dosages up to 0.5 mg/kg (approximately 1 to 3 times the clinical doses adjusted for body surface area). In male rats, there was no significant difference in fertility rate compared to controls at a dosage of 2 mg/kg (approximately 4 to 11 times the clinical doses adjusted for body surface area). Reductions in testicular weights and/or histological lesions (e.g., tubular atrophy and tubular giant cells) were observed in rats following dosages of 0.65 mg/kg (approximately 1 to 3 times the clinical doses adjusted for body surface area) and above and in a monkey study at 0.1 mg/kg (approximately 0.4 to 1 times the clinical doses adjusted for body surface area) and above. Sperm counts were reduced in male rats following the administration of sirolimus for 13 weeks at a dosage of 6 mg/kg (approximately 12 to 32 times the clinical doses adjusted for body surface area), but showed improvement by 3 months after dosing was stopped.

Pregnancy

Pregnancy Category C: Sirolimus was embryo/feto toxic in rats at dosages of 0.1 mg/kg and above (approximately 0.2 to 0.5 the clinical doses adjusted for body surface area). Embryo/feto toxicity was manifested as mortality and reduced fetal weights (with associated delays in skeletal ossification). However, no teratogenesis was evident. In combination with cyclosporine, rats had increased embryo/feto mortality compared to Rapamune alone. There were no effects on rabbit development at the maternally toxic dosage of 0.05 mg/kg (approximately 0.3 to 0.8 times the clinical doses adjusted for body surface area). There are no adequate and well controlled studies in pregnant women. Effective contraception must be initiated before Rapamune therapy, during Rapamune therapy, and for 12 weeks after Rapamune therapy has been stopped. Rapamune should be used during pregnancy only if the potential benefit outweighs the potential risk to the embryo/fetus.

Use during lactation

Sirolimus is excreted in trace amounts in milk of lactating rats. It is not known whether sirolimus is excreted in human milk. The pharmacokinetic and safety profiles of sirolimus in infants are not known. Because many drugs are excreted in human milk and because of the potential for adverse reactions in nursing infants from sirolimus, a decision should be made whether to discontinue nursing or to discontinue the drug, taking into account the importance of the drug to the mother.

Pediatric use

The safety and efficacy of Rapamune in pediatric patients below the age of 13 years have not been established.

Geriatric use

Clinical studies of Rapamune Oral Solution or Tablets did not include sufficient numbers of patients aged 65 years and over to determine whether safety and efficacy differ in this population from younger patients. Data pertaining to sirolimus trough concentrations suggest that dose adjustments based upon age in geriatric renal patients are not necessary.

ADVERSE REACTIONS

Rapamune® Oral Solution: The incidence of adverse reactions was determined in two randomized, double-blind, multicenter controlled trials in which 499 renal transplant patients received Rapamune Oral Solution 2 mg/day, 477 received Rapamune Oral Solution 5 mg/day, 160 received azathioprine, and 124 received placebo. All patients were treated with cyclosporine and corticosteroids. Data (≥ 12 months post-transplant) presented in the table below show the adverse reactions that occurred in any treatment group with an incidence of ≥ 20%.

Specific adverse reactions associated with the administration of Rapamune Oral Solution occurred at a significantly higher frequency than in the respective control group. For both Rapamune Oral Solution 2 mg/day and 5 mg/day these include hypercholesterolemia, hyperlipemia, hypertension, and rash; for Rapamune Oral Solution 2 mg/day acne; and for Rapamune Oral Solution 5 mg/day anemia, arthralgia, diarrhea, hypokalemia, and thrombocytopenia. The elevations of triglycerides and cholesterol and decreases in platelets and hemoglobin occurred in a dose-related manner in patients receiving Rapamune.

Patients maintained on Rapamune Oral Solution 5 mg/day, when compared to patients on Rapamune Oral Solution 2 mg/day, demonstrated an increased incidence of the following adverse events: anemia, leukopenia, thrombocytopenia, hypokalemia, hyperlipemia, fever, and diarrhea.

[See table at bottom of next page]

At 12 months, there were no significant differences in incidence rates for clinically important opportunistic or common transplant-related infections across treatment groups, with the exception of mucosal infections with *Herpes simplex*, which occurred at a significantly greater rate in patients treated with Rapamune 5 mg/day than in both of the comparator groups.

The table below summarizes the incidence of malignancies in the two controlled trials for the prevention of acute rejection. At 12 months following transplantation, there was a very low incidence of malignancies and there were no significant differences among treatment groups.

[See table at bottom of next page]

Among the adverse events that were reported at a rate of ≥3% and <20%, the following were more prominent in patients maintained on Rapamune 5 mg/day, when compared to patients on Rapamune 2 mg/day: epistaxis, lymphocele, insomnia, thrombotic thrombocytopenic purpura (hemolytic-uremic syndrome), skin ulcer, increased LDH, hypotension, facial edema.

The following adverse events were reported with ≥3% and <20% incidence in patients in any Rapamune treatment group in the two controlled clinical trials for the prevention of acute rejection, BODY AS A WHOLE: abdomen enlarged, abscess, ascites, cellulitis, chills, face edema, flu syndrome, generalized edema, hernia, *Herpes zoster* infection, lymphocele, malaise, pelvic pain, peritonitis, sepsis; CARDIOVASCULAR SYSTEM: atrial fibrillation, congestive heart failure, hemorrhage, hypervolemia, hypotension, palpitation, peripheral vascular disorder, postural hypotension, syncope, tachycardia, thrombophlebitis, thrombosis, vasodilatation; DIGESTIVE SYSTEM: anorexia, dysphagia, eructation, esophagitis, flatulence, gastritis, gastroenteritis, gingivitis, gum hyperplasia, ileus, liver function tests abnormal, mouth ulceration, oral moniliasis, stomatitis; ENDOCRINE SYSTEM: Cushing's syndrome, diabetes mellitus, glycosuria; HEMIC AND LYMPHATIC SYSTEM: ecchymosis, leukocytosis, lymphadenopathy, polycythemia, thrombotic thrombocytopenic purpura (hemolytic-uremic syndrome); METABOLIC AND NUTRITIONAL: acidosis, alkaline phosphatase increased, BUN increased, creatine phosphokinase increased, dehydration, healing abnormal, hypercalcemia, hyperglycemia, hyperphosphatemia, hypocalcemia, hypoglycemia, hypomagnesemia, hyponatremia, lactic dehydrogenase increased, SGOT increased, SGPT increased, weight loss; MUSCULOSKELETAL SYSTEM: arthrosis, bone necrosis, leg cramps, myalgia, osteoporosis, tetany; NERVOUS SYSTEM: anxiety, confusion, depression, dizziness, emotional lability, hypertonia, hypesthesia, hypotonia, insomnia, neuropathy, paresthesia, somnolence; RESPIRATORY SYSTEM: asthma, atelectasis, bronchitis, cough increased, epistaxis, hypoxia, lung edema, pleural effusion, pneumonia, rhinitis, sinusitis; SKIN AND APPENDAGES: fungal

dermatitis, hirsutism, pruritus, skin hypertrophy, skin ulcer, sweating; SPECIAL SENSES: abnormal vision, cataract, conjunctivitis, deafness, ear pain, otitis media, tinnitus; UROGENITAL SYSTEM: albuminuria, bladder pain, dysuria, hematuria, hydronephrosis, impotence, kidney pain, kidney tubular necrosis, nocturia, oliguria, pyelonephritis, pyuria, scrotal edema, testis disorder, toxic nephropathy, urinary frequency, urinary incontinence, urinary retention.

Less frequently occurring adverse events included: mycobacterial infections, Epstein-Barr virus infections, and pancreatitis.

Rapamune® Tablets: The safety profile of the tablet did not differ from that of the oral solution formulation. The incidence of adverse reactions up to 12 months was determined in a randomized, multicenter controlled trial (Study 3) in which 229 renal transplant patients received Rapamune Oral Solution 2 mg once daily and 228 patients received Rapamune Tablets 2 mg once daily. All patients were treated with cyclosporine and corticosteroids. The adverse reactions that occurred in either treatment group with an incidence of ≥20% in Study 3 are similar to those reported for Studies 1 & 2. There was no notable difference in the incidence of these adverse events between treatment groups (oral solution versus tablets) in Study 3, with the exception of acne, which occurred more frequently in the oral solution group, and tremor which occurred more frequently in the tablet group, particularly in Black patients.

The adverse events that occurred in patients with an incidence of ≥3% and <20% in either treatment group in Study

3 were similar to those reported in Studies 1 & 2. There was no notable difference in the incidence of these adverse events between treatment groups (oral solution versus tablets) in Study 3, with the exception of hypertonia, which occurred more frequently in the oral solution group and diabetes mellitus which occurred more frequently in the tablet group. Hispanic patients in the tablet group experienced hyperglycemia more frequently than Hispanic patients in the oral solution group. In Study 3 alone, menorrhagia, metrorrhagia, and polyuria occurred with an incidence of ≥3% and <20%.

The clinically important opportunistic or common transplant-related infections were identical in all three studies and the incidences of these infections were similar in Study 3 compared with Studies 1 & 2. The incidence rates of these infections were not significantly different between the oral solution and tablet treatment groups in Study 3.

In Study 3 (at 12 months), there were two cases of lymphoma/lymphoproliferative disorder in the oral solution treatment group (0.8%) and two reported cases of lymphoma/lymphoproliferative disorder in the tablet treatment group (0.8%). These differences were not statistically significant and were similar to the incidences observed in Studies 1 & 2.

Other clinical experience: Cases of pneumonitis with no identified infectious etiology, sometimes with an interstitial pattern, have occurred in patients receiving immunosuppressive regimens including Rapamune. In some cases, the pneumonitis has resolved upon discontinuation of Rapamune. There have been rare reports of pancytopenia.

OVERDOSAGE

There is minimal experience with overdose. During clinical trials, there were two accidental Rapamune ingestions, of 120 mg and 150 mg. One patient, receiving 150 mg, experienced an episode of transient atrial fibrillation. The other patient experienced no adverse effects. General supportive measures should be followed in all cases of overdose. Based on the poor aqueous solubility and high erythrocyte binding of Rapamune, it is anticipated that Rapamune is not dialyzable to any significant extent. In mice and rats, the acute oral lethal dose was greater than 800 mg/kg.

DOSAGE AND ADMINISTRATION

It is recommended that Rapamune Oral Solution and Tablets be used in a regimen with cyclosporine and corticosteroids. Two-mg Rapamune oral solution has been demonstrated to be clinically equivalent to 2-mg Rapamune oral tablets; hence, are interchangeable on a mg to mg basis. However, it is not known if higher doses of Rapamune oral solution are clinically equivalent to higher doses of tablets on a mg to mg basis. (See CLINICAL PHARMACOLOGY: Absorption). Rapamune is to be administered orally once daily. The initial dose of Rapamune should be administered as soon as possible after transplantation. For *de novo* transplant recipients, a loading dose of Rapamune of 3 times the maintenance dose should be given. A daily maintenance dose of 2 mg is recommended for use in renal transplant patients, with a loading dose of 6 mg. Although a daily maintenance dose of 5 mg, with a loading dose of 15 mg was used in clinical trials of the oral solution and was shown to be safe and effective, no efficacy advantage over the 2 mg dose be established for renal transplant patients. Patients receiving 2 mg of Rapamune Oral Solution per day demonstrated an overall better safety profile than did patients receiving 5 mg of Rapamune Oral Solution per day.

To minimize the variability of exposure to Rapamune, this drug should be taken consistently with or without food. Grapefruit juice reduces CYP3A4-mediated metabolism of Rapamune and must not be administered with Rapamune or used for dilution.

It is recommended that sirolimus be taken 4 hours after administration of cyclosporine oral solution (MODIFIED) and/or cyclosporine capsules (MODIFIED).

Dosage Adjustments
The initial dosage in patients ≥13 years who weigh less than 40 kg should be adjusted, based on body surface area, to 1 mg/m²/day. The loading dose should be 3 mg/m².
It is recommended that the maintenance dose of Rapamune be reduced by approximately one third in patients with hepatic impairment. It is not necessary to modify the Rapamune loading dose. Dosage need not be adjusted because of impaired renal function.

Blood Concentration Monitoring
Routine therapeutic drug level monitoring is not required in most patients. Blood sirolimus levels should be monitored in pediatric patients, in patients with hepatic impairment, during concurrent administration of strong CYP3A4 inducers and inhibitors, and/or if cyclosporine dosing is markedly reduced or discontinued. In controlled clinical trials with concomitant cyclosporine, mean sirolimus whole blood trough levels, as measured by immunoassay, were 9 ng/mL (range 4.5 – 14 ng/mL [10th to 90th percentile]) for the 2 mg/day treatment group, and 17 ng/mL (range 10 – 28 ng/mL [10th to 90th percentile]) for the 5 mg/day dose.

Results from other assays may differ from those with an immunoassay. On average, chromatographic methods (HPLC UV or LC/MS/MS) yield results that are approximately 20% lower than the immunoassay for whole blood concentration determinations. Adjustments to the targeted range should be made according to the assay utilized to determine sirolimus trough concentrations. Therefore, comparison between concentrations in the published literature and an in-

ADVERSE EVENTS OCCURRING AT A FREQUENCY OF ≥ 20% IN ANY TREATMENT GROUP IN PREVENTION OF ACUTE RENAL REJECTION TRIALS (%)[a] AT ≥ 12 MONTHS POST-TRANSPLANTATION FOR STUDIES 1 AND 2

Body System Adverse Event	Rapamune® Oral Solution 2 mg/day		Rapamune® Oral Solution 5 mg/day		Azathioprine 2–3 mg/kg/day	Placebo
	Study 1 (n = 281)	Study 2 (n = 218)	Study 1 (n = 269)	Study 2 (n = 208)	Study 1 (n = 160)	Study 2 (n = 124)
Body As A Whole						
Abdominal pain	28	29	30	36	29	30
Asthenia	38	22	40	28	37	28
Back pain	16	23	26	22	23	20
Chest pain	16	18	19	24	16	19
Fever	27	23	33	34	33	35
Headache	23	34	27	34	21	31
Pain	24	33	29	29	30	25
Cardiovascular System						
Hypertension	43	45	39	49	29	48
Digestive System						
Constipation	28	36	34	38	37	31
Diarrhea	32	25	42	35	28	27
Dyspepsia	17	23	23	25	24	34
Nausea	31	25	36	31	39	29
Vomiting	21	19	25	25	31	21
Hemic And Lymphatic System						
Anemia	27	23	37	33	29	21
Leukopenia	9	9	15	13	20	8
Thrombocytopenia	13	14	20	30	9	9
Metabolic And Nutritional						
Creatinine increased	35	39	37	40	28	38
Edema	24	20	16	18	23	15
Hypercholesteremia (See WARNINGS and PRECAUTIONS)	38	43	42	46	33	23
Hyperkalemia	15	17	12	14	24	27
Hyperlipemia (See WARNINGS and PRECAUTIONS)	38	45	44	57	28	23
Hypokalemia	17	11	21	17	11	9
Hypophosphatemia	20	15	23	19	20	19
Peripheral edema	60	54	64	58	58	48
Weight gain	21	11	15	8	19	15
Musculoskeletal System						
Arthralgia	25	25	27	31	21	18
Nervous System						
Insomnia	14	13	22	14	18	8
Tremor	31	21	30	22	28	19
Respiratory System						
Dyspnea	22	24	28	30	23	30
Pharyngitis	17	16	16	21	17	22
Upper respiratory infection	20	26	24	23	13	23
Skin And Appendages						
Acne	31	22	20	22	17	19
Rash	12	10	13	20	6	6
Urogenital System						
Urinary tract infection	20	26	23	33	31	26

a: Patients received cyclosporine and corticosteroids.

INCIDENCE (%) OF MALIGNANCIES IN PREVENTION OF ACUTE RENAL REJECTION TRIALS: AT 12 MONTHS POST-TRANSPLANT[a]

Malignancy	Rapamune® Oral Solution 2 mg/day (n = 511)	Rapamune® Oral Solution 5 mg/day (n = 493)	Azathioprine 2–3 mg/kg/day (n = 161)	Placebo (n = 130)
Lymphoma/lymphoproliferative disease	0.4	1.4	0.6	0
Non-melanoma skin carcinoma	0.4	1.4	1.2	3.1
Other malignancy	0.6	0.6	0	0

a: Patients received cyclosporine and corticosteroids.

Continued on next page

Rapamune—Cont.

dividual patient concentration using current assays must be made with detailed knowledge of the assay methods employed. A discussion of the different assay methods is contained in *Clinical Therapeutics,* Volume 22, Supplement B, April 2000.

Instructions for Dilution and Administration of Rapamune® Oral Solution Bottles

The amber oral dose syringe should be used to withdraw the prescribed amount of Rapamune® Oral Solution from the bottle. Empty the correct amount of Rapamune from the syringe into only a glass or plastic container holding at least two (2) ounces (1/4 cup, 60 mL) of water or orange juice. No other liquids, including grapefruit juice, should be used for dilution. Stir vigorously and drink at once. Refill the container with an additional volume (minimum of four [4] ounces (1/2 cup, 120 mL)) of water or orange juice, stir vigorously, and drink at once.

Pouches

When using the pouch, squeeze the entire contents of the pouch into only a glass or plastic container holding at least two (2) ounces (1/4 cup, 60 mL) of water or orange juice. No other liquids, including grapefruit juice, should be used for dilution. Stir vigorously and drink at once. Refill the container with an additional volume (minimum of four [4] ounces (1/2 cup, 120 mL)) of water or orange juice, stir vigorously, and drink at once.

Handling and Disposal

Since Rapamune is not absorbed through the skin, there are no special precautions. However, if direct contact with the skin or mucous membranes occurs, wash thoroughly with soap and water; rinse eyes with plain water.

HOW SUPPLIED

Rapamune® Oral Solution is supplied at a concentration of 1 mg/mL in:

1. Cartons:
   NDC # 0008-1030-06, containing a 2 oz (60 mL fill) amber glass bottle.
   NDC # 0008-1030-15, containing a 5 oz (150 mL fill) amber glass bottle.

In addition to the bottles, each carton is supplied with an oral syringe adapter for fitting into the neck of the bottle, sufficient disposable amber oral syringes and caps for daily dosing, and a carrying case.

2. Cartons:
   NDC # 0008-1030-03, containing 30 unit-of-use laminated aluminum pouches of 1 mL.
   NDC # 0008-1030-07, containing 30 unit-of-use laminated aluminum pouches of 2 mL.
   NDC # 0008-1030-08, containing 30 unit-of-use laminated aluminum pouches of 5 mL.

Rapamune® Tablets are available as follows: 1 mg, white, triangular-shaped tablets marked "RAPAMUNE 1 mg" on one side.
NDC # 0008-1031-05, bottle of 100 tablets.
NDC # 0008-1031-10, Redipak® cartons of 100 tablets (10 blister cards of 10 tablets each).

Storage

Rapamune® Oral Solution bottles and pouches should be stored protected from light and refrigerated at 2°C to 8°C (36°F to 46°F). Once the bottle is opened, the contents should be used within one month. If necessary, the patient may store both the pouches and the bottles at room temperature up to 25°C (77°F) for a short period of time (e.g., several days, but not longer than 30 days).

An amber syringe and cap are provided for dosing and the product may be kept in the syringe for a maximum of 24 hours at room temperatures up to 25°C (77°F) or refrigerated at 2°C to 8°C (36°F to 46°F). The syringe should be discarded after one use. After dilution, the preparation should be used immediately.

Rapamune Oral Solution provided in bottles may develop a slight haze when refrigerated. If such a haze occurs allow the product to stand at room temperature and shake gently until the haze disappears. The presence of this haze does not affect the quality of the product.

Rapamune® Tablets should be stored at 20° to 25°C (USP Controlled Room Temperature) (68°–77°F). Use cartons to protect blister cards and strips from light. Dispense in a tight, light-resistant container as defined in the USP.

℞ only

US Pat. Nos.: 5,100,899; 5,212,155; 5,308,847; 5,403,833; 5,536,729.

PATIENT INSTRUCTIONS FOR RAPAMUNE® ORAL SOLUTION ADMINISTRATION

Bottles

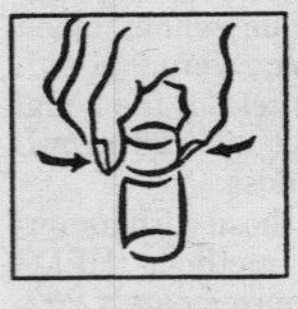

1. Open the solution bottle. Remove the safety cap by squeezing the tabs on the cap and twisting counterclockwise.

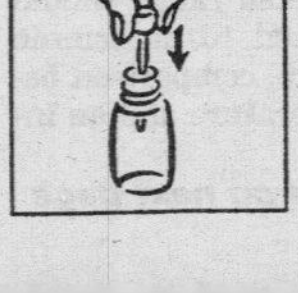

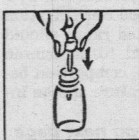

2. On first use, insert the adapter assembly (plastic tube with stopper) tightly into the bottle until it is even with the top of the bottle. Do not remove the adapter assembly from the bottle once inserted.

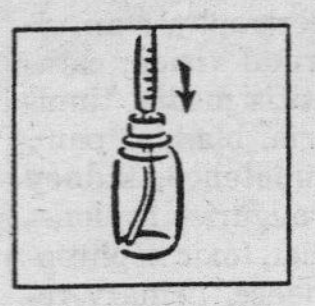

3. For each use, tightly insert one of the amber syringes with the plunger fully depressed into the opening in the adapter.

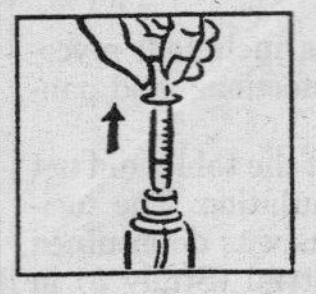

4. Withdraw the prescribed amount of Rapamune® Oral Solution by gently pulling out the plunger of the syringe until the bottom of the black line of the plunger is even with the appropriate mark on the syringe. Always keep the bottle in an upright position. If bubbles form in the syringe, empty the syringe into the bottle and repeat the procedure.

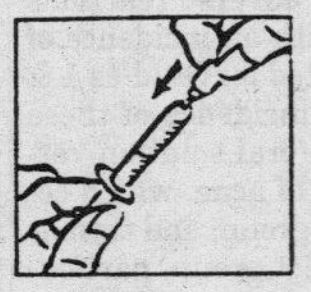

5. You may have been instructed to carry your medication with you. If it is necessary to carry the filled syringe, place a cap securely on the syringe—the cap should snap into place.

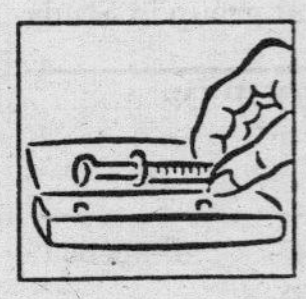

6. Then place the capped syringe in the enclosed carrying case. Once in the syringe, the medication may be kept at room temperature or refrigerated and should be used within 24 hours. Extreme temperature (below 36°F and above 86°F) should be avoided. Remember to keep this medication out of the reach of children.

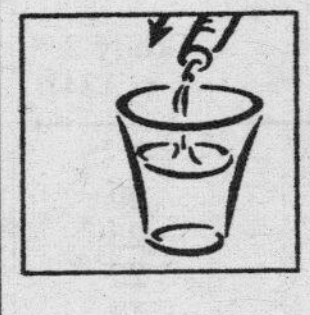

7. Empty the syringe into a glass or plastic cup containing at least 2 ounces (1/4 cup; 60 mL) of water or orange juice, stir vigorously for one (1) minute and drink immediately. Refill the container with at least 4 ounces (1/2 cup; 120 mL) of water or orange juice, stir vigorously again and drink the rinse solution. Apple juice, grapefruit juice, or other liquids are NOT to be used. Only glass or plastic cups should be used to dilute Rapamune® Oral Solution. The syringe and cap should be used once and then discarded.

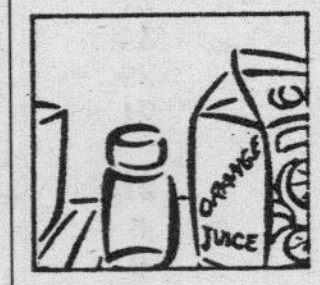

8. Always store the bottles of medication in the refrigerator. When refrigerated, a slight haze may develop in the solution. The presence of a haze does not affect the quality of the product. If this happens, bring the Rapamune® Oral Solution to room temperature and shake until the haze disappears. If it is necessary to wipe clean the mouth of the bottle before returning the product to the refrigerator, wipe with a dry cloth to avoid introducing water, or any other liquid, into the bottle.

PATIENT INSTRUCTIONS FOR RAPAMUNE® ORAL SOLUTION ADMINISTRATION

Pouches

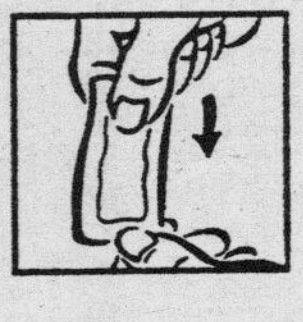

1. Before opening the pouch, squeeze the pouch from the neck area to push the contents into the lower part of the pouch.

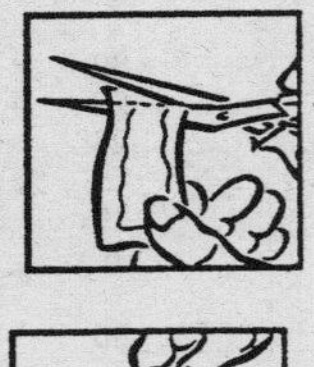

2. Carefully open the pouch by folding the marked area and then cutting with a scissors along the marked line near the top of the pouch.

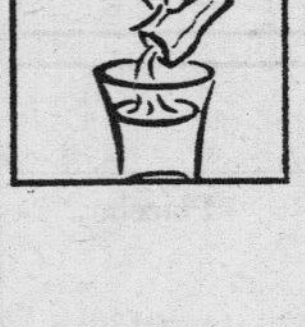

3. Squeeze the entire contents of the pouch into a glass or plastic cup containing at least 2 ounces (1/4 cup; 60 mL) of water or orange juice, stir vigorously for one (1) minute and drink immediately. Refill the container with at least 4 ounces (1/2 cup, 120 mL) of water or orange juice, stir vigorously again and drink the rinse solution. Apple juice, grapefruit juice or other liquids are NOT to be used. Only glass or plastic cups should be used to dilute RAPAMUNE® oral solution.

4. Unused pouches should be stored in the refrigerator.

SYNVISC® ℞

[*sĭn' vĭsk*]

(Hylan G-F 20)

Prescribing information for this product, which appears on pages 3455–3457 of the 2001 PDR, has been revised. Please write "See Supplement A" next to the product heading.

The second bulleted point under **WARNINGS** should be deleted and replaced with the following:

- Do not inject Synvisc extra-articularly or into the synovial tissues and capsule. Local and systemic adverse events, generally in the area of the injection, have occurred following extra-articular injection of Synvisc.

The second bulleted point under the heading **Information for Patients** should be deleted and replaced with the following:

- Transient pain, swelling and/or effusion of the injected joint may occur after intra-articular injection of Synvisc. In some cases the effusion may be considerable and can cause pronounced pain; cases where swelling is extensive should be discussed with the physician.

The four paragraphs in the **ADVERSE REACTIONS** section should be deleted and replaced with the following:

Adverse Events Involving the Injected Joint

Clinical Trials: A total of 511 patients (559 knees) received 1771 injections in seven clinical trials of Synvisc. There were 39 reports in 37 patients (2.2% of injections, 7.2% of patients) of knee pain and/or swelling after these injections. Ten patients (10 knees) were treated with arthrocentesis and removal of joint effusion. Two additional patients (two knees) received treatment with intra-articular steroids. Two patients (two knees) received NSAIDs. One of these patients also received arthrocentesis. One patient was treated with arthroscopy. The remaining patients with adverse events localized to the knee received no treatment or only analgesics.

Postmarket Experience: The most common adverse events reported have been pain, swelling and/or effusion in the injected knee. In some cases the effusion was considerable and caused pronounced pain. In some instances, patients have presented with knees that were tender, warm and red. It is important to rule out infection or crystalline arthropathies in such cases. Synovial fluid aspirates of varying volumes have revealed a range of cell counts, from very few to over 50,000 cells/mm^3. Reported treatments included symptomatic therapy (e.g., rest, ice, heat, elevation, simple analgesics and NSAIDs) and/or arthrocentesis. Intra-articular corticosteroids have been used when infection was excluded. Rarely, arthroscopy has been performed. The occurrence of post-injection effusion may be associated with patient history of efffusion, advanced stage of disease and/or the number of injections a patient receives. Reactions generally abate within a few days. Clinical benefit from the treatment may still occur after such reactions.

Intra-articular infections did not occur in any of the clinical trials and have been reported only rarely during clinical use of Synvisc.

Other Adverse Events

Clinical Trials: In three concurrently controlled clinical trials with a total of 112 patients who received Synvisc and 110 patients who received either saline or arthrocentesis, there were no statistically significant differences in the numbers or types of adverse events between the group of patients that received Synvisc and the group that received control treatments.

Systemic adverse events each occurred in 10 (2.0%) of the Synvisc-treated patients. There was one case each of rash (thorax and back) and itching of the skin following Synvisc injections in these studies. These symptoms did not recur when the patients received additional Synvisc injections. The remaining generalized adverse events reported were calf cramps, hemorrhoid problems, ankle edema, muscle pain, tonsillitis with nausea, tachyarrhythmia, phlebitis with varicosities and low back sprain.

Postmarket Experience: Other adverse events reported include: rash, *hives,* itching, *fever,* nausea, *headache, dizziness, chills,* muscle cramps, *paresthesia,* peripheral edema, *malaise, respiratory difficulties, flushing* and *facial swelling.* There have been rare reports of *thrombocytopenia* coincident with Synvisc injection. These medical events occurred under circumstances where causal relationship to Synvisc is uncertain. (Adverse events reported *only* in worldwide postmarketing experience, not seen in clinical trials, are considered more rare and are *italicized.*)

The words "over a 26-week period" should be added to the end of the second paragraph of the **CLINICAL STUDIES** section.

The words "over a twelve-week period (See Table 3)," which appear at the end of the third paragraph of the **CLINICAL STUDIES** section should be deleted and replaced with "over a 26-week period (see Tables 3A and 3B)."

In the second sentence of the fourth paragraph of the **CLINICAL STUDIES** section, "12-week" should be deleted and replaced with "26-week."

The following sentence should be added to the end of the fourth paragraph of the **CLINICAL STUDIES** section:

In both of these studies the most pain relief and the greatest amount of treatment success occurred 8 to 12 weeks after Synvisc treatment began.

The following paragraph should be added as the new fifth paragraph of the **CLINICAL STUDIES** section:

Investigators obtained data at 26 weeks by telephone interviews. A validation study suggested that the results obtained in telephone interviews are equivalent to those obtained in office visits. Since investigators did not follow patients beyond week 26, the duration of pain relief beyond 26 weeks is not known.

The following paragraph should be added as the ninth entry under **DIRECTIONS FOR USE** just after "Inject Synvisc into the knee joint through an 18 to 22 gauge needle.":

To ensure a tight seal and prevent leakage during administration, secure the needle tightly while firmly holding the luer hub.

The heading **"MANUFACTURED BY"** and the information under the heading should be deleted, and the heading **"DEVELOPED BY"** should be deleted and replaced by **"DEVELOPED AND MANUFACTURED BY"**.